国家科学技术学术著作出版基金资助出版

# 第六次中国总膳食研究

## The Sixth China Total Diet Study

**国家食品安全风险评估中心**

李敬光　吕　冰　邱楠楠　王雨昕　周　爽　主编

吴永宁　赵云峰　主审

国家食品安全风险评估中心高层次人才队伍建设 523 项目

科学出版社

北　京

## 内 容 简 介

总膳食研究是世界卫生组织近年来一直极力推荐适用于研究评价一个国家或地区一般人群或特定人群膳食化学污染物和营养素总摄入量的研究方法。我国自 1990 年以来，已开展了六次总膳食研究，研究结果已经成为膳食暴露评估和法规、标准制定的科学依据，被世界卫生组织誉为发展中国家开展总膳食研究的典范。第六次中国总膳食研究于 2016~2021 年开展，涉及了包括脂肪酸、元素、农药残留、兽药残留、食品加工过程污染物、持久性有机污染物、真菌毒素及其他热点化学物质的分析检测及暴露评估。本书按照总膳食研究成果整体集结出版的模式，参照《第五次中国总膳食研究》体例，全面总结了第六次总膳食研究的最新成果，评价了我国居民多种污染物及营养元素的膳食摄入水平，并与历次总膳食研究结果进行比较，了解其变化趋势。本书数据充分，结论可靠，是定期发布的我国居民膳食营养元素摄入和污染物暴露结果，对食品安全风险评估及标准制修订具有重要意义，亦是世界各国开展总膳食研究工作的重要参考工具。

本研究定期发布我国居民膳食营养素摄入和污染物暴露结果。本书可作为食品卫生相关学科的学生、研究人员，以及从事膳食暴露的专业人员的参考用书，亦是世界各国开展总膳食研究工作的重要参考工具。

---

图书在版编目（CIP）数据

第六次中国总膳食研究/李敬光等主编. —北京：科学出版社，2025.3
ISBN 978-7-03-074851-5

Ⅰ.①第⋯ Ⅱ.①李⋯ Ⅲ.①居民–膳食营养–研究–中国 Ⅳ.① R151.4

中国国家版本馆 CIP 数据核字（2023）第 027135 号

责任编辑：罗　静　岳漫宇　尚　册/责任校对：郑金红
责任印制：肖　兴/封面设计：刘新新

科学出版社 出版
北京东黄城根北街 16 号
邮政编码：100717
http://www.sciencep.com

北京建宏印刷有限公司印刷
科学出版社发行　各地新华书店经销

\*

2025 年 3 月第　一　版　　开本：787×1092　1/16
2025 年 3 月第一次印刷　　印张：59
字数：1 400 000

**定价：598.00 元**
（如有印装质量问题，我社负责调换）

# 编者名单

主　　编　李敬光　吕　冰　邱楠楠　王雨昕　周　爽

副 主 编　张　烁　陈达炜　马　兰　苗宏健　张　磊

编写人员　第一章　吕　冰　李敬光

　　　　　第二章　方从容　裴紫薇　杨　杰　周　爽

　　　　　第三章　尚晓虹　赵　馨　马　兰　周　爽　韦　昱

　　　　　第四章　陈达炜　吕　冰　李少华　刘志斌　辛少鲲

　　　　　第五章　陈达炜　韦　昱　张　晶　赵晓雪　王　轩

　　　　　第六章　徐小民　朱　峰　吉文亮　周萍萍　黄飞飞

　　　　　　　　　吴平谷　苗宏健　王紫菲　王雨昕　邵　兵

　　　　　第七章　张　磊　施致雄　吕　冰　王雨昕　刘嘉颖

　　　　　　　　　高丽荣　裴紫薇　李敬光

　　　　　第八章　邱楠楠　张　烁　周　爽

　　　　　第九章　陈达炜　鲍　彦　张　晶　邵　兵　施致雄

　　　　　　　　　刘嘉颖　苗宏健　李敬光

主　　审　吴永宁　赵云峰

**参与人员名单**（按姓氏笔画为序）：

| | | | | | |
|---|---|---|---|---|---|
| 马晓晨 | 马梦婷 | 王　辛 | 尹晓晨 | 石萌萌 | 田美娜 |
| 付鹏钰 | 丛　源 | 朱珍妮 | 朱谦让 | 任泽萍 | 刘长青 |
| 刘怡娅 | 刘思洁 | 刘　潇 | 闫世春 | 许丽丽 | 李成莲 |
| 李秋娟 | 李绥晶 | 李梓民 | 李　蕾 | 肖培瑞 | 宋壮志 |
| 张　辉 | 张　睿 | 陈子慧 | 陈少威 | 陈莉莉 | 罗宝章 |
| 胡国良 | 钞　凤 | 贺林娟 | 袁秀娟 | 贾海先 | 唐　丽 |
| 黄丽娜 | 黄　峥 | 曹文成 | 崔春霞 | 章荣华 | 梁效成 |
| 蒋玉艳 | 韩澄华 | 赖善榕 | 褚遵华 | 颜　玲 | 戴　月 |

# 序

总膳食研究（Total Diet Study，TDS）是对一个国家或一个地区代表性人群评估膳食污染物暴露量和营养素摄入量的最经济有效的方法，是世界卫生组织极力推荐的一种膳食暴露评估技术。在世界卫生组织鼓励下，我国于1990年首次成功开展中国总膳食研究以来，在国家食品安全风险评估中心的组织下，到2021年为止，共开展了六次中国总膳食研究。

中国总膳食研究在创新中不断发展，覆盖的地区不断扩展，由第一次总膳食研究的12个省（自治区、直辖市），发展至第六次的24个省（自治区、直辖市）。在方法学方面创造了混合膳食样品和单个膳食样品相结合的多快好省方法。自2009年开展的第四次总膳食研究开始，在总膳食研究的相同调查点同步采集了母乳样品，用于《关于持久性有机污染物的斯德哥尔摩公约》履约成效评估和重要污染物的机体负荷研究。分析方法和检测项目不断发展，应用和开发了多元素、多组分测定的同位素稀释的串联质谱技术和高分辨质谱技术，检测的化合物包括持久性有机污染物、真菌毒素、农药残留、兽药残留、食品加工过程产生的污染物、营养元素和有害元素，以及脂肪酸等，并发展了非靶向分析技术用于农药残留和兽药残留的筛查和检测。

中国总膳食研究提供的膳食暴露量数据，为我国食品安全风险评估及食品安全国家标准制定提供了有力的科学数据支持。自第四次中国总膳食研究开始，以中、英文两种语言出版和发布所有研究数据。

2016年启动的第六次中国总膳食研究历时6年，完成了24个省（区、直辖市）膳食样品的烹调加工和混合膳食样品的制备，获得了单个膳食样品1358个和混合膳食样品288个。采用优化的高灵敏高通量的检测方法完成了样品分析，在全面数据审核的基础上，获得了脂肪酸、元素、农药残留、兽药残留、持久性有机污染物、食品加工过程污染物、真菌毒素以及其他热点化合物的含量结果，开展了摄入量分析和暴露评估，解析了膳食暴露水平和主要食物贡献来源并分析了污染物膳食暴露的变化趋势。该书数据详实，分析合理，结论可靠，对于深入了解我国居民膳食污染物的污染状况和变化具有重要的指导意义。

该书理论联系实际，以实际膳食样品中获得的暴露评估数据为基础，对于食品安全公共卫生管理措施的制定提供可靠支持。该书作为食品安全风险分析技术丛书，可供国内外公共卫生领域行政管理和科技人员参考。

陈君石
国家食品安全风险评估中心研究员、总顾问
中国工程院院士

# Preface

Total diet study (TDS) is the most cost-effective method for assessing dietary exposure to contaminants and nutrient intake in a representative population of a country or region, and is highly recommended by the World Health Organization (WHO) as a preferable dietary exposure assessment method. Encouraged by the WHO, China has successfully conducted the first total diet study in 1990. Up to 2021, China National Center for Food Safety Risk Assessment has organized six China total diet studies (CTDSs).

The China total diet study has continued to develop through innovation and its study sites have been expanded from 12 provinces (autonomous regions, municipalities) in the first CTDS to 24 provinces (autonomous regions, municipalities) in the sixth CTDS. In terms of the methodology, CTDS created a more effective and economical approach by combining the composite samples and individual samples. Starting with the 4$^{th}$ CTDS in 2009, breast milk samples were collected simultaneously at the same survey sites as the CTDS for evaluating the effects of the *Stockholm Convention on Persistent Organic Pollutants* (POPs) and body burden of POPs in Chinese population. Along the development of CTDS in China, more advanced analytical methods were used and analytes continue to increase. For multi-component determination, tandem mass spectrometry and high resolution mass spectrometry with isotope dilution have been developed and applied to detect substances including POPs, mycotoxins, pesticide residues, veterinary drug residues, contaminants from food processing, fatty acids, nutrition and hazardous elements. Non-targeted analytical techniques have been developed for the screening and detection of pesticide residues and veterinary drug residues.

The dietary exposure data from the CTDS has provided important scientific support for food safety risk assessment and the development of national food safety standards in China. Beginning from the 4$^{th}$ CTDS, the study results have been published and released in both Chinese and English.

The 6$^{th}$ CTDS launched in 2016, lasted 6 years. The food item samples from 24 provinces (autonomous regions, municipalities) were prepared by cooking and mixing, finally obtained 1358 individual samples and 288 composite samples. Following a comprehensive data review, analytical results were obtained for fatty acids, elemens, pesticide residues, veterinary drug residues, persistent organic pollutants (POPs), process-induced contaminants, mycotoxins, and other emerging compounds of concern. The composite samples were analyzed with validated high-sensitivity and high-throughput methods. Dietary exposure levels and major contributed foods were estimated, and trends in dietary exposure to contaminants were studied. This book provides comprehensive results of the 6$^{th}$ CTDS, including indepth data analysis and appropriate conclusions. It could serve as an important guide to understand the food contamination situation and its trends in China.

This CTDS publication has both theory and application. Because the dietary exposure assessment was based on data from cooked and prepared food samples, it provides reliable technical support for the development of risk management measures. As one of the food safety risk analysis publications, this book can be used as a reference for risk managers and scientists in the field of public health in China and abroad.

Chen Junshi
Professor / Chief Adviser, China National Centre for Food Safety Risk Assessment
Academician, China Academy of Engineering

# 前　言

总膳食研究是我国食品安全风险评估的基础性工作。在中国工程院院士、国家食品安全风险评估中心总顾问陈君石研究员开创下，我国于 1990 年开展了首次总膳食研究，迄今已完成了六次总膳食研究。

第六次中国总膳食研究始于 2016 年，在国家食品安全风险评估中心技术总师吴永宁研究员推动下，其规模进一步发展。根据 4 个"市场菜篮子研究"总体要求，全国共有 24 个省（自治区、直辖市）参加，覆盖了近 90% 人口，并且 5000 万人以上的地区设置 6 个调查点，以进一步反映总膳食研究地区的代表性。按照第四次总膳食研究方式，第六次总膳食研究依然采用分省份研究的模式，制备了分省份的混合膳食样品 288 份，同时制备了分省份的单个膳食样品 1300 余份，这为总膳食研究的溯源分析提供了可靠的样品资源。国家食品安全风险评估中心为保证总膳食研究结果的可靠性，进一步加强精准检测技术的发展，推动多组分、高通量、高灵敏度、高确证以及非靶向筛查的检验技术的应用，并通过与国际权威实验室结果的比较，提高了检测结果的可比性。在检测项目上，第六次总膳食研究进一步得以拓展，增加了热点化合物，如有机磷酸酯、交链孢毒素等检测，并应用高分辨质谱法的非靶向筛查技术，进行了农药残留和兽药残留筛查和确认分析。首次发布了碘、氯化石蜡、全氟烷基化合物、丙烯酰胺、多环芳烃、氨基甲酸乙酯、缩水甘油酯、双酚类化合物、高氯酸盐、有机磷酸酯、交链孢毒素等新兴毒素等混合膳食样品的污染水平及膳食暴露评估数据。通过与以往总膳食研究结果的比较，分析我国混合膳食样品中脂肪酸、营养元素和污染元素、二噁英等持久性有机污染物、农药残留、兽药残留、氯丙醇等食品加工过程产生的污染物、黄曲霉毒素等真菌毒素的污染状况及变化趋势，为我国开展可靠的食品安全风险评估和标准制定提供的重要科学依据，并有助于了解不同省（自治区、直辖市）的污染差异以及膳食暴露的贡献来源。

第六次中国总膳食研究获得了"十三五"国家重点研发计划"食品污染物暴露组解析与中国总膳食研究"（2017YFC1600500）的支持。为使中国总膳食研究结果能够连续、系统地展示，国家食品安全风险评估中心将第六次中国总膳食研究结果进行整理，继续采用专著的方式进行出版发布。

参加本书编写的人员为专门从事我国总膳食研究的技术人员，对总膳食研究具有深刻理解，严格按照中国总膳食研究方法的工作手册进行操作，采用的检测方法进行了系统优化验证，按照形成的标准操作程序和规定的良好质量控制要求进行检测，获得了结果进行的严谨审查，确保发布数据的可靠性。

本书发布的数据，更新了我国混合膳食样品中多种污染物含量和摄入量数据，是我国食品安全风险评估的基础性数据，对我国系统性开展膳食暴露评估具有实用价值，为推动以总膳食研究为方法学的暴露评估技术提供参考。但是，总膳食研究涉及的步骤繁多，技术要求高，本书的不足在所难免，希望读者不吝赐教，批评指正。

李敬光

国家食品安全风险评估中心研究员

# Foreword

Total diet studies (TDSs) are fundamental to food safety risk assessments in China, pioneered by Prof. Chen Junshi, an academician of the Chinese Academy of Engineering and general counsel to China National Center for Food Safety Risk Assessment. China's first TDS was conducted in 1990, and six TDSs have been completed to date.

In 2016, China began its sixth TDS and the method for this was developed further from original protocols by Prof. Wu Yongning, technical chief of China National Center for Food Safety Risk Assessment. Four market basket studies were conducted involving a total of 24 provinces (autonomous regions, municipalities). This covered nearly 90% of the population. In provinces with populations of over 50 million people, six survey sites were set up to represent the entire area. Similar to the fourth TDS approach, 288 composite dietary samples and more than 1300 individual dietary samples were obtained from the provinces for the sixth TDS. This provided reliable sample sources for traceability analysis of the TDS. To ensure the reliability of TDS results, China National Center for Food Safety Risk Assessment developed precision testing methods and promoted the application of multi-component, high-throughput, high-sensitivity, high-confirmation, and non-target screening technologies. Comparability of test results has improved through comparison with results from authoritative international laboratories. In terms of target compounds, the sixth TDS was expanded to include a number of compounds of high interest, such as organophosphates and *Alternaria* toxins. Non-target screening techniques using high-resolution mass spectrometry were developed for screening and confirmation of pesticide residues and veterinary drug residues.

For the first time, contamination levels and dietary exposure assessment data for iodine, chlorinated paraffins, perfluoroalkyl substances, acrylamide, polycyclic aromatic hydrocarbons, ethyl carbamate, glycidyl fatty acid esters, bisphenol analogues, perchlorate, organophosphates, and emerging toxins in the total diet such as *Alternaria* toxins were published. Through comparison with the results of previous TDSs, contamination status and trends were analyzed for fatty acids, nutrients and contaminant elements, persistent organic pollutants (e.g., dioxins, pesticide residues, and veterinary drug residues), contaminants from food processing (e.g., chloropropanols), and mycotoxins (e.g., aflatoxins) in composite dietary samples. The data provide an important scientific basis for reliable food safety risk assessments and setting of standards in China. In addition, this knowledge improves our understanding of the differences in contamination among provinces (autonomous regions, municipalities) and the sources that contribute to dietary exposure.

The sixth China TDS was supported by the National Key Research and Development Program of the 13th Five-Year Plan Characterizing the Exposoure of Food Contamination and Total Diet Study (2017YFC1600500). To present the results of the China TDS in a continuous and systematic manner, China National Center for Food Safety Risk Assessment has collated the results of the sixth China

TDS in a monograph. Technical staff specializing in China TDSs have contributed to this book. Guidelines for the methodology of the China TDS were strictly followed, the testing methods adopted were systematically optimized and validated, the tests were conducted in accordance with standard operating procedures and requirements for good quality control, and the results obtained were critically reviewed to ensure the reliability of the published data.

This book updates fundamental data for food safety risk assessments on the levels and intakes of a wide range of contaminants in mixed dietary samples in China. The data are of practical value to the systematic development of dietary exposure assessments in China, and provide a reference for the promotion of exposure assessment techniques using the TDS. However, as the TDS involves many steps and is technically demanding, shortcomings are inevitable and we appreciate any critiques or constructive feedback from the readers.

Li Jingguang

Professor, China National Center for Food Safety Risk Assessment

# 目 录

| | | |
|---|---|---|
| 概要 | | 1 |
| **第一章** | **中国总膳食研究方法学** | **13** |
| 　第一节 | 膳食调查方法和样品制备步骤 | 13 |
| 　第二节 | 样品分析测定方法及质量控制 | 18 |
| 　第三节 | 膳食暴露评估方法 | 73 |
| **第二章** | **脂肪酸的膳食暴露评估** | **74** |
| **第三章** | **元素的膳食暴露评估** | **89** |
| 　第一部分 | 营养元素 | 89 |
| 　　第一节 | 钠和钾 | 89 |
| 　　第二节 | 钙 | 92 |
| 　　第三节 | 镁 | 95 |
| 　　第四节 | 磷 | 97 |
| 　　第五节 | 锰 | 100 |
| 　　第六节 | 铁 | 102 |
| 　　第七节 | 锌 | 104 |
| 　　第八节 | 铬 | 107 |
| 　　第九节 | 铜 | 109 |
| 　　第十节 | 硒 | 111 |
| 　　第十一节 | 钼 | 114 |
| 　　第十二节 | 碘 | 116 |
| 　第二部分 | 污染元素 | 119 |
| 　　第十三节 | 铅 | 119 |
| 　　第十四节 | 镉 | 122 |
| 　　第十五节 | 汞 | 125 |
| 　　第十六节 | 砷 | 128 |
| 　　第十七节 | 铝 | 132 |
| **第四章** | **农药残留的膳食暴露评估** | **135** |
| **第五章** | **兽药残留的膳食暴露评估** | **196** |

## 第六章　食品加工过程污染物的膳食暴露评估　　**222**

　　第一节　氯丙醇 · · · · · · · · · · · · · · · · · · · · · · · · · · · · · · · · · · · · · · · · · · · · · · · · · · · · · · · · · · · · · · · · · · · · · · · 222
　　第二节　氯丙醇酯 · · · · · · · · · · · · · · · · · · · · · · · · · · · · · · · · · · · · · · · · · · · · · · · · · · · · · · · · · · · · · · · · · · · 226
　　第三节　缩水甘油酯 · · · · · · · · · · · · · · · · · · · · · · · · · · · · · · · · · · · · · · · · · · · · · · · · · · · · · · · · · · · · · · · · 231
　　第四节　丙烯酰胺 · · · · · · · · · · · · · · · · · · · · · · · · · · · · · · · · · · · · · · · · · · · · · · · · · · · · · · · · · · · · · · · · · · · 234
　　第五节　多环芳烃 · · · · · · · · · · · · · · · · · · · · · · · · · · · · · · · · · · · · · · · · · · · · · · · · · · · · · · · · · · · · · · · · · · · 238
　　第六节　氨基甲酸乙酯 · · · · · · · · · · · · · · · · · · · · · · · · · · · · · · · · · · · · · · · · · · · · · · · · · · · · · · · · · · · · · 246
　　第七节　邻苯二甲酸酯 · · · · · · · · · · · · · · · · · · · · · · · · · · · · · · · · · · · · · · · · · · · · · · · · · · · · · · · · · · · · · 250

## 第七章　持久性有机污染物的膳食暴露评估　　**257**

　　第一节　二噁英及其类似物 · · · · · · · · · · · · · · · · · · · · · · · · · · · · · · · · · · · · · · · · · · · · · · · · · · · · · · 257
　　第二节　指示性多氯联苯 · · · · · · · · · · · · · · · · · · · · · · · · · · · · · · · · · · · · · · · · · · · · · · · · · · · · · · · · · · 260
　　第三节　多溴二苯醚 · · · · · · · · · · · · · · · · · · · · · · · · · · · · · · · · · · · · · · · · · · · · · · · · · · · · · · · · · · · · · · · · 263
　　第四节　六溴环十二烷 · · · · · · · · · · · · · · · · · · · · · · · · · · · · · · · · · · · · · · · · · · · · · · · · · · · · · · · · · · · · · 267
　　第五节　持久性有机氯农药 · · · · · · · · · · · · · · · · · · · · · · · · · · · · · · · · · · · · · · · · · · · · · · · · · · · · · · 270
　　第六节　全氟烷基化合物 · · · · · · · · · · · · · · · · · · · · · · · · · · · · · · · · · · · · · · · · · · · · · · · · · · · · · · · · · · 276
　　第七节　短链与中链氯化石蜡 · · · · · · · · · · · · · · · · · · · · · · · · · · · · · · · · · · · · · · · · · · · · · · · · · · · 282

## 第八章　真菌毒素的膳食暴露评估　　**286**

## 第九章　其他化合物的膳食暴露评估　　**320**

　　第一节　高氯酸盐 · · · · · · · · · · · · · · · · · · · · · · · · · · · · · · · · · · · · · · · · · · · · · · · · · · · · · · · · · · · · · · · · · · · 320
　　第二节　硝酸盐与亚硝酸盐 · · · · · · · · · · · · · · · · · · · · · · · · · · · · · · · · · · · · · · · · · · · · · · · · · · · · · · 323
　　第三节　双酚类化合物 · · · · · · · · · · · · · · · · · · · · · · · · · · · · · · · · · · · · · · · · · · · · · · · · · · · · · · · · · · · · · 328
　　第四节　有机磷酸酯 · · · · · · · · · · · · · · · · · · · · · · · · · · · · · · · · · · · · · · · · · · · · · · · · · · · · · · · · · · · · · · · · 334
　　第五节　谷氨酸盐 · · · · · · · · · · · · · · · · · · · · · · · · · · · · · · · · · · · · · · · · · · · · · · · · · · · · · · · · · · · · · · · · · · · 339

## 参考文献　　**343**

## 附录　　**357**

　　第二章　附表 · · · · · · · · · · · · · · · · · · · · · · · · · · · · · · · · · · · · · · · · · · · · · · · · · · · · · · · · · · · · · · · · · · · · · · · · · · · 357
　　第三章　附表 · · · · · · · · · · · · · · · · · · · · · · · · · · · · · · · · · · · · · · · · · · · · · · · · · · · · · · · · · · · · · · · · · · · · · · · · · · · 376
　　第四章　附表 · · · · · · · · · · · · · · · · · · · · · · · · · · · · · · · · · · · · · · · · · · · · · · · · · · · · · · · · · · · · · · · · · · · · · · · · · · · 453
　　第五章　附表 · · · · · · · · · · · · · · · · · · · · · · · · · · · · · · · · · · · · · · · · · · · · · · · · · · · · · · · · · · · · · · · · · · · · · · · · · · · 680
　　第六章　附表 · · · · · · · · · · · · · · · · · · · · · · · · · · · · · · · · · · · · · · · · · · · · · · · · · · · · · · · · · · · · · · · · · · · · · · · · · · · 724
　　第七章　附表 · · · · · · · · · · · · · · · · · · · · · · · · · · · · · · · · · · · · · · · · · · · · · · · · · · · · · · · · · · · · · · · · · · · · · · · · · · · 780
　　第八章　附表 · · · · · · · · · · · · · · · · · · · · · · · · · · · · · · · · · · · · · · · · · · · · · · · · · · · · · · · · · · · · · · · · · · · · · · · · · · · 818
　　第九章　附表 · · · · · · · · · · · · · · · · · · · · · · · · · · · · · · · · · · · · · · · · · · · · · · · · · · · · · · · · · · · · · · · · · · · · · · · · · · · 890

# Contents

| | | |
|---|---|---|
| **Summary** | | **1** |
| **Chapter 1** | **Methodology of China Total Diet Study** | **13** |
| Section 1 | Method of Dietary Research and Steps of Sample Preparation | 13 |
| Section 2 | Methods of Sample Analysis and Quality Control | 18 |
| Section 3 | Dietary Exposure Assessment Method | 73 |
| **Chapter 2** | **Dietary Exposure Assessment of Fatty acids** | **74** |
| **Chapter 3** | **Dietary Exposure Assessment of Elements** | **89** |
| Part 1 | **Nutrient Elements** | 89 |
| Section 1 | Sodium and Potassium | 89 |
| Section 2 | Calcium | 92 |
| Section 3 | Magnesium | 95 |
| Section 4 | Phosphorus | 97 |
| Section 5 | Manganese | 100 |
| Section 6 | Iron | 102 |
| Section 7 | Zinc | 104 |
| Section 8 | Chromium | 107 |
| Section 9 | Copper | 109 |
| Section 10 | Selenium | 111 |
| Section 11 | Molybdenum | 114 |
| Section 12 | Iodine | 116 |
| Part 2 | **Contaminating Elements** | 119 |
| Section 13 | Lead | 119 |
| Section 14 | Cadmium | 122 |
| Section 15 | Mercury | 125 |
| Section 16 | Arsenic | 128 |
| Section 17 | Aluminum | 132 |
| **Chapter 4** | **Dietary Exposure Assessment of Pesticide Residues** | **135** |
| **Chapter 5** | **Dietary Exposure Assessment of Veterinary Drug Residues** | **196** |

## Chapter 6  Dietary Exposure Assessment of Contaminants from Food Processing — 222

- Section 1  Chloropropanols — 222
- Section 2  Chloropropanol Fatty Acid Esters — 226
- Section 3  Glycidyl Fatty Acid Esters — 231
- Section 4  Acrylamide — 234
- Section 5  Polycyclic Aromatic Hydrocarbons — 238
- Section 6  Ethyl Carbamate — 246
- Section 7  Phthalates — 250

## Chapter 7  Dietary Exposure Assessment of Persistent Organic Pollutants — 257

- Section 1  Dioxins and Their Analogues — 257
- Section 2  Indicator PCBs — 260
- Section 3  Polybrominated Diphenyl Ethers — 263
- Section 4  Hexabromocyclododecane — 267
- Section 5  Persistent Organochlorine Pesticides — 270
- Section 6  Perfluoroalkyl Substances — 276
- Section 7  Short- and Medium-Chain Chlorinated Paraffins — 282

## Chapter 8  Dietary Exposure Assessment of Mycotoxins — 286

## Chapter 9  Dietary Exposure Assessment of Other Compounds — 320

- Section 1  Perchlorate — 320
- Section 2  Nitrate and Nitrite — 323
- Section 3  Bisphenolic Analogues — 328
- Section 4  Organophosphate Esters — 334
- Section 5  Glutamate Acid Salt — 339

## References — 343

## Appendix — 357

- Annexed Tables of Chapter 2 — 357
- Annexed Tables of Chapter 3 — 376
- Annexed Tables of Chapter 4 — 453
- Annexed Tables of Chapter 5 — 680
- Annexed Tables of Chapter 6 — 724
- Annexed Tables of Chapter 7 — 780
- Annexed Tables of Chapter 8 — 818
- Annexed Tables of Chapter 9 — 890

# 概 要
## Summary

总膳食研究（TDS）是研究和估计某一人群通过烹调加工的、可食状态的代表性膳食（包括饮水）摄入的各种膳食化学成分（污染物、营养素）的方法。总膳食研究旨在评价一个国家（地区）不同性别/年龄组对某种化学品的平均摄入量。这些数据对于评估特定化学品是否会对健康造成危害十分必要。事实上，总膳食研究可用作确定优先评估清单的工具，使风险管理者能够将有限的资源集中用于那些对公众健康构成最大风险的化学品。本书旨在发布第六次中国总膳食研究结果。

第六次中国总膳食研究的主要研究内容及研究结果如下。

### 1. 中国总膳食研究工作方法

第一部分阐述了总膳食研究中关于调查点的选择、采样单的形成、食物样品聚类、食物样品准备和运输等环节。

### 2. 第六次中国总膳食研究脂肪酸的膳食摄入量评估

我国居民膳食平均每标准人日能量摄入量为 2081 kcal（1 cal=4.184 J）。总脂肪酸摄入量为 30.1% 供能比（% E）；饱和脂肪酸（SFA）摄入量为 7.5% E，低于 10% E 推荐值；单不饱和脂肪酸（MUFA）摄入量为 12.5% E；n-6 多不饱和脂肪酸（n-6 PUFA）摄入量为 8.6% E，符合 2.5%～9.0% E 推荐值范

Total diet study is considered as a most efficient and effective method to evaluate the dietary intakes of certain chemical substances (e.g., contaminates and nutrients) through the ready to eat diet including water for a group of populations. Total diet studies are designed to measure the average amount of each chemical ingested by different age/sex groups living in a country (region). These data are necessary to assess whether or not specific chemicals pose a risk to health. In fact, total diet studies can be used as a priority-setting tool to enable risk managers to focus their limited resources on those chemicals, that pose the greatest risks to public health. This book aims to release the results of $6^{th}$ China total diet study.

The main description of methods and results of $6^{th}$ China total diet study was as following.

### 1. The Establishment of Total Diet Study Procedures

In the first part of the study, the detailed procedures were explained including the principle of selecting the investigated place, design of sampling list, the aggregation of the food samples, the preparation and the transportation of the diet samples.

### 2. The Dietary Intakes of Fatty Acids of the $6^{th}$ CTDS

The average dietary energy intake per standard man per day of China residents was 2081 kcal. The intake of total fatty acids was 30.1 percentage of total energy intake (% E); the intake of saturated fatty acids (SFA) was 7.5% E, which was lower than the recommended value of 10% E; the intake of monounsaturated fatty acids (MUFA) was 12.5% E; the intake of n-6

围；n-3 多不饱和脂肪酸（n-3 PUFA）摄入量为 1.2% E，符合 0.5%～2.0% E 推荐值范围；反式脂肪酸（TFA）摄入量为 0.2% E，低于可耐受最高摄入量（UL）1% E 的推荐值，表明膳食中反式脂肪酸是可接受的；二十碳五烯酸（EPA）+二十二碳六烯酸（DHA）摄入量为 0.067 g/d，低于推荐值下限，摄入量不充分。总脂肪酸和 SFA 的膳食来源主要为肉类、蔬菜类与谷类；MUFA 的膳食来源主要为肉类和蔬菜类；n-6 PUFA 的膳食来源主要为蔬菜类、肉类、谷类和豆类；n-3 PUFA 的膳食来源主要为蔬菜类、肉类、豆类、谷类和薯类；TFA 的膳食来源主要为蔬菜类和肉类、谷类。与第五次中国总膳食研究相比，总脂肪酸、SFA、MUFA、n-6 PUFA、n-3 PUFA 和 TFA 摄入量基本持平，而 EPA+DHA 摄入量明显降低。

**3. 第六次中国总膳食研究元素的膳食摄入量评估**

（1）营养元素

我国居民营养元素膳食摄入量分别为：钠 4485 mg/d，主要膳食来源为蔬菜类、谷类和肉类；钾 2024 mg/d，主要膳食来源为蔬菜类、谷类和肉类；钙 481 mg/d，主要膳食来源为蔬菜类、豆类和谷类；镁 305 mg/d，主要膳食来源为谷类、蔬菜类和豆类；磷 890 mg/d，主要膳食来源为谷类、肉类、蔬菜类和豆类；锰 4.83 mg/d，主要膳食来源为谷类、蔬菜类和豆类；铁 15.7 mg/d，主要膳食来源为谷类和蔬菜类；锌 6.17 mg/d，主要膳食来源为谷类和肉类；铬 139 μg/d，主要膳食来源为谷类、蔬菜类和肉类；铜 1.25 mg/d，主要膳食来源为谷类、豆类和蔬菜类；硒

polyunsaturated fatty acids (PUFA) was 8.6% E, which was in line with the recommended range of 2.5%-9.0% E; the intake of n-3 PUFA was 1.2% E, which was in line with the recommended range of 0.5%-2.0% E; the intake of *trans*-fatty acids (TFA) was 0.2% E, which was lower than the recommendation of the tolerable upper intake level (UL) of 1% E, indicating that the dietary TFA was acceptable; the intake of icosapentaenoic acid (EPA) plus docosahexaenoic acid (DHA) was 0.067 g/d, which was lower than the low end of recommendation, indicating the intake was not sufficient. The primary sources of dietary intake to total fatty acids and SFA in the diet were meats, vegetables and cereals; the primary sources of dietary intake to MUFA in the diet were meats and vegetables; the primary sources of dietary intake to n-6 PUFA in the diet were vegetables, meats, cereals and legumes; the primary sources of dietary intake to n-3 PUFA in the diet were vegetables, meats, legumes, cereals and potatoes, and the primary sources of dietary intake to TFA were vegetables and meats. Compared with the 5th China TDS, the intakes of total fatty acids, SFA, MUFA, n-6 PUFA, n-3 PUFA and TFA were essentially unchanged, and the intakes of EPA plus DHA decreased significantly.

**3. The Dietary Intakes of Elements of 6th China TDS**

(1) Nutrient Elements

The dietary intakes of nutrient elements of China residents were: sodium 4485 mg/d, the main food sources were vegetables, cereals and meats; potassium 2024 mg/d, the main food sources were vegetables, cereals and meats; calcium 481 mg/d, the main food sources were vegetables, legumes and cereals; magnesium 305 mg/d, the main food sources were cereals, vegetables and legumes; phosphorus 890 mg/d, the main food sources were cereals, meats, vegetables and legumes; manganese 4.83 mg/d, the main food sources were cereals, vegetables and legumes; iron 15.7 mg/d, the main food sources were

35.7 μg/d，主要膳食来源为肉类、谷类、水产类和蛋类；钼 161 μg/d，主要膳食来源为谷类、豆类和蔬菜类；碘 497 μg/d，主要膳食来源为蔬菜类。

（2）污染元素

我国居民重金属、有害元素及其形态的膳食暴露量分别为：铅 20.0 μg/d，主要膳食来源为谷类和蔬菜类；镉 17.3 μg/d，主要膳食来源为谷类和蔬菜类；总汞 1.26 μg/d，主要膳食来源为谷类和水产类；甲基汞 0.32 μg/d，主要膳食来源为水产类；总砷 41.5 μg/d，主要膳食来源为蔬菜类、谷类和水产类；无机砷 9.83 μg/d，主要膳食来源为谷类；铝 8.10 mg/d，主要膳食来源为谷类和蔬菜类。

### 4. 第六次中国总膳食研究农药残留的膳食摄入量评估

第六次中国总膳食研究在膳食样品中检测到 59 种农药残留，包括 26 种杀虫剂、28 种杀菌剂、3 种杀螨剂、2 种除草剂和植物生长调节剂。我国居民 26 种杀虫剂的平均膳食摄入量为 0.012～140.35 ng/(kg bw[①]·d)，占各自每日允许摄入量（ADI）的比例为 0.00%～7.80%。我国居民 28 种杀菌剂的平均膳食摄入量为 0.023～326.42 ng/(kg bw·d)，占各自 ADI 的比例为 0.00%～0.62%；3 种杀螨剂的平均膳食摄入量为 1.620～48.31 ng/(kg bw·d)，占各自 ADI 的比例为 0.02%～0.48%；2 种除草剂和植物生长调节剂的平均膳食摄入量为 0.273～1.638 ng/(kg bw·d)，占各自 ADI 的比例为 0.00%～0.01%。

---

① bw 表示体重，bw means body weight

cereals and vegetables; zinc 6.17 mg/d, the main food sources were cereals and meats; chromium 139 μg/d, the main food sources were cereals, vegetables and meats; copper 1.25 mg/d, the main food sources were cereals, legumes and vegetables; selenium 35.7 μg/d, the main food sources were meats, cereals, aquatic foods and eggs; molybdenum 161 μg/d, the main food sources were cereals, legumes and vegetables; iodine 497 μg/d, the main food sources were vegetables.

(2) Contaminating Elements

The dietary exposure to heavy metals and harmful elements and their species of China residents were as follows: lead 20.0 μg/d, the main food sources were cereals and vegetables; cadmium 17.3 μg/d, the main food sources were cereals and vegetables; total mercury 1.26 μg/d, the main food sources were cereals and aquatic foods; methylmercury 0.32 μg/d, the main food sources were aquatic foods; total arsenic 41.5 μg/d, the main food sources were vegetables, cereals and aquatic foods; inorganic arsenic 9.83 μg/d, the main food sources were cereals; aluminum 8.10 mg/d, the main food sources were cereals and vegetables.

### 4. The Dietary Intakes of Pesticide Residues of 6th China TDS

The sixth China total diet study detected 59 pesticide residues in dietary samples, including 26 pesticides, 28 fungicides, 3 acaricides, 2 herbicides and plant growth regulators. The average dietary intake of 26 insecticides in China was between 0.012-140.35 ng/(kg bw·d), accounting for 0.00%-7.80% of the ADI. The average dietary intake of 28 fungicides among China residents was between 0.023 ng/(kg bw·d) and 326.42 ng/(kg bw·d), accounting for 0.00%-0.62% of the ADI. The average dietary intake of three acaricides ranged from 1.620 ng/(kg bw·d) to 48.31 ng/(kg bw·d), accounting for 0.02%-0.48% of the ADI. The average dietary intake of the two herbicides and plant growth regulators ranged from 0.273 ng/(kg bw·d) to

## 5. 第六次中国总膳食研究兽药残留的膳食摄入量评估

在第六次中国总膳食研究的动物源性食品样品中检测到35种兽药及其代谢物,包括抗菌增效剂、喹诺酮类、磺胺类、三苯甲烷类、硝基咪唑类、苯并咪唑类和氯霉素类。我国居民抗菌增效剂的平均膳食摄入量为8.611 ng/(kg bw·d),占ADI的0.205%。喹诺酮类药物的平均膳食摄入量为0.001～35.35 ng/(kg bw·d),其中,恩诺沙星占ADI的0.570%。总磺胺类药物的平均膳食摄入量为15.77 ng/(kg bw·d),占ADI的0.032%。三苯甲烷类药物的平均膳食摄入量为16.31 ng/(kg bw·d)。硝基咪唑类药物的平均膳食摄入量为5.376～10.58 ng/(kg bw·d)。苯并咪唑类药物的平均膳食摄入量为0.039～0.235 ng/(kg bw·d),占ADI的0.000%～0.003%。氯霉素类药物的平均膳食摄入量为0.017～4.413 ng/(kg bw·d),占ADI的0.000%～0.147%。

## 6. 第六次中国总膳食研究生产加工过程污染物的膳食摄入量评估

（1）氯丙醇

我国居民3-氯-1,2-丙二醇（3-MCPD）和2-氯-1,3-丙二醇（2-MCPD）平均膳食摄入量分别为0.144 μg/(kg bw·d)和0.010 μg/(kg bw·d),分别占每日最大耐受摄入量（PMTDI）的3.6%和0.3%。3-MCPD主要来源于蔬菜类（69.2%）、谷类（16.4%）、薯类（5.0%）、肉类（4.3%）,占总摄入量的94.9%。与第五次中国总膳食研究的膳食摄入量0.250 μg/(kg bw·d)相比,第六次中国总膳食研究3-MCPD膳食摄入量呈现明显降低。

1.638 ng/(kg bw·d), accounting for 0.00%-0.01% of the ADI.

## 5. The Dietary Intakes of Veterinary Drug Residues of 6th China TDS

A total of 35 veterinary drugs and their metabolites, including antibacterial synergists, quinolones, sulfonamides, triphenylmethanes, nitroimidazoles, benzimidazoles, and chloramphenicol, were detected in animal-derived dietary samples from the sixth China total diet study. The average dietary intake of antibacterial synergists in China residents was 8.611 ng/(kg bw·d), accounting for 0.205% of the ADI. The average dietary intake of quinolones ranged from 0.001 ng/(kg bw·d) to 35.35 ng/(kg bw·d), of which enrofloxacin accounting for 0.570% of the ADI. The average dietary intake of total sulfonamides was 15.77 ng/(kg bw·d), accounting for 0.032% of the ADI. The average dietary intake of triphenylmethanes was 16.31 ng/(kg bw·d). The average dietary intake of nitroimidazoles was 5.376-10.58 ng/(kg bw·d). The average dietary intake of benzimidazoles was 0.039-0.235 ng/(kg bw·d), accounting for 0.000%-0.003% of the ADI. The average dietary intake of chloramphenicol was 0.017-4.413 ng/(kg bw·d), accounting for 0.000%-0.147% of the ADI.

## 6. The Dietary Intakes of Contaminants from Food Processing of 6th China TDS

(1) Chloropropanols

The average dietary intakes of 3-MCPD and 2-MCPD for China residents were 0.144 μg/(kg bw·d) and 0.010 μg/(kg bw·d), accounting for 3.6% and 0.3% of the PMTDI value for 3-MCPD and 2-MCPD, respectively. The primary sources of 3-MCPD dietary intake identified in the 6th China TDS were vegetables (69.2%), cereals (16.4%), potatoes (5.0%), meats (4.3%), accounting for over 94.9%. The dietary intake of 3-MCPD from the 6th China TDS declined significantly in comparison with that of 5th China TDS [0.250 μg/(kg bw·d)].

（2）氯丙醇酯

我国居民 3-MCPD 酯和 2-MCPD 酯平均膳食摄入量分别为 1.074 μg/(kg bw·d) 和 0.258 μg/(kg bw·d)，分别占 PMTDI 的 26.8% 和 6.4%。3-MCPD 酯主要来源于蔬菜类（43.5%）、谷类（15.1%）、蛋类（12.1%）、肉类（9.3%）、薯类（8.2%）、水及饮料类（5.6%）、豆类（3.1%），占总摄入量的 96.9%；2-MCPD 酯的来源与 3-MCPD 酯类似；3-MCPD 酯与第五次中国总膳食研究的膳食摄入量 1.32 μg/(kg bw·d) 相比，呈现明显降低。

（3）缩水甘油酯

我国居民缩水甘油酯平均膳食摄入量为 0.787 μg/(kg bw·d)，暴露边界值（MOE）为 12 963。缩水甘油酯主要来源于蔬菜类（51.4%）、肉类（11.9%）、谷类（9.4%）、薯类（7.6%）、水及饮料类（6.7%）、蛋类（6.1%）、豆类（4.0%），占总摄入量的 97.1%。

（4）丙烯酰胺

第六次中国总膳食研究的我国居民丙烯酰胺平均膳食摄入量为 0.175 μg/(kg bw·d)，主要来源于蔬菜类（59.0%）、谷类（18.9%）、薯类（10.1%）、豆类（4.7%），占总膳食摄入量的 92.7%。与第五次中国总膳食研究的膳食摄入量 0.319 μg/(kg bw·d) 相比，呈现明显降低。根据无可见不良作用水平（NOAEL），我国居民第六次中国总膳食研究摄入丙烯酰胺的 MOE 为 1143；根据大鼠和小鼠的基准剂量置信下限（$BMDL_{10}$），我国居民膳食摄入丙烯酰胺的 MOE 分别为 1771 和 1029。

（5）多环芳烃（PAH）

我国居民苯并[a]芘的平均膳食摄入量为 2.82 ng/(kg bw·d)，PAH4 的平均膳食摄入量为 16.50 ng/(kg bw·d)，PAH16 的平均膳食摄入量为 28.99 ng/(kg bw·d)。蔬菜类是我国居民膳食摄入多环芳烃的主要来源。

(2) Chloropropanol Fatty Acid Esters

The average dietary intakes of 3-MCPD esters and 2-MCPD esters for China residents were 1.074 μg/(kg bw·d) and 0.258 μg/(kg bw·d), accounting for 26.8% and 6.4% of the PMTDI value for 3-MCPD esters and 2-MCPD esters, respectively. The primary sources of 3-MCPD esters dietary intake identified in the 6$^{th}$ China TDS are vegetables (43.5%), cereals (15.1%), eggs (12.1%), meats (9.3%), potatoes (8.2%), water and beverages (5.6%), legumes (3.1%), accounting for 96.9%. The sources of 2-MCPD esters is similar to 3-MCPD esters. The dietary intake of 3-MCPD from the 6$^{th}$ China TDS declined significantly in comparison with that of 5$^{th}$ China TDS [1.32 μg/(kg bw·d)].

(3) Glycidyl Fatty Acid Esters

The average dietary intake of glycidyl fatty acid esters for China residents was 0.787 μg/(kg bw·d), accounting for the MOE of 12 963. The primary sources of glycidyl fatty acid esters dietary intake identified in the 6$^{th}$ China TDS are vegetables (51.4%), meats (11.9%), cereals (9.4%), potatoes (7.6%), water and beverages (6.7%), eggs (6.1%), legumes (4.0%), accounting for 97.1%.

(4) Acrylamide

The average dietary intake of acrylamide for China residents in the 6$^{th}$ China total diet study (TDS) was 0.175 μg/(kg bw·d). Vegetables (59.0%), cereals (18.9%), potatoes (10.1%) and beans (4.7%) were the predominant contributors of acrylamide intake, accounting for approximately 92.7% of the overall EDIs. Compared with the dietary intake of the 5$^{th}$ China TDS [0.319 μg/(kg bw·d)], it showed a significant decrease. The MOE was 1143 based on NOAEL. The MOEs of rats and mice were 1771 and 1029 based on $BMDL_{10}$, respectively.

(5) Polycyclic Aromatic Hydrocarbons (PAHs)

The average dietary intake of benzo [a] pyrene for China residents in the 6$^{th}$ China total diet study (TDS) was 2.82 ng/(kg bw·d), the average dietary intake of PAH4 of China residents was 16.50 ng/(kg bw·d), the average dietary intake of PAH16 of China residents was

（6）氨基甲酸乙酯

我国居民氨基甲酸乙酯膳食摄入量为 0.05 μg/(kg bw·d)，主要来源于肉类（53.82%）、蔬菜类（24.90%）、水产类（15.14%）和酒类（6.14%）。其与第五次中国总膳食研究的膳食摄入量 0.08 μg/(kg bw·d) 相比，呈现下降趋势。第六次中国总膳食研究我国居民膳食摄入氨基甲酸乙酯的 MOE 为 6000。

（7）邻苯二甲酸酯

我国居民邻苯二甲酸二丁酯（DBP）膳食摄入量为 0.98 μg/(kg bw·d)，主要来源于谷类（34.5%）、水及饮料类（24.9%）和蔬菜类（20.4%）。其与第五次中国总膳食研究的膳食摄入量 5.97 μg/(kg bw·d) 相比，呈现明显下降趋势，同时低于欧洲食品安全局提出的 10 μg/(kg bw·d) 的每日可耐受摄入量（TDI）。邻苯二甲酸二异丁酯（DiBP）膳食摄入量为 0.80 μg/(kg bw·d)，主要来源于水及饮料类（42.3%）、谷类（29.6%）和蔬菜类（13.3%），与第五次中国总膳食研究的膳食摄入量 3.71 μg/(kg bw·d) 相比，呈现明显下降趋势，同时低于我国国家食品安全风险评估中心提出的 30 μg/(kg bw·d) 的 TDI。邻苯二甲酸二(2-乙基)己酯（DEHP）膳食摄入量为 1.16 μg/(kg bw·d)，主要来源为谷类（34.3%）、蔬菜类（30.8%）和水及饮料类（13.9%），与第五次中国总膳食研究的膳食摄入量 6.21 μg/(kg bw·d) 相比，呈现明显下降趋势。第六次中国总膳食研究 DEHP 膳食暴露量未超过 TDI 为 50 μg/(kg bw·d) 的限量。

### 7. 第六次中国总膳食研究持久性有机污染物的膳食摄入量评估

（1）二噁英及其类似物

我国居民 PCDD/Fs 和 dl-PCB 平均膳食摄入量为 7.7 pg TEQ/(kg bw·月)，

28.99 ng/(kg bw·d). The primary sources of PAHs intake identified in the 6$^{th}$ China TDS are vegetables.

(6) Ethyl Carbamate

The dietary intake of ethyl carbamate for China residents was 0.05 μg/(kg bw·d), mainly from meats (53.82%), vegetables (24.90%), aquatic foods (15.14%), and alcohol beverages (6.14%). Compared with the dietary intake of 0.08 μg/(kg bw·d) in the 5$^{th}$ China TDS, it showed a decreasing trend. The MOE of dietary intake of ethyl carbamate for China residents in the 6$^{th}$ China total diet study was 6000.

(7) Phthalates

The dietary intake of dibutyl phthalate (DBP) for China residents was 0.98 μg/(kg bw·d), mainly from cereals (34.5%), water and beverages (24.9%), and vegetables (20.4%). The intake showed a significant downward trend compared to the dietary intake of 5.97 μg/(kg bw·d) in the 5$^{th}$ China TDS. At the same time, it is lower than the TDI of 10 μg/(kg bw·d) proposed by the European Food Safety Authority (EFSA). Diisobutyl phthalate (DiBP) dietary intake was 0.80 μg/(kg bw·d), mainly from water and beverages (42.3%), cereals (29.6%), and vegetables (13.3%), compared with the dietary intake of 3.71 μg/(kg bw·d) in the 5$^{th}$ China TDS, showing a significant downward trend. At the same time, it is lower than the TDI of 30 μg/(kg bw·d) proposed by China National Center for Food Safety Risk Assessment (CFSA). Dietary intake of di (2-ethyl) hexyl phthalate (DEHP) was 1.16 μg/(kg bw·d), mainly from cereals (34.3%), vegetables (30.8%), water and beverages (13.9%), compared with the dietary intake of 6.21 μg/(kg bw·d) in the 5$^{th}$ China TDS, showing a significant decreasing trend. The dietary exposure in the 6$^{th}$ China TDS was not more than the TDI of 50 μg/(kg bw·d) for DEHP.

### 7. The Dietary Intakes of Persistent Organic Pollutants of 6$^{th}$ China TDS

(1) Dioxins and Their Analogues

The average dietary intake of PCDD/Fs and dl-PCBs for China residents was 7.7 pg TEQ/(kg

远低于食品添加剂联合专家委员会（JECFA）规定的 70 pg TEQ/(kg bw·月)的暂定每月可耐受摄入量（PTMI），其膳食来源主要为肉类和水产类，分别占 48.7% 和 32.6%。其与第五次中国总膳食研究的膳食摄入量 15.0 pg TEQ/(kg bw·月)相比，呈现明显降低趋势。

（2）指示性多氯联苯（PCB）

我国居民指示性 PCB 膳食摄入量为 429.9 pg/(kg bw·d)，其膳食来源主要为肉类、水产类和谷类，分别占 25.5%、20.1% 和 19.3%。其与第五次中国总膳食研究的膳食摄入量 666.0 pg/(kg bw·d)相比，呈现明显降低趋势。

（3）多溴二苯醚（PBDE）

我国居民 PBDE 膳食摄入量为 249.0 pg/(kg bw·d)，基于 EFSA 提出的 BMDL$_{10}$，我国居民膳食摄入的 MOE 为 1000~17 000 000，其膳食来源主要为谷类、肉类及蔬菜类，占比分别为 23.4%、24.4% 和 23.2%。其与第五次中国总膳食研究的膳食摄入量 646.0 pg/(kg bw·d)相比，呈现明显降低趋势。

（4）六溴环十二烷

我国居民通过动物性膳食摄入的六溴环十二烷（HBCD）的平均值（EDI）为 3062 pg/(kg bw·d)，明显高于第四次和第五次中国总膳食研究获得的结果 [平均值分别为 432 pg/(kg bw·d) 和 1476 pg/(kg bw·d)]。膳食摄入 HBCD 主要来源于肉类，占总摄入量的 87.7%。根据欧洲食品安全局设定的健康指导值（HBGV）2.35 μg/(kg bw·d)估算，我国居民膳食摄入 HBCD 的暴露边界值（MOE）的中位数为 1590，远高于阈值，提示我国总体上由动物性膳食摄入 HBCD 导致的健康风险较低，但部分高暴露地区的 MOE 已接近阈值，需持续关注。

bw·month) in the 6$^{th}$ China TDS, which was obviously lower than the PTMI, 70 pg TEQ/(kg bw·month), regulated by JECCFA. The main diet sources were attributed to meats and aquatic foods with a percentage contribution of 48.7% and 32.6%, respectively. A significance decrease was observed in dietary intake of PCDD/Fs and dl-PCBs by comparison with that in the 5$^{th}$ China TDS, 15.0 pg TEQ/(kg bw·month).

(2) Indicator PCBs

The average dietary intake of indicator PCBs for China residents was 429.9 pg/(kg bw·d) in the 6$^{th}$ China TDS. The main diet source was attributed to meats, followed by aquatic foods, and cereals, with a percentage contribution of 25.5%, 20.1%, and 19.3%, respectively. A significance decrease was observed in dietary intake of indicator PCBs by comparison with that in the 5$^{th}$ China TDS, 666.0 pg/(kg bw·d).

(3) Polybrominated Diphenyl Ethers (PBDEs)

The average dietary intake of PBDEs for China residents was 249.0 pg/(kg bw·d) in the 6$^{th}$ China TDS. By comparison with the BMDL$_{10}$ recommended by EFSA, the MOE of dietary intakes of PBDEs for China residents were in the range of 1000-17 000 000. The main diet source was attributed to cereals, followed by meats, and vegetables, with a percentage contribution of 23.4%, 24.4%, and 23.2%, respectively. A significance decrease was observed in dietary intake of PBDEs by comparison with that in the 5$^{th}$ China TDS, 646.0 pg/(kg bw·d).

(4) Hexabromocyclododecane

The average estimated daily intake (EDI) of hexabromocyclododecane (HBCD) via animal-based food was 3062 pg/(kg bw·d) for Chinese population, which was significantly higher than the EDIs of HBCD obtained in the 4$^{th}$ and 5$^{th}$ China TDS [averages of 432 pg/(kg bw·d) and 1476 pg/(kg bw·d)]. The dietary intake of HBCD was mainly from meats consumption, and which accounted for 87.7% in total HBCD intake. According to the health-based guidance value [2.35 μg/(kg bw·d)] suggested by European Food Safety Authority (EFSA), the margin of exposure (MOE) of HBCD

（5）持久性有机氯农药

第六次中国总膳食研究中我国居民滴滴涕（DDT）的平均膳食摄入量（EDI）为 2.883 ng/(kg bw·d)，其膳食来源主要为水产类和肉类；六六六的平均膳食摄入量为 1.337 ng/(kg bw·d)，其膳食来源主要为水产类、肉类和蔬菜类；硫丹的平均膳食摄入量为 2.689 ng/(kg bw·d)；五氯苯的平均膳食摄入量为 2.782 ng/(kg bw·d)；六氯苯（HCB）的平均膳食摄入量为 0.713 ng/(kg bw·d)。从膳食暴露评估结果可以得出，我国各地区居民持久性有机氯农药（OCP）的膳食摄入量远远低于各自的健康指导值，健康风险极低。

（6）全氟烷基化合物

我国居民全氟辛醇（PFOA）的平均膳食摄入量（EWI）为 2.17 ng/(kg bw·周)，主要来源于蛋类（34.6%）、谷类（23.1%）、肉类（16.2%）、蔬菜类（13.4%）、水产类（7.0%），占总膳食摄入量的 94.3%。我国居民全氟辛烷磺醇（PFOS）的平均膳食摄入量为 2.72 ng/(kg bw·周)，主要来源于水产类（54.4%）、肉类（23.5%）、蔬菜类（10.0%）、蛋类（7.3%），占总膳食摄入量的 95.2%。依据 EFSA 在 2018 年提出的 PFOA 和 PFOS 的健康指导值每周可耐受摄入量（TWI），目前我国居民 PFOA 和 PFOS 膳食暴露的健康风险依然较低。

intake was calculated. The median level of MOE of HBCD for Chinese population was 1590. This value was significantly higher than the threshold set by EFSA, suggesting that the intake of HBCD via animal-based food consumption for Chinese population was unlikely to cause significant health concerns. However, the MOEs of HBCD in some areas have found to be close to the threshold, which suggested that the monitoring of HBCD should continue.

(5) Persistent Organochlorine Pesticides (OCPs)

The average estimated daily intake (EDI) of DDTs in the 6$^{th}$ China total diet study was 2.883 ng/(kg bw·d), The primary food sources of dietary intake to the DDTs were aquatic foods, followed by meats; The average EDI of HCHs was 1.337 ng/(kg bw·d), The primary food sources of dietary intake to the HCHs were aquatic foods, followed by meats and vegetables; The average EDI of endosulfans was 2.689 ng/(kg bw·d); The average EDI of pentachlorobenzene (PCB) was 2.782 ng/(kg bw·d); The average EDI of hexachlorobenzene (HCB) was 0.713 ng/(kg bw·d). The results of dietary exposure showed that the dietary intakes of OCPs of the Chinese population are far lower than their health-based guidance values and pose little risk.

(6) Perfluoroalkyl Substances

The average estimated weekly intake (EWI) of PFOA was 2.17 ng/(kg bw·week). Eggs were the primary source of dietary intake to PFOA, contributing 34.6% to the total intake, followed by cereals (23.1%), meats (16.2%), vegetables (13.4%), and aquatic foods (7.0%), which totally accounting for 94.3% of the total dietary intake. The average EWI of PFOS was 2.72 ng/(kg bw·week). Aquatic foods were the primary source of dietary intake to PFOS, contributing 54.4% to the total intake, followed by meats (23.5%), vegetables (10.0%), and eggs (7.3%), which totally accounting for 95.2% of the total dietary intake. The EWI of PFOA and PFOS were far below the tolerable weekly intake (TWI) recommended by EFSA in 2018, indicating that low health risks via dietary exposure of PFOA and PFOS for the most population in China.

（7）氯化石蜡

我国居民短链和中链氯化石蜡膳食平均摄入量分别为 1041 ng/(kg bw·d) 和 918 ng/(kg bw·d)，主要来源于谷类（分别为44.8%和45.5%）与蔬菜类（分别为24.2%和22.1%）。与第五次总膳食研究结果相比，除肉类中链氯化石蜡（MCCP）浓度呈现上升趋势外，豆类、谷类和水产类短链氯化石蜡（SCCP）和MCCP的浓度水平均表现出明显的下降趋势。基于 EFSA 推算的 $BMDL_{10}$ 计算，我国居民膳食摄入 SCCP 和 MCCP 的 MOE 分别为 $2 \times 10^3$ 和 $4 \times 10^4$，远大于1000，表明通过膳食摄入 SCCP 和 MCCP 的健康风险较低。

### 8. 第六次中国总膳食研究真菌毒素的膳食摄入量评估

我国居民各类主要真菌毒素的膳食暴露量分别为：黄曲霉毒素 BG 2.55 ng/(kg bw·d)，T-2毒素与HT-2毒素 3.11 ng/(kg bw·d)，脱氧雪腐镰刀菌烯醇（DDN）、3-乙酰-脱氧雪腐镰刀菌烯醇（3-Ac-DON）与15-乙酰-脱氧雪腐镰刀菌烯醇（15-Ac-DON） 0.690 μg/(kg bw·d)，脱氧雪腐镰刀菌烯醇、3-乙酰-脱氧雪腐镰刀菌烯醇、15-乙酰-脱氧雪腐镰刀菌烯醇与3-葡萄糖-脱氧雪腐镰刀菌烯醇（DON-3-G） 0.715 μg/(kg bw·d)，雪腐镰刀菌烯醇（NIV） 0.009 μg/(kg bw·d)，赭曲霉毒素A（OTA） 0.876 ng/(kg bw·d)，玉米赤霉烯酮 7.77 ng/(kg bw·d)，伏马菌素 0.104 μg/(kg bw·d)，交链孢菌酮酸（TeA） 141 ng/(kg bw·d)，腾毒素（TEN） 143 ng/(kg bw·d)，交链孢酚单甲醚（AME） 33.8 ng/(kg bw·d)，交链孢烯（ALT） 16.7 ng/(kg bw·d)，白僵菌素（BEA） 13.5 ng/(kg bw·d)，恩镰孢菌素（ENN）A 5.54 ng/(kg bw·d)，恩镰孢菌素A1 5.73 ng/(kg bw·d)，恩

(7) Chlorinated Paraffins

The total estimated dietary intake of SCCPs and MCCPs in sixth China total diet study, with average values of 1041 ng/(kg bw·d) and 918 ng/(kg bw·d) were mostly contributed by cereals (44.8% and 45.5%, respectively) and vegetables (24.2% and 22.1%, respectively). Compared with the results of the fifth China total diet study, the concentrations of SCCPs and MCCPs in the legumes, cereals and aquatic foods were decreased except that the concentrations of MCCPs in meats were increased. The MOEs of SCCPs and MCCPs based on $BMDL_{10}$ by European Food Safety Authority in all the eight food categories were $2 \times 10^3$ and $4 \times 10^4$, respectively, which were much higher than 1000, indicating that SCCPs and MCCPs may not pose a significant risk to human health in China.

### 8. The Dietary Intakes of Mycotoxins of 6th China TDS

The dietary exposure of major mycotoxins were: aflatoxin BG 2.55 ng/(kg bw·d), T-2 and HT-2 3.11 ng/(kg bw·d), the sum of DON, 3-Ac-DON and 15-Ac-DON 0.690 μg/(kg bw·d), the sum of DON, 3-Ac-DON, 15-Ac-DON, and DON-3-G 0.715 μg/(kg bw·d), NIV 0.009 μg/(kg bw·d), OTA 0.876 ng/(kg bw·d), zearalenone 7.77 ng/(kg bw·d), fumonisins 0.104 μg/(kg bw·d), TeA 141 ng/(kg bw·d), TEN 143 ng/(kg bw·d), AME 33.8 ng/(kg bw·d), ALT 16.7 ng/(kg bw·d), BEA 13.5 ng/(kg bw·d), ENNA 5.54 ng/(kg bw·d), ENNA1 5.73 ng/(kg bw·d), ENNB 50.8 ng/(kg bw·d), ENNB1 15.6 ng/(kg bw·d) and SMC 1.13 ng/(kg bw·d). The dietary intakes of fumonisins, PAT, NIV, ZEN, T-2 and HT-2, TEN and TeA were all lower than 10% of the PMTDI, indicating a low health risk. The national average MOE value of aflatoxin BG was 67, presenting a potential health hazard. Legumes and cereals are the primary food sources of dietary aflatoxin BG. The national average dietary exposure to the sum of DON, 3-Ac-DON, and 15-Ac-DON was 0.690 μg/(kg bw·d), which was 69% of the PMTDI value set by JECFA. Sichuan, Qinghai, Beijing, Shandong, and

镰孢菌素 B 50.8 ng/(kg bw·d)，恩镰孢菌素 B1 15.6 ng/(kg bw·d)，杂色曲霉毒素（SMC）1.13 ng/(kg bw·d)。其中伏马菌素、展青霉素（PAT）、雪腐镰刀菌烯醇、玉米赤霉烯酮（ZEN）、T-2 与 HT-2 毒素、腾毒素、交链孢菌酮酸的膳食暴露量均小于 PMTDI 的 10%，健康风险较低。黄曲霉毒素 BG 的全国平均 MOE 为 67，存在潜在的健康风险。膳食黄曲霉毒素 BG 的主要食物来源是豆类和谷类。脱氧雪腐镰刀菌烯醇、3-乙酰-脱氧雪腐镰刀菌烯醇与 15-乙酰-脱氧雪腐镰刀菌烯醇的全国平均膳食暴露量为 0.690 μg/(kg bw·d)，约为 JECFA 设定 PMTDI [1 μg/(kg bw·d)] 的 69%，四川、青海、北京、山东、黑龙江均超出 PMTDI，该类毒素最主要的膳食暴露来源是谷类，贡献率超过 98%。脱氧雪腐镰刀菌烯醇、3-乙酰-脱氧雪腐镰刀菌烯醇、15-乙酰-脱氧雪腐镰刀菌烯醇与 3-葡萄糖-脱氧雪腐镰刀菌烯醇的全国平均膳食暴露量为 0.715 μg/(kg bw·d)，约为 EFSA 设定 PMTDI [1 μg/(kg bw·d)] 的 72%，四川、青海、北京、山东、山西、湖北、黑龙江均超出 PMTDI，该类毒素最主要的膳食暴露来源是谷类，贡献率超过 95%。一般人群赭曲霉毒素 A 的平均膳食摄入量为 6.13 ng/(kg bw·周)，占 JECFA 设定的暂定每周允许摄入量（PTWI）[100 ng/(kg bw·周)] 的 6.13%，整体风险较低，但内蒙古的摄入量为 102 ng/(kg bw·周)，超过 JECFA 设定的 PTWI，谷类贡献率超过 99%。一般人群 AME 的膳食摄入量为 33.8 ng/(kg bw·d)，约为 EFSA 制定毒理学关注阈值（TTC）[2.5 ng/(kg bw·d)] 的 13.5 倍，20 个省份的摄入量均超过 TTC，健康风险需引起关注。

Heilongjiang exceeded the health-based guidance value. Cereals were the primary source of dietary exposure to DON, 3-Ac-DON and 15-Ac-DON, accounting for more than 98% of the total level. The national average dietary exposure to the sum of DON, 3-Ac-DON, 15-Ac-DON and DON-3-G was 0.715 μg/(kg bw·d), which was 72% of the PMTDI value set by EFSA. Sichuan, Qinghai, Beijing, Shandong, Shanxi, Hubei, and Heilongjiang exceeded the health-based guidance value. Cereals were the primary source of dietary exposure to DON, 3-Ac-DON, 15-Ac-DON, and DON-3-G, accounting for more than 95% of the total level. The national average dietary exposure of OTA was 6.13 ng/(kg bw·week), which was 6.13% of the PTWI value set by JECFA, indicating a low health risk, but Inner Mongolia exceeded the health-based guidance value. Cereals were the primary source, accounting for more than 99%. The national average dietary exposure to AME was 33.8 ng/(kg bw·week), which was 13.5 times the TTC value set by EFSA, 20 provinces exceeded the TTC value, and the health risk should be paid attention to.

## 9. 第六次中国总膳食研究其他化合物的膳食摄入量评估

（1）高氯酸盐

我国居民第六次中国总膳食研究的高氯酸盐膳食摄入量为 0.449 μg/(kg bw·d)，主要来源于蔬菜类（45.9%）、水及饮料类（25.7%）、谷类（18.6%），占总摄入量的 90.2%。我国居民膳食摄入的高氯酸盐占 NAS 设定的健康指导值（HBGV）[0.7 μg/(kg bw·d)] 的 64.1%，占 JECFA 的健康指导值 [10 μg/(kg bw·d)] 的 4.5%，占 EFSA 的健康指导值 [0.3 μg/(kg bw·d)] 的 149.7%。

（2）硝酸盐与亚硝酸盐

我国居民硝酸盐平均膳食摄入量为 6071 μg/(kg bw·d)，范围为 1878～17 371 μg/(kg bw·d)，主要暴露来源为蔬菜类，占总膳食摄入量的 94%。亚硝酸盐摄入量为 0.74 μg/(kg bw·d)，范围为 0.13～4.89 μg/(kg bw·d)，主要暴露来源为水及饮料类（28.3%）。

（3）双酚类化合物

我国居民双酚类化合物的膳食暴露量为：双酚 A（BPA）18.13 ng/(kg bw·d)、双酚 S（BPS）22.20 ng/(kg bw·d)、双酚 F（BPF）0.49 ng/(kg bw·d)、双酚 AF（BPAF）0.38 ng/(kg bw·d)。BPA 膳食摄入的食物来源主要为谷类（40.3%）和水及饮料（17.4%）；BPS 的主要食物来源为谷类（32.4%）和肉类（25.4%）。

（4）有机磷酸酯

我国居民通过动物性膳食摄入有机磷酸酯（OPE）的膳食摄入量平均值为 0.45～18.12 ng/(kg bw·d)。第六次中国总膳食研究的 OPE 膳食摄入主要来源于肉类，占总摄入量的 50% 以上。根据美国环境保护署和欧盟设定的 OPE 健康指导值 [7～100 μg/(kg bw·d)]，我国居民膳食摄入的 OPE 尚不足以引起健康风险。

## 9. The Dietary Intakes of Other Compounds of 6$^{th}$ China TDS

(1) Perchlorate

The dietary intake of perchlorate in the 6$^{th}$ China TDS of China residents is 0.449 μg/(kg bw·d), mainly from vegetables (45.9%), water and beverages (25.7%), and cereals (18.6%), accounting for 90.2% of the total intake. The dietary intake of perchlorate by China residents accounts for 64.1% of the HBGV [0.7 μg/(kg bw·d)] set by NAS, 4.5% of the HBGV [10 μg/(kg bw·d)] set by JECFA, and 149.7% of the HBGV [0.3 μg/(kg bw·d)] set by EFSA.

(2) Nitrate and Nitrite

The average dietary intake of nitrate for China residents was 6071 μg/(kg bw·d), ranging from 1878 μg/(kg bw·d) to 17 371 μg/(kg bw·d). The vegetables were the major sources for the total dietary exposure, accounting for 94% of the total dietary intake. The average dietary intake of nitrite is 0.74 μg/(kg bw·d), ranging from 0.13 μg/(kg bw·d) to 4.89 μg/(kg bw·d). The main source of dietary exposure was water and beverages (28.3%).

(3) Bisphenolic Analogues

The estimated dietary exposures of bisphenol A (BPA), bisphenol S (BPS), bisphenol F (BPF) and bisphenol AF (BPAF) for an average adult were 18.13 ng/(kg bw·d), 22.20 ng/(kg bw·d), 0.49 ng/(kg bw·d) and 0.38 ng/(kg bw·d), respectively. The main dietary contributors for BPA were cereals (40.3%), water and beverages (17.4%), as well as for BPS were cereals (32.4%) and meats (25.4%).

(4) Organophosphate Esters

The average estimated daily intake (EDI) of organophosphate esters (OPEs) via animal-based food consumption was 0.45-18.12 ng/(kg bw·d) for Chinese population. The dietary intake of OPEs was mainly from meats, and which accounted for over 50% in total OPE intake. Compared to the health-based guidance values suggested by European Food Safety Authority (EFSA) and U.S. Environmental Protection Agency (USEPA),

（5）谷氨酸盐

第六次中国总膳食研究的我国居民谷氨酸盐膳食摄入量为 17.63 mg/(kg bw·d)，主要来源于蔬菜（43.9%）、谷类（21.0%）、肉类（14.1%）、豆类（9.4%），占总膳食摄入量的 88.4%。我国居民膳食摄入的谷氨酸盐未超过欧洲食品安全局（EFSA）最新提出的 ADI 30 mg/(kg bw·d)；与第五次中国总膳食研究的膳食摄入量 14.53 mg/(kg bw·d) 相比，呈现明显上升趋势。

which were 7-100 μg/(kg bw·d), the dietary OPEs intake via food for Chinese population was unlikely to cause significant health concerns.

(5) Glutamate Acid Salt

The dietary intake of glutamate acid salt for China residents in the 6th China total diet study was 17.63 mg/(kg bw·d), mainly from vegetables (43.9%), cereals (21.0%), meats (14.1%), and legumes (9.4%), accounting for 88.4% of the total dietary intake. The intake showed a clear increasing trend compared to 14.53 mg/(kg bw·d) dietary intake in the 5th China TDS. Compared with the latest ADI of 30 mg/(kg bw·d) proposed by the European Food Safety Authority (EFSA), the dietary intake of glutamate acid salt for our population was within the EFSA regulation.

# 第一章　中国总膳食研究方法学
# Chapter 1　Methodology of China Total Diet Study

## 第一节　膳食调查方法和样品制备步骤
## Section 1　Method of Dietary Research and Steps of Sample Preparation

### 一、研究方法

简述研究方法，包括：①食物聚类；②样品采集；③烹调及混合膳食样品制备；④混合与单个膳食样品测定；⑤通过混合与单个膳食样品中化学污染物和营养素的测定，计算出成年男子（标准人）每人每日膳食化学污染物和营养素的摄入量。

### 二、调查地点

第六次中国总膳食研究包括24个省（自治区、直辖市）。各大区具体组成如下。

北方一区：黑龙江省、辽宁省、河北省、吉林省、北京市、山西省。

北方二区：河南省、陕西省、宁夏回族自治区、青海省、内蒙古自治区、甘肃省。

南方一区：江西省、福建省、上海市、江苏省、浙江省、山东省。

南方二区：湖北省、四川省、广西壮族自治区、湖南省、广东省、贵州省。

每个区（一个大菜篮子）由6个省（自治区、直辖市）组成，全国24个省（自治区、直辖市）共组成4个区。每省（自治区、直辖市）为一个具体实施单位（一个小菜篮子），按照人口下设3个/6个调查点，即：5000万以上人口

### Ⅰ. Research Method

The research method was simply listed as: ① food aggregation; ② collection of individual samples; ③ cooking and preparation of food composite samples; ④ analysis of composite and individual food samples; ⑤ calculation of daily dietary intake and exposure to chemical contaminants and nutrient elements of adult males (reference man) through measurement of chemical contaminants and nutrient elements in composite and individual food samples.

### Ⅱ. Geographic Scope of TDS

The 6$^{th}$ China total diet study includes 24 provinces (autonomous regions, municipalities). The regions under survey were as follows.

North 1 Region: Heilongjiang, Liaoning, Hebei, Jilin, Shanxi provinces and Beijing Municipality.

North 2 Region: Henan, Shaanxi, Qinghai, Gansu provinces, Ningxia Hui Autonomous Region, Inner Mongolia Autonomous Region.

South 1 Region: Jiangxi, Fujian, Jiangsu, Zhejiang, Shandong provinces and Shanghai Municipality.

South 2 Region: Hubei, Sichuan, Hunan, Guangdong, Guizhou provinces and Guangxi Zhuang Autonomous Region.

Each region (representing a major market basket) is comprised of 6 provinces (autonomous regions, municipalities). The above four regions cover a total of

省份设置6个调查点（包括2个城市点及4个农村点），5000万以下人口省份设置3个调查点（包括1个城市点及2个农村点）。

## 三、食物样品的收集

### 1. 食物样品分类

按目前采用的混合食物样品法将调查所得的人均食物消费量分为13类，即将所消费的各种食品按所属类别（表1-1）进行归类。

24 provinces (autonomous regions, municipalities). Each province (autonomous region, municipality) constitutes an implementation unit (representing a minor market basket), each having three or six survey points according to the population, i.e.: 6 survey points (including 2 urban points and 4 rural points) in provinces with population of more than 50 million, and 3 survey points in provinces with population of less than 50 million (including 1 urban sites and 2 rural sites).

## III. Collection of Food Samples

### 1. Classification of Food Samples

The per capital consumption of foods was classified into 13 categories according to the food composite approach adopted in this study, as shown in Table 1-1.

表 1-1　中国总膳食研究食物分类
Table 1-1　Food categories for China TDS

1. 谷类 Cereals
2. 豆类 Legumes
3. 薯类 Potatoes
4. 肉类 Meats
5. 蛋类 Eggs
6. 水产类 Aquatic foods
7. 乳类 Dairy products
8. 蔬菜类 Vegetables
9. 水果类 Fruits
10. 糖类 Sugar
11. 水及饮料类 Water and beverages
12. 酒类 Alcohol beverages
13. 调味品类（包括烹调用油）Condiments (including cooking oils)

### 2. 食物聚类

根据膳食调查的结果，各省份住户各类食物消费量的聚类按成年男子计算出每个省份各种食品的每日消费量。个体食物消费量的聚类按各年龄组计算出每个省份各种食品的每日消费量，根据聚类原则和方法将各种食品归入相应的

### 2. Food Aggregation

The results of the household dietary survey were aggregated for calculation of average daily consumption of each food category by adult males in each province. The results of the individual dietary consumption were aggregated as per age group for calculation of the daily consumption of each food category in each province,

一类。聚类的目的是使样品的数量有效地减少，同时又不能影响食物消费量的数值，减少样品采集、烹调加工及样品测定的数量，有效提高可操作性并节省经费。

### 3. 采样

按聚类后各类食品的品种和数量并根据分析测定样品所需用量制订采样单。在采样前一定要做好烹调样品制备及烹调的所有准备工作，如安排好洗菜用具、菜刀、菜板、称量用秤、烹调用具以及烹调地点、人员等，以防采集后的样品不能及时烹调，而使样品腐败变质，影响研究的质量和进度。

根据采样单，按采样程序分别在各个调查点所在的居委会或村附近的食物采购场所，如菜市场、副食店、粮店、农贸市场或农民家，采集各种食物样品，实际采样的量应略大于计算的采样量。

采集样品时应选择新鲜的食物，特别是蔬菜、水果、肉、蛋、奶和水产品等，粮食应采集无杂质的粮食。样品采集后应尽快运至烹调加工的地点，如不能立即烹调，应放入4℃冰箱保存，生肉及水产品应贮存在冰箱冷冻室内备用。

with the various food items being classified under their corresponding categories according to the principles and methods of aggregation. The purpose of aggregation is to effectively reduce the number of samples and the amount of work of sample collection, food cooking and processing and sample analysis without affecting the values of food consumption.

### 3. Sampling

The sampling lists were determined in the light of the amounts needed for sample analysis on the basis of the varieties and quantities of food items in various food categories. Emphasis was placed on adequate preparation for the preparation and cooking of food samples. For example: vegetable washing ware, kitchen knives, chopping boards, weighing balances, cooking utensils, and cooking sites and personnel were strictly managed to avoid sample decomposition and degradation caused by delayed cooking of samples and its negative impact on the quality and progress of the study, effectively improve operability and save costs.

The samples of various food items were purchased at food purchase points such as vegetable markets, grocery stores, grain shops, farmer's markets and farmer's homes in amounts slightly greater than the actually needed amounts according to the sampling lists.

Food items purchased were required to be fresh, especially such food items as vegetables, fruits, meats, eggs, milk and aquatic products, and grains should be free from impurities. Food samples were required to be taken to the cooking and processing sites as soon as possible and stored in the refrigerator at 4℃ if they could not be cooked immediately. Raw meats and aquatic products were stored in the freezing chamber for use.

## 四、烹调及样品制备

### 1. 食物样品烹调

（1）烹调用食物样品的确定

根据一个标准人的各种食物类别的人均消费量和实验室分析所需的样品量，计算烹调样品用量。在此基础上制成烹调样品取样表，然后将三个点所采集的同一食物品种按同一比例混合，即为一个省（自治区、直辖市）的某种食物样品，待烹调加工。

（2）烹调用调味品的计算

根据膳食调查结果，将各种调味品分别归入各类主、副食品中，计算出在烹调各种食品时每种调味品的用量。

（3）烹调方法的确定

根据膳食调查得到的食谱，参考当地饮食习惯和菜谱编写出各种食品的烹调方法。

（4）烹调步骤

首先，将各类烹调用食物样品和调味品按各类食物样品烹调前的加工要求制备，再将准备好的各种烹调原料按编写的烹调方法在指定的饭馆、厨房或实验室，用当地习惯使用的炊事用具进行烹调。可直接入口的熟食或成品无需烹调。本次烹调方法不同于平时烹调方法的地方是将肉和菜分开炒，烹调后的食物样品要称重，详细记录烹调用水及烹调后样品熟重。

### 2. 样品制备

将各类已烹调的食物样品按照各自要求进行制备，方法简述如下：

## IV. Cooking and Sample Preparation

### 1. Food Sample Cooking

(1) Determination of Food Samples for Cooking

The amounts of samples for cooking were calculated according to a standard man's consumption of various food categories and the amounts of samples needed for laboratory analysis. On this basis, a sampling sheet of food samples for cooking was prepared. Then food items of each type collected from three sites were mixed equally to form the sample of the food type in the province (autonomous region, municipality) in question, which would then be processed.

(2) Calculation of Condiments for Cooking

According to the results of the dietary survey, various condiments were put under various staple and non-staple food categories, and the amount of each condiment to be used for cooking of each food was calculated.

(3) Determination of Cooking Methods

The cooking methods of various foods were designed according to the recipes collected by the dietary survey and in the light of the local culinary habits and recipes.

(4) Cooking Procedure

First, the various food samples and condiments for cooking were processed according to applicable requirements and then cooked with cooking ware customarily used by local residents in the designated restaurant, kitchen or laboratory according to the designed cooking methods. Cooked foods or finished products that are directly edible did not need to be cooked. One difference of this cooking method from common cooking methods was that meats and vegetables were cooked separately, with post-cooking food samples and the amounts of water used for cooking weighed and recorded.

### 2. Sample Preparation

The various cooked food samples were prepared in their corresponding methods, as introduced briefly below.

1）谷类、豆类、坚果类、蛋类、薯类和蔬菜类样品的制备是将烹调后的各类食品分别混匀、打碎成匀浆。

2）水果类样品制备的方法是将三个点采集的水果样品分别称重，然后按比例混合、削皮、去核，去掉不可食部分，再将可食部分称重、打碎成匀浆。

3）肉类及水产品类除在烹调前去掉不可食部分外，还需在烹调后去掉骨头和鱼刺等不可食的部分，其他方法同上。

4）乳类食品如为鲜奶需煮熟，奶粉按 1 份奶粉加 7 份水配制或按奶粉包装上注明的比例配制。方法是先用少量凉开水将奶粉调成稀糊状，然后用开水冲开。

5）糖类如有红糖、白糖、蜂蜜同时存在时，应分别取样不混合，存放在不同的容器内。

6）水及饮料类的制备方法为：①自来水要烧开；②茶水按 3 g 茶叶加 250 mL 水的比例，将开水放至 70～80℃后加茶叶，将茶叶浸泡 5 min 后，滤去茶叶。将开水①放至室温后与②茶水及其他饮料按各自消费量的比例混合。

a. 酒类按啤酒、果酒和白酒的各自消费量的比例混合。

b. 各省份的总膳食研究按各自的膳食组成和烹调方法烹调、制备各类膳食单样，再将各类膳食单样按成年男性（标准人）膳食组成混成 12 类膳食样品，并保存相对应的单个样品。

## 五、样品的运送及储存

样品要求全程冷链运输到实验室（建议箱子中加入干冰运输），箱子的顶面和侧面及箱内有装箱单，应注明箱号、样品的品种及数量。每个样品瓶上要贴两张标签，以防丢失。所有样品均需保存在≤-20℃下。

1) Cooked food samples in the categories of cereals, legumes, nuts, eggs, potatoes, and vegetables were each evenly blended into homogenates.

2) Fruits samples collected from three points were weighed separately, mixed equally, and then had their peels, stones and inedible parts removed before the edible parts were weighed and blended into homogenates.

3) In the case of meats and aquatic products, inedible parts such as bones were removed before and after cooking, with other procedures the same as above.

4) For dairy products, fresh milk was cooked, and powdered milk was mixed with water (one part powdered milk to seven parts water, or as indicated by the product instruction). In brief, the powdered milk was mixed with cold boiled water to become diluted paste which was then further diluted by boiling water.

5) For sugar, brown sugar, white sugar and honey, if any, were not mixed but stored separately.

6) Water and beverages were prepared as follows: ① drinking water was boiled; ② tea water was prepared by mixing tea and boiling water of 70-80℃ (3 g tea to 250 mL water) for five minutes and then removing tea leaves. The drinking water ① in a room temperature environment was mixed with the tea water ② and/or other beverages in ratios according to their respective amounts of consumption.

a. For alcohol beverages, beer, fruit wine and white liquor were mixed in ratios based on their respective amounts of consumption.

b. For TDS in each province, various food samples were cooked and prepared according to the local dietary patterns and cooking methods, where 12 categories of food samples representing adult males (reference man) were composited, with the individual samples being stored.

## V. Transport and Storage of Samples

All the samples were transferred to the laboratory through the cold chain (dry ice is recommended to be added to the box for transportation). The packing list is required on the top、side and inside of the box, and the box number, the variety and quantity of the samples should be indicated. Apply two labels to each vial to prevent loss. All samples should be stored at −20℃.

## 第二节 样品分析测定方法及质量控制
## Section 2　Methods of Sample Analysis and Quality Control

### 一、脂肪酸分析方法

第六次总膳食研究对膳食样品进行了 62 种脂肪酸含量的测定，采用气相色谱-氢火焰离子化检测器法（GC-FID）。用相对浓度响应因子法进行定量。

**1. 样品的制备**

（1）试样的水解

谷类、豆类、薯类、肉类、蔬菜类、水果类总膳食样品：称取膳食样品 0.5～10 g（含脂肪 0.1～0.2 g）至锥形瓶中，加入 2.0 mL 十一碳酸甘油三酯（TAG）内标溶液，加入约 100 mg 焦性没食子酸，加入 2 mL 95% 乙醇和 4 mL 水混匀后，再加入 10 mL 盐酸溶液，于 70～80℃ 水浴中水解 40～50 min。水解完成后，取出锥形瓶冷却至室温，加入 10 mL 95% 乙醇。

乳类总膳食样品：称取均质乳类样品约 5 g（含脂肪 0.2 g）至锥形瓶中，加入 2.0 mL 十一碳酸甘油三酯内标溶液，加入约 100 mg 焦性没食子酸和 5 mL 氨水，于 70～80℃ 水浴中水解 20 min。水解完成后，取出锥形瓶冷却至室温，加入 10 mL 95% 乙醇。

### I. Analysis Method of Fatty Acids

The contents of 62 fatty acids in dietary samples from the 6$^{th}$ total diet study (TDS) were determined using gas chromatography with flame ionization detector (GC-FID). The relative response factor method was used for the calculation of quantity.

**1. Sample Preparation**

(1) Hydrolysis of Samples

TDS samples of categories of cereals, legumes, potatoes, meats, vegetables and fruits: weigh homogenized sample of 0.5-10 g (containing 0.1 g to 0.2 g of fat) into an Erlenmeyer flask. Add 2.0 mL of C11:0 TAG internal standard solution, add about 100 mg of pyrogallic acid, 2 mL of 95% ethanol and 4 mL of water, and mix well. Then, add 10 mL of hydrochloric acid solution. Put the Erlenmeyer flask in a water bath at 70-80℃ for 40-50 min. After the hydrolysis, put out and cool the Erlenmeyer flask to room temperature, then add 10 mL of 95% ethanol to the hydrolyzed sample.

TDS samples of dairy products: weigh homogenized sample of 5 g (containing 0.2 g of fat) into an Erlenmeyer flask. Add 2.0 mL of C11:0 TAG internal standard solution, add about 100 mg of pyrogallic acid and 5 mL of aqueous ammonia. Put the Erlenmeyer flask in a water bath at 70-80℃ for 20 min. After the hydrolysis, put out and cool the Erlenmeyer flask to room temperature, then add 10 mL of 95% ethanol to the hydrolyzed sample.

（2）脂肪提取

在上述总膳食样品水解完成后，将水解液移入 150 mL 分液漏斗中，以 50 mL 乙醚和石油醚混合溶液冲洗锥形瓶，冲洗液并入分液漏斗中。振摇 3 min，静置 20 min，将醚层提取液收集到 250 mL 烧瓶中。按照以上步骤重复提取水解液 2 次，并收集到 250 mL 烧瓶中。使用旋转蒸发仪浓缩至干，残留物为脂肪提取物。

（3）水产类和蛋类总膳食样品的脂肪提取

称取水产类和蛋类膳食样品 2 g（含脂肪 0.1~0.2 g），加入 2.0 mL 十一碳酸甘油三酯内标溶液，加入 45 mL 氯仿-甲醇混合溶液（2∶1 体积比），浸泡过夜。将浸泡液过滤至分液漏斗中，用氯仿-甲醇混合溶液冲洗滤渣，冲洗液并入分液漏斗中。加入 0.85% 的氯化钠溶液 13 mL，混匀后，再次浸泡过夜。分层后将下层溶液移入烧瓶中，利用旋转蒸发仪浓缩至干，残留物为脂肪提取物。

（4）脂肪的皂化和脂肪酸的甲酯化

在脂肪提取物中加入 2% 氢氧化钠甲醇溶液，于 90℃ 水浴中回流 15~20 min，从回流冷凝器上端加入 14% 三氟化硼甲醇溶液，继续回流 5 min。用少量水冲洗回流冷凝器，停止加热，从水浴上取下烧瓶，迅速冷却至室温。加入 10 mL 正庚烷，振摇 2 min，再加入饱和氯化钠溶液，振摇 30 s，静置分层，吸取正庚烷提取液 2 mL 过装有 2 g 无水硫酸钠的 0.45 μm 有机滤膜，滤液装入进样瓶中待测定。

(2) Extraction of Fat

After the hydrolysis of the above TDS samples, the hydrolysis solution was transferred into a 150 mL separatory funnel, and the conical flask was rinsed with 50 mL of a mixture of ether and petroleum ether, and the rinsing solution was incorporated into the separatory funnel. Shake for 3 min, let stand for 20 min, and collect the ether layer extract into a 250 mL flask. Repeat the above steps to extract the hydrolysate 2 times and collect into a 250 mL flask. The rotary evaporator was used to concentrate to dryness and the residue was fat extract.

(3) Fat Extraction from TDS Samples of Categories of Aquatic Foods and Eggs

Weigh approximately 2 g sample of aquatic foods or eggs (containing 0.1 g to 0.2 g of fat), accurately add 2.0 mL of C11:0 TAG internal standard solution, add 45 mL of chloroform/methanol (2∶1, $V/V$), and soak overnight. Filter the soak solution into a separatory funnel and wash the filter residues with chloroform/methanol, and combine the filtrate and the washing. Add 13 mL of 0.85% sodium chloride solution, and mix, soak again overnight. After stratification, the lower solution was transferred into a flask and concentrated to dryness by rotary evaporator and the residue was fat extract.

(4) Saponification of Fats and Methyl Esterification of Fatty Acids

Add methanol containing 2% sodium hydroxide to the Erlenmeyer flask containing fat extracts, heat flask in water bath for 15-20 min at 90℃, add $BF_3$ reagents (14% in methanol) from the top of the reflux condenser, and reflux was continued for 5 min. Flush the reflux condenser with a little water, stop heating, take off the Erlenmeyer flask from the water bath and quickly cool to room temperature. Add 10 mL of *n*-heptane, shake for 2 min, then add saturated sodium chloride solution, shake for 30 s, and stand until the phases separate. Pipet 2 mL of *n*-heptane extract onto a 0.45 μm organic membrane containing 2 g of anhydrous sodium sulfate, and the filtrate was loaded into the injection bottle for assay.

## 2. 仪器测定

使用配有氢火焰离子化检测器的气相色谱仪（GC-FID）。色谱柱：CP-SIL88 100 m × 0.25 mm × 0.20 μm，进样口温度：240℃，检测器温度：250℃。载气：高纯氦气，流速：1.3 mL/min，氢气流速：40 mL/min，空气流速：400 mL/min。分流比：30∶1，进样量：1.0 μL。升温程序：初始温度120℃，保持10 min，以3℃/min升温至180℃，以1.5℃/min升温至200℃，保持3 min，再以2℃/min升温至225℃，保持20 min。

## 3. 检出限

谷类和水果类检出限：C4:0为6 mg/kg，C6:0为5 mg/kg，C8:0为4 mg/kg，其他脂肪酸为3 mg/kg。豆类和薯类检出限：C4:0为13 mg/kg，C6:0为10 mg/kg，C8:0为9 mg/kg，其他脂肪酸为8 mg/kg。乳类检出限：C4:0为10 mg/kg，C6:0和C8:0为8 mg/kg，其他脂肪酸为6 mg/kg。肉类检出限：C4:0为36 mg/kg，C6:0为28 mg/kg，C8:0为25 mg/kg，其他脂肪酸为20 mg/kg。蔬菜类、水产类和蛋类检出限：C4:0为20 mg/kg，C6:0为15 mg/kg，C8:0为13 mg/kg，其他脂肪酸为10 mg/kg。

## 4. 质量控制

在正式分析样品之前，充分熟悉方法的分析程序及相关的知识背景，并能准确定量一系列质量标准物质[具有证书的参比物（CRM）]。每批次样品测定时至少做方法空白实验，排除试剂污染对测定的干扰。每个分析批次至少分析一种参考物质，参考物质的测定值应在标示值范围内。

## 2. Instrumental Determination

The GC-FID was used. Column: CP-SIL88 of 100 m × 0.25 mm × 0.20 μm; injector temperature: 240℃; detector temperature: 250℃. The carrier gas was high purity helium; column flow was 1.3 mL/min; hydrogen flow rate was 40 mL/min; air flow rate was 400 mL/min. Injection mode was split injection with split ratio of 30∶1 and the injection volume was 1.0 μL. Temperature programming: the initial oven temperature was 120℃, maintained for 10 min, then raised at a rate of 3℃/min up to 180℃, then raised at a rate of 1.5℃/min up to 200℃ for 3 min, and then raised at a rate of 2 /min up to 225 for 20 min.

## 3. Limits of Detection

Limits of detection for cereals and fruits: C4:0 was 6 mg/kg, C6:0 was 5 mg/kg, C8:0 was 4 mg/kg, and other fatty acids were 3 mg/kg. Limits of detection for legumes and potatoes: C4:0 was 13 mg/kg, C6:0 was 10 mg/kg, C8:0 was 9 mg/kg, and other fatty acids were 8 mg/kg. Limits of detection for dairy products: C4:0 was 10 mg/kg, C6:0 and C8:0 were 8 mg/kg, and other fatty acids were 6 mg/kg. Limits of detection for meats: C4:0 was 36 mg/kg, C6:0 was 28 mg/kg, C8:0 was 25 mg/kg, and other fatty acids were 20 mg/kg. Limits of detection for vegetables, aquatic foods and eggs: C4:0 was 20 mg/kg, C6:0 was 15 mg/kg, C8:0 was 13 mg/kg, and other fatty acids were 10 mg/kg.

## 4. Quality Control

Before analyzing samples formally, be familiar with the method analytical procedures and related knowledge background thoroughly, and quantify a series of quality reference materials [certified reference materials (CRM)] accurately. At least one method blank was analyzed to check the interference substances in the reagent per analysis batch. At least one reference material was analyzed per analysis batch. The reference substance results should be within the expected value range.

## 二、多元素分析方法

第六次中国总膳食研究采用电感耦合等离子体质谱法（ICP-MS）对膳食样品中18种元素进行了测定，采用液相色谱-电感耦合等离子体质谱联用方法对膳食样品中甲基汞、无机砷进行了形态测定。

**1. 膳食样品中多元素及碘元素的分析方法**

（1）多元素测定的样品前处理

称取样品0.3～2.0 g（精确至0.001 g）于微波消解内管中，含乙醇或二氧化碳的样品先在控温电热装置上低温加热除去乙醇或二氧化碳，然后加入5 mL浓硝酸，加盖放置过夜，旋紧管盖，次日按照微波消解仪标准操作步骤进行消解。冷却至室温后，将样品放入超声水浴中去除气态氮氧化物，然后转移到塑料离心管中，用超纯水转移至25 mL刻度线，混匀后进行检测。随机取一个微波消解管，只加入试剂，作为整个过程的对照空白（消解条件参考表1-2）。

## II. Analysis Method of Multi-Elements

In the sixth China total diet study, 18 elements in dietary samples were determined by inductively coupled plasma mass spectrometry (ICP-MS). The speciation analysis of methyl mercury and inorganic arsenic was performed using high pressure liquid chromatography (HPLC) coupled ICP-MS.

**1. Analysis Method of Multi-Elements and Iodine in Samples**

(1) Sample Digestion Procedure of Multi-Elements

Dietary samples of 0.3-2.0 g (accurate to 0.001 g) were weighed precisely and placed in microwave digestion tubes. The samples containing ethanol or carbon dioxide were first heated at low temperature on a temperature-controlled electric heating device to remove ethanol or carbon dioxide. Then added 5 mL concentrated nitric acid into the sample, covered the microwave digestion tube and left to stand overnight, and digested in a microwave digestion system on the following day. After cooling at room temperature, the sample was placed in an ultrasonic water bath to remove the gaseous nitrogen oxides, and then transferred into a plastic centrifuge tube, brought to 25 mL with ultrapure water, and evenly mixed before detection. One randomly-selected microwave digestion tube was filled with reagents only and taken through the entire procedure as a blank. The digestion procedure was as follows (Table 1-2).

表1-2 样品消解程序
Table 1-2　Sample digestion procedure

| 步骤 Steps | 最大功率 Maximum power/W | 温度 Temperature/℃ | 升温时间 Time/min | 保温时间 Hold time/min |
|---|---|---|---|---|
| 1 | 1800 | 140 | 10 | 5 |
| 2 | 1800 | 170 | 5 | 5 |
| 3 | 1800 | 200 | 5 | 20 |
| 4 |  | 降温 Cooling | 15 |  |

（2）碘元素测定的样品前处理

称取膳食样品0.5～2 g于50 mL离心管中，加入5 mL提取液[5%四甲基氢氧化铵（TMAH）]混匀，在85℃±5℃烘箱提取3 h，冷却至室温，用水定容至25 mL，大于3000 r/min下离心10 min，取上清液过0.45 μm的滤膜，滤液进ICP-MS进行测定。

（3）仪器测定

用Agilent 8800电感耦合等离子体质谱仪测定。开机后先用调谐液调试仪器各项指标，使仪器灵敏度、氧化物、双电荷、分辨率等各项指标达到测定要求。然后用调谐溶液调谐，直至仪器达最佳测试状态。最后依次测定标准系列溶液及样品。测定条件见表1-3。

(2) Sample Pretreatment for Iodine Detection

A food sample of 0.5-2 g was weighed and placed into a 50 mL centrifuge tube, mixed with 5 mL 5% TMAH. The resulting mixture was heated in an oven at 85℃ ± 5℃ for 3 h. Then cooled down to room temperature, brought to 25 mL with water, and centrifuged at 3000 r/min for 10 min. The supernatant was filtered through a 0.45 μm filter for ICP-MS detection.

(3) Instrument Measurement

Measured with Agilent 8800 ICP-MS. After system startup, tuned liquid was used to calibrate the instrument so that it met requirements in all parameters including sensitivity, oxide, double charge, and resolution. It was then tuned with the tuning solution to reach the best state. At last, the standard solutions and samples were assayed one by one. The assay conditions were shown in Table 1-3.

表1-3 多元素测定条件

Table 1-3 Conditions of multi-element determination

| 名称 Name | 参数 Parameter | 名称 Name | 参数 Parameter |
| --- | --- | --- | --- |
| 射频功率 Radio frequency power | 1550 W | 采样深度 Sampling depth | 10 mm |
| 载气流量 Flow rate of carrier gas | 0.83 L/min | 雾化器 Atomizer | Barbinton |
| 辅助气流量 Makeup gas flow rate | 0.37 L/min | 雾化室温度 Spray chamber temperature | 2℃ |
| 氦气流量 Flow rate of He | 4～5 mL/min | 蠕动泵转速 Peristaltic pump speed | 0.1 r/min |
| 分析方式 Analysis methods | 氦碰撞反应 Helium collision mode | 样品提升速度 Sample uptake speed | 0.3 r/min |
| 采样锥 Sampler cone | 孔径1.0 mm，镍锥 Bore diameter at 1.0 mm, nickel sampler cone | 重复测定次数 Number of repeated determination | 3 |
| 截取锥 Skimmer cone | 孔径0.4 mm，镍锥 Bore diameter at 0.4 mm, nickel sampler cone | 重复取样次数 Number of repeated sampling | 3 |

（4）各种元素的检出限

每个元素的检出限（LOD）是基于10次测定的基线值的标准差的3倍。详细结果如表1-4所示。

(4) The Limits of Detection of Various Elements

The LOD for each element was three times the standard deviation of the baseline values of ten determinations. Detailed results were shown in Table 1-4.

表 1-4　各元素测定的检出限和定量限（单位：μg/kg）

Table 1-4　Limits of detection and limits of quantification of various elements (Unit: μg/kg)

| 元素 Element | 元素符号 Element symbol | 检出限 Limits of detection | 定量限 Limits of quantification |
| --- | --- | --- | --- |
| 钠 Sodium | Na | 125 | 400 |
| 镁 Magnesium | Mg | 15 | 50 |
| 铝 Aluminum | Al | 50 | 150 |
| 磷 Phosphorus | P | 200 | 600 |
| 钾 Potassium | K | 80 | 250 |
| 钙 Calcium | Ca | 150 | 450 |
| 铬 Chromium | Cr | 1.0 | 3.0 |
| 锰 Manganese | Mn | 1.0 | 3.0 |
| 铁 Iron | Fe | 8.0 | 25 |
| 铜 Copper | Cu | 2.0 | 6.0 |
| 锌 Zinc | Zn | 4.0 | 15 |
| 砷 Arsenic | As | 0.25 | 0.8 |
| 硒 Selenium | Se | 0.25 | 1.0 |
| 钼 Molybdenum | Mo | 0.5 | 2.0 |
| 镉 Cadmium | Cd | 0.05 | 0.2 |
| 汞 Mercury | Hg | 0.1 | 0.3 |
| 铅 Lead | Pb | 0.08 | 0.3 |
| 碘 Iodine | I | 14 | 40 |

**2. 膳食样品中甲基汞的分析方法**

（1）样品提取

称取均质样品 1.0～2.0 g（精确至 0.001 g）于 15 mL 塑料离心管中，加入 10 mL 的 5 mol/L 盐酸溶液，混合浸泡 12h。室温下超声提取 60 min（超声过程中如水浴温度升高则在水浴中加入冰块降温），每 15 min 振摇一次。8000 r/min 转速离心 15 min。准确吸取 2.0 mL 上清液至 5 mL 试管，逐滴加入氨水溶液（1＋1），调节样品溶液 pH 为 3～7。加入 0.2 mL 10 g/L 的 L-半胱氨酸溶液，最后用水定容至 5 mL。用 0.45 μm 有机滤膜过滤，待测。同时做空白实验。

（2）仪器测定

**2. Analysis Method of Methylmercury in Food Samples**

(1) Sample Extraction

1.0-2.0 g (accurate to 0.001 g) homogenized sample was weighed and put into 15 mL centrifuge tube with 10 mL of 5 mol/L HCl, mixed and soaked over 12 h. The chemical was extracted by ultrasonication at room temperature for 60 min (shake once every 15 min), followed by high-speed centrifugation at 8000 r/min for 15 min. If the temperature of the water bath rises during ultrasonication, ice can be added to cool it down. 2.0 mL supernatant was transferred into 5 mL testing tube, and ammonia solution (1 + 1) was added until the pH was between 3-7, then 0.2 mL of 10 g/L L-cysteine solution was added and set the final volume to 5 mL with water. The resulting solution was filtered using a 0.45 μm organic filter membrane.

i. 液相色谱条件

色谱柱：MP C18 分析柱（柱长 150 mm，内径 4.6 mm）。流动相组成：3% 甲醇＋3 g/L 乙酸铵＋1 g/L L-半胱氨酸。流速：1.0 mL/min。进样体积：50 μL。

ii. ICP-MS 仪器条件

射频功率 1550 W，载气流量 0.77 L/min，辅助气流速 0.43 L/min，采集时间 4 min，蠕动泵转速 0.5 r/s，采样深度 10 mm，雾化室温度 2℃，检测质量数 202。

（3）检出限

当样品称样量为 1 g 时，甲基汞的检出限为 0.003 mg/kg。

### 3. 膳食样品中无机砷的分析方法

（1）样品提取

称取样品 1.0～2.0 g（准确至 0.001 g）于 50 mL 塑料离心管中，加入 20 mL 的 0.15 mol/L 硝酸溶液，放置过夜。于 90℃恒温箱中热浸提 2.5 h，每半小时振摇一次。提取完毕后，取出冷却至室温，8000 r/min 离心 15 min，取 2 mL 上层清液，经 0.45 mm 有机滤膜过滤上机测定。同时做空白实验（对脂肪含量高的试样，离心后取 5 mL 上层清液，加入 5 mL 正己烷除脂，振摇 1 min 后，8000 r/min 离心 15 min，弃去正己烷层。此过程可重复一次。然后用长颈滴管小心吸取下层清液，经 0.45 mm 有机滤膜过滤上机测定）。

（2）仪器测定

i. 液相色谱测定条件

色谱柱：ZORBAX SB-Aq C18 色谱柱 4.6 mm×250 mm，5 μm 或等效柱。

流动相组成：20 mmol/L 柠檬酸与 5 mmol/L 己烷磺酸钠的混合溶液（pH=4.3）。流速：1.0 mL/min；进样体积：30 μL。

(2) Instrument Measurement

i. Liquid Chromatography Condition

Chromatographic column: MP C18 (4.6 mm × 150 mm); mobile phase: 3% methanol +3 g/L ammonium acetate +1 g/L L-cysteine; flow rate: 1.0 mL/min; injection volume: 50 μL.

ii. ICP-MS Conditions

Radio frequency power: 1550 W; flow rate of carrier gas: 0.77 L/min; makeup gas flow rate: 0.43 L/min; acquisition time: 4 min; peristaltic pump speed: 0.5 r/s; sampling depth: 10 mm; spray chamber temperature: 2℃; mass number: 202.

(3) The Limits of Detection

For 1 g sample analyzed, the limit of detection of methylmercury was 0.003 mg/kg.

### 3. Analysis Method of Inorganic Arsenic in Food Samples

(1) Sample Extraction

Weigh 1.0-2.0 g (accurate to 0.001 g) of the sample in a 50 mL plastic centrifuge tube, add 20 mL of 0.15 mol/L nitric acid solution, and leave overnight. The resulting mixture was heated in an oven at 90℃ for 2.5 h. After cooled down to room temperature, the extract was centrifuged at 8000 r/min for 15 min. 2.0 mL of supernatant was filtered using 0.45 μm organic filter membrane (For samples with high fat content, 5 mL supernatant was taken after centrifugation, and 5 mL n-hexane was added, shaking for 1 min, followed by centrifugation at 8000 r/min for 15 min, then the n-hexane layer was removed, the above process was repeated once. Then the subnatant was carefully absorbed with a long neck dropper, and filtered using 0.45 μm organic filter membrane).

(2) Instrument Measurement

i. Liquid Chromatography Condition

Chromatographic column: ZORBAX SB-Aq C18 (4.6 mm × 250 mm, 5 μm or equivalent columns); mobile phase: 20 mmol/L citric acid +5 mmol/L sodium hexanesulfonate (pH=4.3); flow rate: 1.0 mL/min; injection volume: 30 μL.

ii. ICP-MS 仪器条件

射频功率 1550 W，载气流量 0.77 L/min，辅助气流速 0.43 L/min，采集时间 4 min，蠕动泵转速 0.5 r/s，采样深度 10 mm，雾化室温度 2℃，检测质量数 75。

（3）检出限

当样品称样量为 1 g 时，无机砷检出限为 0.001 mg/kg。

**4. 质控措施**

为了保证样品检测结果的准确可靠，采取如下质控措施。

1）使用具有标准物质证书的标准溶液，保证其量值可溯源；所有试剂均在有效期内。

2）所有消化管和玻璃器皿在 20% 硝酸溶液中浸泡 24 h 以上，然后用自来水冲洗，最后用纯水冲洗 3 次。晾干备用。

3）每批次样品测定时做两个空白实验，排除本底污染对测定的干扰。

4）样品进行双平行样测定；平行测定结果的相对标准偏差（RSD）不大于算术平均值的 10%。

5）每批次样品检测时采用标准参考物质作为质控样品同时进行检测，标准参考物质的测定值应在标示值范围内。

6）方法线性相关系数达到 $R \geqslant 0.999$。

7）样品溶液的上机测定浓度应在标准曲线线性范围内。

8）检测方法通过参加国际实验室分析水平测试得到了验证。

ii. ICP-MS Conditions

Radio frequency power: 1550 W; Flow rate of carrier gas: 0.77 L/min; makeup gas flow rate: 0.43 L/min; acquisition time: 4 min; peristaltic pump speed: 0.5 r/s; sampling depth: 10 mm, spray chamber temperature: 2℃; mass number: 75.

(3) The Limits of Detection

For 1 g sample analyzed, the limit of detection of inorganic arsenic was 0.001 mg/kg.

**4. Quality Control**

In order to ensure the accuracy and reliability of the sample test results, the following quality control measures were taken during the sample analysis.

1) Certificated standard solutions were used to ensure the traceability, all reagents were within the expiration date.

2) All digestion tubes and glassware were soaked in 20% nitric acid solution for over 24 hours, then rinsed with tap water and finally rinsed with distilled water and ultrapure water for 3 times, and then dried for use.

3) Two blanks were determined for each batch of samples to exclude the interference of background contamination on the determination.

4) All samples were tested in duplicate, and the relative standard deviation between the parallel results was not more than 10% of the arithmetic average.

5) Each batch of samples for testing using a standard reference material as a quality control sample at the same time for testing, the determination of the standard reference material should be within the range of the labeled value.

6) The linear correlation coefficient should be greater than 0.999.

7) The concentration of sample solution measured should be within the linear range of the standard curve.

8) The method was validated by participating in international proficiency test.

## 三、农药残留分析方法

农药残留的检测分析采用超高效液相色谱-高分辨质谱（UPLC-HRMS）非靶向筛查和定量分析方法。针对筛查到的常检出农药（75 种），采用 UPLC-HRMS 的全扫描采集（Full Scan）模式，以目标分析物的精确母离子为定量离子，以保留时间和高分辨质谱采集的二级质谱碎片离子作为定性确证，用外标法定量分析。针对热点的典型农药，10 种新烟碱类农药和 4 种氟虫腈及其代谢物分别采用 UPLC-HRMS 的靶向单一离子监测模式（tSIM），以目标分析物的精确母离子为定量离子，以保留时间和高分辨质谱采集的二级质谱碎片离子作为定性确证，用内标法定量分析。

### 1. 样品制备

精确称取 5 g 膳食样品于 50 mL 离心管中，加入内标混合中间液（1 mg/L）50 μL，静置 10 min 后，依据样品含水量，适量加入 3～6 mL 水，涡旋混匀后，加入 10 mL 乙腈，涡旋混匀 5 min，再加入 2 g 氯化钠和 8 g 无水硫酸钠剧烈振荡 2 min，以 8000 r/min 离心 5 min，取乙腈上清液 1.5 mL 加入预先装有分散固相萃取（DSPE）混合净化剂的 2 mL 离心管中，涡旋 30 s，以 10 000 r/min 离心 5 min，取 1.0 mL 上清液，加入 5 mL 离心管中，再加入 1.5 mL 纯净水，混匀，在 –80℃ 冷冻 7 min 诱导相分离后，取上层乙腈相，以 13 000 r/min 离心 5 min 后，待测定。

## III. Analysis Method of Pesticide Residues

Non-targeted screening and quantitative analysis methods were used for the detection and analysis of pesticide residues by ultra-high performance liquid chromatography-high resolution mass spectrometry (UPLC-HRMS). For the common 75 pesticides screened, the Full Scan mode of UPLC-HRMS was adopted. The accurate parent ions of the target analytes were used as the quantitative ions, and the retention time and secondary mass spectrometry fragment ions collected by high-resolution mass spectrometry were used as the qualitative confirmation, and the external standard method was used for quantitative analysis. Focusing on the hot-spots pesticides, including 10 neonicotinoid pesticides and four fipronils and metabolites, targeted single ion monitoring mode (tSIM) by UPLC-HRMS was used for their determinations. The accurate parent ions of the target analytes were used as the quantitative ions, and the retention time and secondary mass spectrometry fragment ions collected by high-resolution mass spectrometry were used as qualitative confirmation. Internal standard method was used for quantitative analysis.

### 1. Sample Preparation

Accurately weigh 5 g of homogenized sample in a 50 mL centrifuge tube, add 50 μL of internal standard mixed intermediate solution (1 mg/L), stand for 10 min, add 3-6 mL of water according to the water content of the sample, then vortex. Add 10 mL of acetonitrile, vortex for 5 min, then add 2 g of sodium chloride and 8 g of anhydrous sodium sulfate, shake violently for 2 min, centrifuge at 8000 r/min for 5 min, take 1.5 mL of acetonitrile supernatant, put it into a 2 mL centrifuge tube with DSPE mixed detergent in advance, vortex for 30 s, centrifuge at 10 000 r/min for 5 min, take 1.0 mL of supernatant, add into a 5 mL centrifuge tube, then add 1.5 mL of water, mix well, freeze at –80℃ for 7 min to induce phase separation, take the upper acetonitrile phase, and centrifuge at 13 000 r/min for 5 min before determination.

## 2. 仪器测定

（1）农药残留的非靶向筛查

流动相A为含0.1%甲酸和5 mmol/L甲酸铵的水溶液，流动相B为含0.1%甲酸和5 mmol/L甲酸铵的甲醇。进样量5 μL；流速400 μL/min；柱温40℃；Accucore aQ C18色谱柱（2.6 μm，2.1 mm × 150 mm）。质谱参数：加热正电喷雾离子源（HESI$^+$）；喷雾电压为3.8 kV，毛细管温度为325℃；鞘气为40 arb，辅助气为10 arb；Full Scan/ddMS2扫描模式；采集范围为10~1000 Da。

（2）新烟碱类农药

流动相A为含0.1%甲酸和5 mmol/L甲酸铵的水溶液，流动相B为含0.1%甲酸和5 mmol/L甲酸铵的甲醇。进样量10 μL；流速400 μL/min；柱温40℃；Accucore aQ C18色谱柱（2.6 μm，2.1 mm × 150 mm）。质谱参数：正电喷雾离子源（HESI$^+$）；喷雾电压为3.8 kV；毛细管温度为325℃；鞘气流速为40 arb，辅助气流速为10 arb；tSIM/ddMS$^2$扫描模式；定量分离宽度4 Da。

（3）氟虫腈及其代谢物

流动相A为含0.1%甲酸的水溶液，流动相B为甲醇。进样量5 μL；流速300 μL/min；柱温40℃；BEH C18色谱柱（100 mm×2.1 mm，1.7 μm）。质谱参数：加热负电喷雾离子源（HESI$^-$）；喷雾电压为3.2 kV；毛细管温度为325℃；鞘气流速为40 arb，辅助气流速为10 arb；tSIM/ddMS$^2$扫描模式：定量分离宽度4 Da。

## 3. 检出限和定量限

各农药在膳食基质中的检出限和定量限见表1-5。

## 2. Instrument Detection

(1) Non-targeted Screening of Pesticide Residues

Solvent A (aqueous solution, 5 mmol/L ammonium formate and 0.1% formic acid, $V/V$) and solvent B (methanol, 5 mmol/L ammonium formate and 0.1% formic acid). The flow rate was 400 μL/min and the injection volume was 5 μL. The oven temperature was maintained at 40℃, equipped with an Accucore aQ C18 analytical column (2.6 μm, 2.1 mm × 150 mm). Mass spectrometry parameters: HESI$^+$; spray voltage, 3.8 kV; capillary temperature, 325℃; sheath gas flow, 40 arb; auxiliary gas flow, 10 arb; scan mode, Full Scan/ddMS$^2$, acquisition range, 100-1000 Da.

(2) Neonicotinoid Pesticides

Solvent A (ammonium formate, 5 mmol/L and 0.1% formic acid, $V/V$) and solvent B (methanol, 5 mmol/L ammonium formate and 0.1% formic acid). The flow rate was 400 μL/min and the injection volume was 10 μL. The oven temperature was maintained at 40℃, equipped with an Accucore aQ C18 analytical column (2.6 μm, 2.1 mm × 150 mm). Mass spectrometry parameters: positive electrospray ion mode (HESI$^+$); spray voltage, 3.8 kV; capillary temperature, 325℃; sheath gas flow, 40 arb; auxiliary gas flow, 10 arb; scan mode, tSIM/ddMS$^2$, quantitative separation width, 4 Da.

(3) Fipronil and Its Metabolites

Solvent A (0.1% formic acid in water) and solvent B (methanol). The flow rate was 300 μL/min and the injection volume was 5 μL. The oven temperature was maintained at 40℃, equipped with a BEH C18 analytical column (100 mm × 2.1 mm, i.d., 1.7 μm). Mass spectrometry parameters: HESI$^-$; spray voltage, 3.2 kV; capillary temperature, 325℃; sheath gas flow, 40 arb; auxiliary gas flow, 10 arb; scan mode, tSIM/ddMS$^2$, quantitative separation width, 4 Da.

## 3. Limits of Detection and LOQs

The specific pesticides, their limits of detection and limits of quantitation are shown in the Table 1-5.

表 1-5 75 种农药的检出限和定量限（单位：μg/kg）
Table 1-5 LODs and LOQs of 75 pesticides (Unit: μg/kg)

| 农药名称 Pesticides | 检出限 LOD | 定量限 LOQ |
| --- | --- | --- |
| 3-羟基克百威 3-hydroxy-carbofuran | 0.1 | 0.3 |
| 乙酰甲胺磷 Acephate | 0.08 | 0.24 |
| 啶虫脒 Acetamiprid | 0.005 | 0.015 |
| 嘧菌酯 Azoxystrobin | 0.05 | 0.15 |
| 联苯三唑醇 Bitertanol | 0.05 | 0.15 |
| 糠菌唑 Bromuconazole | 0.05 | 0.15 |
| 乙嘧酚磺酸酯 Bupirimate | 0.05 | 0.15 |
| 噻嗪酮 Buprofezin | 0.05 | 0.15 |
| 多菌灵 Carbendazim | 0.05 | 0.15 |
| 克百威 Carbofuran | 0.1 | 0.3 |
| 毒死蜱 Chlorpyrifos | 0.1 | 0.3 |
| 甲基毒死蜱 Chlorpyrifos-methyl | 0.1 | 0.3 |
| 噻虫胺 Clothianidin | 0.003 | 0.009 |
| 环唑醇 Cyproconazole | 0.05 | 0.15 |
| 嘧菌环胺 Cyprodinil | 0.05 | 0.15 |
| 二嗪磷 Diazinon | 0.05 | 0.15 |
| 敌敌畏 Dichlorvos | 0.05 | 0.15 |
| 苯醚甲环唑 Difenoconazole | 0.05 | 0.15 |
| 乐果 Dimethoate | 0.04 | 0.12 |
| 烯酰吗啉 Dimethomorph | 0.05 | 0.15 |
| 氟环唑 Epoxiconazole | 0.05 | 0.15 |
| 氯苯嘧啶醇 Fenarimol | 0.05 | 0.15 |
| 腈苯唑 Fenbuconazole | 0.05 | 0.15 |
| 环酰菌胺 Fenhexamid | 0.05 | 0.15 |
| 氟虫腈 Fipronil | 0.001 | 0.003 |
| 氟甲腈 Fipronil desulfinyl | 0.001 | 0.003 |
| 氟虫腈砜 Fipronil sulfone | 0.001 | 0.003 |
| 氟虫腈亚砜 Fipronil sulfide | 0.001 | 0.003 |
| 咯菌腈 Fludioxonil | 0.05 | 0.15 |
| 氟吡菌胺 Fluopicolide | 0.04 | 0.12 |
| 氟喹唑 Fluquinconazole | 0.05 | 0.15 |
| 氟硅唑 Flusilazole | 0.05 | 0.15 |
| 氟酰胺 Flutolanil | 0.05 | 0.15 |
| 粉唑醇 Flutriafol | 0.05 | 0.15 |
| 己唑醇 Hexaconazole | 0.05 | 0.15 |

续表

| 农药名称 Pesticides | 检出限 LOD | 定量限 LOQ |
|---|---|---|
| 抑霉唑 Imazalil | 0.05 | 0.15 |
| 吡虫啉 Imidacloprid | 0.003 | 0.009 |
| 茚虫威 Indoxacarb | 0.05 | 0.15 |
| 利谷隆 Linuron | 0.05 | 0.15 |
| 甲霜灵 Metalaxyl | 0.05 | 0.15 |
| 叶菌唑 Metconazole | 0.05 | 0.15 |
| 甲氧虫酰肼 Methoxyfenozide | 0.05 | 0.15 |
| 腈菌唑 Myclobutanil | 0.05 | 0.15 |
| 氧化乐果 Omethoate | 0.08 | 0.24 |
| 多效唑 Paclobutrazol | 0.05 | 0.15 |
| 戊菌唑 Penconazole | 0.05 | 0.15 |
| 抗蚜威 Pirimicarb | 0.05 | 0.15 |
| 咪鲜胺 Prochloraz | 0.05 | 0.15 |
| 丙溴磷 Profenophos | 0.05 | 0.15 |
| 炔螨特 Propargite | 0.05 | 0.15 |
| 丙环唑 Propiconazole | 0.05 | 0.15 |
| 丙硫唑 Prothioconazole | 0.05 | 0.15 |
| 吡唑醚菌酯 Pyraclostrobin | 0.05 | 0.15 |
| 哒螨灵 Pyridaben | 0.05 | 0.15 |
| 嘧霉胺 Pyrimethanil | 0.03 | 0.09 |
| 蚊蝇醚 Pyriproxyfen | 0.05 | 0.15 |
| 喹氧灵 Quinoxyfen | 0.05 | 0.15 |
| 多杀菌素 A Spinosad A | 0.05 | 0.15 |
| 多杀菌素 D Spinosad D | 0.05 | 0.15 |
| 螺螨酯 Spirodiclofen | 0.05 | 0.15 |
| 螺环菌胺 Spiroxamine | 0.05 | 0.15 |
| 戊唑醇 Tebuconazole | 0.05 | 0.15 |
| 氟醚唑 Tetraconazole | 0.05 | 0.15 |
| 噻菌灵 Thiabendazole | 0.05 | 0.15 |
| 噻虫啉 Thiacloprid | 0.003 | 0.009 |
| 噻虫嗪 Thiamethoxam | 0.005 | 0.015 |
| 三唑酮 Triadimefon | 0.06 | 0.18 |
| 三唑醇 Triadimenol | 0.05 | 0.15 |
| 三唑磷 Triazophos | 0.05 | 0.15 |
| 肟菌酯 Trifloxystrobin | 0.05 | 0.15 |
| 灭菌唑 Triticonazole | 0.05 | 0.15 |

续表

| 农药名称 Pesticides | 检出限 LOD | 定量限 LOQ |
|---|---|---|
| 莠去津 Atrazine | 0.05 | 0.15 |
| 灭蝇胺 Cyromazine | 0.06 | 0.18 |
| 烯啶虫胺 Nitenpyram | 0.005 | 0.015 |
| 呋虫胺 Dinotefuran | 0.005 | 0.015 |
| 氯噻啉 Imidaclothiz | 0.005 | 0.015 |
| 环氧虫啶 Cycloxaprid | 0.005 | 0.015 |
| N-脱甲基啶虫脒 Acetamiprid-N-desmethyl | 0.005 | 0.015 |
| 甲胺磷 Methamidophos | 0.05 | 0.15 |

## 4. 质量控制与质量保证

农药多残留的非靶向筛查和定量分析方法参加了欧盟农药欧盟能力测试（EUPT）国际比对考核的定性筛查和定量考核，均取得了满意的结果。对于典型农药的靶向定量分析方法，其中氟虫腈及其代谢物参加了瓦格宁根大学研究中心组织的动物性样品（鸡蛋、鸡肉、鸡油）中氟虫腈及其代谢物能力验证考核，考核结果满意。

目前，暂未获得相关农药的标准参考物质，为确保实验结果的准确性，每批样品的测定过程中加入空白加标样品作为质量控制样品。每批样品中选择一个无目标化合物检出的膳食样品，进行加标回收实验。其中，加标回收率结果控制在70%~120%，说明试验结果准确、可靠。

## 四、兽药残留分析方法

兽药多残留的检测分析采用超高效液相色谱-高分辨质谱（UPLC-HRMS）非靶向筛查和定量分析方法。在全扫描采集模式下，以目标分析物的精确母离子为定量离子，以保留时间和高分辨质谱采集的二级质谱碎片离子作为定性确证，外标法和内标法相结合进行定量分析。针对检出率较高的典型兽药，如喹

## 4. Quality Control and Quality Assurance

Non-targeted screening and quantitative analysis methods of multi-residues of pesticides have achieved satisfactory results by participating in qualitative screening and quantitative assessment of EU pesticide EUPT international comparison assessment. Targeted quantitative analysis method of typical pesticides, in which fipronil and its metabolites participated in the ability verification assessment of fipronil and its metabolites in animal samples (eggs, chicken, and chicken oil) organized by the research center of Wageningen University, and the assessment results were satisfactory.

At present, the standard reference materials of related pesticides have not been obtained yet. To ensure the accuracy of the experimental results, blank spiked samples were added as quality control samples during the determination of each batch of samples. Select a dietary sample with no target compound detected in each batch of samples, and carry out standard addition recovery test. Among them, the recovery rate of standard addition was controlled at 70%-120%, indicating that the test results were accurate and reliable.

## Ⅳ. Analysis Method of Veterinary Drugs

Non-targeted screening and quantitative analysis methods were used for the detection and analysis of multi-residues of veterinary drugs by ultra-high

诺酮类、磺胺类、硝基咪唑类、苯并咪唑类和氯霉素类等采用 UPLC-HRMS 的靶向单一离子监测模式（tSIM），以目标分析物的精确母离子为定量离子，以保留时间和高分辨质谱采集的二级质谱碎片离子作为定性确证，内标法定量分析。

**1. 样品制备**

（1）多兽药残留

称取 5 g（精确到 0.01 g）膳食样品，加入同位素内标溶液，涡旋混匀，静置 30 min；加入适量水，混匀后再加入 15 mL 乙腈，超声提取 30 min。室温下 9500 r/min 离心 5 min，取上清液 3 mL 于 5 mL 离心管中，置于 –20℃ 冷冻处理 1 h；取 1 mL 上清液转移至装有 250 mg 无水硫酸钠和 50 mg C18 粉末的 2 mL 离心管中，涡旋混匀后 15 000 r/min 离心 5 min。取离心上清液，待检测。

（2）喹诺酮类

称取 5 g（精确到 0.01 g）膳食样品，加入同位素内标溶液，涡旋混匀，静置 30 min；加入适量水，混匀后再加入 15 mL 乙腈，超声提取 30 min。室温下 9500 r/min 离心 5 min，取上清液 4 mL 于 5 mL 离心管中，加入 200 μL 氨水，混合均匀后置于 –20℃ 冷冻处理 1 h；分层后取下层于 1.5 mL 离心管中，涡旋混匀后 15 000 r/min 离心 5 min。取离心上清液，待检测。

performance liquid chromatography-high resolution mass spectrometry (UPLC-HRMS). In the Full-Scan acquisition mode, the accurate parent ions of the target analytes were used as quantitative ions, and the retention time and secondary mass spectrometry fragment ions collected by high-resolution mass spectrometry were used as qualitative confirmations. The external standard method and the internal standard method were combined for quantitative analysis. For typical veterinary drugs with high detection rates, such as quinolones, sulfonamides, nitroimidazoles, benzimidazoles, and chloramphenicols, the targeted single ion monitoring mode (tSIM) by UPLC-HRMS was used to detect target analytes. The accurate parent ions of the target analytes were used as quantitative ions, and the retention time and the fragment ions of the secondary mass spectrometry collected by high-resolution mass spectrometry were used as qualitative confirmation, and the internal standard method was used for quantitative analysis.

**1. Sample Preparation**

(1) Multiple Veterinary Drug Residues

Weigh 5 g (accurate to 0.01 g) dietary sample, add isotope internal standard solution, vortex to mix, and let stand for 30 min; add appropriate amount of water, mix well, then add 15 mL of acetonitrile, and ultrasonically extract for 30 min. Centrifuge at 9500 r/min for 5 min at room temperature, take 3 mL of supernatant into a 5 mL centrifuge tube, and freeze at –20℃ for 1 h; transfer 1 mL of supernatant to a 2 mL centrifuge tube containing 250 mg of anhydrous sodium sulfate and 50 mg C18 powder, vortex to mix, and centrifuge at 15 000 r/min for 5 min. Take the centrifuged supernatant for analysis.

(2) Quinolones

Weigh 5 g (accurate to 0.01 g) dietary sample, add isotope internal standard solution, vortex to mix, and let stand for 30 min; add appropriate amount of water, mix well, and then add 15 mL of acetonitrile for ultrasonic extraction for 30 min. Centrifuge at 9500 r/min for 5 min at room temperature, take 4 mL of the supernatant into a 5 mL centrifuge tube, add 200 μL of ammonia water,

## 2. 仪器测定

正离子采集：流动相 A 为含 0.1% 甲酸的水溶液，流动相 B 为含 0.1% 甲酸的甲醇。负离子采集：流动相 A 为含 0.01% 氨水的水溶液，流动相 B 为乙腈。进样量 5 μL；流速 300 μL/min；柱温 40 ℃；HSS T3 色谱柱（1.8 μm，2.1 mm × 100 mm）。加热电喷雾离子源（HESI）温度为 325 ℃；毛细管电压为 3.8 kV；鞘气流速为 40 arb，辅助气流速为 10 arb；非靶向筛查采用 Full Scan/ddMS$^2$ 扫描模式：采集范围为 100～1000 Da。靶向分析采用 tSIM/ddMS$^2$ 扫描模式：定量分离宽度 5 Da。

## 3. 检出限和定量限

膳食样品中兽药的检出限和定量限见表 1-6。

## 2. Instrumental Determination

Positive ion acquisition: mobile phase A is an aqueous solution containing 0.1% formic acid, and mobile phase B is methanol containing 0.1% formic acid. Negative ion acquisition: mobile phase A is an aqueous solution containing 0.01% ammonia water and mobile phase B is acetonitrile. Injection volume, 5 μL; flow rate, 300 μL/min; column temperature, 40 ℃; HSS T3 column (1.8 μm, 2.1 mm × 100 mm). Heated electrospray ion source (HESI) temperature, 325 ℃; capillary voltage, 3.8 kV; sheath gas flow, 40 arb, auxiliary gas flow, 10 arb; Non-targeted screening was performed using Full Scan/ddMS$^2$ scan mode: range, 100-1000 Da. Targeted analysis was performed using tSIM/ddMS$^2$ scan mode: quantitative separation width of 5 Da.

## 3. LODs and LOQs

LODs and LOQs of veterinary drugs in dietary samples are shown in Table 1-6.

表 1-6　检出兽药的检出限和定量限（单位：μg/kg）
Table 1-6　LODs and LOQs of detected veterinary drugs (Unit: μg/kg)

| 兽药名称 Veterinary drug name | 检出限 LOD | 定量限 LOQ |
|---|---|---|
| 甲氧苄啶 Trimethoprim | 0.008 | 0.03 |
| 麻保沙星 Marbofloxacin | 0.02 | 0.06 |
| 氧氟沙星 Ofloxacin | 0.007 | 0.02 |
| 培氟沙星 Pefloxacin | 0.03 | 0.1 |
| 诺氟沙星 Norfloxacin | 0.01 | 0.03 |
| 环丙沙星 Ciprofloxacin | 0.01 | 0.03 |
| 恩诺沙星 Enrofloxacin | 0.01 | 0.03 |
| 达氟沙星 Danofloxacin | 0.01 | 0.03 |
| 洛美沙星 Lomefloxacin | 0.02 | 0.06 |
| 奥比沙星 Orbifloxacin | 0.02 | 0.06 |
| 沙拉沙星 Sarafloxacin | 0.01 | 0.03 |
| 氟甲喹 Flumequine | 0.01 | 0.03 |

续表

| 兽药名称 Veterinary drug name | 检出限 LOD | 定量限 LOQ |
|---|---|---|
| 磺胺二甲嘧啶 Sulfadimidine | 0.01 | 0.03 |
| 磺胺噻唑 Sulfathiazole | 0.01 | 0.03 |
| 磺胺甲噁唑 Sulfamethoxazole | 0.01 | 0.03 |
| 磺胺间甲氧嘧啶 Sulfamonomethoxine | 0.01 | 0.03 |
| 结晶紫 Crystal violet | 0.006 | 0.02 |
| 左旋咪唑 Levamisole | 0.04 | 0.12 |
| 甲硝唑 Metronidazole | 0.05 | 0.15 |
| 羟基甲硝唑 OH-Metronidazole | 0.05 | 0.15 |
| 地美硝唑 Dimetridazole | 0.05 | 0.15 |
| 2-羟基地美硝唑 2-Hydroxy-dimetridazole | 0.05 | 0.15 |
| 阿苯达唑 Albendazole | 0.01 | 0.03 |
| 阿苯达唑亚砜 Albendazole sulfoxide | 0.01 | 0.03 |
| 阿苯达唑砜 Albendazole sulfone | 0.01 | 0.03 |
| 阿苯达唑-2-氨基砜 Albendazole 2-amino sulfone | 0.01 | 0.03 |
| 芬苯达唑 Fenbendazole | 0.008 | 0.02 |
| 奥芬达唑 Oxfendazole | 0.008 | 0.02 |
| 奥芬达唑砜 Oxfendazole sulfone | 0.008 | 0.02 |
| 氟苯达唑 Flubendazole | 0.003 | 0.01 |
| 甲苯达唑 Mebendazole | 0.003 | 0.01 |
| 氟苯尼考 Florfenicol | 0.02 | 0.06 |
| 氟苯尼考胺 Florfenicol amine | 0.03 | 0.1 |
| 氯霉素 Chloramphenicol | 0.02 | 0.06 |
| 甲砜霉素 Thiamphenicol | 0.03 | 0.1 |

### 4. 质量控制与质量保证

为确保实验结果的准确性，在每批样品的测定过程中加入空白加标样品作为质量控制样品。每批样品中选择一个无目标化合物检出的膳食样品，进行加标回收实验。其中，加标回收率结果控制在70%～120%，说明实验结果准确、可靠。

### 五、氯丙醇分析方法

采用气相色谱-串联质谱法（GC-MS/MS）测定总膳食样品中氯丙醇的

### 4. Quality Control and Quality Assurance

To ensure the accuracy of the experimental results, blank spiked samples were added as quality control samples during the determination of each batch of samples. A blank dietary sample was selected for the spiked recovery test. Among them, the recovery results were controlled at 70%-120%, indicating that the test results are accurate and reliable.

### V. Analysis Method of Chloropropanols

The contents of chloropropanols in TDS samples were analyzed by gas chromatography-tandem mass

含量，内标法定量。

**1. 样品制备**

（1）水及饮料类、酒类和乳类等液体样品

准确称取试样约 2 g（精确至 0.001 g）于 10 mL 离心管中，加入混合内标工作液（10 μg/mL 的 $D_5$-3-MCPD、$D_5$-2-MCPD 和 $D_5$-1,3-DCP）20 μL，混匀，用滴管加到硅藻土柱（2 g/10 mL）中，静置 15 min，用 50% 二氯甲烷/乙酸乙酯（$V/V$）以 1 滴/s 的流速淋洗，收集洗脱液共 14 mL，于室温氮吹浓缩至约 1 mL 后进行 GC-MS/MS 测定。

（2）糖类、蛋类、蔬菜类和水果类等样品

准确称取试样约 2 g（精确至 0.001 g）于 10 mL 离心管中，加入混合内标工作液（10 μg/mL 的 $D_5$-3-MCPD、$D_5$-2-MCPD 和 $D_5$-1,3-DCP）20 μL，混匀，加 20% 溴化钠溶液 2 mL，充分混匀提取 2 min，10 000 r/min 离心 5 min，水相 2 mL 用滴管加到硅藻土柱中，之后操作同（1）。

（3）肉类、水产类和豆类等样品

准确称取试样约 2 g（精确至 0.001 g）于 10 mL 离心管中，加入混合内标工作液（10 μg/mL 的 $D_5$-3-MCPD、$D_5$-2-MCPD 和 $D_5$-1,3-DCP）20 μL，混匀，加 20% 溴化钠溶液 3 mL，充分混匀提取 2 min，10 000 r/min 离心 5 min，水相 2 mL 用滴管加到硅藻土柱中，之后操作同（1），进样前定容到 0.5 mL。

（4）谷类和薯类等样品

准确称取试样约 2 g（精确至 0.001 g）于 10 mL 离心管中，加入混合内标工作液（10 μg/mL 的 $D_5$-3-MCPD、$D_5$-2-MCPD 和 $D_5$-1,3-DCP）20 μL，混匀，加 20% 溴化钠溶液 4 mL，充分混匀提取 2 min，10 000 r/min 离心 5 min，水相 2 mL 用滴管加到硅藻土柱中，之后

spectrometry (GC-MS/MS), and quantified internal standard method.

**1. Sample Preparation**

(1) Liquid Samples such as Water and Beverages, Alcohol Beverages and Liquid Dairy Products

A portion of 2 g (accurate to 0.001 g) TDS sample was weighted into a 10 mL centrifuge tube, spiked with 20 μL internal standard mixture solution (10 μg/L of $D_5$-3-MCPD, $D_5$-2-MCPD and $D_5$-1,3-DCP). The solution was vortex mixed, and then transferred to a diatomite cartridge (2 g/10 mL) and stood for 15 min. The cartridge was then eluted with 50% dichloromethane/ethyl acetate ($V/V$) at a rate of 1 drop/s. A total of 14 mL of the eluent was collected and evaporated to near 1 mL under a gentle stream of nitrogen at room temperature and ready for GC-MS/MS measurement.

(2) Sugar, Eggs, Vegetables and Fruits Samples

A portion of 2 g (accurate to 0.001 g) TDS sample was weighted into a 10 mL centrifuge tube, spiked with 20 μL internal standard mixture solution (10 μg/L of $D_5$-3-MCPD, $D_5$-2-MCPD and $D_5$-1,3-DCP), added with 2 mL of 20% sodium bromide solution and vortex mixed for 2 min. The mixture was then centrifuged for 5 min at 10 000 r/min. 2 mL of the supernatant was then transferred to a diatomite cartridge and the next steps was the same as the section (1).

(3) Meats, Aquatic Foods and Legumes Samples

A portion of 2 g (accurate to 0.001 g) TDS sample was weighted into a 10 mL centrifuge tube, spiked with 20 μL internal standard mixture solution (10 μg/L of $D_5$-3-MCPD, $D_5$-2-MCPD and $D_5$-1,3-DCP), added with 3 mL of 20% sodium bromide solution and vortex mixed for 2 min. The mixture was then centrifuged for 5 min at 10 000 r/min. 2 mL of the supernatant was then transferred to a diatomite cartridge and the next steps was the same as the section (1). The constant volume was 0.5 mL before injection.

(4) Cereals and Potatoes Samples

A portion of 2 g (accurate to 0.001 g) TDS sample was weighted into a 10 mL centrifuge tube, spiked with

操作同（1），进样前定容到 0.5 mL。

## 2. 仪器测定

所使用仪器为气相色谱-串联质谱仪（岛津 GC-MS TQ-8040）。

色谱条件：色谱柱为 Innowax 柱（30 m×0.25 mm×0.25 μm）；进样口温度：250℃；程序升温：50℃保持 3 min，以 10℃/min 升至 170℃，再以 40℃/min 升至 250℃，并保持 5 min；载气：氦气，流速 1 mL/min；碰撞气：氮气；进样方式：不分流进样；进样体积：1.0 μL。

质谱条件：离子化方式：EI；离子源温度：230℃；传输线温度：250℃；四极杆温度：150℃；溶剂延迟：4.0 min；多反应监测模式（MRM）。

## 3. 检出限

本方法 12 类膳食样品的氯丙醇检出限均为 2 μg/kg。

## 4. 质量控制

（1）空白实验

为了评估前处理过程中是否可能引入氯丙醇，造成假阳性结果，本次实验的每一批次样品处理时，均进行了全程空白实验，即在不称样的前提下，按照样品前处理流程进行操作（包括内标的加入等）。结果表明，实验所使用的所有耗材、试剂等均未引入氯丙醇。

20 μL internal standard mixture solution (10 mg/L of $D_5$-3-MCPD, $D_5$-2-MCPD and $D_5$-1,3-DCP), added with 4 mL of 20% sodium bromide solution and vortex mixed for 2 min. The mixture was then centrifuged for 5 min at 10 000 r/min. 2 mL of the supernatant was then transferred to a diatomite cartridge and the next steps was the same as the section (1). The constant volume was 0.5 mL before injection.

## 2. Instrumental Determination

Instrument was GC-MS/MS (Shimadzu GC-MS TQ-8040).

GC conditions: Gas chromatography column, Innowax (30 m × 0.25 mm × 0.25 μm); injector temperatures: 250℃; oven temperature program: started at 50℃ for 3 min, heated to 170℃ at a rate of 10℃/min, then increased to 250℃ at a rate of 40℃/min and held at 250℃ for 5 min; carrier gas: helium, 1 mL/min; collision gas: nitrogen; injection volume: 1 μL with splitless mode.

MS conditions: electron impact ionization (EI) mode; ion source, quadrupole rod and transfer line temperatures: 230℃, 150℃ and 250℃, respectively; solvent delay: 4 min; multiple reaction monitoring (MRM) mode.

## 3. Limits of Detection

The LODs of all chloropropanols in the 12 TDS samples were 2 μg/kg.

## 4. Quality Control

(1) Blank Test

Blank test was performed to evaluate the possibility of introducing chloropropanols during the pretreatment process and avoiding false positive results. During the sample processing of each batch of this experiment, whole blank experiment was carried out, that is, the sample pretreatment process was operated (including the addition of internal standard, etc.) under the premise of not weighing the sample. The results showed that all the consumables and reagents used in the experiment did not introduce chloropropanols.

（2）随行质控

为了保证分析结果的准确，要求每批样品至少做一个加标回收实验，采用空白膳食样品加标 50 μg/kg，要求加标回收率为 70%～120%。

## 六、氯丙醇酯及缩水甘油酯分析方法

### 1. 样品制备

水及饮料类和酒类：准确称取试样约 5 g（精确至 0.001 g），用 5 mL 50% 乙醚/石油醚（V/V）重复提取两次，合并提取液，于 40℃水浴中氮吹至干；糖类：准确称取试样约 5 g（精确至 0.001 g），用 10 mL 水溶解，用 5 mL 50% 乙醚/石油醚（V/V）重复提取两次，合并提取液，于 40℃水浴中氮吹至干；谷类和薯类：准确称取试样约 2 g（精确至 0.001 g），加入 20 g 石英砂，充分搅拌使样品均匀分散，按 GB 5009.6—2016《食品安全国家标准 食品中脂肪的测定》索氏抽提法提取脂肪；其他膳食样品：准确称取试样约 2 g（精确至 0.001 g），加入 10 mL 65℃热水，充分混匀，按 GB 5009.6—2016《食品安全国家标准 食品中脂肪的测定》碱水解法提取脂肪。

准确称取 0.100 g 提取的脂肪（脂肪提取量低于 0.15 g 的样品无需单独称取，可以全部用于后续溴代反应）于 15 mL 离心管中，加入 2 mL 四氢呋喃；准确加入 20 μL 混合内标使用液（10.0 μg/mL），涡旋混匀。准确加入 30 μL 0.70% 溴化钠溶液，涡旋混匀，于烘箱中 50℃保温 15 min，然后加入 3.0 mL 0.60% 碳酸氢钠溶液中和。加入 3 mL 正己烷萃取，充分涡旋，待溶液分层后，将上层液体转移至另一支离心管中，氮吹至干，加入 0.5 mL 四氢呋喃复溶。

## VI. Analysis Method of MCPD Esters and Glycidyl Fatty Acid Esters

### 1. Sample Preparation

Water and beverages and alcohol beverages: a portion of 5 g (accurate to 0.001 g) TDS sample was weighted, extracted with 5 mL of 50% (V/V) ether/petroleum ether mixture twice. The extract was combined and evaporated to dry by a gentle stream of nitrogen at 40℃ water bath. Sugar: a portion of 5 g (accurate to 0.001 g) TDS sample was weighted, dissolved with 10 mL water, extracted with 5 mL of 50% (V/V) ether/petroleum ether mixture twice. The extract was combined and evaporated to dry by a gentle stream of nitrogen at 40℃ water bath. Cereals and potatoes: a portion of 2 g (accurate to 0.001 g) TDS sample was weighted, added with 20 g quartz sand and stir thoroughly to disperse the sample. The fat was extracted by Soxhlet extraction procedure according to GB 5009.6—2016 *National Food Safety Standard-Determination of Fat in Food*. The other TDS samples: a portion of 2 g (accurate to 0.001 g) TDS sample was weighted, added with 10 mL of 65℃ water and vortex mixed. The fat was extracted by alkaline hydrolysis extraction procedure according to GB 5009.6—2016 *National Food Safety Standard-Determination of Fat in Food*.

A portion of 0.100 g fat extracted from TDS sample (samples with a fat amount less than 0.15 g do not need to be weighed separately and can be used entirely for subsequent bromination reaction) was weighted into a 15 mL centrifuge tube, added with 2 mL tetrahydrofuran, spiked with 20 μL internal standard mixture solution and vortex mixed, added with 30 μL of 0.70% sodium bromide solution and vortex mixed. The

复溶后的液体中加入 0.9 mL 1.8% 硫酸甲醇溶液，涡旋混匀，于 40℃下反应 16 h 进行酸水解。反应结束后加入 0.25 mL 9.6% 碳酸氢钠中和，再加入 0.5 mL 水和 0.5 mL 正己烷，混匀，3000 r/min 离心 2 min，弃去正己烷层。

将下层水相转移到硅藻土柱中，静置 15 min，用 50% 二氯甲烷/乙酸乙酯（$V/V$）以 1 滴/s 的流速淋洗，收集洗脱液共 14 mL，于室温氮吹浓缩至约 0.5 mL。

在浓缩液中加 2% 苯硼酸（PBA）乙醚溶液 0.05 mL，混匀，静置 10 min，继续氮吹近干，加异辛烷 0.5 mL，混匀，经超声处理以充分溶解被测物，3000 r/min 离心 5 min，待 GC-MS/MS 测定。

**2. 仪器测定**

所使用仪器为气相色谱-串联质谱仪（岛津 GC-MS TQ-8040）。

色谱条件：色谱柱为 DB-5 ms 柱（30 m × 0.25 mm × 0.25 μm）；进样口温度：250℃；程序升温：50℃保持 1 min，再以 15℃/min 的速度升至 190℃，保持 2 min，再以 70℃/min 的速度升至 280℃，保持 5 min；载气：高纯氦气，流速 1 mL/min；碰撞气：高纯氮气；进样方式：不分流进样；进样体积：1.0 μL。

质谱条件：离子化方式：EI；离子源温度：230℃；传输线温度：250℃；四极杆温度：150℃；溶剂延迟：4.0 min；多反应监测模式（MRM）。

mixture was then incubated at 50℃ for 15 min, after then added with 3 mL of 0.60% sodium bicarbonate solution to neutralize. The resultant mixture was vortex mixed with 3 mL $n$-hexane. The up layer extract was evaporated to dry by a gentle stream of nitrogen. The residue was dissolved with 0.5 mL of tetrahydrofuran.

The redissolved solution was vortex mixed with 0.9 mL of 1.8% sulfuric acid methanol solution, reaction for 16 h at 40℃, and then added 0.25 mL of 9.6% sodium bicarbonate solution to neutralize. The resultant mixture was vortex mixed with 0.5 mL water and 0.5 mL $n$-hexane centrifuged for 2 min at 3000 r/min. The $n$-hexane layer was removed.

The water phase in the under layer was then transferred to a diatomite cartridge and stood for 15 min. The cartridge was then eluted with 50% dichloromethane/ethyl acetate ($V/V$) at a rate of 1 drop/s. A total of 14 mL of the eluent was collected and evaporated to near 0.5 mL under a gentle stream of nitrogen at room temperature and ready for derivatization.

The above concentrate solution was vortex mixed with 0.05 mL of 2% PBA in ether, stood for 10 min, and then evaporated to near dryness. The residue was dissolved with 0.5 mL $iso$-octane by ultrasonic treatment, centrifuged for 5 min at 3000 r/min and ready for GC-MS/MS measurement.

**2. Instrumental Determination**

Instrument was GC-MS/MS (Shimadzu GC-MS TQ-8040).

GC conditions: gas chromatography column: DB-5 ms (30 m × 0.25 mm × 0.25 μm); injector temperatures: 250℃; oven temperature program: started at 50℃ for 1 min, heated to 190℃ at a rate of 15℃/min and held at 190℃ for 2 min, then increased to 280℃ at a rate of 70℃/min and held at 280℃ for 5 min; carrier gas: helium, 1 mL/min; collision gas: nitrogen; injection volume: 1 μL with splitless mode. MS conditions: electron impact ionization (EI) mode; ion source, quadrupole rod and transfer line temperatures: 230℃, 150℃ and 250℃, respectively; solvent delay: 4 min;

## 3. 检出限

本方法12类膳食样品的检出限均为 4 μg/kg。

## 4. 质量控制

（1）空白实验

为了评估前处理过程中是否可能引入氯丙醇酯或缩水甘油酯，造成假阳性结果，本次实验的每一批次样品处理，均进行了全程空白实验，即在不称样的前提下，按照样品前处理流程进行操作（包括内标的加入等），结果表明，实验所使用的所有耗材、试剂等均未引入氯丙醇酯或缩水甘油酯。

（2）随行质控

为了保证分析结果的准确性，要求每批样品至少做一个加标回收实验，采用空白膳食样品加标 50 μg/kg，要求加标回收率为 70%～120%。在处理每一批次的总膳食样品时，使用 3-MCPD 酯、2-MCPD 酯和缩水甘油酯含量分别为 155 μg/kg、99.6 μg/kg 和 74.0 μg/kg 的薯片 FAPAS 质控样，共进行了 18 批次的检测，测得的平均值分别为 154.7 μg/kg、88.7 μg/kg 和 83.5 μg/kg，相对标准偏差分别为 10.0%、7.4% 和 9.4%，表明在进行总膳食样品中氯丙醇酯和缩水甘油酯的测定时，该方法稳定可靠。

## 七、丙烯酰胺分析方法

采用高效液相色谱-串联质谱法测定第六次中国总膳食研究样品中的丙烯酰胺含量，用内标法定量。

multiple reaction monitoring (MRM) mode.

## 3. Limits of Detection

The LODs of all analytes in the 12 TDS samples were 4 μg/kg.

## 4. Quality Control

(1) Blank Test

Blank test was performed to evaluate the possibility of introducing the analytes during the pretreatment process and avoiding false positive results. During the sample processing of each batch of this experiment, whole blank experiment was carried out, that is, the sample pretreatment process was operated (including the addition of internal standard, etc.) under the premise of not weighing the sample. The results showed that all the consumables and reagents used in the experiment did not introduce the analytes.

(2) Accompanying Quality Control

In order to ensure the accuracy of analysis results, each batch of samples was required to do at least one spiked recovery experiment. Blank TDS sample was spiked 50 μg/kg, and the spiking recovery was required to be between 70% and 120%. FAPAS QC of potato chips containing 155 μg/kg of 3-MCPD esters, 99.6 μg/kg of 2-MCPD esters and 74.0 μg/kg of glycidyl fatty acid esters was processed in each batch of TDS samples. The mean values were 154.7 μg/kg of 3-MCPD esters, 88.7 μg/kg of 2-MCPD esters and 83.5 μg/kg of glycidyl fatty acid esters, with relative standard deviations of 10.0%, 7.4% and 9.4%, respectively, indicating that the method was stable and reliable for the determination of MCPD esters and glycidyl fatty acid esters in TDS samples.

## Ⅶ. Analysis Method of Acrylamide

The content of acrylamide in the samples of the sixth China total diet study (TDS) was determined by high performance liquid chromatography-tandem

## 1. 样品制备

称取研细的膳食样品 2.00 g，加入 500 ng/mL 丙烯酰胺-D$_3$ 溶液 0.01 mL，即 5 ng 丙烯酰胺-D$_3$，加水 10 mL，混匀，振荡提取 20 min，提取液于 0℃下以 12 000 r/min 离心 5 min，迅速取上清液 5 mL，经 0.45 μm 聚醚砜滤膜过滤。取上述 1.5 mL 滤液上 Oasis HLB 柱，Oasis HLB 柱使用前用 3 mL 甲醇和 3 mL 水处理。待滤液完全通过柱床，用 0.5 mL 水洗涤，再用 1.5 mL 水洗脱，收集此洗脱液，然后上 Bond Elut-Accucat 柱，Bond Elut-Accucat 柱使用前用 3 mL 甲醇和 3 mL 水处理，弃去前 0.5 mL 洗脱液，收集剩余 1 mL 样品液，用液相色谱-串联质谱仪测定，同位素内标法定量。上述所有净化过程中，样品液依靠重力自然流出，不需加速。

## 2. 仪器测定

所使用仪器为高效液相色谱-串联质谱仪（Qtrap 5500，AB SCIEX 公司）。

色谱条件：色谱柱为 Atlantis dC18 色谱柱（2.1 mm × 150 mm，5 μm），流动相为 0.1% 甲酸水溶液和甲醇，梯度洗脱。流速为 0.20 mL/min，柱温为 40℃，进样量为 20 μL。

质谱条件：离子源为电喷雾电离（ESI）；扫描方式为正离子扫描；监测模式为多反应监测（MRM）；气帘气（curtain gas）为 30 psi；离子源温度（TEM）为 550℃；雾化气（GS1）为 50 psi；辅助气（GS2）为 50 psi；喷雾电压为 5500 V。

mass spectrometry, and quantified by internal standard method.

## 1. Sample Preparation

Weighted 2.00 g homogenized TDS sample into a 50 mL polypropylene centrifuge tube, and 0.01 mL isotope internal standard solution (acrylamide-D$_3$) at the concentration of 500 ng/mL was spiked into the sample, and then 10 mL water as added. The mixture was vortexed for 20 min and then centrifuged at 12 000 r/min for 5 min at 0℃. The supernatant of 5 mL was filtered through a 0.45 μm polyethersulfone filter membrane. Oasis HLB cartridge and Bond Elut-Accucat cartridge were preconditioned with 3 mL methanol and 3 mL water. Then, 1.5 mL supernatant was loaded on a preconditioned Oasis HLB cartridge, and the effluent was discarded. The cartridge was rinsed by 0.5 mL water, then eluted by 1.5 mL water. Elution is collected and loaded on a preconditioned Bond Elut-Accucat cartridge. The initial elution of 0.5 mL was discarded, and the rest elution of 1 mL was collected, which was used for LC-MS/MS analysis and quantified by isotope internal standard method. The extracted solution flows through the cartridge naturally by gravity without acceleration in the all purification process.

## 2. Instrument Measurement

The analysis was performance by a high performance liquid chromatography-tandem mass spectrometry (Qtrap 5500, AB SCIEX).

LC conditions: column: Atlantis dC18 column (2.1 mm × 150 mm, 5 μm); mobile phase: water contained 0.1% formic acid and methanol with gradient elution; flow rate: 0.20 mL/min; column temperature: 40℃; injection volume: 20 μL.

MS conditions: ionization mode, positive electrospray ionization (ESI+) mode with multi-reaction monitoring (MRM); curtain gas: 30 psi: ion source temperature: 550℃; gas 1: 50 psi; gas 2: 50 psi; spray voltage: 5500 V.

## 3. Limits of Detection

The LOD of this method was 0.16 μg/kg.

## 4. Quality Control

(1) Blank Test

During the processing of each batch of samples in this experiment, the whole process blank experiment was carried out. The operation was performed according to the sample pretreatment process (including the addition of internal standard) without weighing the samples. The results showed that all consumables and reagents used in the experiment did not introduce acrylamide.

(2) International Test

This method was used to participated the acrylamide test (Food Chemistry Proficiency Test 3085) in potato chips organized by FAPAS in 2018. Our laboratory result was 223.07 μg/kg (median value was 229 μg/kg), Z value was –0.1.

FAPAS test sample was used as quality control samples during processing each batch of total dietary samples. A total of 16 batches were analyzed, and the average value of FAPAS test sample was 215.9 μg/kg, and the relative standard deviation was 5.0%, which showed that the method was stable and reliable in acrylamide determination.

## Ⅷ. Analysis Method of Polycyclic Aromatic Hydrocarbons

Gas chromatography-mass spectrometry was used to determine the content of 16 kinds of polycyclic aromatic hydrocarbons in the samples of the sixth China total diet study, and the internal standard method was used for quantification.

### 1. Sample Preparation

1) For samples with low oil content such as fruits, sugar, water and beverages, and alcohol beverages, weigh 10.00 g of sample, add 0.2 μg/mL 16 kinds of PAHs internal standard solution 50 μL, add cyclohexane-ethyl acetate (1∶1) to mix 15-20 mL

EZ-2 真空浓缩仪除去有机溶剂。加入 5 mL 0.3 mol/L 氢氧化钾乙醇溶液，超声溶解，室温放置 5 min 后，加 4 mL 水、5 mL 正己烷，涡旋提取 2 min，以 10 000 r/min 离心 2 min，上层正己烷提取液待净化。

2）谷类、豆类、薯类、肉类、蛋类、水产类、蔬菜类等油脂含量高的总膳食样品称取 10.00 g（精确至 0.01 g）试样于 50 mL 具塞离心管中，加入 50 μL 0.2 μg/mL 16 种 PAH 内标使用液、20.0 g 无水硫酸钠（注意要分散，不要结块，脱水不够影响提取效果）、20 mL 的环己烷-乙酸乙酯（1∶1）混合溶剂，涡旋震荡 3 min 后，超声 15 min，以 10 000 r/min 离心 3 min，吸取上层有机相至离心管中，在 35℃用 EZ-2 真空浓缩仪除去有机溶剂。加 5 mL 1.5 mol/L 氢氧化钾乙醇溶液，超声溶解，70℃ 水浴放置 3 min，取出冷却后加 4 mL 水、5 mL 正己烷，涡旋提取 2 min，以 10 000 r/min 离心 2 min，上层正己烷提取液待净化。

3）乳类称取 10.00 g（精确至 0.01 g）于 50 mL 具塞离心管中，加入 50 μL 0.2 μg/mL 16 种 PAH 内标使用液、2 mL 氨水充分混匀，在（65±5）℃水浴中放置 10 min，取出冷却至室温，加入 10 mL 无水乙醇，缓慢混匀，加入 8 mL 无水乙醚，漩涡振荡 5 min，再加入 8 mL 石油醚，漩涡振荡 5 min，以 10 000 r/min 下离心 5 min，吸出上层有机相至离心管中，在 35℃用 EZ-2 真空浓缩仪除去有机溶剂。加 5 mL 1.5 mol/L 氢氧化钾乙醇溶液，超声溶解，70℃ 水浴放置 3 min，取出冷却后加 4 mL 水、5 mL 正己烷，涡旋提取 2 min，以 10 000 r/min 离心 2 min，上层正己烷提取液待净化。

在 EU 多环芳烃专用净化柱上加 1.0 g 无水硫酸钠，依次用 3 mL 二氯

of solvent, vortexed, centrifuged, sucked the organic layer, concentrated, added 5 mL of 0.3 mol/L potassium hydroxide ethanol solution, dissolved by sonication, placed at room temperature, added 4 mL of water, 5 mL of $n$-hexane, vortex for 2 min, centrifuge at 10 000 r/min for 2 min, the upper $n$-hexane extract is to be purified.

2) Grains, beans, potatoes, meats, eggs, aquatic products, vegetables and other samples with high oil content, weigh 10.00 g, add 50 μL 0.2 μg/mL 16 kinds of PAHs internal standard solution, anhydrous sodium sulfate 20.0 g, cyclohexane-ethyl acetate (1∶1) mixed solvent 20 mL, vortexed, sonicated, centrifuged, sucked the organic layer, concentrated, added 5 mL of 1.5 mol/L potassium hydroxide ethanol solution, dissolved by ultrasonic, water bath at 70℃ set aside, add 4 mL of water and 5 mL of $n$-hexane after cooling, vortex for 2 min, centrifuge at 10 000 r/min for 2 min, and the upper $n$-hexane extract is to be purified.

3) Weigh 10.00 g of milk sample, add 50 μL of 0.2 μg/mL 16 kinds of PAHs internal standard solution, add 2 mL of ammonia water, mix well, place in a (65 ± 5)℃ water bath for 10 min, cool to room temperature, add 10 mL of absolute ethanol, and mix slowly, add 8 mL of anhydrous ether, after vortexing for 5 min, add 8 mL of petroleum ether, vortex for 5 min, centrifuge at 10 000 r/min for 5 min, suck the organic layer, after concentration, add 5 mL of 1.5 mol/L potassium hydroxide ethanol solution, dissolve by ultrasonic, 70℃ place in a water bath, add 4 mL of water and 5 mL of $n$-hexane after cooling, vortex for 2 min, centrifuge at 10 000 r/min for 2 min, and the upper $n$-hexane extract is to be purified.

Add 1.0 g of anhydrous sodium sulfate to the special purification column for EU polycyclic aromatic hydrocarbons, rinse the column with 3 mL of dichloromethane and 3 mL of $n$-hexane in turn. After the activation, draw the $n$-hexane extract and transfer it to the purification column. Then, rinse with 4 mL of $n$-hexane to remove impurities, and then eluted with 5 mL of dichloromethane-ethyl acetate (1∶1, $V/V$), collect the eluate, and after concentration, add acetone-

甲烷、3 mL 正己烷淋洗柱子，活化结束后吸取正己烷提取液并转移到净化柱上，待过柱后，用 4 mL 正己烷淋洗除杂，最后用 5 mL 二氯甲烷-乙酸乙酯（1∶1，*V/V*）溶液洗脱并收集，加 0.05 mL 丙酮-异辛烷（1∶1，*V/V*）定容液超声溶解残留物，转移至锥形进样瓶中，待 GC/MS 分析。

**2. 仪器测定**

DB-PAHEU 毛细管色谱柱（Part Number 121-9627）：20 m×0.18 mm（内径）×0.14 μm（膜厚）或相当色谱柱；进样口温度：250℃；电离模式：电子轰击源（EI），能量为 70 eV，自动调谐后电子倍增器电压加 200 V；四极杆温度：150℃；离子源温度：280℃；传输线温度：300℃；溶剂延迟：18 min；进样方式：不分流进样；进样量：2 μL；检测方式：选择离子扫描（SIM）采集。

**3. 定量限和检出限**

本方法 16 种多环芳烃的定量限为 0.05 μg/kg，检出限为 0.02 μg/kg。

**4. 质量控制**

为了保证分析结果的准确性，要求每批样品至少做一个加标回收实验，采用低本底样品加标 0.2 μg/kg（即 10 g 样品加 10 μL 0.2 μg/mL 的 16 种 EU PAH 标准使用液），同时采用低浓度 PAH FAPAS TQ0671 可可脂进行质控跟踪。

## 九、氨基甲酸乙酯分析方法

采用气相色谱-质谱法测定第六次中国总膳食研究样品中的氨基甲酸乙酯（EC）含量，用内标法定量。

*iso*-octane (1∶1, *V/V*) 0.05 mL ultrasonically dissolves the residue and transfers it to a sample vial for GC/MS analysis.

**2. Instrumental Determination**

DB-PAHEU capillary column (Part Number 121-9627): 20 m × 0.18 mm (inner diameter) × 0.14 μm (film thickness) or equivalent column; inlet temperature: 250℃; ionization mode: electron bombardment source (EI), the energy is 70 eV, and the electron multiplier voltage is added 200 V after auto-tuning; quadrupole rod temperature: 150℃; ion source temperature: 280℃; transfer line temperature: 300℃; solvent delay: 18 min; injection mode: splitless injection sample; injection volume: 2 μL; detection mode: selected ion scanning (SIM) acquisition.

**3. LOQs and Limits of Detection**

The limit of quantitation of 16 polycyclic aromatic hydrocarbons in this method is 0.05 μg/kg, and the limit of detection is 0.02 μg/kg.

**4. Quality Control**

In order to ensure the accuracy of the analysis results, it is required to do at least one standard addition recovery experiment for each batch of samples, using low background samples to add 0.2 μg/kg (that is, 10 g samples plus 0.2 μg/mL 10 μL of 16 kinds of EU PAHs standard solution), while using low concentration of PAHs FAPAS TQ0671 cocoa butter was evaluated for quality control.

## Ⅸ. Analysis Method of Ethyl Carbamate

The content of ethyl carbamate in the 6th China TDS was determined by gas chromatography-mass spectrometry (GC-MS) and quantified by internal standard method.

## 1. 样品制备

称取均质的试样1 g（精确到0.01 g），置于15 mL聚丙烯离心管中。加入40 μL的D₅-氨基甲酸乙酯溶液（10 μg/mL）、3 mL去离子水及1 g NaCl，涡旋混匀5 min。加入2 mL乙腈，涡旋混匀5 min，超声提取15 min，以9500 r/min在4℃下离心15 min，吸取上层有机相溶液并保留，下层试样再加入5 mL乙腈，重复提取2次，合并上层有机相溶液，待净化。取Oasis Prime@ HLB固相萃取小柱（500 mg，6 m³），先用3 mL的80%乙腈溶液清洗。上样收集流出液，40℃氮吹至近干，用乙腈定容至2.0 mL，涡旋10 min，10 000 r/min离心5 min，取上清液，过0.22 μm滤膜后待GC-MS测定。

## 2. 仪器测定

气相色谱条件：色谱柱为VF-WAX（30 m×0.25 mm×0.39 μm）；进样口温度为220℃；进样模式为不分流进样；进样体积为1 μL；色谱柱升温程序为初温85℃，保持8 min，以8℃/min升至180℃；载气为高纯氦气（纯度＞99.999%），流速为1 mL/min。

质谱条件：质谱检测模式为选择离子监测（SIM）；EI源为70 eV；离子源温度为230℃；传输线温度为240℃；溶剂延迟时间为8 min。氨基甲酸乙酯选择监测离子（$m/z$）为44、62、74、89，定量离子为62。D₅-氨基甲酸乙酯选择监测离子（$m/z$）为64、76、94，定量离子为64。对于总膳食基质，称取0.5 g样品于10 mL刻度管，加入1.0 g的NaCl，加入5 mL 0.1 mol/L的HCl萃取，涡旋2 min，离心5 min，取1 mL上清液待净化。

## 1. Sample Preparation

The homogenous sample was weighed to 1 g (accurate to 0.01 g) and placed in a 15 mL polypropylene centrifuge tube. In this tube, 40 μL of D₅-ethyl carbamate solution (10 μg/mL), 3 mL of deionized water, and 1 g of NaCl were added and vortexed for 5 min. The sample was extracted with 2 mL of acetonitrile, vortexed for 5 min, sonicated for 15 min, and centrifuged at 9500 r/min for 15 min at 4℃. Then the upper organic phase solution was aspirated and retained. The lower layer was then added to 5 mL of acetonitrile, and the extraction was repeated twice. The upper organic phase was combined and left to purify. The Oasis Prime@HLB solid-phase extraction column (500 mg, 6 m³) was washed with 3 mL of 80% acetonitrile solution. The extract was uploaded into the column, and the effluent was collected. The effluent was concentrated to near dryness at 40℃ under nitrogen, then was resolved to 2.0 mL with acetonitrile, vortexed for 10 min, and centrifuged at 10 000 r/min for 5 min. The supernatant was removed, filtered through a 0.22 μm membrane, and determined by GC-MS.

## 2. Instrument Determination

Gas chromatography conditions: the column was VF-WAX (30 m × 0.25 mm × 0.39 μm). The injection port temperature was 220℃. The injection mode was non-split injection; the injection volume was 1 μL. Initially, the column ramp-up procedure was 85℃, held for 8 min and ramped up to 180℃ at 8℃/min. The carrier gas was high purity helium (purity>99.999%) at a 1 mL/min flow rate.

Mass spectrometry conditions: mass spectrometric detection mode was selected ion monitoring (SIM). EI source was 70 eV. Ion source temperature was 230℃; transmission line temperature was 240℃; solvent delay time was 8 min. Selected monitoring ions ($m/z$) of ethyl carbamate were 44, 62, 74, 89; quantitative ion was for 62. Selected monitoring ions ($m/z$) of D₅-ethyl carbamate were 64, 76, 94; quantitative ion was for 64. For the

### 3. 检出限

以空白样品作为基质，根据不同膳食基质分别加入目标物质，按照样品前处理流程进行操作，上机测定，获得目标物的信噪比数据，以 3 倍信噪比（S/N=3）计算本方法的检出限，本方法的检出限为 2.0～7.6 μg/kg。

### 4. 质量控制

每类基质准确称取空白均质试样 18 份，共 3 组，定量加入氨基甲酸乙酯标准品，每类基质设置三个加标水平（原则上按照每种基质的 1 倍、3 倍、5 倍定量限添加），按前述方法处理样品后进行测定。经检测，不同基质平均加标回收率范围在 78.7%～109.3%，平均相对标准偏差为 5.67%～18.53%（$n$=6）。

## 十、邻苯二甲酸酯分析方法

采用气相色谱-质谱法测定第六次中国总膳食研究样品中的 16 种邻苯二甲酸酯含量，用内标法定量。

### 1. 样品制备

对于固体膳食样品而言，称取 1.0 g 样品于 10 mL 具塞玻璃刻度管，加入内标混合液（50 μg/mL）20 μL，加入 4 mL 去离子水、2.0 g NaCl、4 mL 甲苯涡旋提取 3 min 后，3000 r/min 以上离心 5 min，取 2 mL 上清液待净化。对于液体膳食样品而言，称取 1.0 g 样品于 10 mL 具塞玻璃刻度管，酒类样品需加入 2 mL 水稀释，然后加入内标混合液（50 μg /mL）20 μL，加入 1.0 g NaCl，以 2 mL 甲苯涡旋提取 3 min 后，3000 r/min 以上离心 5 min，取 1 mL 上清液待净化。

dietary matrices, 0.5 g of sample was weighed into a 10 mL graduated tube, 1.0 g of NaCl was added, 5 mL of 0.1 mol/L HCl was added for extraction, vortexed for 2 min, and centrifuged for 5 min. Finally, 1 mL of supernatant was removed for purification.

### 3. Limits of Detection

A blank sample was used as the matrix, and the target substances were added according to different dietary matrices, respectively. The sample was operated according to the sample pretreatment procedure and determined by GC-MS to obtain the signal-to-noise ratio data of the target substances. The limit of detection was calculated by 3 times of the signal-to-noise ratio (S/N=3). The limits of detection for this method were 2.0-7.6 μg/kg.

### 4. Quality Control

A total of three groups of eighteen blank homogenized specimens were accurately weighted for each type of matrix and the standard of EC was added quantitatively. Three spiked levels were set for each matrix (in principle, 1, 3 and 5 times of the limit of quantification for each matrix), and the samples were treated as described above and then determined. The average spiked recoveries of the different matrices ranged from 78.7% to 109.3%, with an average relative standard deviation of 5.67%-18.53% ($n$=6).

## X. Analysis Method of Phthalates

The contents of 16 phthalates in the 6th China TDS were determined by gas chromatography-mass spectrometry (GC-MS) and quantified by internal standard method.

### 1. Sample Preparation

For solid dietary samples, 1.0 g of sample was weighed in a 10 mL glass stoppered tube, and 20 μL of internal standard with a concentration of 50 μg/mL was added. Phthalates were extracted with 4 mL of

将 Silica/PSA 固相萃取（SPE）柱以 5 mL 二氯甲烷和 5 mL 乙腈活化后，以 2 mL 提取液上样，以 6 mL 乙腈洗脱样品并接收。洗脱液在 45℃下用氮气吹至近干后，以 1 mL 正己烷复溶，3000 r/min 以上离心 5 min，取上清液进气相色谱-质谱仪检测。

**2. 仪器测定**

气相色谱条件：色谱柱为 DB-5MS UI 石英毛细管色谱柱，柱长 30 m，内径 0.25 mm，膜厚 0.25 μm；进样口温度为 250℃；升温程序为初温 60℃，保持 1 min，以 20℃/min 升至 220℃，保持 1 min，再以 5℃/min 升至 280℃，保持 1 min；以 20℃/min 升至 300℃，保持 4 min；载气为高纯氦气，纯度≥99.999%，流速 1.0 mL/min；进样方式为柱上不分流进样；进样量为 1 μL。

质谱条件：电离方式：电子轰击源（EI）；电离能量：70 eV；传输线温度：280℃；离子源温度：250℃；监测方式：选择离子扫描（SIM）；溶剂延迟：6 min。

deionized water, 2.0 g of NaCl, and 4 mL of toluene by vortexing for 3 min and then centrifuged at 3000 r/min for 5 min. The supernatant with a volume of 2 mL was removed for purification. 1.0 g of sample was weighed into a 10 mL glass stoppered graduated tube for liquid dietary samples. The alcohol beverages samples should be diluted with 2 mL of water, then 20 μL of internal standard with a 50 μg/mL concentration, and 1.0 g of NaCl should be added into the glass tube. Phthalates were extracted by vortexing with 2 mL of toluene for 3 min, then centrifuged at 3000 r/min for 5 min, and 1 mL of supernatant should be taken for purification.

The SPE column of Silica/PSA was equilibrium before sample loading by 5 mL of dichloromethane and 5 mL of acetonitrile. The sample of 2 mL was loaded with extraction solution, eluted with 6 mL of acetonitrile, and collected. The eluate was evaporated with nitrogen at 45℃ until nearly dry, then redissolved in 1 mL of hexane and centrifuged at 3000 r/min for 5 min. The supernatant was taken into a gas chromatograph-mass spectrometer for detection.

**2. Instrument Determination**

Gas chromatography conditions: the column was a DB-5MS UI quartz capillary column with a column length of 30 m, an inner diameter of 0.25 mm, and a film thickness of 0.25 μm; the inlet temperature was 250℃; the ramp-up procedure was 60℃ at the beginning, held for 1 min, 20℃/min to 220℃, held for 1 min, then 5℃/min to 280℃, held for 1 min, 20℃/min to 300℃, held for 4 min; the carrier gas was high purity helium, purity ≥99.999%, the flow rate was 1.0 mL/min; the injection method was a non-split injection on the column; the injection volume was 1 μL.

Mass spectrometry conditions: ionisation: electron bombardment source (EI); ionisation energy: 70 eV; transmission line temperature: 280℃; ion source temperature: 250℃; monitoring mode: selected ion scan (SIM); solvent delay: 6 min.

### 3. 检出限

以空白样品作为基质,根据不同膳食基质分别加入目标物质,按照样品前处理流程进行操作,上机测定,根据信噪比(S/N)为3和10时的响应值得出本方法16种邻苯二甲酸酯的检出限与定量限分别为 3.0 μg/kg 和 10.0 μg/kg。

### 4. 质量控制

每类基质准确称取空白均质试样 18 份,共 3 组,定量加入邻苯二甲酸酯标准物质,每类基质设置三个加标水平(原则上按照每种基质的 1 倍、3 倍、5 倍定量限添加),按前述方法处理样品后进行测定。经检测,不同基质平均加标回收率范围在 91.5～100.5,平均相对标准偏差为 1.67%～7.32%($n$=6)。

## 十一、二噁英及其类似物、指示性多氯联苯及多溴二苯醚分析方法

采用同位素稀释的高分辨气相色谱-高分辨质谱法(HRGC-HRMS)对第六次中国总膳食研究膳食样品中多氯代二苯并二噁英和多氯代苯并呋喃(PCDD/Fs)、二噁英样多氯联苯(dl-PCB)和指示性 PCB 以及多溴二苯醚(PBDE)的含量进行了测定。

### 1. 样品制备

称取均质化后的膳食样品适量(植物性食品 40～60 g,动物性食品 25～40 g),使用冷冻干燥机干燥,研磨后与硅藻土混合均匀,加入稳定同位素 $^{13}$C 标记的 PCDD/Fs、dl-PCB、指示性 PCB 和 PBDE 的定量内标后,以正己烷:二氯甲烷(1:1)为提取溶剂进行加速溶剂提取。提取条件为:温度,150 ℃;压力,10.3 MPa(1500 psi);循环,2 次;静态时间,7 min。

### 3. Limits of Detection

Using the blank sample as the matrix, adding the target substances to different dietary matrices, the samples were operated according to the sample pretreatment process, and measured on the machine. The limits of detection (LOD) and limits of quantification (LOQ) for each of the 16 phthalates in this method were determined based on the response values of signal-to-noise ratios (S/N) at 3 and 10 for 3.0 μg/kg and 10.0 μg/kg, respectively.

### 4. Quality Control

Eighteen blank homogeneous samples were accurately weighed into 3 groups for each matrix type, and phthalate standards were added quantitatively. 3 spiked levels were set for each matrix type (in principle, 1, 3, and 5 times of limit of quantification of each matrix), and the samples were treated as described above and then measured. The average spiked recoveries of the different matrices were in the range of 91.5%-105.5%, with an average relative standard deviation of 1.67%-7.32% ($n$=6).

## XI. Analysis Method of Dioxins and Their Analogues (DLCs), Indicator Polychlorinated Biphenyls (PCBs), Polybrominated Diphenyl Ethers (PBDEs)

The contents of polychlorinated dibenzo-$p$-dioxins and polychlorinated dibenzofurans (PCDD/Fs), dioxins like polychlorinated biphenyls (dl-PCBs), indicator PCBs, and polybrominated diphenyl ethers (PBDEs) in the samples of the sixth China total diet study (TDS) were determined by a high resolution gas chromatography-high resolution mass spectrometry (HRGC-HRMS) with isotopic dilution techniques.

### 1. Sample Preparation

After homogenization, an aliquot of solid sample, 40-60 g for plant origin samples and 25-40 g for animal origin samples, respectively, was placed in a glass dish,

提取液使用旋转蒸发仪蒸发至近干，残渣使用 150 mL 正己烷进行复溶，加入 20~40 g 44%（质量分数）硫酸硅胶进行除脂处理，取上清液浓缩后，用配备复合硅胶柱、碱性氧化铝柱和活性炭柱的全自动净化系统作进一步净化，分别接收含有 PCDD/Fs、PCB 和 PBDE 组分的洗脱液，浓缩至 20~40 μL 后，分别加入稳定同位素 $^{13}$C 标记的 PCDD/Fs、PCB 和 PBDE 回收内标，涡旋混匀后，以高分辨气相色谱-高分辨质谱仪（HRGC-HRMS）测定。

**2. 仪器测定**

使用高分辨气相色谱-高分辨质谱仪（HRGC-HRMS）（DFS，Thermo Scientific）进行分析测定。

（1）PCDD/Fs 测定

色谱条件：色谱柱为 DB-5MS UI（柱长 60 m、内径 0.25 mm、液膜厚度 0.25 μm），载气为高纯氦气，流速 0.8 mL/min，进样量 2 μL，不分流进样，恒流模式；进样口温度 280℃；接口温度：310℃。升温程序：初始温度 120℃，保持 1 min；以 70℃/min 至 220℃，保持 15 min；以 2℃/min 升至 250℃，再以 1℃/min 至 260℃，再以 20℃/min 升至 310℃，保持 5 min。

质谱条件：离子源温度：280℃；电离模式：EI；电子轰击能量：45 eV；灯丝电流：0.75 mA；参考气：全氟三丁胺（FC43）；参考气温度：100℃；倍增器增益：2E6；分辨率：>10 000。

and then the moisture was removed by lyophilisation. After grinding in a ceramic mortar, the sample was mixed with diatomite. The mixture was placed into the extraction cell, and after spiking $^{13}$C-labeled compounds, including PCDD/Fs, dl-PCBs, indicator PCBs, and PBDEs, accelerate solvent extraction (ASE) was performed by applying a mixture of 1∶1 (V/V) n-hexane and dichloromethane. Recommended conditions are as follows: 150℃, 1500 psi, two circles, and 7 min for static time.

The extraction was evaporated to dryness by using a decompression rotary evaporator. The residue was dissolved in 150 mL n-hexane, then 20-40 g of 44% acid silica gel (m/m) was added to remove the lipids. Then, after condensing, the supernatant was prepared by using automatic clean-up system equipped with commercial columns of mixed silica gel, alkaline alumina, and carbon. The fractions containing PCDD/Fs, PCBs, and PBDEs were collected respectively, and concentrated to a volume of 20-40 μL. After spiking $^{13}$C-labeled recovery internal standards and vortex, analytes were determined by using a high resolution gas chromatography-high resolution mass spectrometry (HRGC-HRMS).

**2. Instrument Determination**

An HRGC-HRMS (DFS, Thermo Scientific) was applied for the determination of PCDD/Fs, dl-PCBs, indicator PCBs, and PBDEs.

(1) PCDD/Fs Determination

GC conditions: DB-5MS UI column (60 m × 0.25 mm × 0.25 μm); carrier gas: high purity helium; column flow: 0.8 mL/min; injection volume: 2 μL, splitless and constant flow mode; injector temperature: 280℃; interface temperature: 310℃; oven temperature program: initial temperature 120℃, hold for 1 min, increased to 220℃ at 70℃/min, hold for 15 min, to 250℃ at 2℃/min, to 260℃ at 1℃/min, to 310℃ at 20℃/min, hold for 5 min.

MS conditions: ion source temperature: 280℃; ionization method: electron impact (EI) at 45 eV; filament

（2）PCB 测定

色谱条件：色谱柱为 DB-5MS UI（柱长 60 m、内径 0.25 mm、液膜厚度 0.25 μm），载气为高纯氦气，流速 0.8 mL/min，进样量 1 μL，不分流进样，恒流模式，进样口温度为 290℃，接口温度为 290℃。升温程序：初始温度：110 ℃，保持 1 min；以 15 ℃/min 升温速率升至 180℃，保持 1 min；再以 3℃/min 升温速率升至 300℃，保持 32 min。

质谱条件：同 3.1。

（3）PBDE 测定

色谱条件：色谱柱为 DB-5MS HT（柱长 15 m、内径 0.25 mm、液膜厚度 0.10 μm），载气为高纯氦气，流速 1.0 mL/min，进样量 1 μL，不分流进样，恒流模式，进样口温度 260℃，接口温度 270℃。升温程序：初始温度 120℃，保持 2 min；以 15 ℃/min 升温速率升至 230℃，以 5℃/min 升温速率升至 270℃，以 9.25℃/min 升温速率升至 325℃，保持 2 min，以 2.5℃/min 升温速率升至 330℃。

质谱条件：离子源温度：265 ℃；电离模式：EI；电子轰击能量：45 eV；灯丝电流：0.75 mA；参考气：全氟化煤油（PFK）；参考气温度：120℃；倍增器增益：2E6；分辨率：>5000。

### 3. 检出限

TCDD/Fs 的检出限为 0.001～0.002 pg/g，OCDD/F 的检出限为 0.002～0.099 pg/g，其他 PCDD/Fs 的检出限为 0.001～0.013 pg/g，PCB 的检出限为 0.005～0.027 pg/g，PBDE 的检出限为 0.01～0.04 pg/g。

### 4. 质量控制

（1）灵敏度

进样 1 pg 的 2,3,7,8-TCDD，其响

current: 0.75 mA; reference gas: perfluorotributylamine (FC43); inlet temperature: 100℃; multiplier gain: 2E6; mass resolution: >10 000.

(2) dl-PCBs and Indicator PCBs Determination

GC conditions: DB-5MS UI column (60 m × 0.25 mm × 0.25 μm); carrier gas: high purity helium; column flow: 0.8 mL/min; injection volume: 1 μL, splitless and constant flow mode; injector temperature: 290℃; interface temperature: 290℃; oven temperature program: initial temperature 110℃, hold for 1 min, increased to 180℃ at 15℃/min, hold for 1 min, to 300℃ at 3℃/min, hold for 32 min.

MS conditions: the same as section (1).

(3) PBDEs Determination

GC conditions: DB-5MS HT column (15 m × 0.25 mm × 0.10 μm); carrier gas: high purity helium; column flow: 1.0 mL/min; injection volume: 1 μL, splitless and constant flow mode; injector temperature: 260℃; interface temperature: 270℃; oven temperature program: initial temperature 120℃, hold for 2 min, increased to 230℃ at 15℃/min, to 270℃ at 5℃/min, increased to 325℃ at 9.25℃/min, hold for 2 min, increased to 330℃ at 2.5℃/min.

MS conditions: ion source temperature: 265℃; ionization method: electron impact (EI) at 45 eV; filament current: 0.75 mA; reference gas: polyfluoro kerosene (PFK); inlet temperature: 120℃; multiplier gain: 2E6; mass resolution: >5000.

### 3. Limits of Detection

LODs of TCDD/Fs were in a range of 0.001-0.002 pg/g. LODs of OCDD/F were in a range of 0.002-0.099 pg/g. LODs of other PCDD/Fs were 0.001-0.013 pg/g. LODs of PCBs were 0.005-0.027 pg/g. LODs of PBDEs were 0.01-0.04 pg/g.

### 4. Quality control

(1) Sensitivity

When 1 pg of 2,3,7,8-TCDD was injected in to HRGC-HRMS, the intensity, peak height, should be comparable to $3 \times 10^3$. Moreover, the difference between

应强度不得低于 $3 \times 10^3$。此外，高端估计（UB 估计）和低端估计（LB 估计）的偏差<20%，符合法规 [Commission Regulation (EU) No 589/2014] 要求。

（2）回收率和检出限

稳定同位素取代定量内标回收率 40%～110%，符合 GB 5009.205—2013 规定。

（3）实验室空白

每批次样品包含一个实验室空白样品，即除不添加任何样品外，其他处理过程与实际样品完全一致，用于测量整个分析过程的本底背景水平，日常工作中应绘制空白结果的质量控制图，以评价实验室可能的污染状况。此外，所用有机溶剂在浓缩 10 000 倍后不得检出 2,3,7,8-TCDD。

（4）质控样品

每批次样品包含一个质控样品，所选质控样品的基质尽量与待分析样品的基质相同或相近，本次研究中所用的标准物质包括乳粉中二噁英、多氯联苯成分分析标准物质（GBW10109，国家食品安全风险评估中心，北京），牛肉粉中二噁英、多氯联苯成分分析标准物质（GBW10132，国家食品安全风险评估中心，北京）以及冻干鱼肉（WMF01，Wellington Laboratories Inc.，加拿大），用于有机污染物分析。

（5）国际比对考核

本实验室自 2005 年起，每年都参加由挪威公共卫生研究所组织的食品中卤代持久性有机污染物测定的国际比对考核，对肉类、蛋类、鱼类、乳制品等 4 类样品中的 PCDD/Fs、dl-PCB、指示性 PCB、PBDE 等开展测定，Z 评分范围为–1.3～1.8，结果优秀。

upperbound (UB) level and lowerbound (LB) level were not exceed 20%, complying with the Commission Regulation (EU) No 589/2014.

(2) Recovery and LODs

The recoveries of the individual internal standards were in the range of 40%-110%, complying with the national standards GB 5009.205—2013.

(3) Blank Test

A method blank was performed in every batch. Method blank sample was prepared though spiking labeled internal standards in to an ASE cell filled diatomite, which was applied to determined the background contamination of the analysis laboratory. Quality control chart was used to evaluate the potential contamination of the laboratory. In addition, 2,3,7,8-TCDD should not be detected in all organic solvents after 10 000 times concentrated.

(4) Quality Control Samples

One quality control sample was included in each batch. The matrix of the selected quality control sample should be the same as or similar to the matrix of the sample to be analyzed. Some reference material or certified reference materials were selected in the current study, including dioxins and polychlorinated biphenyls in milk powder (GBW10109, China National Center for Food Safety Risk Assessment, Beijing, China), dioxins and polychlorinated biphenyls in beef powder (GBW10132, China National Center for Food Safety Risk Assessment, Beijing, China), and freeze-dried fish tissue for organic contaminant analysis (WMF01, Wellington Laboratories Inc., Canada).

(5) International Inter-laboratory Comparison

Our laboratory has participated in the international inter-laboratory comparison study on POPs in foods organized by Norwegian Institute of Public Health since 2005. We determined PCDD/Fs, dl-PCBs, indicator PCBs, and PBDEs in various testing materials including eggs, meats, fishes, and dairy products. The Z-score was in the range of –1.3-1.8, indicating a satisfactory results in our laboratory.

# XII. Analysis Method of Persistent Organochlorine Pesticides

25 persistent organochlorine pesticides (OCPs) were quantified using their own isotopic internal standards, and the other 2 OCPs were quantified using isotope-labeled analogs as internal standards by gas chromatography-tandem mass spectrometry.

## 1. Sample Preparation

Accurately weigh 5 g dietary sample into a 50 mL centrifuge tube, add 40 μL of internal standard mixture (ES-5465-A-5X), and stand for 10 min, add 3-6 mL of water according to the water content of the sample. After vortexing and mixing, add 10 mL of acetonitrile, vortex and mix for 5 min, then add 2 g of sodium chloride and 8 g of anhydrous sodium sulfate, shake vigorously for 2 min, centrifuge at 8000 r/min for 5 min, and take the acetonitrile supernatant. 1.5 mL of supernatant was added, 1.0 mL of *n*-hexane was added for extraction, and the supernatant was filtered through an organic filter membrane to be determined.

## 2. Instrumental Determination

Chromatographic column: DB-5MS (30 m × 0.25 mm × 0.25 μm); carrier gas: helium (purity 99.999%); flow rate: 1.0 mL/min; injection volume: 2 μL. The heating program of the column oven: the initial temperature was kept at 60℃ for 4 min, the temperature was increased to 150℃ at 25℃/min, and then increased to 300℃ at 8℃/min, maintained for 5 min, and the analysis time was 33 min; the PTV injection port heating program: the initial temperature was kept at 65℃ for 1 min, and the temperature was increased to 250℃ at 200℃/min, and held for 10 min. Diverter valve program: 0-0.9 min split ratio is 20∶1, 0.9-3.5 min diverter valve is closed, 3.5 min is opened again, and the split ratio is 20∶1.

Ionization method: EI, ionization energy 70 eV; transfer line temperature 270℃; ion source temperature 200℃; solvent delay 7 min.

### 3. 检出限

顺式环氧七氯、反式环氧七氯及异狄氏剂的检出限为 0.1 μg/kg，其余有机氯农药的检出限为 0.014 μg/kg。

### 4. 质量控制

本实验的每一批次样品处理时，均进行了全程空白实验，即在不称样的前提下，按照样品前处理流程进行操作（包括内标的加入等），结果表明，实验所使用的所有耗材、试剂等均未引入OCP。

## 十三、全氟烷基化合物分析方法

### 1. 样品制备

对于水产类、肉类、蛋类、谷类、薯类、豆类、蔬菜类和水果类食品，取 1.00 g（湿重）样品，加入 20 ng/mL 内标工作液（$^{13}$C-PFOA 和 $^{13}$C-PFOS）10 μL，放置离心管中冷冻干燥 24 h，向干燥好的样品里加入 10 mL 50 mmol/L NaOH 甲醇溶液，超声提取 30 min 后，旋转摇床提取 16 h，离心后取出上清液，氮吹至近干（小于 500 μL），加入 8 mL 水（Milli-Q）混合均匀后，离心后取全部上清液至活化过的 WAX 固相萃取柱（6 mL 9% 氨水甲醇、6 mL 甲醇和 6 mL 水依次活化），用 2 mL 2% 甲酸水溶液、2 mL 2% 甲酸甲醇/水（$V/V$=1/1）和 2 mL 甲醇依次淋洗，用 3 mL 9% 氨水甲醇溶液洗脱，洗脱液氮吹至干，用 0.2 mL 甲醇/水溶液（$V/V$=1/1）复溶，离心后取上清液上机测定。

### 3. Limits of Detection

The limits of detection of *cis*-heptachlor epoxide, *trans*-heptachlor epoxide and endrin were 0.1 μg/kg, and the limits of detection of other OCPs were 0.014 μg/kg.

### 4. Quality Control

For each batch of samples in this experiment, a blank experiment was carried out throughout the whole process, that is, without weighing the samples, according to the sample pretreatment process (including the addition of internal standards, etc.), the results showed that all the consumables, reagents, etc, used in the experiment were not introduced into OCPs.

## XIII. Analysis Method of Perfluoroalkyl Substances (PFASs)

### 1. Sample Preparation

1 g wet weight sample (aquatic foods, meats, eggs, cereals, potatoes, legumes, vegetables, and fruits) was spiked with 10 μL 20 ng/mL internal standards ($^{13}$C-PFOA and $^{13}$C-PFOS) and freeze-dried for 24 h in a PP tube. Then the dried sample was extracted with 10 mL 50 mmol/L sodium hydroxide methanol by sonication for 30 min. After 16 h shaking and centrifugation, the supernatant was transferred to a new PP tube and evaporated to a volume of less than 500 μL under nitrogen. 8 mL water (Milli-Q) was added to redissolve the residue for centrifugation. The supernatant was transferred to the WAX SPE column preconditioned by 6 mL 9% NH$_4$OH in methanol, 6 mL methanol and 6 mL water. After loading the sample, the cartridge was washed with 2 mL 2% aqueous formic acid, 2 mL 2% formic acid solution of water/methanol ($V/V$=1/1), and 2 mL methanol. After washing, the target compounds were eluted with 3 mL 9% NH$_4$OH in methanol. The eluant was concentrated to dryness under nitrogen and reconstituted by 0.2 mL water/methanol ($V/V$=1/1). After centrifugation, the supernatant was taken into the injection vial for analysis.

对于乳类食品，取 2 mL 样品置于离心管中，加入 20 ng/mL 内标工作液（$^{13}$C-PFOA 和 $^{13}$C-PFOS）10 μL，并放置 12 h，涡旋混匀后加入 6 mL 乙腈超声提取 30 min 离心后，收集上清液于另 1 支离心管中。残渣中再加入 6 mL 乙腈，重复该提取过程。将合并的提取液氮吹至近干（小于 500 μL），加入 8 mL 水（Milli-Q）混合均匀，离心后取全部上清液至活化过的 WAX 固相萃取柱净化，后续操作过程同上述膳食样品类型相同。

### 2. 仪器测定

选用超高效液相色谱串联三重四级杆质谱对直链和支链 PFOA 和 PFOS 进行分析。

色谱柱选用 ACQUITY UPLC HSS PFP 柱（2.1 mm × 150 mm × 1.8 μm）；流动相 A：甲醇，流动相 B：甲酸铵水溶液（pH=4），梯度淋洗，流速：0.2 mL/min，柱温：40℃，进样量：10 μL。

目标化合物选用电喷雾离子源负离子模式，多反应模式监测，内标法定量；毛细管电压：0.95 kV；离子源温度：120℃；脱溶剂气温度：400℃；脱溶剂气流量：800 L/h；碰撞气流量：0.30 mL/min。

### 3. 检出限

PFOA 和 PFOS 在不同膳食基质中的检出限详见表 1-7。

2 mL dairy products sample was spiked with 10 μL 20 ng/mL internal standards ($^{13}$C-PFOA and $^{13}$C-PFOS) for 12 h in a PP tube. Then the mixture was extracted with 6 mL acetonitrile by sonication for 30 min and the supernatant was transferred to a new PP tube after centrifugation. The solid remaining was extracted one more time by 6 mL of acetonitrile. The combined supernatant was evaporated to a volume of less than 500 μL under nitrogen. 8 mL water (Milli-Q) was added to re-dissolve the residue for centrifugation. The supernatant was transferred to the WAX SPE column for purification. The purification method and follow-up steps were described in details above for the food samples.

### 2. Instrumental Determination

The linear and branched PFOA and PFOS were analyzed by ultra-performance liquid chromatography and tandem mass spectrometry. The separation was finished by a ACQUITY UPLC HSS PFP column (2.1 mm × 150 mm × 1.8 μm) with 10 μL injection. The temperature of the separation column was kept at 40℃. Methanol (A) and ammonium formate (pH=4) (B) were used for the gradient program, with the flow rate of 0.2 mL/min. The target compounds were analyzed in negative mode with ESI source and MRM mode and quantified using internal standards. The capillary was 0.95 kV. The temperature of ion source and desolvation were 120℃ and 400℃ respectively. In addition, the gas flow of desolvation and collision were 800 L/h and 0.30 mL/min respectively.

### 3. Limits of Detection

The LODs of PFOA and PFOS in different categories were shown in Table 1-7.

表 1-7 PFOA 和 PFOS 的检出限
Table 1-7　The LODs of PFOA and PFOS

| 化合物<br>Compounds | 谷类<br>Cereals | 豆类<br>Legumes | 薯类<br>Potatoes | 乳类<br>Dairy products | 肉类<br>Meats | 蛋类<br>Eggs | 水产类<br>Aquatic foods | 蔬菜类<br>Vegetables | 水果类<br>Fruits |
|---|---|---|---|---|---|---|---|---|---|
| 4m-PFOA | 1 | 5 | 1 | 12 | 6.2 | 0.3 | 2 | 6 | 2 |

续表

| 化合物<br>Compounds | 谷类<br>Cereals | 豆类<br>Legumes | 薯类<br>Potatoes | 乳类<br>Dairy products | 肉类<br>Meats | 蛋类<br>Eggs | 水产类<br>Aquatic foods | 蔬菜类<br>Vegetables | 水果类<br>Fruits |
|---|---|---|---|---|---|---|---|---|---|
| 5m-PFOA | 1 | 5 | 1 | 12 | 6.2 | 0.3 | 2 | 6 | 2 |
| iso-PFOA | 1 | 5 | 1 | 12 | 6.2 | 0.3 | 2 | 6 | 2 |
| n-PFOA | 1 | 5 | 1 | 12 | 6.2 | 0.3 | 2 | 6 | 2 |
| 1m-PFOS | 1 | 5 | 2 | 1.5 | 4.3 | 1.5 | 3.3 | 15 | 2 |
| 3m-PFOS | 1 | 5 | 2 | 1.5 | 4.3 | 1.5 | 3.3 | 15 | 2 |
| 4m-PFOS | 1 | 5 | 2 | 1.5 | 4.3 | 1.5 | 3.3 | 15 | 2 |
| 5m-PFOS | 1 | 5 | 2 | 1.5 | 4.3 | 1.5 | 3.3 | 15 | 2 |
| iso-PFOS | 1 | 5 | 2 | 1.5 | 4.3 | 1.5 | 3.3 | 15 | 2 |
| n-PFOS | 1 | 5 | 2 | 1.5 | 4.3 | 1.5 | 3.3 | 15 | 2 |

#### 4. 质量控制

实验过程中所用的试剂均需监测 PFAS 本底水平，选用无 PFAS 本底的试剂进行样品前处理和样品测定。处理每批样品时需要做 4 个空白样品（Milli-Q 超纯水）来监测本底水平，且各 PFAS 在 0.05～10 ng/mL 范围均呈现良好的线性关系（$R^2>0.99$）。本研究采用加标回收实验（回收率满足 80%～120%）和内标定量法来确保分析方法的准确性。另外，实验室自 2013 年起开始参加食品基质中 PFAS 的国际考核比对项目，样品包括鱼肉、鸡蛋、虾肉和西红柿，组织方包括：联合国环境规划署、挪威公共卫生研究所、澳大利亚国家计量研究院和荷兰瓦格宁根大学，考核结果均为满意，Z 评分均小于 2，验证了分析方法的准确性和实验室的分析能力。

### 十四、六溴环十二烷分析方法

采用同位素稀释的超高效液相色谱-串联质谱法（UPLC-MS/MS）对第六次中国总膳食研究膳食样品中 3 种六溴环十二烷（HBCD）同分异构体进行了测定。

#### 4. Quality Control

Various solvents were examined for PFASs background contamination, and solvents without PFASs were used for sample preparation. Four method blank samples were set in the pretreatment process to check the background concentrations. The standard calibration exhibited excellent linearity ($R^2>0.99$) in the range from 0.05 ng/mL to 10 ng/mL for PFASs. Spiked recovery tests (with recoveries between 80%-120%) and quantification by internal standard were used to ensure the accuracy of the method. In addition, the accuracy of our method and the analyzing capability of our laboratory were verified by participating in global inter-laboratory comparison organized by United Nations Environment Programme, Norwegian Institute of Public Health, National Measurement Institute of Australia, and Wageningen University of Netherlands from 2013. Sample categories of inter-laboratory comparison included fish, eggs, prawns and tomatoes. The Z-score of our method was lower than 2, and the results were all satisfactory.

### XIV. Analysis Method of Hexabromocyclododecane

In the 6$^{th}$ China total diet study (TDS), concentrations of hexabromocyclododecane (HBCD) in TDS samples

## 1. 样品制备

各样品依据脂肪含量称取适量，水产类取约 15 g，肉类取约 5 g，蛋类取约 10 g，奶类取约 30 g，使各样品中脂肪量控制在约 1 g。于冷冻干燥机中冻干 48 h。冻干后的样品经研钵研磨成粉末并与适量硅藻土混匀后装入加速溶剂萃取仪萃取池，随后加入内标溶液（$^{13}$C-α-HBCD、β-HBCD、γ-HBCD）。以正己烷：丙酮（1∶1，V/V）为提取溶剂进行样品提取。加速溶剂萃取仪参考条件为：温度，110℃；压力，10.3 MPa（1500 psi）；循环，3 次。提取液旋转蒸发至近干，并用 10 mL 正己烷复溶，随后上样至自制串联酸化硅胶柱 [由两根独立的玻璃柱组成，每根玻璃柱自下到上填充脱脂棉、5 g 无水硫酸钠、20 g 酸化硅胶（44%，m/m）和 5 g 无水硫酸钠] 净化，先后以 100 mL 正己烷和 150 mL 正己烷：二氯甲烷（1∶1，V/V）洗脱目标物，洗脱液旋转蒸发至干，再复溶于 100 μL 甲醇中待仪器分析。

## 2. 仪器测定

所使用仪器为高效液相色谱-串联质谱仪（UPLC-MS/MS，ACQUITY™-Micromass Xevo TQS，美国 Waters 公司）。

色谱条件：Waters BEH C18 色谱柱（2.1 mm × 50 mm × 1.7 μm），流动相为水（A）-甲醇/乙腈（1∶1，V/V）（B），梯度洗脱，洗脱程序为：起始 10% B 并保持 1 min，3 min 内线性提升至 80% B 并保持 5 min，随后直接调整至 100% B，保持 3 min 后直接返回起始比例。流速为 0.30 mL/min，柱温为 40℃，进样量为 10 μL。

were measured by ultrahigh performance liquid chromatography-tandem mass spectrometry (UPLC-MS/MS).

## 1. Sample Preparation

An appropriate amount of sample with lipid content of approximately 1 g (15 g for aquatic products, 5 g for meats, 10 g for eggs, and 30 g for dairy products) was freeze-dried for 48 hours by a lyophilizer. The lyophilized sample was then ground and transferred to extraction cell of the accelerated solvent extractor (ASE), spiked with $^{13}$C-labeled internal standards ($^{13}$C12-α-, β-, and γ- HBCD) and mixed with diatomite. The mixture was then extracted by a mixture of *n*-hexane：acetone (1∶1, V/V) using ASE. For parameters of the ASE, the extraction temperature was set at 110℃ with a pressure of 10.3 MPa (1500 psi), and three extract cycles were performed. The extract was concentrated to dryness by a rotary evaporator and reconstituted in 10 mL of *n*-hexane. Then, the extract was loaded on a cleanup apparatus which was composed of two self-made acidic silica gel columns. The two columns were both packed with an appropriate amount of absorbent cotton, 5 g of Na$_2$SO$_4$, 20 g of acidic silica gel (44%), and 5 g of Na$_2$SO$_4$ (from bottom to top). After loading the extract, 100 mL of *n*-hexane and 150 mL of *n*-hexane：dichloromethane (1∶1, V/V) were successively loaded to elute all target compounds from the tandem columns. All eluent was combined and evaporated to dryness. The residue was reconstituted in 100 μL of methanol for instrumental analysis.

## 2. Instrumental Determination

Analyte quantification was performed on an UPLC-MS/MS (ACQUITY™-Micromass Xevo TQS, Waters Corporation).

LC conditions: A Waters BEH C18 column (2.1 mm × 50 mm × 1.7 μm) was used with water (A) and methanol/acetonitrile (1∶1, V/V) (B) as mobile phase. The injection volume, mobile phase flow rate and column temperature were set at 10 μL, 0.3 mL/min and

质谱条件：离子源为电喷雾电离（ESI）；扫描方式为负离子扫描；监测模式为多反应监测（MRM）；毛细管电压 3 kV，脱溶剂气温度 350℃，脱溶剂气流量 800 L/h，锥孔气流量 150 L/h。

**3. 检出限**

HBCD 三种异构体的检出限为 2~6 pg/g。

**4. 质量控制**

（1）空白实验

测定每批次食品样时均同时进行一个空白样的前处理与测定，以检测样本分析过程中可能存在的杂质干扰和背景污染。结果表明空白样中均未检出被测物。

（2）回收实验

以巴沙鱼、鸡胸肉、鸡蛋和牛奶作为代表性基质，加标水平为 0.5 ng/g 和 5 ng/g，HBCD 回收率为 80%~120%。

（3）国际考核

采用本方法参加挪威公共卫生研究所组织的国际比对考核，$Z$ 值评分均在 2.0 以下。

40℃, respectively. The gradient elution was applied, and the elution program was as follows: the mobile phase program was as follows: started with 10% B and hold for 1 min, and changed linearly to 80% B in 3 min and maintained for 5 min, and then directly increased to 100% B and hold for 3 min, and returned to the initial conditions (10% B).

MS conditions: The MS was operated in the electrospray ionization (ESI) negative ion mode with a desolvation temperature of 350℃. The desolvation gas and cone gas were set at a flow rate of 800 L/h and 150 L/h, respectively. The capillary voltage was set at 3 kV. Analyte quantification was performed in multiple reaction monitoring (MRM) mode.

**3. Limits of Detection**

The LODs of the three HBCD isomers ranged from 2 pg/g to 6 pg/g.

**4. Quality Control**

(1) Blank Test

A procedural blank sample was pretreated and tested along with every batch of food samples to monitor the possible interference or background contamination during sample analysis. No analytes were detected in the procedural blanks.

(2) Recovery Test

The recovery test was performed using basa fish, chicken breast, chicken eggs, and cow milk as matrix with two spiking levels (0.5 ng/g and 5 ng/g). Recoveries of all analytes in four matrix ranged from 80% to 120%.

(3) Global Inter-calibration

The laboratory performance was validated by participating in an interlaboratory comparison study organized by the Norwegian Institute of Public Health (NIPH). Data from our laboratory were usually within the acceptable range of the consensus values ($Z$<2.0).

## 十五、氯化石蜡分析方法

采用全二维气相色谱-串联质谱技术，测定膳食样品中短链氯化石蜡（SCCP）和中链氯化石蜡（MCCP）的含量，内标法定量。

### 1. 样品制备

准确称量膳食样品（精确到0.01 g），于冷冻干燥仪中干燥处理至恒重，并称量干燥后的干重，据此得出样品的含水量。称取约4.00 g干燥膳食样品，加入2.5 ng的$^{13}C_{10}$-反式氯丹，然后用二氯甲烷和正己烷的混合溶液（1∶1，V/V）进行加速溶剂提取。

将提取液旋转蒸发浓缩，通过重量法测定样品脂重。进一步使用凝胶渗透色谱及多层复合硅胶柱（从下至上依次填充3.00 g弗罗里硅土、2.00 g活化硅胶、5.00 g酸性硅胶和4.00 g无水硫酸钠）依次对样品进行净化。净化后样品经过减压旋转蒸发仪、氮吹仪依次浓缩，加入2.5 ng的进样标ε-六氯环己烷（ε-HCH），使用环己烷定容至50 μL，振荡混匀，进行仪器分析。

### 2. 仪器测定

所使用仪器为全二维气相色谱串联电子捕获负化学电离源质谱仪（GC×GC-ECNI-MS）（美国 Agilent Technologies 公司）环形热调制器 ZX2004（美国 Zoex 公司）。色谱条件：色谱柱为DB-5MS（30 m × 0.25 mm × 0.25 μm）+ BPX-50（1 m × 0.1 mm × 0.1 μm）；进样口温度为280℃；进样模式为不分流进样，恒流模式；进样体积为1 μL；传输线温度为280℃；柱温为起始60℃，以10℃/min升至180℃，再以1.5℃/min升至310℃并保持5 min；调制周期为7 s；载气为高纯氦气（＞99.999%），0.8 mL/min。

## XV. Analysis Method of Chlorinated Paraffins

The concentrations of SCCP and MCCP in the dietary samples were determined by two-dimensional gas chromatography-tandem mass spectrometry. The internal standard quantification method was used.

### 1. Sample Preparation

Before analysis, the sample were weighed and freeze-dried to constant weight. The dry weight after drying was weighed accurately and the water content of the sample was obtained. About 4.00 g of dried dietary samples were weighed and 2.5 ng of $^{13}C_{10}$-*trans*-chlordane as was added, then the sample were extracted with accelerated solvent extraction with a mixture of dichloromethane and *n*-hexane (1∶1, *V/V*).

The extracts were concentrated by rotary evaporation and the lipid weight of the sample was determined by gravimetric method. Then the samples were purified by elution through a gel permeation chromatography column and a multilayer silica gel column (from bottom to top with 3.00 g Florian silica, 2.00 g activated silica gel, 5.00 g acidic silica gel, and 4.00 g anhydrous sodium sulfate). After purification, the extracts were concentrated by a vacuum rotary evaporator, and then concentrated under a gentle stream of high-purity nitrogen. The concentrated extracts were spiked with 2.5 ng of ε-HCH adjusted to approximately 50 μL using cyclohexane before analysis.

### 2. Instrumental Determination

The SCCP and MCCP concentrations in the samples were analyzed by a two-dimensional gas chromatograph coupled with an electron-capture negative-ionization mass spectrometer (Agilent Technologies, USA) equipped with a ZX2004 loop cryogenic modulator (Zoex, USA). The parameter of chromatography were as follows. For two-dimensional gas chromatograph, the first-dimension column was a DB-5MS column (30 m long, 0.25 mm i.d., 0.25 μm film thickness) and the second-dimension column was a BPX-50 column (1 m

质谱条件：电离模式为电子捕获负化学电离源（ECNI）；反应气为甲烷（$CH_4$）；分辨率≥5000；离子源温度为200℃；离子监测模式为选择离子监测。

### 3. 检出限

将采集的膳食样品经过 ASE 提取多次，保证其中的 SCCP 和 MCCP 低于仪器检出限后作为空白样品。取 5 g 空白样品，加入 1 μg SCCP（氯含量为55.5%）、1 μg MCCP（氯含量为52%）和 2.5 ng $^{13}C_{10}$-反式氯丹，按前处理步骤进行提取净化后上机检测。以空白样品中化合物的平均浓度加上三倍相对标准偏差定义为膳食中 SCCP 和 MCCP 的方法检出限（MDL），SCCP 和 MCCP 的 MDL 分别为 3.2 ng/g 和 3.5 ng/g。

### 4. 质量控制

在实验之前，所有玻璃器皿依次用超纯水、甲醇、丙酮和二氯甲烷淋洗三遍。每 10 个样本加一个程序空白样品来监控背景污染。结果表明，空白样品中 SCCP 和 MCCP 含量均小于实际样品浓度的 10%。净化内标 $^{13}C_{10}$-反式氯丹的回收率基于进样内标 ε-HCH 进行计算，平均回收率为 70%～95%。每 10 个样本随机选择一个进行平行实验，相对标准偏差小于 15%。

long, 0.1 mm i.d., 0.1 μm film thickness). The injection mode is non-split injection and constant flow mode. A 1 μL aliquot of an extract was injected in splitless mode. The transfer line temperature was 280℃, The gas chromatograph oven program started at 60℃, increased at 10℃/min to 180℃, and then increased at 1.5℃/min to 310℃, which was held for 5 min. The modulation period is 7 s. High purity helium (>99.999%) was used as carrier gas with a flow rate 0.8 mL/min. The parameters of mass spectrometry were as follows. Electron capture negative chemical ionization source (ECNI) was used and the reaction gas is methane ($CH_4$). The resolution of mass spectrometry were higher than 5000. The ion source temperature were set as 200℃. The SCCPs and MCCPs were analyzed by selective ion monitoring mode.

### 3. Limits of Detection

The dietary samples were extracted by ASE for several times to ensure that the concentrations of SCCP and MCCP in the extracted samples were below the instrumental detection limit. The extracted sample were used as blank sample and 5 g blank sample were weighed. 1 μg SCCPs (chlorine content 55.5%), 1 μg MCCPs (chlorine content 52%) and 2.5 ng $^{13}C_{10}$-*trans*-chlordane were added and then sample were prepared as the real sample. The method limit of detection (MDL) of SCCPs and MCCPs was calculated by the mean concentration of compounds in the blank sample plus three times relative standard deviation (RSD). The MDL of SCCPs and MCCPs were 3.2 ng/g and 3.5 ng/g, respectively.

### 4. Quality Control

In order to eliminate the possible background contamination, all glassware was rinsed with ultrapure water, methanol, acetone and dichloromethane three times before use. One system blank sample was added to every ten samples. The results showed that SCCP and MCCP concentration of blank sample were lower than ten percent of those of dietary samples. The mean recoveries were 70%-95% which were calculated by

## 十六、真菌毒素分析方法

第六次中国总膳食研究对膳食样品进行了43种真菌毒素的测定,采用了同位素稀释的超高效液相色谱-串联质谱法(UPLC-MS/MS)。其中,21种真菌毒素采用目标化合物相应的同位素内标进行定量,其他22种真菌毒素则采用参考同位素内标进行定量(Qiu et al.,2022)。

### 1. 伏马菌素(FB1、FB2、FB3)与赭曲霉毒素(OTA、OTB)的分析

(1)样品制备

准确称取膳食样品2 g(水及饮料类移取2 mL)于40 mL的离心管中,加入同位素内标($^{13}$C-FB1、$^{13}$C-FB2、$^{13}$C-FB3、$^{13}$C-OTA)后,以10 mL乙腈/水溶液($V/V$=50/50)提取,室温下振摇1h后,9000 r/min下离心10 min。准确吸取上层清液5 mL,用NaOH溶液(0.1 mol/L)调pH至6~9,与10 mL甲醇-水溶液($V/V$=75/25)混合。

准确吸取上层清液5 mL,过MultiSep 211 Fum固相萃取柱,用10 mL甲醇/水溶液($V/V$=75/25)淋洗,用10 mL含1%甲酸的甲醇溶液洗脱,洗脱液在40℃下用氮气吹干,用1 mL乙腈和含0.2%的甲酸水溶液($V/V$=20/80)定容,涡旋30 s后,在20 000 r/min下离心30 min,取上清液进样测定。

the ratio of the cleanup standard ($^{13}$C$_{10}$-*trans*-chlordane) to the internal standard (ε-hexachlorocyclohexane) in samples. One sample was randomly selected for parallel experiments from every ten samples, and the relative standard deviation of parallel samples was less than 15%.

## XVI. Analysis Method of Mycotoxins

All the 43 mycotoxins were analyzed using UPLC-MS/MS with isotope internal standard dilution (Qiu et al., 2022). Twenty one mycotoxins were determined using their own isotope internal standards, and the other 22 mycotoxins were determined using the corresponding reference isotope internal standards.

### 1. Analysis of Fumonisins (FB1, FB2, FB3) and Ochratoxins (OTA, OTB) in Samples

(1) Sample Preparation

A food sample of exactly 2 g (2 mL water and beverages) in a 40 mL centrifuge tube was added to isotope internal standards ($^{13}$C-FB1, $^{13}$C-FB2, $^{13}$C-FB3, $^{13}$C-OTA) and soaked with 10 mL acetonitrile/water solution ($V/V$=50/50) for one hour before being homogenized with a high-speed homogenizer for 5 min and centrifugated at 9000 r/min for 10 min. Exactly 5 mL of the supernatant was drawn and adjusted with a NaOH solution (0.1 mol/L) to a pH value of 6-9 before being mixed with 10 mL methanol/water solution ($V/V$=75/25).

Exactly 5 mL of the supernatant was filtered through a MultiSep 211 Fum solid phase extraction column and washed with a 10 mL methanol/water solution ($V/V$=75/25) and eluted with 10 mL methanol containing 1% formic acid. The eluent was nitrogen-dried at 40℃ and diluted with 1 mL of acetonitrile/water containing 0.2% formic acid ($V/V$=20/80). After vortex mixing for 30 s, the solution was centrifuged at 20 000 r/min for 30 min prior to analysis.

（2）仪器测定

使用 Exion LC AD™ System 超高效液相色谱-串联 QTRAP® AB SCIEX 6500+三重四极杆质谱（美国 SCIEX 公司）；色谱柱：Waters CORTECS™ UPLC® C18柱（2.1 mm × 100 mm，1.6 μm）。流动相A：0.2%的甲酸水溶液；流动相B：乙腈。总运行时间 10 min；柱温：50℃；进样体积：5 μL。

质谱条件：采用正离子模式（ESI+）；检测模式：多反应监测（MRM）。具体参数如下：喷撞气（CAD）：9 psi；气帘气（CUR）：25 psi；喷雾气（GS1）：55 psi；辅助加热气（GS2）：65 psi；离子化电压（IS）：5500 V；温度（TEM）：550℃。

**2. 26 种真菌毒素的分析**

测定的 26 种真菌毒素包括 NEO、AFM2、AFM1、AFG2、AFG1、AFB2、AFB1、DAS、HT2、T2、SMC、MON、DON、NIV、3-ADON、15-ADON、Fus X、ZEN、ZAN、α-ZOL、β-ZOL、α-ZAL、β-ZAL、PAT、Deepoxy-DON、3-Glu-DON 等。

（1）样品制备

准确称取膳食样品 2 g（水及饮料类 2 mL）于 50 mL 的离心管中，分别加入 40 μL $^{13}$C-AFB1、$^{13}$C-AFB2、$^{13}$C-AFG1、$^{13}$C-AFG2、$^{13}$C-AFM1、$^{13}$C-T2、$^{13}$C-HT2、$^{13}$C-ZON、$^{13}$C-DON、$^{13}$C-NIV、$^{13}$C-3-ADON、$^{13}$C-PAT、$^{13}$C-SMC 和 $^{13}$C-DAS 同位素内标后，再加入 9 mL 乙腈/水（V/V=84/16）溶液，室温下浸泡 0.5 h，超声波超声 0.5 h，9000 r/min 下离心 10 min。取上清液，待净化。

准确吸取上层清液 5 mL，过 MycoSep 226 净化柱，用 3 mL 乙腈洗脱净化柱，抽干后合并洗脱液于 10 mL 试管中，用氮气在 40℃下吹干。复溶于 1mL 乙腈/0.2% 甲酸水溶液（V/V=10/90）中。

(2) Instrumental Determination

UPLC-MS/MS analysis was performed on an Exion LC AD™ System (SCIEX, USA) coupled with a Triple Quad 6500+ mass spectrometer (SCIEX, USA); CORTECS™ UPLC® C18 Column (2.1 mm × 100 mm, 1.6 μm, Waters). Mobile phase A: 0.2% formic acid solution; mobile phase B: acetonitrile. Taking a total of 10 min, column temperature: 50℃; injection volume: 5 μL.

Mass spectrometry parameters: ESI+; detection model: multiple reaction monitoring (MRM). CAD: 9 psi; curtain gas: 25 psi; sheath gas: 55 psi; drying gas: 65 psi; ion spray voltage: 5500 V; source temperature: 550℃.

**2. Analysis of 26 Mycotoxins in Samples**

The 26 mycotoxins include NEO, AFM2, AFM1, AFG2, AFG1, AFB2, AFB1, DAS, HT2, T2, SMC, MON, DON, NIV, 3-ADON, 15-ADON, Fus X, ZEN, ZAN, α-ZOL, β-ZOL, α-ZAL, β-ZAL, PAT, Deepoxy-DON, 3-Glu-DON, etc.

(1) Sample Preparation

A food sample of 2 g (2 mL water and beverages) in a 40 mL centrifuge tube was added to isotope internal standards ($^{13}$C-AFB1, $^{13}$C-AFB2, $^{13}$C-AFG1, $^{13}$C-AFG2, $^{13}$C-AFM1, $^{13}$C-T2, $^{13}$C-HT2, $^{13}$C-ZON, $^{13}$C-DON, $^{13}$C-NIV, $^{13}$C-3-ADON, $^{13}$C-PAT, $^{13}$C-SMC and $^3$C-DAS) and 9 mL acetonitrile/water solution (V/V=84/16), soaked for 0.5 h at room temperature, ultrasonized for 0.5 h, and centrifuged at 9000 r/min for 10 min. The supernatant was obtained for purification.

Exactly 5 mL of the supernatant was drawn and filtered through a MycoSep 226 purification column. The purification column was washed with 3 mL methanol. The eluents were combined and put into a 10 mL test tube and nitrogen-dried at 40℃. Added to 800 μL acetonitrile/0.2% formic acid solution (V/V= 10/90). The mixture was vortexed for 30 s and then centrifuged at 20 000 r/min for 30 min prior to analysis.

混合液涡旋 30 s 后，20 000 r/min 下离心 30 min，取上清液进样测定。

（2）仪器测定

色谱柱：Waters CORTECS™ UPLC® C18 柱（2.1 mm × 100 mm, 1.6 μm）。流动相 A：水；流动相 B：甲醇/乙腈（1∶1, *V/V*）溶液。总用时 32 min；柱温：50℃；进样体积：5 μL。

质谱条件：采用正离子模式（ESI+）和负离子模式（ESI–）；检测模式：多反应监测（MRM）。具体参数如下：喷撞气（CAD）：9；气帘气（CUR）：20 psi；喷雾气（GS1）：50 psi；辅助加热气（GS2）：40 psi；离子化电压（IS）：–4500 V 和 +5500 V；温度（TEM）：550℃。

## 3. 12 种新兴真菌毒素的分析

测定的 12 种新兴真菌毒素包括 AOH、ALT、AME、TeA、TEN、BEA、ENNA1、ENNA、ENNB、ENNB1、CIT、CPA。

（1）样品制备

准确称取膳食样品 2 g（水及饮料类 2 mL）于 50 mL 离心管中，加入 40 μL 同位素混标（$^{13}$C-TeA 和 TEN-d3 与 $^{13}$C-AFB2），涡旋 30 s 混匀，加入 9 mL 样品提取液（乙腈/甲醇/水=45∶10∶45, *V/V/V*, pH 3.0 NaH$_2$PO$_4$），室温下振荡提取 30 min，再超声提取 30 min，冷却至室温，于 9000 r/min 低温（4℃）离心 10 min，准确移取 5.0 mL 上清液于另一 50mL 离心管中，加入 15 mL 0.05 mol/L 磷酸二氢钠溶液（pH 3.0），涡旋 30 s 混匀，待净化。

使用 HLB 固相萃取柱进行样品净化处理。依次用 5 mL 甲醇和 5 mL 乙腈洗脱，抽干柱子，合并洗脱液于小试管中，于 45℃ 水浴中氮吹至近干，复溶于 1 mL 乙腈/水溶液（10∶90, *V/V*）中，混合涡旋 30s，于 20 000 r/min 低温（4℃）离心 30 min，取上清液进样

(2) Instrumental Determination

Waters CORTECS™ UPLC® C18 Column (2.1 mm × 100 mm, 1.6 μm). Mobile phase A: Water; mobile phase B: methanol/acetonitrile (1∶1, *V/V*). The whole process taking a total of 32 min, column temperature: 50℃; sample volume: 5 μL.

Mass spectrometry parameters: ESI+ and ESI–; detection model: multiple reaction monitoring (MRM). CAD: 9; curtain gas: 20 psi; sheath gas: 50 psi; drying gas: 40 psi; ion spray voltage: –4500 V and +5500 V; source temperature: 550℃.

## 3. Analysis of 12 Emerging Mycotoxins in Samples

The 12 emerging mycotoxins include AOH, AME, TeA, ALT, TEN, BEA, ENNA1, ENNA, ENNB1, ENNB, CIT, and CPA.

(1) Sample Preparation

Food samples of 2 g (2 mL of water and beverages) in a 50 mL centrifuge tube were added to 40 μL of mixed isotope internal standard ($^{13}$C-TeA, TEN-d3, and $^{13}$C-AFB2) and 9 mL of extraction solution (acetonitrile/methanol/water, 45∶10∶45, *V/V/V*, pH 3.0 NaH$_2$PO$_4$), incubated for 0.5 h at room temperature, ultrasonized for 0.5 h, and centrifuged at 9000 r/min for 10 min. Then, 5 mL of the resulting supernatant was added to 15 mL of 0.05 mol/L phosphate buffer (pH 3.0). After vortexing for 30 s, the supernatant was obtained for purification.

Used the HLB SPE column for sample purification treatment. Washed with 5 mL of methanol and 5 mL of acetonitrile in sequence, drained the column, and combined the eluents in a small test tube. The eluate was nitrogen-dried at 45℃, and reconstituted in 1 mL of acetonitrile/water (10∶90, *V/V*). The mixture was vortexed for 30 s and then centrifuged at low temperature (4℃) at 20 000 r/min for 30 min. The supernatant was obtained for analysis.

测定。

（2）仪器测定

色谱柱：Waters CORTECS™ UPLC® C18 柱（2.1 mm×100 mm，1.6 μm）。流动相 A：0.01% 氨水+5 mmol/L 乙酸铵水溶液；流动相 B：乙腈。总用时 10 min；柱温 50℃；进样量 5 μL。

质谱条件：采用正离子模式（ESI+）和负离子模式（ESI–）；检测模式：多反应监测（MRM）。具体参数如下：喷撞气（CAD）：10；气帘气（CUR）：20 psi；喷雾气（GS1）：60 psi；辅助加热气（GS2）：55 psi；离子化电压（IS）：–4500 V 和+5500 V；温度（TEM）：450℃。

4. 检出限

43 种毒素的定量内标和检出限见表 1-8。

(2) Instrumental Determination

CORTECS™ UPLC® C18 Column (2.1 mm × 100 mm, 1.6 μm, Waters). Mobile phase A: 0.01% aqueous ammonia with 5 mmol/L ammonium acetate; mobile phase B: acetonitrile. The whole process taking a total of 10 min. column temperature: 50℃; sample volume: 5 μL.

Mass spectrometry parameters: ESI+ and ESI–; detection model: multiple reaction monitoring (MRM). CAD: 10; curtain gas: 20 psi; sheath gas: 60 psi; drying gas: 55 psi; ion spray voltage: –4500 V and +5500 V; source temperature: 450℃.

4. Limits of Detection

The quantitative internal standards and limits of detection of 43 mycotoxins are shown in Table 1-8.

表 1-8　43 种真菌毒素的定量内标和检出限（单位：μg/kg）

Table 1-8　Quantitative internal standards and limits of detection of 43 mycotoxins (Unit: μg/kg)

| 真菌毒素 | Mycotoxins | 定量内标<br>Quantitative internal standard | 检出限<br>Limits of detection |
|---|---|---|---|
| 新茄病镰刀菌烯醇 | NEO | $^{13}$C-DAS | 0.02 |
| 黄曲霉毒素 M2 | AFM2 | $^{13}$C-AFM1 | 0.004 |
| 黄曲霉毒素 M1 | AFM1 | $^{13}$C-AFM1 | 0.004 |
| 黄曲霉毒素 G2 | AFG2 | $^{13}$C-AFG2 | 0.004 |
| 黄曲霉毒素 G1 | AFG1 | $^{13}$C-AFG1 | 0.004 |
| 黄曲霉毒素 B2 | AFB2 | $^{13}$C-AFB2 | 0.002 |
| 黄曲霉毒素 B1 | AFB1 | $^{13}$C-AFB1 | 0.002 |
| 二乙酰镳草镰刀菌烯醇 | DAS | $^{13}$C-DAS | 0.04 |
| 桔青霉素 | CIT | $^{13}$C-CIT | 0.04 |
| HT-2 毒素 | HT2 | $^{13}$C-HT2 | 0.08 |
| T-2 毒素 | T2 | $^{13}$C-T2 | 0.04 |
| 杂色曲霉毒素 | SMC | $^{13}$C-SMC | 0.002 |
| 赭曲霉毒素 A | OTA | $^{13}$C-OTA | 0.004 |
| 赭曲霉毒素 B | OTB | $^{13}$C-OTA | 0.004 |
| 环匹阿尼酸 | CPA | $^{13}$C-SMC | 0.02 |
| 串珠镰刀菌素 | MON | $^{13}$C-AFB1 | 0.8 |
| 脱氧雪腐镰刀菌烯醇 | DON | $^{13}$C-DON | 0.2 |

续表

| 真菌毒素 | Mycotoxins | 定量内标<br>Quantitative internal standard | 检出限<br>Limits of detection |
|---|---|---|---|
| 雪腐镰刀菌烯醇 | NIV | $^{13}$C-NIV | 0.1 |
| 3-乙酰脱氧雪腐镰刀菌烯醇 | 3-Ac-DON | $^{113}$C-3-ADON | 0.2 |
| 15-乙酰脱氧雪腐镰刀菌烯醇 | 15-Ac-DON | $^{13}$C-3-ADON | 0.1 |
| 镰刀菌烯酮 | Fus X | $^{13}$C-NIV | 0.2 |
| 玉米赤霉烯酮 | ZEN | $^{13}$C-ZEN | 0.02 |
| 玉米赤霉酮 | ZAN | $^{13}$C-ZEN | 0.02 |
| α-玉米赤霉烯醇 | α-ZOL | $^{13}$C-ZEN | 0.01 |
| β-玉米赤霉烯醇 | β-ZOL | $^{13}$C-ZEN | 0.04 |
| α-玉米赤霉醇 | α-ZAL | $^{13}$C-ZEN | 0.02 |
| β-玉米赤霉醇 | β-ZAL | $^{13}$C-ZEN | 0.01 |
| 展青霉素 | PAT | $^{13}$C-PAT | 1 |
| 去环氧-脱氧雪腐镰刀菌烯醇 | Deepoxy-DON | $^{13}$C-DON | 0.2 |
| 3-葡萄糖-脱氧雪腐镰刀菌烯醇 | 3-Glu-DON | $^{13}$C-DON | 0.1 |
| 伏马菌素 B1 | FB1 | $^{13}$C-FB1 | 0.01 |
| 伏马菌素 B2 | FB2 | $^{13}$C-FB2 | 0.02 |
| 伏马菌素 B3 | FB3 | $^{13}$C-FB3 | 0.02 |
| 交链孢酚甲基醚 | AME | $^{13}$C-AFB2 | 0.02 |
| 细交链孢菌酮酸 | TeA | $^{13}$C-TeA | 0.2 |
| 腾毒素 | TEN | TEN-d3 | 0.05 |
| 链格孢酚 | AOH | $^{13}$C-TeA | 0.2 |
| 交链孢烯 | ALT | $^{13}$C-AFB2 | 0.2 |
| 白僵菌素 | BEA | $^{13}$C-TeA | 0.02 |
| 恩镰孢菌素 A | ENNA | $^{13}$C-TeA | 0.02 |
| 恩镰孢菌素 A1 | ENNA1 | $^{13}$C-TeA | 0.02 |
| 恩镰孢菌素 B | ENNB | $^{13}$C-TeA | 0.004 |
| 恩镰孢菌素 B1 | ENNB1 | $^{13}$C-TeA | 0.02 |

### 5. 质量控制

伏马菌素和赭曲霉毒素组以小麦粉BRM003018-M14072F（美国Biopure公司）为标准参考物质，多毒素组以玉米粉BRM003028-M13243A（美国Biopure公司）为标准参考物质，进行质量控制，多次测定结果均在参考值所给出的范围内。目前，暂未获得交链孢毒素和新兴镰刀菌毒素的标准参考物质，为

### 5. Quality Control

For the fumonisins and ochratoxins group, wheat flour BRM003018-M14072F (Biopure, USA) was used as the standard reference material. For multi-mycotoxin group, corn flour BRM003028-M13243A (Biopure, USA) was used as the standard reference material for quality control. Applying the methods mentioned above, the results of multiple determinations were all within the indicated reference range.

确保实验结果的准确性，每批样品的测定过程中加入空白加标样品作为质量控制样品。每批样品中选择一个无目标化合物检出的膳食样品，进行加标回收实验。回收率为80%～130%，说明实验结果准确、可靠。

## 十七、高氯酸盐分析方法

采用液相色谱-轨道阱高分辨质谱法测定膳食样品中的高氯酸盐，内标法定量。

### 1. 样品制备

1）谷类、豆类、薯类、肉类、蛋类、水产类、乳类、蔬菜类、水果类、糖类、水及饮料类样品制备：称取5.0 g（精确至0.01 g）样品于50 mL离心管中，加20 μL同位素内标液（1.0 mg/L），涡旋混匀，静置30 min；依据样品含水量，适量加入5～10 mL水，涡旋混匀后，加入10 mL乙腈，超声提取15 min。室温下8000 r/min离心5 min，取乙腈上清液2 mL于5 mL离心管中，置−20℃冰箱冷冻处理1 h；取上清液13 000 r/min高速离心5 min，收集离心液于进样瓶中待分析。

2）酒类样品制备：称取5.0 g（精确至0.01 g）样品于50 mL离心管中，置水浴锅80℃加热2 h，挥发酒精，放冷后用水定容至10.0 mL，加20 μL同位素内标液（1.0 mg/L），涡旋混匀，静置30 min，加入10 mL乙腈，超声提取15 min。室温下8000 r/min离心5 min，取稀释液2 mL于5 mL离心管中，置−20℃冰箱冷冻处理1 h；取上清液13 000 r/min高速离心5 min，收集离心液于进样瓶中待分析。

At present, the standard reference materials for *Alternaria* mycotoxins and emerging *Fusarium* mycotoxins are not commercially available. To ensure the accuracy of our analysis, blank spiked samples were prepared as quality control samples used in each batch of analysis. We also selected an analytes negative real sample to spiked recovery tests. The recoveries of all the analytes were within 80%-130%, indicating our methods were accurate and reliable.

## XVII. Analysis Method of Perchlorate

Liquid chromatography-Q-orbitrap high resolution mass spectrometry was used for the determination of perchlorate in dietary samples. The quantification of perchlorate was used for internal standard method.

### 1. Sample Preparation

1) For cereals, legumes, potatoes, meats, eggs, aquatic products, dairy products, vegetables, fruits, sugar, water and beverages, accurately weigh 5.0 g (accurate to 0.01 g) of homogenized sample in a 50 mL centrifuge tube, add 20 μL of internal standard solution (1.0 mg/L), vortex to mix, stand for 30 min, add 5-10 mL of water according to the water content of the sample, then vortex. Add 10 mL of acetonitrile and ultrasonic extraction for 15 min. Centrifuge at 8000 r/min for 5 min at room temperature, take 2 mL of acetonitrile supernatant, put it into a 5 mL centrifuge tube, and freeze at −20℃ for 1 hour to induce phase separation. The supernatant was centrifuged at 13 000 r/min for 5 min, and then was collected in the injection vial for analysis.

2) For alcohol beverages, accurately weigh 5.0 g (accurate to 0.01 g) of homogenized sample in a 50 mL centrifuge tube, and heat it in a water bath at 80℃ for 2 hours to volatilize the alcohol. After the cooling, add water to make the volume to 10.0 mL, and add 20 μL of internal standard solution (1.0 mg/L), stand for 30 min. Add 10 mL of acetonitrile and ultrasonic extraction for 15 min, centrifuge at 8000 r/min for 5 min at room

## 2. 仪器测定

所使用仪器为液相色谱-轨道阱高分辨质谱仪（Dionex U3000-Q-Exactive HRMS）。

色谱条件：色谱柱为 Infinitylab Poroshell 120 PFP 色谱柱（1.9 μm，2.1 mm × 50 mm），流动相：A 为 1% 乙酸水溶液，B 为甲醇，梯度洗脱；流速：600 μL/min；柱温：40℃；进样量：2 μL。

质谱参数：加热负电喷雾离子源（HESI⁻）；检测方式：靶向单一离子监测模式（tSIM）；喷雾电压为 3.0 kV；毛细管温度为 320℃；加热温度为 400℃；鞘气流速为 40 arb；辅助气流速为 10 arb；分辨率：70 000 FWHM；母离子（$m/z$）：$^{16}O_4$ 高氯酸根 98.947 90，$^{18}O_4$ 高氯酸根 106.964 80。

## 3. 检出限

本方法 12 类膳食样品的检出限均为 0.2 μg/kg。

## 4. 质量控制

（1）空白实验

为了评估前处理过程中是否可能引入高氯酸盐，造成假阳性结果。本次实验的每一批次样品处理中，均进行了全程空白实验，即在无基质的前提下，按照样品前处理流程进行操作（包括内标的加入等），结果表明，实验所使用的所有耗材、试剂等均未引入高氯酸盐。

temperature, take 2 mL of acetonitrile supernatant, put it into a 5 mL centrifuge tube, and freeze at −20℃ for 1 hour to induce phase separation. The supernatant was centrifuged at 13 000 r/min for 5 min, and then was collected in the injection vial for analysis.

## 2. Instrument Determination

Liquid chromatography-Q-orbitrap high resolution mass spectrometry (Dionex U3000-Q-Exactive HRMS) was used for the determination of perchlorate. Chromatography conditions: the chromatographic column is Infinitylab Poroshell 120 PFP (1.9 μm, 2.1 mm × 50 mm); mobile phase: A is 1% acetic acid aqueous solution, B is methanol, gradient elution; flow rate: 600 μL/min; column temperature: 40℃; injection volume: 2 μL. Mass spectrometry parameters: heated negative electrospray ion scanning (HESI⁻); scan mode, target single ion monitoring (tSIM); spray voltage, 3.0 kV; capillary temperature, 320℃; heated temperature, 400℃; sheath gas flow, 40 arb; auxiliary gas flow, 10 arb; resolution: 70 000 FWHM; parent ion ($m/z$): $Cl^{16}O_4^-$ 98.947 90, $Cl^{18}O_4^-$ 106.964 80.

## 3. Limits of Detection

The limits of detection of 12 dietary samples were 0.2 μg/kg.

## 4. Quality Control

(1) Blank Test

The whole process blank experiment was carried out to evaluate whether perchlorate may be introduced during pretreatment, resulting in false positive results. During the processing of each batch of samples in this experiment, the blank sample without matrix was carried out according to the sample pretreatment process (including the addition of internal standards). The results showed that all consumables and reagents used in the experiment did not introduce perchlorate.

（2）随行质控

为了保证分析结果的准确，要求每批样品至少做一个加标回收实验，采用空白膳食样品加标 1.0 μg/kg，要求加标回收率为 70%～120%。

## 十八、硝酸盐和亚硝酸盐分析方法

参照《食品安全国家标准 食品中亚硝酸盐与硝酸盐的测定》（GB 5009.33—2016），采用离子色谱法对12类膳食样品中的硝酸盐和亚硝酸盐进行定量测定。

**1. 样品制备**

（1）谷类、豆类、薯类、肉类、蛋类、水产类、蔬菜类、水果类

称取试样匀浆 2 g（精确至 0.01 g，下同），以 40 mL 水洗入 50 mL 容量瓶中（蔬菜、水果样品中另加入 0.5 mL 1 mol/L 氢氧化钾溶液），超声提取 30 min，每隔 5 min 振摇一次，保持固相完全分散。于 75℃ 水浴中放置 5 min，取出放置至室温，加水稀释至刻度。10 000 r/min 离心 15 min，蛋类取上清液 3 mL 加入 7 mL 乙腈，10 000 r/min 离心 15 min；其他样品取上清液 5 mL，12 000～15 000 r/min 离心 10 min，上清液备用。

（2）乳类

称取试样 5 g，置于 50 mL 容量瓶中，加水 40 mL，摇匀，超声 30 min，加入 3% 乙酸溶液 1 mL，混匀后于 4℃ 放置 20 min，取出放置至室温，加水稀释至刻度。取上清液 5 mL，12 000～15 000 r/min 离心 10 min，上清液备用。

(2) Accompanying Quality Control

To ensure the accuracy of the analysis results, each batch of samples is required to conduct at least one spiked recovery experiment, and the blank dietary samples were spiked with 1.0 μg/kg. The recovery rate of standard addition is required to be between 70%-120%.

## XVIII. Analysis Method of Nitrate and Nitrite

Nitrate and nitrite in 12 food categories were determined by using ion chromatography according to the modified Chinese national standards analytical method refer to *National food safety standard-Determination of nitrate and nitrite in food* (GB 5009.33—2016).

**1. Sample Preparation**

(1) Cereals, Legumes, Potatoes, Meats, Eggs, Aquatic Products, Vegetables, Fruits

Two grams (accurate to 0.01 g, the same below) of a sample was removed into a 50 mL volumetric flask, then 40 mL deionized water was added (another 0.5 mL of 1 mol/L KOH was added for vegetables and fruits), to conduct ultrasonic extraction for 30 min. The volumetric flask was shook once every 5 min to keep the solid phase completely dispersed. The volumetric flask was heated in a water bath at 75℃ for 5 min, then cooled to room temperature, and made up to a final volume of 50 mL. The extract was centrifuged at 10 000 r/min for 15 min. For eggs sample, 7 mL acetonitrile was added into 3 mL supernatant and centrifuged at 10 000 r/min for 15 min, and for other samples, 5 mL supernatants were taken and centrifuged at 12 000-15 000 r/min for 10 min. Following centrifugation, the supernatant was collected for analysis.

(2) Dairy Products

Five grams of a sample was removed into a 50 mL volumetric flask, then 40 mL deionized water was added. After 30 min ultrasonic extraction, 1 mL of 3% acetic acid was added. Then, the sample was cooled down to 4℃ for 20 min, then remove and equilibrate

（3）糖类

称取试样 1 g，用水定容至 50 mL。10 000 r/min 离心 15 min，取上清液备用。

（4）水及饮料类、酒类

称取 10 mL 样品，12 000～15 000 r/min 离心 10 min，上清液备用。

**2. 仪器测定**

所用仪器为配备了电导检测器与离子抑制器（Dionex AERS）的离子色谱（Dionex ICS-5000）。色谱条件如下：使用色谱柱 Dionex IonPac AS19-4 μm（2 mm × 250 mm）分离硝酸盐与亚硝酸盐；淋洗液为氢氧化钾溶液，洗脱梯度如下：10 mmol/L 20 min，70 mmol/L 5 min，10 mmol/L 5 min；流速 0.3 mL/min；柱温：30℃；进样量：25 μL。

**3. 检出限**

本方法水及饮料类、酒类样品中硝酸盐和亚硝酸盐的检出限分别为 0.003 mg/kg 和 0.001 mg/kg；其他样品中硝酸盐和亚硝酸盐的检出限分别为 0.03 mg/kg 和 0.01 mg/kg。

**4. 质量控制**

每批样品测定时做两个全程空白实验。采用一种肉类基质和两种蔬菜基质的定值参考物验证方法的准确性，硝酸盐和亚硝酸盐的测定值在标示值范围内。样品的平均加标回收率为 70%～120%。

to room temperature, and dilute to volume with water. 5 mL supernatant was taken and centrifuged at 12 000-15 000 r/min for 10 min, and then the supernatant was collected for analysis.

(3) Sugar

1 gram of a sample was weighed into a 50 mL volumetric flask, then diluted and made up to the final volume by deionized water. The sample was centrifuged at 10 000 r/min for 15 min. The supernatant was collected for analysis after centrifugation.

(4) Water and Beverages, Alcohol Beverages

10 mL of a sample was weighed. The sample was centrifuged at 12 000-15 000 r/min for 10 min. After centrifugation, the supernatant was collected for analysis.

**2. Instrument Determination**

The determinations were performed on an ion chromatograph (Dionex ICS-5000) equipped with a conductivity detector, and an ion suppressor (Dionex AERS). The chromatographic conditions were as follows: a Dionex IonPac AS19-4 μm analytical column (2 mm × 250 mm) was used for separation of nitrate and nitrite; the potassium hydroxide was used as eluent for the following elution gradient: 10 mmol/L 20 min, 70 mmol/L 5 min, 10 mmol/L 5 min; the flow rate was 0.3 mL/min; the column temperature was 30℃; the injection volume was 25 μL.

**3. Limits of Detection**

The limits of detection (LODs) were 0.003 mg/kg for nitrate and 0.001 mg/kg for nitrite in water and beverages, and alcohol beverages; and 0.03 mg/kg for nitrate and 0.01 mg/kg for nitrite in other food samples.

**4. Quality Control**

Each food group was accompanied with two procedural blank tests. One meats sample and two vegetables samples of reference materials were applied to validate the method. Levels of nitrate and nitrite in each material were all within the certified reference

## 十九、双酚类化合物分析方法

采用液相色谱-串联质谱法测定第六次总膳食研究复合膳食样品中双酚A、双酚F、双酚S和双酚AF的含量，用同位素稀释内标法定量。

### 1. 样品制备

酒类、水及饮料类试样称取5 g（精确至0.01 g），置于50 mL聚丙烯离心管中，加入50 μL同位素内标混合使用液，静置30 min。再加入20 mL磷酸缓冲液（PBS）混匀，备用。

对于动物源性试样（肉类、蛋类、乳类和水产类），称取1 g（精确至0.01 g）置于50 mL聚丙烯离心管中，加入50 μL同位素内标混合使用液和5 mL乙腈。涡旋30 s，超声提取20 min，10 000 r/min离心10 min。将上清液转移至新的15 mL聚丙烯离心管中，加入3 mL PBS混合液，置于−20℃下60 min。收集上层乙腈层在40℃下缓慢氮吹至近干，用10 mL甲醇和PBS混合液（10∶90，V/V）重新溶解，涡旋30 s，所得溶液进行免疫亲和柱（IAC）净化。

其他试样称取1 g（精确至0.01 g），置于50 mL聚丙烯离心管中，加入50 μL同位素内标混合使用液和5 mL乙腈。涡旋30 s，超声提取20 min，10 000 r/min下4℃离心10 min。将上清液转移至新的15 mL聚丙烯离心管中。用5 mL乙腈对试样进行再次提取，合并提取液后在40℃下缓慢氮吹至近干，用10 mL甲醇和PBS混合液（10∶90，V/V）重新溶解，涡旋30 s，所得溶液进行IAC净化。

ranges. The average spiking recoveries were in the range of 70%-120%.

## XIX. Analysis Method of Bisphenolic Analogues

The levels of bisphenpl A (BPA), bisphenpl F (BPF), bisphenpl S (BPS), and bisphenpl AF (BPAF) in composite TDS samples from the 6$^{th}$ CTDS was determined using isotop-dilution internal standard method with liquid chromatography-tandem mass spectrometry (LC-MS/MS) analysis.

### 1. Sample Preparation

5 g (accurate to 0.01 g) of alcohol beverages, water and beverages TDS samples were weighted into a 50 mL polypropylene centrifuge tube. 50 μL mixed isotope internal standard working solution is added and allowed to stand for 30 min, followed by the addition of 20 mL phosphate buffer solution (PBS). The mixture is vortexed thoroughly for subsequent use.

For animal-derived TDS samples (meats, eggs, dairy products, and aquatic foods), 1 g (accurate to 0.01 g) of samples were weighed in 50 mL polypropylene centrifuge tubes. 50 μL the pooled isotope internal standard solution and 5 mL acetonitrile were added. The mixtures were vortexed for 30 s, ultrasonically extracted for 20 min, and centrifuged at 10 000 r/min for 10 min. The supernatants were transferred to fresh 15 mL polypropylene centrifuge tubes, then 3 mL PBS was added, the mixture was stored at −20℃ for 60 min. The upper acetonitrile layer was then collected and concentrated to near dryness by a gentle stream of $N_2$ at 40℃. The residue was redissolved in 10 mL methanol/PBS (10∶90, V/V), and the solution was vortexed for 30 s. The resultant solution was subjected to IAC cleanup.

For the other TDS samples, 1 g (accurate to 0.01 g) of samples were weighed into 50 mL polypropylene centrifuge tubes. 50 μL the mixed isotope internal standard working solution and 5 mL acetonitrile were added. The mixtures were vortexed for 30 s, ultrasonically extracted for 20 min, and centrifuged at 10 000 r/min for 10 min

将低温保存的IAC（3 mL，200 ng）从冰箱中取出恢复至室温，然后让柱内原有液体自然流尽。取上述备用液全部过柱，自然流干，弃去全部流出液，依次用9 mL PBS和9 mL水对免疫亲和柱进行淋洗。待水滴完后，用洗耳球挤出残留水分。加入3 mL甲醇洗脱，收集洗脱液于玻璃氮吹瓶中，40℃下氮吹至近干，加入300 μL甲醇，涡旋30 s，再加入700 μL水，涡旋混匀，混合液在10 000 r/min下离心5 min，取800 μL上清液于进样小瓶中供液相色谱-串联质谱测定。

## 2. 仪器测定

液相色谱-串联质谱分析采用液相系统（Nexera X2，日本岛津公司），配有日本岛津公司LC-MS 8060三重四极杆质谱仪。

色谱条件：色谱柱为C18色谱柱（2.1 mm × 100 mm，1.7 μm），流动相为水（A）-甲醇（B），梯度洗脱。梯度为0～6 min，30% B～100% B；保持2 min，然后在0.1 min内于下一次进样前降至30% B。流速为0.30 mL/min，柱温为40℃，进样量为5 μL。

质谱条件：离子源为电喷雾电离（ESI）；扫描方式为负离子扫描；监测模式为多反应监测（MRM）；氮气作为雾化气，流速为3 L/min；加热气和干燥气的流速均为10 L/min；接口温度、脱溶剂温度和加热块温度分别为300℃、250℃和400℃。

at 4℃. The supernatants were transferred to fresh 15 mL polypropylene centrifuge tubes. The residues were extracted again by 5 mL acetonitrile, and the combined extractions were concentrated to near dryness by a gentle stream of $N_2$ at 40℃. The residue was redissolved in 10 mL methanol/PBS (10∶90, $V/V$), and the solution was vortexed for 30 s. The resultant solution was subjected to IAC cleanup.

IAC (3 mL, 200 ng) was taken out from refrigerator compartment. Wait it to room temperature and make the preservation solution dripped out naturally. The prepared solution was loading onto the IAC, then washed with 9 mL PBS solution and 9 mL water. After squeezed out most of the residual moisture, 3 mL methanol was used to elute IAC. The eluant was collected and evaporated to near dryness under nitrogen at 40℃. The residue was redissolved with 300 μL methanol and votexed for 30 s, then added 700 μL water and votexed again. The resultants were centrifuged at 10 000 r/min for 5 min. 800 μL supernatant were transferred in vials followed analysis by LC-MS/MS.

## 2. Instrument Determination

LC-MS/MS analysis was carried out using an LC system (Nexera X2, Shimadzu, Japan) coupled with a Shimadzu LC-MS 8060 triple quadrupole mass spectrometer (Japan).

LC conditions: LC separation was performed on an C18 column (2.1 mm × 100 mm, 1.7 μm). Gradient mobile phases consist of water (A) and methanol (B). The gradient was from 30% B to 100% B over 0-6 min, equilibrated for 2 min, and then decreased to 30% B in 0.1 min waiting for the next injection. The column temperature was set at 40℃ with a flow rate of 0.3 mL/min, and the injection volume was 5 μL. MS conditions: The MS/MS detection was operated in negative ionization mode with multiple reaction monitoring. The $N_2$ was used as the nebulizing gas at flow rate of 3 L/min; heating gas and drying gas flow rate were both 10 L/min. Interface temperature, desolvation line temperature, and heat block temperature were 300℃,

## 3. 检出限

在空白添加样品中，各双酚类化合物在检测中信噪比为3∶1的最低添加浓度作为方法的检出限。BPA和BPF的检出限均为0.15 μg/kg；BPS和BPAF的检出限均为0.015 μg/kg。

## 4. 质量控制

（1）空白实验

在痕量检测BPA时，空白污染是一个令人困扰的问题，应尽量避免污染以获得低检出限。过程空白（一份不含基质且经过全部测定过程的样品，该过程包括内标的加入以及与试验样品相同的测定方式）用来评估每种分析物的背景浓度，确保浓度低于其LOD。

（2）加标实验

以空白试样作为基质，设立低、中、高3个加标水平，每个加标水平设6个平行，双酚类化合物的回收率为84.6%~116.3%，日内RSD均低于13.5%，日间RSD均低于14.4%。

## 二十、有机磷酸酯分析方法

第六次中国总膳食研究采用超高效液相色谱-串联质谱法（UPLC-MS/MS）测定总膳食样品中5种有机磷酸酯含量，用同位素内标法定量。

### 1. 样品制备

取适量样品（10~15 g），于冷冻干燥机中冻干48 h。冻干后的样品经研钵研磨成粉末后取0.5 g，转移至15 mL聚丙烯离心管，随后加入内标溶液（含6种同位素内标各5 ng）。以含0.5%甲酸的5 mL乙腈为提取溶剂进行超声萃取，随后离心取上清液净化。

250℃ and 400℃, respectively.

## 3. Limits of Detection

The LODs of the method were determined as the lowest spiked concentration of each of bisphenolic analogues that could be detected with a signal-to-noise ratio of 3∶1 in blank spiked samples. The limits of detection (LOD) of BPA and BPF were 0.15 μg/kg as well as BPS and BPAF were 0.015 μg/kg.

## 4. Quality Control

(1) Blank Test

Blank contamination is a disturbing problem in the ultra-trace analysis of BPA, and should be avoided in order to achieve low limit of detection. procedural blanks (a sample that does not contain the matrix, that is brought through the entire measurement procedure including internal standards spikes and analysed in the same manner as a test sample) were analyzed to evaluate background concentration of each analyte, the concentration was ensured to be below the LODs.

(2) Spiked Test

The recoveries of BPS, BPF, BPA, BPB, and BPAF in the blank matrix sample at three spiked levels (low, middle and high) in six replicates ranged from 84.6% to 116.3%. The intraday RSDs and interday RSDs were all be low 13.5% and 14.4%, respectively.

## XX. Analysis Method of Organophosphate Esters

In the 6$^{th}$ China total diet study (TDS), concentrations of 5 organophosphate esters (OPEs) in TDS samples were measured by using ultrahigh performance liquid chromatography-tandem mass spectrometry and quantified by isotopically labelled internal standard.

### 1. Sample Preparation

10-15 g of food sample was weighted and freeze-dried in a lyophilizer for 48 h. The dried sample was ground into powder, and 0.5 g of sample powder was weighted and transferred into a 15 mL polypropylene

往提取液中添加无水硫酸钠、C18和 N-丙基乙二胺（PSA）吸附剂，振荡去除脂肪类杂质，随后离心取上清液，上样至 Oasis HLB 固相萃取柱，用乙腈洗脱待测物，氮吹至干，200 µL 甲醇复溶待仪器分析。

### 2. 仪器测定

所使用仪器为高效液相色谱-串联质谱仪（ACQUITYTM-Micromass Xevo TQS，美国 Waters 公司）。

色谱条件：Waters BEH C18 色谱柱（2.1 mm × 100 mm，1.7 µm），流动相为水（含 0.01% 甲酸）-甲醇（含 10 mmol/L 乙酸铵），梯度洗脱。流速为 0.20 mL/min，柱温为 40℃，进样量为 5 µL。

质谱条件：离子源为电喷雾电离（ESI）；扫描方式为正离子扫描；监测模式为多反应监测（MRM）；毛细管电压 3 kV，脱溶剂气温度 450℃，脱溶剂气流量 800 L/h，锥孔气流量 80 L/h。

### 3. 检出限

膳食样品中有机磷酸酯的检出限为 1~10 pg/g。

(PP) tube. Internal standard solution which containing 5 ng each of 6 isotopically labelled internal standards was also added. Subsequently, 5 mL of acetonitrile (containing 0.5% formic acid) was added as extraction solvent. The mixture was ultrasonic extracted and centrifuged, and the supernatant was transferred into another PP tube for purification. Sorbents including primary secondary amine (PSA), C18 and anhydrous $Na_2SO_4$ were added and shaken for lipid removal. After centrifuging the supernatant was collected and loaded on an Oasis HLB column, and the analytes was eluted with acetonitrile. The elute was evaporated to dryness under $N_2$, and the residue was redissolved in 200 µL of methanol for instrumental analysis.

### 2. Instrument Determination

A Waters Acquity ultrahigh performance liquid chromatographic system coupled to a Xevo TQS triple quadrupole mass detector (Waters, USA) was used for quantification.

LC conditions: The analytes were separated in a Waters BEH C18 column (100 mm × 2.1 mm, 1.7 µm), and the column temperature was maintained at 40℃. The injection volume was 5 µL. Water (with 0.01% formic acid) (A) and methanol (with 10 mmol/L ammonium acetate) (B) were used as mobile phases at a constant flow rate of 0.2 mL/min, and gradient elution was applied.

MS conditions: The MS detector was equipped with an ESI probe and operated in positive ion mode. Analyte quantification was performed in multiple reaction monitoring (MRM) mode. The capillary voltage was set at 3 kV. The desolvation temperature was set at 450℃, and the desolvation gas and cone gas flows were set at 800 L/h and 80 L/h, respectively.

### 3. Limits of Detection

The limits of detection of OPEs were 1-10 pg/g.

## 4. 质量控制

（1）空白实验

本实验的每一批次样品处理中，均进行了全程空白实验，结果发现部分有机磷酸酯存在微量背景污染，因此在计算膳食样中相应待测物含量时将扣除背景污染。

（2）回收实验

以巴沙鱼、鸡胸肉、鸡蛋和牛奶作为代表性基质，按加标水平 1 ng/g 和 5 ng/g 加入一定量内标及目标物质，按照样品前处理流程测定并获得目标物的回收率数据，OPE 的回收率为 80%～120%。

## 二十一、谷氨酸盐分析方法

采用超高效液相色谱-串联质谱法测定总膳食样品中谷氨酸盐含量，外标法定量。

### 1. 样品制备

对于总膳食基质，称取 0.5 g 样品于 10 mL 刻度管，加入 1.0 g NaCl，加入 5 mL 0.1 mol/L HCl 萃取，涡旋 2 min，离心 5 min，取 1 mL 上清液待净化。

对于 MAX 柱净化的样品，以 1 mL 5% $NH_3H_2O$ 活化 MAX 柱，抽干，1 mL 0.1 mol/L HCl 上清液以 1 mL 0.1 mol/L NaOH 中和后，以 2 mL 中和液上样，0.5 mL 纯水淋洗 2 次，0.5 mL 甲醇淋洗 2 次后，以含 2% 甲酸（$V/V$）的甲醇 0.5 mL 溶液洗脱 2 次后，合并洗脱液，吹干并以 0.1 mol/L HCl 复溶，以水稀释样品 100 倍后上样。

## 4. Quality Control

(1) Blank Test

A procedural blank sample was pretreated and tested along with every batch of food samples to monitor the possible interference or background contamination during sample analysis. Trace levels of some OPEs were found in the procedural blanks, and the blank value has been subtracted from the measurement of corresponding target compound.

(2) Recovery Test

Basa fish, chicken breast, eggs and cow milk were used as representative matrices in recovery test. Recovery test was performed by spiking matrices with internal standard and the target compounds at two levels (1 ng/g and 5 ng/g) and testing based on the analytical method described above. The recoveries of OPEs fell in the range of 80%-120%.

## XXI. Analysis Method of Glutamate acid salt

The glutamate acid salt content in total dietary samples was determined by ultra-high performance liquid chromatography-tandem mass spectrometry (UPLC-MS/MS) and quantified by external standard method.

### 1. Sample Preparation

For TDS matrix, weigh 0.5 g of sample in a 10 mL graduated tube, add 1.0 g NaCl, add 5 mL of 0.1 mol/L HCl extraction, vortex for 2 min, centrifuge for 5 min, remove 1 mL of supernatant for purification. For MAX column clean-up, the MAX column was activated with 1 mL of 5% $NH_3H_2O$. 1 mL of 0.1 mol/L HCl supernatants was neutralized with 1 mL of 0.1 mol/L NaOH. The sample was loaded with 2 mL of the neutralization solution, washed twice with 0.5 mL of pure water, washed twice with 0.5 mL of methanol, eluted twice with 0.5 mL of methanol containing 2% formic acid ($V/V$), and the eluates were combined. The sample was blown dry and redissolved in 0.1 mol/L HCl. The sample was diluted 100 times with water.

## 2. 仪器测定

分析仪器：LC-30A 系统。

色谱条件：色谱柱为 HSS PFP，2.1 mm i.d. × 100 mm l.，1.7 μm。流动相：A 相为 0.2% 甲酸水溶液，B 相为含 0.2% 甲酸的乙腈溶液。梯度洗脱，B 相初始浓度为 40%，时间程序为 0～3 min，B 相 40%；3～6 min，B 相线性升至 100%，保持 2min。流速为 0.35 mL/min，柱温为 40℃，进样量为 1 μL。

质谱条件：离子化模式为 ESI，正离子模式；离子喷雾电压为 +4.5 kV；氮气流速为 3.0 L/min；干燥气流速为 10 L/min；加热气流速为 10 L/min；碰撞气为氩气；脱溶剂气温度为 300℃；加热模块温度为 400℃；扫描模式为多反应监测（MRM）；驻留时间为 8 ms；延迟时间为 3 ms。

## 3. 检出限

以空白样品作为基质，加入 3.0 μg/kg 的目标物质，按照样品前处理流程进行操作，上机测定，获得目标物的信噪比数据，以 3 倍信噪比（S/N=3）计算本方法的检出限，本方法的检出限为 3.0 μg/kg。

## 4. 质量控制

对于添加谷氨酸盐的 7 类膳食食品基质（谷类、豆类、薯类、蛋类、水产类、蔬菜类和肉类），采取样品测试后吹干，并直接在样品中分别加入 10 ng/g、100 ng/g 和 1000 ng/g 浓度标准物质的方式进行加标回收实验。平行测定 6 次后，加标回收率为 77.0%～122.1%，RSD 为 2.3%～14.3%。

## 2. Instrument Determination

Analytical instrumental: LC-30A system.

Chromatographic conditions: the column was HSS PFP, 2.1 mm i.d. × 100 mm l., 1.7 μm. The mobile phase was 0.2% formic acid in water for phase A and 0.2% formic acid in acetonitrile for phase B. The initial concentration of phase B was 40%, the time program was 0-3 min, phase B 40%; 3-6 min, phase B linearly increased to 100%, the flow rate was held for 2 min under gradient elution. The flow rate was 0.35 mL/min. The column temperature was 40℃, and the injection volume was 1 μL.

Mass spectrometry conditions: the ionization mode was ESI, positive ion mode. Ion spray voltage was +4.5 kV. The nitrogen flow rate was 3.0 L/min. The drying gas flow rate was 10 L/min. The heating gas flow rate was 10 L/min. Collision gas was argon. Desolvation line temperature was 300℃. The heating module temperature was 400℃; the scan mode was multiple reaction monitoring (MRM). Dwell time was 8 ms. The delay time was 3 ms.

## 3. Limits of Detection

3.0 μg/kg of the target substance was added into blank samples, the sample was operated according to the sample pre-treatment procedure, the S/N data of the target substance was obtained on the machine, and the limit of detection of the method was calculated with a 3-fold S/N ratio (S/N=3). The limit of detection for this method was 3.0 μg/kg.

## 4. Quality Control

For the seven dietary food matrices (cereals, legumes, potatoes, eggs, aquatics, vegetables, and meats) for which glutamate were added, spiked recovery experiments were performed by blowing the samples dry after testing and adding standards at concentrations of 10 ng/g, 100 ng/g, and 1000 ng/g directly to the samples. The recoveries of the spiked standards after six parallel determinations. They ranged from 77.0%-122.1%, with an RSD of 2.3%-14.3%.

# 第三节 膳食暴露评估方法
# Section 3　Dietary Exposure Assessment Method

## 一、膳食摄入量的计算

**1. 每人每日某类食品某种化学污染物、营养素摄入量计算方法**

$$I_1 = C_1 \times E_1$$

式中，$I_1$ 为每人每日某类食品某膳食化学污染物、营养素摄入量；$C_1$ 为某类食品某膳食化学污染物、营养素含量；$E_1$ 为某类食品某膳食消费量（烹调、制备后）。

**2. 每人每日某膳食化学污染物、营养素总摄入量计算方法**

$$I_T = I_1 + I_2 + I_3 + I_4 + I_5 + \cdots + I_{12}$$

式中，$I_T$ 为每人每日某膳食化学污染物、营养素总摄入量；$I_1 \sim I_{12}$ 为每人每日某类食品某膳食化学污染物、营养素摄入量。

## 二、低水平数据的处理

WHO 推荐：当有小于 60% 的结果低于检出限（LOD）时，所有小于 LOD 的结果均以 1/2 LOD 计；当有大于 60% 的结果低于检出限时，所有小于 LOD 的结果以 0、1/2 LOD 和 LOD 分别计算摄入量。

## 三、数据处理软件

三天入户称量食物结合三天 24 h 膳食回顾的个体调查生成最终的食品采样单。Microsoft® Office Excel 和 SPSS13.0 用于所有数据的处理，包括食物聚类、编制程序以及计算膳食暴露量。

## Ⅰ. Calculation of Dietary Intake

**1. Calculation of Daily Intake Per Person of Certain Chemical Contaminants and Nutrients in Certain Food Categories**

$$I_1 = C_1 \times E_1$$

$I_1$—Dietary intake of chemical contaminant and nutrient from one food group per person per day.

$C_1$—Dietary chemical contaminant and nutrient content of one food type.

$E_1$—Dietary consumption of certain food items (after cooking and preparation).

**2. Calculation of Total Daily Intake of a Dietary Chemical Contaminant and Nutrient Per Person Per Day**

$$I_T = I_1 + I_2 + I_3 + I_4 + I_5 + \cdots + I_{12}$$

$I_T$—Total daily intake of a dietary chemical contaminant and nutrient per person per day.

$I_1$-$I_{12}$—Daily intake of a dietary chemical contaminant, nutrient per person per day for one food group.

## Ⅱ. Treatment of Low-level Data

WHO recommendation: if less than 60% of the results were below the limits of detection (LOD), all the results below LOD were calculated as 1/2 LOD. If more than 60% of the results were below the limits of detection (LOD), all the results below LOD were calculated as 0, 1/2 LOD and LOD separately.

## Ⅲ. Data processing software

The final food list was created by combining the results of the three-day household food weighing and individual recalls of three 24-hour dietary intakes. All data were processed with Microsoft® Office Excel and SPSS13.0, including food aggregation, program formulation, and dietary exposure calculation.

# 第二章  脂肪酸的膳食暴露评估
## Chapter 2  Dietary Exposure Assessment of Fatty acids

## 一、背景

脂肪称为甘油三酯，是人体必需的能量来源之一。脂肪酸是构成甘油三酯、磷脂的重要成分。脂肪酸根据其碳链的长度，分为短链（C4～C6）、中链（C8～C12）、长链（C14～C20）和极长链（>C22）脂肪酸。脂肪酸根据碳链的饱和程度，分为饱和脂肪酸（SFA）和不饱和脂肪酸（UFA）。UFA又分为单不饱和脂肪酸（MUFA）、多不饱和脂肪酸（PUFA）和反式脂肪酸（TFA）。PUFA根据其第一个双键所在碳原子的位置分为n-3和n-6脂肪酸。

SFA是指不含双键的脂肪酸，月桂酸（C12:0）、豆蔻酸（C14:0）、棕榈酸（C16:0）、硬脂酸（C18:0）为典型代表；MUFA是指含有1个双键的脂肪酸，最主要的MUFA为油酸（C18:1n-9）；PUFA是指含有两个或两个以上双键且碳链长度为18～22个碳原子的直链脂肪酸，通常分为n-3和n-6脂肪酸。n-3 PUFA的主要代表为α-亚麻酸（C18:3n-3，ALA）、二十碳五烯酸（C20:5n-3，EPA）、二十二碳六烯酸（C22:6n-3，DHA）；n-6 PUFA的主要代表为亚油酸（C18:2n-6，LA）和花生四烯酸（C20:4n-6，AA）。

构成膳食脂肪的脂肪酸种类不同，其生理功能和健康效应也不同。研究表明，不同种类SFA对血脂浓度的影响不同，如月桂酸、豆蔻酸和棕榈酸会使血清胆固醇值升高，而硬脂酸并不会导致血清胆固醇值升高；用MUFA替

## I . Background

Fat, being an essential energy source of people, is called triglyceride. Fatty acid is a necessary component of triglyceride and phospholipid. According to the carbon chain length, fatty acids are divided into short-chain (C4-C6), medium-chain (C8-C12), long-chain (C14-C20), and very-long-chain (>C22). According to the degree of saturation of the carbon chain, fatty acids are divided into saturated fatty acids (SFA) and unsaturated fatty acids (UFA); and UFA are divided into monounsaturated fatty acids (MUFA), polyunsaturated fatty acids (PUFA), and *trans*-fatty acids (TFA). Polyunsaturated fatty acids are generally divided into n-3 and n-6 fatty acids according to the position of the carbon atom of its first double bond.

SFA have no double bond of carbons with typical representatives of lauric acid (C12:0), myristic acid (C14:0), palmitic acid (C16:0), and stearic acid (C18:0). MUFA contain one double bond, and the predominant form is oleic acid (C18:1n-9). PUFA, generally divided into n-3 and n-6 fatty acids, are straight-chain fatty acids containing more than one double bond with a carbon chain length of 18 to 22 carbons. The prominent representatives of n-3 PUFA are α-linolenic acid (C18:3n-3, ALA), eicosapentaenoic acid (C20:5n-3, EPA), and docosahexaenoic acid (C22:6n-3, DHA), and the prominent representatives of n-6 PUFA are linoleic acid (C18:2n-6, LA) and arachidonic acid (C20:4n-6, AA).

The types of fatty acids that make up dietary fat are different, and their physiological functions and health effects are also different. Researches found that different SFA have different effects on blood lipids. For example,

代碳水化合物，可以提高高密度脂蛋白胆固醇（HDL-C）水平，用 MUFA 替代 SFA 会降低低密度脂蛋白胆固醇（LDL-C）水平和血清总胆固醇/HDL-C 值。PUFA 能够降低冠心病的发生，但 PUFA 不饱和程度较高，容易导致脂质氧化。来自氢化植物油的 TFA 能够增加患冠心病的风险。由于膳食脂肪及其脂肪酸对健康和疾病的影响，2010 年联合国粮食及农业组织（FAO）和美国医学研究所（IOM）膳食营养素参考摄入量（DRI）专家委员会提出使用"宏量营养素可接受范围"（acceptable macronutrient distribution range，AMDR）和"适宜摄入量"（adequate intake，AI）以推荐脂肪与脂肪酸的参考摄入量。AMDR 和 AI 用脂肪供能占总能量的百分比（% E）来表示。EPA、DHA 采用绝对量（g/d）来表示。2013 年，中国营养学会颁布了《中国居民膳食营养素参考摄入量（2013 版）》。

## 二、健康指导值

《中国居民膳食营养素参考摄入量（2013 版）》推荐成人和老年人膳食总脂肪的 AMDR 为 20% E～30% E。推荐成人、老年人、孕妇和乳母膳食的 SFA 膳食摄入量上限（U-AMDR）为 10% E。MUFA 仅提出原则，即在控制总脂肪供能＜30% E，SFA 摄入量＜10% E 或＜8% E，满足 n-6 PUFA、n-3 PUFA 适宜摄入量的前提下，其余膳食脂肪供能由 MUFA 提供。推荐成年人和老年人膳食 n-6 PUFA 的 AMDR 为 2.5% E～9.0% E，其中亚油酸（LA）的 AI 为 4.0% E。推荐成年人和老年人膳食 n-3 PUFA 的 AMDR 为 0.5% E～2.0% E，其中 α-亚油酸（ALA）的 AI 为 0.60% E，EPA + DHA 的 AMDR 为 0.25～2.0 g/d；TFA 的可耐受最高摄入量（UL）＜1% E。

C12:0, C14:0, and C16:0 will raise the serum cholesterol level while C18:0 will not. Substituting carbohydrates with MUFA raises the level of high density lipoprotein-cholesterol (HDL-C), and substituting SFA with MUFA decreases the level of low density lipoprotein-cholesterol (LDL-C) and the ratio of total serum cholesterol (TC)/HDL-C. PUFA can reduce the occurrence of coronary heart disease, however, the high unsaturation are susceptible to lipid oxidation. TFA from hydrogenated vegetable oils can increase the risk of coronary heart disease. Due to the effects of dietary fats and their fatty acids on health and disease, the acceptable macronutrient distribution ranges (AMDR) and adequate intake (AI) were introduced by the the Food and Agriculture Organization of the United Nations (FAO) and the U.S. Expert Committee of the Institute of Medicine (IOM) on Dietary Reference Intakes (DRIs) in 2010 to recommend the referred intakes of fats and fatty acids. The AMDR and AI are expressed as percentage of fat energy supply to total energy intake (% E), and the EPA and DHA are expressed as absolute amount (g/d). In 2013, the Chinese Nutrition Society issued the *Chinese Dietary Reference Intakes (2013 version)*.

## II. HBGV

The AMDR of dietary total fat for adults and the elderly is 20% E-30% E in the *Chinese Dietary Reference Intakes (2013 version)*. The upper limit of dietary intake of SFA (U-AMDR) is 10% E for adults, the elderly, pregnant women, and lactating mothers. MUFA are proposed as a principle merely, that is the rest of the dietary fat supply is provided by MUFA in the condition that the intake of total fat is<30% E, the intake of SFA is<10% E or<8% E, and the appropriate intakes of n-6 PUFA and n-3 PUFA are met. The AI of linoleic acid (LA) for adults and the elderly is 4.0% E, and the AMDR of n-6 PUFA is 2.5% E-9.0% E; the AMDR of n-3 PUFA for adults and the elderly is 0.5% E-2.0% E, and the AI of α-linolenic acid (ALA) is 0.60% E; the AMDR of EPA plus DHA is 0.25-2.0 g/d; the tolerable upper intake level (UL) of TFA is<1% E.

2009年，美国心脏协会营养委员会（American Heart Association Nutrition Committee，AHA）推荐成人膳食 SFA 的 U-AMDR＜7% E，TFA 的 UL＜1% E。

## 三、总膳食研究结果

本次总膳食研究对 24 个省（自治区、直辖市）的 9 类混合膳食样品（谷类、豆类、薯类、肉类、蛋类、水产类、乳类、蔬菜类、水果类）进行了 62 种脂肪酸的测定，具体包括 17 种 SFA：丁酸（C4:0）、己酸（C6:0）、辛酸（C8:0）、癸酸（C10:0）、十一烷酸（C11:0）、月桂酸（C12:0）、十三烷酸（C13:0）、豆蔻酸（C14:0）、十五烷酸（C15:0）、棕榈酸（C16:0）、十七烷酸（C17:0）、硬脂酸（C18:0）、二十烷酸（C20:0）、二十一烷酸（C21:0）、二十二烷酸（C22:0）、二十三烷酸（C23:0）、二十四烷酸（C24:0）；9 种 MUFA：十四碳一烯酸（C14:1）、十五碳一烯酸（C15:1）、十六碳一烯酸（C16:1）、十七碳一烯酸（C17:1）、十八碳一烯酸（C18:1n-9，油酸）、十八碳一烯酸（C18:1n-7）、二十碳一烯酸（C20:1）、二十二碳一烯酸（C22:1，芥酸）、二十四碳一烯酸（C24:1）；14 种 PUFA：十八碳二烯酸（C18:2n-6，亚油酸）、十八碳三烯酸（C18:3n-6，γ-亚麻酸）、十八碳三烯酸（C18:3n-3，α-亚麻酸）、二十碳二烯酸（C20:2n-6）、二十碳三烯酸（C20:3n-6）、二十碳三烯酸（C20:3n-3）、二十碳四烯酸（C20:4n-6，花生四烯酸）、二十碳五烯酸（C20:5n-3，EPA）、二十二碳二烯酸（C22:2n-6）、二十二碳四烯酸（C22:4n-6）、二十二碳五烯酸（C22:5n-6）、二十二碳五烯酸（C22:5n-3，DPA）、二十二碳六烯酸（C22:6n-3，DHA）、顺-9,反-11-十八碳二烯酸（9c11t，C18:2，共轭亚油酸）；22 种 TFA：反-9-十四碳

The American Heart Association Nutrition Committee (AHA) recommends U-AMDR of SFA is <7% E, and the UL of TFA is < 1% E in 2009.

## III. TDS Results

This TDS measured 62 fatty acids in nine categories of composite dietary samples (cereals, legumes, potatoes, meats, eggs, aquatic foods, dairy products, vegetables and fruits) from 24 provinces (autonomous regions, municipalities). The 62 fatty acids include 17 SFA [butyric acid (C4:0), caproic acid (C6:0), caprylic acid (C8:0), decanoic acid (C10:0), undecanoic acid (C11:0), lauric acid (C12:0), tridecanoic acid (C13:0), myristic acid (C14:0), pentadecanoic acid (C15:0), palmitic acid (C16:0), heptadecanoic acid (C17:0), stearic acid (C18:0), eicosanoic acid (C20:0), heneicosanoic acid (C21:0), docosanoic acid (C22:0), tricosanoic acid (C23:0) and lignoceric acid (C24:0)], 9 MUFA [myristoleic acid (C14:1), pentadecenoic acid (C15:1), palmitoleic acid (C16:1), heptadecenoic acid (C17:1), oleic acid (C18:1n-9), vacuum acid (C18:1n-7), eicosenoic acid (C20:1), erucic acid (C22:1) and tetracosenoic acid (C24:1)], 14 PUFA [linoleic acid (C18:2n-6), γ-linolenic acid (C18:3n-6), α-linolenic acid (C18:3n-3), eicosadienoic acid (C20:2n-6), eicosatrienoic acid (C20:3n-6), eicosatrienoic acid (C20:3n-3), arachidonic acid (C20:4n-6), eicosapentaenoic acid (C20:5n-3, EPA), docosadienoic acid (C22:2n-6), docosatetraenoic acid (C22:4n-6), docosapentaenoic acid (C22:5n-6), docosapentaenoic acid (C22:5n-3, DPA), docosahexaenoic acid (C22:6n-3, DHA) and *cis*-9, *trans*-11-octadecadienoate conjugated acids (9c11t, C18:2)], and 22 TFA [*trans*-9-myristolenic acid (9t, C14:1), *trans*-10-pentadecanoic acid (10t, C15:1), *trans*-9-hexadecenoic acid (9t, C16:1), *trans*-10-heptadecenoic acid (10t, C17:1), *trans*-6-oleic acid (6t, C18:1), *trans*-9-oleic acid (9t, C18:1), *trans*-10-oleic acid (10t, C18:1), *trans*-11-oleic acid (11t, C18:1), *trans*-12-oleic acid (12t, C18:1), *trans*-13/14-oleic acid (13t/14t, C18:1), *trans*-9, *trans*-12-linoleic acid (9t12t,

一烯酸（9t，C14:1）、反-10-十五碳一烯酸（10t，C15:1）、反-9-十六碳一烯酸（9t，C16:1）、反-10-十七碳一烯酸（10t，C17:1）、反-6-十八碳一烯酸（6t，C18:1）、反-9-十八碳一烯酸（9t，C18:1）、反-10-十八碳一烯酸（10t，C18:1）、反-11-十八碳一烯酸（11t，C18:1）、反-12-十八碳一烯酸（12t，C18:1）、反-13/14-十八碳一烯酸（13t/14t，C18:1）、反-9，反-12-十八碳二烯酸（9t12t，C18:2）、顺-9，反-12-十八碳二烯酸（9c12t，C18:2）、反-9，顺-12-十八碳二烯酸（9t12c，C18:2）、反-9，反-12，反-15-十八碳三烯酸（9t12t15t，C18:3）、反-9，反-12，顺-15-十八碳三烯酸（9t12t15c，C18:3）、反-9，顺-12，反-15-十八碳三烯酸（9t12c15t，C18:3）、反-9，顺-12，顺-15-十八碳三烯酸（9t12c15c，C18:3）、顺-9，反-12，反-15-十八碳三烯酸（9c12t15t，C18:3）、顺-9，反-12，顺-15-十八碳三烯酸（9c12t15c，C18:3）、顺-9，顺-12，反-15-十八碳三烯酸（9c12c15t，C18:3）、反-11-二十碳一烯酸（11t，C20:1）、反-13-二十二碳一烯酸（13t，C22:1）。

**1. 混合膳食样品中脂肪酸的组成和含量**

在不同膳食样品中脂肪酸含量和脂肪酸构成差异较大，表2-1为不同类别膳食样品中脂肪酸平均含量水平。未烹饪蔬菜类、薯类和谷类的脂肪酸含量应很低，但由于烹调加工时使用了烹调油及其他调味料，因此在总膳食样品中呈现出较高的脂肪酸含量。同理，肉类、蛋类、豆类、水产类的脂肪酸含量也包含烹调加工中所使用的烹调用油及其他调味料。各类膳食样品的总脂肪酸平均含量水平为0.03～27.13 g/100 g，在各类膳食样品中含量水平依次为肉类、蛋类、豆类、水产类、蔬菜类、薯类、乳类、谷类和水果类。各类膳食

C18:2), *cis*-9, *trans*-12-linoleic acid (9c12t, C18:2), *trans*-9, *cis*-12-linoleic acid (9t12c, C18:2), *trans*-9, *trans*-12, *trans*-15-linolenic acid (9t12t15t, C18:3), *trans*-9, *trans*-12, *cis*-15-linolenic acid (9t12t15c, C18:3), *trans*-9, *cis*-12, *trans*-15-linolenic acid (9t12c15t, C18:3), *trans*-9, *cis*-12, *cis*-15-linolenic acid (9t12c15c, C18:3), *cis*-9, *trans*-12, *trans*-15-linolenic acid (9c12t15t, C18:3), *cis*-9, *trans*-12, *cis*-15-linolenic acid (9c12t15c, C18:3) and *cis*-9, *cis*-12, *trans*-15-linolenic acid (9c12c15t, C18:3), *trans*-11-eicosenoic acid (11t, C20:1) and *trans*-13-erucic acid (13t, C22:1)].

**1. Composition and Contents of Fatty Acids in TDS Composite Samples**

The composition and contents of fatty acids varied widely among the different dietary samples, and Table 2-1 shows the average contents of fatty acids of different categories. The fatty acid contents of uncooked vegetables, potatoes, and cereals should be low; however, due to the usage of cooking oil and other condiments in the cooking process, they had a high fatty acid content in the total dietary samples. Similarly, the fatty acid contents of meats, eggs, legumes, and aquatic foods included cooking oils and other condiments used in the cooking process. The average content level of total fatty acids in various dietary samples was 0.03-27.13 g/100 g, with the descending order of meats, eggs, legumes, aquatic foods, vegetables, potatoes, dairy products, cereals and fruits. The average content level of SFA in various dietary samples was 0.01-9.22 g/100 g, and the top three of content level were meats, eggs and dairy products. The average content level of MUFA in various dietary samples was 0.01-12.18 g/100 g, and the top three of content level were meats, eggs and aquatic foods. The average content level of PUFA in various dietary samples was 0.01-5.58 g/100 g, and the top three of content level were meats, legumes and eggs. The average content level of n-6 PUFA in various dietary samples was 0.01-4.99 g/100 g, and the top three of content level were meats, legumes and eggs. The average content level of n-3 PUFA in various dietary

表 2-1　第六次中国总膳食研究中膳食样品脂肪酸平均含量（单位：g/100 g）
Table 2-1　The average contents of fatty acids in dietary samples from the 6$^{th}$ China TDS (Unit: g/100 g)

| 脂肪酸<br>Fatty acid | 谷类<br>Cereals | 豆类<br>Legumes | 薯类<br>Potatoes | 肉类<br>Meats | 蛋类<br>Eggs | 水产类<br>Aquatic foods | 乳类<br>Dairy products | 蔬菜类<br>Vegetables | 水果类<br>Fruits |
|---|---|---|---|---|---|---|---|---|---|
| 饱和脂肪酸（SFA） | 0.33 | 1.53 | 0.83 | 9.22 | 3.65 | 1.57 | 2.24 | 0.98 | 0.01 |
| 单不饱和脂肪酸（MUFA） | 0.38 | 3.15 | 2.29 | 12.18 | 6.60 | 3.48 | 0.76 | 2.73 | 0.01 |
| 多不饱和脂肪酸（PUFA） | 0.56 | 4.23 | 2.01 | 5.58 | 3.86 | 2.82 | 0.12 | 2.27 | 0.01 |
| n-6 多不饱和脂肪酸（n-6 PUFA） | 0.52 | 3.71 | 1.68 | 4.99 | 3.31 | 2.24 | 0.09 | 1.90 | 0.01 |
| n-3 多不饱和脂肪酸（n-3 PUFA） | 0.05 | 0.52 | 0.33 | 0.59 | 0.54 | 0.57 | 0.02 | 0.37 | 0.00 |
| 反式脂肪酸（TFA） | 0.01 | 0.03 | 0.04 | 0.15 | 0.08 | 0.05 | 0.12 | 0.06 | 0.00 |
| 总脂肪酸<br>Total fatty acids | 1.29 | 8.94 | 5.17 | 27.13 | 14.18 | 7.92 | 3.24 | 6.03 | 0.03 |

样品的 SFA 平均含量水平为 0.01～9.22 g/100 g，在各类膳食样品中含量水平前 3 位依次为肉类、蛋类和乳类。各类膳食样品的 MUFA 平均含量水平为 0.01～12.18 g/100 g，在各类膳食样品中含量水平前 3 位依次为肉类、蛋类和水产类。各类膳食样品的 PUFA 平均含量水平为 0.01～5.58 g/100 g，在各类膳食样品中含量水平前 3 位依次为肉类、豆类和蛋类。各类膳食样品的 n-6 PUFA 平均含量水平为 0.01～4.99 g/100 g，在各类膳食样品中含量水平前 3 位依次为肉类、豆类和蛋类。各类膳食样品的 n-3 PUFA 平均含量水平为 0.00～0.59 g/100 g，在各类膳食样品中含量水平前 3 位依次为肉类、水产类和蛋类。各类膳食样品的 TFA 平均含量水平为 0.00～0.15 g/100 g，在各类膳食样品中含量水平前 3 位依次为肉类、乳类和蛋类。TFA 在除水果类外的 8 类食品中普遍检出，但含量都较低。C18:1 TFA 在乳类和蛋类中的检出率为 100%，其余依次为水产类（88%）、蔬菜类

samples was 0.00-0.59 g/100 g, and the top three of content level were meats, aquatic foods and eggs. The average content level of TFA in various dietary samples was 0.00-0.15 g/100 g, and the top three of content level were meats, dairy products and eggs. The TFA were generally detected in 8 food groups except the fruits, but the contents were low relatively. The detection rates of C18:1 TFA in dairy products and eggs were 100%. The detection rates of other food groups were 88% (aquatic foods), 79% (vegetables), 79% (cereals), 67% (meats), 17% (legumes), and 8% (potatoes) averagely. The range of detection rate of C18:2 TFA in 8 food groups was 92%-100%. C18:3 TFA were not detected in dairy products, and the range of detection rate in other food groups was 58%-96%. The content levels of various fatty acids in each category from different provinces (autonomous regions, municipalities) are detailed in Annexed Table 2-1-Annexed Table 2-7.

（79%）、谷类（79%）、肉类（67%）、豆类（17%）、薯类（8%）。C18:2 TFA 在 8 类食品中的检出率为 92%~100%；C18:3 TFA 在乳类中没有检出，在其他膳食样品中的检出率为 58%~96%。不同省（自治区、直辖市）每类膳食样品中总脂肪酸、SFA、MUFA、PUFA（n-6 PUFA、n-3 PUFA）和 TFA 的含量水平详见附表 2-1~附表 2-7。

图 2-1 显示不同类别的膳食样品中脂肪酸的构成情况不尽相同。膳食样品中 SFA 占总脂肪酸的比例为 16.1%~69.0%，乳类最高，肉类次之，为 34.0%；SFA 以棕榈酸和硬脂酸为主，平均含量分别占总脂肪酸含量的 16.9% 和 7.3%。膳食样品中 MUFA 占总脂肪酸的比例为 19.5%~46.5%，蛋类、肉类、薯类、水产类和蔬菜类占总脂肪酸的比例相当（43.9%~46.5%）；MUFA 以油酸为主，平均含量占总脂肪酸含量的 39.1%，芥酸平均含量占总脂肪酸含量的 0.9%。PUFA 占总脂肪酸的比例为 3.6%~47.3%，其中豆类、谷类和水果类均高于 40% 以上，豆类最高，乳

Figure 2-1 shows that the composition of fatty acids in dietary samples varied among different categories. The proportion of SFA to total fatty acids ranged from 16.1% to 69.0%, the dairy products recorded the highest value followed by the meats (34%). SFA were dominated by palmitic acid and stearic acid, which accounted for 16.9% and 7.3% of total fatty acids respectively. The proportion of MUFA to total fatty acids ranged from 19.5% to 46.5%, and the proportion of eggs, meats, potatoes, aquatic foods, and vegetables were comparable from 43.9% to 46.5%. The dominated component of MUFA was oleic acid, accounting for 39.1% of total fatty acids, and the erucic acid accounted for 0.9%. The proportion range of PUFA to total fatty acids was 3.6%-47.3%, and the proportions of legumes, cereals, and fruits were all higher than 40% with legumes being the highest and dairy products being the lowest. The n-6 PUFA were dominated by linoleic acid accounting for 24.0%, and the arachidonic acid accounted for 0.4%. The n-3 PUFA were dominated by α-linolenic acid , accounting for 3.7%. The proportion of TFA to total fatty acids of dietary samples ranged from 0.0% to 3.8% with dairy products being the highest; averagely, the C18:1 TFA, C18:2 TFA and C18:3 TFA

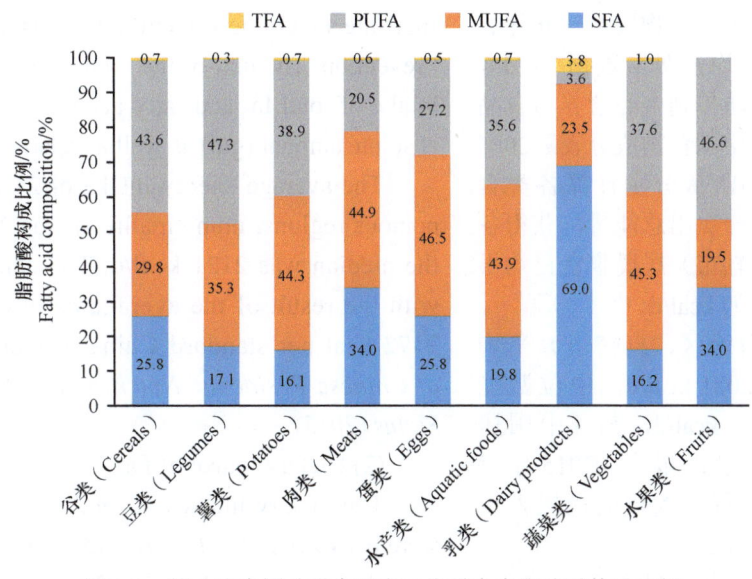

图 2-1 第六次中国总膳食研究 9 类膳食中脂肪酸构成比例

Figure 2-1 The composition of various fatty acids in nine food categories from the 6th China TDS

类最低；n-6 PUFA 以亚油酸为主，平均含量占总脂肪酸含量的 24.0%，花生四烯酸平均含量占总脂肪酸含量的 0.4%。n-3 PUFA 以 α-亚麻酸为主，平均含量占总脂肪酸含量的 3.7%。膳食样品中 TFA 占总脂肪酸的比例为 0.0%～3.8%，乳类最高。C18:1 TFA、C18:2 TFA 和 C18:3 TFA 平均含量分别占总脂肪酸含量的 0.3%、0.2% 和 0.2%。

## 2. 膳食暴露评估

以成年男子的摄入量为代表分析我国居民脂肪、脂肪酸摄入水平，利用能量脂肪折算系数（9 kcal/g）（1 cal= 4.184 J）计算第六次总膳食研究中总脂肪、SFA、MUFA、n-6 PUFA、n-3 PUFA、TFA 摄入能量，并用 24 个省（自治区、直辖市）膳食摄入能量进行供能比（相对总能量摄入，% E）的计算，与《中国居民膳食营养素参考摄入量（2013版）》推荐的脂肪和脂肪酸摄入量进行比较。脂肪和脂肪酸的摄入量以绝对量（g/d）与相对量（% E）表示。

（1）膳食摄入总能量

以 24 个省（自治区、直辖市）的食物消费量数据进行食物聚类，并计算出聚类食物的日均消费量数据（g/d），采用中国疾病预防控制中心营养与食品安全所编制的《中国食物成分表》2004 版、2009 版、2018 版分别计算各类食物能量供给，并计算出总能量，获得各省（自治区、直辖市）居民膳食日均摄入总能量，单位为 kcal/d。

24 个省（自治区、直辖市）平均能量摄入量为 2081 kcal/d，中位数能量摄入量为 2121 kcal/d，与《中国居民营养与慢性病状况报告（2015 年）》中国居民平均每标准人日能量摄入量 2172 kcal 相比持平。

（2）脂肪膳食摄入量

脂肪摄入量范围为 23.5% E～39.5% E

accounted for 0.3%, 0.2% and 0.2% of total fatty acids respectively.

## 2. Dietary Exposure Assessment

This study analyzed the dietary intakes of fat and fatty acids based on the adult males by using an energy/fat factor of 9 kcal/g to calculate the energy intakes from the total fat, the total fatty acids, SFA, MUFA, PUFA, and TFA from the 6th China TDS. Then, the percentages of total energy intake (% E) was calculated using the energy intake values of 24 provinces (autonomous regions, municipalities) and compared with the corresponding values of fat and fatty acids in the dietary nutrient reference intakes for *Chinese Dietary Reference Intakes (2013 version)*.

(1) Dietary Intake of Total Energy

Food clustering was performed based on the food consumption data of 24 provinces (autonomous regions, municipalities), and the average daily consumption data (g/d) of the clustered foods were calculated. The average daily intake of total energy of residents in each province (autonomous region, municipality) was obtained by calculating the energies of various kinds of foods using *Chinese Food Composition Table* (2004, 2009, and 2018 versions) prepared by the Nutrition and Food Safety Institute of Chinese Center for Disease Control and Prevention. The unit of the total energy was kcal/d. The intake of total fat and fatty acids are presented in both absolute amount (g/d) as well as relative amount (% E).

The average energy intake of 24 provinces (autonomous regions, municipalities) was 2081 kcal/d, and the median was 2121 kcal/d. The data is comparable with the result of the average daily energy intake of 2172 kcal per standard China resident in the *Report of Chinese Residents' Nutrition and Chronic Disease Status (2015)*.

(2) Dietary Intake of Fat

The dietary intakes of total fat in various regions were between 23.5% E (39.5 g/d) and 39.5% E (104.0 g/d) with an average of 31.5% E (72.9 g/d) and a median of 30.1% E (71.1 g/d), as shown in Annexed Table 2-8

（39.5～104.0 g/d）（附表 2-8 和图 2-2），平均摄入量为 31.5% E（72.9 g/d），中位数摄入量为 30.1% E（71.1 g/d）。总的来说，膳食平均脂肪提供的能量约占能量摄入量的 1/3（31.5%），略高于脂肪 AMDR 上限 30% E。《中国居民营养与慢性病状况报告（2015 年）》指出，2012 年中国居民脂肪提供的能量比例为 32.9% E，略高于第六次中国总膳食研究结果。

and Figure 2-2. Overall, total fat was responsible for about one-third of the energy intake (31.5%), which slightly exceeded the U-AMDR of 30% E. *Report of Chinese Residents' Nutrition and Chronic Disease Status* (*2015*) pointed out that the proportion of energy from fat of China residents in 2012 was 32.9% E, which was slightly higher than the result from the 6th CTDS.

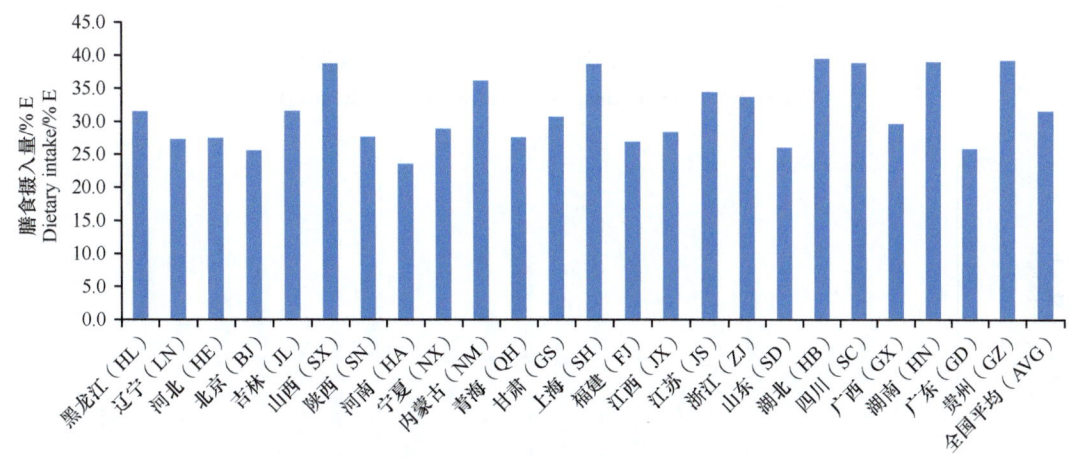

图 2-2　第六次中国总膳食研究脂肪膳食摄入量
Figure 2-2　Dietary intake of total fat from the 6th China TDS

（3）饱和脂肪酸（SFA）膳食摄入量

SFA 摄入量范围为 4.2% E～11.4% E（10.1～28.1 g/d），见附表 2-9 和图 2-3，平均摄入量 7.5% E（17.4 g/d），中位数摄入量 7.4% E（16.7 g/d）。总的来说，SFA 平均摄入量低于 U-AMDR 10% E，但略高于美国心脏病协会的 7% E 推荐值。

（4）单不饱和脂肪酸（MUFA）膳食摄入量

MUFA 摄入量范围为 6.6% E～19.6% E（15.0～52.5 g/d），见附表 2-10 和图 2-4，平均摄入量 12.5% E（29.2 g/d），中位数摄入量 12.1% E（27.4 g/d）。

(3) Dietary Intake of SFA

The dietary intakes of SFA in various regions were between 4.2% E (10.1 g/d) and 11.4% E (28.1 g/d) with an average of 7.5% E (17.4 g/d) and a median of 7.4% E (16.7 g/d), as shown in Annexed Table 2-9 and Figure 2-3. On the whole, the average SFA intake was lower than the U-AMDR of 10% E, while slightly higher than the 7% E recommended by the American Heart Association.

(4) Dietary Intake of MUFA

The dietary intake of MUFA in various regions were between 6.6% E (15.0 g/d) and 19.6% E (52.5 g/d) with an average of 12.5% E (29.2 g/d) and a median of 12.1% E (27.4 g/d), as shown in Annexed Table 2-10 and Figure 2-4.

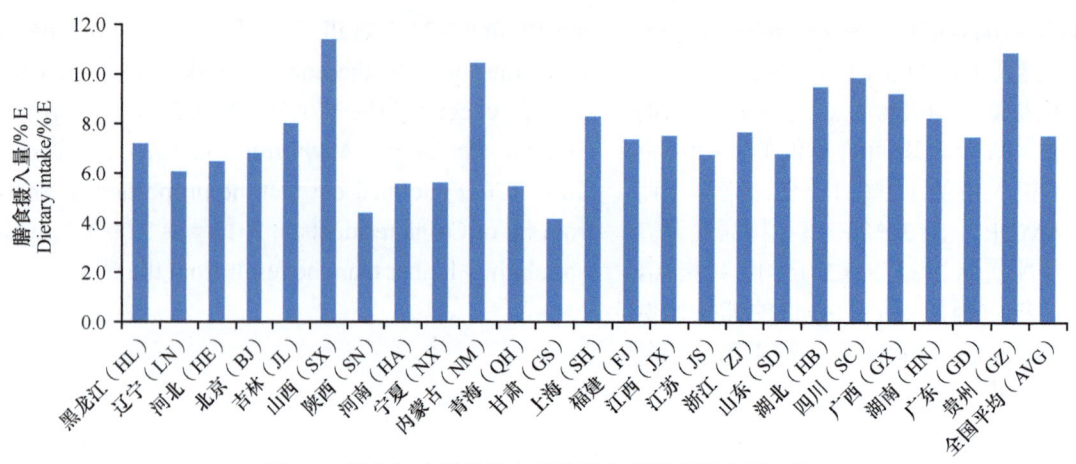

图 2-3　第六次中国总膳食研究饱和脂肪酸膳食摄入量
Figure 2-3　Dietary intake of SFA from the 6th China TDS

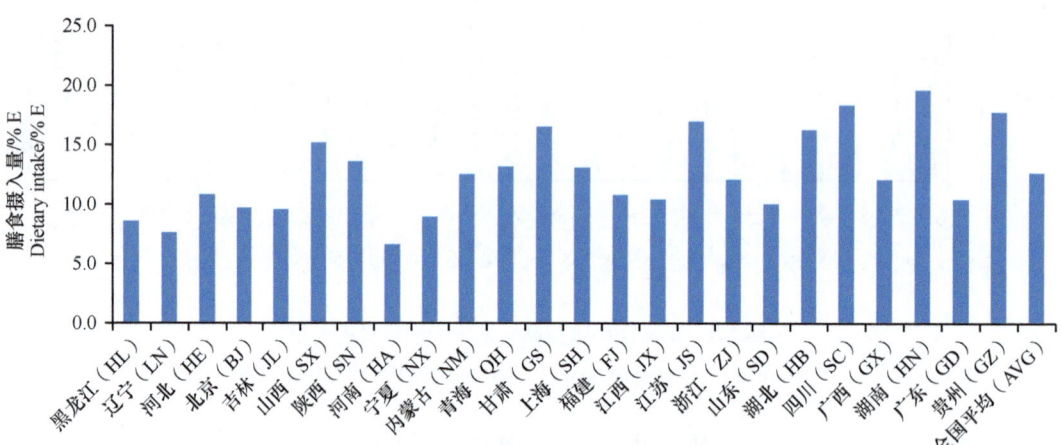

图 2-4　第六次中国总膳食研究单不饱和脂肪酸膳食摄入量
Figure 2-4　Dietary intake of MUFA from the 6th China TDS

（5）n-6 多不饱和脂肪酸（n-6 PUFA）膳食摄入量

n-6 PUFA 摄入量范围为 6.1% E～14.2% E（9.4～28.7 g/d），见附表 2-11 和图 2-5，平均摄入量 8.6% E（19.8 g/d），中位数摄入量 7.5% E（19.3 g/d）。总的来说，LA 摄入量都大于 AI 推荐值（4% E），表明 n-6 PUFA 摄入量充足。

（6）n-3 多不饱和脂肪酸（n-3 PUFA）膳食摄入量

n-3 PUFA 主要包括 ALA、EPA、DHA。n-3 PUFA 的摄入量范围为 0.2% E～5.3% E（0.5～10.7 g/d），见附表 2-12 和

(5) Dietary Intake of n-6 PUFA

The dietary intakes of n-6 PUFA in various regions were between 6.1% E (9.4 g/d) and 14.2% E (28.7 g/d) with an average of 8.6% E (19.8 g/d) and a median of 7.5% E (19.3 g/d), as shown in Annexed Table 2-11 and Figure 2-5. Overall, the intakes of LA exceeded the AI of 4% E, indicating the adequate intake.

(6) Dietary Intake of n-3 PUFA

The n-3 PUFA mainly included ALA, EPA, and DHA. The dietary intakes of n-3 PUFA were between 0.2% E (0.5 g/d) and 5.3% E (10.7 g/d) with an average of 1.2% E (2.7 g/d) and a median of 1.1% E (2.6 g/d), as shown in Annexed Table 2-12 and Figure 2-6.

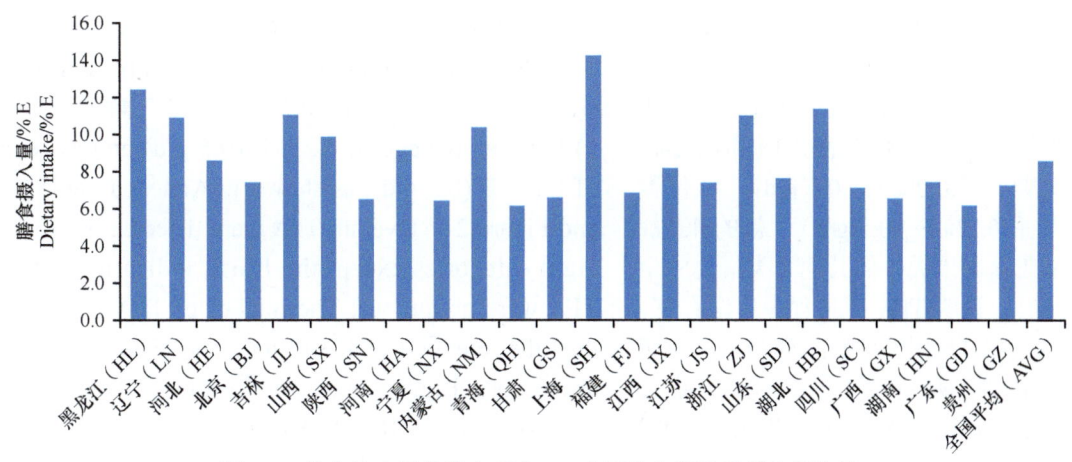

图 2-5　第六次中国总膳食研究 n-6 多不饱和脂肪酸膳食摄入量
Figure 2-5　Dietary intake of n-6 PUFA from the 6<sup>th</sup> China TDS

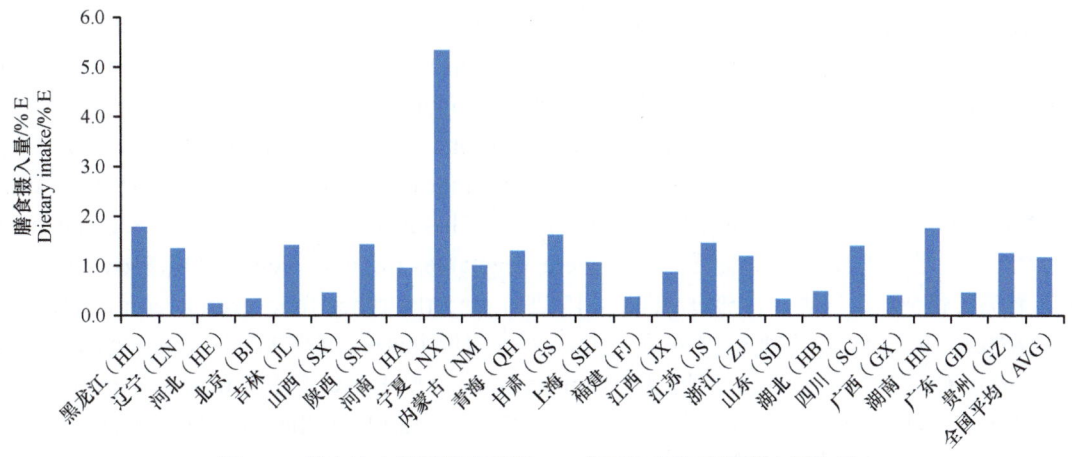

图 2-6　第六次中国总膳食研究 n-3 多不饱和脂肪酸膳食摄入量
Figure 2-6　Dietary intake of n-3 PUFA from the 6<sup>th</sup> China TDS

图 2-6，平均摄入量 1.2% E（2.7 g/d），中位数摄入量 1.1% E（2.6 g/d）。有 19 个地方的 n-3 PUFA 摄入量符合 AMDR 0.5% E～2% E 的推荐量。

EPA、DHA 的摄入量以绝对量（g/d）表示。EPA+DHA 的摄入量范围为 0.011～0.29 g/d，平均摄入量 0.067 g/d，中位数摄入量 0.039 g/d。总的来说，EPA+DHA 的摄入量低于 L-AMDR 0.25 g/d 的推荐量，表明摄入量不充足。EPA+DHA 摄入量的缺乏可导致各种慢性病风险的增加，应加以关注。

The n-3 PUFA intakes in 19 regions met the AMDR recommendation of 0.5% E-2% E.

The dietary intakes of EPA and DHA were presented as the absolute amount (g/d). The dietary intakes of EPA plus DHA in various regions were between 0.011 g/d and 0.29 g/d (average: 0.067 g/d and median: 0.039 g/d). Overall, the average dietary intake of EPA plus DHA was lower than the L-AMDR of 0.25 g/d, indicating an insufficient intake. The lack of EPA and DHA could increase the risk of various chronic diseases.

（7）反式脂肪酸（TFA）膳食摄入量

TFA 摄入量范围为 0.1% E～0.4% E（0.2～1.1 g/d），见附表 2-13 和图 2-7，平均摄入量 0.2% E（0.5 g/d），中位数摄入量 0.2% E（0.5 g/d）。总的来说，TFA 在除水果类外的其他 8 类膳食中全部检出，说明 TFA 在膳食中广泛存在，但 TFA 摄入量＜1% E 的推荐量，表明膳食中 TFA 是可接受的。对 8 类膳食进行了 C18:1 TFA、C18:2 TFA、C18:3 TFA 的分析，C18:1 TFA 摄入量范围为 0.02% E～0.1% E，平均摄入量 0.06% E，C18:1 TFA 摄入量占膳食总 TFA 摄入量的 28.7%，C18:1 TFA 膳食来源主要为肉类（43.2%）、乳类（24.4%）、蔬菜类（18.1%），其他食品类别的贡献率小于 10%。C18:2 TFA 摄入量范围为 0.03% E～0.2% E，平均摄入量 0.06% E，C18:2 TFA 摄入量占膳食总 TFA 摄入量的 28.7%，C18:2 TFA 膳食来源主要为蔬菜类（42.6%）、谷类（17.5%）、肉类（17.2%），其他食品类别的贡献率小于 10%。C18:3 TFA 摄入量范围为 0.00% E～0.3% E，平均摄入量 0.1% E，C18:3 TFA 摄入量占膳食总 TFA 摄入量的 42.8%，C18:3 TFA 膳食来源主要为蔬菜类（49.4%）、谷类（15.0%）、肉类

(7) Dietary Intake of TFA

The dietary intakes of TFA in various regions were between 0.1% E (0.2 g/d) and 0.4% E (1.1 g/d) with an average of 0.2% E (0.5 g/d) and a median of 0.2% E (0.5 g/d), as shown in Annexed Table 2-13 and Figure 2-7. Overall, TFA were detected in all other eight categories except the fruits, indicating that the TFA were ubiquitous. The intakes of TFA were lower than the reference of 1% E, thus, the dietary TFA were acceptable. Eight dietary food groups were analyzed for C18:1 TFA, C18:2 TFA and C18:3 TFA. C18:1 TFA intake ranged from 0.02% E to 0.1% E, with a mean intake of 0.06% E. C18:1 TFA intake accounted for 28.7% of total TFA intake. The main food sources of C18:1 TFA intake were meats (43.2%), dairy products (24.4%), and vegetables (18.1%), and the other food groups contributed less than 10%. The intakes of C18:2 TFA in dietary samples ranged from 0.03% E to 0.2% E with an average of 0.06% E, accounting for 28.7% of the total TFA. The main food sources of C18:2 TFA intake were vegetables (42.6%), cereals (17.5%), and meats (17.2%), and the other food groups contributed less than 10%. The intakes of C18:3 TFA in dietary samples ranged from 0.00% E to 0.3% E with an average of 0.1% E, accounting for 42.8% of the total TFA. The main food sources of C18:3 TFA intake were vegetables (49.4%), cereals (15.0%), meats (12.9%), and potatoes (12.5%), and the other food groups contributed less than 10%.

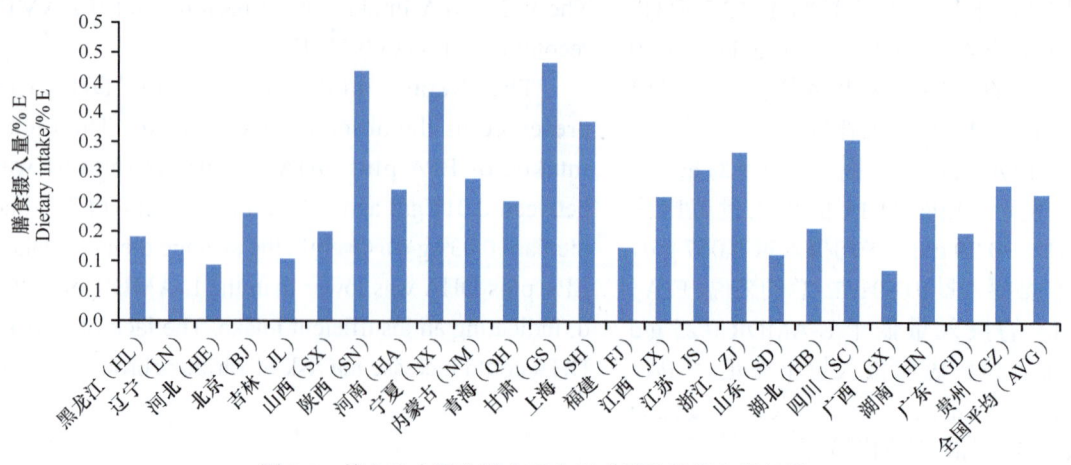

图 2-7　第六次中国总膳食研究反式脂肪酸膳食摄入量

Figure 2-7　Dietary intake of TFA from the 6th China TDS

（12.9%）、薯类（12.5%），其他食品类别的贡献率小于10%。

**3. 各类膳食对总膳食摄入的贡献**

总脂肪酸的主要膳食来源为肉类（33.1%）、蔬菜类（29.5%）和谷类（13.2%），其他食品类别的贡献率小于10%。SFA的主要膳食来源为肉类（45.4%）、蔬菜类（19.6%）和谷类（13.6%），其他食品类别的贡献率小于10%。MUFA的主要膳食来源为肉类（35.5%）和蔬菜类（32.0%），其他食品类别的贡献率小于10%。n-6 PUFA的主要膳食来源为蔬菜类（33.1%）、肉类（21.4%）、谷类（18.5%）和豆类（13.0%），其他食品类别的贡献率小于10%。n-3 PUFA的主要膳食来源为蔬菜类（38.9%）、肉类（15.9%）、豆类（12.7%）、谷类（12.1%）和薯类（10.7%），其他食品类别的贡献率小于10%。TFA的主要膳食来源为蔬菜类（37.9%）、肉类（23.4%）和谷类（13.7%），其他食品类别的贡献率小于10%。总脂肪酸、SFA、MUFA、n-6和n-3 PUFA与TFA的膳食来源见附表2-14～附表2-19和图2-8～图2-13。

**3. Contributions of Food Categories to the Total Dietary Intake**

The primary sources of dietary intake to total fatty acids were meats (33.1%), vegetables (29.5%) and cereals (13.2%), and the other food groups contributed less than 10%. The primary sources of dietary intake to SFA were meats (45.4%), vegetables (19.6%), and cereals (13.6%) and the other food groups contributed less than 10%. The primary sources of dietary intake to MUFA were meats (35.5%) and vegetables (32.0%) and the other food groups contributed less than 10%. The primary sources of dietary intake to n-6 PUFA were vegetables (33.1%), meats (21.4%), cereals (18.5%), and legumes (13.0%) and the other food groups contributed less than 10%. The primary sources of dietary intake to n-3 PUFA were vegetables (38.9%), meats (15.9%), legumes (12.7%), cereals (12.1%) and potatoes (10.7%) and the other food groups contributed less than 10%. The primary sources of dietary intake to TFA were vegetables (37.9%), meats (23.4%), and cereals (13.7%) and the other food groups contributed less than 10%, as shown in Annexed Table 2-14-Annexed Table 2-19 and Figure 2-8-Figure 2-13.

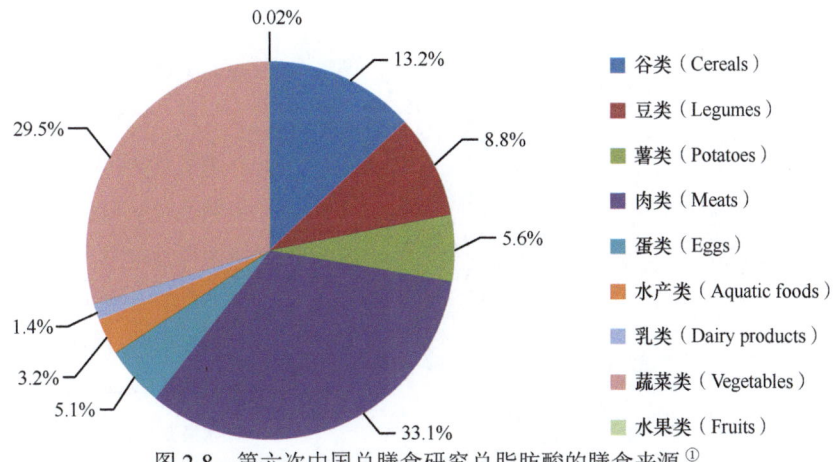

图2-8 第六次中国总膳食研究总脂肪酸的膳食来源[①]

Figure 2-8 Dietary sources of total fatty acids from the 6th China TDS

---

① 比例之和不为100%是因为数据进行过舍入修约，下同

the sum of proportions is not 100% is because the data has been rounded off, the same below

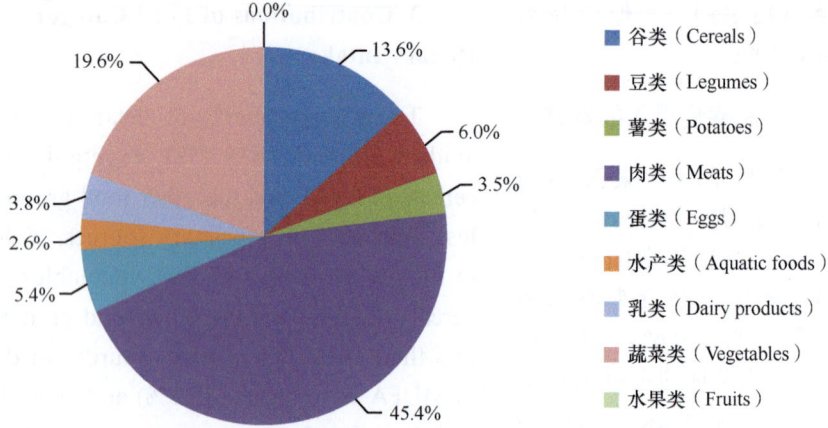

图 2-9　第六次中国总膳食研究饱和脂肪酸的膳食来源
Figure 2-9　Dietary sources of SFA from the 6th China TDS

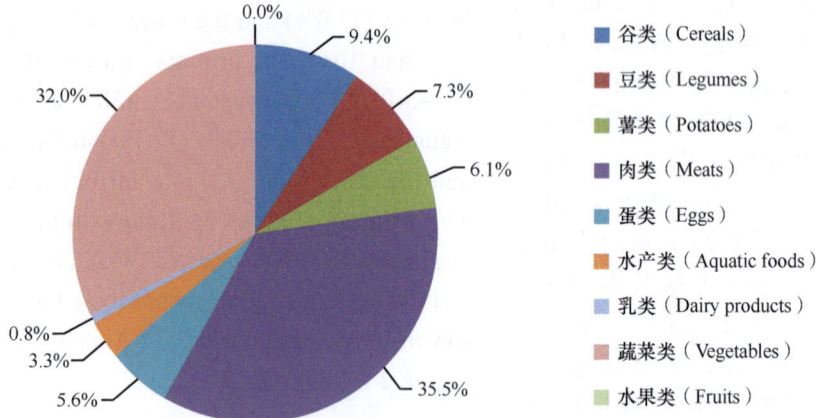

图 2-10　第六次中国总膳食研究单不饱和脂肪酸的膳食来源
Figure 2-10　Dietary sources of MUFA from the 6th China TDS

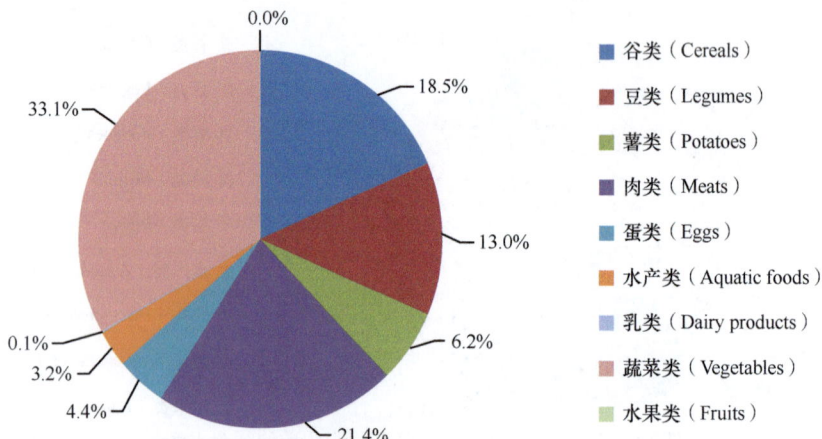

图 2-11　第六次中国总膳食研究单 n-6 多不饱和脂肪酸的膳食来源
Figure 2-11　Dietary sources of n-6 PUFA from the 6th China TDS

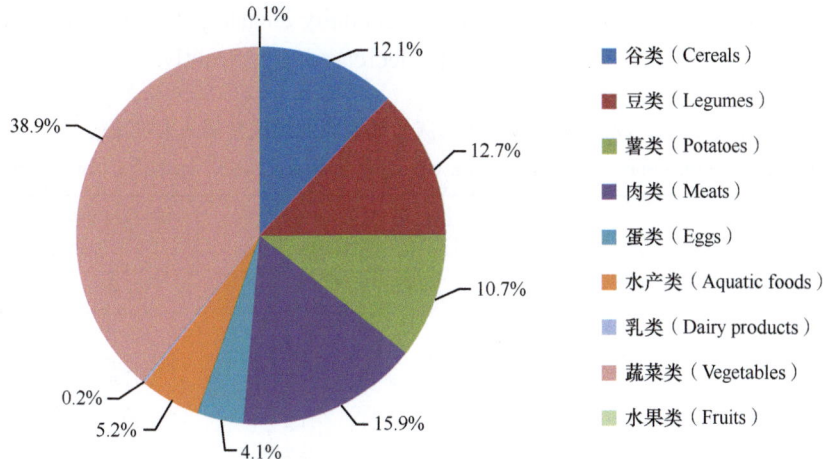

图 2-12 第六次中国总膳食研究单 n-3 多不饱和脂肪酸的膳食来源
Figure 2-12　Dietary sources of n-3 PUFA from the 6$^{th}$ China TDS

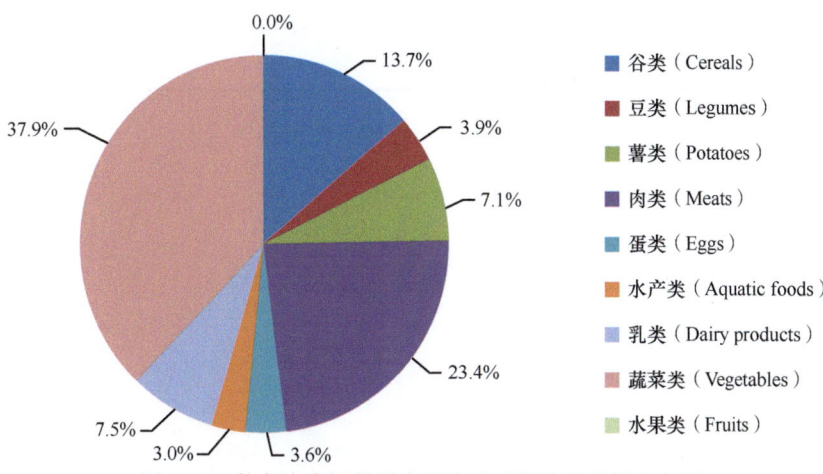

图 2-13 第六次中国总膳食研究反式脂肪酸的膳食来源
Figure 2-13　Dietary sources of *trans*-fatty acids from the 6$^{th}$ China TDS

## 四、与以往中国总膳食研究结果的比较

第五次和第六次 CTDS 的脂肪酸的膳食摄入量比较见表 2-2。第五次 CTDS 使用的是 2012 年中国居民城乡能量摄入值（2172 kcal）进行供能比的计算，而第六次 CTDS 使用的是 24 个省（自治区、直辖市）平均能量摄入值（2081 kcal）进行供能比的计算。与第五次中国总膳食研究相比，总脂肪酸、SFA、MUFA、n-6 和 n-3 PUFA 与 TFA

## Ⅳ. Comparison with Previous China TDSs Results

The comparison of the dietary intakes of fatty acids between the 5$^{th}$ CTDS and 6$^{th}$ CTDS was shown in Table 2-2. For the 5$^{th}$ CTDS, the value of 2172 kcal of the energy intake of China residents in urban and rural areas in 2012 was used to calculate the percentage of total energy intake; and, for the 6$^{th}$ CTDS, the value of 2081 kcal of the average energy intake of 24 regions was used to calculate the percentage of total energy intake. Compared with the 5$^{th}$ China TDS, the intakes of total fatty acids, SFA, MUFA, n-6 PUFA, n-3 PUFA and TFA

摄入量基本持平，而 EPA + DHA 摄入量明显降低。

were essentially unchanged, and the intakes of EPA plus DHA decreased significantly.

表 2-2　第五次和第六次中国总膳食研究脂肪酸膳食摄入情况比较

Table 2-2　Comparison of intakes of fatty acids between the 5th and 6th China TDSs

| 脂肪酸 Fatty acids | 第五次中国总膳食研究摄入量 Intake of 5th CTDS ||  第六次中国总膳食研究摄入量 Intake of 6th CTDS ||
|---|---|---|---|---|
|  | g/d | %E | g/d | %E |
| 总脂肪酸 Total fatty acids | 71.9 | 29.8 | 69.6 | 30.1 |
| 饱和脂肪酸（SFA） | 19.2 | 8.0 | 17.4 | 7.5 |
| 单不饱和脂肪酸（MUFA） | 27.0 | 11.2 | 29.2 | 12.5 |
| 多不饱和脂肪酸（PUFA） | 25.4 | 10.5 | 22.5 | 9.7 |
| n-3 多不饱和脂肪酸（n-3 PUFA） | 3.4 | 1.4 | 2.7 | 1.2 |
| n-6 多不饱和脂肪酸（n-6 PUFA） | 22.0 | 9.1 | 19.8 | 8.6 |
| 反式脂肪酸（TFA） | 0.6 | 0.2 | 0.5 | 0.2 |
| EPA +DHA | 0.16 |  | 0.067 |  |

# 第三章 元素的膳食暴露评估
# Chapter 3  Dietary Exposure Assessment of Elements

## 第一部分 营 养 元 素
## Part 1  Nutrient Elements

食物中的营养元素对人体的许多结构和功能都起着重要的作用。中国膳食指南推荐居民饮食多样化，以便摄入足够的营养成分。从公共健康的角度评估营养成分摄入是否充足是非常重要的，因为营养成分摄入不足或者摄入过量都会对健康造成不利的影响。这与农药残留、兽药残留和污染物所引起的健康隐患不同。

第六次中国总膳食研究对钠、钾、钙、镁、磷、锰、铁、锌、铬、铜、硒、钼和碘元素进行了评估。

Nutritional components in foods play an important role in many structures and functions of the human body. China's national dietary guide recommends dietary diversification for adequate intake of nutrient elements. It is very important to assess the adequacy of dietary intake to nutrient elements from the perspective of public health because both inadequate and excessive intake of nutrient elements will have a negative impact on health. This is different from the health risks caused by pesticides, veterinary drugs and contaminants.

The chemical elements assessed in the 6$^{th}$ China TDS include sodium, potassium, calcium, magnesium, phosphorus, manganese, iron, zinc, chromium, copper, selenium, molybdenum and iodine.

### 第一节 钠 和 钾
### Section 1  Sodium and Potassium

一、背景

钠和钾是人体内极为重要的常量元素。其作为溶解于体液内的电解质，具有维持体液的酸碱平衡、维持细胞内正常渗透压、维持神经肌肉的应激性和正常功能等重要作用。此外，钾还参与细胞新陈代谢和酶促反应。研究证实，膳食中钠摄入量与血压呈正相关。提高膳食钾的摄入量有助于预防高血压等慢性病（柳鹏等，2011；牟建军等，

Ⅰ. Background

Sodium and potassium are extremely important macroelements in human body. As electrolytes dissolved in body fluid, potassium and sodium play important role in maintaining the body fluids' acid-base balance, maintaining normal osmotic pressure in cells, and maintaining neuromuscular stress and normal function. In addition, potassium involves in cell metabolism and enzymatic reactions. Studies have confirmed that dietary sodium intake is positively correlated with

2016)。膳食中钠钾摄入比值是影响人群血压水平和高血压的一个重要因素。

## 二、健康指导值

以《中国居民膳食营养素参考摄入量（2013版）》中的适宜摄入量来评价中国居民膳食钠、钾摄入状况，成人膳食钠的适宜摄入量（AI）为每人1500 mg/d，成人膳食钾的适宜摄入量（AI）为每人2000 mg/d（中国营养学会，2014）。

## 三、总膳食研究结果

### 1. 总膳食研究样品中钠和钾的含量

对24个省（自治区、直辖市）的12类混合膳食样品进行钠含量和钾含量的检测。结果如附表3-1所示，钠含量较高的样品依次为肉类、蛋类、水产类及蔬菜类。附表3-4显示，水产类、肉类、豆类及蔬菜类食物的钾含量较高。

### 2. 膳食暴露评估

我国居民膳食中钠的摄入量（附表3-2，图3-1）平均值为4485 mg/d，范围为2825～6427 mg/d，均远高于钠的AI值（1500 mg/d）。

我国居民钾的膳食摄入量（附表3-5，图3-2）平均值为2024 mg/d，相当于钾AI值的101%。膳食钾摄入量范围为1004～3412 mg/d。

blood pressure. Increasing dietary potassium intake can help prevent chronic diseases such as hypertension (Liu et al., 2011; Mou et al., 2016). The ratio of dietary sodium intake to potassium intake is an important factor affecting blood pressure levels and hypertension.

## Ⅱ. HBGV

The adequate intakes (AI) recommended in *Chinese Dietary Reference Intakes* (*2013 version*) were used to assess the dietary intake of sodium and potassium of China residents. The AI value of sodium is 1500 mg/d per person for adults, and that of potassium is 2000 mg/d per person for adults (Chinese Nutrition Society, 2014).

## Ⅲ. TDS Results

### 1. Levels of Sodium and Potassium in TDS Composite Samples

Composite dietary samples of 12 food categories from 24 provinces (autonomous regions, municipalities) were analyzed for the level of sodium and potassium. Annexed Table 3-1 shows foods that were rich in sodium including meats, eggs, aquatic foods, and vegetables. Annexed Table 3-4 shows foods that were rich in potassium including aquatic foods, meats, legumes, and vegetables.

### 2. Dietary Exposure Assessment

The average dietary sodium intake for China residents (Annexed Table 3-2, Figure 3-1) was 4485 mg/d, ranging from 2825 mg/d to 6427 mg/d, much higher than the AI value for sodium (1500 mg/d).

The average dietary intake of potassium for China residents (Annexed Table 3-5, Figure 3-2) was 2024 mg/d, equivalent to 101% of the AI value for potassium, ranging from 1004 mg/d to 3412 mg/d.

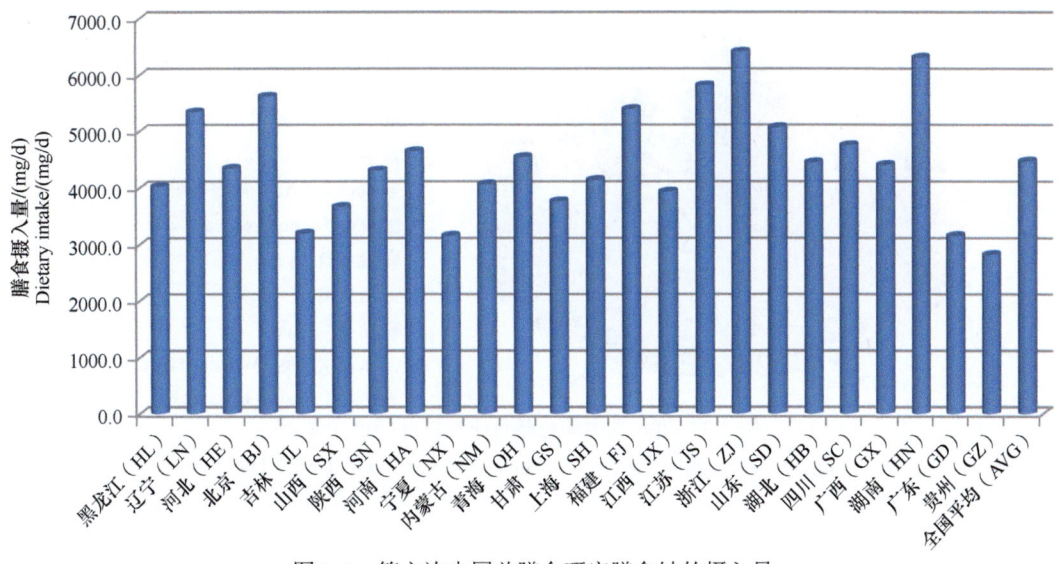

图 3-1 第六次中国总膳食研究膳食钠的摄入量
Figure 3-1 Dietary sodium intakes from 6$^{th}$ China TDS

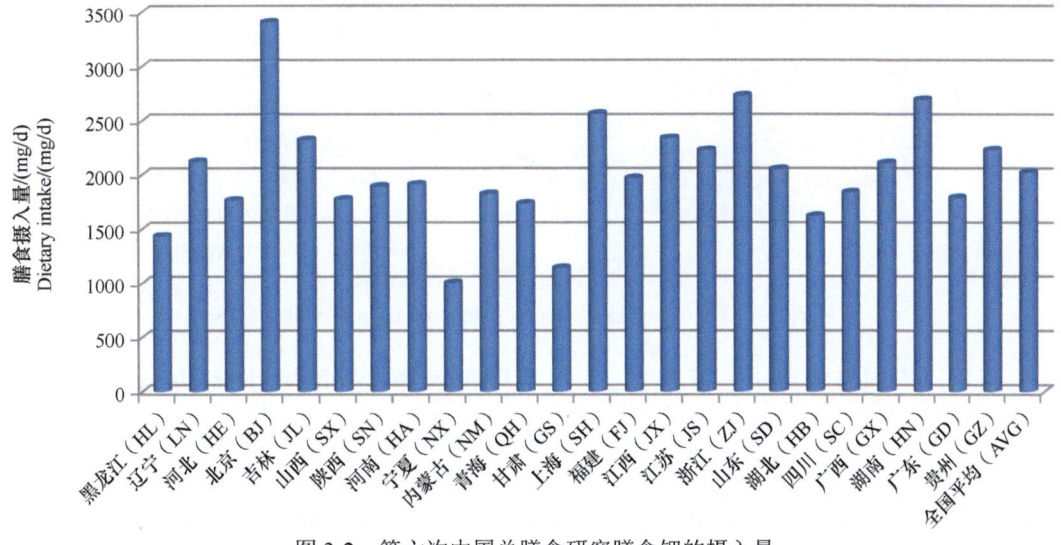

图 3-2 第六次中国总膳食研究膳食钾的摄入量
Figure 3-2 Dietary potassium intakes from 6$^{th}$ China TDS

### 3. 各类膳食对总膳食摄入的贡献

我国居民膳食钠的主要摄入来源（附表 3-3，图 3-3）依次是蔬菜类、谷类和肉类。我国居民膳食钾的主要摄入来源（附表 3-6，图 3-4）和钠类似，依次是蔬菜类、谷类和肉类。

### 3. Contributions of Food Categories to the Total Dietary Intake

The primary sources of sodium and potassium intakes of China residents (Annexed Table 3-3 and Annexed Table 3-6, Figure 3-3 and Figure 3-4) were vegetables, followed by cereals and meats.

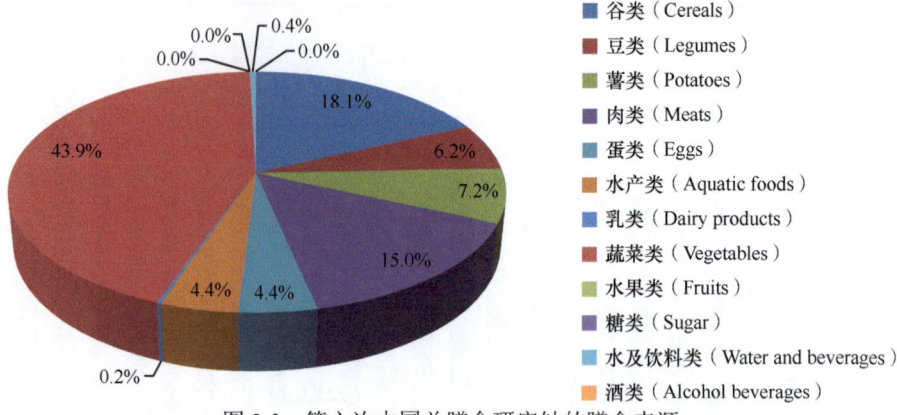

图 3-3　第六次中国总膳食研究钠的膳食来源
Figure 3-3　Food sources of dietary sodium from 6th China TDS

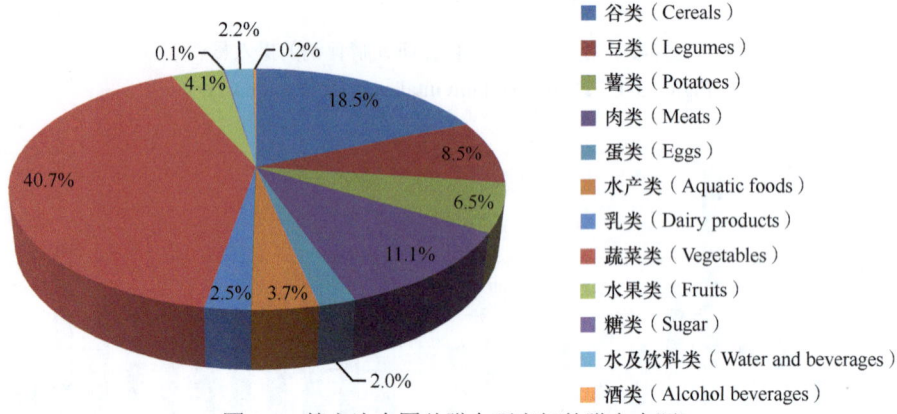

图 3-4　第六次中国总膳食研究钾的膳食来源
Figure 3-4　Food sources of dietary potassium from 6th China TDS

**4. 与以往中国总膳食研究结果的比较**

与 4th CTDS、5th CTDS 比较，6th CTDS 中我国居民膳食钠的平均摄入量分别降低了 26% 和 15%；我国居民膳食钾的平均摄入量分别降低了 8% 和 15%。

**4. Comparison with Previous China TDSs Results**

As compared to the 4th and 5th China TDSs, the average dietary sodium intake of China residents in the 6th CTDS decreased by 26% and 15%, respectively, and the average dietary potassium intake in the 6th CTDS decreased by 8% and 15%, respectively.

## 第二节　钙
## Section 2　Calcium

### 一、背景
### Ⅰ. Background

钙是人体必需的一种重要营养元

Calcium is one of the essential nutrients in the body,

素，维持人体多种生理功能，如参与凝血、肌肉收缩、神经递质合成和释放、激素合成与分泌等生理过程，并对多种酶具有激活作用。绝大部分钙存在于骨骼中，少量存在于牙齿中，其余存在于血液和组织里。钙缺乏会造成佝偻病和成年人骨软化症，导致骨质疏松，甚至发生脊柱压缩性骨折；还会造成肌肉紧张，严重时产生痉挛（WHO，2004；EFSA，2006b）。

## 二、健康指导值

以《中国居民膳食营养素参考摄入量（2013 版）》中的推荐摄入量（RNI）来评价中国居民膳食钙的摄入状况，成人钙的 RNI 为每人 800 mg/d（中国营养学会，2014）。

## 三、总膳食研究结果

### 1. 总膳食研究样品中钙的含量

对 24 个省（自治区、直辖市）的 12 类混合膳食样品进行钙含量的检测，结果如附表 3-7 所示，钙含量较高的样品是豆类和乳类，其次是水产类。

### 2. 膳食暴露评估

我国 24 个省（自治区、直辖市）居民膳食钙摄入量平均为 481 mg/d，范围为 314～755 mg/d（附表 3-8，图 3-5）。我国居民膳食钙的摄入量均低于 RNI，平均钙摄入量相当于 60% RNI。钙摄入量较高的江苏和贵州两个省分别达到 94% RNI 和 93% RNI。中国居民钙摄入量普遍偏低。

maintaining a variety of physiological functions, such as blood coagulation, muscle contraction, neurotransmitter synthesis and release, hormone synthesis and secretion, and other physiological processes, and has an activation effect on a variety of enzymes. The majority of calcium is present in bones, with a little amount in the teeth, and the rest in the blood and tissues. The deficiency of calcium causes rickets, osteomalacia in adults, leading to osteoporosis and even spinal compression fractures. It can also cause muscle tension and, in severe cases, spasms (WHO, 2004; EFSA, 2006b).

## II. HBGV

The recommended nutrient intake (RNI) in the *Chinese Dietary Reference Intakes* (*2013 version*) was used to assess the adequacy of dietary calcium intake of China residents. The RNI of calcium is 800 mg/d per person (Chinese Nutrition Society, 2014).

## III. TDS Results

### 1. Levels of Calcium in TDS Composite Samples

Composite samples of 12 food categories from 24 provinces (autonomous regions, municipalities) were analyzed for the level of calcium. Annexed Table 3-7 shows foods that were rich in calcium, including legumes, dairy products, and aquatic foods.

### 2. Dietary Exposure Assessment

The average dietary intake of calcium for China residents was 481 mg/d, ranging from 314 mg/d to 755 mg/d in 24 provinces (autonomous regions, municipalities) (Annexed Table 3-8, Figure 3-5). The dietary intake of calcium was below the RNI value, and the average calcium intake was only 60% of the RNI. The calcium intakes in Jiangsu and Guizhou were 94% RNI and 93% RNI, respectively. The calcium intakes of China residents were generally low.

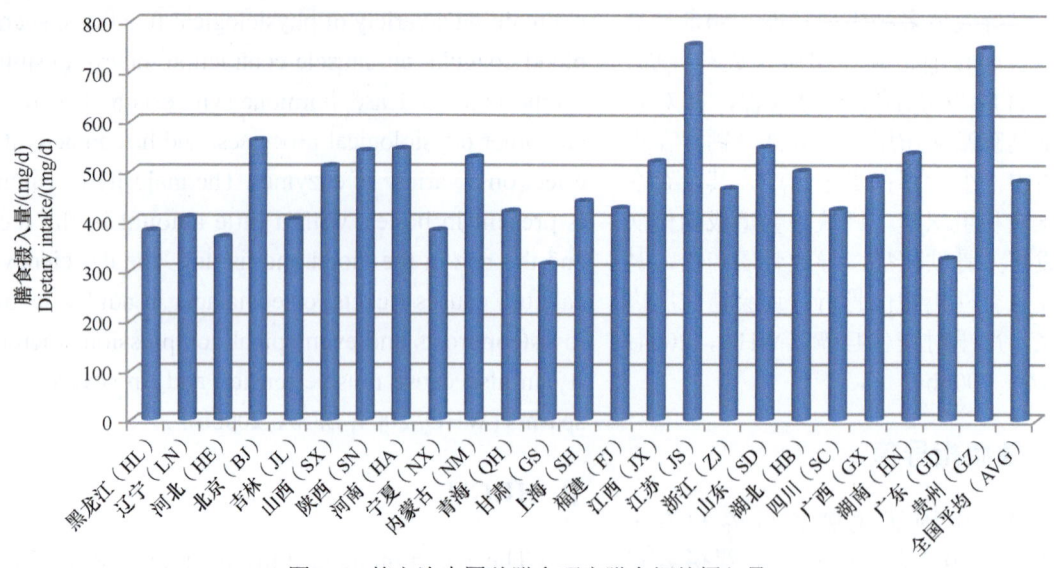

图 3-5 第六次中国总膳食研究膳食钙的摄入量

Figure 3-5 Dietary calcium intakes from 6th China TDS

## 3. 各类膳食对总膳食摄入的贡献

我国居民膳食钙摄入的主要来源（附表 3-9，图 3-6）为蔬菜类（31.9%）、谷类（19.0%）和豆类（18.8%），约占总摄入来源的 70%。因钙含量较高的乳类食物消费量低，致使整体钙的摄入量偏低。这与我国居民的饮食结构密切相关。

## 3. Contributions of Food Categories to the Total Dietary Intake

The main sources of calcium intake for China residents (Annexed Table 3-9, Figure 3-6) were vegetables (31.9%), cereals (19.0%) and legumes (18.8%), accounting for about 70% of the total intake. Due to the low consumption of calcium-rich foods such as dairy products, the overall calcium intake was rather low. This is closely related to the dietary structure of China residents.

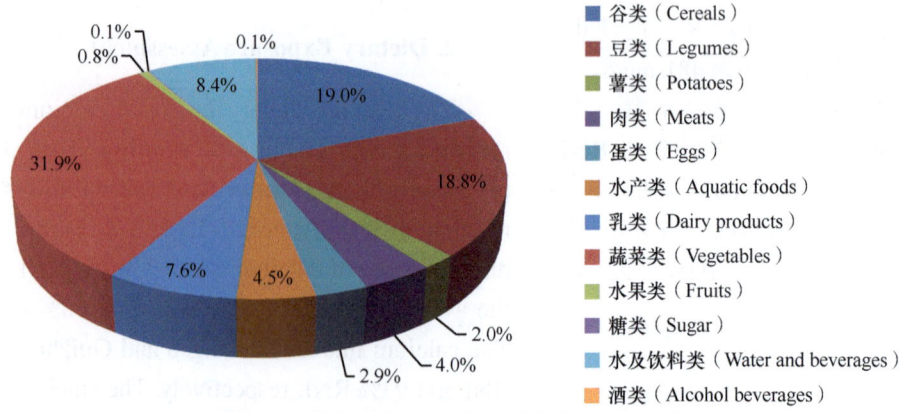

图 3-6 第六次中国总膳食研究钙的膳食来源

Figure 3-6 Food sources of dietary calcium from 6th China TDS

## 4. 与以往中国总膳食研究结果的比较

6<sup>th</sup> CTDS 我国居民平均膳食钙摄入量比 4<sup>th</sup> CTDS 降低了 20%，与 5<sup>th</sup> CTDS 相当。这三次 CTDS 中我国居民平均膳食钙摄入量都没有达到钙的 RNI 值（800 mg/d）。

## 4. Comparison with Previous China TDSs Results

The average calcium intake of China residents in the 6$^{th}$ CTDS was 20% lower than that of the 4$^{th}$ CTDS and similar to that in the 5$^{th}$ CTDS. In these three CTDSs, the average calcium intakes of China residents were all lower than the RNI value of calcium (800 mg/d).

# 第三节　镁
# Section 3　Magnesium

## 一、背景

镁是维持生命活动的必需元素。镁几乎参与了所有的新陈代谢，维持核酸机制的稳定，抑制神经的兴奋性，参与蛋白质合成、肌肉收缩等。镁参与体内 300 多种酶促反应。镁缺乏的早期表现常有厌食、恶心、呕吐等。镁缺乏加重可造成记忆力减退、心律失常、高血压、冠心病等。过量镁摄入会导致四肢软弱无力、心律失常甚至昏迷（张忠诚等，2006）。

## 二、健康指导值

以《中国居民膳食营养素参考摄入量（2013 版）》中的推荐摄入量（RNI）来评价中国居民膳食镁摄入状况，成人膳食镁摄入的 RNI 值为每人 330 mg/d（中国营养学会，2014）。

## 三、总膳食研究结果

### 1. 总膳食研究样品中镁的含量

对 24 个省（自治区、直辖市）的 12 类混合膳食样品进行镁含量检测，结果见附表 3-10，膳食样品中镁含量较高的样品依次为豆类、水产类和肉类食品。

## I. Background

Magnesium is an essential element for life and is widely involved in human metabolic processes, maintaining the stability of nucleic acid mechanism, inhibiting the excitability of nerves, participating in protein synthesis, muscle contraction and so on. Magnesium also takes part in more than 300 enzymatic reactions. Magnesium deficiency early leads to anorexia, nausea, and vomiting. Severe magnesium deficiency can cause memory loss, arrhythmia, hypertension, coronary heart disease, etc. Excessive magnesium intake can cause weakness in the limbs, heart rhythm disturbances and even coma (Zhang et al., 2006).

## II. HBGV

The recommended nutrient intake (RNI) in the *Chinese Dietary Reference Intakes* (*2013 version*) was used to assess the dietary magnesium intake of China residents. The RNI value of magnesium is 330 mg/d per person for adults (Chinese Nutrition Society, 2014).

## III. TDS Results

### 1. Levels of Magnesium in TDS Composite Samples

Composite samples of 12 food categories from 24 provinces (autonomous regions, municipalities) were analyzed for the level of magnesium. Annexed Table

**2. 膳食暴露评估**

我国24个省（自治区、直辖市）居民膳食镁的摄入量（附表3-11，图3-7）范围为182～504 mg/d，平均摄入量为305 mg/d，相当于镁RNI值（330 mg/d）的92%。有17个省（自治区、直辖市）居民膳食镁的摄入量没有达到RNI值。

3-10 shows foods that were rich in magnesium including legumes, aquatic foods, and meats.

**2. Dietary Exposure Assessment**

The average dietary intake of magnesium for China residents was 305 mg/d, ranging from 182 mg/d to 504 mg/d in 24 provinces (autonomous regions, municipalities) (Annexed Table 3-11, Figure 3-7). The average magnesium intake was equivalent to 92% of the RNI. Magnesium intakes were below the RNI in 17 provinces (autonomous regions, municipalities).

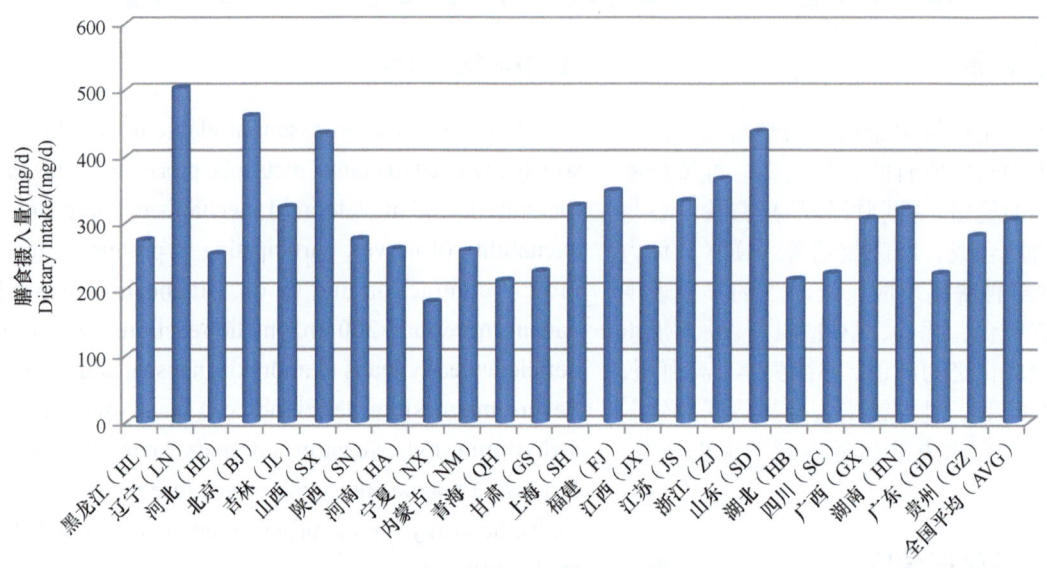

图 3-7　第六次中国总膳食研究膳食镁的摄入量
Figure 3-7　Dietary magnesium intakes from 6th China TDS

**3. 各类膳食对总膳食摄入的贡献**

我国居民膳食镁摄入的主要来源（附表3-12，图3-8）依次是谷类、蔬菜类和豆类，占膳食镁总摄入量的75%以上。

**4. 与以往中国总膳食研究结果的比较**

6th CTDS 中我国居民平均膳食镁摄入量与 4th CTDS 相当，比 5th CTDS 降低了11%。4th CTDS、5th CTDS 和 6th CTDS 的膳食平均镁摄入量分别达到

**3. Contributions of Food Categories to the Total Dietary Intake**

The main sources of magnesium intake for China residents (Annexed Table 3-12, Figure 3-8) were cereals, vegetables, and legumes, accounting for over 75% of all the total intake.

**4. Comparison with Previous China TDSs Results**

The average magnesium intake of China residents in the 6th CTDS was 11%, lower than that of the 5th CTDS and similar to that in the 4th CTDS. The average magnesium intakes in the 4th CTDS, 5th CTDS, and 6th

RNI 值（330 mg/d）的 94%、104% 和 92%。

CTDS were 94%, 104%, and 92% of the RNI value, respectively.

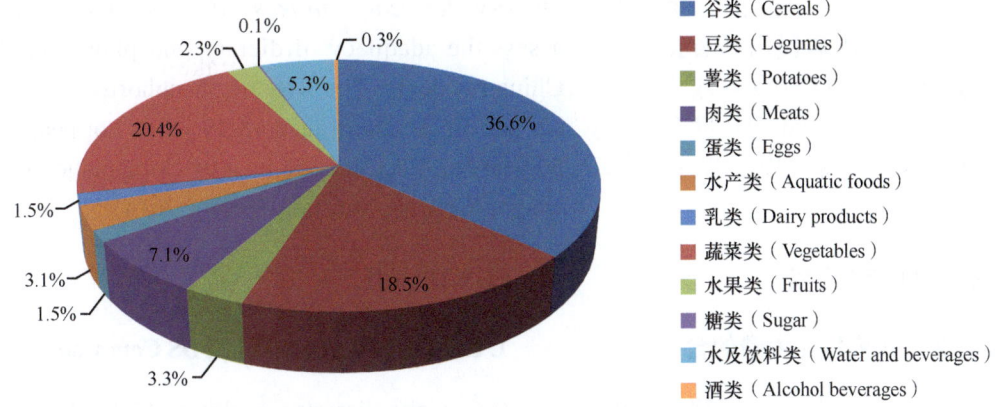

图 3-8　第六次中国总膳食研究镁的膳食来源
Figure 3-8　Food sources of dietary magnesium from 6$^{th}$ China TDS

## 第四节　磷
## Section 4　Phosphorus

### 一、背景

### I. Background

磷是机体极为重要的元素之一，约占成人体重的 1%，其中 85.7% 集中在骨骼和牙齿中，其余的分布在人体的细胞、蛋白质、全身各组织中（贺婷婷和左兆成，2013）。磷缺乏会引起骨骼和牙齿发育不正常、骨质疏松、软骨病、食欲不振等症状，食物中磷含量普遍而丰富，故很少由膳食原因引起营养性磷缺乏。但磷摄入过多会干扰钙的吸收，当膳食中的钙磷比例过低（≤0.5），可致血磷升高、尿钙排出增加，干扰钙代谢（中国营养学会，2014）。因此，我们在关注磷缺乏时应同时防止磷过量引发的危害。

Phosphorus is one of the most important elements in the body, accounting for about 1% of the adult body weight. 85.7% of phosphorus in the human body is contained in bones and teeth, and the rest is distributed in human cells, proteins, and tissues throughout the body (He and Zuo, 2013). Phosphorus deficiency can cause several symptoms, such as abnormal development of bones and teeth, osteoporosis, osteomalacia, and the loss of appetite. The phosphorus content in food is widespread and abundant. So nutritional phosphorus deficiency was rarely due to dietary causes. However, excessive phosphorus intake will interfere with the absorption of calcium. When the proportion of calcium and phosphorus in the diet is too low (≤0.5), it would increase blood phosphorus and increase urinary calcium excretion, interfering with metabolism (Chinese Nutrition Society, 2014). Therefore, when we are concerned about phosphorus deficiency, we should also prevent the harm caused by phosphorus excess.

## 二、健康指导值

以《中国居民膳食营养素参考摄入量（2013版）》中的推荐摄入量（RNI）来评价中国居民由膳食摄入的磷元素是否充足，18~49岁成人磷的RNI值为每人720 mg/d，50岁及以上根据体重外推法计算（中国营养学会，2014）。

## 三、总膳食研究结果

### 1. 总膳食研究样品中磷的含量

对24个省（自治区、直辖市）的12类混合膳食样品进行磷含量检测，结果见附表3-13。膳食样品中磷含量较高的样品为蛋类、水产类、肉类、豆类和乳类食品。膳食样品中磷含量存在地区差异。

### 2. 膳食暴露评估

我国居民磷的膳食摄入量（附表3-14、图3-9）平均为890mg/d，全国24个省（自治区、直辖市）为572~1166 mg/d；我国大部分省份居民膳食

## Ⅱ. HBGV

Recommended nutrient intake (RNI) in the *Chinese Dietary Reference Intakes* (*2013 version*) is used to assess the adequacy of dietary phosphorus intake of China residents. The RNI of phosphorus is 720 mg/d per person for adults aged 18-49 years. For people aged 50 years or older, it is derived by extrapolation of body weight (Chinese Nutrition Society, 2014).

## Ⅲ. TDS Results

### 1. Levels of Phosphorus in TDS Composite Samples

Composite dietary samples of 12 food categories from 24 provinces (autonomous regions, municipalities) were analyzed for the level of phosphorus. Annexed Table 3-13 shows foods that were rich in phosphorus including eggs, aquatic foods, meats, legumes, and dairy products. The levels of phosphorus in food samples varied by region.

### 2. Dietary Exposure Assessment

The average dietary intake of phosphorus for China residents (Annexed Table 3-14, Figure 3-9) was 890 mg/d, ranging from 572 mg/d to 1166 mg/d in 24 provinces

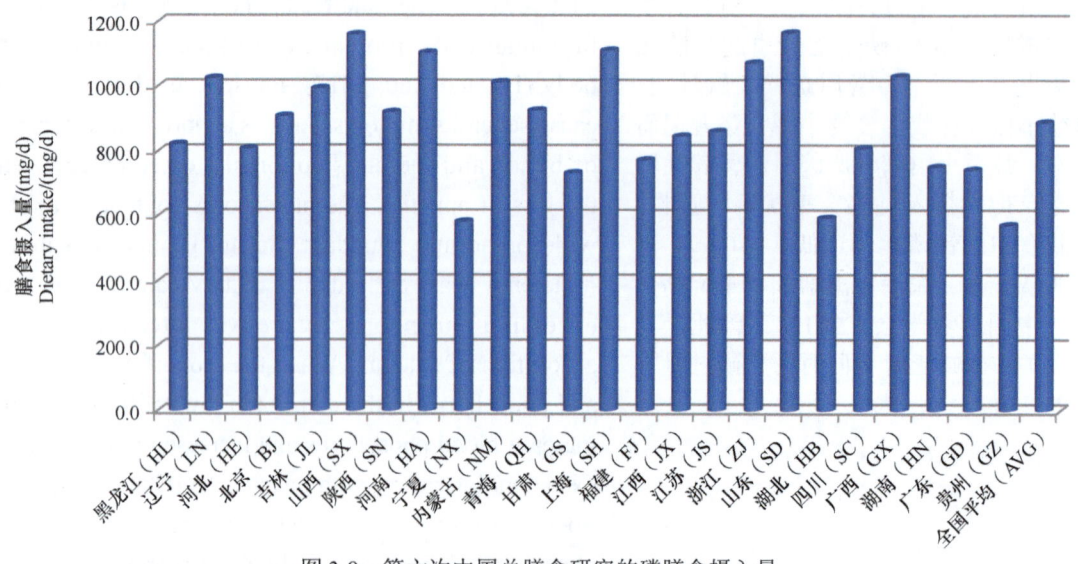

图 3-9　第六次中国总膳食研究的磷膳食摄入量

Figure 3-9　Dietary intake of phosphorus from the 6$^{th}$ China TDS

磷的摄入量高于 RNI 值，仅有 3 个省份居民膳食磷的摄入量略低，约为 RNI 的 80%。

**3. 各类膳食对总膳食摄入的贡献**

6th CTDS 我国居民磷的主要膳食来源（附表 3-15，图 3-10）为谷类、肉类、蔬菜和豆类，约占总摄入来源的 80%。

(autonomous regions, municipalities). In most provinces, the dietary intake of phosphorus was higher than the RNI value for phosphorus. Only three provinces had a slightly lower intake of phosphorus, where the level was equivalent to 80% of the RNI.

**3. Contributions of Food Categories to the Total Dietary Intake**

The primary sources of dietary intake of phosphorus in the 6th CTDS (Annexed Table 3-15, Figure 3-10) were cereals, meats, vegetables, and legumes, accounting for about 80% of the total intake.

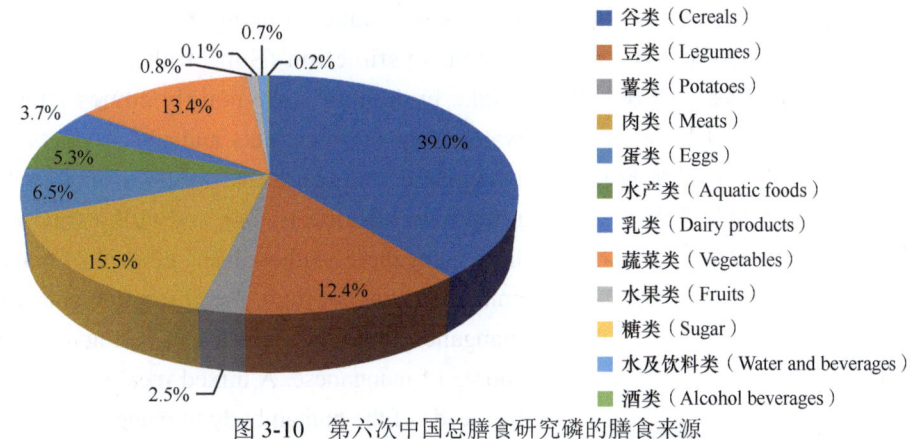

图 3-10　第六次中国总膳食研究磷的膳食来源
Figure 3-10　Dietary sources of phosphorus from the 6th China TDS

**4. 与以往中国总膳食研究结果的比较**

与第五次中国总膳食研究相比，第六次中国总膳食研究磷的平均摄入量有所下降，由第五次中国总膳食研究的 1189.5 mg/d 下降至第六次中国总膳食研究的 890 mg/d。各类膳食对总膳食磷的贡献变化不大。

**4. Comparison with Previous China TDSs Results**

Compared with the 5th China TDS, the dietary intake of phosphorus decreased in the 6th China TDS, the average intake of phosphorus decreased from 1189.5 mg/d in the 5th China TDS to 890 mg/d in the 6th China TDS. There was little change in the contributions of different food categories to total phosphorus intake.

# 第五节 锰
# Section 5　Manganese

## 一、背景

锰广泛存在于自然环境中，是地壳最丰富的金属元素之一，也是人类和其他生物正常生长、发育及维持细胞内环境稳定所必需的微量元素（滕小华等，2021）。锰缺乏会引起生长迟缓、生育力损害以及出生缺陷。过量的锰摄入会造成中枢神经系统损伤（孙中兴等，2011）。人体摄入锰主要来自膳食和水，粗粮、坚果、豆制品中富含锰，茶叶内锰含量最丰富，精制的谷类、肉类、鱼类、奶类中锰含量比较少。虽然动物性食物锰含量不高，但其吸收和存留较高，仍不失为锰的良好来源。一般荤素混杂的膳食基本可以满足人体对锰的需要。

## 二、健康指导值

以《中国居民膳食营养素参考摄入量（2013版）》中的适宜摄入量（AI）来评价中国居民由膳食摄入的锰元素是否充足，18岁以上成年人锰的AI值为每人4.5 mg/d（中国营养学会，2014）。

## 三、总膳食研究结果

### 1. 总膳食研究样品中锰的含量

对24个省（自治区、直辖市）的12类混合膳食样品进行锰含量的检测，结果见附表3-16，膳食样品中锰含量较高的样品为豆类食品，且样品锰含量存在较大的地区差异。

## Ⅰ. Background

Manganese widely exists in the natural environment and is one of the most abundant metal elements in the earth's crust. It is also an essential trace element for normal growth, development, and maintenance in the stability of the intracellular environment in organisms (Teng et al., 2021). Deficiency of manganese leads to growth retardation, subfertility, and birth defect. Excessive intake to manganese may cause nervous system dysfunction (Sun et al., 2011). Manganese intake by human body mainly comes from diet and water. Coarse grains, nuts and soy products are rich in manganese, and tea is the richest in manganese, while refined cereals, meats, fish and milk contain relatively little manganese. Although the content of manganese in animal food is not high, the absorption and retention of manganese are high, which can be regarded as a good source of manganese. A mixed meal can basically meet the needs of the human body to manganese.

## Ⅱ. HBGV

Adequate intake (AI) in the *Chinese Dietary Reference Intakes* (*2013 version*) was used to assess the adequacy of dietary manganese intake of China residents. The AI of manganese is 4.5 mg/d per person for adults aged 18 years or older (Chinese Nutrition Society, 2014).

## Ⅲ. TDS Results

### 1. Levels of Manganese in TDS Composite Samples

Composite dietary samples of 12 food categories from 24 provinces (autonomous regions, municipalities) were analyzed for the levels of manganese. As shown in the Annexed Table 3-16, manganese-rich foods were mainly legumes. And manganese levels in these foods vary from region to region.

## 2. 膳食暴露评估

我国居民锰的膳食摄入量（附表3-17，图3-11）平均为4.83 mg/d，全国24个省（自治区、直辖市）为2.48～6.86 mg/d，存在较大的地区差异，部分地区的居民锰摄入量不足。

## 2. Dietary Exposure Assessment

The average dietary intake of manganese for China residents (Annexed Table 3-17, Figure 3-11) was 4.83 mg/d, ranging from 2.48 mg/d to 6.86 mg/d in 24 provinces (autonomous regions, municipalities) with significant regional differences. The dietary intake of manganese was insufficient in some provinces.

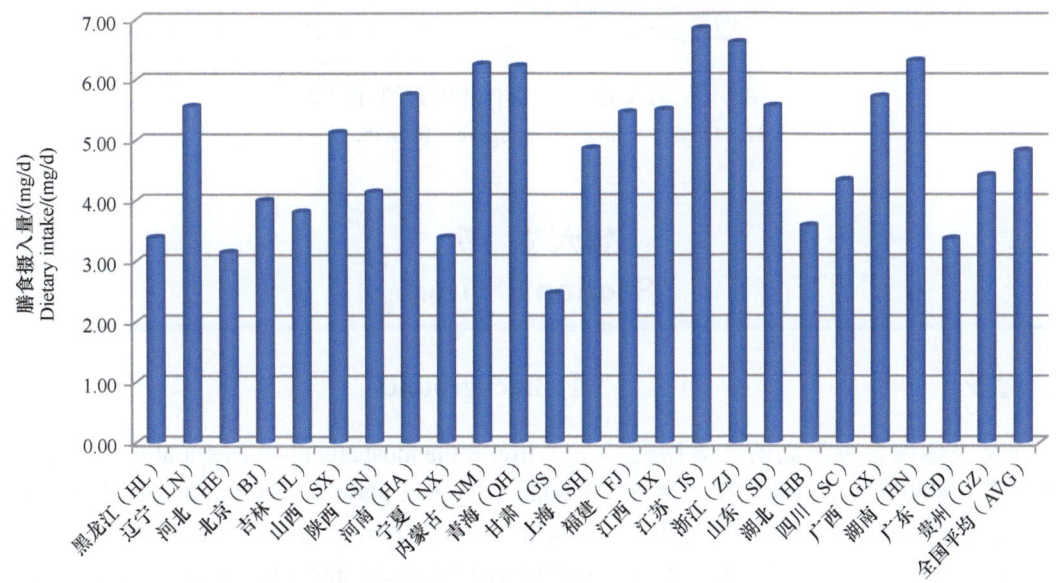

图 3-11 第六次中国总膳食研究的锰膳食摄入量
Figure 3-11 Dietary intake of manganese from the 6th China TDS

## 3. 各类膳食对总膳食摄入的贡献

6th CTDS 我国居民的膳食锰主要来源（附表3-18，图3-12）于谷类、蔬菜和豆类，占总摄入来源的80%以上。大部分省（自治区、直辖市）的锰食物来源也基本相似。

## 4. 与以往中国总膳食研究结果的比较

对比 4th CTDS、5th CTDS 发现，6th CTDS 中我国居民膳食锰的平均摄入量（4.83 mg/d）相较于 4th CTDS（5.58 mg/d）下降了13%，相较于 5th CTDS（6.92 mg/d）下降了30%。

## 3. Contributions of Food Categories to the Total Dietary Intake

The primary sources of dietary intake to manganese for China residents in the 6th CTDS (Annexed Table 3-18, Figure 3-12) were cereals, vegetables and legumes, accounting for over 80% of the total intake. The sources of manganese are basically similar among most of the provinces (autonomous regions, municipalities).

## 4. Comparison with Previous China TDSs Results

Compared with the previous CTDSs, the results of the 6th CTDS showed that the China residents average dietary intake of manganese decreased by 13% compared to the 4th CTDS (5.58 mg/d) and by 30% compared to the 5th CTDS (6.92 mg/d).

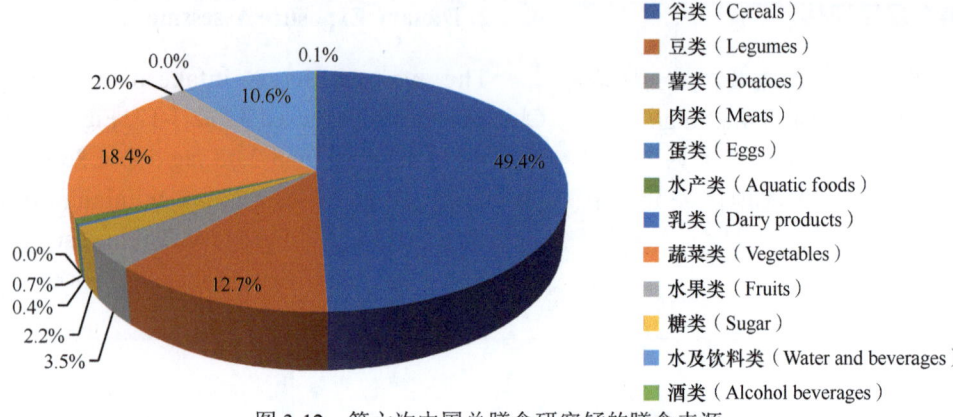

图 3-12　第六次中国总膳食研究锰的膳食来源
Figure 3-12　Dietary sources of manganese from the 6<sup>th</sup> China TDS

# 第六节　铁
# Section 6　Iron

## 一、背景

铁是人体内含量最高的必需微量元素，具有参与氧的运输和贮存，参与合成细胞色素和多种金属酶、增强机体免疫功能等非常重要的生理作用。当机体摄入铁不足时，往往导致缺铁性贫血及电子传递、氧化还原等代谢紊乱（董国力，2013）。铁本身不具有毒性，但有研究提示，铁过量可能诱发一系列神经退行性疾病，铁过度沉积会导致神经元坏死，进而导致脑萎缩（姚蕾和王晓平，2012）。但膳食引起的铁摄入过量极其罕见。铁广泛存在于各种食物中，但动物性食物和植物性食物的吸收利用率相差较大。一般动物性食物铁的含量和吸收率均较高，动物肝脏、血、畜禽肉、鱼类、蛋黄等是铁的良好来源。

## Ⅰ. Background

Iron is the most abundant essential trace element in human body and plays a very important physiological role in the transportation and storage of oxygen, the synthesis of cytochrome and various metal enzymes, enhancing the immune function of the body. When iron intake is insufficient, it often leads to iron deficiency anemia, electron transport, or redox metabolic disorders (Dong, 2013). Iron itself is not toxic, but some studies suggest that excessive iron may induce a series of neurodegenerative diseases. Excessive iron deposition leads to neuronal necrosis, followed by brain atrophy (Yao and Wang, 2012). However, excessive dietary intake of iron is extremely rare. Iron is widely found in a variety of foods, but the absorption and utilization rate of animal and plant foods is quite different. Iron content in animal food is generally higher, and the absorption rate of iron is also very high. Good sources of iron intake include animal livers, blood, poultry and livestock meats, fish, egg yolks, etc.

## 二、健康指导值

以《中国居民膳食营养素参考摄入量（2013 版）》中的推荐摄入量（RNI）来评价中国居民由膳食摄入的铁元素是否充足。成年男子膳食铁的 RNI 为每人 12 mg/d（中国营养学会，2014）。

## 三、总膳食研究结果

### 1. 总膳食研究样品中铁的含量

对 24 个省（自治区、直辖市）的 12 类混合膳食样品进行铁含量的检测，结果见附表 3-19，富含铁的食物主要有豆类、肉类和蛋类。不同地区的食品中铁含量存在差别。

### 2. 膳食暴露评估

我国居民铁的膳食摄入量（附表 3-20，图 3-13）平均为 15.7 mg/d，全国 24 个省（自治区、直辖市）为 9.2～32.7 mg/d，差距较大，约有 29.2% 的省份存在铁摄入不足。

## II. HBGV

Recommended nutrient intake (RNI) in the *Chinese Dietary Reference Intakes (2013 version)* was used to assess the adequacy of dietary iron intake of China residents. The RNI of iron is 12.5 mg/d per person for adult males (Chinese Nutrition Society, 2014).

## III. TDS Results

### 1. Levels of Iron in TDS Composite Samples

The composite dietary samples of 12 food categories from 24 provinces (autonomous regions, municipalities) were analyzed for the level of iron. Annexed Table 3-19 shows foods that are rich in iron, including legumes, meats, and eggs. The levels of iron in food samples varied by region.

### 2. Dietary Exposure Assessment

The average dietary intake of iron for China residents (Annexed Table 3-20, Figure 3-13) was 15.7 mg/d, ranging from 9.2 mg/d to 32.7 mg/d in 24 provinces (autonomous regions, municipalities). About 29.2% of provinces had insufficient iron intake.

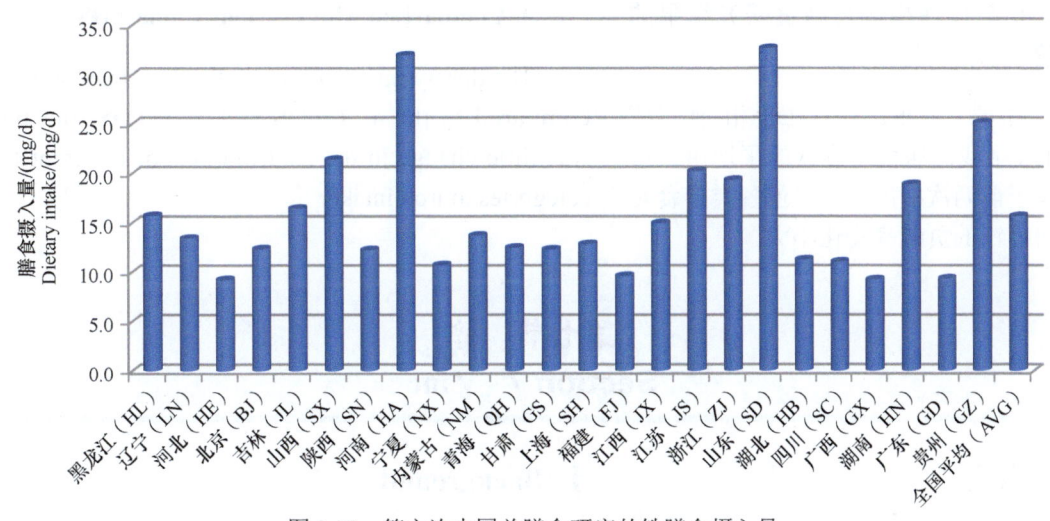

图 3-13 第六次中国总膳食研究的铁膳食摄入量
Figure 3-13 Dietary intake of iron from the 6<sup>th</sup> China TDS

## 3. Contributions of Food Categories to the Total dietary Intake

The primary sources of dietary intake of iron of China residents in the 6th CTDS (Annexed Table 3-21, Figure 3-14) were cereals and vegetables, accounting for over 60% of the total intake. 75% of the dietary iron intake of China residents came from plant-based diets. Food categories with high iron content like legumes, meats, and eggs only accounted for 26.6% of the food sources of China residents.

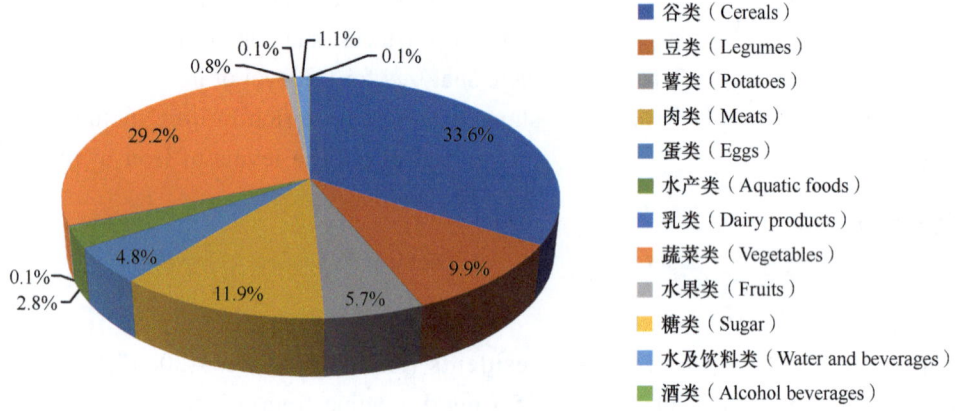

Figure 3-14　Dietary sources of iron from the 6th China TDS

## 4. Comparison with Previous China TDSs Results

The dietary intake of iron in the 6th CTDS decreased compared to the 4th CTDS and 5th CTDS, but there was little change in the contributions of different food categories to iron intake.

# Section 7　Zinc

## Ⅰ. Background

Zinc is an essential trace element in numerous kinds of metabolisms in our body, and plays a significant role in maintaining human physiological activities.

小儿生长发育，进而导致佝偻病；还可使机体免疫力降低，增加感染性疾病发生的风险。孕期母体锌水平较低或缺乏与早产、低出生体重及小于胎龄儿有一定的相关性，孕期补锌对降低不良出生结局有积极作用（向海云和陶芳标，2019）。锌广泛存在于食物中，肉类、鱼类和禽肉是锌摄入的主要来源，谷类和奶制品也含有丰富的锌，保持均衡膳食是预防缺锌的主要措施。母乳，尤其是初乳中锌含量丰富，提倡母乳喂养对预防小儿缺锌具有重要意义。

## 二、健康指导值

以《中国居民膳食营养素参考摄入量（2013 版）》中的推荐摄入量（RNI）来评价中国居民由膳食摄入的锌元素是否充足，成年男子膳食锌的 RNI 为每人 12.5 mg/d（中国营养学会，2014）。

## 三、总膳食研究结果

### 1. 总膳食研究样品中锌的含量

对 24 个省（自治区、直辖市）的 12 类混合膳食样品进行锌含量的检测，结果见附表 3-22，膳食样品中锌含量较高的样品依次为肉类、蛋类、水产类和豆类食品。且样品中锌含量存在地区差异。

### 2. 膳食暴露评估

我国居民锌的平均膳食摄入量（附表 3-23，图 3-15）为 6.17 mg/d，全国 24 个省（自治区、直辖市）为 3.16～9.36 mg/d，差距较大；我国各省份居民锌的平均膳食摄入量均低于锌的 RNI 值。

The deficiency of zinc impairs infantile growth and consequently leads to rhachitis; it can also lead to decreased immunity and greater vulnerability to infectious diseases. Low zinc level or zinc deficiency in pregnant women are associated with premature birth, low birth weight, and small for gestational age. Appropriate zinc supplementation during pregnancy is positive in reducing adverse birth outcomes (Xiang and Tao, 2019). Zinc is widely contained in food. Meats, fish, and poultry are the main sources of zinc intake. Cereals and dairy products are also rich in zinc. Adhering to a balanced diet is a key measure to prevent zinc deficiency. Breast milk, especially colostrum, is rich in zinc, and it is of great significance to promote breastfeeding to prevent zinc deficiency in children.

## II. HBGV

Recommended nutrient intake (RNI) in the *Chinese Dietary Reference Intakes (2013 version)* was used to assess the adequacy of dietary zinc intake of Chinese reference. The RNI of zinc is 12.5 mg/d per person in adult males (Chinese Nutrition Society, 2014).

## III. TDS Results

### 1. Levels of Zinc in TDS Composite Samples

Composite dietary samples of 12 food categories from 24 provinces (autonomous regions, municipalities) were analyzed for the levels of zinc. As shown in the Annexed Table 3-22, zinc-rich foods include, in a descending order, meats, eggs, aquatic products and legumes. And zinc levels in these samples varied from region to region.

### 2. Dietary Exposure Assessment

The average dietary intake of zinc for China residents (Annexed Table 3-23, Figure 3-15) was 6.17 mg/d, ranging from 3.16 mg/d to 9.36 mg/d in 24 provinces (autonomous regions, municipalities). The average dietary intake of zinc for China residents was below the

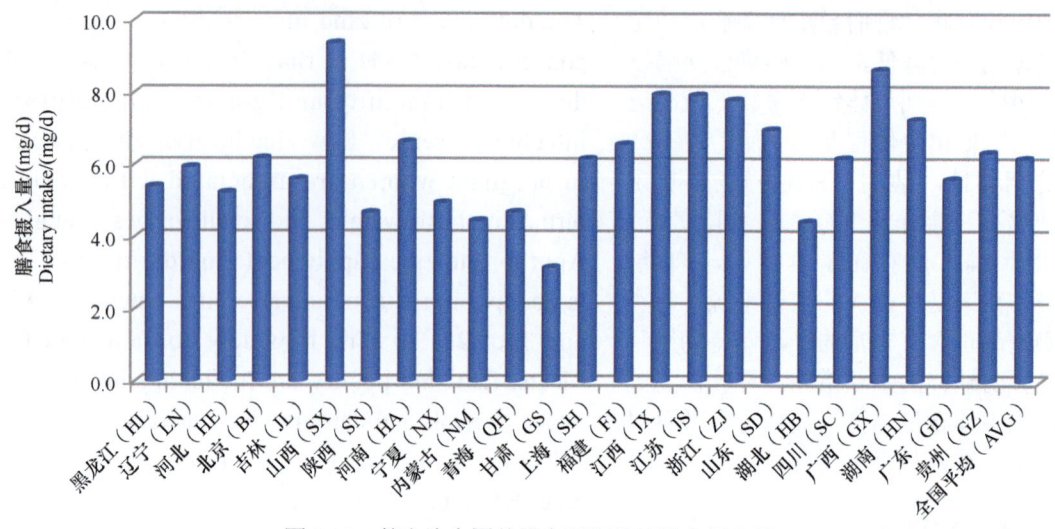

图 3-15　第六次中国总膳食研究的锌膳食摄入量
Figure 3-15　Dietary intake of zinc from the 6th China TDS

### 3. 各类膳食对总膳食摄入的贡献

6th CTDS 中我国居民锌的主要膳食来源（附表 3-24，图 3-16）为谷类，约占总摄入来源的 46%，其次为肉类，约为 21%，各省（自治区、直辖市）的锌食物来源也基本相似。因含锌较高的食物品种，如肉类、蛋类、水产类的消费量较低，导致我国居民膳食锌的摄入量偏低。

### 3. Contributions of Food Categories to the Total Dietary Intake

The primary source of dietary intake for zinc in the 6th CTDS (Annexed Table 3-24, Figure 3-16) was cereals, which accounted for over 46% of the total, followed by meats, at about 21%. The food sources were basically similar among the provinces (autonomous regions, municipalities). Due to the low consumption of foods rich in zinc, such as meats, eggs, and aquatic foods, there was an overall low zinc intake among China's residents.

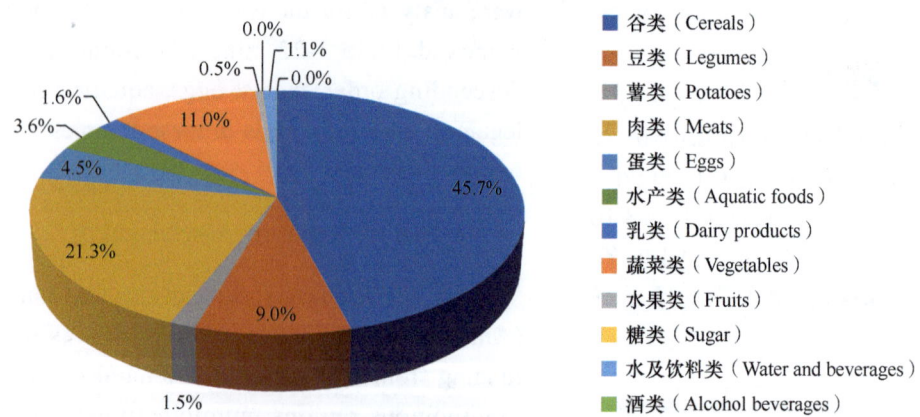

图 3-16　第六次中国总膳食研究锌的膳食来源
Figure 3-16　Dietary sources of zinc from the 6th China TDS

### 4. 与以往中国总膳食研究结果的比较

第六次中国总膳食研究锌的全国平均膳食摄入量与第四次中国总膳食研究的相当，相较于第五次中国总膳食研究下降了48%。

### 4. Comparison with Previous China TDSs Results

The national average dietary intake of zinc in the sixth China total diet study was similar to that in the fourth China total diet study and decreased by 48% compared to the fifth China total diet study.

## 第八节 铬
## Section 8　Chromium

### 一、背景

铬是人体必需的微量元素之一，是维持人体生命活动和胰岛素活性的必需元素。人体对无机铬的吸收利用率极低，只有小部分的铬能被吸收，被吸收的铬与血浆蛋白结合后被转运入肝。

铬以三价铬或者六价铬形态存在于自然界中，铬的毒性与其存在的价态有极大的关系，三价铬是对人体有益的，而六价铬是有毒的。铬在食品中主要以三价铬形态存在。全谷物、奶酪、肉类、小牛肝脏、啤酒酵母、豆类都是三价铬的良好来源（Stipanuk and Caudill, 2012; Wong, 2012）。另外，加工过程和地质因素对铬在食物中的含量有非常大的影响（顾景范等，2003）。

### 二、健康指导值

以《中国居民膳食营养素参考摄入量（2013版）》中的适宜摄入量（AI）来评价中国居民由膳食摄入的铬元素是否充足。成人铬的AI值为每人30 μg/d（中国营养学会，2014）。

### Ⅰ. Background

Chromium is one of the essential trace elements, which is necessary to maintain human life activities and insulin activity. The absorption and utilization rate of inorganic chromium by the human body is very low. Only a small part of chromium can be absorbed by the body and bound to plasma proteins and transferred into the liver.

Chromium typically adopts a $Cr^{3+}$ or $Cr^{6+}$ oxidation state, mainly $Cr^{3+}$ in foods. The toxicity of chromium has a great relationship with its valence state, $Cr^{3+}$ is beneficial to the human body, while $Cr^{6+}$ is toxic. Some of the good sources of $Cr^{3+}$ are whole grains, cheeses, meats, calf livers, brewer's yeast, and beans (Stipanuk and Caudill, 2012; Wong, 2012). Processing and geological factors have a great impact on the chromium level in foods (Gu et al., 2003).

### Ⅱ. HBGV

Adequate intake (AI) in the *Chinese Dietary Reference Intakes* (*2013 version*) is used to assess the adequacy of dietary chromium intake of China residents. The AI of chromium is 30 μg/d per person for adults (Chinese Nutrition Society, 2014).

## 三、总膳食研究结果

### 1. 总膳食研究样品中铬的含量

对 24 个省（自治区、直辖市）的 12 类混合膳食样品进行铬含量的检测，结果见附表 3-25。铬含量较高的样品依次为肉类、薯类和豆类食品，且样品铬含量存在地区差异。

### 2. 膳食暴露评估

我国居民的膳食铬的摄入量（附表 3-26，图 3-17）平均为 139 μg/d，全国 24 个省（自治区、直辖市）为 32～589 μg/d，差距较大；我国居民膳食铬的平均摄入量均高于铬的 AI 值（30 μg/d）。

### 3. 各类膳食对总膳食摄入的贡献

我国居民的膳食铬主要来源（附表 3-27，图 3-18）于谷类、蔬菜类和肉类，占总摄入来源的 80% 以上。各省（自治区、直辖市）的铬膳食来源也基本相似。

## III. TDS Results

### 1. Levels of Chromium in TDS Composite Samples

The composite dietary samples of 12 food categories from 24 provinces (autonomous regions, municipalities) were analyzed for the level of chromium. The detailed results are shown in the Annexed Table 3-25. Chromium-rich foods include, in descending order, meats, potatoes and legumes. And chromium level in these foods varied from region to region.

### 2. Dietary Exposure Assessment

The average dietary intake of chromium for China residents (Figure 3-17) was 139 μg/d, ranging significantly from 32 μg/d to 589 μg/d in 24 provinces (autonomous regions, municipalities). The average dietary intake of chromium for China residents is higher than the AI value for chromium.

### 3. Contributions of Food Categories to the Total Dietary Intake

The primary sources of dietary intake for chromium (Figure 3-18) were cereals, vegetables and meats, accounting for over 80% of the total intake. The food sources of chromium were basically similar among the provinces (autonomous regions, municipalities).

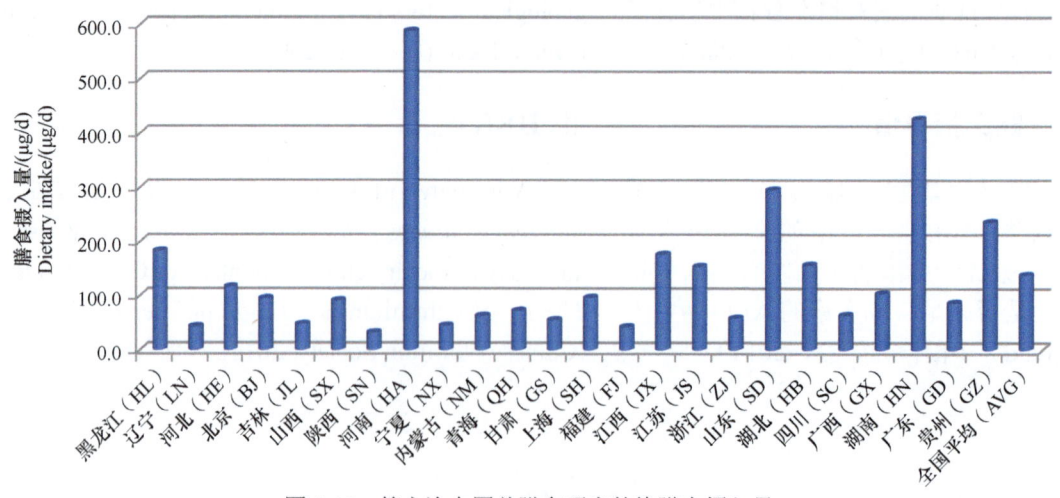

图 3-17 第六次中国总膳食研究的铬膳食摄入量

Figure 3-17 Dietary intake of chromium from the 6th China TDS

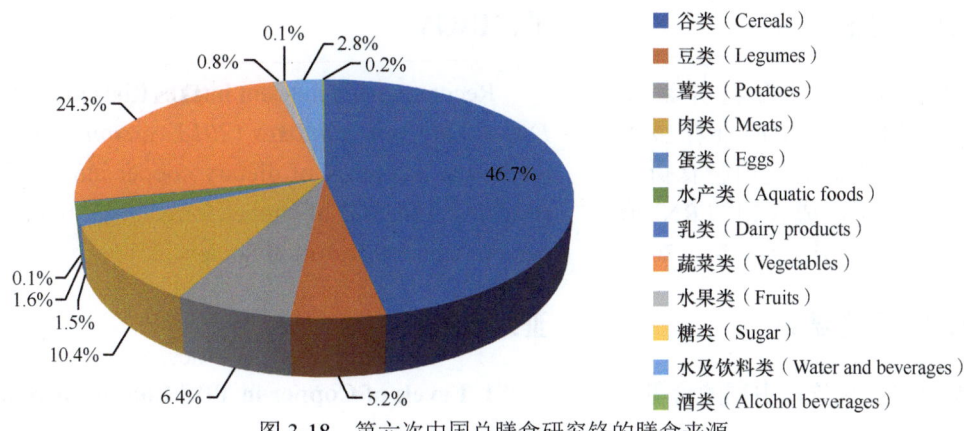

图 3-18　第六次中国总膳食研究铬的膳食来源
Figure 3-18　Dietary sources of chromium from the 6$^{th}$ China TDS

### 4. 与以往中国总膳食研究结果的比较

与第四次和第五次中国总膳食研究中铬的摄入量进行比较，结果发现第六次中国总膳食研究中铬的平均摄入量明显降低。总体而言，中国居民铬的膳食摄入量在持续下降。

### 4. Comparison with Previous China TDSs Results

The dietary intake of chromium in the 6$^{th}$ China TDS significantly decreased compared to the 4$^{th}$ and 5$^{th}$ China TDSs. Overall, the dietary intake of chromium for the Chinese population continued to decline.

## 第九节　铜
## Section 9　Copper

### 一、背景

铜是人体健康所必需的矿物质元素，也是几种金属酶的重要成分，这几种金属酶在多种生物反应中作为氧化酶。同时铜也可能有毒，这取决于摄入的量（Araya et al.，2007）。

大多数食物中都含有铜，含铜量丰富的食物有动物内脏、海产品、豆类、坚果和菜籽、小麦麸皮与全麦食品（顾景范等，2003）。铜的代谢与其他矿物质紧密结合，铜的缺乏会影响铁的转运，导致缺铁（Araya et al.，2007）。

### Ⅰ. Background

Copper is an essential mineral element for human health and is an important component of several metalloenzymes which act as oxidative enzymes in a variety of biological reactions. At the same time, depending on the amount ingested, copper can be poisonous (Araya et al., 2007).

Copper is present in most foods and abundant in animal offals, marine products, beans, nuts, rapeseed, wheat bran and whole-wheat foods (Gu et al., 2003). Copper metabolism is tightly coupled with other minerals and copper deficiency impairs iron mobilization, resulting in iron deficiency (Araya et al., 2007).

## 二、健康指导值

以《中国居民膳食营养素参考摄入量（2013 版）》中的推荐摄入量（RNI）来评价中国居民由膳食摄入的铜元素是否充足，成人铜的 RNI 值为每人 0.8 mg/d（中国营养学会，2014）。

## 三、总膳食研究结果

### 1. 总膳食研究样品中铜的含量

对 24 个省（自治区、直辖市）的 12 类混合膳食样品进行铜含量的检测，结果见附表 3-28，铜含量较高的样品依次为豆类、水产类和肉类食品。

### 2. 膳食暴露评估

我国居民膳食铜的摄入量（附表 3-29，图 3-19）平均为 1.25 mg/d，全国 24 个省（自治区、直辖市）铜的摄入量为 0.83~2.03 mg/d；我国居民膳食铜的平均摄入量基本满足 RNI 水平，但是不同地区间差异较大。

## II. HBGV

Recommended nutrient intake (RNI) in the *Chinese Dietary Reference Intakes* (*2013 version*) was used to assess the adequacy of dietary copper intake of China residents. The RNI of copper for adults is 0.8 mg/d per person (Chinese Nutrition Society, 2014).

## III. TDS Results

### 1. Levels of Copper in TDS Composite Samples

Composite dietary samples of 12 food categories from 24 provinces (autonomous regions, municipalities) were analyzed for the level of copper, with the detailed results shown in the Annexed Table 3-28. Copper-rich foods included legumes, aquatic foods and meats.

### 2. Dietary Exposure Assessment

The average dietary intake of copper for China residents (Figure 3-19) was 1.25 mg/d, ranging from 0.83 mg/d to 2.03 mg/d in 24 provinces (autonomous regions, municipalities). The average dietary intake of copper for China residents was basically in line with the RNI value for copper. However, there is a significant regional difference.

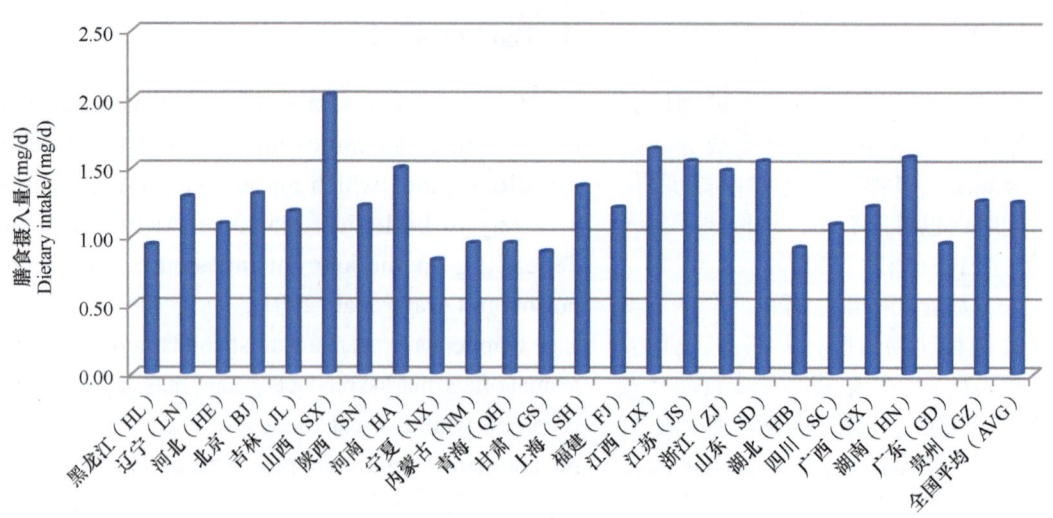

图 3-19　第六次中国总膳食研究的铜膳食摄入量

Figure 3-19　Dietary intake of copper from the 6th China TDS

## 3. 各类膳食对总膳食摄入的贡献

我国居民的膳食铜主要来源（附表3-30，图3-20）于谷类、豆类和蔬菜类，占总摄入来源的80%以上。各省（自治区、直辖市）的铜膳食来源也基本相似。

## 3. Contributions of Food Categories to the Total Dietary Intake

The primary sources of dietary intake of copper (Figure 3-20) were cereals, legumes and vegetables, accounting for over 80% of the total intake. The food sources of copper were basically similar among the provinces (autonomous regions, municipalities).

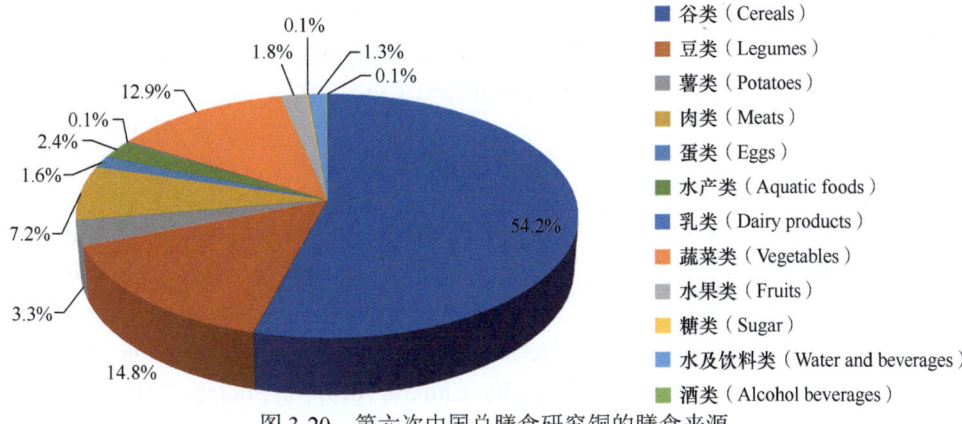

图 3-20　第六次中国总膳食研究铜的膳食来源

Figure 3-20　Dietary sources of copper from the 6th China TDS

## 4. 与以往中国总膳食研究结果的比较

与第四次和第五次中国总膳食研究样品中铜的摄入量进行比较，结果发现第六次中国总膳食研究铜的平均摄入量明显降低。总体而言，中国居民铜的膳食摄入量在持续下降。

## 4. Comparison with Previous China TDSs Results

The dietary intake of copper in the 6th China TDS significantly decreased compared to the 4th and 5th China TDSs. Overall, the dietary intake of copper for the Chinese population continued to decline.

# 第十节　硒
# Section 10　Selenium

## 一、背景

硒是一种人体必需的微量元素，其缺乏与许多疾病如免疫损伤有关。硒是抗氧化酶的重要组成部分，特别是谷胱甘肽过氧化物酶和其他一些硒蛋白，参与各种生理活动，通过调节细胞反应

## Ⅰ. Background

Selenium is an essential trace element, and its deficiency has been linked to a variety of human disorders, including immune impairment. It is an important component of antioxidant enzymes, especially glutathione peroxidase and certain other selenoproteins

保护细胞免受自由基的有害影响（Riaz and Mehmood，2012）。人体中超过 35 种硒蛋白的合成和表达中必须用到硒，这些蛋白质参与氧化还原调节、甲状腺激素调节、能量代谢、细胞膜维持、免疫反应和保护 DNA 不被破坏（顾景范等，2003）。膳食中硒的主要来源是肉类、海鲜及生长在硒含量较高的土壤中的谷物或植物（National Institute of Health，2013）。

## 二、健康指导值

以《中国居民膳食营养素参考摄入量（2013 版）》中的推荐摄入量（RNI）来评价中国居民由膳食摄入的硒元素是否充足，成人硒的 RNI 值为每人 60 μg/d（中国营养学会，2014）。

## 三、总膳食研究结果

### 1. 总膳食研究样品中硒的含量

对 24 个省（自治区、直辖市）的 12 类混合膳食样品进行硒含量的检测，结果见附表 3-31，硒含量较高的样品依次为蛋类、水产类和肉类食品。

### 2. 膳食暴露评估

我国居民膳食硒的摄入量（附表 3-32，图 3-21）平均为 35.7 μg/d，全国 24 个省（自治区、直辖市）为 11.0～61.9 μg/d；我国居民膳食硒的平均摄入量偏低，只有 1 个省份高于 RNI 值，硒摄入量最低的省份，只相当于 RNI 的 18%。这说明我国居民的日常膳食中硒的摄入量明显偏低。

that participate in various physiological processes and protect cells from the harmful effect of free radicals by regulating cell response (Riazand and Mehmood, 2012). Selenium is essential for the synthesis and expression of more than 35 proteins which are involved in redox regulation, thyroid hormone regulation, energy metabolism, cell membrane maintenance, immunoreaction and DNA protection (Gu et al., 2003). Good sources of dietary selenium are meats, seafoods, grains or plants grown in selenium-rich soils (National Institute of Health, 2013).

## II. HBGV

Recommended nutrient intake (RNI) in the *Chinese Dietary Reference Intakes* (*2013 version*) is used to assess the adequacy of dietary selenium intake of China residents. The RNI of selenium is 60 μg/d per person for adults (Chinese Nutrition Society, 2014).

## III. TDS Results

### 1. Levels of Selenium in TDS Composite Samples

Composite dietary samples of 12 food categories from 24 provinces (autonomous regions, municipalities) were analyzed for the level of selenium, with the detailed results shown in the Annexed Table 3-31. Selenium-rich foods include eggs, aquatic foods and meats.

### 2. Dietary Exposure Assessment

The average dietary intake of selenium for China residents (Figure 3-21) was 35.7 μg/d, ranging from 11.0 μg/d to 61.9 μg/d in 24 provinces (autonomous regions, municipalities). The average dietary intake of selenium for China residents was below the RNI value for selenium, only one province having a higher selenium intake than the RNI value. The province with the lowest selenium intake, equivalent to only 18% of the RNI. This indicated that China residents had a low dietary intake of selenium.

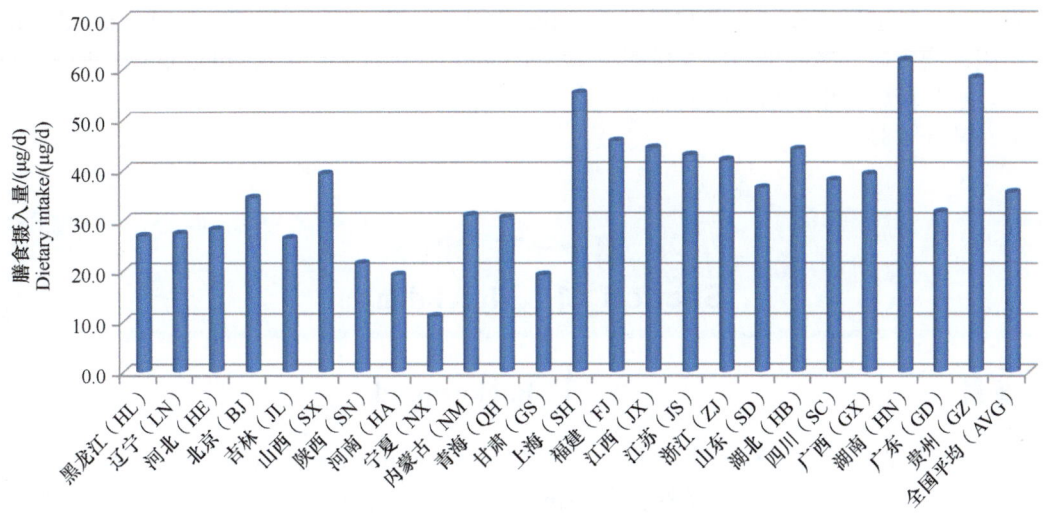

图 3-21 第六次中国总膳食研究的硒膳食摄入量
Figure 3-21　Dietary intake of selenium from the 6th China TDS

**3. 各类膳食对总膳食摄入的贡献**

我国居民的膳食硒主要来源（附表 3-33，图 3-22）于肉类、谷类、水产和蛋类，占总摄入来源的 80% 以上。各省（自治区、直辖市）的硒膳食来源也基本相似。

**3. Contributions of Food Categories to the Total Dietary Intake**

The primary sources of dietary intake of the selenium (Figure 3-22) of China residents were meats, cereals, aquatic foods and eggs, accounting for over 80% of the total intake. The food sources of selenium were generally similar among the provinces (autonomous regions, municipalities).

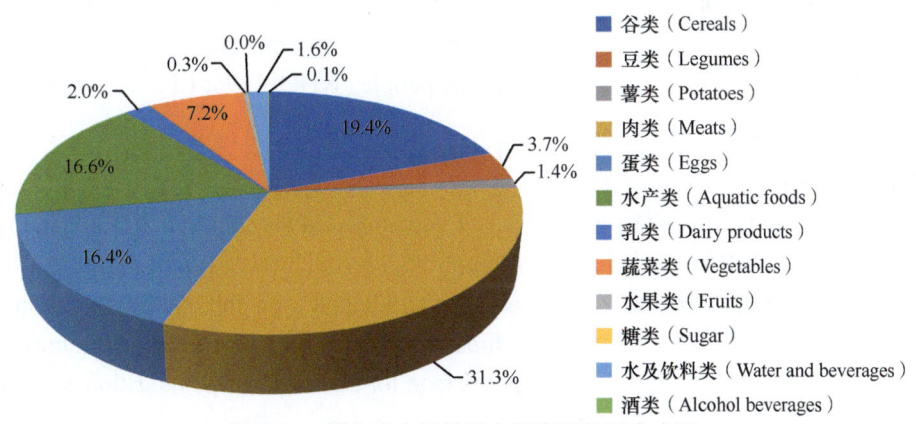

图 3-22 第六次中国总膳食研究硒的膳食来源
Figure 3-22　Dietary sources of selenium from the 6th China TDS

**4. 与以往中国总膳食研究结果的比较**

与第四次和第五次中国总膳食研

**4. Comparison with Previous China TDSs Results**

In comparison with the results from the 4th and 5th China TDSs, the dietary intake of selenium in the 6th

究中硒的摄入量进行比较，结果发现第六次中国总膳食研究硒的平均摄入量明显降低。总体而言，中国居民硒的膳食摄入量在持续下降。

China TDS was significantly lower. Overall, the intake of selenium for the Chinese population was decreasing.

## 第十一节　钼
## Section 11　Molybdenum

### 一、背景

钼是一种过渡元素，存在于人体各种组织中，成人体内钼的总量约为 9 mg，主要以钼酶的形式存在，作为许多酶的辅助因子起作用。钼以多种钼金属酶发挥其生理功能，近年来报道了它们在脂肪细胞线粒体中的作用途径，显示其对脂肪合成至关重要（顾景范等，2003）。

肉类、牛肝、全谷物、荞麦、大麦、小麦胚芽和其他豆类（如豌豆、扁豆、花生）、向日葵种子、牛奶和深绿色叶类蔬菜是钼的主要来源。目前未发现正常饮食会使人体出现缺乏钼的情况（WHO，1996；EFSA，2006b）。

### 二、健康指导值

以《中国居民膳食营养素参考摄入量（2013版）》中的推荐摄入量（RNI）来评价中国居民由膳食摄入的钼元素是否充足，成人钼的 RNI 值为每人 100 μg/d（中国营养学会，2014）。

### Ⅰ. Background

Molybdenum is a kind of transition element, which exists in various tissues of human body. The total amount of molybdenum in the adult body is about 9 mg, mainly in the form of molybdenum enzyme, it functions as a cofactor for a number of enzymes. Molybdenum exerts its physiological function through many kinds of molybdenum metal enzymes. In recent years, it has been reported that they are in the role of mitochondria in fat cells, which shows that it is very important to the synthesis of fat (Gu et al., 2003).

Meats, calf livers, whole grains, buckwheats, barleys, wheat germs and other legumes such as peas, lentils, peanuts, sunflower seeds, milk, and dark green leafy vegetables are good sources of molybdenum. Dietary molybdenum deficiency has never been observed in healthy people (WHO, 1996; EFSA, 2006b).

### Ⅱ. HBGV

Recommended nutrient intake (RNI) in the *Chinese Dietary Reference Intakes* (*2013 version*) was used to assess the adequacy of dietary molybdenum intake of China residents. The RNI of molybdenum is 100 μg/d per person for adults (Chinese Nutrition Society, 2014).

## III. TDS Results

### 1. Levels of Molybdenum in TDS Composite Samples

Composite dietary samples of 12 food categories from 24 provinces (autonomous regions, municipalities) were analyzed for the level of molybdenum, with the detailed results shown in the Annexed Table 3-34. Molybdenum-rich foods included cereals and legumes.

### 2. Dietary Exposure Assessment

The average dietary intake of molybdenum for China residents (Figure 3-23) was 161 μg/d, ranging from 91.3 μg/d to 300 μg/d in 24 provinces (autonomous regions, municipalities). The average dietary intake of molybdenum for China residents was basically in line with the RNI value. Molybdenum intakes were below the RNI in 4 provinces (autonomous regions, municipalities).

### 3. Contributions of Food Categories to the Total Dietary Intake

The primary sources of dietary intake of molybdenum (Figure 3-24) were cereals, legumes and

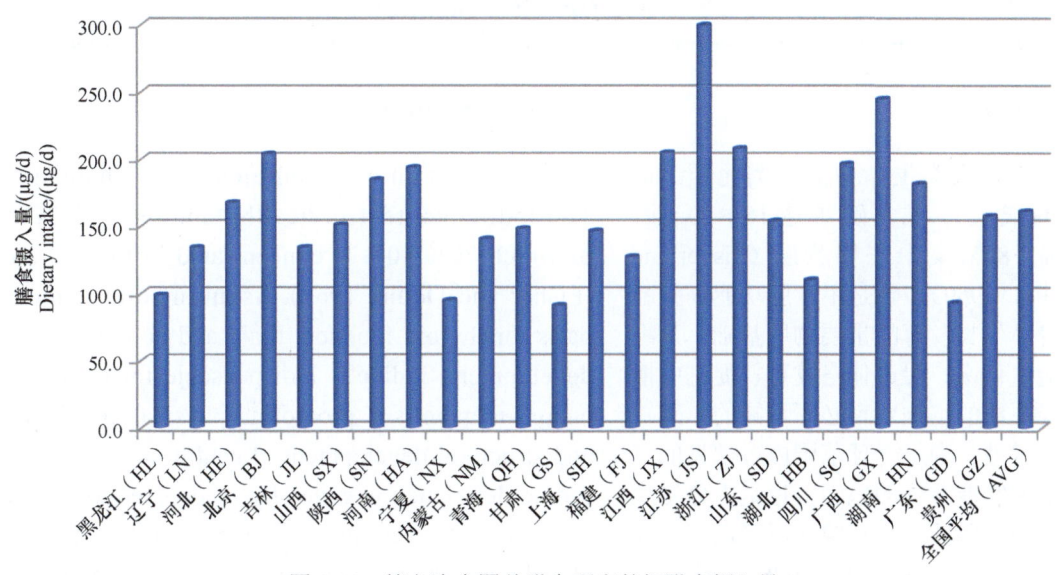

Figure 3-23　Dietary intake of molybdenum from the 6$^{th}$ China TDS

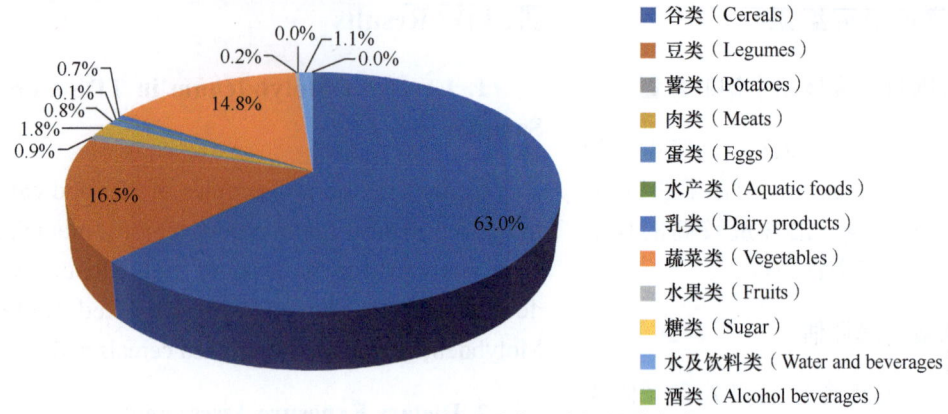

图 3-24 第六次中国总膳食研究钼的膳食来源
Figure 3-24　Dietary sources of molybdenum from the 6th China TDS

**4. 与以往中国总膳食研究结果的比较**

与第五次中国总膳食研究样品中钼的摄入量进行比较，结果发现第六次中国总膳食研究钼的平均摄入量明显降低。

vegetables, accounting for nearly 95% of the total intake. The food sources of molybdenum were generally similar among the provinces (autonomous regions, municipalities).

**4. Comparison with Previous China TDSs Results**

The dietary intake of molybdenum decreased significantly in the 6th China TDS compared to the 5th China TDS.

## 第十二节　碘
## Section 12　Iodine

### 一、背景
### Ⅰ. Background

碘是人类生命中的必需元素。健康的成人体内含碘量达 15～20 mg，70%～80% 集中在甲状腺（Fisher and Oddie, 1969）。碘是甲状腺功能、大脑和身体生长发育的重要物质基础，是维持能量代谢、促进体格发育、促进中枢神经系统的结构发育必不可缺的。碘缺乏通常被认为是全球范围内最常见的可预防的智能障碍的原因，也是内分泌疾病（甲状腺肿和甲状腺功能减退症）最常见的原因（Patrick, 2008）。碘缺乏可导致甲状腺肿，死胎和流产，新生儿

Iodine is an essential element for human life. The iodine content in healthy adults is 15-20 mg, of which 70%-80% is concentrated in thyroid gland (Fisher and Oddie, 1969). As an important material basis for thyroid function, brain and body growth and development, iodine is indispensable for maintaining energy metabolism, promoting physical development and structural development of central nervous system. Iodine deficiency is generally recognized as the most commonly preventable cause of mental retardation globally and the most common cause of endocrinopathy (goiter and hypothyroidism) (Patrick, 2008). Iodine

期和青春期甲状腺功能低下，还会引起聋哑、肌肉痉挛和瘫痪，会导致轻度丧失一定的体力，以及造成一定的智力损伤。碘缺乏发生在胎儿期和婴幼儿期的后期时尤为严重，将出现脑发育滞后，出生后表现不可逆转的智能障碍。人体需要的碘的 80%～90% 来源于食物，通常食物中的碘含量很少，需要在食物加工过程中添加碘盐。全民食盐加碘（universal salt iodization，USI）是全球推荐的最安全、最有效、成本最低且效果最持久的消除碘缺乏病的策略。碘的主要来源是干海藻、鳕鱼、碘盐、乳制品、虾、烤火鸡胸肉和煮鸡蛋（Health Alicious Ness.Com，2008）。

## 二、健康指导值

WHO 和欧盟提出碘长期慢性终生暴露的每日可耐受摄入量（TDI）为 600 μg/d（WHO，1985）。中国营养学会于 2013 年重新修订中国居民营养素膳食参考摄入量，下调了不同年龄组人群碘的推荐摄入量（RNI）和可耐受最高摄入量（UL），将成人碘的 RNI 由每日 150 μg 下降到 120 μg，UL 从每日 1000 μg 下降到 600 μg[《中国居民膳食营养素参考摄入量（2013 版）》]。第六次中国总膳食研究以此进行了膳食摄入量评估。

## 三、总膳食研究结果

### 1. 总膳食研究样品中碘的含量

对 24 个省（自治区、直辖市）的 12 类混合膳食样品进行碘含量的检测，从附表 3-37 的测定结果可以看出，混合膳食样品中碘的平均含量为 0.007～1.021 mg/kg。各地区各类膳食样品的碘含量差异较大，蔬菜类膳食碘的含量较高，为 0.406～3.520 mg/kg，湖北的蔬菜

deficiency can result in goiter, stillbirth and abortion, hypothyroidism in neonatal and adolescent period, deaf-mute, muscle spasm and paralysis, and slight loss of intellectual ability. Iodine deficiency is particularly serious in the late stage of fetus and infancy, which will lead to brain development lag and irreversible mental retardation after birth. 80%-90% of the iodine needed by the human body comes from food. Usually, there is very little iodine in food, unless it has been added during processing, which is now the case with salt. Universal salt iodization (USI) is the globally recommended safest, most effective, lowest cost, and longest lasting strategy to eliminate iodine deficiency disorders. Some of the main sources of iodine are dried seaweeds, cods, iodized salt, dairy products, shrimps, baked turkey breast, and boiled eggs (Health Alicious Ness.Com, 2008).

## II. HBGV

WHO and the EU suggested that the tolerable daily intake (TDI) of long-term chronic lifetime exposure to iodine was 600 μg/d (WHO, 1985). In 2013, the Chinese Nutrition Society revised the dietary reference intake of nutrients for China residents, lowered the recommended nutrient intake (RNI) and the tolerable upper intake level (UL) of iodine in different age groups, decreasing the RNI from 150 μg/d to 120 μg/d and the UL from 1000 μg/d to 600 μg/d for adults [*Chinese Dietary Reference Intakes (2013 version)*]. The 6$^{th}$ China TDS assessed the dietary intake accordingly.

## III. TDS Results

### 1. Levels of Iodine in TDS Composite Samples

Composite dietary samples of 12 food categories from 24 provinces (autonomous regions, municipalities) were analyzed for the level of iodine, with the detailed results shown in the Annexed Table 3-37. The average levels of iodine in composite dietary samples were from 0.007 mg/kg to 1.021 mg/kg. The iodine level of various food categories varied greatly among regions, with

类膳食碘含量（3.520 mg/kg）是混合膳食样品中最高的。

### 2. 膳食暴露评估

从附表 3-38、图 3-25 的摄入量结果可以看出，我国居民平均膳食碘摄入量为 497 μg/d。各地膳食碘的摄入量差异较大，除 5 个省外，其他省（自治区、直辖市）居民的平均膳食碘摄入量均未超过我国调整后的碘 UL。24 个省（自治区、直辖市）的膳食碘摄入水平均达到 RNI（120 μg/d）。

### 3. 各类膳食对总膳食摄入的贡献

如附表 3-39、图 3-26 所示，各省份居民碘的膳食来源主要是蔬菜类（72.9%）、肉类（7.4%）、薯类（4.7%），合计占膳食碘摄入量的 85.0%，其他类别膳食的贡献率均低于 4%。

### 4. 与以往中国总膳食研究结果的比较

在第二次和第四次中国总膳食研究中开展了碘的检测，与第四次中国总膳食研究的碘摄入量 422.8 μg/d 相比，第六次中国总膳食研究碘的平均摄入量

high content in vegetables ranging from 0.406 mg/kg to 3.520 mg/kg. The vegetables sample from Hubei had the highest level at 3.520 mg/kg.

### 2. Dietary Exposure Assessment

As shown in Figure 3-25, the average dietary intake of iodine for China residents was 497 μg/d. There were significant regional differences in dietary intake of iodine. Except for 5 provinces the average dietary iodine intake of residents in other provinces (autonomous regions, municipalities) did not exceed the adjusted UL value. The dietary intake of iodine in 24 provinces (autonomous regions, municipalities) reached RNI (120 μg/d).

### 3. Contributions of Food Categories to the Total Dietary Intake

As shown in Figure 3-26, the primary sources of iodine intake were vegetables (72.9%), meats (7.4%), and potatoes (4.7%), accounting for 85.0% of the total intake, with the contributions of other food categories being all less than 4%.

### 4. Comparison with Previous China TDSs Results

The detection of iodine was carried out in the 2$^{nd}$ and 4$^{th}$ China TDSs. Compared with the iodine intake

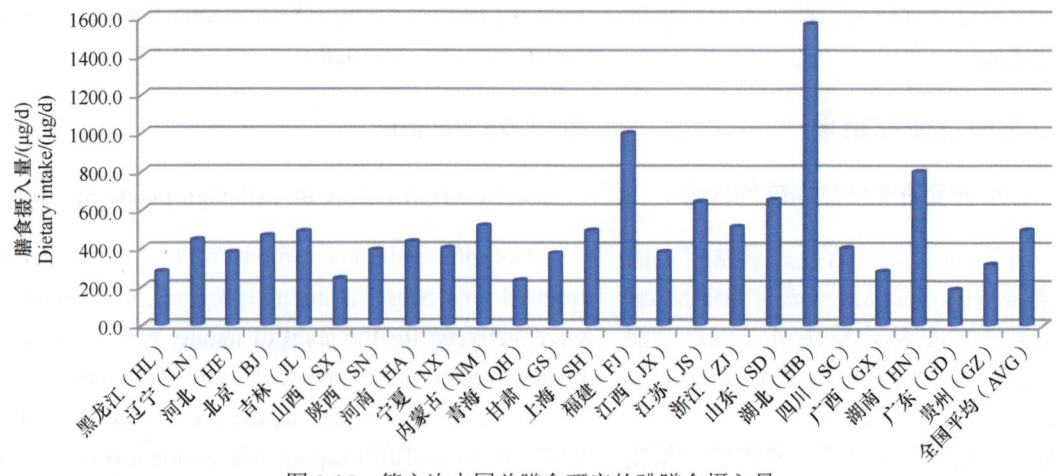

图 3-25　第六次中国总膳食研究的碘膳食摄入量

Figure 3-25　Dietary intake of iodine from the 6$^{th}$ China TDS

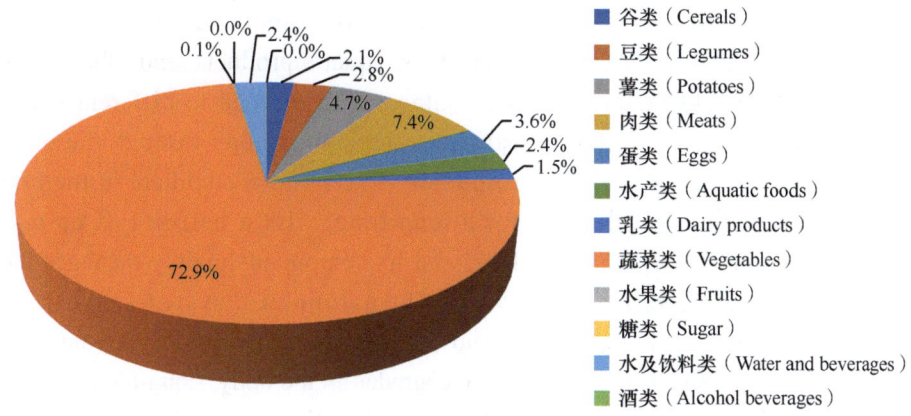

图 3-26 第六次中国总膳食研究碘的膳食来源
Figure 3-26　Dietary sources of iodine from the 6$^{th}$ China TDS

没有明显变化，处于中国营养学会制定的碘 RNI 与 UL 的范围内。

of 422.8 μg/d in the 4$^{th}$ China TDS, the average dietary intake of iodine in the 6$^{th}$ China TDS did not change significantly, which was within the range of RNI and UL formulated by the Chinese Nutrition Society.

## 第二部分　污染元素
## Part 2　Contaminating Elements

污染元素通过环境因素，如空气、土壤和水，或者食品加工烹调过程进入到食品中。关注重金属及有害元素污染物，主要目的是评估公共健康和风险。《食品安全国家标准 食品中污染物限量》（GB 2762—2022）规定了食品中有害元素限量标准，目的是指导食品加工与保护公共健康和安全。本章第二部分污染元素包括铅、镉、汞、砷和铝。

Contaminating elements find their way into foods through environmental factors such as air, soil, and water or in the cooking process. The main purpose of focusing on heavy metals and harmful elements pollution is to assess public health and risk. *National food safety standard-Contaminant Limits in Foods* (GB 2762—2022) establishes standards for maximum limits of contaminants in foods, with the aim of guiding food processing and protecting public health and safety. Contaminating elements in Part 2 include lead, cadmium, mercury, arsenic, and aluminum.

## 第十三节　铅
## Section 13　Lead

一、背景

Ⅰ. Background

铅是一种在自然界广泛存在的重

Lead is a heavy metal contaminant that is widely

金属污染物。饮用水和粮食、蔬菜、水产品等各类食品均不同程度地受到铅污染。铅可通过消化道和呼吸道进入人体,在人体内长期蓄积,半衰期长达14年。铅是人体非必需元素。铅及其化合物可对人体多个系统造成损伤,主要累及神经、造血、消化、心血管等系统和肾脏,铅在体内不能被生物降解。铅在低浓度长期暴露情况下可影响大脑和神经系统发育,尤其损害儿童的认知能力和智力。膳食中的铅摄入情况一直是国际上关注的热点(Callan and hinwood,2011;Nihei 等,2001;董兆敏等,2011)。

2010年JECFA第73次会议指出,根据血铅水平与儿童智力发育降低、成人收缩压升高的剂量反应关系研究结果,认为原暂定每周可耐受摄入量(PTWI)25 μg/(kg bw·周)会引起儿童智商(IQ)下降至少3个点,会导致成人收缩压升高至少3 mm汞柱,对人类健康已不具有保护作用。因此,JECFA在重新评估后撤销了铅的PTWI值,并认为目前尚无法确定一个可有效保护健康的铅暴露阈值。建议各国以尽量减少膳食中的铅暴露为目标(JECFA,2010b)。

## 二、健康指导值

因目前没有可以用于铅的健康指导阈值,采用国际最新的儿童智商下降或成人收缩压升高为评价指标,利用暴露边界值(MOE)评估方法,评估我国居民膳食铅暴露的健康风险。根据2010年JECFA的结论,当铅暴露量为1.2 μg/(kg bw·d)时,成人的血压收缩压上升1 mm汞柱。上述剂量并非健康保护阈值,但铅暴露产生负面影响的风险相对较低。当MOE大于1时,认为膳食铅摄入的健康风险属于可接受

distributed throughout the world. Drinking water, vegetables, aquatic products, and other kinds of food, are contaminated by lead to different degrees. Lead can enter the human body through the digestive and respiratory tracts and accumulate in the human body for a long time, with a half-life of up to 14 years. Lead and its compounds mainly damages the nervous system, hematopoietic system, digestive system, cardiovascular system, and kidney system. Lead cannot be biodegraded in the body. Long-term exposure to lead at low concentrations can affect the development of the brain and nervous system, especially impairing the cognitive ability and intelligence of children. Therefore, the dietary lead intake has always been a major concern around the world. (Callan and hinwood, 2011; Nihei et al., 2001; Dong et al., 2011).

In 2010, based on the results of the dose-response relationships between blood lead levels and reduced intellectual development in children and increased systolic blood pressure in adults, the Joint FAO/WHO Expert Committee on Food Additives (JECFA) in its 73$^{rd}$ meeting report, estimated that a PTWI of 25 μg/(kg bw · week) of lead is associated with a decrease of at least three intelligence quotation (IQ) points in children and an increase in systolic blood pressure (SBP) of approximately 3 mmHg in adults. Therefore, the committee concluded that the PTWI could no longer be considered sufficient to protect health, and it was withdrawn. However, the committee was unable to establish new health-based guidelines, as there is no evidence for a threshold for the key effects of lead. JECFA also recommends that countries try to keep their lead intake as low as possible (JECFA, 2010b).

## II. HBGV

As there is no JECFA threshold for lead exposure, based on the results of the latest international studies on IQ decline in children or systolic blood pressure increase in adults, the margin of exposure (MOE) method is used for risk characterization. The JECFA concluded that for

的低水平,反之则表明存在潜在的健康风险。

### 三、总膳食研究结果

#### 1. 总膳食研究样品中铅的含量

对24个省(自治区、直辖市)的12类混合膳食样品进行铅检测,如附表3-40所示,铅含量较高的食物类别依次为蔬菜类、水产类、豆类、谷类。

#### 2. 膳食暴露评估

我国居民膳食铅的摄入量(附表3-41,图3-27)范围为6.45～47.0 μg/d,铅摄入量平均值为20.0 μg/d。成年男子膳食铅摄入量的MOE值为1.6～11.7,MOE值平均为3.8。MOE值均大于1,说明我国居民膳食铅摄入的健康风险较低。

adults, a lead exposure of 1.2 μg/(kg bw·d) will lead to an increase of 1 mmHg in systolic blood pressure. The above-mentioned dose is not a health-protective threshold but has a relatively lower risk of negative effects of lead exposure. When the MOE is greater than 1, the health risk of dietary lead intake is considered to be at an acceptably low level, while the opposite indicates a potential health risk.

### Ⅲ. TDS Results

#### 1. Levels of Lead in TDS Composite Samples

Composite samples of 12 food categories from 24 provinces (autonomous regions, municipalities) were analyzed for the lead level. Annexed Table 3-40 showed foods that were rich in lead including vegetables, aquatic foods, legumes, and cereals.

#### 2. Dietary Exposure Assessment

The average dietary intake of lead for China residents was 20.0 μg/d, ranging from 6.45 μg/d to 47.0 μg/d in 24 provinces (autonomous regions, municipalities) (Annexed Table 3-41, Figure 3-27). The MOE value ranged from 1.6 to 11.7, with an average of

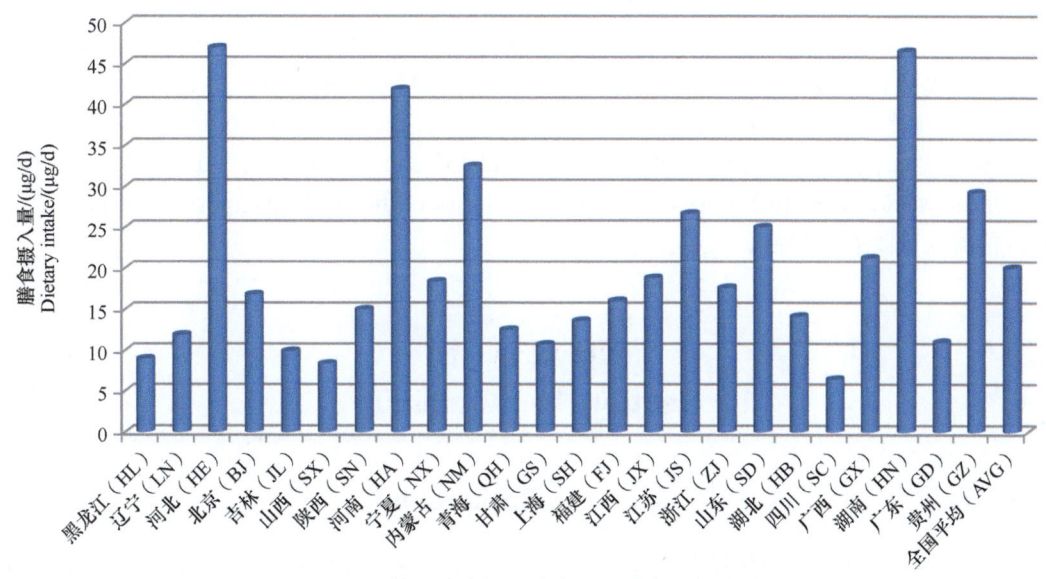

图3-27 第六次中国总膳食研究膳食铅摄入量

Figure 3-27 Dietary intake of lead from the 6th China TDS

**3. 各类膳食对总膳食摄入的贡献**

6th CTDS 我国居民膳食铅主要来源（附表 3-42，图 3-28）于谷类（43.5%）和蔬菜类食物（29.0%），超过总摄入量的 70%。

3.8. The MOE values were all greater than 1, indicating that the health risk of dietary lead intake for China residents was generally low.

**3. Contributions of Food Categories to the Total Dietary Intake**

The primary sources of lead dietary intake for China residents in the 6th CTDS were cereals (43.5%) and vegetables (29.0%), accounting for over 70% of the total intake (Annexed Table 3-42, Figure 3-28).

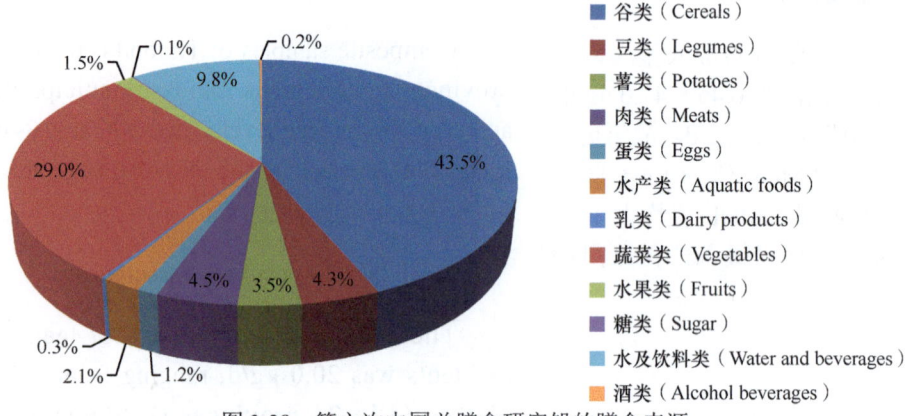

图 3-28 第六次中国总膳食研究铅的膳食来源
Figure 3-28　Dietary sources of lead from 6th China TDS

**4. 与以往中国总膳食研究结果的比较**

我国居民膳食铅摄入量从 1st CTDS 到 3rd CTDS 变化不大，从 3rd CTDS 到 6th CTDS 逐次降低，降低幅度依次是 33%、36%、43%，表明我国居民铅暴露状况的健康风险有所降低。

**4. Comparison with Previous China TDSs Results**

The dietary lead intake of China residents changed little from the 1st CTDS to the 3rd CTDS and gradually decreased from the 3rd CTDS to the 6th CTDS by 33%, 36%, and 43%, respectively. It indicated a reduction in the health risk of dietary lead exposure in China.

## 第十四节　镉
## Section 14　Cadmium

**一、背景**

镉是一种蓄积性很强的有毒重金属元素，早在 1993 年国际癌症研究机

**Ⅰ. Background**

Cadmium is a highly accumulated toxic metal element. As early as 1993, the International Agency

构就将镉定为确证的人类致癌物质（祝白春等，2019）。欧盟将镉列为高危害有毒物质和可致癌物质并予以规管。镉主要通过食物、水和空气进入人体内，可引起多系统损伤，痛痛病是公认的一种镉污染公害病。镉可在农作物内积聚（ATSDR，2008），水稻是典型的"受害作物"，2011年年初反映我国部分地区稻米镉含量超标的一则调查报告，引起社会广泛关注和担忧。

## 二、健康指导值

2010年JECFA第73次会议取消了之前镉的暂定每周可耐受摄入量（PTWI），认定镉的长期终生暴露对人群健康的危害更值得关注，因此改为制定了镉的暂定每月耐受摄入量（PTMI），并降低为25 μg/(kg bw·月)。

## 三、总膳食研究结果

### 1. 总膳食研究样品中镉的含量

对24个省（自治区、直辖市）的12类混合膳食样品进行镉含量的检测，从检测结果（附表3-43）可以看出，膳食中镉含量较高的样品依次为水产类、豆类、谷类、蔬菜类和薯类。膳食中镉含量存在地区差异，南方各省（自治区、直辖市）膳食中镉含量普遍高于北方各省（自治区、直辖市）。

### 2. 膳食暴露评估

我国居民镉的膳食平均摄入量（附表3-44，图3-29）为17.3 μg/d，相当于PTMI的33.0%，摄入量范围为5.46～63.1 μg/d（相当于PTMI的10.4%～120.1%）（计算时体重取63 kg），存在明显的地区差异。我国居民镉的膳食暴露平均值小于JECFA镉的PTMI [25 μg/(kg bw·月)]，对人体健康安全的风险

for Research on Cancer identified cadmium as a confirmed human carcinogen (Zhu et al., 2019). The European Union lists cadmium as a highly hazardous toxic substance and a carcinogen and regulates it. Cadmium enters the body mainly through food, water, and air, which can cause damage to multiple systems of the human body. Itai-itai disease is a public nuisance disease caused by cadmium pollution. Cadmium can accumulate in crops (ATSDR, 2008). Rice is a typical "victimized crop". At the beginning of 2011, a report about cadmium-tainted rice in some parts of China, in particular, received wide attention and much concern from the public.

## II. HBGV

At the 73$^{rd}$ JECFA meeting in 2010, the PTWI value for cadmium was withdrawn on the ground that long-term cadmium exposure poses a greater threat to health and therefore deserves more attention, and the PTWI value was replaced by provisional tolerable monthly intake (PTMI) at the lower value of 25 μg/(kg bw·month).

## III. TDS Results

### 1. Levels of Cadmium in TDS Composite Samples

Composite dietary samples of 12 food categories from 24 provinces (autonomous regions, municipalities) were analyzed for the level of cadmium. Annexed Table 3-43 shows that food categories with high cadmium levels were, in order, aquatic foods, legumes, cereals, vegetables, and potatoes. The levels of cadmium in food samples varied by region, with the southern provinces (autonomous regions, municipalities) having generally higher cadmium levels than the northern provinces (autonomous regions, municipalities).

### 2. Dietary Exposure Assessment

The average dietary intake of cadmium for China residents (Annexed Table 3-44, Figure 3-29) was 17.3 μg/d

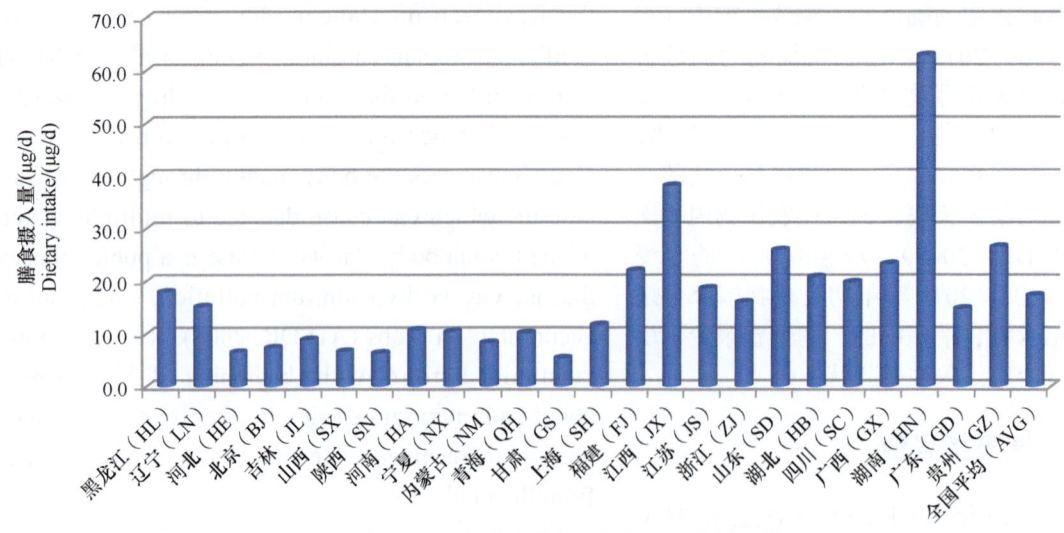

图 3-29　第六次中国总膳食研究的镉膳食摄入量
Figure 3-29　Dietary intake of cadmium from the 6<sup>th</sup> China TDS

较低，但个别地区镉的暴露水平相对较高。

**3. 各类膳食对总膳食摄入的贡献**

6<sup>th</sup> CTDS 中我国居民镉的主要膳食来源（附表 3-45，图 3-30）为谷类和蔬菜类，超过总摄入来源的 80%，重点控制谷类膳食中的镉含量对减少中国居民镉的摄入尤为关键。

(33.0% of PTMI), ranging from 5.46 μg/d to 63.1 μg/d (10.4%-120.1% of PTMI) (weight: 63 kg), which indicated significant regional differences. The average dietary intake of cadmium was below the PTMI value of 25 μg/(kg bw·month) established by JECFA which poses a low risk to human health, but individual areas have relatively high exposure.

**3. Contributions of Food Categories to the Total Dietary Intake**

The primary sources of dietary intake for cadmium for China residents in the 6<sup>th</sup> CTDS (Annexed Table 3-45,

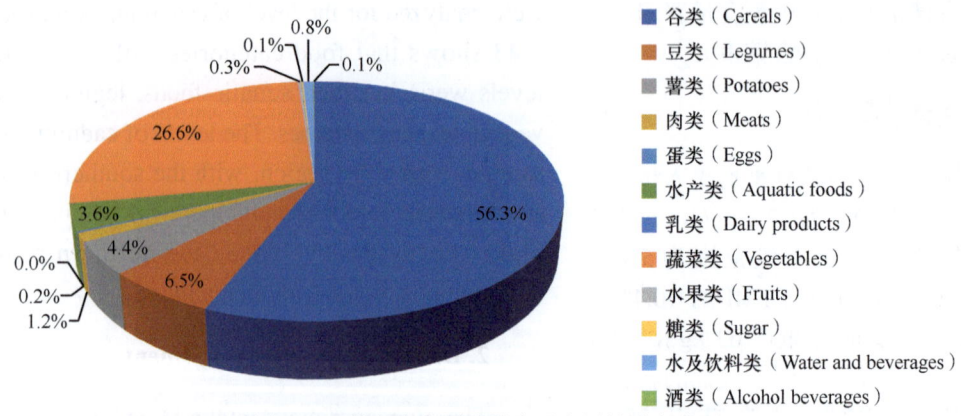

图 3-30　第六次中国总膳食研究镉的膳食来源
Figure 3-30　Dietary sources of cadmium from the 6<sup>th</sup> China TDS

## 4. 与以往中国总膳食研究结果的比较

中国总膳食研究共开展了 6 次镉元素的检测，镉的膳食摄入量在 30 年间处于相对稳定但略有波动的状态。

Figure 3-30) were cereals and vegetables, accounting for more than 80% of the total intake. It is very important to control the cadmium content in the cereals diet to reduce the cadmium intake of China residents.

## 4. Comparison with Previous China TDSs Results

Cadmium was included in six China TDSs. The cadmium intake was in a relatively stable but slightly fluctuating state over a 30-year period.

# 第十五节　汞
# Section 15　Mercury

## 一、背景

汞在自然界中广泛存在，具有生物富集和生物放大效应，对人体健康和动植物生长都有一定的影响（焦君杰等，2018）。汞有多种存在形态，其中对人体危害最大的为甲基汞，可造成神经系统损害，还有致畸和胚胎毒性。世界卫生组织（WHO）估计成年人血汞浓度达到 200 μg/L 会有毒性反应，至今世界上汞的使用与扩散已多次造成人类及动植物"伤害"，其中最严重的就是 20 世纪 50 年代在日本水俣湾发生的甲基汞中毒事件（陈影和邵玉芳，2012）。

大多数食物中所含的汞为无机汞，甲基汞绝大部分是由于微生物对汞的甲基化作用生成的，海洋和淡水中的生物因为食物链的富集作用，使甲基汞在体内进行累积，所以，通常情况下大型食肉鱼类含有更高水平的甲基汞。总体而言，人们日常摄入的水产类是摄入甲基汞的最主要来源。

## I. Background

Mercury widely exists in nature and has bio-accumulation and biomagnification effects. It has a certain impact on human health and the growth of animals and plants (Jiao et al., 2018). Mercury exists in a variety of forms, methylmercury is the most harmful mercury compound to the human body, which can cause damage to the nervous system, as well as teratogenicity and embryotoxicity. The World Health Organization (WHO) estimates that adults with a blood mercury concentration of 200 μg/L will have toxic reactions. So far, the use and diffusion of mercury in the world have caused human, flora and fauna "harm" many times, the most serious of which is the methylmercury poisoning in Minamata Bay, Japan in the 1950s (Chen and Shao, 2012).

The mercury found in most foods is inorganic mercury, methylmercury is mostly formed from methylation of inorganic mercury by microorganisms. Marine and freshwater organisms typically contain higher levels of methyl mereury in large carnivorous fish due to the bioaccumulation of methylmercury in the body as a result of enrichment in the food chain. Overall, people's daily intake of aquatic products are the primary source of methylmercury intake.

## 二、健康指导值

2010年，JECFA第72届会议将无机汞的暂定每周可耐受摄入量（PTWI）降为4 μg/(kg bw·周)，适用于来源于非鱼贝类食品的膳食汞暴露评估，对来源于鱼贝类食品的膳食汞暴露评估仍采用以前设定的甲基汞的PTWI[1.6 μg/(kg bw·周)]。将膳食总汞摄入量扣除来自水产动物的汞摄入量，可作为膳食无机汞摄入量的估计值。

## 三、总膳食研究结果

### 1. 总膳食研究样品中总汞和甲基汞的含量

对24个省（自治区、直辖市）的12类混合膳食样品进行总汞含量的检测，附表3-46列出了总汞的检测结果。总汞含量存在明显的食品类别差异，总汞含量较高的为水产类膳食。由于除水产类膳食外其他类别膳食的总汞含量均低于甲基汞的检出限，因此只检测了水产类膳食样品中的甲基汞含量，结果见附表3-49。甲基汞含量存在明显地区差异。

### 2. 膳食暴露评估

我国居民总汞的平均膳食摄入量（附表3-47，图3-31）为1.26 μg/d，范围为0.29～3.10 μg/d，存在明显的地区差异。我国居民从水产类膳食中摄入甲基汞的量（附表3-50，图3-32）平均为0.32 μg/d，范围为0.00～1.51 μg/d，相当于2.2% PTWI（范围为0.0%～10.5% PTWI）（计算时体重取63 kg）。甲基汞摄入量呈现明显的南方区高于北方区的趋势。

## II. HBGV

At the 72$^{nd}$ JECFA meeting in 2010, the PTWI value for inorganic mercury was lowered to 4 μg/(kg bw·week), applicable to the assessment of dietary exposure to mercury in foods other than fish and shellfish. The assessment of dietary exposure to mercury in fish and shellfish still uses the original PTWI value [1.6 μg/(kg bw·week)]. The dietary intake of inorganic mercury is estimated to be the total mercury intake less the mercury intake from aquatic animals.

## III. TDS Results

### 1. Levels of Total Mercury and Methylmercury in TDS Composite Samples

Composite dietary samples of 12 food categories from 24 provinces (autonomous regions, municipalities) were analyzed for the level of total mercury. As shown in the Annexed Table 3-46. There were category differences in total mercury levels. Aquatic foods were higher in total mercury. Since the total mercury levels in all food categories except aquatic foods were lower than the LOD of methylmercury, only aquatic foods samples were determined for methylmercury, as shown in the Annexed Table 3-49. And there are regional differences in methylmercury content.

### 2. Dietary Exposure Assessment

The average dietary intake of total mercury for China residents (Annexed Table 3-47, Figure 3-31) was 1.26 μg/d, ranging from 0.29 μg/d to 3.10 μg/d, with significant regional differences. The average dietary intake of methylmercury from aquatic foods for China residents (Annexed Table 3-50, Figure 3-32) was 0.32 μg/d, ranging from 0.00 μg/d to 1.51 μg/d, equivalent to 2.2% of the PTWI (0.0%-10.5% of PTWI) (weight: 63 kg). The dietary intake of methylmercury was remarkably higher in the southern region than in the northern region.

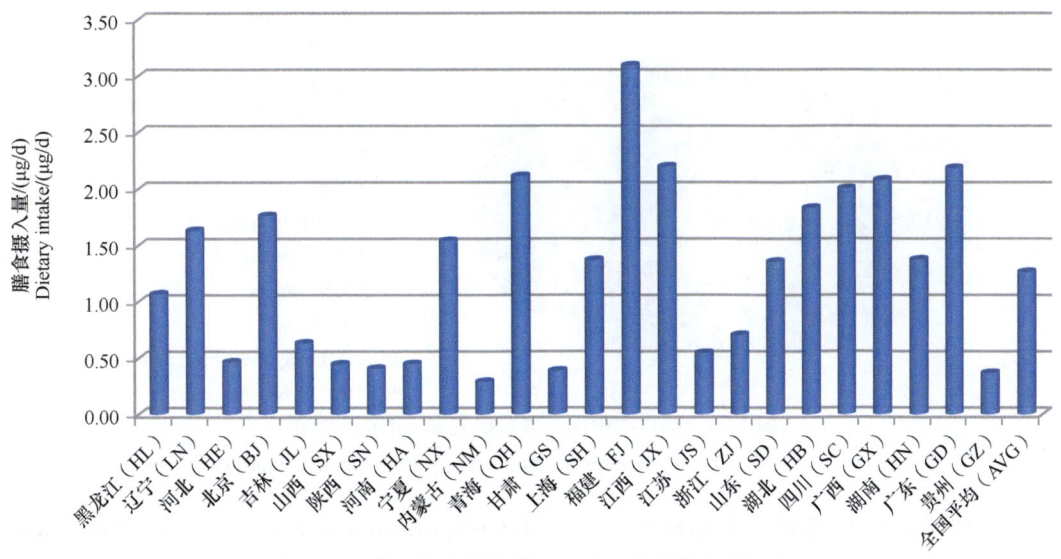

图 3-31　第六次中国总膳食研究的总汞膳食摄入量
Figure 3-31　Dietary intake of total mercury from the 6$^{th}$ China TDS

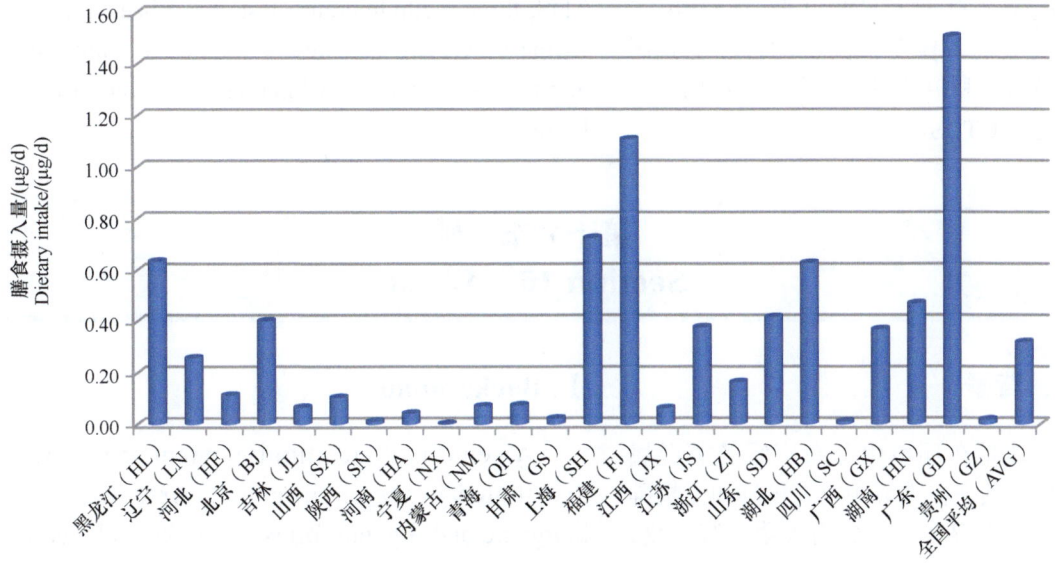

图 3-32　第六次中国总膳食研究的甲基汞膳食摄入量
Figure 3-32　Dietary intake of methylmercury from the 6$^{th}$ China TDS

## 3. 各类膳食对总膳食摄入的贡献

6$^{th}$ CTDS 中我国居民总汞的主要膳食来源（附表 3-48，图 3-33）为谷类和水产类食品。甲基汞几乎全部来源于水产类，甲基汞的暴露量与水产类膳食的消费量密切相关。

## 3. Contributions of Food Categories to the Total Dietary Intake

The primary sources of dietary intake for total mercury for China residents in the 6$^{th}$ CTDS (Annexed Table 3-48, Figure 3-33) were cereals and aquatic foods. The dietary intake of methylmercury almost entirely came from aquatic foods, and methylmercury exposure is closely related to the consumption of aquatic foods.

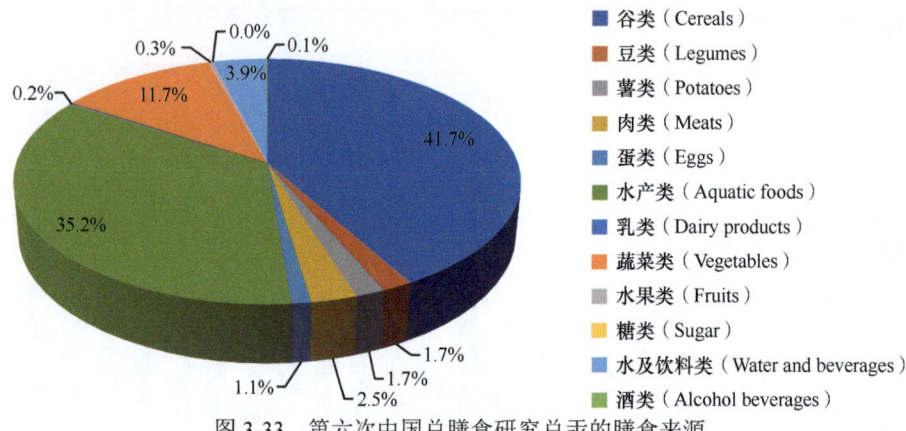

图 3-33 第六次中国总膳食研究总汞的膳食来源
Figure 3-33  Dietary sources of total mercury from the 6th China TDS

**4. 与以往中国总膳食研究结果的比较**

中国总膳食研究共开展了 6 次总汞的检测，自 4th CTDS 以来，已开展了三次甲基汞检测，在 6th CTDS 中我国居民总汞和甲基汞的膳食摄入量均低于前几次 CTDS。

**4. Comparison with Previous China TDSs Results**

A total of six tests of total mercury have been conducted in the China TDSs. Since the fourth China TDS, three methylmercury tests have been carried out. In the 6th CTDS, the dietary intakes of total mercury and methylmercury for China residents were lower than before.

# 第十六节　砷
# Section 16　Arsenic

## 一、背景
## Ⅰ. Background

砷是在环境中分布广泛的类金属元素。其在自然界中以有机砷和无机砷两种状态存在。在岩石土壤、沉积物、水以及陆生植物中主要以亚砷酸、砷酸、一甲基砷酸和二甲基砷酸形态存在；在水产品中主要以砷甜菜碱、砷胆碱以及更为复杂的砷化合物如砷糖、砷酯等形态存在。砷化合物的毒性与其形态密切相关，且相差甚远。无机砷形态具有很强的毒性，已被国际癌症研究机构确认为致癌物（IARC, 2004）。一甲基砷酸和二甲基砷酸形态毒性较弱。而砷甜菜碱、砷胆碱、砷糖、砷脂通常被

Arsenic is a metalloid element that is widely distributed in the environment. Arsenic occurs in inorganic and organic forms. In rocky soil, sediment, water, and terrestrial plants, it exists mainly in the form of arsenous acid, arsenic acid, monomethylarsenic acid, and dimethylarsenic acid; in aquatic products, it exists mainly in the form of arsenic betaine, arsenic choline, and more complex arsenic compounds such as arsenic sugar and arsenic esters. The toxicity of arsenic compounds is closely related to their form and varies widely. The inorganic arsenic form is highly toxic and has been recognized as a carcinogen by the International Agency for Research on Cancer (IARC, 2004). The

认为低毒或无毒。长期摄入无机砷会导致皮肤损害、心血管疾病、发育毒性、糖代谢异常、2型糖尿病、神经毒性和免疫毒性等，还会引发皮肤癌、肺癌、膀胱癌等癌症。大多数食物中含有低浓度的砷。膳食，尤其是海产品，是大多数人群摄入砷的主要来源（JECFA，2011a）。

## 二、健康指导值

JECFA 于 1989 年提出无机砷的暂定每周可耐受摄入量（PTWI）为 15 μg/(kg bw·周)。2010 年，JECFA 第 72 次会议明确了无机砷为致癌物，将其纳入致癌物管理，因此取消了无机砷的 PTWI 值。JECFA（2011a）确定了人类肺癌发病率增加 0.5% 的无机砷基准剂量置信下限（$BMDL_{0.5}$）为 3.0 μg/(kg bw·d)[范围为 2~7 μg/(kg bw·d)]。推荐采用暴露边界值（MOE）方法评估膳食无机砷暴露的健康风险。无机砷的 MOE 值是 $BMDL_{0.5}$ 与无机砷膳食摄入量的比值。当 MOE 大于 1 时，认为无机砷暴露的健康风险属于可接受的低水平，反之则表明可能存在潜在风险。

## 三、总膳食研究结果

### 1. 总膳食研究样品中总砷和无机砷的含量

对 24 个省（自治区、直辖市）的 12 类混合膳食样品进行了总砷及无机砷的检测，总砷结果如附表 3-51 所示，总砷平均含量较高的膳食样品依次是水产类、蔬菜类和谷类。无机砷结果如附表 3-54 所示，无机砷含量较高的样品为谷类、蔬菜类、水产类、糖类。

monomethylarsenic acid and dimethylarsenic acid forms are less toxic. Arsenic betaine, arsenic choline, arsenic sugar, and arsenolipids are usually considered to be low or non-toxic. Long-term intake of inorganic arsenic can cause skin damage, cardiovascular disease, developmental toxicity, abnormal glucose metabolism, type 2 diabetes, neurotoxicity, and immunotoxicity, as well as skin cancer, lung cancer, bladder cancer, and other cancers. Most foods contain arsenic in varying concentrations. Diet, especially seafoods, is the main source of arsenic intake for most of the population (JECFA, 2011a).

## II. HBGV

In 1989, JECFA recommended a provisional tolerable weekly intake (PTWI) of 15 μg/(kg bw·week) for inorganic arsenic. At the 72$^{nd}$ JECFA meeting in 2010, inorganic arsenic was confirmed as a carcinogen and included within the scope of carcinogen management, the PTWI value for inorganic arsenic was withdrawn. JECFA (2011a) determined the inorganic arsenic benchmark dose lower confidence limit for a 0.5% increased incidence of lung cancer in human ($BMDL_{0.5}$) as 3.0 μg/(kg bw·d) [in the region of 2-7 μg/(kg bw·d)]. In order to assess the health risk of dietary exposure for inorganic arsenic, the margin of exposure (MOE) approach is used. The MOE for inorganic arsenic is the ratio of $BMDL_{0.5}$ to the inorganic arsenic dietary exposure estimate. When the MOE value is greater than 1, the health risk of inorganic arsenic intake is at a low level, while the opposite indicates a potential risk may exist.

## III. TDS Results

### 1. Levels of Total Arsenic and Inorganic Arsenic in TDS Composite Samples

Composite samples of 12 food categories from 24 provinces (autonomous regions, municipalities) were analyzed for the level of total arsenic and inorganic

## 2. 膳食暴露评估

我国居民膳食总砷摄入量（附表3-52，图3-34）平均为41.5 μg/d，范围为12.3～137 μg/d。

我国居民膳食无机砷摄入量（附表3-55，图3-35）平均为9.83 μg/d，范围为4.65～26.4 μg/d。膳食无机砷摄入量的MOE值为5～27，平均值为 arsenic. Annexed Table 3-51 showed foods that were rich in total arsenic include aquatic foods, vegetables, and cereals. Annexed Table 3-54 showed foods that were rich in inorganic arsenic include cereals, vegetables, aquatic foods, and sugar.

## 2. Dietary Exposure Assessment

The average dietary intake of total arsenic for China residents was 41.5 μg/d, ranging significantly from 12.3 μg/d

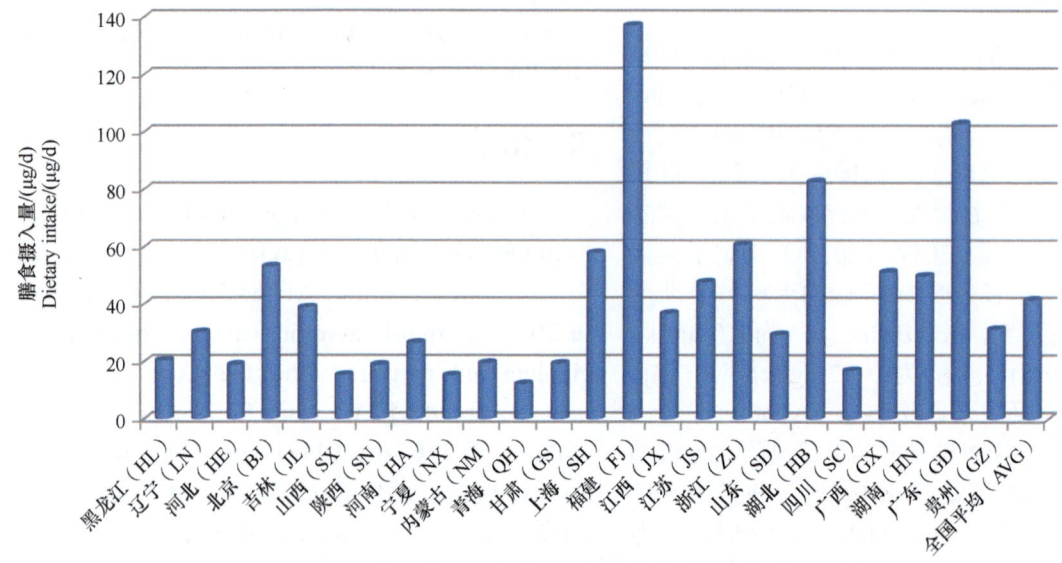

图 3-34 第六次中国总膳食研究膳食总砷的摄入量
Figure 3-34 Dietary total arsenic intakes from 6th China TDS

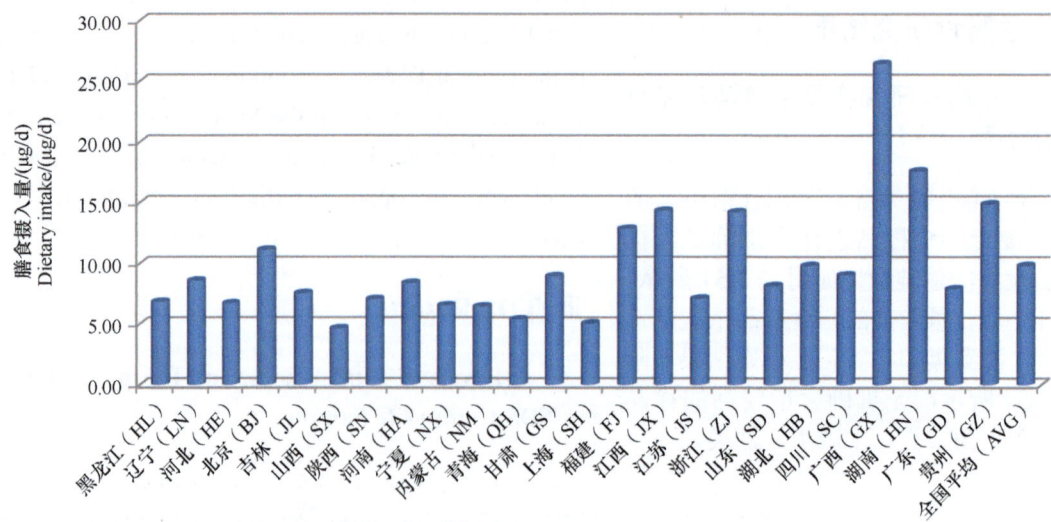

图 3-35 第六次中国总膳食研究膳食无机砷的摄入量
Figure 3-35 Dietary inorganic arsenic intakes from 6th China TDS

13。MOE值均大于1，说明我国居民膳食无机砷暴露的健康风险较低。

**3. 各类膳食对总膳食摄入的贡献**

我国居民膳食总砷摄入主要来源（附表3-53，图3-36）于蔬菜类，其次是谷类和水产类，约占总膳食摄入量的95%。我国居民膳食无机砷摄入主要来源于谷类，占总膳食摄入量的77%（附表3-56，图3-37）。

to 137 μg/d (Annexed Table 3-52, Figure 3-34).

The average dietary intake of inorganic arsenic for China residents was 9.83 μg/d, ranging from 4.65 μg/d to 26.4 μg/d (Annexed Table 3-55, Figure 3-35). The MOE value of dietary inorganic arsenic intake ranged from 5 to 27, with an average of 13. The MOE values were all greater than 1, indicating that the health risk of dietary inorganic arsenic intake for China residents was generally low.

**3. Contributions of Food Categories to the Total Dietary Intake**

The main sources of total arsenic intake for China residents (Annexed Table 3-53, Figure 3-36) were vegetables, cereals, and Aquatic foods, accounting

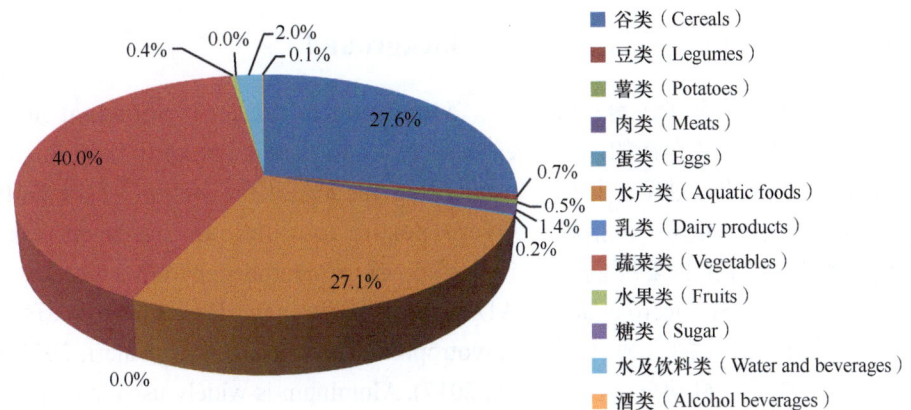

图 3-36　第六次中国总膳食研究总砷摄入的膳食来源
Figure 3-36　Food sources of dietary total arsenic from 6th China TDS

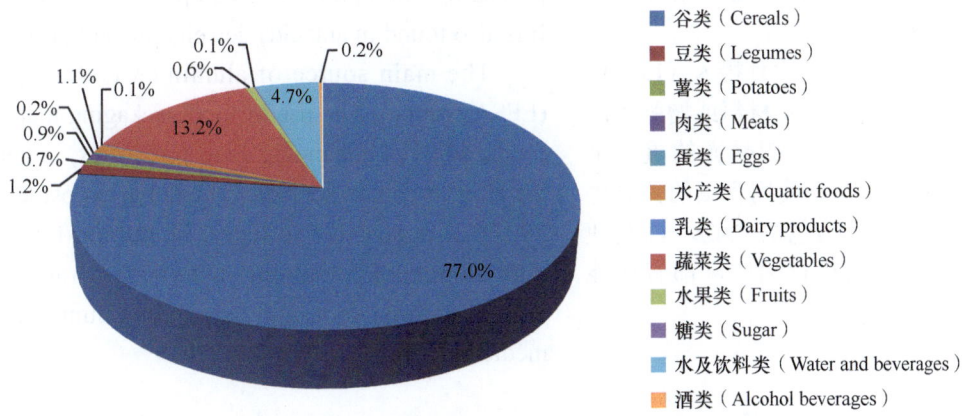

图 3-37　第六次中国总膳食研究无机砷摄入的膳食来源
Figure 3-37　Food sources of dietary inorganic arsenic from 6th China TDS

## 4. 与以往中国总膳食研究结果的比较

我国居民 6th CTDS 中总砷、无机砷摄入量相较 4th CTDS、5th CTDS 都有较大程度下降。6th CTDS 中总砷摄入量分别比 4th CTDS、5th CTDS 降低了 33.4%、64.8%。6th CTDS 中无机砷摄入量相比 4th CTDS、5th CTDS 分别降低了 64.1%、64.5%。

for over 95% of the total intake. The main source of inorganic arsenic for China residents intake was cereals (77%) (Annexed Table 3-56, Figure 3-37).

## 4. Comparison with Previous China TDSs Results

The dietary intakes of total arsenic and inorganic arsenic among China residents decreased significantly in the 6th CTDS. Compared with the 4th CTDS and the 5th CTDS, the intake of total arsenic decreased by 33.4% and 64.8%, and inorganic arsenic intake decreased by 64.1% and 64.5%, respectively, in the 6th CTDS.

# 第十七节 铝
# Section 17  Aluminum

## 一、背景

铝是地壳中最丰富的金属元素，自然界中铝是以复合物的形式存在的，地壳的 8% 都是由铝构成的。过度、长期高铝暴露与神经退行性疾病（包括阿尔茨海默病、帕金森病和肌萎缩侧索硬化症）（Cavaleri，2015；Cicero et al.，2017）的风险增加有关。铝在工业中用途广泛，如飞机、轮船、机动车、建筑和电子应用。另外，铝在食品和饮料包装、食品加工设备与厨房用具中也有大量应用。铝在抗酸药物、首饰和止汗产品中也有应用。

铝的主要来源是饮食摄入（EFSA，2008c）。使用食品包装材料或增强食品特性的食品添加剂是铝暴露的重要来源（WHO，2007）。使用含铝的器具进行烹饪，使用铝箔包裹食物，以及使用含有铝的药品进行治疗，都有可能摄入铝。

## Ⅰ. Background

Aluminum is the most abundant metal in the earth's crust and occurs naturally only in compounds, accounting for 8% of the weight of the earth's crust. Overexposure to aluminum has been related to an increased risk of neurodegenerative diseases, including Alzheimer's disease, Parkinson's disease, and amyotrophic lateral sclerosis (Cavaleri, 2015; Cicero et al., 2017). Aluminum is widely used in many industries, such as aircraft, ships, motor vehicles, buildings and electronics. It is also used in food and beverage packaging, food processing equipment and kitchenware. It is also found in antacids, jewelry and antiperspirants.

The main source of aluminum is dietary intake (EFSA, 2008c). The use of food packaging materials or food additives enhancing food properties, is generally the most important source of aluminum exposure (WHO, 2007). It is possible to ingest aluminum for cooking with aluminum containing table ware, wrapping food with aluminum fool, and using aluminum containing medicines.

## 二、健康指导值

2011年，JECFA对铝的每周可耐受摄入量（PTWI）进行了修订，专家委员会根据实验动物的发育和慢性神经毒性研究，建立了对所有人群的铝的暂定每周可耐受摄入量（PTWI）为2 mg/(kg bw·周)（WHO，2011a）。

## 三、总膳食研究结果

### 1. 总膳食研究样品中铝的含量

对24个省（自治区、直辖市）的12类混合膳食样品进行铝含量的检测，从检测结果（附表3-57）可以看出，铝含量较高的样品依次为薯类、谷类、豆类和蔬菜类食品。

### 2. 膳食暴露评估

我国居民膳食铝的平均摄入量（附表3-58，图3-38）为8.10 mg/d，范围为1.80~22.1 mg/d，相当于PTWI的45.2%（范围为10.2%~123% PTWI）（计算时体重取63 kg）。铝摄入量存在明显的地区差异。我国居民铝的膳食暴露均值均小于JECFA建立的PTWI [2 mg/(kg bw·周)]，对人体的健康风险较低。

## II. HBGV

In 2011, the JECFA Expert Committee revised the provisional tolerable weekly intake (PTWI) for aluminum, establishing a PTWI of 2 mg/(kg bw·week) based on developmental and chronic neurotoxicity studies in experimental animals (WHO, 2011a).

## III. TDS Results

### 1. Levels of Aluminum in TDS Composite Samples

The composite dietary samples of 12 food categories from 24 provinces (autonomous regions, municipalities) were analyzed for the level of aluminum. The detailed results are shown in the Annexed Table 3-57. Food samples with high aluminum levels included, in descending order, potatoes, cereals, legumes and vegetables.

### 2. Dietary Exposure Assessment

The average dietary intake of aluminum for China residents (Figure 3-38) was 8.10 mg/d (45.2% of PTWI), ranging from 1.80 mg/d to 22.1 mg/d (10.2%-123% of PTWI) (weight: 63 kg). There were significant regional differences in aluminum intakes. The aluminum exposures were all below the PTWI value of 2 mg/(kg bw·week) established by JECFA, and the health risk was low.

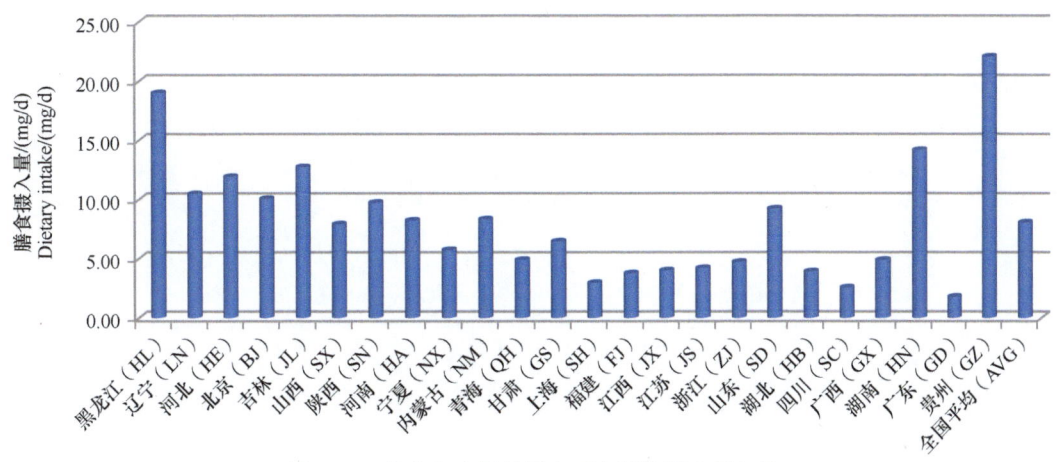

图3-38 第六次中国总膳食研究铝的膳食摄入量

Figure 3-38 Dietary intake of aluminum from the 6th China TDS

**3. 各类膳食对总膳食摄入的贡献**

我国居民膳食铝摄入的主要来源（附表 3-59，图 3-39）为谷类和蔬菜类食物，占总摄入来源的近 80%，其中谷类食物占总摄入来源的 50% 以上。各省（自治区、直辖市）的食物来源也基本相似。

**3. Contributions of Food Categories to the Total Dietary Intake**

The primary sources of dietary aluminum intake (Figure 3-39) were cereals and vegetables, accounting for nearly 80% of the total intake, with cereals accounting for over 50%. The food sources of aluminum were basically similar among provinces (autonomous regions, municipalities).

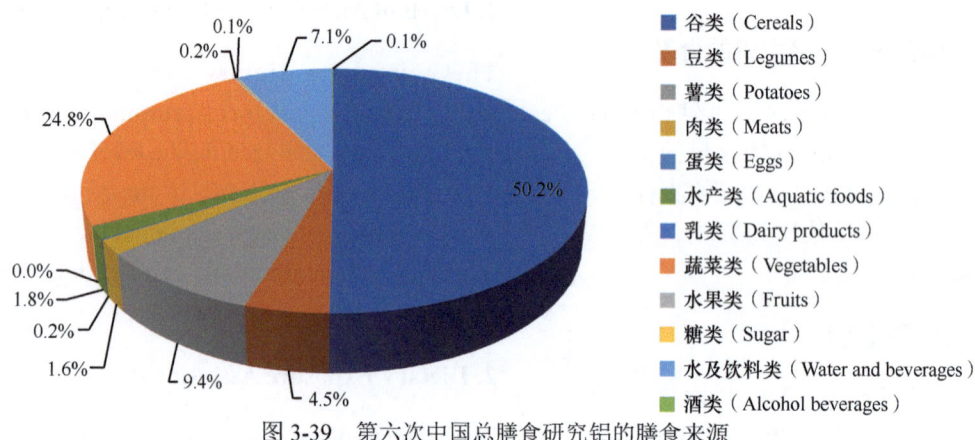

图 3-39 第六次中国总膳食研究铝的膳食来源
Figure 3-39  Dietary sources of aluminum from the 6$^{th}$ China TDS

# 第四章　农药残留的膳食暴露评估
## Chapter 4　Dietary Exposure Assessment of Pesticide Residues

一、背景

农药是一类用于预防和控制危害农作物及农副产品的病虫害、杂草及其他有害生物的药物总称，其是农业生产中不可或缺的，已广泛应用于农业、畜牧业、林业和公共卫生事业等方面。施用于农作物上的农药一部分附着在农作物表面，一部分散落在土壤、大气和水等环境中，环境中残留的农药又会被农作物的根、茎、叶吸收，从而影响农产品品质。残留农药可直接通过农作物或水到达人、畜体内，或通过环境和食物链最终传递给人。农药残留是施药后的必然现象，但如果超过规定的最大残留限量，会对人、畜产生毒害的风险。农药按防治对象可分为杀虫剂、杀螨剂、杀菌剂、杀线虫剂、杀鼠剂、除草剂和植物生长调节剂等；而按结构类型则可分为有机氯类、有机磷类、拟除虫菊酯类、氨基甲酸酯类、苯并咪唑类、三唑类、三嗪类、苯甲酰脲类、新烟碱类等。食品中的农药残留不仅包括农药本身的残留，还包括被认为具有毒理学意义的农药衍生物，如农药转化物、代谢物、反应产物和杂质残留物。

随着农业产业化、工业化和城市化进程的加快，农药使用量逐年增加。随着农药的大量使用以及不合理使用，食品中的农药残留问题日益显露。食品中的农药残留受到诸多因素的影响：①食用作物的农药吸收：一般内吸性农药能进入植物体内，由于其在体内迅速运转，使植物体内部的农药残留量高于植

Ⅰ. Background

Pesticides are a general term for a class of compounds used to prevent and control diseases and pests, weeds, and other harmful organisms that harm crops and agricultural and sideline products. It is indispensable in agricultural production and has been widely used in agriculture, animal husbandry, forestry and public health. Some of the pesticides applied to crops are attached to the surface of crops, while others are scattered in the environment such as soil, atmosphere, and water. The residual pesticides in the environment will be absorbed by the roots, stems and leaves of crops, thus affecting the quality of agricultural products. Pesticide residues can enter into people and livestock directly through crops or water, or finally be transmitted to people through the environment and food chains. Pesticide residue is an inevitable phenomenon after application, but if it exceeds the prescribed maximum residue limit, it will be harmful to human beings and animals. Pesticides can be classified into insecticides, acaricides, fungicides, nematicides, rodenticides, herbicides, and plant growth regulators according to the control objects. According to the structural types, it can be divided into organochlorines, organophosphorus, pyrethroids, carbamates, benzimidazoles, triazoles, triazines, benzoylureas, neonicotinoids and so on. Pesticide residues in food not only include the residues of pesticides themselves, but also pesticide derivatives that are considered to have toxicological significance, such as pesticide transformers, metabolites, reaction products and residue of impurities.

With the acceleration of agricultural industrialization and urbanization, the use of pesticides is

物体外部；而渗透性农药只沾染在植物外表，因此外表的农药浓度高于内部。②喷洒作物：农药在食用作物上的残留受到农药品种、施药次数、施药浓度、施药时间、施药方法和气象条件等多种因素的影响。③植物的种类：农药残留随植物的种类不同和同一种类不同部位而不同，一般叶菜类植物的农药残留量高于果菜类和根菜类。④较低的农药残留认知水平，如未遵守农药的停药期规定而提前采收，造成农药残留；使用不被允许使用在该农作物上的农药，或倾向于使用高毒、高残留甚至国家明令禁止的高毒农药。

食用含有大量高毒、剧毒农药残留的食物，会导致人、畜急性中毒。长期食用农药残留超标的食品，虽不会导致急性中毒，但可能引起人和动物的慢性中毒，导致疾病的发生。目前使用的绝大多数有机合成农药都是脂溶性的，易残留于食品原料中，如有机氯农药。若长期食用农药残留较高的食品，农药则会在人体内逐渐蓄积，最终导致机体生理功能发生变化，引起慢性中毒。另外，通过动物实验证实，部分农药还会引起一些特殊毒性，如致畸、致癌和致突变作用，如涕灭威、久效磷等农药。

increasing year by year. With the large amount and unreasonable use of pesticides, the problem of pesticide residues in food is becoming more and more obvious. Pesticide residues in food are affected by many factors: ① pesticide absorption of edible crops: generally, inhalant pesticides can enter the plant. Due to their rapid operation in the body, the pesticide residues in the plant are higher than those outside the plant. The osmotic pesticide is only contaminated on the plant surface, so the pesticide concentration on the surface is higher than that on the inside. ② Spraying crops: pesticide residues on edible crops are affected by many factors, such as pesticide variety, application times, application concentration, application time, application method, and meteorological conditions. ③ Types of plants: pesticide residues vary with different types of plants and different parts of the same kind. Generally, the pesticide residues of leafy vegetables are higher than those of fruit vegetables and root vegetables. ④ Low awareness level of pesticide residues, such as early harvest without complying with the provisions of pesticide withdrawal period, resulting in pesticide residues; use pesticides that are not allowed to be used in this crop, or tend to use highly toxic, high residue and even highly toxic pesticides banned by the state.

Eating food containing a large amount of highly toxic and severely toxic pesticide residues will lead to acute poisoning of people and livestock. Long-term consumption of food with excessive pesticide residues will not lead to acute poisoning, but it may lead to chronic poisoning of people and animals further causing the outbreak of diseases. At present, most organic synthetic pesticides used are fat-soluble and easy to remain in food raw materials, such as organochlorine pesticides. If people eat foods with high pesticide residues for a long time, pesticides will gradually accumulate in the human body, eventually leading to changes in physiological functions of the body and chronic poisoning. In addition, animal experiments have proved that some pesticides can also cause some special toxicity, such as teratogenic, carcinogenic and

加工过程有助于降低食品中农药残留的含量，常见加工过程方法有：①清水浸泡洗涤法，这有助于对附着于果蔬表面上的农药的去除，以及对极性农药的溶出去除；②加热烹调法，加热有助于部分农药的降解，如有机磷类农药和氨基甲酸酯类农药；③清洗去皮法，对于附着于果蔬表皮的农药可通过去皮初步减少农药。然而，某些加工过程也可能造成农药残留水平提高，如干燥或晾晒，因为食品中水分减少，从而使得农药的残留水平增加，而加热等方式会使某些农药转化成比其自身毒性更大的代谢物，从而造成食品安全隐患。如蒸煮过程中敌百虫会转化为敌敌畏，以及丁硫克百威和丙硫克百威可以转化为克百威，并进一步降解为3-羟基克百威等。因此，加工过程仅是对已残留的农药所采取的一定的应对措施，要降低食品中的农药残留，以便不超过最大残留限量，必须从源头上杜绝农药残留，可采取的控制措施有：①严禁使用国家管控的剧毒或高毒农药；农药在使用中要严格按照《农药合理使用准则》国家标准，采用合理的用药方法，严格控制使用次数和施药浓度；严格执行农药使用安全间隔期。②开展全面、系统的农药残留监测工作，掌握食品中农药残留的状况和规律。③开发易降解、低残留、高活性以及对环境有益、比较安全的新型农药，如使用低毒、低残留的生物农药。

mutagenic effects, such as aldicarb, monocrotophos and other pesticides.

Processing helps to reduce the content of pesticide residues in food. For example, common processing methods include: ① soaking and washing with clear water, which is helpful to remove pesticides attached to the surfaces of fruits and vegetables, and to remove polar pesticides by dissolution; ② heating cooking method, heating is helpful to the degradation of some pesticides, such as organophosphorus pesticides and carbamates pesticides; ③ cleaning and peeling method, pesticides attached to the epidermis of fruits and vegetables, peeling can initially reduce pesticides. However, some processing processes may also increase the level of pesticide residues, such as drying or sun exposure. Because of the decrease of water in food, the level of pesticide residues will increase, while some pesticides will be transformed into metabolites with greater toxicity than their own by heating, which will lead to food safety hazards. For example, trichlorfon will be transformed into dichlorvos during cooking, carbosulfan and benfuracarb can be transformed into carbofuran, and further degraded into 3-hydroxy carbofuran, etc. Therefore, the processing process is only a certain response to pesticide residues. To reduce pesticide residues in food so as not to exceed the maximum residue limit, pesticide residues must be eliminated from the source. The control measures that can be taken are as follows: ① it is strictly forbidden to use severely toxic or highly toxic pesticides controlled by the state. In the use of pesticides, we should strictly follow the national standard of *Guidelines for the Rational Use of Pesticides*, adopt reasonable pesticide use methods, and strictly control the rate of use and the concentration to be applied. Strictly implement the safe interval of pesticide use. ② Carry out comprehensive and systematic monitoring of pesticide residues, and master the status and laws of pesticide residues in food. ③ Develop new pesticides that are easy to degrade, low residue, high activity, beneficial to the environment and relatively safe, such as biological pesticides with low

联合国粮食及农业组织和世界卫生组织专门设置了农药残留联席会议（JMPR），并通过国际食品法典委员会（CAC）制定和颁布了各种农药在不同食品中的残留限量标准，即最大残留限量（MRL）。欧盟也制定和颁布了相关食品中的农药残留限量标准，并且其标准非常严格，甚至超过了CAC的标准，如对尚未确定MRL的农药一律采用0.01 mg/kg的严格限量标准。日本同样建立了系统的食品农药残留限量标准和法规，并在食品中引入"肯定列表制度"，对所有农业化学品在食品中的残留提出了限量要求。中国现行的农药最大残留限量标准《食品安全国家标准 食品中农药最大残留限量》（GB 2763—2021）基本涵盖了在中国获得农药登记的、允许使用的和禁止使用的农药。截至2019年底，中国禁止生产、销售和使用的农药名单达到41种，限制使用的农药有19种。

## 二、健康指导值

我国《食品安全国家标准 食品中农药最大残留限量》（GB 2763—2021）规定了各类农药的每日允许摄入量（ADI），本章列出第六次中国总膳食研究样品中检出的农药ADI值，见表4-1。

toxicity and low residue.

The Food and Agriculture Organization of the United Nations and the World Health Organization specially set up the Joint Conference on Pesticide Residues (JMPR), and through the Codex Alimentarius Commission (CAC), formulated and promulgated the residue limit standards of various pesticides in different foods, namely the maximum residue limit (MRL). The European Union has also formulated and promulgated the pesticide residue limit standard in related foods, and its standard is very strict, even exceeding the CAC standard. For example, the strict limit standard of 0.01 mg/kg is adopted for all pesticides for which MRL has not been determined. Japan has also established systematic standards and regulations for pesticide residue limit in food, and introduced "positive list system" into food, which puts forward the limit requirements for all agricultural chemicals residues in food. China's current pesticide maximum residue limit standard *National Food Safety Standard-The Maximum Residue Limits for Pesticides* (GB 2763—2021) basically covers the pesticides registered, allowed and prohibited in China. By the end of 2019, there were 41 kinds of pesticides banned from production, sale and use in China, and 19 kinds of pesticides restricted in use.

## II. HBGV

The acceptable daily intake (ADI) values for pesticides were specified by the *National Food Safety Standard-The Maximum Residue Limits for Pesticides* (GB 2763—2021) in Food are shown in Table 4-1.

表 4-1 第六次中国总膳食研究样品中检出农药清单及其 ADI
Table 4-1 The pesticide lists detected in 6$^{th}$ CTDS and their respective ADIs

| 农药类别 Pesticide categories | 农药 Pesticides | ADI/[mg/(kg bw · d)] |
|---|---|---|
| 杀虫剂 Insecticides | | |
| 有机磷类 Organophosphorus | 甲胺磷 Methamidophos | 0.004 |
| | 乙酰甲胺磷 Acephate | 0.03 |
| | 氧乐果 Omethoate | 0.0003 |
| | 乐果 Dimethoate | 0.002 |

续表

| 农药类别 Pesticide categories | 农药 Pesticides | ADI/[mg/(kg bw·d)] |
|---|---|---|
| 有机磷类 Organophosphorus | 敌敌畏 Dichlorvos | 0.004 |
| | 三唑磷 Triazophos | 0.001 |
| | 二嗪磷 Diazinon | 0.005 |
| | 丙溴磷 Profenofos | 0.03 |
| | 毒死蜱 Chlorpyrifos | 0.01 |
| 氨基甲酸酯类 Carbamates | 克百威（克百威和3-羟基克百威）Carbofuran (the sum of carbofuran and 3-hydroxycarbofuran) | 0.001 |
| | 茚虫威 Indoxacarb | 0.01 |
| 新烟碱类 Neonicotinoids | 吡虫啉 Imidacloprid | 0.06 |
| | 噻虫嗪 Thiamethoxam | 0.08 |
| | 噻虫胺 Clothianidin | 0.1 |
| | 啶虫脒 Acetamiprid | 0.07 |
| | N-脱甲基啶虫脒 Acetamiprid-N-desmethyl | 0.07 |
| | 烯啶虫胺 Nitenpyram | 0.53 |
| | 呋虫胺 Dinotefuran | 0.2 |
| | 噻虫啉 Thiacloprid | 0.01 |
| | 氯噻啉 Imidaclothiz | 0.025 |
| | 总新烟碱 Total neonicotinoids | 0.06 |
| 苯基吡唑类 Phenylpyrazoles | 氟虫腈（氟虫腈、氟虫腈砜、氟甲腈和氟虫腈亚砜）Total fipronil (the sum of fipronil, fipronil sulfone, fipronil desulfinyl, and fipronil sulfide) | 0.0002 |
| 三嗪类 Triazines | 灭蝇胺 Cyromazine | 0.06 |
| 有机氮类 Organic nitrogens | 甲氧虫酰肼 Methoxyfenozide | 0.1 |
| | 噻嗪酮 Buprofezin | 0.009 |
| 吡啶类 Pyridines | 吡丙醚 Pyriproxyfen | 0.1 |
| 杀菌剂 Fungicides | | |
| 三唑类 Triazoles | 粉唑醇 Flutriafol | 0.01 |
| | 腈菌唑 Myclobutanil | 0.03 |
| | 三唑醇 Triadimenol | 0.03 |
| | 三唑酮 Triadimefon | 0.03 |
| | 四氟醚唑 Tetraconazole | 0.004 |
| | 氟环唑 Epoxiconazole | 0.02 |
| | 腈苯唑 Fenbuconazole | 0.03 |
| | 氟硅唑 Flusilazole | 0.007 |
| | 戊唑醇 Tebuconazole | 0.03 |
| | 戊菌唑 Penconazole | 0.03 |
| | 丙环唑 Propiconazole | 0.07 |

续表

| 农药类别 Pesticide categories | 农药 Pesticides | ADI/[mg/(kg bw·d)] |
|---|---|---|
| 三唑类 Triazoles | 己唑醇 Hexaconazole | 0.005 |
| | 苯醚甲环唑 Difenoconazole | 0.01 |
| 咪唑类 Imidazoles | 多菌灵 Carbendazim | 0.03 |
| | 噻菌灵 Thiabendazole | 0.1 |
| | 抑霉唑 Imazalil | 0.03 |
| | 咪鲜胺 Prochloraz | 0.01 |
| 酰胺类 Amides | 甲霜灵 Metalaxyl | 0.08 |
| | 环酰菌胺 Fenhexamid | 0.2 |
| 嘧啶类 Pyrimidines | 嘧霉胺 Pyrimethanil | 0.2 |
| | 乙嘧酚磺酸酯 Bupirimate | 0.05 |
| | 嘧菌环胺 Cyprodinil | 0.03 |
| 酰胺类 Amides | 氟吡菌胺 Fluopicolide | 0.08 |
| | 烯酰吗啉 Dimethomorph | 0.2 |
| 吡咯类 Pyrroles | 咯菌腈 Fludioxonil | 0.4 |
| 甲氧基丙烯酸酯类 Strobilurins | 嘧菌酯 Azoxystrobin | 0.2 |
| | 吡唑醚菌酯 Pyraclostrobin | 0.03 |
| | 肟菌酯 Trifloxystrobin | 0.04 |
| 杀螨剂 Acaricides | | |
| 有机硫类 Organosulfurs | 炔螨特 Propargite | 0.01 |
| 季酮酸类 Tetronic acids | 螺螨酯 Spirodiclofen | 0.01 |
| 哒嗪类 Pyridazines | 哒螨灵 Pyridaben | 0.01 |
| 除草剂 Herbicides | | |
| 三嗪类 Triazines | 莠去津 Atrazine | 0.02 |
| 植物生长调节剂 Plant growth regulators | | |
| 三唑类 Triazoles | 多效唑 Paclobutrazol | 0.1 |

## 三、总膳食研究结果

### （一）杀虫剂

#### 1. 有机磷类农药

（1）混合膳食样品中有机磷类农药的含量

第六次中国总膳食研究混合膳食样品中检出9种有机磷类农药，分别为甲胺磷、乙酰甲胺磷、氧乐果、乐果、敌敌畏、三唑磷、二嗪磷、丙溴磷和毒

## III. TDS Results

### (I) Insecticides

#### 1. Organophosphorus Pesticides

(1) Levels of Organophosphorus Pesticides in Composite Dietary Samples

Nine organophosphorus pesticides were detected in the 6$^{th}$ China TDS composite samples, including methamidophos, acephate, omethoate, dimethoate, dichlorvos, triazophos, diazinon, profenofos, and

死蜱。其在 12 类膳食样品中均有检出，有机磷类农药的总检出率为 63.9%，其中，蔬菜类检出率最高（100%），其次是水果类和水产类（分别为 87.5% 和 83.3%），乳类、水及饮料类、糖类、酒类检出率较低，分别为 37.5%、33.3%、25.0% 和 25.0%。9 种有机磷类农药的残留水平在 ND[①]～68.75 μg/kg（表 4-2），按检出率由高至低排列分别为毒死蜱（附表 4-1）、敌敌畏（附表 4-2）、乙酰甲胺磷（附表 4-3）、三唑磷（附表 4-4）、丙溴磷（附表 4-5）、氧乐果（附表 4-6）、乐果（附表 4-7）、甲胺磷（附表 4-8）和二嗪磷（附表 4-9）。

chlorpyrifos. The total detection rate of organophosphorus pesticides was 63.9%. Among them, vegetables had the highest detection rate (100%), followed by fruits and aquatic products (87.5% and 83.3%, respectively). The detection rates of dairy products, water and beverages, sugar, and alcohol beverages were low with 37.5%, 33.3%, 25.0%, and 25.0%, respectively. The Residue level of 9 organophosphorus pesticides was ND-68.75 μg/kg (Table 4-2). According to the detection rates from high to low, they were chlorpyrifos (Annexed Table 4-1), dichlorvos (Annexed Table 4-2), acephate (Annexed Table 4-3), triazophos (Annexed Table 4-4), profenofos (Annexed Table 4-5), ometoate (Annexed Table 4-6), dimethoate (Annexed Table 4-7), methamidophos (Annexed Table 4-8), and diazinon (Annexed Table 4-9).

表 4-2　第六次中国总膳食研究有机磷类农药的残留水平和膳食摄入量
Table 4-2　Residue levels and dietary intakes of organophosphorus pesticides in the 6th China TDS

| 农药 Pesticides | 检出率 Detection rates/% | 残留水平 Residue levels/(μg/kg) | 平均水平 Mean/(μg/kg) | 摄入量 Dietary intakes/[ng/(kg bw·d)] | ADI/% |
|---|---|---|---|---|---|
| 甲胺磷 Methamidophos | 1.0 | ND～0.13 | 0.00 | 0.012 | 0.00 |
| 乙酰甲胺磷 Acephate | 17.0 | ND～3.97 | 0.19 | 7.194 | 0.02 |
| 氧乐果 Omethoate | 4.5 | ND～14.45 | 0.10 | 7.106 | 2.37 |
| 乐果 Dimethoate | 3.1 | ND～68.75 | 0.25 | 24.743 | 1.24 |
| 敌敌畏 Dichlorvos | 18.1 | ND～36.48 | 0.55 | 39.306 | 0.98 |
| 三唑磷 Triazophos | 10.8 | ND～3.09 | 0.03 | 1.671 | 0.17 |
| 二嗪磷 Diazinon | 0.7 | ND～0.18 | 0.00 | 0.012 | 0.00 |
| 丙溴磷 Profenofos | 9.4 | ND～15.65 | 0.16 | 6.626 | 0.02 |
| 毒死蜱 Chlorpyrifos | 44.4 | ND～61.73 | 1.32 | 47.99 | 0.48 |

（2）膳食暴露评估

我国居民有机磷类农药的平均膳食摄入量在 0.012～47.99 ng/(kg bw·d)（表 4-2，附表 4-10～附表 4-18，图 4-1～图 4-9），占各自 ADI 的比例在 0.00%～2.37%。平均膳食摄入量最高的是毒死蜱 [47.99 ng/(kg bw·d)]，其次为敌敌畏 [39.306 ng/(kg bw·d)]。

(2) Dietary Exposure Assessment

The average dietary intake of organophosphorus pesticides for China residents ranged from 0.012 ng/(kg bw·d) to 47.99 ng/(kg bw·d) (Table 4-2, Annexed Table 4-10-Annexed Table 4-18, Figure 4-1-Figure 4-9), accounting for 0.00%-2.37% of their respective ADIs. The highest average dietary intake was chlorpyrifos [47.99 ng/(kg bw·d)], followed by dichlorvos [39.306 ng/(kg bw·d)].

---

① ND 表示未检出，ND means not detectable

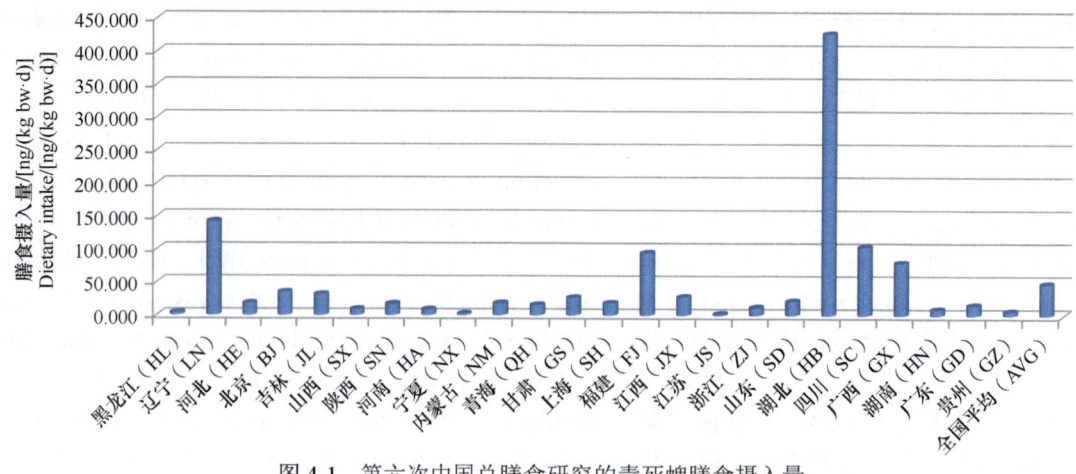

图 4-1 第六次中国总膳食研究的毒死蜱膳食摄入量
Figure 4-1　Dietary intake of chlorpyrifos from the 6$^{th}$ China TDS

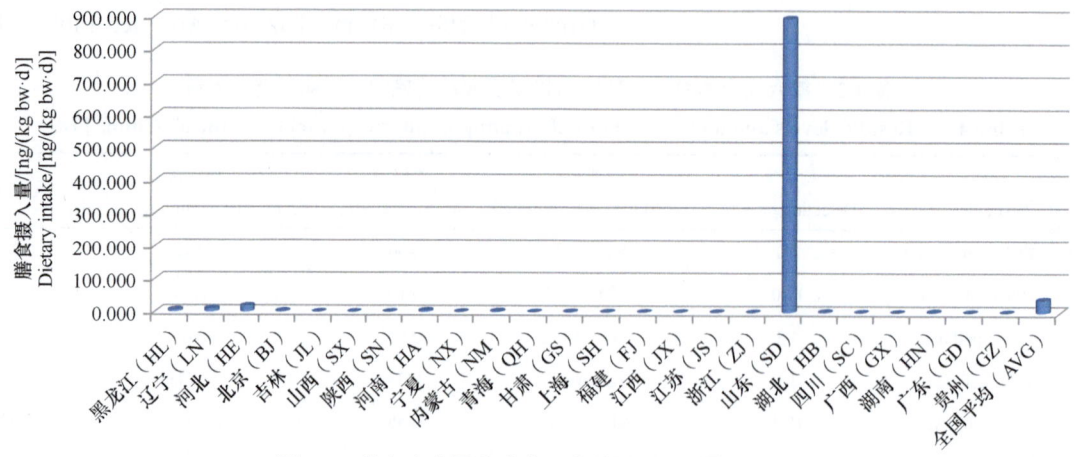

图 4-2 第六次中国总膳食研究的敌敌畏膳食摄入量
Figure 4-2　Dietary intake of dichlorvos from the 6$^{th}$ China TDS

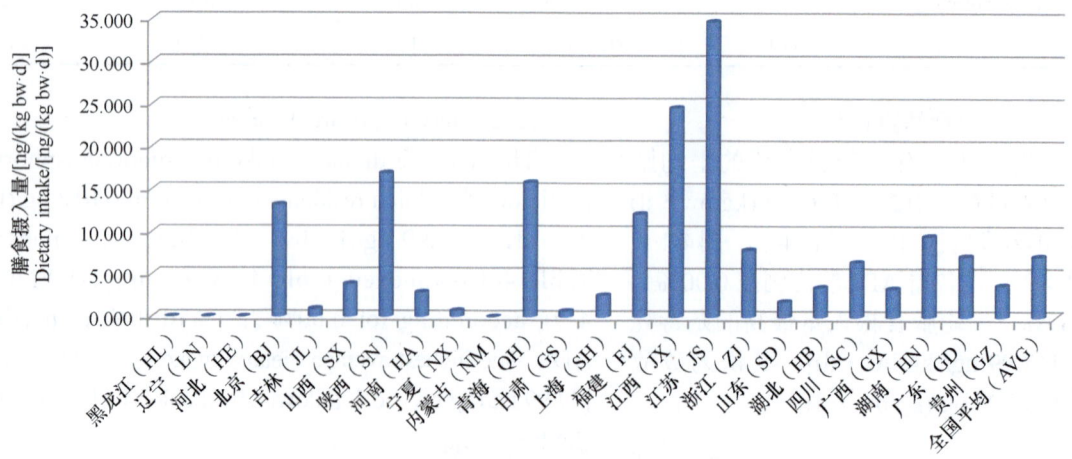

图 4-3 第六次中国总膳食研究的乙酰甲胺磷膳食摄入量
Figure 4-3　Dietary intake of acephate from the 6$^{th}$ China TDS

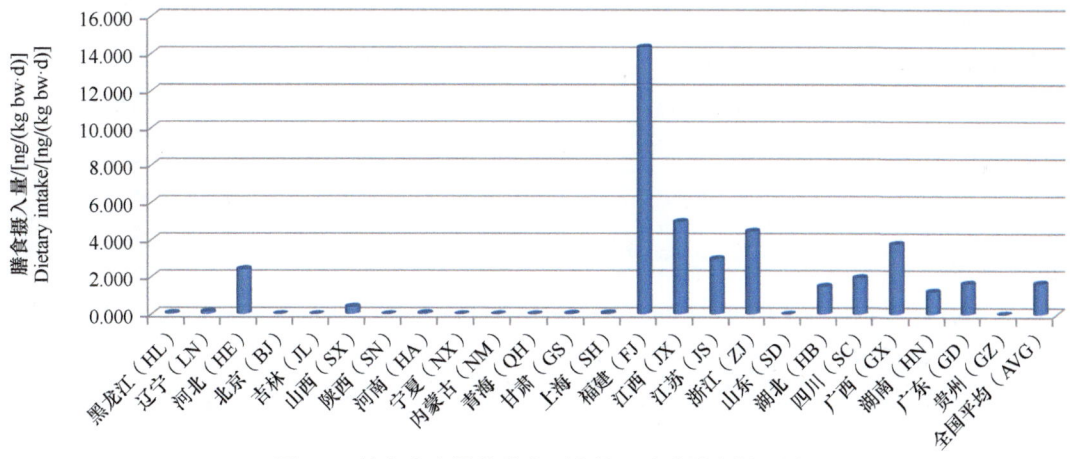

图 4-4　第六次中国总膳食研究的三唑磷膳食摄入量
Figure 4-4　Dietary intake of triazophos from the 6$^{th}$ China TDS

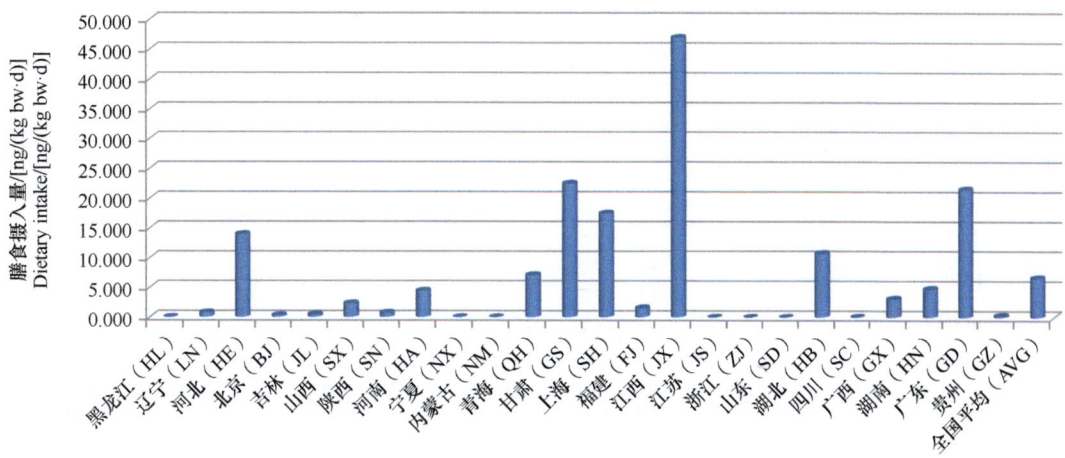

图 4-5　第六次中国总膳食研究的丙溴磷膳食摄入量
Figure 4-5　Dietary intake of profenofos from the 6$^{th}$ China TDS

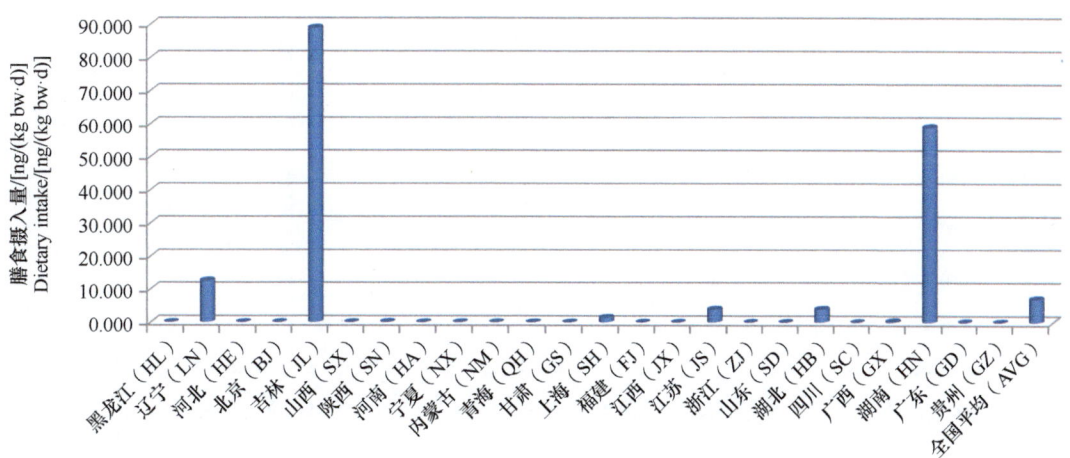

图 4-6　第六次中国总膳食研究的氧乐果膳食摄入量
Figure 4-6　Dietary intake of omethoate from the 6$^{th}$ China TDS

第四章　农药残留的膳食暴露评估　143

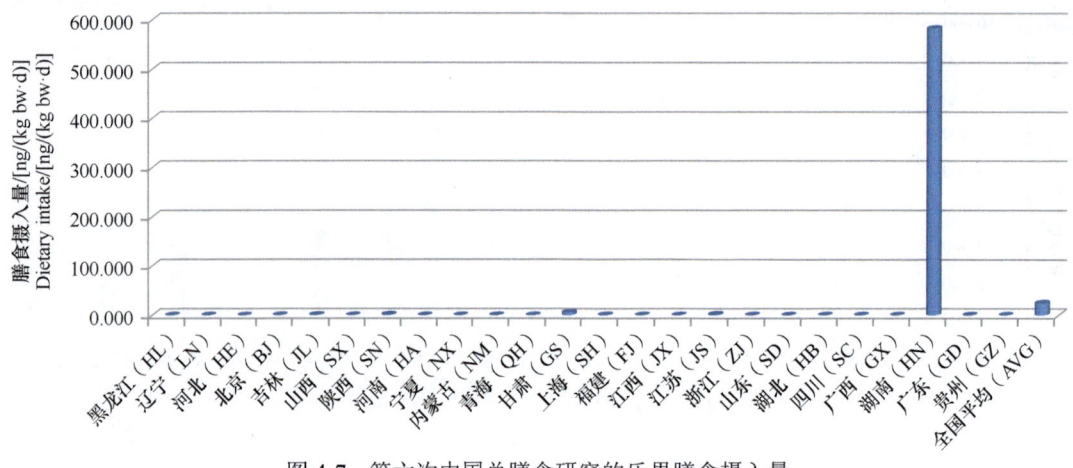

图 4-7　第六次中国总膳食研究的乐果膳食摄入量
Figure 4-7　Dietary intake of dimethoate from the 6<sup>th</sup> China TDS

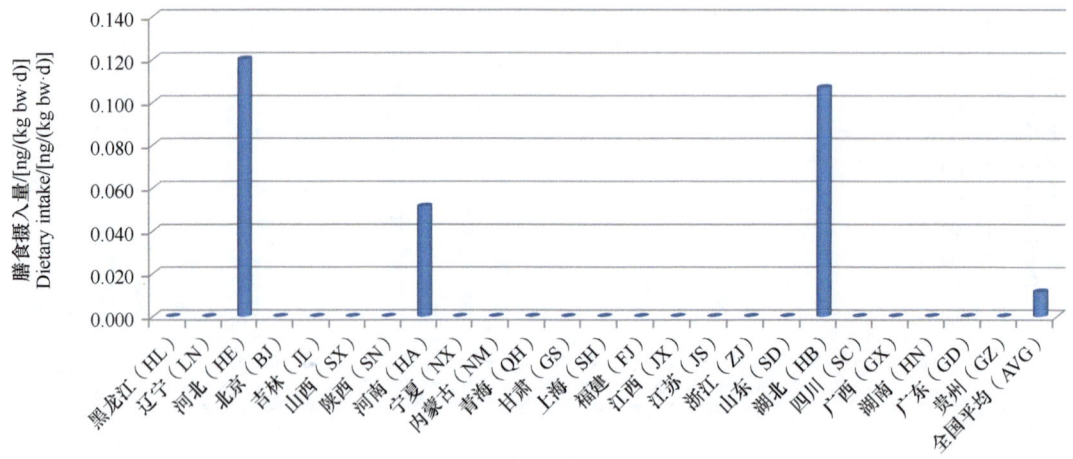

图 4-8　第六次中国总膳食研究的甲胺磷膳食摄入量
Figure 4-8　Dietary intake of methamidophos from the 6<sup>th</sup> China TDS

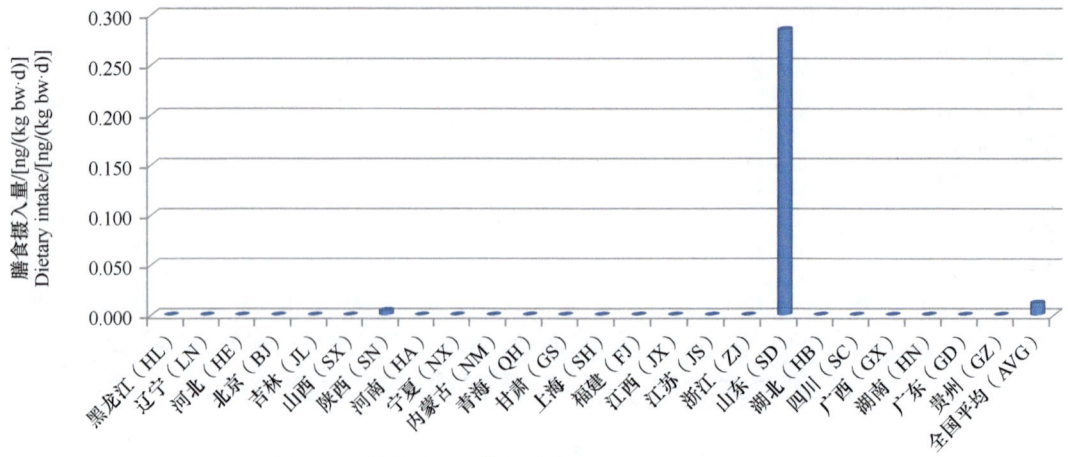

图 4-9　第六次中国总膳食研究的二嗪磷膳食摄入量
Figure 4-9　Dietary intake of diazinon from the 6<sup>th</sup> China TDS

膳食暴露评估结果表明，我国居民有机磷类农药的膳食摄入量较低，有机磷类农药膳食摄入对我国居民的健康风险在可接受水平内，健康风险较低。

（3）各类膳食对总膳食摄入的贡献

各类膳食对我国居民有机磷类农药的膳食摄入的贡献情况见附表4-19～附表4-27和图4-10～图4-18。除敌敌畏外，我国居民有机磷类农药的膳食摄入主要来源于蔬菜类、水果类、谷类等膳食。

From the exposure assessment results, it can be concluded that the dietary intake of organophosphorus pesticides of the China residents was low, and the health risk of the China residents to organophosphorus pesticides was low and in the acceptable level.

(3) Contributions of Food Categories to the Total Dietary Intake

The contribution of various dietary samples to the dietary intake of organophosphorus pesticides by China residents is shown in Annexed Table 4-19-Annexed Table 4-27 and Figure 4-10-Figure 4-18. In addition to dichlorvos, the primary sources of dietary intake to organophosphorus pesticides for China residents were vegetables, fruits, cereals, and other meals.

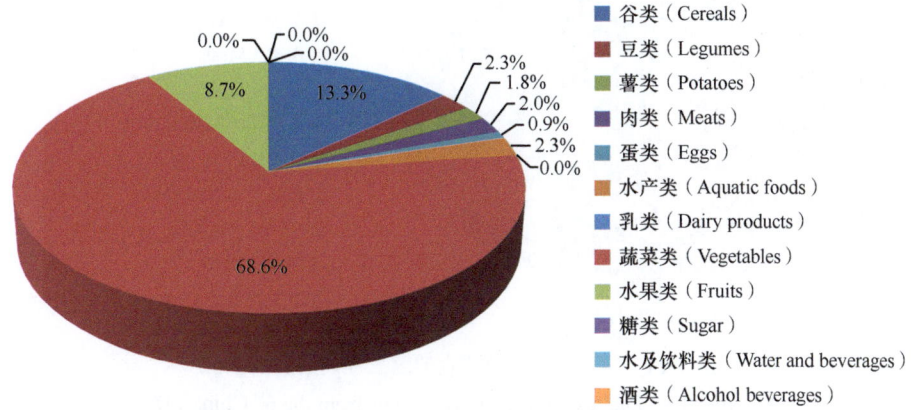

图4-10　第六次中国总膳食研究毒死蜱的膳食来源

Figure 4-10　Dietary sources of chlorpyrifos from the 6$^{th}$ China TDS

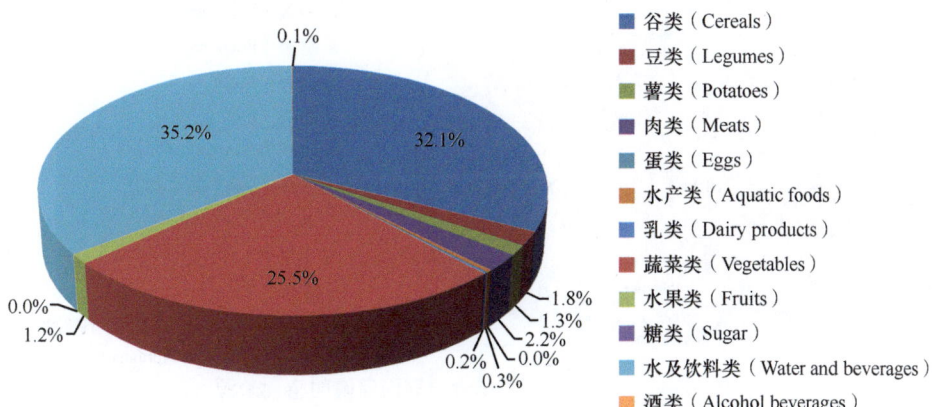

图4-11　第六次中国总膳食研究敌敌畏的膳食来源

Figure 4-11　Dietary sources of dichlorvos from the 6$^{th}$ China TDS

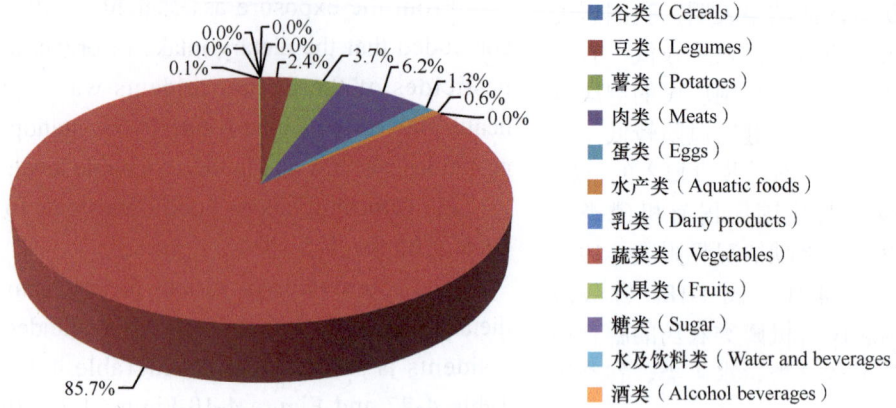

图 4-12　第六次中国总膳食研究乙酰甲胺磷的膳食来源

Figure 4-12　Dietary sources of acephate from the 6<sup>th</sup> China TDS

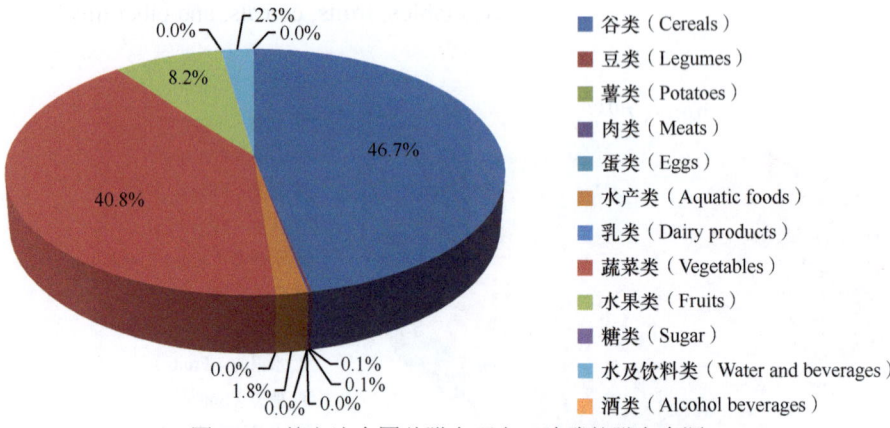

图 4-13　第六次中国总膳食研究三唑磷的膳食来源

Figure 4-13　Dietary sources of triazophos from the 6<sup>th</sup> China TDS

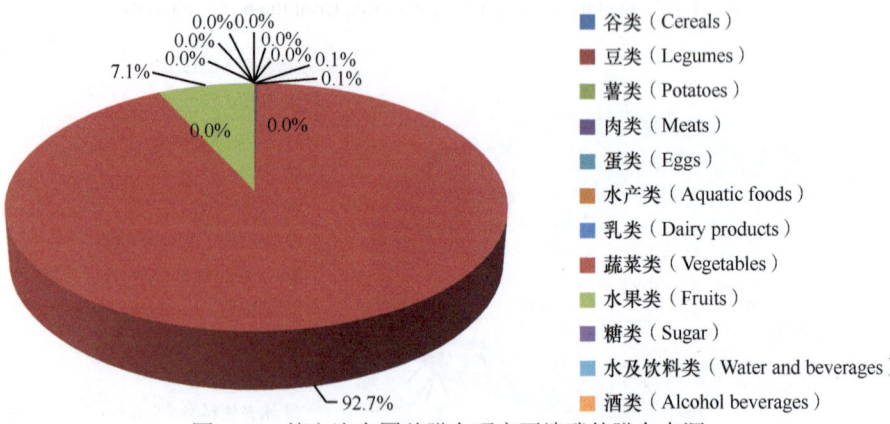

图 4-14　第六次中国总膳食研究丙溴磷的膳食来源

Figure 4-14　Dietary sources of profenofos from the 6<sup>th</sup> China TDS

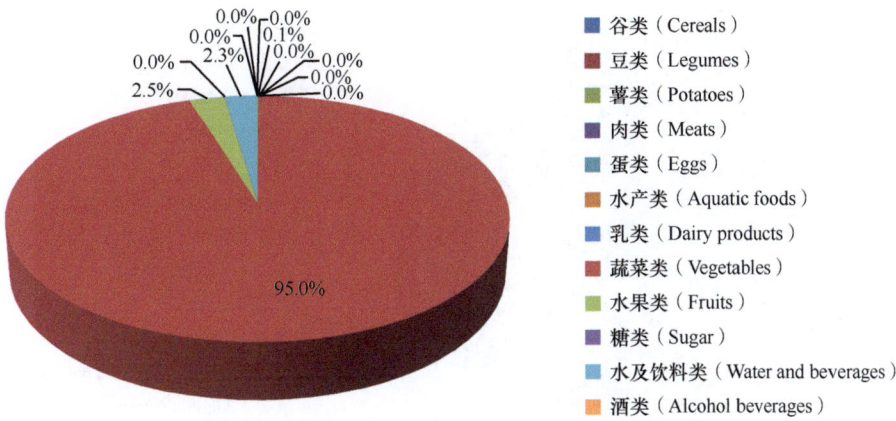

图 4-15　第六次中国总膳食研究氧乐果的膳食来源

Figure 4-15　Dietary sources of omethoate from the 6th China TDS

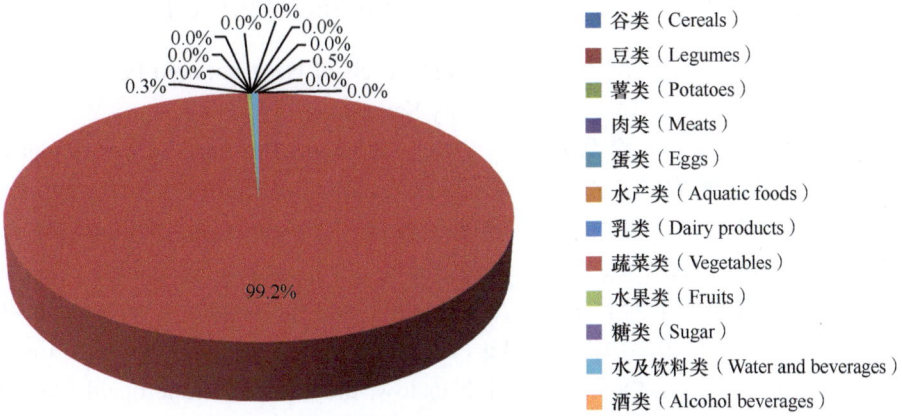

图 4-16　第六次中国总膳食研究乐果的膳食来源

Figure 4-16　Dietary sources of dimethoate from the 6th China TDS

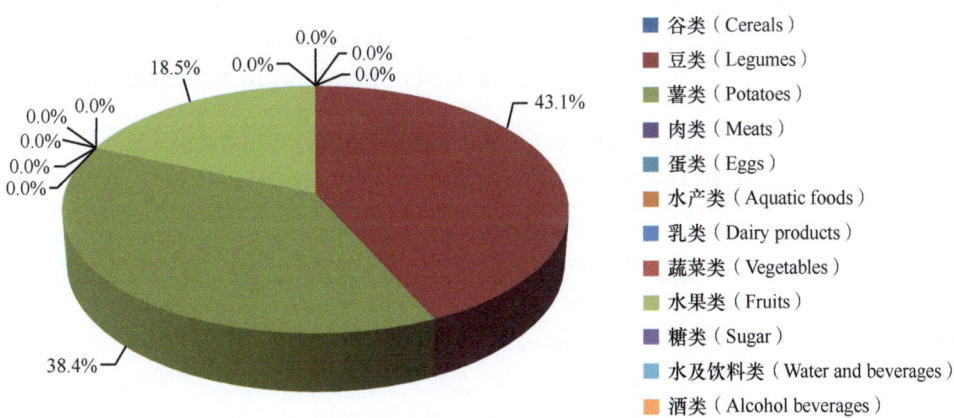

图 4-17　第六次中国总膳食研究甲胺磷的膳食来源

Figure 4-17　Dietary sources of methamidophos from the 6th China TDS

第四章　农药残留的膳食暴露评估

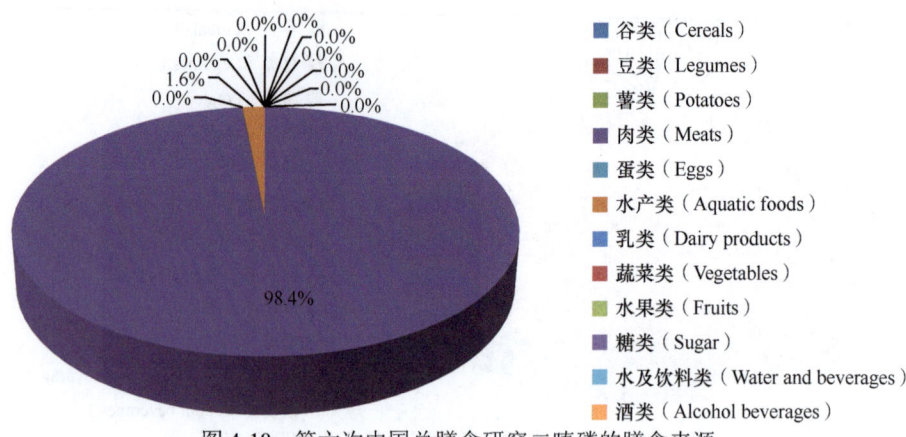

图 4-18　第六次中国总膳食研究二嗪磷的膳食来源
Figure 4-18　Dietary sources of diazinon from the 6th China TDS

## 2. 新烟碱类农药

（1）混合膳食样品中新烟碱类农药的含量

第六次中国总膳食研究混合膳食样品中检出 9 种新烟碱类农药，分别为啶虫脒、吡虫啉、噻虫嗪、噻虫胺、噻虫啉、呋虫胺、烯啶虫胺、氯噻啉和 N- 脱甲基啶虫脒，残留水平为 ND～185.53 μg/kg（表 4-3），按检出率由高至低排列分别为吡虫啉（附表 4-28）、啶虫脒（附表 4-29）、噻虫嗪（附表 4-30）、噻虫胺（附表 4-31）、N- 脱甲基啶虫脒（附表 4-32）、呋虫胺（附表 4-33）、烯啶虫胺（附表 4-34）、噻虫啉（附表 4-35）和氯噻啉（附表 4-36）。

## 2. Neonicotinoid Pesticides

(1) Levels of Neonicotinoid Pesticides in Composite Dietary Samples

Nine neonicotinoid pesticides were detected in the 6th CTDS composite samples, including acetamiprid, imidacloprid, thiamethoxam, clothianidin, thiacloprid, dinotefuran, nitenpyram, imidaclothiz, and acetamiprid-N-desmethyl, and the residue level was ND-185.53 μg/kg (Table 4-3). According to the detection rates from high to low, they were imidacloprid (Annexed Table 4-28), acetamiprid (Annexed Table 4-29), thiamethoxam (Annexed Table 4-30), clothianidin (Annexed Table 4-31), acetamiprid-N-desmethyl (Annexed Table 4-32), dinotefuran (Annexed Table 4-33), nitenpyram (Annexed Table 4-34), thiacloprid (Annexed Table 4-35), and

表 4-3　第六次中国总膳食研究新烟碱类农药的残留水平和膳食摄入量
Table 4-3　Residue levels and dietary intakes of neonicotinoid pesticides in the 6th China TDS

| 农药 Pesticides | 检出率 Detection rates/% | 残留水平 Residue levels/(μg/kg) | 平均水平 Mean/(μg/kg) | 摄入量 Dietary intakes/[ng/(kg bw·d)] | ADI/% |
|---|---|---|---|---|---|
| 啶虫脒 Acetamiprid | 56.9 | ND～185.53 | 2.59 | 140.35 | 0.20 |
| 吡虫啉 Imidacloprid | 61.8 | ND～28.05 | 0.92 | 33.50 | 0.06 |
| 噻虫嗪 Thiamethoxam | 54.9 | ND～71.31 | 1.03 | 42.57 | 0.05 |
| 噻虫胺 Clothianidin | 52.8 | ND～39.01 | 0.48 | 22.88 | 0.02 |
| 噻虫啉 Thiacloprid | 2.4 | ND～1.42 | 0.01 | 0.442 | 0.00 |
| 呋虫胺 Dinotefuran | 7.3 | ND～1.70 | 0.02 | 1.217 | 0.00 |
| 烯啶虫胺 Nitenpyram | 6.9 | ND～2.34 | 0.03 | 1.762 | 0.00 |

续表

| 农药<br>Pesticides | 检出率<br>Detection rates/% | 残留水平<br>Residue levels/(μg/kg) | 平均水平<br>Mean/(μg/kg) | 摄入量<br>Dietary intakes/[ng/(kg bw·d)] | ADI/% |
|---|---|---|---|---|---|
| 氯噻啉 Imidaclothiz | 0.3 | ND～0.90 | 0.00 | 0.242 | 0.00 |
| N-脱甲基啶虫脒<br>Acetamiprid-N-desmethyl | 44.8 | ND～14.98 | 0.28 | 10.735 | 0.02 |
| 总新烟碱<br>Total neonicotinoids |  |  |  | 703.0 | 1.17 |

（2）膳食暴露评估

我国居民新烟碱类农药的平均膳食摄入量为 0.242～140.35 ng/(kg bw·d)（表4-3，附表4-37～附表4-45，图4-19～图4-27），占各自 ADI 的比例为 0.00%～0.20%。平均膳食摄入量最高的是啶虫脒 [140.35 ng/(kg bw·d)]，其次为噻虫嗪 [42.57 ng/(kg bw·d)]。采用相对效能因子方法，对总新烟碱类农药进行整体评估，并以吡虫啉的 ADI 作为评估基准值，结果显示，我国居民总新烟碱类农药的平均膳食摄入量为 703.0 ng/(kg bw·d)（表4-3，附表4-46，图4-28），占 ADI 的比例为 1.17%。

imidaclothiz (Annexed Table 4-36).

(2) Dietary Exposure Assessment

The average dietary intake of neonicotinoid pesticides for China residents was from 0.242 ng/(kg bw·d) to 140.35 ng/(kg bw·d) (Table 4-3, Annexed Table 4-37-Annexed Table 4-45, Figure 4-19-Figure 4-27), accounting for 0.00%-0.20% of their respective ADIs. The highest average dietary intake was acetamiprid [140.35 ng/(kg bw·d)], followed by thiamethoxam [42.57 ng/(kg bw·d)]. The relative efficacy factor method was used to evaluate the total neonicotinoid pesticides as a whole, and the ADI of imidacloprid was used as the benchmark value. The results showed that the average dietary intake of total neonicotinoid pesticides of China residents was 703.0 ng/(kg bw·d) (Table 4-3, Annexed Table 4-46, Figure 4-28), accounting for 1.17% of the ADI.

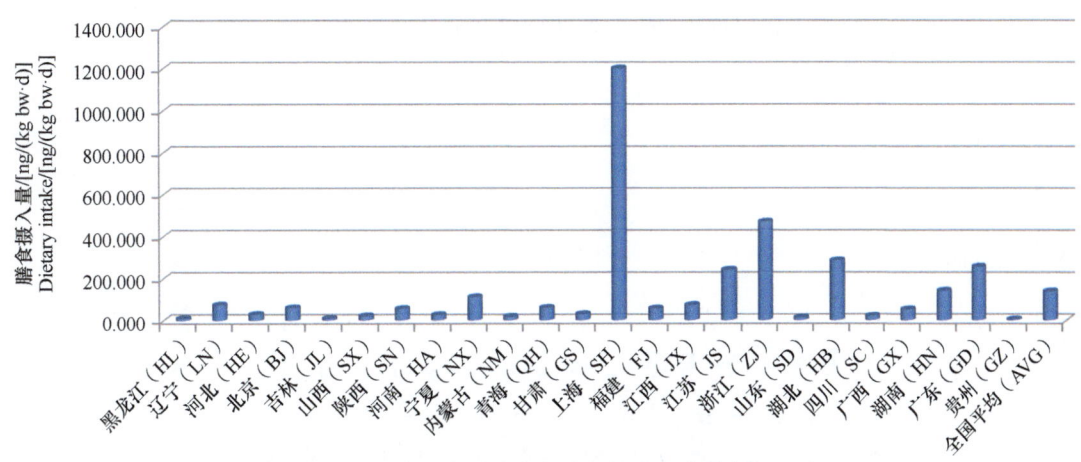

图 4-19 第六次中国总膳食研究的啶虫脒膳食摄入量
Figure 4-19 Dietary intake of acetamiprid from the 6th China TDS

第四章 农药残留的膳食暴露评估

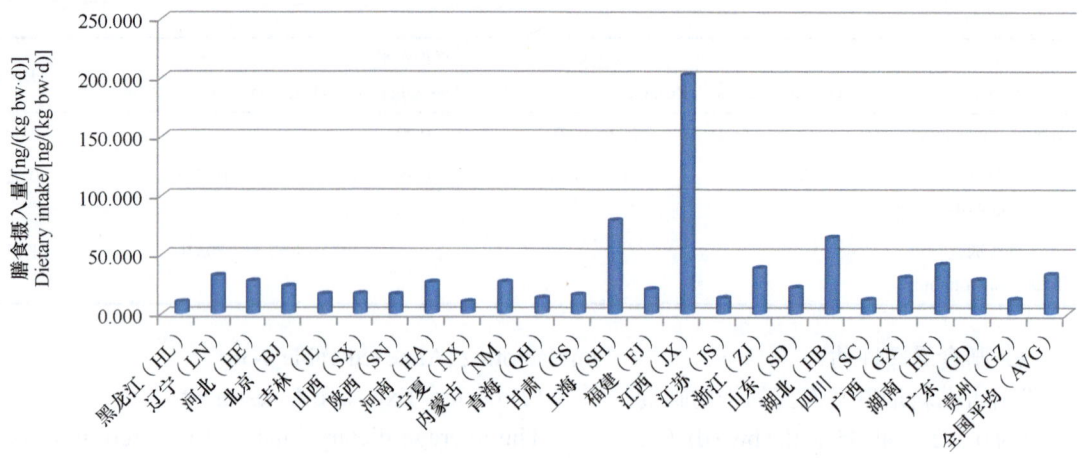

图 4-20　第六次中国总膳食研究的吡虫啉膳食摄入量
Figure 4-20　Dietary intake of imidacloprid from the 6$^{th}$ China TDS

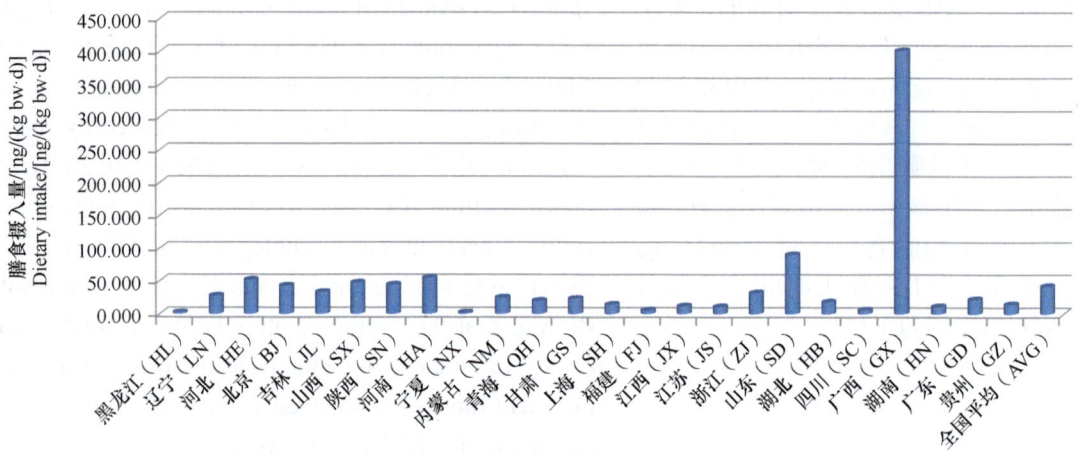

图 4-21　第六次中国总膳食研究的噻虫嗪膳食摄入量
Figure 4-21　Dietary intake of thiamethoxam from the 6$^{th}$ China TDS

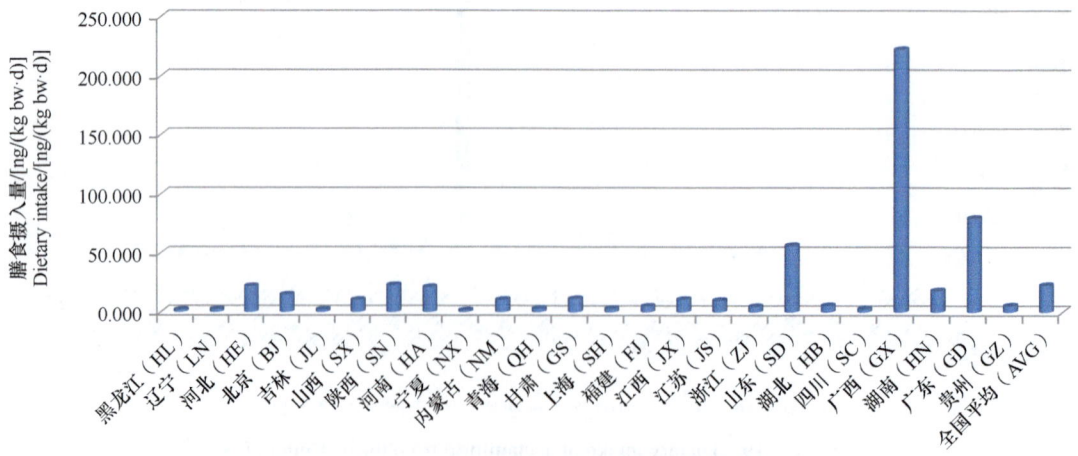

图 4-22　第六次中国总膳食研究的噻虫胺膳食摄入量
Figure 4-22　Dietary intake of clothianidin from the 6$^{th}$ China TDS

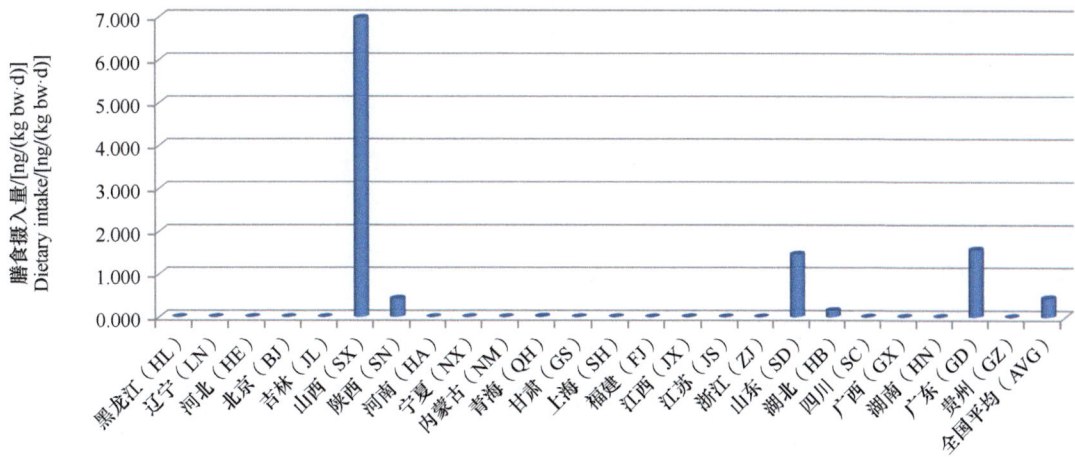

图 4-23 第六次中国总膳食研究的噻虫啉膳食摄入量
Figure 4-23　Dietary intake of thiacloprid from the 6th China TDS

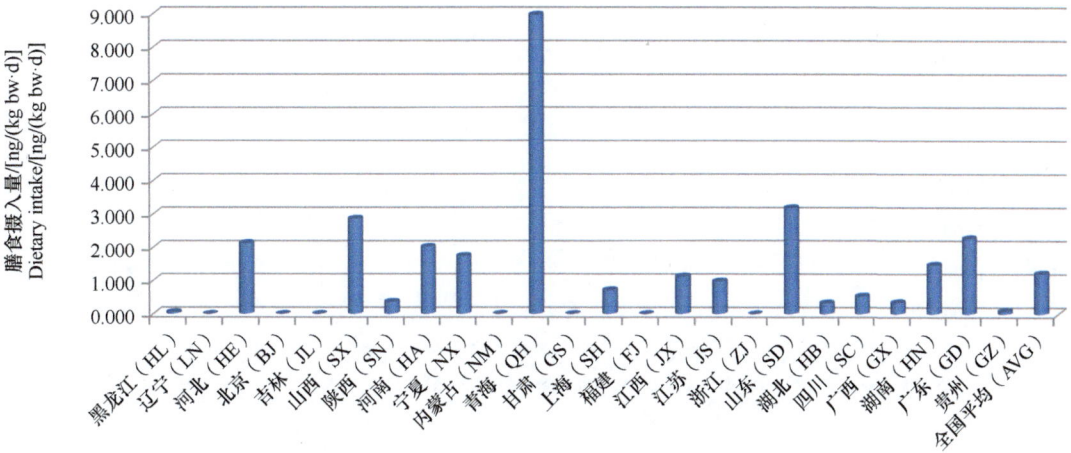

图 4-24 第六次中国总膳食研究的呋虫胺膳食摄入量
Figure 4-24　Dietary intake of dinotefuran from the 6th China TDS

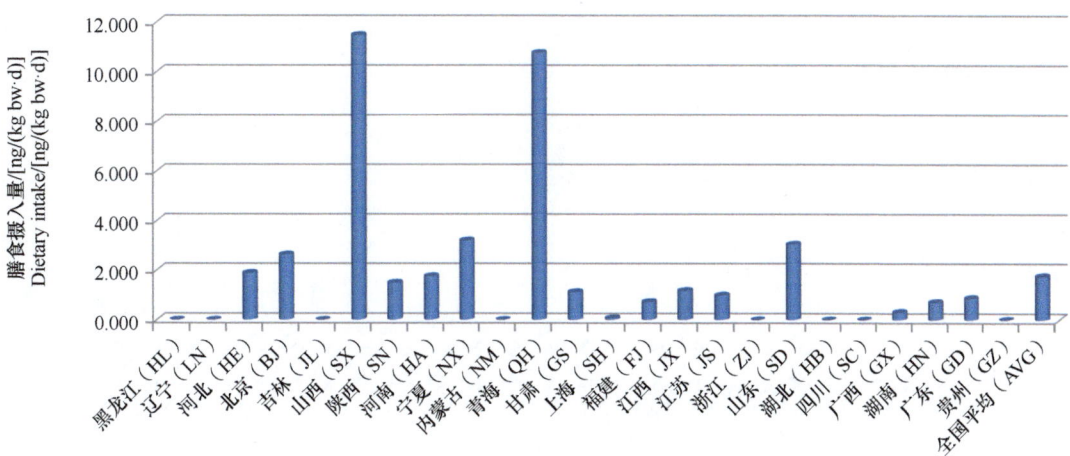

图 4-25 第六次中国总膳食研究的烯啶虫胺膳食摄入量
Figure 4-25　Dietary intake of nitenpyram from the 6th China TDS

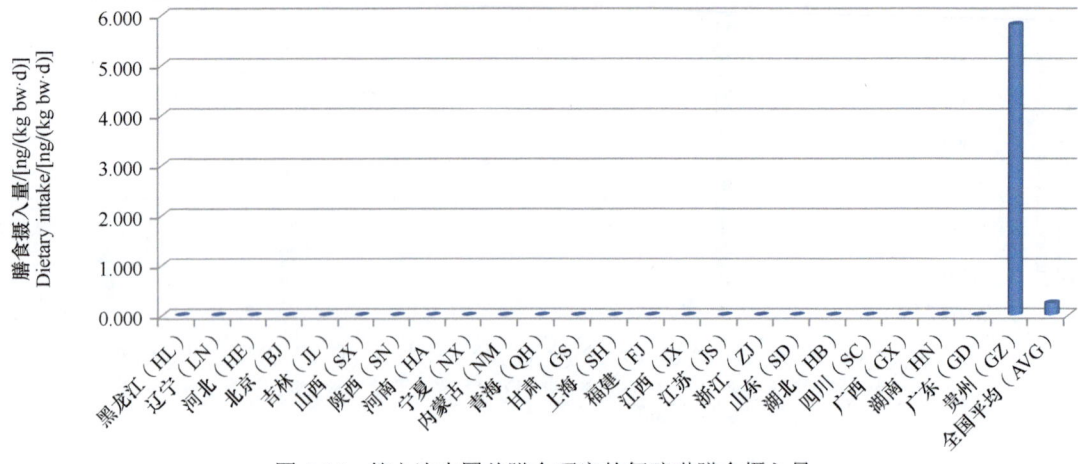

图 4-26　第六次中国总膳食研究的氯噻啉膳食摄入量

Figure 4-26　Dietary intake of imidaclothiz from the 6<sup>th</sup> China TDS

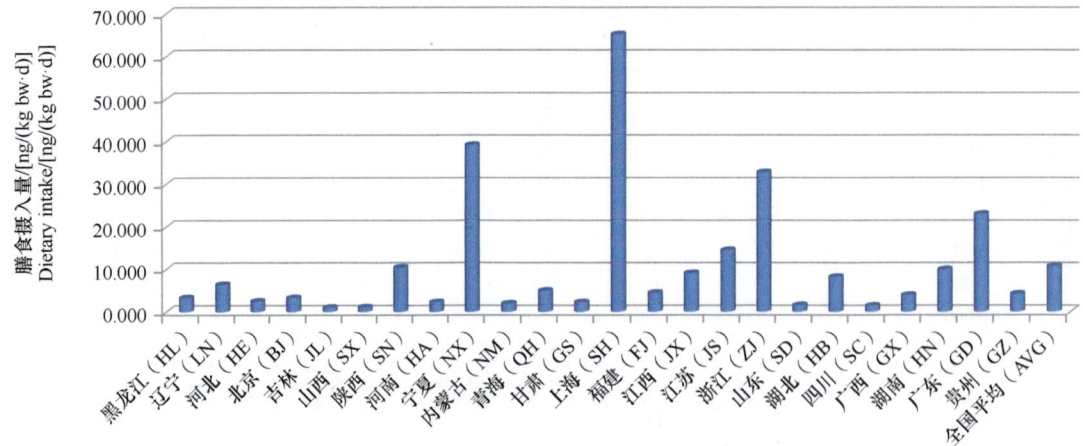

图 4-27　第六次中国总膳食研究的 N-脱甲基啶虫脒膳食摄入量

Figure 4-27　Dietary intake of acetamiprid-*N*-desmethyl from the 6<sup>th</sup> China TDS

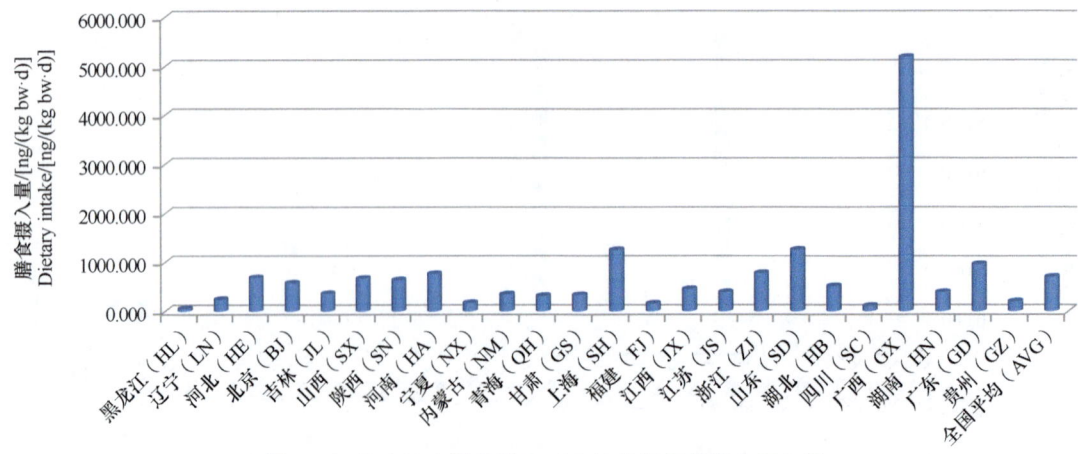

图 4-28　第六次中国总膳食研究的总新烟碱膳食摄入量

Figure 4-28　Dietary intake of total neonicotinoids from the 6<sup>th</sup> China TDS

膳食暴露评估结果表明，我国居民新烟碱类农药的膳食摄入量较低，新烟碱类农药膳食摄入对我国居民的健康风险在可接受水平内，健康风险较低。

（3）各类膳食对总膳食摄入的贡献

各类膳食对我国居民新烟碱类农药的膳食摄入的贡献情况见附表4-47～附表4-55和图4-29～图4-37。我国居民新烟碱类农药的膳食摄入主要来源于蔬菜类、水果类、谷类等膳食。从我国居民总新烟碱类农药的膳食摄入贡献来看，蔬菜类为我国居民新烟碱类农药膳食摄入的主要来源（85.2%），其他食物类别的贡献率均小于5%（附表4-56和图4-38）。

### 3. 苯基吡唑类农药

（1）混合膳食样品中苯基吡唑类农药的含量

第六次中国总膳食研究混合膳食样品中检出氟虫腈及其代谢物（氟甲腈、氟虫腈砜和氟虫腈亚砜），其中氟虫腈及其代谢物农药的残留含量以氟虫腈及其代谢物的总和计。氟虫腈的检出率为79.5%，残留水平为ND～383.4 μg/kg（附表4-57）。

From the exposure assessment results, it can be concluded that the dietary intake of neonicotinoid pesticides of the China residents was low, and the health risk of the China residents to neonicotinoid pesticides was low and in the acceptable level.

(3) Contributions of Food Categories to the Total Dietary Intake

The contribution of various dietary samples to the dietary intake of neonicotinoid pesticides in China residents is shown in Annexed Table 4-47-Annexed Table 4-55 and Figure 4-29-Figure 4-37. The dietary intake of neonicotinoid pesticides in China residents was mainly from vegetables, fruits, cereals, and other diets. From the perspective of the dietary intake contribution of total neonicotinoid pesticides in China residents, vegetables was the main source of dietary intake of neonicotinoid pesticides in China (85.2%), and the contribution of other food categories was less than 5% (Annexed Table 4-56 and Figure 4-38).

### 3. Phenylpyrazole Pesticides

(1) Levels of Phenylpyrazole in Composite Dietary Samples

Fipronil and its metabolites (fipronil desulfinyl, fipronil sulfone and fipronil sulfide) were detected in the 6$^{th}$ CTDS composite samples. The residue level of total fipronils was calculated by the sum of fipronil and its metabolites. The detection rate of fipronils was 79.5%,

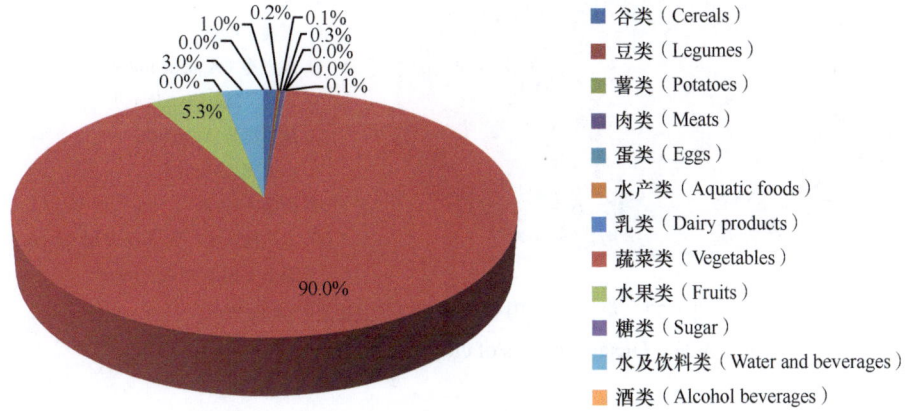

图4-29　第六次中国总膳食研究啶虫脒的膳食来源

Figure 4-29　Dietary sources of acetamiprid from the 6$^{th}$ China TDS

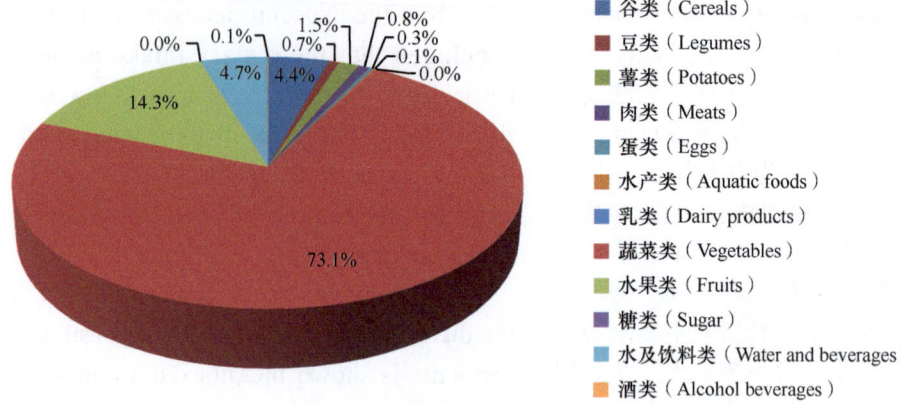

图 4-30 第六次中国总膳食研究吡虫啉的膳食来源

Figure 4-30　Dietary sources of imidacloprid from the 6$^{th}$ China TDS

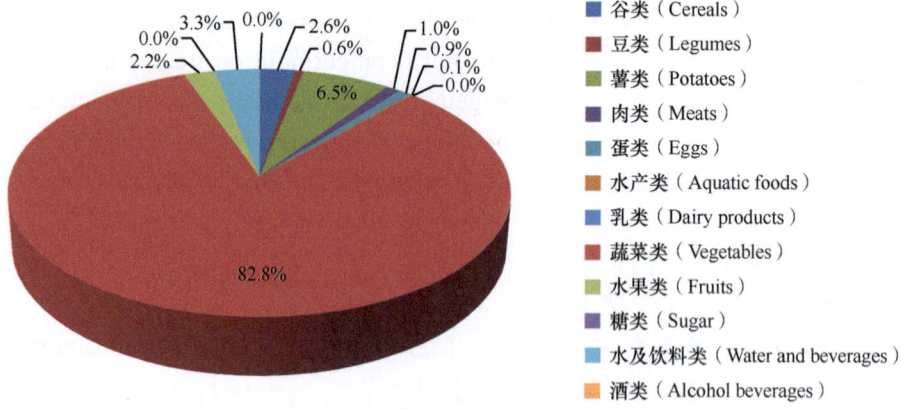

图 4-31 第六次中国总膳食研究噻虫嗪的膳食来源

Figure 4-31　Dietary sources of thiamethoxam from the 6$^{th}$ China TDS

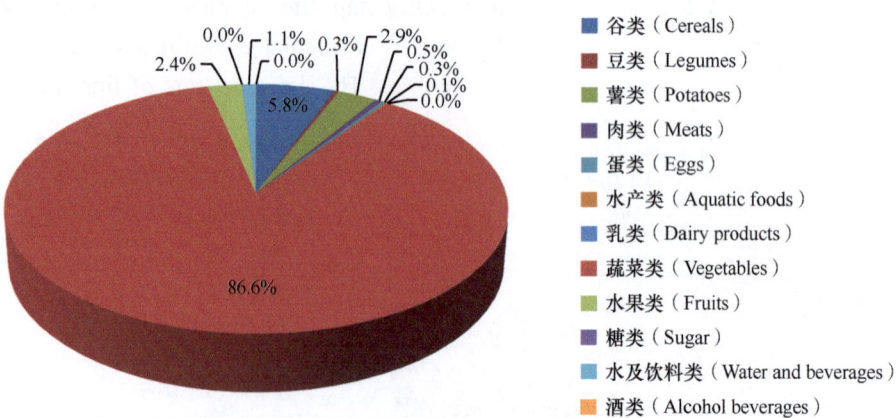

图 4-32 第六次中国总膳食研究噻虫胺的膳食来源

Figure 4-32　Dietary sources of clothianidin from the 6$^{th}$ China TDS

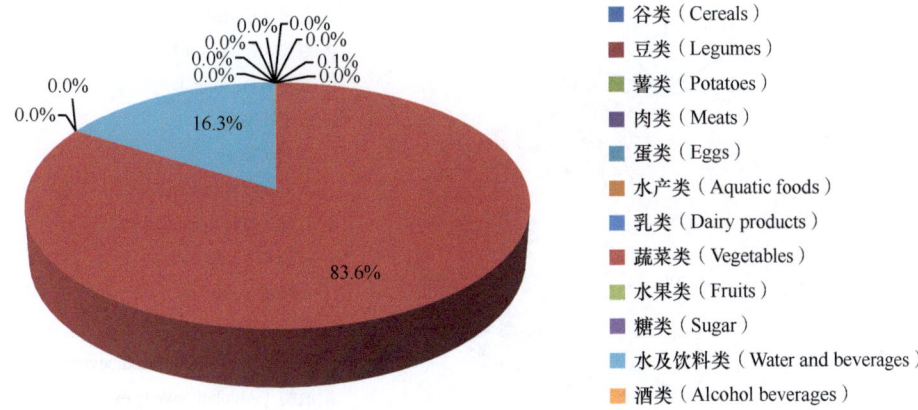

图 4-33 第六次中国总膳食研究噻虫啉的膳食来源
Figure 4-33 Dietary sources of thiacloprid from the 6th China TDS

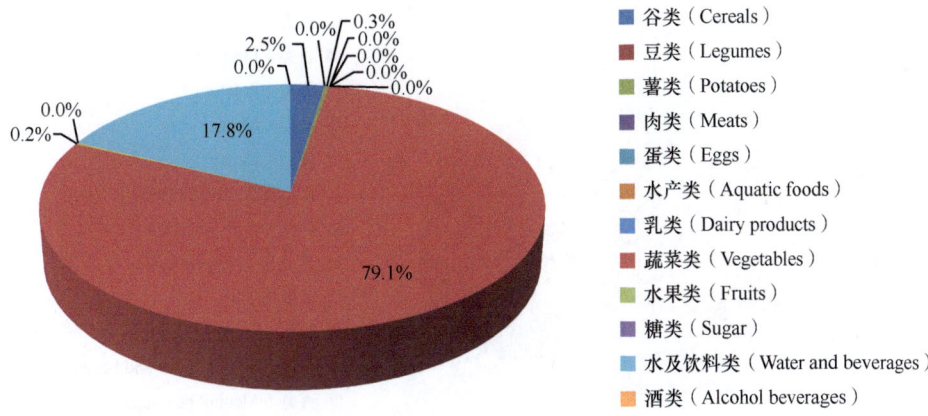

图 4-34 第六次中国总膳食研究呋虫胺的膳食来源
Figure 4-34 Dietary sources of dinotefuran from the 6th China TDS

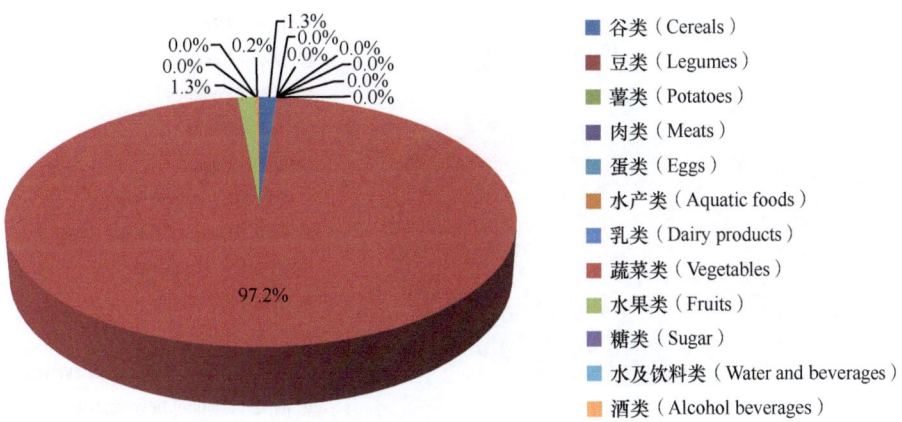

图 4-35 第六次中国总膳食研究烯啶虫胺的膳食来源
Figure 4-35 Dietary sources of nitenpyram from the 6th China TDS

第四章 农药残留的膳食暴露评估

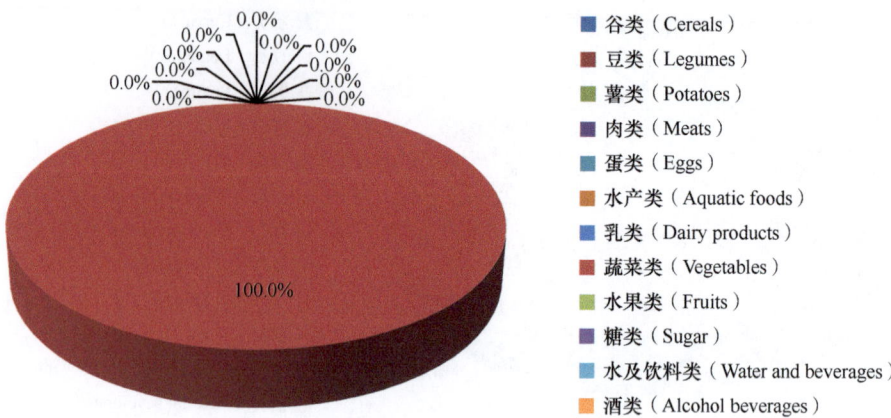

图 4-36　第六次中国总膳食研究氯噻啉的膳食来源
Figure 4-36　Dietary sources of imidaclothiz from the 6th China TDS

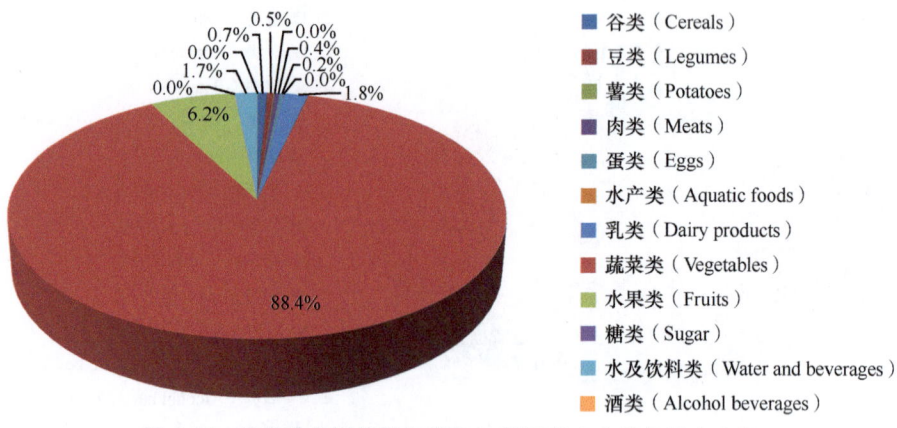

图 4-37　第六次中国总膳食研究 N-脱甲基啶虫脒的膳食来源
Figure 4-37　Dietary sources of acetamiprid-N-desmethyl from the 6th China TDS

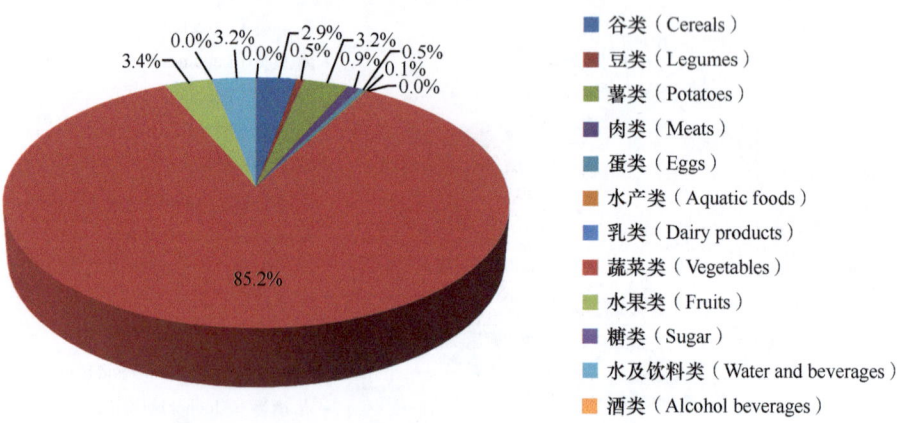

图 4-38　第六次中国总膳食研究总新烟碱的膳食来源
Figure 4-38　Dietary sources of total neonicotinoids from the 6th China TDS

（2）膳食暴露评估

我国居民氟虫腈及其代谢物农药的平均膳食摄入量为 15.6 ng/(kg bw·d)（附表 4-58），占 ADI 的比例为 7.80%。我国各地区居民的总氟虫腈农药的膳食摄入量为 0.358～135.7 ng/(kg bw·d)（图 4-39），其中，甘肃平均膳食摄入量为 135.7 ng/(kg bw·d)，广西为 65.37 ng/(kg bw·d)。

and the residue level was ND-383.4 µg/kg (Annexed Table 4-57).

(2) Dietary Exposure Assessment

The average dietary intake of fipronil and its metabolites among China residents was 15.6 ng/(kg bw·d) (Annexed Table 4-58), accounting for 7.80% of the ADI. The dietary intake of total fipronils by residents in various regions of China ranged from 0.358 ng/(kg bw·d) to 135.7 ng/(kg bw·d) (Figure 4-39), among which Gansu had the highest average dietary intake [135.7 ng/(kg bw·d)], followed by Guangxi [65.37 ng/(kg bw·d)].

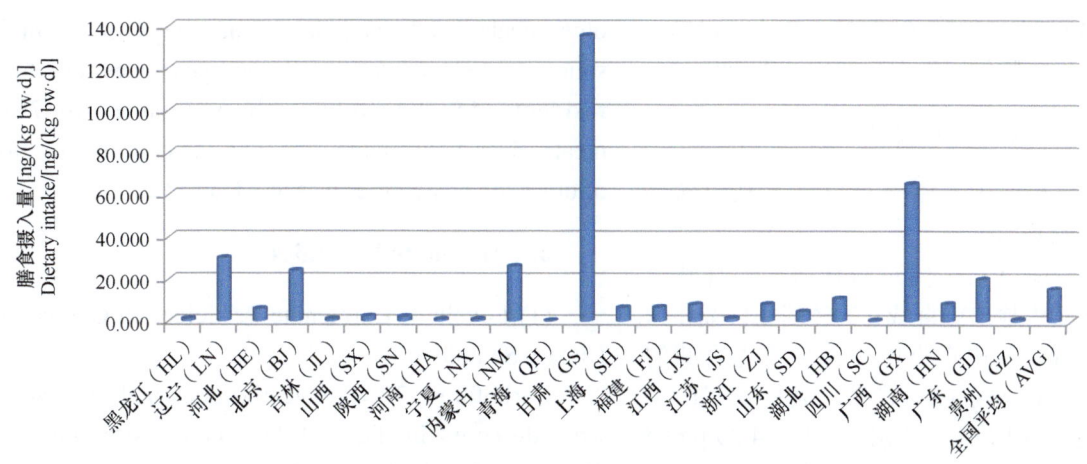

图 4-39　第六次中国总膳食研究的氟虫腈膳食摄入量

Figure 4-39　Dietary intake of fipronil from the 6th China TDS

膳食暴露评估结果表明，我国居民氟虫腈农药的膳食摄入量较低，氟虫腈农药膳食摄入对我国居民的健康风险在可接受水平内，健康风险较低，但甘肃省的氟虫腈农药膳食摄入量占 ADI 的 67.8%，值得关注。

（3）各类膳食对总膳食摄入的贡献

各类膳食对我国居民氟虫腈农药的膳食摄入的贡献情况见附表 4-59 和图 4-40。我国居民氟虫腈农药的膳食摄入主要来源于蛋类、蔬菜类、肉类、谷类等膳食。从全国平均水平来看，蛋类为我国居民氟虫腈农药膳食摄入的主要来源（55.3%），其次为蔬菜类

From the dietary exposure assessment results, it can be concluded that the dietary intake of total fipronils of the China residents was low, and the health risk to fipronil pesticides was low and in the acceptable level. However, the dietary intake of fipronil pesticides in Gansu accounted for 67.8% of the ADI, which was worthy of attention.

(3) Contributions Food Categories to the Total Dietary Intake

The contribution of various dietary samples to the dietary intake of total fipronils by China residents is shown in Annexed Table 4-59 and Figure 4-40. The dietary intake of fipronil pesticides for China residents was mainly from eggs, vegetables, meats, cereals and

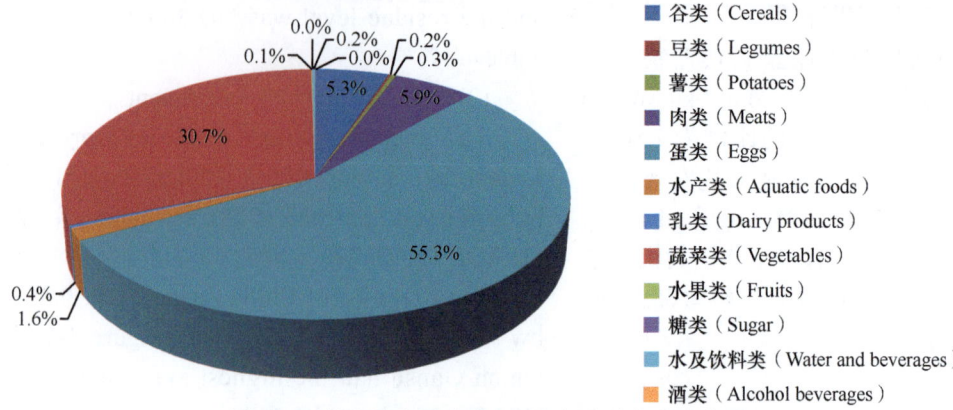

图 4-40　第六次中国总膳食研究氟虫腈的膳食来源

Figure 4-40　Dietary sources of fipronil from the 6$^{th}$ China TDS

(30.7%)、肉类（5.9%）、谷类（5.3%），其他食物类别的贡献率均小于 5%。

**4. 氨基甲酸酯类农药**

（1）混合膳食样品中氨基甲酸酯类农药的含量

第六次中国总膳食研究混合膳食样品中检出克百威、3-羟基克百威和茚虫威。其中克百威和 3-羟基克百威的总和计为克百威总量。克百威和茚虫威的残留水平分别为 ND～4.20 μg/kg 和 ND～24.26 μg/kg，其检出率分别为 5.9% 和 4.2%。膳食样品中克百威和茚虫威的含量状况具体详见附表 4-60 和附表 4-61。

（2）膳食暴露评估

我国居民克百威和茚虫威农药的平均膳食摄入量分别为 3.117 ng/(kg bw·d)（占 ADI 的 0.31%）和 19.522 ng/(kg bw·d)（占 ADI 的 0.20%），均远低于各自的 ADI 值（附表 4-62～附表 4-63，图 4-41～图 4-42）。

other meals. On the national average, eggs was the main source of dietary intake of fipronil pesticides for China residents (55.3%), followed by vegetables (30.7%), meats (5.9%), cereals (5.3%), and the contribution rate of other food categories was less than 5%.

**4. Carbamate Pesticides**

(1) Levels of Carbamate Pesticides in Composite Dietary Samples

Carbofuran, 3-hydroxycarbofuran, and indoxacarb were detected in the 6$^{th}$ CTDS composite samples. The sum of carbofuran and 3-hydroxycarbofuran was calculated as the total carbofuran. The residue levels of carbofuran and indoxacarb were ND-4.20 μg/kg and ND-24.26 μg/kg, respectively, and the detection rates were 5.9% and 4.2%, respectively. See Annexed Table 4-60 and Annexed Table 4-61 for the content of carbofuran and indoxacarb in dietary samples.

(2) Dietary Exposure Assessment

The average dietary intake of carbofuran and indoxacarb pesticides for China residents was 3.117 ng/(kg bw·d) (accounting for 0.31% of the ADI) and 19.522 ng/(kg bw·d) (accounting for 0.20% of the ADI), respectively, which was far lower than their respective ADI values (Annexed Table 4-62-Annexed Table 4-63, Figure 4-41-Figure 4-42).

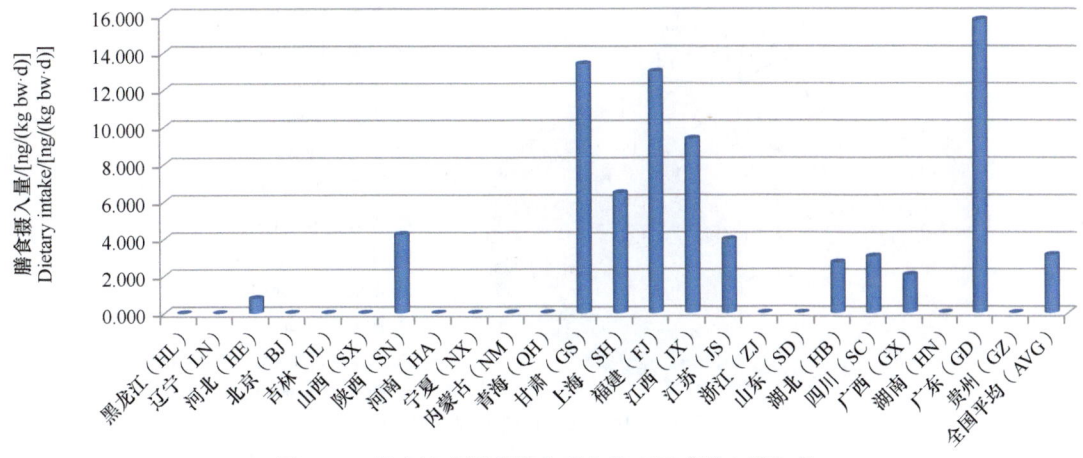

图 4-41　第六次中国总膳食研究的克百威膳食摄入量
Figure 4-41　Dietary intake of carbofuran from the 6th China TDS

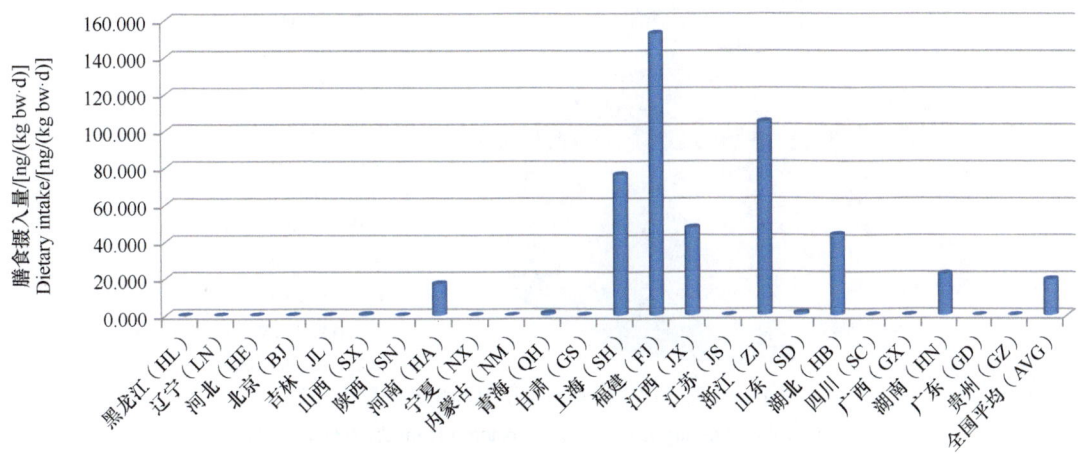

图 4-42　第六次中国总膳食研究的茚虫威膳食摄入量
Figure 4-42　Dietary intake of indoxacarb from the 6th China TDS

膳食暴露评估结果表明，我国居民氨基甲酸酯类农药的膳食摄入量较低，对我国居民的健康风险在可接受水平内，健康风险较低。

（3）各类膳食对总膳食摄入的贡献

各类膳食对我国居民氨基甲酸酯类农药的膳食摄入的贡献情况见附表4-64～附表4-65和图4-43～图4-44。我国居民氨基甲酸酯类农药的膳食摄入主要来源于蔬菜类等膳食。

From the exposure assessment results, it can be concluded that the dietary intake of carbamate pesticides of the China residents was low, and the health risk to carbamate pesticides was low and in the acceptable level.

(3) Contributions of Food Categories to the Total Dietary Intake

The contribution of various dietary samples to the dietary intake of carbamate pesticides by China residents is shown in Annexed Table 4-64 and Annexed Table 4-65, Figure 4-43 and Figure 4-44. The dietary intake of carbamate pesticides for China residents was mainly from vegetables and other meals.

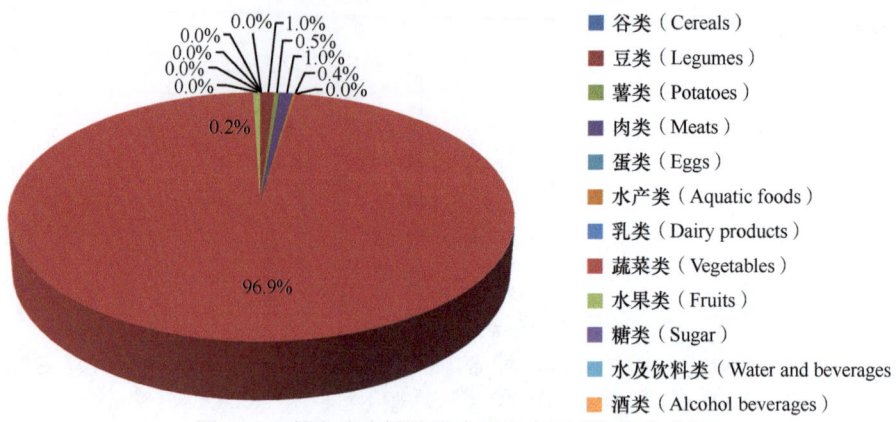

图 4-43  第六次中国总膳食研究克百威的膳食来源
Figure 4-43  Dietary sources of carbofuran from the 6th China TDS

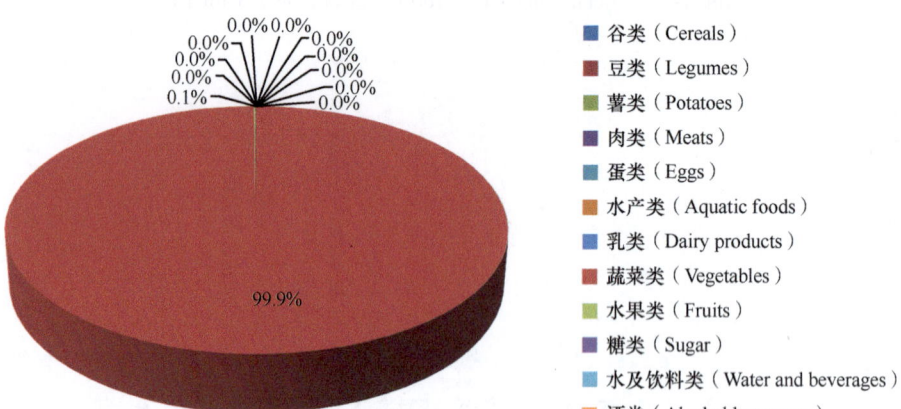

图 4-44  第六次中国总膳食研究茚虫威的膳食来源
Figure 4-44  Dietary sources of indoxacarb from the 6th China TDS

### 5. 三嗪类农药

（1）混合膳食样品中灭蝇胺的含量

第六次中国总膳食研究混合膳食样品中检出三嗪类杀虫剂灭蝇胺，其检出率为12.2%，残留水平为ND～4.66 μg/kg。总膳食样品中灭蝇胺的含量状况具体详见附表4-66。

（2）膳食暴露评估

我国居民灭蝇胺农药的平均膳食摄入量为3.923 ng/(kg bw·d)，占ADI的比例低于0.01%（附表4-67和图4-45）。

### 5. Triazine Pesticides

(1) Levels of Triazine Pesticides in Composite Dietary Samples

Triazine insecticide cyromazine was detected in the 6th CTDS composite samples, the detection rate was 12.2%, and the residue level was ND-4.66 μg/kg. See Annexed Table 4-66 for the content of cyromazine in dietary samples.

(2) Dietary Exposure Assessment

The average dietary intake of cyromazine pesticide among China residents was 3.923 ng/(kg bw·d), accounting for less than 0.01% of the ADI (Annexed Table 4-67 and Figure 4-45).

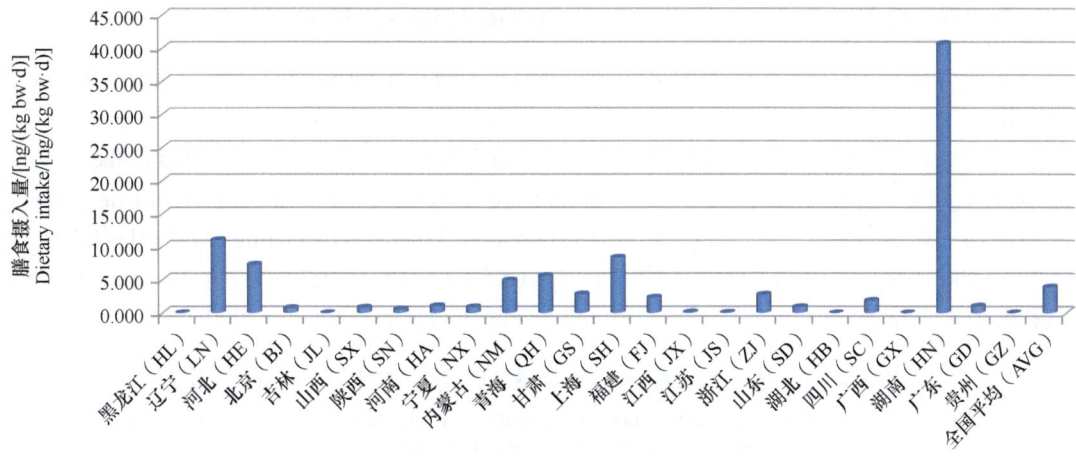

图 4-45　第六次中国总膳食研究的灭蝇胺膳食摄入量

Figure 4-45　Dietary intake of cyromazine from the 6th China TDS

膳食暴露评估结果表明，我国居民三嗪类农药的膳食摄入量较低，对我国居民的健康风险在可接受水平内，健康风险较低。

（3）各类膳食对总膳食摄入的贡献

各类膳食对我国居民三嗪类农药的膳食摄入的贡献情况见附表 4-68 和图 4-46。我国居民三嗪类农药的膳食摄入主要来源于蔬菜类、蛋类和肉类。

From the dietary exposure assessment results, the dietary intake of triazine pesticides for China residents was lower, and the dietary intake to triazine pesticides posed low health risk that was within acceptable level.

(3) Contributions of Food Categories to the Total Dietary Intake

The contribution of various dietary samples to the dietary intake of triazine pesticides by China residents is shown in Annexed Table 4-68 and Figure 4-46. The dietary intake of triazine pesticides in China was mainly from vegetables, eggs, and meats.

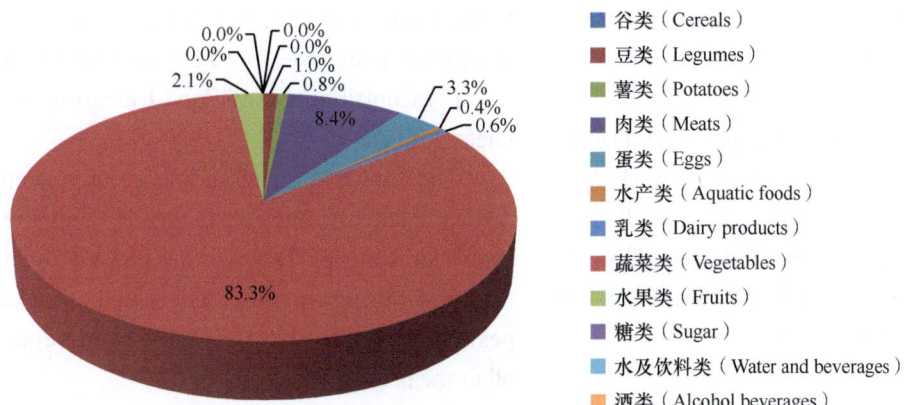

图 4-46　第六次中国总膳食研究灭蝇胺的膳食来源

Figure 4-46　Dietary sources of cyromazine from the 6th China TDS

第四章　农药残留的膳食暴露评估

## 6. 其他类杀虫剂

### 6. Other Insecticides

（1）混合膳食样品中其他类杀虫剂的含量

第六次中国总膳食研究混合膳食样品中检出3种其他类杀虫剂，分别为甲氧虫酰肼（附表4-69）、噻嗪酮（附表4-70）和吡丙醚（附表4-71），其检出率和残留水平见表4-4。

(1) Levels of Other Insecticides in Composite Dietary Samples

Three other pesticides were detected in the 6$^{th}$ CTDS composite samples, namely methoxyfenozide (Annexed Table 4-69), buprofezin (Annexed Table 4-70), and pyriproxyfen (Annexed Table 4-71). The detection rates and residue levels are shown in Table 4-4.

表4-4　第六次中国总膳食研究其他类杀虫剂的残留水平和膳食摄入量
Table 4-4　Residue levels and dietary intakes of other insecticides in the 6$^{th}$ China TDS

| 农药<br>Pesticides | 检出率<br>Detection rates/% | 残留水平<br>Residue levels/(μg/kg) | 平均水平<br>Mean/(μg/kg) | 平均膳食摄入量<br>Average dietary intakes/[ng/(kg bw·d)] | ADI/% |
|---|---|---|---|---|---|
| 甲氧虫酰肼 Methoxyfenozide | 4.9 | ND～38.50 | 0.15 | 11.092 | 0.01 |
| 噻嗪酮 Buprofezin | 14.6 | ND～6.70 | 0.05 | 2.308 | 0.03 |
| 吡丙醚 Pyriproxyfen | 6.9 | ND～20.34 | 0.14 | 6.254 | 0.01 |

（2）膳食暴露评估

我国居民其他类杀虫剂农药的平均膳食摄入量在2.308～11.092 ng/(kg bw·d)（附表4-72～附表4-74，图4-47～图4-49），占各自ADI的比例为0.01%～0.03%。

膳食暴露评估结果表明，我国居民其他类杀虫剂农药的膳食摄入量较低，其他类杀虫剂农药膳食摄入对我国居民的健康风险在可接受水平内，健康风险较低。

（3）各类膳食对总膳食摄入的贡献

各类膳食对我国居民其他类杀虫剂的膳食摄入的贡献情况见附表4-75～附表4-77和图4-50～图4-52。我国居民其他类杀虫剂的膳食摄入主要来源于蔬菜类等膳食。

(2) Dietary Exposure Assessment

The average dietary intake of other insecticides among China residents ranged from 2.308 ng/(kg bw·d) to 11.092 ng/(kg bw·d) (Annexed Table 4-72-Annexed Table 4-74, Figure 4-47-Figure 4-49), accounting for 0.01%-0.03% of their respective ADIs.

From the dietary exposure assessment results, it can be concluded that the dietary intake of other insecticides of the China residents was low, and the health risk to other insecticides was low and in the acceptable level.

(3) Contributions of Food Categories to the Total Dietary Intake

The contribution of various dietary samples to the dietary intake of other pesticides by China residents is shown in Annexed Table 4-75-Annexed Table 4-77 and Figure 4-50-Figure 4-52. The dietary intake of other pesticides in China was mainly from vegetables and other meals.

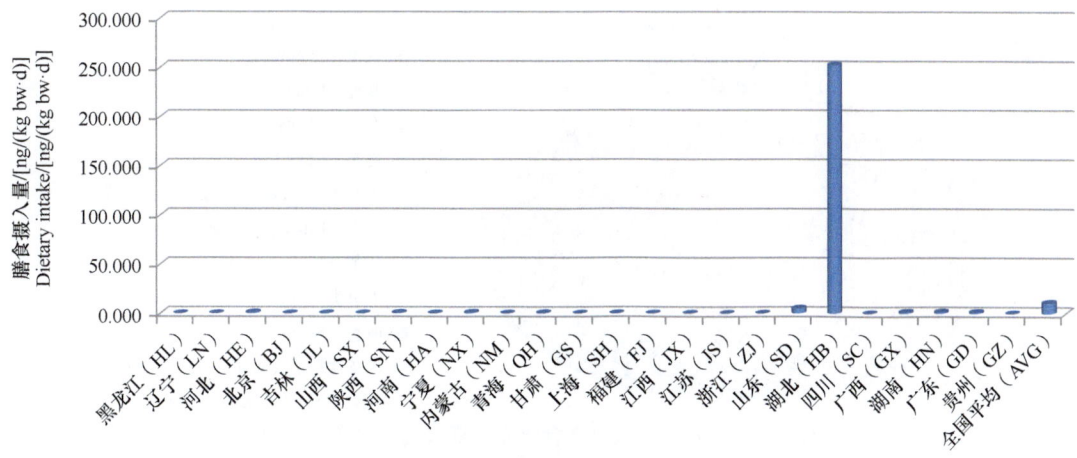

图 4-47　第六次中国总膳食研究的甲氧虫酰肼膳食摄入量
Figure 4-47　Dietary intake of methoxyfenozide from the 6th China TDS

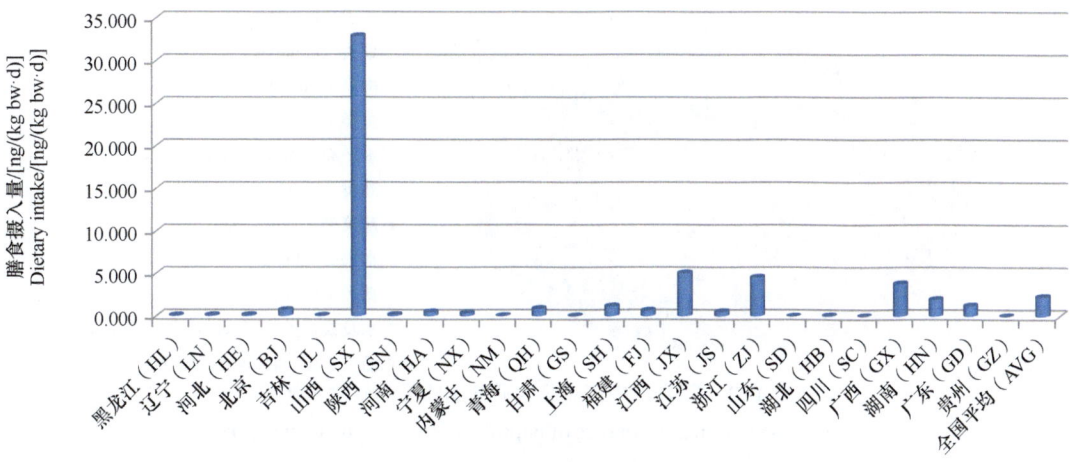

图 4-48　第六次中国总膳食研究的噻嗪酮膳食摄入量
Figure 4-48　Dietary intake of buprofezin from the 6th China TDS

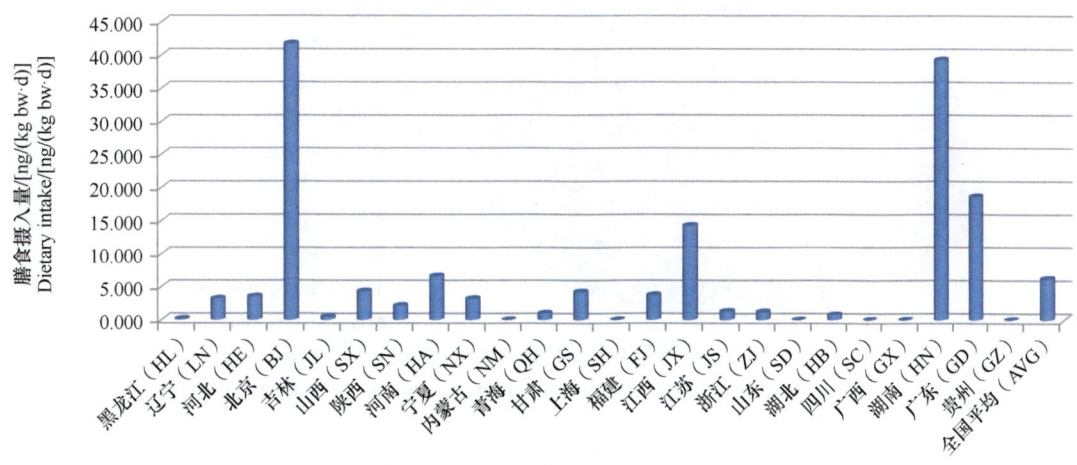

图 4-49　第六次中国总膳食研究的吡丙醚膳食摄入量
Figure 4-49　Dietary intake of pyriproxyfen from the 6th China TDS

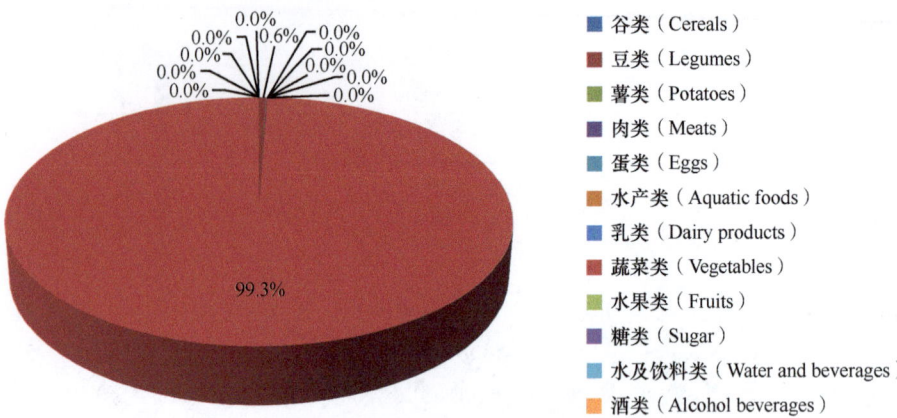

图 4-50　第六次中国总膳食研究甲氧虫酰肼的膳食来源

Figure 4-50　Dietary sources of methoxyfenozide from the 6th China TDS

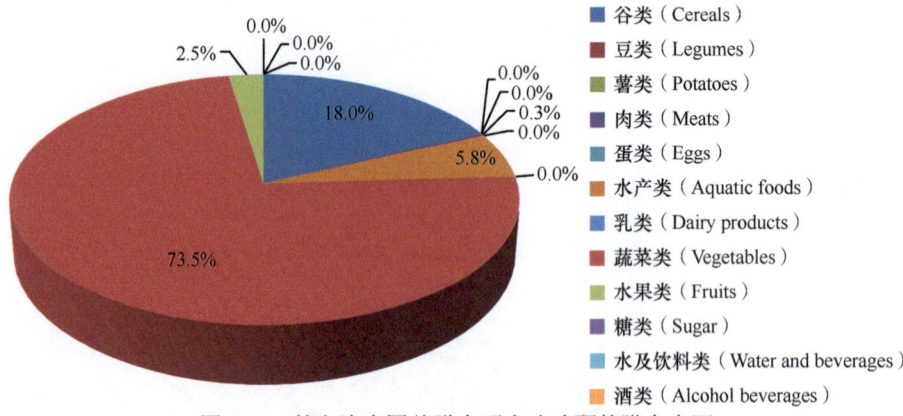

图 4-51　第六次中国总膳食研究噻嗪酮的膳食来源

Figure 4-51　Dietary sources of buprofezin from the 6th China TDS

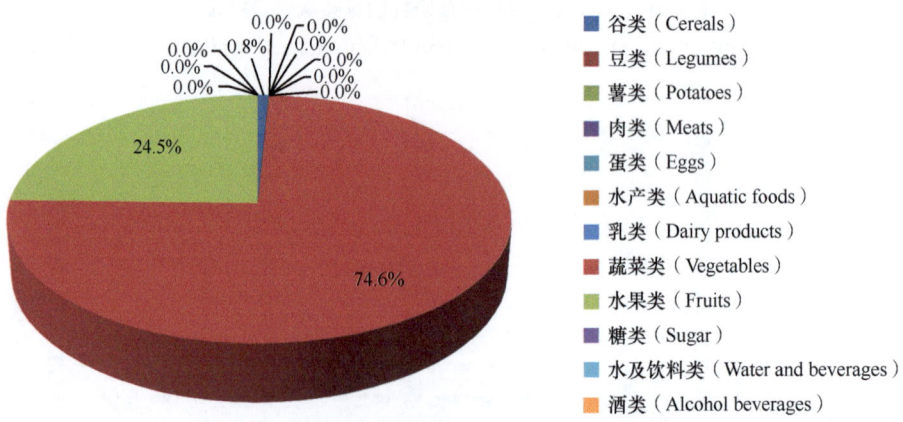

图 4-52　第六次中国总膳食研究吡丙醚的膳食来源

Figure 4-52　Dietary sources of pyriproxyfen from the 6th China TDS

## （二）杀菌剂

### 1. 三唑类农药

（1）混合膳食样品中三唑类农药的含量

第六次中国总膳食研究混合膳食样品中检出13种三唑类农药，分别为粉唑醇（附表4-78）、腈菌唑（附表4-79）、三唑醇（附表4-80）、三唑酮（附表4-81）、四氟醚唑（附表4-82）、氟环唑（附表4-83）、腈苯唑（附表4-84）、氟硅唑（附表4-85）、戊唑醇（附表4-86）、戊菌唑（附表4-87）、丙环唑（附表4-88）、己唑醇（附表4-89）和苯醚甲环唑（附表4-90），残留水平为ND～249.10 μg/kg（表4-5），按检出率由高至低排列分别为戊唑醇、腈苯唑、三唑酮、苯醚甲环唑、三唑醇、丙环唑、腈菌唑、氟硅唑、己唑醇、粉唑醇、氟环唑、四氟醚唑和戊菌唑。

## （Ⅱ）Fungicides

### 1. Triazole Pesticides

(1) Levels of Triazole Pesticides in Composite Dietary Samples

Thirteen triazole pesticides were detected in the composite dietary samples from the sixth China TDS, including flutriafol (Annexed Table 4-78), myclobutanil (Annexed Table 4-79), triadimenol (Annexed Table 4-80), triadimefon (Annexed Table 4-81), tetraconazole (Annexed Table 4-82), epoxiconazole (Annexed Table 4-83), fenbuconazole (Annexed Table 4-84), flusilazole (Annexed Table 4-85), tebuconazole (Annexed Table 4-86) penconazole (Annexed Table 4-87), propiconazole (Annexed Table 4-88), hexaconazole (Annexed Table 4-89), and difenoconazole (Annexed Table 4-90), and the residue level was ND-249.10 μg/kg (Table 4-5). According to the detection rates from high to low, they were tebuconazole, fenbuconazole, triadimefon, difenoconazole, triadimenol, propiconazole, myclobutanil, flusilazole, hexaconazole, flutriafol, epoxiconazole, tetraconazole, and pentaconazole.

表4-5 第六次中国总膳食研究三唑类农药的残留水平和膳食摄入量
Table 4-5 Residue levels and dietary intakes of triazole pesticides in the 6th China TDS

| 农药 Pesticides | 检出率 Detection rates/% | 残留水平 Residue levels/(μg/kg) | 平均水平 Mean/(μg/kg) | 平均膳食摄入量 Average dietary intakes/[ng/(kg bw·d)] | ADI/% |
|---|---|---|---|---|---|
| 粉唑醇 Flutriafol | 3.8 | ND～0.86 | 0.01 | 0.425 | 0.00 |
| 腈菌唑 Myclobutanil | 9.4 | ND～1.74 | 0.04 | 1.397 | 0.01 |
| 三唑醇 Triadimenol | 11.5 | ND～10.76 | 0.19 | 9.406 | 0.03 |
| 三唑酮 Triadimefon | 18.1 | ND～17.78 | 0.24 | 12.581 | 0.04 |
| 四氟醚唑 Tetraconazole | 1.7 | ND～0.40 | 0.00 | 0.119 | 0.00 |
| 氟环唑 Epoxiconazole | 3.8 | ND～1.44 | 0.01 | 0.202 | 0.00 |
| 腈苯唑 Fenbuconazole | 18.8 | ND～29.16 | 0.41 | 3.053 | 0.01 |
| 氟硅唑 Flusilazole | 6.6 | ND～165.14 | 0.79 | 43.512 | 0.62 |
| 戊唑醇 Tebuconazole | 32.3 | ND～37.21 | 0.50 | 24.553 | 0.08 |
| 戊菌唑 Penconazole | 1.0 | ND～1.25 | 0.01 | 0.064 | 0.00 |
| 丙环唑 Propiconazole | 10.8 | ND～249.10 | 2.72 | 80.739 | 0.12 |
| 己唑醇 Hexaconazole | 6.3 | ND～40.97 | 0.16 | 11.095 | 0.22 |
| 苯醚甲环唑 Difenoconazole | 13.9 | ND～92.07 | 0.72 | 33.876 | 0.34 |

## （2）膳食暴露评估

我国居民三唑类农药的平均膳食摄入量为 0.064～80.739 ng/(kg bw·d)（附表 4-91～附表 4-103，图 4-53～图 4-65），占各自 ADI 的比例为 0.00%～0.62%。平均膳食摄入量最高的是丙环唑 [80.739 ng/(kg bw·d)]，其次为氟硅唑 [43.512 ng/(kg bw·d)]。

膳食暴露评估结果表明，我国居民三唑类农药的膳食摄入量较低，三唑类农药膳食摄入对我国居民的健康风险在可接受水平内，健康风险较低。

## (2) Dietary Exposure Assessment

The average dietary intake of triazole pesticides for China residents ranged from 0.064 ng/(kg bw·d) to 80.739 ng/(kg bw·d) (Annexed Table 4-91-Annexed Table 4-103, Figure 4-53-Figure 4-65), accounting for 0.00%-0.62% of their respective ADIs. The highest average dietary intake was propiconazole [80.739 ng/(kg bw·d)], followed by flusilazole [43.512 ng/(kg bw·d)].

From the dietary exposure assessment results, it can be concluded that the dietary intake of triazole pesticides of the China residents was low, and the health risk to triazole pesticides was low and in the acceptable level.

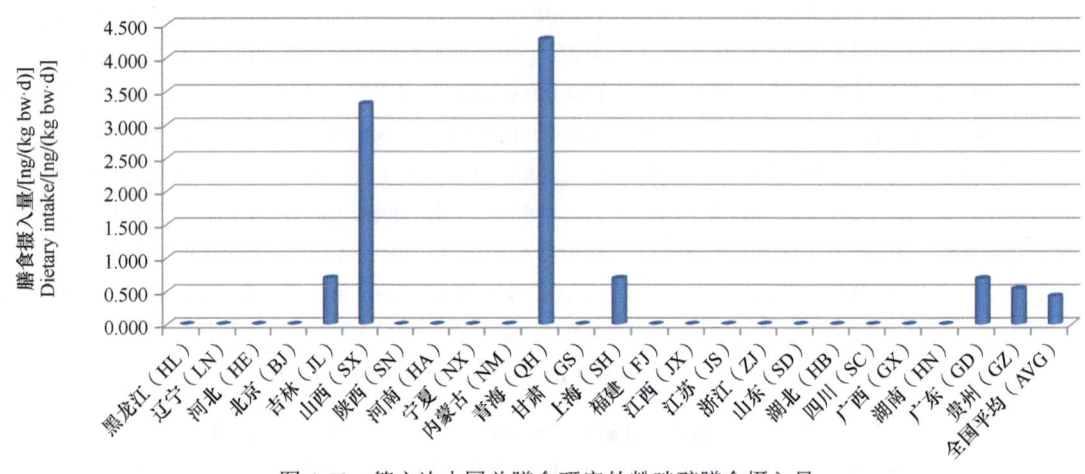

图 4-53　第六次中国总膳食研究的粉唑醇膳食摄入量
Figure 4-53　Dietary intake of flutriafol from the 6$^{th}$ China TDS

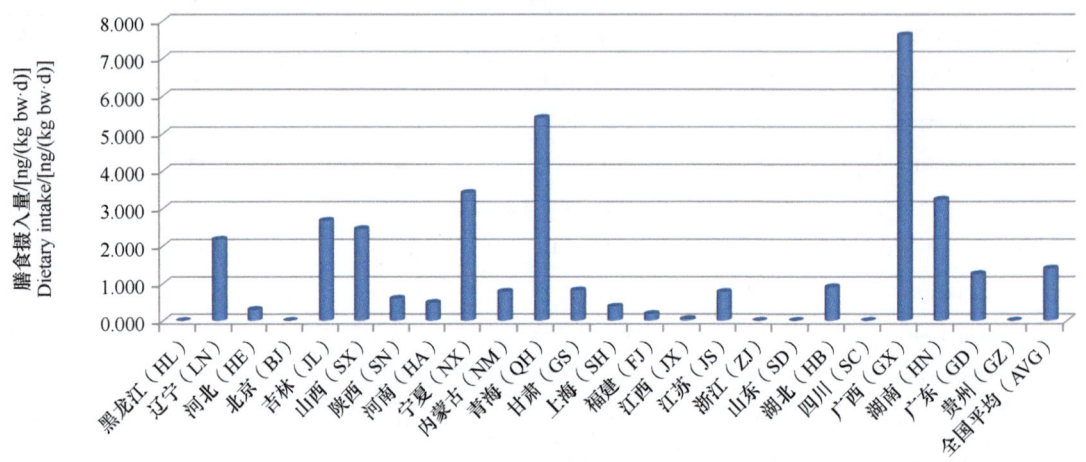

图 4-54　第六次中国总膳食研究的腈菌唑膳食摄入量
Figure 4-54　Dietary intake of myclobutanil from the 6$^{th}$ China TDS

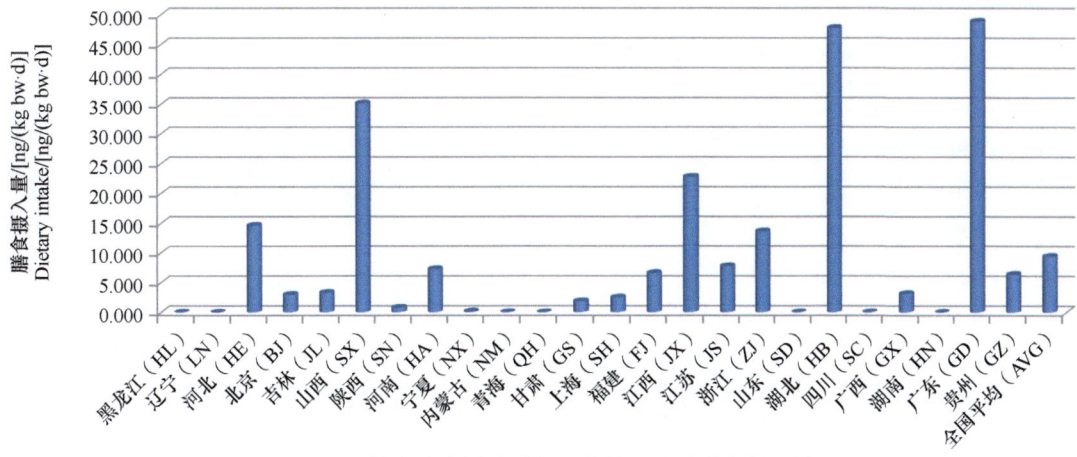

图 4-55　第六次中国总膳食研究的三唑醇膳食摄入量
Figure 4-55　Dietary intake of triadimenol from the 6th China TDS

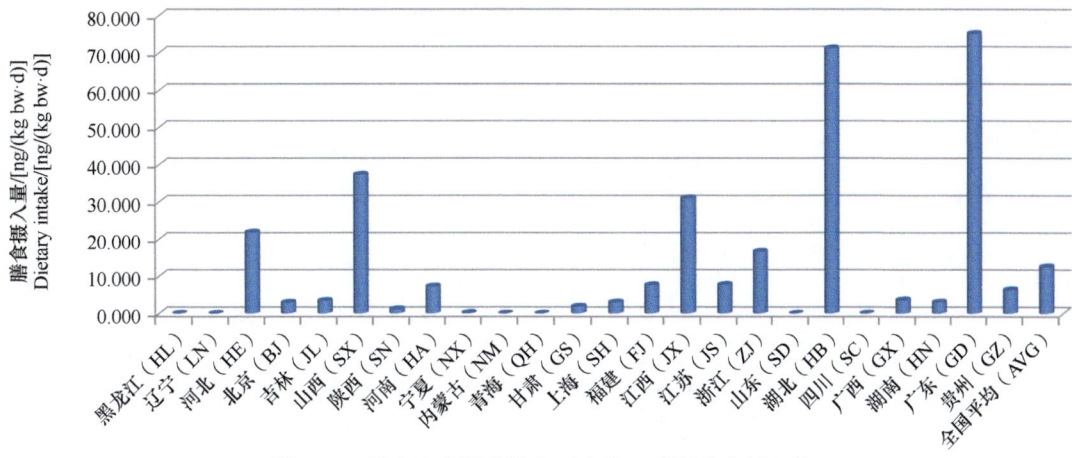

图 4-56　第六次中国总膳食研究的三唑酮膳食摄入量
Figure 4-56　Dietary intake of triadimefon from the 6th China TDS

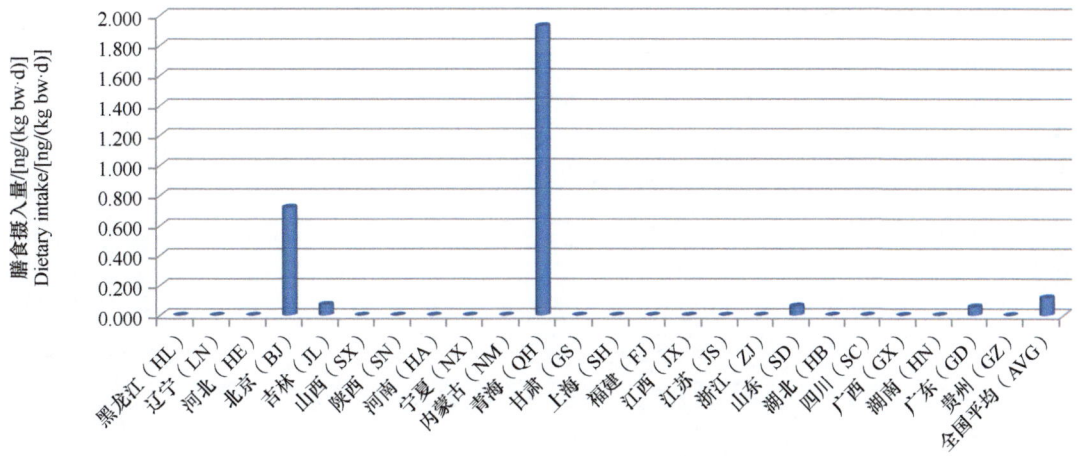

图 4-57　第六次中国总膳食研究的四氟醚唑膳食摄入量
Figure 4-57　Dietary intake of tetraconazole from the 6th China TDS

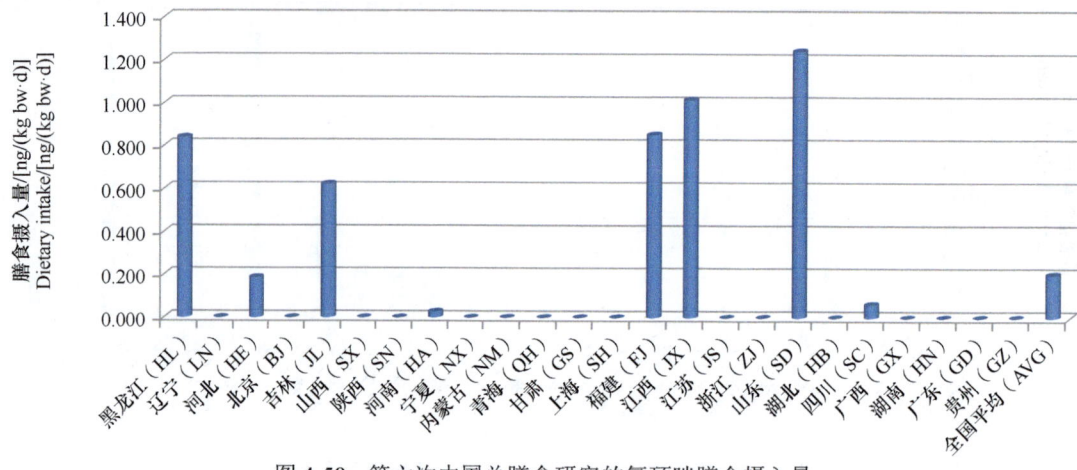

图 4-58　第六次中国总膳食研究的氟环唑膳食摄入量

Figure 4-58　Dietary intake of epoxiconazole from the 6th China TDS

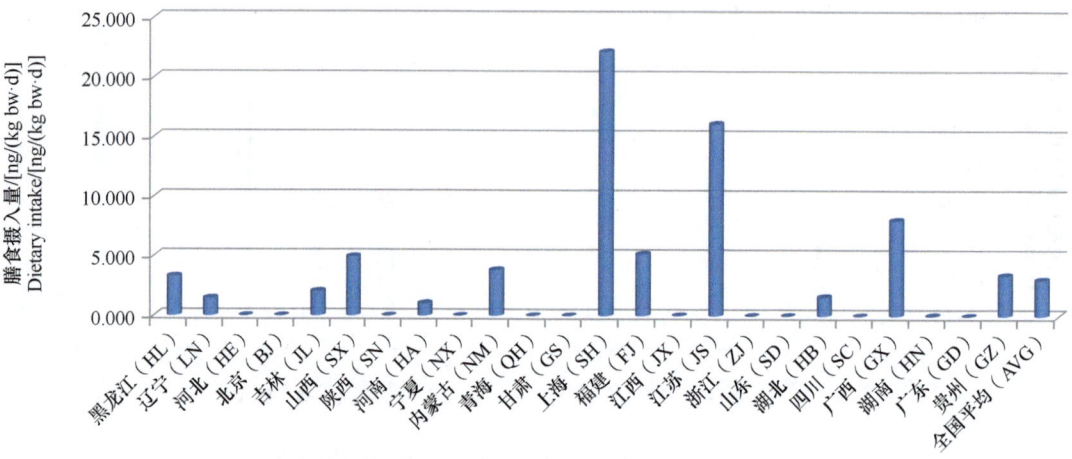

图 4-59　第六次中国总膳食研究的腈苯唑膳食摄入量

Figure 4-59　Dietary intake of fenbuconazole from the 6th China TDS

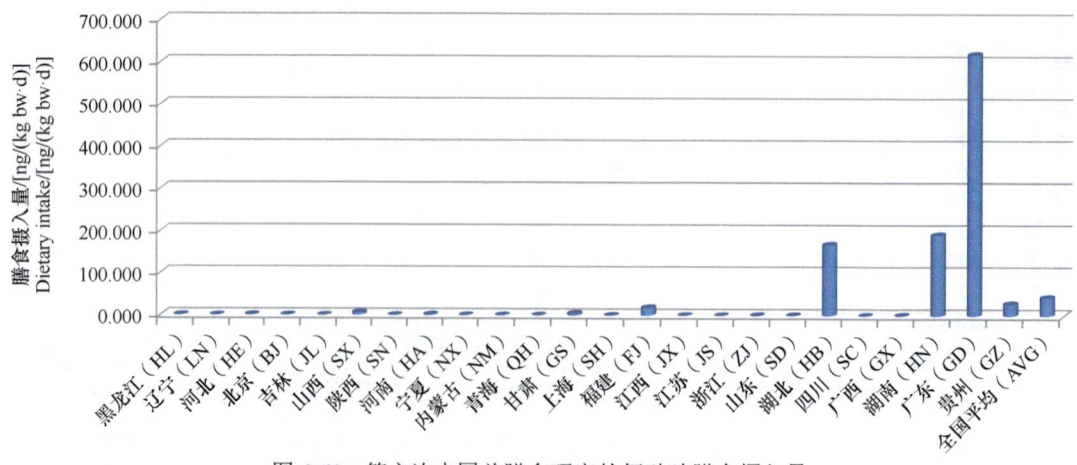

图 4-60　第六次中国总膳食研究的氟硅唑膳食摄入量

Figure 4-60　Dietary intake of flusilazole from the 6th China TDS

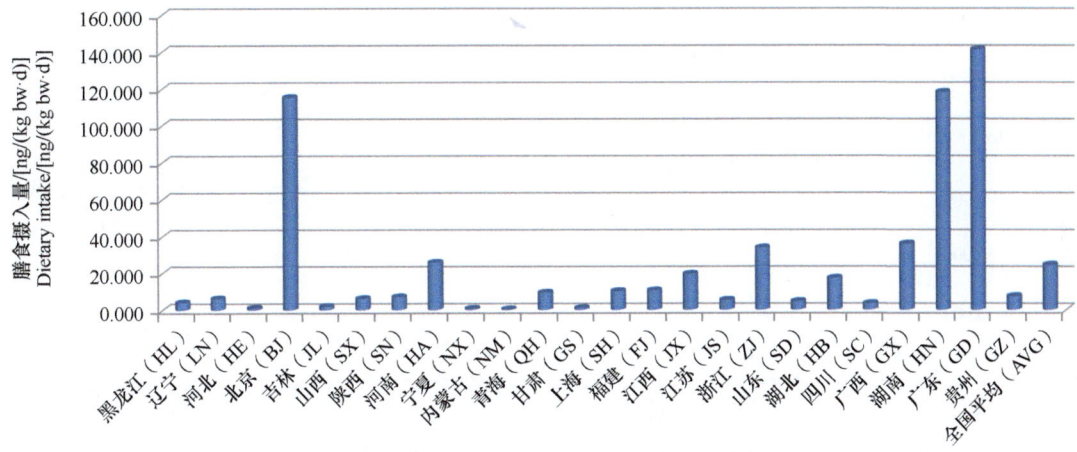

图 4-61　第六次中国总膳食研究的戊唑醇膳食摄入量

Figure 4-61　Dietary intake of tebuconazole from the 6$^{th}$ China TDS

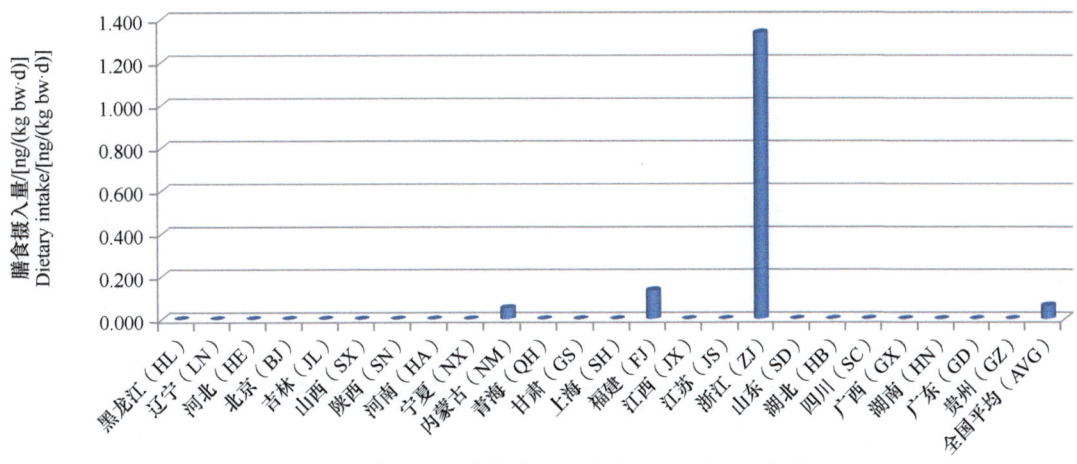

图 4-62　第六次中国总膳食研究的戊菌唑膳食摄入量

Figure 4-62　Dietary intake of penconazole from the 6$^{th}$ China TDS

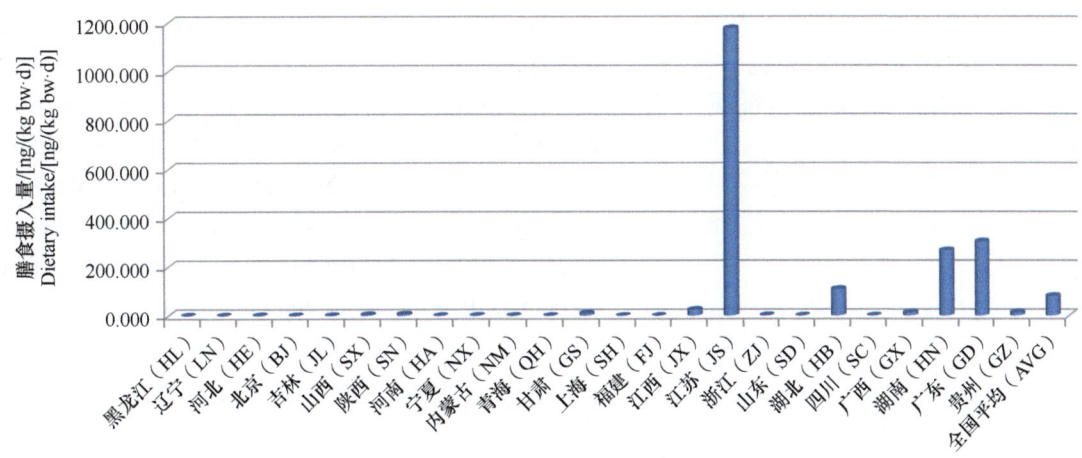

图 4-63　第六次中国总膳食研究的丙环唑膳食摄入量

Figure 4-63　Dietary intake of propiconazole from the 6$^{th}$ China TDS

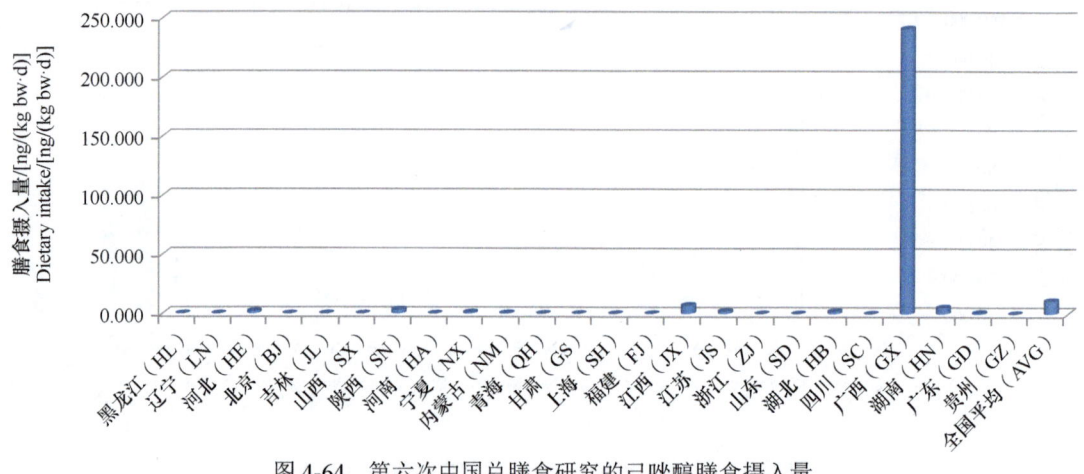

图 4-64　第六次中国总膳食研究的己唑醇膳食摄入量
Figure 4-64　Dietary intake of hexaconazole from the 6$^{th}$ China TDS

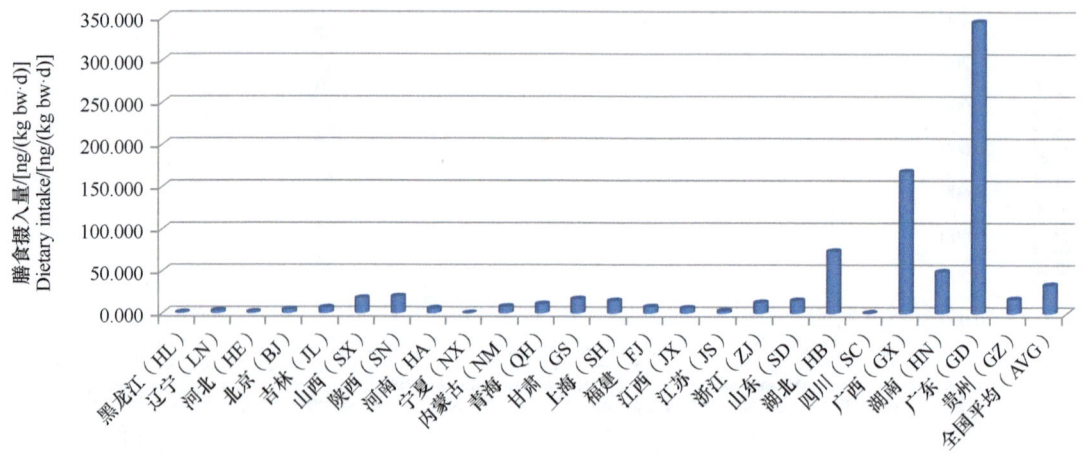

图 4-65　第六次中国总膳食研究的苯醚甲环唑膳食摄入量
Figure 4-65　Dietary intake of difenoconazole from the 6$^{th}$ China TDS

（3）各类膳食对总膳食摄入的贡献

各类膳食对我国居民三唑类农药的膳食摄入的贡献情况见附表4-104～附表4-116和图4-66～图4-78。我国居民三唑类农药的膳食摄入主要来源于蔬菜类、水果类、谷类等膳食。

(3) Contributions of Food Categories to the Total Dietary Intake

The contribution of various dietary samples to the dietary intake of triazole pesticides by China residents is shown in Annexed Table 4-104-Annexed Table 4-116 and Figure 4-66-Figure 4-78. The dietary intake of triazole pesticides for China residents was mainly from vegetables, fruits, cereals, and other meals.

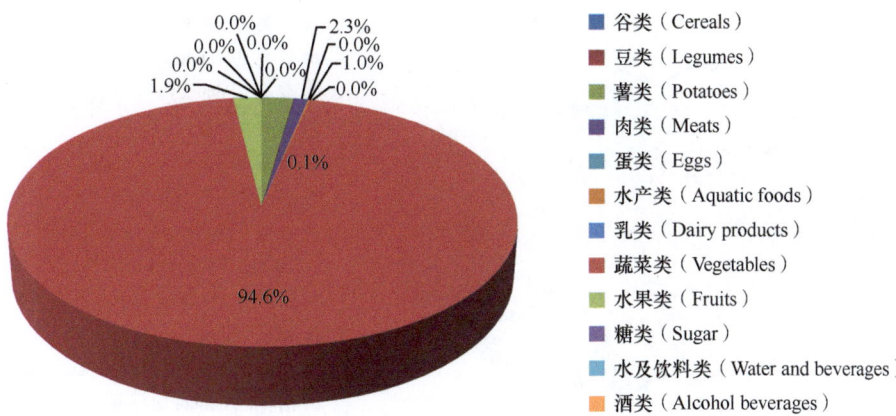

图 4-66　第六次中国总膳食研究粉唑醇的膳食来源

Figure 4-66　Dietary sources of flutriafol from the 6th China TDS

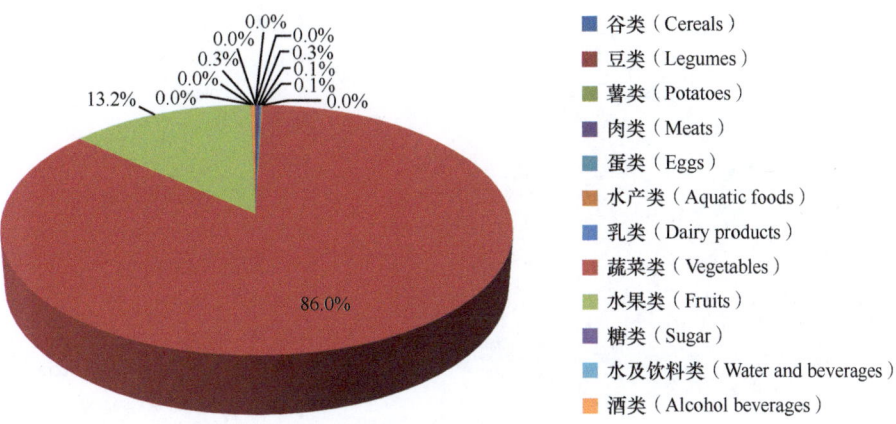

图 4-67　第六次中国总膳食研究腈菌唑的膳食来源

Figure 4-67　Dietary sources of myclobutanil from the 6th China TDS

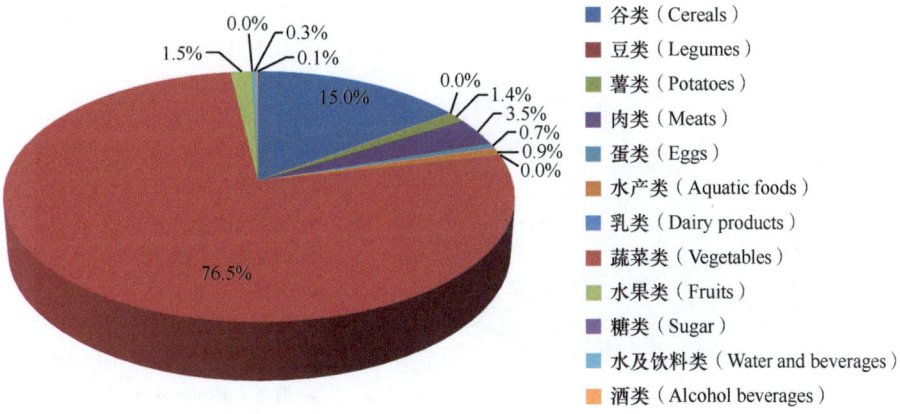

图 4-68　第六次中国总膳食研究三唑醇的膳食来源

Figure 4-68　Dietary sources of triadimenol from the 6th China TDS

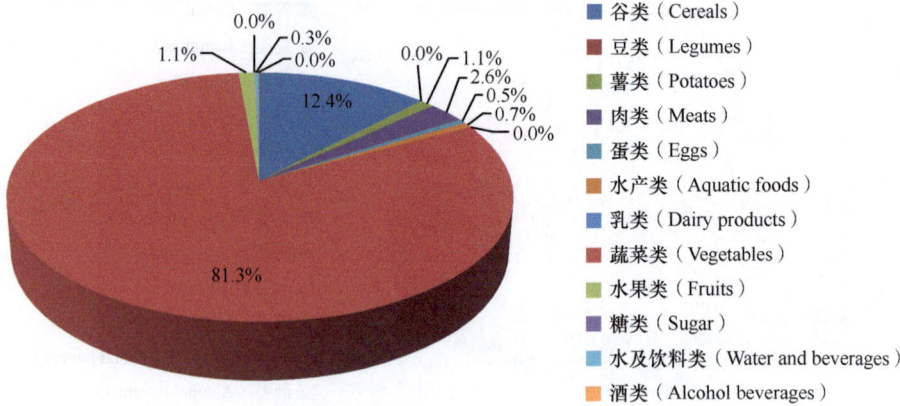

图 4-69　第六次中国总膳食研究三唑酮的膳食来源

Figure 4-69　Dietary sources of triadimefon from the 6$^{th}$ China TDS

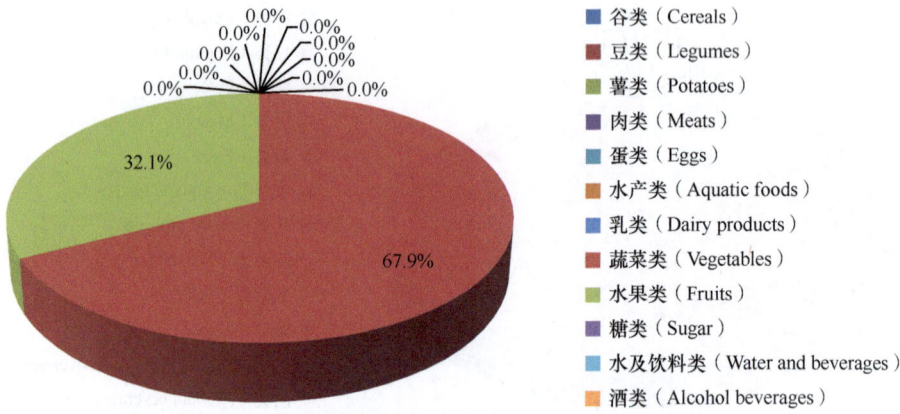

图 4-70　第六次中国总膳食研究四氟醚唑的膳食来源

Figure 4-70　Dietary sources of tetraconazole from the 6$^{th}$ China TDS

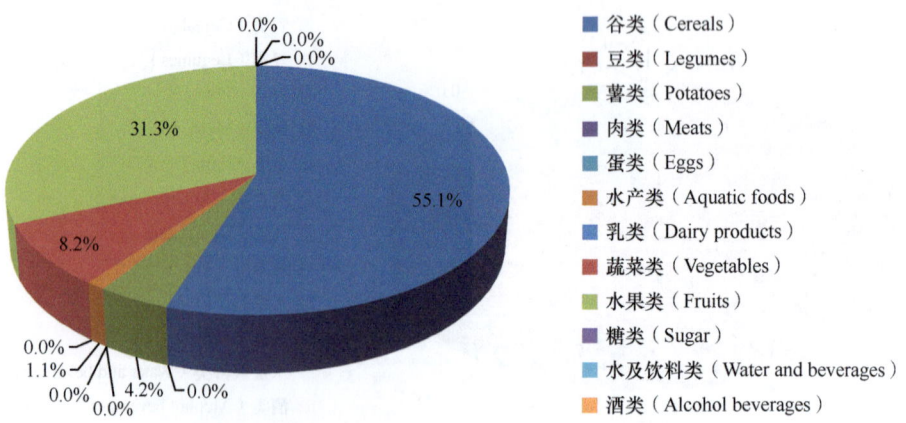

图 4-71　第六次中国总膳食研究氟环唑的膳食来源

Figure 4-71　Dietary sources of epoxiconazole from the 6$^{th}$ China TDS

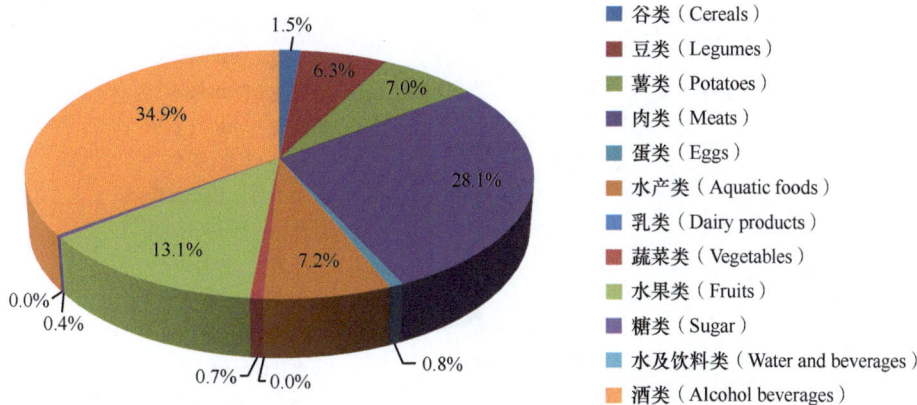

图 4-72　第六次中国总膳食研究腈苯唑的膳食来源

Figure 4-72　Dietary sources of fenbuconazole from the 6th China TDS

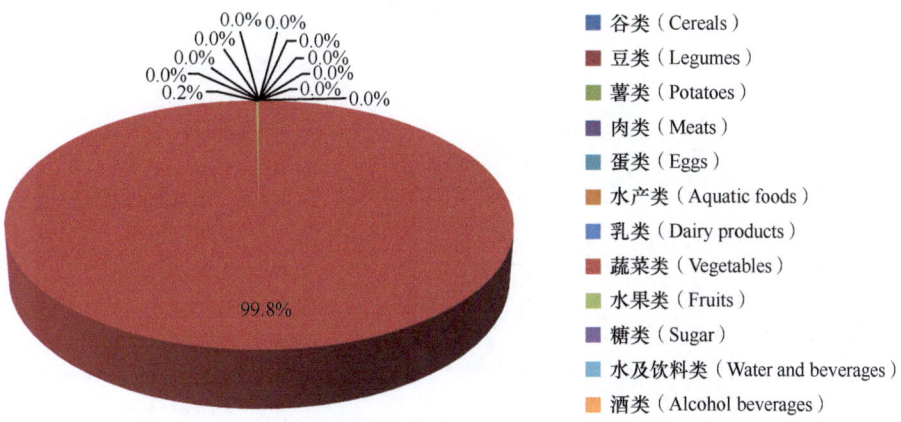

图 4-73　第六次中国总膳食研究氟硅唑的膳食来源

Figure 4-73　Dietary sources of flusilazole from the 6th China TDS

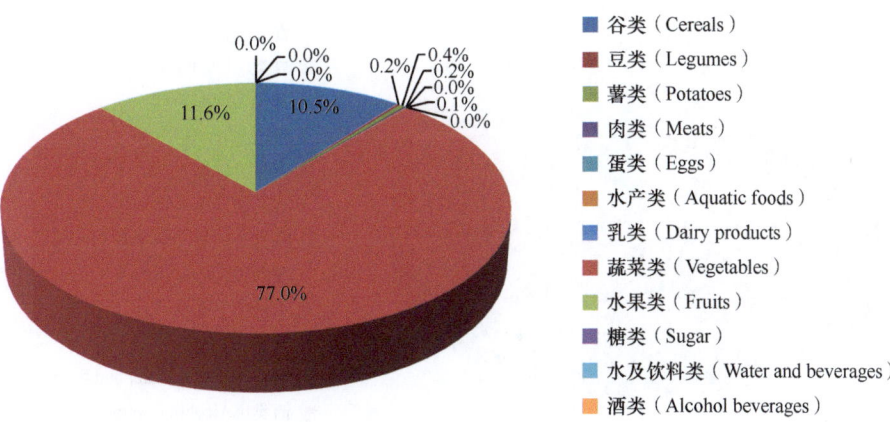

图 4-74　第六次中国总膳食研究戊唑醇的膳食来源

Figure 4-74　Dietary sources of tebuconazole from the 6th China TDS

第四章　农药残留的膳食暴露评估

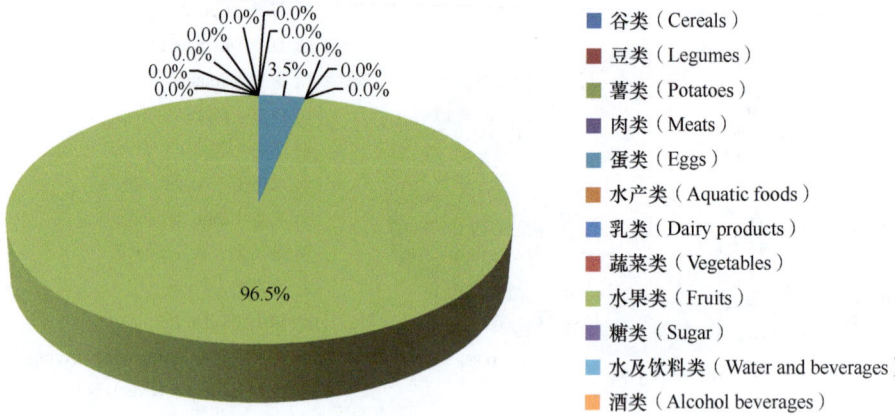

图 4-75　第六次中国总膳食研究戊菌唑的膳食来源

Figure 4-75　Dietary sources of penconazole from the 6$^{th}$ China TDS

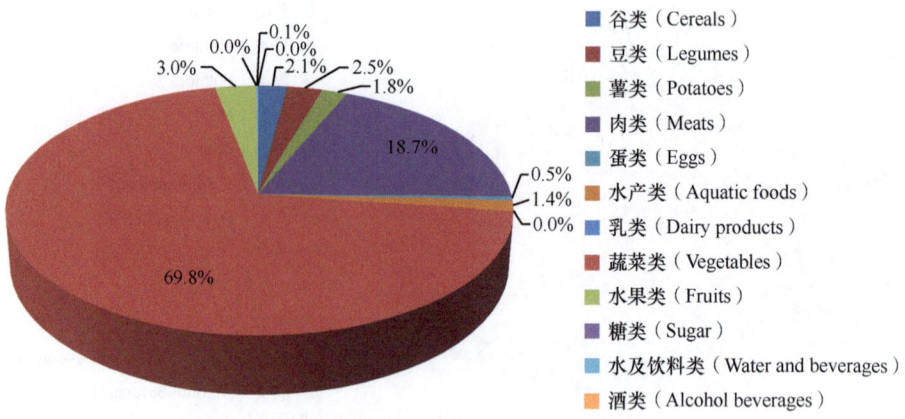

图 4-76　第六次中国总膳食研究丙环唑的膳食来源

Figure 4-76　Dietary sources of propiconazole from the 6$^{th}$ China TDS

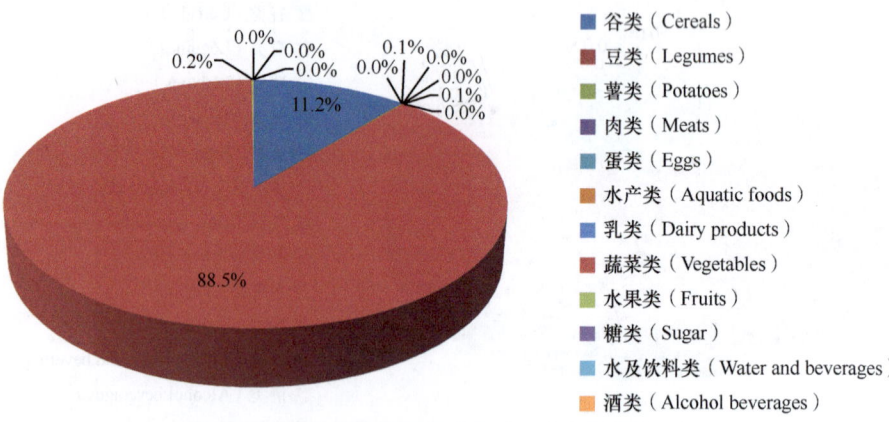

图 4-77　第六次中国总膳食研究己唑醇的膳食来源

Figure 4-77　Dietary sources of hexaconazole from the 6$^{th}$ China TDS

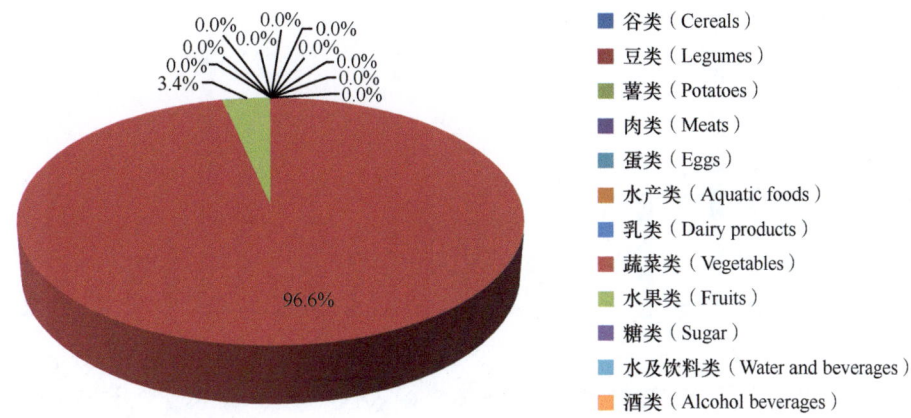

图 4-78 第六次中国总膳食研究苯醚甲环唑的膳食来源
Figure 4-78 Dietary sources of difenoconazole from the 6th China TDS

## 2. 咪唑类农药

（1）混合膳食样品中咪唑类农药的含量

第六次中国总膳食研究混合膳食样品中检出 4 种三唑类农药，分别为多菌灵（附表 4-117）、噻菌灵（附表 4-118）、抑霉唑（附表 4-119）和咪鲜胺（附表 4-120），其残留水平和膳食摄入量见表 4-6，按检出率由高至低排列分别为多菌灵、咪鲜胺、抑霉唑和噻菌灵。

## 2. Imidazole Pesticides

(1) Levels of Imidazole Pesticides in Composite Dietary Samples

Four triazole pesticides were detected in the composite dietary samples from the sixth China TDS, namely carbendazim (Annexed Table 4-117), thiabendazole (Annexed Table 4-118), imazalil (Annexed Table 4-119), and prochloraz (Annexed Table 4-120). The residue levels are shown in Table 4-6. According to the detection rates from high to low, they were carbendazim, prochloraz, imazalil, and thiabendazole.

表 4-6 第六次中国总膳食研究咪唑类农药的残留水平和膳食摄入量
Table 4-6 Residue levels and dietary intakes of imidazole pesticides in the 6th China TDS

| 农药 Pesticides | 检出率 Detection rates/% | 残留水平 Residue levels/(μg/kg) | 平均水平 Mean/(μg/kg) | 平均膳食摄入量 Average dietary intakes/[ng/(kg bw·d)] | ADI/% |
|---|---|---|---|---|---|
| 多菌灵 Carbendazim | 50.7 | ND～63.66 | 3.01 | 83.13 | 0.28 |
| 噻菌灵 Thiabendazole | 9.7 | ND～47.29 | 0.49 | 6.166 | 0.01 |
| 抑霉唑 Imazalil | 18.8 | ND～33.46 | 0.41 | 4.648 | 0.02 |
| 咪鲜胺 Prochloraz | 28.1 | ND～28.54 | 0.34 | 11.626 | 0.12 |

（2）膳食暴露评估

我国居民咪唑类农药的平均膳食摄入量为 4.648～83.13 ng/(kg bw·d)（附表 4-121～附表 4-124，图 4-79～图 4-82），占各自 ADI 的比例为 0.01%～0.28%。平均膳食摄入量最高的是多菌灵 [83.13 ng/(kg bw·d)]，其次为咪鲜

(2) Dietary Exposure Assessment

The average dietary intake of imidazole pesticides among China residents ranged from 4.648 ng/(kg bw·d) to 83.13 ng/(kg bw·d) (Annexed Table 4-121-Annexed Table 4-124, Figure 4-79-Figure 4-82), accounting for 0.01%-0.28% of their respective ADIs. The highest average dietary intake was carbendazim

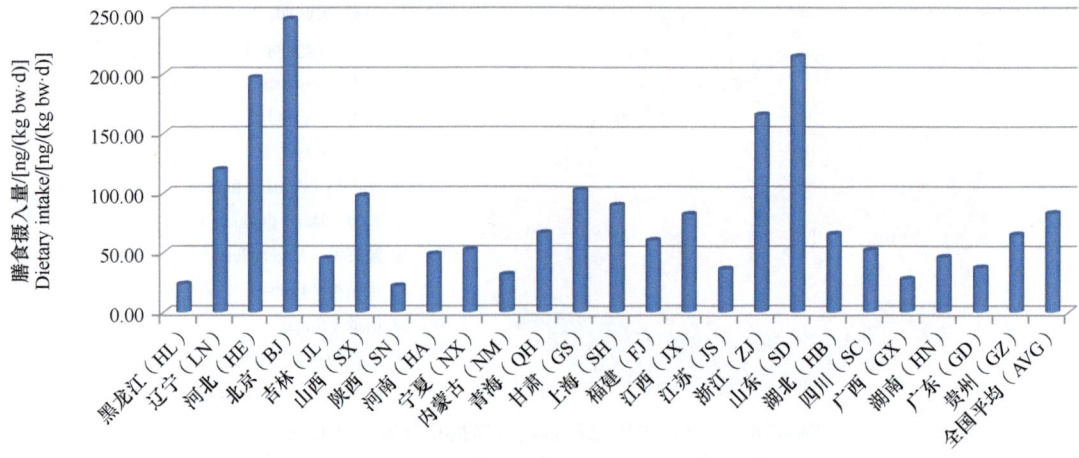

图 4-79　第六次中国总膳食研究的多菌灵膳食摄入量

Figure 4-79　Dietary intake of carbendazim from the 6$^{th}$ China TDS

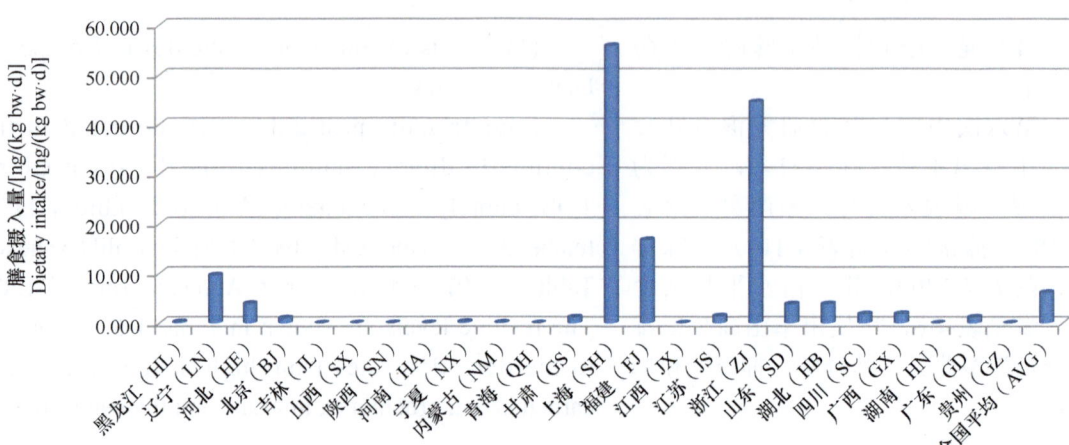

图 4-80　第六次中国总膳食研究的噻菌灵膳食摄入量

Figure 4-80　Dietary intake of thiabendazole from the 6$^{th}$ China TDS

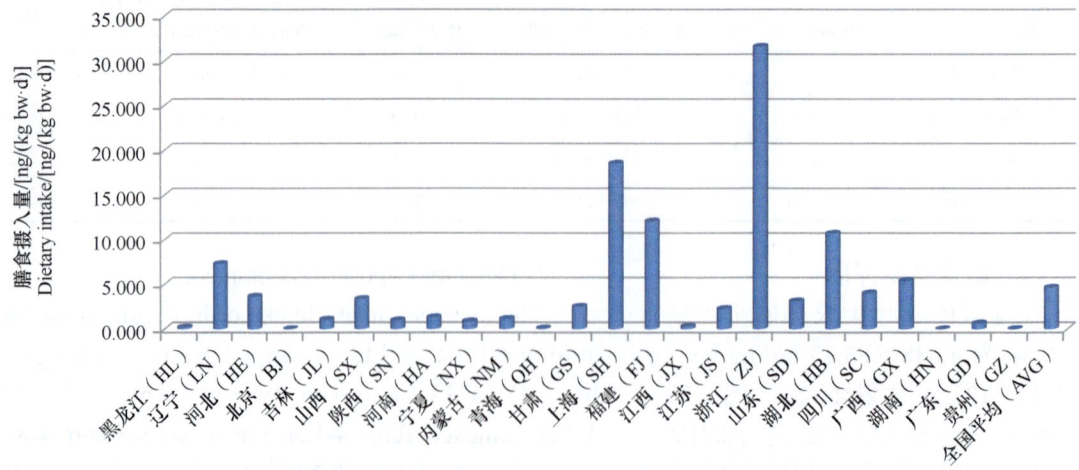

图 4-81　第六次中国总膳食研究的抑霉唑膳食摄入量

Figure 4-81　Dietary intake of imazalil from the 6$^{th}$ China TDS

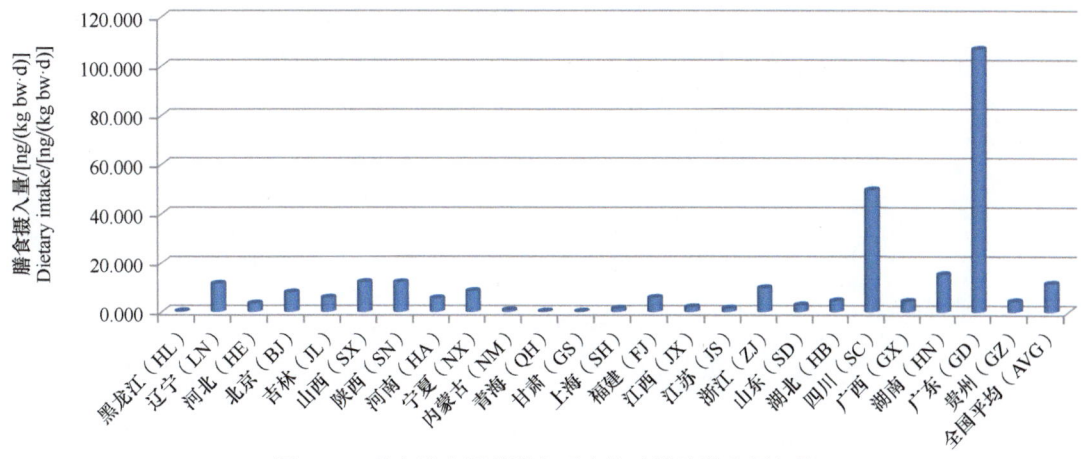

图 4-82 第六次中国总膳食研究的咪鲜胺膳食摄入量
Figure 4-82　Dietary intake of prochloraz from the 6th China TDS

胺 [11.626 ng/(kg bw·d)]。

（3）各类膳食对总膳食摄入的贡献

各类膳食对我国居民咪唑类农药的膳食摄入的贡献情况见附表 4-125～附表 4-128 和图 4-83～图 4-86。我国居民咪唑类农药的膳食摄入主要来源于蔬菜类、水果类、谷类等膳食。其中，多菌灵和咪鲜胺主要来源于蔬菜类和水果类，而噻菌灵和抑霉唑则主要来源于水果类，且抑霉唑还有部分来源于动物性样品。

[83.13 ng/(kg bw·d)], followed by prochloraz [11.626 ng/(kg bw·d)].

From the dietary exposure assessment results, it can be concluded that the dietary intake of imidazole pesticides of the China residents was low, and the health risk to imidazole pesticides was low and in the acceptable level.

(3) Contributions of Food Categories to the Total Dietary Intake

The contribution of various diets to the dietary intake of imidazole pesticides by China residents is shown in Annexed Table 4-125-Annexed Table 4-128 and Figure 4-83-Figure 4-86. The dietary intake of imidazole pesticides for China residents was mainly from vegetables, fruits, cereals, and other meals. Among

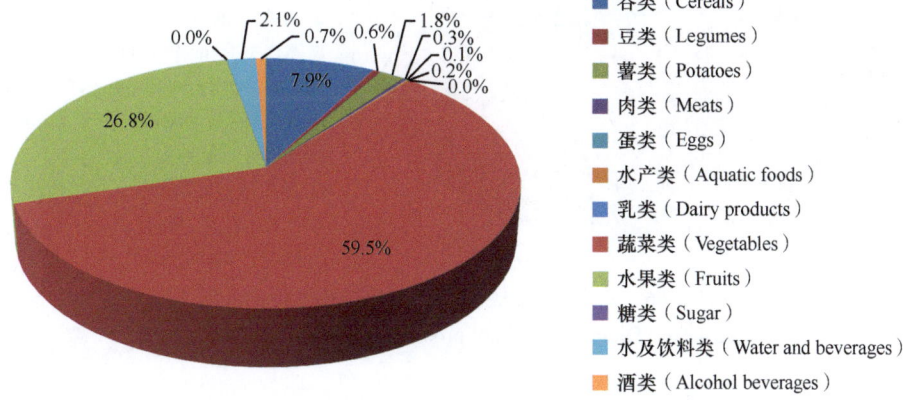

图 4-83 第六次中国总膳食研究多菌灵的膳食来源
Figure 4-83　Dietary sources of carbendazim from the 6th China TDS

第四章　农药残留的膳食暴露评估　177

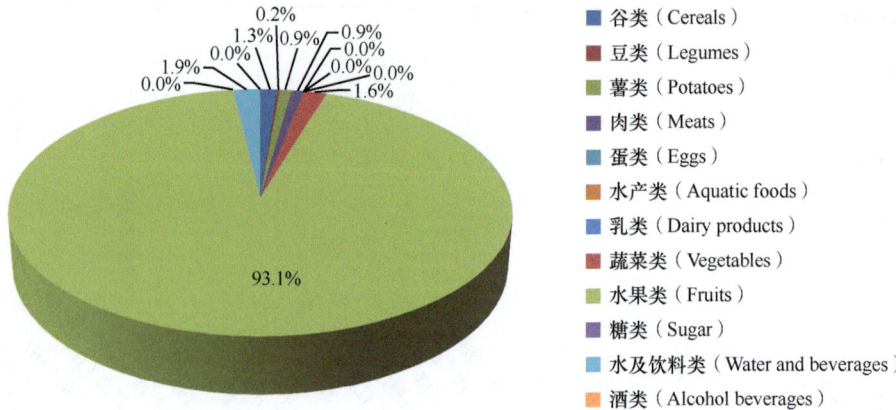

图 4-84　第六次中国总膳食研究噻菌灵的膳食来源
Figure 4-84　Dietary sources of thiabendazole from the 6th China TDS

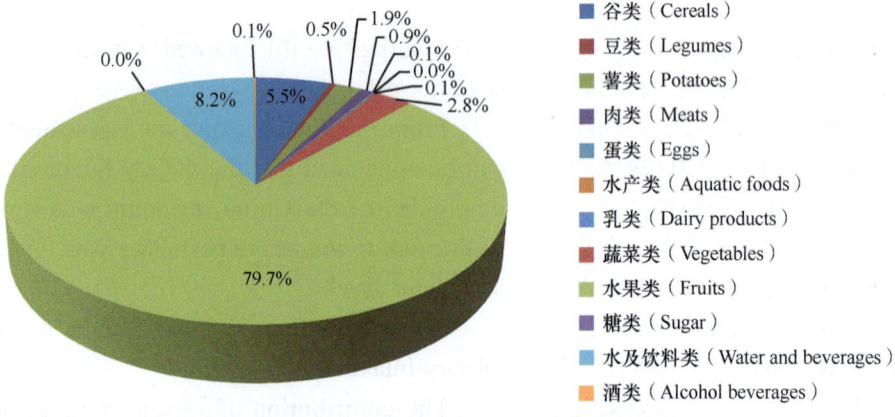

图 4-85　第六次中国总膳食研究抑霉唑的膳食来源
Figure 4-85　Dietary sources of imazalil from the 6th China TDS

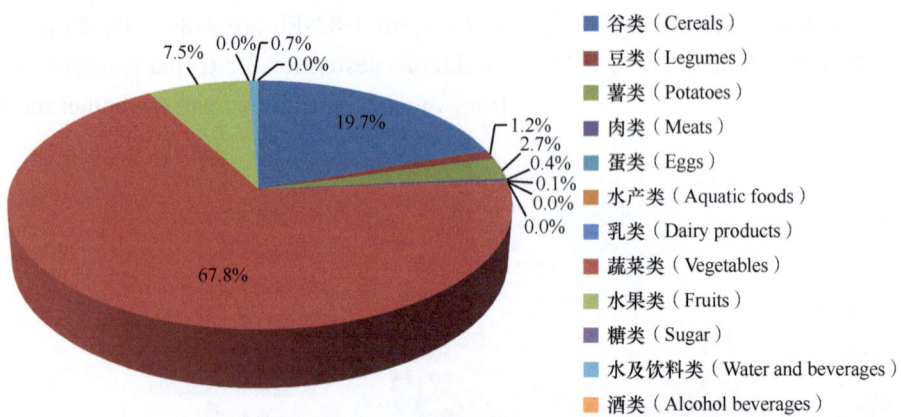

图 4-86　第六次中国总膳食研究咪鲜胺的膳食来源
Figure 4-86　Dietary sources of prochloraz from the 6th China TDS

## 3. 甲氧基丙烯酸酯类农药

（1）混合膳食样品中甲氧基丙烯酸酯类农药的含量

第六次中国总膳食研究混合膳食样品中检出3种甲氧基丙烯酸酯类农药，分别为嘧菌酯（附表4-129）、吡唑醚菌酯（附表4-130）和肟菌酯（附表4-131），其残留水平见表4-7。其中，嘧菌酯和吡唑醚菌酯的检出率均为28.8%，而肟菌酯的检出率为9.4%。

them, carbendazim and prochloraz were mainly from vegetables and fruits, while thiabendazole and imazalil were mainly from fruits, and imazalil was also partially from animal-derived samples.

## 3. Strobilurin Pesticides

(1) Levels of Strobilurin Pesticides in Composite Dietary Samples

Three strobilurin pesticides were detected in the composite dietary samples from the Sixth China TDS, namely azoxystrobin (Annexed Table 4-129), pyraclostrobin (Annexed Table 4-130), and trifloxystrobin (Annexed Table 4-131). See Table 4-7 for their residue levels. Among them, the detection rates of azoxystrobin and pyraclostrobin were 28.8%, while the detection rate of trifloxystrobin was 9.4%.

表 4-7　第六次中国总膳食研究甲氧基丙烯酸酯类农药的残留水平和膳食摄入量
Table 4-7　Residue levels and dietary intakes of strobilurin pesticides in the 6$^{th}$ China TDS

| 农药 Pesticides | 检出率 Detection rates/% | 残留水平 Residue levels/(μg/kg) | 平均水平 Mean/(μg/kg) | 平均膳食摄入量 Average dietary intakes/[ng/(kg bw·d)] | ADI/% |
|---|---|---|---|---|---|
| 嘧菌酯 Azoxystrobin | 28.8 | ND～24.39 | 0.49 | 19.364 | 0.01 |
| 吡唑醚菌酯 Pyraclostrobin | 28.8 | ND～47.10 | 0.67 | 37.417 | 0.13 |
| 肟菌酯 Trifloxystrobin | 9.4 | ND～19.46 | 0.11 | 3.010 | 0.01 |

（2）膳食暴露评估

我国居民甲氧基丙烯酸酯类农药的平均膳食摄入量为3.010～37.417 ng/(kg bw·d)（表4-7，附表4-132～附表4-134，图4-87～图4-89），占各自ADI的比例为0.01%～0.13%。平均膳食摄入量最高的是吡唑醚菌酯[37.417 ng/(kg bw·d)]，其次为嘧菌酯[19.364 ng/(kg bw·d)]。

膳食暴露评估结果表明，我国居民甲氧基丙烯酸酯类农药的膳食摄入量较低，甲氧基丙烯酸酯类农药膳食摄入对我国居民的健康风险在可接受水平内，健康风险较低。

(2) Dietary Exposure Assessment

The average dietary intake of strobilurin pesticides for China residents ranged from 3.010 ng/(kg bw·d) to 37.417 ng/(kg bw·d) (Table 4-8, Annexed Table 4-132-Annexed Table 4-134, Figure 4-87-Figure 4-89), accounting for 0.01%-0.13% of their respective ADIs. The highest average dietary intake was pyraclostrobin [37.417 ng/(kg bw·d)], followed by azoxystrobin [19.364 ng/(kg bw·d)].

From the exposure assessment results, it can be concluded that the dietary intake of strobilurin pesticides of the China residents was low, and the health risk to strobilurin pesticides was low and in the acceptable level.

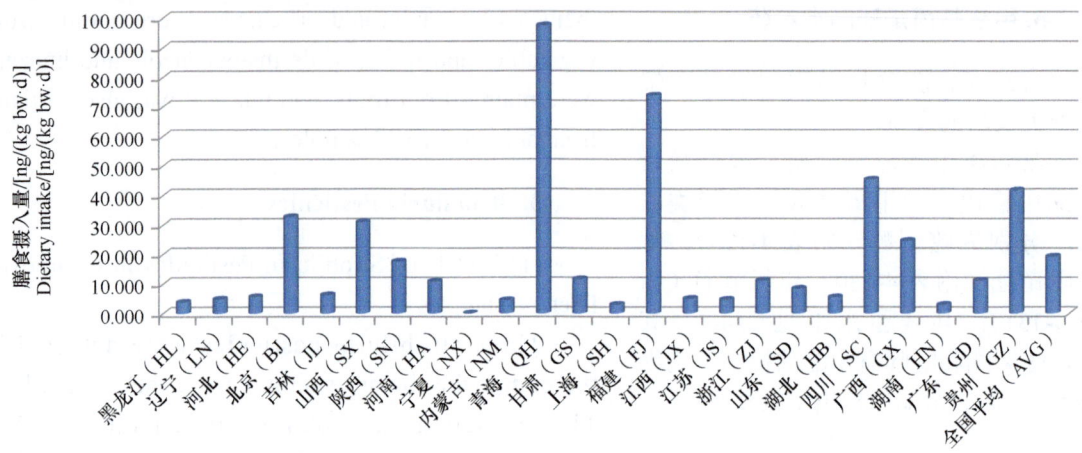

图 4-87　第六次中国总膳食研究的嘧菌酯膳食摄入量
Figure 4-87　Dietary intake of azoxystrobin from the 6$^{th}$ China TDS

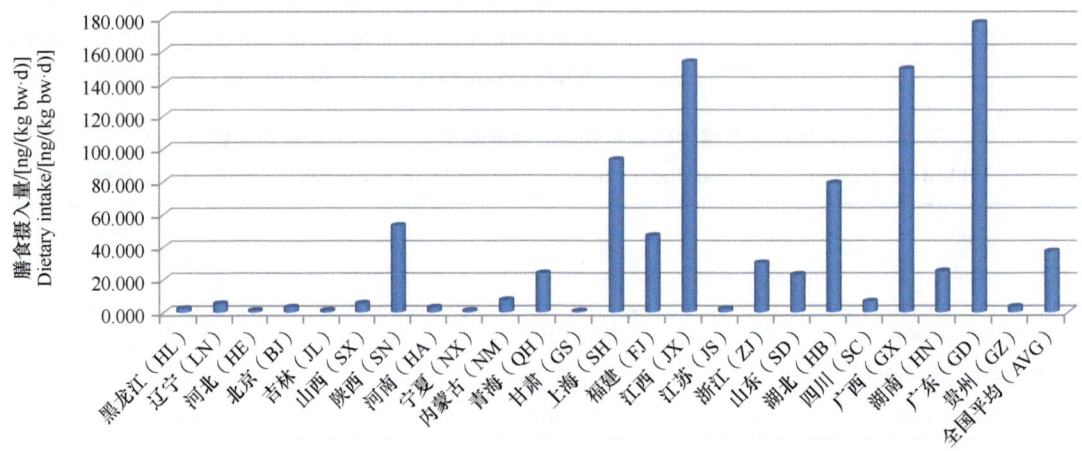

图 4-88　第六次中国总膳食研究的吡唑醚菌酯膳食摄入量
Figure 4-88　Dietary intake of pyraclostrobin from the 6$^{th}$ China TDS

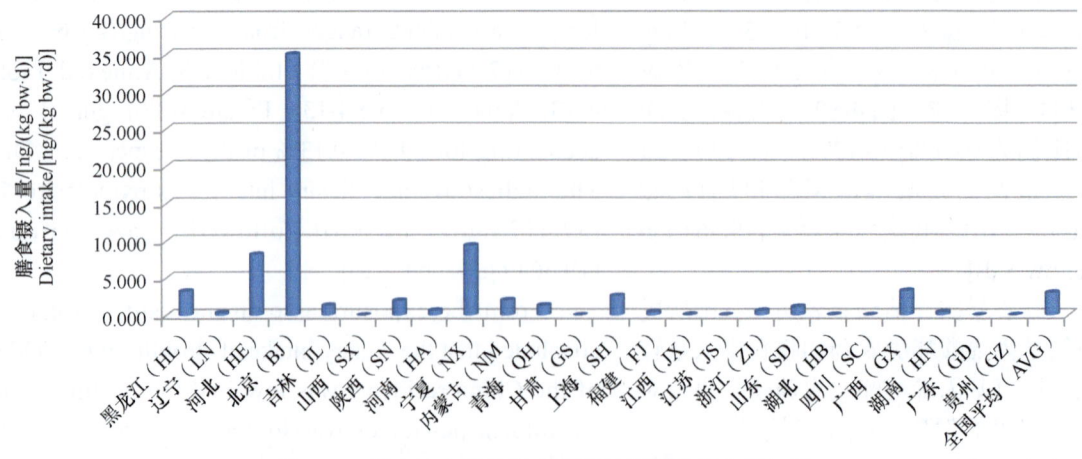

图 4-89　第六次中国总膳食研究的肟菌酯膳食摄入量
Figure 4-89　Dietary intake of trifloxystrobin from the 6$^{th}$ China TDS

（3）各类膳食对总膳食摄入的贡献

各类膳食对我国居民甲氧基丙烯酸酯类农药的膳食摄入的贡献情况见附表4-135～附表4-137和图4-90～图4-92。我国居民甲氧基丙烯酸酯类农药的膳食摄入主要来源于蔬菜类、水果类、谷类等膳食。

**4. 其他类杀菌剂**

（1）混合膳食样品中其他类杀菌剂的含量

第六次中国总膳食研究混合膳食样品中检出8种其他类杀菌剂，分别为甲霜灵（附表4-138）、环酰菌胺（附表4-139）、嘧霉胺（附表4-140）、乙

(3) Contributions of Food Categories to the Total Dietary Intake

The contribution of various diets to the dietary intake of strobilurin pesticides by China residents is shown in Annexed Table 4-135-Annexed Table 4-137 and Figure 4-90-Figure 4-92. The dietary intake of strobilurin pesticides for China residents was mainly from vegetables, fruits, cereals, and other meals.

**4. Other Fungicides**

(1) Levels of Other Fungicides in Composite Dietary Samples

Eight other fungicides were detected in the 6th CTDS composite samples, including metalaxyl (Annexed Table 4-138), fenhexamid (Annexed Table

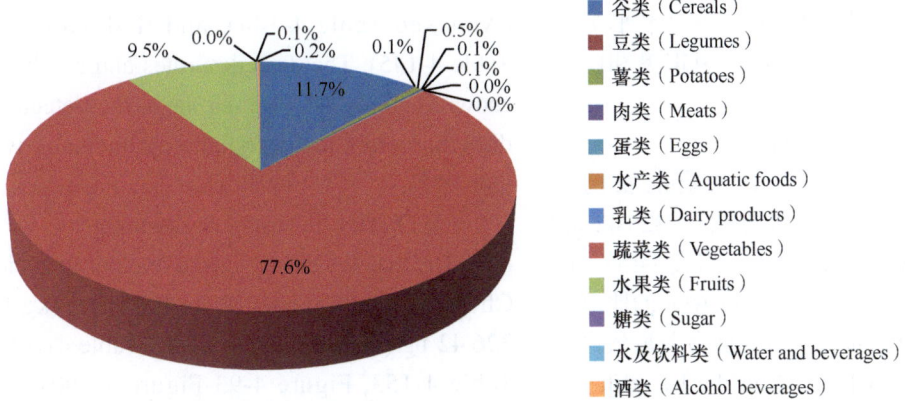

图4-90 第六次中国总膳食研究嘧菌酯的膳食来源

Figure 4-90 Dietary sources of azoxystrobin from the 6th China TDS

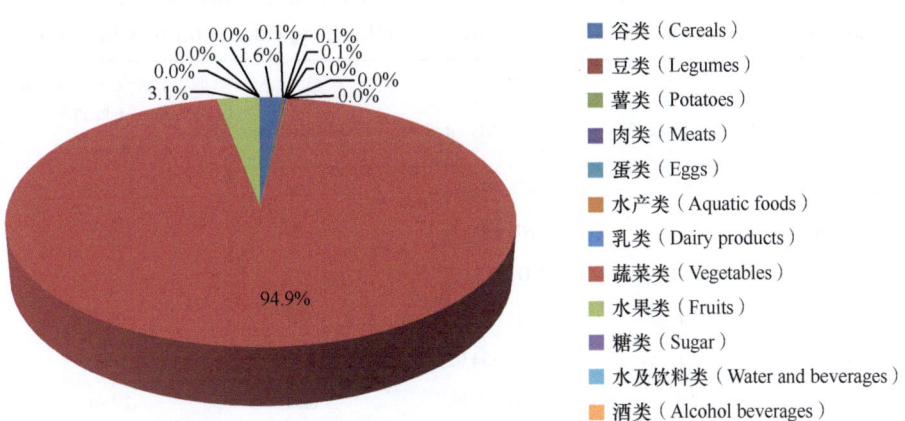

图4-91 第六次中国总膳食研究吡唑醚菌酯的膳食来源

Figure 4-91 Dietary sources of pyraclostrobin from the 6th China TDS

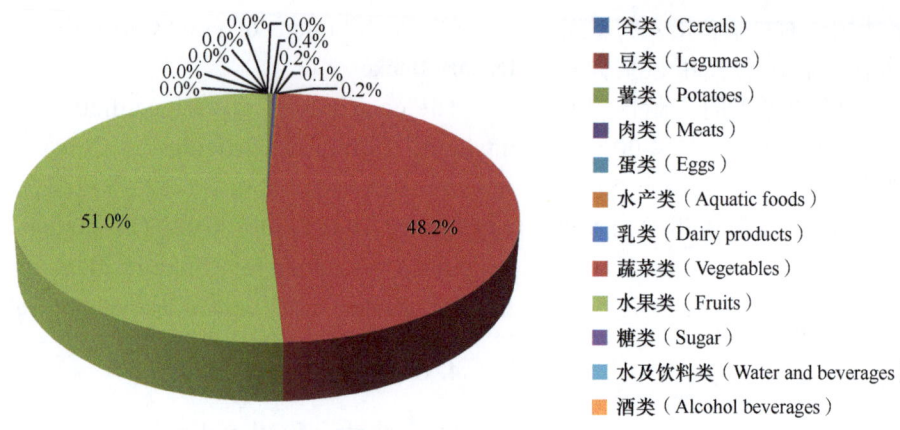

图 4-92 第六次中国总膳食研究肟菌酯的膳食来源
Figure 4-92 Dietary sources of trifloxystrobin from the 6th China TDS

嘧酚磺酸酯（附表 4-141）、嘧菌环胺（附表 4-142）、氟吡菌胺（附表 4-143）、烯酰吗啉（附表 4-144）和咯菌腈（附表 4-145），其检出率和残留水平见表 4-8。其中，烯酰吗啉、甲霜灵和嘧霉胺的检出率高于 10%。

（2）膳食暴露评估

我国居民其他类杀菌剂农药的平均膳食摄入量在 0.023～326.42 ng/(kg bw·d)（附表 4-146～附表 4-153，图 4-93～图 4-100），占各自 ADI 的比例在 0.00%～0.16%。平均膳食摄入量最高的是烯酰吗啉 [326.42 ng/(kg bw·d)]，其次为嘧霉胺 [33.043 ng/(kg bw·d)]。

4-139), pyrimethanil (Annexed Table 4-140), bupirimate (Annexed Table 4-141), cyprodinil (Annexed Table 4-142), fluopicolide (Annexed Table 4-143), dimethomorph (Annexed Table 4-144), and fludioxonil (Annexed Table 4-145). The detection rates and residue levels are shown in Table 4-8. Among them, the detection rates of dimethomorph, metalaxyl and pyrimethanil were higher than 10%.

(2) Dietary Exposure Assessment

The average dietary intake of other fungicides among China residents ranged from 0.023 ng/(kg bw·d) to 326.42 ng/(kg bw·d) (Annexed Table 4-146-Annexed Table 4-153, Figure 4-93-Figure 4-100), accounting for 0.00%-0.16% of their respective ADIs. The highest

表 4-8 第六次中国总膳食研究其他类杀菌剂的残留水平和膳食摄入量
Table 4-8 Residue levels and dietary intakes of other fungicides in the 6th China TDS

| 农药 Pesticides | 检出率 Detection rates/% | 残留水平 Residue levels/(μg/kg) | 平均水平 Mean/(μg/kg) | 平均膳食摄入量 Average dietary intakes/[ng/(kg bw·d)] | ADI/% |
|---|---|---|---|---|---|
| 甲霜灵 Metalaxyl | 21.2 | ND～25.50 | 0.36 | 19.979 | 0.03 |
| 环酰菌胺 Fenhexamid | 0.3 | ND～0.47 | 0.00 | 0.023 | 0.00 |
| 嘧霉胺 Pyrimethanil | 18.8 | ND～130.61 | 0.82 | 33.043 | 0.02 |
| 乙嘧酚磺酸酯 Bupirimate | 1.7 | ND～1.79 | 0.01 | 0.482 | 0.00 |
| 嘧菌环胺 Cyprodinil | 3.1 | ND～34.03 | 0.15 | 2.052 | 0.01 |
| 氟吡菌胺 Fluopicolide | 7.6 | ND～2.39 | 0.04 | 2.180 | 0.00 |
| 烯酰吗啉 Dimethomorph | 36.1 | ND～516.98 | 5.17 | 326.42 | 0.16 |
| 咯菌腈 Fludioxonil | 1.0 | ND～1.80 | 0.01 | 0.098 | 0.00 |

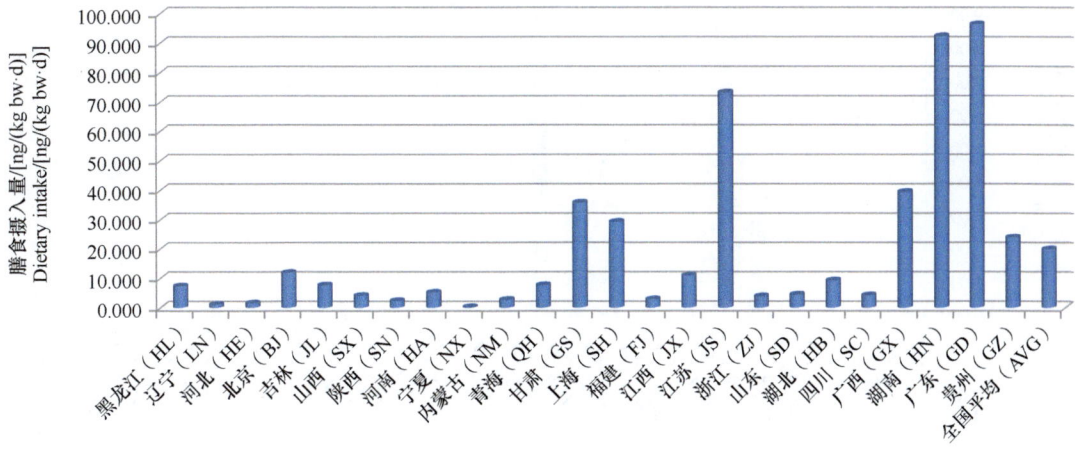

图 4-93　第六次中国总膳食研究的甲霜灵膳食摄入量
Figure 4-93　Dietary intake of metalaxyl from the 6th China TDS

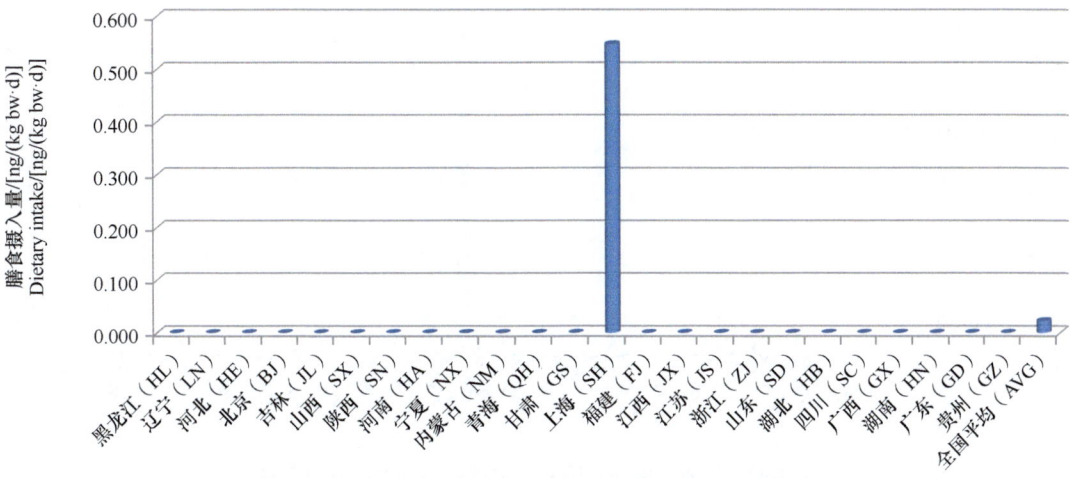

图 4-94　第六次中国总膳食研究的环酰菌胺膳食摄入量
Figure 4-94　Dietary intake of fenhexamid from the 6th China TDS

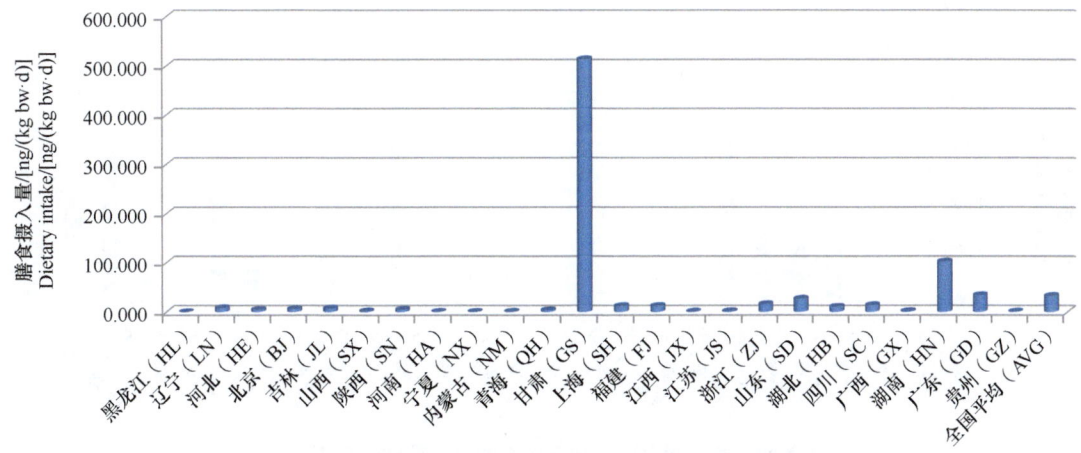

图 4-95　第六次中国总膳食研究的嘧霉胺膳食摄入量
Figure 4-95　Dietary intake of pyrimethanil from the 6th China TDS

第四章　农药残留的膳食暴露评估　183

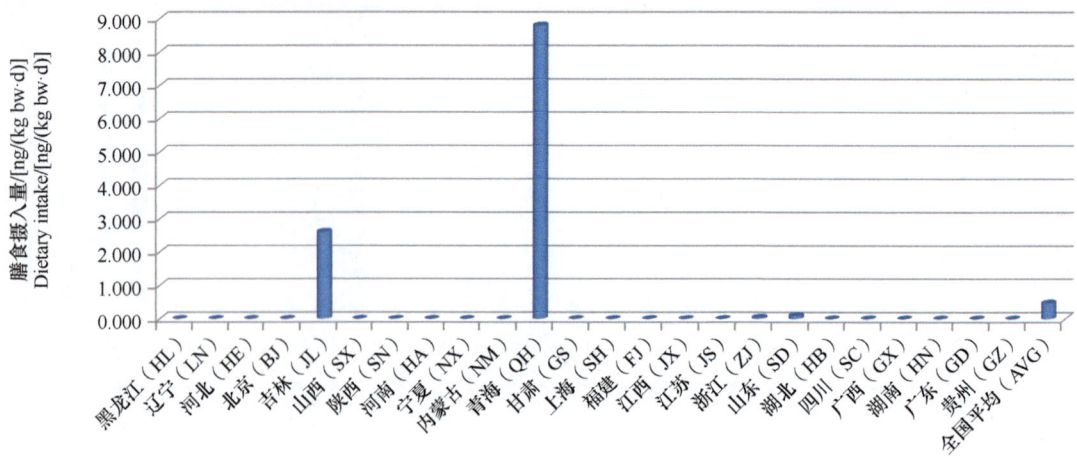

图 4-96 第六次中国总膳食研究的乙嘧酚磺酸酯膳食摄入量
Figure 4-96 Dietary intake of bupirimate from the 6<sup>th</sup> China TDS

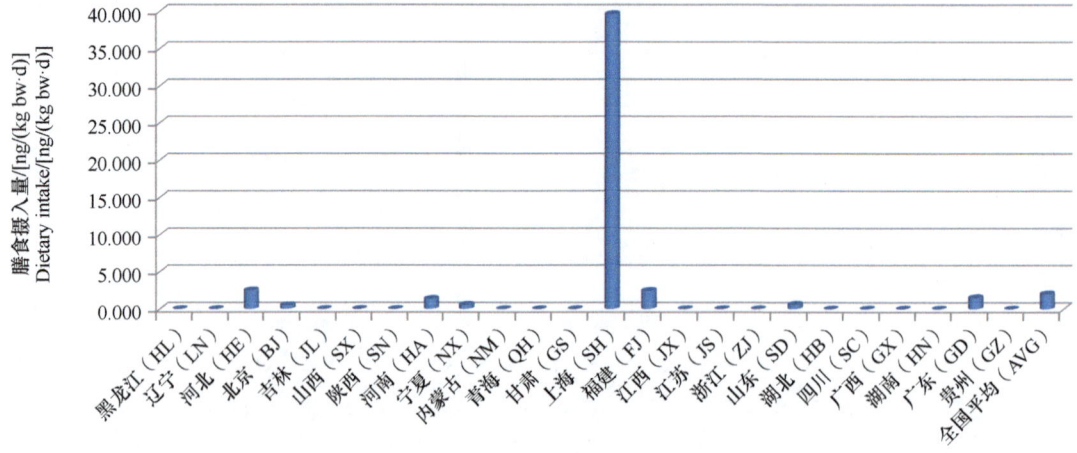

图 4-97 第六次中国总膳食研究的嘧菌环胺膳食摄入量
Figure 4-97 Dietary intake of cyprodinil from the 6<sup>th</sup> China TDS

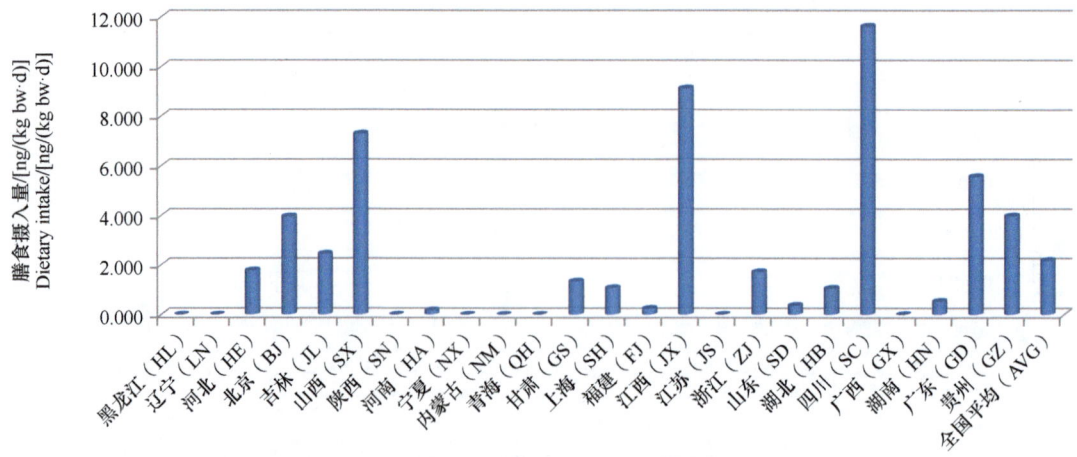

图 4-98 第六次中国总膳食研究的氟吡菌胺膳食摄入量
Figure 4-98 Dietary intake of fluopicolide from the 6<sup>th</sup> China TDS

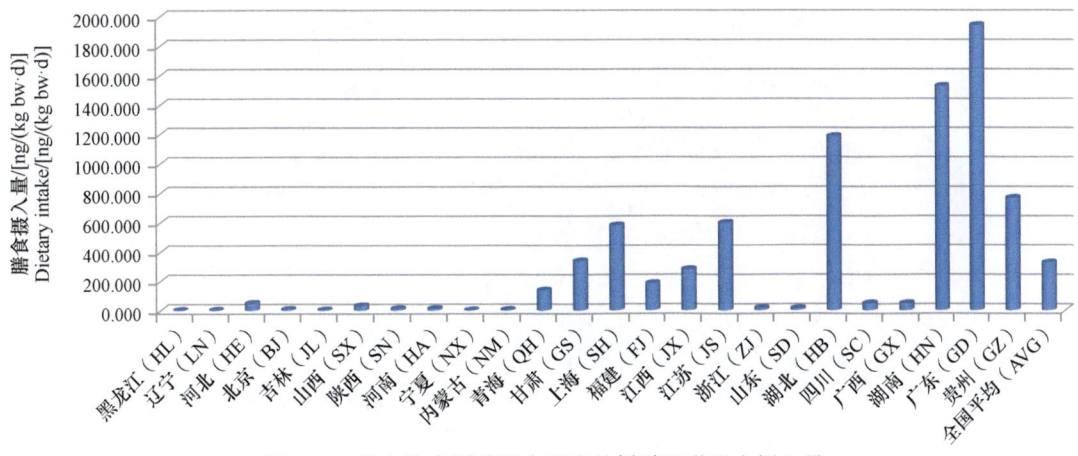

图 4-99　第六次中国总膳食研究的烯酰吗啉膳食摄入量
Figure 4-99　Dietary intake of dimethomorph from the 6th China TDS

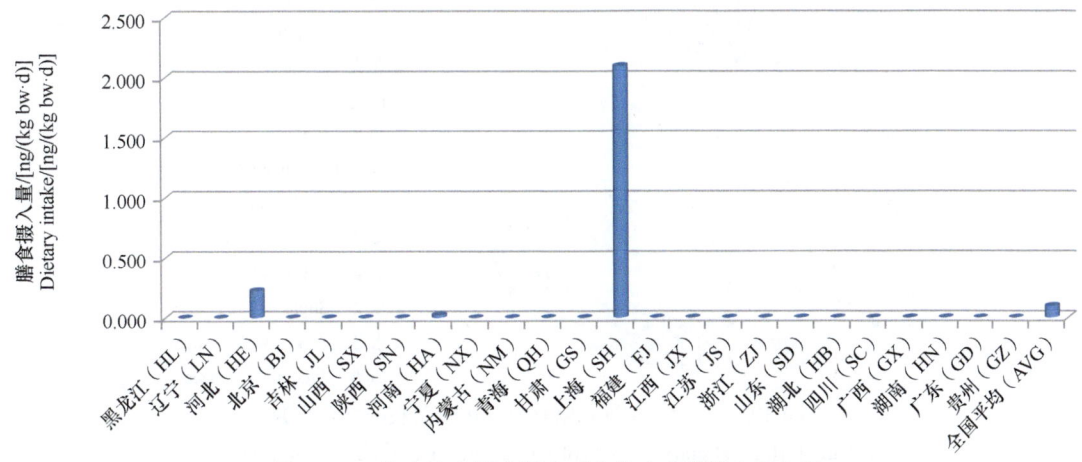

图 4-100　第六次中国总膳食研究的咯菌腈膳食摄入量
Figure 4-100　Dietary intake of fludioxonil from the 6th China TDS

膳食暴露评估结果表明，我国居民其他类杀菌剂农药的膳食摄入量较低，其他类杀菌剂农药膳食摄入对我国居民的健康风险在可接受水平内，健康风险较低。

（3）各类膳食对总膳食摄入的贡献

各类膳食对我国居民其他类杀菌剂的膳食摄入的贡献情况见附表4-154～附表4-161和图4-101～图4-108。我国居民其他类杀菌剂的膳食摄入主要来源于蔬菜类等膳食。

average dietary intake was dimethomorph [326.42 ng/(kg bw·d)], followed by pyrimethanil [33.043 ng/(kg bw·d)].

From the dietary exposure assessment results, it can be concluded that the dietary intake of other fungicides of the China residents was low, and the health risk to other fungicides was low and in the acceptable level.

(3) Contributions of Food Categories to the Total Dietary Intake

The contribution of various diets to the dietary intake of other fungicides by China residents is shown in Annexed Table 4-154-Table 4-161 and Figure 4-101-Figure 4-108. The dietary intake of other fungicides in China was mainly from vegetables and other meals.

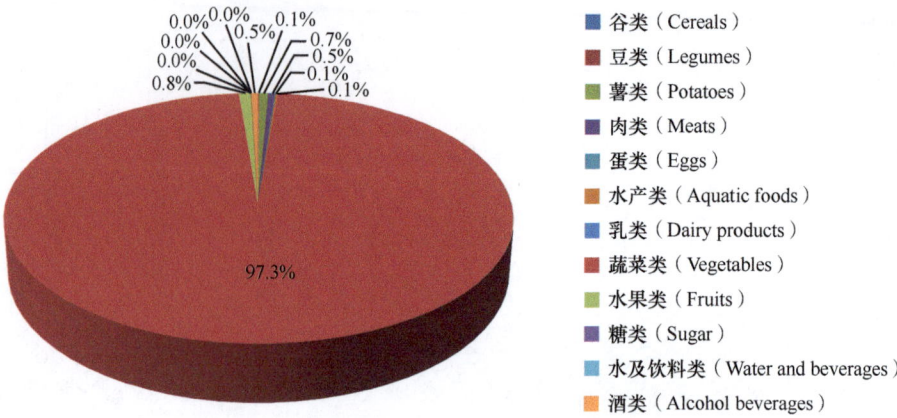

图 4-101　第六次中国总膳食研究甲霜灵的膳食来源
Figure 4-101　Dietary sources of metalaxyl from the 6th China TDS

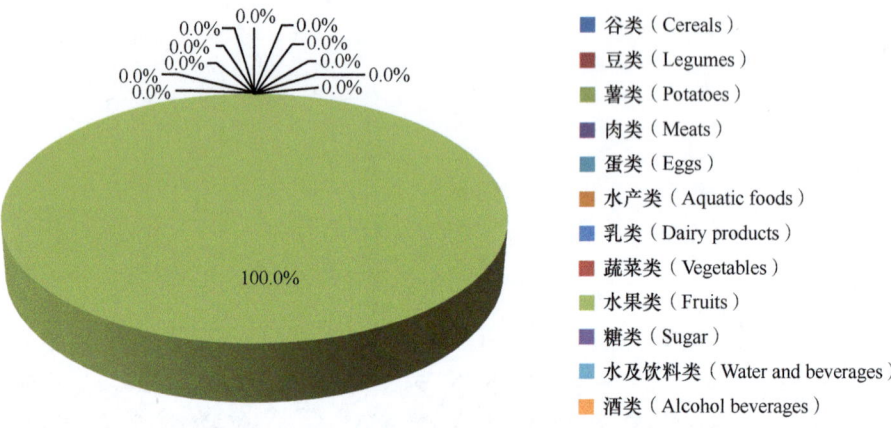

图 4-102　第六次中国总膳食研究环酰菌胺的膳食来源
Figure 4-102　Dietary sources of fenhexamid from the 6th China TDS

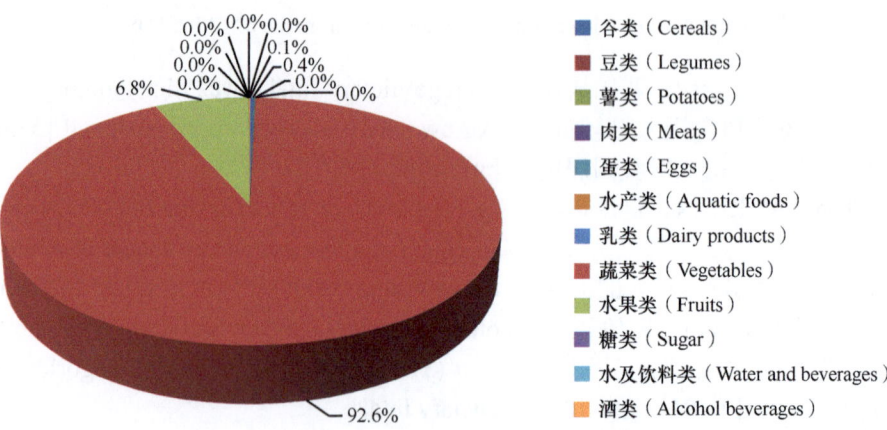

图 4-103　第六次中国总膳食研究嘧霉胺的膳食来源
Figure 4-103　Dietary sources of pyrimethanil from the 6th China TDS

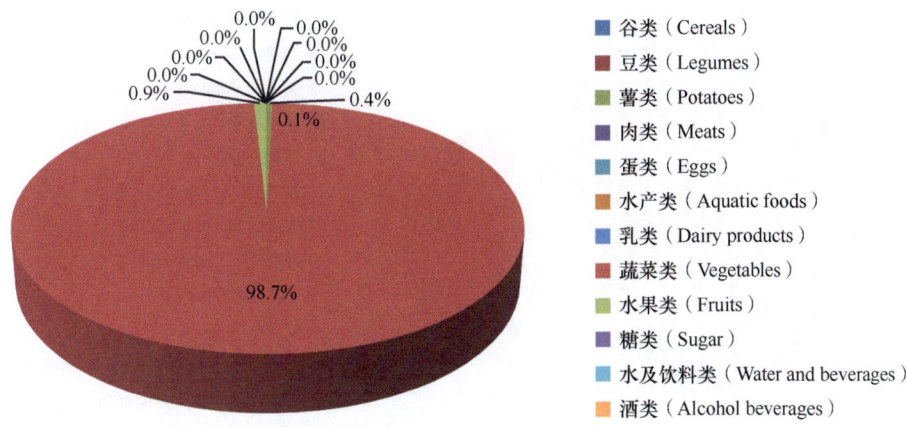

图 4-104　第六次中国总膳食研究乙嘧酚磺酸酯的膳食来源
Figure 4-104　Dietary sources of bupirimate from the 6$^{th}$ China TDS

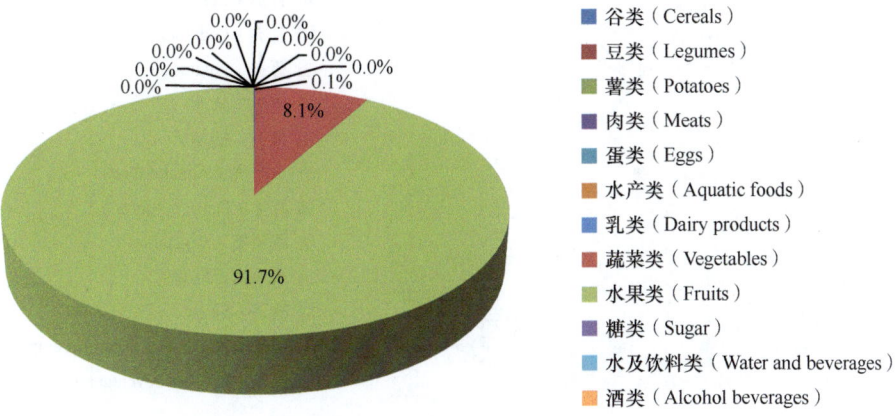

图 4-105　第六次中国总膳食研究嘧菌环胺的膳食来源
Figure 4-105　Dietary sources of cyprodinil from the 6$^{th}$ China TDS

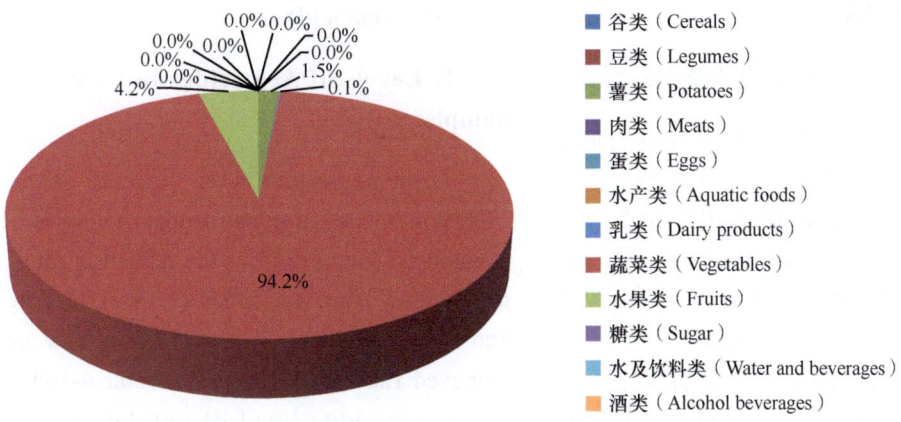

图 4-106　第六次中国总膳食研究氟吡菌胺的膳食来源
Figure 4-106　Dietary sources of fluopicolide from the 6$^{th}$ China TDS

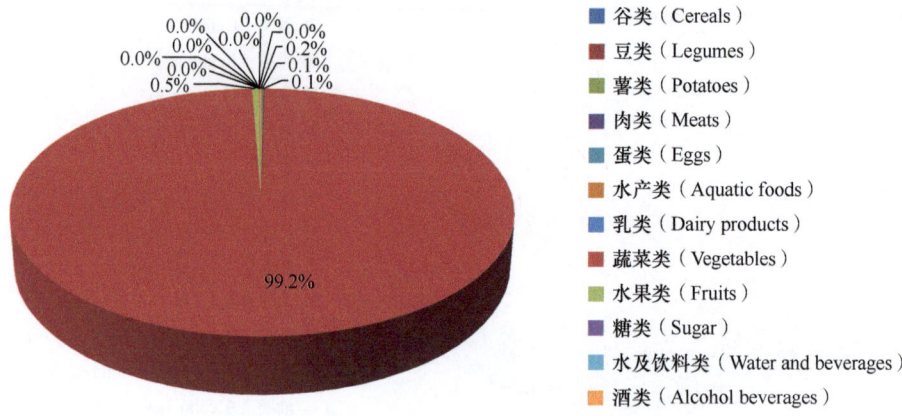

图 4-107　第六次中国总膳食研究烯酰吗啉的膳食来源
Figure 4-107　Dietary sources of dimethomorph from the 6$^{th}$ China TDS

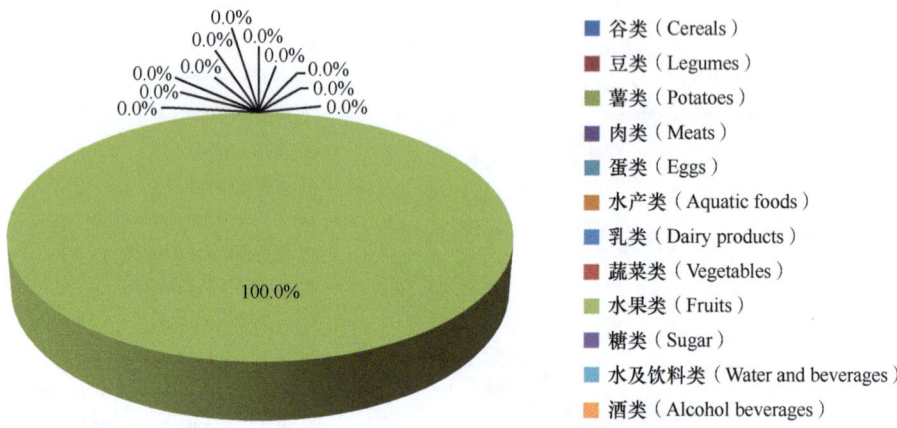

图 4-108　第六次中国总膳食研究咯菌腈的膳食来源
Figure 4-108　Dietary sources of fludioxonil from the 6$^{th}$ China TDS

（三）杀螨剂

**1. 混合膳食样品中杀螨剂的含量**

第六次中国总膳食研究混合膳食样品中检出 3 种杀螨剂（炔螨特、螺螨酯和哒螨灵），按检出率由高至低排列分别为哒螨灵（11.8%）、炔螨特（8.7%）和螺螨酯（6.3%），检测结果见附表 4-162～附表 4-164。

第六次中国总膳食研究膳食样品中哒螨灵的残留水平为 ND～60.42 μg/kg。哒螨灵在各类膳食样品中的检出主要集中于蔬菜类与水果类，肉类、薯类和水产类亦有部分检出。蔬

**(Ⅲ) Acaricides**

**1. Levels of Acaricides in Composite Dietary Samples**

Three acaricides were detected in the 6$^{th}$ China TDS composite samples (propargite, spirodiclofen and pyridaben). According to the detection rates from high to low, they were pyridaben (11.8%), propargite (8.7%) and spirodiclofen (6.3%), and the results are shown in Annexed Table 4-162-Annexed Table 4-164.

The residue level of pyridaben in the dietary samples of the sixth China TDS was ND-60.42 μg/kg. Pyridaben was mainly detected in vegetables and fruits, and some were also detected in meats, potatoes and

菜类的平均残留水平为 7.31 μg/kg，显著高于水果类（0.19 μg/kg）、薯类（0.02 μg/kg）、肉类（0.01 μg/kg）和水产类（0.01 μg/kg）的平均残留水平。

第六次中国总膳食研究膳食样品中炔螨特的残留水平为 ND～15.23 μg/kg。炔螨特在各类膳食样品中分布广泛，除豆类、蛋类、乳类、糖类、酒类和水及饮料类外均有检出。除水果类的平均残留水平（0.71 μg/kg）相对较高外，其他类别膳食样品的平均残留水平均较低。

第六次中国总膳食研究膳食样品中螺螨酯的残留水平为 ND～4.62 μg/kg。在蔬菜类和水果类膳食样品中检出螺螨酯，蔬菜类膳食中的平均残留水平（0.34 μg/kg）高于水果类膳食中的平均残留水平（0.16 μg/kg）。

**2. 膳食暴露评估**

我国居民第六次中国总膳食研究炔螨特的平均膳食摄入量为 1.620 ng/(kg bw·d)，是炔螨特 ADI 的 0.02%；螺螨酯为 2.249 ng/(kg bw·d)，是螺螨酯 ADI 的 0.02%；哒螨灵为 48.313 ng/(kg bw·d)，是哒螨灵 ADI 的 0.48%。哒螨灵、炔螨特和螺螨酯的平均膳食摄入量结果分别见附表 4-165～附表 4-167 和图 4-109～图 4-111。

膳食暴露评估结果表明，我国居民杀螨剂的膳食摄入量较低，杀螨剂膳食摄入对我国居民的健康风险在可接受水平内，健康风险较低。

**3. 各类膳食对总膳食摄入的贡献**

各类膳食对我国居民杀螨剂的膳食摄入的贡献情况见附表 4-168～附表 4-170 和图 4-112～图 4-114。我国居民哒螨灵的膳食摄入的 99.5% 来源于蔬菜类，0.4% 来源于水果类；螺螨酯的膳食摄入的 94.5% 来源于蔬菜类，5.5%

aquatic products. The average residue level of vegetables was 7.31 μg/kg, which was significantly higher than that of fruits (0.19 μg/kg), potatoes (0.02 μg/kg), meats (0.01 μg/kg), and aquatic products (0.01 μg/kg).

The residue level of propargite in the dietary samples of the sixth China TDS was between ND and 15.23 μg/kg. Propargite was widely distributed in all kinds of dietary samples, except legumes, eggs, dairy products, sugar, alcohol beverages, water and beverages. Except that the average residue level of fruits was relatively high (0.71 μg/kg), the average residue level of other dietary samples was low.

The residue level of spirodiclofen in the dietary samples of the sixth China TDS was ND-4.62 μg/kg. Spirodiclofen was detected in vegetables and fruits. The average residue level in vegetables (0.34 μg/kg) was higher than that in fruits (0.16 μg/kg).

**2. Dietary Exposure Assessment**

The average dietary intake of propargite in the 6th China TDS of China residents was 1.620 ng/(kg bw·d), accounting for 0.02% of the ADI. The average dietary intake of spirodiclofen was 2.249 ng/(kg bw·d), accounting for 0.02% of the ADI. The average dietary intake of pyridaben was 48.313 ng/(kg bw·d), accounting for 0.48% of the ADI. The average dietary intake results of pyridaben, propargite and spirodiclofen are shown in Annexed Table 4-165-Annexed Table 4-167 and Figure 4-109-Figure 4-111, respectively.

From the dietary exposure assessment results, it can be concluded that the dietary intake of acaricides of the China residents was low, and the health risk to acaricides was low and in the acceptable level.

**3. Contributions of Food Categories to the Total Dietary Intake**

The contribution of various diets to the dietary intake of acaricides by China residents is shown in Annexed Table 4-168-Annexed Table 4-170 and Figure 4-112-Figure 4-114. 99.5% of the dietary intake of pyridaben for China residents was from vegetables

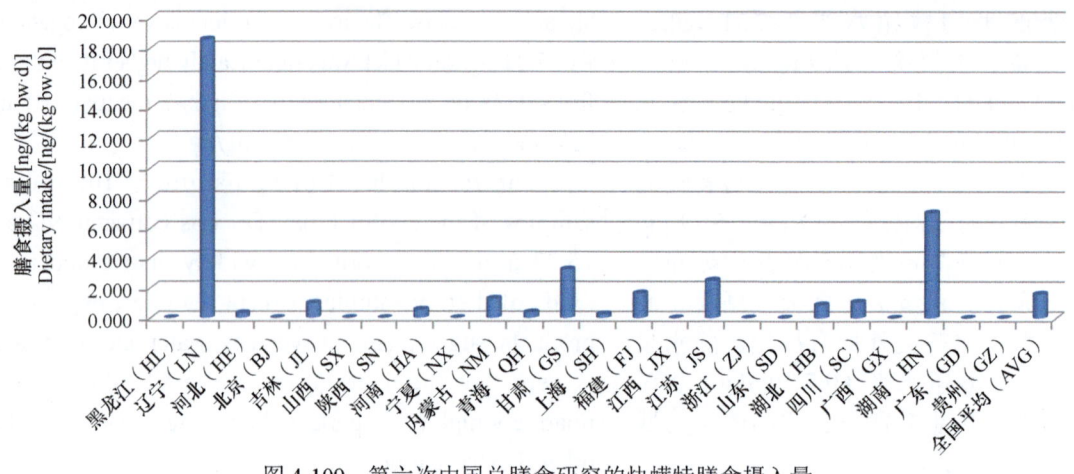

图 4-109　第六次中国总膳食研究的炔螨特膳食摄入量
Figure 4-109　Dietary intake of propargite from the 6th China TDS

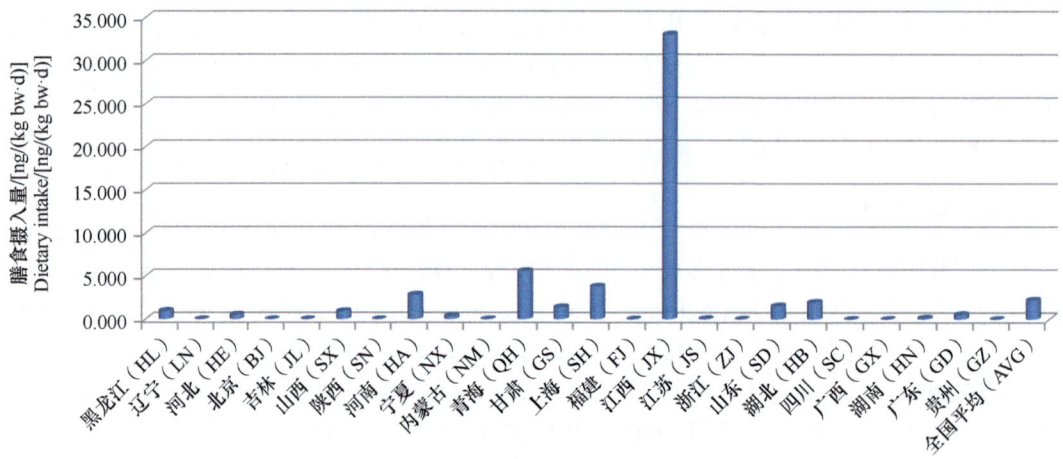

图 4-110　第六次中国总膳食研究的螺螨酯膳食摄入量
Figure 4-110　Dietary intake of spirodiclofen from the 6th China TDS

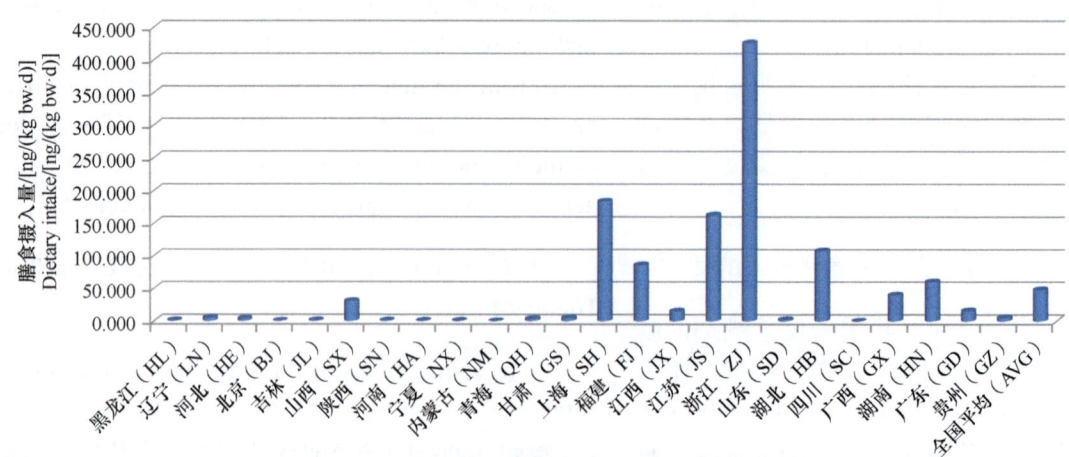

图 4-111　第六次中国总膳食研究的哒螨灵膳食摄入量
Figure 4-111　Dietary intake of pyridaben from the 6th China TDS

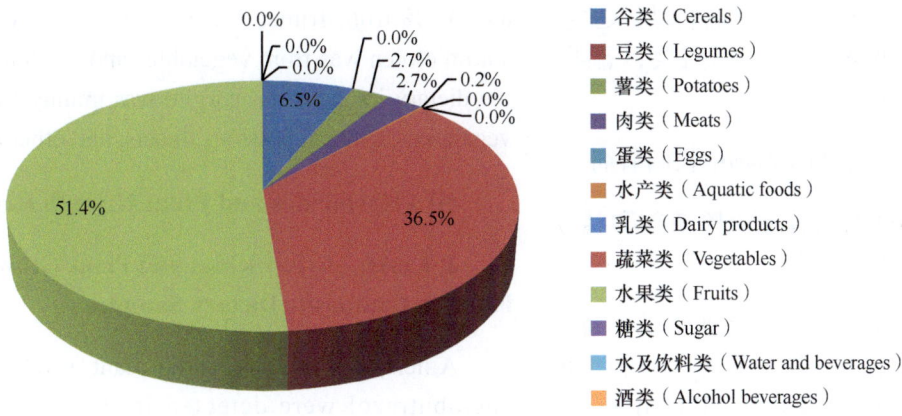

图 4-112　第六次中国总膳食研究炔螨特的膳食来源

Figure 4-112　Dietary sources of propargite from the 6th China TDS

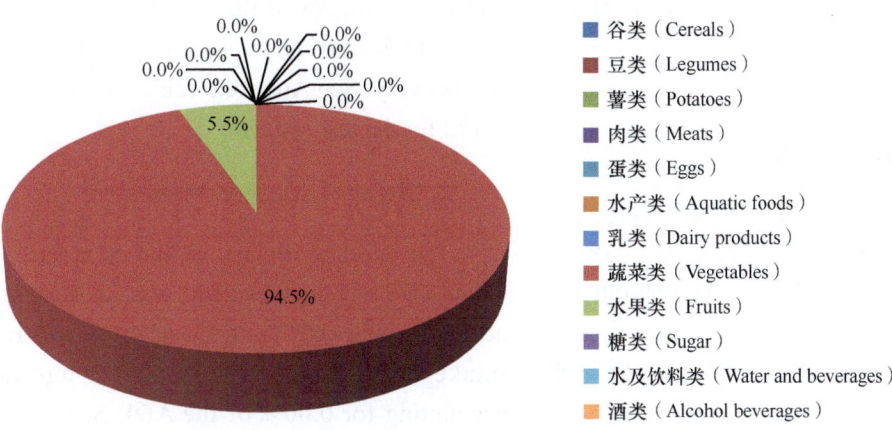

图 4-113　第六次中国总膳食研究螺螨酯的膳食来源

Figure 4-113　Dietary sources of spirodiclofen from the 6th China TDS

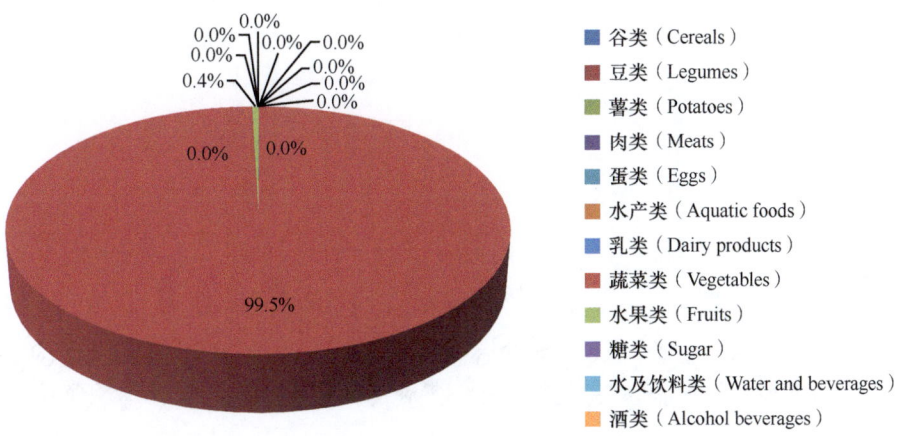

图 4-114　第六次中国总膳食研究哒螨灵的膳食来源

Figure 4-114　Dietary sources of pyridaben from the 6th China TDS

第四章　农药残留的膳食暴露评估

来源于水果类；炔螨特的膳食摄入主要来源于水果类、蔬菜类、谷类、薯类、肉类等膳食。

### （四）除草剂和植物生长调节剂

**1. 混合膳食样品中除草剂和植物生长调节剂的含量**

第六次中国总膳食研究混合膳食样品中检出 1 种除草剂莠去津和 1 种植物生长调节剂多效唑，其检出率分别为 20.1% 和 3.8%。第六次中国总膳食研究膳食样品中莠去津和多效唑的残留水平分别为 ND～1.12 μg/kg 和 ND～2.70 μg/kg，检测结果见附表 4-171～附表 4-172。

**2. 膳食暴露评估**

我国居民第六次中国总膳食研究莠去津的平均膳食摄入量为 1.638 ng/(kg bw·d)，是莠去津 ADI 的 0.01%；多效唑为 0.273 ng/(kg bw·d)，是多效唑 ADI 的 0.00%，详细结果分别见附表 4-173～附表 4-174 和图 4-115～图 4-116。

and 0.4% from fruits; 94.5% of the dietary intake of spirodiclofen was from vegetables and 5.5% from fruits; the dietary intake of propargite was mainly from fruits, vegetables, cereals, potatoes, meats, and other meals.

### (IV) Herbicides and Plant Growth Regulators

**1. Levels of Herbicides and Plant Growth Regulators in Composite Dietary Samples**

A herbicide atrazine and a plant growth regulator paclobutrazol were detected in the 6th China TDS composite samples, and the detection rates were 20.1% and 3.8%, respectively. The residue levels of atrazine and paclobutrazol in the dietary samples of the sixth China TDS were ND-1.12 μg/kg and ND-2.70 μg/kg, respectively. See Annexed Table 4-171-Annexed Table 4-172 for the test results.

**2. Dietary Exposure Assessment**

The average dietary intake of atrazine in the 6th China TDS of China residents was 1.638 ng/(kg bw·d), accounting for 0.01% of the ADI. The average dietary intake of paclobutrazol was 0.273 ng/(kg bw·d), accounting for 0.00% of the ADI. See Annexed Table 4-173-Annexed Table 4-174 and Figure 4-115-Figure 4-116 for detailed results.

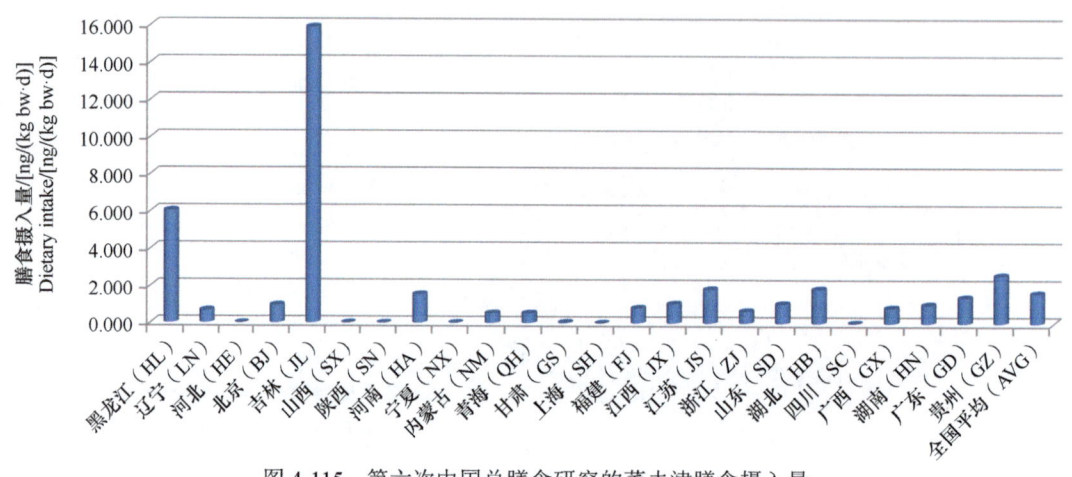

图 4-115 第六次中国总膳食研究的莠去津膳食摄入量
Figure 4-115　Dietary intake of atrazine from the 6th China TDS

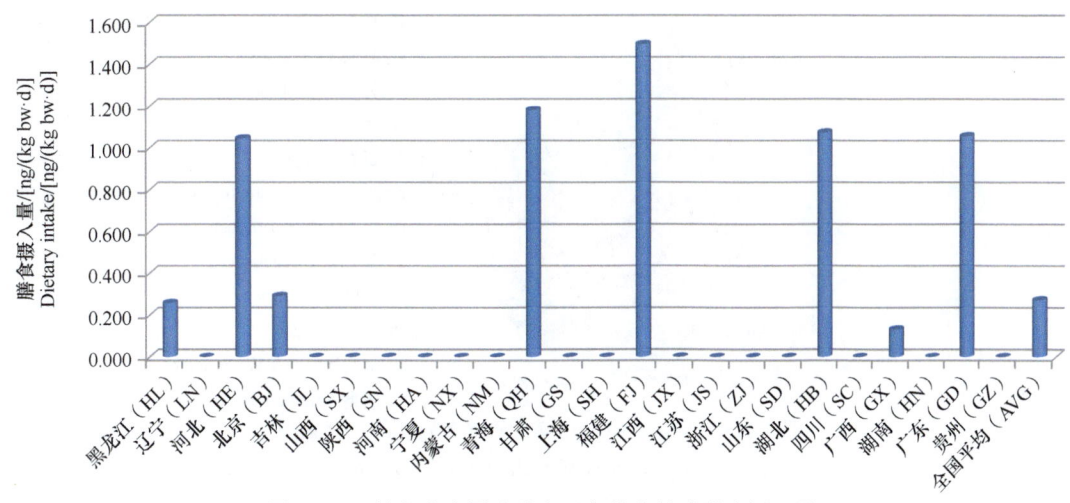

图 4-116　第六次中国总膳食研究的多效唑膳食摄入量
Figure 4-116　Dietary intake of paclobutrazol from the 6<sup>th</sup> China TDS

膳食暴露评估结果表明，我国居民除草剂和植物生长调节剂的膳食摄入量较低，除草剂和植物生长调节剂膳食摄入对我国居民的健康风险在可接受水平内，健康风险较低。

**3. 各类膳食对总膳食摄入的贡献**

各类膳食对我国居民除草剂和植物生长调节剂的膳食摄入的贡献情况见附表 4-175～附表 4-176 和图 4-117～图 4-118。我国居民莠去津的膳食摄入的 41.8% 来源于蔬菜类，27.3% 来源于水及饮料类；多效唑的膳食摄入主要来源

From the dietary exposure assessment results, it can be concluded that the dietary intake of herbicides and plant growth regulators of the China residents was low, and the health risk to herbicides and plant growth regulators was low and in the acceptable level.

**3. Contributions of Food Categories to the Total Dietary Intake**

The contribution of various diets to the dietary intake of herbicides and plant growth regulators for China residents is shown in Annexed Table 4-175-Annexed Table 4-176 and Figure 4-117-Figure 4-118. 41.8% of the dietary intake of atrazine for China

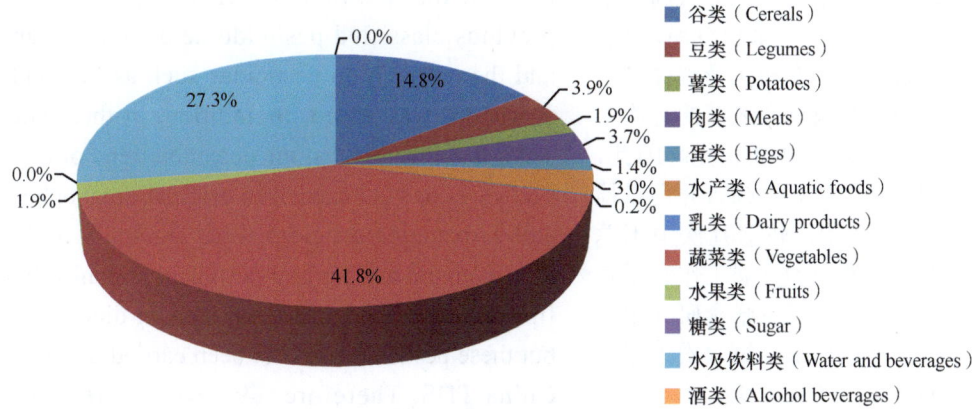

图 4-117　第六次中国总膳食研究莠去津的膳食来源
Figure 4-117　Dietary sources of atrazine from the 6<sup>th</sup> China TDS

第四章　农药残留的膳食暴露评估　193

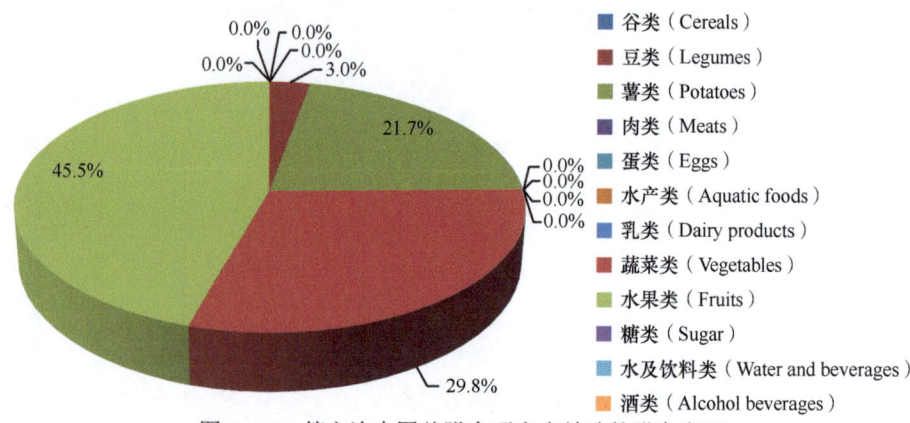

图 4-118　第六次中国总膳食研究多效唑的膳食来源

Figure 4-118　Dietary sources of paclobutrazol from the 6<sup>th</sup> China TDS

于水果类、蔬菜类、薯类等膳食。

## 四、以往中国总膳食研究结果的比较

第四次和第五次中国总膳食研究对农药的研究主要集中于杀虫剂，且采取的方式是以农药类别进行的，如有机氯类、有机磷类、菊酯类和氨基甲酸酯类等农药。第六次中国总膳食研究对农药残留的研究首次采用了非靶向筛查技术结合精准靶向定量分析方法，与以前开展的分类别农药检测分析有所不同，并新增了杀菌剂和杀螨剂等农药的研究。此外，第六次中国总膳食研究发现杀虫剂类农药的检出趋势有所改变，原先的有机磷类和氨基甲酸酯类农药逐渐被新烟碱类和氟虫腈类杀虫剂所取代，新烟碱类和氟虫腈类农药在膳食样品中普遍存在，而这些农药在之前的几次中国总膳食研究中均未开展研究。因此，第六次中国总膳食研究共筛查并定量检出了 59 种农药残留，较前几次中国总膳食研究对农药残留的开展工作有了较大的进步。前两次中国总膳食研究中开展的农药类别检出情况与第六次中国总膳食研究的结果比较见表 4-9。

residents was from vegetables and 27.3% from water and beverages. The dietary intake of paclobutrazol was mainly from fruits, vegetables, potatoes, and other meals.

## IV. Comparison with Previous China TDSs Results

The research on pesticides in the fourth and fifth China TDS mainly focused on insecticides, and the methods adopted were carried out according to the types of pesticides, such as organochlorines, organophosphorus, pyrethroids, carbamates and other pesticides. In the sixth China TDS on pesticide residues, the non-targeted screening technique combined with accurate targeted quantitative analysis methods were used for the first time, which was different from the previous classified pesticide detection and analysis, and the research on pesticides such as fungicides and acaricides was added. In addition, in the sixth China TDS, it was found that the detection trend of insecticide pesticides had changed. The original organophosphorus and carbamate pesticides were gradually replaced by neonicotinoid and fipronil pesticides. Neonicotinoid and fipronil pesticides were common in dietary samples, but these pesticides had not been carried out in previous China TDS. Therefore, 59 pesticide residues were screened and quantitatively detected in the sixth China

TDS, which has made great progress compared with the previous work on pesticide residues in China TDS. See Table 4-9 for the comparison between the detection of pesticide categories carried out in the previous two CTDS and the results of the sixth CTDS.

表 4-9 三次中国总膳食研究农药膳食摄入情况比较

Table 4-9 Pesticide dietary intakes from 4$^{th}$, 5$^{th}$ and 6$^{th}$ China TDSs

| 农药 Pesticides | 膳食摄入 Dietary intake/[ng/(kg bw·d)] | | |
|---|---|---|---|
| | 第四次中国总膳食研究 4$^{th}$ CTDS | 第五次中国总膳食研究 5$^{th}$ CTDS | 第六次中国总膳食研究 6$^{th}$ CTDS |
| 有机磷类 Organophosphorus | 0～226 | 0～3.97 | 0～47.99 |
| 菊酯类 Pyrethroids | 0～160 | 0～41.1 | — |
| 三嗪类 Triazines | 0～88.3 | 0～843 | 0～3.923 |
| 氨基甲酸酯类 Carbamates | 0～341 | * | 0～19.52 |

注："—"表示未检测;"*"表示未检出

Note: "—" means not analysis; "*" means not detectable

# 第五章 兽药残留的膳食暴露评估
# Chapter 5　Dietary Exposure Assessment of Veterinary Drug Residues

## 一、背景

兽药在防治动物疾病、提高养殖效益、促进养殖业发展和提高人们生活水平方面发挥了重要作用。兽药残留是指动物在应用兽药或饲料添加剂后，在动物的细胞、组织、器官或可食性产品中蓄积或贮存的原型药物及代谢物。

动物源性食品中的兽药残留不仅对人类健康构成威胁，还会对环境造成日益严重的危害，主要表现为人体直接中毒、过敏反应、细菌耐药性、致畸、致突变和致癌等。在动物源性食品中较容易引起残留超标的兽药主要有抗生素类、磺胺类、呋喃类、抗寄生虫类和激素类药物等。

美国、欧盟、澳大利亚、加拿大、日本等国家和地区对食品中的兽药残留均有最大残留限量规定。在我国，《食品安全国家标准 食品中兽药最大残留限量》（GB 31650—2019）明确规定最大残留限量（MRL）的兽药有104种，允许用于食品动物但不需要制定残留限量的兽药有154种，不再收载禁止药物及化合物清单；允许治疗使用但不得在食品中检出的镇静剂、抗生素与激素等共9种。

由于兽药是在食用动物养殖及运输过程中使用的，一般只在动物源性食品中残留，因此，仅对中国总膳食研究混合样品中的肉类、蛋类、水产类和乳类4类膳食共96份混合膳食样品进行了兽药残留的检测及膳食暴露评估。在进行污染水平评价和膳食暴露评估

## Ⅰ. Background

Veterinary drugs have played an important role in preventing and treating animal diseases, improving breeding efficiency, promoting the development of the breeding industry, and improving people's living standards. Veterinary drug residues refer to the prototype drugs and metabolites accumulated or stored in the cells, tissues, organs or edible products of animals after the application of veterinary drugs or feed additives.

Veterinary drug residues in animal-derived foods not only pose a threat to human health, but also cause more and more serious harm to the environment, mainly manifested as direct human poisoning, allergic reactions, bacterial resistance, teratogenicity, mutagenicity, and carcinogenicity, etc. The veterinary drugs that are more likely to cause excessive residues in animal-derived foods include mainly antibiotics, sulfonamides, furans, antiparasitic drugs, and hormone drugs.

The United States, the European Union, Australia, Canada, Japan, and other countries and regions have regulations on maximum residue limits for veterinary drug residues in foods. In China, *National Food Safety Standard-Maximum Residue Limits for Veterinary Drugs in Foods* (GB 31650—2019) clearly stipulates that there are 104 veterinary drugs with MRLs, and 154 veterinary drugs that are allowed to be used in food animals but do not require residue limits, and no longer contain the list of prohibited drugs and compounds. A total of 9 kinds of sedatives, antibiotics, and hormones are allowed for therapeutic use but not detected in foods.

Since veterinary drugs are used in the breeding and transportation of edible animals, they generally only remain in animal-derived foods. Therefore, only the

时，膳食样品中未检出的兽药的含量均以 0 计。

## 二、健康指导值

《食品安全国家标准 食品中兽药最大残留限量》（GB 31650—2019）规定了各类兽药的每日允许摄入量（ADI），本章列出第六次中国总膳食研究样品中检出的兽药的 ADI 值，见表 5-1。

four types of diets of meats, eggs, aquatic foods, and dairy products in the composite samples of the China total diet study were collected. A total of 96 composite dietary samples were tested for veterinary drug residues and dietary exposure assessment. During the evaluation of contamination level and dietary exposure, the content of undetected veterinary drugs in dietary samples was treated as 0.

## II. HBGV

The ADI values for various veterinary drugs were provided by the *National Food Safety Standard-Maximum Residue Limits for Veterinary Drugs in Foods* (GB 31650—2019). This chapter lists the ADI values of veterinary drugs detected in the sixth China total diet study samples, see Table 5-1.

表 5-1　第六次中国总膳食研究样品中检出的兽药清单及其 ADI
Table 5-1　The veterinary drug lists detected in 6th CTDS and their respective ADIs

| 兽药类别 Category | 兽药名称 Veterinary drugs name | | ADI/[μg/(kg bw·d)] |
|---|---|---|---|
| 抗菌增效剂 Antibacterial synergist | 甲氧苄啶 | Trimethoprim | 4.2 |
| 喹诺酮类 Quinolones | 麻保沙星 | Marbofloxacin | — |
| | 氧氟沙星 | Ofloxacin | — |
| | 培氟沙星 | Pefloxacin | — |
| | 诺氟沙星 | Norfloxacin | — |
| | 恩诺沙星（恩诺沙星和环丙沙星之和） | Enrofloxacin (Sum of enrofloxacin and ciprofloxacin) | 6.2 |
| | 达氟沙星 | Danofloxacin | 20 |
| | 洛美沙星 | Lomefloxacin | — |
| | 奥比沙星 | Orbifloxacin | — |
| | 沙拉沙星 | Sarafloxacin | 0.3 |
| | 氟甲喹 | Flumequine | 30 |
| 磺胺类 Sulfonamides | 磺胺二甲嘧啶 | Sulfadimidine | 50 |
| | 总磺胺类 | Total sulfonamides | 50 |
| 三苯甲烷类 Triphenylmethanes | 结晶紫 | Crystal violet | — |
| 咪唑类 Imidazoles | 左旋咪唑 | Levamisole | 6 |

续表

| 兽药类别 Category | 兽药名称 Veterinary drugs name | | ADI/[μg/(kg bw·d)] |
|---|---|---|---|
| 硝基咪唑类 Nitroimidazoles | 甲硝唑 | Metronidazole | — |
| | 羟基甲硝唑 | OH-Metronidazole | — |
| | 地美硝唑 | Dimetridazole | — |
| | 2-羟基地美硝唑 | 2-Hydroxy-dimetridazole | — |
| 苯并咪唑类 Benzimidazoles | 阿苯达唑（阿苯达唑亚砜、阿苯达唑砜、阿苯达唑-2-氨基砜和阿苯达唑之和） | Albendazole (Sum of albendazole sulfoxide, albendazole sulfone, albendazole 2-amino sulfone, and albendazole) | 50 |
| | 芬苯达唑/奥芬达唑（芬苯达唑、奥芬达唑和奥芬达唑砜之和） | Fenbendazole/oxfendazole (Sum of fenbendazole, oxfendazole, and oxfendazole sulfone) | 7 |
| | 氟苯达唑 | Flubendazole | 12 |
| | 甲苯达唑 | Mebendazole | 12.5 |
| 氯霉素类 Chloramphenicols | 氟苯尼考（氟苯尼考和氟苯尼考胺之和） | Florfenicol (Sum of florfenicol and florfenicol amine) | 3 |
| | 氯霉素 | Chloramphenicol | — |
| | 甲砜霉素 | Thiamphenicol | 5 |

注："—"表示该兽药暂未制定健康指导值
Note: "—" means HBGV of this veterinary drug has not established

## 三、总膳食研究结果

### （一）抗菌增效剂

#### 1. 混合膳食样品中甲氧苄啶的含量

第六次中国总膳食研究 96 份动物源性混合膳食样品中抗菌增效剂甲氧苄啶的检出率为 54.2%，最高残留水平来自山东省的蛋类样品（173.15 μg/kg，附表 5-1）。

#### 2. 膳食暴露评估

我国各地区居民动物源性膳食甲氧苄啶的膳食摄入量为 0～122.317 ng/(kg bw·d)，占 ADI 的百分比为 0%～2.91%，平均值为 8.611 ng/(kg bw·d)，占 ADI 的 0.205%（图 5-1 和附表 5-2）。我国居民动物源性膳食甲氧苄啶的膳食摄入量均很低，健康风险亦较低。

## III. TDS Results

### (I) Antibacterial Synergist

#### 1. Levels of Trimethoprim in Composite Dietary Samples

The detection rate of the antibacterial synergist trimethoprim in 96 composite samples of animal-derived dietary samples in the sixth China total diet study was 54.2%, and the highest residue level was from eggs samples from Shandong (173.15 μg/kg, Annexed Table 5-1).

#### 2. Dietary Exposure Assessment

The animal-derived dietary intake of China residents in various regions of China to trimethoprim ranged from 0 ng/(kg bw·d) to 122.317 ng/(kg bw·d), accounting for 0%-2.91% of the ADI, with an average value at 8.611 ng/(kg bw·d), accounting for 0.205% of the ADI (Figure 5-1 and Annexed Table 5-2). The trimethoprim from animal-derived dietary intake of China residents was quite low, as well as the health risk.

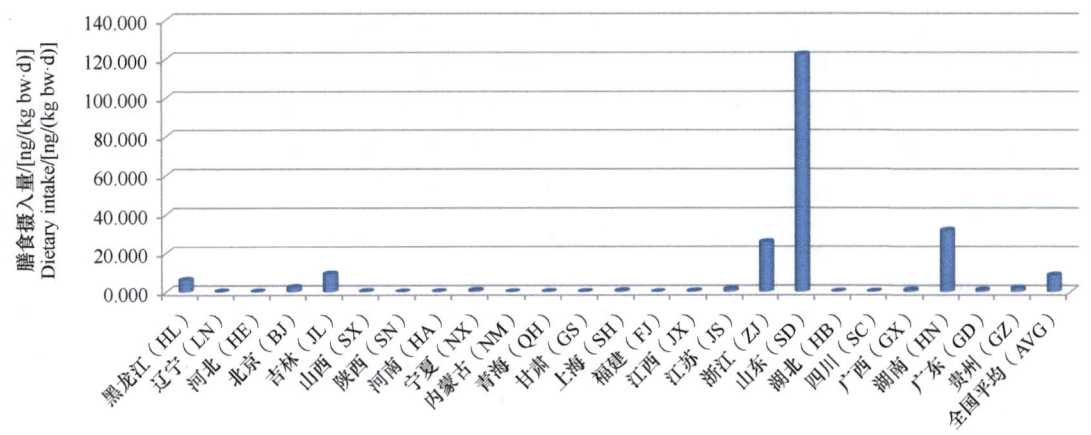

图 5-1 第六次中国总膳食研究的甲氧苄啶膳食摄入量

Figure 5-1　Dietary intake of trimethoprim from the 6th China TDS

## 3. 各类膳食对总膳食摄入的贡献

在肉类、水产类、蛋类和乳类混合膳食中，甲氧苄啶的膳食摄入贡献主要来自蛋类（66.8%）和肉类（32.8%）（图 5-2 和附表 5-3）。

## 3. Contributions of Food Categories to the Total Dietary Intake

Of the four categories of animal food composite samples, i.e. meats, aquatic foods, eggs, and dairy products, the dietary intake of trimethoprim was mainly contributed by eggs (66.8%) and meats (32.8%) (Figure 5-2 and Annexed Table 5-3).

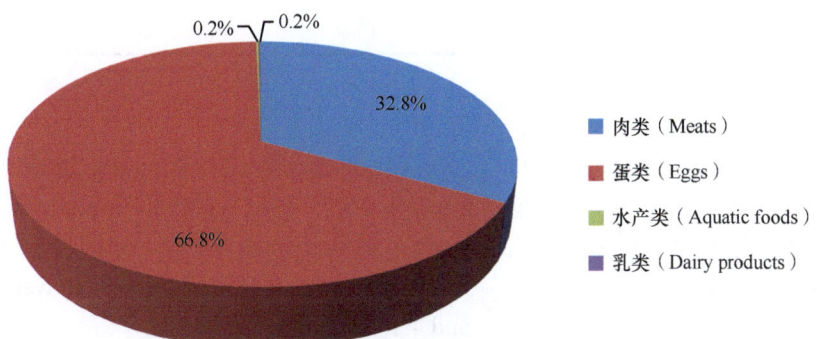

图 5-2 第六次中国总膳食研究甲氧苄啶的膳食来源

Figure 5-2　Dietary sources of trimethoprim from the 6th China TDS

## （二）喹诺酮类药物

### 1. 混合膳食样品中喹诺酮类药物的含量

我国动物源性膳食样品中检出的喹诺酮类药物包括麻保沙星、氧氟沙星、培氟沙星、诺氟沙星、恩诺沙星（以恩诺沙星和环丙沙星之和计）、达氟

## (Ⅱ) Quinolones

### 1. Levels of Quinolones in Composite Dietary Samples

The quinolones detected in animal-derived dietary samples in China included mabrofloxacin, ofloxacin, pefloxacin, norfloxacin, enrofloxacin (calculated as the sum of enrofloxacin and ciprofloxacin), danfloxacin,

沙星、洛美沙星、奥比沙星、沙拉沙星和氟甲喹，残留水平为 ND～475.10 μg/kg。其中，各个药物的检出率和残留水平结果见表 5-2 和附表 5-4～附表 5-31。

lomefloxacin, orbifloxacin, sarafloxacin, and flumequine, with a residue level ranging from ND-475.10 μg/kg. Among them, the detection rate and residue level of each drug are shown in Table 5-2 and Annexed Table 5-4-Annexed Table 5-31.

表 5-2　喹诺酮类药物的检出率、最大残留水平和膳食摄入量
Table 5-2　Detection rates, maximum residue levels, and dietary intakes of quinolones

| 喹诺酮<br>Quinolones | 检出率<br>Detection rates/% | 最大残留水平<br>Maximum residue levels/(μg/kg) | 膳食摄入量<br>Dietary intakes/[ng/(kg bw·d)] | ADI/% |
|---|---|---|---|---|
| 麻保沙星 mabrofloxacin | 4.2 | 0.38 | 0.011 | — |
| 氧氟沙星 ofloxacin | 20.8 | 4.10 | 0.545 | — |
| 培氟沙星 pefloxacin | 9.4 | 0.27 | 0.038 | — |
| 诺氟沙星 norfloxacin | 1.0 | 0.32 | 0.007 | — |
| 恩诺沙星（恩诺沙星和环丙沙星之和计）<br>enrofloxacin (calculated as the sum of enrofloxacin and ciprofloxacin) | 65.6 | 475 | 35.35 | 0.570 |
| 达氟沙星 danfloxacin | 2.1 | 0.13 | 0.001 | 0.000 |
| 洛美沙星 lomefloxacin | 2.1 | 0.05 | 0.001 | — |
| 奥比沙星 orbifloxacin | 1.0 | 2.43 | 0.029 | — |
| 沙拉沙星 sarafloxacin | 5.2 | 6.78 | 0.104 | — |
| 氟甲喹 flumequine | 6.3 | 0.06 | 0.003 | 0.000 |

注："—"表示该药物暂未制定健康指导值
Note: "—" means HBGV of this drug has not established

恩诺沙星和氧氟沙星的检出率与残留水平相对较高，其中，恩诺沙星和氧氟沙星残留水平最高的均是来自北京的肉类样品，分别为 475.10 μg/kg 和 4.10 μg/kg。

The detection rates and residue levels of enrofloxacin and ofloxacin were relatively high, among which, the highest residue levels of enrofloxacin and ofloxacin were from meats samples of Beijing, which were 475.10 μg/kg and 4.10 μg/kg, respectively.

**2. 喹诺酮类药物的膳食暴露评估**

我国各地区居民喹诺酮类药物的平均膳食摄入量为 0.001～35.35 ng/(kg bw·d)（表5-2）。其中，恩诺沙星的膳食摄入量为 0.195～507.9 ng/(kg bw·d)，占 ADI 的 0.003%～8.19%，平均摄入量为 35.35 ng/(kg bw·d)，占 ADI 的 0.570%（附表 5-17 和图 5-3），其他喹诺酮类药物的膳食摄入量及相关结果见附表 5-5～附表 5-32 和图 5-4～图 5-12。

**2. Dietary Exposure Assessment of Quinolones**

The average dietary intake of quinolones among residents of various regions in China ranged from 0.001 ng/(kg bw·d) to 35.35 ng/(kg bw·d) (Table 5-2). Of the total intakes of quinolones, the dietary intake of enrofloxacin ranged from 0.195 ng/(kg bw·d) to 507.9 ng/(kg bw·d), accounting for 0.003%-8.19% of the ADI, with an average value of 35.35 ng/(kg bw·d), accounting for 0.570% of the ADI (Annexed Table 5-17 and Figure 5-3). The dietary intake of other quinolone

我国居民动物源性膳食恩诺沙星、达氟沙星和氟甲喹的暴露量均很低,健康风险亦较低。

**3. 各类膳食对总膳食摄入的贡献**

恩诺沙星的膳食摄入贡献来自肉类(88.1%)、蛋类(0.9%)和水产类(11.0%)(图5-13和附表5-18);氧氟沙星的膳食摄入贡献来自肉类(62.9%)、蛋类(7.7%)和乳类(29.4%)(图5-14和附表5-9);培氟沙星的膳食摄入贡献来自肉类(86.2%)、蛋类(10.5%)和乳类(3.4%)(图5-15和附表5-12);洛美

drugs and related results are shown in Annexed Table 5-5-Annexed Table 5-32 and Figure 5-4-Figure 5-12. The exposure of China residents to enrofloxacin, danfloxacin, and flumequine through animal-derived dietary samples was very low, and the health risk was also low.

**3. Contributions of Food Categories to the Total Dietary Intake**

The dietary intake of enrofloxacin was contributed by meats (88.1%), eggs (0.9%), and aquatic foods (11.0%) (Figure 5-13 and Annexed Table 5-18). The dietary intake of ofloxacin was contributed by meats

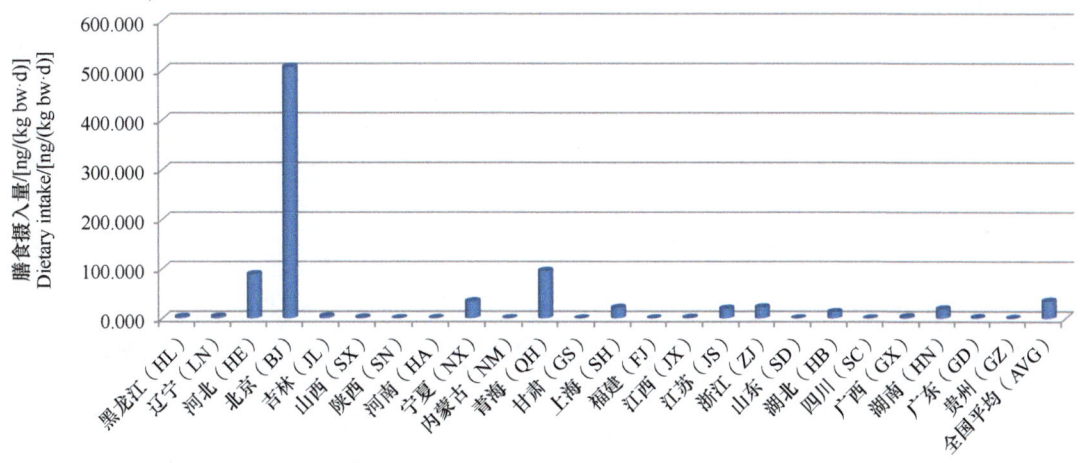

图 5-3 第六次中国总膳食研究的恩诺沙星膳食摄入量

Figure 5-3 Dietary intake of enrofloxacin from the 6$^{th}$ China TDS

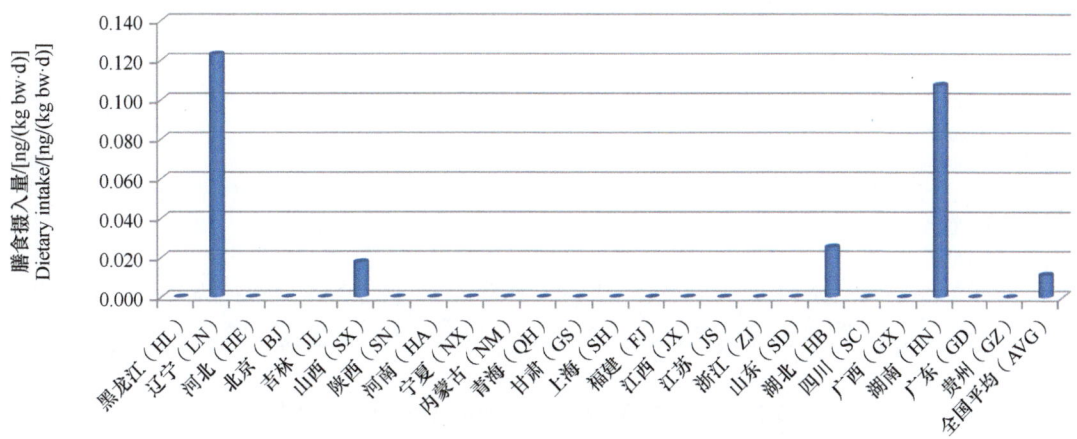

图 5-4 第六次中国总膳食研究的麻保沙星膳食摄入量

Figure 5-4 Dietary intake of marbofloxacin from the 6$^{th}$ China TDS

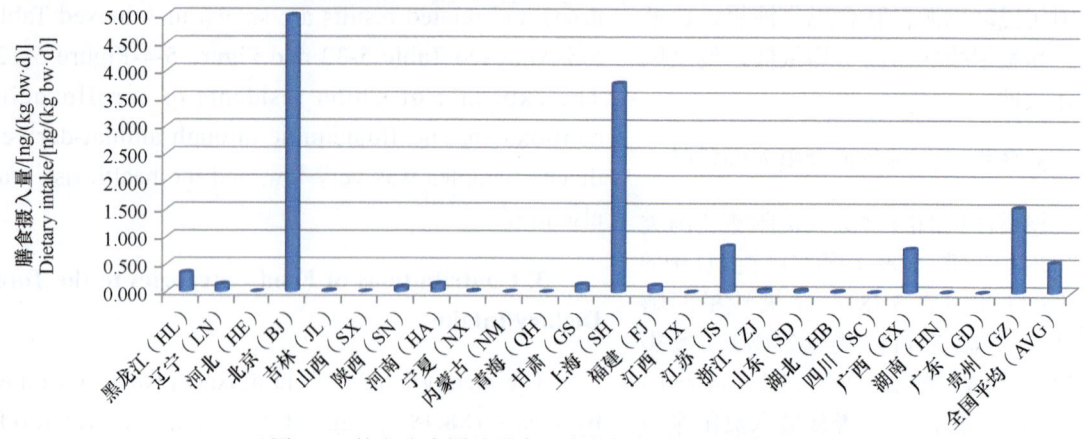

图 5-5　第六次中国总膳食研究的氧氟沙星膳食摄入量

Figure 5-5　Dietary intake of ofloxacin from the 6$^{th}$ China TDS

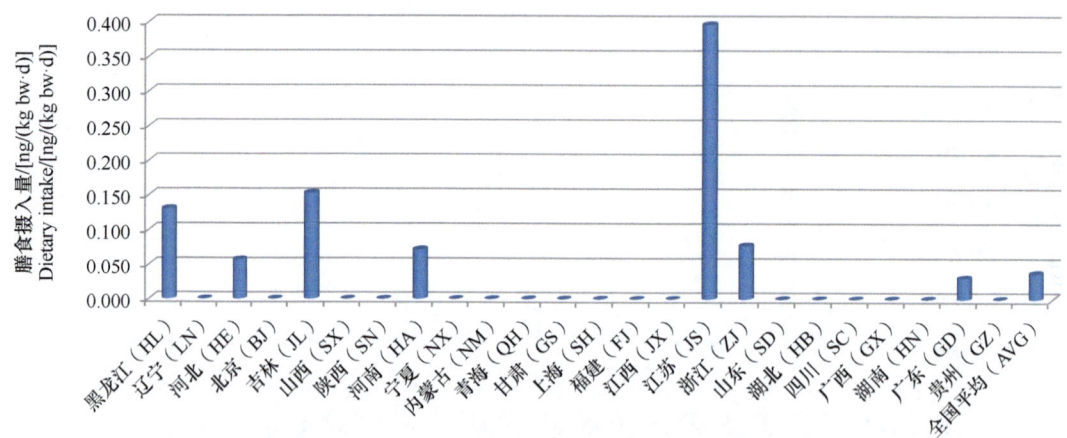

图 5-6　第六次中国总膳食研究的培氟沙星膳食摄入量

Figure 5-6　Dietary intake of pefloxacin from the 6$^{th}$ China TDS

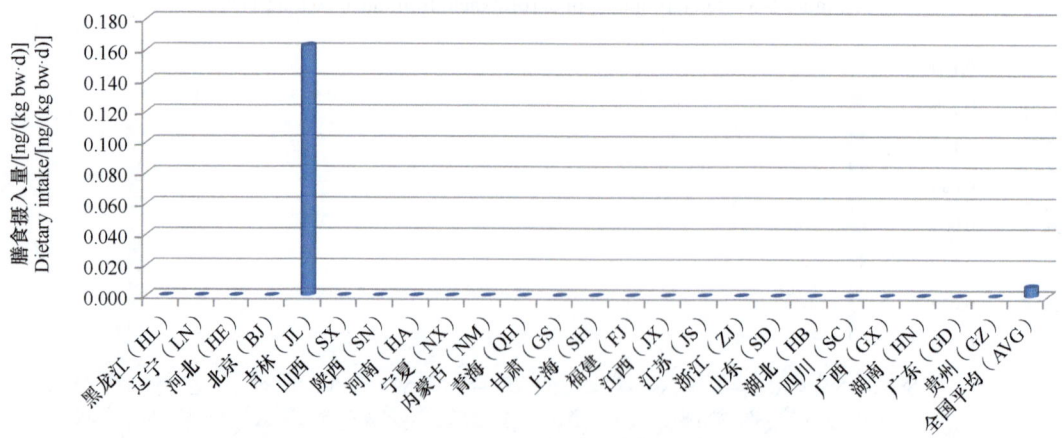

图 5-7　第六次中国总膳食研究的诺氟沙星膳食摄入量

Figure 5-7　Dietary intake of norfloxacin from the 6$^{th}$ China TDS

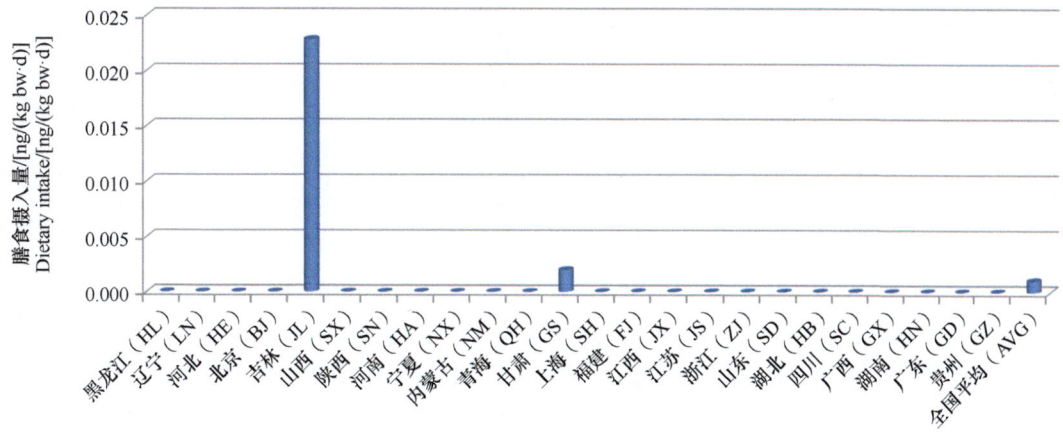

图 5-8　第六次中国总膳食研究的达氟沙星膳食摄入量
Figure 5-8　Dietary intake of danofloxacin from the 6$^{th}$ China TDS

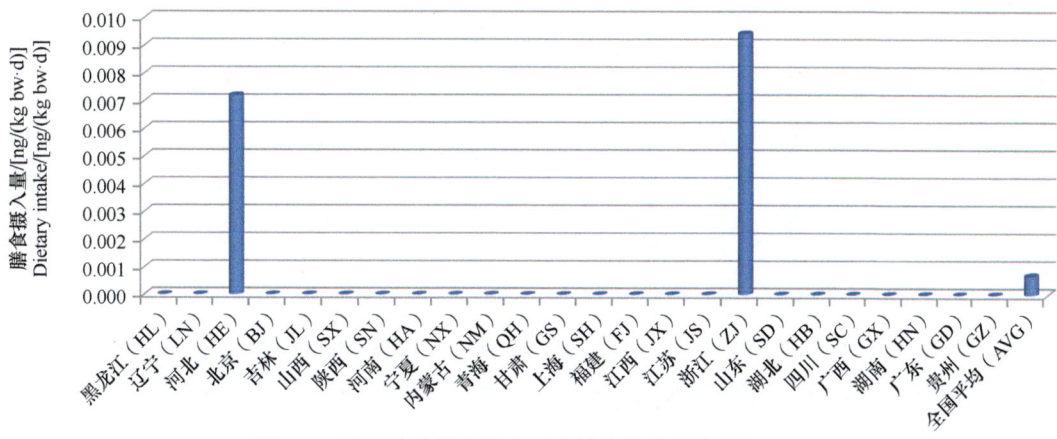

图 5-9　第六次中国总膳食研究的洛美沙星膳食摄入量
Figure 5-9　Dietary intake of lomefloxacin from the 6$^{th}$ China TDS

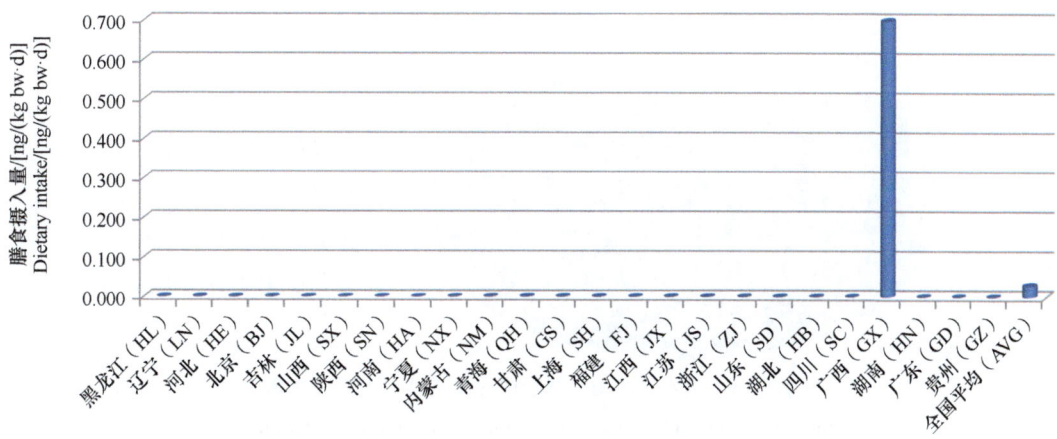

图 5-10　第六次中国总膳食研究的奥比沙星膳食摄入量
Figure 5-10　Dietary intake of orbifloxacin from the 6$^{th}$ China TDS

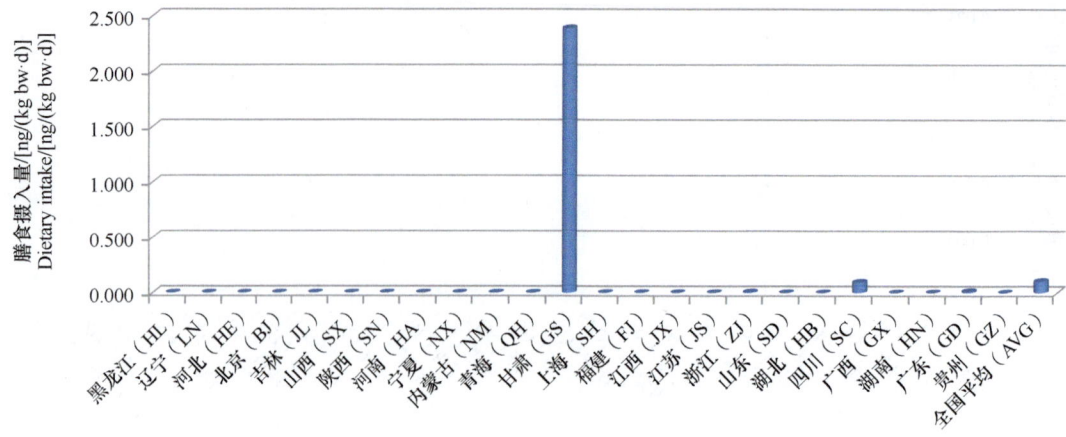

图 5-11　第六次中国总膳食研究的沙拉沙星膳食摄入量
Figure 5-11　Dietary intake of sarafloxacin from the 6th China TDS

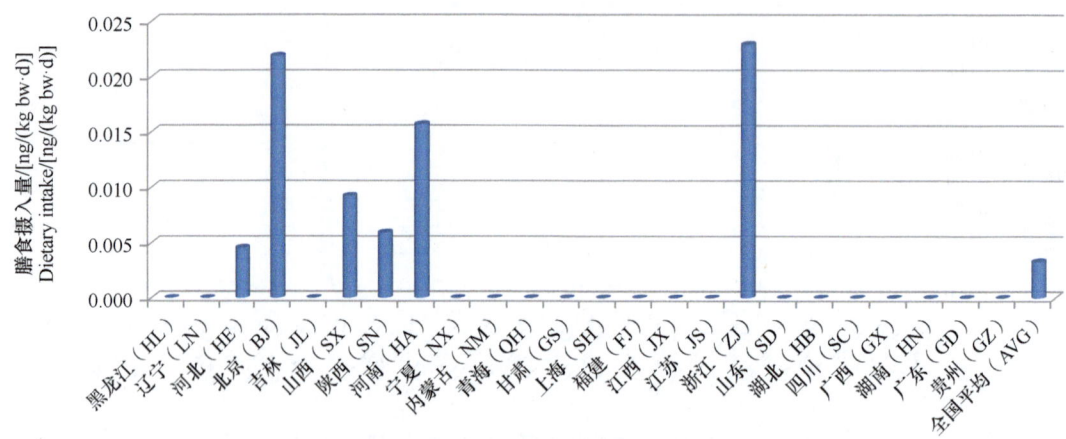

图 5-12　第六次中国总膳食研究的氟甲喹膳食摄入量
Figure 5-12　Dietary intake of flumequine from the 6th China TDS

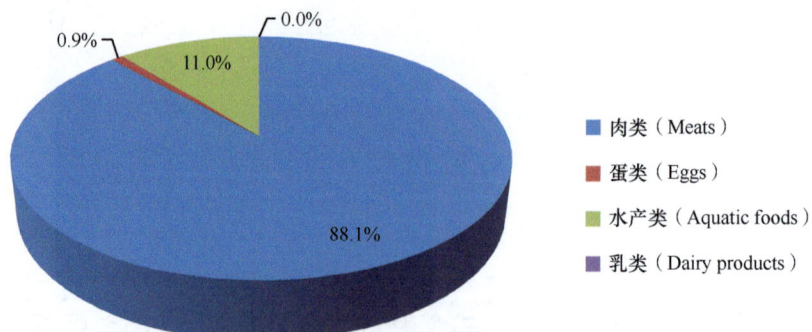

图 5-13　第六次中国总膳食研究恩诺沙星的膳食来源
Figure 5-13　Dietary sources of enrofloxacin from the 6th China TDS

沙星的膳食贡献来自蛋类（56.7%）和水产类（43.3%）（图5-16和附表5-24）；沙拉沙星的膳食摄入贡献来自肉类（3.5%）、蛋类（96.2%）和乳类（0.3%）（图5-17和附表5-30）；氟甲喹的膳食摄入贡献来自肉类（27.3%）、蛋类

(62.9%), eggs (7.7%), and dairy products (29.4%) (Figure 5-14 and Annexed Table 5-9). The dietary intake of pefloxacin was contributed by meats (86.2%), eggs (10.5%), and dairy products (3.4%) (Figure 5-15 and Annexed Table 5-12). The dietary intake of lomefloxacin was contributed by eggs (56.7%) and

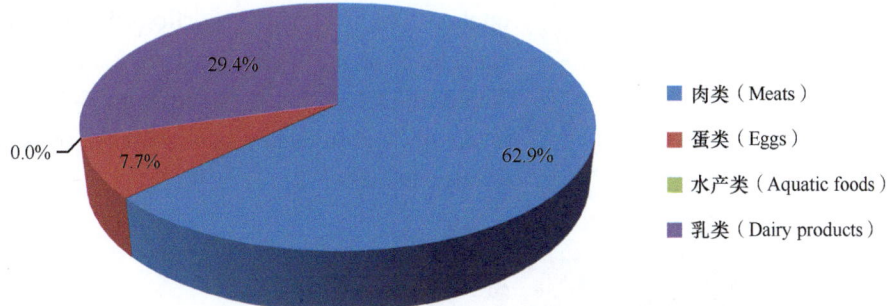

图 5-14　第六次中国总膳食研究氧氟沙星的膳食来源
Figure 5-14　Dietary sources of ofloxacin from the 6th China TDS

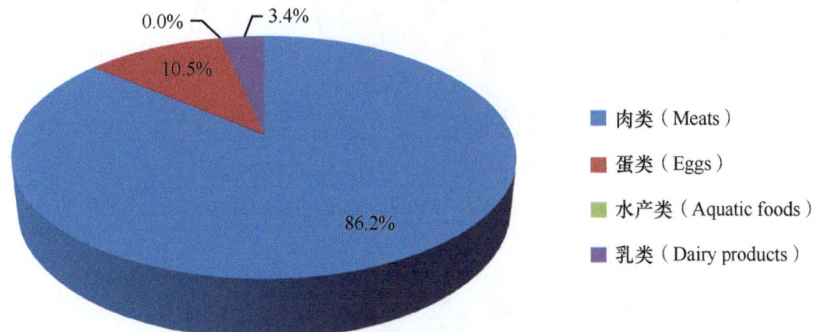

图 5-15　第六次中国总膳食研究培氟沙星的膳食来源
Figure 5-15　Dietary sources of pefloxacin from the 6th China TDS

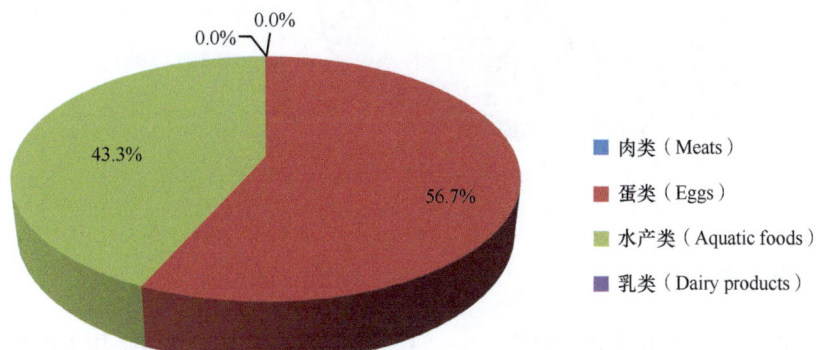

图 5-16　第六次中国总膳食研究洛美沙星的膳食来源
Figure 5-16　Dietary sources of lomefloxacin from the 6th China TDS

（67.0%）和乳类（5.7%）（图 5-18 和附表 5-33）；麻保沙星、诺氟沙星、奥比沙星的膳食摄入贡献来自乳类（附表 5-7、附表 5-15、附表 5-27）；达氟沙星的膳食摄入贡献来自水产类（附表 5-21）。

aquatic foods (43.3%) (Figure 5-16 and Annexed Table 5-24). The dietary intake of sarafloxacin was contributed by meats (3.5%), eggs (96.2%), and dairy products (0.3%) (Figure 5-17 and Annexed Table 5-30). The dietary intake of flumequine was contributed by meats (27.3%), eggs (67.0%), and dairy products (5.7%) (Figure 5-18 and Annexed Table 5-33). The dietary intake of mabrofloxacin, norfloxacin, and orbifloxacin was contributed by dairy products (Annexed Table 5-7, Annexed Table 5-15, Annexed Table 5-27). The dietary intake of danofloxacin was contributed by aquatic foods (Annexed Table 5-21).

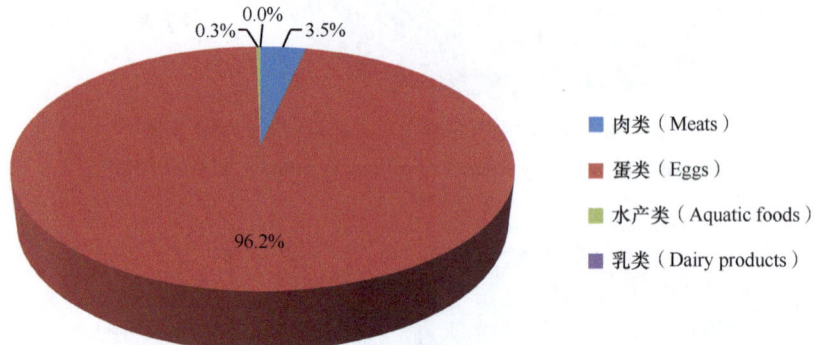

图 5-17　第六次中国总膳食研究沙拉沙星的膳食来源
Figure 5-17　Dietary sources of sarafloxacin from the 6th China TDS

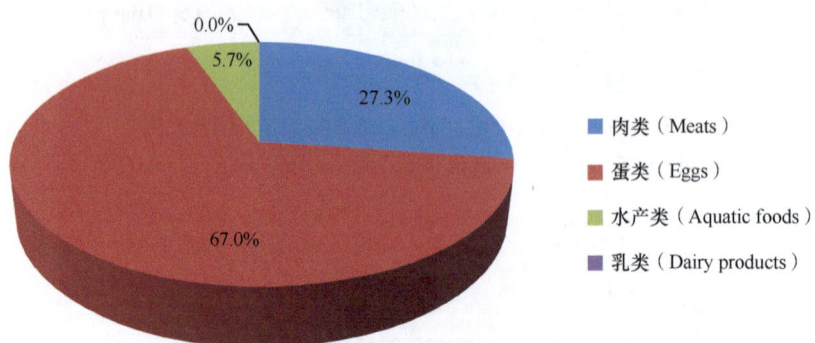

图 5-18　第六次中国总膳食研究氟甲喹的膳食来源
Figure 5-18　Dietary sources of flumequine from the 6th China TDS

（三）磺胺类药物

**1. 混合膳食样品中磺胺类药物的含量**

第六次中国总膳食研究动物源性膳食样品中检出的磺胺类药物包括磺

(Ⅲ) Sulfonamides

**1. Levels of Sulfonamides in Composite Dietary Samples**

The sulfonamides detected in animal-derived dietary samples in the 6th CTDS included sulfamethazine,

胺二甲嘧啶、磺胺噻唑、磺胺甲噁唑和磺胺间甲氧嘧啶，其残留水平分别为ND～3.11 μg/kg（附表5-34）、ND～0.04 μg/kg（附表5-39）、ND～373.07 μg/kg（附表5-40）、ND～87.20 μg/kg（附表5-41）。其中，总磺胺类药物的残留水平为ND～374.09 μg/kg（附表5-42）。

磺胺二甲嘧啶、磺胺噻唑、磺胺甲噁唑和磺胺间甲氧嘧啶的检出率分别为14.6%、7.3%、31.3%和12.5%。其中，磺胺二甲嘧啶残留水平最高的是来自广东的肉类混合样品（3.11 μg/kg），磺胺甲噁唑残留水平最高的是来自山东的蛋类混合样品（373.07 μg/kg），磺胺间甲氧嘧啶残留水平最高的是来自黑龙江的蛋类混合样品（87.20 μg/kg）。

**2. 磺胺类药物的膳食暴露评估**

我国各地区居民动物源性膳食磺胺二甲嘧啶膳食摄入量为0～5.144 ng/(kg bw·d)，占ADI的百分比为0%～0.010%，平均值为0.511 ng/(kg bw·d)，占ADI的0.001%（图5-19和附表5-35）。我国各地区居民动物源性膳食磺胺噻唑摄入量为0～0.015 ng/(kg bw·d)，平均值为0.003 ng/(kg bw·d)（附表5-40）。我国各地区居民动物源性膳食磺胺甲噁唑摄入量为0～263.0 ng/(kg bw·d)，平

sulfathiazole, sulfamethoxazole, and sulfamonomethoxine, with a residue level ranging from ND-3.11 μg/kg (Annexed Table 5-34), ND-0.04 μg/kg (Annexed Table 5-39), ND-373.07 μg/kg (Annexed Table 5-40), ND-87.20 μg/kg (Annexed Table 5-41), respectively. Among them, the residue level of total sulfonamides was ND-374.09 μg/kg (Annexed Table 5-42).

The detection rates of sulfamethazine, sulfathiazole, sulfamethoxazole, and sulfamonomethoxine were 14.6%, 7.3%, 31.3%, and 12.5%, respectively. Among them, the highest residue level of sulfamethazine was from meats composite samples of Guangdong (3.11 μg/kg). The highest residue level of sulfamethoxazole was from eggs composite samples of Shandong (373.07 μg/kg). The highest residue level of sulfamonomethoxine was from eggs composite samples of Heilongjiang (87.20 μg/kg).

**2. Dietary Exposure Assessment of Sulfonamides**

The dietary intake of sulfamethazine among residents of various regions in China ranged from 0 ng/(kg bw·d) to 5.144 ng/(kg bw·d), accounting for 0%-0.010% of the ADI, with an average value of 0.511 ng/(kg bw·d), accounting for 0.001% of the ADI (Figure 5-19 and Annexed Table 5-35). The dietary intake of sulfathiazole in China ranged from 0 ng/(kg bw·d) to 0.015 ng/(kg bw·d), with an average value of 0.003 ng/(kg bw·d) (Annexed Table 5-40). The dietary intake of sulfamethoxazole in China ranged from 0 ng/(kg bw·d)

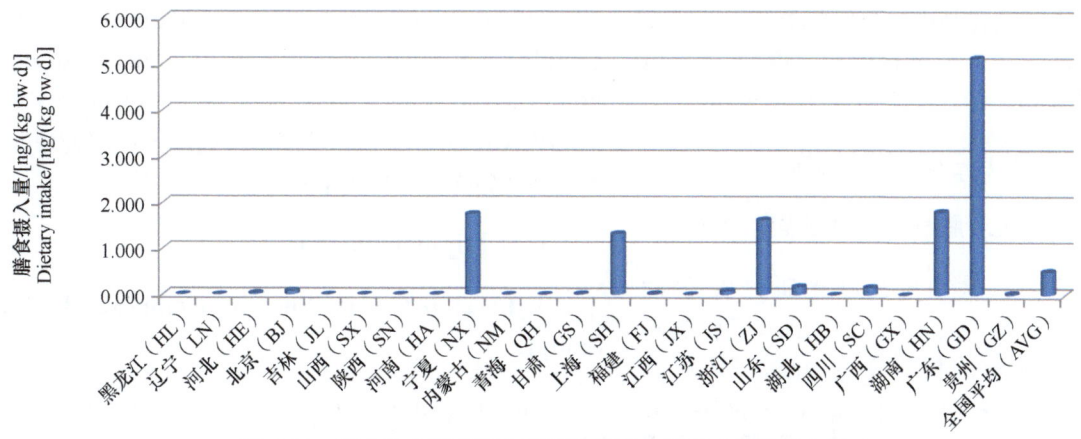

图5-19 第六次中国总膳食研究的磺胺二甲嘧啶膳食摄入量

Figure 5-19 Dietary intake of sulfamethazine from the 6th China TDS

均值为 11.01 ng/(kg bw·d)（附表 5-41）。我国各地区居民动物源性膳食磺胺间甲氧嘧啶摄入量为 0～72.57 ng/(kg bw·d)，平均值为 4.246 ng/(kg bw·d)（附表 5-42）。我国各地区居民动物源性膳食总磺胺类药物摄入量为 0～264.0 ng/(kg bw·d)，占 ADI 的百分比为 0%～0.528%，平均值为 15.77 ng/(kg bw·d)，占 ADI 的 0.032%（图 5-20 和附表 5-43）。我国居民动物源性膳食磺胺类药物暴露量很低，健康风险亦较低。

to 263.0 ng/(kg bw·d), with an average value of 11.01 ng/(kg bw·d) (Annexed Table 5-41). The dietary intake of sulfamonomethoxine in China ranged from 0 ng/(kg bw·d) to 72.57 ng/(kg bw·d), with an average value of 4.246 ng/(kg bw·d) (Annexed Table 5-42). The dietary intake of total sulfonamides in China ranged from 0 ng/(kg bw·d) to 264.0 ng/(kg bw·d), accounting for 0%-0.528% of the ADI, with an average value of 15.77 ng/(kg bw·d), accounting for 0.032% of the ADI (Figure 5-20 and Annexed Table 5-43). The exposure of China residents to animal-derived dietary sulfonamides was very low, and the health risk was also low.

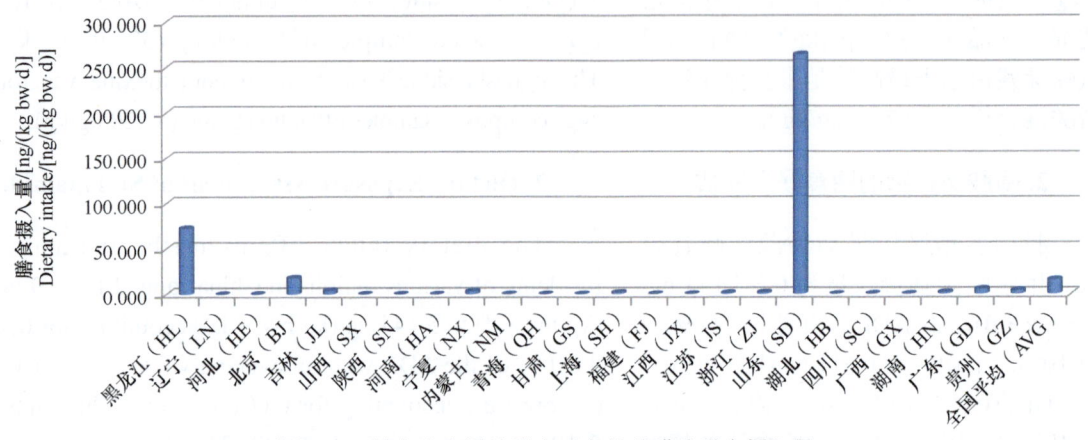

图 5-20　第六次中国总膳食研究的总磺胺膳食摄入量

Figure 5-20　Dietary intake of total sulfonamides from the 6th China TDS

**3. 各类膳食对总膳食摄入的贡献**

在肉类、水产类、蛋类和乳类 4 类混合膳食样品中，总磺胺类药物的膳食摄入贡献主要来自肉类（13.3%）和蛋类（86.6%）（图 5-21 和附表 5-44）。

**（四）三苯甲烷类药物**

**1. 混合膳食样品中结晶紫的含量**

第六次中国总膳食研究 96 份动物源性混合膳食样品中三苯甲烷类药物结晶紫的检出率为 100%，残留水平为 0.09～47.51 μg/kg（附表 5-45）。其中，较高残留水平来自广西的蛋类样品（47.51 μg/kg）和水产类样品

**3. Contributions of Food Categories to the Total Dietary Intake**

Of the four categories of animal-derived composite samples, i.e. meats, aquatic foods, eggs, and dairy products, the dietary intake of total sulfonamides was contributed by meats (13.3%) and eggs (86.6%) (Figure 5-21 and Annexed Table 5-44).

**(Ⅳ) Triphenylmethanes**

**1. Level of Crystal Violet in Composite Dietary Samples**

The detection rate of triphenylmethane crystal violet in 96 composite samples of animal-derived dietary samples in the sixth China TDS was 100%, and the

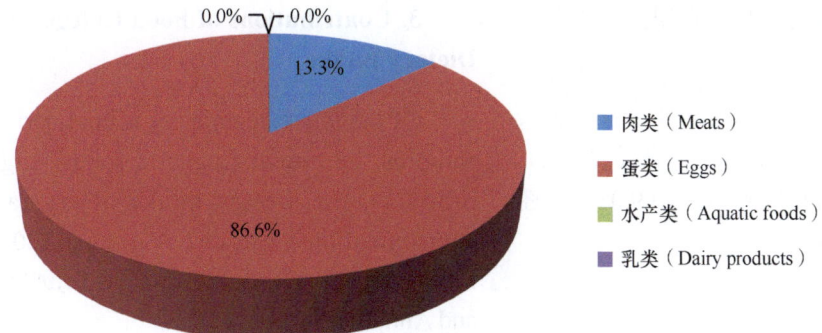

图 5-21 第六次中国总膳食研究总磺胺的膳食来源

Figure 5-21　Dietary sources of total sulfonamides from the 6th China TDS

（45.43 μg/kg），肉类样品最高的来自四川省（21.32 μg/kg），乳类样品最高的来自广东省（30.62 μg/kg）。

**2. 结晶紫的膳食暴露评估**

我国各地区居民动物源性膳食结晶紫膳食摄入量为 1.446～82.01 ng/(kg bw·d)，平均值为 16.31 ng/(kg bw·d)（图 5-22 和附表 5-46）。

residue level was between 0.09 μg/kg and 47.51 μg/kg (Annexed Table 5-45). Among them, the higher residue levels of crystal violet were from eggs samples (47.51 μg/kg) and aquatic foods (45.43 μg/kg) in Guangxi. The highest residue level in meats samples was from Sichuan (21.32 μg/kg). The highest residue level in dairy products was from Guangdong (30.62 μg/kg).

**2. Dietary Exposure Assessment of Crystal Violet**

The animal-derived dietary intake of China residents among various regions to crystal violet ranged from 1.446 ng/(kg bw·d) to 82.01 ng/(kg bw·d), with an average value of 16.31 ng/(kg bw·d) (Figure 5-22 and Annexed Table 5-46).

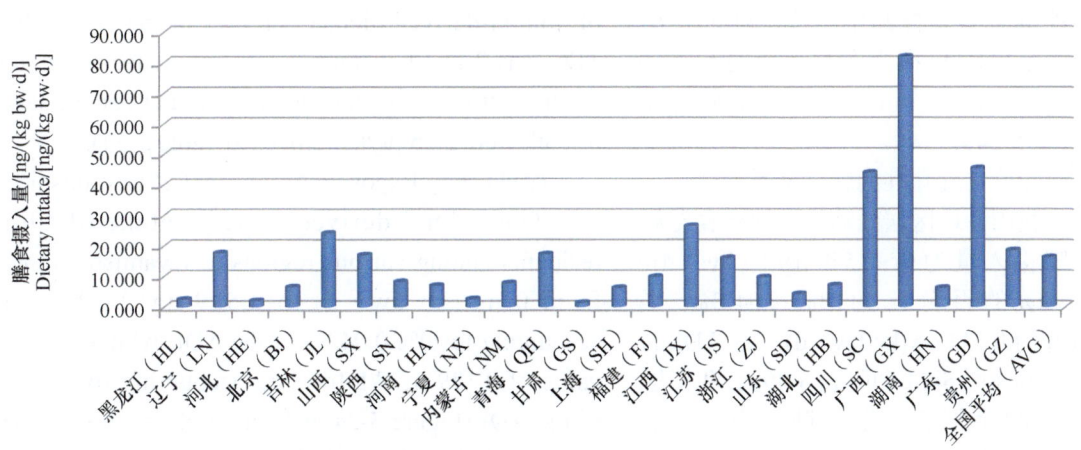

图 5-22 第六次中国总膳食研究的结晶紫膳食摄入量

Figure 5-22　Dietary intake of crystal violet from the 6th China TDS

## 3. Contributions of Food Categories to the Total Dietary Intake

Of the four categories of animal-derived composite samples, i.e., meats, aquatic foods, eggs, and dairy products, the dietary intake of crystal violet was contributed by meats (51.5%), eggs (20.7%), aquatic foods (18.7%) and dairy products (9.0%) (Figure 5-23 and Annexed Table 5-47).

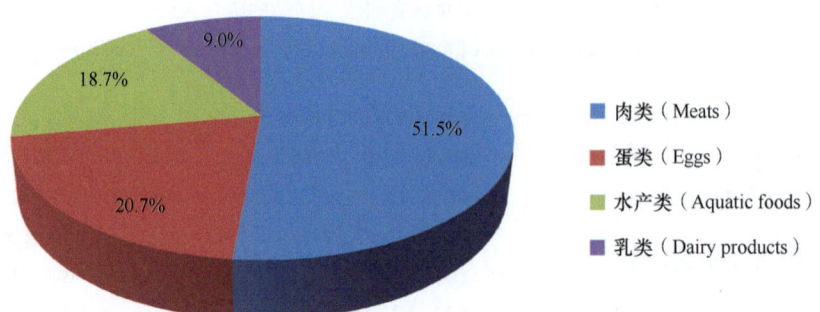

Figure 5-23　Dietary sources of crystal violet from the 6$^{th}$ China TDS

### (V) Imidazoles

#### 1. Levamisole

(1) Level of Levamisole in Composite Dietary Samples

The detection rate of levamisole in 96 samples of animal-derived dietary samples in the sixth China TDS was 2.1%. Levamisole was only detected in dairy products from Shanghai and Jiangxi, and residue levels of both were 2.25 μg/kg (Annexed Table 5-54).

(2) Dietary Exposure Assessment of Levamisole

The animal-derived dietary intake of China residents among various regions to levamisole ranged from 0 ng/(kg bw · d) to 2.549 ng/(kg bw · d), accounting for 0%-0.042% of the ADI, with an average value of 0.139 ng/(kg bw · d), accounting for 0.002% of the ADI (Figure 5-24 and Annexed Table 5-49). The levamisole from animal-derived dietary exposure of China residents was quite low, as well as the health risk.

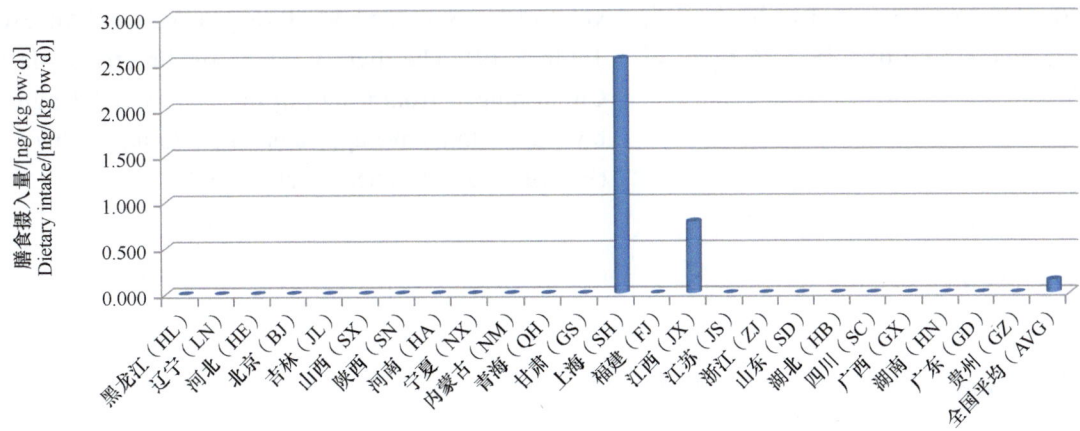

图 5-24　第六次中国总膳食研究的左旋咪唑膳食摄入量
Figure 5-24　Dietary intake of levamisole from the 6$^{th}$ China TDS

（3）各类膳食对总膳食摄入的贡献

左旋咪唑的膳食摄入贡献来自乳类（附表 5-56）。

**2. 硝基咪唑类药物**

（1）混合膳食样品中硝基咪唑类药物的含量

第六次中国总膳食研究动物源性膳食样品中检出的硝基咪唑类药物包括甲硝唑（以甲硝唑和羟基甲硝唑之和计）与地美硝唑（以地美硝唑和 2-羟基地美硝唑之和计），其残留水平分别为 ND～602.90 μg/kg（附表 5-48）和 ND～169.22 μg/kg（附表 5-51）。

甲硝唑和地美硝唑的检出率分别为 20.8% 和 2.1%。其中，甲硝唑的最大残留水平来自湖南的蛋类样品（602.90 μg/kg），而地美硝唑仅在上海和内蒙古的蛋类样品检出，残留水平分别为 169.22 μg/kg 和 51.41 μg/kg。

（2）硝基咪唑类药物的膳食暴露评估

我国各地区居民动物源性膳食甲硝唑膳食摄入量为 0～218.2 ng/(kg bw·d)，平均值为 10.58 ng/(kg bw·d)（图 5-25 和附表 5-49）。我国各地区居民动物源性膳食地美硝唑膳食摄入量

(3) Contributions of Food Categories to the Total Dietary Intake

The dietary intake of levamisole was contributed by dairy products (Annexed Table 5-56).

**2. Nitroimidazoles**

(1) Level of Nitroimidazoles in Composite Dietary Samples

The nitroimidazoles detected in animal-derived dietary samples in the 6$^{th}$ CTDS included metronidazole (calculated as the sum of metronidazole and hydroxy-metronidazole) and dimenidazole (calculated as the sum of dimenidazole and 2-hydroxy-dimenidazole). Their residue levels were ND-602.90 μg/kg (Annexed Table 5-48) and ND-169.22 μg/kg, respectively (Annexed Table 5-51).

The detection rates of metronidazole and dimetridazole were 20.8% and 2.1%, respectively. Among them, the maximum residue levels of metronidazole were from eggs samples in Hunan (602.90 μg/kg), while dimenidazole was only detected in eggs samples from Shanghai and Inner Mongolia, with residue levels of 169.22 μg/kg and 51.41 μg/kg, respectively.

(2) Dietary Exposure Assessment of Nitroimidazole

The dietary intake of metronidazole among residents of various regions in China ranged from 0 ng/(kg bw·d) to 218.2 ng/(kg bw·d), with an average

为 0~104.8 ng/(kg bw·d)，平均值为 5.376 ng/(kg bw·d)（图 5-26 和附表 5-52）。

value of 10.58 ng/(kg bw·d) (Figure 5-25 and Annexed Table 5-49). The dietary intake of dimetridazole in China ranged from 0 ng/(kg bw·d) to 104.8 ng/(kg bw·d), with an average value of 5.376 ng/(kg bw·d) (Figure 5-26 and Annexed Table 5-52).

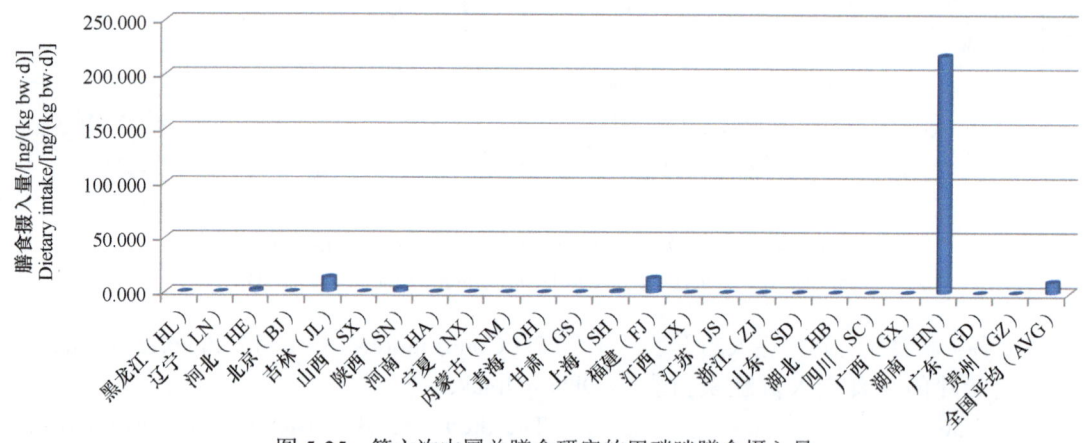

图 5-25　第六次中国总膳食研究的甲硝唑膳食摄入量
Figure 5-25　Dietary intake of metronidazole from the 6$^{th}$ China TDS

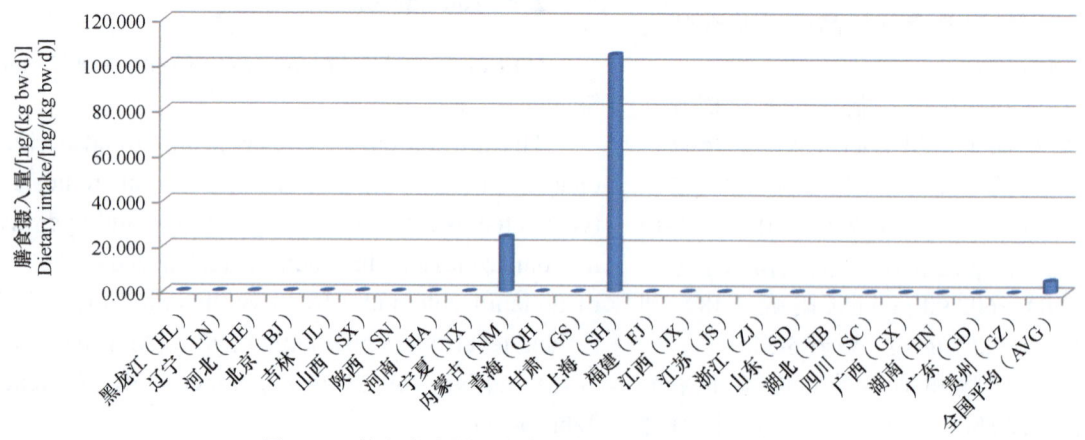

图 5-26　第六次中国总膳食研究的地美硝唑膳食摄入量
Figure 5-26　Dietary intake of dimetridazole from the 6$^{th}$ China TDS

（3）各类膳食对总膳食摄入的贡献

在肉类、水产类、蛋类和乳类 4 类混合膳食样品中，甲硝唑的膳食摄入贡献来自蛋类（94.6%）和肉类（5.4%）（图 5-27 和附表 5-50）；地美硝唑的膳食摄入贡献来自蛋类（附表 5-53）。

(3) Contributions of Food Categories to the Total Dietary Intake

Of the four categories of animal-derived composite samples, i.e., meats, aquatic foods, eggs, and dairy products, the dietary intake of metronidazole was contributed by eggs (94.6%) and meats (5.4%) (Figure 5-27 and Annexed Table 5-50). The dietary intake of dimetridazole was contributed by eggs (Annexed Table 5-53).

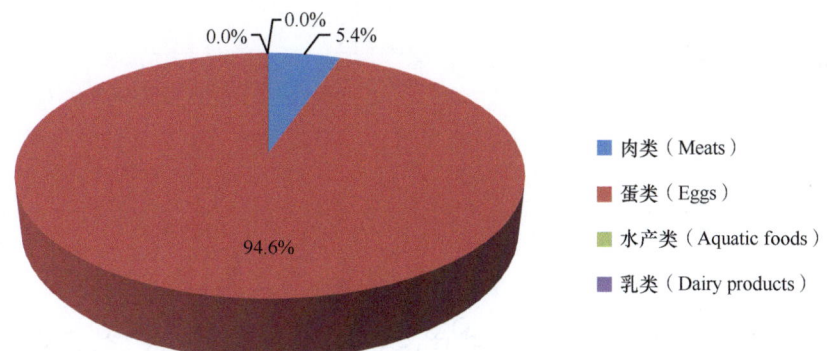

图 5-27　第六次中国总膳食研究甲硝唑的膳食来源
Figure 5-27　Dietary sources of metronidazole from the 6th China TDS

### 3. 苯并咪唑类药物

（1）混合膳食样品中苯并咪唑类药物的含量

检出的苯并咪唑类药物包括阿苯达唑（以阿苯达唑亚砜、阿苯达唑砜、阿苯达唑-2-氨基砜和阿苯达唑之和计）、芬苯达唑/奥芬达唑（以芬苯达唑、奥芬达唑和奥芬达唑砜之和计）、氟苯达唑和甲苯达唑，其残留水平分别为 ND～4.29 μg/kg（附表 5-57）、ND～0.52 μg/kg（附表 5-60）、ND～0.12 μg/kg（附表 5-63）和 ND～0.05 μg/kg（附表 5-66），检出率分别为 21.9%、76.0%、81.3% 和 68.8%。

（2）苯并咪唑类药物的膳食暴露评估

我国各地区居民动物源性膳食阿苯达唑膳食摄入量为 0～3.422 ng/(kg bw·d)，平均值为 0.235 ng/(kg bw·d)（图 5-28 和附表 5-58）。我国各地区居民动物源性膳食芬苯达唑膳食摄入量为 0～1.067 ng/(kg bw·d)，平均值为 0.206 ng/(kg bw·d)（图 5-29 和附表 5-61）。我国各地区居民动物源性膳食氟苯达唑膳食摄入量为 0～0.278 ng/(kg bw·d)，平均值为 0.080 ng/(kg bw·d)（图 5-30 和附表 5-64）。我国各地区居民动物源性膳食甲苯达唑暴露量为 0～

### 3. Benzimidazoles

(1) Level of Benzimidazoles in Composite Dietary Samples

Detected benzimidazoles included albendazole (calculated as the sum of albendazole sulfoxide, albendazole sulfone, albendazole-2-aminosulfone, and albendazole), fenbendazole/oxfendazole (calculated as the sum of fenbendazole, oxfendazole and oxfendazole sulfone), flubendazole, and mebendazole, with residue levels of ND-4.29 μg/kg (Annexed Table 5-57), ND-0.52 μg/kg (Annexed Table 5-60), ND-0.12 μg/kg (Annexed Table 5-63), and ND-0.05 μg/kg (Annexed Table 5-66), and with the detection rates of 21.9%, 76.0%, 81.3%, and 68.8%, respectively.

(2) Dietary Exposure Assessment of Benzimidazoles

The animal-derived dietary intake of China residents among various regions to albendazole ranged from 0 ng/(kg bw·d) to 3.422 ng/(kg bw·d), with an average value of 0.235 ng/(kg bw·d) (Figure 5-28 and Annexed Table 5-58). The animal-derived dietary intake of China residents to fenbendazole ranged from 0 ng/(kg bw·d) to 1.067 ng/(kg bw·d), with an average value of 0.206 ng/(kg bw·d) (Figure 5-29 and Annexed Table 5-61). The animal-derived dietary intake of China residents to flubendazole ranged from 0 ng/(kg bw·d) to 0.278 ng/(kg bw·d), with an average value of 0.080 ng/(kg bw·d) (Figure 5-30 and Annexed Table 5-64). The animal-derived dietary intake of China residents to

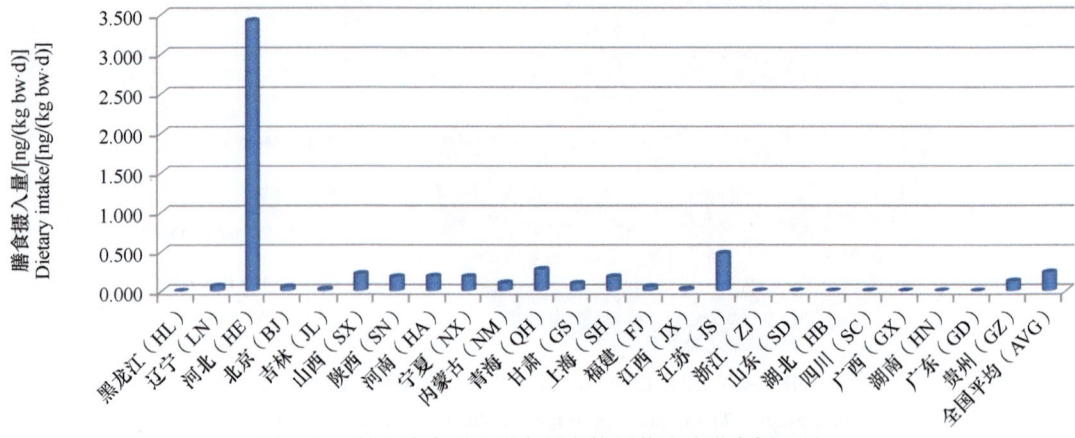

图 5-28 第六次中国总膳食研究的阿苯达唑膳食摄入量
Figure 5-28 Dietary intake of albendazole from the 6$^{th}$ China TDS

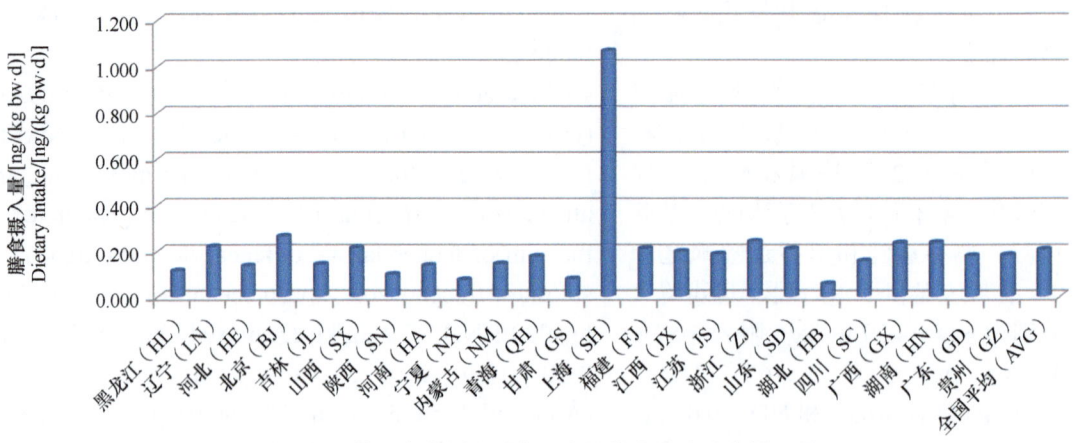

图 5-29 第六次中国总膳食研究的芬苯达唑膳食摄入量
Figure 5-29 Dietary intake of fenbendazole from the 6$^{th}$ China TDS

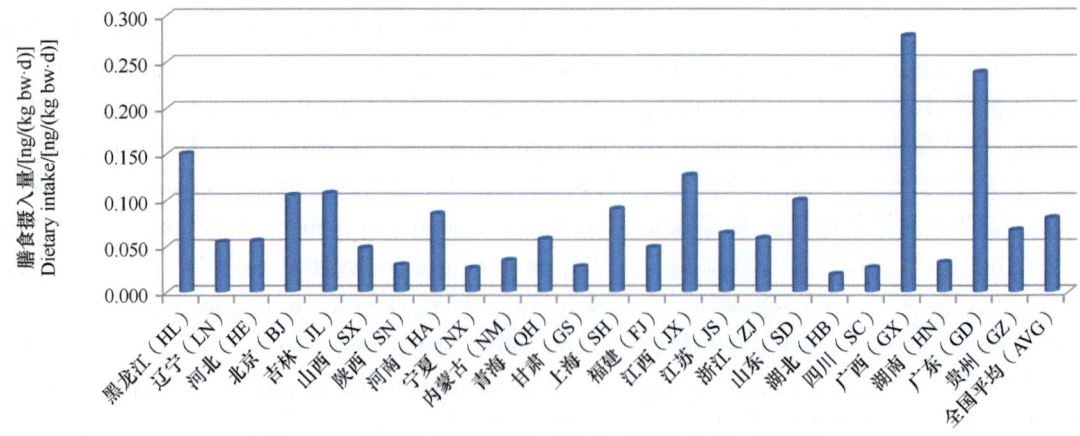

图 5-30 第六次中国总膳食研究的氟苯达唑膳食摄入量
Figure 5-30 Dietary intake of flubendazole from the 6$^{th}$ China TDS

0.094 ng/(kg bw·d)，平均值为 0.039 ng/(kg bw·d)（图 5-31 和附表 5-67）；以上药物的暴露量均占各自 ADI 的 0.1% 以下，表明我国居民动物源性膳食苯并咪唑类药物的暴露量很低，健康风险亦较低。

mebendazole ranged from 0 ng/(kg bw·d) to 0.094 ng/(kg bw·d), with an average value of 0.039 ng/(kg bw·d) (Figure 5-31 and Annexed Table 5-67). The exposures of the above drugs all accounted for less than 0.1% of their respective ADIs, indicating that the benzimidazoles intake of China residents from animal-derived dietary samples was quite low, as well as the health risk.

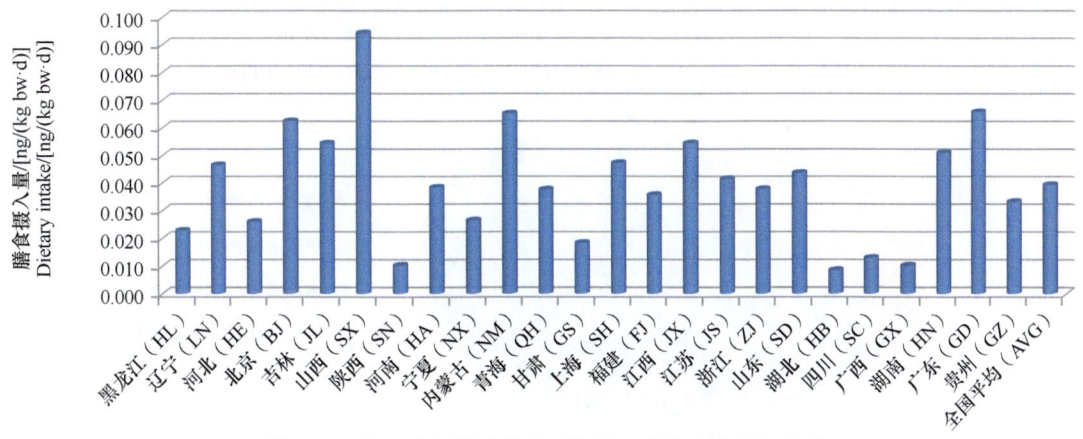

图 5-31 第六次中国总膳食研究的甲苯达唑膳食摄入量
Figure 5-31 Dietary intake of mebendazole from the 6th China TDS

（3）各类膳食对总膳食摄入的贡献

在肉类、水产类、蛋类和乳类 4 类混合膳食样品中，阿苯达唑的膳食摄入贡献来自肉类（76.9%）、蛋类（19.4%）、水产类（3.3%）和乳类（0.4%）（图 5-32 和附表 5-59）；芬苯达唑的膳食摄入贡献来自肉类（62.6%）、蛋类（17.3%）、水产类（0.9%）和乳类（19.2%）（图 5-33 和附表 5-62）；氟苯达唑的膳食摄入贡献来自肉类（58.6%）、蛋类（17.8%）、水产类（2.0%）和乳类（21.7%）（图 5-34 和附表 5-65）；甲苯达唑的膳食摄入贡献来自肉类（42.7%）、蛋类（23.2%）和乳类（34.1%）（图 5-35 和附表 5-68）。

(3) Contributions of Food Categories to the Total Dietary Intake

Of the four categories of animal-derived composite samples, i.e. meats, aquatic foods, eggs, and dairy products, the dietary intake of albendazole was contributed by meats (76.9%), eggs (19.4%), aquatic foods (3.3%), and dairy products (0.4%) (Figure 5-32 and Annexed Table 5-59). The dietary intake of fenbendazole was contributed by meats (62.6%), eggs (17.3%), aquatic foods (0.9%), and dairy products (19.2%) (Figure 5-33 and Annexed Table 5-62). The dietary intake of flubendazole was contributed by meats (58.6%), eggs (17.8%), aquatic foods (2.0%), and dairy products (21.7%) (Figure 5-34 and Annexed Table 5-65). The dietary intake of mebendazole was contributed by meats (42.7%), eggs (23.2%), and dairy products (34.1%) (Figure 5-35 and Annexed Table 5-68).

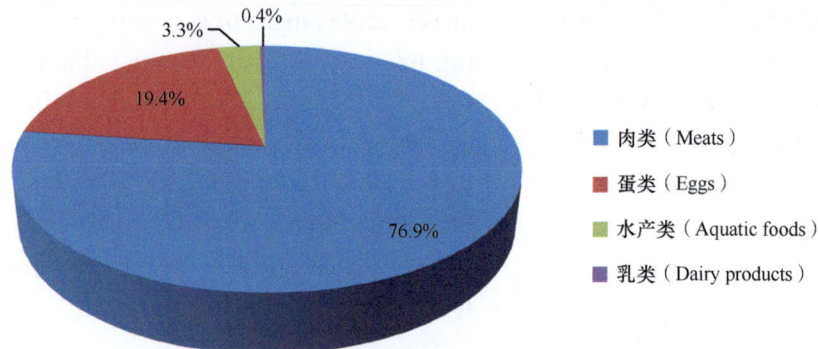

图 5-32　第六次中国总膳食研究阿苯达唑的膳食来源
Figure 5-32　Dietary sources of albendazole from the 6th China TDS

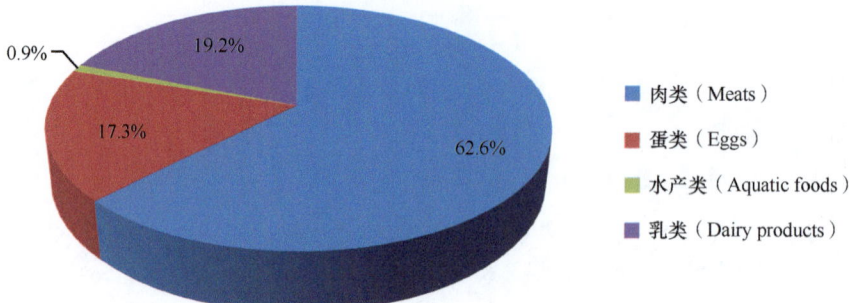

图 5-33　第六次中国总膳食研究芬苯达唑的膳食来源
Figure 5-33　Dietary sources of fenbendazole from the 6th China TDS

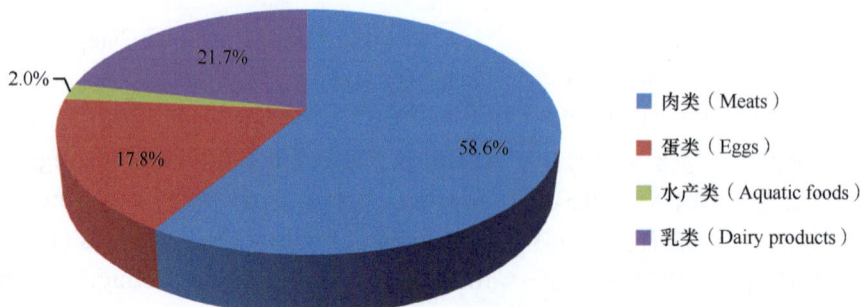

图 5-34　第六次中国总膳食研究氟苯达唑的膳食来源
Figure 5-34　Dietary sources of flubendazole from the 6th China TDS

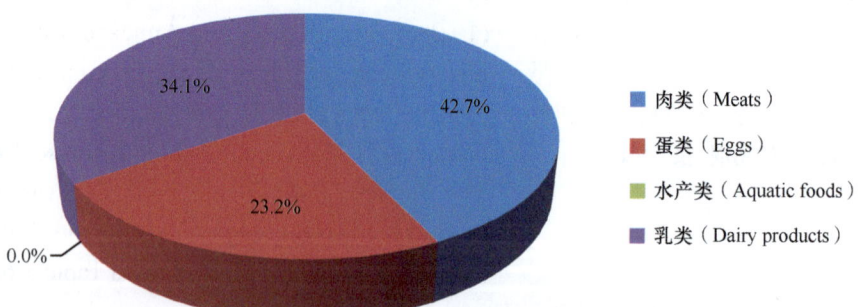

图 5-35　第六次中国总膳食研究甲苯达唑的膳食来源
Figure 5-35　Dietary sources of mebendazole from the 6th China TDS

## （六）氯霉素类药物

### 1. 混合膳食样品中氯霉素类药物的含量

第六次中国总膳食研究动物源性膳食样品中检出的氯霉素类药物包括氟苯尼考（以氟苯尼考和氟苯尼考胺之和计）、氯霉素和甲砜霉素，其残留水平分别为 ND～49.85 μg/kg（附表 5-69）、ND～0.23 μg/kg（附表 5-72）和 ND～0.27 μg/kg（附表 5-75）。其中，氟苯尼考、氯霉素和甲砜霉素的检出率分别为 38.5%、4.2% 和 4.2%。

### 2. 氯霉素类药物的膳食暴露评估

我国各地区居民动物源性膳食氟苯尼考膳食摄入量为 0～45.924 ng/(kg bw·d)，占 ADI 的 0%～1.531%，平均值为 4.413 ng/(kg bw·d)，占 ADI 的 0.147%（图 5-36 和附表 5-70）。我国各地区居民动物源性膳食氯霉素暴露量为 0～0.374 ng/(kg bw·d)，平均值为 0.019 ng/(kg bw·d)（图 5-37 和附表 5-73）。我国各地区居民动物源性膳食甲砜霉素暴露量为 0～0.252 ng/(kg bw·d)，占 ADI 的 0%～0.005%，平均值为 0.017 ng/(kg bw·d)（图 5-38 和附表 5-76）。我国居

## (VI) Chloramphenicol

### 1. Level of Chloramphenicol in Composite Dietary Samples

The chloramphenicols detected in animal-derived dietary samples in the 6th CTDS included florfenicol (calculated as the sum of florfenicol and florfenicol amine), chloramphenicol, and thiamphenicol, with residue levels of ND-49.85 μg/kg (Annexed Table 5-69), ND-0.23 μg/kg (Annexed Table 5-72), and ND-0.27 μg/kg (Annexed Table 5-75), respectively. Among them, the detection rates of florfenicol, chloramphenicol, and thiamphenicol were 38.5%, 4.2%, and 4.2%, respectively.

### 2. Dietary Exposure Assessment of Chloramphenicol

The animal-derived dietary intake of China residents among various regions to florfenicol ranged from 0 ng/(kg bw·d) to 45.924 ng/(kg bw·d), accounting for 0%-1.531% of the ADI, with an average value of 4.413 ng/(kg bw·d), accounting for 0.147% of the ADI (Figure 5-36 and Annexed Table 5-70). The animal-derived dietary intake of China residents to chloramphenicol ranged from 0 ng/(kg bw·d) to 0.374 ng/(kg bw·d), with an average value of 0.019 ng/(kg bw·d) (Figure 5-37 and Annexed Table 5-73).

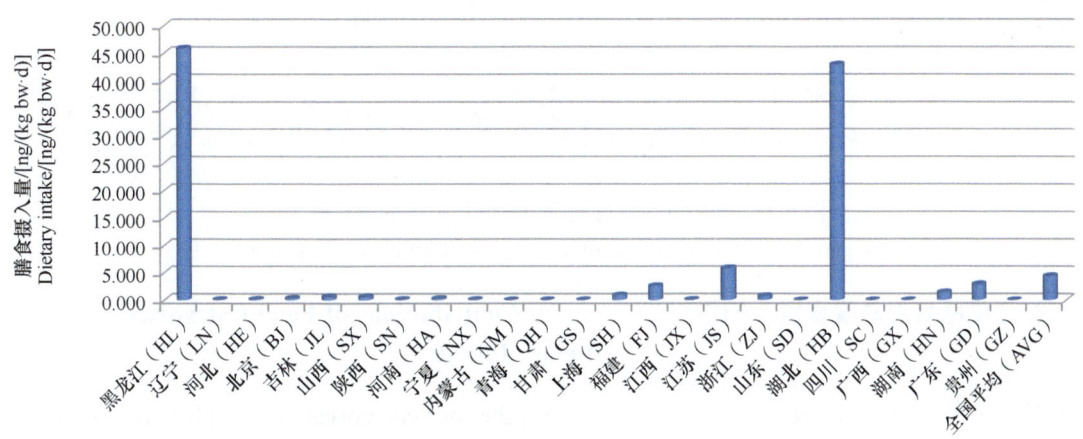

图 5-36　第六次中国总膳食研究的氟苯尼考膳食摄入量

Figure 5-36　Dietary intake of florfenicol from the 6th China TDS

民动物源性膳食氟苯尼考、氯霉素和甲砜霉素膳食暴露量很低，健康风险亦较低。

The animal-derived dietary intake of China residents to thiamphenicol ranged from 0 ng/(kg bw·d) to 0.252 ng/(kg bw·d), accounting for 0%-0.005% of the ADI, with an average value of 0.017 ng/(kg bw·d), accounting for 0.000% of the ADI (Figure 5-38 and Annexed Table 5-76). The florfenicol, chloramphenicol and thiamphenicol animal-derived dietary exposure of China residents was quite low, as well as the health risk.

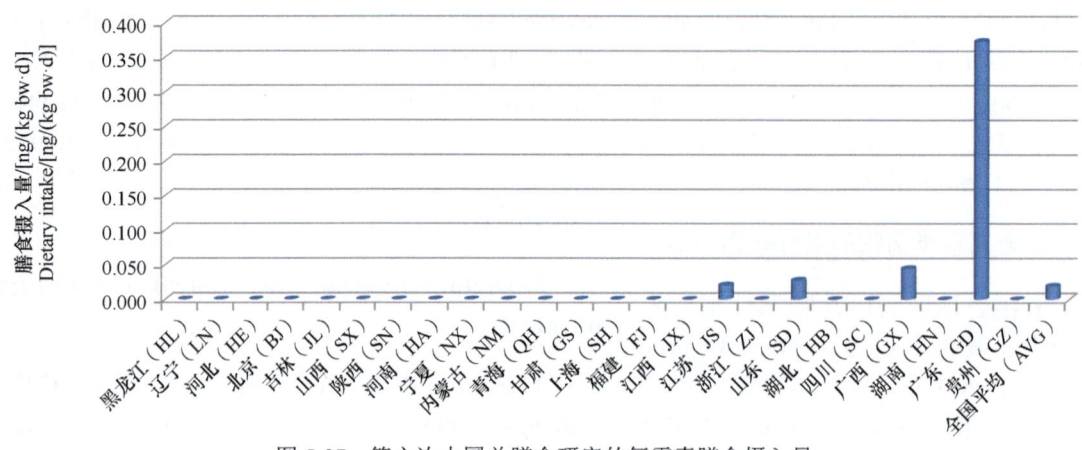

图 5-37　第六次中国总膳食研究的氯霉素膳食摄入量
Figure 5-37　Dietary intake of chloramphenicol from the 6th China TDS

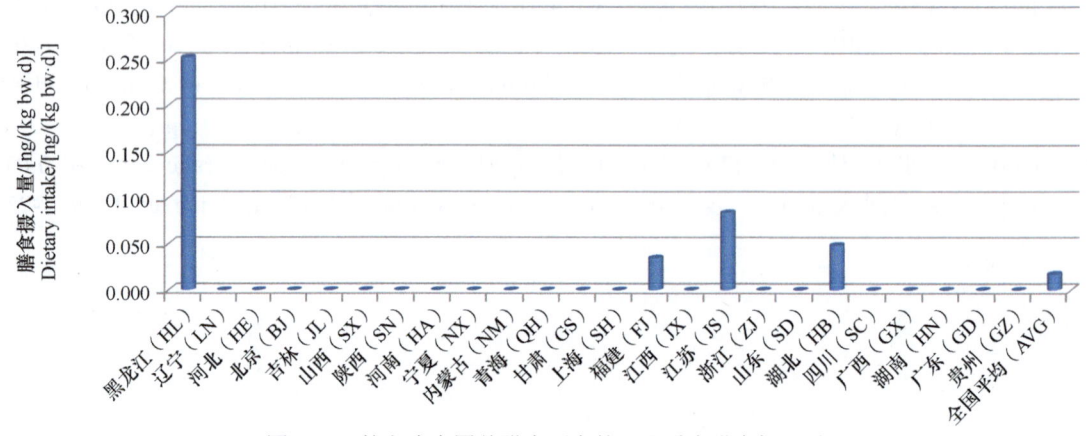

图 5-38　第六次中国总膳食研究的甲砜霉素膳食摄入量
Figure 5-38　Dietary intake of thiamphenicol from the 6th China TDS

### 3. 各类膳食对总膳食摄入的贡献

在肉类、水产类、蛋类和乳类4类混合膳食样品中，氟苯尼考的膳食摄入贡献来自肉类（94.0%）、蛋类（5.5%）、水产类（0.4%）和乳类（0.1%）（图5-39和附表5-71）；氯霉素

### 3. Contributions of Food Categories to the Total Dietary Intake

Of the four categories of animal-derived composite samples, i.e., meats, aquatic foods, eggs, and dairy products, the dietary intake of florfenicol was contributed by meats (94.0%), eggs (5.5%), aquatic

的膳食摄入贡献来自肉类（80.0%）和水产类（20.0%）（图 5-40 和附表 5-74）；甲砜霉素的膳食摄入贡献来自肉类（91.7%）和蛋类（8.3%）（图 5-41 和附表 5-77）。

foods (0.4%), and dairy products (0.1%) (Figure 5-39 and Annexed Table 5-71). The dietary intake of chloramphenicol was contributed by meats (80.0%), and aquatic foods (20.0%) (Figure 5-40 and Annexed Table 5-74). The dietary intake of thiamphenicol was contributed by meats (91.7%) and eggs (8.3%) (Figure 5-41 and Annexed Table 5-77).

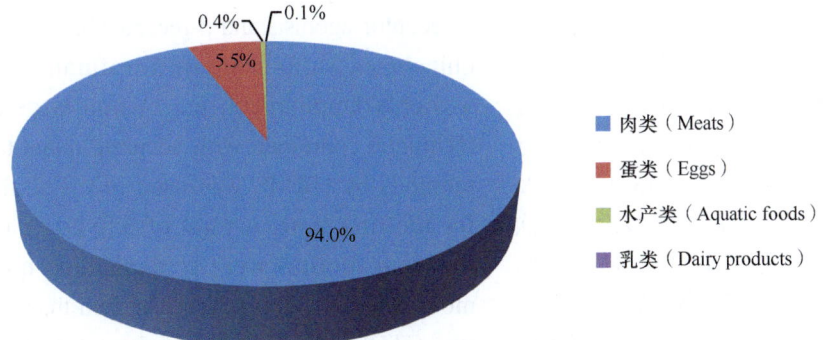

图 5-39　第六次中国总膳食研究氟苯尼考的膳食来源
Figure 5-39　Dietary sources of florfenicol from the 6$^{th}$ China TDS

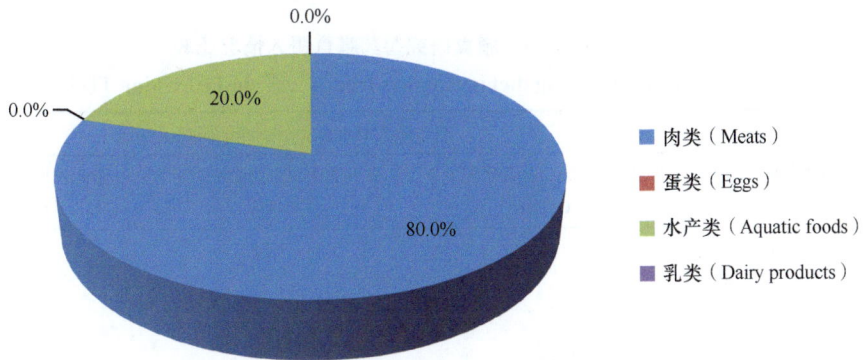

图 5-40　第六次中国总膳食研究氯霉素的膳食来源
Figure 5-40　Dietary sources of chloramphenicol from the 6$^{th}$ China TDS

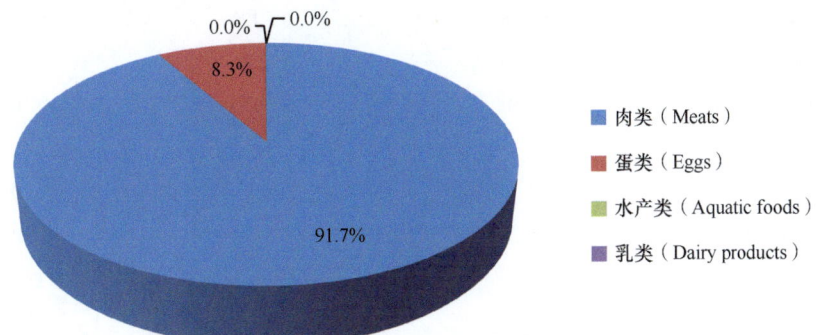

图 5-41　第六次中国总膳食研究甲砜霉素的膳食来源
Figure 5-41　Dietary sources of thiamphenicol from the 6$^{th}$ China TDS

## 四、与以往中国总膳食研究结果的比较

近三次中国总膳食研究的兽药摄入情况如表 5-3 所示。第四次和第五次中国总膳食研究中，采用液相色谱三重四极杆质谱方法对兽药进行分类定向检测，包括 β-受体激动剂和 β-受体阻断剂、四环素类、喹诺酮类、磺胺类、硝基呋喃类、甲硝唑和氯霉素等药物。第六次中国总膳食研究首次采用了以高分辨质谱非靶向筛查技术结合精准定量分析方法，共筛查并定量了 35 种药物及其代谢产物，检出药物种类多于前两次总膳食研究。三次中国总膳食研究的结果表明喹诺酮类、磺胺类、硝基咪唑类药物检出较多，且与磺胺类一同使用的抗菌增效剂甲氧苄啶也普遍检出。此外，值得关注的是氟苯尼考和结晶紫，

## IV. Comparison with Previous China TDSs Results

The veterinary drug intake of three China total diet studies is shown in Table 5-3. In the 4$^{th}$ and 5$^{th}$ China TDSs, liquid chromatography triple quadrupole mass spectrometry was used to conduct classification-directed detection of veterinary drugs, including β-receptor agonists and β-receptor blockers, tetracyclines, quinolones, sulfonamides, nitrofurans, metronidazole and chloramphenicol, etc. A non-targeted screening technique combined with accurate quantitative analysis methods by HRMS was used in the sixth China TDS for the first time. A total of 35 veterinary drugs and their metabolites were screened and quantified, and more veterinary drugs were detected than in the previous two CTDSs. The results of three CTDSs showed that quinolones, sulfonamides, and nitroimidazoles were more frequently detected, and trimethoprim, an

表 5-3 三次中国总膳食研究兽药膳食摄入情况比较
Table 5-3 Veterinary drug dietary intakes from 4$^{th}$, 5$^{th}$ and 6$^{th}$ China TDSs

| 兽药 Veterinary drugs | 膳食摄入 Dietary intakes/[ng/(kg bw·d)] | | |
|---|---|---|---|
| | 第四次中国总膳食研究 4$^{th}$ CTDS | 第五次中国总膳食研究 5$^{th}$ CTDS | 第六次中国总膳食研究 6$^{th}$ CTDS |
| β-受体激动剂和 β-受体阻断剂 β-receptor agonists and β-receptor blockers | 0～7.46 | 0～1.24 | * |
| 四环素类 Tetracyclines | 0～2.86 | 0～0.59 | * |
| 喹诺酮类 Quinolones | 0～72.2 | 2.22～119 | 0～35.4 |
| 磺胺类 Sulfonamides | 0～84.6 | 0～3.01 | 0～264 |
| 硝基咪唑类 Nitroimidazoles | 0～20.8 | 0～120 | 0～218 |
| 硝基呋喃类 Nitrofurans | 0～2.06 | 0～2.06 | — |
| 氯霉素 Chloramphenicol | 0～0.048 | 0～0.15 | 0～0.37 |
| 氟苯尼考 Florfenicol | — | — | 0～45.9 |
| 左旋咪唑 Levamisole | — | — | 0～2.55 |
| 苯并咪唑类 Benzimidazoles | — | — | 0～3.42 |
| 抗菌增效剂 Antibacterial synergist | — | — | 0～122 |
| 三苯甲烷类 Triphenylmethanes | — | — | 1.45～82.0 |

注："—"表示未开展检测；"*"表示未检出
Note: "—" indicates that this work was not carried out; "*" indicates that these drugs was not detected

前者在肉类和蛋类样品中有一定检出，而结晶紫则普遍存在于各类动物源性膳食食品中。与前两次中国总膳食研究相比，第六次中国总膳食研究的兽药摄入水平有一定的变化，但均处于很低的水平。

antibacterial synergist used together with sulfonamides, were also commonly detected. In addition, the veterinary drugs of florfenicol and crystal violet deserves attention. Florfenicol had certain detection in meats and eggs samples, while crystal violet was commonly found in various animal-derived dietary foods. Compared with the previous two China TDSs, the veterinary drug intake levels had some changes in the sixth China TDS, but all were at very low levels.

# 第六章　食品加工过程污染物的膳食暴露评估
# Chapter 6　Dietary Exposure Assessment of Contaminants from Food Processing

## 第一节　氯丙醇
## Section 1　Chloropropanols

### 一、背景

氯丙醇是丙三醇中的羟基被氯原子取代的一类化合物，包括3-氯-1,2-丙二醇（3-MCPD）与2-氯-1,3-丙二醇（2-MCPD）和1,3-二氯-2-丙醇（1,3-DCP）与2,3-二氯-1-丙醇（2,3-DCP）。酸水解植物蛋白（acid-HVP）可产生高浓度的氯丙醇，主要以3-MCPD和2-MCPD的形式存在。添加酸水解植物蛋白的调味产品如酱油、鸡精等可能造成氯丙醇的污染（Nyman et al.，2003）。热加工食品中也可能含有低水平的氯丙醇（Wenzl et al.，2007；Baer et al.，2010）。食品中污染水平最高的是3-MCPD。

2009年，国际食品法典委员会（CAC）建立了含有酸水解植物蛋白的液态调味料（不包括天然发酵酱油）中3-MCPD的最大残留限量为0.4 mg/kg。我国《食品安全国家标准 食品中污染物限量》（GB 2762—2022）规定了含有酸水解植物蛋白的液态调味品和固态调味品中3-MCPD的最大残留限量分别为0.4 mg/kg和1.0 mg/kg。

### 二、健康指导值

3-MCPD在大鼠中经口半数致死剂量（LD$_{50}$）为150 mg/(kg bw·d)；1 mg/(kg bw·d)的重复剂量可使动物精子

### I. Background

Chloropropanols are chemicals formed when the hydroxyl groups of glycerol are substituted by chlorine atoms, including 3-chloro-1,2-propanediol (3-MCPD), 2-chloro-1,3-propanediol (2-MCPD), 1,3-dichloro-2-propanol (1,3-DCP) and 2,3-dichloro-1-propanol (2,3-DCP). High concentration of chloropropanols, mainly in the form of 3-MCPD and 2-MCPD, can be found in the acid hydrolyzed vegetable protein (HVP). Condiments containing acid-HVP, such as soy sauce and chicken essence, may cause the contamination of chloropropanols (Nyman et al., 2003). Low levels of chloropropanols can also be found in hot-processed food (Wenzl et al. 2007; Baer et al. 2010). Among the 4 chloropropanols, the contamination level of 3-MCPD is the highest in food.

Codex Alimentarius Commission (CAC) established the maximum residue limit (MRL) for 3-MCPD in liquid condiments containing acid-HVP (excluding naturally fermented soy sauce) at the level of 0.4 mg/kg in 2009. The Chinese *National Food Safety Standard-Contaminant Limits in Foods* (GB 2762—2022) also has provisions on the maximum residue limits of 3-MCPD in liquid (0.4 mg/kg) and solid (1.0 mg/kg) condiments containing acid-HVP.

### II. HBGV

The oral LD$_{50}$ of 3-MCPD is 150 mg/(kg bw·d)

活性降低，导致雄性生殖能力受到损害；3-MCPD 还具有肾脏毒性和神经毒性（JECFA，2002b，2006）。1,3-DCP 在大鼠中经口 LD$_{50}$ 为 120～140 mg/(kg bw·d)；1,3-DCP 具有肾脏及肝脏毒性，在大鼠体内可诱发肝脏、肾脏、甲状腺等不同器官的肿瘤，体外试验表明 1,3-DCP 具有致突变作用和遗传毒性。JECFA 基于其本身的毒性认为不适合评估其容许摄入量（JECFA，2002b，2006）。1,3-DCP 和 2,3-DCP 均可引起小鼠的肝脏与肾脏损伤，2,3-DCP 引起的肾脏损伤比 1,3-DCP 严重（Omura et al.，1995）。2,3-DCP 可使大鼠附睾重量明显降低，2,3-DCP 和 1,3-DCP 可使精子数量减少（JECFA，2002b，2006）。

2001 年，JECFA 第 57 次会议以肾小管增生作为最低可见作用水平（LOEL），确定 3-MCPD 的暂定每日最大耐受摄入量（PMTDI）为 2 μg/(kg bw·d)。2018 年，JECFA 第 83 次会议根据最新毒理学研究结果，将 3-MCPD 的 PMTDI 由 2 μg/(kg bw·d) 修改为 4 μg/(kg bw·d)。2-MCPD 的毒性研究数据较为缺乏。第六次中国总膳食研究基于 2-MCPD 毒性与 3-MCPD 相同的假设，以 4 μg/(kg bw·d) 作为健康指导值来评估 2-MCPD 的暴露风险。

## 三、总膳食研究结果

对 24 个省（自治区、直辖市）的 12 类共 288 份混合膳食样品中 4 种氯丙醇 3-MCPD、2-MCPD、1,3-DCP 和 2,3-DCP 的含量进行测定，对未检出的样品以 1/2LOD 值进行污染水平分析和膳食暴露评估。

in rats; when 3-MCPD was given to rats at repeated doses in excess of 1 mg/(kg bw·d), it decreased sperm motility and impaired male fertility; in addition, 3-MCPD has nephrotoxicity and neurotoxicity(JECFA, 2002b, 2006). The oral LD$_{50}$ of 1,3-DCP ranged from 120 mg/(kg bw·d) to 140 mg/(kg bw·d) in rats, and research clearly indicated that 1,3-DCP was nephrotoxic, hepatotoxic, and induced a variety of tumours in various organs including liver, kidney and thyroid gland in rats, and was mutagenic and genotoxic *in vitro* (JECFA, 2002b, 2006). The committee concluded that it would be inappropriate to estimate a tolerable intake because of the nature of the toxicity. It was reported that both 1,3-DCP and 2,3-DCP cause damage to the kidney and liver in rats, but the damage caused by 2,3-DCP is far more serious (Omura et al., 1995). It has been found that 2,3-DCP can significantly reduce the weight of epididymis of rats, and that 2,3-DCP and 1,3-DCP can reduce the amount of sperms (JECFA, 2002b, 2006).

At the 57th JECFA meeting in 2001, JECFA established the provisional maximum tolerable daily intake (PMTDI) of 2 μg/(kg bw·d) for 3-MCPD on the basis of the lowest observed effect level (LOEL) for tubule hyperplasia. At the 83rd JECFA meeting in 2018, JECFA modified the PMTDI from 2 μg/(kg bw·d) to 4 μg/(kg bw·d) for 3-MCPD based on the latest toxicology studies. Toxicity data of 2-MCPD are relatively insufficient. The PMTDI of 4 μg/(kg bw·d) is used as HBGV in the 6th China TDS for 2-MCPD exposure risk based on the assumption that the toxicity of 2-MCPD was the same as that of 3-MCPD.

## III. TDS Results

A total of 288 TDS composite dietary samples of 12 categories from 24 provinces (autonomous regions, municipalities) were analyzed for the levels of 3-MCPD, 2-MCPD, 1,3-DCP and 2,3-DCP. The values of those sample with no detectable were assigned the value of half of the LOD in the contamination levels evaluation and the dietary exposure assessment.

**1. 混合膳食样品中氯丙醇的含量**

第六次中国总膳食研究的混合膳食样品中 3-MCPD 的污染水平为 ND～88.9 µg/kg，检出率为 30.6%，污染水平最高的是贵州的蔬菜类膳食样品；各类膳食的平均污染水平为 ND～17.4 µg/kg，总的平均污染水平为 3.5 µg/kg（附表 6-1）。在各类被 3-MCPD 污染的膳食中，污染水平的排序为蔬菜类（17.4 µg/kg）、薯类（6.1 µg/kg）、蛋类（4.8 µg/kg）、肉类（4.0 µg/kg）等，乳类、水果类、糖类和水及饮料类均未检出。各类膳食中 2-MCPD 的污染水平为 ND～19.2 µg/kg，检出率为 1.7%，仅在蔬菜、肉类、薯类和蛋类中检出，污染水平最高的是四川的蛋类膳食样品，总的平均污染水平为 0.4 µg/kg（附表 6-2）。各类膳食中 1,3-DCP 和 2,3-DCP 均未检出。

**2. 膳食暴露评估**

基于 3-MCPD 和 2-MCPD 的 PMTDI [4 µg/(kg bw·d)] 进行暴露评估。对均未检出 3-MCPD 的乳类、水果类、糖类和水及饮料类膳食样品，未进行摄入量评估。我国居民 3-MCPD 的平均膳食摄入量为 0.144 µg/(kg bw·d)，占 3-MCPD 的 PMTDI 的 3.6%（附表 6-3）。2-MCPD 的膳食摄入量评估仅针对检出的蔬菜类、薯类、肉类和蛋类进行，其平均膳食摄入量为 0.010 µg/(kg bw·d)，占 PMTDI 的 0.3%（附表 6-4）。我国各地区居民 3-MCPD 的膳食摄入量为 0.046～0.640 µg/(kg bw·d)，其中，膳食摄入量最高的是贵州，占 PMTDI 的 16.0%，最低的是辽宁，占 PMTDI 的 1.2%（图 6-1）。

**1. Levels of Chloropropanols in TDS Composite Samples**

In the 6$^{th}$ China TDS study, the contamination levels of 3-MCPD in the composite dietary samples were in the range of ND-88.9 µg/kg with the detection rate of 30.6%. The highest level of contamination for 3-MCPD was found in vegetables from Guizhou. The average contamination levels of each food category ranged from ND to 17.4 µg/kg with the total average contamination level of 3.5 µg/kg (Annexed Table 6-1). The food categories that were found to be contaminated by 3-MCPD, in a descending order of contamination level, were vegetables (17.4 µg/kg), potatoes (6.1 µg/kg), eggs (4.8 µg/kg) and meats (4.0 µg/kg), et al. 3-MCPD was not detected in dairy products, fruits, sugar and water and beverages. The contamination levels of 2-MCPD in the composite dietary samples were in the range of ND-19.2 µg/kg with the detection rate of 1.7%. 2-MCPD was only found in vegetables, potatoes, meats and eggs with the highest level of contamination in eggs from Sichuan. The total average contamination level was of 0.4 µg/kg (Annexed Table 6-2). 1,3-DCP and 2,3-DCP were not found in all the TDS composite samples.

**2. Dietary Exposure Assessment**

The exposure assessment was based on the PMTDI of 4 µg/(kg bw·d) for 3-MCPD and 2-MCPD. The intake assessment was not performed for samples without 3-MCPD detection such as dairy products, fruits, sugar, water and beverages.

The average dietary intake of 3-MCPD for China residents was 0.144 µg/(kg bw·d), accounting for 3.6% of the PMTDI value for 3-MCPD as shown in Annexed Table 6-3. The intake assessment of 2-MCPD was performed for samples such as vegetables, potatoes, meats and eggs. The average dietary intake of 2-MCPD for China residents was 0.010 µg/(kg bw·d), accounting for 0.3% of the PMTDI value for 2-MCPD as shown in Annexed Table 6-4. The dietary exposure of 3-MCPD for the population from the 24 provinces (autonomous

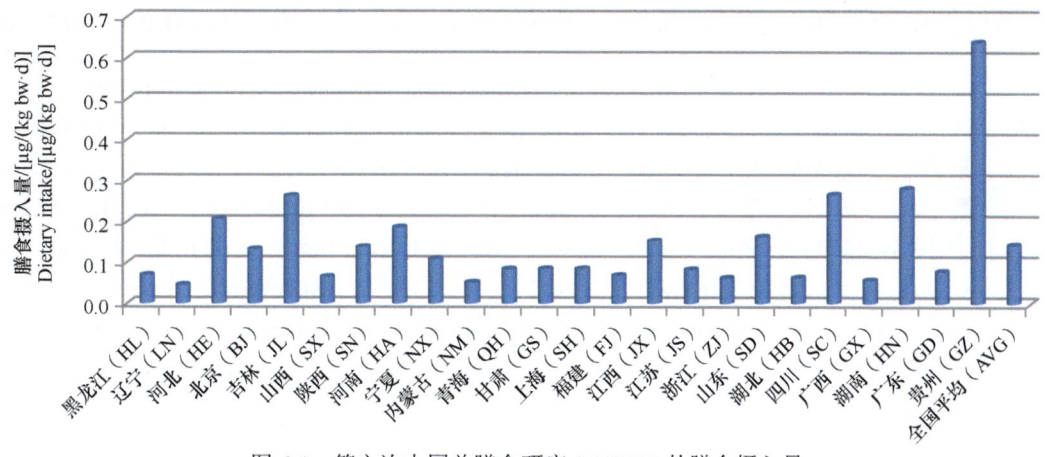

图 6-1 第六次中国总膳食研究 3-MCPD 的膳食摄入量
Figure 6-1　Dietary intake of 3-MCPD from the 6th China TDS

**3. 各类膳食对总膳食摄入的贡献**

第六次中国总膳食研究的膳食 3-MCPD 主要来源于蔬菜类（69.2%）、谷类（16.4%）、薯类（5.0%）、肉类（4.3%），其占总摄入量的 94.9%，其余膳食样品的贡献率均小于 3%（附表 6-5，图 6-2）。

regions, municipalities) ranged from 0.046 μg/(kg bw·d) to 0.640 μg/(kg bw·d) (Figure 6-1), with the highest level in Guizhou accounting for 16.0% of PMTDI and the lowest level in Liaoning accounting for 1.2% of PMTDI.

**3. Contributions of Food Categories to the Total Dietary Intake**

The primary sources of 3-MCPD dietary intake identified in the 6th CTDS are vegetables (69.2%), cereals (16.4%), potatoes (5.0%) and meats (4.3%), accounting for over 94.9%, the contribution of other dietary samples was less than 3% as shown in Annexed Table 6-5 and Figure 6-2.

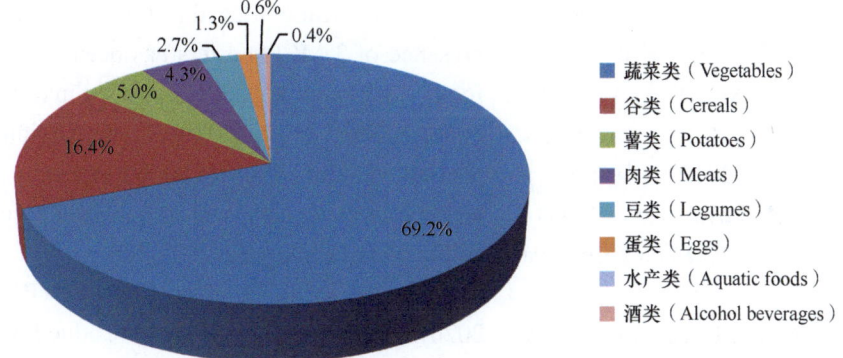

图 6-2 第六次中国总膳食研究 3-MCPD 的膳食来源
Figure 6-2　Dietary sources of 3-MCPD from the 6th China TDS

## 四、与以往中国总膳食研究结果的比较

自第四次中国总膳食研究以来，我国连续开展膳食样品 3-MCPD 的检测，第四次、第五次、第六次中国总膳食研究的我国居民 3-MCPD 膳食摄入量分别为 0.398 μg/(kg bw·d)、0.250 μg/(kg bw·d) 和 0.144 μg/(kg bw·d)。与第五次结果相比，第六次中国总膳食研究的膳食摄入量下降了 42.4%。

## Ⅳ. Comparison with the Previous China TDSs

China has continuously carried out 3-MCPD detection in dietary samples since the 4th China TDS. The dietary intakes of 3-MCPD for the general Chinese population were 0.398 μg/(kg bw·d), 0.250 μg/(kg bw·d) and 0.144 μg/(kg bw·d) in the 4th, the 5th and the 6th China TDSs, respectively. The dietary intakes of 3-MCPD from the 6th China TDS declined 42.4% in comparison with that of 5th China TDS.

# 第二节　氯丙醇酯
# Section 2　Chloropropanol Fatty Acid Esters

## 一、背景

氯丙醇脂肪酸酯（氯丙醇酯）是近年来发现的存在于含脂肪食品中的一类新型污染物，其主要在食品加工过程中，尤其是在油脂精炼过程中形成（Franke et al., 2009）。氯丙醇酯包括单氯取代的 3-氯-1,2-丙二醇脂肪酸酯（3-MCPD 酯）和 2-氯-1,3-丙二醇脂肪酸酯（2-MCPD 酯），以及双氯取代的 1,3-二氯-2-丙醇脂肪酸酯（1,3-DCP 酯）和 2,3-二氯-1-丙醇脂肪酸酯（2,3-DCP 酯）。其中，在食品中含量较高、比较典型的是 3-MCPD 酯（Zelinková et al., 2006）。近年来在许多食品中发现的不同水平的 3-MCPD 酯（Doležal et al., 2005，2009；Zelinková et al., 2006；Küsters et al., 2010），甚至母乳中也有存在（Zelinková et al., 2008），尤以精炼食用油中含量最高（Zelinková et al., 2006）。

2020 年，欧盟 EU2020/1322 号法令规定了食用植物油脂和婴幼儿食品中 3-MCPD 酯的最大残留限量，其中椰子、玉米、菜籽、橄榄（橄榄渣油

## Ⅰ. Background

Chloropropanol fatty acid esters (CPFAEs) are a new group of contaminants found in fat-containing foods in recent years, which are mainly created during food processing, especially in the process of oil refining (Franke et al., 2009). CPFAEs include 3-monochloropropane-1,2-diol esters (3-MCPD esters), 2-monochloropropane-1,3-diol esters (2-MCPD esters), 1,3-dichloropropan-2-molesters (1,3-DCP esters) and 2,3-dichloropropan-1-molesters (2,3-DCP esters). Among these four classes of CPFAEs, 3-MCPD esters are typical detected with a higher contamination level in foods (Zelinková et al., 2006). In recent years the presence of 3-MCPD esters has been observed in many foods (Doležal et al., 2005, 2009; Zelinková et al., 2006, 2008; Küsters et al., 2010) even including breast milk (Zelinková et al., 2008) with the varying contamination levels in recent years, with the highest levels in refined edible oils (Zelinková et al., 2006).

The European Union directive (EU2020/1322, 2020) established the maximum residue limit (MRL) for 3-MCPD esters in edible vegetable oils and infant foods. The MRL is 1250 μg/kg in unrefined/refined oil and fats of coconut, corn, rapeseed, olive (excluding pomace

除外）、葵花、大豆和棕榈仁的未精炼油、精炼油与脂肪，以及这类油脂的混合物中 3-MCPD 酯的最大残留限量为 1250 μg/kg，其他精炼植物油（包括橄榄渣油）、鱼油和其他海洋生物油脂的最大残留限量为 2500 μg/kg，用于生产婴幼儿食品（婴幼儿谷类加工食品和幼儿配方奶粉）的植物油和脂肪的限量为 750 μg/kg，粉状和液状婴幼儿配方奶粉、婴幼儿特医食品中的限量分别为 125 μg/kg 和 15 μg/kg。

## 二、健康指导值

氯丙醇酯的直接毒性尚不明确，对氯丙醇酯的风险评估主要基于其在体内 100% 水解为相应氯丙醇的假设。2018年，JECFA 基于 3-MCPD 酯完全水解为 3-MCPD 并以肾小管增生作为最低可见作用水平，提出 3-MCPD 酯的暂定每日最大耐受摄入量（PMTDI）为 4 μg/(kg bw·d)。2-MCPD 酯的毒性研究数据较为缺乏，第六次中国总膳食研究基于 2-MCPD 酯毒性与 3-MCPD 酯相同的假设，以 4 μg/(kg bw·d) 作为健康指导值来评估 2-MCPD 酯的暴露风险。

## 三、总膳食研究结果

对 24 个省（自治区、直辖市）的 12 类共 288 份混合膳食样品中 3-MCPD 酯和 2-MCPD 酯的含量进行测定，对未检出的样品以 1/2 LOD 值进行污染水平分析和膳食暴露评估。

**1. 混合膳食样品中 3-氯丙醇酯和 2-氯丙醇酯的含量**

第六次中国总膳食研究的混合膳食样品中 3-MCPD 酯的污染水平为 ND～4390 μg/kg，检出率为 87.2%，污染水平最高的是浙江的蛋类膳食样品；各类膳食的平均污染水平为 2.6～279.4 μg/kg，

olive oil), sunflower, soybean and palm kernel, and the mixtures. The MRL is 2500 μg/kg in the other refined vegetable oils (include pomace olive oil), fish oils and the other marine organism fats. The MRL is 750 μg/kg in the vegetable oils and fats used in the production of infant foods, processed infant cereals and infant formula. The MRLs are 125 μg/kg in powdered and 15 μg/kg in liquid infant formula, special medical foods for infants.

## II. HBGV

The direct toxicity of CPFAEs is not clear, and the risk assessment is based on the assumption of its 100% *in vivo* hydrolysis to the corresponding chloropropanol. In 2018, JECFA proposed that the provisional PMTDI of 3-MCPD esters was 4 μg/(kg bw·d) based on the complete hydrolysis of 3-MCPD esters to 3-MCPD and renal tubule proliferation as the lowest observed effect level. Toxicity data of 2-MCPD esters are relatively insufficient. The PMTDI of 4 μg/(kg bw·d) is used as HBGV in the 6th China TDS for 2-MCPD esters exposure risk based on the assumption that the toxicity of 2-MCPD esters was the same as that of 3-MCPD esters.

## III. TDS Results

A total of 288 TDS composite dietary samples of 12 categories from 24 provinces (autonomous regions, municipalities) were analyzed for the levels of 3-MCPD esters and 2-MCPD esters. The values of those samples with no detectable were assigned the value of half of the LOD in the contamination levels evaluation and the dietary exposure assessment.

**1. Levels of 3-MCPD Esters and 2-MCPD Esters in TDS Composite Samples**

In the 6th China TDS, the contamination levels of 3-MCPD esters in the composite dietary samples were in the range of ND-4390 μg/kg with the detection rate of 87.2%. The highest contamination level for 3-MCPD esters was found in eggs from Zhejiang. The

总的平均污染水平为52.9 μg/kg（附表6-6）。在各类被3-MCPD酯污染的膳食中，污染水平的排序为蛋类（279.4 μg/kg）、蔬菜类（85.0 μg/kg）、肉类（80.8 μg/kg）、薯类（58.9 μg/kg）、水产类（58.2 μg/kg）、豆类（28.9 μg/kg）等。

第六次中国总膳食研究的混合膳食样品中2-MCPD酯的污染水平为ND～837.0 μg/kg，检出率为41.3%，污染水平最高的是浙江的蛋类膳食样品；各类膳食的平均污染水平为ND～58.8 μg/kg，总的平均污染水平为11.9 μg/kg（附表6-7）。在各类膳食中，2-MCPD酯污染水平的排序为蛋类（58.8 μg/kg）、蔬菜类（23.3 μg/kg）、肉类（16.8 μg/kg）、水产类（16.6 μg/kg）、薯类（15.6 μg/kg）、豆类（7.6 μg/kg）等。乳类、水果类、酒类、水及饮料类均未检出2-MCPD酯。

**2. 膳食暴露评估**

基于3-MCPD酯和2-MCPD酯PMTDI [4 μg/(kg bw·d)]进行暴露评估，对均未检出2-MCPD的乳类、水果类、酒类、水及饮料类膳食样品，未进行摄入量评估。我国居民3-MCPD酯的平均膳食摄入量为1.074 μg/(kg bw·d)，占3-MCPD的PMTDI的26.8%（附表6-8）；2-MCPD酯的平均膳食摄入量为0.258 μg/(kg bw·d)，占PMTDI的6.4%（附表6-9）。我国各地区居民3-MCPD酯的膳食摄入量为0.364～3.513 μg/(kg bw·d)，其中，膳食摄入量最高的是浙江，占PMTDI的87.8%，最低的是山西，占PMTDI的9.1%（图6-3）；2-MCPD酯的膳食摄入量为0.056～0.898 μg/(kg bw·d)，其中，膳食摄入量最高的是福建，占PMTDI的22.5%，最低的是辽宁，占PMTDI的1.4%（图6-4）。

average contamination levels of each food category ranged from 2.6 μg/kg to 279.4 μg/kg with the total average contamination level of 52.9 μg/kg (Annexed Table 6-6). The food categories that were found to be contaminated by 3-MCPD esters, in a descending order of contamination level, were eggs (279.4 μg/kg), vegetables (85.0 μg/kg), meats (80.8 μg/kg), potatoes (58.9 μg/kg), aquatic foods (58.2 μg/kg) and legumes (28.9 μg/kg), et al.

In the 6th China TDS, the contamination levels of 2-MCPD esters in the composite dietary samples were in the range of ND-837.0 μg/kg with the detection rate of 41.3%. The highest level of contamination for 2-MCPD esters was found in eggs from Zhejiang. The average contamination levels of each food category ranged from ND to 58.8 μg/kg with the total average contamination level of 11.9 μg/kg (Annexed Table 6-7). The food categories that were found to be contaminated by 2-MCPD esters, in a descending order of contamination level, were eggs (58.8 μg/kg), vegetables (23.3 μg/kg), meats (16.8 μg/kg), aquatic foods (16.6 μg/kg), potatoes (15.6 μg/kg) and legumes (7.6 μg/kg), et al. 2-MCPD esters were not detected in dairy products, fruits, alcohol beverages, and water and beverages.

**2. Dietary Exposure Assessment**

The exposure assessment was based on the PMTDI of 4 μg/(kg bw·d) for 3-MCPD esters and 2-MCPD esters. The intake assessment was not performed for samples without 2-MCPD esters detection such as dairy products, fruits, alcohol beverages, water and beverages. The average dietary intake of 3-MCPD esters for China residents was 1.074 μg/(kg bw·d), accounting for 26.8% of the PMTDI value for 3-MCPD esters as shown in Annexed Table 6-8. The average dietary intake of 2-MCPD esters for China residents was 0.258 μg/(kg bw·d), accounting for 6.4% of the PMTDI value for 2-MCPD esters as shown in Annexed Table 6-9. The dietary 3-MCPD esters exposure for the population from the 24 provinces (autonomous regions, municipalities) ranged from 0.364 μg/(kg bw·d) to 3.513 μg/(kg bw · d) (Figure 6-3), with the highest level in Zhejiang accounting for 87.8% of PMTDI and the lowest level in Shanxi accounting for 9.1% of PMTDI. The dietary 2-MCPD esters exposure for the population from the 24 provinces (autonomous regions, municipalities) ranged from 0.056 μg/(kg bw · d) to 0.898 μg/(kg bw · d) (Figure 6-4), with the highest level in Fujian accounting for 22.5% of PMTDI and the lowest level in Liaoning accounting for 1.4% of PMTDI.

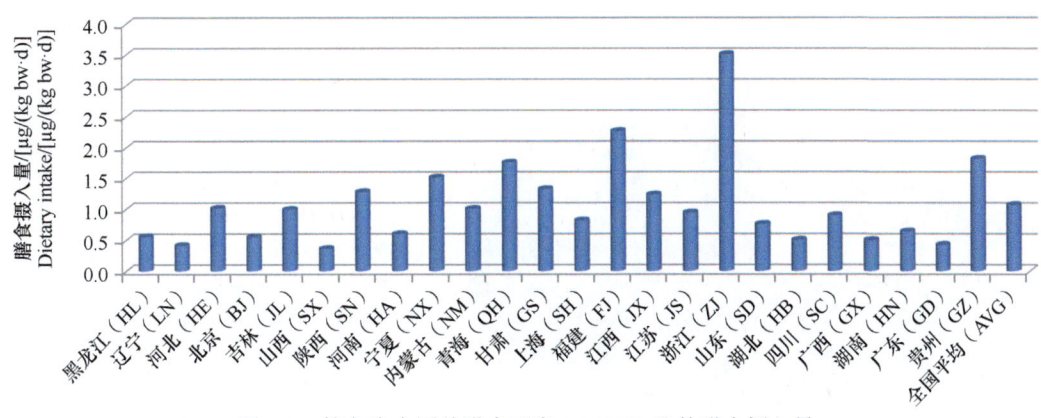

图 6-3　第六次中国总膳食研究 3-MCPD 酯的膳食摄入量

Figure 6-3　Dietary intake of 3-MCPD esters from the 6$^{th}$ China TDS

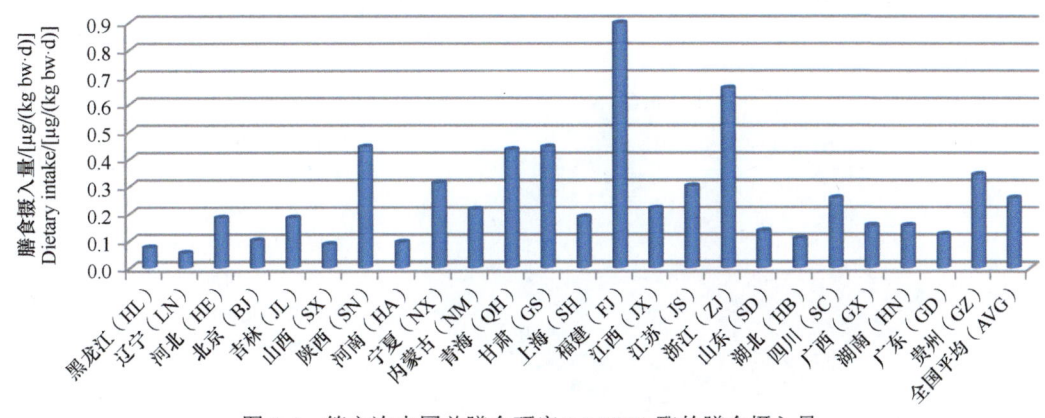

图 6-4　第六次中国总膳食研究 2-MCPD 酯的膳食摄入量

Figure 6-4　Dietary intake of 2-MCPD esters from the 6$^{th}$ China TDS

### 3. 各类膳食对总膳食摄入的贡献

第六次中国总膳食研究的膳食 3-MCPD 酯主要来源于蔬菜类（43.5%）、谷类（15.1%）、蛋类（12.1%）、肉类（9.3%）、薯类（8.2%）、水及饮料类（5.6%）、豆类（3.1%），占总摄入量的

### 3. Contributions of Food Categories to the Total Dietary Intake

The primary sources of 3-MCPD esters dietary intake identified in the 6$^{th}$ China TDS are vegetables (43.5%), cereals (15.1%), eggs (12.1%), meats (9.3%), potatoes (8.2%), water and beverages (5.6%), legumes

96.9%，其余5类膳食样品的贡献率均小于3%（附表6-10，图6-5）。

第六次中国总膳食研究的膳食 2-MCPD 酯主要来源于蔬菜类（49.4%）、谷类（15.9%）、蛋类（10.6%）、薯类（9.4%）、肉类（8.0%）、水产类（3.4%）、豆类（3.3%），占总摄入量的100%（附表6-11，图6-6）。

(3.1%), accounting for over 96.9%, each of other 5 food categories is lower than 3%, as shown in Annexed Table 6-10 and Figure 6-5.

The primary sources of 2-MCPD esters dietary intake identified in the 6th China TDS are vegetables (49.4%), cereals (15.9%), eggs (10.6%), potatoes (9.4%), meats (8.0%), aquatic foods (3.4%), legumes (3.3%), accounting for 100% of total intake, as shown in Annexed Table 6-11 and Figure 6-6.

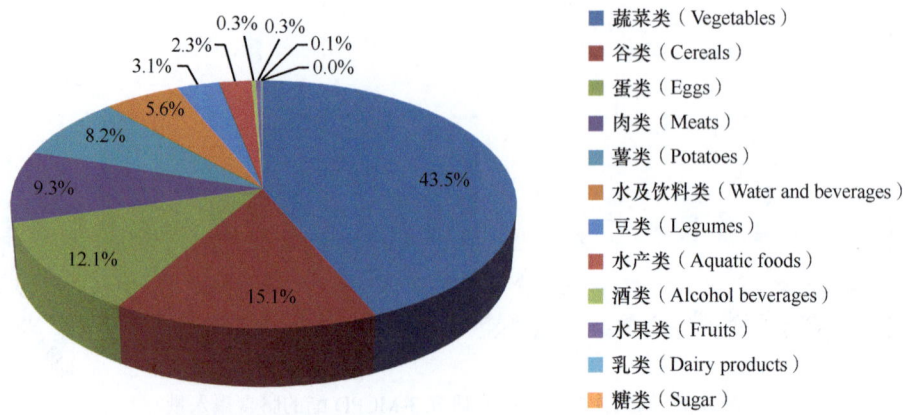

图 6-5　第六次中国总膳食研究 3-MCPD 酯的膳食来源
Figure 6-5　Dietary sources of 3-MCPD esters from the 6th China TDS

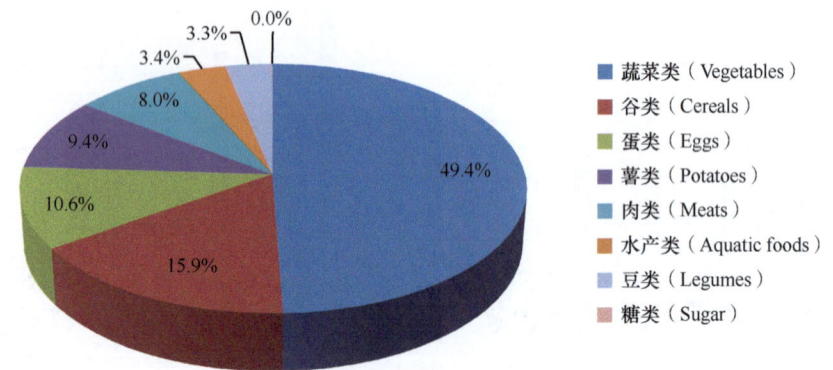

图 6-6　第六次中国总膳食研究 2-MCPD 酯的膳食来源
Figure 6-6　Dietary sources of 2-MCPD esters from the 6th China TDS

## 四、与以往中国总膳食研究结果的比较

我国从第五次中国总膳食研究开始开展膳食样品 3-MCPD 酯的检测，第五次、第六次中国总膳食研究的

## Ⅳ. Comparison with the Previous China TDSs Results

China has continuously carried out 3-MCPD esters detection in dietary samples since the 5th China TDS. The dietary intakes of 3-MCPD esters for the general

3-MCPD 酯的膳食摄入量分别为 1.32 μg/(kg bw·d) 和 1.07 μg/(kg bw·d)。与第五次中国总膳食研究结果相比，第六次中国总膳食研究的膳食摄入量下降了 18.9%。

Chinese population were 1.32 μg/(kg bw · d) and 1.07 μg/(kg bw · d) in the 5$^{th}$ and the 6$^{th}$ China TDS, respectively. The dietary intake of 3-MCPD esters from the 6$^{th}$ China TDS declined 18.9% in comparison with that of 5$^{th}$ China TDS.

## 第三节　缩水甘油酯
## Section 3　Glycidyl Fatty Acid Esters

### 一、背景

缩水甘油脂肪酸酯（缩水甘油酯）是近年来发现的一类新型食品污染物，其主要在食品加工过程中，尤其是在油脂高温精炼过程中形成。缩水甘油酯是缩水甘油（glycidol）的羟基被长链脂肪酸取代的一类单酯化合物。缩水甘油酯主要存在于高温精炼食用油，以及以其为原料加工的食品中（Küsters et al., 2011；Yan et al., 2018）。

2018 年，欧盟 EU2018/290 号法令规定了植物油脂和婴幼儿食品中缩水甘油酯的最大残留限量，其中食用植物油脂中缩水甘油酯的最大残留限量为 1000 μg/kg，用于生产婴儿食品和婴幼儿谷类加工食品的植物油脂的最大残留限量为 500 μg/kg，粉状和液状婴幼儿配方奶粉、婴幼儿特医食品的最大残留限量分别为 50 μg/kg 和 6.0 μg/kg。

### 二、健康指导值

对缩水甘油酯的风险评估主要基于其在体内 100% 水解为缩水甘油的假设。缩水甘油具有遗传毒性和致癌性，国际癌症研究机构（IARC）将其列为 2A 类致癌物，急性经口毒性试验表明，大鼠的 LD$_{50}$ 为 20～850 mg/kg bw，小鼠的 LD$_{50}$ 为 450 mg/kg bw。JECFA 和 EFSA 等均未制定缩水甘油酯的健康指

### I. Background

Glycidyl fatty acid esters (GFAEs) are a group of new food contaminants in recent years, which are mainly created during food processing, especially in the process of oil refining at high temperature. GFAEs are a monoester compounds in which the hydroxyl group of glycidol is replaced by long chain fatty acids. GFAEs is mainly found in high-temperature refined edible oil and food processed with it as raw material (Küsters et al., 2011; Yan et al., 2018).

The European Union directive (EU2018/290) established the MRLs for GFAEs in edible vegetable oils and infant foods. The MRL is 1000 μg/kg in edible vegetable oil. The MRL is 500 μg/kg in the vegetable oils and fats used in the production of infant foods and processed infant cereals foods. The MRLs are 50 μg/kg in powdered and 6.0 μg/kg in liquid infant formula, special medical foods for infants.

### II. HBGV

The risk assessment for GFAEs is based on the assumption of its 100% *in vivo* hydrolysis to glycidol. Glycidol has genotoxicity and carcinogenicity, and has been classified as a class 2A carcinogen by the International Agency for Research on Cancer (IARC). Acute oral toxicity test showed that its LD$_{50}$ was 20-850 mg/kg bw in rats and 450 mg/kg bw in mice. JECFA and EFSA have not established the HBGV of GFAEs. Currently, the evaluation of GFAEs is mainly based on

导值，目前对缩水甘油酯的评估主要基于暴露边界值（MOE）方法。MOE 的计算是缩水甘油暴露水平除以基准剂量 T25（使 25% 动物在特定组织部位发生肿瘤的慢性剂量，10.2 mg/kg bw）。EFSA（2016）认为，当 MOE＞25 000 时，该物质具有较低的公共卫生关注度。

## 三、总膳食研究结果

对 24 个省（自治区、直辖市）的 12 类共 288 份混合膳食样品中缩水甘油酯的含量进行测定，对未检出的样品以 1/2 LOD 值进行污染水平分析和膳食暴露评估。

### 1. 混合膳食样品中缩水甘油酯的含量

第六次中国总膳食研究的混合膳食样品中缩水甘油酯的污染水平为 ND～1294 μg/kg，检出率为 74.3%，污染水平最高的是浙江的蛋类膳食样品；各类膳食的平均污染水平为 ND～103.1 μg/kg，总的平均污染水平为 31.8 μg/kg（附表 6-12）。在各类膳食中，缩水甘油酯污染水平的排序为蛋类（103.1 μg/kg）、蔬菜类（78.7 μg/kg）、肉类（71.0 μg/kg）、水产类（38.5 μg/kg）、薯类（37.6 μg/kg）、豆类（26.8 μg/kg）等，水果类未检出。

### 2. 膳食暴露评估

我国居民缩水甘油酯的平均膳食摄入量为 0.787 μg/(kg bw·d)，MOE 为 12 963（附表 6-13）。我国各地区居民缩水甘油酯的膳食摄入量为 0.261～2.039 μg/(kg bw·d)，其中，膳食摄入量最高的是陕西，MOE 为 39 112，最低的是辽宁，MOE 为 5002（图 6-7）。

the margin of exposure (MOE) approach. The MOE value was calculated by dividing the exposure level of glycidol by the baseline dose of T25 (10.2 mg/kg bw, the chronic dose that causes tumours at specific tissue sites in 25% of animals). EFSA (2016) considers the substance to be of low public health concern when MOE>25 000.

## III. TDS Results

A total of 288 TDS composite dietary samples of 12 categories from 24 provinces (autonomous regions, municipalities) were analyzed for the levels of GFAEs. The values of those samples with no detectable were assigned the value of half of the LOD in the contamination levels evaluation and the dietary exposure assessment.

### 1. Levels of GFAEs in TDS Composite Samples

In the 6$^{th}$ China TDS study, the contamination levels of GFAEs in the composite dietary samples were in the range of ND-1294 μg/kg with the detection rate of 74.3%. The highest level of contamination for GFAEs was found in eggs from Zhejiang. The average contamination levels of each food category ranged from ND to 103.1 μg/kg with the total average contamination level of 31.8 μg/kg (Annexed Table 6-12). The food categories that were found to be contaminated by GFAEs, in a descending order of contamination level, were eggs (103.1 μg/kg), vegetables (78.7 μg/kg), meats (71.0 μg/kg), aquatic foods (38.5 μg/kg), potatoes (37.6 μg/kg) and legumes (26.8 μg/kg), et al. GFAEs were not detected in fruits.

### 2. Dietary Exposure Assessment

The average dietary intake of GFAEs for China residents was 0.787 μg/(kg bw·d), accounting for the MOE of 12 963 as shown in Annexed Table 6-13. The dietary GFAEs exposure for the population from the 24 provinces (autonomous regions, municipalities) ranged from 0.261 μg/(kg bw·d) to 2.039 μg/(kg

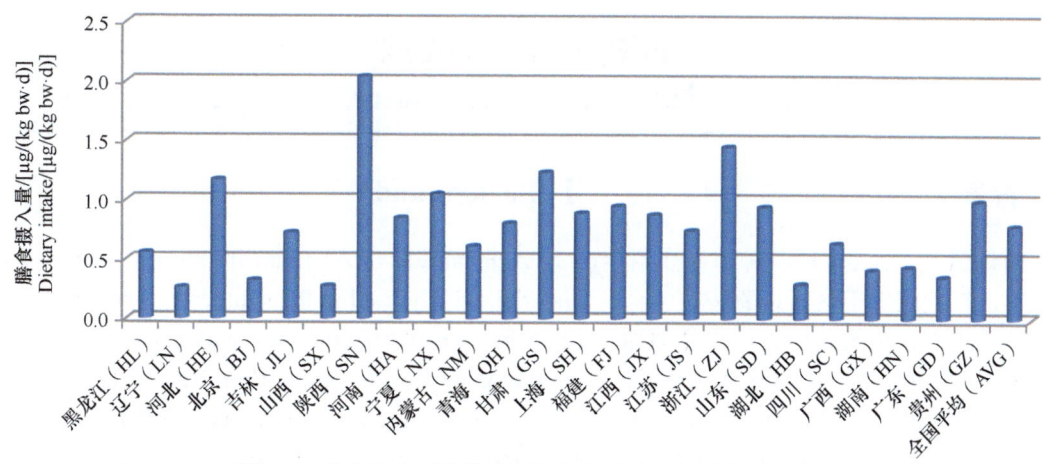

图 6-7 第六次中国总膳食研究缩水甘油酯的膳食摄入量

Figure 6-7 Dietary intake of glycidyl fatty acid esters from the 6$^{th}$ China TDS

### 3. 各类膳食对总膳食摄入量的贡献

第六次中国总膳食研究的膳食缩水甘油酯主要来源于蔬菜类（51.4%）、肉类（11.9%）、谷类（9.4%）、薯类（7.6%）、水及饮料类（6.7%）、蛋类（6.1%）、豆类（4.0%），占总摄入量的97.1%，其余5类膳食样品的贡献率均小于3%（附表6-14，图6-8）。

bw·d) (Figure 6-7), with the highest level in Shaanxi accounting for the MOE of 39 112 and the lowest level in Liaoning accounting for the MOE of 5002.

### 3. Contributions of Food Categories to the Total Dietary Intake

The primary sources of GFAEs dietary intake identified in the 6$^{th}$ China TDS are vegetables (51.4%), meats (11.9%), cereals (9.4%), potatoes (7.6%), water and beverages (6.7%), eggs (6.1%), legumes (4.0%), accounting for over 97.1%, each of other 5 food categories is lower than 3%, as shown in Annexed Table 6-14 and Figure 6-8.

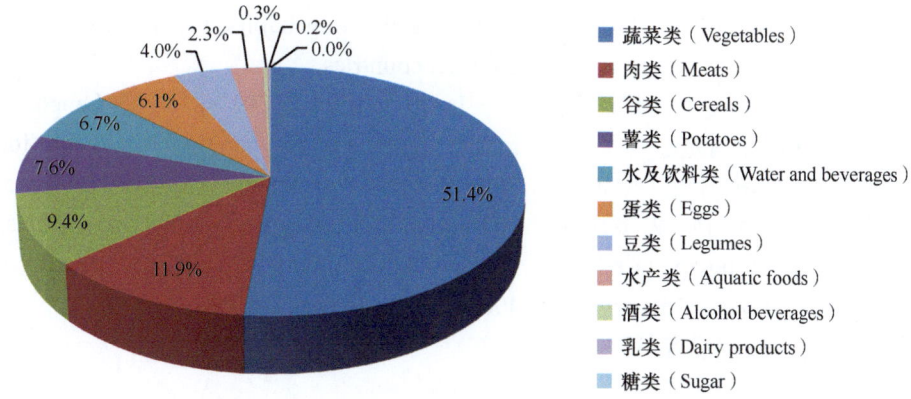

图 6-8 第六次中国总膳食研究缩水甘油酯的膳食来源

Figure 6-8 Dietary sources of glycidyl fatty acid esters from the 6$^{th}$ China TDS

# 第四节 丙烯酰胺
# Section 4　Acrylamide

## 一、背景

丙烯酰胺（AA）是一种重要的化工原料，广泛应用于聚丙烯酰胺塑料合成、油漆生产、污水处理、化妆品添加剂等领域。2002年，瑞典国家食品管理局（NFA）和斯德哥尔摩大学率先报道，淀粉类食物中检出相当含量的丙烯酰胺。研究表明，在某些食品烹制过程中，食品中氨基酸（主要是天冬酰胺）和羰基化合物（主要是还原糖如葡萄糖）加热到100℃以上时发生美拉德反应（Maillard reaction），可以形成丙烯酰胺。

2005年2月，联合国粮食及农业组织（FAO）和世界卫生组织（WHO）食品添加剂联合专家委员会（JECFA）第64次会议对食品中丙烯酰胺进行了系统的危险性评估。2011年，FAO/WHO食品添加剂联合专家委员会对丙烯酰胺膳食摄入量进行评估，结果表明普通人群的日摄入量平均约为1 μg/(kg bw·d)，最高摄入量约为4 μg/(kg bw·d)。由于不同国家烹饪、饮食习惯的不同，各国的丙烯酰胺摄入量有所差异。

2018年，欧盟实施关于丙烯酰胺的法案EU 2017/2158，规定了某些包装食品中丙烯酰胺的基准含量，限定范围在300～850 μg/kg，其中，大多数谷类早餐食品设定为300 μg/kg，饼干和曲奇为350 μg/kg，薯片为750 μg/kg，速溶咖啡为850 μg/kg，烘焙咖啡为400 μg/kg。

## Ⅰ. Background

Acrylamide (AA) is an important chemical raw material, widely used in the synthesis of polyacrylamide plastics, paint production, wastewater treatment, cosmetic additives, and other fields. The Swedish National Food Agency and Stockholm University firstly revealed the considerable presence of acrylamide in starchy foods in 2002. Researches found that acrylamide can be formed in the cooking process at a temperature up to 100°C by Maillard reaction, especially amino acids (mainly asparagine) and carbonyl compounds (mainly reducing sugar such as glucose) existed.

In February 2005, United Nations Food and Agriculture Organization (FAO) and World Health Organization (WHO) conducted a systematic risk assessment of acrylamide in food in the 64$^{th}$ meeting of the Joint FAO / WHO Expert Committee on Food Additives (JECFA). In 2011, the Joint FAO / WHO Expert Committee on Food Additives (JECFA) evaluated the dietary intake of acrylamide, and the results showed that the average daily intake of the general population was approximately 1 μg/(kg bw·d), and the maximum intake was about 4 μg/(kg bw·d). Due to different cooking and eating habits, the dietary intake varies in different countries.

In 2018, the EU 2017/2158 set benchmark levels for the presence of acrylamide in packaging foods (300-850 μg/kg). Most cereals breakfast foods are set to 300 μg/kg, 350 μg/kg for biscuits and cookies, 750 μg/kg for potato chips, 850 μg/kg for instant coffee, and 400 μg/kg for roasted coffee.

## 二、健康指导值

JECFA 和欧洲食品安全局（EFSA）等均未制定丙烯酰胺的健康指导值，目前对丙烯酰胺的健康风险评估主要基于暴露边界值（MOE）方法。丙烯酰胺被国际癌症研究机构（IARC）列为 2A 类致癌物，JECFA（2011a）确定的丙烯酰胺无可见不良作用水平（NOAEL）为 0.2 mg/(kg bw·d)，且 JECFA 提出丙烯酰胺诱导大鼠乳腺肿瘤的 $BMDL_{10}$（10% 反应的基准计量）为 0.31 mg/(kg bw·d)，诱导小鼠哈德氏腺肿瘤的 $BMDL_{10}$ 为 0.18 mg/(kg bw·d)。2015 年，EFSA 采用基准剂量（BMD）法得到丙烯酰胺致癌性的 $BMDL_{10}$ 为 0.17 mg/(kg bw·d)。在本次暴露评估中，基于 JECFA 的 $BMDL_{10}$ 值，通过 MOE 方法，评估丙烯酰胺的暴露风险，当 MOE<10 000 时，认为致癌风险需要优先关注，MOE≥10 000 时，则致癌风险无需优先关注。

## 三、总膳食研究结果

对 24 个省（自治区、直辖市）的 12 类共 288 份混合膳食样品中丙烯酰胺的含量进行测定，对未检出的样品，以 1/2 LOD 值进行污染水平分析和膳食暴露评估。

### 1. 混合膳食样品中丙烯酰胺的含量

第六次中国总膳食研究的混合样品中丙烯酰胺污染水平为 ND～176.90 μg/kg，检出率为 73.3%；各类膳食的平均污染水平为 0.50～18.53 μg/kg，总的平均污染水平为 6.08 μg/kg（附表 6-15）。在各类膳食中，丙烯酰胺污染水平的排序为蔬菜类（18.53 μg/kg）、薯类（17.74 μg/kg）、糖类（14.60 μg/kg）、豆类（7.28 μg/kg）等，水及饮料类最低（0.50 μg/kg）。

## II. HBGV

The health-based guidance value of acrylamide has not been formulated by JECFA, EFSA and other organizations. The risk to health of acrylamide is evaluated by the margin of exposure (MOE) method. Acrylamide is listed as 2A carcinogen by the International Agency for Research on Cancer (IARC). JECFA (2011a) noted that the no observed adverse effect level (NOAEL) for acrylamide was 0.2 mg/(kg bw·d). Moreover, JECFA proposed two different $BMDL_{10}$ (lower limit on the benchmark dose for a 10% response) for acrylamide: 0.31 mg/(kg bw·d) for the induction of mammary tumours in rats and 0.18 mg/(kg bw·d) for Harderian gland tumours in mice. In 2015, EFSA obtained $BMDL_{10}$ of acrylamide carcinogenicity by BMD method, which was 0.17 mg/(kg bw·d). In this exposure assessment, based on the $BMDL_{10}$ value of JECFA, the exposure risk of acrylamide was evaluated by the MOE. When the MOE is less than 10 000, it is considered that the carcinogenic risk needs to be paid priority attention, while when the MOE is ≥10 000, the carcinogenic risk doesn't need to be given priority attention.

## III. TDS Results

A total of 288 composite dietary samples of 12 categories from 24 provinces (autonomous regions, municipalities) were analyzed for the levels of AA. The values of those samples with no detectable AA were assigned the value of half of the LOD in the contamination levels evaluation and the dietary exposure assessment.

### 1. Levels of AA in TDS Composite Samples

In the 6$^{th}$ China TDS, the contamination levels of AA in dietary samples were in the range of ND-176.90 μg/kg with the detection rate of 73.3%. The average contamination levels of each food category ranged from 0.50 μg/kg to 18.53 μg/kg with the average level of 6.08 μg/kg (Annexed Table 6-15). The food categories that were

## 2. 膳食暴露评估

我国居民丙烯酰胺的平均膳食摄入量为175.057 ng/(kg bw·d)（附表6-16）。我国各地区居民的丙烯酰胺膳食摄入量在61.348～1049.005 ng/(kg bw·d)，其中，膳食摄入量最低的是广西[61.348 ng/(kg bw·d)]（图6-9）。根据NOAEL，我国居民膳食摄入丙烯酰胺的平均MOE为1142，广西最高（3260）。此外，大多数省份均高于1000。根据大鼠和小鼠的BMDL$_{10}$ [0.31 mg/(kg bw·d)和0.18 mg/(kg bw·d)]，我国居民膳食摄入丙烯酰胺的平均MOE分别为1771和1029。

found to be contaminated by AA, in a descending order of contaminated level, were vegetables (18.53 μg/kg), potatoes (17.74 μg/kg), sugar (14.60 μg/kg), legumes (7.28 μg/kg), water and beverages was the lowest (0.50 μg/kg).

## 2. Dietary Exposure Assessment

The average dietary intake (ADI) of AA for Chinese residents was 175.057 ng/(kg bw·d) (Annexed Table 6-16). The dietary intake of AA for population from various regions of China ranged from 61.348-1049.005 ng/(kg bw·d), with Guangxi having the lowest level of 61.348 ng/(kg bw·d) of ADI (Figure 6-9). Based on NOAEL, the MOE was 1142, with Guangxi recording the highest level of 3260. In addition, the MOE values of most provinces were higher than 1000. Moreover, the MOE values calculated based on the BMDL$_{10}$ [0.31 mg/(kg bw·d) and 0.18 mg/(kg bw·d)] of rats and mice were 1771 and 1029.

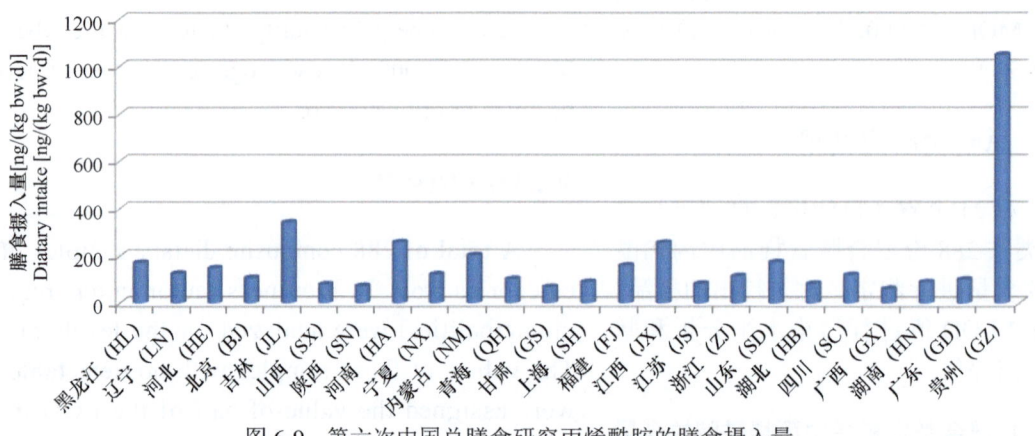

图6-9　第六次中国总膳食研究丙烯酰胺的膳食摄入量
Figure 6-9　Dietary intake of acrylamide from the 6$^{th}$ China TDS

## 3. 各类膳食对总膳食摄入的贡献

第六次中国总膳食研究的膳食丙烯酰胺主要来源于蔬菜类（59.0%）、谷类（18.9%）、薯类（10.1%）、豆类（4.7%），占总摄入量的92.7%，其余8类膳食样品的贡献率均小于3%（附表6-17，图6-10）。

## 3. Contributions of Food Categories to the Total Dietary Intake

The primary sources of dietary intake to the AA in the 6$^{th}$ China TDS were vegetables (59.0%), cereals (18.9%), potatoes (10.1%) and legumes (4.7%), accounting for 92.7% of the total intake, and each of other 8 food categories is lower than 3%, as is shown in Annexed Table 6-17 and Figure 6-10.

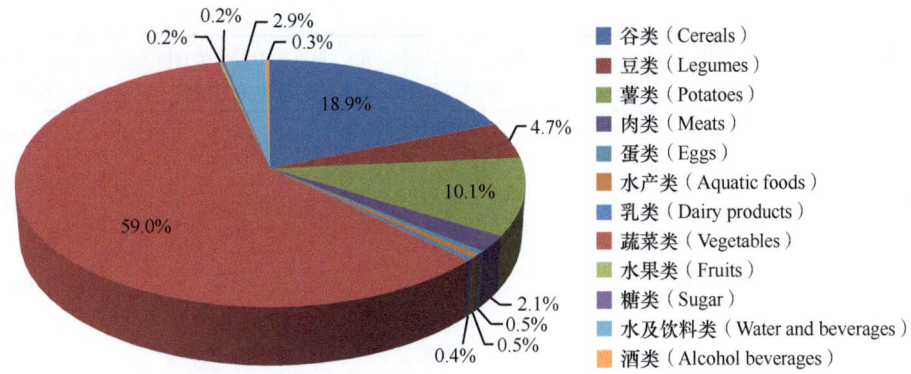

图 6-10 第六次中国总膳食研究丙烯酰胺的膳食来源
Figure 6-10 Dietary sources of acrylamide from the 6th China TDS

## 四、与以往中国总膳食研究结果的比较

自第三次中国总膳食研究以来，我国连续开展了膳食样品丙烯酰胺的检测，第三次、第四次、第五次、第六次中国总膳食研究的丙烯酰胺膳食摄入量分别为 0.188 μg/(kg bw·d)、0.286 μg/(kg bw·d)、0.319 μg/(kg bw·d) 和 0.175 μg/(kg bw·d)（表 6-1）。蔬菜类是我国居民丙烯酰胺摄入量的主要来源，摄入量大于 0.1 μg/(kg bw·d)。与第五次结果相比，第六次中国总膳食研究的膳食摄入量下降了 45.1%。

## IV. Comparison with Previous China TDSs Results

Since the 3rd China TDS, AA has been continuously detected. The dietary intake of acrylamide of the 3rd, 4th, 5th and 6th China TDS were 0.188 μg/(kg bw·d), 0.286 μg/(kg bw·d), 0.319 μg/(kg bw·d) and 0.175 μg/(kg bw·d) (Annexed Table 6-1). Vegetables are the main source of acrylamide intake of China residents, more than 0.1 μg/(kg bw·d). The dietary intakes of AA for the average Chinese population decreased 45.1% compared with the 5th CTDS.

表 6-1 中国总膳食研究中丙烯酰胺摄入量比较 [单位：μg/(kg bw·d)]
Table 6-1 Comparison of the Dietary intake of acrylamide from the 3rd to 6th China TDS [Unit: μg/(kg bw·d)]

| 膳食类别<br>Category | 第三次中国总膳食研究<br>The 3rd CTDS | 第四次中国总膳食研究<br>The 4th CTDS | 第五次中国总膳食研究<br>The 5th CTDS | 第六次中国总膳食研究<br>The 6th CTDS |
|---|---|---|---|---|
| 谷类<br>Cereals | 0.049 | 0.076 | 0.109 | 0.033 |
| 豆类<br>Legumes | 0.013 | 0.016 | 0.018 | 0.008 |
| 薯类<br>Potatoes | 0.023 | 0.023 | 0.050 | 0.018 |
| 肉类<br>Meats | 0.001 | 0.019 | 0.015 | 0.004 |
| 蛋类<br>Eggs | <0.001 | <0.001 | 0.002 | 0.001 |

续表

| 膳食类别<br>Category | 第三次中国总膳食研究<br>The 3rd CTDS | 第四次中国总膳食研究<br>The 4th CTDS | 第五次中国总膳食研究<br>The 5th CTDS | 第六次中国总膳食研究<br>The 6th CTDS |
|---|---|---|---|---|
| 水产类 Aquatic foods | 0.001 | 0.006 | 0.007 | 0.001 |
| 乳类 Diary products | <0.001 | <0.001 | 0.001 | 0.001 |
| 蔬菜类 Vegetables | 0.101 | 0.136 | 0.112 | 0.102 |
| 水果类 Fruits | 0.001 | 0.001 | <0.001 | <0.001 |
| 糖类 Sugar | <0.001 | 0.002 | 0.001 | <0.001 |
| 水及饮料类 Water and beverages | <0.001 | 0.001 | 0.002 | 0.006 |
| 酒类 Alcohol beverages | 0.002 | <0.001 | <0.001 | <0.001 |
| 合计 SUM | 0.188 | 0.286 | 0.319 | 0.175 |

注：摄入量合计时，摄入量<0.001 的结果按 0 计
Note: when the total intake was reached, values <0.001 were treated as 0

## 第五节　多环芳烃
## Section 5　Polycyclic Aromatic Hydrocarbons

### 一、背景

多环芳烃（PAH）是具有两个或两个以上稠环芳香烃环的一类碳氢化合物，是广泛存在于环境和食品中的污染物，迄今已发现几百种 PAH。PAH 主要来源于有机物质如煤、石油、天然气、木材、烟草等的不完全燃烧和热解。人群暴露 PAH 有多种途径，其中最主要的途径是膳食暴露和吸入暴露。对于非吸烟普通人群来说，膳食暴露是最重要的暴露途径，而对于吸烟人群来说，膳食暴露和吸入暴露的贡献相当。空气、土壤、水中的 PAH 作为环境污染物，可能通过沉降和富集进入食物链，食品加工、储存和烹饪过程中也可能产生 PAH 污染。

### Ⅰ. Background

Polycyclic aromatic hydrocarbons (PAHs) constitute a large class of hydrocarbons that are composed of two or more fused aromatic rings, which are pollutants widely present in the environment and food. More than hundreds PAHs have been found so far. PAHs mainly come from incomplete combustion and pyrolysis of organic materials such as coal, petroleum, natural gas, wood and tobacco. Humans are exposed to PAHs by various pathways. The most important ways are dietary exposure and inhalation exposure. While for non-smokers the major route of exposure is consumption of food, for smokers dietary and inhalation exposures contribute equally. Environmental pollution of PAHs in air, soil, and water may enter the food chain through sedimentation and enrichment. PAHs contamination

PAH对人类具有致癌、致畸、致突变的"三致毒性"，并可损害中枢神经系统，对内分泌系统也有一定干扰作用以及具免疫抑制作用，抑制体液免疫和细胞免疫。对PAH关注较多的是其致癌性，其中，苯并[a]芘已被国际癌症研究机构（IARC）认定为I类致癌物。同时，一些PAH还具有遗传毒性，可通过胎盘诱导DNA损伤。PAH暴露对人群的肺脏功能、儿童的生长发育及男性的生殖健康等存在潜在的影响。

迄今为止，许多国际机构对PAH的污染及毒性进行了评估。欧洲食品安全局（EFSA）指出，EPA优先监控的16种PAH（包括萘、二氢苊、苊、芴、菲、蒽、荧蒽、芘、苯并[a]芘、䓛、苯并[a]蒽、苯并[b]荧蒽、苯并[k]荧蒽、二苯并[a,h]蒽、苯并[g,h,i]苝、茚并[1,2,3-cd]芘）并不能真实反映出食品中PAH混合物的总体毒性效应，因此EFSA提出了新的欧盟优先监控的16种PAH（包括苯并[a]芘、䓛、苯并[a]蒽、苯并[b]荧蒽、苯并[k]荧蒽、二苯并[a,h]蒽、苯并[g,h,i]苝、茚并[1,2,3-cd]芘、5-甲基䓛、苯并[j]荧蒽、苯并[c]芴、二苯并[a,e]芘、二苯并[a,h]芘、二苯并[a,i]芘、二苯并[a,l]芘和环戊并[c,d]芘）名单，其中包含了更多的毒性较大的5-甲基䓛、苯并[j]荧蒽等8种重质PAH。

2011年8月，欧盟委员会发布了Regulation (EC) No 835/2011法规，对Regulation (EC) No 1881/2006进行了修订，更新了食品中的PAH限量规定。新法规规定，以食物中苯并[a]芘、䓛、苯并[a]蒽和苯并[b]荧蒽4种PAH（4种化合物合计为PAH4）污染物的总含量作为评价PAH污染的一个指标，同时继续保留苯并[a]芘的含量作为另一个评价指标。欧盟[Regulation

may also be produced during food processing, storage and cooking.

PAHs are carcinogenic, teratogenic and mutagenic to humans, which is called "3R toxicity". PAHs can also damage the central nervous system, interfere with the endocrine system to a certain extent, and inhibit immune suppression, inhibiting humoral and cellular immunity. More attention has been paid to the carcinogenicity of PAHs, among which benzo [a] pyrene has been classified by International Agency for Research on Cancer (IARC) as carcinogenic to humans (group I). Meanwhile, some PAHs are genotoxic and can induce DNA damage through the placenta. PAHs exposure has potential effects on lung function in the population, growth and development of children and male reproductive health.

So far, the pollution and toxicity of PAHs have been evaluated by many international organizations. The European Food Safety Authority (EFSA) pointed out that the 16 PAHs (naphthalene, acenaphthylene, acenaphthene, fluorene, phenanthrene, anthracene, fluoranthene, pyrene, benzo [a] pyrene, perylene, benzo [a] anthracene, benzo [b] fluoranthene, benzo [k] fluoranthene, dibenzo [a,h] pyrene, benzo [g,h,i] perylene, indeno [1,2,3-cd] pyrene) prioritized for monitoring by EPA do not reflect the overall toxic effects of PAHs mixtures in food. As a result, the EFSA proposed a new EU list of 16 PAHs (benzo [a] pyrene, perylene, benzo [a] anthracene, benzo [b] fluoranthene, benzo [k] fluoranthene, dibenzo [a,h] pyrene, benzo [g,h,i] perylene, indeno [1,2,3-cd] pyrene, 5-methylchrysene, benzo [j] fluoranthene, benzo [c] fluorene, dibenzo [a,e] pyrene, dibenzo [a,h] pyrene, dibenzo [a,i] pyrene, dibenzo [a,l] pyrene, cyclopenta [c,d] pyrene) for priority monitoring, including 8 heavy PAHs such as more toxic 5-methylchrysene, benzo [j] fluoranthene.

In August 2011, the European Commission issued Regulation (EC) No 835/2011 regulations, revising Regulation (EC) No 1881/2006 and updating maximum levels for PAHs in food. In 2015, the EU

(EC) No 835/2011] 为10类食品制定了苯并 [a] 芘及 PAH4 的最大限量值。2015年，欧盟 [Commission Regulation (EU) 2015/1933] 进一步增加了食品营养补充剂、干制药材等多环芳烃的限量规定。目前，我国对食品中 PAH 的监管，仍以苯并 [a] 芘作为评价指标。《食品安全国家标准 食品中污染物限量》（GB 2762—2022）制定了谷类及其制品（5 μg/kg）、熏烧烤肉类（5 μg/kg）、熏烤水产品（5 μg/kg）、油脂及其制品（10 μg/kg）的苯并 [a] 芘限量。

## 二、健康指导值

PAH 是遗传毒性致癌物，与造成 DNA 损伤呈非线性关系，通常认为 PAH 对人群的健康影响无阈值，因此无健康指导值。遗传毒性致癌物的健康风险评估通常有线性外推法（linear extrapolation method）、暴露边界值（MOE）和毒理学关注阈值（TTC）等方法。用 MOE 法计算有害效应观察终点（如基准剂量置信下限 BMDL）与人群 PAH 暴露量的比值，当 MOE 值高于 10 000 时，通常认为引起健康危害的风险在公共卫生意义上不属于优先关注，而低于 10 000 时，认为需要在公共卫生学上优先关注。

PAH 是较为复杂的混合物，属于多物质联合暴露，评估其健康风险的常用方法有类别 ADI/TDI、替代物（surrogate）法和毒性当量因子法（TEF）等。替代物法的核心是选择合适的替代物，即以混合物中某一种或几种成分的浓度来衡量整个混合物的毒性效应。

[Communication Regulation (EU) 2015/1933] further setting maximum levels for polycyclic aromatic hydrocarbons in nutritional supplements and dried medicinal materials. According to the new regulations, the total content of four PAHs pollutants (PAH4) of benzo [a] pyrene, perylene, benzo [a] anthracene and benzo [b] fluoranthene in food was used as an index to evaluate PAHs pollution, while the content of benzo [a] pyrene was retained as another evaluation index. Regulation (EC) No 835/2011 set maximum levels for benzo [a] pyrene and PAH4 for 10 food categories. At present, benzo [a] pyrene is still used as the evaluation index in the supervision of PAHs in food in China. The maximum levels for benzo [a] pyrene in cereals and its products (5 μg/kg), smoked and grilled meats (5 μg/kg), smoked and grilled aquatic products (5 μg/kg), oil and its products (10 μg/kg) were set in the *National Food Safety Standard-Contaminant Limits in Foods* (GB 2762—2022).

## II. HBGV

PAHs are genotoxic carcinogens, causing DNA damage in a non-linear relationship. It is generally considered that there is no threshold value, so there is no health-based guidance value for the health impact of PAHs on the population. Linear extrapolation method, margin of exposure (MOE) and the threshold of toxicological concern (TTC) are commonly used for health risk assessment of genotoxic carcinogens. MOE method is used to calculate the ratio of the observed endpoints of harmful effects [such as benchmark dose lower confidence limit (BMDL)] to the population exposure to PAHs. When MOE value is higher than 10 000, health hazard risk is generally considered as not a priority concern in public health, while MOE value is lower than 10 000, it is considered as a priority concern.

PAHs is a complex mixture of multi-substance combined exposure. Common methods to assess their health risks include the category ADI/TDI, surrogate and toxicity equivalency factor (TEF) method. The core of surrogate is the selection of appropriate indicators,

EFSA 在 2008 年发布了最新的食品中 PAH 评估报告，报告中关注了 EU 优先监控的 16 种 PAH，尤其关注其中 8 种具有致癌性和遗传毒性的 PAH。欧盟认为苯并 [a] 芘不再适合作为单一的指示物，而是提出了以 PAH2（苯并 [a] 芘+苉）、PAH4 和 PAH8(PAH4+苯并 [k] 荧蒽+苯并 [g,h,i] 芘+二苯并 [a,h] 蒽+茚并 [1,2,3-cd] 芘 ) 作为指示物，其中以 PAH4 为最优。EFSA 基于 MOE 法的评估结果显示，平均消费水平的膳食 PAH 暴露对人类健康的影响不属于优先关注，而高消费水平的膳食暴露健康风险为优先关注，可能需要采取进一步风险管理措施。第六次中国总膳食研究基于 EFSA 的评估方法，分别对我国居民膳食苯并 [a] 芘和 PAH4（苯并 [a] 芘、苉、苯并 [a] 蒽和苯并 [b] 荧蒽）进行膳食暴露评估。

## 三、总膳食研究结果

### 1. 混合膳食样品中多环芳烃的含量

对 24 个省（直辖市、自治区）的 12 类混合膳食样品中 EU 优先监控的 16 种多环芳烃的含量进行测定。对未检出的样品，以 1/2 LOD 值进行污染水平评价和膳食暴露评估（12 类膳食样品中 16 种多环芳烃的 LOD 值均为 0.01 μg/kg）。结果显示，苯并 [a] 芘在各类膳食样品中均有检出，其中在豆类、水产类及蔬菜类样品中的检出率均为 100%，在蛋类、肉类、薯类样品中的检出率也较高，均超过 90%，在水及饮料类和酒类样品中的检出率较低，仅在一个省份样品中检出。12 类 288 份膳食样品中，肉类的苯并 [a] 芘平均污染水平最高，为 0.32 μg/kg，其中青海省肉类样品苯并 [a] 芘的污染水平最高，为 2.24 μg/kg。豆类和蔬菜类样品苯并 [a] 芘的平均污染水平仅次于肉类

which measure the toxic effect of a mixture based on the concentration of one or more ingredients in the mixture.

The EFSA published its latest assessment report on PAHs in food in 2008, which focused on 16 PAHs under EU superior control, especially 8 of them with carcinogenicity and genotoxicity. The EU considered that benzo [a] pyrene was no longer suitable as a single indicator, but proposed PAH2 (benzo [a] pyrene + perylene), PAH4, and PAH8 (benzo [a] pyrene + perylene + benzo [a] anthracene + benzo [b] fluoranthene + benzo [k] fluoranthene + dibenzo [a,h] pyrene + benzo [g,h,i] perylene + indeno [1,2,3-cd] pyrene) as indicators, with PAH4 being the best. The results of EFSA assessment based on MOE method showed that dietary PAHs exposure at average consumption levels was not a priority concern for human health effects, while dietary exposure at high consumption levels was a priority concern for health risks and might require further risk management measures. The sixth China total diet study assessed the dietary exposure of benzo [a] pyrene and PAH4 (benzo [a] pyrene, perylene, benzo [a] anthracene and benzo [b] fluoranthene) of China residents based on the EFSA assessment methods.

## III. TDS Results

### 1. Levels of Polycyclic Aromatic Hydrocarbons in TDS Composite Dietary Intake

The levels of 16 PAHs under EU priority monitoring were detected in 12 categories of mixed dietary samples from 24 provinces (autonomous regions, municipalities). For the undetected samples, 1/2 LOD value was used to evaluate the contamination level and dietary exposure (the LOD values of 16 PAHs in 12 categories dietary samples were 0.01 μg/kg). According to the results, benzo [a] pyrene was detected in all kinds of dietary samples, among which the detection rate was 100% in legumes, aquatic foods and vegetables samples, and was also higher in eggs, meats and potatoes samples, all of which exceeded 90%. While the detection rate was lower in water and beverages and alcohol beverages

类，均为 0.25 μg/kg。各省份样品中苯并 [a] 芘平均污染水平为 0.36～4.50 μg/kg，其中青海省平均污染水平最高（附表 6-18）。

苯并 [c] 芴、5-甲基䓛、二苯并 [a,l] 芘、二苯并 [a,e] 芘、二苯并 [a,i] 芘、二苯并 [a,h] 芘在所有 12 类膳食样品中均未检出。12 类膳食样品中其余 9 种 PAH 单体的含量分别见附表 6-19～附表 6-27。

以苯并 [a] 芘、䓛、苯并 [a] 蒽和苯并 [b] 荧蒽之和计的 PAH4（未检出样品以 1/2 LOD 值计）在各类膳食样品中的检出率均较高，均大于 60%，仅在水及饮料类和酒类样品中检出率较低，均为 17%。PAH4 在豆类、肉类及蔬菜类样品中的平均污染水平较高，分别为 1.84 μg/kg、1.50 μg/kg、1.33 μg/kg，三类样品中 PAH4 最高水平分别为 5.96 μg/kg、7.11 μg/kg 及 4.03 μg/kg。各省份样品中 PAH4 平均污染水平为 2.70～17.9 μg/kg，其中青海省平均污染水平最高，辽宁省最低（附表 6-28）。

以检测的 16 个化合物之和计的 PAH16（未检出样品以 1/2 LOD 值计）在 97.3% 的样品中有检出，仅在 8 份样品（3 份酒类，2 份水及饮料类，乳类、水果类、糖类各 1 份）无检出。与 PAH4 类似，PAH16 是在肉类、豆类及蔬菜类样品中平均污染水平较高，分别为 2.79 μg/kg、2.60 μg/kg、2.31μg/kg，三类样品中 PAH16 最高水平分别为 17.84 μg/kg、8.13 μg/kg 及 10.1 μg/kg。各省份样品中 PAH16 平均污染水平为 4.21～37.18 μg/kg，其中青海省平均污染水平最高，辽宁省最低（附表 6-29）。

samples, only detected in one province samples. Among the 288 of 12 categories dietary samples, the average contamination level of benzo [a] pyrene in meats was the highest (0.32 μg/kg), among which the highest contamination level of benzo [a] pyrene in meats samples was 2.24 μg/kg in Qinghai province. The average level of benzo [a] pyrene in legumes and vegetables was second only to that in meats, with both averaging at 0.25 μg/kg. The average contamination level of benzo [a] pyrene in the samples from various provinces ranged from 0.36 μg/kg to 4.50 μg/kg, with the highest average contamination level in Qinghai province (Annexed Table 6-18).

Benzo [c] fluorene, 5-methylchrysene, dibenzo [a,l] pyrene, dibenzo [a,e] pyrene, dibenzo [a,i] pyrene, dibenzo [a,h] pyrene were not detected in all 12 categories of dietary samples. The contents of the other 9 PAHs monomers in the 12 categories of dietary samples are shown in Annexed Table 6-19-Annexed Table 6-27.

PAH4 measured as the sum of benzo [a] pyrene, perylene, benzo [a] anthracene and benzo [b] fluoranthene (non-detected samples were calculated by 1/2 LOD value), was detected at a high rate of more than 60% in all categories of dietary samples, but the detection rate of PAH4 in water and beverages and alcohol beverages samples was lower than 17%. The average contamination levels of PAH4 in legumes, meats and vegetables were relatively high, at 1.84 μg/kg, 1.50 μg/kg and 1.33 μg/kg, respectively. The highest levels of PAH4 in legumes, meats and vegetables were 5.96 μg/kg, 7.11 μg/kg and 4.03 μg/kg, respectively. The average contamination level of PAH4 in the samples of each province was 2.70-17.9 μg/kg, with the highest average contamination level in Qinghai province and the lowest in Liaoning province (Annexed Table 6-28).

PAH16 measured by the sum of 16 compounds detected (undetected samples were calculated by the value of 1/2 LOD) was detected in 97.3% of the samples, and only 8 samples (3 samples of alcohol beverages, 2 samples of water and beverages, 1 sample of dairy products, fruits and sugar) were not detected. Similar to

## 2. 膳食暴露评估

我国居民苯并[a]芘的平均膳食摄入量为 2.82 ng/(kg bw·d)，其中贵州省居民苯并[a]芘的平均膳食摄入量最高，为 11.81 ng/(kg bw·d)，其次是青海省，为 6.33 ng/(kg bw·d)（附表 6-30 及图 6-11）。PAH4 的平均膳食摄入量为 16.50 ng/(kg bw·d)，也是以贵州省居民 PAH4 的平均膳食摄入量最高，为 44.67 ng/(kg bw·d)，其次是青海省，为 25.75 ng/(kg bw·d)（附表 6-31 及图 6-12）。PAH16 的平均膳食摄入量为 28.82 ng/(kg bw·d)，也是以贵州省居民 PAH16 的平均膳食摄入量最高，为 95.92 ng/(kg bw·d)，其次是青海省，为 53.07 ng/(kg bw·d)，PAH16 平均膳食摄入量最低的为辽宁省，为 9.98 ng/(kg bw·d)（附表 6-32 和图 6-13）。

PAH4, the average contamination levels of PAH16 in meats, legumes and vegetables were relatively high, at 2.79 μg/kg, 2.60 μg/kg and 2.31 μg/kg, respectively. The highest levels of PAH16 in three kinds of samples were 17.8 μg/kg, 8.13 μg/kg and 10.1 μg/kg, respectively. The average contamination level of PAH16 in the samples of different provinces ranged from 4.21 μg/kg to 37.18 μg/kg, with the highest average pollution level in Qinghai province and the lowest in Liaoning province (Annexed Table 6-29).

### 2. Dietary Exposure Assessment

The average dietary intake of benzo [a] pyrene in China residents was 2.82 ng/(kg bw·d), Guizhou province was the highest [11.81 ng/(kg bw·d)], followed by Qinghai province [6.33 ng/(kg bw·d)] (Annexed Table 6-30 and Figure 6-11). The average dietary intake of PAH4 was 16.50 ng/(kg bw·d), also the highest in Guizhou province [44.67 ng/(kg bw·d)], followed by Qinghai province [25.75 ng/(kg bw·d)] (Annexed Table 6-31 and Figure 6-12). The average dietary intake of PAH16 was 28.82 ng/(kg bw·d), the highest in Guizhou province [95.92 ng/(kg bw·d)], followed by Qinghai province [53.07 ng/(kg bw·d)],

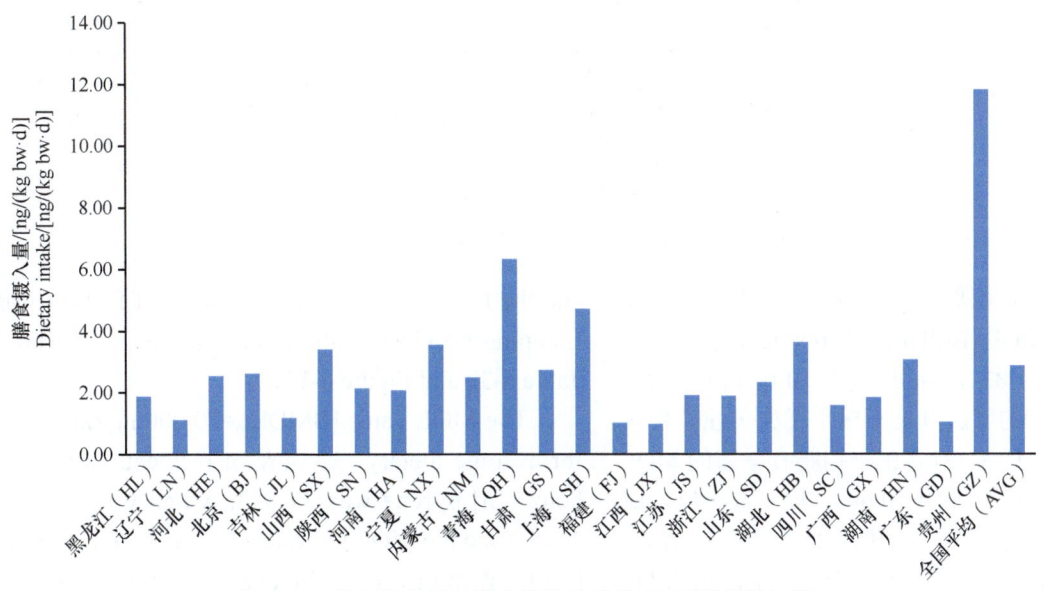

图 6-11 第六次中国总膳食研究的苯并[a]芘膳食摄入量

Figure 6-11 Dietary intake of benzo [a] pyrene from the 6$^{th}$ China TDS

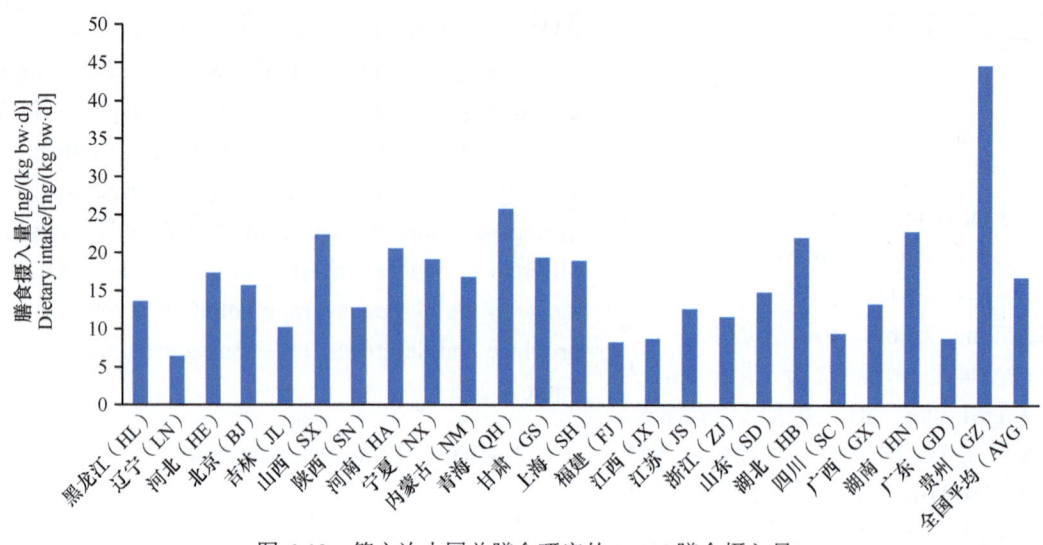

图 6-12　第六次中国总膳食研究的 PAH4 膳食摄入量
Figure 6-12　Dietary intake of PAH4 from the 6th China TDS

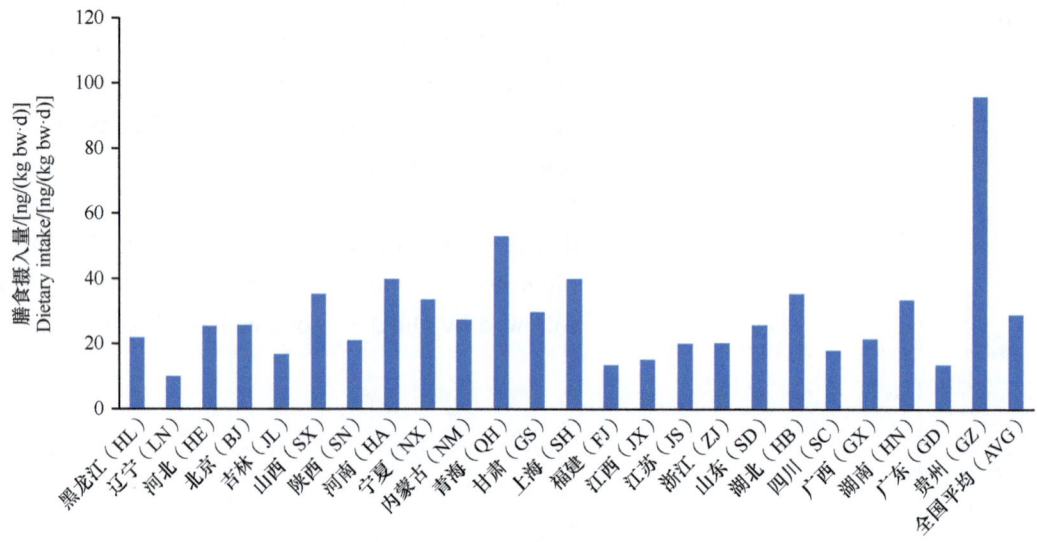

图 6-13　第六次中国总膳食研究的 PAH16 膳食摄入量
Figure 6-13　Dietary intake of PAH16 from the 6th China TDS

我国居民苯并 [a] 芘平均膳食暴露的 MOE [$BMDL_{10}$=70 000 ng/(kg bw·d)] 为 24 823，MOE 大于 10 000 时，膳食暴露的健康风险不属于优先关注。贵州省居民苯并 [a] 芘平均膳食暴露的 MOE 为 5927，小于 10 000，提示健康风险属于优先关注；而其余 23 个省（自治区、直辖市）居民苯并 [a] 芘暴露的 MOE 均大于 10 000，健康风险不属于优先关

and the lowest average dietary intake of PAH16 was in Liaoning province with 9.98 ng/(kg bw·d) (Annexed Table 6-32 and Figure 6-13).

The MOE value [$BMDL_{10}$=70 000 ng/(kg bw·d)] for average dietary exposure of residents in China for benzo [a] pyrene was 24 823, which was more than 10 000 and the MOE indicate a low concern for residents health at the average dietary exposures. In Guizhou province, the MOE value for benzo [a] pyrene exposure

注。同时，将 PAH4 作为健康风险评价指标，我国居民 PAH4 平均膳食暴露的 MOE [BMDL$_{10}$=340 000 ng/(kg bw·d)] 为 20 606，大于 10 000，健康风险不属于优先关注。除贵州省 PAH4 暴露的 MOE 为 7611，小于 10 000，其健康风险属于优先关注外，其他各省份 PAH4 暴露的 MOE 均大于 10 000，健康风险不属于优先关注。

**3. 各类膳食对总膳食摄入的贡献**

将第六次中国总膳食研究我国居民 12 大类膳食暴露来源的苯并 [a] 芘、PAH4 和 PAH16 摄入量分别除以其对应的膳食摄入总量就可以得到苯并 [a] 芘、PAH4 和 PAH16 的膳食来源贡献。

我国居民苯并 [a] 芘的膳食摄入总量中，蔬菜类贡献率最高，为 49%，其次为肉类（15%）和谷类（13%）（图 6-14）。

was 5927, which was less than 10 000, indicating that a potential concern for residents health. The MOEs for benzo [a] pyrene exposure in the remaining 23 provinces (autonomous regions, municipalities) was greater than 10 000 and the health risk was low concern. Meanwhile, taking PAH4 as health risk indicator, MOE [BMDL$_{10}$=340 000 ng/(kg bw·d)] to PAH4 for the average dietary exposure of residents in China was 20 606, which was more than 10 000, and the health risk was a low concern. The MOEs for PAH4 for all of provinces residents were all greater than 10 000 except for Guizhou province residents and the MOEs indicate a low concern. The MOE for PAH4 exposure was 7611 for Guizhou province residents, which was less than 10 000 indicating a potential concern for Guizhou province residents health.

**3. Contributions of Food Categories to Total Dietary Intake**

The dietary source of benzo [a] pyrene, PAH4 and PAH16 can be calculated by dividing the benzo [a] pyrene, PAH4 and PAH16 from 12 categories of dietary exposure sources of China residents in the sixth China total diet study by their corresponding total dietary intake, respectively.

Among the total dietary intake of benzo [a] pyrene in China residents, vegetables contributed the highest proportion (49%), followed by meats (15%) and cereals (13%) (Figure 6-14).

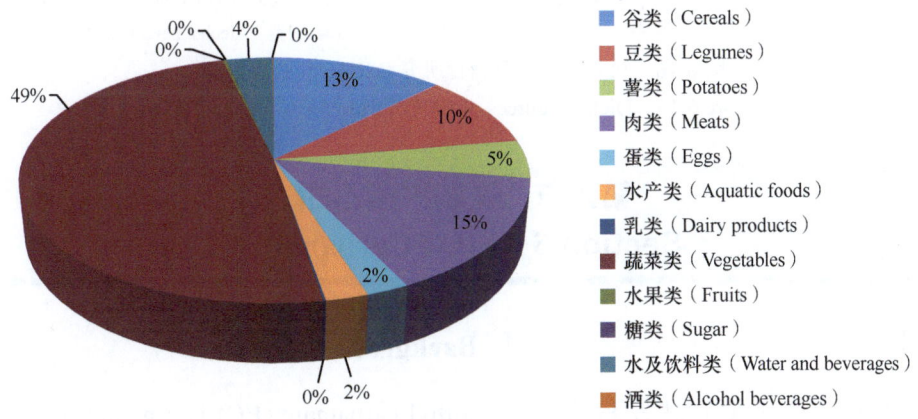

图 6-14　第六次中国总膳食研究苯并 [a] 芘的膳食来源

Figure 6-14　Dietary sources of benzo [a] pyrene from the 6$^{th}$ China TDS

PAH4 膳食摄入总量中，蔬菜类样品同样贡献最高，为 44%，其次为谷类（20%）和肉类（12%）（图 6-15）。

PAH16 膳食摄入总量中，蔬菜类样品仍为贡献最高的食品种类，贡献率为 43.9%，其次为谷类（18.3%）和肉类（13.0%）（图 6-16）。

Of the total dietary intake of PAH4, vegetables samples also contributed the highest (44%), followed by cereals (20%) and meats (12%) (Figure 6-15).

Among the total dietary intake of PAH16, vegetables samples still made the highest contribution, accounting for 43.9%, followed by cereals (18.3%) and meats (13.0%) (Figure 6-16).

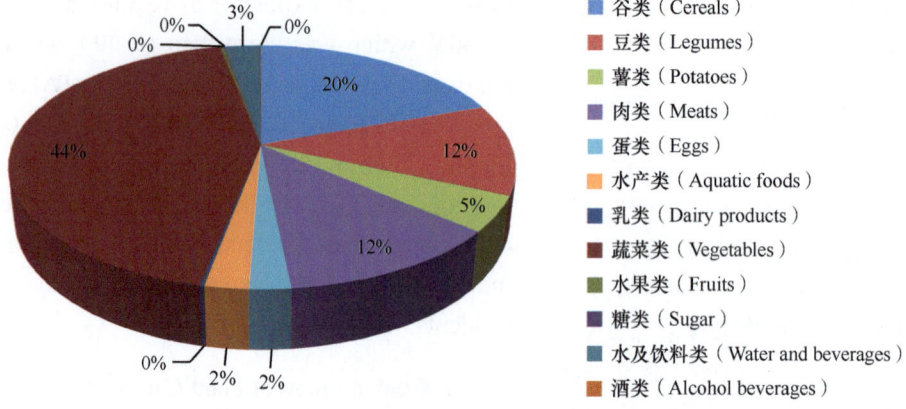

图 6-15　第六次中国总膳食研究 PAH4 的膳食来源
Figure 6-15　Dietary sources of PAH4 from the 6th China TDS

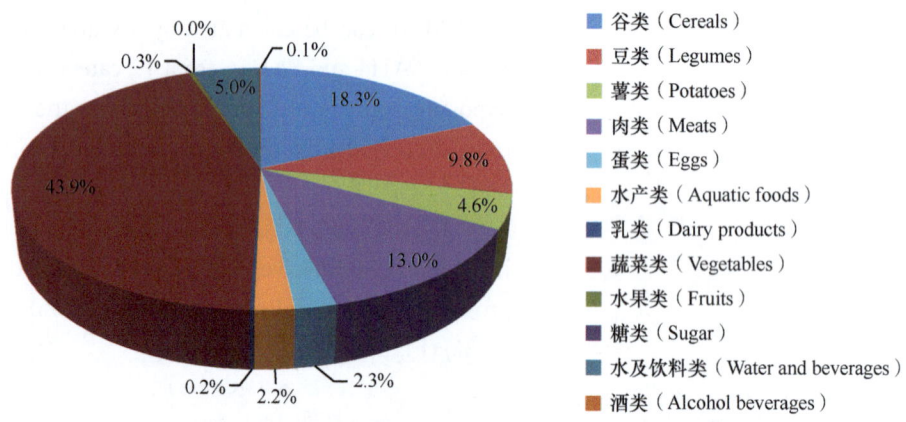

图 6-16　第六次中国总膳食研究 PAH16 的膳食来源
Figure 6-16　Dietary sources of PAH16 from the 6th China TDS

## 第六节　氨基甲酸乙酯
## Section 6　Ethyl Carbamate

### 一、背景
### I. Background

氨基甲酸乙酯（EC）是发酵食品（如酱油、腐乳、泡菜等）和酒类

Ethyl carbamate (EC) is a natural product found in fermented foods (e.g., soy sauce, curd, kimchi,

中存在的天然产物，具有遗传毒性和致癌性（如肺癌、肝癌等）。2007年，国际癌症研究机构（IARC）将氨基甲酸乙酯等级由"Group 2B"提升到"Group 2A"类，属于"很可能对人类致癌的物质"（probably carcinogenic to humans）。膳食摄入的氨基甲酸乙酯主要来自发酵食物和酒精饮料。目前，国际上对氨基甲酸乙酯的限量制定主要集中在酒类产品中，不同品种的酒类产品的限量为30～1000 μg/L。如加拿大规定佐餐葡萄酒中氨基甲酸乙酯的限量为30 μg/kg，加强葡萄酒为100 μg/kg，蒸馏酒为150 μg/kg，日本清酒为200 μg/kg，水果白兰地和烈性甜酒为400 μg/kg。我国尚未制定食品基质中氨基甲酸乙酯的限量标准。

## 二、健康指导值

目前，国际上未针对氨基甲酸乙酯制定每日允许摄入量（ADI）。联合国粮食及农业组织（FAO）/世界卫生组织（WHO）食品添加剂联合专家委员会（JECFA）根据动物致癌性试验结果，按最保守的估计推算引起动物肺癌的基准剂量置信下限（BMDL）为每天0.3 mg/kg bw。JECFA对氨基甲酸乙酯的评估方法为，以0.3 mg/kg bw与标准人每日每千克体重摄入量相除得出暴露边界值（MOE），当被评估物质的MOE＞10 000时，暂时不需要关注该物质。当被评估物质的MOE＜10 000时，需要关注该物质对人体健康的风险。

## 三、总膳食研究结果

对24个省（自治区、直辖市）的12类共288份混合膳食样品中氨基甲酸乙酯的含量进行测定。当一类膳食样品中氨基甲酸乙酯的含量水平低于对应的检出限时，则不进行摄入量计算和分

etc.) and alcohol beverages that is genotoxic and carcinogenic (e.g., lung cancer, liver cancer, etc.). In 2007, the International Agency for Research on Cancer (IARC) upgraded the classification of EC from "Group 2B" to "Group 2A", which is "probably carcinogenic to humans". Dietary exposure to EC is mainly from fermented foods and alcohol beverages. Currently, international limits for EC are mainly set for alcohol beverages, ranging from 30 μg/L to 1000 μg/L for different varieties of alcohol beverages, e.g., 30 μg/kg for table wines in Canada, 100 μg/kg for fortified wines, 150 μg/kg for distilled spirits, 200 μg/kg for Japanese sake, and 400 μg/kg for fruit brandies and strong liqueurs. No limit standard for ethyl carbamate in food matrices has been established in China.

## II. HBGV

Currently, there is no internationally established acceptable daily intake (ADI) for ethyl carbamate. The Joint Food and Agriculture Organization (FAO)/World Health Organization (WHO) Expert Committee on Food Additives (JECFA) has estimated a benchmark dose lower confidence limit (BMDL) of 0.3 mg/kg bw per day for lung cancer in animals based on the results of animal carcinogenicity tests, as the most conservative estimate. Ethyl carbamate was assessed by JECFA by eliminating 0.3 mg/kg bw from the standard human daily intake per kilogram of body weight to derive a margin of exposure (MOE). When the MOE of the substance under assessment is >10 000, the substance is not of concern for the time being. When the MOE of the substance under assessment is less than 10 000, the risk to human health is of concern.

## III. TDS Results

The levels of ethyl carbamate were determined in 288 mixed dietary samples of 12 categories from 24 provinces (autonomous regions, municipalities). No intake calculations and analyses were performed for the type of dietary samples with levels below the corresponding limits

析，对于在 LOD 和 LOQ 之间的检出结果，则以实际检测值进行摄入量计算和分析。

### 1. 混合膳食样品中氨基甲酸乙酯的含量

第六次中国总膳食研究的混合膳食样品中氨基甲酸乙酯的含量水平为 ND～145.16 μg/kg，平均含量为 5.00 μg/kg，谷类、豆类、薯类、蛋类、乳类、水果类、糖类、水及饮料类膳食样品中氨基甲酸乙酯的含量全部低于相对应的检出限，记为未检出。所有样品的检出率为 20.1%（附表 6-33）。在检出的 4 类膳食样品中，肉类的氨基甲酸乙酯平均含量最高（24.40 μg/kg），其次是水产类（22.93 μg/kg）、酒类（10.24 μg/kg）、蔬菜类（2.42 μg/kg）。

### 2. 膳食暴露评估

第六次中国总膳食研究中，由肉类、水产类、酒类和蔬菜类膳食摄入的氨基甲酸乙酯的全国平均值为 0.05 μg/(kg bw·d)。其中，辽宁省平均标准人膳食摄入量最高，为 0.135 μg/(kg bw·d)，上海市和广东省最低，未见摄入（附表 6-34 和图 6-17）。各类膳食的摄入量最高的为肉类，摄入量为 0.027 μg/(kg bw·d)，最低的为酒类，摄入量为 0.003 μg/(kg bw·d)。按照 JECFA 评估方法，以 0.3 mg/(kg bw·d) 与氨基甲酸乙酯的全国平均值 0.05 μg/(kg bw·d) 相除，得出 MOE 为 6000。

根据 JECFA 的评估结果，当被评估物质的 MOE＞10 000 时，在评估其对人类造成的健康危害时，暂时不需要关注该物质。在第六次膳食研究中，膳食摄入的平均 MOE 为 6000。

### 1. Levels of Ethyl Carbamate in TDS Composite Dietary Samples

The levels of ethyl carbamate in the mixed dietary samples of the 6$^{th}$ CTDS ranged from ND to 145.16 μg/kg, with a mean level of 5.00 μg/kg. The levels of ethyl carbamate in the dietary samples of cereals, legumes, potatoes, eggs, dairy products, fruits, sugar, water and beverages were all below the corresponding LODs and were recorded as non-detect. The detection rate for all samples was 20.1% (Annexed Table 6-33). Among the four dietary samples detected, the meats had the highest mean EC level (24.40 μg/kg), followed by aquatic foods (22.93 μg/kg), alcohol beverages (10.24 μg/kg), and vegetables (2.42 μg/kg).

### 2. Dietary Exposure Assessment

The national mean dietary exposure to EC from meats, aquatic foods, alcohol beverages and vegetables in the 6$^{th}$ China total diet study was 0.05 μg/(kg bw·d). Among them, the highest mean standard human dietary intake was found in Liaoning at 0.135 μg/(kg bw·d), and the lowest was seen in Shanghai and Guangdong (Annexed Table 6-34 and Figure 6-17). The highest intake for all dietary categories was meats with 0.027 μg/(kg bw·d), and the lowest was alcohol beverages with 0.003 μg/(kg bw·d). The MOE of 6000 was obtained by dividing 0.3 mg/(kg bw·d) with the national mean of 0.05 μg/(kg bw·d) of ethyl carbamate, according to the JECFA assessment method.

According to the JECFA assessment, when the MOE value of the substance under assessment was ＞ 10 000, the substance was not of concern for the time being when assessing the health risk posed to humans. In the 6$^{th}$ CTDS, the average MOE value for dietary intake was 6000.

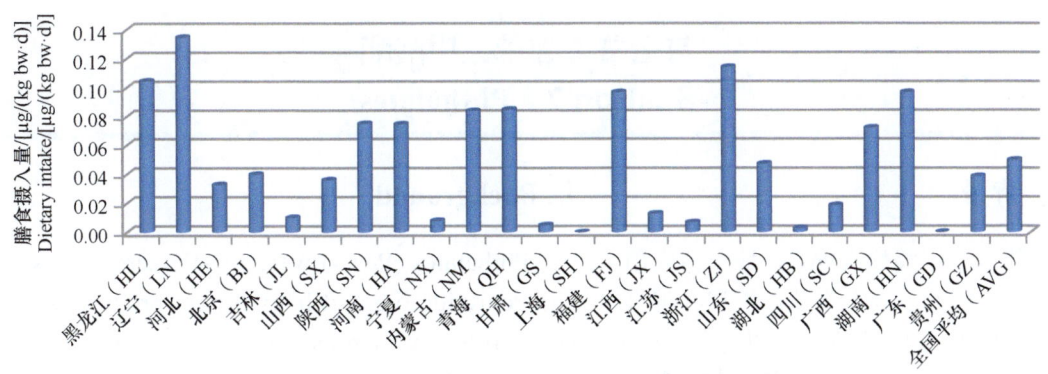

图 6-17 第六次中国总膳食研究的氨基甲酸乙酯膳食摄入量

Figure 6-17 Dietary intake of ethyl carbamate from the 6th China TDS

### 3. 各类膳食对总膳食摄入的贡献

第六次中国总膳食研究的膳食氨基甲酸乙酯主要来源于肉类（53.82%）、蔬菜类（24.90%）、水产类（15.14%）以及酒类（6.14%）（附表6-35，图6-18）。

### 3. Contributions of Food Categories to Total Dietary Intake

Dietary intake of ethyl carbamate in the 6th CTDS was mainly derived from meats (53.82%), vegetables (24.90%), aquatic foods (15.14%) and alcohol beverages (6.14%) (Annexed Table 6-35 and Figure 6-18).

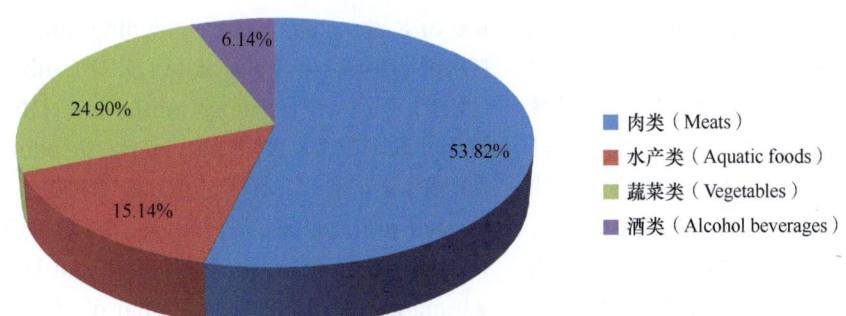

图 6-18 第六次中国总膳食研究氨基甲酸乙酯的膳食来源

Figure 6-18 Dietary sources of ethyl carbamate from the 6th China TDS

### 四、与以往中国总膳食研究结果的比较

自第五次中国总膳食研究以来，我国连续开展了膳食样品氨基甲酸乙酯的检测，第五次、第六次中国总膳食研究的氨基甲酸乙酯的膳食摄入量分别为 0.08 μg/(kg bw·d) 和 0.05 μg/(kg bw·d)。

### IV. Comparison with the Results of the Previous China TDS

Since the fifth China total diet study, dietary samples for ethyl carbamate have been continuously tested in China. The dietary intakes of ethyl carbamate in the fifth and sixth CTDS were 0.08 μg/(kg bw·d) and 0.05 μg/(kg bw·d), respectively.

# 第七节　邻苯二甲酸酯
# Section 7　Phthalates

## 一、背景

邻苯二甲酸酯（PAE）是一种应用广泛的塑化剂，具有生殖毒性和肝脏毒性等。PAE 与塑料等材质以分子间作用力混合，缺少化学键的键合力，极易通过迁移、挥发和溶解等作用进入食品和环境，通过人体摄入影响人体健康。中国、欧盟和美国等对 PAE 的使用种类与迁移限量进行了规定。我国《食品安全国家标准 食品接触材料及制品用添加剂使用标准》（GB 9685—2016）中规定了 8 种邻苯二甲酸酯的使用，包括邻苯二甲酸二甲酯（DMP）、邻苯二甲酸二异丁酯（DiBP）、邻苯二甲酸二丁酯（DBP）、邻苯二甲酸二 (2-乙基) 己酯（DEHP）、邻苯二甲酸二烯丙酯（DAP）、DAP 聚合物、邻苯二甲酸二异壬酯（DINP）和邻苯二甲酸二异辛酯（DIOP）。其中 DEHP 的特定迁移限量为 1.5 mg/kg，DBP 为 0.3 mg/kg，DAP、DAP 聚合物的总迁移量均为 6.0 mg/kg，DINP 的总迁移量为 9.0 mg/kg，所有 PAE 的总迁移量之和不得高于 60 mg/kg。

## 二、健康指导值

欧洲食品安全局（EFSA）基于 DEHP 的生殖毒性提出 DEHP 的每日可耐受摄入量（TDI）为 0.05 mg/(kg bw·d)；根据大鼠发育毒性实验研究，提出 DBP 的 TDI 为 0.01 mg/(kg bw·d)。除此以外，我国国家食品安全风险评估中心提出 DiBP 的 TDI 为 0.03 mg/(kg bw·d)。

## I. Background

Phthalates (PAEs) were plasticizers widely used with reproductive and hepatotoxic properties. PAEs were mixed with plastics and other materials by intermolecular forces. They could easily be introduced to food and the environment through migration, volatilization, and dissolution because they lack the binding force of chemical bonds between plastic and these molecules. They were affecting human health through the human intake. PAEs were regulated in China, the EU, and the USA, regarding the types of usage and migration limits. China's *National Food Safety-the Use Standard of Additives in Food Contact Materials and Products* (GB 9685—2016) specifies the use of 8 phthalate esters, including dimethyl phthalate (DMP), di-isobutyl phthalate (DiBP), dibutyl phthalate (DBP), di(2-ethyl) hexyl phthalate (DEHP), diallyl phthalate (DAP), DAP polymers, diisononyl phthalate (DINP) and di-isooctyl phthalate (DIOP). The specific migration limits are 1.5 mg/kg for DEHP, 0.3 mg/kg for DBP, 6.0 mg/kg for both DAP and DAP polymers, 9.0 mg/kg for DINP and the sum of all PAEs must not exceed 60 mg/kg.

## II. HBGV

The European Food Safety Authority (EFSA) had proposed a tolerable daily intake (TDI) of 0.05 mg/(kg bw·d) for DEHP based on the reproductive toxicity and a TDI of 0.01 mg/(kg bw·d) for DBP based on experimental studies of developmental toxicity in rats. In addition to these, China National Center for Food Safety Risk Assessment (CFSA) proposed a TDI of 0.03 mg/(kg bw·d) for DiBP.

## 三、总膳食研究结果

### 1. 混合膳食样品中邻苯二甲酸酯的含量

对24个省（自治区、直辖市）的12类共288份混合膳食样品中的16种邻苯二甲酸酯进行含量检测，其中检出率最高的是DBP（93.4%），其次是DiBP（91.7%）和DEHP（87.2%）。邻苯二甲酸二(2-乙氧基)乙酯（DEEP）（31.9%）、邻苯二甲酸二(2-甲氧基)乙酯（DMEP）（31.9%）、邻苯二甲酸二(2-丁氧基)乙酯（DBEP）（23.3%）、邻苯二甲酸二乙酯（DEP）（22.2%）、邻苯二甲酸二戊酯（DPP）（14.2%）、DMP（11.8%）、邻苯二甲酸丁苄酯（BBP）（11.8%）、邻苯二甲酸二(4-甲基-2-戊基)酯（BMPP）（9.0%）、邻苯二甲酸二环己酯（DCHP）（2.8%）的检出率均低于50%，而邻苯二甲酸二辛酯（DNOP）、邻苯二甲酸二苯酯（DBzP）、邻苯二甲酸二己酯（DHXP）、邻苯二甲酸二壬酯（DNP）的检出率均小于0.1%。对未检出的膳食样品，则以1/2 LOD进行摄入量计算和分析；对于在LOD和LOQ之间的检出结果，则以实际检测值进行摄入量计算和分析。

第六次中国总膳食研究的混合样品中各地区DBP的含量水平为13.24~97.49 μg/kg，总体平均含量为30.05 μg/kg（附表6-36）；水产类平均含量最高（46.41 μg/kg），其次是肉类（38.43 μg/kg）和酒类（36.70 μg/kg）。

DiBP的含量水平为5.31~48.69 μg/kg，总体平均含量为20.27 μg/kg（附表6-37）；水产类平均含量最高（46.41 μg/kg）（附表6-37）。

DEHP的含量水平为11.68~119.97 μg/kg，总体平均含量为27.86 μg/kg（附表6-38）；蔬菜类平均含量最高，为74.10 μg/kg（附表6-38）。

## III. TDS Results

### 1. Levels of Phthalates in TDS Composite Samples

A total of 288 samples from 12 categories of composite dietary samples in 24 provinces (autonomous regions, municipalities) were tested for 16 phthalates, the highest detection rate was 93.4% for DBP, followed by DiBP (91.7%) and DEHP (87.2%). Bis (2-ethoxyethyl) phthalate (DEEP) (31.9%), bis (2-methylglycol) phthalate (DMEP) (31.9%), bis (2-butoxyethyl) phthalate (DBEP) (23.3%), diethyl phthalate (DEP) (22.2%), dipentyl phthalate (DPP) (14.2%), DMP (11.8%), benzyl butyl phthalate (BBP) (11.8%), bis (4-methyl-2-pentanyl) phthalate (BMPP) (9.0%) and dicyclohexyl phthalate (DCHP) (2.8%) were all detected less than 50%, while dioctyl phthalate (DNOP), diphenyl phthalate (DBzP), dihexyl phthalate (DHXP) and dinonyl phthalate (DNP) were all detected at less than 0.1%. For "not detected" dietary samples, the intake was calculated and analyzed using 1/2 LOD; for detection results between LOD and LOQ, the intake was calculated and analyzed using actual detection values.

The levels of DBP in the composite samples of the 6$^{th}$ China TDS was ranged from 13.24 μg/kg to 97.49 μg/kg. The average was 30.05 μg/kg (Annexed Table 6-36); the highest average level was found in aquatic products (46.41 μg/kg), followed by alcohol beverages (38.43 μg/kg) and vegetables (36.70 μg/kg).

DiBP levels ranged from 5.31 μg/kg to 48.69 μg/kg, with an overall average of 20.27 μg/kg (Annexed Table 6-37); the highest average level was found in alcohol beverages (36.70 μg/kg) (Annexed Table 6-37).

DEHP levels ranged from 11.68 μg/kg to 119.97 μg/kg with an overall mean of 27.86 μg/kg (Annexed Table 6-38); vegetables had the highest mean level of 74.10 μg/kg (Annexed Table 6-38).

## 2. 膳食暴露评估

## 2. Dietary Exposure Assessment

DBP 的标准人平均膳食摄入量为 0.99 μg/(kg bw·d)，其中，北京市平均膳食摄入量最高，陕西省最低，分别为 3.52 μg/(kg bw·d) 和 0.35 μg/(kg bw·d)。谷类的平均摄入量最高，为 0.33 μg/(kg bw·d)，其次是水及饮料类和蔬菜类，平均摄入量分别为 0.26 μg/(kg bw·d) 和 0.21 μg/(kg bw·d)。最低的为糖类，平均摄入量小于 0.001 μg/(kg bw·d)（附表 6-39，图 6-19）。DBP 的全国平均膳食摄入量，未超过 TDI 为 10 μg/(kg bw·d) 的限量。

The average dietary intake of DBP for standard man was 0.99 μg/(kg bw·d), with the highest average dietary intake in Beijing and the lowest in Shaanxi province, at 3.52 μg/(kg bw·d) and 0.35 μg/(kg bw·d), respectively. The highest mean intake was 0.33 μg/(kg bw·d) for cereals, followed by water and beverages and vegetables with an average intake of 0.26 μg/(kg bw·d) and 0.21 μg/(kg bw·d), respectively. The lowest was sugar, with an average intake of fewer than 0.001 μg/(kg bw·d) (Annexed Table 6-39, Figure 6-19). The dietary intake of DBP did not exceed the TDI of 10 μg/(kg bw·d).

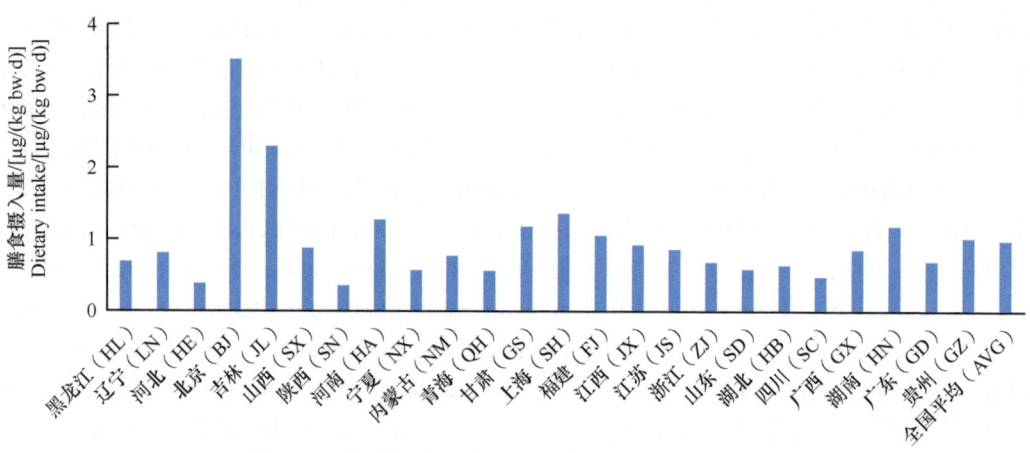

图 6-19 第六次中国总膳食研究的 DBP 膳食摄入量

Figure 6-19 Dietary intake of DBP from the 6$^{th}$ China TDS

DiBP 标准人的平均膳食摄入量为 0.80 μg/(kg bw·d)，其中，福建省膳食摄入量最高，黑龙江省最低，分别为 1.92 μg/(kg bw·d) 和 0.18 μg/(kg bw·d)。水及饮料类的平均摄入量最高，为 0.36 μg/(kg bw·d)，其次是谷类和蔬菜类，平均摄入量分别为 0.23 μg/(kg bw·d) 和 0.10 μg/(kg bw·d)。最低的为糖类，平均摄入量小于 0.001 μg/(kg bw·d)（附表 6-40，图 6-20）。DiBP 平均膳食摄入量未超过 TDI 为 30 μg/(kg bw·d) 的限量。

The average dietary intake of DiBP for standard man was 0.80 μg/(kg bw·d), with the highest dietary intake in Fujian province and the lowest in Heilongjiang province, at 1.92 μg/(kg bw·d) and 0.18 μg/(kg bw·d), respectively. The highest average intake was 0.36 μg/(kg bw·d) for water and beverages, followed by cereals and vegetables with an average intake of 0.23 μg/(kg bw·d) and 0.10 μg/(kg bw·d), respectively. The lowest was sugar, with an average of fewer than 0.001 μg/(kg bw·d) (Annexed Table 6-40, Figure 6-20). The DiBP dietary intake did not exceed the TDI of 30 μg/(kg bw·d).

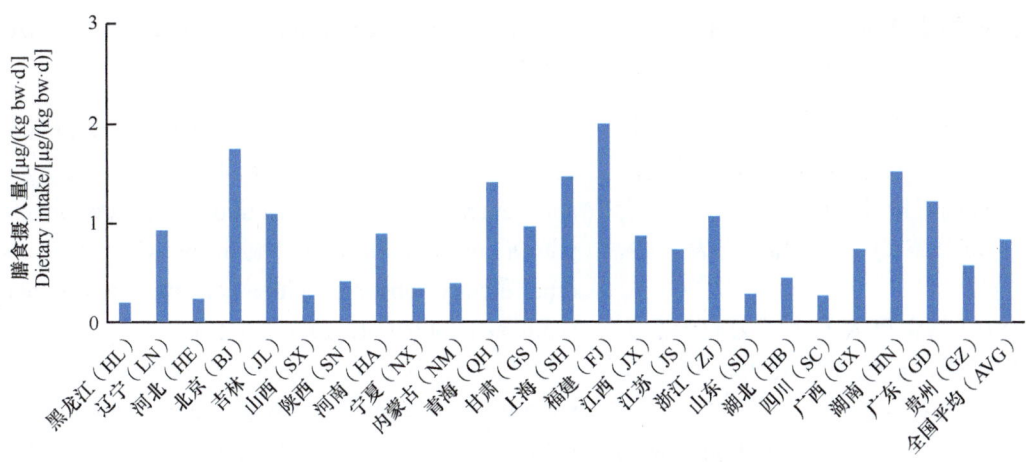

图 6-20　第六次中国总膳食研究的 DiBP 膳食摄入量
Figure 6-20　Dietary intake of DiBP from the 6th China TDS

DEHP 标准人的平均膳食摄入量为 1.16 μg/(kg bw·d)，其中，内蒙古摄入量最高，江苏省最低，分别为 7.97 μg/(kg bw·d) 和 0.39 μg/(kg bw·d)。摄入量较高的为谷类、蔬菜类和水及饮料类，平均摄入量分别为 0.46 μg/(kg bw·d)、0.36 μg/(kg bw·d) 和 0.17 μg/(kg bw·d)。最低的为糖类，平均摄入量小于 0.001 μg/(kg bw·d)（附表 6-41，图 6-21）。DEHP 平均膳食摄入量未超过 TDI 为 50 μg/(kg bw·d) 的限量。

The average dietary intake of DEHP for standard man was 1.16 μg/(kg bw·d), with the highest intake in Inner Mongolia and the lowest in Jiangsu province at 7.97 μg/(kg bw·d) and 0.39 μg/(kg bw·d), respectively. Higher intakes were found in cereals, vegetables, and water and beverages, with average intakes of 0.46 μg/(kg bw·d), 0.36 μg/(kg bw·d), and 0.17 μg/(kg bw·d), respectively. The lowest intake was for sugar, with a mean intake of less than 0.001 μg/(kg bw·d) (Annexed Table 6-41, Figure 6-21). The dietary intake of DEHP was not more than the TDI of 50 μg/(kg bw·d).

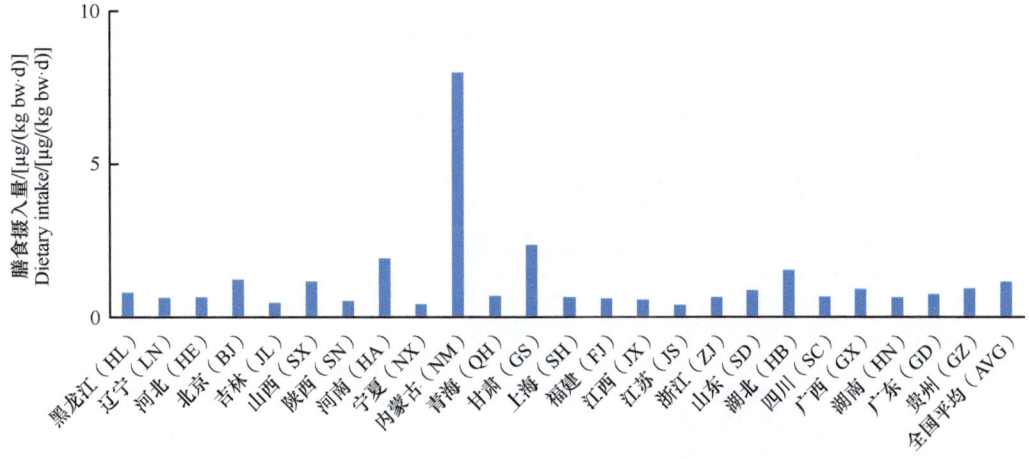

图 6-21　第六次中国总膳食研究的 DEHP 膳食摄入量
Figure 6-21　Dietary intake of DEHP from the 6th China TDS

第六章　食品加工过程污染物的膳食暴露评估　253

## 3. Contributions of Food Categories to Total Dietary Intake

The main source food of DBP dietary intake was cereals with a contribution of 34.5%, followed by water and beverages with a contribution of 24.9%, vegetables with a contribution of 20.4%, meats with 5.0%, and all other dietary substrates with a contribution less than 5% (Annexed Table 6-42, Figure 6-22).

The main source foods of DiBP dietary intake were water and beverages with a contribution of 42.3%, followed by cereals with a contribution of 29.6%, vegetables with a contribution of 13.3%, and other dietary substrates with a contribution of less than 5% (Annexed Table 6-43, Figure 6-23).

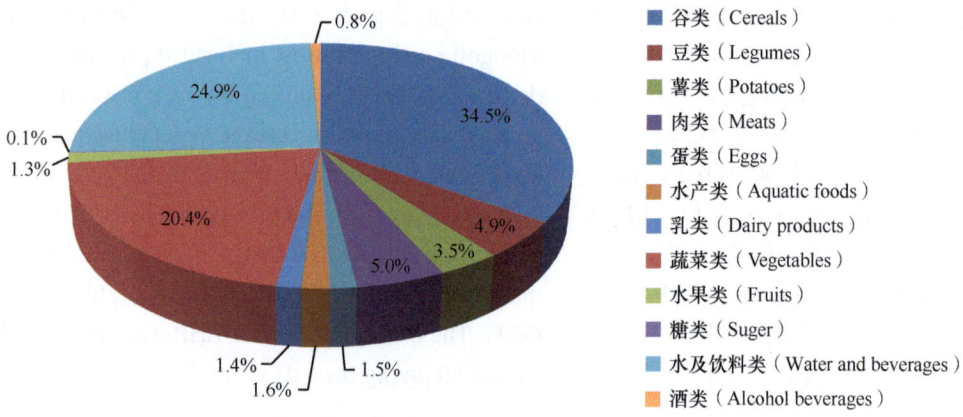

Figure 6-22　Dietary sources of DBP from the 6th China TDS

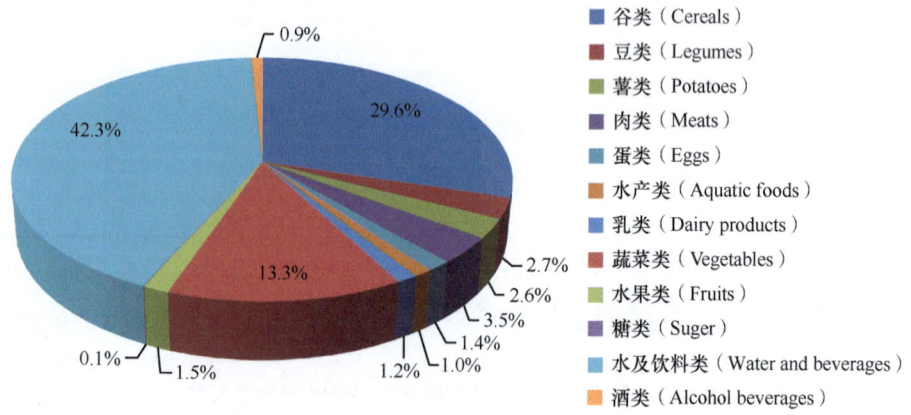

Figure 6-23　Dietary sources of DiBP from the 6th China TDS

DEHP 膳食摄入的主要来源为谷类（34.3%）、蔬菜类（30.8%）、水及饮料类（13.9%）、肉类（9.1%），其他膳食基质的贡献率均小于 5%（附表 6-44，图 6-24）。

The main sources of DEHP dietary intake were cereals (34.3%), vegetables (30.8%), water and beverages (13.9%), and meats (9.1%), with all other dietary substrates contributing less than 5% (Annexed Table 6-44, Figure 6-24).

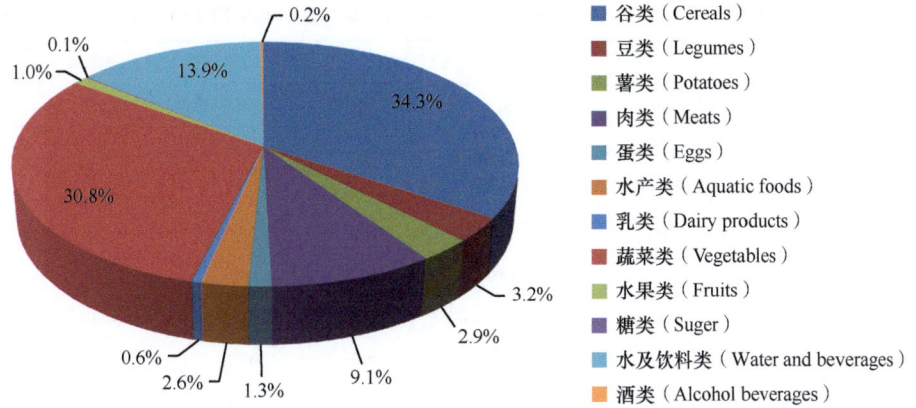

图 6-24　第六次中国总膳食研究 DEHP 的膳食来源
Figure 6-24　Dietary sources of DEHP from the 6th China TDS

## 四、与以往中国总膳食研究结果的比较

自第五次中国总膳食研究以来，我国连续开展了膳食样品中邻苯二甲酸酯类化合物的检测，第五次、第六次中国总膳食研究的 DBP 膳食摄入量分别为 5.97 μg/(kg bw·d) 和 0.98 μg/(kg bw·d)，谷类是我国居民 DBP 膳食摄入量的主要来源，摄入量为 0.33 μg/(kg bw·d)。与第五次结果相比，第六次 DBP 膳食摄入量下降了 83.6%。第五次、第六次中国总膳食研究的 DiBP 膳食摄入量分别为 3.71 μg/(kg bw·d) 和 0.80 μg/(kg bw·d)，水及饮料类是我国居民 DiBP 膳食摄入量的主要来源，摄入量为 0.36 μg/(kg bw·d)。与第五次结果相比，第六次 DiBP 膳食摄入量下降了 78.4%。第五次、第六次中国总膳食研究的 DEHP 膳食摄入量分别为 6.21 μg/(kg bw·d) 和 1.16 μg/(kg bw·d)，谷类是我国居民 DEHP 膳食

## IV. Comparison with the Results of Previous China TDS

Since the 5th China total diet study (TDS), dietary samples have been continuously tested for phthalates in China. The dietary intakes of DBP in the 5th and 6th CTDSs were 5.97 μg/(kg bw·d) and 0.98 μg/(kg bw·d), respectively, and cereals were the main sources of DBP dietary intake for China residents, with an intake of 0.33 μg/(kg bw·d). Dietary intake of DiBP decreased by 83.6% compared to the 5th result. The dietary intakes of DiBP in the 5th and 6th CTDSs were 3.71 μg/(kg bw·d) and 0.80 μg/(kg bw·d), respectively, while water and beverages were the main sources of DiBP intake in China, with an intake of 0.36 μg/(kg bw·d). Dietary intake of DEHP decreased by 78.4% in the 6th CTDS compared with the 5th CTDS results. The dietary intakes of DEHP in the 5th and 6th CTDSs were 6.21 μg/(kg bw·d) and 1.16 μg/(kg bw·d), respectively, while the cereals were the main sources of DEHP intake for China residents with an intake of 0.46 μg/(kg bw·d). Compared with the fifth result, the sixth dietary intake

摄入量的主要来源，摄入量为 0.46 μg/(kg bw·d)。与第五次结果相比，第六次 DEHP 膳食摄入量下降了 81.3%（表 6-2）。

of DEHP decreased by 81.3% (Table 6-2).

表 6-2 中国总膳食研究中邻苯二甲酸酯摄入量比较 [ 单位：μg/(kg bw·d)]
Table 6-2 Comparison of dietary intakes of phthalates from the China TDSs [Unit: μg/(kg bw·d)]

| 膳食类别 Category | 第五次中国总膳食研究 5<sup>th</sup> CTDS |  |  | 第六次中国总膳食研究 6<sup>th</sup> CTDS |  |  |
|---|---|---|---|---|---|---|
|  | DBP | DiBP | DEHP | DBP | DiBP | DEHP |
| 谷类 Cereals | 1.44 | 1.15 | 3.02 | 0.33 | 0.23 | 0.46 |
| 豆类 Legumes | 0.09 | 0.09 | 0.44 | 0.04 | 0.02 | 0.02 |
| 薯类 Potatoes | 0.02 | 0.02 | 0.38 | 0.03 | 0.02 | 0.04 |
| 肉类 Meats | 0.22 | 0.18 | 0.08 | 0.05 | 0.02 | 0.07 |
| 蛋类 Eggs | 0.01 | 0.01 | 0.01 | 0.01 | 0.01 | 0.01 |
| 水产类 Aquatic foods | 0.04 | 0.02 | 0.09 | 0.02 | 0.01 | 0.02 |
| 乳类 Dairy products | 0.01 | 0.01 | 0.01 | 0.01 | 0.01 | <0.01 |
| 蔬菜类 Vegetables | 3.96 | 2.05 | 2.03 | 0.21 | 0.10 | 0.36 |
| 水果类 Fruits | 0.02 | 0.03 | 0.01 | 0.02 | 0.01 | 0.01 |
| 糖类 Sugar | <0.01 | <0.01 | <0.01 | <0.01 | <0.01 | <0.01 |
| 水及饮料类 Water and beverages | 0.15 | 0.14 | 0.09 | 0.26 | 0.36 | 0.17 |
| 酒类 Alcohol beverages | 0.01 | 0.01 | 0.03 | 0.01 | 0.01 | <0.01 |
| 合计 SUM | 5.97 | 3.71 | 6.21 | 0.98 | 0.80 | 1.16 |

# 第七章 持久性有机污染物的膳食暴露评估
## Chapter 7  Dietary Exposure Assessment of Persistent Organic Pollutants

## 第一节 二噁英及其类似物
## Section 1  Dioxins and Their Analogues

### 一、背景

二噁英及其类似物包括多氯代苯并二噁英和多氯代苯并呋喃（PCDD/Fs）与二噁英样多氯联苯（dl-PCB），是典型的持久性有机污染物（POP），在环境中普遍存在，具有半挥发性，可通过大气环境长距离传输。其难溶于水，log Kow 为 5.6~8.2，具有强脂溶性，可通过食物链富集，膳食摄入尤其是动物性食品摄入，是普通（非职业暴露）人群二噁英类物质暴露的主要来源，可占人体全部暴露的 90% 以上。

PCDD/Fs 不是人类有目的生产的化学品，而是在含氯化学品如农药或 PCB 等生产过程以及燃烧过程中的副产品。研究显示，我国二噁英类物质的排放主要来源于金属冶炼、发电和供热、废弃物焚烧，这三者合计占总排放量的 81%。而 PCB 则属于人工合成的精细化工产品，在 1881 年首次合成至最终于 20 世纪 80 年代全球禁止生产期间，曾经大规模工业生产和使用，主要用作电介质、液压油、塑料和油漆添加剂等，在其生产和使用过程中排放及泄漏而进入环境造成污染。此外，有研究显示燃烧过程也会有 dl-PCB 的生成。

### I. Background

Dioxins and their analogues, including polychlorinated dibenzo-*p*-dioxins and polychlorinated dibenzofurans (PCDD/Fs), and dioxin like polychlorinated biphenyls (dl-PCBs), are classical POPs. PCDD/Fs and dl-PCBs are ubiquitous in the environment. They have semi-volatile and could be transported over long distance through the atmosphere. They are insoluble in water and high lipophilic with log Kow 5.6-8.2, and could be bio-accumulated through the food chain. Many studies have been revealed that the main source of human exposure to PCDD/Fs and dl-PCBs for non-occupational population was dietary intake, especially animal origin foods, accounting for over 90%.

PCDD/Fs are not produced intentionally but occur frequently as unwanted by-products in chemical processes, such as the synthesis of pesticides or PCBs. Combustion processes are recognized as the major sources of PCDD/Fs. In China, dioxins emissions mainly come from metal smelting, power generation and heating, and waste incineration, which together account for 81% of the total emissions. PCBs are synthetic chemical products. They were first synthesized in 1881 and finally banned from production in the 1980s globally. PCBs were used to be large-volume of fabrication and widely used as dielectrics, hydraulic fluids, plastic and paint additives. Emissions and leaks during production and usage caused widespread

## 二、健康指导值

基于动物实验获得观察到有害作用的最低剂量（LOAEL），WHO 确立了人类 1～4 pg TEQ/(kg bw·d) 的每日可耐受摄入量（TDI）。考虑到二噁英及其类似物的持久性和蓄积性，联合国粮食及农业组织和世界卫生组织食品添加剂联合专家委员会（JECFA）设立了二噁英及其类似物长期慢性暴露的暂定每月可耐受摄入量（PTMI）为 70 pg TEQ/(kg bw·月)。

## 三、总膳食研究结果

对第六次中国总膳食研究的肉类、蛋类、水产类、乳类等 4 类样品的代表性混合膳食样品中的二噁英及其类似物含量进行测定，对未检出的样品，以 LOD 值进行污染水平评价和膳食暴露评估。采用 WHO-TEF-1998 折算毒性当量（TEQ）。

**1. 混合膳食样品中二噁英及其类似物的含量**

平均含量最高的是水产类样品，总二噁英及其类似物的含量为 0.16 pg TEQ/g，次之为肉类样品，0.09 pg TEQ/g，再次为蛋类样品，为 0.07 pg TEQ/g，含量最低的为乳类样品，为 0.03 pg TEQ/g（附表 7-1）。

**2. 膳食暴露评估**

我国居民经膳食摄入二噁英及其类似物的暴露量为 7.7 pg TEQ/(kg bw·月)（附表 7-2），远低于 JECFA 规定的 70 pg TEQ/(kg bw·月) 的 PTMI。其中，膳食摄入量最高的是广西，为 22.6 pg TEQ/(kg bw·月)，次之是湖南、浙江和上海，膳食摄入量分别为 16.2 pg TEQ/(kg bw·月)、15.8 pg TEQ/(kg bw·月)、15.2 pg TEQ/(kg

environmental pollution. In addition, combustion could also result in the synthesis of some congeners of dl-PCBs.

## II. HBGV

According to the lowest observed adverse effect level (LOAEL) obtained from animal study, WHO set 1-4 pg TEQ/(kg bw·d) as tolerable daily intake (TDI). Moreover, due to the persistence and bioaccumulation of PCDD/Fs and dl-PCBs, the provisional tolerable monthly intake (PTMI) 70 pg TEQ/(kg bw·month) was set by Joint FAO/WHO Expert Committee on Food Additives (JECFA) for long-life chronic exposure to PCDD/Fs and dl-PCBs.

## III. TDS Results

We determined PCDD/Fs and dl-PCBs in various composite samples from four categories including meats, eggs, aquatic foods, dairy products from 6$^{th}$ CTDS. The value of concentration was set as "LOD" for "not detected" congener to perform the evaluation of contamination levels and dietary exposure. TEF values evaluated by WHO in 1998 (WHO-TEF-1998) was applied to calculate the TEQ.

**1. Concentrations of PCDD/Fs and dl-PCBs in TDS Composite Samples**

The highest concentrations of PCDD/Fs and dl-PCBs were found in aquatic foods with 0.16 pg TEQ/g, followed by meats, and eggs with the concentrations of 0.09 pg TEQ/g, and 0.07 pg TEQ/g, respectively. And the lowest concentrations were found in dairy products with 0.03 pg TEQ/g. Detailed information was listed in Annexed Table 7-1.

**2. Dietary Exposure Assessment**

Estimated dietary intake of PCDD/Fs and dl-PCBs for China residents were listed in Annexed Table 7-2. The levels of dietary intake were 7.7 pg TEQ/(kg

bw·月），最低的是宁夏，为 1.7 pg TEQ/(kg bw·月)（图 7-1）。

bw·month) which was greatly lower than PTMI set by JECFA, 70 pg TEQ/(kg bw·month). Residents from Guangxi, China, ingested the highest PCDD/Fs and dl-PCBs with 22.6 pg TEQ/(kg bw·month), followed by Hunan, Zhejiang, and Shanghai, with 16.2 pg TEQ/(kg bw·month), 15.8 pg TEQ/(kg bw·month), and 15.2 pg TEQ/(kg bw·month), respectively, and the lowest dietary intake attributed to Ningxia was 1.7 pg TEQ/(kg bw·month) (Figure 7-1).

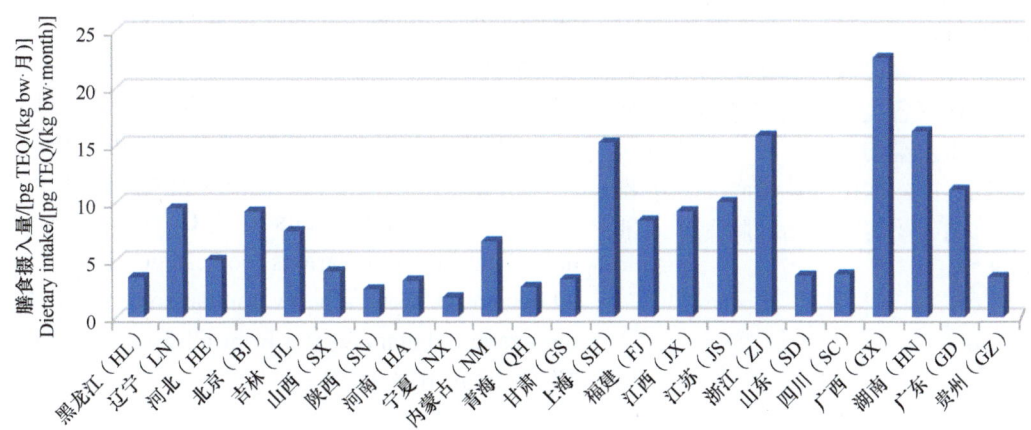

图 7-1　第六次中国总膳食研究二噁英及其类似物的膳食摄入量
Figure 7-1　Dietary intake of PCDD/Fs and dl-PCBs from the 6$^{th}$ China TDS

### 3. 各类膳食对总膳食摄入的贡献

根据第六次中国总膳食研究的结果，膳食摄入的二噁英及其类似物主要来源于肉类（48.7%），其次为水产类（32.6%），蛋类（11.8%）和乳类（6.9%）的贡献较小（图 7-2 和附表 7-3）。

### 3. Contributions of Food Categories to the Total Dietary Intake

According to the results of the 6$^{th}$ China TDS, meats are the main source of dietary intake to the PCDD/Fs and dl-PCBs, accounting for 48.7%, followed by aquatic foods, accounting for 32.6%. The percentage contribution from eggs and dairy products are relatively

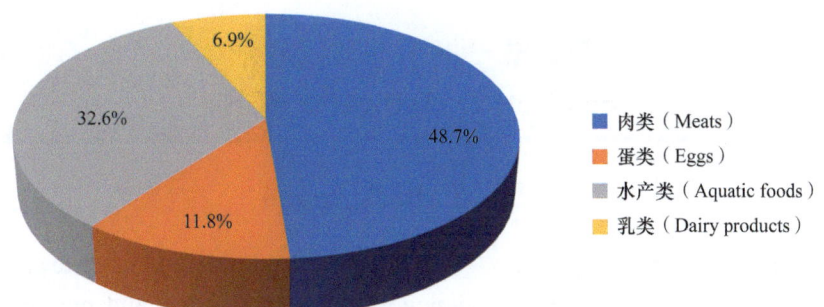

图 7-2　第六次中国总膳食研究二噁英及其类似物的膳食来源
Figure 7-2　Dietary sources of PCDD/Fs and dl-PCBs from the 6$^{th}$ China TDS

## 四、与以往中国总膳食研究结果的比较

自第三次中国总膳食研究以来，我国连续开展二噁英及其类似物的膳食暴露评估工作。第三次、第四次、第五次、第六次中国总膳食研究的二噁英及其类似物的膳食摄入量分别为 15.7 pg TEQ/(kg bw·月)、16.1 pg TEQ/(kg bw·月)、15.0 pg TEQ/(kg bw·月) 和 7.7 pg TEQ/(kg bw·月)（表7-1）。与第五次中国总膳食研究膳食摄入量相比，第六次中国总膳食研究各类食品的二噁英及其类似物膳食摄入量均有所下降。与第五次结果相比，第六次中国总膳食研究中我国居民二噁英及其类似物的膳食摄入量下降 48.7%。

lower, accounting for 11.8% and 6.9%, respectively. Detail information is shown in Figure 7-2 and Annexed Table 7-3.

## IV. Comparison with Previous China TDSs Results

Assessment on dietary intake of PCDD/Fs and dl-PCBs has been continuously carried out at national level based on China TDS since the 3$^{rd}$ CTDS in 2000. The average of estimated dietary intake of PCDD/Fs and dl-PCBs in 3$^{rd}$ CTDS, 4$^{th}$ CTDS, 5$^{th}$ CTDS, and 6$^{th}$ CTDS was 15.7 pg TEQ/(kg bw·month), 16.1 pg TEQ/(kg bw·month), 15.0 pg TEQ/(kg bw·month), and 7.7 pg TEQ/(kg bw·month), respectively (Table 7-1). Compared with the results in 5$^{th}$ CTDS, the estimated dietary intakes from various food categories in 6$^{th}$ CTDS all decreased. Generally, by comparison with 5$^{th}$ CTDS, the average dietary intake from all foods decreased by 48.7% in the 6$^{th}$ CTDS.

表 7-1　中国总膳食研究中二噁英及其类似物的摄入量比较 [ 单位：pg TEQ/(kg bw·月)]

Table 7-1　Comparison of the levels of dietary intakes of PCDD/Fs and dl-PCBs from China TDSs [Unit: pg TEQ/(kg bw·month)]

| 食物类别 Category | 第三次中国总膳食研究 3$^{rd}$ CTDS | 第四次中国总膳食研究 4$^{th}$ CTDS | 第五次中国总膳食研究 5$^{th}$ CTDS | 第六次中国总膳食研究 6$^{th}$ CTDS |
|---|---|---|---|---|
| 肉类 Meats | 6.3 | 5.0 | 4.6 | 3.8 |
| 蛋类 Eggs | 2.6 | 2.5 | 1.3 | 0.9 |
| 水产类 Aquatic Foods | 5.8 | 5.4 | 7.0 | 2.5 |
| 乳类 Dairy products | 1.1 | 3.1 | 2.2 | 0.5 |
| 合计 SUM | 15.7 | 16.1 | 15.0 | 7.7 |

## 第二节　指示性多氯联苯
## Section 2　Indicator PCBs

### 一、背景

多氯联苯（PCB）为典型的持久性有机污染物，根据氯原子取代数目及取代位置的不同共有 209 种同类物。食品污染监测中通常采用检测特定种类

### I. Background

PCBs are classical POPs and there are 209 congeners depending on the number and position of chlorine atoms on aromatic rings. There are specific congeners of PCBs that are determined for representing the total

PCB 来表征整体污染水平，这些特定PCB 称为指示性 PCB（MPCB），参考欧盟相关监测规定，本研究对 PCB 28、PCB 52、PCB 101、PCB 138、PCB 153、PCB 180 共 6 种化合物开展测定。

PCB 被广泛用于多种工业和商业目的，主要包括在液压和传热系统中以及变压器与电容器中作为冷却和绝缘流体，以及用作增塑剂广泛应用于颜料、染料、驱虫剂、无碳复写纸、油漆、密封剂、塑料和橡胶产品中。我国 PCB 的生产始于 1965 年，至 20 世纪 80 年代初停止生产，其累计产量 7000～10 000 t。大量研究显示我国环境中 PCB 含量水平显著低于欧美日等国家。

## 二、总膳食研究结果

对 24 个省（自治区、直辖市）的肉类、蛋类、水产类、乳类、谷类、豆类、薯类、蔬菜类等 8 类样品共 192 份混合膳食样品中的指示性多氯联苯含量进行测定，对未检出的样品，以 LOD 值进行污染水平和膳食暴露评估。

**1. 混合膳食样品中指示性多氯联苯的含量**

以 6 种指示性 PCB 之和（∑MPCB）表示膳食样品的污染水平。不同膳食样品间以及来自不同地区的同种类样品间的污染水平存在极大差别，见附表 7-4。在平均水平上，水产类样品含量最高，为 158.0 pg/g，次之为肉类样品，含量为 100.7 pg/g。

PCBs in foods. And these specific PCB congeners are so-called marker PCBs or indicator PCBs. According to the EU regulation, six congeners of indicator PCBs were determined, including PCB 28, PCB 52, PCB 101, PCB 138, PCB 153, and PCB 180.

PCBs are widely used for a variety of industrial and commercial purposes, including used as cooling and insulating fluids in hydraulic and heat transfer systems as well as in transformers and capacitors, and as plasticizers in pigments, dyes, insect repellents, carbonless papers, paints, sealants, plastics and rubber products. The production of PCBs in China started in 1965 and stopped in the early 1980s, with output of about 7000-10 000 tons.

A large number of studies have shown that the level of PCBs in the environment of our country is significantly lower than that of countries such as Europe, America and Japan.

## II. TDS Results

We determined indicator PCBs in 192 composite samples from eight categories including cereals, legumes, potatoes, meats, eggs, aquatic foods, dairy products, and vegetables from 24 provinces (autonomous regions, municipalities) in China. The value of concentration was set as "LOD" for "not detected" congener to perform the evaluation of contamination levels and dietary exposure.

**1. Concentrations of Indicator PCBs in TDS Composite Samples**

The summation of 6 congeners of indicator PCBs (ΣMPCBs), was calculate to represent the contamination level in food samples. There are big differences in concentrations of PCBs among different food categories as well as among foods with the same category from various regions. Detail information is listed in Annexed Table 7-4. On average, the highest concentrations of indicator PCBs were found in aquatic foods with 158.0 pg/g (mean ± standard deviation), followed by meats with the concentrations of 100.7 pg/g.

## 2. 膳食暴露评估

我国居民指示性 PCB 的平均膳食摄入量为 429.9 pg/(kg bw·d)，中位数为 248.1 pg/(kg bw·d)（图 7-3 和附表 7-5）。其中，膳食摄入量最高的为广西壮族自治区居民，达 3804.7 pg/(kg bw·d)，次之为广东省居民，为 1066.3 pg/(kg bw·d)，具体见图 7-3 和附表 7-5。

## 2. Dietary Exposure Assessment

Mean dietary intake of indicator PCBs for China residents were elucidated in Figure 7-3 and Annexed Table 7-5. The levels of dietary intake were 429.9 pg/(kg bw·d) with a median of 248.1 pg/(kg bw·d). Residents from Guangxi, China, ingested the highest indicator PCBs with 3804.7 pg/(kg bw·d), followed by Guangdong with 1066.3 pg/(kg bw·d).

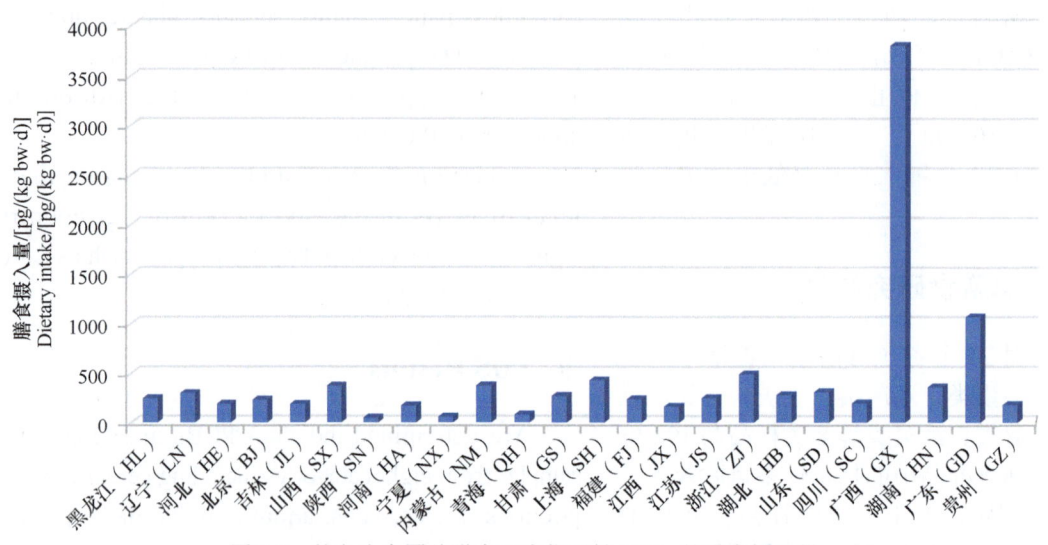

图 7-3　第六次中国总膳食研究指示性 PCBs 的膳食摄入量
Figure 7-3　Dietary intake of indicator PCBs from the 6th China TDS

## 3. 各类膳食对总膳食摄入的贡献

我国居民各类食品中贡献最高的是肉类食品，占 25.5%，次之为水产类、谷类和蔬菜类，分别占 20.1%、19.3% 和 16.1%。植物性食品与动物性食品对膳食暴露的贡献分别为 43.8% 和 56.2%，见图 7-4 和附表 7-6。

## 三、与以往中国总膳食研究结果的比较

第四次、第五次、第六次中国总膳食研究的指示性 PCB 的膳食摄入量分别为 2058.1 pg/(kg bw·d)、666.0 pg/(kg bw·d) 和 429.9 pg/(kg bw·d)（表 7-2）。

## 3. Contributions of Food Categories to the Total Dietary Intake

Meats are the main source of dietary intake for residents in China, accounting for 25.5%, followed by aquatic foods, cereals, and vegetables, accounting for 20.1%, 19.3% and 16.1%, respectively. The total percentage contribution of plant origin foods and animal origin foods is 43.8% and 56.2%, respectively. Detail information is listed in Figure 7-4 and Annex Table 7-6.

## III. Comparison with Previous China TDSs Results

The average of dietary intake of indicator PCBs in 4th CTDS, 5th CTDS, and 6th CTDS was 2058.1 pg/

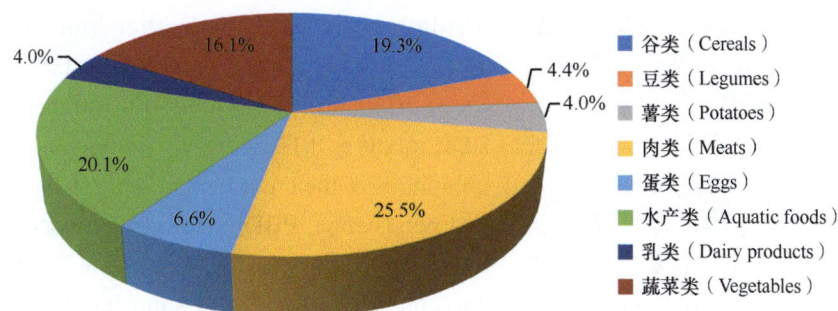

图 7-4 第六次中国总膳食研究指示性 PCBs 的膳食来源
Figure 7-4　Dietary sources of indicator PCBs from the 6th China TDS

表 7-2　中国总膳食研究中指示性 PCB 的膳食摄入量比较 [单位：pg/(kg bw·d)]
Table 7-2　Comparison of the levels of dietary intakes of indicator PCBs from China TDSs [Unit: pg/(kg bw·d)]

| 食物类别 Category | 第四次 CTDS 4th CTDS | 第五次 CTDS 5th CTDS | 第六次 CTDS 6th CTDS |
|---|---|---|---|
| 谷类 Cereals | 827.6 | 74.2 | 67.7 |
| 豆类 Legumes | 68.2 | 13.1 | 11.4 |
| 薯类 Potatoes | 40.0 | 10.1 | 9.1 |
| 肉类 Meats | 279.8 | 86.3 | 195.0 |
| 蛋类 Eggs | 124.1 | 33.8 | 15.2 |
| 水产类 Aquatic foods | 397.9 | 321.2 | 78.0 |
| 乳类 Dairy products | 42.8 | 13.5 | 10.3 |
| 蔬菜类 Vegetables | 277.8 | 113.8 | 43.4 |
| 合计 SUM | 2058.1 | 666.0 | 429.9 |

与第五次中国 TDS 结果相比，第六次中国总膳食研究中我国居民指示性 PCB 的膳食摄入量下降 35.5%。

(kg bw·d), 666.0 pg/(kg bw·d), and 429.9 pg/(kg bw·d), respectively (Table 7-2). By comparison with 5th CTDS, the average dietary intake for China residents decreased by 35.5% in the current CTDS.

## 第三节　多溴二苯醚
## Section 3　Polybrominated Diphenyl Ethers

### 一、背景
### Ⅰ. Background

多溴二苯醚（PBDE）曾大量生产，主要用作添加型阻燃剂，广泛应用在各种消费类产品上，包括电脑、各种电子电气类产品、电视机、纺织品、泡沫填充类家具、绝缘材料以及其他建筑

Polybrominated diphenyl ethers (PBDEs) were used to be produces in huge volume and widely used as additive flame retardants in various consumer products, including computers, various electrical and electronic products, televisions, textiles, and foam-filled furniture,

材料等。其商业化产品主要为3种多溴二苯醚商业性混合物，包括五溴二苯醚混合物、八溴二苯醚混合物和十溴二苯醚混合物。PBDE作为环境污染物，在环境中普遍存在，由于其亲脂性和持久性，可通过食物链富集，在食品样品中也普遍检出。食品中主要检测7种同类物，即BDE-28、BDE-47、BDE-99、BDE-100、BDE-153、BDE-154和BDE-183，用于指示PBDE的总体污染情况。

## 二、健康指导值

EFSA以神经发育毒性为关键终点来评估人体慢性膳食摄入，BDE-47、BDE-99、BDE-153的$BMDL_{10}$分别为172 ng/(kg bw·d)、4.2 ng/(kg bw·d)和9.6 ng/(kg bw·d)。EFSA规定MOE＞2.5即提示无健康风险。

## 三、总膳食研究结果

对24个省（自治区、直辖市）的谷类、豆类、薯类、肉类、蛋类、水产类、乳类、蔬菜类等8类样品共192份混合膳食样品中的多溴二苯醚含量进行测定，对未检出的样品，以LOD值进行污染水平和膳食暴露评估。

**1. 混合膳食样品中多溴二苯醚的含量**

以7种PBDE之和（∑PBDE）表示膳食样品污染水平。按平均含量计，水产类样品含量最高，为39.9 pg/g，次之为肉类样品，含量为29.8 pg/g（附表7-7）。

insulating materials and other building materials. There are three main commercial mixtures, including Penta-BDE mixture, Octa-BDE mixture, and Deca-BDE mixture. PBDEs are environmental pollutants and ubiquitous in the environment. Due to high lipophilicity and persistence, PBDEs could be bioaccumulated and biomagnified through the food chain. PBDEs have been detected in various food samples. Generally, seven congeners of PBDEs are determined to represent the contamination in foods, including BDE-28, BDE-47, BDE-99, BDE-100, BDE-153, BDE-154, and BDE-183.

## II. HBGV

On the basis of the adverse effects on neuro-development as the critical end point and an estimation of chronic human dietary intake, $BMDL_{10}$ recommended by the European Food Safety Authority (EFSA) of BDE-47, BDE-99, and BDE-153 was 172 ng/(kg bw·d), 4.2 ng/(kg bw·d), and 9.6 ng/(kg bw·d), respectively. EFSA regulate MOE>2.5 might indicate that there is no health risk.

## III. TDS Results

We determined PBDEs in 192 composite samples from eight categories including cereals, legumes, potatoes, meats, eggs, aquatic foods, dairy products, and vegetables from 24 provinces (autonomous regions, municipalities) in China. The value of concentration was set as "LOD" for "not detected" congener to perform the evaluation of contamination levels and dietary exposure.

**1. Concentrations of PBDEs in TDS Composite Samples**

The summation of 7 congeners of PBDEs, ∑PBDEs, was calculate to represent the contamination level in food samples. On average, the highest concentrations were found in aquatic foods with 39.9 pg/g, followed by meats with 29.8 pg/g (Annex Table 7-7).

## 2. 膳食暴露评估

我国居民 PBDE 膳食摄入量为 249.0 pg/(kg bw·d)，中位数为 185.7 pg/(kg bw·d)。摄入水平最高的为浙江省居民，达 1959.9 pg/(kg bw·d)，次之为内蒙古自治区和广西壮族自治区居民，分别为 388.0 pg/(kg bw·d) 和 378.2 pg/(kg bw·d)（图 7-5 和附表 7-8）。

基于 EFSA 的 $BMDL_{10}$ 开展风险暴露评估，出于保守估计，以总 PBDE 暴露量与 EFSA 规定的各 PBDE 化合物的 $BMDL_{10}$ 计算暴露边界值（MOE），范围为 1000～17 000 000。

## 2. Dietary Exposure Assessment

Estimated dietary intake of PBDEs for China residents were elucidated in Figure 7-5 and Annexed Table 7-8. The levels of dietary intake were 249.0 pg/(kg bw·d) with a median of 185.7 pg/(kg bw·d). Residents from Zhejiang, China, ingested the highest PBDEs with 1959.9 pg/(kg bw·d), followed by Neimenggu and Guangxi with 388.0 pg/(kg bw·d) and 378.2 pg/(kg bw·d), respectively (Figure 7-5 and Annex Table 7-8).

Risk assessment was conducted using MOE approach by comparison with $BMDL_{10}$ recommended by EFSA. Conservatively, the values of MOE were calculated by dividing each $BMDL_{10}$ of individual PBDEs by estimated dietary intake of ∑PBDEs. The values of MOE are in the rang of 1000-17 000 000.

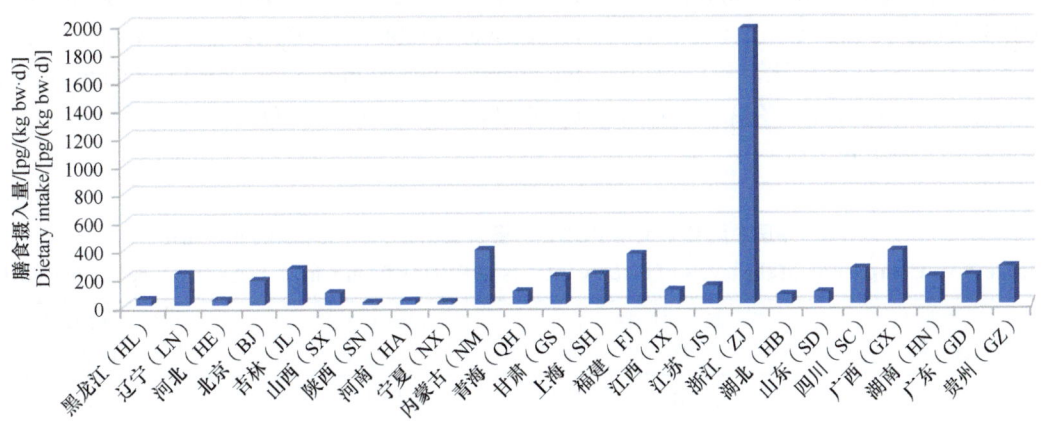

图 7-5　第六次中国总膳食研究 PBDE 的膳食摄入量
Figure 7-5　Dietary intake of PBDEs from the 6th China TDS

## 3. 各类膳食对总膳食摄入的贡献

根据第六次中国总膳食研究的结果，膳食摄入的多溴二苯醚主要来源于谷类（23.4%）、肉类（24.4%）、蔬菜类（23.2%）和水产类（12.7%），合计占总膳食摄入量的 83.7%（图 7-6 和附表 7-9）。

## 3. Contributions of Food Categories to the Total Dietary Intake

According to the results of the 6th China TDS, the average source of dietary intake of PBDEs for residents in China. On average, the main dietary sources attributed to cereals, meats, and vegetables. The percentage contributions of these food categories are comparable, accounting for 23.4%, 24.4%, and 23.2%, respectively, followed by aquatic foods with a percentage contribution of 12.7%. These four categories accounted for 83.7% in totally. Detail information is listed in Figure 7-6 and Annex Table 7-9.

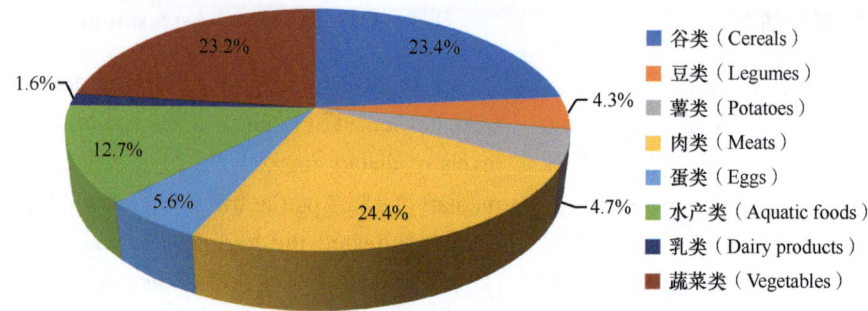

图 7-6 第六次中国总膳食研究 PBDE 的膳食来源
Figure 7-6 Dietary sources of PBDEs from the 6<sup>th</sup> China TDS

## 四、与以往中国总膳食研究结果的比较

第四次、第五次、第六次中国总膳食研究的多溴二苯醚的膳食摄入量分别为 700.7 pg/(kg bw·d)、646.0 pg/(kg bw·d) 和 240.9 pg/(kg bw·d)（表 7-3）。与第五次 CTDS 结果相比，第六次中国总膳食研究中我国居民多溴二苯醚的膳食摄入量下降了 62.7%。

## IV. Comparison with Previous China TDSs Results

The average of dietary intake of PBDEs in 4<sup>th</sup> CTDS, 5<sup>th</sup> CTDS, and 6<sup>th</sup> CTDS was 700.7 pg/(kg bw·d), 646.0 pg/(kg bw·d), and 240.9 pg/(kg bw·d), respectively (Table 7-3). By comparison with 5<sup>th</sup> CTDS, the average dietary intake for China residents decreased by 62.7% in the current CTDS.

表 7-3 中国总膳食研究中 PBDE 的摄入量比较 [单位：pg/(kg bw·d)]
Table 7-3 Comparison of the levels of dietary intakes of PBDEs from China TDSs [Unit: pg/(kg bw·d)]

| 食物类别<br>Category | 第四次 CTDS<br>4<sup>th</sup> CTDS | 第五次 CTDS<br>5<sup>th</sup> CTDS | 第六次 CTDS<br>6<sup>th</sup> CTDS |
|---|---|---|---|
| 谷类 Cereals | 187.7 | 96.0 | 81.0 |
| 豆类 Legumes | 16.9 | 10.0 | 10.7 |
| 薯类 Potatoes | 13.3 | 10.0 | 7.8 |
| 肉类 Meats | 222.0 | 145.0 | 51.8 |
| 蛋类 Eggs | 32.3 | 101.0 | 10.5 |
| 水产类 Aquatic foods | 106.9 | 149.0 | 24.5 |
| 乳类 Dairy products | 7.0 | 9.0 | 2.0 |
| 蔬菜类 Vegetables | 114.5 | 126.0 | 52.5 |
| 合计 SUM | 700.7 | 646.0 | 240.9 |

# 第四节 六溴环十二烷
# Section 4　Hexabromocyclododecane

## 一、背景

六溴环十二烷（HBCD）是自 20 世纪 90 年代以来较常用的一种溴系阻燃剂（BFR）。商用 HBCD 主要由三种异构体（α-HBCD、β-HBCD 和 γ-HBCD）构成。研究表明 HBCD 暴露可引起多种毒性效应。鉴于其较强的毒性及环境持久性，HBCD 已于 2013 年被列入《关于持久性有机污染物的斯德哥尔摩公约》，但我国允许其在 2022 年之前用于建筑物保温材料。膳食是普通人群摄入 HBCD 的主要途径，我国已先后在第四次和第五次中国总膳食研究中开展了 HBCD 膳食暴露评估工作。

## 二、健康指导值

欧洲食品安全局（EFSA）于 2011 年首次设定了 HBCD 的基准剂量置信下限值（benchmark dose lower confidence limit，BMDL）[0.79 mg/(kg bw·d)]。但在 2021 年最新报告中，EFSA 采用人类慢性膳食摄入量（CHDI）代替了 BMDL，并将其用于计算 MOE。EFSA 规定的 HBCD 的 CHDI 为 2.35 μg/(kg bw·d)，MOE 阈值为 24。

## 三、总膳食研究结果

**1. 混合膳食样品中六溴环十二烷的含量**

在第六次 CTDS 中，对 4 类动物性膳食进行了 HBCD 含量分析，包括肉类、水产类、蛋类和乳类，各省（自治区、直辖市）样品中 HBCD（3 种异构体之和）的含量结果见附表 7-10。

## Ⅰ. Background

Hexabromocyclododecane (HBCD) belongs to brominated flame retardants (BFRs) and has been frequently used since 1990s. Commercial HBCD is composed of three isomers (α-HBCD、β-HBCD and γ-HBCD). Studies have shown that the exposure of HBCD would cause toxic effects. Due to its relatively high toxicity and environmental persistence, HBCD has been listed as persistent organic pollutants under the *Stockholm Convention on Persistent Organic Pollutants* since 2013, however, its usage in heat insulating building material was still permitted in China before 2022. Intake of HBCD via food consumption is the major intake pathway for HBCD in general population, and the dietary exposure assessment of HBCD for Chinese population has conducted twice on the basis of the 4$^{th}$ and 5$^{th}$ China total diet study (TDS).

## Ⅱ. HBGV

For HBCD, benchmark dose lower confidence limit (BMDL) of 0.79 mg/(kg bw·d) was set by European Food Safety Authority (EFSA) in 2011. However, in a update report released in 2021, BMDL was replaced by chronic human dietary intake (CHDI), and CHDI was then used to calculate the MOE of HBCD. In the report of EFSA, the value of CHDI and threshold of MOE of HBCD were set as 2.35 μg/(kg bw·d) and 24, respectively.

## Ⅲ. TDS Results

**1. Levels of HBCD in TDS Composite Samples**

In the 6$^{th}$ CTDS, the contamination levels of HBCD (sum of three isomers) were measured in four animal-based CTDS composite samples (meats, aquatic

在来自 24 个省（自治区、直辖市）的所有 96 个动物性膳食样本中均可检出 HBCD。4 类动物性食品中 HBCD 含量均值从高到低为肉类（1840 pg/g）、水产类（441.1 pg/g）、蛋类（93.7 pg/g）和乳类（41.9 pg/g）。由此可见肉类食品中 HBCD 含量明显高于其他类食品。

**2. 膳食暴露评估**

我国各省（自治区、直辖市）标准人经膳食摄入 HBCD 的情况见附表 7-11 和图 7-7。经膳食摄入 HBCD 的均值为 3062 pg/(kg bw·d)，但各地存在明显差异。膳食摄入量较高的三个地区分别为辽宁省 [18 439.6 pg/(kg bw·d)]、四川省 [12 749.2 pg/(kg bw·d)] 和北京市 [11 323.6 pg/(kg bw·d)]。基于 CHDI，采用 EFSA 推荐的 MOE 法对我国居民膳食摄入 HBCD 的健康风险进行评估。我国居民经膳食的 HBCD 暴露的 MOE 值中位数为 1590，远高于 EFSA 设定的 24 这一阈值，表明我国居民经动物性膳食的 HBCD 摄入尚不足以引起显著的健康风险。但部分具有较高 HBCD 暴露的地区，如辽宁（MOE=127）、四川（MOE=184）和北京（MOE=207）

products, eggs and dairy products), and the results are shown in Annexed Table 7-10.

HBCD was detected in all the 96 TDS composite samples collected from 24 provinces (autonomous regions, municipalities) in China. In meats, aquatic products, eggs and dairy products, the average concentrations of HBCD in a descending order were meats (1840 pg/g), aquatic products (441.1 pg/g), eggs (93.7 pg/g), and dairy products (41.9 pg/g). It can be seen that the HBCD level in meats is far higher than that in other food categories.

**2. Dietary Exposure Assessment**

The dietary intake of HBCD for a Chinese standard man in the 24 provinces (autonomous regions, municipalities) are shown in Annexed Table 7-11 and Figure 7-7. The average dietary HBCD intake was 3062 pg/(kg bw·d), and large variety could be observed among different areas. High dietary HBCD intakes were found in Liaoning [18 439.6 pg/(kg bw·d)], Sichuan [12 749.2 pg/(kg bw·d)] and Beijing [11 323.6 pg/(kg bw·d)]. Based on CHDI, the MOE approach suggested by the EFSA was used to assess the health risk caused by dietary HBCD intake for the Chinese population. The median MOE level of HBCD's dietary exposure for Chinese population was 1590. This value was significantly higher than the threshold of 24 set by

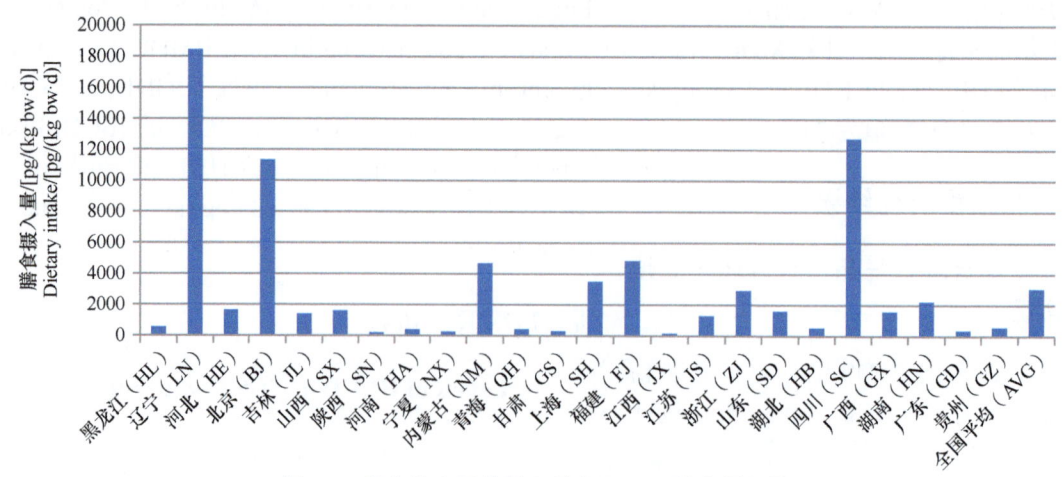

图 7-7 第六次中国总膳食研究 HBCD 膳食摄入量
Figure 7-7 Dietary intake of HBCD in the 6$^{th}$ China total diet study

的 MOE 值已接近阈值，需持续关注。

**3. 各类膳食对总膳食摄入的贡献**

在第六次 CTDS 中，肉类是摄入 HBCD 的最主要膳食来源，占总膳食摄入量的比例平均为 87.7%，其次是水产类，占 9.9%，而来自蛋类和乳类的贡献仅分别为 1.7% 和 0.7%（图 7-8）。在 24 个省（自治区、直辖市）中，肉类是除福建省和广西壮族自治区以外其他地区居民膳食 HBCD 的主要摄入来源，占总摄入量的比例从 53.8%（江西省）到 99.6%（四川省）。对于福建省和广西壮族自治区，水产类食品是当地居民摄入 HBCD 的主要来源，占总摄入量的比例分别为 97.9% 和 58.6%。

EFSA, suggesting that the intake of HBCD via animal-based food consumption for Chinese population was unlikely to cause significant health concerns. However, dietary exposure of HBCD in some areas were relatively high, such as Liaoning (MOE=127), Sichuang (MOE=184) and Beijing (MOE=207), and their MOEs have found to be close to the threshold.

**3. Contributions of Food Categories to the Total Dietary Intake**

The primary sources of dietary intake to HBCD in the 6$^{th}$ CTDS was meats, and which accounted for 87.7% in total intake of HBCD, followed by aquatic foods (9.9%), and the contributions from eggs and dairy products were only 1.7% and 0.7%, respectively (Figure 7-8). In the 24 provinces (autonomous regions, municipalities), meats was the major contributor in dietary intake of HBCD in all areas except for Fujian and Guangxi, and proportions of meats were from 53.8% in Jiangxi to 99.6% in Sichuan. Especially, in Fujian and Guangxi, the dietary intake of HBCD for local people was mainly from aquatic foods, and proportions were 97.9% and 58.6%, respectively.

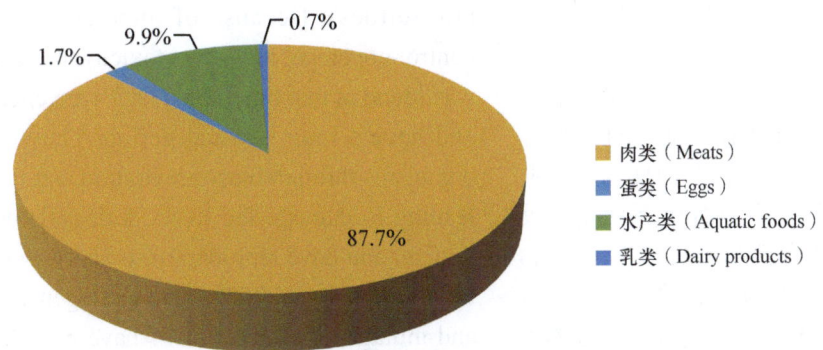

图 7-8　第六次中国总膳食研究 HBCD 的膳食来源
Figure 7-8　Dietary sources of HBCD in the 6$^{th}$ China total diet study

## 四、与以往中国总膳食研究结果的比较

我国从第四次中国总膳食研究开始开展 HBCD 的检测与人群暴露评估。

## IV. Comparison with Previous China TDSs Results

The measurement of HBCD in CTDS samples and exposure assessment of HBCD for Chinese population

第四次、第五次和第六次中国总膳食研究动物性食品中 HBCD 的平均含量分别为 61.5 pg/g、325.3 pg/g 和 604.2 pg/g，呈现逐次上升趋势。第四次、第五次、第六次中国总膳食研究中我国标准人的 HBCD 平均摄入量分别为 432 pg/(kg bw·d)、1476 pg/(kg bw·d) 和 3062 pg/(kg bw·d)，同样呈现逐次上升趋势。

was firstly conducted in the 4th CTDS. The average concentrations of HBCD in animal-based food samples in the 4th, 5th and 6th CTDSs were respectively 61.5 pg/g、325.3 pg/g and 604.2 pg/g, and a successive uptrend can be observed from the 4th to 6th CTDSs. Accordingly, the average dietary HBCD intake for the Chinese standard man in the 4th, 5th and 6th CTDSs were respectively 432 pg/(kg bw · d)、1476 pg/(kg bw · d) and 3062 pg/(kg bw · d), which also presented a successive uptrend.

## 第五节　持久性有机氯农药
## Section 5　Persistent Organochlorine Pesticides

### 一、背景

有机氯农药（OCP）是一类人工合成的广谱、残效期长的化学杀虫剂。OCP 大多数属于含氯烃类、碳环或杂环化合物。从 20 世纪 40 年代开始，人类就开始使用滴滴涕和六六六作为杀虫剂，由于其药效好、防治面广、急性毒性低，而且当时尚未发现其残留毒性，因此被广泛应用于防治农田、森林的害虫，控制传播传染病的害虫（如疟蚊）。大部分 OCP 的化学性质稳定、残留期长，能通过生物富集作用和食物链进入生物体内，会损害肝脏、肾脏、中枢神经系统等，具有一定的生殖毒性和遗传毒性。此外，有些 OCP 还具有致畸、致癌、致突变作用。鉴于 OCP 对环境和生物体有严重危害性，如今已经被禁用。2001年，《关于持久性有机污染物的斯德哥尔摩公约》决定在全世界范围内禁用或严格限用的 12 种持久性有机污染物（POP）中 9 种为有机氯农药，包括艾氏剂（aldrin）、狄氏剂（dieldrin）、异狄氏剂（endrin）、氯丹（chlordane）、七氯（heptachlor）、六氯苯（HCB）、

### I. Background

Organochlorine pesticides (OCPs) are a group of synthetic wide-spectrum chemical pesticides with a long residual life. Most OCPs are chlorinated hydrocarbons, carbocyclic or heterocyclic compounds. Since the 1940s, DDTs and HCHs were widely used as insecticides for the control of farmland and forest pests, also the pests which transmit infectious diseases (such as malaria mosquitoes). Because of their good efficacy, wide control coverage, low acute toxicity, no residual toxicity was found at that time. Most OCPs are chemically stable and have a long residual period. They can enter into organisms through bioconcentration and food chain, and leading to damage the livers, kidneys, central nervous system, and have reproductive toxicity and genotoxicity. In addition, some OCPs have teratogenic, carcinogenic, and mutagenic effects. OCPs have been banned due to their serious environmental and biological hazards. In 2001, the *Stockholm Convention on Persistent Organic Pollutants* decided to ban or strictly limit the use of 12 kinds of persistent organic pollutants (POPs) worldwide, 9 of which were OCPs, including aldrin, dieldrin, endrin, chlordane, heptachlor, hexachlorobenzene (HCB), mirex, toxaphene, and DDT. In 2009, the isomers of hexachlorocyclohexane including α-HCH, β-HCH,

灭蚁灵（mirex）、毒杀芬（toxaphene）和滴滴涕（DDT）。2009 年，六六六的同分异构体包括 α-六六六（α-HCH）、β-六六六（β-HCH）和林丹（lindane）及五氯苯（pentachlorobenzene）被增补到优先控制名单中。近年又新增硫丹及其异构体（endosulfan and its isomers）到新的 POP 清单中。

## 二、健康指导值

FAO/WHO 农药残留联席会议（JMPR）规定了部分持久性有机氯农药的暂定每日可耐受摄入量（PTDI）或每日允许摄入量（ADI），我国《食品安全国家标准 食品中农药最大残留限量》（GB 2763—2021）亦规定了部分持久性有机氯农药的每日允许摄入量（ADI），五氯苯和六氯苯选择加拿大卫生部规定的每日可耐受摄入量（TDI）。具体见表 7-4。

lindane, and pentachlorobenzene (PCB) were added to the priority control list. In recent years, endosulfan and its isomers have been added to the new list of POPs.

## II. HBGV

The provisional tolerable daily intake (PTDI) and acceptable daily intake (ADI) values for OCPs specified by FAO/WHO Joint Meeting of Pesticide Residues (JMPR) and ADI values also specified by the *National Food Safety Standard-The Maximum Residue Limits for Pesticides* in Food are shown in Table 7-4 (GB 2763—2021). For PCB and HCB, the tolerated daily intake (TDI) specified by Health Canada was selected.

表 7-4　持久性有机氯农药的健康指导值
Table 7-4　The HBGVs of OCPs

| 序号 | 农药名称 | Pesticides | PTDI 或 ADI 或 TDI/（mg/kg bw） |
|---|---|---|---|
| 1 | 五氯苯 | Pentachlorobenzene | 0.000 5 |
| 2 | 六六六 | Hexachlorocyclohexane | 0.002 |
| 3 | 六氯苯 | Hexachlorobenzene | 0.000 27 |
| 4 | 七氯 | Heptachlor | 0.000 1 |
| 5 | 氯丹 | Chlordane | 0.000 5 |
| 6 | 艾试剂和狄氏剂 | Aldrin and Dieldrin | 0.000 1 |
| 7 | 滴滴涕 | DDT | 0.01 |
| 8 | 异狄氏剂 | Endrin | 0.000 2 |
| 9 | 硫丹 | Endosulfan | 0.006 |

## 三、总膳食研究结果

**1. 混合膳食样品中持久性有机氯农药的含量**

对 24 个省（自治区、直辖市）的谷类、豆类、薯类、肉类、蛋类、水产

## III. TDS Results

**1. Levels of OCPs in Dietary TDS Composite Samples**

OCPs in various composite samples from nine categories including cereals, legumes, potatoes, meats,

类、乳类、蔬菜类及水果类等9类混合膳食样品中的持久性有机氯农药含量进行测定，对低于检出限的样品，以0进行污染水平评价和膳食暴露评估。第六次总膳食研究混合膳食样品中检出的持久性有机氯农药包括滴滴涕、六六六、硫丹、五氯苯、六氯苯、艾氏剂和狄氏剂、氯丹以及七氯。各种持久性有机氯农药的检出率由高至低分别为五氯苯（97.7%）、六六六（52.8%）、滴滴涕（51.4%）、六氯苯（39.4%）、硫丹（16.7%）、艾氏剂和狄氏剂（6.0%）、氯丹（3.7%）与七氯（2.8%）。

第六次中国总膳食研究的混合膳食样品中五氯苯的污染水平为ND～1.06 μg/kg（附表7-16）。各类膳食样品中均检出五氯苯，水产类和肉类检出污染水平较高，为0.07~0.23 μg/kg。

第六次中国总膳食研究的混合膳食样品中滴滴涕的污染水平为ND～9.83 μg/kg（附表7-13）。除水果类外8类膳食中均检出滴滴涕。水产类膳食中的平均污染水平最高（2.25 μg/kg），其次为肉类和蛋类（均为0.57 μg/kg）、乳类（0.34 μg/kg），其他类膳食中滴滴涕污染水平相对较低。

第六次中国总膳食研究的混合膳食样品中六六六的污染水平为ND～6.62 μg/kg（附表7-14）。除水果类外8类膳食中均检出六六六，水产类膳食中的平均污染水平最高（0.89 μg/kg），其次为肉类（0.33 μg/kg），其他类膳食中六六六污染水平相对较低。

第六次中国总膳食研究的混合膳食样品中硫丹的污染水平为ND～8.19 μg/kg（附表7-15）。薯类、肉类、蛋类、水产类、乳类、蔬菜类、水果类样品中均检出硫丹，其中水产类的平均污染水平最高，为1.16 μg/kg，其他均低于1 μg/kg。

第六次中国总膳食研究的混合膳

eggs, aquatic foods, dairy products, vegetables, and fruits from 6$^{th}$ CTDS were determined. The value of the sample with no detectable OCPs was assigned the value of zero in the contamination levels evaluation and the dietary exposure assessment. The OCPs detected in the 6$^{th}$ CTDS dietary samples included DDTs, HCHs, endosulfans, PCB, HCB, aldrin and dieldrin, chlordanes, and heptachlor with the detection rate of each OCPs was PCB (97.7%), HCHs (52.8%), DDTs (51.4%), HCB (39.4%), endosulfans (16.7%), aldrin and dieldrin (6.0%), chlordanes (3.7%), and heptachlor (2.8%).

In the 6$^{th}$ CTDS, the contamination levels of PCB in dietary samples were in the range of ND-1.06 μg/kg (Annexed Table 7-16). PCB was detected in all kinds of dietary samples, and the higher contamination levels were detected in aquatic foods and meats, ranging from 0.07 μg/kg to 0.23 μg/kg.

In the 6$^{th}$ CTDS, the contamination levels of DDTs in dietary samples were in the range of ND-9.83 μg/kg (Annexed Table 7-13). DDTs were detected in 8 categories dietary samples except fruits. The average contamination level of aquatic foods samples was highest (2.25 μg/kg), followed by meats and eggs (0.57 μg/kg), dairy products (0.34 μg/kg), and contamination levels of DDTs in other categories were lower.

In the 6$^{th}$ CTDS, the contamination levels of HCHs in dietary samples were in the range of ND-6.62 μg/kg (Annexed Table 7-14). HCHs were detected in 8 categories dietary samples except fruits, The average contamination level of aquatic foods samples was highest (0.89 μg/kg), followed by meats (0.33 μg/kg), and contamination levels of HCH in other categories were lower.

In the 6$^{th}$ CTDS, the contamination levels of endosulfans in dietary samples were in the range of ND-8.19 μg/kg (Annexed Table 7-15). Endosulfans were detected in potatoes, meats, eggs, aquatic foods, dairy products, vegetables, fruits. The average contamination level of aquatic foods samples was highest (1.16 μg/kg), and the contamination levels of endosulfans in other categories were all lower than 1 μg/kg.

In the 6$^{th}$ CTDS, the contamination levels of HCB

食样品中六氯苯的污染水平为ND～2.78 μg/kg（附表7-12）。除水果类外8类膳食中均检出六氯苯，平均污染水平均低于0.5 μg/kg。

第六次中国总膳食研究的混合膳食样品中艾氏剂和狄氏剂的污染水平为ND～0.17 μg/kg（附表7-17）。仅在肉类、蛋类、乳类与水产类4类动物膳食样品中检出艾氏剂和狄氏剂，平均污染水平均低于0.03 μg/kg。

第六次中国总膳食研究的混合膳食样品中氯丹的污染水平为ND～0.08 μg/kg（附表7-18）。仅在肉类、蛋类、乳类和水产类4类动物膳食样品中检出氯丹，平均含量均低于0.01 μg/kg。

第六次中国总膳食研究的混合膳食样品中七氯的污染水平为ND～0.09 μg/kg（附表7-19）。仅在薯类、肉类、蛋类及水产类4类膳食中检出七氯，平均含量均低于0.02 μg/kg。

**2. 膳食暴露评估**

第六次中国总膳食研究我国居民滴滴涕的平均膳食摄入量为2.883 ng/(kg bw·d)，占滴滴涕PTDI的0.03%（附表7-20）；六六六的平均膳食摄入量为1.337 ng/(kg bw·d)，占六六六PTDI的0.07%（附表7-21）；硫丹的平均膳食摄入量为2.689 ng/(kg bw·d)，占硫丹PTDI的0.04%（附表7-22）；五氯苯的平均膳食摄入量为2.782 ng/(kg bw·d)，占五氯苯TDI（Canada）的0.55%（附表7-23）；六氯苯的平均膳食摄入量为0.713 ng/(kg bw·d)，占六氯苯PTDI的0.27%（附表7-24）；艾氏剂和狄氏剂的平均膳食摄入量为0.044 ng/(kg bw·d)，占艾氏剂和狄氏剂PTDI的0.05%（附表7-25）；氯丹的平均膳食摄入量为0.009 ng/(kg bw·d)，占氯丹PTDI的0.002%（附表7-26）；七氯的平均膳食摄入量为

in dietary samples were in the range of ND-2.78 μg/kg (Annexed Table 7-12). HCB was detected in 8 categories dietary samples except fruits, and the contamination levels of HCB in all kinds of dietary samples were all lower than 0.5 μg/kg.

In the 6$^{th}$ CTDS, the contamination levels of aldrin and dieldrin in dietary samples were in the range of ND-0.17 μg/kg (Annexed Table 7-17). Aldrin and dieldrin were detected only in meats, eggs, aquatic foods, and dairy products, but the contamination levels of aldrin and dieldrin in all kinds of dietary samples were all lower than 0.03 μg/kg.

In the 6$^{th}$ CTDS, the contamination levels of chlordanes in dietary samples were in the range of ND-0.08 μg/kg (Annexed Table 7-18). Chlordanes were detected only in meats, eggs, aquatic foods, dairy products, but the contamination levels of chlordanes in all kinds of dietary samples were all lower than 0.01 μg/kg.

In the 6$^{th}$ CTDS, the contamination levels of heptachlor in dietary samples were in the range of ND-0.09 μg/kg (Annexed Table 7-19). Heptachlor were detected only in potatoes, meats, eggs, and aquatic foods, but the contamination levels of heptachlor in all kinds of dietary samples were all lower than 0.02 μg/kg.

**2. Dietary Exposure Assessment**

The average dietary intake of DDTs for China residents from the 6$^{th}$ China TDS is 2.883 ng/(kg bw·d), which is 0.03% of the provisional tolerable daily intake (PTDI) value of DDTs (Annexed Table 7-20); The average dietary intake of HCHs is 1.337 ng/(kg bw·d), or 0.07% of PTDI (Annexed Table 7-21); The average dietary intake of endosulfans is 2.689 ng/(kg bw·d), or 0.04% of PTDI (Annexed Table 7-22); The average dietary intake of pentachlorobenzene is 2.782 ng/(kg bw·d), or 0.55% of TDI (Canada) (Annexed Table 7-23); The average dietary intake of HCB is 0.713 ng/(kg bw·d), or 0.27% of PTDI (Annexed Table 7-24); The average dietary intake of aldrin and dieldrin is 0.044 ng/(kg bw·d), or 0.05% of PTDI (Annexed Table 7-25); The average dietary intake of chlordanes is 0.009 ng/

0.017 ng/(kg bw·d)，占七氯 PTDI 的 0.02%（附表 7-27）。

从膳食暴露评估结果可以得出，我国各地区居民持久性有机氯农药的膳食摄入量远远低于各自的健康指导值，健康风险很低。

**3. 各类膳食对总膳食摄入的贡献**

对有较高检出率的滴滴涕和六六六进行膳食暴露来源分析（附表 7-28，附表 7-29，图 7-9 和图 7-10），第六次中国总膳食研究中水产类是我国居民滴滴涕膳食摄入的主要贡献来源（49.2%），其次为肉类（27.6%）。对于六六六，主要的贡献膳食是水产类（25.9%）、肉类（24.6%）和蔬菜类（21.0%）。

(kg bw·d), or 0.002% of PTDI (Annexed Table 7-26); The average dietary intake of heptachlor is 0.017 ng/(kg bw·d), or 0.02% of PTDI (Annexed Table 7-27).

The results of dietary exposure showed that the dietary intakes of OCPs of the Chinese population are far lower than their health-based guidance values and pose little risk.

**3. Contributions of Food Categories to the Total Dietary Intake**

Contributions of food categories to the total dietary intake were performed for DDTs and HCHs with higher detection rates (Annexed Table 7-28, Annexed Table 7-29, Figure 7-9 and Figure 7-10). The primary food sources of dietary intake to the DDTs in the 6$^{th}$ China TDS were aquatic foods (49.2%), followed by meats (27.6%). The primary food sources of dietary intake

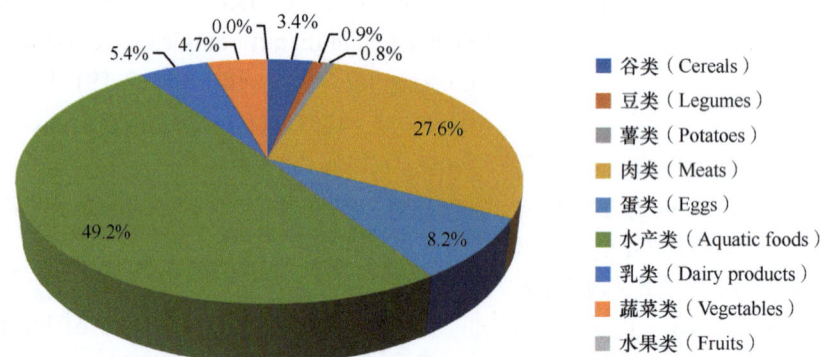

图 7-9　第六次中国总膳食研究滴滴涕的膳食来源

Figure 7-9　Dietary sources of DDTs from the 6$^{th}$ China TDS

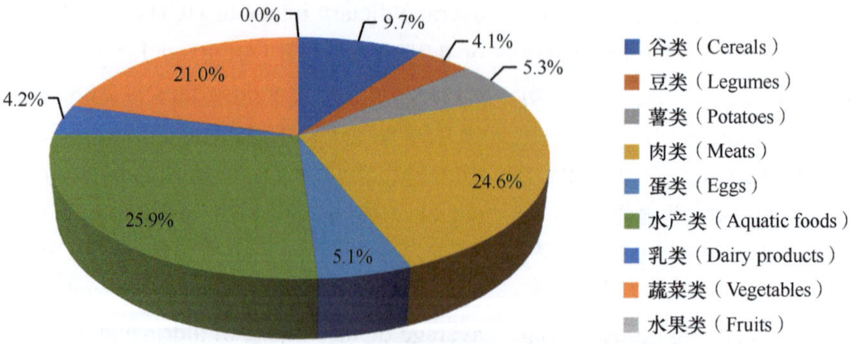

图 7-10　第六次中国总膳食研究六六六的膳食来源

Figure 7-10　Dietary sources of HCHs from the 6$^{th}$ China TDS

## 四、与以往中国总膳食研究结果的比较

第一次、第二次和第三次中国总膳食研究仅检测了滴滴涕与六六六两种持久性有机氯农药。第四次中国总膳食研究检测了19种持久性有机氯农药（35个组分）。第五次中国总膳食研究检测了14种持久性有机氯农药（30个组分）。第六次中国总膳食研究重点关注了10种持久性有机氯农药（27个组分）（表7-5）。

to the HCHs in the 6$^{th}$ China TDS were aquatic foods (25.9%), followed by meats (24.6%) and vegetables (21.0%).

## Ⅳ. Comparison with Previous China TDSs Results

In the 1$^{st}$, 2$^{nd}$, and 3$^{rd}$ China TDS, only two OCPs, HCHs and DDTs, were detected. Nineteen OCPs (35 components) were detected for the 4$^{th}$ China TDS, and fourteen OCPs (30 components) were detected for the 5$^{th}$ China TDS. The 6$^{th}$ China TDS focused on ten OCPs (27 components) (Table 7-5).

表 7-5 六次中国总膳食研究持久性有机氯农药的膳食摄入情况
Table 7-5 The results of OCPs dietary intakes from the six China TDSs

| 中国总膳食研究 China TDS | 采样时间 Sampling period | 滴滴涕 DDT | 六六六 HCH | 硫丹 Endosulfan | 六氯苯 HCB | 氯丹 CHL | 七氯 Heptachlor | 五氯苯（Pentachlo-robenzene） | 艾氏剂和狄氏剂（Aldrin and Dieldrin） |
|---|---|---|---|---|---|---|---|---|---|
| 第一次中国总膳食研究（1$^{st}$ CTDS） | 1990 | 20.48 | 5.04 | — | — | — | — | — | — |
| 第二次中国总膳食研究（2$^{nd}$ CTDS） | 1992 | 4.93 | 9.28 | — | — | — | — | — | — |
| 第三次中国总膳食研究（3$^{rd}$ CTDS） | 2000 | 2.15 | 3.14 | — | — | — | — | — | — |
| 第四次中国总膳食研究（4$^{th}$ CTDS） | 2007 | 0.016 | 0.002 | 0.018 | 0.009 | 0.006 | 0.001 | — | * |
| 第五次中国总膳食研究（5$^{th}$ CTDS） | 2009~2012 | 0.016 | 0.008 | 0.030 | 0.001 | 0.001 | 0.006 | — | 0.007 |
| 第六次中国总膳食研究（6$^{th}$ CTDS） | 2016~2019 | 0.003 | 0.001 | 0.003 | 0.001 | <0.001 | <0.001 | 0.003 | <0.001 |

注："—" 表示未检测；"*" 表示未检出
Note: "—" means not analysis; "*" means not detectable

与第五次中国总膳食研究相比，我国居民第六次中国总膳食研究的各类持久性有机氯农药的膳食暴露量均有明显下降，鉴于第五次中国总膳食研究与第四次中国总膳食研究相比，滴滴涕、六六六、硫丹和七氯的膳食摄入量均有小幅增加，但第六次中国总膳食研究比

In comparison with the results of the 5$^{th}$ China TDS, the dietary exposures of various OCPs in the sixth China TDS of China residents decreased significantly. Although the dietary intakes of DDTs, HCHs, endosulfans, and heptachlor from the 5$^{th}$ China TDS were slightly increased in comparison with the results of the 4$^{th}$ China TDS. However, the results of the 6$^{th}$ China

第四次总膳食研究的结果仍是普遍下降的，因此可以判断我国居民有机氯农药的膳食摄入在持续下降。

与第四次中国总膳食研究结果相似，与第五次中国总膳食研究结果略有不同的是，动物源性食品是我国居民膳食摄入持久性有机氯农药的主要来源，其实是植物源性食品对持久性有机氯农药的膳食暴露贡献率较低。

TDS intakes for all OCPs were lower than the 4$^{th}$ China TDS. On the whole, the intakes of OCPs for Chinese population continues to decline.

Similar to the results of the 4$^{th}$ CTDS and slightly different from the results of the 5$^{th}$ CTDS, animal-derived foods were the main source of dietary intake of OCPs in China. In fact, plant-derived foods contributed less to the dietary exposure to OCPs.

## 第六节　全氟烷基化合物
## Section 6　Perfluoroalkyl Substances

### 一、背景

全氟烷基化合物（PFAS）是指至少含有一个全氟化碳原子的有机化合物（即至少含有一个—$CF_2$或—$CF_3$脂肪链结构单元），20 世纪 40 年代由美国 3M 公司率先研制成功。由于 PFAS 卓越的表面活性，被广泛应用于工业和生活用品中，如消防泡沫、半导体工业的清洁和表面处理液、纺织品与皮革的整理剂、纸张的表面处理剂、不粘锅涂层和食品包装材料等，其中应用最广泛的是全氟辛酸（PFOA）和全氟辛基磺酸（PFOS）。PFOA 和 PFOS 已经在世界范围内的环境、生物体和人体中检出。由于其具有多脏器毒性，包括肝脏毒性、神经毒性、心血管毒性、免疫毒性、胚胎发育与生殖毒性、内分泌干扰等，且其在人体内的半衰期长达数年，2009 年，PFOS 及其盐类和全氟辛基磺酰氟作为严重危害人类健康与自然环境的新持久性有机污染物被增列为《关于持久性有机污染物的斯德哥尔摩公约》优先管控物质。随后，PFOA 及其盐类和相关化合物在 2019 年也被增列入《关于持久性有机污染物的斯德哥尔摩公约》优先管控物质。另外，全氟辛基磺酸及

### Ⅰ. Background

Perfluoroalkyl substances (PFASs) are organic compounds containing at least one perfluorocarbon atom, including at least one —$CF_2$ or —$CF_3$ fatly chain unit. PFASs were first successfully developed by the American 3M Company in the 1940s. Due to their unique surface activity, PFASs have been widely used in industrial and consumer products, such as firefighting foams, cleaning and surface treatment fluids for the semiconductor industry, finishing agents for textiles and leather, surface treatments for paper, non-stick pan coatings and food packaging materials. Perfluorooctanoic acid (PFOA) and perfluorooctane sulfonate (PFOS) are the most widely used PFASs, which were detected in various environment, biota and human tissues in the world. However, PFOA and PFOS have multi-organ toxicity, such as hepatotoxicity, neurotoxicity, cardiovascular toxicity, immunotoxicity, embryonic developmental and reproductive toxicity, endocrine disruption. In addition, the half-life of PFOA and PFOS in the body is up to several years. PFOS and its salts, and perfluorooctanesulfonyl fluoride, PFOA and its salts and related compounds as the new persistent organic pollutants were added to the priority monitoring compounds of the *Stockholm Convention on Persistent Organic Pollutants* in 2009 and 2019,

其盐类和全氟辛基磺酰氟在 2017 年被列入我国环境保护部（现生态环境部）第一批优先控制化学品，随后，全氟辛酸及其盐类和相关化合物在 2020 年也被列入我国生态环境部第二批优先控制化学品。关于 PFAS 的研究已成为国际上环境健康领域的研究热点，其暴露来源大致上分为两类：一类为膳食和水摄入、空气吸入、皮肤接触等直接来源，其中膳食是人体暴露于 PFAS 的最主要来源；另一类为间接来源，即由 PFAS 前体物质的代谢转化而来。

我国自 2014 年 3 月 26 日起，禁止全氟辛基磺酸及其盐类和全氟辛基磺酰氟除特定豁免和可接受用途外的生产、流通、使用和进出口。对于特定豁免用途的，应抓紧研发替代品，确保豁免到期前全部淘汰；对于可接受用途的，应加强管理及风险防范，并努力逐步淘汰其生产和使用。自 2019 年 3 月 26 日起，禁止全氟辛基磺酸及其盐类和全氟辛基磺酰氟除可接受用途外的生产、流通、使用和进出口，已无特定豁免用途。可接受用途的生产和使用仅包括：照片成像、半导体器件的光阻剂和防反射涂层、化合物半导体和陶瓷滤芯的刻蚀剂、航空液压油、只用于闭环系统的金属电镀（硬金属电镀）、某些医疗设备 [ 如乙烯四氟乙烯共聚物（ETFE）层和无线电屏蔽 ETFE 的生产，体外诊断医疗设备与 CCD 滤色仪 ] 和灭火泡沫。

## 二、健康指导值

目前，不同的国家和机构对 PFAS 的健康指导值还没有统一共识。德国联邦风险评估研究所（BfR）、欧盟食品安全局（EFSA）等机构对 PFOS 和 PFOA 的慢性暴露提出了每日可耐受摄入量（TDI）或每周可耐受摄入量（TWI）。由于这些物质对人体健康影响

respectively. In addition, they are the first and second batch of priority control chemicals by the Ministry of Environment Protection of the People's Republic of China and Ministry of Ecology and Environment of the People's Republic of China in 2017 and 2020, respectively. Research on PFASs has gradually become a hotspot in the environmental health in the world. The human exposure to PFASs includes direct exposure and indirect exposure. Diet, water, air, and skin contact are direct exposure sources of PFASs, diet was the most important exposed source of PFASs in human. While the indirect exposure is from the metabolism of the PFASs precursor.

Since March 26, 2014, China has prohibited the production, circulation, use and import and export of PFOS and its salts, and perfluorooctanesulfonyl fluoride, except for specific exemptions and acceptable uses. For specific exemptions uses products, alternatives should be rapidly developed to ensure that the products are all eliminated before the expiration of the exemption. For the acceptable uses products, strengthen management and risk prevention should be implemented, and their production and use should also be gradually eliminated. Since March 26, 2019, China has prohibited the production, circulation, use and import and export of PFOS and its salts, and perfluorooctanesulfonyl fluoride, except for acceptable uses. The production and use of the acceptable uses only include photo imaging, photoresist and anti-reflection coatings for semiconductor devices, etchants for compound semiconductors and ceramic filter elements, aviation hydraulic oil, metal plating for closed loop systems only (hard metal plating), certain medical devices [e.g., production of ethylene tetrafluoroethylene copolymer (ETFE) layers and radio shielding ETFE, *in vitro* diagnostic medical devices and CCD color filters] and fire extinguishing foams.

## II. HBGV

The health-based guidance values for PFASs have not been unified in different countries and institutions.

的不确定性，不同机构提出的数值有所不同。2006 年，德国联邦风险评估研究所以及德国联邦卫生部饮用水委员会提出的 PFOS 和 PFOA 的 TDI 均为 100 ng/(kg bw·d)，英国食品、消费品及环境中化学品毒性委员会提出的 PFOS 和 PFOA 的 TDI 分别为 300 ng/(kg bw·d) 和 3000 ng/(kg bw·d)。EFSA 在 2008 年提出的 PFOS 和 PFOA 的 TDI 分别为 150 ng/(kg bw·d) 和 1500 ng/(kg bw·d)，但在 2018 年 3 月，EFSA 基于人群血清胆固醇水平升高、儿童接种疫苗后抗体反应下降、血清谷丙转氨酶水平增高的流行病学数据，将 PFOS 和 PFOA 的每日可耐受摄入量改为了每周可耐受摄入量，分别为 13 ng/(kg bw·周) 和 6 ng/(kg bw·周)，其与 2008 年提出的 TDI 相比，分别下降到 1/81 和 1/1750，是目前最为严苛的健康指导值。美国毒物和疾病登记署（ATSDR）也在 2018 年提出 PFOA、PFOS、全氟己烷磺酸（PFHxS）和全氟壬酸（PFNA）的 MRL 分别为 3 ng/(kg bw·d)、2 ng/(kg bw·d)、2 ng/(kg bw·d)、3 ng/(kg bw·d)。

## 三、总膳食研究结果

对 24 个省（自治区、直辖市）的 4 类动物源性食品与 5 类植物源性食品进行了 PFOA 和 PFOS 含量分析，包括水产类、肉类、蛋类、乳类、谷类、薯类、豆类、蔬菜类和水果类膳食。对含量低于检出限的样品，按 1/2 LOD 赋值用于膳食暴露评估。

The German Federal Institute for Risk Assessment (BfR), European Food Safety Authority (EFSA) and other institutions have already established the tolerable daily intake or tolerable weekly intake for PFOS and PFOA. Due to the uncertainty of the effects of PFASs on human health, the guidance values recommended by different institutions are different. The TDI of PFOS and PFOA proposed by the BfR and the Drinking Water Committee of the German Federal Ministry of Health are both 100 ng/(kg bw·d) in 2006. Moreover the Committee on Toxicity of Chemicals in Food, Consumer Products and the Environment in UK have also established the TDI for PFOS and PFOA of 300 ng/(kg bw·d) and 3000 ng/(kg bw·d) respectively in 2006. EFSA have established the TDI for PFOS [150 ng/(kg bw·d)] and PFOA [1500 ng/(kg bw·d)] respectively in 2008. However, EFSA have established TWI for PFOS [13 ng/(kg bw·week)] and PFOA [6 ng/(kg bw·week)] based on the epidemiological evidence of increase in serum total cholesterol in adults, the decrease in antibody response at vaccination in children, and the increase in serum alanine aminotransferase in March, 2018. Compared with the TDI recommended by EFSA in 2008, the TWIs of PFOS and PFOA established in 2018 have dropped to 1/81 and 1/1750 respectively, which are the most stringent health-based guidance values at present. In addition, the Agency for Toxic Substances and Disease Registry (ATSDR) of U.S. also established the oral minimal risk levels (MRLs) for PFOA [3 ng/(kg bw·d)], PFOS [2 ng/(kg bw·d)], perfluorohexanesulfonate [PFHxS, 2 ng/(kg bw·d)], and perfluorononanoic acid [PFNA, 3 ng/(kg bw·d)] in 2018.

## III. TDS Results

PFOA and PFOS were analyzed in food composite dietary samples including aquatic foods, meats, eggs, dairy products, cereals, potatoes, legumes, vegetables, and fruits from 24 provinces (autonomous regions, municipalities). The concentrations of samples below the LOD were set to be LOD/2 for dietary exposure assessment.

**1. 混合膳食样品中 PFOA 和 PFOS 的含量**

第六次中国总膳食研究混合膳食样品中 PFOA 的检出率为 39.8%，含量范围为 ND～2.97 µg/kg（附表 7-30）。按平均含量计，在各类膳食中排名前三位的分别是蛋类（0.18 µg/kg）、水产类（0.05 µg/kg）和肉类（0.04 µg/kg）。所有乳类和水果类样品中 PFOA 含量均低于检出限。对于 PFOA 支链异构体（br-PFOA），仅在北京市蛋类样品中检出 br-PFOA，br-PFOA 占 PFOA 的比例为 5.6%。

第六次中国总膳食研究混合膳食样品中 PFOS 的检出率为 31.5%，含量范围为 ND～4.30 µg/kg（附表 7-31）。按平均含量计，在各类膳食中排名前三位的分别是水产类（0.48 µg/kg）、蛋类（0.07 µg/kg）和肉类（0.06 µg/kg）。所有薯类、乳类、蔬菜类和水果类样品中 PFOS 含量均低于检出限。对于 PFOS 支链异构体，肉类样品中仅浙江检出 br-PFOS，占 PFOS 的比例为 5.2%；水产类样品中除辽宁省、福建省、广西壮族自治区和贵州省外，其余省份均检出 br-PFOS，占 PFOS 的比例为 3.3%～21.2%；其余膳食类别中 br-PFOS 的含量均低于检出限。

**2. 膳食暴露评估**

按成年男子计，我国居民 PFOA 的平均每周膳食摄入量为 2.17 ng/(kg bw·周)，范围为 0.18～13.73 ng/(kg bw·周)（附表 7-32，图 7-11）。

我国居民 PFOS 的平均膳食摄入量为 2.72 ng/(kg bw·周)，范围为 0.41～14.28 ng/(kg bw·周)（附表 7-33，图 7-12）。

以 EFSA 在 2018 年最新提出的 PFOA 和 PFOS 的 TWI 为健康指导值，

**1. Levels of PFOA and PFOS in TDS Composite Samples**

The detection rate of PFOA in the 6$^{th}$ China TDS food composite dietary samples was 39.8%. The contamination levels of PFOA ranged from ND to 2.97 µg/kg (Annexed Table 7-30). The highest average contamination level was found in eggs (0.18 µg/kg), followed by aquatic foods (0.05 µg/kg) and meats (0.04 µg/kg). The levels of PFOA were below the LOD in dairy products and fruits. The br-PFOA was only detected in eggs from Beijing with a contribution of 5.6% to total PFOA levels in that sample.

The detection rate of PFOS in the 6$^{th}$ China TDS food composites was 31.5%. The contamination levels of PFOS ranged from ND to 4.30 µg/kg (Annexed Table 7-31). The highest average contamination level was found in aquatic foods (0.48 µg/kg), followed by eggs (0.07 µg/kg) and meats (0.06 µg/kg). The levels of PFOS were below the LOD in potatoes, dairy products, vegetables and fruits. The br-PFOS was only detected in meats from Zhejiang with a contribution of 5.2% to total PFOS levels in that sample. In addition, br-PFOS were detected in most provinces except for Liaoning, Fujian, Guangxi, and Guizhou for aquatic foods, with the contribution ranged from 3.3% to 21.2% to total PFOS. The levels of br-PFOS were below the LOD in other food categories.

**2. Dietary Exposure Assessment**

For the standard Chinese man, the average EWI of PFOA in 6$^{th}$ CTDS were 2.17 ng/(kg bw·week), ranged from 0.18 ng/(kg bw·week) to 13.73 ng/(kg bw·week) (Annexed Table 7-32, Figure 7-11).

The average EWI of PFOS in 6$^{th}$ CTDS were 2.72 ng/(kg bw·week), ranged from 0.41 ng/(kg bw·week) to 14.28 ng/(kg bw·week) (Annexed Table 7-33, Figure 7-12).

The TWI of PFOS established by EFSA in 2018 were used to assess the health risks for general population. The average EWIs of PFOA and PFOS accounted for 36.2%

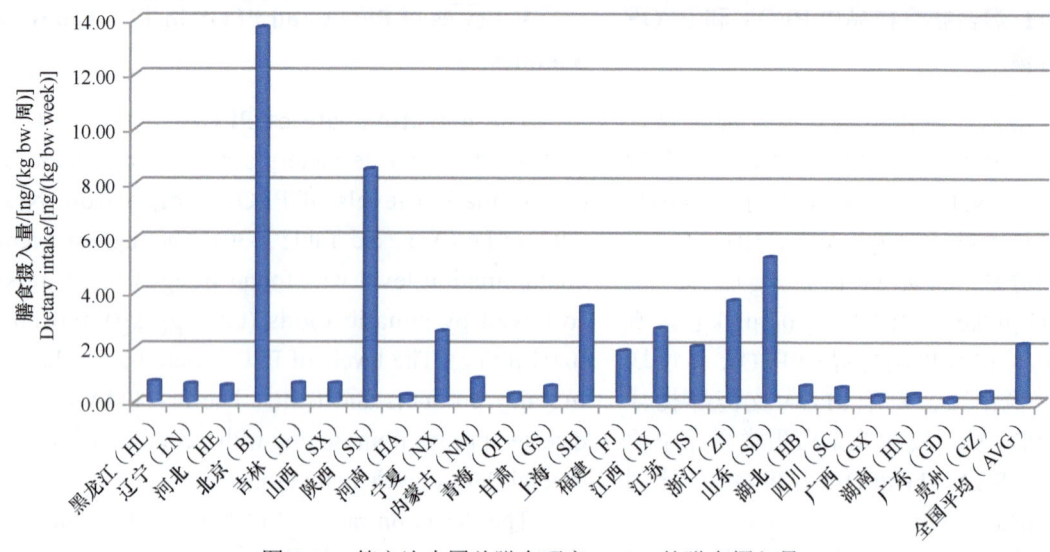

图 7-11　第六次中国总膳食研究 PFOA 的膳食摄入量
Figure 7-11　Dietary intake of PFOA from the 6$^{th}$ China TDS

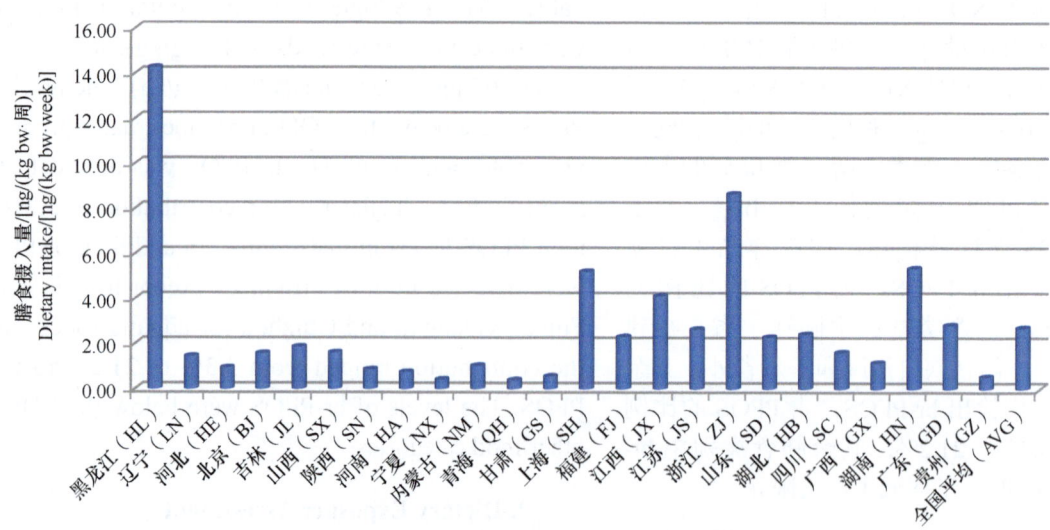

图 7-12　第六次中国总膳食研究 PFOS 的膳食摄入量
Figure 7-12　Dietary intake of PFOS from the 6$^{th}$ China TDS

评价我国居民膳食中 PFOA 和 PFOS 暴露的健康风险，我国居民 PFOA 的平均膳食摄入量为 EFSA 制定的 TWI 的 36.2%，PFOS 的平均膳食摄入量为 EFSA 制定的 TWI 的 20.9%。

### 3. 各类膳食对总膳食摄入的贡献

根据第六次中国总膳食研究的结果，膳食摄入的 PFOA 主要来源于蛋类

and 20.9% of the TWIs, respectively.

### 3. Contributions of Food Categories to the Total Dietary Intake

According to the results of the 6$^{th}$ China TDS, eggs are the primary source of dietary intake to the PFOA, with the contribution of 34.6%, and then followed by cereals (23.1%), meats (16.2%), vegetables (13.4%) and aquatic foods (7.0%). The contributions of these food

(34.6%)、谷类（23.1%）、肉类（16.2%）、蔬菜类（13.4%）、水产类（7.0%），合计占总膳食摄入量的94.3%，其余4类膳食样品的总贡献率小于6%（附表7-34，图7-13）。

categories are 94.3% to the total dietary intake. The contributions of the other four food categories are less than 6% (Annexed Table 7-34 and Figure 7-13).

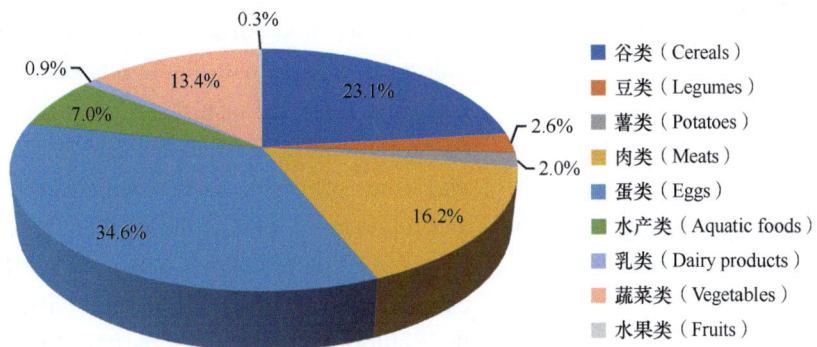

图 7-13　第六次中国总膳食研究 PFOA 的膳食来源
Figure 7-13　Dietary sources of PFOA from the 6th China TDS

第六次中国总膳食研究的膳食 PFOS 主要来源于水产类（54.4%）、肉类（23.5%）、蔬菜类（10.0%）、蛋类（7.3%），占总摄入量的95.2%，其余5类膳食样品的总贡献率小于5%（附表7-35，图7-14）。

Aquatic foods are the primary source of dietary intake to the PFOS, with the contribution of 54.4%, and then followed by meats (23.5%), vegetables (10.0%) and eggs (7.3%). The contributions of these food categories are 95.2% to the total dietary intake. The contributions of the other five food categories are less than 5% (Annexed Table 7-35 and Figure 7-14).

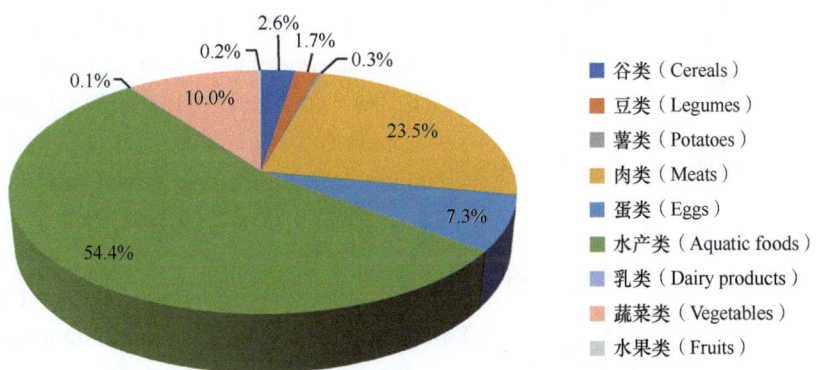

图 7-14　第六次中国总膳食研究 PFOS 的膳食来源
Figure 7-14　Dietary sources of PFOS from the 6th China TDS

第七章　持久性有机污染物的膳食暴露评估　281

# 第七节 短链与中链氯化石蜡
# Section 7　Short- and Medium-Chain Chlorinated Paraffins

## 一、背景

氯化石蜡（CP）是一类高度复杂的工业混合物，具有阻燃性、低挥发性、良好电绝缘性等优点，广泛用于阻燃剂、增塑剂、橡胶、人造革等制品以及涂料、润滑油等的添加剂中。根据氯含量不同 CP 商用产品主要分为 CP-42、CP-52、CP-70 三类。短链氯化石蜡（SCCP，$C_{10-13}$）因具有持久性、长距离迁移性、生物蓄积性和高毒性，已于 2017 年 5 月列入《关于持久性有机污染物的斯德哥尔摩公约》附件 A 名单。中链氯化石蜡（MCCP，$C_{14-17}$）也已被建议列入《关于持久性有机污染物的斯德哥尔摩公约》。中国是目前世界上最大的 CP 生产国，膳食摄入是非职业人群暴露于 SCCP 和 MCCP 的主要途径。

## 二、健康指导值

国际化学品安全计划提出的每日可耐受摄入量为 100 μg/(kg bw·d)。欧洲食品安全局（EFSA）提出 SCCP 和 MCCP 的 $BMDL_{10}$ 分别为 2.3 mg/(kg bw·d) 和 36 mg/(kg bw·d)，作为风险表征的参考点。

考虑到物种之间的变异性、人类个体内部的变异性和从亚慢性研究到长期暴露等各种因素，EFSA 采用暴露边界值（MOE）方法评估 CP 膳食暴露可能对人体产生的健康风险。

## 三、总膳食研究结果

对 24 个省（自治区、直辖市）的谷类、豆类、薯类、蔬菜类、肉类、蛋类、水产类和乳类 8 类共 192 份混合膳

## Ⅰ. Background

Chlorinated paraffins (CPs) are highly complex industrial mixture with flame retardancy, low volatility and good electrical insulation. They are widely used as flame retardants, plasticizers, rubbers, artificial leather and other products, as well as additives in coatings and lubricants. China is the world's largest producer of CPs. CP commercial products are classified into three categories——CP-42, CP-52, and CP-70 according to their chlorine contents. Short-chain CPs (SCCPs $C_{10-13}$) were listed in Annex A of the *Stockholm Convention on Persistent Organic Pollutants* in May 2017 because of their persistence, high toxicity, bioaccumulation, and long-range transportation. Medium-chain chlorinated paraffins (MCCPs, $C_{14-17}$) have also been proposed for inclusion in this convention. Dietary intake is the main way for non-occupational people to be exposed to SCCPs and MCCPs.

## Ⅱ. HBGV

The tolerable daily intakes proposed by the International Programme on Chemical Safety were 100 μg/(kg bw·d). The $BMDL_{10}$ of SCCP and MCCP were set 2.3 mg/(kg bw·d) and 36 mg/(kg bw·d) as the minimum value of risk, respectively recommend by EFSA.

The possible health risks of dietary exposure to CPs in humans were assessed using the margin of exposure (MOE) method recommended by the European Food Safety Authority (EFSA), taking into account variability between species, variability within human individuals, and extrapolation from subchronic studies to chronic exposure duration.

## Ⅲ. TDS Results

SCCPs and MCCPs were determined in 192 composite dietary samples from 8 categories of cereals,

食样品中 SCCP 和 MCCP 的含量进行了测定，对含量低于检出限的样品，以 1/2 LOD 值进行短链和中链氯化石蜡的暴露量计算。

**1. 混合膳食样品中 SCCP 和 MCCP 的含量**

在第六次中国总膳食研究的混合样品中，SCCP 和 MCCP 的含量分别为 5～265 ng/g 和 4～306 ng/g，其中，肉类中 SCCP 和 MCCP 平均含量最高，分别为 63 ng/g 和 70 ng/g（附表 7-36 和附表 7-37）。谷类、蔬菜类、薯类、豆类、乳类和水产类中 SCCP 的平均含量比 MCCP 高 6%～53%，然而在蛋类和肉类中 SCCP 的平均含量分别比 MCCP 低 2% 和 10%。

**2. 膳食暴露评估**

我国居民膳食 SCCP 和 MCCP 平均估计每日摄入量分别为 1041 ng/(kg bw·d) 和 918 ng/(kg bw·d)，估计每日摄入量范围分别为 270～2844 ng/(kg bw·d) 和 192～2927 ng/(kg bw·d)（附表 7-38 和附表 7-39）。如图 7-15 和图 7-16 所示，不同地区居民 SCCP 和 MCCP 膳食摄入量存在较大差异。在第六次中国总膳食研究中，我国居民 SCCP 和 MCCP 的最高估计每日摄入量（EDI）低于国际化学品安全计划提出的可耐受最高摄入量 [100 μg/(kg bw·d)]。基于 EFSA 提出的 $BMDL_{10}$，我国居民膳食摄入的 SCCP 和 MCCP 的 MOE 分别为 $2 \times 10^3$ 和 $4 \times 10^4$，均明显高于 EFSA 提出的风险特征临界值 1000，表明我国居民膳食摄入 SCCP 和 MCCP 的健康风险较低。

legumes, potatoes, vegetables, meats, eggs, aquatic products and dairy products from 24 provinces (autonomous regions, municipalities). The concentrations of SCCPs and MCCPs were calculated with 1/2 LOD when those were below the LOD.

**1. Concentrations of SCCPs and MCCPs in Dietary Samples**

Concentrations of SCCPs and MCCPs in the 6$^{th}$ China TDS composite samples ranged from 5-265 ng/g and 4-306 ng/g, respectively. Among the eight categories dietary, meats had the highest mean concentrations of SCCPs and MCCPs (63 ng/g and 70 ng/g, respectively) (Annexed Table 7-36 and Annexed Table 7-37). The average concentrations of SCCPs in cereals, vegetables, potatoes, legumes, dairy products and aquatic foods were 6%-53% higher than those of MCCPs, while the mean concentrations of SCCPs in eggs and meats were 2% and 10% lower than those of MCCPs, respectively.

**2. Dietary Exposure Assessment**

The estimated daily intake (EDI) of SCCPs and MCCPs in China were 1041 ng/(kg bw·d) [270-2844 ng/(kg bw·d)] and 918 ng/(kg bw·d) [192-2927 ng/(kg bw·d)], respectively (Annexed Table 7-38 and Annexed Table 7-39). From Figure 7-15 and Figure 7-16, it can be seen that the estimated daily intake (EDI) of residents in different provinces were significantly different. The highest EDI values for SCCPs and MCCPs in the sixth China total diet study were still below the tolerable daily intakes proposed by the International Programme on Chemical Safety [100 μg/(kg bw·d)]. The MOE of SCCPs and MCCPs in eight dietary categories calculated by $BMDL_{10}$ based on EFSA were $2 \times 10^3$ and $4 \times 10^4$, respectively, higher than 1000 that proposed by EFSA, indicating that dietary intake of SCCPs and MCCPs may not pose a significant risk to the health of residents.

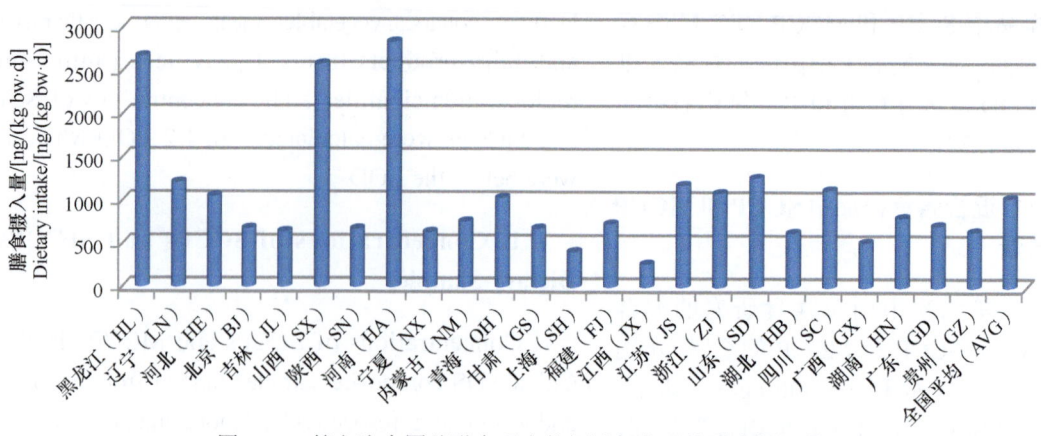

图 7-15　第六次中国总膳食研究的短链氯化石蜡膳食摄入量
Figure 7-15　Dietary intake of SCCPs from the 6th China TDS

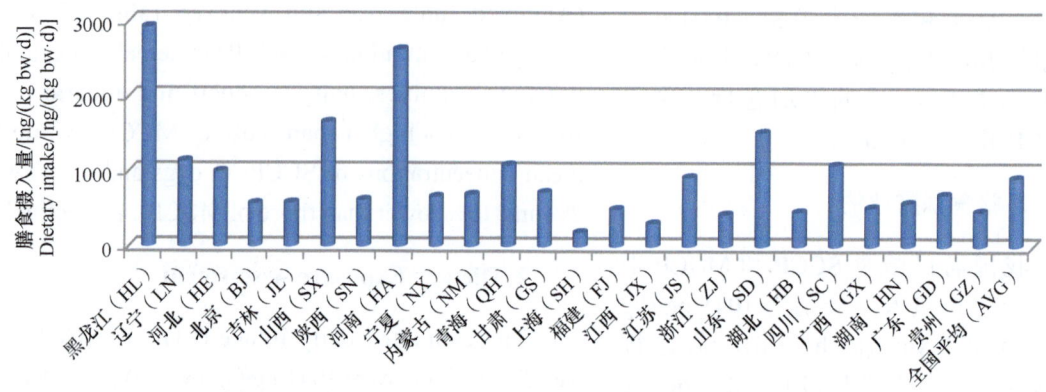

图 7-16　第六次中国总膳食研究的中链氯化石蜡膳食摄入量
Figure 7-16　Dietary intake of MCCPs from the 6th China TDS

### 3. 各类膳食对总膳食摄入的贡献

不同省（自治区、直辖市）的各类膳食对居民 SCCP 和 MCCP 总膳食摄入量的贡献情况不尽相同（附表 7-40 和附表 7-41）。总体上来看，谷类与蔬菜类是我国居民 SCCP 和 MCCP 膳食摄入量的主要来源。我国居民各类膳食中 SCCP 的贡献率均值依次为：谷类（44.8%）＞蔬菜类（24.2%）＞肉类（10.7%）＞豆类（7.3%）＞水产类（3.8%）＞薯类（3.7%）＞乳类（2.8%）＞蛋类（2.7%）（图 7-17）。各类膳食中 MCCP 的贡献率均值依次为：谷类（45.5%）＞蔬菜类（22.1%）＞肉类（13.7%）＞豆类（6.3%）＞水产类

### 3. Contributions of Food Categories to the Total Dietary Intake

The contributions of SCCPs and MCCPs in the different categories to the total dietary intake in different provinces are varied (Annexed Table 7-40 and Annexed Table 7-41). In general, cereals and vegetables are the main sources of dietary intake of SCCPs and MCCPs. According to general population of China, the average contribution rates of SCCPs in different categories were as follows: cereals (44.8%)>vegetables (24.2%)>meats (10.7%)>legumes (7.3%)>aquatic foods (3.8%)>potatoes (3.7%)>dairy products (2.8%)>eggs (2.7%) (Figure 7-17). For MCCPs, the contributions in different categories to total dietary intake were as follows: cereals (45.5%)>vegetables (22.1%)>meats

（3.5%）＞蛋类（3.1%）＞薯类（3.0%）＞乳类（2.7%）（图7-18）。

(13.7%)>legumes (6.3%)>aquatic foods (3.5%)>eggs (3.1%)>potatoes (3.0%)>dairy products (2.7%) (Figure 7-18).

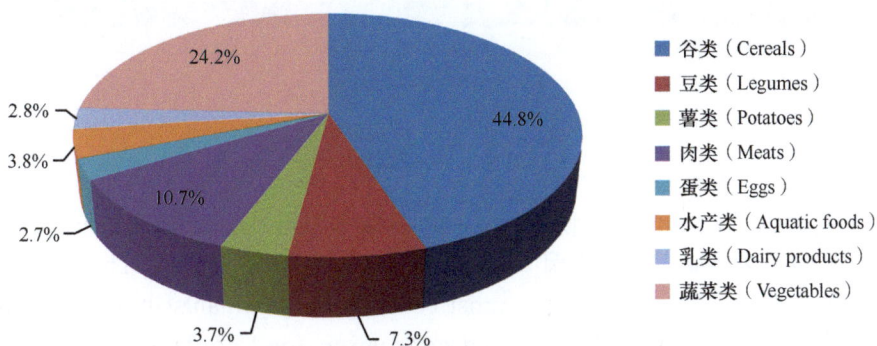

图7-17 第六次中国总膳食研究短链氯化石蜡的膳食来源
Figure 7-17　Dietary sources of SCCPs from the 6th China TDS

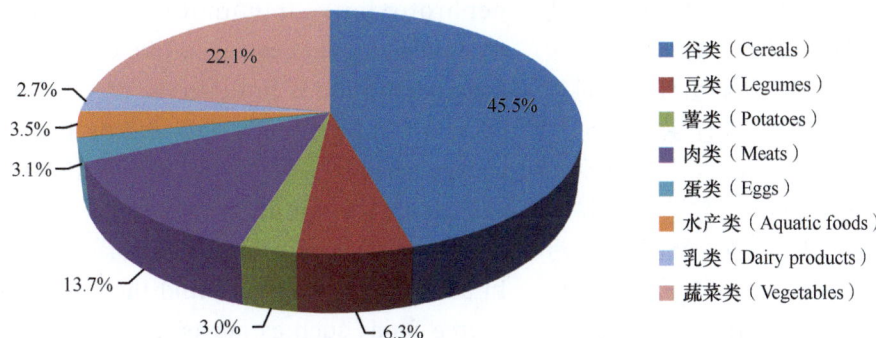

图7-18 第六次中国总膳食研究中链氯化石蜡的膳食来源
Figure 7-18　Dietary sources of MCCPs from the 6th China TDS

## 四、与以往中国总膳食研究结果的比较

第五次中国总膳食研究对豆类、谷类、肉类和水产类中的氯化石蜡进行了检测和暴露评估。与第五次总膳食研究的4类膳食样品相比，除肉类中MCCP含量呈现上升趋势外，其他3类膳食样品中SCCP和MCCP的含量呈现明显的下降趋势。由各类膳食样品中MCCP与SCCP的比值可见，第六次中国总膳食研究的比值大于第五次，提示MCCP的使用和生产占比有所增加。

## IV. Comparison with Previous China TDSs Results

Concentrations of chlorinated paraffins were analyzed and health risks were assessed in dietary sample of legumes, cereals, meats and aquatic foods of the fifth China total diet study. And the results of four categories dietary in the sixth China total diet study were compared with those of the fifth China total diet study. Except the MCCPs concentration in meats increased, the concentrations of SCCPs and MCCPs in the other three categories dietaries decreased. The ratio of MCCPs to SCCPs in each categories dietary was calculated, and it was found that the ratios in the sixth China total diet study was higher than those in the fifth China total diet study, indicating an increase usage and production of MCCPs.

# 第八章 真菌毒素的膳食暴露评估
## Chapter 8　Dietary Exposure Assessment of Mycotoxins

一、背景

真菌毒素是真菌的次级代谢产物，其生物转换物质也称为真菌毒素。真菌毒素是农产品的主要污染物之一，进食被其污染的食品可导致急、慢性中毒，主要表现为致癌性、致突变性、肝毒性、肾毒性、免疫毒性、神经毒性、致畸性及类雌激素样作用。真菌毒素可通过多种途径污染食品：产毒真菌可直接感染谷类等农作物，从而造成真菌毒素污染；使用污染原料进行生产可导致咖啡、果汁等加工食品被真菌毒素污染；此外，污染饲料中毒素的迁移也会造成肉、蛋、奶等动物源性食品的污染。因此，由真菌毒素引起的食源性疾病和贸易争端一直是全球关注的热点。2018 年，欧盟食品和饲料快速预警系统（RASFF）通报真菌毒素食品污染共 569 次，位列所有危害物之首。

目前已知的真菌毒素有 300 多种，但研究主要集中于对人类和动物健康有确定毒性作用的约 20 种化合物上。按照真菌毒素的化学结构及其与人类和动物健康的相关性，可将其划分为主要真菌毒素（包括黄曲霉毒素、赭曲霉毒素、单端孢霉烯毒素、伏马菌素、展青霉素和玉米赤霉烯酮类毒素）、新兴真菌毒素（交链孢毒素、新兴镰刀菌毒素）和其他真菌毒素。一些国家或地区已开展了真菌毒素的总膳食研究，如法国第一次总膳食研究（21 种真菌毒素）、法国第二次总膳食研究（25 种真菌毒素）、西班牙总膳食研究（18 种真

Ⅰ. Background

Mycotoxins are secondary metabolites or biotransformation products of fungi. They are among the most common contaminants in agricultural products and consuming food contaminated with them can lead to acute and chronic toxicity, mainly shown as carcinogenicity, mutagenicity, hepatotoxicity, nephrotoxicity, immunotoxicity, neurotoxicity, teratogenicity, and estrogen-like effects. Mycotoxins contaminate foods in different ways. Crops such as cereals can be directly infested by toxic fungi and contaminated by mycotoxins. Mycotoxin contamination can also occur in processed foods, such as coffee and fruit juice, by using contaminated raw materials. In addition, mycotoxins find their way into animal source foods such as meats, eggs, and milk through contaminated feed. In fact, mycotoxin-caused foodborne diseases and trade disputes have become prominent international issues. In 2018, the EU food and feed rapid warning system (RASFF) reported mycotoxin food contamination 569 times, ranking first among all hazards.

Currently, more than 300 mycotoxins are known, but research has largely focused on approximately 20 mycotoxins that have toxic effects on human and animal health. According to chemical structure and relevance to human and animal health, mycotoxins can be divided into major mycotoxins (including aflatoxin, ochratoxin, trichothecene, fumonisin, patulin, and zearalenones), emerging mycotoxins (*Alternaria* mycotoxins and emerging *Fusarium* toxins) and other mycotoxins. Mycotoxins have been included in previous national or regional TDSs, such as the 1st

菌毒素）、黎巴嫩总膳食研究（4种真菌毒素）、中国香港地区第一次总膳食研究（13种真菌毒素）、中国第四次和第五次总膳食研究（分别38种真菌毒素）。本次中国总膳食研究共对43种真菌毒素进行了含量分析，包括黄曲霉毒素B1、黄曲霉毒素B2、黄曲霉毒素G1、黄曲霉毒素G2、黄曲霉毒素M1、黄曲霉毒素M2、赭曲霉毒素A、赭曲霉毒素B、脱氧雪腐镰刀菌烯醇、雪腐镰刀菌烯醇、3-乙酰脱氧雪腐镰刀菌烯醇、15-乙酰脱氧雪腐镰刀菌烯醇、镰刀菌烯酮、3-葡萄糖-脱氧雪腐镰刀菌烯醇、去环氧-脱氧雪腐镰刀菌烯醇、HT-2毒素、T-2毒素、二乙酰镳草镰刀菌烯醇、新茄病镰刀菌烯醇、玉米赤霉烯酮、玉米赤霉酮、α-玉米赤霉烯醇、β-玉米赤霉烯醇、α-玉米赤霉醇、β-玉米赤霉醇、伏马菌素B1、伏马菌素B2、伏马菌素B3、展青霉素、交链孢酚、交链孢烯、交链孢酚单甲醚、细交链孢菌酮酸、腾毒素、恩镰孢菌素A、恩镰孢菌素A1、恩镰孢菌素B、恩镰孢菌素B1、白僵菌素、串珠镰刀菌素、桔青霉素、霉酚酸和杂色曲霉毒素。这些真菌毒素在各类食品中天然污染并广泛存在，通过膳食摄入是一般人群摄入真菌毒素的主要途径。

## 二、健康指导值

1992年，IARC将黄曲霉毒素B1、黄曲霉毒素B2、黄曲霉毒素G1、黄曲霉毒素G2列为一类致癌物，将黄曲霉毒素M1列为二类致癌物（IARC，1993）。由于具有基因毒性和致癌性的物质不存在效应阈值，SCF（1994）和JECFA（1999）认为无法计算其可耐受膳食摄入量，即使暴露量小于1 ng/(kg bw·d)，仍然有引发肝癌的风险，应尽可能减少对该类物质的暴露。

French TDS (21 mycotoxins), the 2nd French TDS (25 mycotoxins), the Spanish TDS (18 mycotoxins), the Lebanese TDS (4 mycotoxins), the 1st Hong Kong (China) TDS (13 mycotoxins) and the 4th and 5th China TDSs (38 mycotoxins). In total, 43 mycotoxins were analyzed in the 6th China TDS, and they were: aflatoxin B1, aflatoxin B2, aflatoxin G1, aflatoxin G2, aflatoxin M1, aflatoxin M2, ochratoxin A, ochratoxin B, deoxynivalenol, nivalenol, 3-acetyl deoxynivalenol, 15-acetyl-deoxynivalenol, fusarenon X, 3-glucoside-deoxynivalenol, deepoxy-deoxynivalenol, HT-2 toxin, T-2 toxin, diacetoxyscirpenol, neosolaniol, zearalenone, zearalanone, α-zearalenol, β-zearalenol, α-zearalanol, β-zearalanol, fumonisin B1, fumonisin B2, fumonisin B3, patulin, alternariol, altenuene, alternariol monomethyl ether, tenuazonic acid, tentoxin, enniatin A, enniatin A1, enniatin B, enniatin B1, beauvericin, moniliformin, citrinin, mycophenolic acid, and sterigmatocystin. These mycotoxins are common natural contaminants in foods and find their way into the human body mainly through diets.

## II. HBGV

In 1992, the International Agency for Research on Cancer classified aflatoxins B1, aflatoxins B2, aflatoxins G1 and aflatoxins G2 as Group 1 carcinogens and aflatoxin M1 as a Group 2 carcinogen (IARC, 1993). There are no thresholds for chemicals with genotoxic or carcinogenic effects. According to SCF (1994) and JECFA (1999), TDI is not applicable to these chemicals because even low levels of exposure [less than 1 ng/(kg bw·d)] pose a risk of liver cancer, and thus exposure to such chemicals should be minimized.

目前，暂无实验室或流行病学证据表明DON对人类有致癌性。IARC于1993年将DON划分为3类致癌物。JECFA于2001年制定DON的暂定每日最大耐受摄入量（PMTDI）为1 μg/(kg bw·d)，与SCF于2002年制定的DON的暂定每日耐受摄入量（t-TDI）一致。2010年，JECFA将DON、3-Ac-DON和15-Ac-DON合并考虑，设定其总量的PMTDI为1 μg/(kg bw·d)。由于数据不充分，暂时没有设定3-Glu-DON的健康指导值。2017年，EFSA评估了食品和饲料中的DON、3-Ac-DON、15-Ac-DON及3-Glu-DON对动物与人类的健康风险，将DON的TDI值修订为针对DON、3-Ac-DON、15-Ac-DON和3-Glu-DON化合物组的TDI，取值仍为1 μg/(kg bw·d)。

2002年，SCF设立了NIV的暂定每日耐受摄入量（t-PTI）为0.7 μg/(kg bw·d)。2010年，日本食品安全委员会（FSCJ）设定了NIV的TDI为0.4 μg/(kg bw·d)。2013年，EFSA设定NIV的TDI为1.2 μg/(kg bw·d)。

由于HT-2为T-2的代谢产物，T-2与HT-2的毒理学作用无法区分，因此在制定健康指导值时将T-2与HT-2合并计算。JECFA于2001年制定T-2与HT-2单独以及总量的PMTDI为0.06 μg/(kg bw·d)，与2002年SCF设定的T-2与HT-2总量的TDI一致。2011年，EFSA采用基准剂量分析方法将T-2与HT-2总量的TDI设定为100 ng/(kg bw·d)（EFSA，2011b）。

JECFA于1991年对OTA进行了评估，设定其暂定每周耐受摄入量（PTWI）为112 ng/(kg bw·周)。1995年，根据毒理学数据将PTWI值修正为100 ng/(kg bw·周)。此后，经过数次讨论，JECFA认为对OTA的毒理作用与作用机理尚需进一步讨论，因

Up to now, there is no laboratory or epidemiological evidence showing that DON is carcinogenic to humans. IARC classified DON as a Group 3 carcinogen in 1993. JECFA established a provisional maximum tolerable daily intake (PMTDI) of 1 μg/(kg bw·d) for DON in 2001, the same as the temporary tolerable daily intake (t-TDI) set by SCF for DON in 2002. In 2010, JECFA set the PMTDI of the sum of DON, 3-Ac-DON, and 15-Ac-DON at 1 μg/(kg bw·d). Due to inadequacy of data, the HBGV for 3-Glu-DON was not determined. In 2017, EFSA assessed the health risks of DON, 3-Ac-DON, 15-Ac-DON, and 3-Glu-DON in food and feed to animals and humans, and revise the TDI of the sum of DON, 3-Ac-DON, 15-Ac-DON and 3-Glu-DON at 1 μg/(kg bw·d).

In 2002, SCF set the t-PTI value for NIV at 0.7 μg/(kg bw·d). In 2010, the Food Safety Commission of Japan (FSCJ) set the TDI value for NIV at 0.4 μg/(kg bw·d). In 2013, EFSA set the TDI value for NIV at 1.2 μg/(kg bw·d).

As HT-2 is a metabolite of T-2 and their toxicological effects cannot be differentiated, HBGV is determined on the basis of the sum of T-2 and HT-2. The PMTDI value set by JECFA in 2001 for the sum and each of T-2 and HT-2 was 0.06 μg/(kg bw·d), the same as the TDI value set by SCF for the sum of T-2 and HT-2 in 2002. Using a benchmark dose analysis, the EFSA established TDI of 100 ng/(kg bw·d) for the sum of T-2 and HT-2 toxins (EFSA, 2011b).

In 1991, JECFA assessed OTA and set its PTWI value at 112 ng/(kg bw·week), which was then revised to be 100 ng/(kg bw·week) according to toxicological data in 1995. After several rounds of discussion, JECFA concluded that the toxicological effect and mechanism of action of OTA needed to be further ascertained and decided to continue to use the PTWI value of 100 ng/(kg bw·week) in 2008. The tolerable weekly intake (TWI) of OTA set by EFSA in 2006 was 120 ng/(kg bw·week), but in 2020, a margin of exposure (MOE) method was used to assess the health risks of OTA.

而于 2008 年决定暂时继续使用 100 ng/(kg bw·周) 的 PTWI 值。EFSA 曾于 2006 年确定 OTA 的每周可耐受摄入量（TWI）为 120 ng/(kg bw·周)，但 2020 年，EFSA 决定使用暴露边界值（MOE）方法来表征 OTA 的风险。

JECFA 于 2000 年设定了玉米赤霉烯酮的 PMTDI 为 0.5 μg/(kg bw·d)。SCF 于 2000 年设定玉米赤霉烯酮的暂定每日耐受摄入量（t-PTI）为 0.2 μg/(kg bw·d)。EFSA 于 2011 年根据详细的评估结果设定每日耐受摄入量为 0.25 μg/(kg bw·d)。2016 年，EFSA 将玉米赤霉烯酮的 TDI 值修订为针对玉米赤霉烯酮及其衍生物（ZENGlcs、ZENSulfs、α-ZEL、α-ZELGlcs、α-ZELSulfs、β-ZEL、β-ZELGlcs、β-ZELSulfs、ZAN、ZANGlcs、ZANSulfs、α-ZAL、α-ZALGlcs、α-ZALSulfs、β-ZAL、β-ZALGlcs、β-ZALSulfs、cis-ZEN、cis-ZENGlcs、cis-ZENSulfs、cis-α-ZEL、cis-α-ZELGlcs、cis-α-ZELSulfs、cis-β-ZEL、cis-β-ZELGlcs、cis-β-ZELSulfs）化合物组的 TDI，取值仍为 0.25 μg/(kg bw·d)。该 TDI 基于对猪的雌激素作用。ZEN 的衍生物包括其 I 相代谢物和 II 相代谢物，I 相代谢物主要通过还原反应产生，大多数 I 相代谢物具有雌激素活性，因此假设它们的联合作用将是累加的。II 相代谢物主要是 ZEN 及其 I 相代谢物与葡萄糖和硫酸盐（植物中）或葡萄糖醛酸（动物中）的结合物，因此 EFSA 将 ZEN 及其衍生物组（包括 I 相和 II 相代谢物）的 TDI 设定为 0.25 μg/(kg bw·d)。

为了解释体内雌激素效力的差异，每个 I 相代谢物都被设定了一个相对 ZEN 的相对效应因子（RPF），用来进行 ZEN 代谢物的暴露评估。ZENGlcs 和 ZENSulfs 的 RPF 为 1.0；α-ZEL、

In 2000, JECFA set the PMTDI value for zearalenone at 0.5 μg/(kg bw·d). In 2000, SCF set the t-PTI value for zearalenone at 0.2 μg/(kg bw·d). In 2011, EFSA set the TDI value for zearalenone at 0.25 μg/(kg bw·d) according to the results of a detailed assessment. In 2016, EFSA revised the TDI value for zearalenone and its modified forms (ZENGlcs, ZENSulfs, α-ZEL, α-ZELGlcs, α-ZELSulfs, β-ZEL, β-ZELGlcs, β-ZELSulfs, ZAN, ZANGlcs, ZANSulfs, α-ZAL, α-ZALGlcs, α-ZALSulfs, β-ZAL, β-ZALGlcs, β-ZALSulfs, cis-ZEN, cis-ZENGlcs, cis-ZENSulfs, cis-α-ZEL, cis-α-ZELGlcs, and cis-α-ZELSulfs, cis-β-ZEL, cis-β-ZELGlcs, cis-β-ZELSulfs) at 0.25 μg/(kg bw·d). This TDI is based on estrogenicity in pigs, and the modified forms of ZEN identified are phase I and phase II metabolites. Phase I metabolites are mainly formed through reduction. Phase II metabolites are formed by the conjugation of ZEN and its phase I metabolites with glucose or sulfate (in plant), and glucuronic acid (in animals). Most of the phase I metabolites have oestrogenic activity and it is assumed that their combined action will be additive. EFSA found it appropriate to set a group TDI of 0.25 μg/(kg bw·d) expressed as ZEN equivalents for ZEN and its modified forms (phase I and phase II metabolites).

To account for differences in *in vivo* oestrogenic potency, each phase I metabolite was assigned a relative potency factor relative to ZEN to be applied to exposure estimates of the respective ZEN metabolites. The relative potency factors (RPFs) are 1.0 for ZENGlcs and ZENSulfs; 60 for α-ZEL, α-ZELGlcs and α-ZELSulfs; 0.2 for β-ZEL, β-ZELGlcs and β-ZELSulfs; 1.5 for ZAN, ZANGlcs and ZANSulfs; 4.0 for α-ZAL, α-ZALGlcs and α-ZALSulfs; 2.0 for β-ZAL, β-ZALGlcs and β-ZALSulfs; 1.0 for cis-ZEN, cis-ZENGlcs and cis-ZENSulfs; 8.0 for cis-α-ZEL, cis-α-ZELGlcs and cis-α-ZELSulfs; 1.0 for cis-β-ZEL, cis-β-ZELGlcs and cis-β-ZELSulfs. In addition, it is assumed that glucuronides of ZEN and its phase I metabolites have the same RPFs as their aglycones.

α-ZELGlcs 和 α-ZELSulfs 的 RPF 为 60；β-ZEL、β-ZELGlcs 和 β-ZELSulfs 的 RPF 为 0.2；ZAN、ZANGlcs 和 ZANSulfs 的 RPF 为 1.5；α-ZAL、α-ZALGlcs 和 α-ZALSulfs 的 RPF 为 4.0；β-ZAL、β-ZALGlcs 和 β-ZALSulfs 的 RPF 为 2.0；cis-ZEN、cis-ZENGlcs 和 cis-ZENSulfs 的 RPF 为 1.0；cis-α-ZEL、cis-α-ZELGlcs 和 cis-α-ZELSulfs 的 RPF 为 8.0；cis-β-ZEL、cis-β-ZELGlcs 和 cis-β-ZELSulfs 的 RPF 为 1.0。此外，认为 ZEN 及其 Ⅰ 相代谢物的葡萄糖醛酸结合物具有与其苷元相同的 RPF。

JECFA 于 2002 年根据毒理学评估结果，将伏马菌素 FB1、FB2 和 FB3 作为一组，其中单个物质以及其总量的 PMTDI 均为 2 μg/(kg bw·d)。欧盟于 2003 年同样将这组物质的 TDI 设定为 2 μg/(kg bw·d)。

JECFA 于 1990 年设定展青霉素的 PTWI 为 7 μg/(kg bw·d)，1995 年修订 PMTDI 为 0.4 μg/(kg bw·d)。

根据 EFSA 的 2016 年报告，采用毒理学关注阈值（threshold of toxicological concern，TTC）方法对部分交链孢毒素的膳食暴露情况进行评估。TTC 方法是指当污染物的暴露水平低于某个阈值水平时，该污染物对人体健康造成负面影响的可能性很低。EFSA 给出了 4 种交链孢毒素的 TTC 值，TeA 与 TEN 的 TTC 值为 1500 ng/(kg bw·d)，AOH 与 AME 的 TTC 值为 2.5 ng/(kg bw·d)。

由于暂时缺乏数据，EFSA 暂未对桔青霉素制定健康指导值。EFSA 认为在摄入量为每天 0.2 μg/(kg bw·d) 时，不会对人造成肾毒性危害。但是这一阈值不能排除造成基因毒性与致癌性的可能。

In 2002, based on the results of toxicological assessment, JECFA set the PMTDI value for the sum and each of FB1, FB2 and FB3 at 2 μg/(kg bw·d). In 2003, EC set the TDI value for the same group of chemicals at 2 μg/(kg bw·d).

In 1990, JECFA set the PTWI value for patulin at 7 μg/(kg bw·d), which was revised to be the PMTDI value of 0.4 μg/(kg bw·d) in 1995.

In 2016, the threshold of toxicological concern (TTC) approach was used to assess the dietary exposure level of *Alternaria* toxins by EFSA. TTC approach means that when the exposure level of a contaminant is lower than a certain threshold level, the possibility of adverse effect of the contaminant on human health is very low. The TTC values of four *Alternaria* toxins were given by EFSA. TeA and TEN had TTC values of 1500 ng/(kg bw·d), while AOH and AME had TTC values of 2.5 ng/(kg bw·d).

The stance of EFSA as is that it is not appropriate to specify a HBGV for citrin due to a temporary lack of data. EFSA stated that even though a daily intake of 0.2 μg/(kg bw·d) is not nephrotoxic to humans, the threshold cannot exclude the possibility of genotoxicity and carcinogenicity.

## 三、总膳食研究结果

### （一）黄曲霉毒素

第六次中国总膳食研究对12类食品进行了黄曲霉毒素B1、黄曲霉毒素B2、黄曲霉毒素G1、黄曲霉毒素G2、黄曲霉毒素M1、黄曲霉毒素M2以及黄曲霉毒素的总量（AFBG）的分析。黄曲霉毒素的总检出率为21.9%，在不同膳食种类中的检出率差异较大，豆类检出率最高（58.3%），其次是谷类（50%），在水果类、水及饮料类中未检出。在12类膳食样品中，各种黄曲霉毒素的总检出率差别也较大，由高到低依次为：AFB1（19.8%）、AFB2（6.3%）、AFM1（3.8%）、AFG1（2.1%）、AFM2和AFG2（未检出）。各黄曲霉毒素的检出含量见附表8-1～附表8-5。

附表8-1为总膳食研究样品中黄曲霉毒素B1的含量。从全国看，豆类中黄曲霉毒素B1含量最高。《食品安全国家标准 食品中真菌毒素限量》（GB 2761—2017）中关于豆类及其制品中的黄曲霉毒素限量，仅规定了发酵豆制品中AFB1的限量值为5 μg/kg。附表8-2和附表8-3分别为总膳食研究样品中黄曲霉毒素B2和黄曲霉毒素G1的含量。

附表8-4为总膳食研究样品中黄曲霉毒素M1的含量，AFM1在2份乳类样品中检出，其含量分别为0.135 μg/kg和0.020 μg/kg。《食品安全国家标准 食品中真菌毒素限量》（GB 2761—2017）中规定乳及乳制品和特殊膳食用食品中的AFM1限量标准为0.5 μg/kg。

附表8-5为总膳食研究样品中黄曲霉毒素BG的含量状况，从全国看，豆类中的总黄曲霉毒素含量最高（0.703 μg/kg），其次为薯类、蛋类和蔬菜类，其余各类膳食的全国平均含量

## III. TDS Results

### (I) Aflatoxins

In the 6$^{th}$ China TDS, a total of 12 food categories were analyzed for the levels of aflatoxins B1, aflatoxins B2, aflatoxins G1, aflatoxins G2, aflatoxins M1, aflatoxins M2 and the sum of aflatoxin B and G. The total detection rate of aflatoxins was 21.9%, with significant differences among the food categories, where legumes had the highest detection rate at 58.3%, followed by cereals at 50%, and no aflatoxin was detected in the samples of fruits, water and beverages. The various aflatoxins had significantly different detection rates and were ordered in descending order as follows: AFB1 19.8%, AFB2 6.3%, AFM1 3.8%, AFG1 2.1%, AFG2 and AFM2 were not detected.

The levels of aflatoxin B1 in TDS samples are shown in Annexed Table 8-1. For food samples nationwide, legumes had a high level of aflatoxin B1. With respect to the limits of aflatoxins in legumes and legume products, *National Food Safety Standard-Maximum Levels of Fungal Toxins in Food* (GB 2761—2017) has provisions on the limit for fermented legume products, which stands at 5 μg/kg. The levels of aflatoxin B2 and G1 in TDS samples are shown in Annexed Table 8-2 and Annexed Table 8-3.

The levels of aflatoxin M1 in TDS samples are shown in Annexed Table 8-4. AFM1 was detected in two dairy products samples, at a level of 0.135 μg/kg and 0.020 μg/kg, respectively. The maximum limit specified in China national standard GB 2761—2017 for AFM1 in milk and dairy products is 0.5 μg/kg.

The total levels of aflatoxin BG in TDS samples are shown in Annexed Table 8-5. For food samples, nationwide, legumes had the highest total levels of aflatoxins (0.703 μg/kg), followed by potatoes, eggs, and vegetables, with the national average levels of all the other food categories being less than 0.1 μg/kg. The contamination of aflatoxins in legumes deserves more attention. The dietary exposures of adult males

均<0.1 μg/kg。豆类中黄曲霉毒素的污染问题应引起关注。以成年男子为代表，分析我国不同地区居民黄曲霉毒素BG的膳食暴露量，见附表8-6和图8-1。从全国看，一般人群的黄曲霉毒素BG膳食暴露量为2.55 ng/(kg bw·d)。根据SCF（1994）和JECFA（1997，2001）的研究结果，即使暴露量小于1 ng/(kg bw·d)，仍然有引发肝癌的风险。采用暴露边界值（MOE）方法对各省（自治区、直辖市）居民黄曲霉毒素BG的膳食暴露情况进行分析，其中基准剂量置信下限（BMDL）值采用170 ng/(kg bw·d)（EFSA，2007），MOE值低于10 000则表示可能出现公共健康问题。全国平均MOE值为67。这一结果表明，我国居民通过膳食摄入黄曲霉毒素BG存在潜在的健康风险。

从毒素种类分析，黄曲霉毒素B1对膳食暴露的贡献率最高，为79.4%；黄曲霉毒素B2、黄曲霉毒素G1、黄曲霉毒素G2对膳食暴露的贡献率均低于11%。

各食物类别对黄曲霉毒素BG膳食暴露的贡献率见图8-2。总体上，豆类、谷类、蔬菜类是黄曲霉毒素BG膳食暴露的最主要来源，超过总暴露量的75%；其他食物类别的贡献率均小于10%。

to aflatoxins BG in China by provinces are shown in Annexed Table 8-6 and Figure 8-1. The national average daily dietary exposure to aflatoxin BG in China was 2.55 ng/(kg bw·d). According to the findings of SCF (1994) and JECFA (1997, 2001), even an exposure below 1 ng/(kg bw·d) has the risk of liver cancer. The MOE (margin of exposure) method was used to analyze the total exposure to aflatoxins BG for residents in the provinces (autonomous regions, municipalities) under the study, where the BMDL value of 170 ng/(kg bw·d) (EFSA, 2007) was adopted. An MOE value below 10 000 indicates a possible public health issue. The national average MOE value was 67. This revealed that the dietary intake of aflatoxins BG was a potential health hazard in China.

Of the various aflatoxins, aflatoxin B1 had the highest contribution to the dietary exposure at 79.4%, with the contributions of aflatoxins B2, aflatoxins G1 and aflatoxins G2 being all below 11%.

Figure 8-2 depicts the contributions of various food categories to dietary exposure to aflatoxins BG. Overall, legumes, cereals and vegetables were the primary sources of exposure to aflatoxins BG, with a contribution rate of more than 75%; the contributions of other food categories are all less than 10%.

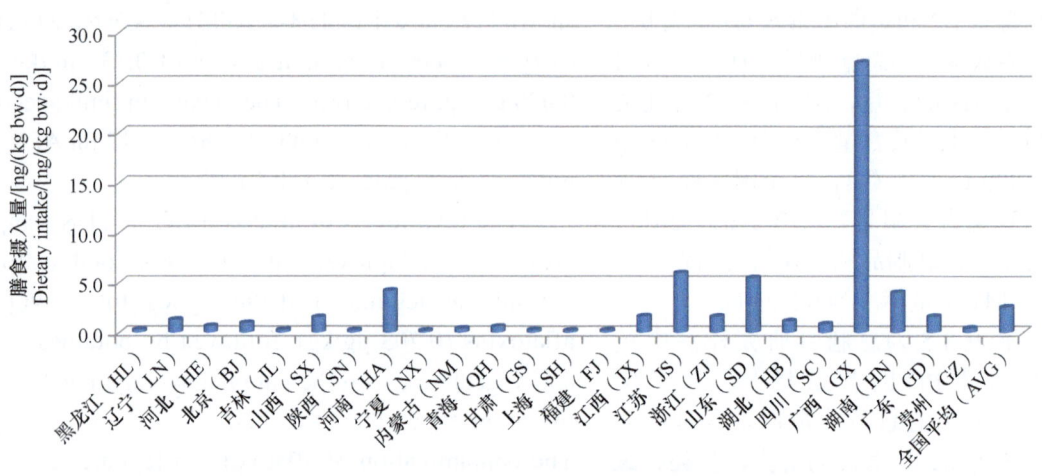

图8-1　第六次中国总膳食研究的黄曲霉毒素BG膳食摄入量

Figure 8-1　Dietary intake of aflatoxin BG from the 6th China TDS

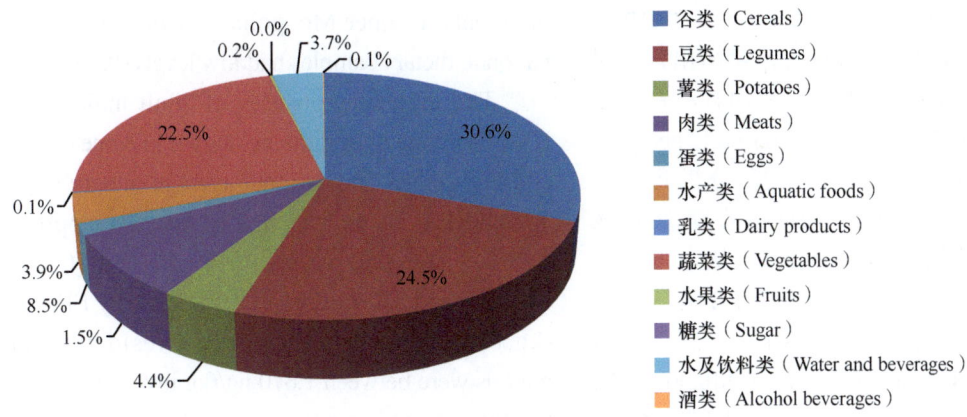

图 8-2　第六次中国总膳食研究黄曲霉毒素 BG 的膳食来源
Figure 8-2　Dietary sources of aflatoxin BG from the 6$^{th}$ China TDS

## （二）单端孢霉烯毒素

根据单端孢霉烯毒素的结构，可将其分为 A、B、C、D 4 种类型，其中 A 型和 B 型较为常见。本次总膳食研究对 12 类食品进行了 11 种单端孢霉烯族真菌毒素的分析，包括 4 种 A 型毒素（T-2、HT-2、NEO、DAS）和 7 种 B 型毒素（DON、3-Ac-DON、15-Ac-DON、3-Glu-DON、deepoxy-DON、NIV、Fus X）。

该类毒素的总检出率为 29.2%。从食品种类看，谷类检出率最高（100%），其次由高到低依次为酒类（70.8%）、水产类（45.8%）、豆类（41.7%）、薯类（29.2%）、肉类（29.2%）、蔬菜类（25.0%）、蛋类（4.2%）、糖类（4.2%），在乳类、水果类、水及饮料中未检出。

不同种类毒素的检出率分别为 DON（27.4%）、3-Glu-DON（7.6%）、T-2（0.3%）、NIV（5.2%）、3-Ac-DON（2.1%）、Fus X（1.4%）、15-Ac-DON（1.7%）、deepoxy-DON（1.4%）、HT-2（0.3%）。DAS 和 NEO 未检出。

### 1. A 型单端孢霉烯毒素

（1）T-2 和 HT-2
附表 8-7 为总膳食研究样品中 T-2

## (Ⅱ) Trichothecenes

Trichothecenes are divided into four (A, B, C, and D) groups according to their chemical structures, with groups A and B being the most common. In the 5$^{th}$ China TDS, 12 food categories were analyzed for the levels of 11 trichothecenes, including four from group A (T-2, HT-2, NEO, and DAS) and seven from group B (DON, 3-Ac-DON, 15-Ac-DON, 3-Glu-DON, deepoxy-DON, NIV, and Fus X).

The total detection rate of trichothecenes was 29.2%. Of the food categories, cereals had the highest detection rate at 100%, followed by alcohol beverages (70.8%), aquatic foods (45.8%), legumes (41.7%), potatoes (29.2%), meats (29.2%), vegetables (25.0%), eggs (4.2%), and sugar (4.2%), with no trichothecene detected in the categories of fruits, dairy products, water and beverages.

The detection rates of the various trichothecenes are 27.4% for DON, 7.6% for 3-Glu-DON, 0.3% for T-2, 5.2% for NIV, 2.1% for 3-Ac-DON, 1.4% for Fus X, 1.7% for 15-Ac-DON, 1.4% for deepoxy-DON, 0.3% for HT-2, and 0% for NEO and DAS.

### 1. Type A Trichothecenes

(1) T-2 and HT-2
The total levels of T-2 and HT-2 in TDS samples are shown in Annexed Table 8-7. T-2 was only found

与HT-2总量的含量状况。本次T-2毒素仅在内蒙古的谷类样品中检出，含量为0.79 μg/kg。从全国平均看，食品中T-2与HT-2含量较低（0.06～0.12 μg/kg）。

以成年男子为代表，分析我国不同地区居民T-2与HT-2的膳食暴露量，见附表8-8和图8-3。从全国平均看，一般人群的T-2与HT-2膳食暴露量为3.11 ng/(kg bw·d)，达到JECFA制定的T-2与HT-2总量TDI[0.06 μg/(kg bw·d)]的5.2%，达到EFSA制定的T-2与HT-2总量TDI[0.1 μg/(kg bw·d)]的3.1%。不同地区居民的暴露量为1.670～12.873 ng/(kg bw·d)，风险较低。

in cereals in Inner Mongolia at 0.79 μg/kg. In terms of national, dietary samples had low levels (0.06-0.14 μg/kg).

The dietary exposures of adult males to T-2 and HT-2 in China by region are shown in Annexed Table 8-8 and Figure 8-3.The national average dietary exposure to T-2 and HT-2 was 3.11 ng/(kg bw·d), approximately 5.2% of the TDI value set by JECFA [0.06 μg/(kg bw·d)] and 3.1% of the TDI value set by EFSA [0.1 μg/(kg bw·d)]. The exposures of residents in studied regions were between 1.670 ng/(kg bw·d) and 12.873 ng/(kg bw·d), at low risk.

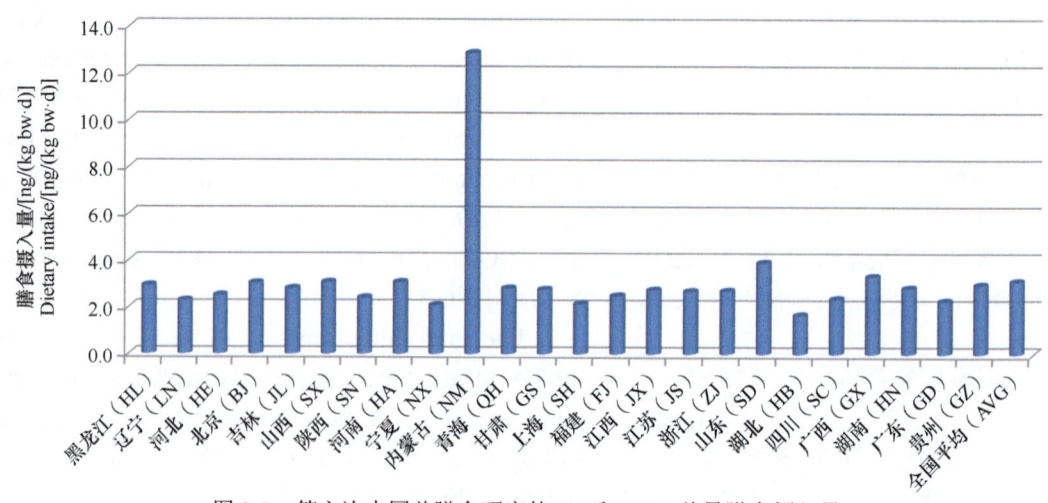

图8-3　第六次中国总膳食研究的T-2和HT-2总量膳食摄入量
Figure 8-3　Dietary intake of T-2 and HT-2 from the 6th China TDS

各食物类别对T-2和HT-2膳食暴露的贡献见图8-4。总体上，谷类是T-2和HT-2膳食暴露的主要来源，约占总暴露量的45.6%。其次是水及饮料类（30.4%）以及蔬菜类（11.1%）。

（2）其他A型单端孢霉烯毒素

本次总膳食研究对另外两种A型单端孢霉烯毒素NEO和DAS进行了测定。但NEO和DAS均无检出。

The contributions of various food categories to the dietary exposure of T-2 and HT-2 are shown in Figure 8-4. Overall, cereals were the main sources of dietary exposure to T-2 and HT-2, accounting for approximately 45.6% of the total exposure, followed by water and beverages (30.4%) and vegetables (11.1%).

(2) Other Type A Trichothecenes

Two other type A trichothecenes, i.e. NEO and DAS, were also analyzed in this TDS. However, they were not detected in all samples.

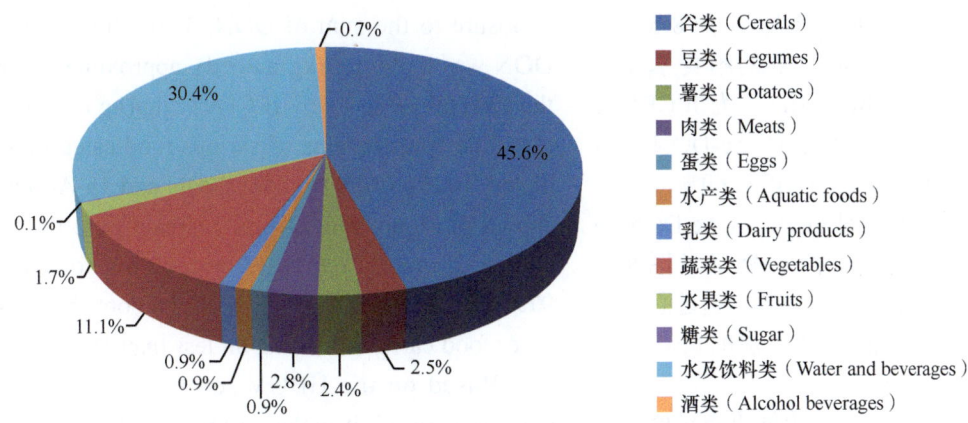

图 8-4 第六次中国总膳食研究 T-2 和 HT-2 总量的膳食来源
Figure 8-4 Dietary sources of T-2 and HT-2 from the 6$^{th}$ China TDS

## 2. B 型单端孢霉烯毒素

（1）DON 及其衍生物

本次总膳食研究对 12 类食品进行了 DON 及其衍生物（3-Ac-DON、15-Ac-DON、3-Glu-DON、deepoxy-DON）的分析。总检出率为 29.5%；其中，谷类、酒类、豆类、薯类、肉类、蛋类、水产类、蔬菜类、水果类、糖类有检出，检出率分别为 100%、70.2%、41.7%、29.2%、29.2%、8.3%、45.8%、20.8%、4.2%、4.2%；乳类、水及饮料类中均未检出。各毒素检出率分别为：DON（27.4%）、3-Glu-DON（6.6%）、3-Ac-DON（2.1%）、15-Ac-DON（1.7%）、deepoxy-DON（1.4%）。总膳食研究样品各毒素含量见附表 8-14。

附表 8-9 为总膳食研究样品中 DON、3-Ac-DON 与 15-Ac-DON 总量的含量状况。从全国平均来看，谷类含量最高（58.39 μg/kg），其次为酒类（3.83 μg/kg）、薯类（2.40 μg/kg）、豆类（2.13 μg/kg）、水产类（1.77 μg/kg）、肉类（1.43 μg/kg），其他各类食品的平均含量均 <1 μg/kg。

依据 JECFA 制定的健康指导值，以成年男子为代表，分析我国不同地区居民 DON、3-Ac-DON 与 15-Ac-DON 膳

## 2. Type B Trichothecenes

(1) DON and Its Derivatives

In this TDS, a total of 12 food categories were analyzed for DON and its derivatives, 3-Ac-DON, 15-Ac-DON, 3-Glu-DON, and deepoxy-DON. The total detection rate was 29.5%, with the highest rates found in cereals (100%), alcohol beverages (70.2%), legumes (41.7%), potatoes (29.2%), meats (29.2%), eggs (8.3%), aquatic foods (45.8%), vegetables (20.8%), fruits (4.2%), sugar (4.2%), and dairy products, water and beverages were not detected. The detection rates for the various analytes were 27.4% for DON, 6.6% for 3-Glu-DON, 2.1% for 3-Ac-DON, 1.7% for 15-Ac-DON, and 1.4% for deepoxy-DON. The levels of these mycotoxins in TDS samples are shown in Annexed Table 8-14.

The total levels of DON, 3-Ac-DON and 15-Ac-DON in TDS samples are shown in Annexed Table 8-9. In terms of national averages, cereals had the highest level at 58.39 μg/kg, followed by alcohol beverages at 3.83 μg/kg, potatoes at 2.40 μg/kg, legumes at 2.13 μg/kg, aquatic foods at 1.77 μg/kg, meats at 1.43 μg/kg, with the average levels in other food categories being all less than 1 μg/kg.

Based on the HBGV set by JECFA, the dietary exposures of adult males to DON, 3-Ac-DON and 15-Ac-DON in China by region are shown in Annexed Table 8-15 and Figure 8-5. The national average dietary

食暴露量，见附表 8-15 和图 8-5。从全国平均看，一般人群的膳食暴露量为 0.690 μg/(kg bw·d)，约为 JECFA 设定 DON、3-Ac-DON、15-Ac-DON 总量 PMTDI[1 μg/(kg bw·d)] 的 69%。

各食物类别对 DON、3-Ac-DON 与 15-Ac-DON 摄入量的贡献率见图 8-6，谷类是最主要的暴露来源，超过总暴露量的 97%；其他食物类别的贡献率均小于 1%。

依据 EFSA 制定的健康指导值，以成年男子为代表，分析我国不同地区居民 DON、3-Ac-DON、15-Ac-DON 与 3-Glu-DON 的膳食暴露量，见附表

exposure to the sum of DON, 3-Ac-DON and 15-Ac-DON was 0.690 μg/(kg bw·d), approximately 69% of the PMTDI value set by JECFA [1 μg/(kg bw·d)].

The contributions of various food categories to the dietary intake of DON, 3-Ac-DON and 15-Ac-DON are shown in Figure 8-6. Overall, cereals were the primary source of dietary exposure, accounting for more than 97% of the total exposure, with the contributions from other food categories being all less than 1%.

Based on the HBGV set by EFSA, the dietary exposures of adult males to DON, 3-Ac-DON, 15-Ac-DON and 3-Glu-DON in China by region are shown in Annexed Table 8-16 and Figure 8-7. The national average dietary exposure in general population to the

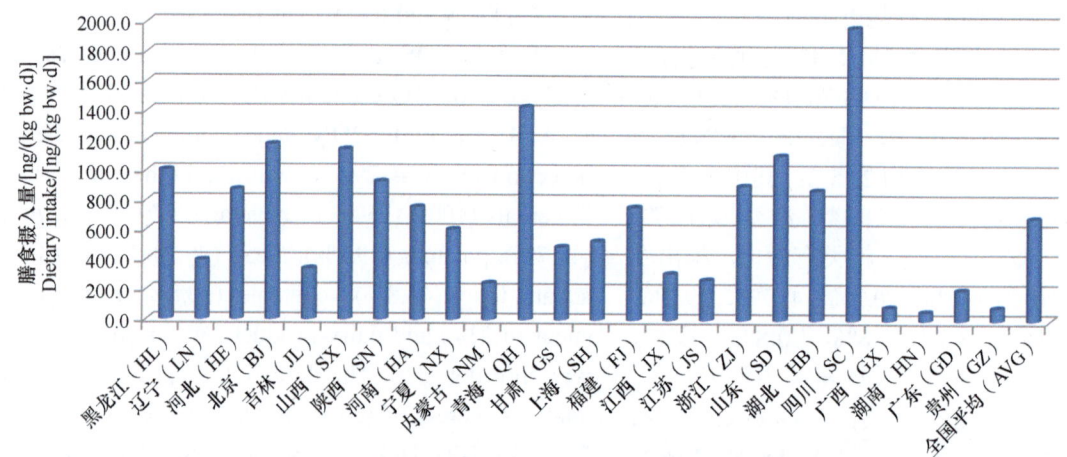

图 8-5　第六次中国总膳食研究的 DON、3-Ac-DON 与 15-Ac-DON 总量膳食摄入量
Figure 8-5　Dietary intake of DON, 3-Ac-DON and 15-Ac-DON from the 6$^{th}$ China TDS

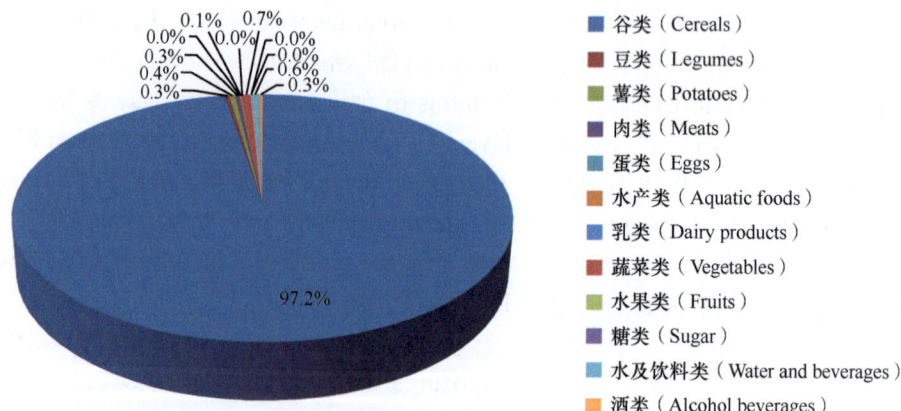

图 8-6　第六次中国总膳食研究 DON、3-Ac-DON 与 15-Ac-DON 总量的膳食来源
Figure 8-6　Dietary sources of DON, 3-Ac-DON and 15-Ac-DON from the 6$^{th}$ China TDS

8-16 和图 8-7。从全国看，一般人群的膳食暴露量为 0.714 μg/(kg bw·d)，约为 EFSA 制定的 TDI（DON、3-Ac-DON、15-Ac-DON 与 3-Glu-DON 总量）[1 μg/(kg bw·d)] 的 72%。从毒素种类分析，DON 对膳食暴露量的贡献率最高，达 95.3%；3-Glu-DON 对膳食暴露量的贡献率为 3.5%，3-Ac-DON 和 15-Ac-DON 贡献率较低，分别为 0.8% 和 0.4%。

各食物类别对 DON、3-Ac-DON、15-Ac-DON 与 3-Glu-DON 摄入量的贡献率见图 8-8，谷类是最主要的暴露来源，为总暴露量的 96.8%；其次为蔬菜

sum of DON, 3-Ac-DON, 15-Ac-DON and 3-Glu-DON was 0.714 μg/(kg bw·d), approximately 72% of the TDI value set by EFSA [1 μg/(kg bw·d)]. DON had the highest contribution to the total exposure, accounting for nearly 95.3%, followed by 3-Glu-DON 3.5%, 3-Ac-DON 0.8%, and 15-Ac-DON 0.4%.

The contributions of various food categories to the dietary intake of DON, 3-Ac-DON, 15-Ac-DON, and 3-Glu-DON are shown in Figure 8-8. Overall, cereals were the primary source of dietary exposure, accounting for more than 96.8% of the total exposure, followed by vegetables (1.0%), with the contributions from other food categories being all less than 1.0%.

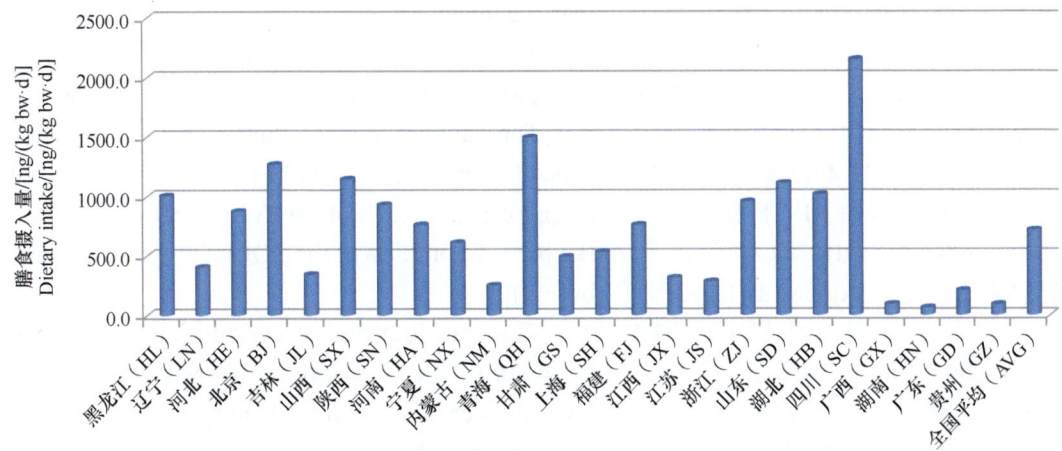

图 8-7 第六次中国总膳食研究的 DON、3-Ac-DON、15-Ac-DON 与 3-Glu-DON 总量膳食摄入量

Figure 8-7 Dietary intake of DON, 3-Ac-DON, 15-Ac-DON and 3-Glu-DON from the 6th China TDS

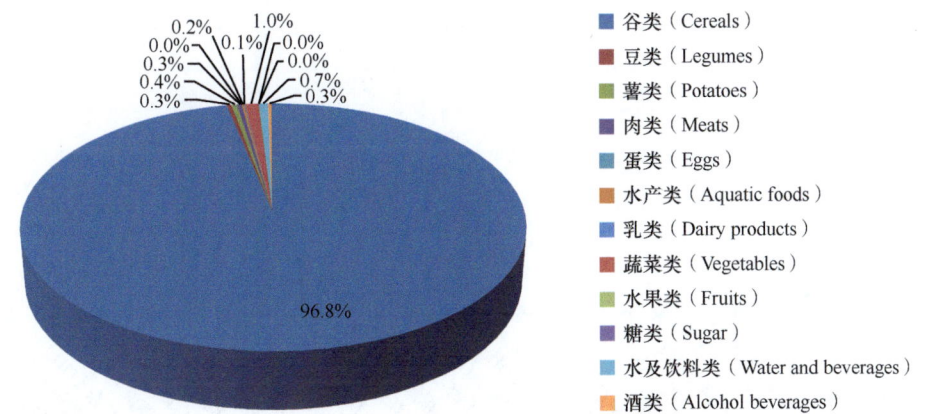

图 8-8 第六次中国总膳食研究 DON、3-Ac-DON、15-Ac-DON 与 3-Glu-DON 总量的膳食来源

Figure 8-8 Dietary sources of DON, 3-Ac-DON, 15-Ac-DON and 3-Glu-DON from the 6th China TDS

类（1.0%），其他食物类别的贡献率均小于1.0%。

（2）NIV

本次总膳食研究对12类食品进行了NIV的测定，在15份样品中检出，检出率为5.2%。从食品类别上看，谷类样品检出率为12.5%，豆类样品检出率为4.2%，薯类样品检出率为8.3%，肉类样品检出率为8.3%，水产样品检出率为8.3%，蔬菜样品检出率为12.5%，酒类样品检出率为12.5%，其他类样品无检出。

附表8-17为总膳食研究样品中NIV的含量状况，从全国平均看，谷类中NIV含量为0.70 μg/kg，酒类中NIV含量为0.29 μg/kg，其他各类食品含量均不超过0.2 μg/kg。以成年男子为代表，分析我国不同地区居民NIV膳食暴露量，见附表8-18和图8-9。从全国平均看，一般人群的NIV膳食暴露量为0.009 μg/(kg bw·d)，约为EFSA制定的PMTDI [1.2 μg/(kg bw·d)]的0.8%，是日本食品安全委员会制定的TDI [0.4 μg/(kg bw·d)]的2.3%。

各食物类别对NIV膳食暴露的贡献率见图8-10，以全国平均水平计，谷类是NIV膳食暴露的最主要来源，贡

(2) NIV

In this TDS, a total of 12 food categories were analyzed for the levels of NIV, with NIV detected in 15 food samples, representing a detection rate of 5.2%. Of the food categories, cereals had a detection rate of 12.5%, legumes at 4.2%, potatoes at 8.3%, meats at 8.3%, aquatic foods at 8.3%, vegetables at 12.5%, alcohol beverages at 12.5%, and other food categories were not detected.

The total levels of NIV in TDS samples are shown in Annexed Table 8-17. In terms of national averages, cereals had the highest NIV level at 0.70 μg/kg, followed by alcohol beverages at 0.29 μg/kg, with the average levels in all other food categories being less than 0.2 μg/kg.

The dietary NIV exposures of adult males in China by region are shown in Annexed Table 8-18 and Figure 8-9. The national average dietary exposure to NIV in general population was 0.009 μg/(kg bw·d), equivalent to approximately 0.8% of the PMTDI set by EFSA [1.2 μg/(kg bw·d)] or 2.3% of the TDI set by FSCJ [0.4 μg/(kg bw·d)].

The contributions of various food categories to the dietary NIV exposure are shown in Figure 8-10. Overall, cereals are the primary source of dietary exposure to NIV, accounting for 75.4% of the total exposure, followed by water and beverages (8.6%) and

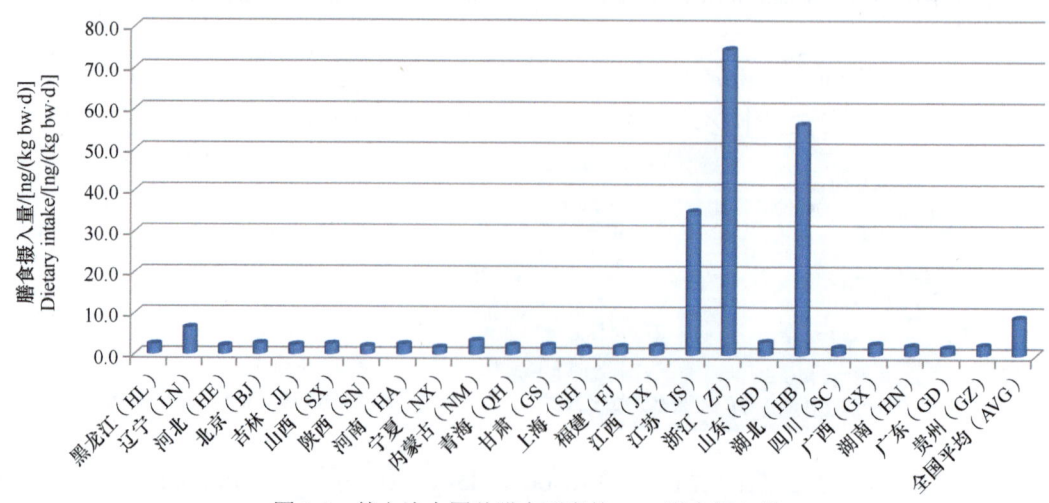

图8-9 第六次中国总膳食研究的NIV膳食摄入量

Figure 8-9 Dietary intake of NIV from the 6th China TDS

献率达到 75.4%；水及饮料类、蔬菜类其次，均占 8.6%；其他食物类别的贡献率均不超过 3%。

vegetables (8.6%), with the contributions from other food categories being all insignificant at less than 3%.

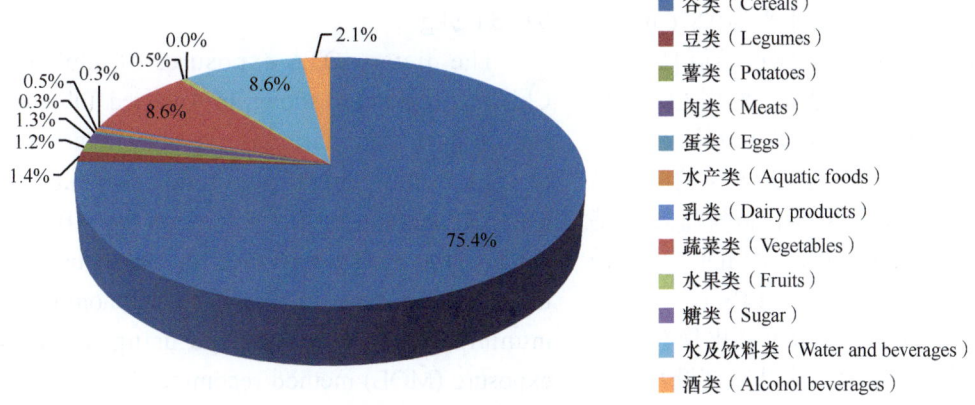

图 8-10 第六次中国总膳食研究 NIV 的膳食来源
Figure 8-10　Dietary sources of NIV from the 6th China TDS

（3）Fus X

在本次总膳食研究中，仅 4 份蔬菜类样品检出 Fus X，检出率为 1.4%。

(3) Fus X

Fus X was detected in four vegetables samples, representing a detection rate of 1.4% in this TDS.

## （三）赭曲霉毒素

本次总膳食研究对 12 类共 288 份食品进行了 OTA 和 OTB 的检测，共在 14 份样品中检出赭曲霉毒素，总检出率为 4.9%。其中 OTA 在 4 份样品中检出，检出率为 1.4%，OTB 在 10 份样品中检出，检出率为 3.5%。不同膳食种类的检出率差异较大，豆类检出率最高（25.0%），其次是谷类（12.5%）、水产类（8.3%），以及肉类、蔬菜类、水果类（均为 4.2%），其他各类中均未检出。各毒素含量见附表 8-19 和附表 8-20。

附表 8-19 为总膳食研究样品中 OTA 的含量状况。从全国平均看，豆类和谷类中 OTA 含量较高，分别为 0.093 μg/kg 和 0.062 μg/kg，其余均＜0.01 μg/kg。附表 8-20 为总膳食研究样品中 OTB 的含量状况。从全国平均看，豆类中 OTB 含量最高，为 0.480 μg/kg，其次为水产类和薯类，分别为 0.219 μg/kg

## (Ⅲ) Ochratoxins

In the 6th CTDS, a total of 288 food samples in 12 categories were analyzed for the levels of OTA and OTB, which were detected in 14 samples, representing a detection rate of 4.9%. OTA was detected in 4 samples with a detection rate of 1.4%, and OTB was detected in 10 samples with a detection rate of 3.5%. The detection rate varied greatly among different food categories. The detection rate of legumes was the highest (25.0%), followed by cereals (12.5%) and aquatic foods (8.3%). The detection rates of meats, vegetables, and fruits were 4.2%, respectively. OTA and OTB were not detected in other food categories. The levels of ochratoxins are shown in Annexed Table 8-19 and Annexed Table 8-20.

The OTA levels in TDS samples are shown in Annexed Table 8-19. In terms of the national averages, legumes (0.093 μg/kg) and cereals (0.062 μg/kg) had the higher OTA levels. In other food categories, the levels of OTA were lower than 0.01 μg/kg. Annexed Table 8-20 shows the levels of OTB in TDS samples.

和 0.183 μg/kg，其余均＜0.015 μg/kg。

以成年男子为代表，分析我国不同地区居民 OTA 的膳食暴露量，见附表 8-21 和图 8-11。从全国平均看，一般人群的 OTA 膳食暴露量水平为 0.876 ng/(kg bw·d)，占 JECFA 健康指导值 [100 ng/(kg bw·周)] 的 6.13%。采用 EFSA 建议的暴露边界值（MOE）方法对各省（自治区、直辖市）居民 OTA 的膳食暴露情况进行分析，其中非肿瘤效应基准剂量置信下限 10%（BMDL$_{10}$）值采用 4.73 μg/(kg bw·d)（EFSA，2020），MOE 低于 200 则表示可能出现公共健康问题；其中肿瘤效应基准剂量置信下限 10%（BMDL$_{10}$）值采用 14.5 μg/(kg bw·d)（EFSA，2020），MOE 低于 10 000 则表示可能出现公共健康问题。全国平均非肿瘤效应和肿瘤效应 MOE 值分别为 5402 和 16 561。

各食物类别对 OTA 膳食暴露的贡献率见图 8-12，总体上，谷类是 OTA 膳食暴露的最主要来源，超过总暴露量的 80%；豆类其次，占 11.7%；其他食物类别的贡献率均小于 5%。

In terms of the national averages, the level of OTB in legumes was the highest at 0.480 μg/kg, followed by aquatic foods and potatoes, at 0.219 μg/kg and 0.183 μg/kg, respectively, and in other categories, it was all below 0.015 μg/kg.

The dietary OTA exposures of adult males in China by region are shown in Annexed Table 8-21 and Figure 8-11. The national average dietary exposure to OTA in the general population was 0.876 ng/(kg bw·d), accounting for 6.13% of the HBGV set by JECFA [100 ng/(kg bw·week)]. The dietary exposure to OTA of residents in provinces (autonomous regions, municipalities) was analyzed using the margin of exposure (MOE) method recommended by EFSA. The benchmark dose lower confidence limit 10% (BMDL$_{10}$) for non-neoplastic effects was 4.73 μg/(kg bw·d), and an MOE value below 200 indicates a possible public health issue (EFSA, 2020). The benchmark dose lower confidence limit 10% (BMDL$_{10}$) for neoplastic effects was 14.5 μg/(kg bw·d), and an MOE value below 10 000 indicates a possible public health issue (EFSA, 2020). The national average non-neoplastic effect and neoplastic effect MOE values were 5402 and 16 561, respectively.

The contributions of various food categories to dietary OTA exposure are shown in Figure 8-12. Overall, cereals were the primary source of dietary exposure

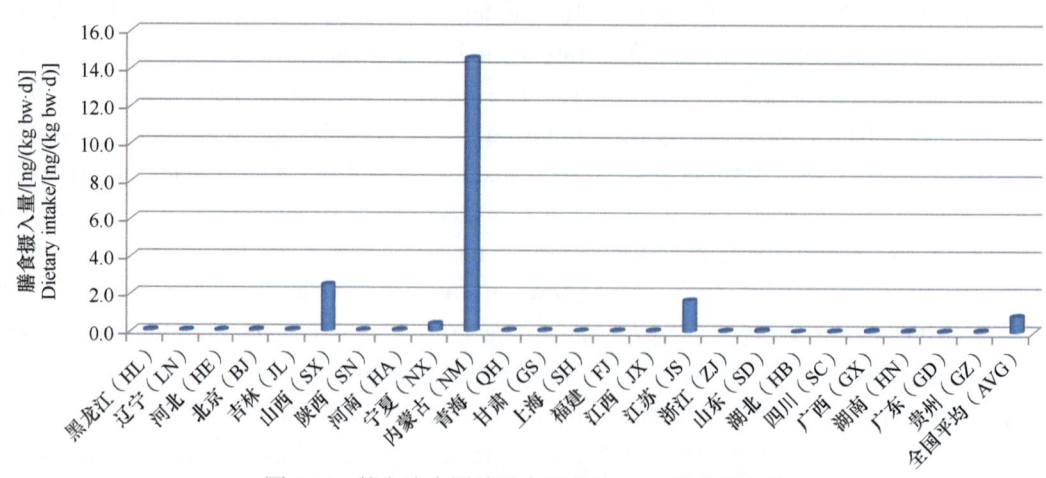

图 8-11　第六次中国总膳食研究的 OTA 膳食摄入量

Figure 8-11　Dietary intake of OTA from the 6$^{th}$ China TDS

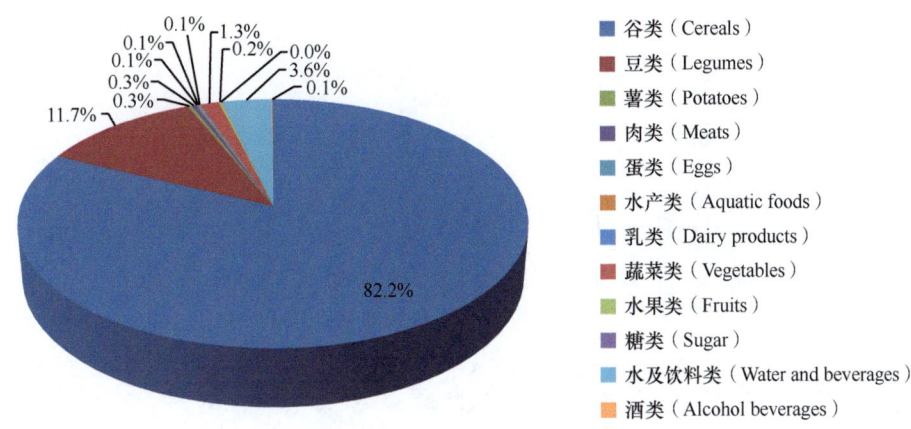

图 8-12 第六次中国总膳食研究 OTA 的膳食来源
Figure 8-12 Dietary sources of OTA from the 6th China TDS

## （四）玉米赤霉烯酮类毒素

本次总膳食研究对 12 类食品进行了玉米赤霉烯酮（ZEN）、玉米赤霉酮（ZAN）、α-玉米赤霉烯醇（α-ZOL）、β-玉米赤霉烯醇（β-ZOL）、α-玉米赤霉醇（α-ZAL）、β-玉米赤霉醇（β-ZAL）6 种毒素含量的分析。该类毒素的总检出率为 47.9%，在各类膳食中均有检出。各种毒素的检出率差异较大，ZEN 为 44.79%、ZAN 为 0.35%、α-ZAL 为 1.39%、β-ZAL 为 6.60%、α-ZOL 为 7.29%、β-ZOL 为 4.51%。各毒素含量见附表 8-23～附表 8-28。

附表 8-23 为总膳食样品中 ZEN 的含量，12 类膳食样品全国平均含量均 < 1 μg/kg。

依据 JECFA 制定的健康指导值，以成年男子为代表，分析我国不同地区居民 ZEN 的膳食暴露量，见附表 8-29 和图 8-13。从全国平均看，一般人群的 ZEN 膳食暴露量水平为 7.772 ng/(kg bw·d)，约为 JECFA 制定的 PMTDI [0.5 μg/(kg bw·d)] 的 1.6%。不同地区居民的 ZEN 膳食暴露水平为 1.019～18.89 ng/(kg bw·d)。

to OTA, contributing over 80% of the total exposure, followed by legumes (11.7%), with the contributions from other food categories being all insignificant at less than 5%.

### (Ⅳ) Zearalenone and Its Derivatives

In this TDS, a total of 12 food categories were analyzed for the levels of the six toxins of zearalenone (ZEN), zearalanone (ZAN), α-zearalenol (α-ZOL), β-zearalenol (β-ZOL), α-zearalanol (α-ZAL), β-zearalanol (β-ZAL). The total detection rate of this group of toxins was 47.9%. They were detected in all food samples. The various toxins had significantly different detection rates and are ordered in descending order as follows: 44.79% for ZEN, 0.35% for ZAN, 1.39% for α-ZAL, 6.60% for β-ZAL, 7.29% for α-ZOL and 4.51% for β-ZOL. The total levels of ZEN and its derivatives in TDS samples are shown in Annexed Table 8-23-Annexed Table 8-28.

The levels of ZEN in TDS samples are shown in Annexed Table 8-23. For food samples, the national average levels in the 12 food categories were all less than 1 μg/kg.

The dietary ZEN exposures of adult males in China by region are shown in Annexed Table 8-29 and Figure 8-13. The national average dietary exposure to ZEN in general population was 7.772 ng/(kg bw·d), equivalent

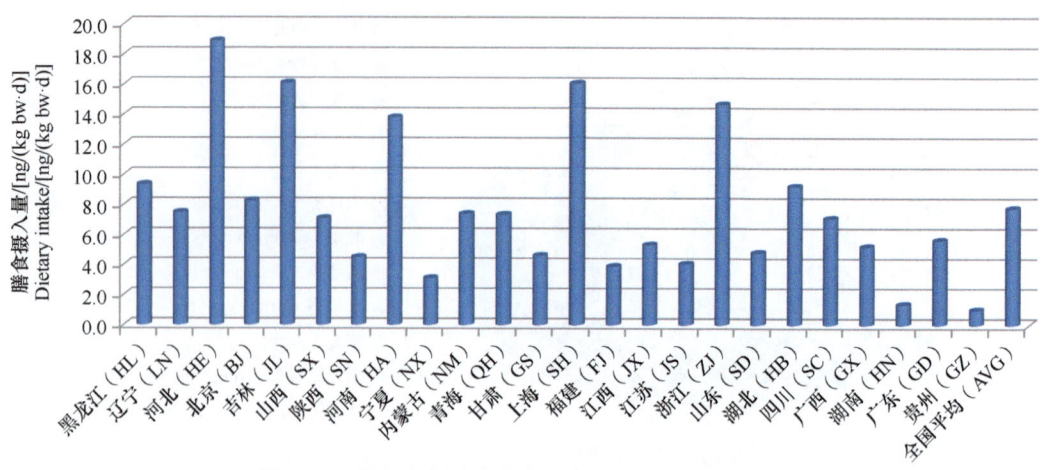

图 8-13 第六次中国总膳食研究的 ZEN 膳食摄入量
Figure 8-13　Dietary intake of ZEN from the 6th China TDS

各食物类别对 ZEN 膳食暴露的贡献率见图 8-14，从全国平均水平来看，谷类为 ZEN 膳食暴露的最主要来源，超过 60%；其次为蔬菜类（15.2%）、豆类（10.0%），其他食物类别的贡献率均小于 5%。

各食物类别对 ZEN 及其衍生物膳食暴露的贡献率见图 8-15，从全国平均水平来看，蔬菜类为 ZEN 类毒素膳食暴露的最主要来源，为 37.6%；其次为谷类（24.2%）、豆类（20.6%）、水及饮料类（11.2%），其他食物类别的贡献率均小于 3%。

to approximately 1.6% of the PMTDI set by JECFA [0.5 μg/(kg bw・d)]. The ZEN exposure of residents in the 24 provinces (autonomous regions, municipalities) ranged from 1.019 ng/(kg bw・d) to 18.89 ng/(kg bw・d).

The contributions of various food categories to the dietary ZEN exposure are shown in Figure 8-14. In terms of national averages, cereals are the primary source of dietary exposure to ZEN, contributing more than 60% of the total exposure, followed by vegetables (15.2%) and legumes (10.0%), with the contributions from other food categories all being insignificant at less than 5%.

The contributions of various food categories to the dietary ZEN and its modified forms exposure are shown

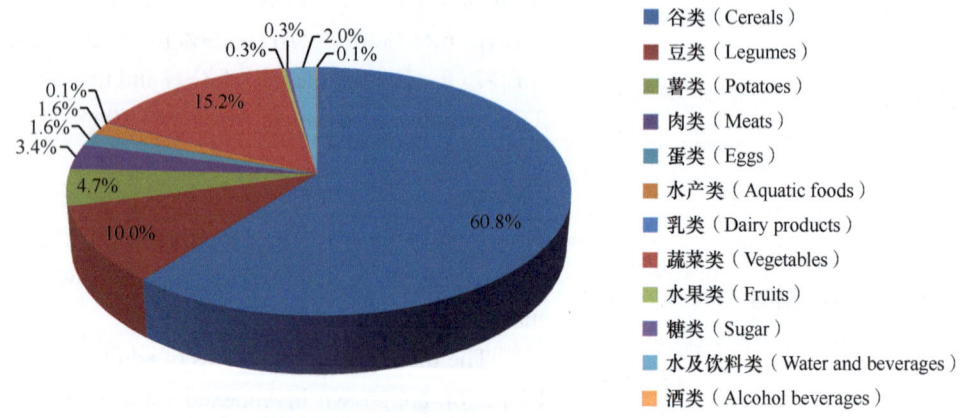

图 8-14　第六次中国总膳食研究 ZEN 的膳食来源
Figure 8-14　Dietary sources of ZEN from the 6th China TDS

in Figure 8-15. In terms of national averages, vegetables are the primary source of dietary exposure to ZEN and its modified forms, contributing 37.6% of the total exposure, followed by cereals (24.2%), legumes (20.6%), water and beverages (11.2%), with the contributions from other food categories being all insignificant at less than 3%.

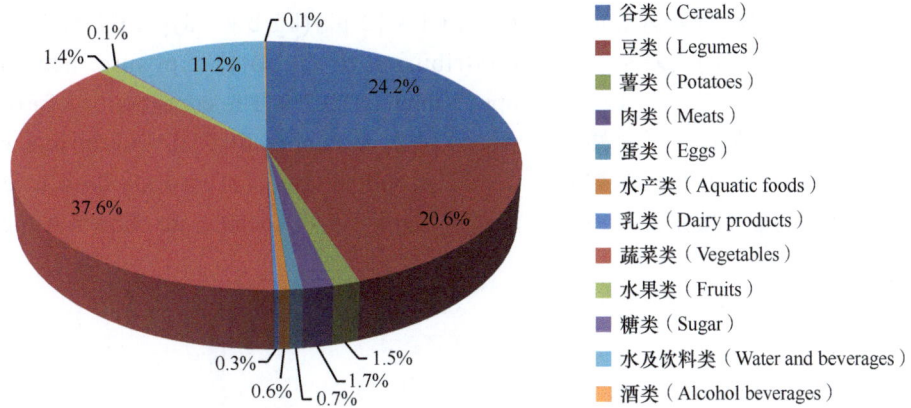

图 8-15　第六次中国总膳食研究 ZEN 及其衍生物的膳食来源

Figure 8-15　Dietary sources of ZEN and its modified from the 6th China TDS

## （五）伏马菌素

本次总膳食研究对 12 类食品进行了伏马菌素 B1、伏马菌素 B2、伏马菌素 B3 的分析。总检出率为 32.6%，FB1、FB2、FB3 的检出率分别为 30.6%、5.9% 和 4.9%。各毒素含量见附表 8-30～附表 8-33。

附表 8-30 为第六次中国总膳食研究样品中伏马菌素的总量（FB1+FB2+FB3），从全国平均看，谷类样品的含量最高，为 7.59 μg/kg，肉类为 1.13 μg/kg，酒类为 1.17 μg/kg，其他各类食品均 <1 μg/kg。目前，我国尚无食品中伏马菌素的限量规定。欧盟对 FB1 和 FB2 的总量作了限量规定，其中玉米中的限量值为 4 mg/kg，玉米基质早餐及玉米基质点心中的限量值为 800 μg/kg，其他用于人类直接消费的玉米及玉米基质食品中的限量值为 1 mg/kg。美国 FDA 规定，玉米中伏马菌素总量的限

## (V) Fumonisins

In this CTDS, a total of 12 food categories were analyzed for the levels of fumonisin B1, fumonisin B2, and fumonisin B3. The total detection rate of this group of toxins was 32.6%. The detection rates of fumonisin B1, fumonisin B2, and fumonisin B3 were 30.6%, 5.9%, and 4.9%, respectively. The levels of fumonisins are shown in Annexed Table 8-30 to Annexed Table 8-33.

The total levels of fumonisins (FB1+FB2+FB3) in the 6th CTDS samples are shown in Annexed Table 8-30. In terms of national averages, cereals had the highest level at 7.59 μg/kg, followed by meats and alcohol beverages with the average levels at 1.13 μg/kg and 1.17 μg/kg, respectively. The fumonisins levels in other food categories were all less than 1 μg/kg. At present, there is no regulatory limit for fumonisins in food in China. The EU has limits on the sum of FB1 and FB2, where the limit in maize is 4 mg/kg, the limit in maize-based breakfast and maize-based snacks is 800 μg/kg, and the limit in maize and maize-based foods intended

量值为 2 mg/kg。

以成年男子为代表，分析我国不同地区居民伏马菌素的膳食暴露量，见附表 8-34 和图 8-16。从全国平均看，一般人群的伏马菌素膳食暴露量水平为 0.104 μg/(kg bw·d)，约为 JECFA 制定的 PMTDI [2 μg/(kg bw·d)] 的 5.2%。从毒素种类分析，FB1 对膳食暴露的贡献率最高，为 70.7%，FB3 的贡献率超过 FB2，占 21.8%。

各食物类别对伏马菌素膳食暴露的贡献率见图 8-17。总体上，谷类是伏马菌素膳食暴露的最主要来源，占总

for humans consumption is 1 mg/kg. The FDA limit for fumonisins in maize is 2 mg/kg.

Annexed Table 8-34 and Figure 8-16 show the dietary fumonisins exposures of adult males in China by region. The national average dietary exposure to fumonisins in general population was 0.104 μg/(kg bw·d), approximately 5.2% of the PMTDI value set by JECFA [2 μg/(kg bw·d)]. FB1 had the highest contribution to the total exposure, accounting for approximately 70.7%. The contribution of FB3 exceeds that of FB2, accounting for 21.8% of the total exposure.

The contributions of various food categories to dietary fumonisins exposure are shown in Figure 8-17.

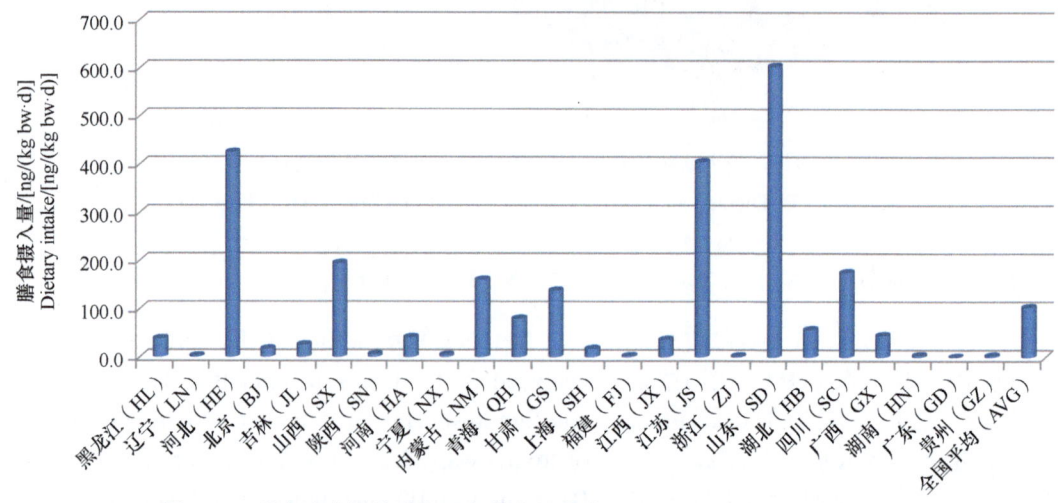

图 8-16　第六次中国总膳食研究的伏马菌素（FB1+FB2+FB3) 膳食摄入量
Figure 8-16　Dietary intake of FB1+FB2+FB3 from the 6th China TDS

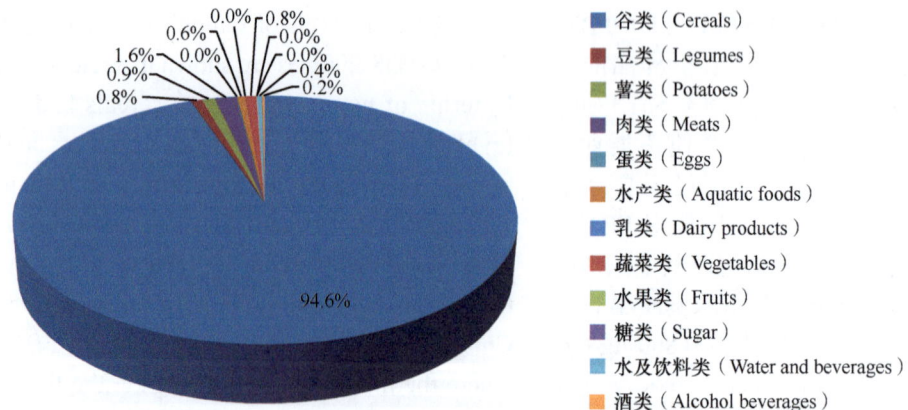

图 8-17　第六次中国总膳食研究伏马菌素（FB1+FB2+FB3) 的膳食来源
Figure 8-17　Dietary sources of FB1+FB2+FB3 from the 6th China TDS

暴露量的94.6%；其他食物类别的贡献率均小于2%。

### （六）展青霉素

本次总膳食研究对12类288份食品样品进行了展青霉素的含量测定，在本次采集的样本中均未检出，表明我国居民通过膳食摄入展青霉素的健康风险较低。

### （七）交链孢毒素

本次总膳食研究对12类288份膳食混合样品进行了交链孢酚（AOH）、交链孢烯（ALT）、交链孢酚单甲醚（AME）、交链孢菌酮酸（TeA）和腾毒素（TEN）含量的测定。总检出率为61.5%，其中，谷类、酒类、豆类、水产类、乳类、蔬菜类、薯类、肉类、蛋类、水果类、糖类、水及饮料类的检出率分别为100%、87.5%、83.3%、75%、70.8%、66.7%、66.7%、54.2%、54.2%、54.2%、16.7%、8.35%。各毒素的检出率分别为：TeA 35.8%、TEN 39.9%、AME 22.6%、ALT 6.9%，AOH未检出。检出的各毒素含量见附表8-35～附表8-38。

#### 1. 交链孢菌酮酸

附表8-35为总膳食研究样品中TeA的含量，从全国平均看，12类膳食样品中谷类的平均含量最高，为10.77 μg/kg，其次为酒类（5.90 μg/kg）；其他类别的含量均<3 μg/kg。

以成年男子为代表，分析我国不同地区居民TeA的膳食暴露量，见附表8-39和图8-18。从全国平均看，一般人群的TeA膳食暴露量水平为140.6 ng/(kg bw·d)。根据EFSA在2016年的报告，采用毒理学关注阈值（threshold of toxicological concern，TTC）方法对居

Overall, cereals were the primary source of dietary exposure to fumonisins, accounting for nearly 94.6% of the total exposure, with the contributions from other food categories being all less than 2%.

### (VI) Patulin

In this TDS, a total of 288 food samples in 12 categories were analyzed for patulin levels, with no patulin detected in any of the samples. This indicated a low health risk from patulin exposure for general population.

### (VII) *Alternaria* Mycotoxins

In the 6$^{th}$ China TDS, a total of 288 food samples in 12 categories were analyzed for the levels of AOH, ALT, AME, TeA and TEN. The total detection rate of *Alternaria* mycotoxins was 61.5%, where cereals had the highest detection rate at 100%, followed by alcohol beverages at 87.5%, legumes at 83.3%, aquatic foods at 75%, dairy products at 70.8%, vegetables at 66.7%, potatoes at 66.7%, meats at 54.2%, eggs at 54.2%, fruits at 54.2%, sugar at 16.7%, water and beverages at 8.35%. The detection rates of various *Alternaria* toxins are as follows: TeA 35.8%, TEN 39.9%, AME 22.6%, ALT 6.9%, AOH not detected. The levels of *Alternaria* toxins in TDS samples are shown in Annexed Table 8-35 to Annexed Table 8-38.

#### 1. TeA

The levels of TeA in TDS samples are shown in Annexed Table 8-35. In terms of national averages, cereals had the highest level at 10.77 μg/kg, followed by alcohol beverages (5.90 μg/kg), with the average levels in other food categories being all less than 3 μg/kg.

The dietary TeA exposures of adult males in China by region are shown in Annexed Table 8-39 and Figure 8-18. The national average dietary exposure to TeA in general population was 140.6 ng/(kg bw·d). The TTC method was used to analyze the total exposure to TeA in the provinces (autonomous regions, municipalities)

民 TeA 的膳食暴露情况进行分析评估。TeA 的 TTC 值为 1500 ng/(kg bw·d)。本次 TeA 膳食暴露量约为 EFSA 制定的 TTC 值的 9.4%。

under the study, where the TTC value of TeA was 1500 ng/(kg bw·d) (EFSA, 2016) was adopted. The national average dietary exposure to TeA was approximately 9.4% of the TTC value set by EFSA.

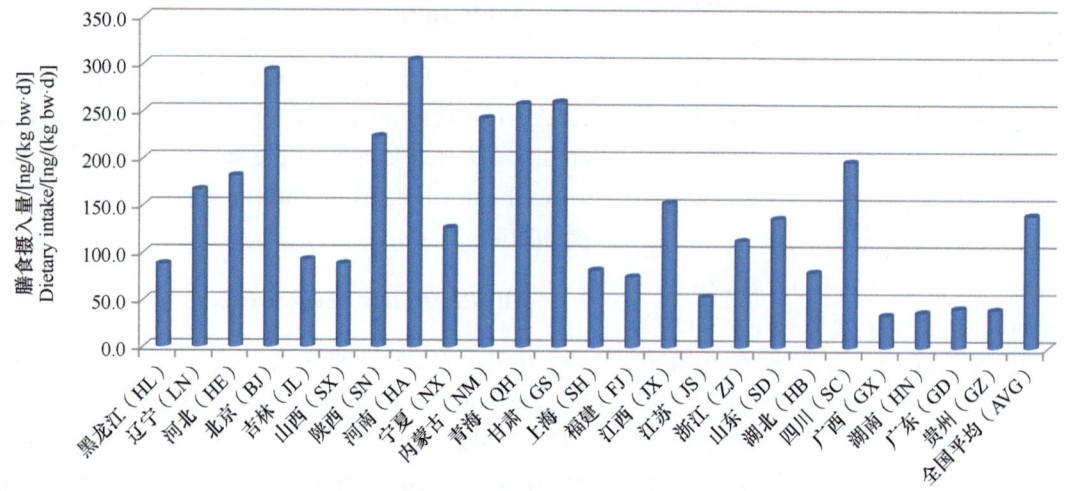

图 8-18　第六次中国总膳食研究的 TeA 膳食摄入量
Figure 8-18　Dietary intake of TeA from the 6<sup>th</sup> China TDS

各食物类别对 TeA 膳食暴露的贡献率见图 8-19，总体上，谷类是 TeA 膳食暴露的最主要来源，超过总暴露量的 85%；其他食物类别的贡献率均小于 5%。

The contributions of various food categories to the dietary TeA exposure are shown in Figure 8-19. Overall, cereals were the primary source of dietary exposure to TeA, accounting for more than 85% of the total exposure, with the contributions from other food categories all being less than 5%.

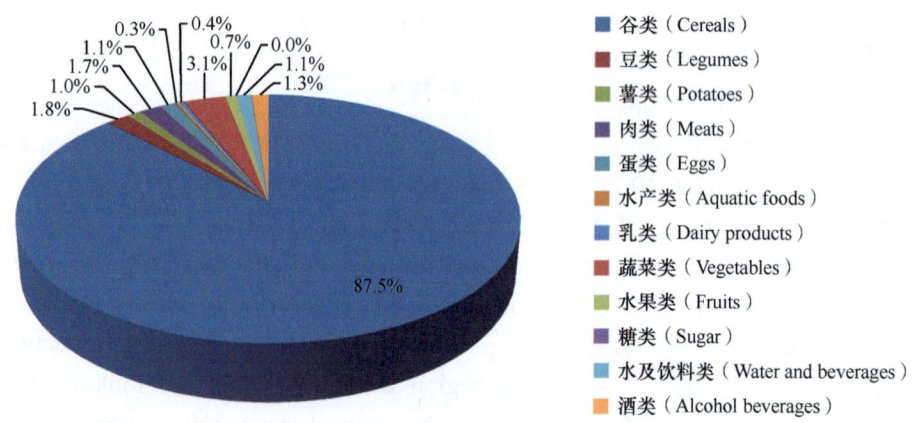

图 8-19　第六次中国总膳食研究 TeA 的膳食来源
Figure 8-19　Dietary sources of TeA from the 6<sup>th</sup> China TDS

**2. 腾毒素**

附表 8-36 为总膳食研究样品中 TEN 的含量，从全国平均看，12 类膳食样品中谷类含量最高，为 11.35 μg/kg，其他类别的含量均＜2 μg/kg。

以成年男子为代表，分析我国不同地区居民 TEN 的膳食暴露量，见附表 8-40 和图 8-20，从全国平均看，一般人群的 TEN 膳食暴露量水平为 143.4 ng/(kg bw·d)。TEN 的 TTC 值为 1500 ng/(kg bw·d)。本次 TEN 膳食暴露量约为 EFSA 制定的 TTC 值的 9.6%。

**2. TEN**

The levels of TEN in TDS samples are shown in Annexed Table 8-36. In terms of national averages, cereals had the highest level at 11.35 μg/kg, with the average levels in other food categories being all less than 2 μg/kg.

The dietary TEN exposures of adult males in China by region are shown in Annexed Table 8-40 and Figure 8-20. The national average dietary exposure to TEN was 143.4 ng/(kg bw·d). The TTC value of TEN was 1500 ng/(kg bw·d) was adopted. The national average dietary exposure to TEN was approximately 9.6% of the TTC value set by EFSA.

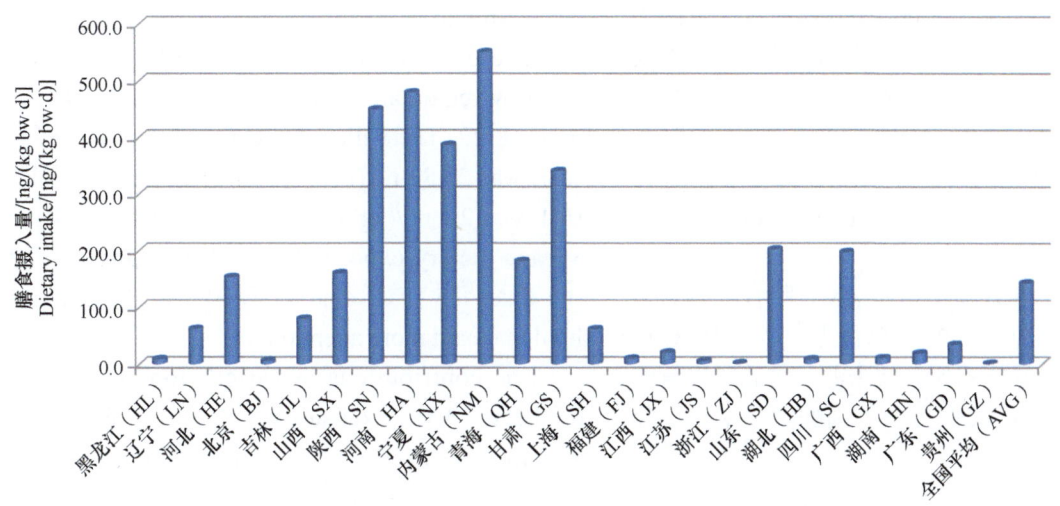

图 8-20 第六次中国总膳食研究的 TEN 膳食摄入量
Figure 8-20 Dietary intake of TEN from the 6th China TDS

各食物类别对 TEN 膳食暴露的贡献率见图 8-21，总体上，谷类是 TEN 膳食暴露的最主要来源，超过总暴露量的 95%；其他食物类别的贡献率均小于 2%。

**3. 交链孢酚单甲醚**

附表 8-37 为总膳食样品中 AME 的含量，从全国平均看，12 类膳食样品中谷类平均含量最高，为 2.65 μg/kg，其他类别的平均含量均＜0.3 μg/kg。

The contributions of various food categories to the dietary TEN exposure are shown in Figure 8-21. Overall, cereals were the primary source of dietary exposure to TEN, accounting for more than 95% of the total exposure, with the contributions from other food categories all being less than 2%.

**3. AME**

The levels of AME in TDS samples are shown in Annexed Table 8-37. In terms of national averages, cereals had the highest level at 2.65 μg/kg, with the

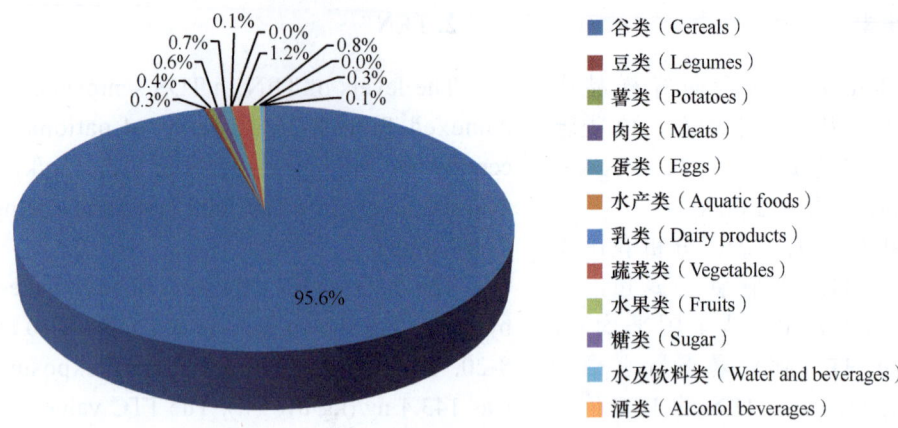

图 8-21　第六次中国总膳食研究 TEN 的膳食来源
Figure 8-21　Dietary sources of TEN from the 6<sup>th</sup> China TDS

以成年男子为代表，分析我国不同地区居民 AME 膳食暴露量，见附表 8-41 和图 8-22，从全国平均看，一般人群的 AME 膳食暴露量水平为 33.82 ng/(kg bw·d)。AME 的 TTC 值为 2.5 ng/(kg bw·d)。本次 AME 膳食暴露量约为 EFSA 制定的 TTC 值的 13.5 倍。健康风险需引起关注。

各食物类别对 AME 膳食暴露的贡献率见图 8-23，总体上，谷类是 AME 膳食暴露的最主要来源，占总暴露量的 94.0%；其他食物类别的贡献率均不超过 2%。

average levels in other food categories all being less than 0.3 μg/kg.

The dietary AME exposures of adult males in China by region are shown in Annexed Table 8-41 and Figure 8-22. The national average dietary exposure to AME was 33.82 ng/(kg bw·d). And the TTC value of AME was 2.5 ng/(kg bw·d) was adopted. The national average dietary exposure to AME was approximately 13.5 times the TTC value set by EFSA. The health risks should be paid more attention to.

The contributions of various food categories to the dietary AME exposure are shown in Figure 8-23. Overall, cereals were the primary source of dietary

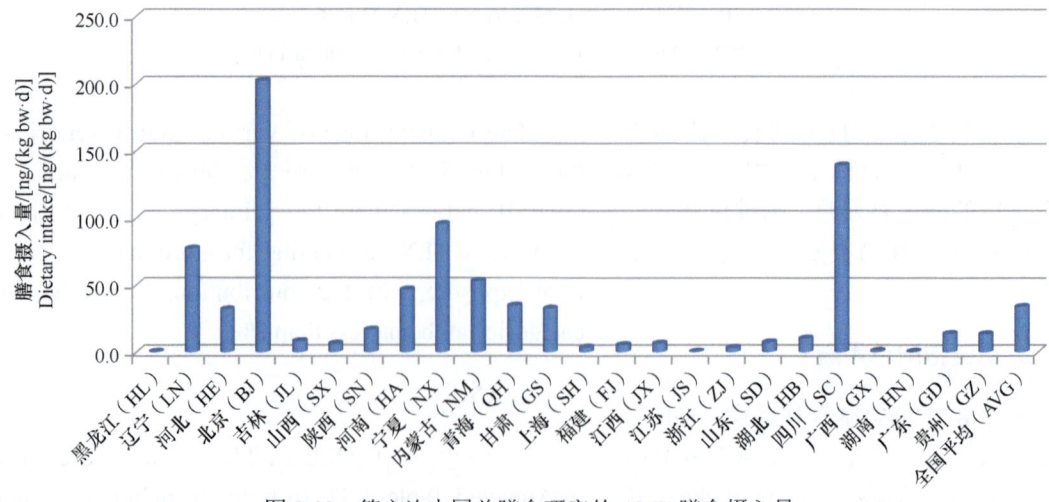

图 8-22　第六次中国总膳食研究的 AME 膳食摄入量
Figure 8-22　Dietary intake of AME from the 6<sup>th</sup> China TDS

exposure to AME, accounting for 94.0% of the total exposure, with the contributions from other food categories being all less than 2%.

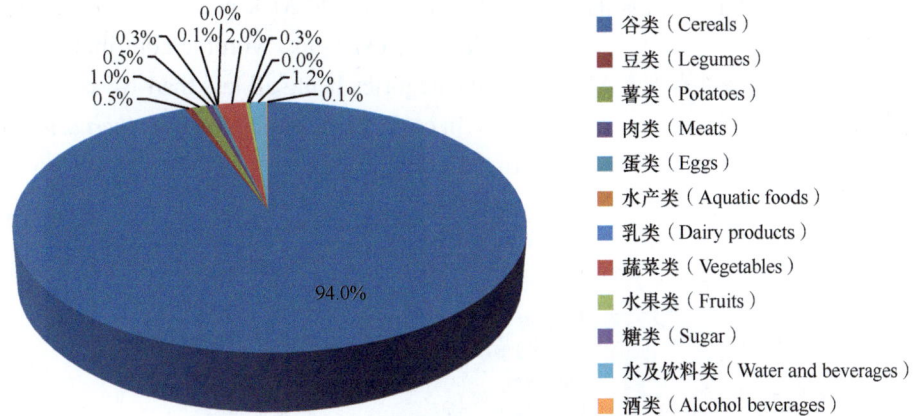

图 8-23 第六次中国总膳食研究 AME 的膳食来源
Figure 8-23 Dietary sources of AME from the 6$^{th}$ China TDS

#### 4. 交链孢烯

附表 8-38 为总膳食研究样品中 ALT 的含量，从全国平均看，12 类膳食样品中蔬菜类平均含量最高，为 1.01 μg/kg，谷类其次（0.68 μg/kg）。

以成年男子为代表，分析我国不同地区居民 ALT 的膳食暴露量，见附表 8-42 和图 8-24，从全国平均看，一般人群的 ALT 膳食暴露量水平为 16.7 ng/(kg bw·d)。

#### 4. ALT

The levels of ALT in TDS samples are shown in Annexed Table 8-38. In terms of national averages, vegetables had the highest level at 1.01 μg/kg, followed by cereals (0.68 μg/kg).

The dietary ALT exposures of adult males in China by region are shown in Annexed Table 8-42 and Figure 8-24. The national average dietary exposure to ALT was 16.7 ng/(kg bw·d).

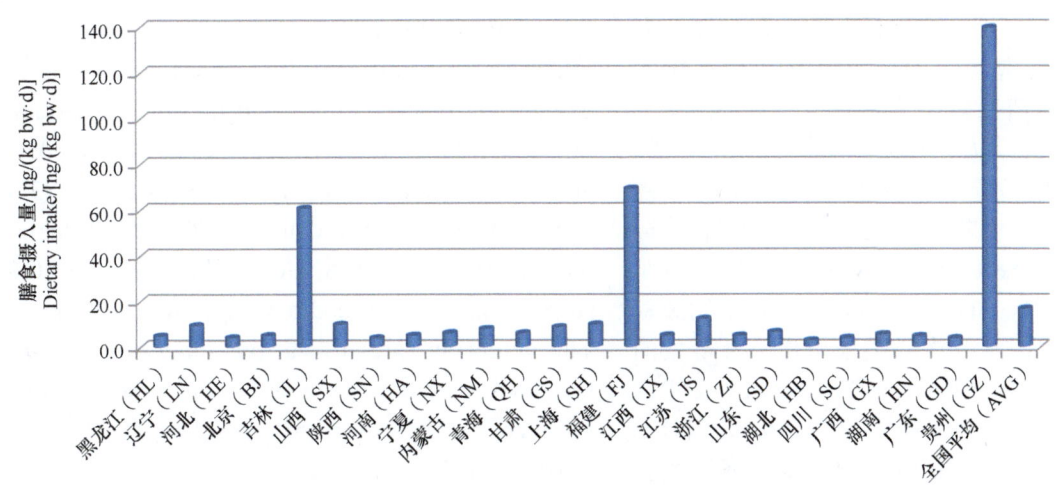

图 8-24 第六次中国总膳食研究的 ALT 膳食摄入量
Figure 8-24 Dietary intake of ALT from the 6$^{th}$ China TDS

各食物类别对 ALT 膳食暴露的贡献率见图 8-25，总体上，谷类、蔬菜类是 ALT 膳食暴露的主要来源，超过总暴露量的 80%，其他食物类别的贡献率均小于 10%。

综上，在 5 种交链孢毒素中，AME 的膳食暴露问题应引起关注。

The contributions of various food categories to the dietary ALT exposure are shown in Figure 8-25. Overall, cereals and vegetables were the primary sources of dietary exposure to ALT, accounting for more than 80% of the total exposure, with the contributions from other food categories being all less than 10%.

In conclusion, among the five *Alternaria* mycotoxins, the dietary exposure of AME should be paid more attention to.

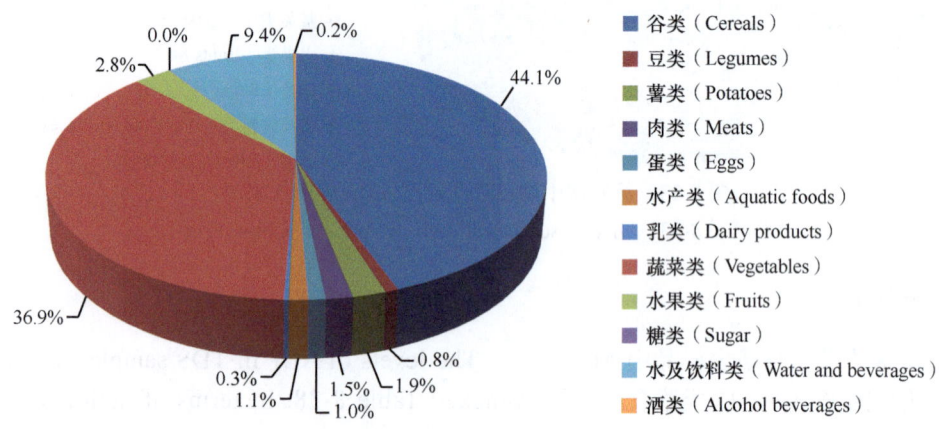

图 8-25　第六次中国总膳食研究 ALT 的膳食来源
Figure 8-25　Dietary sources of ALT from the 6th China TDS

## （八）新兴镰刀菌毒素

本次总膳食研究对 12 类 288 份混样进行了白僵菌素（BEA）、恩镰孢菌素 A（ENNA）、恩镰孢菌素 A1（ENNA1）、恩镰孢菌素 B（ENNB）和恩镰孢菌素 B1（ENNB1）5 种新兴镰刀菌毒素水平的测定。总检出率为 59.7%，从食品类别看，谷类、豆类、薯类、水产类、肉类、蛋类、乳类、蔬菜类、水果类、酒类、糖类的检出率分别为 95.8%、91.7%、87.5%、83.3%、83.3%、83.3%、70.8%、66.7%、25.0%、20.8%、8.3%，水及饮料类未检出。各毒素的检出率分别为：BEA（26.7%）、ENNA（13.5%）、ENNA1（11.1%）、ENNB（55.6%）、ENNB1（19.1%）。各毒素含量见附表 8-43～附表 8-47。

## (Ⅷ) Emerging *Fusarium* Mycotoxins

In the 6th China TDS, a total of 288 food samples in 12 categories were analyzed for the levels of BEA, ENNA, ENNA1, ENNB, and ENNB1. The total detection rate of emerging *Fusarium* mycotoxins was 59.7%, with significant differences among the food categories, where cereals had the highest detection rate at 95.8%, followed by legumes at 91.7%, potatoes at 87.5%, aquatic foods at 83.3%, meats at 83.3%, eggs at 83.3%, dairy products at 70.8%, vegetables at 66.7%, fruits at 25.0%, alcohol beverages at 20.8%, sugar at 8.3%, water and beverages were not detected. The detection rates of various emerging *Fusarium* mycotoxins are ordered in descending order as follows: BEA 26.7%, ENNA 13.5%, ENNA1 11.1%, ENNB 55.6%, ENNB1 19.1%. The levels of emerging *Fusarium* mycotoxins in TDS samples are shown in Annexed Table 8-43 to Annexed Table 8-47.

**1. 白僵菌素**

附表 8-43 为总膳食研究样品中 BEA 的含量，全国 12 类膳食样品中蛋类含量最高，为 1.22 μg/kg，谷类（0.88 μg/kg）、豆类（0.72 μg/kg）其次。

以成年男子为代表，分析我国不同地区居民 BEA 的膳食暴露量，见附表 8-48 和图 8-26，从全国平均看，一般人群的 BEA 膳食暴露量水平为 13.48 ng/(kg bw·d)。BEA 尚无健康指导值。

各食物类别对 BEA 膳食暴露的贡献率见图 8-27，总体上，谷类是 BEA 膳食暴露的主要来源，占总暴露量的

**1. BEA**

The levels of BEA in TDS samples are shown in Annexed Table 8-43. For food samples nationwide, eggs had a high level of BEA at 1.22 μg/kg, followed by cereals (0.88 μg/kg), legumes (0.72 μg/kg).

The dietary BEA exposures of adult males in China by region are shown in Annexed Table 8-48 and Figure 8-26. The national average dietary exposure to BEA was 13.48 ng/(kg bw·d). BEA has no HBGV.

The contributions of various food categories to the dietary BEA exposure are shown in Figure 8-27. Overall, cereals were the primary source of dietary exposure to BEA, accounting for 72.5% of the total exposure,

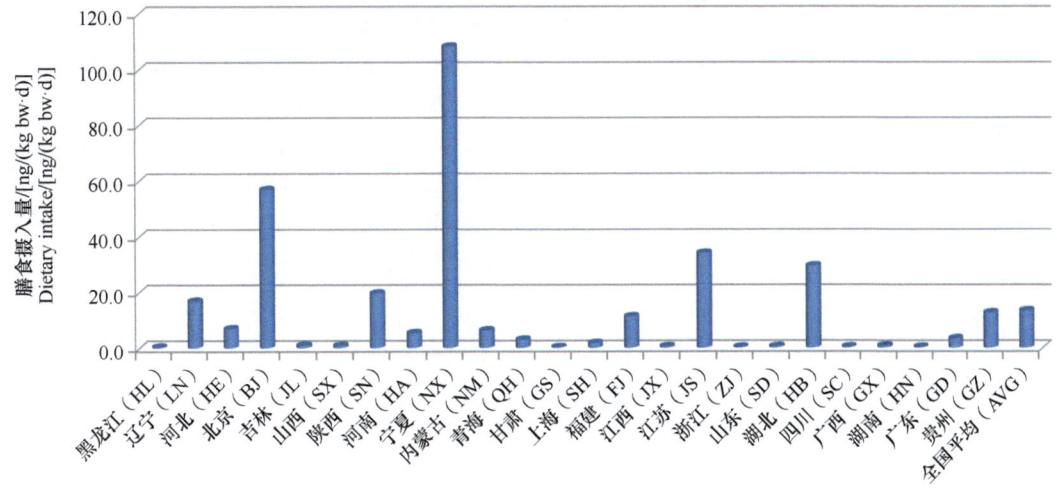

图 8-26 第六次中国总膳食研究的 BEA 膳食摄入量
Figure 8-26 Dietary intake of BEA from the 6$^{th}$ China TDS

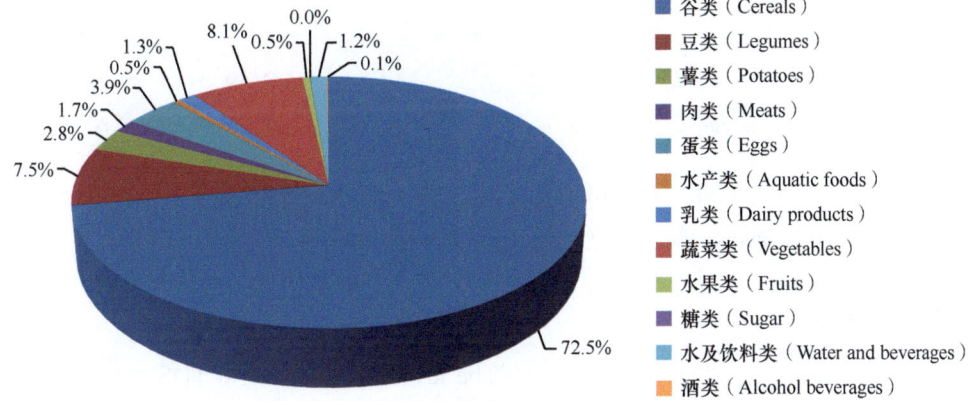

图 8-27 第六次中国总膳食研究 BEA 的膳食来源
Figure 8-27 Dietary sources of BEA from the 6$^{th}$ China TDS

72.5%；其次是蔬菜类 8.1%、豆类 7.5%，其他食物类别的贡献率均小于 5%。

### 2. 恩镰孢菌素 A

总膳食研究样品中 ENNA 的检出率为 14.6%，含量见附表 8-44，全国 12 类膳食样品中谷类平均含量最高，为 0.43 μg/kg，其次为蛋类 0.22 μg/kg，其他类别的含量均＜0.2 μg/kg。

以成年男子为代表，分析我国不同地区居民 ENNA 的膳食暴露量，见附表 8-49 和图 8-28，从全国平均看，一般人群的 ENNA 膳食暴露量水平为 5.534 ng/(kg bw·d)。ENNA 尚无健康指导值。

各食物类别对 ENNA 膳食暴露的贡献率见图 8-29，总体上，谷类是 ENNA 膳食暴露的主要来源，占总暴露量的 84.0%，其他食物类别的贡献率均小于 5%。

followed by vegetables (8.1%), legumes (7.5%), with the contributions from other food categories being all less than 5%.

### 2. ENNA

The levels of ENNA in TDS samples are shown in Annexed Table 8-44, and the detection rate was 14.6%. For food samples nationwide, cereals had a high level of ENNA at 0.43 μg/kg, followed by eggs (0.22 μg/kg), with the average levels in other food categories all being less than 0.2 μg/kg.

The dietary ENNA exposures of adult males in China by region are shown in Annexed Table 8-49 and Figure 8-28. The national average dietary exposure to ENNA was 5.534 ng/(kg bw·d). ENNA has no HBGV.

The contributions of various food categories to the dietary ENNA exposure are shown in Figure 8-29. Overall, cereals were the primary sources of dietary exposure to ENNA, accounting for 84.0% of the total exposure, with the contributions from other food categories all being less than 5%.

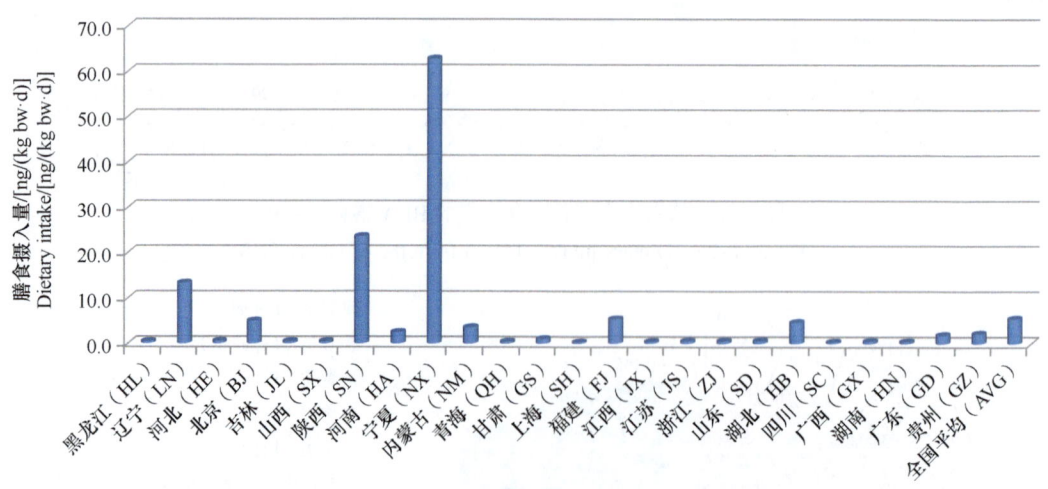

图 8-28　第六次中国总膳食研究的 ENNA 膳食摄入量
Figure 8-28　Dietary intake of ENNA from the 6th China TDS

### 3. 恩镰孢菌素 A1

附表 8-45 为总膳食研究样品中 ENNA1 的含量，全国 12 类膳食样品中谷类含量最高，为 0.46 μg/kg，其他类

### 3. ENNA1

The levels of ENNA1 in TDS samples are shown in Annexed Table 8-45. For food samples nationwide, cereals had a high level of ENNA1 at 0.46 μg/kg, with

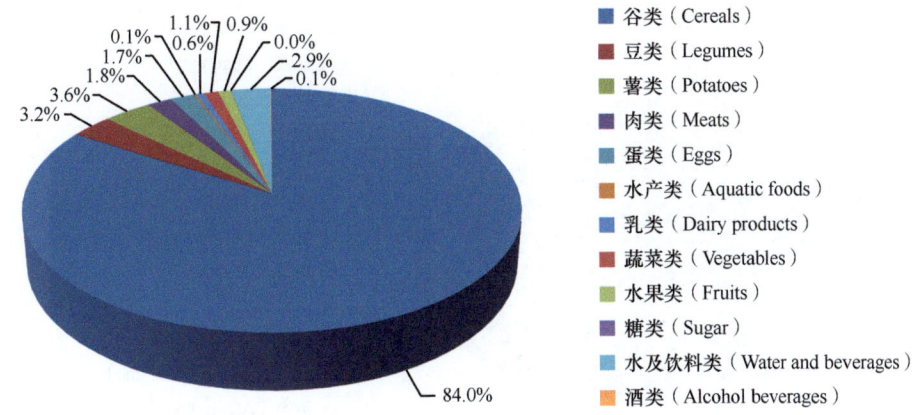

图 8-29　第六次中国总膳食研究 ENNA 的膳食来源

Figure 8-29　Dietary sources of ENNA from the 6$^{th}$ China TDS

别的含量均＜0.1 μg/kg。

以成年男子为代表,分析我国不同地区居民 ENNA1 的膳食暴露量,见附表 8-50 和图 8-30,从全国平均看,一般人群的 ENNA1 膳食暴露量水平为 5.741 ng/(kg bw·d)。ENNA1 尚无健康指导值。

各食物类别对 ENNA1 膳食暴露的贡献率见图 8-31,总体上,谷类是 ENNA1 膳食暴露的主要来源,超过总暴露量的 92%;其他食物类别的贡献率均小于 5%。

the average levels in other food categories all being less than 0.1 μg/kg.

The dietary ENNA1 exposures of adult males in China by region are shown in Annexed Table 8-50 and Figure 8-30. The national average dietary exposure to ENNA1 in general population was 5.741 ng/(kg bw·d). ENNA1 has no HBGV.

The contributions of various food categories to the dietary ENNA1 exposure are shown in Figure 8-31. Overall, cereals were the primary source of dietary exposure to ENNA1, accounting for more than 92% of the total exposure, with the contributions from other food categories all being less than 5%.

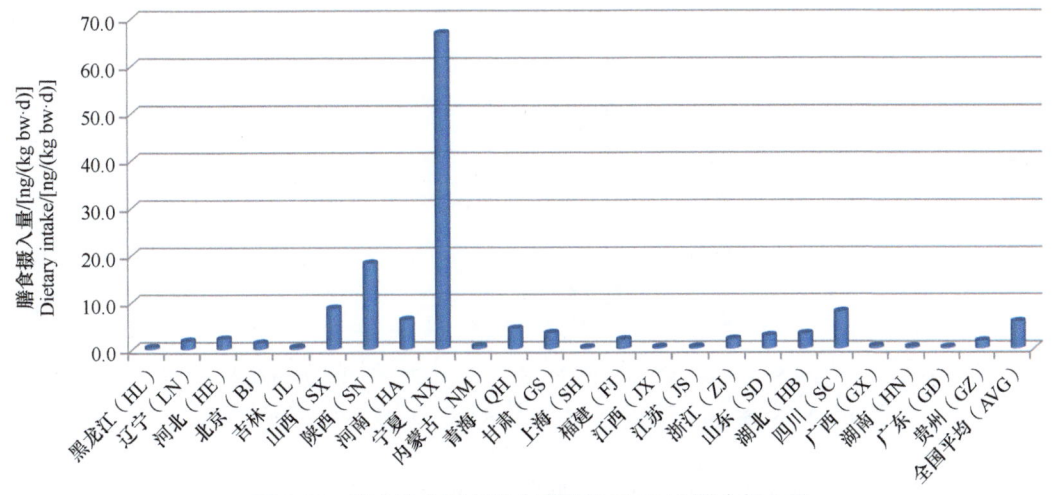

图 8-30　第六次中国总膳食研究的 ENNA1 膳食摄入量

Figure 8-30　Dietary intake of ENNA1 from the 6$^{th}$ China TDS

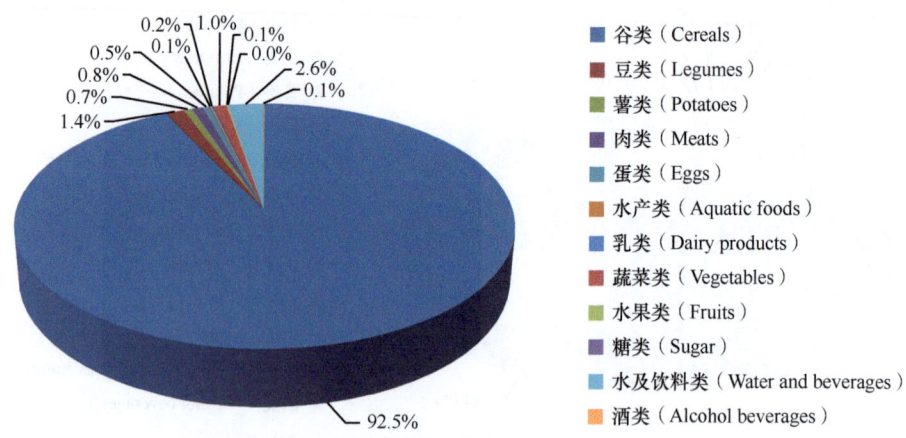

图 8-31　第六次中国总膳食研究 ENNA1 的膳食来源
Figure 8-31　Dietary sources of ENNA1 from the 6$^{th}$ China TDS

#### 4. 恩镰孢菌素 B

附表 8-46 为总膳食研究样品中 ENNB 的含量，全国 12 类膳食样品中谷类平均含量最高，为 4.006 μg/kg，其他类别的平均含量均 <1 μg/kg，水及饮料类样品中未检出。

以成年男子为代表，分析我国不同地区居民 ENNB 的膳食暴露量，见附表 8-51 和图 8-32，从全国平均看，一般人群的 ENNB 膳食暴露量水平为 50.75 ng/(kg bw·d)。ENNB 尚无健康指导值。

#### 4. ENNB

The levels of ENNB in TDS samples are shown in Annexed Table 8-46. For food samples nationwide, cereals had a high level of ENNB at 4.006 μg/kg, with the average levels in other food categories all being less than 1 μg/kg, water and beverages were not detected.

The dietary ENNB exposures of adult males in China by region are shown in Annexed Table 8-51 and Figure 8-32. The national average dietary exposure to ENNB in general population was 50.75 ng/(kg bw·d). ENNB has no HBGV.

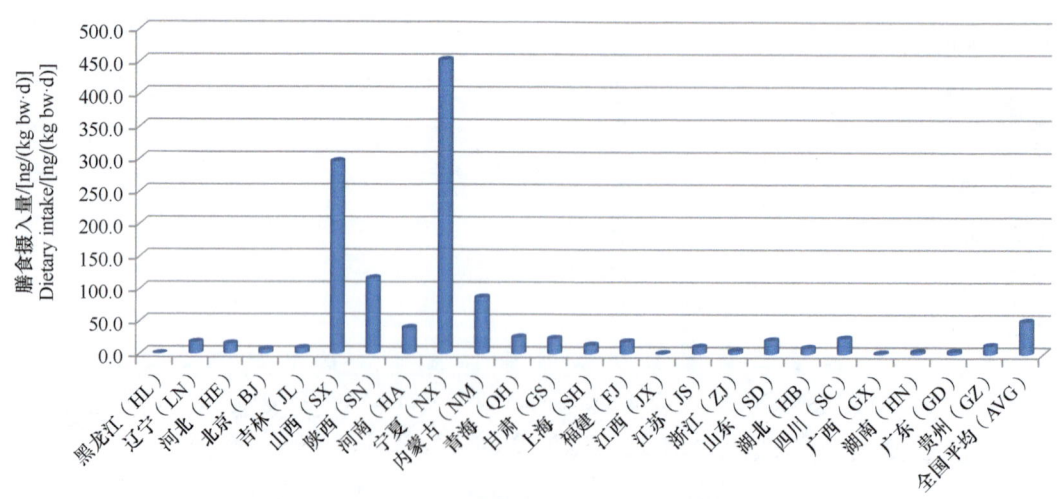

图 8-32　第六次中国总膳食研究的 ENNB 膳食摄入量
Figure 8-32　Dietary intake of ENNB from the 6$^{th}$ China TDS

各食物类别对 ENNB 膳食暴露的贡献率见图 8-33，总体上，谷类是 ENNB 膳食暴露的主要来源，超过总暴露量的 95%；其他食物类别的贡献率均小于 2%。

The contributions of various food categories to the dietary ENNB exposure are shown in Figure 8-33. Overall, cereals were the primary sources of dietary exposure to ENNB, accounting for more than 95% of the total exposure, with the contributions from other food categories all being less than 2%.

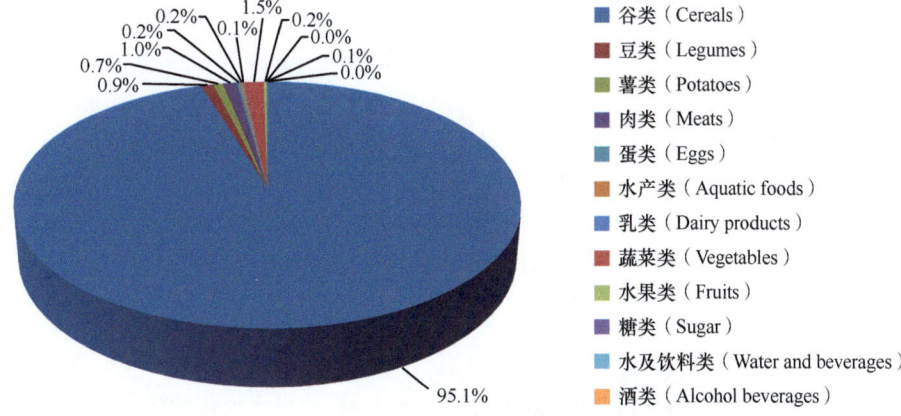

图 8-33　第六次中国总膳食研究 ENNB 的膳食来源
Figure 8-33　Dietary sources of ENNB from the 6th China TDS

**5. 恩镰孢菌素 B1**

附表 8-47 为总膳食研究样品中 ENNB1 的含量，全国 12 类膳食样品中谷类含量最高，为 1.26 μg/kg，其他类别的含量均＜0.2 μg/kg。

以成年男子为代表，分析我国不同地区居民 ENNB1 的膳食暴露量，见附表 8-52 和图 8-34，从全国平均看，一般人群的 ENNB1 膳食暴露量水平为 15.63 ng/(kg bw·d)。ENNB1 尚无健康指导值。

各食物类别对 ENNB1 膳食暴露的贡献率见图 8-35，总体上，谷类是 ENNB1 膳食暴露的主要来源，约占总暴露量的 95%；其他食物类别的贡献率均小于 2%。

BEA 与 ENN 暂无相关健康指导值。新兴镰刀菌毒素的检出率较高，其在谷类中的污染应引起关注。ENN 主要存在于北方区，特别是北方二区。

**5. ENNB1**

The levels of ENNB1 in TDS samples are shown in Annexed Table 8-47. For food samples nationwide, cereals had a high level of ENNB1 at 1.26 μg/kg, with the average levels in other food categories all being less than 0.2 μg/kg.

The dietary ENNB1 exposures of adult males in China by region are shown in Annexed Table 8-54 and Figure 8-34. The national average dietary exposure to ENNB1 was 15.63 ng/(kg bw·d). ENNB1 has no HBGV.

The contributions of various food categories to the dietary ENNB1 exposure are shown in Figure 8-35. Overall, cereals were the primary sources of dietary exposure to ENNB, accounting for 95% of the total exposure, with the contributions from other food categories all being less than 2%.

BEA and ENNs have no relevant health-based guidance values. The detection rate of emerging *Fusarium* mycotoxins were high, and the pollution in

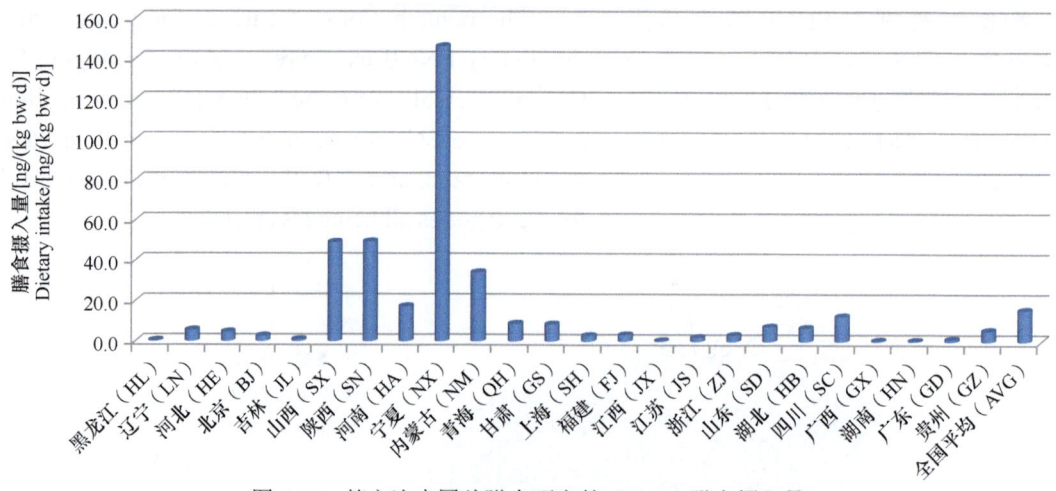

图 8-34 第六次中国总膳食研究的 ENNB1 膳食摄入量
Figure 8-34 Dietary intake of ENNB1 from the 6th China TDS

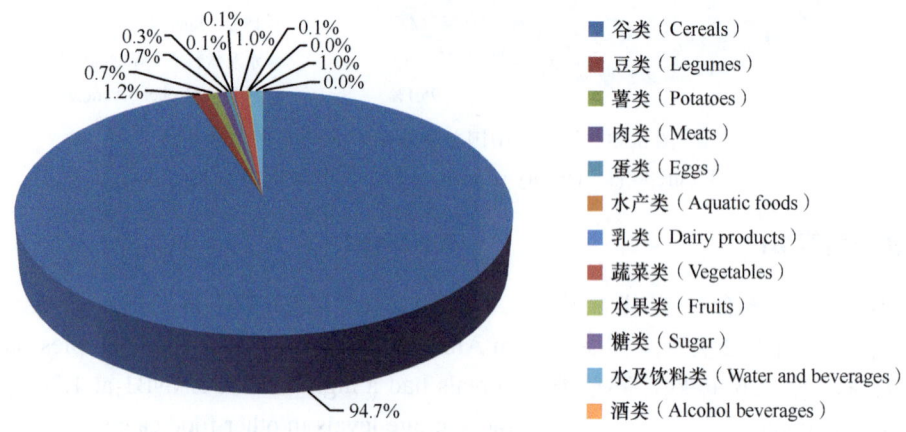

图 8-35 第六次中国总膳食研究 ENNB1 的膳食来源
Figure 8-35 Dietary sources of ENNB1 from the 6th China TDS

## （九）其他真菌毒素

除上述几类主要真菌毒素外，本次总膳食研究对12类食品进行了串珠镰刀菌素（MON）、桔青霉素（CIT）、霉酚酸（CPA）、杂色曲霉毒素（SMC）4种真菌毒素的含量测定，MON、CIT、CPA 在所有种类食品中均未检出，SMC 检出率较高，为27.1%。从食品类别看，谷类中 SMC 检出率较高（62.5%），其次依次为薯类54.2%、肉类45.8%、蔬菜类45.8%、豆类41.7%、蛋类41.7%、水产类29.2%、糖类4.2%；乳类、水果

cereals should be paid attention to. ENNs mainly existed in the northern region, especially the northern region Ⅱ.

### (IX) Other Mycotoxins

In addition to the several groups of mycotoxins mentioned above, this TDS also analyzed the 12 food categories for the levels of 4 other mycotoxins, including MON, CIT, CPA, SMC, MON, CIT, and CPA were not detected in samples collected in this study, and the detection rate of SMC was 27.1%.

In terms of food categories, cereals had the highest detection rate of SMC (62.5%), followed by potatoes at 54.2%, meats at 45.8%, vegetables at 45.8%, legumes at

类、水及饮料类、酒类中 SMC 未检出。

附表 8-53 为总膳食样品中 SMC 的含量，豆类最高，为 0.218 μg/kg，其他 11 类样品中的含量均小于 0.1 μg/kg。

以成年男子为代表，分析我国不同地区居民 SMC 的膳食暴露量，见附表 8-54 和图 8-36，从全国平均看，一般人群的 SMC 平均暴露水平为 1.127 ng/(kg bw·d)。SMC 目前尚无健康指导值。

各食品类别对 SMC 膳食暴露的贡献率见图 8-37，总体上，由于消费量的差异，谷类、豆类、蔬菜类是 SMC 膳食暴露最主要的潜在来源，接近总量的 85%；其次为肉类（5.8%）和薯类

41.7%, eggs at 41.7%, aquatic foods at 29.2%, sugar at 4.2%. Dairy products, fruits, alcohol and beverages, water and beverages were not detected in any food categories.

The levels of SMC in TDS samples are shown in Annexed Table 8-53, legumes had a high level of SMC at 0.218 μg/kg, with the average levels in other food categories all being less than 0.1 μg/kg.

The dietary SMC exposures of adult males in China by region are shown in Annexed Table 8-54 and Figure 8-36. The national average dietary exposure to SMC was 1.127 ng/(kg bw·d). SMC has no HBGV.

The contributions of various food categories to the dietary SMC exposure are shown in Figure 8-37. Overall, due to the difference in food consumptions,

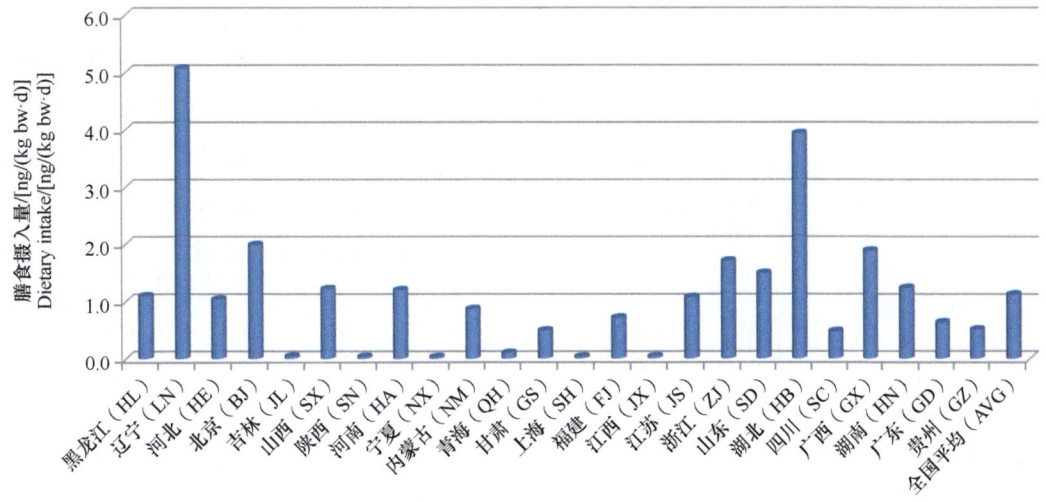

图 8-36　第六次中国总膳食研究的 SMC 膳食摄入量

Figure 8-36　Dietary intake of SMC from the 6th China TDS

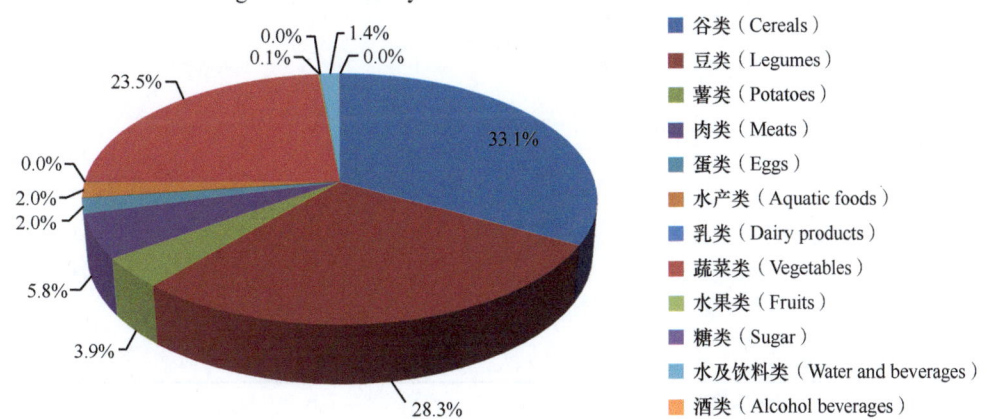

图 8-37　第六次中国总膳食研究 SMC 的膳食来源

Figure 8-37　Dietary sources of SMC from the 6th China TDS

（3.9%）；其他食物类别的贡献率均不超过2%。

## 四、与以往中国总膳食研究结果的比较

第四次和第五次中国总膳食研究共检测了38种真菌毒素，而第六次总膳食研究共检测了43种真菌毒素。第六次中国总膳食研究剔除了5种检出率和污染水平均很低且无明确健康指导值的次要毒素。同时参考JECFA及EFSA近期评估报告，第六次中国总膳食研究增加了5种交链孢毒素和5种新兴镰孢菌毒素。主要毒素历次膳食摄入量比较见表8-1。

cereals, legumes, and vegetables were the primary sources of dietary exposure to SMC, accounting for 85% of the total exposure, followed by meats (5.8%) and potatoes (3.9%), with the contributions from other food categories being all less than 2%.

## IV. Comparison with Previous China TDSs Results

A total of 38 mycotoxins were analyzed in the 4th and 5th China TDSs, while 43 mycotoxins were analyzed in the 6th China TDS. The 6th China TDS eliminated 5 minor mycotoxins with low detection rates and levels without health-based guidance value. With reference to recent reports from JECFA and EFSA, five *Alternaria* mycotoxins and 5 emerging *Fusarium* mycotoxins were added to the 6th CTDS. The comparison of the results of dirtary exposure in China TDSs is shown in Table 8-1.

表 8-1　三次中国总膳食研究真菌毒素的膳食摄入情况比较
Table 8-1　Mycotoxin dietary intakes from 4th, 5th and 6th China TDSs

| 真菌毒素 Mycotoxins | 膳食摄入 Dietary intakes/[ng/(kg bw · d)] |||
|---|---|---|---|
| | 第四次中国总膳食研究 4th CTDS | 第五次中国总膳食研究 5th CTDS | 第六次中国总膳食研究 6th CTDS |
| 黄曲霉毒素 | 22.3 | 9.53 | 2.55 |
| T-2 和 HT-2 | 70 | 52.2 | 3.11 |
| DON、3-Ac-DON 和 15-Ac-DON | 217 | 434 | 690 |
| NIV | 16 | 43.2 | 9.17 |
| OTA | 5.3 | 0.58 | 0.88 |
| ZEN | 15.4 | 21.7 | 7.77 |
| 伏马菌素 | 199 | 54.9 | 104 |
| 展青霉素 | 3.8 | * | * |
| 交链孢菌酮酸 | — | — | 141 |
| 腾毒素 | — | — | 143 |
| 交链孢酚单甲醚 | — | — | 33.8 |
| 交链孢酚 | — | — | * |
| 交链孢烯 | — | — | 16.7 |
| 恩镰孢菌素 | — | — | 77.7 |

注："—"表示未检测；"*"表示未检出
Note: "—" indicates that this work was not carried out; "*" indicates that these mycotoxins was not detected

黄曲霉毒素的膳食摄入量在近三次中国总膳食研究中呈明显下降趋势。T-2 和 HT-2 毒素的膳食摄入量在第六次 CTDS 中显著降低，主要原因是检测技术的改进导致 T-2 和 HT-2 检测灵敏度的提高；第六次 CTDS 中 T-2 和 HT-2 的检出限分别为 0.04 μg/kg 和 0.08 μg/kg，T-2 和 HT-2 检出限的显著降低，使根据 1/2 LOD 代替未检出值计算的膳食摄入量也显著降低，能够较真实地反映暴露情况。DON 及其衍生物的膳食摄入量有逐渐上升的趋势，该类毒素的污染日趋严重，应着重关注，谷类一直是该类毒素最主要的食物来源，占 90% 以上。OTA 的膳食摄入量在第五次和第六次 CTDS 显著下降。NIV、ZEN、伏马菌素的膳食摄入量无明显变化趋势，且总体水平较低，均不到健康指导值的 10%，风险很低。

The dietary intakes of aflatoxin showed a significant downward trend during the three China TDSs. The dietary intakes of T-2 and HT-2 toxins decreased significantly in the sixth CTDS. The main reason is that the improvement of detection technology lead to the improvement of the detection sensitivity of T-2 and HT-2, with the limits of detection to 0.04 μg/kg and 0.08 μg/kg, respectively. As a result, calculating wih these much lower 1/2 LODs to replace the not detected value, the result in a significantly lower dietary intakes of T-2 and HT-2 in the $6^{th}$ CTDS, which more accurately reflect the true exposure level. The intake of DON and its derivatives is gradually increasing, and this should be given more attention. Cereals are the primary sources of dietary exposure to DON and its derivatives, accounting for more than 90% of the total. The dietary exposure of OTA decreased significantly in $5^{th}$ and $6^{th}$ China TDSs. Moreover, the dietary exposures to NIV, ZEN, and fumonisins showed no significant change, with low levels of less than 10% of their individual health-based guidance values, indicating their low health risks to China residents.

# 第九章　其他化合物的膳食暴露评估
# Chapter 9　Dietary Exposure Assessment of Other Compounds

## 第一节　高氯酸盐
## Section 1　Perchlorate

### 一、背景

高氯酸根离子（$ClO_4^-$）中的氯原子被4个氧原子包围，呈现四面体结构，其物理化学性质极其稳定，水溶性高，可在自然水系中持续迁移。高氯酸盐通常是以 $NH_4ClO_4$、$KClO_4$、$NaClO_4$ 的形式存在。高氯酸盐用作强氧化剂，用于火箭推进剂、烟火制作、军火工业、爆破作业等领域，以及将其作为添加剂的润滑油、织物固定剂、电镀液、皮革鞣剂、橡胶制品、染料涂料、冶炼铝和镁电池等产品的生产过程。环境中的高氯酸盐除自然来源外（主要产生于一些肥料和草木灰中），主要来自人为污染。

目前，高氯酸盐对人体健康的影响主要集中在对甲状腺功能的作用。研究显示，高氯酸盐可干扰甲状腺中碘化物的运输系统。由于高氯酸盐与碘的结构形状非常相似，高氯酸盐可通过与碘离子竞争转运蛋白而抑制碘的吸收，削弱甲状腺的功能，干扰甲状腺素的合成和分泌，从而影响人体正常的新陈代谢和生长、发育，对儿童、孕妇、胎儿和新生儿的影响尤为严重。有研究认为，一旦婴幼儿体内的高氯酸盐过量，儿童期会出现智商偏低、学习障碍、发育迟缓、多动症（ADHD）、注意力分散甚至智力低下等症状。此外，过量的高氯酸盐

### I. Background

The chlorine atom in perchlorate ion ($ClO_4^-$) is surrounded by four oxygen atoms, showing a tetrahedral structure. Perchlorate has extremely physicochemical stability and high water solubility, resulting in continuous migration in natural water systems. Perchlorate usually exists in the form of $NH_4ClO_4$, $KClO_4$, and $NaClO_4$. Perchlorate is used as a strong oxidant in the fields of rocket propellant, pyrotechnics, arms industry, and blasting operation, as well as the production process of lubricating oil, fabric fixing agent, electroplating solution, leather tanning agent, rubber products, dye coatings, smelting aluminum and magnesium batteries. Perchlorate in the environment mainly comes from artificial pollution in addition to natural sources (mainly from some fertilizers and plant ash).

At present, studies of perchlorate on human health mainly focus on the effect on the thyroid function. Studies show that perchlorate can interfere with the transport system of iodide in the thyroid. Due to the similar structure shape between perchlorate and iodine, perchlorate can inhibit the absorption of iodine by competing with iodine ion transporter, weaken thyroid function, and interfere with the synthesis and secretion of thyroxine, thus affecting the normal metabolism and growth and development of human body, especially for children, pregnant women, fetuses, and newborns. Some studies report that once the perchlorate intake in

造成甲状腺激素分泌不足，影响血红蛋白的生成，进而影响心肺功能和骨骼发育，甚至影响听觉功能与免疫力维持。

固态的高氯酸盐可以以粉尘的形式通过呼吸系统、皮肤接触进入人和动物体内，而溶解于水中的高氯酸盐会通过饮水和食物经消化道进入人体，后者是人体暴露于高氯酸盐的主要途径。高氯酸盐对婴儿的暴露途径主要是通过母乳暴露，还可通过胎盘和脐带血作用于胎儿，也就是胚胎暴露。

## 二、健康指导值

美国国家科学院（NAS）基于 Greer 等（2002）的研究确定的无可见作用水平（NOEL），提出包括婴幼儿及孕妇等敏感人群在内的高氯酸盐摄入的每日参考剂量（RfD）为 0.7 μg/(kg bw·d)。联合国粮食及农业组织（FAO）/世界卫生组织（WHO）食品添加剂联合专家委员会（JECFA）由剂量-反应分析获得的暂定每日最大耐受摄入量（PMTDI）为 10 μg/(kg bw·d)。EFSA 基于 Greer 等（2002）的研究制定的每日可耐受摄入量（TDI）为 0.3 μg/(kg bw·d)。

## 三、总膳食研究结果

对 24 个省（自治区、直辖市）的 288 份混合膳食样品中高氯酸盐的含量进行了测定。对未检出的样品，以 1/2 LOD 值进行污染水平评价和膳食暴露评估（12 类膳食样品的 LOD 值均为 0.2 μg/kg）。

infants is excessive, children will have low IQ, learning disabilities, growth retardation, ADHD, distraction, and even mental retardation. In addition, excessive perchlorate intake causes insufficient thyroid hormone secretion, which affects hemoglobin production, lung and heart function, bone development, maintenance of immunity and function of auditory organs.

Solid form of perchlorate can enter human and animal bodies in the form of dust from respiratory system and skin contact, while perchlorate dissolved in water will enter human body through drinking water and food through the digestive tract. The latter is the main pathway of human exposure to perchlorate. The exposure pathway of perchlorate to infants is mainly through breast milk exposure, and can also act on the fetus through placenta and umbilical cord blood, that is, embryo exposure.

## II. HBGV

Based on the NOEL value determined by Greer et al. (2002), the National Academy of Sciences (NAS) of USA proposed that the daily reference dose (RfD) of perchlorate intake was 0.7 μg/(kg bw·d), including sensitive populations, such as pregnant women and infants. The PMTDI obtained by the Joint FAO/WHO Expert Committee on Food Additives (JECFA) from the dose-response analysis was 10 μg/(kg bw·d). Based on Greer et al. (2002), EFSA established a tolerable daily intake (TDI) of 0.3 μg/(kg bw·d).

## III. TDS Results

The concentration of perchlorate in 288 composite dietary samples from 24 provinces (autonomous regions, municipalities) was determined. For the undetected samples, the contamination level and dietary exposure were evaluated with half of the LOD value (the LOD value of 12 dietary samples was 0.2 μg/kg).

**1. 混合膳食样品中高氯酸盐的含量**

第六次中国总膳食研究的混合样品中高氯酸盐的污染水平为 ND～128.88 μg/kg，检出率为 94.8%；各类膳食的平均污染水平为 1.67～34.92 μg/kg（附表 9-1）。在各类膳食中，污染水平的排序为：蔬菜类（34.92 μg/kg）、蛋类（14.09 μg/kg）、薯类（9.65 μg/kg）、豆类（8.14 μg/kg）等，糖类最低（1.67 μg/kg）。

**2. 膳食暴露评估**

我国居民高氯酸盐的平均膳食摄入量为 0.449 μg/(kg bw·d)（附表 9-2），占 NAS 设定的健康指导值 [0.7 μg/(kg bw·d)] 的 64.1%，占 JECFA 的健康指导值 [10 μg/(kg bw·d)] 的 4.5%，占 EFSA 的健康指导值 [0.3 μg/(kg bw·d)] 的 149.7%。我国各地区居民的高氯酸盐膳食摄入量为 0.082～1.449 μg/(kg bw·d)（图 9-1），其中，吉林省平均膳食摄入量为 1.449 μg/(kg bw·d)，贵州省为 1.063 μg/(kg bw·d)、湖南省为 0.865 μg/(kg bw·d)、江西省为 0.857 μg/(kg bw·d)、湖北省为 0.759 μg/(kg bw·d)，这些省份的膳食摄入量虽未超

## 1. Levels of Perchlorate in TDS Composite Samples

In the 6$^{th}$ CTDS, the contamination levels of perchlorate in dietary samples were in the range of ND-128.88 μg/kg. The detection rate of perchlorate was 94.8%. The average contamination level of various dietary samples was 1.67-34.92 μg/kg (Annexed Table 9-1). Among all kinds of dietary samples, the order of contamination level was vegetables (34.92 μg/kg), eggs (14.09 μg/kg), potatoes (9.65 μg/kg), legumes (8.14 μg/kg), and the lowest sugar (1.67 μg/kg).

## 2. Dietary Exposure Assessment

The average dietary intake of perchlorate for China residents was 0.449 μg/(kg bw·d) (Annexed Table 9-2), accounting for 64.1% of the HBGV [0.7 μg/(kg bw·d)] set by NAS, 4.5% of the HBGV [10 μg/(kg bw·d)] set by JECFA, and 149.7% of the HBGV [0.3 μg/(kg bw·d)] set by EFSA. The dietary intake of perchlorate of residents in various regions of China ranged from 0.082 μg/(kg bw·d) to 1.449 μg/(kg bw·d) (Figure 9-1). Among them, the average dietary intake of Jilin was the highest [1.449 μg/(kg bw·d)], followed by Guizhou [1.063 μg/(kg bw·d)], Hunan [0.865 μg/(kg bw·d)], Jiangxi [0.857 μg/(kg bw·d)], and Hubei [0.759 μg/(kg bw·d)]. Although the dietary intake of

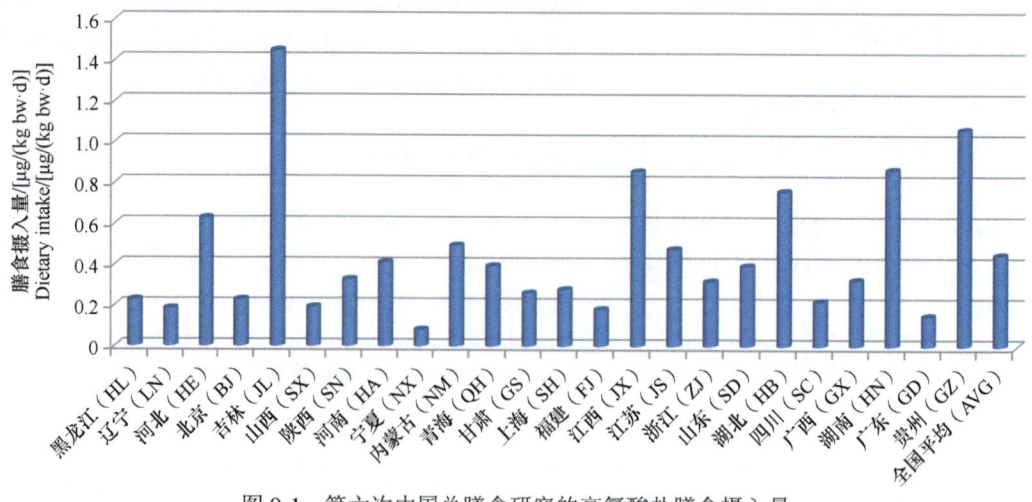

图 9-1 第六次中国总膳食研究的高氯酸盐膳食摄入量

Figure 9-1　Dietary intake of perchlorate from the 6$^{th}$ China TDS

过 JECFA 制定的 PMTDI，但均已超过 NAS 设定的 RfD 和 EFSA 制定的 TDI。此外，我国人均每日摄入量低于 RfD 和 PMTDI，但超过了 TDI，因此，为及时应对可能发生的健康风险，我国应制定相应的管理和控制措施。

**3. 各类膳食对总膳食摄入的贡献**

第六次中国总膳食研究的膳食高氯酸盐主要来源于蔬菜类（45.9%）、水及饮料类（25.7%）、谷类（18.6%），占总摄入量的 90.2%，其余 9 类膳食样品的贡献率均小于 3%（附表 9-3，图 9-2）。

perchlorate in these provinces have not exceeded the PMTDI set by JECFA, they have exceeded the RfD set by NAS and the TDI set by EFSA. In addition, Chinese average daily intake was lower than RfD and PMTDI, but higher than TDI. Therefore, China should formulate corresponding management and control measures to deal with the possible health risk.

**3. Contributions of Food Categories to the Total Dietary Intake**

The primary sources of dietary intake to the perchlorate in the 6$^{th}$ China TDS were vegetables (45.9%), water and beverages (25.7%), and cereals (18.6%), accounting for 90.2% of the total intake. The contribution of the other dietary samples was less than 3% (Annexed Table 9-3, Figure 9-2).

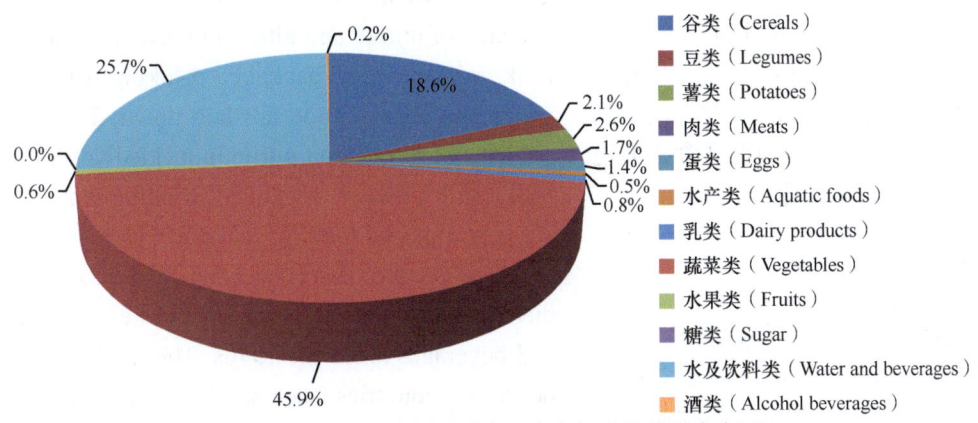

图 9-2　第六次中国总膳食研究高氯酸盐的膳食来源

Figure 9-2　Dietary sources of perchlorate from the 6$^{th}$ China TDS

## 第二节　硝酸盐与亚硝酸盐
## Section 2　Nitrate and Nitrite

### 一、背景

硝酸盐和亚硝酸盐在环境中普遍存在，由枯死腐败的植物和动物的有机残留物在固氮过程中产生。硝酸盐在现代农业中被用作肥料以代替传统的动物粪便；硝酸盐和亚硝酸盐也经常在食

### Ⅰ. Background

Nitrate and nitrite are ions naturally occurring in the environment, resulting from nitrogen fixation of dead and decaying plant and animal matter. Nitrate is used in agriculture as a fertilizer to replace the traditional use of livestock manure; nitrate and nitrite are also commonly

品加工过程中被用作肉类与鱼类的抗菌剂、保存剂及发色剂。人体主要通过膳食摄入硝酸盐，WHO 的数据表明，硝酸盐的主要膳食来源为蔬菜类，其贡献率可高达 90% 以上；亚硝酸盐的暴露则主要来源于硝酸盐的内源性转换。

硝酸盐对人体毒性低，但亚硝酸盐可引发高铁血红蛋白症。鉴于硝酸盐和亚硝酸盐的膳食暴露可能对人造成的健康危害，欧盟对某些叶菜中的硝酸盐含量设定了限量值；中国、美国与欧盟分别对饮用水中的硝酸盐和亚硝酸盐设定了限量。我国现行《食品安全国家标准 食品中污染物限量》（GB 2762—2022）规定了腌渍蔬菜、生乳、乳粉、包装饮用水、矿泉水及特殊膳食用食品中的硝酸盐与亚硝酸盐的限量。

英国从 20 世纪 70 年代开始对食品和饮料中的硝酸盐及亚硝酸盐含量开展持续的调查与膳食评估。芬兰、澳大利亚等发达国家随后开展的总膳食研究也都包含了硝酸盐与亚硝酸盐。

## 二、健康指导值

联合国粮食及农业组织和世界卫生组织食品添加剂联合专家委员会（JECFA）于 1961 年首次对硝酸盐与亚硝酸盐的暴露风险进行了评估。欧盟食品科学委员会（SCF）于 1990 年评估了硝酸盐和亚硝酸盐的毒性作用，并将硝酸盐的 ADI 值上限设定为 3700 μg/(kg bw·d)，1995 年的评估保留了此值，并由此推导出亚硝酸盐的 ADI 为 60 μg/(kg bw·d)。JECFA 于 2002 年完成的评估再次肯定了硝酸盐的 ADI 为 3700 μg/(kg bw·d)，并设定亚硝酸盐的 ADI 为 70 μg/(kg bw·d)。

used in food processing as antibiotics, preservatives, and colorants for meats and fish. People's exposure to nitrate is mainly through diet. The largest source of dietary intake for nitrate is vegetables. According to the data from WHO, vegetables contribute up to over 90% of the average dietary intake for nitrate around the world. People's exposure to nitrite is primarily through endogenous conversion from nitrate.

Nitrate itself is a low-toxic compound, while nitrite is associated with methemoglobinemia. Considering adverse health implications for humans, resulting from dietary exposure to nitrate and nitrite, EU established regulatory limits for nitrates in some leafy vegetables; China, US and EU set standards on the nitrate and nitrite contents in drinking water. *National Food Safety Standard Contaminant Limits in Foods* (GB 2762—2022) was established in China, in which the maximum contents of nitrate and nitrite in pickled vegetables, raw milk, milk powder, packaged drinking water, mineral water and special food are laid down. The maximum contents of nitrate and nitrite in pickled vegetables, raw milk, milk powder, packaged drinking water, mineral water and special food are laid down in this standard.

The UK has been conducting continuous surveys and dietary assessments of nitrate and nitrite contents in food and beverages since the 1970s. The TDS conducted by developed countries, such as Finland and Australia, also surveyed nitrate and nitrite.

## II. HBGV

The Joint FAO/WHO Expert Committee on Food Additives (JECFA) conducted the first international evaluation of the risks associated with the exposure of nitrate and nitrite in 1961. The Scientific Committee for Food (SCF) of the EU reviewed the toxicological effects of nitrate and nitrite and established an ADI as 3700 μg/(kg bw·d) for nitrate in 1990, retained the ADI in 1995 and derived an ADI as 60 μg/(kg bw·d) for nitrite. The JECFA completed its most recent review in 2002 and reconfirmed an ADI as 3700 μg/(kg bw·d) for nitrate and set an ADI as 70 μg/(kg bw·d) for nitrite.

## 三、总膳食研究结果

对24个省（自治区、直辖市）的288份混合膳食样品中硝酸盐和亚硝酸盐的含量进行了测定。对未检出的样品，以1/2 LOD值进行污染水平评价和膳食暴露评估。

### （一）混合膳食样品中硝酸盐和亚硝酸盐的含量

#### 1. 硝酸盐

硝酸盐在12类膳食样品中均有检出（附表9-4）。平均含量较高的膳食样品为蔬菜类（992 mg/kg）、薯类（73 mg/kg）和乳类（52 mg/kg），含量较低的样品为蛋类（2.7 mg/kg）、肉类（4.1 mg/kg）和酒类（4.9 mg/kg）。水及饮料类样品的平均硝酸盐含量为9.2 mg/kg。

#### 2. 亚硝酸盐

亚硝酸盐检出率较高的膳食样品为糖类（58%）和水及饮料类（21%）。平均含量水平较高的膳食样品为糖类（1.15 mg/kg）、水产类（0.16 mg/kg）和水果类（0.16 mg/kg）（附表9-5）。

### （二）膳食暴露评估

#### 1. 硝酸盐

我国居民硝酸盐的平均膳食摄入量为6071 μg/(kg bw·d)，范围为1878～17 371 μg/(kg bw·d)（附表9-6）。按照JECFA制定的ADI[3700 μg/(kg bw·d)]进行评估，我国居民的硝酸盐膳食摄入量相当于ADI的51%～469%（图9-3）。

## III. TDS Results

The contents of nitrate and nitrite in 288 composite dietary samples from 24 provinces (autonomous regions, municipalities) were analyzed. The values of samples with no detectable nitrate and nitrite were assigned the values of half of the LOD to evaluate contamination levels and dietary exposure.

### (I) Levels of Nitrate and Nitrite in TDS Composite Samples

#### 1. Nitrate

Nitrate was detected in all 12 food categories (Annexed Table 9-4). Vegetables had the highest average level of nitrate (992 mg/kg), followed by potatoes (73 mg/kg) and dairy products (52 mg/kg). The relatively low concentrations were found in eggs (2.7 mg/kg), meats (4.1 mg/kg) and alcohol beverages (4.9 mg/kg). The average concentration of nitrate in water and beverages was 9.2 mg/kg.

#### 2. Nitrite

Sugar had the highest detection rate (58%) of nitrite, followed by water and beverages (21%). Food categories with relatively high levels of nitrite were sugar (1.15 mg/kg), aquatic foods (0.16 mg/kg), and fruits (0.16 mg/kg) (Annexed Table 9-5).

### (II) Dietary Exposure Assessment

#### 1. Nitrate

The average dietary intake of nitrate for China residents was 6071 μg/(kg bw·d), ranging from 1878 μg/(kg bw·d) to 17 371 μg/(kg bw·d) (Annexed Table 9-6), accounting for 51%-469% of the ADI [3700 μg/(kg bw·d)] set by JECFA (Figure 9-3).

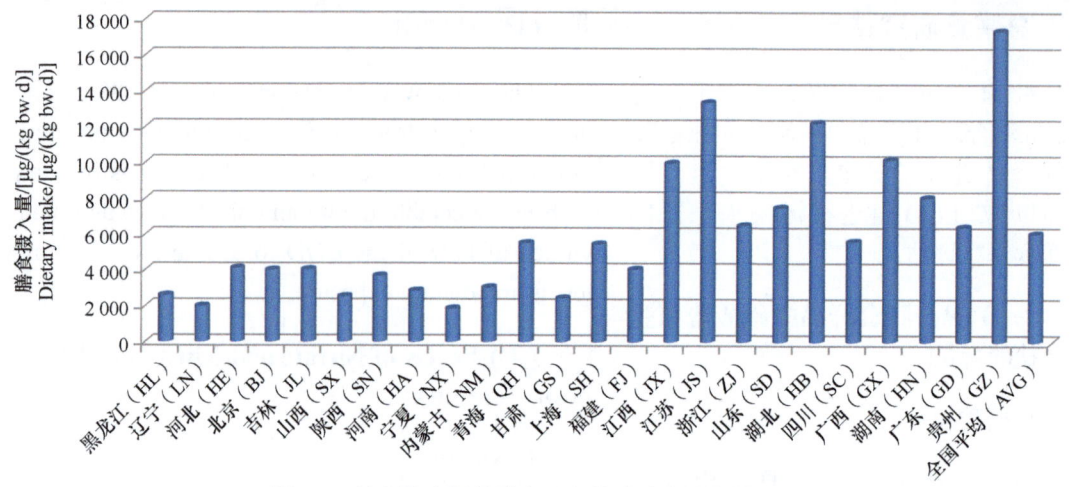

图 9-3  第六次中国总膳食研究的硝酸盐膳食摄入量
Figure 9-3  Dietary intake of nitrate from the 6$^{th}$ China TDS

## 2. 亚硝酸盐

我国居民亚硝酸盐的膳食平均摄入量为 0.74 μg/(kg bw·d)，范围为 0.13～4.89 μg/(kg bw·d)（附表 9-7）。按照 JECFA 制定的 ADI [70 μg/(kg bw·d)] 进行暴露评估，我国居民的亚硝酸盐平均膳食摄入量相当于 ADI 的 1.1%（图 9-4）。

## 2. Nitrite

The average dietary intake of nitrite for China residents was 0.83 μg/(kg bw·d), ranging from 0.13 μg/(kg bw·d) to 4.89 μg/(kg bw·d) (Annexed Table 9-7). According to the ADI [70 μg/(kg bw·d)] set by the JECFA, the average dietary intake of nitrite for China residents was 1.2% of this ADI (Figure 9-4).

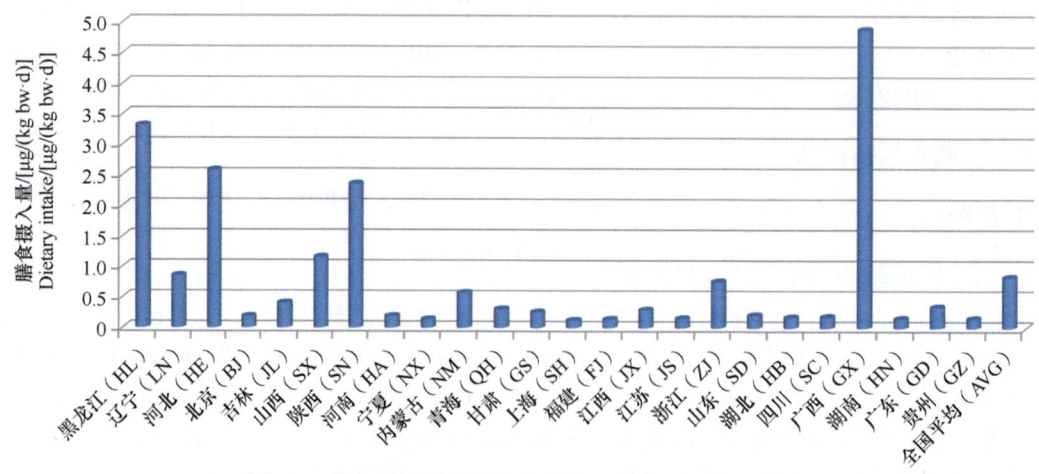

图 9-4  第六次中国总膳食研究的亚硝酸盐膳食摄入量
Figure 9-4  Dietary intake of nitrite from the 6$^{th}$ China TDS

## （三）各类膳食对总膳食摄入的贡献

第六次CTDS我国居民硝酸盐膳食暴露的主要来源为蔬菜类（94%）、水及饮料类（2.7%）和薯类（1.2%）、谷类（1.2%），其余各类食物的贡献率均小于1%（附表9-8，图9-5）。亚硝酸盐的主要膳食暴露来源为水及饮料类（32%）（附表9-9，图9-6）。

## (Ⅲ) Contributions of Food Categories to the Total Dietary Intake

The primary sources of dietary intake for the nitrate in the 6th CTDS were vegetables (94%), water and beverages (2.7%), potatoes (1.2%) and cereals (1.2%), and the contributions of the other dietary samples were all less than 1% (Annexed Table 9-8, Figure 9-5). The primary sources of dietary intake for the nitrite in the 6th CTDS were water and beverages (32%) (Annexed Table 9-9, Figure 9-6).

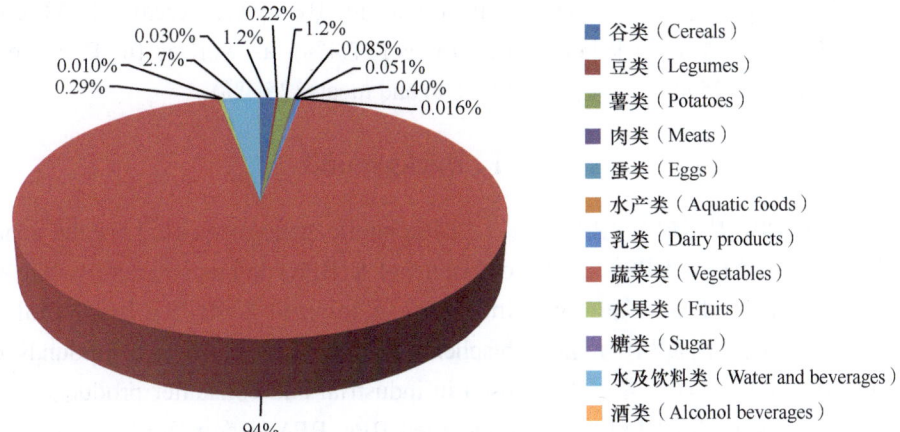

图 9-5 第六次中国总膳食研究硝酸盐的膳食来源
Figure 9-5 Dietary sources of nitrate from the 6th China TDS

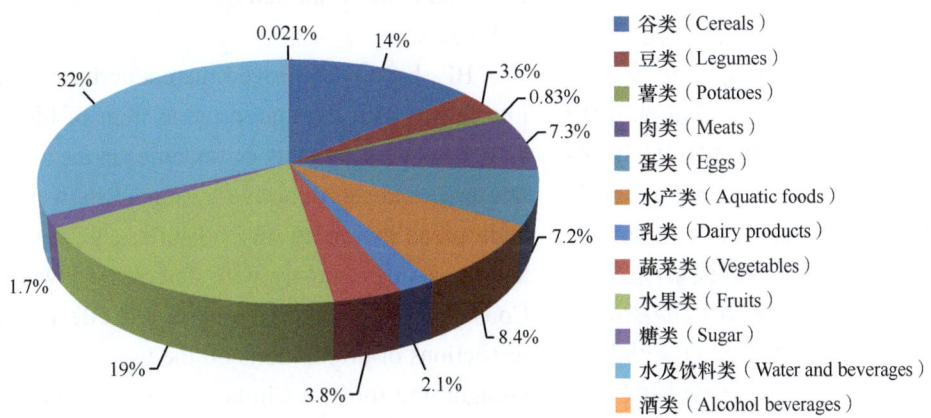

图 9-6 第六次中国总膳食研究亚硝酸盐的膳食来源
Figure 9-6 Dietary sources of nitrite from the 6th China TDS

## 第三节　双酚类化合物
## Section 3　Bisphenolic Analogues

我国居民双酚类化合物的膳食暴露量为：双酚 A（BPA）18.1 ng/(kg bw·d)、双酚 S（BPS）22.2 ng/(kg bw·d)、双酚 F（BPF）0.49 ng/(kg bw·d)、双酚 AF（BPAF）0.38 ng/(kg bw·d)。与第五次中国总膳食研究的结果相比，双酚类化合物呈现出显著下降趋势。BPA 膳食摄入的食物来源主要为谷类（40.3%）和水及饮料类（17.4%）；BPS 的主要食物来源为谷类（32.4%）和肉类（25.4%）。

The dietary exposures of bisphenol A (BPA), bisphenol S (BPS), bisphenol F (BPF) and bisphenol AF (BPAF) for residents in China were 18.1 ng/(kg bw·d), 22.2 ng/(kg bw·d), 0.49 ng/(kg bw·d) and 0.38 ng/(kg bw·d), respectively. Compared with the results of 5th China TDS, bisphenolic analogues (BPs) showed a significant decreasing trend. The main dietary contributors for BPA were cereals (40.3%), water and beverages (17.4%), as well as for BPS were cereals (32.4%) and meats (25.4%).

## 一、背景
## I. Background

双酚类化合物（BP）是双酚 A（BPA）及其结构类似物如双酚 S（BPS）、双酚 F（BPF）、双酚 AF（BPAF）等的统称，这类物质在工业品和消费品中广泛使用。其中，BPA 最受关注，常被用来合成聚碳酸酯和环氧树脂等材料，广泛应用于食品包装材料、食品贮藏容器以及工业洗涤剂、塑料增塑剂和稳定剂等。

BP 可通过干扰人体内分泌系统，导致内分泌失衡，对神经、免疫、生殖等系统产生各种毒性。报道显示 BP 在谷物、肉类及蔬菜等食品中广泛存在，检测水平多为 μg/kg。鉴于 BPA 潜在的不良影响，我国和其他国家均采取了一系列 BPA 的使用限制或禁用措施。我国于 2011 年禁止生产聚碳酸酯婴幼儿奶瓶和其他任何含 BPA 的婴幼儿奶瓶；同年禁止进口和销售聚碳酸酯婴幼儿奶瓶和其他任何含 BPA 的婴幼儿奶瓶。欧盟 EU No.10/2011 规定食品接触塑料中 BPA 的迁移量≤0.6 mg/kg；EU No.321/2011 规定 1 岁以下儿童用聚碳酸酯婴儿奶瓶中禁止含有 BPA。

Bisphenolic analogues (BPs) are the general name of bisphenol A (BPA) and its structurally-like analogues, including bisphenol S (BPS), bisphenol F (BPF), bisphenol AF (BPAF), etc. These compounds are widely used in industrial and consumer products. As the most concerned BPs, BPA is commonly used to synthesize polycarbonate, epoxy resin and other materials, which is widely used in food packaging materials, food storage containers, industrial detergents, plastic plasticizers and stabilizers.

BPs have been proved the endocrine imbalance by interfering with the endocrine system of human body, associated with a variety of toxicities in the neurological, immune, and reproductive system. BPs were reported widespread in variety of foodstuffs, e.g., cereals, meats and vegetables, mostly with detectable level of μg/kg. Considering the potential undesirable effects, a series of restrictions or prohibitions on the use of BPA have been brought into force in China and several other countries. In 2011, China banned the production, import, and sale of baby bottles of polycarbonate and any other baby bottles containing BPA. EU No.10/2011 stipulates that the migration of BPA from food contact plastics is less than 0.6 mg/kg; EU No.321/2011 stipulates that

## 二、健康指导值

2006年，欧洲食品安全局将BPA的每日可耐受摄入量（TDI）设定为50 μg/(kg bw·d)；2008年，加拿大卫生部将BPA的临时TDI（t-TDI）设定为25 μg/(kg bw·d)；2015年，欧洲食品安全局根据新的毒理学研究数据将BPA的t-TDI降至4 μg/(kg bw·d)。

目前暂无BPS、BPF和BPAF的健康指导值。

## 三、总膳食研究结果

对24个省（自治区、直辖市）的12类共288份混合膳食样品中双酚类化合物的含量进行测定。在进行污染水平评价和膳食暴露评估时，膳食样品中未检出的BPA和BPS的含量均以1/2 LOD计，未检出的BPF和BPAF的含量均以0计。

### 1. 混合膳食样品中双酚类化合物的含量

在第六次中国总膳食研究样品中，BPA、BPS、BPF和BPAF的总检出率分别为75.3%、78.5%、8.3%和27.1%。各类样品中BPA的平均含量为0.13~1.68 μg/kg（附表9-10），其中，肉类、水果类和糖类的平均含量较高，乳类、水及饮料类、酒类的平均含量较低。BPS的平均含量为0.02~5.83 μg/kg（附表9-11），其中，肉类的平均含量较高，乳类、糖类、水及饮料类、酒类的平均含量较低。BPF的平均含量为ND~0.15 μg/kg（附表9-12），其中豆类的平均含量最高。BPAF的平均含量为ND~0.12 μg/kg（附表9-13），其中水产类平均含量最高。

polycarbonate infant bottles for children under age 1 are prohibited from containing BPA.

## II. HBGV

In 2006, the European Food Safety Authority set a tolerable daily intake (TDI) of of BPA 50 μg/(kg bw·d); In 2008, the temporary TDI (t-TDI) of 25 μg/(kg bw·d) has been pre-established by Health Canada. In 2015, EFSA reduced the t-TDI from 50 μg/(kg bw·d) to 4 μg/(kg bw·d) based on toxicological research data.

Currently there are no health-based guidance values for BPS, BPF and BPAF.

## III. TDS Results

The concentration of BPs in 288 composite dietary samples from 24 provinces (autonomous regions, municipalities) was determined. For the undetected samples of BPA and BPS, the level and dietary exposure were evaluated with a half of LOD value. For the undetected samples of BPF and BPAF, the level and dietary exposure were evaluated with zero.

### 1. Levels of BPs in Composite TDS Samples

In the 6th CTDS samples, the detection rate of BPA, BPS, BPF and BPAF were 75.3%, 78.5%, 8.3% and 27.1%, respectively. The average level of BPA in various dietary samples was 0.13-1.68 μg/kg (Annexed Table 9-10). BPA in meats, fruits, and sugar presented relatively higher levels; while BPA in dairy products, water and beverages as well as alcohol beverages were quite low. The average level of BPS in various dietary samples was 0.02-5.83 μg/kg (Annexed Table 9-11), among which meats posed high level while the mean concentration of dairy products, sugar, water and beverages as well as alcohol beverages were low. The average level of BPF in various dietary samples was ND-0.15 μg/kg (Annexed Table 9-12) and legumes exhibited highest level. The average level of BPAF in various dietary samples was ND-0.12 μg/kg (Annexed Table 9-13) and the maximum level was from the aquatic foods.

## 2. 膳食暴露评估

我国居民双酚类化合物的平均膳食摄入量如下：BPA 为 18.13 ng/(kg bw·d)（占 EFSA 设定的 t-TDI 的 0.45%，附表 9-14，图 9-7），BPS 为 22.19 ng/(kg bw·d)（附表 9-15，图 9-8），BPF 为 0.49 ng/(kg bw·d)（附表 9-16，图 9-9），BPAF 为 0.38 ng/(kg bw·d)（附表 9-17，图 9-10）。BPA、BPS、BPF 和 BPAF 膳食摄入量最高分别为 56.86 ng/(kg bw·d)、

## 2. Dietary Exposure Assessment

The average dietary intake of BPs for China residents was as follows: the average dietary intake of BPA was 18.13 ng/(kg bw·d) (Annexed Table 9-14, Figure 9-7), accounting for 0.45% of the t-TDI [4 μg/(kg bw·d)] set by EFSA. The average dietary intakes of BPS, BPF and BPAF were 22.19 ng/(kg bw·d) (Annexed Table 9-15, Figure 9-8), 0.49 ng/(kg bw·d) (Annexed Table 9-16, Figure 9-9) and 0.38 ng/(kg bw·d) (Annexed Table 9-17, Figure 9-10),

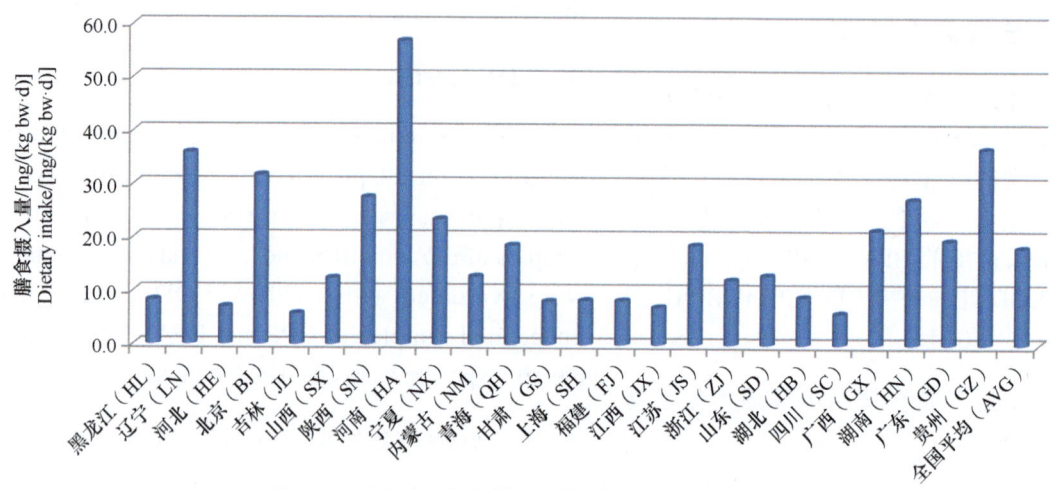

图 9-7　第六次中国总膳食研究的 BPA 膳食摄入量
Figure 9-7　Dietary intake of BPA from the 6th China TDS

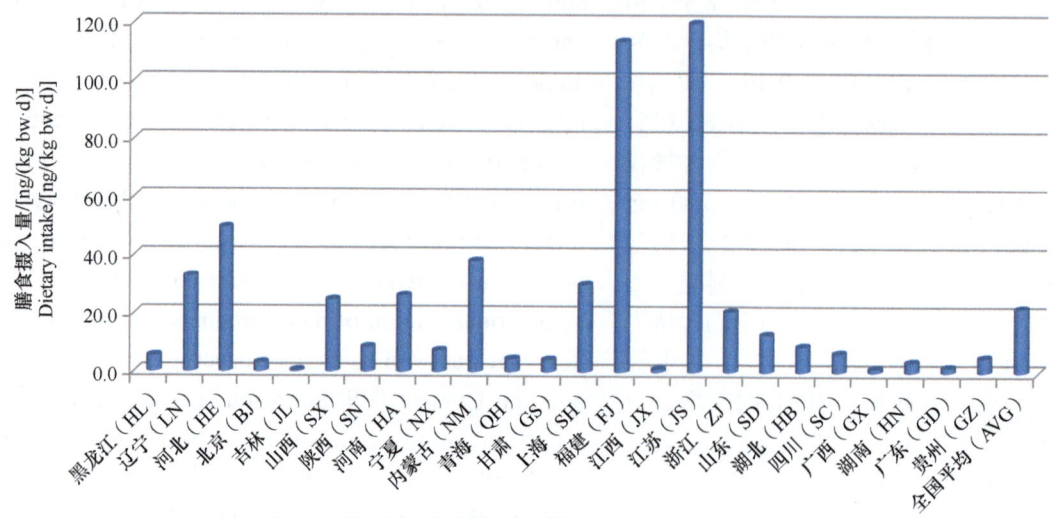

图 9-8　第六次中国总膳食研究的 BPS 膳食摄入量
Figure 9-8　Dietary intake of BPS from the 6th China TDS

119.96 ng/(kg bw・d)、2.92 ng/(kg bw・d) 和 1.87 ng/(kg bw・d)。总体上,各省(自治区、直辖市)BPA 的膳食摄入量都远低于 EFSA 于 2015 年推荐的临时健康指导值 [4 μg/(kg bw・d)]。

respectively. For these four BPs (BPA, BPS, BPF, and BPAF), the maximum dietary intakes were 56.86 ng/(kg bw・d), 119.96 ng/(kg bw・d), 2.92 ng/(kg bw・d), and 1.87 ng/(kg bw・d)], respectively. Generally, the dietary intakes of BPA from provinces (autonomous regions, municipalities) is far less than the t-TDI [4 μg/(kg bw・d)] set by EFSA in 2015.

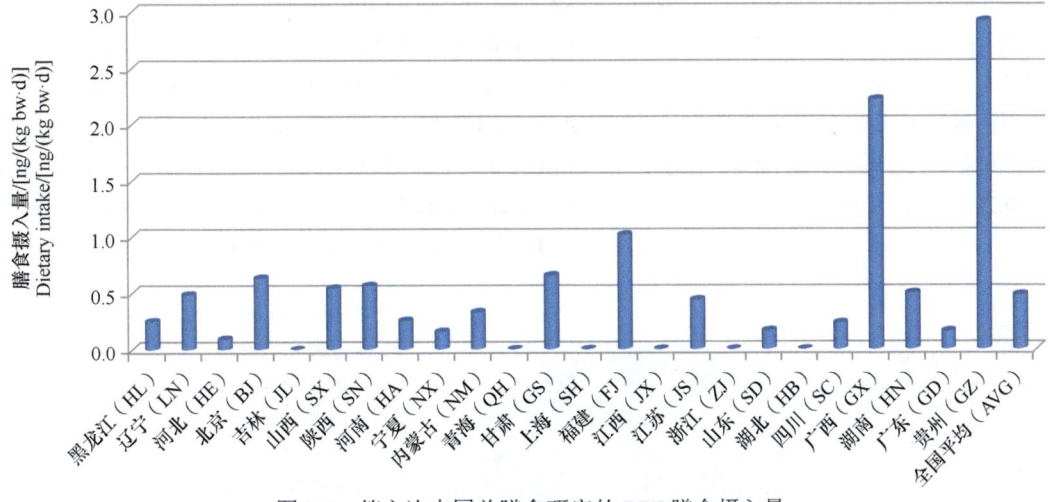

图 9-9　第六次中国总膳食研究的 BPF 膳食摄入量
Figure 9-9　Dietary intake of BPF from the 6$^{th}$ China TDS

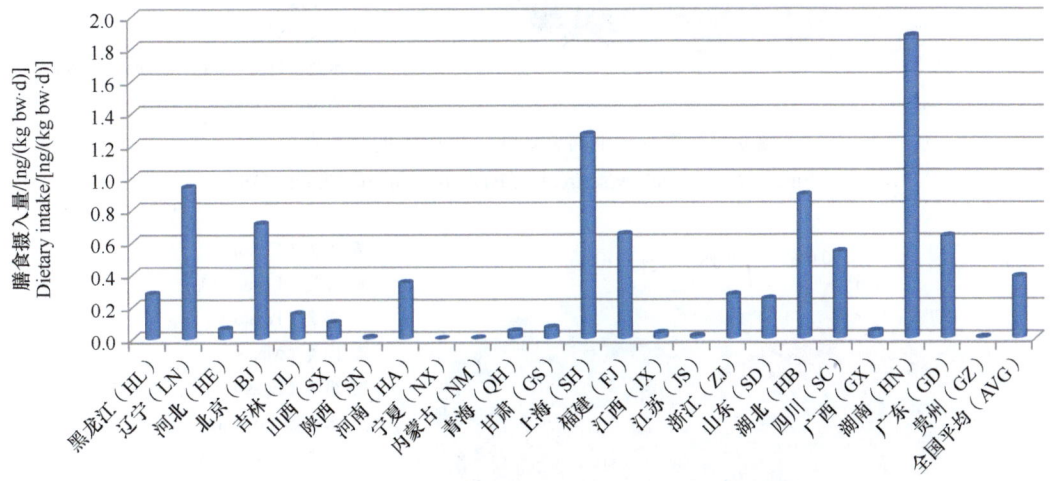

图 9-10　第六次中国总膳食研究的 BPAF 膳食摄入量
Figure 9-10　Dietary intake of BPAF from the 6$^{th}$ China TDS

## 3. 各类膳食对总膳食摄入的贡献

第六次中国总膳食研究中我国居民BPA的膳食摄入主要来源于谷类（40.3%）、水及饮料类（17.4%）、蔬菜类（13.7%）（附表9-18，图9-11）；BPS的主要来源为谷类（32.4%）、肉类（25.4%）、豆类（11.7%）和蔬菜类（11.7%）（附表9-19，图9-12）；BPF的主要来源为豆类（41.2%）、肉类（20.7%）和水果类（11.3%）（附表9-20，图9-13）；BPAF的主要来源为谷类（22.6%）、蔬菜类（21.2%）和水产类（20.2%）（附表9-21，图9-14）。

## 3. Contributions of Food Categories to the Total Dietary Intake

The main dietary contributors in the 6$^{th}$ CTDS for BPA were from the cereals (40.3%), water and beverages (17.4%) as well as vegetables (13.7%) (Annexed Table 9-18, Figure 9-11). As for BPS, the dominant contribution food categories were cereals (32.4%), followed by meats (25.4%), legumes (11.7%), vegetables (11.7%) (Annexed Table 9-19, Figure 9-12). Legumes (41.2%), meats (20.7%) and fruits (11.3%) (Annexed Table 9-20, Figure 9-13) were the top three contributors of BPF. Exposure of BPAF was mainly from cereals (22.6%), vegetables (21.2%) and aquatic foods (20.2%) (Annexed Table 9-21, Figure 9-14).

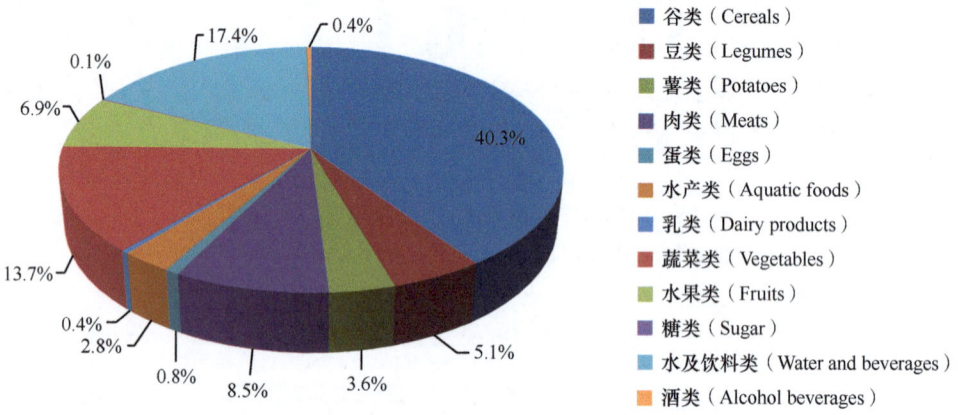

图 9-11 第六次中国总膳食研究 BPA 的膳食来源
Figure 9-11 Dietary sources of BPA from the 6$^{th}$ China TDS

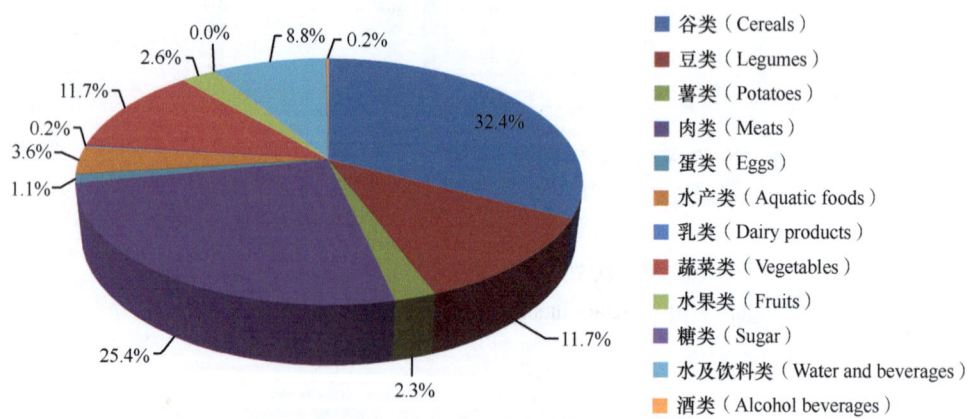

图 9-12 第六次中国总膳食研究 BPS 的膳食来源
Figure 9-12 Dietary sources of BPS from the 6$^{th}$ China TDS

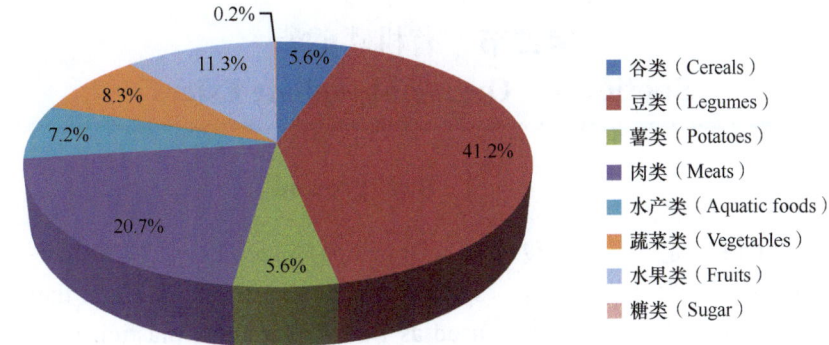

图 9-13 第六次中国总膳食研究 BPF 的膳食来源
Figure 9-13　Dietary sources of BPF from the 6th China TDS

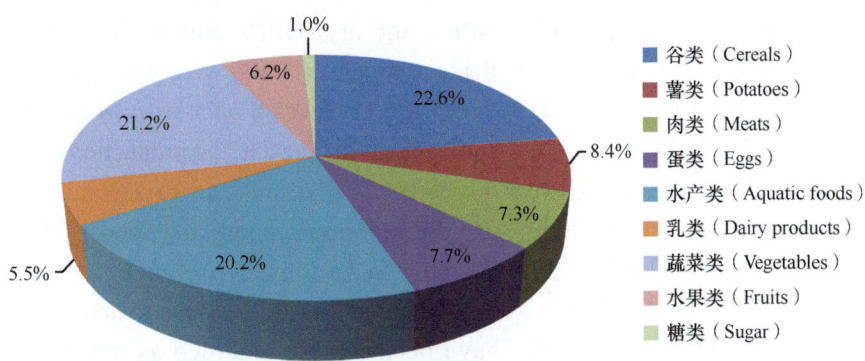

图 9-14 第六次中国总膳食研究 BPAF 的膳食来源
Figure 9-14　Dietary sources of BPAF from the 6th China TDS

## 四、与以往中国总膳食研究结果的比较

第四次中国总膳食研究仅检测了 BPA，平均暴露量为 43.0 ng/(kg bw·d)，第五次中国总膳食研究检测了 BPA、BPS、BPF 和 BPAF，其平均暴露量分别为 217 ng/(kg bw·d)、25.6 ng/(kg bw·d)、25.1 ng/(kg bw·d) 和 0.499 ng/(kg bw·d)。与第五次中国总膳食研究相比，第六次中国总膳食研究的 BPA 暴露量为 18.13 ng/(kg bw·d)，下降了 95.8%，可能与自 2011 年起我国对 BPA 的限制使用有关；BPS、BPF 和 BPAF 暴露量与第五次中国总膳食研究相比分别下降了 14.1%、98.0% 和 23.8%。

## IV. Comparison with Previous China TDSs Results

In the 4th CTDS, BPA as the only concerned BPs shows an average dietary intake for China residents was 43.0 ng/(kg bw·d). In the 5th CTDS, the average dietary intakes of BPA, BPS, BPF and BPAF were 217 ng/(kg bw·d), 25.6 ng/(kg bw·d), 25.1 ng/(kg bw·d) and 0.499 ng/(kg bw·d), respectively. The exposure of BPA in the 6th CTDS was 18.13 ng/(kg bw·d), which was 95.8% less than that in the 5th CTDS, which may be related to the measures and restrictions of BPA use in China from 2011. The exposures of BPS, BPF and BPAF in the 6th CTDS were also decreased 14.1%, 98.0% and 23.8%, respectively compared to that in the 5th CTDS.

# 第四节 有机磷酸酯
# Section 4  Organophosphate Esters

## 一、背景

有机磷酸酯（OPE）是一系列磷酸酯类化学助剂的统称，作为阻燃剂、增塑剂、润滑剂和消泡剂广泛应用于各类产品中。按照取代基的不同，有机磷酸酯可分为卤代磷酸酯、烷基磷酸酯和芳基磷酸酯三大类。随着以往最常用的溴代阻燃剂不断被列入《关于持久性有机污染物的斯德哥尔摩公约》名单而被禁用，有机磷酸酯作为溴代阻燃剂的替代品，其产量和使用量迅速增长，同时也带来了严重的环境与食品污染。OPE在各类环境基质中均有检出，并可在动物体内引起多种毒性效应，已成为备受关注的新污染物。膳食是普通人群摄入OPE的主要途径，特别是对于非职业暴露人群。欧洲和北美洲已陆续开展食品中OPE的监测与人群膳食暴露评估，欧洲食品安全局和美国环境保护署已陆续开展了OPE的暴露风险评估，并设定了若干种常用OPE的健康指导值。第六次中国总膳食研究首次开展了膳食样品中OPE的检测和膳食暴露评估。根据已在我国环境中发现的典型OPE，并参考欧洲食品安全局和美国环境保护署已设定健康指导值的OPE，本次研究针对5个OPE进行检测，包括三(2-氯乙基)磷酸酯（TCEP）、2-乙基己基二苯基磷酸酯（EHDPP）、三(2-氯丙基)磷酸酯（TCIPP）、三丁基磷酸酯（TnBP）、三(2-乙基己基)磷酸酯（TEHP）。

## Ⅰ. Background

Organophosphate esters (OPEs) are a class of phosphates and chemical additive and they are normally used as flame retardants, plasticizers, lubricants, and antifoaming agents in various products. According to different substituent group, OPEs can be classified to three categories, including halogenated-OPEs, alkyl-OPEs, and aryl-OPEs. Since traditional brominated flame retardants (BFRs) were gradually listed under the *Stockholm Convention on Persistent Organic Pollutants* and banned. As a result, the production and use of OPEs increase rapidly and lead to serious contamination of OPEs in environment and foods. OPEs have been detected in various environmental matrices, and its exposure could cause multiple toxicities in biota. OPEs have been widely regarded as novel environmental pollutant. It is generally known that dietary intake is a major pathway for the exposure of OPEs to human beings, especially in the general population without occupational exposure. The monitoring of OPEs in foods and dietary exposure assessment have been conducted in Europe and North America, and European Food Safety Authority (EFSA) and U.S. Environmental Protection Agency (USEPA) have performed exposure risk assessment of OPEs and set the health-based guidance values for several commonly used OPEs. In the 6th China total diet study (TDS), the measurement and dietary exposure assessment of OPEs were firstly conducted. According to the occurrence of OPEs measured in environmental matrices from China, and OPEs which have health-based guidance values set EFSA and USEPA, five commonly used OPEs, including tris (2-chloroethyl) phosphate (TCEP), 2-ethylhexyl diphenyl phosphate (EHDPP), tri (2-chloropropyl) phosphate (TCIPP), tri-n-butyl phosphate (TnBP), and tris (2-ethylhexyl) phosphate (TEHP), were tested in the 6th China TDS.

## 二、健康指导值

美国环境保护署提出了 OPE 摄入参考剂量（RfD），包括 TCIPP [10 μg/(kg bw·d)]、TCEP [7 μg/(kg bw·d)]、TnBP [10 μg/(kg bw·d)] 和 TEHP [100 μg/(kg bw·d)]，欧盟则提出了 EHDPP 的摄入参考剂量 [15 μg/(kg bw·d)]。

## 三、总膳食研究结果

### 1. 混合膳食样品中 OPE 的含量

第六次中国总膳食研究对 24 省（自治区、直辖市）的 96 份动物性膳食样品（肉类、水产类、蛋类和乳类）进行 5 种 OPE 含量的检测，结果见附表 9-22～附表 9-26。肉类、水产类、蛋类和乳类的膳食样品中 OPE 的检出率均在 90% 以上。4 类动物性膳食中，TCIPP 含量平均值从高到低为水产类（1.99 ng/g）、肉类（1.96 ng/g）、蛋类（1.78 ng/g）和乳类（0.71 ng/g）；TCEP 含量平均值从高到低为蛋类（1.41 ng/g）、肉类（1.11 ng/g）、水产类（0.91 ng/g）和乳类（0.28 ng/g）；TnBP 含量平均值从高到低为肉类（0.18 ng/g）、水产类（0.13 ng/g）、乳类（0.13 ng/g）和蛋类（0.09 ng/g）；TEHP 含量平均值从高到低为水产类（1.21 ng/g）、乳类（0.82 ng/g）、肉类（0.80 ng/g）和蛋类（0.54 ng/g）；EHDPP 含量平均值从高到低为肉类（8.62 ng/g）、水产类（5.32 ng/g）、蛋类（4.56 ng/g）和乳类（2.03 ng/g）。5 种 OPE 在 4 类动物性膳食中的污染并无明确规律。TCIPP、TCEP、TnBP、TEHP 和 EHDPP 在所检测的全部动物性膳食中的含量平均值分别为 1.61 ng/g、0.928 ng/g、0.134 ng/g、0.843 ng/g 和 5.13 ng/g，可见 EHDPP 的含量最高。

## II. HBGV

USEPA has set reference doses (RfDs) for TCIPP [10 μg/(kg bw·d)], TCEP [7 μg/(kg bw·d)], TnBP [10 μg/(kg bw·d)] and TEHP [100 μg/(kg bw·d)]. EFSA has set a RfD for EHDPP [15 μg/(kg bw·d)].

## III. TDS Results

### 1. Levels of OPEs in TDS Composite Samples

In the 6$^{th}$ CTDS, the levels of the five target OPEs were measured in 96 animal-based TDS composite samples from four food categories (meats, aquatic foods, eggs and dairy products), and the results are shown in Annexed Table 9-22-Annexed Table 9-26. The detection rates of OPEs in all the four food categories were over 90%. In meats, aquatic foods, eggs and dairy products, the average levels of TCIPP in a descending order were aquatic foods (1.99 ng/g), meats (1.96 ng/g), eggs (1.78 ng/g), and dairy products (0.71 ng/g); those of TCEP in a descending order were eggs (1.41 ng/g), meats (1.11 ng/g), aquatic foods (0.91 ng/g) and dairy products (0.28 ng/g); those of TnBP in a descending order were meats (0.18 ng/g), aquatic foods (0.13 ng/g), dairy products (0.13 ng/g) and eggs (0.09 ng/g); those of TEHP in a descending order were aquatic foods (1.21 ng/g), dairy products (0.82 ng/g), meats (0.80 ng/g) and eggs (0.54 ng/g); and those of EHDPP in a descending order were meats (8.62 ng/g), aquatic foods (5.32 ng/g), eggs (4.56 ng/g) and dairy products (2.03 ng/g). No significant regularity could be found in the contamination pattern of OPEs in the four food categories. The average concentrations of TCIPP, TCEP, TnBP, TEHP, and EHDPP in the whole animal-based food samples were 1.61 ng/g, 0.928 ng/g, 0.134 ng/g, 0.843 ng/g and 5.13 ng/g, respectively. It is obvious that EHDPP presented the highest levels in the five OPEs.

## 2. 膳食暴露评估

24 个省（自治区、直辖市）成年男子经膳食摄入 OPE 的结果如附表 9-27～附表 9-31 所示，通过动物性膳食摄入 TCIPP、TCEP、TnBP、TEHP 和 EHDPP 的平均量分别为 5.20 ng/(kg bw·d)、2.88 ng/(kg bw·d)、0.45 ng/(kg bw·d)、1.91 ng/(kg bw·d) 和 18.12 ng/(kg bw·d)。我国居民的 OPE 摄入量存在明显地区差异，以膳食中含量最高的 EHDPP 为例，摄入量最高值为 60.01 ng/(kg bw·d)，最低值为 0.47 ng/(kg bw·d)，相差近 130 倍（图 9-15～图 9-19）。第六次中国总膳食研究的结果显示，我国居民当前的 TCIPP、TCEP、TnBP、TEHP 和 EHDPP 膳食摄入量远低于美国环境保护署和欧盟提出的参考剂量。

## 3. 各类膳食对总膳食摄入的贡献

第六次中国总膳食研究 OPE 的主要膳食来源是肉类，在 5 种 OPE 的总膳食摄入量中占比为 49.2%～66.1%（附表 9-32～附表 9-36）。水产类和蛋类膳食的贡献较为接近，一般为 10%～20%，乳

## 2. Dietary Exposure Assessment

Dietary intake of OPEs for Chinese male adult in 24 provinces (autonomous regions, municipalities) are shown in Annexed Table 9-27-Annexed Table 9-31 and Figure 9-15-Figure 9-19. The average dietary intakes of TCIPP, TCEP, TnBP, TEHP and EHDPP via animal-based food consumption were 5.20 ng/(kg bw·d), 2.88 ng/(kg bw·d), 0.45 ng/(kg bw·d), 1.91 ng/(kg bw·d) and 18.12 ng/(kg bw·d), respectively. Large variety was found in EDIs of OPEs among provinces. When EHDPP was taken as an example, it can be seen that the highest EDI of EHDPP was 60.01 ng/(kg bw·d), whereas the lowest EDI of EHDPP was only 0.47 ng/(kg bw·d), which was roughly 130 times lower. Based on results of the 6$^{th}$ China TDS, the EDIs of TCIPP, TCEP, TnBP, TEHP and EHDPP for Chinese population were much lower than RfDs set by USEPA and EFSA.

## 3. Contributions of Food Categories to the Total Dietary Intake

Meats was the primary source of dietary OPE intake in the 6$^{th}$ China TDS. In the dietary intake of the five OPEs, the contributions from meats ranged from 49.2% to 66.1% (Annexed Table 9-32-Annexed Table 9-36). The contributions from aquatic foods and eggs

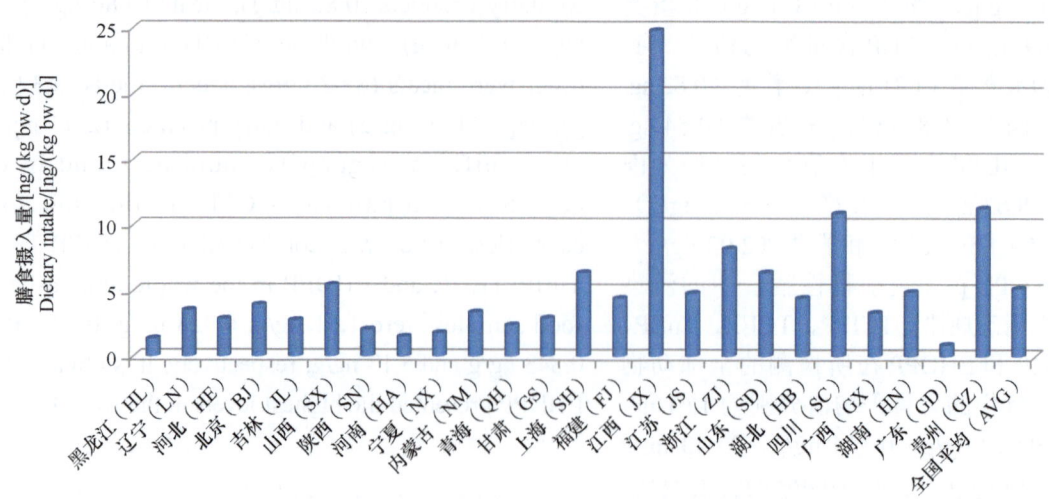

图 9-15　第六次中国总膳食研究 TCIPP 的膳食摄入量

Figure 9-15　Dietary intake of TCIPP from the 6$^{th}$ China TDS

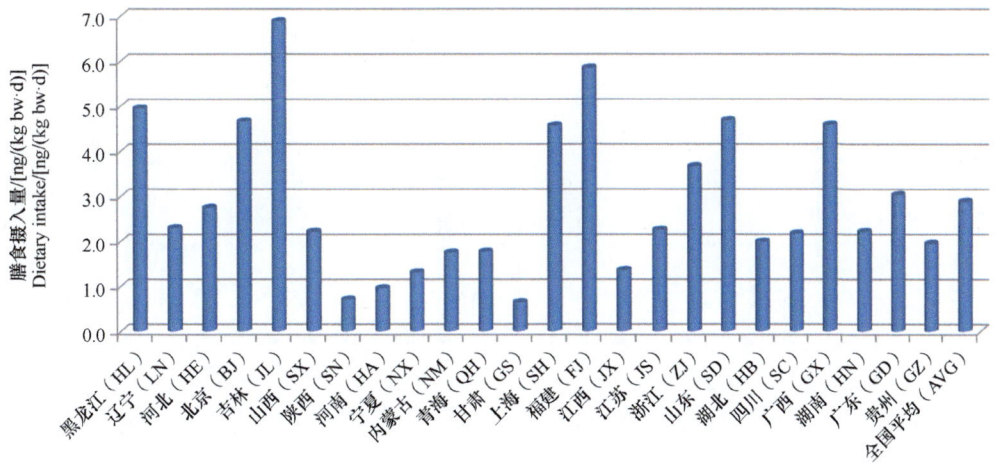

图 9-16　第六次中国总膳食研究 TCEP 的膳食摄入量
Figure 9-16　Dietary intake of TCEP from the 6$^{th}$ China TDS

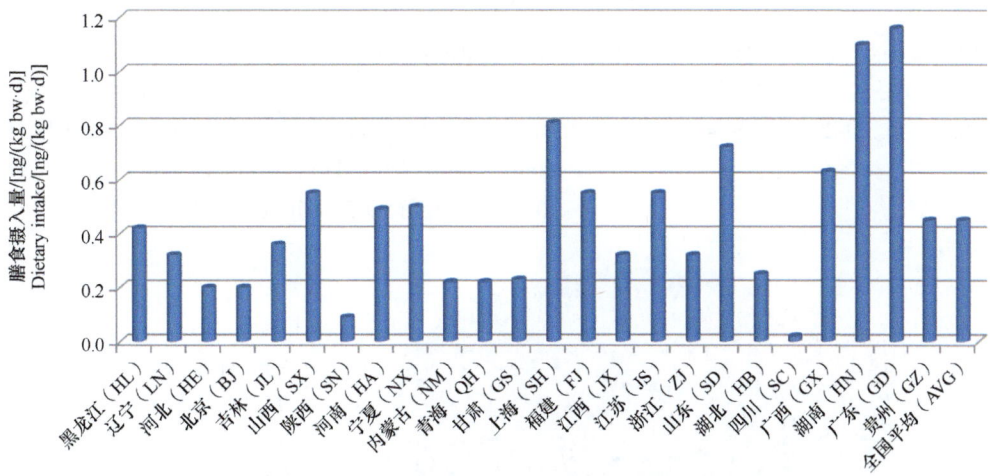

图 9-17　第六次中国总膳食研究 TnBP 的膳食摄入量
Figure 9-17　Dietary intake of TnBP from the 6$^{th}$ China TDS

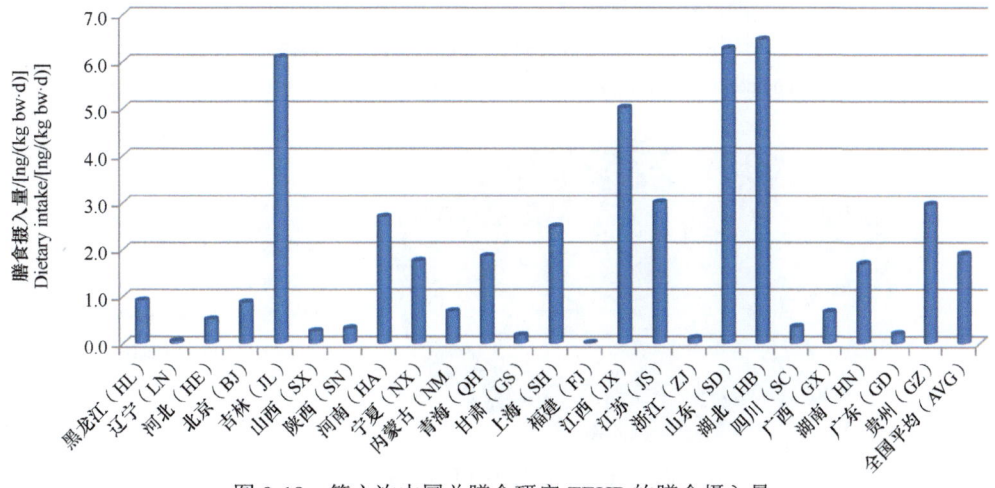

图 9-18　第六次中国总膳食研究 TEHP 的膳食摄入量
Figure 9-18　Dietary intake of TEHP from the 6$^{th}$ China TDS

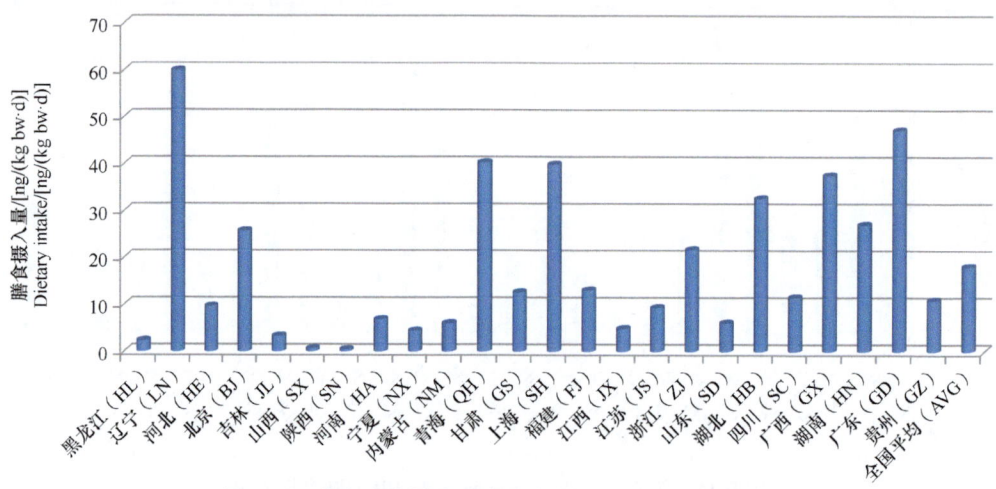

图 9-19　第六次中国总膳食研究 EHDPP 的膳食摄入量
Figure 9-19　Dietary intake of EHDPP from the 6th China TDS

类膳食的贡献较小，如 TCIPP、TCEP 和 EHDPP 的膳食摄入中乳类贡献仅为 4.4%～6.3%（图 9-20～图 9-24）。

were similar and with a proportion of 10%-20%. The contribution from dairy products was relatively small. In the dietary intake of TCIPP, TECP and EHDPP, the contributions from dairy products only ranged from 4.4% to 6.3% (Figure 9-20-Figure 9-24).

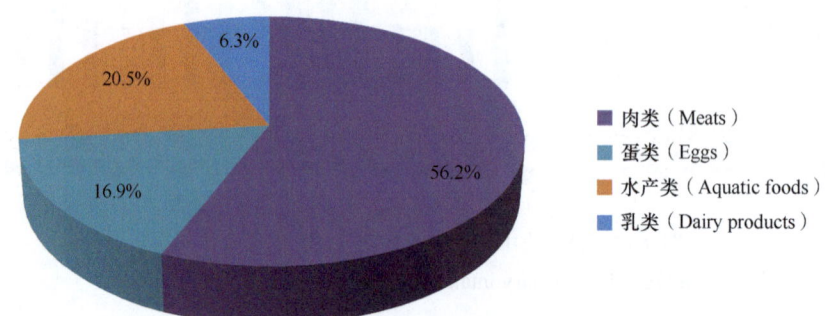

图 9-20　各类膳食对 TCIPP 膳食摄入的贡献
Figure 9-20　The contribution to the dietary intake of TCIPP from different food categories

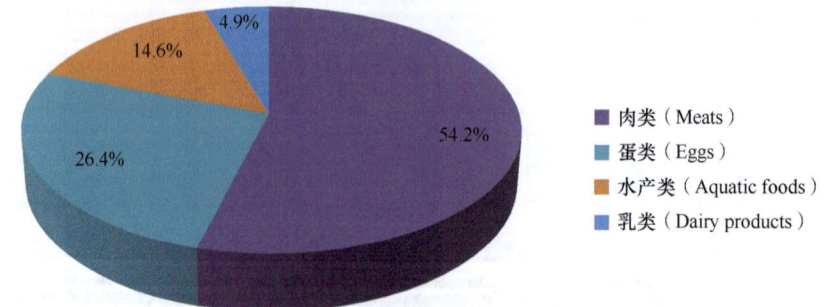

图 9-21　各类膳食对 TCEP 膳食摄入的贡献
Figure 9-21　The contribution to the dietary intake of TCEP from different food categories

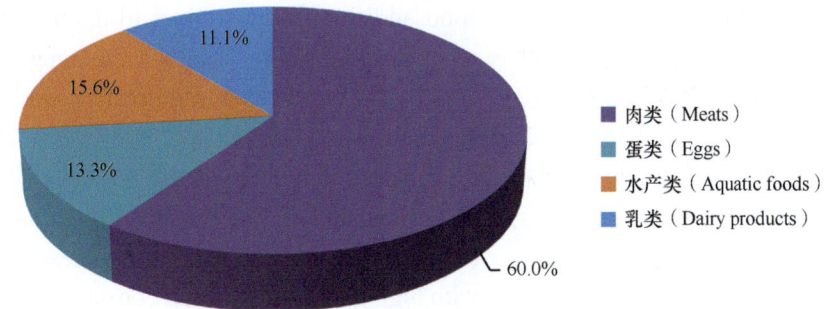

图 9-22　各类膳食对 TnBP 膳食摄入的贡献
Figure 9-22　The contribution to the dietary intake of TnBP from different food categories

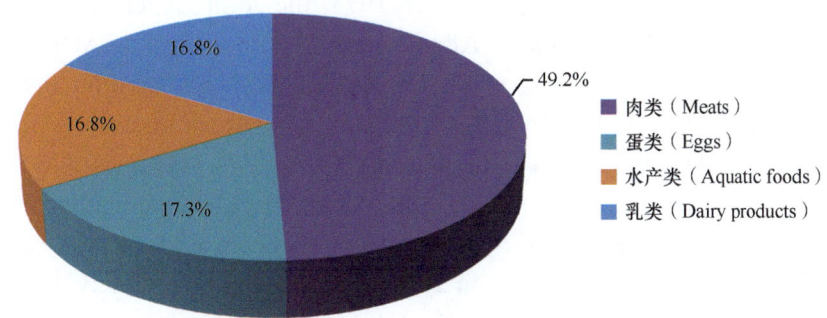

图 9-23　各类膳食对 TEHP 膳食摄入的贡献
Figure 9-23　The contribution to the dietary intake of TEHP from different food categories

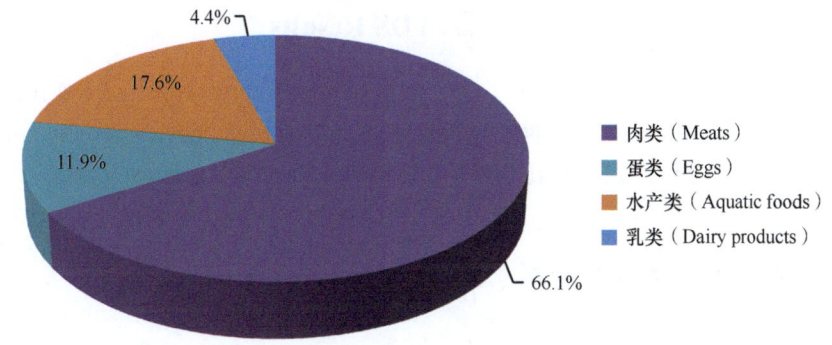

图 9-24　各类膳食对 EHDPP 膳食摄入的贡献
Figure 9-24　The contribution to the dietary intake of EHDPP from different food categories

## 第五节　谷氨酸盐
## Section 5　Glutamate Acid Salt

一、背景

谷氨酸盐（glutamate acid salt）为

Ⅰ. Background

Glutamate acid salt was commonly used as a

一种常用的食品添加剂。其中，谷氨酸钠是最为常用的食品调味剂。目前，世界各国均未对食品加工中谷氨酸盐的使用量采取限制用量的措施，但是大量摄入谷氨酸盐可能引发哮喘、肥胖、糖尿病和炎症等。2017年，欧洲食品安全局通过调研认为谷氨酸盐高消费量人群的暴露量值得关注。

## 二、健康指导值

1973年，食品添加剂联合专家委员会（JECFA）基于大鼠NOAEL（3000 mg/kg bw），不确定系数为50的结果，提出谷氨酸盐的ADI为0～120 mg/kg bw。1987年和2004年再评估认为谷氨酸作为食品添加剂，其ADI修订为"不作具体规定"，2017年，欧洲食品安全局（EFSA）基于大鼠神经发育毒性试验结果，修改谷氨酸及其盐的ADI为0～30 mg/kg bw。

## 三、总膳食研究结果

对24个省（自治区、直辖市）的7类（谷类、豆类、薯类、蛋类、水产类、蔬菜类和肉类）共168份混合膳食样品中谷氨酸盐的含量进行测定，检出率为100.0%。

### 1. 混合膳食样品中谷氨酸盐的含量

第六次中国总膳食研究的混合样品中谷氨酸盐全国平均含量为0.22～2.28 g/kg，平均含量为1.16 g/kg（附表9-37），检出率为100.0%；各类膳食中，污染水平的排序为：水产类（2.28 g/kg）、肉类（1.71 g/kg）、蔬菜类（1.41 g/kg）、豆类（1.38 g/kg）、薯类（0.77 g/kg）、谷类（0.34 g/kg）、蛋类（0.22 g/kg）。

food additive. Monosodium glutamate was the most widely used food flavoring agent among these salts. No country has adopted dosage restrictions on glutamate acid salt in food processing. However, a high intake of glutamate acid salt may cause asthma, obesity, diabetes, and inflammation. The European Food Safety Authority (EFSA) concluded in 2017 that the exposure of people with high glutamate acid salt consumption is of concern.

## II. HBGV

In 1973, the Joint Expert Committee on Food Additives (JECFA) proposed an ADI of 0-120 mg/kg bw for glutamate acid salt based on a NOAEL for rats (3000 mg/kg bw) with an uncertainty factor of 50. In 1987 and 2004, the ADI was revised to "not specified" after reassessed that glutamic acid as a food additive did not warrant concern about its safety at intake levels. In 2017, the European Food Safety Authority (EFSA) revised the ADI for glutamate and its salts to 0-30 mg/kg bw based on a neurodevelopmental toxicity test in rats.

## III. TDS Results

One hundred sixty-eight mixed dietary samples from 24 provinces (autonomous regions, municipalities) in 7 categories (cereals, legumes, potatoes, eggs, aquatic foods, vegetables, and meats) were measured for the levels of glutamate acid salt . The detection rate was 100.0%.

### 1. Levels of Glutamate Acid Salt in TDS Composite Samples

The levels of glutamate acid salt in the mixed samples of the 6th China total diet study ranged from 0.22 g/kg to 2.28 g/kg, with an average level of 1.16 g/kg (Table 9-37) and a detection rate of 100.0%; among the dietary categories, the contamination levels were ranked as follows: aquatic foods (2.28 g/kg), meats (1.71 g/kg), vegetables (1.41 g/kg), legumes (1.38 g/kg), potatoes (0.77 g/kg), cereals (0.34 g/kg) and eggs (0.22 g/kg).

## 2. Dietary Exposure Assessment

Our population's average dietary glutamate acid salt intake was 17.63 mg/(kg bw·d) (Annexed Table 9-38). The dietary intake of glutamate acid salt for residents in various regions of China ranged from 4.26 mg/(kg bw·d) to 32.34 mg/(kg bw·d), with the highest dietary intake in Shanghai and the lowest in Shandong (Figure 9-25, Annexed Table 9-38).

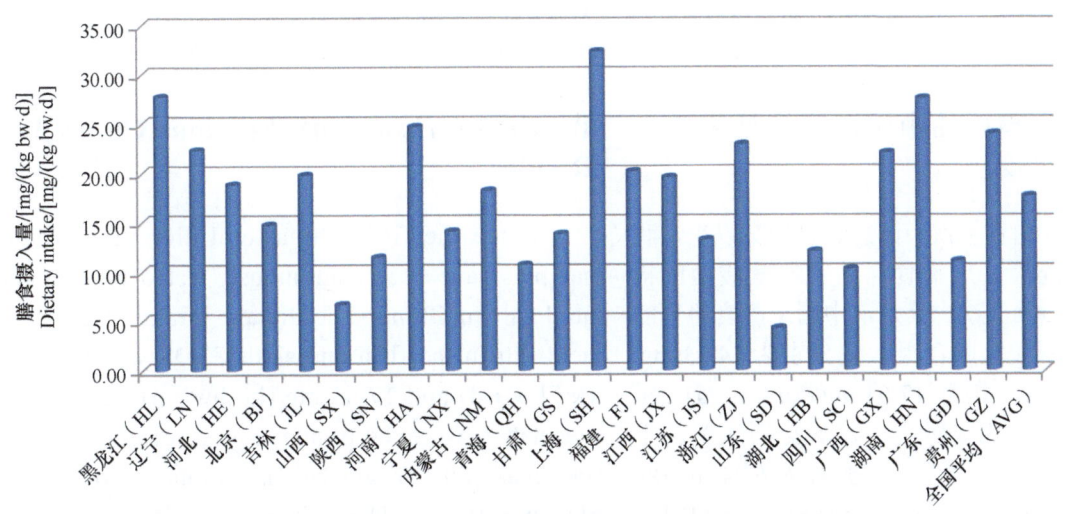

Figure 9-25 Dietary intake of glutamate acid salt from the 6th China TDS

The dietary intake of glutamate acid salt for residents in China was a ratio of 0.59 compared to the ADI proposed by EFSA, with the highest in Shanghai (1.08) and the lowest in Shandong (0.14).

### 3. Contributions of Food Categories to the Total Dietary Intake

The top three primary sources dietary intake to the glutamate acid salt in the 6th CTDS were vegetables (43.88%), cereals (20.96%), and meats (14.09%) (Annexed Table 9-39, Figure 9-26).

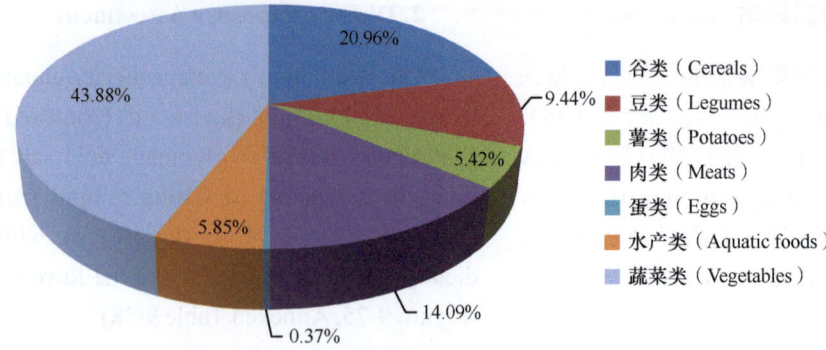

图 9-26 第六次中国总膳食研究谷氨酸盐的膳食来源
Figure 9-26　Dietary sources of glutamate acid salt from the 6th China TDS

## 四、与以往中国总膳食研究结果的比较

自第五次中国总膳食研究以来，我国连续开展膳食样品中谷氨酸盐的检测，第五次、第六次中国总膳食研究的谷氨酸盐膳食摄入量分别为 14.53 mg/(kg bw·d) 和 17.63 mg/(kg bw·d)。蔬菜类是我国居民谷氨酸盐摄入量的主要来源，摄入量分别为 6.94 mg/(kg bw·d) 和 7.74 mg/(kg bw·d)（表 9-1）。

## IV. Comparison with Previous China TDSs Results

Since the fifth China total diet study, dietary samples have been continuously tested for glutamate acid salt in China. The dietary intake of glutamate acid salt in the fifth and sixth CTDS was 14.53 mg/(kg bw·d) and 17.63 mg/(kg bw·d), respectively. Vegetables were the primary source of glutamate acid salt intake for our population, with intakes of 6.94 mg/(kg bw·d) and 7.74 mg/(kg bw·d) (Table 9-1).

表 9-1　中国总膳食研究中谷氨酸盐摄入量比较 [ 单位：mg/(kg bw·d)]
Table 9-1　Comparison of dietary intake of glutamate acid salt from the China TDSs [Unit: mg/(kg bw·d)]

| 膳食类别 Category | 第五次中国总膳食研究 5th CTDS | 第六次中国总膳食研究 6th CTDS |
| --- | --- | --- |
| 谷类 Cereals | 2.80 | 3.70 |
| 豆类 Legumes | 1.06 | 1.66 |
| 薯类 Potatoes | 1.01 | 0.97 |
| 肉类 Meats | 1.93 | 2.49 |
| 蛋类 Eggs | 0.22 | 0.06 |
| 水产类 Aquatic foods | 0.55 | 1.03 |
| 蔬菜类 Vegetables | 6.94 | 7.74 |
| 合计 SUM | 14.53 | 17.63 |

# 参 考 文 献
## References

鲍彦 (Bao Y), 尹帅星 (Yin S X), 张磊 (Zhang L), 等. 2016. 中国居民多溴联苯醚的膳食暴露水平和风险评估. 环境化学, 36: 1172-1179.

陈影 (Chen Y), 邵玉芳 (Shao Y F). 2012. 汞污染及人体负荷研究进展. 环境化学, 31(12): 1934-1941.

董国力 (Dong G L). 2013. 微量元素铁、锌、碘、硒、氟与人体健康的相关性探究. 中国当代医药, 20(6): 183-184.

董兆敏 (Dong Z M), 吴世闽 (Wu S M), 胡建英 (Hu J Y). 2011. 中国部分地区铅暴露儿童健康风险评价. 中国环境科学, 31(11): 1910-1916.

顾景范 (Gu J F), 杜寿玢 (Du S F), 查良锭 (Zha L D), 等. 2003. 现代临床营养学. 北京: 科学出版社.

国家卫生和计划生育委员会 (National Health and Family Planning Commission). 2015. 中国居民营养与慢性病状况报告 (2015 年). 北京: 人民卫生出版社.

国家卫生和计划生育委员会 (National Health and Family Planning Commission). 2017. GB 9685—2016 食品安全国家标准 食品接触材料及制品用添加剂使用标准.

国家卫生和计划生育委员会 (National Health and Family Planning Commission), 国家食品药品监督管理总局 (China Food and Drug Administration). 2017. GB 2762—2017 食品安全国家标准 食品中污染物限量.

国家卫生健康委员会 (National Health Commission). 2020. 中国居民营养与慢性病状况报告 (2020 年). 北京: 人民卫生出版社.

国家卫生健康委员会 (National Health Commission), 农业农村部 (Ministry of Agriculture and Rural Affairs), 国家市场监督管理总局 (National Medical Products Administration). 2021. GB 2763—2021 食品安全国家标准 食品中农药最大残留限量.

韩雪 (Han X). 2011. 重庆及三峡库区多环芳烃和邻苯二甲酸酯类物质环境暴露对男性生殖器损害的研究. 重庆: 第三军医大学博士学位论文.

贺婷婷 (He T T), 左兆成 (Zuo Z C). 2013. 浅谈磷与人体健康的关系. 微量元素与健康研究, 30(5): 73-74.

环境保护部 (Ministry of Environmental Protection), 外交部 (Ministry of Foreign Affairs), 国家发展和改革委员会 (National Development and Reform Commission), 等. 2014. 关于《关于持久性有机污染物的斯德哥尔摩公约》新增列九种持久性有机污染物的《关于附件 A、附件 B 和附件 C 修正案》和新增列硫丹的《关于附件 A 修正案》生效的公告.

焦君杰 (Jiao J J), 张坤 (Zhang K), 张黎 (Zhang L). 2018. 汞污染的环境效应及人体暴露研究进展. 四川地质学报, 38(3): 484-487, 492.

李敬光 (Li J G). 2015. 全氟有机化合物: 具有潜在健康风险的新型环境污染物. 中华预防医学杂志, 49: 467-469.

刘太秀 (Liu T X). 2017. PAHs、PAEs 内暴露与男性精子 DNA 损伤关系的研究. 银川: 宁夏医科大学硕士学位论文.

柳鹏 (Liu P), 王勃诗 (Wang B S). 2011. 膳食中营养成分与高血压关系的研究进展. 中国食物与营养, 17(2): 75-78.

牟建军 (Mou J J), 褚超 (Chu C). 2016. 盐敏感性高血压研究进展与展望. 中华高血压杂志, 24(8): 706-708.

邵懿 (Shao Y), 尹帅星 (Yin S X), 张磊 (Zhang L), 等. 2016. 中国居民指示性多氯联苯膳食摄入水平研究. 中华预防医学杂志, 50: 503-507.

生态环境部 (Ministry of Ecology and Environment), 外交部 (Ministry of Foreign Affairs), 国家发展和改革委员会 (National Development and Reform Commission), 等. 2019. 关于禁止生产、流通、使用和进出口林丹等持久性有机污染物的公告.

孙中兴 (Sun Z X), 姜永根 (Jiang Y G), 王海银 (Wang H Y). 2011. 锰的人体暴露水平与控制措施. 环境与职业医学, 28(6): 379-382.

滕小华 (Teng X H), 刘宇昊 (Liu Y H), 李克非 (Li K F), 等. 2021. 环境锰污染对生物健康的威胁. 东北农业大学学报, 52(1): 90-96.

吴永宁 (Wu Y N), 李敬光 (Li Y G). 2008. 加强持久性有机污染物监测能力开展履行斯德哥尔摩公约成效评估. 中华预防医学杂志, 42: 293-295.

向海云 (Xiang H Y), 陶芳标 (Tao F B). 2019. 孕期锌水平与出生结局综述. 现代预防医学, 46(15): 2749-2752.

姚蕾 (Yao L), 王晓平 (Wang X P). 2012. 关注铁过量与神经退行性疾病. 中国神经免疫学和神经病学杂志, 19(5): 388-390.

于冬梅 (Yu D M), 赵丽云 (Zhao L Y), 琚腊红 (Ju L H), 等. 2021. 2015-2017 年中国居民能量和主要营养素的摄入状况. 中国食物与营养, 27(4): 5-10.

张兵 (Zhang B), 王惠君 (Wang H J), 杜文雯 (Du W W), 等. 2011. 1989-2009 年中国九省区居民膳食营养素摄入状况及变化趋势 (二): 18~49 岁成年居民膳食能量摄入状况及变化趋势. 营养学报, 33(3): 237-242.

张坚 (Zhang J), 孟丽苹 (Meng L P), 姜元荣 (Jiang Y R), 等. 2009. 中国成人膳食脂肪酸摄入和食物来源状况分析. 营养学报, 31(5): 424-427.

张永慧 (Zhang Y H), 马文君 (Ma W J). 2016. 广东省居民膳食营养与健康状况十年变化分析. 北京: 中国质检出版社, 中国标准出版社.

张忠诚 (Zhang Z C), 徐祗云 (Xu Z Y), 张素洁 (Zhang S J). 2006. 镁与人体健康. 微量元素与健康研究, 23(4): 67-69.

郑明辉 (Zheng M H), 孙阳昭 (Sun Y Z), 刘文彬 (Liu W B). 2008. 中国二噁英类持久性有机污染物排放清单研究. 北京: 中国环境科学出版社.

中国营养学会 (Chinese Nutrition Society). 2014. 中国居民膳食营养素参考摄入量 (2013 版). 北京: 中国轻工业出版社.

祝白春 (Zhu B C), 王艳莉 (Wang Y L), 郭宝福 (Guo B F), 等. 2019. 2013-2016 年南京市民膳食中镉暴露风险评估. 实用预防医学, 26(9): 1027-1030.

Airaodion A I. 2019. Toxicological effect of monosodium glutamate in seasonings on human health. Global Journal of Nutrition & Food Science, 1(5): 1-9.

Al-Agili Z H. 2020. The effect of food additives (monosodium glutamate - MSG) on human health - a critical review. Journal of AlMaarif University College, 31(1): 362-369.

Almeida S, Raposo A, Almeida-González M, et al. 2018. Bisphenol A: food exposure and impact on human health. Compr Rev Food Sci Food Saf, 17(6): 1503-1517.

Anderson G H, Fabek H, Akilen R, et al. 2018. Acute effects of monosodium glutamate addition to whey protein on appetite, food intake, blood glucose, insulin and gut hormones in healthy young men. Appetite, 120: 92-99.

Aranceta J, Rodrigo C. 2012. Recommended dietary reference intakes, nutritional goals and dietary guidelines for fat and fatty acids: a systematic review. British Journal of Nutrition, 107(2): S8-S22.

Araya M, Olivares M, Pizarro F. 2007. Copper in human health. Int J Environ Health, 1: 608-620.

ATSDR (Agency for Toxic Substances and Disease Registry). Draft Toxicological Profile For Cadmium. U.S. Department of Health and Human Services. Atlanta, GA: Public Health Service Agency for Toxic Substances and

Disease Registry.

Baars A, Bakker M, Baumann R, et al. 2004. Dioxins, dioxin-like PCBs and non-dioxin-like PCBs in foodstuffs: Occurrence and dietary intake in the netherlands. Toxicology Letters, 151: 51-61.

Baer I, de la Calle B, Taylor P. 2010. 3-MCPD in food other than soy sauce or hydrolysed vegetable protein (HVP). Anal Bioanal Chem, 396: 443-456.

Bahadoran Z, Mirmiran P, Jeddi S, et al. 2016. Nitrate and nitrite content of vegetables, fruits, grains, legumes, dairy products, meats and processed meats. Journal of Food Composition and Analysis, 51: 93-105.

Barlow S, Renwick A G, Kleiner J, et al. 2006. Risk assessment of substances that are both genotoxic and carcinogenic: report of an international conference organized by EFSA and WHO with support of ILSI Europe. Food and Chemical Toxicology, 44(10): 1636-1650.

Beltrán E, Ibáñez M, Portolés T, et al. 2013. Development of sensitive and rapid analytical methodology for food analysis of 18 mycotoxins included in a total diet study. Anal Chim Acta, 783: 39-48.

Blekkenhorst L C, Prince R L, Ward N C, et al. 2017. Development of a reference database for assessing dietary nitrate in vegetables. Molecular Nutrition & Food Research, 61(8): 1600982.

Bradley L E, Burden A R, Bentayeb K, et al. 2013. Exposure to phthalic acid, phthalate diesters and phthalate monoesters from foodstuffs: UK total diet study results. Food Additives & Contaminants: Part A, 30(4): 735-742.

CAC (Codex Alimentarius Commission). 2014. Joint FAO/WHO Standards Programme, Codex Committee on Contaminants in Foods. 8th Session, Discussion Paper on Aflatoxins in Cereals. The Hague, Netherlands.

Cai Y, Shi Y, Zhang P, et al. 2006. Perchlorate related environmental problems. Progress in Chemistry, 18(15): 54-59.

Callan A C, Hinwood A L. 2011. Exposures to lead. Reviews on Environmental Health, 26(1): 13-15.

Cao X L, Zhao W, Dabeka R. 2015. Di-(2-ethylhexyl) adipate and 20 phthalates in composite food samples from the 2013 Canadian Total Diet Study. Food Additives & Contaminants: Part A, 32(11): 1893-1901.

Carere A. 2006. Genotoxicity and carcinogenicity of acrylamide: a critical review. Ann Ist Super Sanita, 422: 144-155.

Cavaleri F. 2015. Review of amyotrophic lateral sclerosis, Parkinson's and Alzheimer's diseases helps further define pathology of the novel paradigm for Alzheimer's with heavy metals as primary disease cause. Med Hypotheses, 85(6): 779-790.

Cebi N, Dogan C E, Olgun E O, et al. 2018. A survey of free glutamic acid in foods using a robust LC-MS/MS method. Food Chem, 248: 8-13.

Charles A S, Dennis R P, Thomsa F P, et al. 1997. The environmental fate of phthalate esters: a literature review. Chemosphere, 35: 667-749.

Chen D, Kannan K, Tan H, et al. 2016. Bisphenol analogues other than BPA: environmental occurrence, human exposure, and toxicity-a review. Environ Sci Technol, 50(11): 5438-5453.

Chen D, Ren Y, Zhong Q, et al. 2017. Ethyl carbamate in alcoholic beverages from China: levels, dietary intake, and risk assessment. Food Control, 72: 283-288.

Chen X L, Fan S, Lyu B, et al. 2021a. Occurrence and Dietary intake of organophosphate esters via animal-origin food consumption in China: results of a Chinese total diet study, J Agric Food Chem, 69: 13964-13973.

Chen X L, Li W, Li J G, et al. 2021b. Rapid determination of 13 organophosphorus flame retardants in milk by using modified quick, easy, cheap, effective, rugged, and safe technique, solid-phase extraction, and HPLC-MS/MS. J Sep Sci, 44(11): 2269-2278.

Cicero C E, Mostile G, Vasta R, et al. 2017. Metals and neurodegenerative diseases. A systematic review. Environ Res,

159: 82-94.

Collison K S, Maqbool Z, Saleh S M, et al. 2009. Effect of dietary monosodium glutamate on *trans* fat-induced nonalcoholic fatty liver disease. J Lipid Res, 50(8): 1521-1537.

Correia M, Barroso Â, Barroso M F, et al. 2010. Contribution of different vegetable types to exogenous nitrate and nitrite exposure. Food Chemistry, 120(4): 960-966.

Darrow L, Stein C, Kyle S. 2013. Serum perfluorooctanoic acid and perfluorooctane sulfonate concentrations in relation to birth outcomes in the Mid-Ohio Valley, 2005-2010. Environ Health Persp, 121: 1207-1213.

Doležal M, Chaloupská M, Divinová V, et al. 2005. Occurrence of 3-chloropropane-1, 2-diol and its esters in coffee. European Food Research and Technology, 221(3): 221-225.

Doležal M, KertISoVá J, ZelInKoVá Z, et al. 2009. Analysis of bread lipids for 3-MCPD esters. Czech J Food Sci, 27: S417-S420.

EC (European Commission)/ESIS (European Chemical Substances Information System). 2000. IUCLID dataset, 2-ethylhexyl diphenyl phosphate (1241-94-7). http://esis.jrc.ec.europa.eu[2018-10-10].

EC (European Commission). 2011. Commission Regulation (EU) No 10/2011 of 14 January 2011 on plastic materials and articles intended to come into contact with food. Off J Eur Comm L, 12: 1-89.

EFSA (European Food Safety Authority). 2005a. Opinion of the scientific committee on a request from EFSA related to a harmonised approach for risk assessment of substances which are both genotoxic and carcinogenic.

EFSA (European Food Safety Authority). 2005b. Opinion of the scientific panel on contaminants in the food chain [contam] related to the presence of non dioxin-like polychlorinated biphenyls (PCB) in feed and food.

EFSA (European Food Safety Authority). 2005c. Opinion of the scientific panel on food additives, flavourings, processing aids and materials in contact with food (AFC) on a request from the commission related to bis (2-ethylhexyl) phthalate (DEHP) for use in food contact materials. EFSA Journal, 243: 1-20.

EFSA (European Food Safety Authority). 2005d. Opinion of the scientific panel on food additives, flavourings, processing aids and materials in contact with food (AFC) on a request from the commission related to butyl benzyln phthalate (BBP) for use in food contact materials. EFSA Journal, 241: 1-14.

EFSA (European Food Safety Authority). 2005e. Opinion of the scientific panel on food additives, flavourings, processing aids and material in contact with food (AFC) on a request from the commission related to di - butyl phthalate (DBP) for use in food contact materials. EFSA Journal, 242: 1-17.

EFSA (European Food Safety Authority). 2005f. Opinion of the scientific panel on food additives, flavourings, processing aids and materials in contact with food (AFC) on a request from the commission related to di-isononylphthalate (DINP) for use in food contact materials. EFSA Journal, 244: 1-18.

EFSA (European Food Safety Authority). 2006a. Opinion of the Scientific Panel on Contaminants in the Food Chain on a request from the Commission related to ochratoxin A in food. EFSA Journal, 365: 1-56.

EFSA (European Food Safety Authority). 2006b. Tolerable Upper Intake Levels for Vitamins and Minerals. http://www.efsa.europa.eu/en/ndatopics/docs/ndatolerableuil.pdf[2020-10-12].

EFSA (European Food Safety Authority). 2007. Opioion of the sciencefic panel on contaminants in the food chain on a request from the commission related to the potential increase of consumer health risk by a possible increase of the existing maximum levels for aflatoxins in almonds, hazelnuts and pistachios and derived products. EFSA Journal, 446: 1-127.

EFSA (European Food Safety Authority). 2008a. Perfluorooctane sulfonate (PFOS), perfluorooctanoic acid (PFOA) and their salts. EFSA Journal, 653: 1-131.

EFSA (European Food Safety Authority). 2008b. Polycyclic Aromatic Hydrocarbons in Food Scientific Opinion of the Panel on Contaminants in the Food Chain. (Question NoEFSA-Q-2007-136). Eur Food Saf Auth J, 724: 1-114.

EFSA (European Food Safety Authority). 2008c. Safety of aluminum from dietary intake. Scientific Opinion of the Panel on Food Additives, Flavourings, Processing Aids and Food Contact Materials (AFC). EFSA Journal, 754: 1-34.

EFSA (European Food Safety Authority). 2008d. The setting of nutrient profiles for foods bearing nutrition and health claims pursuant to Article 4 of the Regulation (EC) No 1924/2006 - Scientific Opinion of the Panel on Dietetic Products, Nutrition and Allergies. EFSA Journal, 644: 1-44.

EFSA (European Food Safety Authority). 2011a. Scientific opinion on the risks for animal and public health related to the presence of T-2 and HT-2 toxin in food and feed. EFSA Journal, 9(12): 2481.

EFSA (European Food Safety Authority). 2011b. Scientific opinion on the risks for public health related to the presence of zearalenone in food. EFSA Journal, 9(6): 2197.

EFSA (European Food Safety Authority). 2011c. Scientific opinion on polybrominated diphenyl ethers (PBDEs) in food. EFSA Journal, 9(5): 2156.

EFSA (European Food Safety Authority). 2012a. Scientific opinion on the applicability of the margin of exposure approach for the safety assessment of impurities which are both genotoxic and carcinogenic in substances added to food/feed. EFSA Journal, 10: 2578-2582.

EFSA (European Food Safety Authority). 2012b. Scientific opinion on the risks for public and animal health related to the presence of citrinin in food and feed. EFSA Journal, 10(3): 2605.

EFSA (European Food Safety Authority). 2012c. Update of the monitoring of levels of dioxins and PCBs in food and feed. EFSA Journal, 10(7): 82.

EFSA (European Food Safety Authority). 2013. Scientific opinion on risks for animal and public health related to the presence of nivalenol in food and feed. EFSA Journal, 11(6): 3262.

EFSA (European Food Safety Authority). 2014a. Scientific opinion on the risks to human and animal health related to the presence of beauvericin and enniatins in food and feed. EFSA Journal, 12(8): 3802.

EFSA (European Food Safety Authority). 2014b. Evaluation of monitoring data on levels of ethyl carbamate in the years 2010–2012. EFSA Supporting Publications, 11(4): 578E.

EFSA (European Food Safety Authority). 2016. Risks for human health related to the presence of 3- and 2-monochloropropanediol (MCPD), and their fatty acid esters, and glycidyl fatty acid esters in food EFSA Panel on ontaminants in the Food Chain (CONTAM). EFSA Journal, 14(5): 4426.

EFSA (European Food Safety Authority). 2017. Risks to human and animal health related to the presence of deoxynivalenol and its acetylated and modified forms in food and feed. EFSA Journal, 15(9): 4718.

EFSA (European Food Safety Authority). 2018a. Risk to human health related to the presence of perfluorooctane sulfonic acid and perfluorooctanoic acid in food. EFSA Journal, 16(12): 5194.

EFSA (European Food Safety Authority). 2018b. Scientific and technical assistance on *trans* fatty acids. https://www.efsa.europa.eu/en/supporting/pub/en-1433[2021-1-10].

EFSA (European Food Safety Authority). 2020. Risk assessment of ochratoxin A in food. EFSA Journal, 18(5): e06113.

EFSA Panel on Contaminants in the Food Chain (CONTAM). 2016. Appropriateness to set a group health-based guidance value for zearalenone and its modified forms. EFSA Journal, 14(4): 4425.

EFSA Panel on Contaminants in the Food Chain (CONTAM). 2020. Risk assessment of ochratoxin A in food. EFSA

Journal, 18(5): 6113.

EFSA Panel on Dietetic Products, Nutrition, and Allergies (NDA). 2010. Scientific opinion on dietary reference values for fats, including saturated fatty acids, polyunsaturated fatty acids, monounsaturated fatty acids, *trans* fatty acids, and cholesterol. EFSA Journal, 8(3): 1461.

EFSA Panel on Food Contact Materials, Enzymes Flavouring and Processing. 2015. Scientific opinion on the risks to public health related to the presence of bisphenol A (BPA) in foodstuffs. EFSA Journal, 13(1): e3978.

EPA (U.S. Environmental Protection Agency). 2005. Guidelines for carcinogen risk assessment. Washington, DC.

EPA (U.S. Environmental Protection Agency).2024. Risk assessment: regional screening levels (RSLs). Washington, DC: U.S. Environmental Protection Agency. https://www.epa.gov/risk/regional-screening-levels-rsls[2014-7-31].

EPA (U.S. Environmental Protection Agency). 1996. PCBs: Cancer dose-response assessment and application to environmental mixtures. Washington, DC.

EU (European Union). 2011a. Commission Regulation (EU) No 1259/2011 of 2 December 2011.

EU (European Union). 2011b. Commission Regulation No 835/2011 of 19 August 2011 amending Regulation (EC) No 1881/2006 as regards maximum levels for polycyclic aromatic hydrocarbons in foodstuffs. Off J Eur Union, L215: 4-8.

EU (European Union). 2017. Commission Regulation (EU) 2017/2158 of 20 November 2017 establishing mitigation measures and benchmark levels for the reduction of the presence of acrylamide in food. https://eurlex.europa.eu/legalcontent/EN/TXT/PDF/?uri=CELEX:32017R2158&from=EN[2018-10-3].

Fang F, Qiu Y, Du G, et al. 2018. Evaluation of ethyl carbamate formation in Luzhou-flavor spirit during distillation and storage processes. Food Bioscience, 23: 137-141.

FAO/WHO. 2005. Evaluation of certain food contaminants. Sixty-fourth report of the Joint FAO/WHO Expert Committee on Food Additives. Geneva: World Health Organization. WHO Technical Report Series, 930. http://whqlibdoc.who.int/trs/WHO_TRS_930_eng.pdf[2020-6-8].

Fisher D A, Oddie T H. 1969. Thyroid iodine content and turnover in euthyroid subjects: validity of estimation of thyroid iodine accumulation from short-term clearance studies. J Clin Endocrinol Metab, 29(5): 721-727.

Franke K, Strijowski U, Fleck G, et al. 2009. Influence of chemical refining process and oil type on bound 3-chloro-1, 2-propanediol contents in palm oil and rapeseed oil. LWT-Food Science and Technology, 42(10): 1751-1754.

Fromme H, Tittlemier S, Völkel W, et al. 2009. Perfluorinated compounds-exposure assessment for the general population in western countries. Int J Hyg Envir Heal, 212(3): 239-270.

FSA (Food Standards Agency). 2006. Brominated chemicals: UK dietary intakes.

FSAI (Food Safety Authority of Ireland). 2016. Report on a total diet study carried out by the Food Safety Authority of Ireland in the period 2012–2014. https://www.fsai.ie/publications_TDS_2012-2014/[2022-5-16].

FSANZ (Food Standards Australia New Zealand). 2001. The 19th Australian total diet study. Canberra: food standards Australia New Zealand. http://www.foodstandards.gov.au/publications/Pages/19thaustraliantotaldietsurveyapril2001/19thaustraliantotaldietsurvey/Default.aspx[2021-12-10].

FSANZ (Food Standards Australia New Zealand). 2003. The 20th Australian total diet study. Canberra: food standards Australia New Zealand. http://www.foodstandards.gov.au/publications/Pages/20thaustraliantotaldietsurveyjanuary2003/20thaustraliantotaldietsurveyfullreport/Default.aspx[2022-9-20].

FSANZ (Food Standards Australia New Zealand). 2011. The 23rd Australian total diet study. Canberra: food standards Australia New Zealand. http://www.foodstandards.gov.au/publications/pages/23rdaustraliantotald5367.aspx[2022-8-20].

Gao J, Zhao Y, Zhu F, et al. 2016. Dietary exposure of acrylamide from the fifth Chinese Total Diet Study. Food Chem Toxicol, 87: 97-102.

Geens T, Goeyens L, Covaci A. 2011. Are potential sources for human exposure to bisphenol-a overlooked? Int J Hyg Environ Health, 214: 339-347.

Gowd V, Su H, Karlovsky P, et al. 2018. Ethyl carbamate: an emerging food and environmental toxicant. Food chemistry, 248: 312-321.

Greer M A, Goodman G, Pleus R C, et al. 2002. Health effects assessment for environmental perchlorate contamination: the dose response for inhibition of thyroidal radioiodine uptake in humans. Environmental Health Perspectives, 110(9): 27-34.

Guo F, Zhong Y, Wang Y, et al. 2011. Perfluorinated compounds in human blood around Bohai Sea, China. Chemosphere, 85: 156-162.

He C, Wang X Y, Tang S Y, et al. 2018. Concentrations of organophosphate esters and their specific metabolites in food in Southeast Queensland, Australia: is dietary exposure an important pathway of organophosphate esters and their metabolites? Environ Sci Technol, 52(21): 12765-12773.

He K, Du S, Xun P, et al. 2011. Consumption of monosodium glutamate in relation to incidence of overweight in Chinese adults: China health and nutrition survey (CHNS). Am J Clin Nutr, 93(6): 1328-1336.

Hernandez-Ojeda M, Urena-Guerrero M E, Gutierrez-Barajas P E, et al. 2017. KB-R7943 reduces 4-aminopyridine-induced epileptiform activity in adult rats after neuronal damage induced by neonatal monosodium glutamate treatment. J Biomed Sci, 24(1): 27.

Hossain M, Haque M, Aziz M, et al. 2020. Monosodium glutamate level in kid's food and its dietary effects on liver and kidney functions in adult rats. American Journal of Food and Nutrition, 8(2): 32-36.

Hsu J, Arcot J, Lee N A. 2009. Nitrate and nitrite quantification from cured meat and vegetables and their estimated dietary intake in Australians. Food Chemistry, 115(1): 334-339.

Huang H, Gao L, Zheng M, et al. 2018. Dietary exposure to short- and medium-chain chlorinated paraffins in meat and meat products from 20 provinces of China. Environ Pollut, 233: 439-445.

Huong B T M, Brimer L, Dalsgaard A. 2016. Dietary exposure to aflatoxin B 1, ochratoxin A and fuminisins of adults in Lao Cai province, Viet Nam: a total dietary study approach. Food Chem Toxicol, 98: 127-133.

IARC (International Agency for Research on Cancer). 1993. Monographs on the evaluation of carcinogenic risks to humans. Some naturally occurring substances: food items and constituents, heterocyclic aromatic amines and mycotoxins.

IARC (International Agency for Research on Cancer). 2004. Some Drinking-water Disinfectants and Contaminants, including Arsenic. IARC Monographs on the Evaluation of Carcinogenic Risks to Humans, 84: 269-477. Available from URL: http://monographs.iarc. fr/ENG/ Monographs /vol84/mono84.pdf[2022-5-6].

IARC (International Agency for Research on Cancer). 2010. Working Group on the Evaluation of Carcinogenic Risks to Humans. Some non-heterocyclic polycyclic aromatic hydrocarbons and some related exposures. IARC Monographs on the Evaluation of Carcinogenic Risks to Humans, 92: 1-853.

IPCS (International Programme on Chemical Safety). 1990. Selected Mycotoxins: Ochratoxins, Trichothecenes, Egrot. Environmental Health Criteria 105. Geneva (Switzerland). https://apps.who.int/iris/bitstream/handle/10665/39552/9241571055_eng.pdf[2020-5-10].

Ismail N H, Jamil N M, Samsulrizal N. 2014. Gonadotoxic and cytotoxic effect of induced obesity via monosodium glutamate on *Mus musculus* testis cytoarchitecture and sperm parameter. World Academy of Science, Engineering and Technology, 8: 1000-1003.

JECFA (Joint FAO/WHO Expert Committee on Food Additives). 1990. Evaluation of certain food additives and contaminants: thirty-fifth report of the Joint FAO/WHO Expert Committee on Food Additives.

JECFA (Joint FAO/WHO Expert Committee on Food Additives). 1995. Evaluation of certain food additives and contaminants, forty-fourth report of the Joint FAO/WHO Expert Committee on Food Additives (JECFA).

JECFA (Joint FAO/WHO Expert Committee on Food Additives). 1998. Evaluation of certain food additives and contaminants: forty-ninth report of the Joint FAO/WHO Expert Committee on Food Additives. WHO Food Additives Series, 40: 73. http://apps.who.int/iris/bitstream/10665/42142/1/WHO_TRS_884.pdf[2021-6-7].

JECFA (Joint FAO/WHO Expert Committee on Food Additives). 1999. Evaluation of certain food additives and contaminants. Forty-nine report. WHO Technical Report Series, 884: 69-77.

JECFA (Joint FAO/WHO Expert Committee on Food Additives). 2000. Zearalenone. Safety Evaluation of Certain Food Additives and Contaminants. WHO Food Additives Series, 44.

JECFA (Joint FAO/WHO Expert Committee on Food Additives). 2001. Evaluation of certain food additives and contaminants. Fifty-seventh report of the Joint FAO/WHO Expert Committee on Food Additives. WHO Technical Report Series, 909: 139-146.

JECFA (Joint FAO/WHO Expert Committee on Food Additives). 2002a. Evaluation of certain mycotoxins in food. Fifty-sixth report of the Joint FAO/WHO Expert Committee on Food Additives. WHO Technical Report Series, 906: 1-62.

JECFA (Joint FAO/WHO Expert Committee on Food Additives). 2002b. Safety evaluation of certain food additives and contaminants prepared by the fifty-seventh meeting of the Joint FAO/WHO Expert Committee on Food Additives. WHO Food Additives Series, 48: 401-432.

JECFA (Joint FAO/WHO Expert Committee on Food Additives). 2006. Safety evaluation of certain food additives and contaminants prepared by the sixty-seventh meeting of the Joint FAO/WHO Expert Committee on Food Additives. WHO Food Additives Series, 58: 209-239.

JECFA (Joint FAO/WHO Expert Committee on Food Additives). 2008. Safety evaluation of certain food additives and contaminants. Prepared by the sixty-eighth meeting of the Joint FAO/WHO Expert Committee on Food Additives (JEFCA). http://apps.who.int/iris/bitstream/10665/43823/1/9789241660594_eng.pdf[2021-8-19].

JECFA (Joint FAO/WHO Expert Committee on Food Additives). 2010a. Seventy-second meeting Rome, 16-25 February 2010, Summary and conclusions. http://apps.who.int/iris/handle/10665/44514[2021-12-10].

JECFA (Joint FAO/WHO Expert Committee on Food Additives). 2010b. Joint FAO/WHO Expert Committee on Food Additives Seventy-third meeting. http://www.who.int/foodsafety/publications/chem/summary73.pdf[2022-6-25].

JECFA (Joint FAO/WHO Expert Committee on Food Additives). 2011a. Evaluation of certain contaminants in food:Seventy-second Report of the Joint FAO /WHO Expert Committee on food additives. Geneva, WHO Technical Report Series, 959. http://whqlibdoc.who.int/trs/WHO_TRS_959_eng.pdf[2021-3-5].

JECFA (Joint FAO/WHO Expert Committee on Food Additives). 2011b. Safety evaluation of certain contaminants in food: prepared by the seventy-second meeting of the Joint FAO/WHO Expert Committee on Food Additives (JECFA) Geneva, Switzerland: World Health Organization; Rome, Italy: Food and Agriculture Organization of the United Nations.

JECFA (Joint FAO/WHO Expert Committee on Food Additives). 2018. Evaluation of certain food additives and contaminants. Eighty-third report of the Joint FAO/WHO Expert Committee on Food Additives. WHO Technical Report Series, 1002.

Jin L, Lin L, Li G Y, et al. 2018. Monosodium glutamate exposure during the neonatal period leads to cognitive deficits in adult Sprague-Dawley rats. Neurosci Lett, 682: 39-44.

Joensen U, Bossi R, Leffers H, et al. 2009. Do perfluoroalkyl compounds impair human semen quality? Environ. Health Persp, 117: 923-927.

Kayode O T, Rotimi D E, Olaolu T D, et al. 2020. Ketogenic diet improves and restores redox status and biochemical indices in monosodium glutamate-induced rat testicular toxicity. Biomed Pharmacother, 127: 110227.

Küsters M, Bimber U, Reeser S, et al. 2011. Simultaneous determination and differentiation of glycidyl esters and 3-monochloropropane-1, 2-diol (MCPD) esters in different foodstuffs by GC-MS. J Agr Food Chem, 59(11): 6263-6270.

Lau O W, Mok C S. 1995. Indirect conductometric detection of amino acids after liquid chromatographic separation. Part II. determination of monosodium glutamate in foods. Analytica Chimica Acta, 302(1): 45-52.

Leblanc J C, Tard A, Volatier J L. 2005. Estimated dietary exposure to principal food mycotoxins from the first French Total Diet Study. Food Addit Contam, 22: 652-672.

Li J G, Wu Y N, Zhang L, et al. 2007. Dietary intake of polychlorinated dioxins, furans and dioxin-like polychlorinated biphenyls from foods of animal origin in China. Food Additives and Contaminants, 24(2): 186-193.

Li P C, Li X N, Du Z H, et al. 2018. Di (2-ethyl hexyl) phthalate (DEHP)-induced kidney injury in quail (Coturnix japonica) via inhibiting HSF1/HSF3-dependent heat shock response. Chemosphere, 209: 981-988.

Li S H, Chen D, Lv B, et al. 2019. Enhanced sensitivity and effective cleanup strategy for analysis of neonicotinoids in complex dietary samples and the application in the Total Diet Study. Journal of Agricultural and Food Chemistry, 67: 2732-2740.

Li S H, Chen D, Lv B, et al. 2020. One-step cold-induced aqueous two-phase system for the simultaneous determination of fipronil and its metabolites in dietary samples by liquid chromatography–high resolution mass spectrometry and the application in Total Diet Study. Food Chemistry. 309: 125748.

Lovekamp-Swan T, Davis B J. 2007. Mechanisms of phthalate ester toxicity in the female reproductive system. Environ Health Perspect, 111(2): 139-146.

Luo L, Lei H T, Yang J Y, et al. 2017. Development of an indirect ELISA for the determination of ethyl carbamate in Chinese rice wine. Analytica Chimica Acta, 950: 162-169.

Küsters M, Bimber U, Ossenbrüggen A, et al. 2010. Rapid and simple micromethod for the simultaneous determination of 3-MCPD and 3-MCPD esters in different foodstuffs. Journal of Agricultural and Food Chemistry, 58: 6570-6577.

Mensinga T T, Speijers G J A, Meulenbelt J. 2003. Health implications of exposure to environmental nitrogenous compounds. Toxicological Reviews, 22(1): 41-51.

Miralles-Marco A, Harrad S. 2015. Perfluorooctane sulfonate: a review of human exposure, biomonitoring and the environmental forensics utility of its chirality and isomer distribution. Environ Int, 77: 148-159.

Mortensen A, Aguilar F, Crebelli R, et al. 2017. Re-evaluation of glutamic acid (E 620), sodium glutamate (E 621), potassium glutamate (E 622), calcium glutamate (E 623), ammonium glutamate (E 624) and magnesium glutamate (E 625) as food additives. EFSA Journal, 15(7): 4910.

Motzer W E. 2001. Perchlorate: problems, detection, and solutions. Environmental Forensics, 2(3): 1-11.

National Institute of Health. 2013. Dietary supplement fact sheet: selenium. http://ods.od.nih.gov/factsheets/Selenium-HealthProfessional[2020-10-9].

NHC (National Health Commission). 2017. National Food Safety Standard-Maximum Levels of Contaminants in Food. National Health Commission, PRC. China Food and Drug Administration.

Nihei M K, McGlothan J L, Toscano C D, et al. 2001. Low level Pb ($2^+$) exposure affects hippocampal protein kinase C gamma gene and protein expression in rats. Neuroscience Letters, 298(3): 212-216.

Niu Y, Zhang J, Duan H, et al. 2015. Bisphenol A and nonylphenol in foodstuffs: Chinese dietary exposure from the 2007 total diet study and infant health risk from formulas. Food Chem, 167(15): 320-325.

Nyman P J, Diachenko G W, Perfetti G A. 2003. Determination of 1, 3-dichloropropanol in soy and related sauces by using gas chromatography/mass spectrometry. Food Additives and Contaminants, 20(10): 903-908.

O'Brien E, Heussner H, Dietrich D R. 2001. Species-, sex-, and cell type-specific effects of ochratoxin A and B. Toxicol Sci, 63(2): 256-264.

Olsen G, Burris J, Ehresman D, et al. 2007. Half-Life of serum elimination of perfluorooctanesulfonate, perfluorohexanesulfonate, and perfluorooctanoate in retired fluorochemical production workers. Environ Health Persp, 115: 1298-1305.

Omura M, Hirata M, Zhao M, et al. 1995. Comparative testicular toxicities of two isomers of dichloropropanol, 2, 3-dichloro-l-propanol, and 1, 3-dichlo-ro-2-propanol, and their metabolites alpha-chlorohydrin and epichlorohydrin, and the potent testicular toxicant 1, 2-dibromo-3-chloropropane. Bulletin of Environmental Contamination Toxicology, 55(1): 127.

Onobrudu D A, Nwiloh B I. 2020. Monosodium glutamate alter hepatic functions, redox potential and lipid metabolism: Omega 3 fatty acids ameliorative intervention. GSC Biological and Pharmaceutical Sciences, 13(1): 101-110.

Patrick L. 2008. Iodine: deficiency and therapeutic considerations. Altern Med Rev, 13: 116-127.

Penttilä P L, Räsänen L, Kimppa S. 1990. Nitrate, nitrite, and N-nitroso compounds in finnish foods and the estimation of the dietary intakes. Zeitschrift für Lebensmittel-Untersuchung und Forschung, 190(4): 336-340.

Petersen A, Stoltze S. 1999. Nitrate and nitrite in vegetables on the Danish market: content and intake. Food Additives & Contaminants, 16(7): 291-299.

Pirjo P, Merja P, Heli R, et al. 2010. FInDIET 2007 Survey: energy and nutrient intakes. Public Health Nutrition, 13(6A): 920-924.

POPRC. 2017. Eighth meeting of the conference of the parties to the stockholm convention.

Praveena S M, Teh S W, Rajendran R K, et al. 2018. Recent updates on phthalate exposure and human health: a special focus on liver toxicity and stem cell regeneration. Environ Sci Pollut Res Int, 25(7): 1-10.

Qiu N N, Sun D, Zhou S, et al. 2005. Rapid and sensitive UHPLC-MS/MS methods for dietary sample analysis of 43 mycotoxins in China total diet study. J Adv Res, 39: 15-47.

Raad F, Nasreddine L, Hilan C, et al. 2014. Dietary exposure to aflatoxins, ochratoxin A and deoxynivalenol from a total diet study in an adult urban Lebanese population. Food Chem Toxicol, 73: 35-43.

Reddy A K, Ghoshal J A K, Sankaran P K, et al. 2021. Histomorphometric study on effects of monosodium glutamate in liver tissue of Wistar rats. Journal of Basic and Clinical Physiology and Pharmacology, 32(5): 1007-1012.

Reinik M, Tamme T, Roasto M. 2008. Naturally occurring nitrates and nitrites in foods. Bioactive Compounds in Foods, 2008: 225-253.

Renata M, Shulkin M L, Peñalvo J L, et al. 2017. Etiologic effects and optimal intakes of foods and nutrients for risk of cardiovascular diseases and diabetes: systematic reviews and meta-analyses from the nutrition and Chronic Diseases Expert Group (nutriCoDE). PLoS One, 12(4): 1-25.

Rhodes J, Titherley A C, Norman J A, et al. 1991. A survey of the monosodium glutamate content of foods and an estimation of the dietary intake of monosodium glutamate. Food Additives and Contaminants, 8(3): 265-274.

Riaz M, Mehmood K T. 2012. Selenium in human health and disease: a review. J Postgrad Med Inst, 26: 120-133.

Rivera-Carvantes M C, Jarero-Basulto J J, Feria-Velasco A I, et al. 2017. Changes in the expression level of MAPK pathway components induced by monosodium glutamate-administration produce neuronal death in the hippocampus from neonatal rats. Neuroscience, 365: 57-69.

Roos P, Angerer J, Wilhelm M, et al. 2008. Perfluorinated compounds (PFC) hit the headlines: meeting report on a satellite symposium of the annual meeting of the german society of toxicology. Arch Toxicol, 82(1): 57-59.

Ryu D, Choi B, Kim N, et al. 2016. Validation of analytical methods for ethyl carbamate in nine food matrices. Food Chemistry, 211: 770-775.

Santamaria P. 2006. Nitrate in vegetables: toxicity, content, intake and EC regulation. Journal of the Science of Food and Agriculture, 86(1): 10-17.

SCF (Scientific Committee for Food). 1994. European Commission DG XXIV Unit B3. Thirty-fifth report. Opinion on Aflatoxins B1, B2, G1, G2 and M1, Expressed on 23 September.

SCF (Scientific Committee for Food). 2000. Opinion of the Scientific Committee on Food on Fusarium toxins. Part 2: Zearalenone (ZEA).

SCF (Scientific Committee for Food). 2002. Opinion of the Scientific Committee on Food on Fusarium toxins. Part 6: Group evaluation of T-2 toxin, HT-2 toxin, nivalenol and deoxynivalenol. http://ec.europa.eu/food/fs/sc/scf/out123_en.pdf[2022-6-10].

SCF (Scientific Committee for Food). 2003. Updated opinion of the Scientific Committee on Food on Fumonisin B1, B2 and B3.

Schecter A, Harris T R, Shah N, et al. 2008. Brominated flame retardants in us food. Molecular Nutrition & Food Research, 52: 266-272.

Schettler T. 2006. Human exposure to phthalates via consumer products. Int J Androl, 29(1): 134-139.

Schlatter J, DiNovi M, Setzer R W. 2010. Application of the margin of exposure (MoE) approach to substances in food that are genotoxic and carcinogenic: example: ethyl carbamate (CAS 51-79-6). Food and Chemical Toxicology, 48: S63-S68.

Schrenk D, Bignami M, Bodin L, et al. 2020. Risk assessment of chlorinated paraffins in feed and food. EFSA Journal, 18(3): e05991.

Schrenk D, Bignami M, Bodin L, et al. 2021. Update of the risk assessment of hexabromocyclododecanes (HBCDDs) in food. EFSA Journal, 19: e06421.

Scippo M L, Eppe G, Saegerman C, et al. 2008. Chapter 14 persistent organochlorine pollutants, dioxins and polychlorinated biphenyls. Comprehensive Analytical Chemistry, 51: 457-506.

Shi Y, Vestergren R, Xu L, et al. 2016. Human exposure and elimination kinetics of chlorinated polyfluoroalkyl ether sulfonic acids (Cl-PFESAs). Environ Sci Technol, 50: 2396-2404.

Shi Z, Yuan B, Wittert G A, et al. 2012. Monosodium glutamate intake, dietary patterns and asthma in Chinese adults. PLoS One, 7(12): e51567.

Shi Z X, Wu Y N, Li J G, et al. 2009. Dietary exposure assessment of Chinese adults and nursing infants to tetrabromobisphenol-A and hexabromocyclododecanes: occurrence measurements in foods and human milk. Environ Sci Technol, 43(12): 4314-4319.

Shi Z X, Zhang L, Zhao Y F, et al. 2017. Dietary exposure assessment of Chinese population to tetrabromobisphenol-A, hexabromocyclododecane and decabrominated diphenyl ether: results of the 5th Chinese total diet study. Environl Pollut, 229: 539-547.

Singh A, Nair K C, Kamal R, et al. 2016. Assessing hazardous risks of indoor airborne polycyclic aromatic hydrocarbons in the kitchen and its association with lung functions and urinary PAH metabolites in kitchen workers. Clinica Chimica Acta, 452: 204-213.

Sirot V, Fremy J, Leblanc J. 2013. Dietary exposure to mycotoxins and health risk assessment in the second French total diet study. Food Chem Toxicol, 52: 1-11.

Sprong R C, De Wit-Bos L, TeBiesebeek J D, et al. 2016a. A mycotoxin-dedicated total diet study in the Netherlands in 2013: part III–exposure and risk assessment. World Mycotoxin J, 9(1): 109-128.

Sprong R C, De Wit-Bos L, Zeilmaker M J, et al. 2016a. A mycotoxin-dedicated total diet study in the Netherlands in 2013: part I–design. World Mycotoxin J, 9(1): 73-88.

Steenland K, Fletcher T, Savitz D. 2010. Epidemiologic evidence on the health effects of perfluorooctanoic acid (PFOA). Environ Health Persp, 118: 1100-1108.

Stipanuk M H, Caudill M A. 2012. Biochemical, Physiological, and Molecular Aspects of Human Nutrition. 3rd Edition. Philadelphia: Elsevier Saundre Publishing.

Stockholm Convention on Persistent Organic Pollutants (POPs). http://chm.pops.int/-Convention/Media/Pressreleases/COP4Geneva9May2009/tabid/542/language/en-US/Default.aspx2009[2009-5-8].

Tam J, Pantazopoulos P, Scott P M, et al. 2011. Application of isotope dilution mass spectrometry: determination of ochratoxin A in the Canadian total diet study. Food Addit Contam, 28(6): 754-761.

Tang A S P, Chung S W C, Kwong K, et al. 2011. Ethyl carbamate in fermented foods and beverages: dietary exposure of the Hong Kong population in 2007–2008. Food Additives and Contaminants: Part B, 4(3): 195-204.

Urbansky E T. 1998. Perchlorate chemistry: implications for analysis and remediation. Bioremediation Journal, 2(8): 81-95.

US Department of Health and Human Services, Agency for Toxic Substances and Disease Registry. 2018. Toxicological Profile for Perfluoroalkyls.

Van den Berg M, Birnbaum L, Denison M, et al. 2006. The 2005 World Health Organization reevaluation of human and mammalian toxic equivalency factors for dioxins and dioxin-like compounds. Toxicological Sciences, 93(2): 223-241.

Wan Y, Huo W, Xu S, et al. 2018. Relationship between maternal exposure to bisphenol S and pregnancy duration. Environ Pollut, 238: 717-724.

Wang Q, Afshin A, Yakoob M Y, et al. 2016. Impact of nonoptimal intakes of saturated, polyunsaturated, and *trans* fat on global burdens of coronary heart disease. J Am Heart Assoc, 5(1): e002891.

Wang R, Gao L, Zheng M, et al. 2018. Short- and medium-chain chlorinated paraffins in aquatic foods from 18 Chinese provinces: occurrence, spatial distributions, and risk assessment. Sci Total Environ, 615: 1199-1206.

Wang R, Gao L, Zheng M, et al. 2019. Characterization of short- and medium-chain chlorinated paraffins in cereals and legumes from 19 Chinese provinces. Chemosphere, 226: 282-289.

Wenzl T, Lachenmeier D W, Gokmen V. 2007. Analysis of heat-induced contaminants (acrylamide, chloropropanols and furan) in carbohydrate-rich food. Anal Bioanal Chem, 389: 119-137.

WHO (World Health Organization). 1985. Guidelines for the study of dietary intakes of chemical contaminants. Geneva, Switzerland: World Health Organization.

WHO (World Health Organization). 1996. Trace elements in human nutrition and health. URL:http://whqlibdoc.who.int/publications/1996/9241561734_eng.pdf[2021-10-12].

WHO (World Health Organization). 1998. Assessment of the health risk of dioxins: re-evaluation of the tolerable daily intake (TDI). Geneva, Switzerland.

WHO (World Health Organization). 2004. Vitamin and mineral requirements in human nutrition, second edition. URL: http://whqlibdoc.who.int/publications/2004/9241546123.pdf[2022-1-23].

WHO (World Health Organization). 2006. GEMS/Food Total Diet Studies. Food safety consultations. Report of the 4th International Workshop on Total Diet Studies Beijing, China 23–27 October 2006. http://www.who.int/foodsafety/publications/chem/TDS_Beijing_2006_en.pdf[2020-6-15].

WHO (World Health Organization). 2007. Evaluation of certain food additives and contaminants: sixty-seventh report of the Joint FAO/WHO Expert Committee on Food Additives. WHO Technical Report Series 940. Geneva: WHO. URL: http://whqlibdoc.who.int/trs/WHO_TRS_940_eng.pdf[2021-1-21].

WHO (World Health Organization). 2011a. Evaluation of certain food additives and contaminants: seventy-fourth report of the Joint FAO/WHO Expert Committee on Food Additives. WHO Technical Report Series 966. Geneva: WHO.URL: http://whqlibdoc.who.int/trs/WHO_TRS_966_eng.pdf[2022-1-2].

WHO (World Health Organization). 2011b. Safety evaluation of certain food additives and contaminants (WHO food additives series 64). Geneva: World Health Organization.

Wong C. 2012. Chromium picolinate side effects. http://altmedicine.about.com/od/herbsupplementguide/a/chromiumsideeff.htm[2020-10-21].

Wu Y, Wang Y, Li J, et al. 2012. Perfluorinated compounds in seafood from coastal areas in China. Environ Int, 42: 67-71.

Xia Q, Yang C, Wu C, et al. 2018. Quantitative strategies for detecting different levels of ethyl carbamate (EC) in various fermented food matrices: an overview. Food Control, 84: 499-512.

Xu X J, Liu J X, Huang C Y, et al. 2015. Association of polycyclic aromatic hydrocarbons (PAHs) and lead co-exposure with child physical growth and development in an e-waste recycling town. Chemosphere, 139: 295-302.

Yan J, Oey S B, van Leeuwen S P J, et al. 2018. Discrimination of processing grades of olive oil and other vegetable oils by monochloropropanediol esters and glycidyl esters. Food Chem, 248: 93-100.

Yao K, Zhang J, Yin J, et al. 2020. Bisphenol A and its analogues in Chinese total diets: contaminated levels and risk assessment. Oxid Med Cell Longev, 2020: e8822321.

Yau A T C, Chen M Y Y, Lam C H, et al. 2016. Dietary exposure to mycotoxins of the Hong Kong adult population from a total diet study. Food Addit Contam A, 33(6): 1026-1035.

Ysart G, Miller P, Barrett G, et al. 1999. Dietary exposures to nitrate in the UK. Food Additives & Contaminants, 16(12): 521-532.

Zanfirescu A, Ungurianu A, Tsatsakis A M, et al. 2019. A review of the alleged health hazards of monosodium glutamate. Compr Rev Food Sci Food Safe, 18(4): 1111-1134.

Zelinková Z, Novotný O, Schůrek J, et al. 2008. Occurrence of 3-MCPD fatty acid esters in human breast milk. Food Additives and Contaminants, 25(6): 669-676.

Zelinková Z, Svejkovská B, Velíšek J, et al. 2006. Fatty acid esters of 3-chloropropane-1, 2-diol in edible oils. Food Additives and Contaminants, 23(12): 1290-1298.

Zhang L, Li J G, Liu X, et al. 2013a. Dietary intake of PCDD/Fs and dioxin-like PCBs from the Chinese total diet study in 2007. Chemosphere, 90(5): 1625-1630.

Zhang L, Li J G, Zhao Y F, et al. 2013b. PBDEs and indicator PCBs in foods from China: levels, dietary intake and risk assessment. Journal of Agricultural and Food Chemistry, 61: 6544-6551.

Zhang P, Shi Y, Cai Y, et al. 2007. Analysis of perchlorate, bromate and iodide in milk using ion chromatography-electrospray tandem mass spectrometry. Journal of Instrumental Analysis, 26(6): 90-98.

Zhao Y G, Wong C K C, Wong M H. 2012. Environmental contamination, human exposure and body loadings of perfluorooctane sulfonate (PFOS), focusing on Asian countries. Chemosphere, 89: 355-368.

Zhong W, Hu C, Wang M. 2002. Nitrate and nitrite in vegetables from north China: content and intake. Food Additives & Contaminants, 19(12): 1125-1129.

Zhou K, Liu Y, Li W Q, et al. 2017. An improved HPLC-FLD for fast and simple detection of ethyl carbamate in soy sauce and prediction of precursors. Food Analytical Methods, 10(12): 3856-3865.

Zhou K, Siroli L, Patrignani F, et al. 2019a. Formation of ethyl carbamate during the production process of cantonese soy sauce. Molecules, 24(8): 1474.

Zhou M, Wang H, Zeng X, et al. 2019b. Mortality, morbidity, and risk factors in China and its provinces, 1990-2017: a systematic analysis for the Global Burden of Disease Study 2017. Lancet, 394(10204): 1145-1158.

Zhou P, Zhao Y, Liu H, et al. 2013. Dietary exposure of the Chinese population to acrylamide. Biomed Environ Sci, 26: 421-429.

# 附 录
# Appendix

## 第二章 附 表
## Annexed Tables of Chapter 2

附表 2-1　第六次中国总膳食研究膳食样品中总脂肪酸的含量（单位：g/100g）

Annexed Table 2-1　Levels of total fatty acids in food samples from the 6th China TDS (Unit: g/100g)

| 膳食类别<br>Category | 黑龙江<br>HL | 辽宁<br>LN | 河北<br>HE | 北京<br>BJ | 吉林<br>JL | 山西<br>SX | 陕西<br>SN | 河南<br>HA | 宁夏<br>NX | 内蒙古<br>NM | 青海<br>QH | 甘肃<br>GS | 上海<br>SH | 福建<br>FJ | 江西<br>JX | 江苏<br>JS | 浙江<br>ZJ | 山东<br>SD | 湖北<br>HB | 四川<br>SC | 广西<br>GX | 湖南<br>HN | 广东<br>GD | 贵州<br>GZ | 全国平均<br>AVG |
|---|---|---|---|---|---|---|---|---|---|---|---|---|---|---|---|---|---|---|---|---|---|---|---|---|---|
| 谷类 Cereals | 2.56 | 0.74 | 1.67 | 1.48 | 1.25 | 1.28 | 1.53 | 1.41 | 1.10 | 3.88 | 1.21 | 1.16 | 1.42 | 0.90 | 0.96 | 0.83 | 0.90 | 1.06 | 1.35 | 1.19 | 0.70 | 0.64 | 0.99 | 0.75 | 1.29 |
| 豆类 Legumes | 9.98 | 15.84 | 9.01 | 4.91 | 9.73 | 7.60 | 12.79 | 8.52 | 8.81 | 10.05 | 6.37 | 10.89 | 3.80 | 7.73 | 10.88 | 10.33 | 6.21 | 9.30 | 11.12 | 7.97 | 7.41 | 8.76 | 9.10 | 7.49 | 8.94 |
| 薯类 Potatoes | 6.74 | 5.35 | 6.39 | 5.00 | 3.47 | 3.02 | 5.30 | 2.21 | 8.97 | 6.30 | 6.84 | 9.82 | 7.81 | 2.11 | 2.93 | 3.15 | 1.33 | 2.79 | 5.24 | 8.30 | 2.82 | 6.34 | 0.13 | 11.59 | 5.17 |
| 肉类 Meats | 32.16 | 17.08 | 21.47 | 22.13 | 32.13 | 37.70 | 30.09 | 23.79 | 33.08 | 32.50 | 27.87 | 36.39 | 20.27 | 18.14 | 22.57 | 32.53 | 25.32 | 20.63 | 28.40 | 36.23 | 24.34 | 27.53 | 14.02 | 34.79 | 27.13 |
| 蛋类 Eggs | 12.04 | 11.34 | 14.63 | 15.37 | 10.82 | 15.69 | 16.55 | 12.61 | 26.46 | 13.27 | 23.63 | 18.07 | 11.83 | 12.44 | 11.25 | 13.61 | 11.47 | 12.33 | 15.98 | 15.72 | 11.63 | 14.11 | 5.09 | 14.42 | 14.18 |
| 水产类 Aquatic foods | 9.14 | 4.14 | 4.62 | 6.58 | 11.05 | 4.44 | 9.69 | 6.69 | 7.82 | 6.58 | 10.71 | 6.83 | 8.80 | 6.89 | 7.18 | 7.53 | 9.36 | 6.52 | 8.94 | 9.88 | 7.04 | 9.58 | 7.59 | 12.36 | 7.92 |
| 乳类 Dairy products | 3.14 | 3.14 | 3.39 | 3.30 | 3.33 | 2.84 | 4.41 | 3.27 | 3.35 | 2.65 | 3.24 | 2.89 | 2.98 | 3.28 | 3.24 | 3.05 | 3.14 | 3.09 | 4.17 | 3.21 | 3.04 | 3.31 | 3.00 | 3.36 | 3.24 |

附录　357

续表

| 膳食类别 Category | 黑龙江 HL | 辽宁 LN | 河北 HE | 北京 BJ | 吉林 JL | 山西 SX | 陕西 SN | 河南 HA | 宁夏 NX | 内蒙古 NM | 青海 QH | 甘肃 GS | 上海 SH | 福建 FJ | 江西 JX | 江苏 JS | 浙江 ZJ | 山东 SD | 湖北 HB | 四川 SC | 广西 GX | 湖南 HN | 广东 GD | 贵州 GZ | 全国平均 AVG |
|---|---|---|---|---|---|---|---|---|---|---|---|---|---|---|---|---|---|---|---|---|---|---|---|---|---|
| 蔬菜类 Vegetables | 5.85 | 4.76 | 6.91 | 3.24 | 4.13 | 4.08 | 7.24 | 4.92 | 9.21 | 4.68 | 8.79 | 11.60 | 6.41 | 5.43 | 5.49 | 6.41 | 5.63 | 4.85 | 8.80 | 6.23 | 3.15 | 6.50 | 4.19 | 6.29 | 6.03 |
| 水果类 Fruits | 0.02 | 0.04 | 0.03 | 0.02 | 0.02 | 0.04 | 0.03 | 0.02 | 0.02 | 0.02 | 0.02 | 0.02 | 0.03 | 0.03 | 0.03 | 0.03 | 0.02 | 0.03 | 0.03 | 0.04 | 0.03 | 0.04 | 0.02 | 0.06 | 0.03 |

注：由于数据进行过舍入修约，平均值和总和的计算略有差异。下同

Note: due to rounding and rounding of the data, there is a slight difference in the calculation of the average and total values. The same applies below

附表 2-2 第六次中国总膳食研究膳食样品中饱和脂肪酸的含量（单位：g/100g）

Annexed Table 2-2 Levels of saturated fatty acids in food samples from the 6$^{th}$ China TDS (Unit: g/100g)

| 膳食类别 Category | 黑龙江 HL | 辽宁 LN | 河北 HE | 北京 BJ | 吉林 JL | 山西 SX | 陕西 SN | 河南 HA | 宁夏 NX | 内蒙古 NM | 青海 QH | 甘肃 GS | 上海 SH | 福建 FJ | 江西 JX | 江苏 JS | 浙江 ZJ | 山东 SD | 湖北 HB | 四川 SC | 广西 GX | 湖南 HN | 广东 GD | 贵州 GZ | 全国平均 AVG |
|---|---|---|---|---|---|---|---|---|---|---|---|---|---|---|---|---|---|---|---|---|---|---|---|---|---|
| 谷类 Cereals | 0.52 | 0.22 | 0.39 | 0.36 | 0.30 | 0.30 | 0.28 | 0.33 | 0.25 | 0.98 | 0.38 | 0.29 | 0.36 | 0.30 | 0.25 | 0.22 | 0.26 | 0.28 | 0.33 | 0.35 | 0.26 | 0.18 | 0.31 | 0.28 | 0.33 |
| 豆类 Legumes | 1.79 | 2.88 | 1.78 | 0.90 | 1.75 | 1.43 | 1.41 | 1.60 | 1.34 | 2.28 | 0.93 | 1.36 | 0.64 | 1.60 | 1.93 | 1.64 | 1.08 | 1.78 | 2.15 | 1.00 | 1.44 | 1.15 | 1.88 | 1.04 | 1.53 |
| 薯类 Potatoes | 1.12 | 0.98 | 1.29 | 1.05 | 0.57 | 0.63 | 0.41 | 0.37 | 1.04 | 1.97 | 0.56 | 0.72 | 0.99 | 0.45 | 0.58 | 0.27 | 0.35 | 0.58 | 1.11 | 1.09 | 0.60 | 0.86 | 0.05 | 2.34 | 0.83 |
| 肉类 Meats | 11.32 | 5.38 | 7.09 | 7.54 | 12.15 | 13.65 | 9.47 | 8.26 | 11.12 | 12.46 | 9.13 | 10.24 | 6.17 | 6.25 | 8.27 | 9.95 | 7.98 | 7.18 | 9.80 | 13.28 | 8.92 | 8.66 | 4.89 | 12.17 | 9.22 |
| 蛋类 Eggs | 3.29 | 3.04 | 4.17 | 4.35 | 3.03 | 4.48 | 3.58 | 3.56 | 5.81 | 3.76 | 4.81 | 3.27 | 3.06 | 3.54 | 3.05 | 3.14 | 3.23 | 3.50 | 4.54 | 3.88 | 3.66 | 3.32 | 1.81 | 3.79 | 3.65 |
| 水产类 Aquatic foods | 1.93 | 1.08 | 1.01 | 1.46 | 2.11 | 1.24 | 1.38 | 1.33 | 1.47 | 1.21 | 1.60 | 1.37 | 1.71 | 1.55 | 1.50 | 1.18 | 1.88 | 1.67 | 1.27 | 1.68 | 2.05 | 1.32 | 2.05 | 2.54 | 1.57 |
| 乳类 Dairy products | 2.17 | 2.18 | 2.37 | 2.25 | 2.31 | 1.94 | 3.07 | 2.23 | 2.30 | 1.83 | 2.28 | 2.01 | 2.06 | 2.25 | 2.17 | 2.07 | 2.17 | 2.07 | 2.84 | 2.24 | 2.15 | 2.23 | 2.06 | 2.40 | 2.24 |

续表

| 膳食类别 Category | 黑龙江 HL | 辽宁 LN | 河北 HE | 北京 BJ | 吉林 JL | 山西 SX | 陕西 SN | 河南 HA | 宁夏 NX | 内蒙古 NM | 青海 QH | 甘肃 GS | 上海 SH | 福建 FJ | 江西 JX | 江苏 JS | 浙江 ZJ | 山东 SD | 湖北 HB | 四川 SC | 广西 GX | 湖南 HN | 广东 GD | 贵州 GZ | 全国平均 AVG |
|---|---|---|---|---|---|---|---|---|---|---|---|---|---|---|---|---|---|---|---|---|---|---|---|---|---|
| 蔬菜类 Vegetables | 0.97 | 0.84 | 1.43 | 0.67 | 0.69 | 0.87 | 0.75 | 0.81 | 1.09 | 1.24 | 0.78 | 0.94 | 0.83 | 1.39 | 1.29 | 0.58 | 0.77 | 1.02 | 2.05 | 0.50 | 0.66 | 0.88 | 0.91 | 1.49 | 0.98 |
| 水果类 Fruits | 0.01 | 0.01 | 0.01 | 0.01 | 0.01 | 0.01 | 0.01 | 0.01 | 0.01 | 0.01 | 0.01 | 0.01 | 0.01 | 0.01 | 0.01 | 0.01 | 0.01 | 0.01 | 0.01 | 0.01 | 0.01 | 0.02 | 0.01 | 0.01 | 0.01 |

附表 2-3 第六次中国总膳食研究膳食样品中单不饱和脂肪酸的含量（单位：g/100g）

Annexed Table 2-3　Levels of monounsaturated fatty acids in food samples from the 6$^{th}$ China TDS (Unit: g/100g)

| 膳食类别 Category | 黑龙江 HL | 辽宁 LN | 河北 HE | 北京 BJ | 吉林 JL | 山西 SX | 陕西 SN | 河南 HA | 宁夏 NX | 内蒙古 NM | 青海 QH | 甘肃 GS | 上海 SH | 福建 FJ | 江西 JX | 江苏 JS | 浙江 ZJ | 山东 SD | 湖北 HB | 四川 SC | 广西 GX | 湖南 HN | 广东 GD | 贵州 GZ | 全国平均 AVG |
|---|---|---|---|---|---|---|---|---|---|---|---|---|---|---|---|---|---|---|---|---|---|---|---|---|---|
| 谷类 Cereals | 0.57 | 0.16 | 0.54 | 0.43 | 0.28 | 0.36 | 0.66 | 0.34 | 0.36 | 1.28 | 0.25 | 0.25 | 0.38 | 0.26 | 0.27 | 0.32 | 0.25 | 0.28 | 0.46 | 0.50 | 0.22 | 0.26 | 0.33 | 0.23 | 0.38 |
| 豆类 Legumes | 2.89 | 4.66 | 3.43 | 1.96 | 2.57 | 2.51 | 4.55 | 2.40 | 2.69 | 3.22 | 2.18 | 4.96 | 1.10 | 2.63 | 4.18 | 4.23 | 1.85 | 3.30 | 4.07 | 3.82 | 2.64 | 3.48 | 3.26 | 3.09 | 3.15 |
| 薯类 Potatoes | 1.41 | 1.32 | 2.88 | 2.23 | 0.81 | 1.32 | 3.41 | 0.52 | 2.56 | 2.30 | 4.24 | 6.30 | 2.57 | 0.98 | 1.01 | 2.02 | 0.48 | 1.22 | 2.34 | 3.89 | 1.25 | 3.46 | 0.01 | 6.36 | 2.29 |
| 肉类 Meats | 12.75 | 6.52 | 9.58 | 9.90 | 14.12 | 16.75 | 15.22 | 9.47 | 13.56 | 13.53 | 12.79 | 18.60 | 8.54 | 8.37 | 10.03 | 15.96 | 10.62 | 9.33 | 12.63 | 16.71 | 10.97 | 13.45 | 6.33 | 16.62 | 12.18 |
| 蛋类 Eggs | 4.39 | 4.18 | 6.92 | 6.87 | 4.28 | 7.25 | 8.99 | 4.87 | 9.39 | 5.54 | 13.17 | 10.43 | 4.93 | 5.78 | 4.59 | 7.45 | 5.05 | 5.71 | 7.22 | 8.40 | 5.50 | 7.56 | 2.35 | 7.50 | 6.60 |
| 水产类 Aquatic foods | 3.43 | 1.42 | 1.95 | 2.80 | 3.59 | 1.67 | 5.35 | 2.07 | 2.88 | 2.24 | 5.65 | 3.50 | 3.24 | 3.17 | 2.98 | 3.78 | 3.79 | 2.66 | 4.90 | 4.89 | 2.86 | 5.34 | 3.13 | 6.17 | 3.48 |
| 乳类 Dairy products | 0.71 | 0.77 | 0.79 | 0.78 | 0.78 | 0.69 | 1.00 | 0.80 | 0.82 | 0.62 | 0.75 | 0.67 | 0.68 | 0.76 | 0.80 | 0.75 | 0.72 | 0.77 | 0.97 | 0.74 | 0.67 | 0.82 | 0.71 | 0.74 | 0.76 |

续表

| 膳食类别 Category | 黑龙江 HL | 辽宁 LN | 河北 HE | 北京 BJ | 吉林 JL | 山西 SX | 陕西 SN | 河南 HA | 宁夏 NX | 内蒙古 NM | 青海 QH | 甘肃 GS | 上海 SH | 福建 FJ | 江西 JX | 江苏 JS | 浙江 ZJ | 山东 SD | 湖北 HB | 四川 SC | 广西 GX | 湖南 HN | 广东 GD | 贵州 GZ | 全国平均 AVG |
|---|---|---|---|---|---|---|---|---|---|---|---|---|---|---|---|---|---|---|---|---|---|---|---|---|---|
| 蔬菜类 Vegetables | 1.22 | 1.15 | 3.08 | 1.41 | 0.94 | 1.77 | 4.50 | 1.15 | 2.70 | 1.57 | 5.40 | 7.69 | 2.07 | 2.45 | 1.94 | 3.94 | 2.06 | 2.09 | 3.90 | 4.01 | 1.40 | 3.94 | 1.90 | 3.27 | 2.73 |
| 水果类 Fruits | 0.00 | 0.01 | 0.01 | 0.00 | 0.01 | 0.01 | 0.01 | 0.00 | 0.00 | 0.00 | 0.00 | 0.00 | 0.01 | 0.01 | 0.00 | 0.01 | 0.00 | 0.01 | 0.01 | 0.01 | 0.01 | 0.01 | 0.00 | 0.01 | 0.01 |

附表 2-4  第六次中国总膳食研究膳食样品中多不饱和脂肪酸的含量（单位：g/100g）

Annexed Table 2-4  Levels of polyunsaturated fatty acids in food samples from the 6th China TDS (Unit: g/100g)

| 膳食类别 Category | 黑龙江 HL | 辽宁 LN | 河北 HE | 北京 BJ | 吉林 JL | 山西 SX | 陕西 SN | 河南 HA | 宁夏 NX | 内蒙古 NM | 青海 QH | 甘肃 GS | 上海 SH | 福建 FJ | 江西 JX | 江苏 JS | 浙江 ZJ | 山东 SD | 湖北 HB | 四川 SC | 广西 GX | 湖南 HN | 广东 GD | 贵州 GZ | 全国平均 AVG |
|---|---|---|---|---|---|---|---|---|---|---|---|---|---|---|---|---|---|---|---|---|---|---|---|---|---|
| 谷类 Cereals | 1.46 | 0.36 | 0.73 | 0.68 | 0.66 | 0.62 | 0.57 | 0.72 | 0.47 | 1.61 | 0.55 | 0.62 | 0.66 | 0.33 | 0.43 | 0.29 | 0.38 | 0.50 | 0.55 | 0.34 | 0.22 | 0.20 | 0.34 | 0.24 | 0.56 |
| 豆类 Legumes | 5.28 | 8.28 | 3.78 | 2.05 | 5.40 | 3.66 | 6.72 | 4.49 | 4.72 | 4.54 | 3.25 | 4.48 | 2.04 | 3.47 | 4.73 | 4.42 | 3.26 | 4.21 | 4.90 | 3.10 | 3.32 | 4.10 | 3.93 | 3.32 | 4.23 |
| 薯类 Potatoes | 4.19 | 3.04 | 2.20 | 1.71 | 2.08 | 1.08 | 1.36 | 1.29 | 5.21 | 2.01 | 2.00 | 2.61 | 4.18 | 0.68 | 1.30 | 0.85 | 0.49 | 0.98 | 1.79 | 3.28 | 0.96 | 1.99 | 0.07 | 2.82 | 2.01 |
| 肉类 Meats | 7.91 | 5.02 | 4.73 | 4.52 | 5.85 | 7.14 | 5.08 | 5.89 | 7.93 | 6.11 | 5.73 | 7.36 | 5.49 | 3.49 | 4.21 | 6.52 | 6.61 | 4.04 | 5.91 | 5.98 | 4.39 | 5.37 | 2.73 | 5.82 | 5.58 |
| 蛋类 Eggs | 4.32 | 4.09 | 3.51 | 4.12 | 3.47 | 3.91 | 3.77 | 4.10 | 10.99 | 3.92 | 5.54 | 4.14 | 3.77 | 3.08 | 3.54 | 2.93 | 3.12 | 3.09 | 4.19 | 3.33 | 2.44 | 3.16 | 0.92 | 3.07 | 3.86 |
| 水产类 Aquatic foods | 3.75 | 1.62 | 1.66 | 2.31 | 5.31 | 1.51 | 2.80 | 3.21 | 3.41 | 3.10 | 3.42 | 1.89 | 3.78 | 2.14 | 2.63 | 2.52 | 3.60 | 2.17 | 2.63 | 3.23 | 2.10 | 2.86 | 2.38 | 3.59 | 2.82 |
| 乳类 Dairy products | 0.12 | 0.02 | 0.12 | 0.12 | 0.12 | 0.11 | 0.15 | 0.12 | 0.12 | 0.09 | 0.11 | 0.11 | 0.12 | 0.13 | 0.13 | 0.11 | 0.12 | 0.12 | 0.18 | 0.12 | 0.09 | 0.13 | 0.11 | 0.11 | 0.12 |

续表

| 膳食类别 Category | 黑龙江 HL | 辽宁 LN | 河北 HE | 北京 BJ | 吉林 JL | 山西 SX | 陕西 SN | 河南 HA | 宁夏 NX | 内蒙古 NM | 青海 QH | 甘肃 GS | 上海 SH | 福建 FJ | 江西 JX | 江苏 JS | 浙江 ZJ | 山东 SD | 湖北 HB | 四川 SC | 广西 GX | 湖南 HN | 广东 GD | 贵州 GZ | 全国平均 AVG |
|---|---|---|---|---|---|---|---|---|---|---|---|---|---|---|---|---|---|---|---|---|---|---|---|---|---|
| 蔬菜类 Vegetables | 3.63 | 2.76 | 2.38 | 1.15 | 2.48 | 1.42 | 1.83 | 2.89 | 5.26 | 1.86 | 2.58 | 2.74 | 3.42 | 1.57 | 2.18 | 1.81 | 2.71 | 1.72 | 2.81 | 1.63 | 1.08 | 1.63 | 1.35 | 1.48 | 2.27 |
| 水果类 Fruits | 0.01 | 0.02 | 0.01 | 0.01 | 0.01 | 0.02 | 0.01 | 0.01 | 0.01 | 0.01 | 0.01 | 0.01 | 0.02 | 0.02 | 0.01 | 0.02 | 0.01 | 0.01 | 0.01 | 0.02 | 0.01 | 0.01 | 0.01 | 0.03 | 0.01 |

附表 2-5 第六次中国总膳食研究膳食样品中 n-6 多不饱和脂肪酸的含量（单位：g/100g）

Annexed Table 2-5　Levels of n-6 polyunsaturated fatty acids in food samples from the 6th China TDS (Unit: g/100g)

| 膳食类别 Category | 黑龙江 HL | 辽宁 LN | 河北 HE | 北京 BJ | 吉林 JL | 山西 SX | 陕西 SN | 河南 HA | 宁夏 NX | 内蒙古 NM | 青海 QH | 甘肃 GS | 上海 SH | 福建 FJ | 江西 JX | 江苏 JS | 浙江 ZJ | 山东 SD | 湖北 HB | 四川 SC | 广西 GX | 湖南 HN | 广东 GD | 贵州 GZ | 全国平均 AVG |
|---|---|---|---|---|---|---|---|---|---|---|---|---|---|---|---|---|---|---|---|---|---|---|---|---|---|
| 谷食类 Cereals | 1.31 | 0.34 | 0.71 | 0.64 | 0.61 | 0.59 | 0.51 | 0.68 | 0.43 | 1.35 | 0.51 | 0.53 | 0.62 | 0.32 | 0.40 | 0.26 | 0.36 | 0.48 | 0.52 | 0.30 | 0.21 | 0.17 | 0.33 | 0.23 | 0.52 |
| 豆类 Legumes | 4.65 | 7.52 | 3.55 | 1.90 | 4.74 | 3.33 | 5.62 | 4.02 | 3.09 | 4.21 | 2.69 | 3.73 | 1.84 | 3.20 | 4.32 | 3.87 | 2.91 | 3.92 | 4.53 | 2.55 | 3.03 | 3.39 | 3.62 | 2.75 | 3.71 |
| 薯类 Potatoes | 3.63 | 2.69 | 2.19 | 1.70 | 1.84 | 1.06 | 1.02 | 1.16 | 2.23 | 1.98 | 1.46 | 1.90 | 4.00 | 0.67 | 1.18 | 0.63 | 0.45 | 0.98 | 1.78 | 2.77 | 0.95 | 1.70 | 0.06 | 2.27 | 1.68 |
| 肉类 Meats | 7.08 | 4.47 | 4.60 | 4.34 | 5.33 | 6.81 | 4.36 | 5.38 | 4.37 | 5.83 | 4.96 | 6.23 | 5.17 | 3.31 | 3.93 | 5.75 | 6.11 | 3.89 | 5.69 | 5.39 | 4.20 | 4.71 | 2.65 | 5.21 | 4.99 |
| 蛋类 Eggs | 3.82 | 3.66 | 3.44 | 4.03 | 3.13 | 3.81 | 3.15 | 3.70 | 6.22 | 3.83 | 4.40 | 3.25 | 3.58 | 2.97 | 3.01 | 2.41 | 2.87 | 3.00 | 4.10 | 2.72 | 2.36 | 2.57 | 0.86 | 2.58 | 3.31 |
| 水产类 Aquatic foods | 3.06 | 1.15 | 1.42 | 2.10 | 4.54 | 1.14 | 2.12 | 2.70 | 2.08 | 2.88 | 2.65 | 1.35 | 3.11 | 1.98 | 2.32 | 1.95 | 3.01 | 1.70 | 1.97 | 2.13 | 1.86 | 1.92 | 1.90 | 2.82 | 2.24 |
| 乳类 Dairy products | 0.10 | 0.13 | 0.10 | 0.08 | 0.09 | 0.08 | 0.10 | 0.09 | 0.10 | 0.08 | 0.09 | 0.09 | 0.10 | 0.10 | 0.09 | 0.09 | 0.10 | 0.10 | 0.14 | 0.10 | 0.06 | 0.10 | 0.08 | 0.09 | 0.09 |
| 蔬菜类 Vegetables | 3.09 | 2.39 | 2.34 | 1.13 | 2.15 | 1.39 | 1.38 | 2.55 | 2.37 | 1.82 | 2.00 | 2.18 | 3.23 | 1.51 | 1.94 | 1.41 | 2.42 | 1.68 | 2.76 | 1.16 | 1.02 | 1.22 | 1.25 | 1.20 | 1.90 |
| 水果类 Fruits | 0.01 | 0.01 | 0.01 | 0.01 | 0.01 | 0.02 | 0.01 | 0.01 | 0.01 | 0.01 | 0.01 | 0.01 | 0.01 | 0.01 | 0.01 | 0.01 | 0.01 | 0.01 | 0.01 | 0.02 | 0.01 | 0.01 | 0.01 | 0.01 | 0.01 |

附表 2-6  第六次中国总膳食研究膳食样品中 n-3 多不饱和脂肪酸的含量（单位：g/100g）

Annexed Table 2-6  Levels of n-3 polyunsaturated fatty acids in food samples from the 6th China TDS (Unit: g/100g)

| 膳食类别 Category | 黑龙江 HL | 辽宁 LN | 河北 HE | 北京 BJ | 吉林 JL | 山西 SX | 陕西 SN | 河南 HA | 宁夏 NX | 内蒙古 NM | 青海 QH | 甘肃 GS | 上海 SH | 福建 FJ | 江西 JX | 江苏 JS | 浙江 ZJ | 山东 SD | 湖北 HB | 四川 SC | 广西 GX | 湖南 HN | 广东 GD | 贵州 GZ | 全国平均 AVG |
|---|---|---|---|---|---|---|---|---|---|---|---|---|---|---|---|---|---|---|---|---|---|---|---|---|---|
| 谷类 Cereals | 0.14 | 0.02 | 0.02 | 0.04 | 0.05 | 0.02 | 0.07 | 0.05 | 0.04 | 0.25 | 0.04 | 0.09 | 0.03 | 0.02 | 0.03 | 0.03 | 0.02 | 0.02 | 0.02 | 0.04 | 0.01 | 0.02 | 0.01 | 0.01 | 0.05 |
| 豆类 Legumes | 0.63 | 0.76 | 0.23 | 0.15 | 0.66 | 0.33 | 1.11 | 0.48 | 1.62 | 0.33 | 0.56 | 0.75 | 0.20 | 0.27 | 0.41 | 0.56 | 0.35 | 0.29 | 0.37 | 0.54 | 0.29 | 0.71 | 0.31 | 0.58 | 0.52 |
| 薯类 Potatoes | 0.56 | 0.35 | 0.01 | 0.01 | 0.24 | 0.01 | 0.33 | 0.13 | 2.98 | 0.03 | 0.54 | 0.71 | 0.19 | 0.01 | 0.12 | 0.22 | 0.04 | 0.01 | 0.01 | 0.50 | 0.01 | 0.29 | 0.01 | 0.55 | 0.33 |
| 肉类 Meats | 0.83 | 0.55 | 0.13 | 0.18 | 0.52 | 0.33 | 0.71 | 0.50 | 3.56 | 0.28 | 0.76 | 1.13 | 0.31 | 0.18 | 0.28 | 0.77 | 0.50 | 0.15 | 0.22 | 0.60 | 0.20 | 0.66 | 0.08 | 0.61 | 0.59 |
| 蛋类 Eggs | 0.49 | 0.44 | 0.07 | 0.09 | 0.34 | 0.10 | 0.62 | 0.40 | 4.77 | 0.09 | 1.14 | 0.89 | 0.19 | 0.11 | 0.54 | 0.52 | 0.25 | 0.09 | 0.09 | 0.60 | 0.07 | 0.58 | 0.06 | 0.49 | 0.54 |
| 水产类 Aquatic foods | 0.70 | 0.47 | 0.23 | 0.21 | 0.77 | 0.37 | 0.68 | 0.51 | 1.33 | 0.21 | 0.77 | 0.53 | 0.67 | 0.16 | 0.32 | 0.57 | 0.59 | 0.47 | 0.65 | 1.10 | 0.24 | 0.93 | 0.47 | 0.77 | 0.57 |
| 乳类 Dairy products | 0.01 | 0.11 | 0.01 | 0.02 | 0.01 | 0.02 | 0.03 | 0.01 | 0.01 | 0.01 | 0.01 | 0.01 | 0.01 | 0.01 | 0.02 | 0.01 | 0.01 | 0.01 | 0.02 | 0.01 | 0.02 | 0.01 | 0.01 | 0.01 | 0.02 |
| 蔬菜类 Vegetables | 0.54 | 0.36 | 0.04 | 0.02 | 0.33 | 0.04 | 0.45 | 0.33 | 2.89 | 0.04 | 0.57 | 0.56 | 0.19 | 0.06 | 0.24 | 0.40 | 0.29 | 0.04 | 0.05 | 0.47 | 0.06 | 0.40 | 0.09 | 0.28 | 0.37 |
| 水果类 Fruits | 0.00 | 0.00 | 0.00 | 0.00 | 0.00 | 0.00 | 0.00 | 0.00 | 0.00 | 0.00 | 0.00 | 0.00 | 0.00 | 0.00 | 0.00 | 0.00 | 0.00 | 0.00 | 0.00 | 0.00 | 0.00 | 0.00 | 0.00 | 0.02 | 0.00 |

附表 2-7 第六次中国总膳食研究膳食样品中反式脂肪酸的含量（单位：g/100g）

Annexed Table 2-7　Levels of *trans*-fatty acids in food samples from the 6th China TDS (Unit: g/100g)

| 膳食类别<br>Category | 黑龙江<br>HL | 辽宁<br>LN | 河北<br>HE | 北京<br>BJ | 吉林<br>JL | 山西<br>SX | 陕西<br>SN | 河南<br>HA | 宁夏<br>NX | 内蒙古<br>NM | 青海<br>QH | 甘肃<br>GS | 上海<br>SH | 福建<br>FJ | 江西<br>JX | 江苏<br>JS | 浙江<br>ZJ | 山东<br>SD | 湖北<br>HB | 四川<br>SC | 广西<br>GX | 湖南<br>HN | 广东<br>GD | 贵州<br>GZ | 全国平均<br>AVG |
|---|---|---|---|---|---|---|---|---|---|---|---|---|---|---|---|---|---|---|---|---|---|---|---|---|---|
| 谷类 Cereals | 0.01 | 0.00 | 0.01 | 0.01 | 0.01 | 0.01 | 0.02 | 0.01 | 0.01 | 0.02 | 0.02 | 0.01 | 0.02 | 0.01 | 0.01 | 0.01 | 0.01 | 0.01 | 0.01 | 0.01 | 0.00 | 0.00 | 0.01 | 0.00 | 0.01 |
| 豆类 Legumes | 0.01 | 0.02 | 0.02 | 0.00 | 0.01 | 0.01 | 0.10 | 0.03 | 0.06 | 0.01 | 0.02 | 0.10 | 0.02 | 0.03 | 0.03 | 0.03 | 0.03 | 0.01 | 0.01 | 0.05 | 0.01 | 0.03 | 0.03 | 0.03 | 0.03 |
| 薯类 Potatoes | 0.03 | 0.02 | 0.01 | 0.00 | 0.01 | 0.00 | 0.12 | 0.03 | 0.16 | 0.01 | 0.05 | 0.19 | 0.06 | 0.01 | 0.04 | 0.01 | 0.01 | 0.00 | 0.01 | 0.04 | 0.01 | 0.03 | ND | 0.07 | 0.04 |
| 肉类 Meats | 0.17 | 0.16 | 0.08 | 0.18 | 0.02 | 0.16 | 0.32 | 0.17 | 0.47 | 0.41 | 0.19 | 0.20 | 0.08 | 0.03 | 0.05 | 0.10 | 0.10 | 0.08 | 0.06 | 0.26 | 0.06 | 0.05 | 0.07 | 0.18 | 0.15 |
| 蛋类 Eggs | 0.04 | 0.03 | 0.03 | 0.04 | 0.03 | 0.04 | 0.21 | 0.08 | 0.28 | 0.05 | 0.11 | 0.23 | 0.07 | 0.04 | 0.06 | 0.08 | 0.08 | 0.03 | 0.03 | 0.10 | 0.04 | 0.07 | 0.01 | 0.07 | 0.08 |
| 水产类 Aquatic foods | 0.03 | 0.02 | 0.01 | 0.01 | 0.04 | 0.02 | 0.16 | 0.07 | 0.07 | 0.03 | 0.04 | 0.07 | 0.07 | 0.03 | 0.07 | 0.06 | 0.09 | 0.03 | 0.14 | 0.08 | 0.03 | 0.06 | 0.03 | 0.07 | 0.05 |
| 乳类 Dairy products | 0.14 | 0.06 | 0.12 | 0.16 | 0.13 | 0.11 | 0.18 | 0.12 | 0.11 | 0.10 | 0.10 | 0.10 | 0.12 | 0.13 | 0.13 | 0.12 | 0.13 | 0.13 | 0.18 | 0.11 | 0.13 | 0.13 | 0.13 | 0.11 | 0.12 |
| 蔬菜类 Vegetables | 0.02 | 0.02 | 0.02 | 0.01 | 0.01 | 0.01 | 0.15 | 0.07 | 0.16 | 0.02 | 0.04 | 0.22 | 0.08 | 0.03 | 0.07 | 0.09 | 0.09 | 0.02 | 0.04 | 0.09 | 0.01 | 0.05 | 0.02 | 0.05 | 0.06 |
| 水果类 Fruits | ND | ND | ND | ND | ND | ND | ND | ND | ND | ND | ND | ND | ND | ND | ND | ND | ND | ND | ND | ND | ND | ND | ND | ND | 0.00 |

注：未检出（ND）按 0 检出限（LOD）计

Note: values not detected (ND) were treated as being 0 of the limit of detection (LOD)

附表 2-8 第六次中国总膳食研究的脂肪膳食摄入量（单位：g/d）
Annexed Table 2-8  Dietary intakes of fat from the 6th China TDS (Unit: g/d)

| 膳食类别 Category | 黑龙江 HL | 辽宁 LN | 河北 HE | 北京 BJ | 吉林 JL | 山西 SX | 陕西 SN | 河南 HA | 宁夏 NX | 内蒙古 NM | 青海 QH | 甘肃 GS | 上海 SH | 福建 FJ | 江西 JX | 江苏 JS | 浙江 ZJ | 山东 SD | 湖北 HB | 四川 SC | 广西 GX | 湖南 HN | 广东 GD | 贵州 GZ | 全国平均 AVG |
|---|---|---|---|---|---|---|---|---|---|---|---|---|---|---|---|---|---|---|---|---|---|---|---|---|---|
| 谷类 Cereals | 14.68 | 4.77 | 13.29 | 12.33 | 7.66 | 13.86 | 12.21 | 13.66 | 7.58 | 29.33 | 9.67 | 8.34 | 6.66 | 5.96 | 6.31 | 6.74 | 5.95 | 11.03 | 7.43 | 12.01 | 6.91 | 3.86 | 4.73 | 5.27 | 9.59 |
| 豆类 Legumes | 4.63 | 20.19 | 5.37 | 5.22 | 7.67 | 5.52 | 11.07 | 4.81 | 3.21 | 4.19 | 0.43 | 4.69 | 4.67 | 6.77 | 8.18 | 9.11 | 9.15 | 5.10 | 7.76 | 5.62 | 3.20 | 6.71 | 2.65 | 7.95 | 6.41 |
| 薯类 Potatoes | 5.48 | 4.06 | 4.07 | 3.06 | 4.39 | 3.75 | 6.40 | 1.87 | 10.69 | 8.06 | 7.30 | 14.82 | 2.94 | 0.94 | 0.99 | 1.11 | 0.51 | 1.35 | 4.87 | 5.50 | 0.38 | 3.58 | 0.03 | 4.17 | 4.18 |
| 肉类 Meats | 20.21 | 11.93 | 10.64 | 15.58 | 22.36 | 54.11 | 11.35 | 13.78 | 16.15 | 24.98 | 20.83 | 11.81 | 23.48 | 16.31 | 22.17 | 31.22 | 31.34 | 20.99 | 16.09 | 48.85 | 38.33 | 43.05 | 15.27 | 38.75 | 24.15 |
| 蛋类 Eggs | 5.10 | 4.85 | 4.83 | 6.24 | 4.55 | 3.44 | 3.80 | 3.92 | 3.60 | 4.12 | 3.25 | 4.20 | 4.83 | 2.47 | 2.41 | 4.00 | 2.87 | 5.73 | 4.15 | 2.40 | 1.70 | 3.37 | 1.27 | 2.45 | 3.73 |
| 水产类 Aquatic foods | 2.56 | 0.69 | 0.46 | 1.12 | 1.27 | 0.30 | 0.41 | 0.32 | 0.19 | 0.71 | 0.40 | 0.20 | 6.26 | 4.62 | 3.25 | 3.03 | 4.87 | 1.55 | 3.73 | 0.86 | 7.07 | 6.53 | 4.06 | 0.44 | 2.29 |
| 乳类 Dairy products | 0.44 | 1.46 | 0.87 | 2.98 | 1.13 | 1.24 | 0.90 | 0.67 | 0.54 | 0.96 | 1.83 | 0.43 | 2.24 | 1.24 | 0.74 | 0.88 | 1.11 | 0.75 | 0.29 | 0.42 | 0.58 | 0.63 | 1.15 | 1.00 | 1.02 |
| 蔬菜类 Vegetables | 19.61 | 16.26 | 21.25 | 13.31 | 16.74 | 13.20 | 21.90 | 14.36 | 15.58 | 12.60 | 28.53 | 30.04 | 26.83 | 22.53 | 25.90 | 28.49 | 26.12 | 20.65 | 38.09 | 19.89 | 11.65 | 36.24 | 10.35 | 27.00 | 21.55 |
| 水果类 Fruits | 0.02 | 0.03 | 0.01 | 0.03 | 0.02 | 0.02 | 0.01 | 0.01 | 0.02 | 0.03 | 0.00 | 0.01 | 0.03 | 0.02 | 0.02 | 0.01 | 0.02 | 0.02 | 0.01 | 0.01 | 0.02 | 0.03 | 0.01 | 0.01 | 0.02 |
| 合计 SUM | 72.73 | 64.25 | 60.79 | 59.87 | 65.80 | 95.42 | 68.05 | 53.38 | 57.57 | 84.98 | 72.25 | 74.54 | 77.94 | 60.88 | 69.97 | 84.60 | 81.93 | 67.16 | 82.43 | 95.57 | 69.85 | 104.00 | 39.53 | 87.05 | 72.94 |

附表 2-9　第六次中国总膳食研究的饱和脂肪酸膳食摄入量（单位：g/d）

Annexed Table 2-9　Dietary intakes of saturated fatty acids from the 6th China TDS (Unit: g/d)

| 膳食类别 Category | 黑龙江 HL | 辽宁 LN | 河北 HE | 北京 BJ | 吉林 JL | 山西 SX | 陕西 SN | 河南 HA | 宁夏 NX | 内蒙古 NM | 青海 QH | 甘肃 GS | 上海 SH | 福建 FJ | 江西 JX | 江苏 JS | 浙江 ZJ | 山东 SD | 湖北 HB | 四川 SC | 广西 GX | 湖南 HN | 广东 GD | 贵州 GZ | 全国平均 AVG |
|---|---|---|---|---|---|---|---|---|---|---|---|---|---|---|---|---|---|---|---|---|---|---|---|---|---|
| 谷类 Cereals | 2.87 | 1.35 | 2.97 | 2.85 | 1.75 | 3.10 | 2.15 | 3.08 | 1.66 | 7.06 | 2.94 | 1.96 | 1.62 | 1.91 | 1.59 | 1.68 | 1.67 | 2.79 | 1.77 | 3.35 | 2.44 | 1.04 | 1.43 | 1.87 | 2.37 |
| 豆类 Legumes | 0.81 | 3.51 | 1.01 | 0.91 | 1.32 | 0.99 | 1.17 | 0.86 | 0.47 | 0.91 | 0.06 | 0.56 | 0.75 | 1.26 | 1.43 | 1.36 | 1.52 | 0.94 | 1.43 | 0.68 | 0.61 | 0.84 | 0.52 | 1.06 | 1.04 |
| 薯类 Potatoes | 0.86 | 0.71 | 0.79 | 0.61 | 0.69 | 0.74 | 0.47 | 0.29 | 1.04 | 2.41 | 0.56 | 1.04 | 0.36 | 0.19 | 0.19 | 0.09 | 0.13 | 0.27 | 0.98 | 0.68 | 0.08 | 0.46 | 0.01 | 0.80 | 0.60 |
| 肉类 Meats | 6.78 | 3.60 | 3.36 | 5.07 | 8.08 | 18.73 | 3.42 | 4.57 | 5.19 | 9.15 | 6.48 | 3.17 | 6.83 | 5.37 | 7.77 | 9.13 | 9.45 | 6.99 | 5.32 | 17.12 | 13.45 | 12.95 | 5.09 | 12.96 | 7.92 |
| 蛋类 Eggs | 1.33 | 1.24 | 1.32 | 1.69 | 1.22 | 0.94 | 0.79 | 1.06 | 0.76 | 1.12 | 0.63 | 0.73 | 1.19 | 0.67 | 0.63 | 0.88 | 0.77 | 1.56 | 1.14 | 0.57 | 0.51 | 0.76 | 0.43 | 0.62 | 0.94 |
| 水产类 Aquatic foods | 0.52 | 0.17 | 0.10 | 0.24 | 0.24 | 0.08 | 0.06 | 0.06 | 0.04 | 0.12 | 0.06 | 0.04 | 1.17 | 0.99 | 0.66 | 0.46 | 0.95 | 0.38 | 0.52 | 0.14 | 1.98 | 0.88 | 1.05 | 0.09 | 0.46 |
| 乳类 Dairy products | 0.29 | 0.97 | 0.57 | 1.93 | 0.75 | 0.80 | 0.59 | 0.44 | 0.35 | 0.63 | 1.22 | 0.28 | 1.47 | 0.81 | 0.47 | 0.57 | 0.73 | 0.48 | 0.19 | 0.28 | 0.39 | 0.40 | 0.75 | 0.68 | 0.67 |
| 蔬菜类 Vegetables | 3.11 | 2.73 | 4.20 | 2.63 | 2.67 | 2.70 | 2.17 | 2.25 | 1.71 | 3.19 | 2.42 | 2.34 | 3.33 | 5.51 | 5.84 | 2.45 | 3.43 | 4.14 | 8.49 | 1.51 | 2.34 | 4.69 | 2.16 | 6.09 | 3.42 |
| 水果类 Fruits | 0.00 | 0.01 | 0.00 | 0.01 | 0.01 | 0.00 | 0.00 | 0.00 | 0.00 | 0.01 | 0.00 | 0.00 | 0.01 | 0.01 | 0.00 | 0.00 | 0.00 | 0.01 | 0.00 | 0.00 | 0.01 | 0.01 | 0.00 | 0.00 | 0.01 |
| 合计 SUM | 16.60 | 14.29 | 14.32 | 15.95 | 16.71 | 28.10 | 10.81 | 12.62 | 11.22 | 24.60 | 14.38 | 10.12 | 16.73 | 16.72 | 18.57 | 16.63 | 18.65 | 17.54 | 19.83 | 24.33 | 21.81 | 22.01 | 11.45 | 24.16 | 17.42 |

附表 2-10 第六次中国总膳食研究的单不饱和脂肪酸膳食摄入量（单位：g/d）

Annexed Table 2-10 Dietary intakes of monounsaturated fatty acids from the 6th China TDS (Unit: g/d)

| 膳食类别 Category | 黑龙江 HL | 辽宁 LN | 河北 HE | 北京 BJ | 吉林 JL | 山西 SX | 陕西 SN | 河南 HA | 宁夏 NX | 内蒙古 NM | 青海 QH | 甘肃 GS | 上海 SH | 福建 FJ | 江西 JX | 江苏 JS | 浙江 ZJ | 山东 SD | 湖北 HB | 四川 SC | 广西 GX | 湖南 HN | 广东 GD | 贵州 GZ | 全国平均 AVG |
|---|---|---|---|---|---|---|---|---|---|---|---|---|---|---|---|---|---|---|---|---|---|---|---|---|---|
| 谷类 Cereals | 3.11 | 0.99 | 4.09 | 3.44 | 1.62 | 3.70 | 5.00 | 3.16 | 2.40 | 9.25 | 1.94 | 1.69 | 1.73 | 1.66 | 1.69 | 2.47 | 1.57 | 2.74 | 2.43 | 4.81 | 2.11 | 1.51 | 1.53 | 1.53 | 2.76 |
| 豆类 Legumes | 1.32 | 5.68 | 1.96 | 2.00 | 1.94 | 1.74 | 3.77 | 1.29 | 0.95 | 1.28 | 0.14 | 2.04 | 1.30 | 2.07 | 3.08 | 3.51 | 2.60 | 1.73 | 2.72 | 2.58 | 1.12 | 2.53 | 0.91 | 3.14 | 2.14 |
| 薯类 Potatoes | 1.09 | 0.95 | 1.76 | 1.30 | 0.97 | 1.56 | 3.91 | 0.42 | 2.55 | 2.82 | 4.30 | 9.07 | 0.92 | 0.42 | 0.33 | 0.68 | 0.18 | 0.56 | 2.07 | 2.45 | 0.16 | 1.86 | 0.00 | 2.18 | 1.77 |
| 肉类 Meats | 7.64 | 4.35 | 4.54 | 6.66 | 9.39 | 22.98 | 5.49 | 5.24 | 6.33 | 9.94 | 9.08 | 5.77 | 9.45 | 7.20 | 9.42 | 14.65 | 12.57 | 9.08 | 6.86 | 21.54 | 16.55 | 20.11 | 6.59 | 17.70 | 10.38 |
| 蛋类 Eggs | 1.77 | 1.71 | 2.18 | 2.67 | 1.72 | 1.52 | 1.98 | 1.45 | 1.22 | 1.65 | 1.73 | 2.32 | 1.92 | 1.10 | 0.94 | 2.10 | 1.21 | 2.54 | 1.80 | 1.23 | 0.77 | 1.72 | 0.56 | 1.22 | 1.63 |
| 水产类 Aquatic foods | 0.93 | 0.23 | 0.19 | 0.46 | 0.40 | 0.11 | 0.22 | 0.10 | 0.07 | 0.23 | 0.20 | 0.10 | 2.22 | 2.03 | 1.30 | 1.47 | 1.91 | 0.61 | 1.99 | 0.41 | 2.77 | 3.55 | 1.60 | 0.21 | 0.97 |
| 乳类 Dairy products | 0.10 | 0.34 | 0.19 | 0.67 | 0.25 | 0.29 | 0.19 | 0.16 | 0.12 | 0.21 | 0.40 | 0.09 | 0.48 | 0.27 | 0.18 | 0.21 | 0.24 | 0.18 | 0.06 | 0.09 | 0.12 | 0.15 | 0.26 | 0.21 | 0.23 |
| 蔬菜类 Vegetables | 3.92 | 3.75 | 9.05 | 5.52 | 3.65 | 5.49 | 12.93 | 3.21 | 4.21 | 4.03 | 16.76 | 19.08 | 8.31 | 9.71 | 8.77 | 16.76 | 9.13 | 8.50 | 16.14 | 12.13 | 4.95 | 21.03 | 4.50 | 13.32 | 9.37 |
| 水果类 Fruits | 0.00 | 0.00 | 0.00 | 0.00 | 0.01 | 0.00 | 0.00 | 0.00 | 0.00 | 0.00 | 0.00 | 0.00 | 0.00 | 0.00 | 0.00 | 0.00 | 0.00 | 0.00 | 0.00 | 0.00 | 0.00 | 0.01 | 0.00 | 0.00 | 0.00 |
| 合计 SUM | 19.87 | 18.01 | 23.95 | 22.72 | 19.96 | 37.39 | 33.50 | 15.03 | 17.86 | 29.41 | 34.56 | 40.16 | 26.34 | 24.45 | 25.71 | 41.84 | 29.41 | 25.94 | 34.08 | 45.25 | 28.55 | 52.46 | 15.95 | 39.51 | 29.25 |

附表 2-11　第六次中国总膳食研究的 n-6 多不饱和脂肪酸膳食摄入量（单位：g/d）

Annexed Table 2-11　Dietary intakes of n-6 polyunsaturated fatty acids from the 6th China TDS (Unit: g/d)

| 膳食类别 Category | 黑龙江 HL | 辽宁 LN | 河北 HE | 北京 BJ | 吉林 JL | 山西 SX | 陕西 SN | 河南 HA | 宁夏 NX | 内蒙古 NM | 青海 QH | 甘肃 GS | 上海 SH | 福建 FJ | 江西 JX | 江苏 JS | 浙江 ZJ | 山东 SD | 湖北 HB | 四川 SC | 广西 GX | 湖南 HN | 广东 GD | 贵州 GZ | 全国平均 AVG |
|---|---|---|---|---|---|---|---|---|---|---|---|---|---|---|---|---|---|---|---|---|---|---|---|---|---|
| 谷类 Cereals | 7.20 | 2.07 | 5.34 | 5.05 | 3.58 | 6.16 | 3.86 | 6.24 | 2.86 | 9.79 | 3.94 | 3.62 | 2.79 | 2.01 | 2.49 | 2.00 | 2.25 | 4.78 | 2.76 | 2.93 | 1.98 | 0.98 | 1.49 | 1.53 | 3.65 |
| 豆类 Legumes | 2.11 | 9.17 | 2.02 | 1.93 | 3.58 | 2.31 | 4.65 | 2.17 | 1.09 | 1.68 | 0.17 | 1.54 | 2.16 | 2.51 | 3.19 | 3.21 | 4.10 | 2.06 | 3.02 | 1.72 | 1.28 | 2.46 | 1.01 | 2.79 | 2.58 |
| 薯类 Potatoes | 2.81 | 1.94 | 1.34 | 1.00 | 2.21 | 1.26 | 1.17 | 0.93 | 2.22 | 2.42 | 1.48 | 2.73 | 1.44 | 0.28 | 0.38 | 0.21 | 0.17 | 0.45 | 1.57 | 1.75 | 0.12 | 0.91 | 0.02 | 0.78 | 1.23 |
| 肉类 Meats | 4.24 | 2.99 | 2.18 | 2.92 | 3.55 | 9.34 | 1.57 | 2.98 | 2.04 | 4.28 | 3.52 | 1.93 | 5.73 | 2.84 | 3.69 | 5.27 | 7.23 | 3.78 | 3.09 | 6.94 | 6.33 | 7.05 | 2.75 | 5.54 | 4.24 |
| 蛋类 Eggs | 1.55 | 1.50 | 1.09 | 1.57 | 1.26 | 0.80 | 0.69 | 1.10 | 0.81 | 1.14 | 0.58 | 0.72 | 1.40 | 0.56 | 0.62 | 0.68 | 0.69 | 1.33 | 1.03 | 0.40 | 0.33 | 0.59 | 0.21 | 0.42 | 0.88 |
| 水产类 Aquatic foods | 0.83 | 0.19 | 0.14 | 0.34 | 0.51 | 0.07 | 0.09 | 0.13 | 0.05 | 0.30 | 0.09 | 0.04 | 2.13 | 1.27 | 1.01 | 0.76 | 1.51 | 0.39 | 0.80 | 0.18 | 1.79 | 1.28 | 0.97 | 0.10 | 0.62 |
| 乳类 Dairy products | 0.01 | 0.06 | 0.02 | 0.07 | 0.03 | 0.03 | 0.02 | 0.02 | 0.02 | 0.03 | 0.05 | 0.01 | 0.07 | 0.04 | 0.02 | 0.02 | 0.03 | 0.02 | 0.01 | 0.01 | 0.01 | 0.02 | 0.03 | 0.03 | 0.03 |
| 蔬菜类 Vegetables | 9.92 | 7.82 | 6.87 | 4.43 | 8.35 | 4.29 | 3.95 | 7.10 | 3.71 | 4.68 | 6.22 | 5.40 | 12.94 | 5.98 | 8.76 | 5.98 | 10.76 | 6.82 | 11.43 | 3.52 | 3.61 | 6.54 | 2.96 | 4.90 | 6.54 |
| 水果类 Fruits | 0.00 | 0.01 | 0.00 | 0.01 | 0.01 | 0.01 | 0.00 | 0.00 | 0.01 | 0.01 | 0.00 | 0.00 | 0.01 | 0.01 | 0.01 | 0.00 | 0.00 | 0.01 | 0.00 | 0.00 | 0.00 | 0.00 | 0.00 | 0.00 | 0.01 |
| 合计 SUM | 28.67 | 25.73 | 19.00 | 17.32 | 23.06 | 24.27 | 16.01 | 20.67 | 12.80 | 24.32 | 16.07 | 16.00 | 28.67 | 15.51 | 20.17 | 18.14 | 26.75 | 19.64 | 23.72 | 17.45 | 15.46 | 19.83 | 9.44 | 16.09 | 19.78 |

附表 2-12　第六次中国总膳食研究的 n-3 多不饱和脂肪酸膳食摄入量（单位：g/d）

Annexed Table 2-12　Dietary intakes of n-3 polyunsaturated fatty acids from the 6<sup>th</sup> China TDS (Unit: g/d)

| 膳食类别 Category | 黑龙江 HL | 辽宁 LN | 河北 HE | 北京 BJ | 吉林 JL | 山西 SX | 陕西 SN | 河南 HA | 宁夏 NX | 内蒙古 NM | 青海 QH | 甘肃 GS | 上海 SH | 福建 FJ | 江西 JX | 江苏 JS | 浙江 ZJ | 山东 SD | 湖北 HB | 四川 SC | 广西 GX | 湖南 HN | 广东 GD | 贵州 GZ | 全国平均 AVG |
|---|---|---|---|---|---|---|---|---|---|---|---|---|---|---|---|---|---|---|---|---|---|---|---|---|---|
| 谷类 Cereals | 0.78 | 0.13 | 0.16 | 0.34 | 0.32 | 0.25 | 0.50 | 0.44 | 0.27 | 1.82 | 0.30 | 0.65 | 0.16 | 0.10 | 0.20 | 0.25 | 0.15 | 0.21 | 0.12 | 0.37 | 0.07 | 0.14 | 0.04 | 0.09 | 0.33 |
| 豆类 Legumes | 0.28 | 0.93 | 0.13 | 0.15 | 0.50 | 0.23 | 0.92 | 0.26 | 0.57 | 0.13 | 0.04 | 0.31 | 0.24 | 0.22 | 0.30 | 0.46 | 0.50 | 0.15 | 0.25 | 0.37 | 0.12 | 0.52 | 0.09 | 0.59 | 0.34 |
| 薯类 Potatoes | 0.43 | 0.25 | 0.01 | 0.00 | 0.28 | 0.01 | 0.38 | 0.10 | 2.98 | 0.04 | 0.54 | 1.02 | 0.07 | 0.00 | 0.04 | 0.07 | 0.01 | 0.00 | 0.01 | 0.32 | 0.00 | 0.16 | 0.00 | 0.19 | 0.29 |
| 肉类 Meats | 0.50 | 0.37 | 0.06 | 0.12 | 0.34 | 0.46 | 0.26 | 0.28 | 1.66 | 0.21 | 0.54 | 0.35 | 0.35 | 0.16 | 0.26 | 0.71 | 0.59 | 0.15 | 0.12 | 0.77 | 0.30 | 0.98 | 0.09 | 0.65 | 0.43 |
| 蛋类 Eggs | 0.20 | 0.18 | 0.02 | 0.04 | 0.14 | 0.02 | 0.14 | 0.12 | 0.62 | 0.03 | 0.15 | 0.20 | 0.07 | 0.02 | 0.11 | 0.15 | 0.06 | 0.04 | 0.02 | 0.09 | 0.01 | 0.13 | 0.01 | 0.08 | 0.11 |
| 水产类 Aquatic foods | 0.19 | 0.08 | 0.02 | 0.03 | 0.09 | 0.02 | 0.03 | 0.02 | 0.03 | 0.02 | 0.03 | 0.01 | 0.46 | 0.10 | 0.14 | 0.22 | 0.30 | 0.11 | 0.27 | 0.09 | 0.24 | 0.62 | 0.24 | 0.03 | 0.14 |
| 乳类 Dairy products | 0.00 | 0.05 | 0.00 | 0.02 | 0.00 | 0.01 | 0.01 | 0.00 | 0.00 | 0.00 | 0.01 | 0.00 | 0.01 | 0.00 | 0.00 | 0.00 | 0.00 | 0.00 | 0.00 | 0.00 | 0.00 | 0.00 | 0.00 | 0.00 | 0.01 |
| 蔬菜类 Vegetables | 1.73 | 1.19 | 0.13 | 0.09 | 1.28 | 0.11 | 1.30 | 0.93 | 4.51 | 0.10 | 1.78 | 1.39 | 0.78 | 0.24 | 1.10 | 1.71 | 1.28 | 0.17 | 0.21 | 1.43 | 0.21 | 2.15 | 0.22 | 1.16 | 1.05 |
| 水果类 Fruits | 0.00 | 0.00 | 0.00 | 0.00 | 0.00 | 0.00 | 0.00 | 0.00 | 0.00 | 0.00 | 0.00 | 0.00 | 0.00 | 0.00 | 0.00 | 0.00 | 0.00 | 0.00 | 0.00 | 0.00 | 0.00 | 0.00 | 0.00 | 0.00 | 0.00 |
| 合计 SUM | 4.12 | 3.18 | 0.53 | 0.79 | 2.95 | 1.11 | 3.52 | 2.15 | 10.65 | 2.35 | 3.39 | 3.94 | 2.13 | 0.84 | 2.15 | 3.59 | 2.89 | 0.83 | 1.00 | 3.43 | 0.95 | 4.71 | 0.71 | 2.78 | 2.70 |

附表 2-13 第六次中国总膳食研究的反式脂肪酸膳食摄入量（单位：g/d）

Annexed Table 2-13 Dietary intakes of *trans*-fatty acids from the 6th China TDS (Unit: g/d)

| 膳食类别<br>Category | 黑龙江<br>HL | 辽宁<br>LN | 河北<br>HE | 北京<br>BJ | 吉林<br>JL | 山西<br>SX | 陕西<br>SN | 河南<br>HA | 宁夏<br>NX | 内蒙古<br>NM | 青海<br>QH | 甘肃<br>GS | 上海<br>SH | 福建<br>FJ | 江西<br>JX | 江苏<br>JS | 浙江<br>ZJ | 山东<br>SD | 湖北<br>HB | 四川<br>SC | 广西<br>GX | 湖南<br>HN | 广东<br>GD | 贵州<br>GZ | 全国平均<br>AVG |
|---|---|---|---|---|---|---|---|---|---|---|---|---|---|---|---|---|---|---|---|---|---|---|---|---|---|
| 谷类 Cereals | 0.07 | 0.03 | 0.05 | 0.12 | 0.07 | 0.05 | 0.16 | 0.13 | 0.07 | 0.14 | 0.14 | 0.05 | 0.08 | 0.04 | 0.06 | 0.06 | 0.04 | 0.08 | 0.04 | 0.06 | 0.01 | 0.02 | 0.03 | 0.03 | 0.07 |
| 豆类 Legumes | 0.01 | 0.03 | 0.01 | 0.00 | 0.01 | 0.01 | 0.08 | 0.02 | 0.02 | 0.00 | 0.00 | 0.04 | 0.02 | 0.02 | 0.02 | 0.03 | 0.04 | 0.00 | 0.00 | 0.04 | 0.00 | 0.02 | 0.01 | 0.03 | 0.02 |
| 薯类 Potatoes | 0.02 | 0.01 | 0.01 | 0.00 | 0.01 | 0.00 | 0.14 | 0.02 | 0.16 | 0.02 | 0.05 | 0.28 | 0.02 | 0.00 | 0.01 | 0.00 | 0.00 | 0.00 | 0.00 | 0.03 | 0.00 | 0.02 | 0.00 | 0.02 | 0.03 |
| 肉类 Meats | 0.10 | 0.11 | 0.04 | 0.12 | 0.01 | 0.22 | 0.12 | 0.09 | 0.22 | 0.30 | 0.14 | 0.06 | 0.09 | 0.03 | 0.05 | 0.09 | 0.12 | 0.08 | 0.03 | 0.33 | 0.09 | 0.07 | 0.07 | 0.20 | 0.12 |
| 蛋类 Eggs | 0.02 | 0.01 | 0.01 | 0.01 | 0.01 | 0.01 | 0.05 | 0.02 | 0.04 | 0.01 | 0.01 | 0.05 | 0.03 | 0.01 | 0.01 | 0.01 | 0.02 | 0.01 | 0.01 | 0.01 | 0.01 | 0.02 | 0.00 | 0.01 | 0.02 |
| 水产类 Aquatic foods | 0.01 | 0.00 | 0.00 | 0.00 | 0.00 | 0.00 | 0.01 | 0.00 | 0.00 | 0.00 | 0.00 | 0.00 | 0.05 | 0.02 | 0.03 | 0.02 | 0.05 | 0.01 | 0.06 | 0.01 | 0.02 | 0.04 | 0.02 | 0.00 | 0.01 |
| 乳类 Dairy products | 0.02 | 0.03 | 0.03 | 0.14 | 0.04 | 0.04 | 0.04 | 0.02 | 0.02 | 0.03 | 0.06 | 0.01 | 0.08 | 0.05 | 0.03 | 0.03 | 0.04 | 0.03 | 0.01 | 0.01 | 0.02 | 0.02 | 0.05 | 0.03 | 0.04 |
| 蔬菜类 Vegetables | 0.08 | 0.06 | 0.06 | 0.03 | 0.06 | 0.04 | 0.44 | 0.18 | 0.25 | 0.05 | 0.13 | 0.55 | 0.31 | 0.12 | 0.30 | 0.37 | 0.39 | 0.08 | 0.17 | 0.27 | 0.04 | 0.27 | 0.05 | 0.19 | 0.19 |
| 水果类 Fruits | 0.00 | 0.00 | 0.00 | 0.00 | 0.00 | 0.00 | 0.00 | 0.00 | 0.00 | 0.00 | 0.00 | 0.00 | 0.00 | 0.00 | 0.00 | 0.00 | 0.00 | 0.00 | 0.00 | 0.00 | 0.00 | 0.00 | 0.00 | 0.00 | 0.00 |
| 合计 SUM | 0.32 | 0.28 | 0.21 | 0.42 | 0.22 | 0.37 | 1.03 | 0.50 | 0.77 | 0.56 | 0.53 | 1.05 | 0.68 | 0.28 | 0.52 | 0.63 | 0.69 | 0.29 | 0.33 | 0.75 | 0.21 | 0.49 | 0.23 | 0.51 | 0.49 |

附表 2-14 第六次中国总膳食研究总脂肪酸的膳食来源（单位：%）

Annexed Table 2-14 Dietary sources of total fatty acids from the 6$^{th}$ China TDS (Unit: %)

| 膳食类别<br>Category | 黑龙江<br>HL | 辽宁<br>LN | 河北<br>HE | 北京<br>BJ | 吉林<br>JL | 山西<br>SX | 陕西<br>SN | 河南<br>HA | 宁夏<br>NX | 内蒙古<br>NM | 青海<br>QH | 甘肃<br>GS | 上海<br>SH | 福建<br>FJ | 江西<br>JX | 江苏<br>JS | 浙江<br>ZJ | 山东<br>SD | 湖北<br>HB | 四川<br>SC | 广西<br>GX | 湖南<br>HN | 广东<br>GD | 贵州<br>GZ | 全国平均<br>AVG |
|---|---|---|---|---|---|---|---|---|---|---|---|---|---|---|---|---|---|---|---|---|---|---|---|---|---|
| 谷类 Cereals | 20.2 | 7.4 | 21.8 | 20.6 | 11.7 | 14.5 | 18.0 | 25.6 | 13.6 | 34.5 | 13.4 | 11.2 | 8.5 | 9.9 | 9.0 | 8.0 | 7.3 | 16.5 | 9.0 | 12.6 | 9.9 | 3.7 | 12.0 | 6.1 | 13.2 |
| 豆类 Legumes | 6.5 | 31.4 | 8.9 | 8.7 | 11.7 | 5.8 | 16.3 | 9.0 | 5.8 | 4.9 | 0.6 | 6.3 | 6.0 | 10.5 | 11.9 | 10.6 | 11.2 | 7.6 | 9.4 | 5.9 | 4.7 | 6.4 | 6.7 | 9.2 | 8.8 |
| 薯类 Potatoes | 7.5 | 6.3 | 6.7 | 5.1 | 6.6 | 3.9 | 9.4 | 3.5 | 16.8 | 9.5 | 10.1 | 19.8 | 3.8 | 1.5 | 1.4 | 1.3 | 0.6 | 2.0 | 5.9 | 5.7 | 0.5 | 3.4 | 0.1 | 4.8 | 5.6 |
| 肉类 Meats | 27.7 | 18.6 | 17.5 | 26.0 | 34.0 | 56.7 | 16.7 | 25.8 | 29.0 | 29.4 | 28.7 | 15.8 | 30.1 | 27.0 | 31.6 | 36.9 | 38.2 | 31.2 | 19.5 | 51.2 | 54.8 | 41.4 | 38.6 | 44.6 | 33.1 |
| 蛋类 Eggs | 7.0 | 7.6 | 8.0 | 10.4 | 6.9 | 3.6 | 5.6 | 7.4 | 6.5 | 4.9 | 4.5 | 5.6 | 6.2 | 4.1 | 3.4 | 4.7 | 3.5 | 8.5 | 5.1 | 2.5 | 2.4 | 3.2 | 3.2 | 2.8 | 5.1 |
| 水产类 Aquatic foods | 3.6 | 1.1 | 0.8 | 1.9 | 2.0 | 0.3 | 0.6 | 0.6 | 0.4 | 0.8 | 0.6 | 0.3 | 8.1 | 7.6 | 4.7 | 3.6 | 6.0 | 2.3 | 4.6 | 0.9 | 10.2 | 6.4 | 10.3 | 0.5 | 3.2 |
| 乳类 Dairy products | 0.6 | 2.3 | 1.4 | 4.9 | 1.7 | 1.3 | 1.3 | 1.3 | 1.0 | 1.1 | 2.5 | 0.6 | 2.8 | 2.0 | 1.1 | 1.0 | 1.3 | 1.1 | 0.4 | 0.4 | 0.8 | 0.6 | 2.9 | 1.1 | 1.4 |
| 蔬菜类 Vegetables | 27.0 | 25.3 | 35.0 | 22.2 | 25.5 | 13.8 | 32.0 | 26.8 | 27.0 | 14.8 | 39.6 | 40.4 | 34.4 | 37.3 | 36.9 | 33.8 | 31.9 | 30.7 | 46.2 | 20.7 | 16.6 | 34.9 | 26.2 | 30.9 | 29.5 |
| 水果类 Fruits | 0.0 | 0.0 | 0.0 | 0.0 | 0.0 | 0.0 | 0.0 | 0.0 | 0.0 | 0.0 | 0.0 | 0.0 | 0.0 | 0.0 | 0.0 | 0.0 | 0.0 | 0.0 | 0.0 | 0.0 | 0.0 | 0.0 | 0.0 | 0.0 | 0.0 |

附表 2-15　第六次中国总膳食研究饱和脂肪酸的膳食来源（单位：%）

Annexed Table 2-15　Dietary sources of saturated fatty acids from the 6$^{th}$ China TDS (Unit: %)

| 膳食类别<br>Category | 黑龙江<br>HL | 辽宁<br>LN | 河北<br>HE | 北京<br>BJ | 吉林<br>JL | 山西<br>SX | 陕西<br>SN | 河南<br>HA | 宁夏<br>NX | 内蒙古<br>NM | 青海<br>QH | 甘肃<br>GS | 上海<br>SH | 福建<br>FJ | 江西<br>JX | 江苏<br>JS | 浙江<br>ZJ | 山东<br>SD | 湖北<br>HB | 四川<br>SC | 广西<br>GX | 湖南<br>HN | 广东<br>GD | 贵州<br>GZ | 全国平均<br>AVG |
|---|---|---|---|---|---|---|---|---|---|---|---|---|---|---|---|---|---|---|---|---|---|---|---|---|---|
| 谷类 Cereals | 17.3 | 9.4 | 20.8 | 17.9 | 10.4 | 11.0 | 19.9 | 24.4 | 14.8 | 28.7 | 20.5 | 19.4 | 9.7 | 11.4 | 8.6 | 10.1 | 9.0 | 15.9 | 8.9 | 13.8 | 11.2 | 4.7 | 12.5 | 7.7 | 13.6 |
| 豆类 Legumes | 4.9 | 24.5 | 7.1 | 5.7 | 7.9 | 3.5 | 10.8 | 6.9 | 4.2 | 3.7 | 0.4 | 5.5 | 4.5 | 7.5 | 7.7 | 8.2 | 8.2 | 5.3 | 7.2 | 2.8 | 2.8 | 3.8 | 4.6 | 4.4 | 6.0 |
| 薯类 Potatoes | 5.2 | 4.9 | 5.5 | 3.8 | 4.1 | 2.6 | 4.4 | 2.3 | 9.3 | 9.8 | 3.9 | 10.3 | 2.1 | 1.1 | 1.0 | 0.5 | 0.7 | 1.5 | 4.9 | 2.8 | 0.4 | 2.1 | 0.1 | 3.3 | 3.5 |
| 肉类 Meats | 40.9 | 25.2 | 23.4 | 31.8 | 48.4 | 66.7 | 31.6 | 36.2 | 46.3 | 37.2 | 45.1 | 31.4 | 40.8 | 32.1 | 41.8 | 54.9 | 50.6 | 39.8 | 26.8 | 70.4 | 61.7 | 58.8 | 44.4 | 53.6 | 45.4 |
| 蛋类 Eggs | 8.0 | 8.7 | 9.2 | 10.6 | 7.3 | 3.3 | 7.3 | 8.4 | 6.7 | 4.5 | 4.4 | 7.2 | 7.1 | 4.0 | 3.4 | 5.3 | 4.1 | 8.9 | 5.7 | 2.3 | 2.4 | 3.4 | 3.8 | 2.6 | 5.4 |
| 水产类 Aquatic foods | 3.2 | 1.2 | 0.7 | 1.5 | 1.4 | 0.3 | 0.5 | 0.5 | 0.3 | 0.5 | 0.4 | 0.4 | 7.0 | 5.9 | 3.5 | 2.8 | 5.1 | 2.2 | 2.6 | 0.6 | 9.1 | 4.0 | 9.1 | 0.4 | 2.6 |
| 乳类 Dairy products | 1.8 | 6.8 | 4.0 | 12.1 | 4.5 | 2.9 | 5.5 | 3.5 | 3.1 | 2.6 | 8.5 | 2.8 | 8.8 | 4.8 | 2.6 | 3.4 | 3.9 | 2.7 | 1.0 | 1.2 | 1.8 | 1.8 | 6.6 | 2.8 | 3.8 |
| 蔬菜类 Vegetables | 18.8 | 19.1 | 29.3 | 16.5 | 16.0 | 9.6 | 20.0 | 17.8 | 15.2 | 13.0 | 16.8 | 23.1 | 19.9 | 33.0 | 31.4 | 14.8 | 18.4 | 23.6 | 42.8 | 6.2 | 10.7 | 21.3 | 18.9 | 25.2 | 19.6 |
| 水果类 Fruits | 0.0 | 0.1 | 0.0 | 0.1 | 0.0 | 0.0 | 0.0 | 0.0 | 0.0 | 0.0 | 0.0 | 0.0 | 0.1 | 0.0 | 0.0 | 0.0 | 0.0 | 0.0 | 0.0 | 0.0 | 0.0 | 0.0 | 0.0 | 0.0 | 0.0 |

附表 2-16　第六次中国总膳食研究单不饱和脂肪酸的膳食来源（单位：%）

Annexed Table 2-16　Dietary sources of monounsaturated fatty acids from the 6<sup>th</sup> China TDS (Unit: %)

| 膳食类别 Category | 黑龙江 HL | 辽宁 LN | 河北 HE | 北京 BJ | 吉林 JL | 山西 SX | 陕西 SN | 河南 HA | 宁夏 NX | 内蒙古 NM | 青海 QH | 甘肃 GS | 上海 SH | 福建 FJ | 江西 JX | 江苏 JS | 浙江 ZJ | 山东 SD | 湖北 HB | 四川 SC | 广西 GX | 湖南 HN | 广东 GD | 贵州 GZ | 全国平均 AVG |
|---|---|---|---|---|---|---|---|---|---|---|---|---|---|---|---|---|---|---|---|---|---|---|---|---|---|
| 谷类 Cereals | 15.7 | 5.5 | 17.1 | 15.1 | 8.1 | 9.9 | 14.9 | 21.0 | 13.5 | 31.4 | 5.6 | 4.2 | 6.6 | 6.8 | 6.6 | 5.9 | 5.4 | 10.6 | 7.1 | 10.6 | 7.4 | 2.9 | 9.6 | 3.9 | 9.4 |
| 豆类 Legumes | 6.6 | 31.6 | 8.2 | 8.8 | 9.7 | 4.7 | 11.3 | 8.6 | 5.3 | 4.4 | 0.4 | 5.1 | 4.9 | 8.5 | 12.0 | 8.4 | 8.9 | 6.7 | 8.0 | 5.7 | 3.9 | 4.8 | 5.7 | 8.0 | 7.3 |
| 薯类 Potatoes | 5.5 | 5.3 | 7.3 | 5.7 | 4.8 | 4.2 | 11.7 | 2.8 | 14.3 | 9.6 | 12.4 | 22.6 | 3.5 | 1.7 | 1.3 | 1.6 | 0.6 | 2.2 | 6.1 | 5.4 | 0.6 | 3.5 | 0.0 | 5.5 | 6.1 |
| 肉类 Meats | 38.4 | 24.2 | 18.9 | 29.3 | 47.1 | 61.5 | 16.4 | 34.9 | 35.4 | 33.8 | 26.3 | 14.4 | 35.9 | 29.4 | 36.6 | 35.0 | 42.7 | 35.0 | 20.1 | 47.6 | 58.0 | 38.3 | 41.3 | 44.8 | 35.5 |
| 蛋类 Eggs | 8.9 | 9.5 | 9.1 | 11.7 | 8.6 | 4.1 | 5.9 | 9.6 | 6.8 | 5.6 | 5.0 | 5.8 | 7.3 | 4.5 | 3.7 | 5.0 | 4.1 | 9.8 | 5.3 | 2.7 | 2.7 | 3.3 | 3.5 | 3.1 | 5.6 |
| 水产类 Aquatic foods | 4.7 | 1.3 | 0.8 | 2.0 | 2.0 | 0.3 | 0.7 | 0.6 | 0.4 | 0.8 | 0.6 | 0.2 | 8.4 | 8.3 | 5.1 | 3.5 | 6.5 | 2.3 | 5.8 | 0.9 | 9.7 | 6.8 | 10.0 | 0.5 | 3.3 |
| 乳类 Dairy products | 0.5 | 1.9 | 0.8 | 2.9 | 1.3 | 0.8 | 0.6 | 1.0 | 0.7 | 0.7 | 1.2 | 0.2 | 1.8 | 1.1 | 0.7 | 0.5 | 0.8 | 0.7 | 0.2 | 0.2 | 0.4 | 0.3 | 1.6 | 0.5 | 0.8 |
| 蔬菜类 Vegetables | 19.7 | 20.8 | 37.8 | 24.3 | 18.3 | 14.7 | 38.6 | 21.4 | 23.6 | 13.7 | 48.5 | 47.5 | 31.5 | 39.7 | 34.1 | 40.1 | 31.0 | 32.8 | 47.4 | 26.8 | 17.3 | 40.1 | 28.2 | 33.7 | 32.0 |
| 水果类 Fruits | 0.0 | 0.0 | 0.0 | 0.0 | 0.0 | 0.0 | 0.0 | 0.0 | 0.0 | 0.0 | 0.0 | 0.0 | 0.0 | 0.0 | 0.0 | 0.0 | 0.0 | 0.0 | 0.0 | 0.0 | 0.0 | 0.0 | 0.0 | 0.0 | 0.0 |

附表 2-17 第六次中国总膳食研究 n-6 多不饱和脂肪酸的膳食来源（单位：%）

Annexed Table 2-17 Dietary sources of n-6 polyunsaturated fatty acids from the 6th China TDS (Unit: %)

| 膳食类别 Category | 黑龙江 HL | 辽宁 LN | 河北 HE | 北京 BJ | 吉林 JL | 山西 SX | 陕西 SN | 河南 HA | 宁夏 NX | 内蒙古 NM | 青海 QH | 甘肃 GS | 上海 SH | 福建 FJ | 江西 JX | 江苏 JS | 浙江 ZJ | 山东 SD | 湖北 HB | 四川 SC | 广西 GX | 湖南 HN | 广东 GD | 贵州 GZ | 全国平均 AVG |
|---|---|---|---|---|---|---|---|---|---|---|---|---|---|---|---|---|---|---|---|---|---|---|---|---|---|
| 谷类 Cereals | 25.1 | 8.0 | 28.1 | 29.2 | 15.5 | 25.4 | 24.1 | 30.2 | 22.3 | 40.2 | 24.5 | 22.6 | 9.7 | 12.9 | 12.4 | 11.0 | 8.4 | 24.3 | 11.6 | 16.8 | 12.8 | 5.0 | 15.7 | 9.5 | 18.5 |
| 豆类 Legumes | 7.4 | 35.6 | 10.6 | 11.2 | 15.5 | 9.5 | 29.0 | 10.5 | 8.5 | 6.9 | 1.1 | 9.6 | 7.5 | 16.2 | 15.8 | 17.7 | 15.3 | 10.5 | 12.8 | 9.9 | 8.3 | 12.4 | 10.7 | 17.4 | 13.0 |
| 薯类 Potatoes | 9.8 | 7.5 | 7.0 | 5.8 | 9.6 | 5.2 | 7.3 | 4.5 | 17.4 | 9.9 | 9.2 | 17.1 | 5.0 | 1.8 | 1.9 | 1.2 | 0.6 | 2.3 | 6.6 | 10.0 | 0.8 | 4.6 | 0.2 | 4.8 | 6.2 |
| 肉类 Meats | 14.8 | 11.6 | 11.5 | 16.9 | 15.4 | 38.5 | 9.8 | 14.4 | 15.9 | 17.6 | 21.9 | 12.1 | 20.0 | 18.3 | 18.3 | 29.1 | 27.0 | 19.3 | 13.0 | 39.8 | 40.9 | 35.6 | 29.2 | 34.5 | 21.4 |
| 蛋类 Eggs | 5.4 | 5.8 | 5.7 | 9.0 | 5.5 | 3.3 | 4.3 | 5.3 | 6.3 | 4.7 | 3.6 | 4.5 | 4.9 | 3.6 | 3.1 | 3.7 | 2.6 | 6.8 | 4.3 | 2.3 | 2.1 | 3.0 | 2.2 | 2.6 | 4.4 |
| 水产类 Aquatic foods | 2.9 | 0.7 | 0.1 | 2.0 | 2.2 | 0.3 | 0.5 | 0.6 | 0.4 | 1.2 | 0.6 | 0.2 | 7.4 | 8.2 | 5.0 | 4.2 | 5.7 | 2.0 | 3.4 | 1.0 | 11.6 | 6.4 | 10.3 | 0.6 | 3.2 |
| 乳类 Dairy products | 0.0 | 0.2 | 0.1 | 0.4 | 0.1 | 0.1 | 0.1 | 0.1 | 0.1 | 0.1 | 0.3 | 0.1 | 0.2 | 0.2 | 0.1 | 0.1 | 0.1 | 0.1 | 0.0 | 0.1 | 0.1 | 0.1 | 0.3 | 0.2 | 0.1 |
| 蔬菜类 Vegetables | 34.6 | 30.4 | 36.2 | 25.6 | 36.2 | 17.7 | 24.7 | 34.4 | 29.0 | 19.3 | 38.7 | 33.8 | 45.1 | 38.6 | 43.5 | 33.0 | 40.2 | 34.7 | 48.2 | 20.2 | 23.3 | 33.0 | 31.4 | 30.4 | 33.1 |
| 水果类 Fruits | 0.0 | 0.0 | 0.0 | 0.0 | 0.0 | 0.0 | 0.0 | 0.0 | 0.1 | 0.0 | 0.0 | 0.0 | 0.0 | 0.0 | 0.0 | 0.0 | 0.0 | 0.0 | 0.0 | 0.0 | 0.0 | 0.0 | 0.0 | 0.0 | 0.0 |

附表 2-18 第六次中国总膳食研究 n-3 多不饱和脂肪酸的膳食来源（单位：%）

Annexed Table 2-18 Dietary sources of n-3 polyunsaturated fatty acids from the 6th China TDS (Unit: %)

| 膳食类别 Category | 黑龙江 HL | 辽宁 LN | 河北 HE | 北京 BJ | 吉林 JL | 山西 SX | 陕西 SN | 河南 HA | 宁夏 NX | 内蒙古 NM | 青海 QH | 甘肃 GS | 上海 SH | 福建 FJ | 江西 JX | 江苏 JS | 浙江 ZJ | 山东 SD | 湖北 HB | 四川 SC | 广西 GX | 湖南 HN | 广东 GD | 贵州 GZ | 全国平均 AVG |
|---|---|---|---|---|---|---|---|---|---|---|---|---|---|---|---|---|---|---|---|---|---|---|---|---|---|
| 谷类 Cereals | 18.9 | 4.2 | 30.7 | 43.0 | 10.7 | 22.2 | 14.2 | 20.4 | 2.5 | 77.4 | 8.9 | 16.5 | 7.3 | 11.6 | 9.2 | 7.1 | 5.2 | 25.4 | 12.3 | 10.6 | 6.9 | 3.0 | 6.3 | 3.1 | 12.1 |
| 豆类 Legumes | 6.9 | 29.3 | 24.5 | 18.8 | 16.9 | 20.7 | 26.0 | 12.0 | 5.4 | 5.7 | 1.1 | 7.8 | 11.1 | 25.5 | 13.9 | 12.9 | 17.2 | 18.3 | 24.9 | 10.7 | 12.9 | 11.0 | 12.4 | 21.1 | 12.7 |
| 薯类 Potatoes | 10.5 | 8.0 | 1.1 | 0.6 | 9.6 | 1.3 | 10.8 | 4.8 | 28.0 | 1.6 | 16.0 | 25.9 | 3.2 | 0.4 | 1.8 | 2.0 | 0.5 | 0.4 | 1.0 | 9.2 | 0.1 | 3.3 | 0.3 | 6.8 | 10.7 |
| 肉类 Meats | 12.1 | 11.5 | 11.2 | 15.3 | 11.6 | 41.3 | 7.3 | 13.0 | 15.6 | 8.8 | 16.0 | 8.9 | 16.3 | 18.5 | 12.2 | 19.8 | 20.5 | 17.5 | 11.7 | 22.4 | 31.6 | 20.8 | 12.4 | 23.3 | 15.9 |
| 蛋类 Eggs | 4.8 | 5.6 | 4.0 | 4.5 | 4.6 | 1.9 | 3.9 | 5.6 | 5.8 | 1.1 | 4.4 | 5.0 | 3.4 | 2.5 | 5.1 | 4.1 | 2.0 | 4.6 | 2.2 | 2.6 | 1.1 | 2.8 | 2.0 | 2.8 | 4.1 |
| 水产类 Aquatic foods | 4.6 | 2.4 | 4.2 | 4.3 | 2.9 | 2.1 | 0.8 | 1.1 | 0.3 | 0.9 | 0.8 | 0.4 | 21.7 | 12.3 | 6.5 | 6.2 | 10.2 | 12.8 | 26.6 | 2.7 | 24.8 | 13.2 | 34.2 | 1.0 | 5.2 |
| 乳类 Dairy products | 0.0 | 1.6 | 0.5 | 1.9 | 0.1 | 0.6 | 0.1 | 0.1 | 0.0 | 0.1 | 0.2 | 0.1 | 0.5 | 0.6 | 0.2 | 0.1 | 0.1 | 0.3 | 0.1 | 0.0 | 0.3 | 0.0 | 0.7 | 0.1 | 0.2 |
| 蔬菜类 Vegetables | 42.0 | 37.3 | 23.5 | 11.2 | 43.5 | 9.9 | 36.8 | 43.0 | 42.4 | 4.2 | 52.6 | 35.4 | 36.3 | 28.4 | 51.1 | 47.8 | 44.1 | 20.6 | 21.2 | 41.7 | 22.0 | 45.7 | 31.7 | 41.7 | 38.9 |
| 水果类 Fruits | 0.0 | 0.1 | 0.2 | 0.3 | 0.1 | 0.1 | 0.0 | 0.0 | 0.0 | 0.1 | 0.0 | 0.0 | 0.1 | 0.3 | 0.1 | 0.0 | 0.1 | 0.2 | 0.1 | 0.0 | 0.2 | 0.0 | 0.1 | 0.1 | 0.1 |

附表 2-19　第六次中国总膳食研究反式脂肪酸的膳食来源（单位：%）

Annexed Table 2-19　Dietary sources of *trans*-fatty acids from the 6$^{th}$ China TDS (Unit: %)

| 膳食类别<br>Category | 黑龙江<br>HL | 辽宁<br>LN | 河北<br>HE | 北京<br>BJ | 吉林<br>JL | 山西<br>SX | 陕西<br>SN | 河南<br>HA | 宁夏<br>NX | 内蒙古<br>NM | 青海<br>QH | 甘肃<br>GS | 上海<br>SH | 福建<br>FJ | 江西<br>JX | 江苏<br>JS | 浙江<br>ZJ | 山东<br>SD | 湖北<br>HB | 四川<br>SC | 广西<br>GX | 湖南<br>HN | 广东<br>GD | 贵州<br>GZ | 全国平均<br>AVG |
|---|---|---|---|---|---|---|---|---|---|---|---|---|---|---|---|---|---|---|---|---|---|---|---|---|---|
| 谷类<br>Cereals | 21.9 | 10.8 | 26.3 | 28.0 | 32.8 | 14.2 | 15.4 | 26.5 | 8.6 | 25.0 | 26.5 | 4.9 | 11.6 | 13.3 | 11.2 | 9.0 | 5.1 | 28.5 | 11.2 | 7.5 | 5.9 | 5.1 | 12.8 | 5.8 | 13.7 |
| 豆类<br>Legumes | 1.9 | 10.5 | 6.3 | 0.6 | 3.1 | 1.5 | 8.2 | 3.1 | 2.7 | 0.8 | 0.2 | 4.0 | 2.8 | 7.7 | 4.3 | 4.6 | 5.2 | 1.5 | 1.3 | 4.7 | 1.1 | 4.2 | 3.8 | 5.4 | 3.9 |
| 薯类<br>Potatoes | 6.4 | 4.7 | 2.6 | 0.5 | 6.3 | 1.1 | 13.8 | 4.7 | 20.3 | 3.0 | 8.7 | 26.3 | 3.2 | 0.8 | 2.4 | 0.4 | 0.7 | 0.6 | 1.4 | 3.7 | 0.4 | 3.4 | 0.0 | 4.6 | 7.1 |
| 肉类<br>Meats | 32.3 | 38.2 | 18.6 | 28.4 | 5.1 | 59.1 | 11.2 | 18.8 | 28.8 | 53.2 | 25.6 | 5.8 | 13.2 | 9.8 | 9.6 | 14.4 | 17.3 | 26.0 | 9.8 | 43.7 | 44.8 | 15.2 | 31.5 | 38.5 | 23.4 |
| 蛋类<br>Eggs | 5.1 | 4.3 | 4.9 | 3.2 | 5.9 | 2.2 | 4.6 | 4.8 | 4.8 | 2.5 | 2.6 | 4.9 | 4.2 | 2.4 | 2.5 | 3.8 | 2.6 | 4.8 | 2.1 | 2.0 | 2.6 | 3.3 | 1.4 | 2.2 | 3.6 |
| 水产类<br>Aquatic foods | 2.3 | 1.1 | 0.6 | 0.3 | 1.8 | 0.3 | 0.6 | 0.6 | 0.2 | 0.5 | 0.3 | 0.2 | 7.3 | 6.4 | 5.5 | 3.5 | 6.9 | 2.2 | 17.9 | 0.9 | 12.1 | 8.4 | 7.5 | 0.5 | 3.0 |
| 乳类<br>Dairy products | 5.8 | 9.1 | 14.0 | 32.3 | 18.7 | 11.9 | 3.4 | 4.7 | 2.3 | 6.0 | 10.6 | 1.3 | 12.4 | 16.2 | 5.7 | 5.3 | 6.4 | 10.3 | 3.6 | 1.9 | 11.3 | 4.9 | 20.6 | 6.0 | 7.5 |
| 蔬菜类<br>Vegetables | 24.3 | 21.3 | 26.7 | 6.8 | 26.4 | 9.7 | 42.9 | 36.8 | 32.3 | 9.0 | 25.5 | 52.6 | 45.4 | 43.4 | 58.7 | 58.8 | 55.8 | 26.0 | 52.7 | 35.7 | 21.9 | 55.5 | 22.4 | 37.0 | 37.9 |
| 水果类<br>Fruits | 0.0 | 0.0 | 0.0 | 0.0 | 0.0 | 0.0 | 0.0 | 0.0 | 0.0 | 0.0 | 0.0 | 0.0 | 0.0 | 0.0 | 0.0 | 0.0 | 0.0 | 0.0 | 0.0 | 0.0 | 0.0 | 0.0 | 0.0 | 0.0 | 0.0 |

# 第三章 附 表
# Annexed Tables of Chapter 3

附表 3-1 第六次中国总膳食研究膳食样品中钠的含量（单位：mg/g）

Annexed Table 3-1 Levels of sodium in food samples from the 6$^{th}$ China TDS (Unit: mg/g)

| 膳食类别<br>Category | 黑龙江<br>HL | 辽宁<br>LN | 河北<br>HE | 北京<br>BJ | 吉林<br>JL | 山西<br>SX | 陕西<br>SN | 河南<br>HA | 宁夏<br>NX | 内蒙古<br>NM | 青海<br>QH | 甘肃<br>GS | 上海<br>SH | 福建<br>FJ | 江西<br>JX | 江苏<br>JS | 浙江<br>ZJ | 山东<br>SD | 湖北<br>HB | 四川<br>SC | 广西<br>GX | 湖南<br>HN | 广东<br>GD | 贵州<br>GZ | 全国平均<br>AVG |
|---|---|---|---|---|---|---|---|---|---|---|---|---|---|---|---|---|---|---|---|---|---|---|---|---|---|
| 谷类 Cereals | 1.41 | 1.18 | 1.90 | 1.11 | 0.78 | 0.87 | 1.97 | 1.56 | 1.92 | 2.21 | 2.16 | 0.76 | 0.86 | 0.69 | 0.82 | 0.73 | 0.55 | 1.02 | 1.27 | 0.71 | 0.44 | 0.66 | 1.32 | 0.45 | 1.14 |
| 豆类 Legumes | 4.61 | 7.10 | 3.39 | 2.41 | 3.93 | 3.00 | 4.41 | 2.09 | 3.08 | 2.83 | 1.89 | 4.96 | 2.66 | 3.64 | 5.18 | 4.97 | 5.61 | 2.95 | 4.53 | 5.73 | 2.37 | 3.87 | 2.73 | 2.74 | 3.78 |
| 薯类 Potatoes | 3.94 | 5.48 | 8.38 | 4.81 | 3.07 | 4.25 | 5.91 | 3.34 | 5.69 | 4.36 | 3.75 | 6.77 | 4.58 | 3.04 | 3.30 | 4.83 | 3.80 | 4.68 | 4.19 | 4.51 | 5.49 | 3.24 | 0.60 | 5.22 | 4.47 |
| 肉类 Meats | 9.83 | 8.19 | 8.13 | 11.25 | 6.31 | 6.24 | 5.77 | 10.56 | 10.32 | 7.61 | 8.98 | 9.66 | 7.48 | 9.06 | 6.80 | 10.69 | 9.24 | 7.38 | 7.46 | 7.53 | 7.44 | 6.64 | 6.49 | 5.69 | 8.11 |
| 蛋类 Eggs | 6.86 | 9.51 | 9.76 | 7.19 | 5.61 | 5.73 | 6.40 | 8.10 | 6.29 | 1.45 | 9.93 | 7.00 | 6.17 | 8.00 | 5.69 | 10.15 | 14.78 | 8.90 | 8.35 | 6.45 | 9.06 | 7.93 | 5.40 | 4.81 | 7.48 |
| 水产类 Aquatic foods | 5.28 | 3.50 | 4.63 | 8.98 | 7.88 | 5.31 | 4.55 | 7.65 | 4.98 | 7.34 | 6.80 | 9.30 | 6.03 | 10.77 | 6.80 | 5.18 | 10.96 | 5.80 | 7.67 | 6.74 | 5.48 | 7.22 | 7.27 | 4.65 | 6.70 |
| 乳类 Dairy products | 0.39 | 0.37 | 0.35 | 0.44 | 0.36 | 0.41 | 0.52 | 0.32 | 0.35 | 0.30 | 0.31 | 0.33 | 0.28 | 0.36 | 0.32 | 0.30 | 0.33 | 0.40 | 0.41 | 0.38 | 0.42 | 0.33 | 0.40 | 0.31 | 0.36 |
| 蔬菜类 Vegetables | 5.36 | 7.14 | 4.97 | 7.61 | 3.42 | 3.27 | 4.83 | 7.00 | 3.96 | 4.14 | 5.46 | 6.30 | 4.42 | 7.35 | 4.12 | 7.47 | 7.04 | 5.91 | 5.27 | 7.50 | 5.71 | 7.15 | 5.35 | 3.29 | 5.59 |
| 水果类 Fruits | 0.01 | 0.02 | 0.02 | 0.03 | 0.01 | 0.01 | 0.02 | 0.01 | 0.02 | 0.01 | 0.01 | 0.01 | 0.01 | 0.01 | 0.00 | 0.01 | 0.02 | 0.00 | 0.01 | 0.02 | 0.03 | 0.03 | 0.01 | 0.00 | 0.01 |

续表

| 膳食类别<br>Category | 黑龙江<br>HL | 辽宁<br>LN | 河北<br>HE | 北京<br>BJ | 吉林<br>JL | 山西<br>SX | 陕西<br>SN | 河南<br>HA | 宁夏<br>NX | 内蒙古<br>NM | 青海<br>QH | 甘肃<br>GS | 上海<br>SH | 福建<br>FJ | 江西<br>JX | 江苏<br>JS | 浙江<br>ZJ | 山东<br>SD | 湖北<br>HB | 四川<br>SC | 广西<br>GX | 湖南<br>HN | 广东<br>GD | 贵州<br>GZ | 全国平均<br>AVG |
|---|---|---|---|---|---|---|---|---|---|---|---|---|---|---|---|---|---|---|---|---|---|---|---|---|---|
| 糖类<br>Sugar | 0.03 | 0.01 | 0.01 | 0.39 | 0.00 | 0.03 | 0.01 | 0.47 | 0.01 | 0.17 | 0.02 | 0.03 | 0.20 | 0.00 | 0.00 | 0.00 | 0.34 | 0.03 | 0.01 | 0.00 | 0.00 | 0.00 | 0.01 | 0.02 | 0.08 |
| 水及饮料类<br>Water and beverages | 0.01 | 0.05 | 0.01 | 0.02 | 0.01 | 0.03 | 0.02 | 0.02 | 0.04 | 0.03 | 0.01 | 0.02 | 0.02 | 0.01 | 0.02 | 0.04 | | 0.02 | 0.02 | 0.02 | 0.02 | 0.01 | 0.01 | 0.01 | 0.02 |
| 酒类<br>Alcohol beverages | 0.01 | 0.01 | 0.02 | 0.03 | 0.01 | 0.01 | 0.02 | 0.03 | 0.00 | 0.03 | 0.02 | 0.03 | 0.04 | 0.01 | 0.01 | 0.01 | 0.02 | 0.07 | 0.02 | 0.01 | 0.01 | 0.01 | 0.04 | 0.03 | 0.02 |

附表 3-2 第六次中国总膳食研究钠的膳食摄入量（单位：mg/d）

Annexed Table 3-2 Dietary intakes of sodium from the 6$^{th}$ China TDS (Unit: mg/d)

| 膳食类别<br>Category | 黑龙江<br>HL | 辽宁<br>LN | 河北<br>HE | 北京<br>BJ | 吉林<br>JL | 山西<br>SX | 陕西<br>SN | 河南<br>HA | 宁夏<br>NX | 内蒙古<br>NM | 青海<br>QH | 甘肃<br>GS | 上海<br>SH | 福建<br>FJ | 江西<br>JX | 江苏<br>JS | 浙江<br>ZJ | 山东<br>SD | 湖北<br>HB | 四川<br>SC | 广西<br>GX | 湖南<br>HN | 广东<br>GD | 贵州<br>GZ | 全国平均<br>AVG |
|---|---|---|---|---|---|---|---|---|---|---|---|---|---|---|---|---|---|---|---|---|---|---|---|---|---|
| 谷类<br>Cereals | 774.5 | 728.2 | 1438.7 | 882.9 | 454.5 | 903.7 | 1503.3 | 1444.0 | 1267.4 | 1594.9 | 1654.2 | 523.4 | 384.9 | 438.9 | 514.2 | 564.0 | 349.2 | 1011.5 | 673.0 | 690.2 | 415.0 | 382.1 | 604.7 | 304.8 | 812.6 |
| 豆类<br>Legumes | 209.3 | 865.9 | 193.3 | 244.7 | 296.6 | 208.2 | 365.4 | 112.6 | 108.4 | 112.8 | 12.2 | 204.4 | 312.3 | 285.9 | 382.0 | 412.1 | 790.8 | 154.8 | 302.8 | 387.3 | 100.3 | 281.0 | 76.1 | 278.4 | 279.0 |
| 薯类<br>Potatoes | 304.8 | 395.0 | 511.0 | 281.4 | 368.4 | 504.1 | 678.2 | 268.0 | 568.8 | 532.9 | 380.3 | 974.7 | 164.5 | 128.8 | 106.1 | 161.6 | 139.5 | 216.4 | 371.4 | 283.8 | 70.5 | 173.8 | 14.9 | 178.9 | 324.1 |
| 肉类<br>Meats | 588.5 | 547.1 | 385.1 | 757.2 | 420.0 | 856.4 | 208.0 | 584.6 | 481.7 | 559.3 | 637.6 | 299.6 | 828.3 | 778.9 | 638.3 | 980.8 | 1092.8 | 717.6 | 405.0 | 970.3 | 1122.7 | 992.1 | 676.0 | 605.8 | 672.2 |
| 蛋类<br>Eggs | 277.4 | 389.0 | 307.9 | 279.2 | 225.4 | 120.1 | 140.7 | 240.7 | 81.9 | 43.0 | 130.5 | 155.5 | 240.8 | 151.9 | 116.7 | 285.6 | 353.5 | 395.4 | 208.8 | 94.4 | 126.9 | 180.8 | 129.2 | 78.2 | 198.1 |

续表

| 膳食类别<br>Category | 黑龙江<br>HL | 辽宁<br>LN | 河北<br>HE | 北京<br>BJ | 吉林<br>JL | 山西<br>SX | 陕西<br>SN | 河南<br>HA | 宁夏<br>NX | 内蒙古<br>NM | 青海<br>QH | 甘肃<br>GS | 上海<br>SH | 福建<br>FJ | 江西<br>JX | 江苏<br>JS | 浙江<br>ZJ | 山东<br>SD | 湖北<br>HB | 四川<br>SC | 广西<br>GX | 湖南<br>HN | 广东<br>GD | 贵州<br>GZ | 全国平均<br>AVG |
|---|---|---|---|---|---|---|---|---|---|---|---|---|---|---|---|---|---|---|---|---|---|---|---|---|---|
| 水产类 Aquatic foods | 143.3 | 56.2 | 44.0 | 147.5 | 87.8 | 34.0 | 18.7 | 35.4 | 12.1 | 75.8 | 24.2 | 26.2 | 413.7 | 691.2 | 297.1 | 202.2 | 551.7 | 132.1 | 312.2 | 56.4 | 530.2 | 479.6 | 372.3 | 16.2 | 198.3 |
| 乳类 Dairy products | 5.2 | 16.4 | 8.5 | 37.6 | 11.6 | 17.0 | 10.0 | 6.3 | 5.4 | 10.3 | 16.6 | 4.7 | 20.0 | 13.0 | 7.0 | 8.3 | 11.0 | 9.2 | 2.7 | 4.8 | 7.6 | 5.9 | 14.6 | 8.7 | 10.9 |
| 蔬菜类 Vegetables | 1718.6 | 2332.8 | 1457.9 | 2982.0 | 1328.7 | 1012.3 | 1386.8 | 1946.2 | 618.7 | 1065.8 | 1695.5 | 1562.7 | 1770.6 | 2916.2 | 1860.6 | 3176.6 | 3125.5 | 2401.0 | 2182.3 | 2271.4 | 2019.5 | 3819.9 | 1265.4 | 1341.5 | 1969.1 |
| 水果类 Fruits | 0.6 | 1.2 | 0.8 | 2.8 | 0.9 | 0.3 | 0.8 | 0.2 | 1.3 | 1.1 | 0.2 | 0.3 | 0.7 | 0.3 | 0.2 | 0.3 | 1.6 | 0.0 | 0.2 | 0.3 | 1.9 | 1.9 | 0.3 | 0.0 | 0.8 |
| 糖类 Sugar | 0.1 | 0.0 | 0.0 | 0.8 | 0.0 | 0.0 | 0.2 | 0.2 | 0.0 | 0.2 | 0.0 | 0.0 | 1.5 | 0.0 | 0.0 | 0.0 | 0.4 | 0.0 | 0.0 | 0.0 | 0.0 | 0.0 | 0.0 | 0.0 | 0.1 |
| 水及饮料类 Water and beverages | 12.2 | 25.9 | 7.8 | 20.0 | 13.0 | 22.4 | 7.9 | 23.8 | 20.2 | 77.3 | 6.2 | 23.6 | 14.1 | 7.6 | 23.6 | 40.4 | 10.2 | 36.0 | 5.7 | 6.3 | 26.0 | 10.6 | 11.9 | 12.5 | 19.4 |
| 酒类 Alcohol beverages | 0.2 | 0.5 | 0.2 | 0.7 | 0.1 | 0.0 | 0.0 | 0.1 | 0.0 | 0.6 | 0.1 | 0.1 | 0.9 | 0.2 | 0.2 | 0.4 | 1.2 | 8.0 | 0.3 | 0.1 | 0.3 | 0.2 | 0.1 | 0.1 | 0.6 |
| 合计 SUM | 4035 | 5358 | 4355 | 5637 | 3207 | 3679 | 4320 | 4662 | 3166 | 4074 | 4558 | 3775 | 4152 | 5413 | 3946 | 5832 | 6427 | 5082 | 4465 | 4765 | 4421 | 6328 | 3165 | 2825 | 4485 |

附表 3-3　第六次中国总膳食研究钠的膳食来源（单位：%）

Annexed Table 3-3　Dietary sources of sodium from the 6<sup>th</sup> China TDS (Unit: %)

| 膳食类别<br>Category | 黑龙江<br>HL | 辽宁<br>LN | 河北<br>HE | 北京<br>BJ | 吉林<br>JL | 山西<br>SX | 陕西<br>SN | 河南<br>HA | 宁夏<br>NX | 内蒙古<br>NM | 青海<br>QH | 甘肃<br>GS | 上海<br>SH | 福建<br>FJ | 江西<br>JX | 江苏<br>JS | 浙江<br>ZJ | 山东<br>SD | 湖北<br>HB | 四川<br>SC | 广西<br>GX | 湖南<br>HN | 广东<br>GD | 贵州<br>GZ | 全国平均<br>AVG |
|---|---|---|---|---|---|---|---|---|---|---|---|---|---|---|---|---|---|---|---|---|---|---|---|---|---|
| 谷类 Cereals | 19.2 | 13.6 | 33.0 | 15.7 | 14.2 | 24.6 | 34.8 | 31.0 | 40.0 | 39.1 | 36.3 | 13.9 | 9.3 | 8.1 | 13.0 | 9.7 | 5.4 | 19.9 | 15.1 | 14.5 | 9.4 | 6.0 | 19.1 | 10.8 | 18.1 |

续表

| 膳食类别<br>Category | 黑龙江<br>HL | 辽宁<br>LN | 河北<br>HE | 北京<br>BJ | 吉林<br>JL | 山西<br>SX | 陕西<br>SN | 河南<br>HA | 宁夏<br>NX | 内蒙古<br>NM | 青海<br>QH | 甘肃<br>GS | 上海<br>SH | 福建<br>FJ | 江西<br>JX | 江苏<br>JS | 浙江<br>ZJ | 山东<br>SD | 湖北<br>HB | 四川<br>SC | 广西<br>GX | 湖南<br>HN | 广东<br>GD | 贵州<br>GZ | 全国平均<br>AVG |
|---|---|---|---|---|---|---|---|---|---|---|---|---|---|---|---|---|---|---|---|---|---|---|---|---|---|
| 豆类<br>Legumes | 5.2 | 16.2 | 4.4 | 4.3 | 9.2 | 5.7 | 8.5 | 2.4 | 3.4 | 2.8 | 0.3 | 5.4 | 7.5 | 5.3 | 9.7 | 7.1 | 12.3 | 3.0 | 6.8 | 8.1 | 2.3 | 4.4 | 2.4 | 9.9 | 6.2 |
| 薯类<br>Potatoes | 7.6 | 7.4 | 11.7 | 5.0 | 11.5 | 13.7 | 15.7 | 5.7 | 18.0 | 13.1 | 8.3 | 25.8 | 4.0 | 2.4 | 2.7 | 2.8 | 2.2 | 4.3 | 8.3 | 6.0 | 1.6 | 2.7 | 0.5 | 6.3 | 7.2 |
| 肉类<br>Meats | 14.6 | 10.2 | 8.8 | 13.4 | 13.1 | 23.3 | 4.8 | 12.5 | 15.2 | 13.7 | 14.0 | 7.9 | 19.9 | 14.4 | 16.2 | 16.8 | 17.0 | 14.1 | 9.1 | 20.4 | 25.4 | 15.7 | 21.4 | 21.4 | 15.0 |
| 蛋类<br>Eggs | 6.9 | 7.3 | 7.1 | 5.0 | 7.0 | 3.3 | 3.3 | 5.2 | 2.6 | 1.1 | 2.9 | 4.1 | 5.8 | 2.8 | 3.0 | 4.9 | 5.5 | 7.8 | 4.7 | 2.0 | 2.9 | 2.9 | 4.1 | 2.8 | 4.4 |
| 水产类<br>Aquatic foods | 3.6 | 1.0 | 1.0 | 2.6 | 2.7 | 0.9 | 0.4 | 0.8 | 0.4 | 1.9 | 0.5 | 0.7 | 10.0 | 12.8 | 7.5 | 3.5 | 8.6 | 2.6 | 7.0 | 1.2 | 12.0 | 7.6 | 11.8 | 0.6 | 4.4 |
| 乳类<br>Dairy products | 0.1 | 0.3 | 0.2 | 0.7 | 0.4 | 0.5 | 0.2 | 0.1 | 0.2 | 0.3 | 0.4 | 0.1 | 0.5 | 0.2 | 0.2 | 0.1 | 0.2 | 0.2 | 0.1 | 0.1 | 0.2 | 0.1 | 0.5 | 0.3 | 0.2 |
| 蔬菜类<br>Vegetables | 42.6 | 43.5 | 33.5 | 52.9 | 41.4 | 27.5 | 32.1 | 41.7 | 19.5 | 26.2 | 37.2 | 41.4 | 42.6 | 53.9 | 47.1 | 54.5 | 48.6 | 47.2 | 48.9 | 47.7 | 45.7 | 60.4 | 40.0 | 47.5 | 43.9 |
| 水果类<br>Fruits | 0.0 | 0.0 | 0.0 | 0.1 | 0.0 | 0.0 | 0.0 | 0.0 | 0.0 | 0.0 | 0.0 | 0.0 | 0.0 | 0.0 | 0.0 | 0.0 | 0.0 | 0.0 | 0.0 | 0.0 | 0.0 | 0.0 | 0.0 | 0.0 | 0.0 |
| 糖类<br>Sugar | 0.0 | 0.0 | 0.0 | 0.0 | 0.0 | 0.0 | 0.0 | 0.0 | 0.0 | 0.0 | 0.0 | 0.0 | 0.0 | 0.0 | 0.0 | 0.0 | 0.0 | 0.0 | 0.0 | 0.0 | 0.0 | 0.0 | 0.0 | 0.0 | 0.0 |
| 水及饮料类<br>Water and beverages | 0.3 | 0.5 | 0.2 | 0.4 | 0.4 | 0.6 | 0.2 | 0.5 | 0.6 | 1.9 | 0.1 | 0.6 | 0.3 | 0.1 | 0.6 | 0.7 | 0.2 | 0.7 | 0.1 | 0.1 | 0.6 | 0.2 | 0.4 | 0.4 | 0.4 |
| 酒类<br>Alcohol beverages | 0.0 | 0.0 | 0.0 | 0.0 | 0.0 | 0.0 | 0.0 | 0.0 | 0.0 | 0.0 | 0.0 | 0.0 | 0.0 | 0.0 | 0.0 | 0.0 | 0.0 | 0.2 | 0.0 | 0.0 | 0.0 | 0.0 | 0.0 | 0.0 | 0.0 |

附表 3-4 第六次中国总膳食研究膳食样品中钾的含量（单位：mg/g）

Annexed Table 3-4 Levels of potassium in food samples from the 6th China TDS (Unit: mg/g)

| 膳食类别 Category | 黑龙江 HL | 辽宁 LN | 河北 HE | 北京 BJ | 吉林 JL | 山西 SX | 陕西 SN | 河南 HA | 宁夏 NX | 内蒙古 NM | 青海 QH | 甘肃 GS | 上海 SH | 福建 FJ | 江西 JX | 江苏 JS | 浙江 ZJ | 山东 SD | 湖北 HB | 四川 SC | 广西 GX | 湖南 HN | 广东 GD | 贵州 GZ | 全国平均 AVG |
|---|---|---|---|---|---|---|---|---|---|---|---|---|---|---|---|---|---|---|---|---|---|---|---|---|---|
| 谷类 Cereals | 0.74 | 0.77 | 0.56 | 0.85 | 0.74 | 0.35 | 0.92 | 0.89 | 0.36 | 0.51 | 0.66 | 0.47 | 0.51 | 0.43 | 0.38 | 0.34 | 0.49 | 0.44 | 0.41 | 0.35 | 0.32 | 0.38 | 0.45 | 0.31 | 0.53 |
| 豆类 Legumes | 2.51 | 3.02 | 2.58 | 2.38 | 3.29 | 1.81 | 1.22 | 2.46 | 1.46 | 1.43 | 4.67 | 1.13 | 3.45 | 2.52 | 1.74 | 3.23 | 2.70 | 2.62 | 2.64 | 1.94 | 2.93 | 2.95 | 2.88 | 1.94 | 2.48 |
| 薯类 Potatoes | 0.60 | 1.78 | 1.38 | 2.88 | 2.04 | 1.03 | 2.29 | 1.43 | 1.82 | 2.55 | 1.15 | 1.47 | 1.55 | 1.81 | 3.43 | 2.93 | 1.55 | 2.05 | 2.15 | 1.86 | 2.89 | 2.65 | 2.45 | 3.29 | 2.04 |
| 肉类 Meats | 2.03 | 3.07 | 2.96 | 4.48 | 2.79 | 2.05 | 1.51 | 2.75 | 1.63 | 2.38 | 2.97 | 2.27 | 2.36 | 2.84 | 2.83 | 2.79 | 2.79 | 2.71 | 2.56 | 2.39 | 2.57 | 2.51 | 3.25 | 2.33 | 2.62 |
| 蛋类 Eggs | 1.29 | 1.40 | 1.43 | 2.56 | 1.15 | 1.36 | 1.39 | 1.26 | 1.58 | 1.64 | 1.65 | 0.99 | 1.46 | 1.30 | 1.32 | 1.73 | 2.25 | 1.33 | 1.41 | 1.21 | 1.54 | 2.05 | 1.36 | 1.29 | 1.50 |
| 水产类 Aquatic foods | 2.30 | 3.05 | 3.24 | 3.94 | 3.90 | 3.14 | 2.16 | 2.56 | 2.82 | 2.45 | 3.19 | 2.48 | 2.46 | 2.71 | 3.09 | 2.21 | 2.78 | 2.75 | 2.23 | 3.21 | 2.26 | 2.48 | 3.62 | 2.65 | 2.82 |
| 乳类 Dairy products | 1.89 | 1.79 | 1.71 | 1.71 | 1.67 | 1.62 | 2.22 | 1.56 | 1.56 | 1.60 | 1.61 | 1.62 | 1.32 | 2.09 | 1.69 | 1.57 | 1.63 | 1.71 | 2.27 | 2.02 | 1.63 | 1.62 | 1.55 | 1.70 | 1.72 |
| 蔬菜类 Vegetables | 1.65 | 1.84 | 2.63 | 3.82 | 2.22 | 2.26 | 2.11 | 2.01 | 1.92 | 1.96 | 1.99 | 1.57 | 2.49 | 1.92 | 2.85 | 2.40 | 2.76 | 1.98 | 1.70 | 2.74 | 2.36 | 2.46 | 2.98 | 3.26 | 2.33 |
| 水果类 Fruits | 1.22 | 1.74 | 1.88 | 1.74 | 1.57 | 1.75 | 1.24 | 1.59 | 1.23 | 1.46 | 1.61 | 1.08 | 1.43 | 1.99 | 1.50 | 1.54 | 1.65 | 1.90 | 1.71 | 1.74 | 1.68 | 1.65 | 1.66 | 1.61 | 1.59 |
| 糖类 Sugar | 0.04 | 0.10 | 0.03 | 1.67 | 0.07 | 0.05 | 0.09 | 4.15 | 0.08 | 4.01 | 0.01 | 0.22 | 3.13 | 0.14 | 0.09 | 0.04 | 1.13 | 2.50 | 0.08 | 0.10 | 0.06 | 0.10 | 0.05 | 0.09 | 0.75 |
| 水及饮料类 Water and beverages | 0.00 | 0.05 | 0.01 | 0.01 | 0.06 | 0.00 | 0.12 | 0.01 | 0.01 | 0.04 | 0.18 | 0.01 | 0.24 | 0.03 | 0.02 | 0.10 | 0.07 | 0.01 | 0.07 | 0.07 | 0.03 | 0.08 | 0.06 | 0.02 | 0.05 |

续表

| 膳食类别 Category | 黑龙江 HL | 辽宁 LN | 河北 HE | 北京 BJ | 吉林 JL | 山西 SX | 陕西 SN | 河南 HA | 宁夏 NX | 内蒙古 NM | 青海 QH | 甘肃 GS | 上海 SH | 福建 FJ | 江西 JX | 江苏 JS | 浙江 ZJ | 山东 SD | 湖北 HB | 四川 SC | 广西 GX | 湖南 HN | 广东 GD | 贵州 GZ | 全国平均 AVG |
|---|---|---|---|---|---|---|---|---|---|---|---|---|---|---|---|---|---|---|---|---|---|---|---|---|---|
| 酒类 Alcohol beverages | 0.13 | 0.21 | 0.14 | 0.29 | 0.19 | 0.00 | 0.13 | 0.21 | 0.00 | 0.18 | 0.16 | 0.21 | 0.21 | 0.20 | 0.10 | 0.13 | 0.21 | 0.24 | 0.11 | 0.13 | 0.34 | 0.07 | 0.28 | 0.07 | 0.16 |

附表 3-5 第六次中国总膳食研究钾的膳食摄入量（单位：mg/d）

Annexed Table 3-5 Dietary intakes of potassium from the 6<sup>th</sup> China TDS (Unit: mg/d)

| 膳食类别 Category | 黑龙江 HL | 辽宁 LN | 河北 HE | 北京 BJ | 吉林 JL | 山西 SX | 陕西 SN | 河南 HA | 宁夏 NX | 内蒙古 NM | 青海 QH | 甘肃 GS | 上海 SH | 福建 FJ | 江西 JX | 江苏 JS | 浙江 ZJ | 山东 SD | 湖北 HB | 四川 SC | 广西 GX | 湖南 HN | 广东 GD | 贵州 GZ | 全国平均 AVG |
|---|---|---|---|---|---|---|---|---|---|---|---|---|---|---|---|---|---|---|---|---|---|---|---|---|---|
| 谷类 Cereals | 403.2 | 470.9 | 425.4 | 671.9 | 432.2 | 368.2 | 699.7 | 823.1 | 235.8 | 372.1 | 505.0 | 325.7 | 227.5 | 269.7 | 241.6 | 262.6 | 309.6 | 442.5 | 217.1 | 337.4 | 301.0 | 220.8 | 206.3 | 206.8 | 374.0 |
| 豆类 Legumes | 113.9 | 368.2 | 147.0 | 242.2 | 248.4 | 125.7 | 100.7 | 132.6 | 51.4 | 57.0 | 30.2 | 46.7 | 405.6 | 198.1 | 128.2 | 268.3 | 380.1 | 137.4 | 176.6 | 131.2 | 124.1 | 214.0 | 80.4 | 197.3 | 171.0 |
| 薯类 Potatoes | 46.0 | 128.6 | 84.0 | 168.6 | 244.9 | 121.6 | 262.4 | 115.2 | 181.4 | 312.0 | 116.2 | 212.2 | 55.7 | 76.7 | 110.3 | 97.9 | 56.8 | 94.9 | 190.6 | 117.2 | 37.1 | 142.0 | 60.5 | 112.9 | 131.1 |
| 肉类 Meats | 121.8 | 204.9 | 140.0 | 301.2 | 185.6 | 281.6 | 54.4 | 152.2 | 76.3 | 174.7 | 210.8 | 70.4 | 261.3 | 243.8 | 265.6 | 255.9 | 330.3 | 263.6 | 139.1 | 308.2 | 387.8 | 374.5 | 338.2 | 248.0 | 224.6 |
| 蛋类 Eggs | 52.0 | 57.4 | 45.1 | 99.6 | 46.2 | 28.4 | 30.5 | 37.4 | 20.6 | 48.8 | 21.7 | 22.0 | 56.8 | 24.7 | 27.0 | 48.8 | 53.8 | 59.2 | 35.3 | 17.8 | 21.6 | 46.8 | 32.5 | 21.0 | 39.8 |
| 水产类 Aquatic foods | 62.5 | 48.9 | 30.8 | 64.6 | 43.4 | 20.1 | 8.9 | 11.9 | 6.8 | 25.3 | 11.4 | 7.0 | 168.8 | 173.8 | 135.0 | 86.4 | 140.1 | 62.7 | 90.8 | 26.9 | 218.5 | 165.0 | 185.3 | 9.2 | 75.2 |
| 乳类 Dairy products | 25.3 | 79.7 | 41.5 | 146.5 | 53.9 | 67.2 | 43.0 | 30.5 | 23.9 | 54.9 | 86.1 | 22.9 | 94.2 | 75.2 | 36.9 | 43.2 | 54.7 | 39.3 | 15.2 | 25.4 | 29.5 | 29.2 | 56.6 | 47.9 | 50.9 |

附录 381

续表

| 膳食类别 Category | 黑龙江 HL | 辽宁 LN | 河北 HE | 北京 BJ | 吉林 JL | 山西 SX | 陕西 SN | 河南 HA | 宁夏 NX | 内蒙古 NM | 青海 QH | 甘肃 GS | 上海 SH | 福建 FJ | 江西 JX | 江苏 JS | 浙江 ZJ | 山东 SD | 湖北 HB | 四川 SC | 广西 GX | 湖南 HN | 广东 GD | 贵州 GZ | 全国平均 AVG |
|---|---|---|---|---|---|---|---|---|---|---|---|---|---|---|---|---|---|---|---|---|---|---|---|---|---|
| 蔬菜类 Vegetables | 529.4 | 601.5 | 773.4 | 1496.5 | 860.0 | 700.1 | 605.7 | 558.9 | 299.6 | 503.7 | 618.0 | 389.4 | 997.5 | 761.7 | 1287.0 | 1019.0 | 1227.8 | 804.5 | 704.0 | 829.3 | 834.1 | 1315.5 | 705.8 | 1328.9 | 823.0 |
| 水果类 Fruits | 76.6 | 133.4 | 70.8 | 198.2 | 138.2 | 61.1 | 47.2 | 38.4 | 103.8 | 165.4 | 25.1 | 35.8 | 105.0 | 119.1 | 85.0 | 41.9 | 110.9 | 103.5 | 32.8 | 26.1 | 108.2 | 104.6 | 48.6 | 33.8 | 83.9 |
| 糖类 Sugar | 0.1 | 0.1 | 0.0 | 3.3 | 0.1 | 0.1 | 3.4 | 1.6 | 0.1 | 4.2 | 0.0 | 0.1 | 23.8 | 0.0 | 0.1 | 0.0 | 1.2 | 1.2 | 0.0 | 0.0 | 0.0 | 0.1 | 0.0 | 0.0 | 1.6 |
| 水及饮料类 Water and beverages | 2.4 | 23.2 | 7.8 | 11.1 | 72.9 | 2.2 | 39.7 | 11.9 | 4.1 | 103.0 | 111.3 | 11.8 | 168.6 | 26.0 | 23.6 | 100.9 | 58.2 | 18.0 | 20.0 | 22.0 | 39.1 | 85.0 | 76.3 | 25.0 | 44.3 |
| 酒类 Alcohol beverages | 2.9 | 6.9 | 1.5 | 7.9 | 1.8 | 0.0 | 0.2 | 0.7 | 0.0 | 3.7 | 0.7 | 0.7 | 4.7 | 2.9 | 2.2 | 4.9 | 13.0 | 27.3 | 1.6 | 0.7 | 10.9 | 1.2 | 0.4 | 0.2 | 4.0 |
| 合计 SUM | 1436 | 2124 | 1767 | 3412 | 2328 | 1776 | 1896 | 1914 | 1004 | 1825 | 1737 | 1145 | 2569 | 1972 | 2343 | 2230 | 2736 | 2054 | 1623 | 1842 | 2112 | 2698 | 1791 | 2231 | 2024 |

附表 3-6 第六次中国总膳食研究钾的膳食来源（单位：%）

Annexed Table 3-6 Dietary sources of potassium from the 6$^{th}$ China TDS (Unit: %)

| 膳食类别 Category | 黑龙江 HL | 辽宁 LN | 河北 HE | 北京 BJ | 吉林 JL | 山西 SX | 陕西 SN | 河南 HA | 宁夏 NX | 内蒙古 NM | 青海 QH | 甘肃 GS | 上海 SH | 福建 FJ | 江西 JX | 江苏 JS | 浙江 ZJ | 山东 SD | 湖北 HB | 四川 SC | 广西 GX | 湖南 HN | 广东 GD | 贵州 GZ | 全国平均 AVG |
|---|---|---|---|---|---|---|---|---|---|---|---|---|---|---|---|---|---|---|---|---|---|---|---|---|---|
| 谷类 Cereals | 28.1 | 22.2 | 24.1 | 19.7 | 18.6 | 20.7 | 36.9 | 43.0 | 23.5 | 20.4 | 29.1 | 28.5 | 8.9 | 13.7 | 10.3 | 11.8 | 11.3 | 21.5 | 13.4 | 18.3 | 14.3 | 8.2 | 11.5 | 9.3 | 18.5 |
| 豆类 Legumes | 7.9 | 17.3 | 8.3 | 7.1 | 10.7 | 7.1 | 5.3 | 6.9 | 5.1 | 3.1 | 1.7 | 4.1 | 15.8 | 10.0 | 5.5 | 12.0 | 13.9 | 6.7 | 10.9 | 7.1 | 5.9 | 7.9 | 4.5 | 8.8 | 8.5 |
| 薯类 Potatoes | 3.2 | 6.1 | 4.8 | 4.9 | 10.5 | 6.8 | 13.8 | 6.0 | 18.1 | 17.1 | 6.7 | 18.5 | 2.2 | 3.9 | 4.7 | 4.4 | 2.1 | 4.6 | 11.7 | 6.4 | 1.8 | 5.3 | 3.4 | 5.1 | 6.5 |

续表

| 膳食类别<br>Category | 黑龙江<br>HL | 辽宁<br>LN | 河北<br>HE | 北京<br>BJ | 吉林<br>JL | 山西<br>SX | 陕西<br>SN | 河南<br>HA | 宁夏<br>NX | 内蒙古<br>NM | 青海<br>QH | 甘肃<br>GS | 上海<br>SH | 福建<br>FJ | 江西<br>JX | 江苏<br>JS | 浙江<br>ZJ | 山东<br>SD | 湖北<br>HB | 四川<br>SC | 广西<br>GX | 湖南<br>HN | 广东<br>GD | 贵州<br>GZ | 全国平均<br>AVG |
|---|---|---|---|---|---|---|---|---|---|---|---|---|---|---|---|---|---|---|---|---|---|---|---|---|---|
| 肉类 Meats | 8.5 | 9.6 | 7.9 | 8.8 | 8.0 | 15.9 | 2.9 | 8.0 | 7.6 | 9.6 | 12.1 | 6.1 | 10.2 | 12.4 | 11.3 | 11.5 | 12.1 | 12.8 | 8.6 | 16.7 | 18.4 | 13.9 | 18.9 | 11.1 | 11.1 |
| 蛋类 Eggs | 3.6 | 2.7 | 2.6 | 2.9 | 2.0 | 1.6 | 1.6 | 2.0 | 2.1 | 2.7 | 1.3 | 1.9 | 2.2 | 1.3 | 1.2 | 2.2 | 2.0 | 2.9 | 2.2 | 1.0 | 1.0 | 1.7 | 1.8 | 0.9 | 2.0 |
| 水产类 Aquatic foods | 4.4 | 2.3 | 1.7 | 1.9 | 1.9 | 1.1 | 0.5 | 0.6 | 0.7 | 1.4 | 0.7 | 0.6 | 6.6 | 8.8 | 5.8 | 3.9 | 5.1 | 3.1 | 5.6 | 1.5 | 10.3 | 6.1 | 10.3 | 0.4 | 3.7 |
| 乳类 Dairy products | 1.8 | 3.8 | 2.3 | 4.3 | 2.3 | 3.8 | 2.3 | 1.6 | 2.4 | 3.0 | 5.0 | 2.0 | 3.7 | 3.8 | 1.6 | 1.9 | 2.0 | 1.9 | 0.9 | 1.4 | 1.4 | 1.1 | 3.2 | 2.1 | 2.5 |
| 蔬菜类 Vegetables | 36.9 | 28.3 | 43.8 | 43.9 | 36.9 | 39.4 | 32.0 | 29.2 | 29.8 | 27.6 | 35.6 | 34.0 | 38.8 | 38.6 | 54.9 | 45.7 | 44.9 | 39.2 | 43.4 | 45.0 | 39.5 | 48.7 | 39.4 | 59.6 | 40.7 |
| 水果类 Fruits | 5.3 | 6.3 | 4.0 | 5.8 | 5.9 | 3.4 | 2.5 | 2.0 | 10.3 | 9.1 | 1.4 | 3.1 | 4.1 | 6.0 | 3.6 | 1.9 | 4.1 | 5.0 | 2.0 | 1.4 | 5.1 | 3.9 | 2.7 | 1.5 | 4.1 |
| 糖类 Sugar | 0.0 | 0.0 | 0.0 | 0.1 | 0.0 | 0.0 | 0.2 | 0.1 | 0.0 | 0.2 | 0.0 | 0.0 | 0.9 | 0.0 | 0.0 | 0.0 | 0.0 | 0.1 | 0.0 | 0.0 | 0.0 | 0.0 | 0.0 | 0.0 | 0.1 |
| 水及饮料类 Water and beverages | 0.2 | 1.1 | 0.4 | 0.3 | 3.1 | 0.1 | 2.1 | 0.6 | 0.4 | 5.6 | 6.4 | 1.0 | 6.6 | 1.3 | 1.0 | 4.5 | 2.1 | 0.9 | 1.2 | 1.2 | 1.8 | 3.1 | 4.3 | 1.1 | 2.2 |
| 酒类 Alcohol beverages | 0.2 | 0.3 | 0.1 | 0.2 | 0.1 | 0.0 | 0.0 | 0.0 | 0.0 | 0.2 | 0.0 | 0.1 | 0.2 | 0.1 | 0.1 | 0.2 | 0.5 | 1.3 | 0.1 | 0.0 | 0.5 | 0.0 | 0.0 | 0.0 | 0.2 |

附表 3-7 第六次中国总膳食研究膳食样品中钙的含量（单位：mg/g）

Annexed Table 3-7 Levels of calcium in food samples from the 6th China TDS (Unit: mg/g)

| 膳食类别 Category | 黑龙江 HL | 辽宁 LN | 河北 HE | 北京 BJ | 吉林 JL | 山西 SX | 陕西 SN | 河南 HA | 宁夏 NX | 内蒙古 NM | 青海 QH | 甘肃 GS | 上海 SH | 福建 FJ | 江西 JX | 江苏 JS | 浙江 ZJ | 山东 SD | 湖北 HB | 四川 SC | 广西 GX | 湖南 HN | 广东 GD | 贵州 GZ | 全国平均 AVG |
|---|---|---|---|---|---|---|---|---|---|---|---|---|---|---|---|---|---|---|---|---|---|---|---|---|---|
| 谷类 Cereals | 0.23 | 0.13 | 0.15 | 0.14 | 0.13 | 0.16 | 0.19 | 0.19 | 0.24 | 0.16 | 0.18 | 0.12 | 0.08 | 0.07 | 0.07 | 0.09 | 0.12 | 0.13 | 0.08 | 0.11 | 0.04 | 0.06 | 0.08 | 0.06 | 0.13 |
| 豆类 Legumes | 0.99 | 0.74 | 0.75 | 0.53 | 0.73 | 1.29 | 2.18 | 2.13 | 1.81 | 2.72 | 1.11 | 1.47 | 0.53 | 0.73 | 1.63 | 1.72 | 0.51 | 1.58 | 1.69 | 2.03 | 1.02 | 2.04 | 1.12 | 2.49 | 1.40 |
| 薯类 Potatoes | 0.07 | 0.15 | 0.22 | 0.13 | 0.08 | 0.19 | 0.11 | 0.15 | 0.17 | 0.10 | 0.17 | 0.11 | 0.11 | 0.11 | 0.30 | 0.16 | 0.08 | 0.12 | 0.09 | 0.09 | 0.21 | 0.23 | 0.19 | 0.10 | 0.14 |
| 肉类 Meats | 0.13 | 0.08 | 0.08 | 0.11 | 0.08 | 0.07 | 1.47 | 0.19 | 0.17 | 0.22 | 0.26 | 0.34 | 0.45 | 0.24 | 0.06 | 1.12 | 0.12 | 0.12 | 0.08 | 0.09 | 0.18 | 0.13 | 0.12 | 0.24 | 0.26 |
| 蛋类 Eggs | 0.53 | 0.49 | 0.51 | 0.65 | 0.59 | 0.70 | 0.51 | 0.55 | 0.64 | 0.59 | 0.71 | 0.33 | 0.42 | 0.52 | 0.60 | 0.52 | 0.53 | 0.52 | 0.55 | 0.65 | 0.54 | 0.54 | 0.35 | 0.52 | 0.54 |
| 水产类 Aquatic foods | 0.82 | 1.94 | 0.36 | 1.77 | 0.56 | 0.72 | 0.25 | 0.83 | 1.27 | 0.52 | 0.26 | 0.29 | 0.62 | 0.76 | 0.64 | 1.45 | 0.82 | 0.46 | 0.81 | 0.40 | 0.30 | 0.75 | 1.15 | 0.34 | 0.75 |
| 乳类 Dairy products | 1.32 | 1.22 | 1.14 | 1.22 | 1.17 | 1.18 | 1.74 | 1.07 | 1.20 | 1.09 | 1.22 | 1.15 | 0.91 | 1.44 | 1.26 | 1.16 | 1.17 | 1.28 | 1.84 | 1.44 | 1.22 | 1.21 | 0.96 | 1.27 | 1.24 |
| 蔬菜类 Vegetables | 0.33 | 0.28 | 0.36 | 0.35 | 0.33 | 0.37 | 0.32 | 0.44 | 0.42 | 0.30 | 0.42 | 0.29 | 0.32 | 0.43 | 0.52 | 0.66 | 0.42 | 0.35 | 0.63 | 0.36 | 0.80 | 0.35 | 0.46 | 0.82 | 0.43 |
| 水果类 Fruits | 0.05 | 0.05 | 0.07 | 0.04 | 0.07 | 0.06 | 0.05 | 0.33 | 0.05 | 0.06 | 0.06 | 0.03 | 0.06 | 0.08 | 0.06 | 0.07 | 0.09 | 0.07 | 0.15 | 0.12 | 0.09 | 0.13 | 0.04 | 0.14 | 0.08 |
| 糖类 Sugar | 0.01 | 0.07 | 0.03 | 0.45 | 0.04 | 0.02 | 0.03 | 0.95 | 0.04 | 0.03 | 0.01 | 0.03 | 0.48 | 0.14 | 0.11 | 0.04 | 0.28 | 0.50 | 0.07 | 0.05 | 0.07 | 0.12 | 0.04 | 0.04 | 0.15 |
| 水及饮料类 Water and beverages | 0.02 | 0.04 | 0.05 | 0.07 | 0.04 | 0.05 | 0.04 | 0.05 | 0.06 | 0.05 | 0.05 | 0.04 | 0.04 | 0.01 | 0.03 | 0.05 | 0.02 | 0.06 | 0.03 | 0.06 | 0.02 | 0.04 | 0.02 | 0.03 | 0.04 |

续表

| 膳食类别 Category | 黑龙江 HL | 辽宁 LN | 河北 HE | 北京 BJ | 吉林 JL | 山西 SX | 陕西 SN | 河南 HA | 宁夏 NX | 内蒙古 NM | 青海 QH | 甘肃 GS | 上海 SH | 福建 FJ | 江西 JX | 江苏 JS | 浙江 ZJ | 山东 SD | 湖北 HB | 四川 SC | 广西 GX | 湖南 HN | 广东 GD | 贵州 GZ | 全国平均 AVG |
|---|---|---|---|---|---|---|---|---|---|---|---|---|---|---|---|---|---|---|---|---|---|---|---|---|---|
| 酒类 Alcohol beverages | 0.02 | 0.04 | 0.02 | 0.03 | 0.03 | ND | 0.02 | 0.33 | ND | 0.03 | 0.02 | 0.03 | 0.04 | 0.03 | 0.01 | 0.03 | 0.03 | 0.03 | 0.02 | 0.02 | 0.06 | 0.02 | 0.04 | 0.02 | 0.04 |

注：ND 表示未检出。计算平均值时，ND 按 1/2 LOD 代入

Note: ND means not to be detected. When calculating the average, ND was substituted at 1/2 LOD

附表 3-8　第六次中国总膳食研究的钙的膳食摄入量（单位：mg/d）

Annexed Table 3-8　Dietary intakes of calcium from the 6$^{th}$ China TDS (Unit: mg/d)

| 膳食类别 Category | 黑龙江 HL | 辽宁 LN | 河北 HE | 北京 BJ | 吉林 JL | 山西 SX | 陕西 SN | 河南 HA | 宁夏 NX | 内蒙古 NM | 青海 QH | 甘肃 GS | 上海 SH | 福建 FJ | 江西 JX | 江苏 JS | 浙江 ZJ | 山东 SD | 湖北 HB | 四川 SC | 广西 GX | 湖南 HN | 广东 GD | 贵州 GZ | 全国平均 AVG |
|---|---|---|---|---|---|---|---|---|---|---|---|---|---|---|---|---|---|---|---|---|---|---|---|---|---|
| 谷类 Cereals | 127.3 | 79.1 | 112.6 | 112.0 | 78.6 | 167.4 | 141.1 | 173.3 | 161.5 | 117.0 | 139.3 | 81.4 | 35.0 | 46.5 | 43.1 | 68.1 | 73.4 | 126.4 | 43.4 | 107.4 | 41.5 | 34.0 | 36.8 | 43.5 | 91.2 |
| 豆类 Legumes | 44.8 | 89.9 | 42.9 | 54.2 | 55.1 | 89.4 | 180.1 | 114.9 | 63.6 | 108.5 | 7.2 | 60.8 | 62.2 | 57.7 | 119.8 | 142.8 | 72.4 | 82.9 | 112.8 | 137.4 | 43.2 | 148.0 | 31.1 | 252.9 | 90.6 |
| 薯类 Potatoes | 5.5 | 10.9 | 13.5 | 7.5 | 10.1 | 22.2 | 12.5 | 12.2 | 17.0 | 12.5 | 16.9 | 16.3 | 4.0 | 4.7 | 9.7 | 5.2 | 3.1 | 5.4 | 8.1 | 5.9 | 2.7 | 12.3 | 4.8 | 3.3 | 9.4 |
| 肉类 Meats | 7.8 | 5.6 | 3.6 | 7.6 | 5.0 | 10.1 | 52.9 | 10.4 | 8.1 | 16.5 | 18.7 | 10.5 | 49.8 | 20.4 | 5.7 | 102.9 | 14.1 | 11.5 | 4.5 | 11.7 | 27.2 | 19.6 | 12.1 | 25.2 | 19.2 |
| 蛋类 Eggs | 21.3 | 19.9 | 16.1 | 25.1 | 23.7 | 14.7 | 11.2 | 16.4 | 8.3 | 17.6 | 9.3 | 7.2 | 16.5 | 9.9 | 12.3 | 14.7 | 12.7 | 23.0 | 13.8 | 9.5 | 7.6 | 12.3 | 8.5 | 8.5 | 14.2 |
| 水产类 Aquatic foods | 22.3 | 31.2 | 3.5 | 29.0 | 6.3 | 4.6 | 1.0 | 3.9 | 3.1 | 5.4 | 0.9 | 0.8 | 42.5 | 48.8 | 28.0 | 56.5 | 41.1 | 10.5 | 33.0 | 3.4 | 29.3 | 49.6 | 59.1 | 1.2 | 21.5 |
| 乳类 Dairy products | 17.7 | 54.1 | 27.7 | 104.6 | 37.8 | 49.0 | 33.5 | 20.9 | 18.3 | 37.4 | 65.2 | 16.2 | 65.0 | 51.8 | 27.5 | 31.9 | 39.1 | 29.4 | 12.3 | 18.1 | 22.1 | 21.8 | 35.0 | 35.8 | 36.3 |

附录　385

续表

| 膳食类别<br>Category | 黑龙江<br>HL | 辽宁<br>LN | 河北<br>HE | 北京<br>BJ | 吉林<br>JL | 山西<br>SX | 陕西<br>SN | 河南<br>HA | 宁夏<br>NX | 内蒙古<br>NM | 青海<br>QH | 甘肃<br>GS | 上海<br>SH | 福建<br>FJ | 江西<br>JX | 江苏<br>JS | 浙江<br>ZJ | 山东<br>SD | 湖北<br>HB | 四川<br>SC | 广西<br>GX | 湖南<br>HN | 广东<br>GD | 贵州<br>GZ | 全国平均<br>AVG |
|---|---|---|---|---|---|---|---|---|---|---|---|---|---|---|---|---|---|---|---|---|---|---|---|---|---|
| 蔬菜类 Vegetables | 106.7 | 90.9 | 106.7 | 138.6 | 129.0 | 113.5 | 93.1 | 123.6 | 66.0 | 76.9 | 130.4 | 71.9 | 128.2 | 172.4 | 234.8 | 279.1 | 187.4 | 143.7 | 260.9 | 109.8 | 281.3 | 187.1 | 109.4 | 336.4 | 153.2 |
| 水果类 Fruits | 3.1 | 4.2 | 2.6 | 4.8 | 6.0 | 2.1 | 1.7 | 8.0 | 4.0 | 6.9 | 1.0 | 1.0 | 4.4 | 4.9 | 3.4 | 1.9 | 5.9 | 3.8 | 2.9 | 1.8 | 5.8 | 8.2 | 1.3 | 2.9 | 3.9 |
| 糖类 Sugar | 0.0 | 0.1 | 0.0 | 0.9 | 0.0 | 0.0 | 1.3 | 0.4 | 0.0 | 0.0 | 0.0 | 0.0 | 3.6 | 0.0 | 0.1 | 0.0 | 0.3 | 0.3 | 0.0 | 0.0 | 0.0 | 0.1 | 0.0 | 0.0 | 0.3 |
| 水及饮料类 Water and beverages | 24.5 | 21.2 | 38.8 | 77.5 | 52.1 | 37.3 | 12.4 | 59.6 | 31.5 | 128.8 | 30.9 | 47.2 | 28.1 | 8.7 | 35.5 | 50.5 | 14.2 | 108.0 | 8.6 | 18.8 | 26.0 | 42.5 | 27.9 | 37.6 | 40.3 |
| 酒类 Alcohol beverages | 0.4 | 1.3 | 0.2 | 0.8 | 0.3 | 0.0 | 0.0 | 1.1 | 0.0 | 0.6 | 0.1 | 0.1 | 0.9 | 0.4 | 0.2 | 1.1 | 2.1 | 3.4 | 0.3 | 0.1 | 1.9 | 0.3 | 0.1 | 0.0 | 0.7 |
| 合计 SUM | 381.4 | 408.3 | 368.1 | 562.6 | 403.9 | 510.3 | 540.9 | 544.5 | 381.4 | 527.9 | 419.9 | 313.5 | 440.2 | 426.2 | 520.1 | 754.8 | 465.7 | 548.3 | 500.6 | 423.7 | 488.6 | 535.9 | 326.1 | 747.4 | 480.8 |

附表 3-9 第六次中国总膳食研究钙的膳食来源（单位：%）

Annexed Table 3-9 Dietary sources of calcium from the 6$^{th}$ China TDS (Unit: %)

| 膳食类别<br>Category | 黑龙江<br>HL | 辽宁<br>LN | 河北<br>HE | 北京<br>BJ | 吉林<br>JL | 山西<br>SX | 陕西<br>SN | 河南<br>HA | 宁夏<br>NX | 内蒙古<br>NM | 青海<br>QH | 甘肃<br>GS | 上海<br>SH | 福建<br>FJ | 江西<br>JX | 江苏<br>JS | 浙江<br>ZJ | 山东<br>SD | 湖北<br>HB | 四川<br>SC | 广西<br>GX | 湖南<br>HN | 广东<br>GD | 贵州<br>GZ | 全国平均<br>AVG |
|---|---|---|---|---|---|---|---|---|---|---|---|---|---|---|---|---|---|---|---|---|---|---|---|---|---|
| 谷类 Cereals | 33.4 | 19.4 | 30.6 | 19.9 | 19.5 | 32.8 | 26.1 | 31.8 | 42.3 | 22.2 | 33.2 | 26.0 | 7.9 | 10.9 | 8.3 | 9.0 | 15.8 | 23.1 | 8.7 | 25.3 | 8.5 | 6.3 | 11.3 | 5.8 | 19.0 |
| 豆类 Legumes | 11.7 | 22.0 | 11.6 | 9.6 | 13.7 | 17.5 | 33.3 | 21.1 | 16.7 | 20.5 | 1.7 | 19.4 | 14.1 | 13.5 | 23.0 | 18.9 | 15.6 | 15.1 | 22.5 | 32.4 | 8.8 | 27.6 | 9.5 | 33.8 | 18.8 |

续表

| 膳食类别<br>Category | 黑龙江<br>HL | 辽宁<br>LN | 河北<br>HE | 北京<br>BJ | 吉林<br>JL | 山西<br>SX | 陕西<br>SN | 河南<br>HA | 宁夏<br>NX | 内蒙古<br>NM | 青海<br>QH | 甘肃<br>GS | 上海<br>SH | 福建<br>FJ | 江西<br>JX | 江苏<br>JS | 浙江<br>ZJ | 山东<br>SD | 湖北<br>HB | 四川<br>SC | 广西<br>GX | 湖南<br>HN | 广东<br>GD | 贵州<br>GZ | 全国平均<br>AVG |
|---|---|---|---|---|---|---|---|---|---|---|---|---|---|---|---|---|---|---|---|---|---|---|---|---|---|
| 薯类<br>Potatoes | 1.4 | 2.7 | 3.7 | 1.3 | 2.5 | 4.4 | 2.3 | 2.2 | 4.5 | 2.4 | 4.0 | 5.2 | 0.9 | 1.1 | 1.9 | 0.7 | 0.7 | 1.0 | 1.6 | 1.4 | 0.6 | 2.3 | 1.5 | 0.4 | 2.0 |
| 肉类<br>Meats | 2.0 | 1.4 | 1.0 | 1.3 | 1.2 | 2.0 | 9.8 | 1.9 | 2.1 | 3.1 | 4.4 | 3.3 | 11.3 | 4.8 | 1.1 | 13.6 | 3.0 | 2.1 | 0.9 | 2.8 | 5.6 | 3.7 | 3.7 | 3.4 | 4.0 |
| 蛋类<br>Eggs | 5.6 | 4.9 | 4.4 | 4.5 | 5.9 | 2.9 | 2.1 | 3.0 | 2.2 | 3.3 | 2.2 | 2.3 | 3.8 | 2.3 | 2.4 | 1.9 | 2.7 | 4.2 | 2.8 | 2.2 | 1.5 | 2.3 | 2.6 | 1.1 | 2.9 |
| 水产类<br>Aquatic foods | 5.8 | 7.6 | 0.9 | 5.2 | 1.5 | 0.9 | 0.2 | 0.7 | 0.8 | 1.0 | 0.2 | 0.3 | 9.7 | 11.5 | 5.4 | 7.5 | 8.8 | 1.9 | 6.6 | 0.8 | 6.0 | 9.3 | 18.1 | 0.2 | 4.5 |
| 乳类<br>Dairy products | 4.6 | 13.2 | 7.5 | 18.6 | 9.4 | 9.6 | 6.2 | 3.8 | 4.8 | 7.1 | 15.5 | 5.2 | 14.8 | 12.2 | 5.3 | 4.2 | 8.4 | 5.4 | 2.5 | 4.3 | 4.5 | 4.1 | 10.7 | 4.8 | 7.6 |
| 蔬菜类<br>Vegetables | 28.0 | 22.3 | 29.0 | 24.6 | 31.9 | 22.2 | 17.2 | 22.7 | 17.3 | 14.6 | 31.1 | 22.9 | 29.1 | 40.4 | 45.2 | 37.0 | 40.2 | 26.2 | 52.1 | 25.9 | 57.6 | 34.9 | 33.6 | 45.0 | 31.9 |
| 水果类<br>Fruits | 0.8 | 1.0 | 0.7 | 0.9 | 1.5 | 0.4 | 0.3 | 1.5 | 1.1 | 1.3 | 0.2 | 0.3 | 1.0 | 1.2 | 0.7 | 0.3 | 1.3 | 0.7 | 0.6 | 0.4 | 1.2 | 1.5 | 0.4 | 0.4 | 0.8 |
| 糖类<br>Sugar | 0.0 | 0.0 | 0.0 | 0.2 | 0.0 | 0.0 | 0.2 | 0.1 | 0.0 | 0.0 | 0.0 | 0.0 | 0.8 | 0.0 | 0.0 | 0.0 | 0.1 | 0.0 | 0.0 | 0.0 | 0.0 | 0.0 | 0.0 | 0.0 | 0.1 |
| 水及饮料类<br>Water and beverages | 6.4 | 5.2 | 10.5 | 13.8 | 12.9 | 7.3 | 2.3 | 11.0 | 8.3 | 24.4 | 7.4 | 15.1 | 6.4 | 2.0 | 6.8 | 6.7 | 3.0 | 19.7 | 1.7 | 4.4 | 5.3 | 7.9 | 8.6 | 5.0 | 8.4 |
| 酒类<br>Alcohol beverages | 0.1 | 0.3 | 0.1 | 0.1 | 0.1 | 0.0 | 0.0 | 0.2 | 0.0 | 0.1 | 0.0 | 0.0 | 0.2 | 0.1 | 0.0 | 0.1 | 0.5 | 0.6 | 0.1 | 0.0 | 0.4 | 0.1 | 0.0 | 0.0 | 0.1 |

附表 3-10 第六次中国总膳食研究膳食样品中镁的含量（单位：mg/g）

Annexed Table 3-10 Levels of magnesium in food samples from the 6<sup>th</sup> China TDS (Unit: mg/g)

| 膳食类别<br>Category | 黑龙江<br>HL | 辽宁<br>LN | 河北<br>HE | 北京<br>BJ | 吉林<br>JL | 山西<br>SX | 陕西<br>SN | 河南<br>HA | 宁夏<br>NX | 内蒙古<br>NM | 青海<br>QH | 甘肃<br>GS | 上海<br>SH | 福建<br>FJ | 江西<br>JX | 江苏<br>JS | 浙江<br>ZJ | 山东<br>SD | 湖北<br>HB | 四川<br>SC | 广西<br>GX | 湖南<br>HN | 广东<br>GD | 贵州<br>GZ | 全国平均<br>AVG |
|---|---|---|---|---|---|---|---|---|---|---|---|---|---|---|---|---|---|---|---|---|---|---|---|---|---|
| 谷类 Cereals | 0.23 | 0.24 | 0.17 | 0.21 | 0.18 | 0.29 | 0.24 | 0.14 | 0.15 | 0.15 | 0.14 | 0.18 | 0.10 | 0.13 | 0.08 | 0.09 | 0.10 | 0.21 | 0.08 | 0.09 | 0.13 | 0.07 | 0.12 | 0.10 | 0.15 |
| 豆类 Legumes | 1.26 | 1.69 | 0.79 | 0.71 | 1.09 | 0.77 | 0.39 | 0.60 | 0.49 | 0.42 | 1.02 | 0.43 | 0.79 | 0.73 | 0.94 | 0.89 | 0.80 | 0.89 | 0.82 | 0.43 | 0.77 | 0.86 | 0.90 | 0.57 | 0.79 |
| 薯类 Potatoes | 0.05 | 0.18 | 0.14 | 0.17 | 0.14 | 0.08 | 0.11 | 0.13 | 0.15 | 0.14 | 0.09 | 0.14 | 0.15 | 0.13 | 0.21 | 0.20 | 0.13 | 0.18 | 0.15 | 0.12 | 0.20 | 0.39 | 0.24 | 0.24 | 0.16 |
| 肉类 Meats | 0.21 | 0.33 | 0.20 | 0.39 | 0.24 | 0.13 | 0.12 | 0.30 | 0.15 | 0.21 | 0.29 | 0.24 | 0.26 | 0.32 | 0.24 | 0.29 | 0.25 | 0.26 | 0.23 | 0.21 | 0.24 | 0.33 | 0.34 | 0.19 | 0.25 |
| 蛋类 Eggs | 0.17 | 0.21 | 0.15 | 0.19 | 0.17 | 0.12 | 0.10 | 0.17 | 0.12 | 0.20 | 0.23 | 0.12 | 0.16 | 0.23 | 0.16 | 0.18 | 0.21 | 0.19 | 0.19 | 0.17 | 0.20 | 0.20 | 0.14 | 0.15 | 0.17 |
| 水产类 Aquatic foods | 0.21 | 0.53 | 0.31 | 0.46 | 0.30 | 0.28 | 0.13 | 0.33 | 0.30 | 0.27 | 0.39 | 0.26 | 0.33 | 0.47 | 0.32 | 0.34 | 0.44 | 0.37 | 0.24 | 0.30 | 0.27 | 0.29 | 0.42 | 0.27 | 0.33 |
| 乳类 Dairy products | 0.17 | 0.15 | 0.15 | 0.17 | 0.14 | 0.14 | 0.22 | 0.12 | 0.14 | 0.12 | 0.12 | 0.15 | 0.12 | 0.29 | 0.11 | 0.14 | 0.13 | 0.15 | 0.18 | 0.15 | 0.15 | 0.14 | 0.16 | 0.14 | 0.15 |
| 蔬菜类 Vegetables | 0.13 | 0.21 | 0.11 | 0.26 | 0.15 | 0.09 | 0.10 | 0.15 | 0.14 | 0.11 | 0.17 | 0.14 | 0.20 | 0.29 | 0.18 | 0.27 | 0.25 | 0.14 | 0.17 | 0.18 | 0.18 | 0.19 | 0.24 | 0.15 | 0.17 |
| 水果类 Fruits | 0.11 | 0.14 | 0.14 | 0.14 | 0.14 | 0.14 | 0.09 | 0.11 | 0.08 | 0.15 | 0.09 | 0.11 | 0.14 | 0.17 | 0.08 | 0.11 | 0.13 | 0.15 | 0.12 | 0.11 | 0.17 | 0.15 | 0.18 | 0.15 | 0.13 |
| 糖类 Sugar | 0.00 | 0.01 | 0.00 | 0.26 | 0.01 | 0.00 | 0.01 | 0.47 | 0.02 | 0.57 | 0.01 | 0.02 | 1.04 | 0.02 | 0.02 | 0.06 | 0.09 | 0.08 | 0.00 | 0.02 | 0.02 | 0.14 | 0.00 | 0.01 | 0.12 |
| 水及饮料类 Water and beverages | 0.01 | 0.02 | 0.02 | 0.03 | 0.02 | 0.02 | 0.01 | 0.02 | 0.02 | 0.02 | 0.02 | 0.02 | 0.03 | 0.00 | 0.00 | 0.02 | 0.01 | 0.03 | 0.02 | 0.02 | 0.00 | 0.02 | 0.01 | 0.05 | 0.02 |

续表

| 膳食类别<br>Category | 黑龙江<br>HL | 辽宁<br>LN | 河北<br>HE | 北京<br>BJ | 吉林<br>JL | 山西<br>SX | 陕西<br>SN | 河南<br>HA | 宁夏<br>NX | 内蒙古<br>NM | 青海<br>QH | 甘肃<br>GS | 上海<br>SH | 福建<br>FJ | 江西<br>JX | 江苏<br>JS | 浙江<br>ZJ | 山东<br>SD | 湖北<br>HB | 四川<br>SC | 广西<br>GX | 湖南<br>HN | 广东<br>GD | 贵州<br>GZ | 全国平均<br>AVG |
|---|---|---|---|---|---|---|---|---|---|---|---|---|---|---|---|---|---|---|---|---|---|---|---|---|---|
| 酒类<br>Alcohol beverages | 0.03 | 0.07 | 0.03 | 0.08 | 0.03 | 0.01 | 0.03 | 0.05 | 0.00 | 0.05 | 0.05 | 0.06 | 0.05 | 0.06 | 0.02 | 0.03 | 0.04 | 0.06 | 0.03 | 0.03 | 0.05 | 0.02 | 0.08 | 0.03 | 0.04 |

附表 3-11 第六次中国总膳食研究的膳食摄入量（单位：mg/d）

Annexed Table 3-11 Dietary intakes of magnesium from the 6th China TDS (Unit: mg/d)

| 膳食类别<br>Category | 黑龙江<br>HL | 辽宁<br>LN | 河北<br>HE | 北京<br>BJ | 吉林<br>JL | 山西<br>SX | 陕西<br>SN | 河南<br>HA | 宁夏<br>NX | 内蒙古<br>NM | 青海<br>QH | 甘肃<br>GS | 上海<br>SH | 福建<br>FJ | 江西<br>JX | 江苏<br>JS | 浙江<br>ZJ | 山东<br>SD | 湖北<br>HB | 四川<br>SC | 广西<br>GX | 湖南<br>HN | 广东<br>GD | 贵州<br>GZ | 全国平均<br>AVG |
|---|---|---|---|---|---|---|---|---|---|---|---|---|---|---|---|---|---|---|---|---|---|---|---|---|---|
| 谷类 Cereals | 127.3 | 149.5 | 131.4 | 170.0 | 104.0 | 301.2 | 184.9 | 130.0 | 99.0 | 111.6 | 104.5 | 122.1 | 43.7 | 83.7 | 51.8 | 72.9 | 62.0 | 213.4 | 43.4 | 92.0 | 124.5 | 38.2 | 52.9 | 65.3 | 111.6 |
| 豆类 Legumes | 57.3 | 206.0 | 44.9 | 72.3 | 82.6 | 53.2 | 32.2 | 32.4 | 17.1 | 16.7 | 6.6 | 17.8 | 93.3 | 57.7 | 69.1 | 73.8 | 113.4 | 46.6 | 54.6 | 29.1 | 32.4 | 62.2 | 25.2 | 58.1 | 56.4 |
| 薯类 Potatoes | 4.1 | 13.2 | 8.5 | 10.1 | 16.2 | 8.9 | 12.6 | 10.5 | 15.1 | 16.8 | 9.5 | 20.0 | 5.4 | 5.6 | 6.8 | 6.6 | 4.6 | 8.1 | 13.4 | 7.8 | 2.5 | 20.6 | 5.8 | 8.2 | 10.0 |
| 肉类 Meats | 12.7 | 22.1 | 9.3 | 26.5 | 16.1 | 17.3 | 4.4 | 16.4 | 7.1 | 15.7 | 20.4 | 7.3 | 28.2 | 27.9 | 22.8 | 26.4 | 29.8 | 25.1 | 12.7 | 27.3 | 36.2 | 49.8 | 35.4 | 19.8 | 21.5 |
| 蛋类 Eggs | 6.8 | 8.5 | 4.8 | 7.5 | 6.9 | 2.6 | 2.3 | 4.9 | 1.5 | 5.9 | 3.0 | 2.7 | 6.4 | 4.4 | 3.3 | 4.9 | 5.0 | 8.2 | 4.9 | 2.5 | 2.8 | 4.5 | 3.4 | 2.4 | 4.6 |
| 水产类 Aquatic foods | 5.7 | 8.5 | 3.0 | 7.6 | 3.3 | 1.8 | 0.5 | 1.5 | 0.7 | 2.8 | 1.4 | 0.7 | 22.6 | 30.1 | 13.8 | 13.1 | 22.2 | 8.4 | 9.8 | 2.5 | 26.4 | 19.1 | 21.6 | 0.9 | 9.5 |
| 乳类 Dairy products | 2.2 | 6.5 | 3.6 | 14.1 | 4.4 | 5.6 | 4.2 | 2.3 | 2.1 | 4.1 | 6.4 | 2.1 | 8.6 | 10.3 | 2.3 | 3.7 | 4.4 | 3.4 | 1.2 | 1.9 | 2.7 | 2.4 | 5.9 | 3.8 | 4.5 |

续表

| 膳食类别 Category | 黑龙江 HL | 辽宁 LN | 河北 HE | 北京 BJ | 吉林 JL | 山西 SX | 陕西 SN | 河南 HA | 宁夏 NX | 内蒙古 NM | 青海 QH | 甘肃 GS | 上海 SH | 福建 FJ | 江西 JX | 江苏 JS | 浙江 ZJ | 山东 SD | 湖北 HB | 四川 SC | 广西 GX | 湖南 HN | 广东 GD | 贵州 GZ | 全国平均 AVG |
|---|---|---|---|---|---|---|---|---|---|---|---|---|---|---|---|---|---|---|---|---|---|---|---|---|---|
| 蔬菜类 Vegetables | 41.5 | 69.0 | 31.1 | 101.0 | 58.8 | 28.4 | 28.9 | 42.1 | 21.6 | 27.8 | 51.2 | 33.5 | 78.1 | 114.3 | 81.3 | 113.0 | 108.9 | 55.4 | 68.3 | 54.9 | 64.9 | 99.1 | 56.0 | 63.1 | 62.2 |
| 水果类 Fruits | 6.6 | 10.8 | 5.1 | 16.3 | 11.9 | 4.7 | 3.2 | 2.5 | 6.5 | 17.1 | 1.4 | 3.5 | 9.9 | 10.2 | 4.3 | 2.9 | 8.9 | 8.2 | 2.3 | 1.7 | 10.6 | 9.5 | 5.3 | 3.2 | 6.9 |
| 糖类 Sugar | 0.0 | 0.0 | 0.0 | 0.5 | 0.0 | 0.0 | 0.3 | 0.2 | 0.0 | 0.6 | 0.0 | 0.0 | 7.9 | 0.0 | 0.0 | 0.0 | 0.1 | 0.0 | 0.0 | 0.0 | 0.0 | 0.1 | 0.0 | 0.0 | 0.4 |
| 水及饮料类 Water and beverages | 9.2 | 7.4 | 11.6 | 33.2 | 19.5 | 11.2 | 2.6 | 17.9 | 10.9 | 38.6 | 9.3 | 17.7 | 21.1 | 3.9 | 5.3 | 15.1 | 4.7 | 54.0 | 4.3 | 4.7 | 2.0 | 15.9 | 12.5 | 56.4 | 16.2 |
| 酒类 Alcohol beverages | 0.7 | 2.2 | 0.3 | 2.1 | 0.3 | 0.0 | 0.0 | 0.1 | 0.0 | 0.9 | 0.2 | 0.2 | 1.0 | 0.9 | 0.3 | 1.1 | 2.7 | 6.8 | 0.4 | 0.2 | 1.4 | 0.3 | 0.1 | 0.1 | 0.9 |
| 合计 SUM | 274.1 | 503.6 | 253.7 | 461.2 | 324.0 | 434.9 | 276.0 | 260.9 | 181.6 | 258.8 | 214.0 | 227.7 | 326.2 | 348.9 | 260.9 | 333.7 | 366.7 | 437.8 | 215.3 | 224.6 | 306.5 | 321.8 | 224.1 | 281.2 | 304.9 |

附表 3-12 第六次中国总膳食研究的膳食镁来源（单位：%）

Annexed Table 3-12 Dietary sources of magnesium from the 6<sup>th</sup> China TDS (Unit: %)

| 膳食类别 Category | 黑龙江 HL | 辽宁 LN | 河北 HE | 北京 BJ | 吉林 JL | 山西 SX | 陕西 SN | 河南 HA | 宁夏 NX | 内蒙古 NM | 青海 QH | 甘肃 GS | 上海 SH | 福建 FJ | 江西 JX | 江苏 JS | 浙江 ZJ | 山东 SD | 湖北 HB | 四川 SC | 广西 GX | 湖南 HN | 广东 GD | 贵州 GZ | 全国平均 AVG |
|---|---|---|---|---|---|---|---|---|---|---|---|---|---|---|---|---|---|---|---|---|---|---|---|---|---|
| 谷类 Cereals | 46.5 | 29.7 | 51.8 | 36.9 | 32.1 | 69.3 | 67.0 | 49.8 | 54.5 | 43.1 | 48.8 | 53.6 | 13.4 | 24.0 | 19.8 | 21.9 | 16.9 | 48.7 | 20.2 | 41.0 | 40.6 | 11.9 | 23.6 | 23.2 | 36.6 |
| 豆类 Legumes | 20.9 | 40.9 | 17.7 | 15.7 | 25.5 | 12.2 | 11.6 | 12.4 | 9.4 | 6.5 | 3.1 | 7.8 | 28.6 | 16.5 | 26.5 | 22.1 | 30.9 | 10.7 | 25.3 | 13.0 | 10.6 | 19.3 | 11.3 | 20.7 | 18.5 |

续表

| 膳食类别 Category | 黑龙江 HL | 辽宁 LN | 河北 HE | 北京 BJ | 吉林 JL | 山西 SX | 陕西 SN | 河南 HA | 宁夏 NX | 内蒙古 NM | 青海 QH | 甘肃 GS | 上海 SH | 福建 FJ | 江西 JX | 江苏 JS | 浙江 ZJ | 山东 SD | 湖北 HB | 四川 SC | 广西 GX | 湖南 HN | 广东 GD | 贵州 GZ | 全国平均 AVG |
|---|---|---|---|---|---|---|---|---|---|---|---|---|---|---|---|---|---|---|---|---|---|---|---|---|---|
| 薯类 Potatoes | 1.5 | 2.6 | 3.4 | 2.2 | 5.0 | 2.0 | 4.6 | 4.0 | 8.3 | 6.5 | 4.4 | 8.8 | 1.7 | 1.6 | 2.6 | 2.0 | 1.3 | 1.9 | 6.2 | 3.5 | 0.8 | 6.4 | 2.6 | 2.9 | 3.3 |
| 肉类 Meats | 4.7 | 4.4 | 3.7 | 5.7 | 5.0 | 4.0 | 1.6 | 6.3 | 3.9 | 6.1 | 9.6 | 3.2 | 8.7 | 8.0 | 8.7 | 7.9 | 8.1 | 5.7 | 5.9 | 12.2 | 11.8 | 15.5 | 15.8 | 7.0 | 7.1 |
| 蛋类 Eggs | 2.5 | 1.7 | 1.9 | 1.6 | 2.1 | 0.6 | 0.8 | 1.9 | 0.8 | 2.3 | 1.4 | 1.2 | 1.9 | 1.3 | 1.2 | 1.5 | 1.4 | 1.9 | 2.3 | 1.1 | 0.9 | 1.4 | 1.5 | 0.9 | 1.5 |
| 水产类 Aquatic foods | 2.1 | 1.7 | 1.2 | 1.6 | 1.0 | 0.4 | 0.2 | 0.6 | 0.4 | 1.1 | 0.6 | 0.3 | 6.9 | 8.6 | 5.3 | 3.9 | 6.0 | 1.9 | 4.5 | 1.1 | 8.6 | 5.9 | 9.6 | 0.3 | 3.1 |
| 乳类 Dairy products | 0.8 | 1.3 | 1.4 | 3.1 | 1.3 | 1.3 | 1.5 | 0.9 | 1.1 | 1.6 | 3.0 | 0.9 | 2.6 | 2.9 | 0.9 | 1.1 | 1.2 | 0.8 | 0.6 | 0.8 | 0.9 | 0.8 | 2.6 | 1.4 | 1.5 |
| 蔬菜类 Vegetables | 15.1 | 13.7 | 12.3 | 21.9 | 18.1 | 6.5 | 10.5 | 16.1 | 11.9 | 10.8 | 23.9 | 14.7 | 23.9 | 32.7 | 31.2 | 33.9 | 29.7 | 12.7 | 31.7 | 24.4 | 21.2 | 30.8 | 25.0 | 22.4 | 20.4 |
| 水果类 Fruits | 2.4 | 2.1 | 2.0 | 3.5 | 3.7 | 1.1 | 1.2 | 1.0 | 3.6 | 6.6 | 0.7 | 1.5 | 3.0 | 2.9 | 1.6 | 0.9 | 2.4 | 1.9 | 1.1 | 0.8 | 3.5 | 3.0 | 2.3 | 1.1 | 2.3 |
| 糖类 Sugar | 0.0 | 0.0 | 0.0 | 0.1 | 0.0 | 0.0 | 0.1 | 0.1 | 0.0 | 0.2 | 0.0 | 0.0 | 2.4 | 0.0 | 0.0 | 0.0 | 0.0 | 0.0 | 0.0 | 0.0 | 0.0 | 0.0 | 0.0 | 0.0 | 0.1 |
| 水及饮料类 Water and beverages | 3.3 | 1.5 | 4.6 | 7.2 | 6.0 | 2.6 | 0.9 | 6.9 | 6.0 | 14.9 | 4.3 | 7.8 | 6.5 | 1.1 | 2.0 | 4.5 | 1.3 | 12.3 | 2.0 | 2.1 | 0.6 | 4.9 | 5.6 | 20.0 | 5.3 |
| 酒类 Alcohol beverages | 0.2 | 0.4 | 0.1 | 0.4 | 0.1 | 0.0 | 0.0 | 0.1 | 0.0 | 0.4 | 0.1 | 0.1 | 0.3 | 0.2 | 0.1 | 0.3 | 0.7 | 1.6 | 0.2 | 0.1 | 0.5 | 0.1 | 0.0 | 0.0 | 0.3 |

附表 3-13　第六次中国总膳食研究膳食样品中磷的含量（单位：mg/g）

Annexed Table 3-13　Levels of phosphorus in food samples from the 6$^{th}$ China TDS (Unit: mg/g)

| 膳食类别<br>Category | 黑龙江<br>HL | 辽宁<br>LN | 河北<br>HE | 北京<br>BJ | 吉林<br>JL | 山西<br>SX | 陕西<br>SN | 河南<br>HA | 宁夏<br>NX | 内蒙古<br>NM | 青海<br>QH | 甘肃<br>GS | 上海<br>SH | 福建<br>FJ | 江西<br>JX | 江苏<br>JS | 浙江<br>ZJ | 山东<br>SD | 湖北<br>HB | 四川<br>SC | 广西<br>GX | 湖南<br>HN | 广东<br>GD | 贵州<br>GZ | 全国平均<br>AVG |
|---|---|---|---|---|---|---|---|---|---|---|---|---|---|---|---|---|---|---|---|---|---|---|---|---|---|
| 谷类 Cereals | 0.67 | 0.50 | 0.50 | 0.38 | 0.57 | 0.60 | 0.70 | 0.72 | 0.49 | 0.75 | 0.71 | 0.55 | 0.46 | 0.35 | 0.33 | 0.25 | 0.45 | 0.57 | 0.35 | 0.35 | 0.39 | 0.25 | 0.37 | 0.20 | 0.48 |
| 豆类 Legumes | 2.06 | 2.17 | 1.70 | 0.95 | 2.13 | 1.62 | 1.50 | 2.21 | 1.30 | 1.64 | 1.83 | 1.66 | 1.74 | 1.21 | 1.86 | 1.52 | 1.32 | 1.86 | 1.51 | 1.16 | 1.56 | 2.15 | 1.59 | 0.99 | 1.63 |
| 薯类 Potatoes | 0.21 | 0.44 | 0.38 | 0.29 | 0.38 | 0.25 | 0.34 | 0.22 | 0.31 | 0.36 | 0.27 | 0.39 | 0.32 | 0.28 | 0.47 | 0.36 | 0.25 | 0.31 | 0.24 | 0.26 | 0.43 | 0.38 | 0.52 | 0.40 | 0.33 |
| 肉类 Meats | 1.40 | 1.85 | 1.63 | 1.78 | 2.08 | 1.24 | 1.38 | 1.91 | 1.46 | 1.22 | 1.93 | 2.26 | 1.71 | 1.63 | 1.75 | 1.72 | 1.89 | 1.65 | 1.45 | 1.50 | 1.73 | 1.09 | 1.98 | 1.27 | 1.65 |
| 蛋类 Eggs | 2.11 | 2.02 | 2.18 | 2.45 | 2.22 | 2.69 | 2.20 | 2.34 | 2.52 | 2.62 | 2.65 | 2.09 | 2.07 | 2.15 | 2.28 | 1.86 | 2.28 | 2.00 | 1.81 | 2.84 | 2.53 | 2.06 | 1.55 | 1.58 | 2.21 |
| 水产类 Aquatic foods | 1.62 | 3.03 | 1.85 | 1.68 | 2.16 | 1.93 | 1.13 | 1.94 | 2.04 | 1.88 | 1.64 | 1.93 | 1.68 | 1.60 | 1.78 | 1.65 | 1.79 | 1.78 | 1.33 | 1.78 | 1.38 | 1.08 | 2.67 | 1.33 | 1.78 |
| 乳类 Dairy products | 1.20 | 1.03 | 1.15 | 0.91 | 1.10 | 1.02 | 1.67 | 1.00 | 1.07 | 1.11 | 1.04 | 1.56 | 1.00 | 1.19 | 1.01 | 0.83 | 1.34 | 1.18 | 1.40 | 1.32 | 1.18 | 0.78 | 0.97 | 1.08 | 1.13 |
| 蔬菜类 Vegetables | 0.35 | 0.30 | 0.36 | 0.39 | 0.38 | 0.35 | 0.28 | 0.35 | 0.32 | 0.42 | 0.32 | 0.33 | 0.45 | 0.27 | 0.35 | 0.51 | 0.35 | 0.38 | 0.23 | 0.34 | 0.34 | 0.23 | 0.38 | 0.30 | 0.34 |
| 水果类 Fruits | 0.09 | 0.13 | 0.16 | 0.14 | 0.17 | 0.12 | 0.09 | 0.10 | 0.07 | 0.15 | 0.10 | 0.10 | 0.15 | 0.14 | 0.11 | 0.09 | 0.15 | 0.16 | 0.12 | 0.13 | 0.13 | 0.11 | 0.13 | 0.10 | 0.12 |
| 糖类 Sugar | 0.00 | 0.00 | 0.02 | 0.00 | 0.00 | 0.00 | 0.01 | 0.00 | 0.01 | 0.00 | 0.00 | 0.05 | 1.56 | 0.00 | 0.00 | 0.00 | 0.01 | 0.02 | 0.00 | 0.03 | 0.00 | 0.00 | 0.00 | 0.00 | 0.07 |
| 水及饮料类 Water and beverages | 0.00 | 0.02 | 0.01 | 0.00 | 0.01 | 0.00 | 0.01 | 0.01 | 0.00 | 0.00 | 0.01 | 0.01 | 0.04 | 0.00 | 0.01 | 0.01 | 0.01 | 0.00 | 0.01 | 0.01 | 0.01 | 0.01 | 0.01 | 0.00 | 0.01 |

续表

| 膳食类别<br>Category | 黑龙江<br>HL | 辽宁<br>LN | 河北<br>HE | 北京<br>BJ | 吉林<br>JL | 山西<br>SX | 陕西<br>SN | 河南<br>HA | 宁夏<br>NX | 内蒙古<br>NM | 青海<br>QH | 甘肃<br>GS | 上海<br>SH | 福建<br>FJ | 江西<br>JX | 江苏<br>JS | 浙江<br>ZJ | 山东<br>SD | 湖北<br>HB | 四川<br>SC | 广西<br>GX | 湖南<br>HN | 广东<br>GD | 贵州<br>GZ | 全国平均<br>AVG |
|---|---|---|---|---|---|---|---|---|---|---|---|---|---|---|---|---|---|---|---|---|---|---|---|---|---|
| 酒类<br>Alcohol beverages | 0.05 | 0.08 | 0.07 | 0.12 | 0.11 | 0.00 | 0.06 | 0.08 | ND | 0.08 | 0.07 | 0.13 | 0.16 | 0.10 | 0.04 | 0.05 | 0.09 | 0.08 | 0.04 | 0.06 | 0.07 | 0.02 | 0.13 | 0.03 | 0.07 |

注：ND 表示未检出。计算平均值时，ND 按 1/2 LOD 代入

Note: ND means not to be detected. When calculating the average, ND was substituted at 1/2 LOD

附表 3-14 第六次中国总膳食研究磷的膳食摄入量（单位：mg/d）

Annexed Table 3-14　Dietary intakes of phosphorus from the 6$^{th}$ China TDS (Unit: mg/d)

| 膳食类别<br>Category | 黑龙江<br>HL | 辽宁<br>LN | 河北<br>HE | 北京<br>BJ | 吉林<br>JL | 山西<br>SX | 陕西<br>SN | 河南<br>HA | 宁夏<br>NX | 内蒙古<br>NM | 青海<br>QH | 甘肃<br>GS | 上海<br>SH | 福建<br>FJ | 江西<br>JX | 江苏<br>JS | 浙江<br>ZJ | 山东<br>SD | 湖北<br>HB | 四川<br>SC | 广西<br>GX | 湖南<br>HN | 广东<br>GD | 贵州<br>GZ | 全国平均<br>AVG |
|---|---|---|---|---|---|---|---|---|---|---|---|---|---|---|---|---|---|---|---|---|---|---|---|---|---|
| 谷类<br>Cereals | 364.8 | 308.4 | 381.1 | 302.8 | 331.9 | 624.8 | 537.2 | 664.2 | 326.5 | 544.2 | 544.8 | 374.2 | 207.0 | 219.9 | 205.7 | 192.1 | 287.2 | 563.1 | 183.5 | 341.0 | 365.1 | 144.8 | 170.0 | 133.5 | 346.6 |
| 豆类<br>Legumes | 93.5 | 264.6 | 97.0 | 96.2 | 160.9 | 112.2 | 123.9 | 119.3 | 45.8 | 65.5 | 11.9 | 68.2 | 204.4 | 94.8 | 136.9 | 126.3 | 185.9 | 97.8 | 101.0 | 78.2 | 65.9 | 156.5 | 44.4 | 100.5 | 110.5 |
| 薯类<br>Potatoes | 16.0 | 31.9 | 23.0 | 16.8 | 45.1 | 29.8 | 38.5 | 17.3 | 30.9 | 43.7 | 27.1 | 55.9 | 11.3 | 12.0 | 15.1 | 11.9 | 9.1 | 14.4 | 21.0 | 16.1 | 5.5 | 20.2 | 12.8 | 13.7 | 22.5 |
| 肉类<br>Meats | 83.6 | 123.7 | 77.1 | 119.8 | 138.1 | 170.5 | 49.9 | 105.9 | 68.2 | 89.4 | 137.2 | 69.9 | 189.3 | 140.4 | 164.6 | 158.0 | 224.1 | 160.5 | 78.6 | 193.5 | 261.2 | 163.7 | 206.0 | 134.9 | 137.8 |
| 蛋类<br>Eggs | 85.3 | 82.6 | 68.7 | 95.3 | 89.2 | 56.5 | 48.5 | 69.6 | 32.8 | 77.7 | 34.9 | 46.5 | 80.6 | 40.9 | 46.8 | 52.3 | 54.6 | 89.0 | 45.3 | 41.6 | 35.4 | 46.9 | 37.0 | 25.7 | 57.6 |
| 水产类<br>Aquatic foods | 44.0 | 48.6 | 17.6 | 27.6 | 24.0 | 12.4 | 4.6 | 9.0 | 4.9 | 19.5 | 5.8 | 5.5 | 115.3 | 102.5 | 77.9 | 64.4 | 90.2 | 40.4 | 54.2 | 14.9 | 133.0 | 71.8 | 136.9 | 4.6 | 47.1 |
| 乳类<br>Dairy products | 16.1 | 45.7 | 27.9 | 78.3 | 35.7 | 42.2 | 32.3 | 19.6 | 16.4 | 38.1 | 55.4 | 22.0 | 71.3 | 42.9 | 22.1 | 22.8 | 44.9 | 27.1 | 9.4 | 16.6 | 21.4 | 14.1 | 35.5 | 30.6 | 32.8 |

续表

| 膳食类别 Category | 黑龙江 HL | 辽宁 LN | 河北 HE | 北京 BJ | 吉林 JL | 山西 SX | 陕西 SN | 河南 HA | 宁夏 NX | 内蒙古 NM | 青海 QH | 甘肃 GS | 上海 SH | 福建 FJ | 江西 JX | 江苏 JS | 浙江 ZJ | 山东 SD | 湖北 HB | 四川 SC | 广西 GX | 湖南 HN | 广东 GD | 贵州 GZ | 全国平均 AVG |
|---|---|---|---|---|---|---|---|---|---|---|---|---|---|---|---|---|---|---|---|---|---|---|---|---|---|
| 蔬菜类 Vegetables | 111.1 | 98.5 | 105.0 | 152.8 | 146.4 | 107.7 | 79.1 | 96.8 | 50.1 | 106.9 | 99.8 | 82.1 | 182.1 | 107.6 | 158.9 | 218.7 | 155.0 | 153.2 | 96.2 | 101.7 | 120.7 | 122.0 | 90.5 | 122.6 | 119.4 |
| 水果类 Fruits | 5.9 | 10.3 | 6.1 | 15.7 | 14.6 | 4.2 | 3.5 | 2.4 | 6.2 | 16.5 | 1.6 | 3.3 | 10.9 | 8.2 | 6.5 | 2.4 | 10.1 | 8.5 | 2.3 | 1.9 | 8.5 | 7.0 | 4.0 | 2.0 | 6.8 |
| 糖类 Sugar | 0.0 | 0.0 | 0.0 | 0.0 | 0.0 | 0.0 | 0.0 | 0.0 | 0.0 | 0.0 | 0.0 | 0.0 | 11.9 | 0.0 | 0.0 | 0.0 | 0.0 | 0.0 | 0.0 | 0.0 | 0.0 | 0.0 | 0.0 | 0.0 | 0.5 |
| 水及饮料类 Water and beverages | 1.1 | 8.9 | 4.7 | 0.7 | 7.5 | 0.7 | 3.7 | 1.2 | 1.6 | 10.5 | 7.8 | 6.1 | 25.0 | 3.2 | 11.7 | 11.0 | 6.7 | 3.7 | 2.6 | 3.9 | 13.6 | 5.5 | 6.9 | 4.2 | 6.3 |
| 酒类 Alcohol beverages | 1.1 | 2.8 | 0.7 | 3.2 | 1.0 | 0.0 | 0.1 | 0.2 | 0.0 | 1.6 | 0.3 | 0.4 | 3.6 | 1.4 | 0.9 | 2.0 | 5.9 | 8.7 | 0.6 | 0.3 | 2.4 | 0.4 | 0.2 | 0.1 | 1.6 |
| 合计 SUM | 822.6 | 1026.0 | 808.9 | 909.3 | 994.5 | 1161.0 | 921.2 | 1105.5 | 583.5 | 1013.6 | 926.7 | 734.0 | 1112.6 | 774.0 | 847.2 | 861.9 | 1073.6 | 1166.5 | 594.7 | 809.6 | 1032.7 | 752.8 | 744.1 | 572.3 | 889.5 |

附表 3-15 第六次中国总膳食研究磷的膳食来源（单位：%）

Annexed Table 3-15 Dietary sources of phosphorus from the 6$^{th}$ China TDS (Unit: %)

| 膳食类别 Category | 黑龙江 HL | 辽宁 LN | 河北 HE | 北京 BJ | 吉林 JL | 山西 SX | 陕西 SN | 河南 HA | 宁夏 NX | 内蒙古 NM | 青海 QH | 甘肃 GS | 上海 SH | 福建 FJ | 江西 JX | 江苏 JS | 浙江 ZJ | 山东 SD | 湖北 HB | 四川 SC | 广西 GX | 湖南 HN | 广东 GD | 贵州 GZ | 全国平均 AVG |
|---|---|---|---|---|---|---|---|---|---|---|---|---|---|---|---|---|---|---|---|---|---|---|---|---|---|
| 谷类 Cereals | 44.4 | 30.1 | 47.1 | 33.3 | 33.4 | 53.8 | 58.3 | 60.1 | 56.0 | 53.7 | 58.8 | 51.0 | 18.6 | 28.4 | 24.3 | 22.3 | 26.7 | 48.3 | 30.9 | 42.1 | 35.4 | 19.2 | 22.8 | 23.3 | 39.0 |
| 豆类 Legumes | 11.4 | 25.8 | 12.0 | 10.6 | 16.2 | 9.7 | 13.4 | 10.8 | 7.9 | 6.5 | 1.3 | 9.3 | 18.4 | 12.2 | 16.2 | 14.7 | 17.3 | 8.4 | 17.0 | 9.7 | 6.4 | 20.8 | 6.0 | 17.6 | 12.4 |

续表

| 膳食类别 Category | 黑龙江 HL | 辽宁 LN | 河北 HE | 北京 BJ | 吉林 JL | 山西 SX | 陕西 SN | 河南 HA | 宁夏 NX | 内蒙古 NM | 青海 QH | 甘肃 GS | 上海 SH | 福建 FJ | 江西 JX | 江苏 JS | 浙江 ZJ | 山东 SD | 湖北 HB | 四川 SC | 广西 GX | 湖南 HN | 广东 GD | 贵州 GZ | 全国平均 AVG |
|---|---|---|---|---|---|---|---|---|---|---|---|---|---|---|---|---|---|---|---|---|---|---|---|---|---|
| 薯类 Potatoes | 2.0 | 3.1 | 2.8 | 1.8 | 4.5 | 2.6 | 4.2 | 1.6 | 5.3 | 4.3 | 2.9 | 7.6 | 1.0 | 1.6 | 1.8 | 1.4 | 0.8 | 1.2 | 3.5 | 2.0 | 0.5 | 2.7 | 1.7 | 2.4 | 2.5 |
| 肉类 Meats | 10.2 | 12.1 | 9.5 | 13.2 | 13.9 | 14.7 | 5.4 | 9.6 | 11.7 | 8.8 | 14.8 | 9.5 | 17.0 | 18.1 | 19.4 | 18.3 | 20.9 | 13.8 | 13.2 | 23.9 | 25.3 | 21.7 | 27.7 | 23.6 | 15.5 |
| 蛋类 Eggs | 10.4 | 8.1 | 8.5 | 10.5 | 9.0 | 4.9 | 5.3 | 6.3 | 5.6 | 7.7 | 3.8 | 6.3 | 7.2 | 5.3 | 5.5 | 6.1 | 5.1 | 7.6 | 7.6 | 5.1 | 3.4 | 6.2 | 5.0 | 4.5 | 6.5 |
| 水产类 Aquatic foods | 5.3 | 4.7 | 2.2 | 3.0 | 2.4 | 1.1 | 0.5 | 0.8 | 0.8 | 1.9 | 0.6 | 0.7 | 10.4 | 13.2 | 9.2 | 7.5 | 8.4 | 3.5 | 9.1 | 1.8 | 12.9 | 9.5 | 18.4 | 0.8 | 5.3 |
| 乳类 Dairy products | 2.0 | 4.5 | 3.4 | 8.6 | 3.6 | 3.6 | 3.5 | 1.8 | 2.8 | 3.8 | 6.0 | 3.0 | 6.4 | 5.5 | 2.6 | 2.6 | 4.2 | 2.3 | 1.6 | 2.1 | 2.1 | 1.9 | 4.8 | 5.3 | 3.7 |
| 蔬菜类 Vegetables | 13.5 | 9.6 | 13.0 | 16.8 | 14.7 | 9.3 | 8.6 | 8.8 | 8.6 | 10.5 | 10.8 | 11.2 | 16.4 | 13.9 | 18.8 | 25.4 | 14.4 | 13.1 | 16.2 | 12.6 | 11.7 | 16.2 | 12.2 | 21.4 | 13.4 |
| 水果类 Fruits | 0.7 | 1.0 | 0.8 | 1.7 | 1.5 | 0.4 | 0.4 | 0.2 | 1.1 | 1.6 | 0.2 | 0.4 | 1.0 | 1.1 | 0.8 | 0.3 | 0.9 | 0.7 | 0.4 | 0.2 | 0.8 | 0.9 | 0.5 | 0.3 | 0.8 |
| 糖类 Sugar | 0.0 | 0.0 | 0.0 | 0.0 | 0.0 | 0.0 | 0.0 | 0.0 | 0.0 | 0.0 | 0.0 | 0.0 | 1.1 | 0.0 | 0.0 | 0.0 | 0.0 | 0.3 | 0.0 | 0.0 | 0.0 | 0.0 | 0.0 | 0.0 | 0.1 |
| 水及饮料类 Water and beverages | 0.1 | 0.9 | 0.6 | 0.1 | 0.8 | 0.1 | 0.4 | 0.1 | 0.3 | 1.0 | 0.8 | 0.8 | 2.2 | 0.4 | 1.4 | 1.3 | 0.6 | 0.3 | 0.4 | 0.5 | 1.3 | 0.7 | 0.9 | 0.7 | 0.7 |
| 酒类 Alcohol beverages | 0.1 | 0.3 | 0.1 | 0.4 | 0.1 | 0.0 | 0.0 | 0.0 | 0.0 | 0.2 | 0.0 | 0.1 | 0.3 | 0.2 | 0.1 | 0.2 | 0.6 | 0.7 | 0.1 | 0.0 | 0.2 | 0.1 | 0.0 | 0.0 | 0.2 |

附表 3-16 第六次中国总膳食研究膳食样品中锰的含量（单位：mg/kg）

Annexed Table 3-16 Levels of manganese in food samples from the 6th China TDS (Unit: mg/kg)

| 膳食类别 Category | 黑龙江 HL | 辽宁 LN | 河北 HE | 北京 BJ | 吉林 JL | 山西 SX | 陕西 SN | 河南 HA | 宁夏 NX | 内蒙古 NM | 青海 QH | 甘肃 GS | 上海 SH | 福建 FJ | 江西 JX | 江苏 JS | 浙江 ZJ | 山东 SD | 湖北 HB | 四川 SC | 广西 GX | 湖南 HN | 广东 GD | 贵州 GZ | 全国平均 AVG |
|---|---|---|---|---|---|---|---|---|---|---|---|---|---|---|---|---|---|---|---|---|---|---|---|---|---|
| 谷类 Cereals | 4.05 | 3.20 | 2.50 | 2.86 | 3.06 | 3.41 | 2.85 | 4.49 | 3.54 | 3.85 | 3.61 | 2.11 | 2.74 | 4.39 | 4.22 | 2.92 | 4.06 | 3.84 | 2.78 | 2.98 | 3.38 | 3.28 | 2.94 | 2.74 | 3.33 |
| 豆类 Legumes | 11.60 | 15.11 | 8.34 | 4.01 | 12.38 | 9.21 | 9.31 | 11.02 | 3.71 | 8.40 | 9.10 | 5.84 | 6.20 | 6.45 | 12.56 | 10.99 | 7.57 | 10.45 | 9.34 | 5.96 | 7.03 | 10.34 | 6.96 | 7.92 | 8.74 |
| 薯类 Potatoes | 0.59 | 4.47 | 2.16 | 2.02 | 1.16 | 1.18 | 1.87 | 1.25 | 2.93 | 3.54 | 1.41 | 1.53 | 0.86 | 2.31 | 8.59 | 6.86 | 2.56 | 1.39 | 2.18 | 1.63 | 4.36 | 7.32 | 5.70 | 2.95 | 2.95 |
| 肉类 Meats | 1.33 | 1.98 | 1.21 | 1.05 | 1.17 | 1.52 | 1.37 | 1.13 | 2.02 | 1.53 | 2.45 | 2.12 | 1.95 | 0.69 | 1.16 | 2.76 | 1.36 | 0.49 | 1.49 | 0.99 | 0.24 | 0.82 | 0.59 | 0.49 | 1.33 |
| 蛋类 Eggs | 0.43 | 0.62 | 0.69 | 0.60 | 0.44 | 0.62 | 0.63 | 0.64 | 0.61 | 0.42 | 1.15 | 0.29 | 0.30 | 0.91 | 0.48 | 1.28 | 0.70 | 0.98 | 1.67 | 0.61 | 0.54 | 0.69 | 0.40 | 0.49 | 0.67 |
| 水产类 Aquatic foods | 0.32 | 1.54 | 0.63 | 2.30 | 0.91 | 0.87 | 0.17 | 0.93 | 0.18 | 1.64 | 1.73 | 0.84 | 1.06 | 1.94 | 1.16 | 2.26 | 2.71 | 0.89 | 2.13 | 0.47 | 0.16 | 0.80 | 0.80 | 1.26 | 1.15 |
| 乳类 Dairy products | 0.04 | 0.05 | 0.05 | 0.03 | 0.03 | 0.03 | 0.04 | 0.03 | 0.03 | 0.05 | 0.04 | 0.03 | 0.03 | 0.05 | 0.07 | 0.02 | 0.04 | 0.03 | 0.08 | 0.04 | 0.03 | 0.07 | 0.04 | 0.03 | 0.04 |
| 蔬菜类 Vegetables | 1.43 | 3.15 | 1.41 | 2.34 | 1.91 | 1.71 | 2.11 | 2.01 | 2.50 | 1.59 | 1.80 | 1.77 | 2.26 | 3.21 | 3.17 | 4.51 | 4.07 | 2.01 | 1.80 | 1.92 | 3.70 | 2.70 | 2.36 | 3.81 | 2.47 |
| 水果类 Fruits | 0.44 | 0.71 | 2.14 | 0.85 | 0.81 | 1.54 | 0.88 | 2.31 | 1.35 | 2.34 | 0.41 | 0.72 | 1.94 | 4.94 | 0.47 | 1.32 | 1.55 | 2.97 | 1.76 | 1.40 | 6.82 | 0.88 | 2.18 | 1.46 | 1.76 |
| 糖类 Sugar | 0.03 | 0.04 | 3.16 | 0.21 | 0.09 | 0.04 | 0.07 | 0.34 | 0.09 | 0.38 | 0.04 | 2.39 | 4.71 | 0.29 | 0.09 | 0.16 | 0.12 | 0.81 | 0.08 | 0.28 | 0.05 | 0.28 | 0.03 | 0.18 | 0.58 |
| 水及饮料类 Water and beverages | 0.01 | 0.32 | 0.09 | 0.05 | 0.02 | 0.01 | 0.82 | 0.18 | 0.05 | 0.73 | 4.04 | 0.02 | 2.09 | 0.37 | 0.02 | 1.09 | 0.83 | 0.01 | 1.10 | 0.66 | 0.26 | 1.50 | 0.81 | 0.01 | 0.63 |

续表

| 膳食类别<br>Category | 黑龙江<br>HL | 辽宁<br>LN | 河北<br>HE | 北京<br>BJ | 吉林<br>JL | 山西<br>SX | 陕西<br>SN | 河南<br>HA | 宁夏<br>NX | 内蒙古<br>NM | 青海<br>QH | 甘肃<br>GS | 上海<br>SH | 福建<br>FJ | 江西<br>JX | 江苏<br>JS | 浙江<br>ZJ | 山东<br>SD | 湖北<br>HB | 四川<br>SC | 广西<br>GX | 湖南<br>HN | 广东<br>GD | 贵州<br>GZ | 全国平均<br>AVG |
|---|---|---|---|---|---|---|---|---|---|---|---|---|---|---|---|---|---|---|---|---|---|---|---|---|---|
| 酒类<br>Alcohol beverages | 0.05 | 0.11 | 0.13 | 0.25 | 0.11 | 0.00 | 0.09 | 0.19 | 0.01 | 0.11 | 0.11 | 0.11 | 1.13 | 0.20 | 0.06 | 0.40 | 0.28 | 0.19 | 0.06 | 0.07 | 1.29 | 0.11 | 0.52 | 0.19 | 0.24 |

附表 3-17　第六次中国总膳食研究锰的膳食摄入量（单位：mg/d）
Annexed Table 3-17　Dietary intakes of manganese from the 6$^{th}$ China TDS (Unit: mg/d)

| 膳食类别<br>Category | 黑龙江<br>HL | 辽宁<br>LN | 河北<br>HE | 北京<br>BJ | 吉林<br>JL | 山西<br>SX | 陕西<br>SN | 河南<br>HA | 宁夏<br>NX | 内蒙古<br>NM | 青海<br>QH | 甘肃<br>GS | 上海<br>SH | 福建<br>FJ | 江西<br>JX | 江苏<br>JS | 浙江<br>ZJ | 山东<br>SD | 湖北<br>HB | 四川<br>SC | 广西<br>GX | 湖南<br>HN | 广东<br>GD | 贵州<br>GZ | 全国平均<br>AVG |
|---|---|---|---|---|---|---|---|---|---|---|---|---|---|---|---|---|---|---|---|---|---|---|---|---|---|
| 谷类<br>Cereals | 2.22 | 1.97 | 1.89 | 2.27 | 1.79 | 3.54 | 2.18 | 4.15 | 2.34 | 2.79 | 2.77 | 1.45 | 1.23 | 2.77 | 2.66 | 2.27 | 2.57 | 3.83 | 1.47 | 2.89 | 3.18 | 1.89 | 1.34 | 1.85 | 2.39 |
| 豆类<br>Legumes | 0.53 | 1.84 | 0.48 | 0.41 | 0.93 | 0.64 | 0.77 | 0.59 | 0.13 | 0.34 | 0.06 | 0.24 | 0.73 | 0.51 | 0.93 | 0.91 | 1.07 | 0.55 | 0.62 | 0.40 | 0.30 | 0.75 | 0.19 | 0.80 | 0.61 |
| 薯类<br>Potatoes | 0.05 | 0.32 | 0.13 | 0.12 | 0.14 | 0.14 | 0.21 | 0.10 | 0.29 | 0.43 | 0.14 | 0.22 | 0.03 | 0.10 | 0.28 | 0.23 | 0.09 | 0.06 | 0.19 | 0.10 | 0.06 | 0.39 | 0.14 | 0.10 | 0.17 |
| 肉类<br>Meats | 0.08 | 0.13 | 0.06 | 0.07 | 0.08 | 0.21 | 0.05 | 0.06 | 0.09 | 0.11 | 0.17 | 0.07 | 0.22 | 0.06 | 0.11 | 0.25 | 0.16 | 0.05 | 0.08 | 0.13 | 0.04 | 0.12 | 0.06 | 0.05 | 0.10 |
| 蛋类<br>Eggs | 0.02 | 0.03 | 0.02 | 0.02 | 0.02 | 0.01 | 0.01 | 0.02 | 0.01 | 0.01 | 0.02 | 0.01 | 0.01 | 0.02 | 0.01 | 0.04 | 0.02 | 0.04 | 0.04 | 0.01 | 0.01 | 0.02 | 0.01 | 0.01 | 0.02 |
| 水产类<br>Aquatic foods | 0.01 | 0.02 | 0.01 | 0.04 | 0.01 | 0.01 | 0.00 | 0.00 | 0.00 | 0.02 | 0.01 | 0.00 | 0.07 | 0.12 | 0.05 | 0.09 | 0.14 | 0.02 | 0.09 | 0.00 | 0.02 | 0.05 | 0.04 | 0.00 | 0.03 |
| 乳类<br>Dairy products | 0.00 | 0.00 | 0.00 | 0.00 | 0.00 | 0.00 | 0.00 | 0.00 | 0.00 | 0.00 | 0.00 | 0.00 | 0.00 | 0.00 | 0.00 | 0.00 | 0.00 | 0.00 | 0.00 | 0.00 | 0.00 | 0.00 | 0.00 | 0.00 | 0.00 |

续表

| 膳食类别<br>Category | 黑龙江<br>HL | 辽宁<br>LN | 河北<br>HE | 北京<br>BJ | 吉林<br>JL | 山西<br>SX | 陕西<br>SN | 河南<br>HA | 宁夏<br>NX | 内蒙古<br>NM | 青海<br>QH | 甘肃<br>GS | 上海<br>SH | 福建<br>FJ | 江西<br>JX | 江苏<br>JS | 浙江<br>ZJ | 山东<br>SD | 湖北<br>HB | 四川<br>SC | 广西<br>GX | 湖南<br>HN | 广东<br>GD | 贵州<br>GZ | 全国平均<br>AVG |
|---|---|---|---|---|---|---|---|---|---|---|---|---|---|---|---|---|---|---|---|---|---|---|---|---|---|
| 蔬菜类 Vegetables | 0.46 | 1.03 | 0.41 | 0.92 | 0.74 | 0.53 | 0.60 | 0.56 | 0.39 | 0.41 | 0.56 | 0.44 | 0.91 | 1.27 | 1.43 | 1.92 | 1.81 | 0.82 | 0.75 | 0.58 | 1.31 | 1.44 | 0.56 | 1.56 | 0.89 |
| 水果类 Fruits | 0.03 | 0.05 | 0.08 | 0.10 | 0.07 | 0.05 | 0.03 | 0.06 | 0.11 | 0.26 | 0.01 | 0.02 | 0.14 | 0.30 | 0.03 | 0.04 | 0.10 | 0.16 | 0.03 | 0.02 | 0.44 | 0.06 | 0.06 | 0.03 | 0.10 |
| 糖类 Sugar | 0.00 | 0.00 | 0.00 | 0.00 | 0.00 | 0.00 | 0.00 | 0.00 | 0.00 | 0.00 | 0.00 | 0.00 | 0.04 | 0.00 | 0.00 | 0.00 | 0.00 | 0.00 | 0.00 | 0.00 | 0.00 | 0.00 | 0.00 | 0.00 | 0.00 |
| 水及饮料类 Water and beverages | 0.01 | 0.16 | 0.07 | 0.06 | 0.03 | 0.01 | 0.28 | 0.21 | 0.03 | 1.88 | 2.50 | 0.03 | 1.47 | 0.32 | 0.02 | 1.10 | 0.65 | 0.02 | 0.31 | 0.21 | 0.34 | 1.59 | 0.96 | 0.02 | 0.51 |
| 酒类 Alcohol beverages | 0.00 | 0.00 | 0.00 | 0.01 | 0.00 | 0.00 | 0.00 | 0.00 | 0.00 | 0.00 | 0.00 | 0.00 | 0.03 | 0.00 | 0.00 | 0.02 | 0.02 | 0.02 | 0.00 | 0.00 | 0.04 | 0.00 | 0.00 | 0.00 | 0.01 |
| 合计 SUM | 3.39 | 5.56 | 3.15 | 4.01 | 3.81 | 5.13 | 4.15 | 5.76 | 3.40 | 6.26 | 6.23 | 2.48 | 4.87 | 5.47 | 5.51 | 6.86 | 6.62 | 5.57 | 3.59 | 4.35 | 5.73 | 6.32 | 3.38 | 4.43 | 4.83 |

附表 3-18 第六次中国总膳食研究锰的膳食来源（单位：%）

Annexed Table 3-18 Dietary sources of manganese from the 6$^{th}$ China TDS (Unit: %)

| 膳食类别<br>Category | 黑龙江<br>HL | 辽宁<br>LN | 河北<br>HE | 北京<br>BJ | 吉林<br>JL | 山西<br>SX | 陕西<br>SN | 河南<br>HA | 宁夏<br>NX | 内蒙古<br>NM | 青海<br>QH | 甘肃<br>GS | 上海<br>SH | 福建<br>FJ | 江西<br>JX | 江苏<br>JS | 浙江<br>ZJ | 山东<br>SD | 湖北<br>HB | 四川<br>SC | 广西<br>GX | 湖南<br>HN | 广东<br>GD | 贵州<br>GZ | 全国平均<br>AVG |
|---|---|---|---|---|---|---|---|---|---|---|---|---|---|---|---|---|---|---|---|---|---|---|---|---|---|
| 谷类 Cereals | 65.4 | 35.4 | 60.0 | 56.7 | 47.0 | 68.9 | 52.5 | 72.0 | 68.9 | 44.5 | 44.4 | 58.5 | 25.3 | 50.7 | 48.2 | 33.1 | 38.8 | 68.7 | 40.9 | 66.5 | 55.5 | 29.9 | 39.8 | 41.8 | 49.4 |
| 豆类 Legumes | 15.5 | 33.1 | 15.1 | 10.2 | 24.5 | 12.5 | 18.6 | 10.3 | 3.8 | 5.4 | 0.9 | 9.7 | 15.0 | 9.3 | 16.8 | 13.3 | 16.1 | 9.8 | 17.4 | 9.3 | 5.2 | 11.9 | 5.8 | 18.2 | 12.7 |
| 薯类 Potatoes | 1.4 | 5.8 | 4.2 | 2.9 | 3.6 | 2.7 | 5.2 | 1.7 | 8.6 | 6.9 | 2.3 | 8.9 | 0.6 | 1.8 | 5.0 | 3.3 | 1.4 | 1.2 | 5.4 | 2.4 | 1.0 | 6.2 | 4.2 | 2.3 | 3.5 |

续表

| 膳食类别 Category | 黑龙江 HL | 辽宁 LN | 河北 HE | 北京 BJ | 吉林 JL | 山西 SX | 陕西 SN | 河南 HA | 宁夏 NX | 内蒙古 NM | 青海 QH | 甘肃 GS | 上海 SH | 福建 FJ | 江西 JX | 江苏 JS | 浙江 ZJ | 山东 SD | 湖北 HB | 四川 SC | 广西 GX | 湖南 HN | 广东 GD | 贵州 GZ | 全国平均 AVG |
|---|---|---|---|---|---|---|---|---|---|---|---|---|---|---|---|---|---|---|---|---|---|---|---|---|---|
| 肉类 Meats | 2.3 | 2.4 | 1.8 | 1.8 | 2.0 | 4.1 | 1.2 | 1.1 | 2.8 | 1.8 | 2.8 | 2.6 | 4.4 | 1.1 | 2.0 | 3.7 | 2.4 | 0.9 | 2.3 | 2.9 | 0.6 | 1.9 | 1.8 | 1.2 | 2.2 |
| 蛋类 Eggs | 0.5 | 0.5 | 0.7 | 0.6 | 0.5 | 0.3 | 0.3 | 0.3 | 0.2 | 0.2 | 0.2 | 0.3 | 0.2 | 0.3 | 0.2 | 0.5 | 0.3 | 0.8 | 1.2 | 0.2 | 0.1 | 0.2 | 0.3 | 0.2 | 0.4 |
| 水产类 Aquatic foods | 0.3 | 0.4 | 0.2 | 0.9 | 0.3 | 0.1 | 0.0 | 0.1 | 0.0 | 0.3 | 0.1 | 0.1 | 1.5 | 2.3 | 0.9 | 1.3 | 2.1 | 0.4 | 2.4 | 0.1 | 0.3 | 0.8 | 1.2 | 0.1 | 0.7 |
| 乳类 Dairy products | 0.0 | 0.0 | 0.0 | 0.1 | 0.0 | 0.0 | 0.0 | 0.0 | 0.0 | 0.0 | 0.0 | 0.0 | 0.0 | 0.0 | 0.0 | 0.0 | 0.0 | 0.0 | 0.0 | 0.0 | 0.0 | 0.0 | 0.0 | 0.0 | 0.0 |
| 蔬菜类 Vegetables | 13.5 | 18.5 | 13.1 | 22.8 | 19.4 | 10.3 | 14.6 | 9.7 | 11.5 | 6.6 | 9.0 | 17.8 | 18.6 | 23.3 | 26.0 | 28.0 | 27.3 | 14.6 | 20.8 | 13.3 | 22.8 | 22.8 | 16.5 | 35.2 | 18.4 |
| 水果类 Fruits | 0.8 | 1.0 | 2.6 | 2.4 | 1.9 | 1.0 | 0.8 | 1.0 | 3.4 | 4.2 | 0.1 | 1.0 | 2.9 | 5.4 | 0.5 | 0.5 | 1.6 | 2.9 | 0.9 | 0.5 | 7.7 | 0.9 | 1.9 | 0.7 | 2.0 |
| 糖类 Sugar | 0.0 | 0.0 | 0.0 | 0.0 | 0.0 | 0.0 | 0.0 | 0.0 | 0.0 | 0.0 | 0.0 | 0.0 | 0.7 | 0.0 | 0.0 | 0.0 | 0.0 | 0.0 | 0.0 | 0.0 | 0.0 | 0.0 | 0.0 | 0.0 | 0.0 |
| 水及饮料类 Water and beverages | 0.3 | 2.9 | 2.2 | 1.4 | 0.8 | 0.1 | 6.8 | 3.7 | 0.8 | 30.1 | 40.1 | 1.1 | 30.2 | 5.8 | 0.4 | 16.1 | 9.8 | 0.3 | 8.7 | 4.8 | 6.0 | 25.2 | 28.5 | 0.4 | 10.6 |
| 酒类 Alcohol beverages | 0.0 | 0.1 | 0.0 | 0.2 | 0.0 | 0.0 | 0.0 | 0.0 | 0.0 | 0.0 | 0.0 | 0.0 | 0.5 | 0.1 | 0.0 | 0.2 | 0.3 | 0.4 | 0.0 | 0.0 | 0.7 | 0.0 | 0.0 | 0.0 | 0.1 |

附表 3-19 第六次中国总膳食研究膳食样品中铁的含量（单位：mg/kg）

Annexed Table 3-19  Levels of iron in food samples from the 6$^{th}$ China TDS (Unit: mg/kg)

| 膳食类别<br>Category | 黑龙江<br>HL | 辽宁<br>LN | 河北<br>HE | 北京<br>BJ | 吉林<br>JL | 山西<br>SX | 陕西<br>SN | 河南<br>HA | 宁夏<br>NX | 内蒙古<br>NM | 青海<br>QH | 甘肃<br>GS | 上海<br>SH | 福建<br>FJ | 江西<br>JX | 江苏<br>JS | 浙江<br>ZJ | 山东<br>SD | 湖北<br>HB | 四川<br>SC | 广西<br>GX | 湖南<br>HN | 广东<br>GD | 贵州<br>GZ | 全国平均<br>AVG |
|---|---|---|---|---|---|---|---|---|---|---|---|---|---|---|---|---|---|---|---|---|---|---|---|---|---|
| 谷类 Cereals | 10.53 | 4.01 | 6.07 | 4.56 | 7.28 | 10.49 | 6.14 | 23.89 | 7.87 | 8.49 | 9.73 | 8.60 | 2.70 | 2.96 | 4.36 | 3.72 | 2.87 | 20.52 | 1.72 | 5.61 | 1.44 | 0.69 | 5.08 | 3.12 | 6.77 |
| 豆类 Legumes | 20.35 | 23.50 | 15.54 | 14.88 | 41.31 | 17.90 | 28.19 | 25.40 | 11.77 | 15.13 | 28.92 | 21.12 | 22.52 | 13.50 | 29.88 | 32.93 | 22.40 | 25.71 | 20.00 | 14.86 | 18.59 | 29.17 | 18.45 | 22.49 | 22.27 |
| 薯类 Potatoes | 10.71 | 27.63 | 9.74 | 11.57 | 12.37 | 14.56 | 12.69 | 19.51 | 13.07 | 11.38 | 9.18 | 11.67 | 10.76 | 11.69 | 9.45 | 12.70 | 14.03 | 16.74 | 7.35 | 5.29 | 9.59 | 20.33 | 6.35 | 14.95 | 12.64 |
| 肉类 Meats | 36.67 | 14.63 | 8.97 | 19.31 | 32.72 | 22.63 | 20.85 | 18.63 | 24.57 | 18.14 | 17.16 | 26.16 | 20.47 | 13.33 | 18.95 | 27.22 | 24.43 | 17.58 | 16.95 | 18.33 | 10.50 | 28.80 | 31.90 | 34.22 | 21.80 |
| 蛋类 Eggs | 44.01 | 25.54 | 29.45 | 27.58 | 24.83 | 31.39 | 25.93 | 31.76 | 33.01 | 32.14 | 22.99 | 22.17 | 21.87 | 26.53 | 29.50 | 38.56 | 33.83 | 26.07 | 23.22 | 25.07 | 20.00 | 40.14 | 15.90 | 23.91 | 28.14 |
| 水产类 Aquatic foods | 21.72 | 24.54 | 10.24 | 16.26 | 19.39 | 15.09 | 6.54 | 22.70 | 8.67 | 28.45 | 13.04 | 8.61 | 12.08 | 21.27 | 8.22 | 19.26 | 45.39 | 20.55 | 9.27 | 9.64 | 5.28 | 12.50 | 7.37 | 19.74 | 16.08 |
| 乳类 Dairy products | 0.49 | 0.32 | 0.20 | 0.30 | 0.27 | 0.34 | 0.33 | 0.09 | 0.74 | 0.18 | 0.37 | 2.13 | 0.78 | 0.31 | 0.71 | 0.16 | 0.34 | 0.38 | 7.58 | 0.40 | 0.18 | 0.99 | 0.56 | 0.23 | 0.77 |
| 蔬菜类 Vegetables | 10.55 | 10.31 | 5.34 | 9.08 | 10.00 | 11.34 | 8.07 | 16.66 | 11.16 | 9.64 | 6.97 | 9.36 | 9.55 | 7.18 | 14.96 | 22.81 | 17.24 | 15.56 | 15.46 | 4.68 | 12.39 | 15.09 | 7.78 | 39.40 | 12.52 |
| 水果类 Fruits | 1.40 | 2.66 | 3.24 | 1.93 | 1.51 | 1.72 | 0.88 | 8.14 | 2.08 | 1.68 | 2.77 | 1.20 | 2.34 | 1.34 | 1.48 | 1.24 | 1.23 | 1.95 | 1.84 | 1.74 | 1.01 | 8.75 | 2.44 | 4.79 | 2.47 |
| 糖类 Sugar | 1.37 | 2.48 | 6.69 | 1.44 | 1.54 | 0.92 | 0.36 | 1.64 | 1.59 | 1.58 | 1.01 | 5.89 | 51.58 | 1.15 | 1.61 | 2.82 | 2.17 | 6.10 | 0.37 | 1.97 | 1.09 | 8.03 | 1.50 | ND | 4.37 |
| 水及饮料类 Water and beverages | 0.15 | 0.26 | 0.03 | 0.09 | 0.16 | 0.18 | 0.18 | 0.08 | 0.50 | 0.14 | 0.18 | 0.10 | 0.25 | 0.28 | 0.13 | 0.13 | 0.17 | 0.19 | 0.07 | 0.11 | 0.08 | 0.61 | 0.30 | ND | 0.18 |

续表

| 膳食类别 Category | 黑龙江 HL | 辽宁 LN | 河北 HE | 北京 BJ | 吉林 JL | 山西 SX | 陕西 SN | 河南 HA | 宁夏 NX | 内蒙古 NM | 青海 QH | 甘肃 GS | 上海 SH | 福建 FJ | 江西 JX | 江苏 JS | 浙江 ZJ | 山东 SD | 湖北 HB | 四川 SC | 广西 GX | 湖南 HN | 广东 GD | 贵州 GZ | 全国平均 AVG |
|---|---|---|---|---|---|---|---|---|---|---|---|---|---|---|---|---|---|---|---|---|---|---|---|---|---|
| 酒类 Alcohol beverages | 0.12 | 0.12 | 0.05 | 0.24 | 0.19 | 0.18 | 0.13 | 0.40 | 0.39 | 0.03 | 0.17 | 0.16 | 1.61 | 0.22 | 0.08 | 0.30 | 0.31 | 0.52 | 0.06 | 0.26 | 1.84 | 0.53 | 1.16 | 0.15 | 0.38 |

注: ND 表示未检出。计算平均值时, ND 按 1/2 LOD 代入
Note: ND means not to be detected. When calculating the average, ND was substituted at 1/2 LOD

附表 3-20 第六次中国总膳食研究铁的膳食摄入量（单位: mg/d）

Annexed Table 3-20 Dietary intakes of iron from the 6th China TDS (Unit: mg/d)

| 膳食类别 Category | 黑龙江 HL | 辽宁 LN | 河北 HE | 北京 BJ | 吉林 JL | 山西 SX | 陕西 SN | 河南 HA | 宁夏 NX | 内蒙古 NM | 青海 QH | 甘肃 GS | 上海 SH | 福建 FJ | 江西 JX | 江苏 JS | 浙江 ZJ | 山东 SD | 湖北 HB | 四川 SC | 广西 GX | 湖南 HN | 广东 GD | 贵州 GZ | 全国平均 AVG |
|---|---|---|---|---|---|---|---|---|---|---|---|---|---|---|---|---|---|---|---|---|---|---|---|---|---|
| 谷类 Cereals | 5.77 | 2.47 | 4.59 | 3.62 | 4.26 | 10.88 | 4.69 | 22.08 | 5.21 | 6.14 | 7.45 | 5.90 | 1.21 | 1.87 | 2.75 | 2.89 | 1.82 | 20.43 | 0.91 | 5.44 | 1.36 | 0.40 | 2.32 | 2.11 | 5.27 |
| 豆类 Legumes | 0.92 | 2.87 | 0.89 | 1.51 | 3.12 | 1.24 | 2.33 | 1.37 | 0.41 | 0.60 | 0.19 | 0.87 | 2.65 | 1.06 | 2.20 | 2.73 | 3.16 | 1.35 | 1.34 | 1.00 | 0.79 | 2.12 | 0.51 | 2.29 | 1.56 |
| 薯类 Potatoes | 0.83 | 1.99 | 0.59 | 0.68 | 1.48 | 1.73 | 1.46 | 1.57 | 1.31 | 1.39 | 0.93 | 1.68 | 0.39 | 0.49 | 0.30 | 0.42 | 0.51 | 0.77 | 0.65 | 0.33 | 0.12 | 1.09 | 0.16 | 0.51 | 0.89 |
| 肉类 Meats | 2.20 | 0.98 | 0.42 | 1.30 | 2.18 | 3.10 | 0.75 | 1.03 | 1.15 | 1.33 | 1.22 | 0.81 | 2.27 | 1.15 | 1.78 | 2.50 | 2.89 | 1.71 | 0.92 | 2.36 | 1.59 | 4.30 | 3.32 | 3.64 | 1.87 |
| 蛋类 Eggs | 1.78 | 1.04 | 0.93 | 1.07 | 1.00 | 0.66 | 0.57 | 0.94 | 0.43 | 0.95 | 0.30 | 0.49 | 0.85 | 0.50 | 0.60 | 1.08 | 0.81 | 1.16 | 0.58 | 0.37 | 0.28 | 0.92 | 0.38 | 0.39 | 0.75 |
| 水产类 Aquatic foods | 0.59 | 0.39 | 0.10 | 0.27 | 0.22 | 0.10 | 0.03 | 0.11 | 0.02 | 0.29 | 0.05 | 0.02 | 0.83 | 1.37 | 0.36 | 0.75 | 2.28 | 0.47 | 0.38 | 0.08 | 0.51 | 0.83 | 0.38 | 0.07 | 0.44 |
| 乳类 Dairy products | 0.01 | 0.01 | 0.00 | 0.03 | 0.01 | 0.01 | 0.01 | 0.00 | 0.01 | 0.01 | 0.02 | 0.03 | 0.06 | 0.01 | 0.02 | 0.00 | 0.01 | 0.01 | 0.05 | 0.00 | 0.00 | 0.02 | 0.02 | 0.01 | 0.01 |

续表

附表 3-21 第六次中国总膳食研究铁的膳食来源（单位：%）

Annexed Table 3-21 Dietary sources of iron from the 6th China TDS (Unit: %)

| 膳食类别 Category | 黑龙江 HL | 辽宁 LN | 河北 HE | 北京 BJ | 吉林 JL | 山西 SX | 陕西 SN | 河南 HA | 宁夏 NX | 内蒙古 NM | 青海 QH | 甘肃 GS | 上海 SH | 福建 FJ | 江西 JX | 江苏 JS | 浙江 ZJ | 山东 SD | 湖北 HB | 四川 SC | 广西 GX | 湖南 HN | 广东 GD | 贵州 GZ | 全国平均 AVG |
|---|---|---|---|---|---|---|---|---|---|---|---|---|---|---|---|---|---|---|---|---|---|---|---|---|---|
| 蔬菜类 Vegetables | 3.38 | 3.37 | 1.57 | 3.56 | 3.88 | 3.51 | 2.32 | 4.63 | 1.74 | 2.48 | 2.17 | 2.32 | 3.83 | 2.85 | 6.76 | 9.70 | 7.66 | 6.32 | 6.40 | 1.42 | 4.38 | 8.06 | 1.84 | 16.07 | 4.59 |
| 水果类 Fruits | 0.09 | 0.20 | 0.12 | 0.22 | 0.13 | 0.06 | 0.03 | 0.20 | 0.18 | 0.19 | 0.04 | 0.04 | 0.17 | 0.08 | 0.08 | 0.03 | 0.08 | 0.11 | 0.04 | 0.03 | 0.07 | 0.55 | 0.07 | 0.10 | 0.12 |
| 糖类 Sugar | 0.00 | 0.00 | 0.00 | 0.00 | 0.00 | 0.00 | 0.00 | 0.00 | 0.00 | 0.00 | 0.00 | 0.00 | 0.39 | 0.00 | 0.00 | 0.00 | 0.00 | 0.00 | 0.00 | 0.00 | 0.00 | 0.00 | 0.00 | 0.00 | 0.02 |
| 水及饮料类 Water and beverages | 0.18 | 0.13 | 0.02 | 0.10 | 0.21 | 0.14 | 0.06 | 0.09 | 0.26 | 0.35 | 0.11 | 0.12 | 0.17 | 0.24 | 0.15 | 0.13 | 0.14 | 0.34 | 0.02 | 0.04 | 0.10 | 0.64 | 0.36 | 0.01 | 0.17 |
| 酒类 Alcohol beverages | 0.00 | 0.00 | 0.00 | 0.01 | 0.00 | 0.00 | 0.00 | 0.00 | 0.00 | 0.00 | 0.00 | 0.00 | 0.04 | 0.00 | 0.00 | 0.01 | 0.02 | 0.06 | 0.00 | 0.00 | 0.06 | 0.01 | 0.00 | 0.00 | 0.01 |
| 合计 SUM | 15.76 | 13.46 | 9.24 | 12.37 | 16.48 | 21.43 | 12.24 | 32.02 | 10.72 | 13.74 | 12.48 | 12.29 | 12.85 | 9.63 | 15.01 | 20.27 | 19.38 | 32.72 | 11.28 | 11.07 | 9.26 | 18.94 | 9.37 | 25.19 | 15.72 |

| 膳食类别 Category | 黑龙江 HL | 辽宁 LN | 河北 HE | 北京 BJ | 吉林 JL | 山西 SX | 陕西 SN | 河南 HA | 宁夏 NX | 内蒙古 NM | 青海 QH | 甘肃 GS | 上海 SH | 福建 FJ | 江西 JX | 江苏 JS | 浙江 ZJ | 山东 SD | 湖北 HB | 四川 SC | 广西 GX | 湖南 HN | 广东 GD | 贵州 GZ | 全国平均 AVG |
|---|---|---|---|---|---|---|---|---|---|---|---|---|---|---|---|---|---|---|---|---|---|---|---|---|---|
| 谷类 Cereals | 36.6 | 18.3 | 49.6 | 29.3 | 25.8 | 50.8 | 38.2 | 69.0 | 48.6 | 44.7 | 59.7 | 48.0 | 9.4 | 19.5 | 18.3 | 14.3 | 9.4 | 62.4 | 8.0 | 49.1 | 14.7 | 2.1 | 24.8 | 8.4 | 33.6 |
| 豆类 Legumes | 5.9 | 21.3 | 9.6 | 12.2 | 18.9 | 5.8 | 19.0 | 4.3 | 3.9 | 4.4 | 1.5 | 7.1 | 20.6 | 11.0 | 14.7 | 13.5 | 16.3 | 4.1 | 11.8 | 9.1 | 8.5 | 11.2 | 5.5 | 9.1 | 9.9 |

续表

| 膳食类别<br>Category | 黑龙江<br>HL | 辽宁<br>LN | 河北<br>HE | 北京<br>BJ | 吉林<br>JL | 山西<br>SX | 陕西<br>SN | 河南<br>HA | 宁夏<br>NX | 内蒙古<br>NM | 青海<br>QH | 甘肃<br>GS | 上海<br>SH | 福建<br>FJ | 江西<br>JX | 江苏<br>JS | 浙江<br>ZJ | 山东<br>SD | 湖北<br>HB | 四川<br>SC | 广西<br>GX | 湖南<br>HN | 广东<br>GD | 贵州<br>GZ | 全国平均<br>AVG |
|---|---|---|---|---|---|---|---|---|---|---|---|---|---|---|---|---|---|---|---|---|---|---|---|---|---|
| 薯类<br>Potatoes | 5.3 | 14.8 | 6.4 | 5.5 | 9.0 | 8.1 | 11.9 | 4.9 | 12.2 | 10.1 | 7.5 | 13.7 | 3.0 | 5.1 | 2.0 | 2.1 | 2.7 | 2.4 | 5.8 | 3.0 | 1.3 | 5.8 | 1.7 | 2.0 | 5.7 |
| 肉类<br>Meats | 13.9 | 7.3 | 4.6 | 10.5 | 13.2 | 14.5 | 6.1 | 3.2 | 10.7 | 9.7 | 9.8 | 6.6 | 17.6 | 11.9 | 11.9 | 12.3 | 14.9 | 5.2 | 8.2 | 21.3 | 17.1 | 22.7 | 35.5 | 14.5 | 11.9 |
| 蛋类<br>Eggs | 11.3 | 7.8 | 10.1 | 8.7 | 6.1 | 3.1 | 4.7 | 2.9 | 4.0 | 6.9 | 2.4 | 4.0 | 6.6 | 5.2 | 4.0 | 5.4 | 4.2 | 3.5 | 5.1 | 3.3 | 3.0 | 4.8 | 4.1 | 1.5 | 4.8 |
| 水产类<br>Aquatic foods | 3.7 | 2.9 | 1.1 | 2.2 | 1.3 | 0.5 | 0.2 | 0.3 | 0.2 | 2.1 | 0.4 | 0.2 | 6.4 | 14.2 | 2.4 | 3.7 | 11.8 | 1.4 | 3.3 | 0.7 | 5.5 | 4.4 | 4.0 | 0.3 | 2.8 |
| 乳类<br>Dairy products | 0.0 | 0.1 | 0.1 | 0.2 | 0.1 | 0.1 | 0.1 | 0.0 | 0.1 | 0.0 | 0.2 | 0.2 | 0.4 | 0.1 | 0.1 | 0.0 | 0.1 | 0.0 | 0.5 | 0.0 | 0.0 | 0.1 | 0.2 | 0.0 | 0.1 |
| 蔬菜类<br>Vegetables | 21.5 | 25.0 | 17.0 | 28.8 | 23.5 | 16.4 | 18.9 | 14.5 | 16.3 | 18.0 | 17.4 | 18.9 | 29.8 | 29.6 | 45.0 | 47.9 | 39.5 | 19.3 | 56.7 | 12.8 | 47.3 | 42.5 | 19.7 | 63.8 | 29.2 |
| 水果类<br>Fruits | 0.6 | 1.5 | 1.3 | 1.8 | 0.8 | 0.3 | 0.3 | 0.6 | 1.6 | 1.4 | 0.3 | 0.3 | 1.3 | 0.8 | 0.6 | 0.2 | 0.4 | 0.3 | 0.3 | 0.2 | 0.7 | 2.9 | 0.8 | 0.4 | 0.8 |
| 糖类<br>Sugar | 0.0 | 0.0 | 0.0 | 0.0 | 0.0 | 0.0 | 0.0 | 0.0 | 0.0 | 0.0 | 0.0 | 0.0 | 3.0 | 0.0 | 0.0 | 0.0 | 0.0 | 0.0 | 0.0 | 0.0 | 0.0 | 0.0 | 0.0 | 0.0 | 0.1 |
| 水及饮料类<br>Water and beverages | 1.2 | 0.9 | 0.3 | 0.8 | 1.2 | 0.6 | 0.5 | 0.3 | 2.4 | 2.5 | 0.9 | 1.0 | 1.3 | 2.5 | 1.0 | 0.6 | 0.7 | 1.0 | 0.2 | 0.3 | 1.1 | 3.4 | 3.8 | 0.0 | 1.1 |
| 酒类<br>Alcohol beverages | 0.0 | 0.0 | 0.0 | 0.1 | 0.0 | 0.0 | 0.0 | 0.0 | 0.0 | 0.0 | 0.0 | 0.0 | 0.3 | 0.0 | 0.0 | 0.1 | 0.1 | 0.2 | 0.0 | 0.0 | 0.6 | 0.0 | 0.0 | 0.0 | 0.1 |

附表 3-22 第六次中国总膳食研究膳食样品中锌的含量（单位：mg/kg）

Annexed Table 3-22 Levels of zinc in food samples from the 6th China TDS (Unit: mg/kg)

| 膳食类别 Category | 黑龙江 HL | 辽宁 LN | 河北 HE | 北京 BJ | 吉林 JL | 山西 SX | 陕西 SN | 河南 HA | 宁夏 NX | 内蒙古 NM | 青海 QH | 甘肃 GS | 上海 SH | 福建 FJ | 江西 JX | 江苏 JS | 浙江 ZJ | 山东 SD | 湖北 HB | 四川 SC | 广西 GX | 湖南 HN | 广东 GD | 贵州 GZ | 全国平均 AVG |
|---|---|---|---|---|---|---|---|---|---|---|---|---|---|---|---|---|---|---|---|---|---|---|---|---|---|
| 谷类 Cereals | 4.45 | 3.53 | 3.95 | 3.51 | 3.33 | 5.96 | 3.46 | 4.63 | 4.35 | 2.71 | 3.39 | 2.47 | 3.81 | 4.15 | 4.60 | 3.92 | 4.34 | 3.81 | 3.66 | 3.15 | 4.66 | 4.55 | 3.77 | 3.85 | 3.92 |
| 豆类 Legumes | 9.27 | 9.98 | 8.36 | 5.45 | 9.88 | 6.28 | 7.05 | 9.15 | 3.52 | 6.59 | 7.97 | 6.05 | 7.67 | 6.29 | 13.06 | 9.73 | 7.47 | 9.65 | 9.09 | 5.55 | 8.05 | 10.37 | 7.38 | 7.22 | 7.96 |
| 薯类 Potatoes | 0.42 | 1.79 | 1.53 | 1.36 | 1.32 | 0.71 | 1.00 | 0.74 | 1.54 | 2.06 | 0.81 | 1.26 | 1.01 | 1.13 | 1.86 | 2.10 | 0.94 | 1.38 | 1.30 | 0.90 | 3.04 | 2.48 | 3.61 | 2.18 | 1.52 |
| 肉类 Meats | 16.93 | 15.01 | 12.65 | 14.33 | 17.31 | 13.02 | 14.69 | 15.97 | 27.07 | 10.63 | 15.70 | 14.38 | 13.74 | 17.27 | 20.16 | 17.31 | 16.79 | 11.61 | 11.67 | 13.51 | 15.08 | 13.49 | 20.24 | 15.82 | 15.60 |
| 蛋类 Eggs | 9.65 | 8.76 | 10.86 | 12.99 | 10.78 | 12.57 | 10.47 | 10.51 | 14.00 | 12.99 | 13.20 | 7.74 | 8.48 | 11.78 | 12.92 | 10.32 | 10.68 | 9.38 | 11.05 | 12.73 | 10.56 | 10.58 | 7.58 | 10.03 | 10.86 |
| 水产类 Aquatic foods | 13.57 | 10.55 | 9.47 | 10.08 | 22.51 | 7.81 | 5.29 | 6.39 | 9.29 | 6.78 | 6.06 | 5.44 | 7.40 | 7.87 | 7.34 | 9.68 | 11.31 | 9.16 | 4.98 | 7.12 | 5.23 | 4.48 | 10.25 | 8.60 | 8.61 |
| 乳类 Dairy products | 3.55 | 3.33 | 3.36 | 3.04 | 3.70 | 3.11 | 4.77 | 2.96 | 3.64 | 3.33 | 3.05 | 3.78 | 2.65 | 3.91 | 3.78 | 3.42 | 3.54 | 4.12 | 5.01 | 3.71 | 3.05 | 3.37 | 2.76 | 3.68 | 3.53 |
| 蔬菜类 Vegetables | 2.05 | 1.94 | 1.72 | 2.01 | 1.81 | 1.33 | 1.46 | 1.69 | 1.52 | 1.26 | 1.25 | 1.35 | 1.91 | 2.45 | 2.93 | 3.25 | 2.14 | 1.76 | 1.42 | 2.10 | 1.96 | 1.85 | 2.16 | 2.28 | 1.90 |
| 水果类 Fruits | 0.34 | 0.51 | 0.55 | 0.49 | 0.44 | 0.41 | 0.25 | 0.27 | 0.19 | 2.05 | 0.27 | 0.27 | 0.35 | 0.49 | 0.33 | 0.40 | 0.39 | 0.46 | 0.44 | 0.23 | 0.35 | 0.65 | 0.50 | 0.37 | 0.46 |
| 糖类 Sugar | ND | 0.04 | 0.73 | 0.09 | 0.01 | ND | ND | 0.15 | 0.03 | 0.16 | ND | 0.45 | 7.39 | 0.04 | 0.04 | 0.04 | 0.04 | 0.58 | 0.08 | 0.11 | 0.02 | 0.09 | 0.02 | 0.12 | 0.43 |
| 水及饮料类 Water and beverages | 0.01 | 0.13 | 0.05 | 0.02 | 0.04 | 0.01 | 0.12 | 0.04 | 0.05 | 0.03 | 0.17 | 0.01 | 0.14 | 0.05 | 0.12 | 0.25 | 0.06 | 0.01 | 0.13 | 0.07 | 0.13 | 0.08 | 0.13 | 0.01 | 0.08 |

续表

| 膳食类别<br>Category | 黑龙江<br>HL | 辽宁<br>LN | 河北<br>HE | 北京<br>BJ | 吉林<br>JL | 山西<br>SX | 陕西<br>SN | 河南<br>HA | 宁夏<br>NX | 内蒙古<br>NM | 青海<br>QH | 甘肃<br>GS | 上海<br>SH | 福建<br>FJ | 江西<br>JX | 江苏<br>JS | 浙江<br>ZJ | 山东<br>SD | 湖北<br>HB | 四川<br>SC | 广西<br>GX | 湖南<br>HN | 广东<br>GD | 贵州<br>GZ | 全国平均<br>AVG |
|---|---|---|---|---|---|---|---|---|---|---|---|---|---|---|---|---|---|---|---|---|---|---|---|---|---|
| 酒类<br>Alcohol beverages | ND | 0.02 | 0.01 | 0.04 | 0.01 | ND | 0.01 | 0.06 | 0.02 | 0.02 | 0.01 | 0.03 | 0.83 | 0.09 | 0.03 | 0.22 | 0.12 | 0.02 | 0.02 | 0.01 | 0.13 | 0.07 | 0.47 | 0.11 | 0.10 |

注：ND 表示未检出。计算平均值时，ND 按 1/2 LOD 代入

Note: ND means not to be detected. When calculating the average, ND was substituted at 1/2 LOD

附表 3-23　第六次中国总膳食研究锌的膳食摄入量（单位：mg/d）

Annexed Table 3-23　Dietary intakes of zinc from the 6th China TDS (Unit: mg/d)

| 膳食类别<br>Category | 黑龙江<br>HL | 辽宁<br>LN | 河北<br>HE | 北京<br>BJ | 吉林<br>JL | 山西<br>SX | 陕西<br>SN | 河南<br>HA | 宁夏<br>NX | 内蒙古<br>NM | 青海<br>QH | 甘肃<br>GS | 上海<br>SH | 福建<br>FJ | 江西<br>JX | 江苏<br>JS | 浙江<br>ZJ | 山东<br>SD | 湖北<br>HB | 四川<br>SC | 广西<br>GX | 湖南<br>HN | 广东<br>GD | 贵州<br>GZ | 全国平均<br>AVG |
|---|---|---|---|---|---|---|---|---|---|---|---|---|---|---|---|---|---|---|---|---|---|---|---|---|---|
| 谷类 Cereals | 2.44 | 2.18 | 2.99 | 2.79 | 1.95 | 6.18 | 2.64 | 4.28 | 2.88 | 1.96 | 2.60 | 1.69 | 1.71 | 2.63 | 2.90 | 3.05 | 2.75 | 3.79 | 1.93 | 3.05 | 4.38 | 2.63 | 1.72 | 2.60 | 2.82 |
| 豆类 Legumes | 0.42 | 1.22 | 0.48 | 0.55 | 0.74 | 0.44 | 0.58 | 0.49 | 0.12 | 0.26 | 0.05 | 0.25 | 0.90 | 0.49 | 0.96 | 0.81 | 1.05 | 0.51 | 0.61 | 0.37 | 0.34 | 0.75 | 0.21 | 0.73 | 0.56 |
| 薯类 Potatoes | 0.03 | 0.13 | 0.09 | 0.08 | 0.16 | 0.08 | 0.11 | 0.06 | 0.15 | 0.25 | 0.08 | 0.18 | 0.04 | 0.05 | 0.06 | 0.07 | 0.03 | 0.06 | 0.12 | 0.06 | 0.04 | 0.13 | 0.09 | 0.07 | 0.09 |
| 肉类 Meats | 1.01 | 1.00 | 0.60 | 0.96 | 1.15 | 1.79 | 0.53 | 0.88 | 1.26 | 0.78 | 1.11 | 0.45 | 1.52 | 1.49 | 1.89 | 1.59 | 1.99 | 1.13 | 0.63 | 1.74 | 2.28 | 2.02 | 2.11 | 1.68 | 1.32 |
| 蛋类 Eggs | 0.39 | 0.36 | 0.34 | 0.50 | 0.43 | 0.26 | 0.23 | 0.31 | 0.18 | 0.39 | 0.17 | 0.17 | 0.33 | 0.22 | 0.26 | 0.29 | 0.26 | 0.42 | 0.28 | 0.19 | 0.15 | 0.24 | 0.18 | 0.16 | 0.28 |
| 水产类 Aquatic foods | 0.37 | 0.17 | 0.09 | 0.17 | 0.25 | 0.05 | 0.02 | 0.03 | 0.02 | 0.07 | 0.02 | 0.02 | 0.51 | 0.51 | 0.32 | 0.38 | 0.57 | 0.21 | 0.20 | 0.06 | 0.51 | 0.30 | 0.52 | 0.03 | 0.22 |
| 乳类 Dairy products | 0.05 | 0.15 | 0.08 | 0.26 | 0.12 | 0.13 | 0.09 | 0.06 | 0.06 | 0.11 | 0.16 | 0.05 | 0.19 | 0.14 | 0.08 | 0.09 | 0.12 | 0.09 | 0.03 | 0.05 | 0.06 | 0.06 | 0.10 | 0.10 | 0.10 |

续表

| 膳食类别<br>Category | 黑龙江<br>HL | 辽宁<br>LN | 河北<br>HE | 北京<br>BJ | 吉林<br>JL | 山西<br>SX | 陕西<br>SN | 河南<br>HA | 宁夏<br>NX | 内蒙古<br>NM | 青海<br>QH | 甘肃<br>GS | 上海<br>SH | 福建<br>FJ | 江西<br>JX | 江苏<br>JS | 浙江<br>ZJ | 山东<br>SD | 湖北<br>HB | 四川<br>SC | 广西<br>GX | 湖南<br>HN | 广东<br>GD | 贵州<br>GZ | 全国平均<br>AVG |
|---|---|---|---|---|---|---|---|---|---|---|---|---|---|---|---|---|---|---|---|---|---|---|---|---|---|
| 蔬菜类 Vegetables | 0.66 | 0.63 | 0.51 | 0.79 | 0.70 | 0.41 | 0.42 | 0.47 | 0.24 | 0.33 | 0.39 | 0.33 | 0.77 | 0.97 | 1.32 | 1.38 | 0.95 | 0.72 | 0.59 | 0.64 | 0.69 | 0.99 | 0.51 | 0.93 | 0.68 |
| 水果类 Fruits | 0.02 | 0.04 | 0.02 | 0.06 | 0.04 | 0.01 | 0.01 | 0.01 | 0.02 | 0.23 | 0.00 | 0.01 | 0.03 | 0.03 | 0.02 | 0.01 | 0.03 | 0.02 | 0.01 | 0.00 | 0.02 | 0.04 | 0.01 | 0.01 | 0.03 |
| 糖类 Sugar | 0.00 | 0.00 | 0.00 | 0.00 | 0.00 | 0.00 | 0.00 | 0.00 | 0.00 | 0.00 | 0.00 | 0.00 | 0.06 | 0.00 | 0.00 | 0.00 | 0.00 | 0.00 | 0.00 | 0.00 | 0.00 | 0.00 | 0.00 | 0.00 | 0.00 |
| 水及饮料类 Water and beverages | 0.01 | 0.07 | 0.04 | 0.03 | 0.05 | 0.01 | 0.04 | 0.05 | 0.03 | 0.09 | 0.11 | 0.01 | 0.10 | 0.05 | 0.14 | 0.25 | 0.05 | 0.01 | 0.04 | 0.02 | 0.17 | 0.09 | 0.15 | 0.01 | 0.07 |
| 酒类 Alcohol beverages | 0.00 | 0.00 | 0.00 | 0.00 | 0.00 | 0.00 | 0.00 | 0.00 | 0.00 | 0.00 | 0.00 | 0.00 | 0.02 | 0.00 | 0.00 | 0.01 | 0.01 | 0.00 | 0.00 | 0.00 | 0.00 | 0.00 | 0.00 | 0.00 | 0.00 |
| 合计 SUM | 5.40 | 5.94 | 5.24 | 6.18 | 5.61 | 9.36 | 4.68 | 6.63 | 4.96 | 4.47 | 4.70 | 3.16 | 6.17 | 6.57 | 7.96 | 7.93 | 7.80 | 6.97 | 4.43 | 6.18 | 8.63 | 7.25 | 5.61 | 6.34 | 6.17 |

附表 3-24　第六次中国总膳食研究锌的膳食来源（单位：%）
Annexed Table 3-24　Dietary sources of zinc from the 6th China TDS (Unit: %)

| 膳食类别<br>Category | 黑龙江<br>HL | 辽宁<br>LN | 河北<br>HE | 北京<br>BJ | 吉林<br>JL | 山西<br>SX | 陕西<br>SN | 河南<br>HA | 宁夏<br>NX | 内蒙古<br>NM | 青海<br>QH | 甘肃<br>GS | 上海<br>SH | 福建<br>FJ | 江西<br>JX | 江苏<br>JS | 浙江<br>ZJ | 山东<br>SD | 湖北<br>HB | 四川<br>SC | 广西<br>GX | 湖南<br>HN | 广东<br>GD | 贵州<br>GZ | 全国平均<br>AVG |
|---|---|---|---|---|---|---|---|---|---|---|---|---|---|---|---|---|---|---|---|---|---|---|---|---|---|
| 谷类 Cereals | 45.1 | 36.6 | 57.0 | 45.0 | 34.8 | 66.0 | 56.4 | 64.5 | 58.0 | 43.8 | 55.2 | 53.5 | 27.7 | 40.0 | 36.4 | 38.5 | 35.2 | 54.4 | 43.6 | 49.4 | 50.8 | 36.3 | 30.7 | 41.0 | 45.7 |
| 豆类 Legumes | 7.8 | 20.5 | 9.1 | 9.0 | 13.3 | 4.7 | 12.5 | 7.4 | 2.5 | 5.9 | 1.1 | 7.9 | 14.6 | 7.5 | 12.1 | 10.2 | 13.5 | 7.3 | 13.7 | 6.1 | 4.0 | 10.4 | 3.7 | 11.6 | 9.0 |

续表

| 膳食类别 Category | 黑龙江 HL | 辽宁 LN | 河北 HE | 北京 BJ | 吉林 JL | 山西 SX | 陕西 SN | 河南 HA | 宁夏 NX | 内蒙古 NM | 青海 QH | 甘肃 GS | 上海 SH | 福建 FJ | 江西 JX | 江苏 JS | 浙江 ZJ | 山东 SD | 湖北 HB | 四川 SC | 广西 GX | 湖南 HN | 广东 GD | 贵州 GZ | 全国平均 AVG |
|---|---|---|---|---|---|---|---|---|---|---|---|---|---|---|---|---|---|---|---|---|---|---|---|---|---|
| 薯类 Potatoes | 0.6 | 2.2 | 1.8 | 1.3 | 2.8 | 0.9 | 2.4 | 0.9 | 3.1 | 5.6 | 1.7 | 5.7 | 0.6 | 0.7 | 0.8 | 0.9 | 0.4 | 0.9 | 2.6 | 0.9 | 0.5 | 1.8 | 1.6 | 1.2 | 1.5 |
| 肉类 Meats | 18.8 | 16.9 | 11.4 | 15.6 | 20.5 | 19.1 | 11.3 | 13.3 | 25.5 | 17.5 | 23.7 | 14.1 | 24.7 | 22.6 | 23.8 | 20.0 | 25.5 | 16.2 | 14.3 | 28.2 | 26.4 | 27.8 | 37.6 | 26.6 | 21.3 |
| 蛋类 Eggs | 7.2 | 6.0 | 6.5 | 8.2 | 7.7 | 2.8 | 4.9 | 4.7 | 3.7 | 8.6 | 3.7 | 5.4 | 5.4 | 3.4 | 3.3 | 3.7 | 3.3 | 6.0 | 6.2 | 3.0 | 1.7 | 3.3 | 3.2 | 2.6 | 4.5 |
| 水产类 Aquatic foods | 6.8 | 2.9 | 1.7 | 2.7 | 4.5 | 0.5 | 0.5 | 0.4 | 0.5 | 1.6 | 0.5 | 0.5 | 8.2 | 7.7 | 4.0 | 4.8 | 7.3 | 3.0 | 4.6 | 1.0 | 5.9 | 4.1 | 9.4 | 0.5 | 3.6 |
| 乳类 Dairy products | 0.9 | 2.5 | 1.6 | 4.2 | 2.1 | 1.4 | 2.0 | 0.9 | 1.1 | 2.6 | 3.5 | 1.7 | 3.1 | 2.1 | 1.0 | 1.2 | 1.5 | 1.4 | 0.8 | 0.8 | 0.6 | 0.8 | 1.8 | 1.6 | 1.6 |
| 蔬菜类 Vegetables | 12.2 | 10.7 | 9.6 | 12.7 | 12.6 | 4.4 | 8.9 | 7.1 | 4.8 | 7.3 | 8.3 | 10.6 | 12.4 | 14.8 | 16.6 | 17.4 | 12.2 | 10.3 | 13.3 | 10.3 | 8.0 | 13.6 | 9.1 | 14.7 | 11.0 |
| 水果类 Fruits | 0.4 | 0.7 | 0.4 | 0.9 | 0.7 | 0.2 | 0.2 | 0.1 | 0.3 | 5.2 | 0.1 | 0.3 | 0.4 | 0.4 | 0.2 | 0.1 | 0.3 | 0.4 | 0.2 | 0.1 | 0.3 | 0.6 | 0.3 | 0.1 | 0.5 |
| 糖类 Sugar | 0.0 | 0.0 | 0.0 | 0.0 | 0.0 | 0.0 | 0.0 | 0.0 | 0.0 | 0.0 | 0.0 | 0.0 | 0.9 | 0.0 | 0.0 | 0.0 | 0.0 | 0.0 | 0.0 | 0.0 | 0.0 | 0.0 | 0.0 | 0.0 | 0.0 |
| 水及饮料类 Water and beverages | 0.2 | 1.1 | 0.8 | 0.4 | 1.0 | 0.1 | 0.9 | 0.7 | 0.6 | 1.9 | 2.2 | 0.3 | 1.7 | 0.7 | 1.7 | 3.2 | 0.6 | 0.2 | 0.8 | 0.4 | 2.0 | 1.2 | 2.7 | 0.2 | 1.1 |
| 酒类 Alcohol beverages | 0.0 | 0.0 | 0.0 | 0.0 | 0.0 | 0.0 | 0.0 | 0.0 | 0.0 | 0.0 | 0.0 | 0.0 | 0.3 | 0.0 | 0.0 | 0.1 | 0.1 | 0.0 | 0.0 | 0.0 | 0.0 | 0.0 | 0.0 | 0.0 | 0.0 |

附表 3-25 第六次中国总膳食研究膳食样品中铬的含量（单位：μg/kg）

Annexed Table 3-25　Levels of chromium in food samples from the 6$^{th}$ China TDS (Unit: μg/kg)

| 膳食类别 Category | 黑龙江 HL | 辽宁 LN | 河北 HE | 北京 BJ | 吉林 JL | 山西 SX | 陕西 SN | 河南 HA | 宁夏 NX | 内蒙古 NM | 青海 QH | 甘肃 GS | 上海 SH | 福建 FJ | 江西 JX | 江苏 JS | 浙江 ZJ | 山东 SD | 湖北 HB | 四川 SC | 广西 GX | 湖南 HN | 广东 GD | 贵州 GZ | 全国平均 AVG |
|---|---|---|---|---|---|---|---|---|---|---|---|---|---|---|---|---|---|---|---|---|---|---|---|---|---|
| 谷类 Cereals | 278.5 | 21.2 | 102.5 | 55.6 | 27.0 | 22.4 | 4.7 | 430.8 | 24.7 | 33.3 | 57.9 | 42.2 | 79.1 | 27.4 | 79.6 | 79.3 | 18.1 | 208.0 | 52.2 | 39.4 | 62.5 | 112.7 | 41.2 | 184.1 | 86.8 |
| 豆类 Legumes | 57.9 | 88.7 | 70.4 | 24.2 | 85.0 | 22.6 | 110.8 | 234.6 | 25.9 | 28.7 | 59.8 | 83.6 | 25.0 | 29.4 | 667.9 | 210.1 | 26.3 | 182.7 | 119.2 | 53.0 | 24.8 | 86.9 | 35.8 | 121.6 | 103.1 |
| 薯类 Potatoes | 48.0 | 84.7 | 121.9 | 85.6 | 35.9 | 208.9 | 61.6 | 736.6 | 83.8 | 30.7 | 40.6 | 70.4 | 51.8 | 79.1 | 66.9 | 120.7 | 51.7 | 104.5 | 40.2 | 45.5 | 37.3 | 756.3 | 19.9 | 128.0 | 129.6 |
| 肉类 Meats | 81.0 | 28.3 | 69.8 | 147.6 | 82.5 | 158.9 | 60.1 | 183.7 | 74.1 | 47.3 | 73.8 | 47.0 | 33.5 | 44.0 | 73.6 | 117.9 | 76.7 | 130.5 | 169.5 | 64.6 | 47.1 | 856.0 | 504.8 | 201.6 | 140.6 |
| 蛋类 Eggs | 70.3 | 15.6 | 106.0 | 18.1 | 41.3 | 70.3 | 24.4 | 381.6 | 84.7 | ND | 25.5 | 84.9 | 22.5 | 52.2 | 90.7 | 59.9 | 49.7 | 156.2 | 38.9 | 30.2 | 27.5 | 192.3 | 56.4 | 147.7 | 77.0 |
| 水产类 Aquatic foods | 41.8 | 35.4 | 103.7 | 57.0 | 40.6 | 34.2 | 20.9 | 235.5 | 19.0 | 71.6 | 69.6 | 51.3 | 11.2 | 53.7 | 42.3 | 204.9 | 41.3 | 76.4 | 264.3 | 26.8 | 35.3 | 191.8 | 39.1 | 178.9 | 81.1 |
| 乳类 Dairy products | 4.5 | 3.0 | 2.4 | 1.8 | ND | ND | ND | ND | 1.7 | ND | 1.1 | ND | 17.5 | 2.2 | 4.1 | ND | 2.4 | 6.1 | 12.4 | 1.7 | 3.5 | 21.2 | ND | 27.0 | 4.9 |
| 蔬菜类 Vegetables | 45.1 | 23.9 | 61.5 | 74.4 | 32.7 | 53.5 | 31.1 | 292.8 | 64.3 | 70.1 | 53.8 | 35.0 | 108.5 | 20.6 | 138.5 | 115.0 | 62.3 | 120.5 | 229.1 | 33.0 | 79.1 | 223.2 | 33.7 | 169.6 | 90.5 |
| 水果类 Fruits | 9.3 | 11.1 | 50.4 | 9.9 | 4.6 | 13.5 | 6.3 | 316.0 | 29.8 | 10.6 | 26.5 | 8.6 | 7.7 | 2.4 | 15.0 | 20.2 | 7.7 | 14.7 | 85.5 | 7.6 | 16.9 | 48.5 | 5.9 | 12.7 | 30.9 |
| 糖类 Sugar | 8.7 | 5.2 | 39.2 | 23.0 | 16.1 | 14.2 | 15.6 | 97.9 | 1.1 | 23.4 | 36.2 | 13.1 | 356.0 | ND | 19.2 | 16.8 | 8.1 | 41.4 | 5.3 | 13.8 | ND | 585.7 | ND | ND | 55.9 |
| 水及饮料类 Water and beverages | ND | 3.4 | ND | 1.5 | ND | 1.9 | ND | 6.0 | 4.6 | 4.2 | 1.5 | ND | 4.3 | 3.6 | 1.0 | 1.1 | 1.3 | 1.1 | 2.2 | 1.1 | ND | 43.8 | 2.2 | ND | 3.7 |

续表

| 膳食类别 Category | 黑龙江 HL | 辽宁 LN | 河北 HE | 北京 BJ | 吉林 JL | 山西 SX | 陕西 SN | 河南 HA | 宁夏 NX | 内蒙古 NM | 青海 QH | 甘肃 GS | 上海 SH | 福建 FJ | 江西 JX | 江苏 JS | 浙江 ZJ | 山东 SD | 湖北 HB | 四川 SC | 广西 GX | 湖南 HN | 广东 GD | 贵州 GZ | 全国平均 AVG |
|---|---|---|---|---|---|---|---|---|---|---|---|---|---|---|---|---|---|---|---|---|---|---|---|---|---|
| 酒类 Alcohol beverages | 2.7 | 3.9 | ND | 6.1 | 3.8 | 2.1 | 2.0 | 23.1 | 3.7 | ND | 5.4 | ND | 5.4 | 2.2 | 1.0 | 5.4 | 3.0 | 3.1 | 9.7 | 4.1 | 108.3 | 17.8 | 8.4 | 4.3 | 9.5 |

注: ND 表示未检出。计算平均值时，ND 按 1/2 LOD 代入

Note: ND means not to be detected. When calculating the average, ND was substituted at 1/2 LOD

附表 3-26　第六次中国总膳食研究的铬膳食摄入量（单位: μg/d）

Annexed Table 3-26　Dietary intakes of chromium from the 6$^{th}$ China TDS (Unit: μg/d)

| 膳食类别 Category | 黑龙江 HL | 辽宁 LN | 河北 HE | 北京 BJ | 吉林 JL | 山西 SX | 陕西 SN | 河南 HA | 宁夏 NX | 内蒙古 NM | 青海 QH | 甘肃 GS | 上海 SH | 福建 FJ | 江西 JX | 江苏 JS | 浙江 ZJ | 山东 SD | 湖北 HB | 四川 SC | 广西 GX | 湖南 HN | 广东 GD | 贵州 GZ | 全国平均 AVG |
|---|---|---|---|---|---|---|---|---|---|---|---|---|---|---|---|---|---|---|---|---|---|---|---|---|---|
| 谷类 Cereals | 152.6 | 13.0 | 77.4 | 44.2 | 15.8 | 23.2 | 3.6 | 398.2 | 16.4 | 24.0 | 44.4 | 29.0 | 35.5 | 17.3 | 50.1 | 61.7 | 11.4 | 207.1 | 27.6 | 38.2 | 58.8 | 65.1 | 18.8 | 124.3 | 64.9 |
| 豆类 Legumes | 2.6 | 10.8 | 4.0 | 2.5 | 6.4 | 1.6 | 9.2 | 12.7 | 0.9 | 1.1 | 0.4 | 3.4 | 2.9 | 2.3 | 49.2 | 17.4 | 3.7 | 9.6 | 8.0 | 3.6 | 1.0 | 6.3 | 1.0 | 12.4 | 7.2 |
| 薯类 Potatoes | 3.7 | 6.1 | 7.4 | 5.0 | 4.3 | 24.8 | 7.1 | 59.2 | 8.4 | 3.8 | 4.1 | 10.1 | 1.9 | 3.3 | 2.2 | 4.0 | 1.9 | 4.8 | 3.6 | 2.9 | 0.5 | 40.5 | 0.5 | 4.4 | 8.9 |
| 肉类 Meats | 4.8 | 1.9 | 3.3 | 9.9 | 5.5 | 21.8 | 2.2 | 10.2 | 3.5 | 3.5 | 5.2 | 1.5 | 3.7 | 3.8 | 6.9 | 10.8 | 9.1 | 12.7 | 9.2 | 8.3 | 7.1 | 128.0 | 52.5 | 21.5 | 14.5 |
| 蛋类 Eggs | 2.8 | 0.6 | 3.3 | 0.7 | 1.7 | 1.5 | 0.5 | 11.3 | 1.1 | 0.0 | 0.3 | 1.9 | 0.9 | 1.0 | 1.9 | 1.7 | 1.2 | 6.9 | 1.0 | 0.4 | 0.4 | 4.4 | 1.3 | 2.4 | 2.1 |
| 水产类 Aquatic foods | 1.1 | 0.6 | 1.0 | 0.9 | 0.5 | 0.2 | 0.1 | 1.1 | 0.0 | 0.7 | 0.2 | 0.1 | 0.8 | 3.4 | 1.8 | 8.0 | 2.1 | 1.7 | 10.8 | 0.2 | 3.4 | 12.7 | 2.0 | 0.6 | 2.3 |
| 乳类 Dairy products | 0.1 | 0.1 | 0.1 | 0.2 | 0.0 | 0.0 | 0.0 | 0.0 | 0.0 | 0.0 | 0.1 | 0.0 | 1.3 | 0.1 | 0.1 | 0.0 | 0.1 | 0.1 | 0.1 | 0.0 | 0.1 | 0.4 | 0.0 | 0.8 | 0.1 |

续表

| 膳食类别<br>Category | 黑龙江<br>HL | 辽宁<br>LN | 河北<br>HE | 北京<br>BJ | 吉林<br>JL | 山西<br>SX | 陕西<br>SN | 河南<br>HA | 宁夏<br>NX | 内蒙古<br>NM | 青海<br>QH | 甘肃<br>GS | 上海<br>SH | 福建<br>FJ | 江西<br>JX | 江苏<br>JS | 浙江<br>ZJ | 山东<br>SD | 湖北<br>HB | 四川<br>SC | 广西<br>GX | 湖南<br>HN | 广东<br>GD | 贵州<br>GZ | 全国平均<br>AVG |
|---|---|---|---|---|---|---|---|---|---|---|---|---|---|---|---|---|---|---|---|---|---|---|---|---|---|
| 蔬菜类 Vegetables | 14.5 | 7.8 | 18.1 | 29.2 | 12.7 | 16.6 | 8.9 | 81.4 | 10.0 | 18.0 | 16.7 | 8.7 | 43.5 | 8.2 | 62.5 | 48.9 | 27.7 | 49.0 | 94.9 | 10.0 | 27.9 | 119.2 | 8.0 | 69.2 | 33.8 |
| 水果类 Fruits | 0.6 | 0.8 | 1.9 | 1.1 | 0.4 | 0.5 | 0.2 | 7.6 | 2.5 | 1.2 | 0.4 | 0.3 | 0.6 | 0.1 | 0.9 | 0.6 | 0.5 | 0.8 | 1.6 | 0.1 | 1.1 | 3.1 | 0.2 | 0.3 | 1.1 |
| 糖类 Sugar | 0.0 | 0.0 | 0.0 | 0.0 | 0.0 | 0.0 | 0.0 | 0.0 | 0.0 | 0.0 | 0.0 | 0.0 | 2.7 | 0.0 | 0.0 | 0.0 | 0.0 | 0.0 | 0.0 | 0.0 | 0.0 | 0.3 | 0.0 | 0.0 | 0.1 |
| 水及饮料类 Water and beverages | 0.6 | 1.7 | 0.4 | 1.6 | 0.7 | 1.4 | 0.2 | 7.1 | 2.4 | 10.9 | 0.9 | 0.6 | 3.0 | 3.1 | 1.2 | 1.1 | 1.0 | 2.5 | 0.6 | 0.4 | 0.7 | 46.5 | 2.6 | 0.6 | 3.8 |
| 酒类 Alcohol beverages | 0.1 | 0.1 | 0.0 | 0.2 | 0.0 | 0.0 | 0.0 | 0.1 | 0.0 | 0.0 | 0.0 | 0.0 | 0.1 | 0.0 | 0.0 | 0.2 | 0.2 | 0.4 | 0.1 | 0.0 | 3.5 | 0.3 | 0.0 | 0.0 | 0.2 |
| 合计 SUM | 183.6 | 43.7 | 117.0 | 95.5 | 48.0 | 91.5 | 32.0 | 588.9 | 45.2 | 63.4 | 72.9 | 55.6 | 96.8 | 42.8 | 176.9 | 154.5 | 58.8 | 295.7 | 157.4 | 64.2 | 104.4 | 426.7 | 87.0 | 236.3 | 139.1 |

附表 3-27　第六次中国总膳食研究铬的膳食来源（单位：%）

Annexed Table 3-27　Dietary sources of chromium from the 6$^{th}$ China TDS (Unit: %)

| 膳食类别<br>Category | 黑龙江<br>HL | 辽宁<br>LN | 河北<br>HE | 北京<br>BJ | 吉林<br>JL | 山西<br>SX | 陕西<br>SN | 河南<br>HA | 宁夏<br>NX | 内蒙古<br>NM | 青海<br>QH | 甘肃<br>GS | 上海<br>SH | 福建<br>FJ | 江西<br>JX | 江苏<br>JS | 浙江<br>ZJ | 山东<br>SD | 湖北<br>HB | 四川<br>SC | 广西<br>GX | 湖南<br>HN | 广东<br>GD | 贵州<br>GZ | 全国平均<br>AVG |
|---|---|---|---|---|---|---|---|---|---|---|---|---|---|---|---|---|---|---|---|---|---|---|---|---|---|
| 谷类 Cereals | 83.1 | 29.8 | 66.2 | 46.3 | 33.0 | 25.4 | 11.2 | 67.6 | 36.2 | 38.0 | 60.9 | 52.1 | 36.7 | 40.5 | 28.3 | 40.0 | 19.4 | 70.0 | 17.5 | 59.5 | 56.3 | 15.2 | 21.6 | 52.6 | 46.7 |
| 豆类 Legumes | 1.4 | 24.8 | 3.4 | 2.6 | 13.4 | 1.7 | 28.7 | 2.1 | 2.0 | 1.8 | 0.5 | 6.2 | 3.0 | 5.4 | 27.8 | 11.3 | 6.3 | 3.2 | 5.1 | 5.6 | 1.0 | 1.5 | 1.1 | 5.2 | 5.2 |

续表

| 膳食类别<br>Category | 黑龙江<br>HL | 辽宁<br>LN | 河北<br>HE | 北京<br>BJ | 吉林<br>JL | 山西<br>SX | 陕西<br>SN | 河南<br>HA | 宁夏<br>NX | 内蒙古<br>NM | 青海<br>QH | 甘肃<br>GS | 上海<br>SH | 福建<br>FJ | 江西<br>JX | 江苏<br>JS | 浙江<br>ZJ | 山东<br>SD | 湖北<br>HB | 四川<br>SC | 广西<br>GX | 湖南<br>HN | 广东<br>GD | 贵州<br>GZ | 全国平均<br>AVG |
|---|---|---|---|---|---|---|---|---|---|---|---|---|---|---|---|---|---|---|---|---|---|---|---|---|---|
| 薯类 Potatoes | 2.0 | 14.0 | 6.4 | 5.2 | 9.0 | 27.1 | 22.1 | 10.0 | 18.5 | 5.9 | 5.7 | 18.2 | 1.9 | 7.8 | 1.2 | 2.6 | 3.2 | 1.6 | 2.3 | 4.5 | 0.5 | 9.5 | 0.6 | 1.9 | 6.4 |
| 肉类 Meats | 2.6 | 4.3 | 2.8 | 10.4 | 11.4 | 23.8 | 6.8 | 1.7 | 7.6 | 5.5 | 7.2 | 2.6 | 3.8 | 8.8 | 3.9 | 7.0 | 15.4 | 4.3 | 5.8 | 13.0 | 6.8 | 30.0 | 60.4 | 9.1 | 10.4 |
| 蛋类 Eggs | 1.5 | 1.5 | 2.9 | 0.7 | 3.5 | 1.6 | 1.7 | 1.9 | 2.4 | 0.0 | 0.5 | 3.4 | 0.9 | 2.3 | 1.1 | 1.1 | 2.0 | 2.3 | 0.6 | 0.7 | 0.4 | 1.0 | 1.5 | 1.0 | 1.5 |
| 水产类 Aquatic foods | 0.6 | 1.3 | 0.8 | 1.0 | 0.9 | 0.2 | 0.3 | 0.2 | 0.1 | 1.2 | 0.3 | 0.3 | 0.8 | 8.1 | 1.0 | 5.2 | 3.5 | 0.6 | 6.8 | 0.3 | 3.3 | 3.0 | 2.3 | 0.3 | 1.6 |
| 乳类 Dairy products | 0.0 | 0.3 | 0.0 | 0.2 | 0.0 | 0.0 | 0.0 | 0.0 | 0.1 | 0.0 | 0.1 | 0.0 | 1.3 | 0.2 | 0.1 | 0.0 | 0.1 | 0.0 | 0.1 | 0.0 | 0.1 | 0.1 | 0.0 | 0.3 | 0.1 |
| 蔬菜类 Vegetables | 7.9 | 17.9 | 15.4 | 30.5 | 26.5 | 18.1 | 27.9 | 13.8 | 22.2 | 28.4 | 22.9 | 15.6 | 44.9 | 19.1 | 35.3 | 31.7 | 47.0 | 16.6 | 60.3 | 15.6 | 26.8 | 27.9 | 9.1 | 29.3 | 24.3 |
| 水果类 Fruits | 0.3 | 1.9 | 1.6 | 1.2 | 0.8 | 0.5 | 0.7 | 1.3 | 5.6 | 1.9 | 0.6 | 0.5 | 0.6 | 0.3 | 0.5 | 0.4 | 0.9 | 0.3 | 1.0 | 0.2 | 1.0 | 0.7 | 0.2 | 0.1 | 0.8 |
| 糖类 Sugar | 0.0 | 0.0 | 0.0 | 0.0 | 0.0 | 0.0 | 0.0 | 0.0 | 0.0 | 0.0 | 0.0 | 0.0 | 2.8 | 0.0 | 0.0 | 0.0 | 0.0 | 0.0 | 0.1 | 0.0 | 0.0 | 0.1 | 0.0 | 0.0 | 0.1 |
| 水及饮料类 Water and beverages | 0.3 | 3.9 | 0.3 | 1.7 | 1.4 | 1.5 | 0.5 | 1.2 | 5.3 | 17.2 | 1.3 | 1.1 | 3.1 | 7.4 | 0.7 | 0.7 | 1.7 | 0.9 | 0.4 | 0.6 | 0.6 | 10.9 | 3.0 | 0.3 | 2.8 |
| 酒类 Alcohol beverages | 0.0 | 0.3 | 0.0 | 0.2 | 0.1 | 0.0 | 0.0 | 0.0 | 0.0 | 0.0 | 0.0 | 0.0 | 0.1 | 0.1 | 0.0 | 0.1 | 0.3 | 0.1 | 0.1 | 0.0 | 3.3 | 0.1 | 0.0 | 0.0 | 0.2 |

附表 3-28  第六次中国总膳食研究膳食样品中铜的含量（单位：mg/kg）

Annexed Table 3-28  Levels of copper in food samples from the 6$^{th}$ China TDS (Unit: mg/kg)

| 膳食类别<br>Category | 黑龙江<br>HL | 辽宁<br>LN | 河北<br>HE | 北京<br>BJ | 吉林<br>JL | 山西<br>SX | 陕西<br>SN | 河南<br>HA | 宁夏<br>NX | 内蒙古<br>NM | 青海<br>QH | 甘肃<br>GS | 上海<br>SH | 福建<br>FJ | 江西<br>JX | 江苏<br>JS | 浙江<br>ZJ | 山东<br>SD | 湖北<br>HB | 四川<br>SC | 广西<br>GX | 湖南<br>HN | 广东<br>GD | 贵州<br>GZ | 全国平均<br>AVG |
|---|---|---|---|---|---|---|---|---|---|---|---|---|---|---|---|---|---|---|---|---|---|---|---|---|---|
| 谷类 Cereals | 0.99 | 0.90 | 0.88 | 0.80 | 0.78 | 1.52 | 0.94 | 1.08 | 0.83 | 0.67 | 0.86 | 0.80 | 1.07 | 1.04 | 1.30 | 0.91 | 1.00 | 1.07 | 0.86 | 0.68 | 0.74 | 1.16 | 0.88 | 0.93 | 0.94 |
| 豆类 Legumes | 2.55 | 2.98 | 2.63 | 2.18 | 2.72 | 2.13 | 3.36 | 3.49 | 1.34 | 2.69 | 3.10 | 2.03 | 2.93 | 2.07 | 3.58 | 3.44 | 2.14 | 3.30 | 2.97 | 1.90 | 2.62 | 3.39 | 2.48 | 2.30 | 2.68 |
| 薯类 Potatoes | 0.25 | 0.73 | 0.52 | 0.57 | 0.62 | 0.27 | 0.31 | 0.34 | 0.83 | 0.62 | 0.42 | 0.76 | 0.47 | 0.61 | 1.31 | 0.96 | 0.39 | 0.60 | 0.63 | 0.45 | 0.85 | 1.41 | 1.23 | 0.68 | 0.66 |
| 肉类 Meats | 0.66 | 1.00 | 0.61 | 0.78 | 2.31 | 0.67 | 0.75 | 1.95 | 0.71 | 0.64 | 0.67 | 0.74 | 0.77 | 0.85 | 2.05 | 1.04 | 1.92 | 0.47 | 0.85 | 0.92 | 0.88 | 1.64 | 0.62 | 1.12 | 1.03 |
| 蛋类 Eggs | 0.67 | 0.68 | 0.69 | 1.03 | 0.76 | 0.80 | 0.76 | 0.69 | 0.82 | 0.93 | 0.87 | 0.60 | 0.72 | 0.88 | 0.91 | 0.72 | 0.72 | 0.62 | 0.81 | 0.86 | 0.77 | 0.72 | 0.46 | 0.80 | 0.76 |
| 水产类 Aquatic foods | 0.36 | 2.89 | 2.20 | 3.65 | 0.64 | 0.47 | 0.24 | 0.85 | 0.44 | 0.45 | 0.45 | 0.39 | 1.74 | 1.25 | 0.42 | 1.02 | 1.06 | 1.40 | 0.37 | 0.42 | 0.63 | 0.38 | 2.28 | 1.00 | 1.04 |
| 乳类 Dairy products | 0.05 | 0.04 | 0.04 | 0.03 | 0.04 | 0.03 | 0.05 | 0.04 | 0.04 | 0.05 | 0.03 | 0.05 | 0.04 | 0.04 | 0.05 | 0.04 | 0.04 | 0.04 | 0.07 | 0.05 | 0.05 | 0.05 | 0.02 | 0.04 | 0.04 |
| 蔬菜类 Vegetables | 0.49 | 0.43 | 0.48 | 0.51 | 0.52 | 0.44 | 0.39 | 0.49 | 0.44 | 0.43 | 0.41 | 0.37 | 0.45 | 0.39 | 0.57 | 0.79 | 0.44 | 0.33 | 0.28 | 0.42 | 0.45 | 0.45 | 0.46 | 0.56 | 0.46 |
| 水果类 Fruits | 0.34 | 0.38 | 0.55 | 0.51 | 0.37 | 0.47 | 0.42 | 0.49 | 0.38 | 0.41 | 0.32 | 0.49 | 0.52 | 0.45 | 0.38 | 0.43 | 0.38 | 0.50 | 0.53 | 0.37 | 0.30 | 0.64 | 0.48 | 0.44 | 0.44 |
| 糖类 Sugar | 0.04 | ND | 0.07 | 0.02 | ND | 0.02 | 0.06 | 0.01 | 0.05 | 0.01 | 0.01 | 0.35 | 5.09 | 0.01 | 0.05 | 0.10 | 0.01 | 0.10 | 0.02 | 0.04 | 0.14 | 0.01 | ND | 0.17 | 0.27 |
| 水及饮料类 Water and beverages | 0.00 | 0.02 | 0.01 | ND | 0.01 | 0.01 | 0.02 | 0.00 | 0.01 | 0.02 | 0.05 | ND | 0.05 | 0.01 | ND | 0.01 | 0.02 | 0.01 | 0.02 | 0.01 | 0.01 | 0.02 | 0.11 | 0.00 | 0.02 |

续表

| 膳食类别<br>Category | 黑龙江<br>HL | 辽宁<br>LN | 河北<br>HE | 北京<br>BJ | 吉林<br>JL | 山西<br>SX | 陕西<br>SN | 河南<br>HA | 宁夏<br>NX | 内蒙古<br>NM | 青海<br>QH | 甘肃<br>GS | 上海<br>SH | 福建<br>FJ | 江西<br>JX | 江苏<br>JS | 浙江<br>ZJ | 山东<br>SD | 湖北<br>HB | 四川<br>SC | 广西<br>GX | 湖南<br>HN | 广东<br>GD | 贵州<br>GZ | 全国平均<br>AVG |
|---|---|---|---|---|---|---|---|---|---|---|---|---|---|---|---|---|---|---|---|---|---|---|---|---|---|
| 酒类<br>Alcohol beverages | 0.01 | 0.02 | 0.01 | 0.02 | 0.02 | ND | 0.02 | 0.02 | ND | 0.02 | 0.02 | 0.03 | 0.17 | 0.02 | 0.01 | 0.09 | 0.03 | 0.02 | 0.04 | 0.04 | 0.06 | 0.01 | 0.17 | 0.09 | 0.04 |

注：ND 表示未检出。计算平均值时，ND 按 1/2 LOD 代入

Note: ND means not to be detected. When calculating the average, ND was substituted at 1/2 LOD

附表 3-29　第六次中国总膳食研究的铜膳食摄入量（单位：mg/d）

Annexed Table 3-29　Dietary intakes of copper from the 6<sup>th</sup> China TDS (Unit: mg/d)

| 膳食类别<br>Category | 黑龙江<br>HL | 辽宁<br>LN | 河北<br>HE | 北京<br>BJ | 吉林<br>JL | 山西<br>SX | 陕西<br>SN | 河南<br>HA | 宁夏<br>NX | 内蒙古<br>NM | 青海<br>QH | 甘肃<br>GS | 上海<br>SH | 福建<br>FJ | 江西<br>JX | 江苏<br>JS | 浙江<br>ZJ | 山东<br>SD | 湖北<br>HB | 四川<br>SC | 广西<br>GX | 湖南<br>HN | 广东<br>GD | 贵州<br>GZ | 全国平均<br>AVG |
|---|---|---|---|---|---|---|---|---|---|---|---|---|---|---|---|---|---|---|---|---|---|---|---|---|---|
| 谷类 Cereals | 0.55 | 0.55 | 0.67 | 0.64 | 0.46 | 1.58 | 0.72 | 1.00 | 0.55 | 0.48 | 0.66 | 0.55 | 0.48 | 0.66 | 0.82 | 0.71 | 0.63 | 1.06 | 0.45 | 0.66 | 0.70 | 0.67 | 0.40 | 0.63 | 0.68 |
| 豆类 Legumes | 0.12 | 0.36 | 0.15 | 0.22 | 0.21 | 0.15 | 0.28 | 0.19 | 0.05 | 0.11 | 0.02 | 0.08 | 0.34 | 0.16 | 0.26 | 0.29 | 0.30 | 0.17 | 0.20 | 0.13 | 0.11 | 0.25 | 0.07 | 0.23 | 0.19 |
| 薯类 Potatoes | 0.02 | 0.05 | 0.03 | 0.03 | 0.07 | 0.03 | 0.04 | 0.03 | 0.08 | 0.08 | 0.04 | 0.11 | 0.02 | 0.03 | 0.04 | 0.03 | 0.01 | 0.03 | 0.06 | 0.03 | 0.01 | 0.08 | 0.03 | 0.02 | 0.04 |
| 肉类 Meats | 0.04 | 0.07 | 0.03 | 0.05 | 0.15 | 0.09 | 0.03 | 0.11 | 0.03 | 0.05 | 0.05 | 0.02 | 0.09 | 0.07 | 0.19 | 0.10 | 0.23 | 0.05 | 0.05 | 0.12 | 0.13 | 0.25 | 0.06 | 0.12 | 0.09 |
| 蛋类 Eggs | 0.03 | 0.03 | 0.02 | 0.04 | 0.03 | 0.02 | 0.02 | 0.02 | 0.01 | 0.03 | 0.01 | 0.01 | 0.03 | 0.02 | 0.02 | 0.02 | 0.02 | 0.03 | 0.02 | 0.01 | 0.01 | 0.02 | 0.01 | 0.01 | 0.02 |
| 水产类 Aquatic foods | 0.01 | 0.05 | 0.02 | 0.06 | 0.01 | 0.00 | 0.00 | 0.00 | 0.00 | 0.00 | 0.00 | 0.00 | 0.12 | 0.08 | 0.02 | 0.04 | 0.05 | 0.00 | 0.01 | 0.00 | 0.06 | 0.03 | 0.12 | 0.00 | 0.03 |
| 乳类 Dairy products | 0.00 | 0.00 | 0.00 | 0.00 | 0.00 | 0.00 | 0.00 | 0.00 | 0.00 | 0.00 | 0.00 | 0.00 | 0.00 | 0.00 | 0.00 | 0.00 | 0.00 | 0.00 | 0.00 | 0.00 | 0.00 | 0.00 | 0.00 | 0.00 | 0.00 |

续表

| 膳食类别<br>Category | 黑龙江<br>HL | 辽宁<br>LN | 河北<br>HE | 北京<br>BJ | 吉林<br>JL | 山西<br>SX | 陕西<br>SN | 河南<br>HA | 宁夏<br>NX | 内蒙古<br>NM | 青海<br>QH | 甘肃<br>GS | 上海<br>SH | 福建<br>FJ | 江西<br>JX | 江苏<br>JS | 浙江<br>ZJ | 山东<br>SD | 湖北<br>HB | 四川<br>SC | 广西<br>GX | 湖南<br>HN | 广东<br>GD | 贵州<br>GZ | 全国平均<br>AVG |
|---|---|---|---|---|---|---|---|---|---|---|---|---|---|---|---|---|---|---|---|---|---|---|---|---|---|
| 蔬菜类 Vegetables | 0.16 | 0.14 | 0.14 | 0.20 | 0.20 | 0.14 | 0.11 | 0.14 | 0.07 | 0.11 | 0.13 | 0.09 | 0.18 | 0.16 | 0.26 | 0.34 | 0.20 | 0.13 | 0.12 | 0.13 | 0.16 | 0.24 | 0.11 | 0.23 | 0.16 |
| 水果类 Fruits | 0.02 | 0.03 | 0.02 | 0.06 | 0.03 | 0.02 | 0.02 | 0.01 | 0.03 | 0.05 | 0.01 | 0.02 | 0.04 | 0.03 | 0.02 | 0.01 | 0.03 | 0.03 | 0.01 | 0.01 | 0.02 | 0.04 | 0.01 | 0.01 | 0.02 |
| 糖类 Sugar | 0.00 | 0.00 | 0.00 | 0.00 | 0.00 | 0.00 | 0.00 | 0.00 | 0.00 | 0.00 | 0.00 | 0.00 | 0.04 | 0.00 | 0.00 | 0.00 | 0.00 | 0.00 | 0.00 | 0.00 | 0.00 | 0.00 | 0.00 | 0.00 | 0.00 |
| 水及饮料类 Water and beverages | 0.00 | 0.01 | 0.01 | 0.00 | 0.00 | 0.01 | 0.01 | 0.01 | 0.00 | 0.05 | 0.03 | 0.00 | 0.04 | 0.01 | 0.00 | 0.01 | 0.01 | 0.01 | 0.00 | 0.00 | 0.02 | 0.02 | 0.13 | 0.00 | 0.02 |
| 酒类 Alcohol beverages | 0.00 | 0.00 | 0.00 | 0.00 | 0.02 | 0.00 | 0.00 | 0.00 | 0.00 | 0.00 | 0.00 | 0.00 | 0.00 | 0.00 | 0.00 | 0.00 | 0.00 | 0.00 | 0.00 | 0.00 | 0.00 | 0.00 | 0.00 | 0.00 | 0.00 |
| 合计 SUM | 0.94 | 1.29 | 1.09 | 1.31 | 1.18 | 2.03 | 1.22 | 1.50 | 0.83 | 0.95 | 0.95 | 0.89 | 1.37 | 1.21 | 1.64 | 1.55 | 1.48 | 1.55 | 0.92 | 1.09 | 1.22 | 1.58 | 0.95 | 1.26 | 1.25 |

附表 3-30 第六次中国总膳食研究铜的膳食来源（单位：%）

Annexed Table 3-30 Dietary sources of copper from the 6$^{th}$ China TDS (Unit: %)

| 膳食类别<br>Category | 黑龙江<br>HL | 辽宁<br>LN | 河北<br>HE | 北京<br>BJ | 吉林<br>JL | 山西<br>SX | 陕西<br>SN | 河南<br>HA | 宁夏<br>NX | 内蒙古<br>NM | 青海<br>QH | 甘肃<br>GS | 上海<br>SH | 福建<br>FJ | 江西<br>JX | 江苏<br>JS | 浙江<br>ZJ | 山东<br>SD | 湖北<br>HB | 四川<br>SC | 广西<br>GX | 湖南<br>HN | 广东<br>GD | 贵州<br>GZ | 全国平均<br>AVG |
|---|---|---|---|---|---|---|---|---|---|---|---|---|---|---|---|---|---|---|---|---|---|---|---|---|---|
| 谷类 Cereals | 58.1 | 42.8 | 61.3 | 48.8 | 38.8 | 77.7 | 59.2 | 66.5 | 66.1 | 50.8 | 69.7 | 61.5 | 34.8 | 54.1 | 50.0 | 45.9 | 42.5 | 68.9 | 49.1 | 60.5 | 57.1 | 42.3 | 42.2 | 49.7 | 54.2 |
| 豆类 Legumes | 12.3 | 28.2 | 13.8 | 17.0 | 17.4 | 7.3 | 22.9 | 12.5 | 5.7 | 11.3 | 2.1 | 9.4 | 25.1 | 13.5 | 16.1 | 18.4 | 20.3 | 11.2 | 21.6 | 11.8 | 9.1 | 15.6 | 7.3 | 18.5 | 14.8 |

续表

| 膳食类别<br>Category | 黑龙江<br>HL | 辽宁<br>LN | 河北<br>HE | 北京<br>BJ | 吉林<br>JL | 山西<br>SX | 陕西<br>SN | 河南<br>HA | 宁夏<br>NX | 内蒙古<br>NM | 青海<br>QH | 甘肃<br>GS | 上海<br>SH | 福建<br>FJ | 江西<br>JX | 江苏<br>JS | 浙江<br>ZJ | 山东<br>SD | 湖北<br>HB | 四川<br>SC | 广西<br>GX | 湖南<br>HN | 广东<br>GD | 贵州<br>GZ | 全国平均<br>AVG |
|---|---|---|---|---|---|---|---|---|---|---|---|---|---|---|---|---|---|---|---|---|---|---|---|---|---|
| 薯类 Potatoes | 2.1 | 4.1 | 2.9 | 2.5 | 6.4 | 1.6 | 2.9 | 1.8 | 10.1 | 8.0 | 4.5 | 12.4 | 1.2 | 2.1 | 2.6 | 2.1 | 1.0 | 1.8 | 6.1 | 2.6 | 0.9 | 4.8 | 3.2 | 1.9 | 3.3 |
| 肉类 Meats | 4.2 | 5.2 | 2.6 | 4.0 | 13.0 | 4.5 | 2.2 | 7.2 | 4.0 | 4.9 | 5.0 | 2.6 | 6.2 | 6.0 | 11.8 | 6.2 | 15.3 | 3.0 | 5.0 | 11.0 | 10.9 | 15.6 | 6.8 | 9.4 | 7.2 |
| 蛋类 Eggs | 2.9 | 2.2 | 2.0 | 3.0 | 2.6 | 0.8 | 1.4 | 1.4 | 1.3 | 2.9 | 1.2 | 1.5 | 2.0 | 1.4 | 1.1 | 1.3 | 1.2 | 1.8 | 2.2 | 1.2 | 0.9 | 1.0 | 1.2 | 1.0 | 1.6 |
| 水产类 Aquatic foods | 1.0 | 3.6 | 1.9 | 4.6 | 0.6 | 0.1 | 0.1 | 0.3 | 0.1 | 0.5 | 0.2 | 0.1 | 8.7 | 6.6 | 1.1 | 2.6 | 3.6 | 2.1 | 1.6 | 0.3 | 5.0 | 1.6 | 12.3 | 0.3 | 2.4 |
| 乳类 Dairy products | 0.1 | 0.1 | 0.1 | 0.2 | 0.1 | 0.1 | 0.1 | 0.1 | 0.1 | 0.2 | 0.2 | 0.1 | 0.2 | 0.1 | 0.1 | 0.1 | 0.1 | 0.1 | 0.1 | 0.1 | 0.1 | 0.1 | 0.1 | 0.1 | 0.1 |
| 蔬菜类 Vegetables | 16.7 | 10.9 | 12.9 | 15.4 | 17.0 | 6.7 | 9.2 | 9.1 | 8.3 | 11.5 | 13.3 | 10.4 | 13.2 | 12.9 | 15.8 | 21.7 | 13.2 | 8.6 | 12.6 | 11.6 | 13.1 | 15.3 | 11.6 | 18.0 | 12.9 |
| 水果类 Fruits | 2.3 | 2.2 | 1.9 | 4.4 | 2.7 | 0.8 | 1.3 | 0.8 | 3.9 | 4.9 | 0.5 | 1.8 | 2.8 | 2.2 | 1.3 | 0.8 | 1.7 | 1.7 | 1.1 | 0.5 | 1.6 | 2.6 | 1.5 | 0.7 | 1.8 |
| 糖类 Sugar | 0.0 | 0.0 | 0.0 | 0.0 | 0.0 | 0.0 | 0.0 | 0.0 | 0.0 | 0.0 | 0.0 | 0.0 | 2.8 | 0.0 | 0.0 | 0.0 | 0.0 | 0.0 | 0.0 | 0.0 | 0.0 | 0.0 | 0.0 | 0.0 | 0.1 |
| 水及饮料类 Water and beverages | 0.3 | 0.7 | 0.5 | 0.1 | 1.4 | 0.3 | 0.7 | 0.3 | 0.4 | 5.1 | 3.2 | 0.1 | 2.7 | 1.0 | 0.1 | 0.9 | 0.9 | 0.7 | 0.5 | 0.3 | 1.2 | 1.2 | 13.7 | 0.3 | 1.3 |
| 酒类 Alcohol beverages | 0.0 | 0.1 | 0.0 | 0.0 | 0.0 | 0.0 | 0.0 | 0.0 | 0.0 | 0.0 | 0.0 | 0.0 | 0.3 | 0.0 | 0.0 | 0.2 | 0.1 | 0.2 | 0.1 | 0.0 | 0.1 | 0.0 | 0.0 | 0.0 | 0.1 |

附表 3-31　第六次中国总膳食研究膳食样品中硒的含量（单位：μg/kg）

Annexed Table 3-31　Levels of selenium in food samples from the 6th China TDS (Unit: μg/kg)

| 膳食类别 Category | 黑龙江 HL | 辽宁 LN | 河北 HE | 北京 BJ | 吉林 JL | 山西 SX | 陕西 SN | 河南 HA | 宁夏 NX | 内蒙古 NM | 青海 QH | 甘肃 GS | 上海 SH | 福建 FJ | 江西 JX | 江苏 JS | 浙江 ZJ | 山东 SD | 湖北 HB | 四川 SC | 广西 GX | 湖南 HN | 广东 GD | 贵州 GZ | 全国平均 AVG |
|---|---|---|---|---|---|---|---|---|---|---|---|---|---|---|---|---|---|---|---|---|---|---|---|---|---|
| 谷类 Cereals | 10.5 | 6.3 | 12.1 | 8.0 | 5.8 | 12.8 | 7.0 | 4.2 | ND | 10.5 | 15.2 | 7.9 | 14.5 | 5.4 | 6.5 | 7.0 | 0.4 | 5.4 | 35.4 | 11.6 | 0.4 | 23.8 | 2.0 | 30.2 | 10.1 |
| 豆类 Legumes | 16.2 | 13.0 | 21.0 | 12.6 | 14.0 | 14.9 | 31.8 | 17.3 | 13.3 | 49.7 | 9.6 | 18.6 | 8.5 | 10.8 | 12.9 | 22.6 | 3.2 | 16.3 | 20.6 | 12.5 | 31.0 | 28.1 | ND | 65.0 | 19.3 |
| 薯类 Potatoes | 3.3 | 4.1 | 9.3 | 1.1 | 0.3 | 10.2 | 6.9 | ND | ND | 19.4 | 9.0 | 5.9 | 7.2 | 3.6 | ND | 14.9 | 0.3 | 1.6 | 12.3 | 6.1 | 6.3 | 15.7 | ND | 22.7 | 6.7 |
| 肉类 Meats | 84.9 | 89.5 | 111.7 | 117.0 | 136.3 | 98.3 | 122.6 | 82.5 | 112.8 | 101.9 | 129.5 | 142.8 | 167.1 | 143.7 | 186.4 | 185.3 | 171.0 | 98.4 | 131.7 | 131.2 | 106.9 | 137.7 | 123.3 | 159.8 | 128.0 |
| 蛋类 Eggs | 205.4 | 199.7 | 199.4 | 260.3 | 212.8 | 274.2 | 198.5 | 205.6 | 316.6 | 190.6 | 320.6 | 226.3 | 211.0 | 247.5 | 410.2 | 213.5 | 251.3 | 152.0 | 266.5 | 220.5 | 226.0 | 209.5 | 118.0 | 180.8 | 229.9 |
| 水产类 Aquatic foods | 165.9 | 325.3 | 188.2 | 284.8 | 233.4 | 326.6 | 109.0 | 166.2 | 147.2 | 123.4 | 336.2 | 211.0 | 229.7 | 309.2 | 239.5 | 173.7 | 245.7 | 279.6 | 125.1 | 147.1 | 153.8 | 133.1 | 280.2 | 224.1 | 214.9 |
| 乳类 Dairy products | 39.1 | 21.1 | 21.8 | 18.1 | 30.0 | 13.3 | 31.9 | 13.7 | 15.3 | 21.6 | 20.4 | 25.1 | 26.0 | 26.7 | 29.4 | 35.4 | 27.2 | 26.6 | 51.0 | 28.7 | 25.3 | 31.2 | 15.9 | 26.7 | 25.9 |
| 蔬菜类 Vegetables | 5.1 | 4.0 | 10.2 | 4.9 | 1.7 | 4.9 | 8.7 | 6.5 | 2.1 | 7.3 | 6.7 | 6.4 | 6.6 | 7.3 | 4.8 | 9.2 | 3.2 | 9.0 | 8.1 | 11.2 | 5.0 | 15.8 | 0.6 | 18.6 | 7.0 |
| 水果类 Fruits | 1.4 | ND | 2.9 | 3.2 | 0.7 | 4.5 | 2.6 | ND | ND | 3.2 | 2.9 | 0.7 | 1.6 | 2.1 | ND | 4.3 | ND | 0.7 | 5.7 | 5.0 | ND | 10.1 | ND | 9.3 | 2.6 |
| 糖类 Sugar | ND | ND | 13.7 | 3.8 | ND | 0.6 | 3.7 | 4.0 | ND | 4.0 | 0.4 | 0.8 | 21.1 | ND | ND | ND | 3.8 | 3.8 | ND | 1.2 | 1.3 | 4.6 | ND | 5.8 | 3.1 |
| 水及饮料类 Water and beverages | ND | ND | 0.5 | 0.3 | ND | 0.3 | 0.3 | 0.7 | ND | 0.6 | 0.3 | ND | 0.4 | 0.5 | ND | 0.3 | 0.3 | 1.6 | 0.9 | 0.9 | 0.8 | 1.4 | ND | 1.1 | 0.5 |

续表

| 膳食类别 Category | 黑龙江 HL | 辽宁 LN | 河北 HE | 北京 BJ | 吉林 JL | 山西 SX | 陕西 SN | 河南 HA | 宁夏 NX | 内蒙古 NM | 青海 QH | 甘肃 GS | 上海 SH | 福建 FJ | 江西 JX | 江苏 JS | 浙江 ZJ | 山东 SD | 湖北 HB | 四川 SC | 广西 GX | 湖南 HN | 广东 GD | 贵州 GZ | 全国平均 AVG |
|---|---|---|---|---|---|---|---|---|---|---|---|---|---|---|---|---|---|---|---|---|---|---|---|---|---|
| 酒类 Alcohol beverages | 0.8 | 1.3 | 1.4 | 1.2 | 0.4 | 0.3 | 1.2 | 1.1 | ND | 1.6 | 1.3 | 1.3 | 1.7 | 2.1 | ND | 0.9 | 1.4 | 2.1 | 1.1 | 1.6 | 0.5 | 1.5 | 1.2 | 1.3 | 1.1 |

注：ND 表示未检出。计算平均值时，ND 按 1/2 LOD 代入

Note: ND means not to be detected. When calculating the average, ND was substituted at 1/2 LOD

附表 3-32　第六次中国总膳食研究的硒膳食摄入量（单位：µg/d）

Annexed Table 3-32　Dietary intakes of selenium from the 6$^{th}$ China TDS (Unit: µg/d)

| 膳食类别 Category | 黑龙江 HL | 辽宁 LN | 河北 HE | 北京 BJ | 吉林 JL | 山西 SX | 陕西 SN | 河南 HA | 宁夏 NX | 内蒙古 NM | 青海 QH | 甘肃 GS | 上海 SH | 福建 FJ | 江西 JX | 江苏 JS | 浙江 ZJ | 山东 SD | 湖北 HB | 四川 SC | 广西 GX | 湖南 HN | 广东 GD | 贵州 GZ | 全国平均 AVG |
|---|---|---|---|---|---|---|---|---|---|---|---|---|---|---|---|---|---|---|---|---|---|---|---|---|---|
| 谷类 Cereals | 5.7 | 3.9 | 9.1 | 6.3 | 3.4 | 13.3 | 5.4 | 3.9 | 0.1 | 7.6 | 11.7 | 5.4 | 6.5 | 3.4 | 4.1 | 5.5 | 0.3 | 5.4 | 18.7 | 11.3 | 0.4 | 13.7 | 0.9 | 20.4 | 6.9 |
| 豆类 Legumes | 0.7 | 1.6 | 1.2 | 1.3 | 1.1 | 1.0 | 2.6 | 0.9 | 0.5 | 2.0 | 0.1 | 0.8 | 1.0 | 0.8 | 1.0 | 1.9 | 0.5 | 0.9 | 1.4 | 0.8 | 1.3 | 2.0 | 0.0 | 6.6 | 1.3 |
| 薯类 Potatoes | 0.3 | 0.3 | 0.6 | 0.1 | 0.0 | 1.2 | 0.8 | 0.0 | 0.0 | 2.4 | 0.9 | 0.9 | 0.3 | 0.2 | 0.0 | 0.5 | 0.0 | 0.1 | 1.1 | 0.4 | 0.1 | 0.8 | 0.0 | 0.8 | 0.5 |
| 肉类 Meats | 5.1 | 6.0 | 5.3 | 7.9 | 9.1 | 13.5 | 4.4 | 4.6 | 5.3 | 7.5 | 9.2 | 4.4 | 18.5 | 12.4 | 17.5 | 17.0 | 20.2 | 9.6 | 7.2 | 16.9 | 16.1 | 20.6 | 12.8 | 17.0 | 11.2 |
| 蛋类 Eggs | 8.3 | 8.2 | 6.3 | 10.1 | 8.6 | 5.8 | 4.4 | 6.1 | 4.1 | 5.7 | 4.2 | 5.0 | 8.2 | 4.7 | 8.4 | 6.0 | 6.0 | 6.8 | 6.7 | 3.2 | 3.2 | 4.8 | 2.8 | 2.9 | 5.8 |
| 水产类 Aquatic foods | 4.5 | 5.2 | 1.8 | 4.7 | 2.6 | 2.1 | 0.4 | 0.8 | 0.4 | 1.3 | 1.2 | 0.6 | 15.8 | 19.8 | 10.5 | 6.8 | 12.4 | 6.4 | 5.1 | 1.2 | 14.9 | 8.8 | 14.3 | 0.8 | 5.9 |
| 乳类 Dairy products | 0.5 | 0.9 | 0.5 | 1.6 | 1.0 | 0.6 | 0.6 | 0.3 | 0.2 | 0.7 | 1.1 | 0.4 | 1.9 | 1.0 | 0.6 | 1.0 | 0.9 | 0.6 | 0.3 | 0.4 | 0.5 | 0.6 | 0.6 | 0.8 | 0.7 |

附录　417

续表

| 膳食类别<br>Category | 黑龙江<br>HL | 辽宁<br>LN | 河北<br>HE | 北京<br>BJ | 吉林<br>JL | 山西<br>SX | 陕西<br>SN | 河南<br>HA | 宁夏<br>NX | 内蒙古<br>NM | 青海<br>QH | 甘肃<br>GS | 上海<br>SH | 福建<br>FJ | 江西<br>JX | 江苏<br>JS | 浙江<br>ZJ | 山东<br>SD | 湖北<br>HB | 四川<br>SC | 广西<br>GX | 湖南<br>HN | 广东<br>GD | 贵州<br>GZ | 全国平均<br>AVG |
|---|---|---|---|---|---|---|---|---|---|---|---|---|---|---|---|---|---|---|---|---|---|---|---|---|---|
| 蔬菜类 Vegetables | 1.6 | 1.3 | 3.0 | 1.9 | 0.6 | 1.5 | 2.5 | 1.8 | 0.3 | 1.9 | 2.1 | 1.6 | 2.6 | 2.9 | 2.2 | 3.9 | 1.4 | 3.7 | 3.3 | 3.4 | 1.8 | 8.4 | 0.1 | 7.6 | 2.6 |
| 水果类 Fruits | 0.1 | 0.0 | 0.1 | 0.4 | 0.1 | 0.2 | 0.1 | 0.0 | 0.0 | 0.4 | 0.0 | 0.0 | 0.1 | 0.1 | 0.0 | 0.1 | 0.0 | 0.0 | 0.0 | 0.1 | 0.0 | 0.6 | 0.0 | 0.2 | 0.1 |
| 糖类 Sugar | 0.0 | 0.0 | 0.0 | 0.0 | 0.0 | 0.0 | 0.0 | 0.0 | 0.0 | 0.0 | 0.0 | 0.0 | 0.2 | 0.0 | 0.0 | 0.0 | 0.0 | 0.0 | 0.0 | 0.0 | 0.0 | 0.0 | 0.0 | 0.0 | 0.0 |
| 水及饮料类 Water and beverages | 0.2 | 0.1 | 0.4 | 0.3 | 0.2 | 0.2 | 0.1 | 0.9 | 0.1 | 1.7 | 0.2 | 0.1 | 0.3 | 0.5 | 0.1 | 0.3 | 0.3 | 3.0 | 0.2 | 0.3 | 1.1 | 1.4 | 0.1 | 1.4 | 0.6 |
| 酒类 Alcohol beverages | 0.0 | 0.0 | 0.0 | 0.0 | 0.0 | 0.0 | 0.0 | 0.0 | 0.0 | 0.0 | 0.0 | 0.0 | 0.0 | 0.0 | 0.0 | 0.0 | 0.1 | 0.2 | 0.0 | 0.0 | 0.0 | 0.0 | 0.0 | 0.0 | 0.0 |
| 合计 SUM | 27.0 | 27.5 | 28.3 | 34.6 | 26.6 | 39.3 | 21.3 | 19.2 | 11.0 | 31.1 | 30.6 | 19.2 | 55.4 | 45.8 | 44.4 | 43.0 | 42.0 | 36.5 | 44.1 | 38.0 | 39.2 | 61.9 | 31.8 | 58.5 | 35.7 |

附表 3-33　第六次中国总膳食研究硒的膳食来源（单位：%）

Annexed Table 3-33　Dietary sources of selenium from the 6$^{th}$ China TDS (Unit: %)

| 膳食类别<br>Category | 黑龙江<br>HL | 辽宁<br>LN | 河北<br>HE | 北京<br>BJ | 吉林<br>JL | 山西<br>SX | 陕西<br>SN | 河南<br>HA | 宁夏<br>NX | 内蒙古<br>NM | 青海<br>QH | 甘肃<br>GS | 上海<br>SH | 福建<br>FJ | 江西<br>JX | 江苏<br>JS | 浙江<br>ZJ | 山东<br>SD | 湖北<br>HB | 四川<br>SC | 广西<br>GX | 湖南<br>HN | 广东<br>GD | 贵州<br>GZ | 全国平均<br>AVG |
|---|---|---|---|---|---|---|---|---|---|---|---|---|---|---|---|---|---|---|---|---|---|---|---|---|---|
| 谷类 Cereals | 21.2 | 14.1 | 32.3 | 18.3 | 12.8 | 33.8 | 25.1 | 20.1 | 1.3 | 24.5 | 38.0 | 28.2 | 11.8 | 7.4 | 9.3 | 12.7 | 0.6 | 14.7 | 42.4 | 29.7 | 0.9 | 22.2 | 2.8 | 34.9 | 19.4 |
| 豆类 Legumes | 2.7 | 5.8 | 4.2 | 3.7 | 4.0 | 2.6 | 12.3 | 4.9 | 4.3 | 6.4 | 0.2 | 4.0 | 1.8 | 1.9 | 2.2 | 4.4 | 1.1 | 2.4 | 3.1 | 2.2 | 3.4 | 3.3 | 0.0 | 11.3 | 3.7 |

续表

| 膳食类别 Category | 黑龙江 HL | 辽宁 LN | 河北 HE | 北京 BJ | 吉林 JL | 山西 SX | 陕西 SN | 河南 HA | 宁夏 NX | 内蒙古 NM | 青海 QH | 甘肃 GS | 上海 SH | 福建 FJ | 江西 JX | 江苏 JS | 浙江 ZJ | 山东 SD | 湖北 HB | 四川 SC | 广西 GX | 湖南 HN | 广东 GD | 贵州 GZ | 全国平均 AVG |
|---|---|---|---|---|---|---|---|---|---|---|---|---|---|---|---|---|---|---|---|---|---|---|---|---|---|
| 薯类 Potatoes | 1.0 | 1.1 | 2.0 | 0.2 | 0.1 | 3.1 | 3.7 | 0.1 | 0.1 | 7.6 | 3.0 | 4.5 | 0.5 | 0.3 | 0.0 | 1.2 | 0.0 | 0.2 | 2.5 | 1.0 | 0.2 | 1.4 | 0.0 | 1.3 | 1.4 |
| 肉类 Meats | 18.8 | 21.8 | 18.7 | 22.8 | 34.2 | 34.3 | 20.7 | 23.8 | 47.8 | 24.1 | 30.0 | 23.1 | 33.4 | 27.0 | 39.4 | 39.6 | 48.1 | 26.2 | 16.2 | 44.5 | 41.2 | 33.2 | 40.4 | 29.1 | 31.3 |
| 蛋类 Eggs | 30.7 | 29.7 | 22.2 | 29.2 | 32.2 | 14.6 | 20.4 | 31.8 | 37.4 | 18.2 | 13.8 | 26.2 | 14.9 | 10.3 | 18.9 | 14.0 | 14.3 | 18.5 | 15.1 | 8.5 | 8.1 | 7.7 | 8.9 | 5.0 | 16.4 |
| 水产类 Aquatic foods | 16.7 | 19.0 | 6.3 | 13.5 | 9.8 | 5.3 | 2.1 | 4.0 | 3.2 | 4.1 | 3.9 | 3.1 | 28.5 | 43.3 | 23.6 | 15.8 | 29.4 | 17.4 | 11.5 | 3.2 | 37.9 | 14.3 | 45.1 | 1.3 | 16.6 |
| 乳类 Dairy products | 1.9 | 3.4 | 1.9 | 4.5 | 3.7 | 1.4 | 2.9 | 1.4 | 2.1 | 2.4 | 3.6 | 1.9 | 3.4 | 2.1 | 1.5 | 2.3 | 2.2 | 1.7 | 0.8 | 1.0 | 1.2 | 0.9 | 1.8 | 1.3 | 2.0 |
| 蔬菜类 Vegetables | 6.0 | 4.7 | 10.5 | 5.6 | 2.4 | 3.9 | 11.8 | 9.4 | 3.0 | 6.1 | 6.8 | 8.3 | 4.8 | 6.4 | 4.9 | 9.1 | 3.4 | 10.1 | 7.6 | 8.9 | 4.5 | 13.6 | 0.4 | 13.0 | 7.2 |
| 水果类 Fruits | 0.3 | 0.0 | 0.4 | 1.1 | 0.3 | 0.4 | 0.5 | 0.0 | 0.1 | 1.2 | 0.2 | 0.1 | 0.2 | 0.3 | 0.0 | 0.3 | 0.0 | 0.1 | 0.3 | 0.2 | 0.0 | 1.0 | 0.0 | 0.3 | 0.3 |
| 糖类 Sugar | 0.0 | 0.0 | 0.0 | 0.0 | 0.0 | 0.0 | 0.0 | 0.0 | 0.0 | 0.0 | 0.0 | 0.0 | 0.3 | 0.0 | 0.0 | 0.0 | 0.0 | 0.0 | 0.0 | 0.0 | 0.0 | 0.0 | 0.0 | 0.0 | 0.0 |
| 水及饮料类 Water and beverages | 0.6 | 0.2 | 1.4 | 1.0 | 0.6 | 0.5 | 0.4 | 4.6 | 0.6 | 5.4 | 0.6 | 0.8 | 0.5 | 1.0 | 0.3 | 0.8 | 0.6 | 8.1 | 0.6 | 0.8 | 2.7 | 2.3 | 0.5 | 2.4 | 1.6 |
| 酒类 Alcohol beverages | 0.1 | 0.2 | 0.1 | 0.1 | 0.0 | 0.0 | 0.0 | 0.0 | 0.0 | 0.1 | 0.0 | 0.0 | 0.1 | 0.1 | 0.0 | 0.1 | 0.2 | 0.6 | 0.0 | 0.0 | 0.0 | 0.0 | 0.0 | 0.0 | 0.1 |

附表 3-34 第六次中国总膳食研究膳食样品中钼的含量（单位：μg/kg）

Annexed Table 3-34 Levels of molybdenum in food samples from the 6$^{th}$ China TDS (Unit: μg/kg)

| 膳食类别 Category | 黑龙江 HL | 辽宁 LN | 河北 HE | 北京 BJ | 吉林 JL | 山西 SX | 陕西 SN | 河南 HA | 宁夏 NX | 内蒙古 NM | 青海 QH | 甘肃 GS | 上海 SH | 福建 FJ | 江西 JX | 江苏 JS | 浙江 ZJ | 山东 SD | 湖北 HB | 四川 SC | 广西 GX | 湖南 HN | 广东 GD | 贵州 GZ | 全国平均 AVG |
|---|---|---|---|---|---|---|---|---|---|---|---|---|---|---|---|---|---|---|---|---|---|---|---|---|---|
| 谷类 Cereals | 141.5 | 126.2 | 126.4 | 120.4 | 133.0 | 100.1 | 156.9 | 151.9 | 101.4 | 128.9 | 157.6 | 91.8 | 157.8 | 144.8 | 245.6 | 111.2 | 166.7 | 97.3 | 134.7 | 161.4 | 209.7 | 189.6 | 150.9 | 142.5 | 143.7 |
| 豆类 Legumes | 185.6 | 256.1 | 603.3 | 525.8 | 198.1 | 362.9 | 376.9 | 257.9 | 339.0 | 364.8 | 383.0 | 341.9 | 423.4 | 142.9 | 241.6 | 550.7 | 440.8 | 680.8 | 257.4 | 320.5 | 487.9 | 630.1 | 261.9 | 470.2 | 379.3 |
| 薯类 Potatoes | ND | 47.9 | 15.5 | 30.3 | 6.8 | 14.5 | 43.1 | 16.1 | 41.6 | 11.6 | 26.1 | 20.8 | 10.2 | 20.3 | 31.6 | 5.8 | 10.6 | 18.2 | 1.5 | 12.0 | 57.6 | 48.2 | 31.9 | 14.6 | 22.4 |
| 肉类 Meats | 6.4 | 35.5 | 24.9 | 61.4 | 57.6 | 29.2 | 29.8 | 46.4 | 43.3 | 20.3 | 9.2 | 20.7 | 20.7 | 16.8 | 60.6 | 31.9 | 62.8 | 10.7 | 34.8 | 74.2 | 14.2 | 21.4 | 33.8 | 32.3 | 33.3 |
| 蛋类 Eggs | 39.7 | 41.7 | 55.3 | 32.8 | 37.7 | 33.0 | 36.5 | 34.8 | 126.0 | 117.8 | 88.8 | 39.1 | 32.8 | 40.7 | 64.5 | 42.1 | 49.2 | 41.9 | 102.8 | 35.0 | 65.8 | 34.4 | 33.5 | 45.1 | 53.0 |
| 水产类 Aquatic foods | ND | 8.9 | 7.1 | 24.9 | 15.8 | ND | 13.4 | 9.9 | 8.2 | 15.9 | 2.1 | ND | 3.6 | 20.2 | 8.4 | ND | 17.5 | 3.4 | ND | 3.0 | 6.9 | ND | 8.9 | 1.4 | 7.5 |
| 乳类 Dairy products | 35.3 | 30.7 | 36.2 | 27.4 | 34.0 | 34.2 | 48.0 | 32.1 | 43.0 | 34.1 | 36.8 | 40.0 | 30.6 | 41.1 | 36.4 | 31.7 | 35.4 | 37.4 | 48.0 | 42.8 | 38.9 | 32.6 | 38.9 | 32.8 | 36.6 |
| 蔬菜类 Vegetables | 31.1 | 45.3 | 104.6 | 103.4 | 82.9 | 42.1 | 84.3 | 101.2 | 33.6 | 62.6 | 58.3 | 33.3 | 42.7 | 42.0 | 46.1 | 378.5 | 61.3 | 18.9 | 40.5 | 22.0 | 56.7 | 35.8 | 37.7 | 19.1 | 66.0 |
| 水果类 Fruits | 3.7 | 8.8 | 10.5 | 12.1 | 3.1 | 2.4 | 13.0 | 5.9 | 7.4 | 11.7 | 11.6 | ND | 1.5 | 9.9 | 5.4 | ND | 5.2 | 9.0 | ND | 2.2 | 17.9 | ND | 8.3 | ND | 6.3 |
| 糖类 Sugar | ND | 1.1 | 7.1 | 4.0 | 0.6 | ND | 3.7 | 1.9 | ND | 1.4 | ND | ND | 41.9 | 1.2 | 2.0 | ND | 0.5 | 0.8 | ND | 1.8 | ND | ND | ND | ND | 2.9 |
| 水及饮料类 Water and beverages | ND | 1.7 | 2.6 | 2.4 | 1.2 | 1.4 | 4.0 | 4.7 | 3.1 | 2.9 | ND | 0.7 | 2.1 | 1.6 | 1.5 | 1.1 | 1.7 | 4.6 | 0.7 | ND | ND | ND | 0.7 | ND | 1.7 |

续表

| 膳食类别 Category | 黑龙江 HL | 辽宁 LN | 河北 HE | 北京 BJ | 吉林 JL | 山西 SX | 陕西 SN | 河南 HA | 宁夏 NX | 内蒙古 NM | 青海 QH | 甘肃 GS | 上海 SH | 福建 FJ | 江西 JX | 江苏 JS | 浙江 ZJ | 山东 SD | 湖北 HB | 四川 SC | 广西 GX | 湖南 HN | 广东 GD | 贵州 GZ | 全国平均 AVG |
|---|---|---|---|---|---|---|---|---|---|---|---|---|---|---|---|---|---|---|---|---|---|---|---|---|---|
| 酒类 Alcohol beverages | ND | 1.2 | 1.1 | 4.1 | 1.4 | ND | 1.0 | 2.1 | 1.3 | 1.7 | 0.6 | 2.3 | 16.6 | 5.0 | 1.8 | 2.5 | 3.2 | 0.6 | ND | 1.4 | 3.1 | ND | 25.9 | 4.6 | 3.4 |

注：ND 表示未检出。计算平均值时，ND 按 1/2 LOD 代入

Note: ND means not to be detected. When calculating the average, ND was substituted at 1/2 LOD

附表 3-35 第六次中国总膳食研究的钼膳食摄入量（单位：μg/d）

Annexed Table 3-35 Dietary intakes of molybdenum from the 6$^{th}$ China TDS (Unit: μg/d)

| 膳食类别 Category | 黑龙江 HL | 辽宁 LN | 河北 HE | 北京 BJ | 吉林 JL | 山西 SX | 陕西 SN | 河南 HA | 宁夏 NX | 内蒙古 NM | 青海 QH | 甘肃 GS | 上海 SH | 福建 FJ | 江西 JX | 江苏 JS | 浙江 ZJ | 山东 SD | 湖北 HB | 四川 SC | 广西 GX | 湖南 HN | 广东 GD | 贵州 GZ | 全国平均 AVG |
|---|---|---|---|---|---|---|---|---|---|---|---|---|---|---|---|---|---|---|---|---|---|---|---|---|---|
| 谷类 Cereals | 77.5 | 77.7 | 95.5 | 95.8 | 77.9 | 103.9 | 119.6 | 140.4 | 67.1 | 93.2 | 120.8 | 63.0 | 70.9 | 91.6 | 154.7 | 86.5 | 105.5 | 96.9 | 71.1 | 156.6 | 197.2 | 109.5 | 68.9 | 96.1 | 101.6 |
| 豆类 Legumes | 8.4 | 31.2 | 34.4 | 53.5 | 14.9 | 25.2 | 31.2 | 13.9 | 11.9 | 14.5 | 2.5 | 14.1 | 49.8 | 11.2 | 17.8 | 45.7 | 62.1 | 35.7 | 17.2 | 21.7 | 20.7 | 45.7 | 7.3 | 47.8 | 26.6 |
| 薯类 Potatoes | 0.0 | 3.4 | 0.9 | 1.8 | 0.8 | 1.7 | 4.9 | 1.3 | 4.2 | 1.4 | 2.6 | 3.0 | 0.4 | 0.9 | 1.0 | 0.2 | 0.4 | 0.8 | 0.1 | 0.8 | 0.7 | 2.6 | 0.8 | 0.5 | 1.5 |
| 肉类 Meats | 0.4 | 2.4 | 1.2 | 4.1 | 3.8 | 4.0 | 1.1 | 2.6 | 2.0 | 1.5 | 0.7 | 0.6 | 2.3 | 1.4 | 5.7 | 2.9 | 7.4 | 1.0 | 1.9 | 9.6 | 2.1 | 3.2 | 3.5 | 3.4 | 2.9 |
| 蛋类 Eggs | 1.6 | 1.7 | 1.7 | 1.3 | 1.5 | 0.7 | 0.8 | 1.0 | 1.6 | 3.5 | 1.2 | 0.9 | 1.3 | 0.8 | 1.3 | 1.2 | 1.2 | 1.9 | 2.6 | 0.5 | 0.9 | 0.8 | 0.8 | 0.7 | 1.3 |
| 水产类 Aquatic foods | 0.0 | 0.1 | 0.1 | 0.4 | 0.2 | 0.0 | 0.1 | 0.0 | 0.0 | 0.2 | 0.0 | 0.0 | 0.2 | 1.3 | 0.4 | 0.0 | 0.9 | 0.1 | 0.3 | 0.0 | 0.7 | 0.0 | 0.5 | 0.0 | 0.2 |
| 乳类 Dairy products | 0.5 | 1.4 | 0.9 | 2.3 | 1.1 | 1.4 | 0.9 | 0.6 | 0.7 | 1.2 | 2.0 | 0.6 | 2.2 | 1.5 | 0.8 | 0.9 | 1.2 | 0.9 | 0.3 | 0.5 | 0.7 | 0.6 | 1.4 | 0.9 | 1.1 |

续表

| 膳食类别 Category | 黑龙江 HL | 辽宁 LN | 河北 HE | 北京 BJ | 吉林 JL | 山西 SX | 陕西 SN | 河南 HA | 宁夏 NX | 内蒙古 NM | 青海 QH | 甘肃 GS | 上海 SH | 福建 FJ | 江西 JX | 江苏 JS | 浙江 ZJ | 山东 SD | 湖北 HB | 四川 SC | 广西 GX | 湖南 HN | 广东 GD | 贵州 GZ | 全国平均 AVG |
|---|---|---|---|---|---|---|---|---|---|---|---|---|---|---|---|---|---|---|---|---|---|---|---|---|---|
| 蔬菜类 Vegetables | 10.0 | 14.8 | 30.7 | 40.5 | 32.2 | 13.0 | 24.2 | 28.1 | 5.2 | 16.1 | 18.1 | 8.3 | 17.1 | 16.7 | 20.8 | 161.0 | 27.2 | 7.7 | 16.8 | 6.7 | 20.0 | 19.1 | 8.9 | 7.8 | 23.8 |
| 水果类 Fruits | 0.2 | 0.7 | 0.4 | 1.4 | 0.3 | 0.1 | 0.5 | 0.1 | 0.6 | 1.3 | 0.2 | 0.0 | 0.1 | 0.6 | 0.3 | 0.0 | 0.4 | 0.5 | 0.0 | 0.0 | 1.2 | 0.0 | 0.2 | 0.0 | 0.4 |
| 糖类 Sugar | 0.0 | 0.0 | 0.0 | 0.0 | 0.0 | 0.0 | 0.0 | 0.0 | 0.0 | 0.0 | 0.0 | 0.0 | 0.3 | 0.0 | 0.0 | 0.0 | 0.0 | 0.0 | 0.0 | 0.0 | 0.0 | 0.0 | 0.0 | 0.0 | 0.0 |
| 水及饮料类 Water and beverages | 0.3 | 0.9 | 2.0 | 2.6 | 1.5 | 1.0 | 1.4 | 5.6 | 1.6 | 7.5 | 0.2 | 0.9 | 1.5 | 1.4 | 1.8 | 1.1 | 1.4 | 8.3 | 0.2 | 0.1 | 0.3 | 0.3 | 0.8 | 0.3 | 1.8 |
| 酒类 Alcohol beverages | 0.0 | 0.0 | 0.0 | 0.1 | 0.0 | 0.0 | 0.0 | 0.0 | 0.0 | 0.0 | 0.0 | 0.0 | 0.4 | 0.1 | 0.0 | 0.1 | 0.2 | 0.1 | 0.0 | 0.0 | 0.1 | 0.0 | 0.0 | 0.0 | 0.1 |
| 合计 SUM | 99.0 | 134.3 | 167.8 | 203.8 | 134.3 | 151.0 | 184.7 | 193.8 | 95.0 | 140.5 | 148.1 | 91.3 | 146.5 | 127.4 | 204.7 | 299.6 | 207.8 | 153.8 | 110.2 | 196.4 | 244.7 | 181.8 | 93.2 | 157.7 | 161.1 |

附表 3-36 第六次中国总膳食研究钼的膳食来源（单位：%）

Annexed Table 3-36　Dietary sources of molybdenum from the 6<sup>th</sup> China TDS (Unit: %)

| 膳食类别 Category | 黑龙江 HL | 辽宁 LN | 河北 HE | 北京 BJ | 吉林 JL | 山西 SX | 陕西 SN | 河南 HA | 宁夏 NX | 内蒙古 NM | 青海 QH | 甘肃 GS | 上海 SH | 福建 FJ | 江西 JX | 江苏 JS | 浙江 ZJ | 山东 SD | 湖北 HB | 四川 SC | 广西 GX | 湖南 HN | 广东 GD | 贵州 GZ | 全国平均 AVG |
|---|---|---|---|---|---|---|---|---|---|---|---|---|---|---|---|---|---|---|---|---|---|---|---|---|---|
| 谷类 Cereals | 78.3 | 57.8 | 56.9 | 47.0 | 58.0 | 68.8 | 64.8 | 72.5 | 70.6 | 66.4 | 81.5 | 69.0 | 48.4 | 71.9 | 75.6 | 28.9 | 50.8 | 63.0 | 64.5 | 79.7 | 80.6 | 60.2 | 73.9 | 61.0 | 63.0 |
| 豆类 Legumes | 8.5 | 23.3 | 20.5 | 26.2 | 11.1 | 16.7 | 16.9 | 7.2 | 12.5 | 10.4 | 1.7 | 15.4 | 34.0 | 8.8 | 8.7 | 15.3 | 29.9 | 23.2 | 15.6 | 11.0 | 8.5 | 25.2 | 7.8 | 30.3 | 16.5 |

续表

| 膳食类别 Category | 黑龙江 HL | 辽宁 LN | 河北 HE | 北京 BJ | 吉林 JL | 山西 SX | 陕西 SN | 河南 HA | 宁夏 NX | 内蒙古 NM | 青海 QH | 甘肃 GS | 上海 SH | 福建 FJ | 江西 JX | 江苏 JS | 浙江 ZJ | 山东 SD | 湖北 HB | 四川 SC | 广西 GX | 湖南 HN | 广东 GD | 贵州 GZ | 全国平均 AVG |
|---|---|---|---|---|---|---|---|---|---|---|---|---|---|---|---|---|---|---|---|---|---|---|---|---|---|
| 薯类 Potatoes | 0.0 | 2.6 | 0.6 | 0.9 | 0.6 | 1.1 | 2.7 | 0.7 | 4.4 | 1.0 | 1.8 | 3.3 | 0.2 | 0.7 | 0.5 | 0.1 | 0.2 | 0.5 | 0.1 | 0.4 | 0.3 | 1.4 | 0.8 | 0.3 | 0.9 |
| 肉类 Meats | 0.4 | 1.8 | 0.7 | 2.0 | 2.9 | 2.7 | 0.6 | 1.3 | 2.1 | 1.1 | 0.4 | 0.7 | 1.6 | 1.1 | 2.8 | 1.0 | 3.6 | 0.7 | 1.7 | 4.9 | 0.9 | 1.8 | 3.8 | 2.2 | 1.8 |
| 蛋类 Eggs | 1.6 | 1.3 | 1.0 | 0.6 | 1.1 | 0.5 | 0.4 | 0.5 | 1.7 | 2.5 | 0.8 | 1.0 | 0.9 | 0.6 | 0.6 | 0.4 | 0.6 | 1.2 | 2.3 | 0.3 | 0.4 | 0.4 | 0.9 | 0.5 | 0.8 |
| 水产类 Aquatic foods | 0.0 | 0.1 | 0.0 | 0.2 | 0.1 | 0.0 | 0.0 | 0.0 | 0.0 | 0.1 | 0.0 | 0.0 | 0.2 | 1.0 | 0.2 | 0.0 | 0.4 | 0.1 | 0.0 | 0.0 | 0.3 | 0.0 | 0.5 | 0.0 | 0.1 |
| 乳类 Dairy products | 0.5 | 1.0 | 0.5 | 1.2 | 0.8 | 0.9 | 0.5 | 0.3 | 0.7 | 0.8 | 1.3 | 0.6 | 1.5 | 1.2 | 0.4 | 0.3 | 0.6 | 0.6 | 0.3 | 0.3 | 0.3 | 0.3 | 1.5 | 0.6 | 0.7 |
| 蔬菜类 Vegetables | 10.1 | 11.0 | 18.3 | 19.9 | 24.0 | 8.6 | 13.1 | 14.5 | 5.5 | 11.5 | 12.2 | 9.1 | 11.7 | 13.1 | 10.2 | 53.7 | 13.1 | 5.0 | 15.2 | 3.4 | 8.2 | 10.5 | 9.6 | 4.9 | 14.8 |
| 水果类 Fruits | 0.2 | 0.5 | 0.2 | 0.7 | 0.2 | 0.1 | 0.3 | 0.1 | 0.7 | 0.9 | 0.1 | 0.0 | 0.1 | 0.5 | 0.1 | 0.0 | 0.2 | 0.3 | 0.0 | 0.0 | 0.5 | 0.0 | 0.3 | 0.0 | 0.2 |
| 糖类 Sugar | 0.0 | 0.0 | 0.0 | 0.0 | 0.0 | 0.0 | 0.0 | 0.0 | 0.0 | 0.0 | 0.0 | 0.0 | 0.2 | 0.0 | 0.0 | 0.0 | 0.0 | 0.0 | 0.0 | 0.0 | 0.0 | 0.0 | 0.0 | 0.0 | 0.0 |
| 水及饮料类 Water and beverages | 0.3 | 0.6 | 1.2 | 1.3 | 1.1 | 0.7 | 0.7 | 2.9 | 1.7 | 5.4 | 0.1 | 0.9 | 1.0 | 1.1 | 0.9 | 0.4 | 0.7 | 5.4 | 0.2 | 0.0 | 0.1 | 0.1 | 0.9 | 0.2 | 1.1 |
| 酒类 Alcohol beverages | 0.0 | 0.0 | 0.0 | 0.1 | 0.0 | 0.0 | 0.0 | 0.0 | 0.0 | 0.0 | 0.0 | 0.0 | 0.3 | 0.1 | 0.0 | 0.0 | 0.1 | 0.0 | 0.0 | 0.0 | 0.0 | 0.0 | 0.0 | 0.0 | 0.0 |

附表 3-37 第六次中国总膳食研究膳食样品中碘的含量（单位：mg/kg）

Annexed Table 3-37 Levels of iodine in food samples from the 6th China TDS (Unit: mg/kg)

| 膳食类别 Category | 黑龙江 HL | 辽宁 LN | 河北 HE | 北京 BJ | 吉林 JL | 山西 SX | 陕西 SN | 河南 HA | 宁夏 NX | 内蒙古 NM | 青海 QH | 甘肃 GS | 上海 SH | 福建 FJ | 江西 JX | 江苏 JS | 浙江 ZJ | 山东 SD | 湖北 HB | 四川 SC | 广西 GX | 湖南 HN | 广东 GD | 贵州 GZ | 全国平均 AVG |
|---|---|---|---|---|---|---|---|---|---|---|---|---|---|---|---|---|---|---|---|---|---|---|---|---|---|
| 谷类 Cereals | ND | 0.050 | ND | 0.023 | ND | ND | ND | ND | ND | ND | ND | ND | ND | ND | ND | ND | ND | ND | ND | 0.035 | ND | ND | ND | ND | 0.014 |
| 豆类 Legumes | 0.234 | 0.295 | 0.236 | 0.088 | 0.217 | 0.149 | 0.463 | 0.157 | 0.288 | 0.291 | 0.120 | 0.414 | 0.110 | ND | 0.230 | 0.295 | 0.075 | 0.217 | 0.270 | 0.279 | 0.165 | 0.177 | 0.187 | 0.155 | 0.213 |
| 薯类 Potatoes | 0.306 | 0.331 | 0.485 | 0.235 | 0.159 | 0.122 | 0.481 | 0.200 | 0.561 | 0.432 | 0.266 | 0.680 | 0.342 | 0.170 | 0.184 | 0.334 | 0.181 | 0.235 | 0.283 | 0.309 | 0.406 | 0.252 | 0.065 | 0.297 | 0.305 |
| 肉类 Meats | 0.492 | 0.301 | 0.549 | 0.380 | 0.348 | 0.250 | 0.697 | 0.419 | 1.087 | 0.607 | 0.414 | 0.804 | 0.327 | 0.378 | 0.499 | 0.615 | 0.484 | 0.338 | 0.466 | 0.512 | 0.336 | 0.384 | 0.342 | 0.320 | 0.473 |
| 蛋类 Eggs | 0.699 | 0.729 | 1.036 | 0.567 | 0.517 | 0.596 | 0.919 | 0.635 | 1.086 | 0.266 | 1.048 | 0.925 | 0.688 | 1.110 | 0.607 | 0.815 | 0.851 | 0.529 | 0.602 | 0.660 | 0.681 | 0.531 | 0.332 | 0.482 | 0.705 |
| 水产类 Aquatic foods | 0.432 | 0.266 | 0.464 | 0.649 | 1.060 | 0.233 | 0.492 | 0.416 | 0.374 | 0.505 | 0.440 | 0.966 | 0.460 | 0.658 | 0.303 | 0.362 | 0.366 | 0.432 | 0.437 | 0.332 | 0.308 | 0.388 | 0.396 | 0.295 | 0.460 |
| 乳类 Dairy products | 0.266 | 0.181 | 0.323 | 0.126 | 0.245 | 0.194 | 0.303 | 0.192 | 0.317 | 0.349 | 0.199 | 0.292 | 0.249 | 0.240 | 0.228 | 0.344 | 0.362 | 0.499 | 0.399 | 0.334 | 0.134 | 0.445 | 0.196 | 0.183 | 0.275 |
| 蔬菜类 Vegetables | 0.491 | 0.882 | 0.858 | 0.894 | 0.971 | 0.471 | 0.812 | 1.246 | 1.623 | 1.399 | 0.431 | 0.774 | 0.867 | 2.204 | 0.593 | 1.153 | 0.849 | 1.077 | 3.520 | 0.813 | 0.436 | 1.228 | 0.406 | 0.500 | 1.021 |
| 水果类 Fruits | ND | ND | ND | ND | ND | ND | ND | ND | ND | ND | ND | ND | ND | ND | ND | ND | ND | ND | ND | ND | ND | ND | ND | ND | 0.000 |
| 糖类 Sugar | ND | ND | 0.014 | ND | ND | ND | ND | ND | ND | ND | ND | ND | 0.022 | ND | ND | ND | ND | ND | ND | ND | ND | ND | ND | ND | 0.000 |
| 水及饮料类 Water and beverages | ND | 0.014 | ND | ND | ND | ND | ND | ND | ND | ND | ND | ND | ND | ND | ND | ND | ND | 0.058 | ND | ND | ND | ND | ND | 0.025 | 0.004 |

续表

| 膳食类别<br>Category | 黑龙江<br>HL | 辽宁<br>LN | 河北<br>HE | 北京<br>BJ | 吉林<br>JL | 山西<br>SX | 陕西<br>SN | 河南<br>HA | 宁夏<br>NX | 内蒙古<br>NM | 青海<br>QH | 甘肃<br>GS | 上海<br>SH | 福建<br>FJ | 江西<br>JX | 江苏<br>JS | 浙江<br>ZJ | 山东<br>SD | 湖北<br>HB | 四川<br>SC | 广西<br>GX | 湖南<br>HN | 广东<br>GD | 贵州<br>GZ | 全国平均<br>AVG |
|---|---|---|---|---|---|---|---|---|---|---|---|---|---|---|---|---|---|---|---|---|---|---|---|---|---|
| 酒类<br>Alcohol beverages | ND | ND | ND | ND | ND | ND | ND | 0.015 | ND | ND | ND | 0.015 | ND | ND | ND | ND | ND | ND | ND | ND | 0.054 | ND | 0.081 | 0.029 | 0.008 |
| 食盐消费量<br>Consumption of salt (g) | 9.17 | 9.00 | 13.63 | 11.13 | 6.56 | 11.40 | 12.80 | 10.61 | 9.30 | 11.08 | 9.47 | 11.13 | 7.13 | 7.74 | 9.87 | 11.65 | 12.52 | 13.63 | 11.10 | 8.70 | 9.37 | 13.08 | 7.36 | 8.10 | 10.23 |

注：ND 表示未检出。计算平均值时，ND 按 1/2 LOD 代入

Note: ND means not to be detected. When calculating the average, ND was substituted at 1/2 LOD

附表 3-38　第六次中国总膳食研究的碘膳食摄入量（单位：μg/d）

Annexed Table 3-38　Dietary intakes of iodine from the 6$^{th}$ China TDS (Unit: μg/d)

| 膳食类别<br>Category | 黑龙江<br>HL | 辽宁<br>LN | 河北<br>HE | 北京<br>BJ | 吉林<br>JL | 山西<br>SX | 陕西<br>SN | 河南<br>HA | 宁夏<br>NX | 内蒙古<br>NM | 青海<br>QH | 甘肃<br>GS | 上海<br>SH | 福建<br>FJ | 江西<br>JX | 江苏<br>JS | 浙江<br>ZJ | 山东<br>SD | 湖北<br>HB | 四川<br>SC | 广西<br>GX | 湖南<br>HN | 广东<br>GD | 贵州<br>GZ | 全国平均<br>AVG |
|---|---|---|---|---|---|---|---|---|---|---|---|---|---|---|---|---|---|---|---|---|---|---|---|---|---|
| 谷类<br>Cereals | 7.43 | 30.94 | 8.76 | 18.31 | 5.39 | 11.71 | 10.40 | 10.11 | 8.25 | 7.44 | 12.19 | 8.14 | 4.08 | 6.51 | 6.04 | 6.81 | 5.90 | 11.06 | 5.07 | 34.02 | 9.68 | 5.94 | 4.32 | 7.62 | 10.26 |
| 豆类<br>Legumes | 10.65 | 35.95 | 13.46 | 8.95 | 16.39 | 10.34 | 38.32 | 8.45 | 10.12 | 11.58 | 0.77 | 17.06 | 12.98 | 0.56 | 16.98 | 24.47 | 10.53 | 11.38 | 18.02 | 18.87 | 6.98 | 12.88 | 5.23 | 15.75 | 14.03 |
| 薯类<br>Potatoes | 23.67 | 23.83 | 29.56 | 13.75 | 19.14 | 14.45 | 55.10 | 16.02 | 56.02 | 52.82 | 27.01 | 97.84 | 12.27 | 7.20 | 5.93 | 11.19 | 6.64 | 10.86 | 25.07 | 19.42 | 5.21 | 13.49 | 1.59 | 10.17 | 23.26 |
| 肉类<br>Meats | 29.48 | 20.07 | 26.02 | 25.54 | 23.13 | 34.26 | 25.14 | 23.20 | 50.71 | 44.59 | 29.39 | 24.95 | 36.26 | 32.53 | 46.88 | 56.46 | 57.28 | 32.93 | 25.29 | 65.93 | 50.75 | 57.44 | 35.64 | 34.07 | 37.00 |
| 蛋类<br>Eggs | 28.29 | 29.81 | 32.69 | 22.04 | 20.79 | 12.51 | 20.19 | 18.88 | 14.14 | 7.91 | 13.77 | 20.55 | 26.85 | 21.09 | 12.45 | 22.95 | 20.34 | 23.48 | 15.06 | 9.66 | 9.54 | 12.11 | 7.94 | 7.84 | 17.95 |
| 水产类<br>Aquatic foods | 11.74 | 4.28 | 4.41 | 10.66 | 11.81 | 1.49 | 2.02 | 1.93 | 0.91 | 5.22 | 1.57 | 2.72 | 31.54 | 42.23 | 13.26 | 14.14 | 18.42 | 9.85 | 17.78 | 2.78 | 29.76 | 25.80 | 20.28 | 1.03 | 11.90 |

续表

| 膳食类别 Category | 黑龙江 HL | 辽宁 LN | 河北 HE | 北京 BJ | 吉林 JL | 山西 SX | 陕西 SN | 河南 HA | 宁夏 NX | 内蒙古 NM | 青海 QH | 甘肃 GS | 上海 SH | 福建 FJ | 江西 JX | 江苏 JS | 浙江 ZJ | 山东 SD | 湖北 HB | 四川 SC | 广西 GX | 湖南 HN | 广东 GD | 贵州 GZ | 全国平均 AVG |
|---|---|---|---|---|---|---|---|---|---|---|---|---|---|---|---|---|---|---|---|---|---|---|---|---|---|
| 乳类 Dairy products | 3.56 | 8.05 | 7.83 | 10.80 | 7.92 | 8.06 | 5.85 | 3.76 | 4.84 | 11.99 | 10.63 | 4.12 | 17.80 | 8.64 | 4.99 | 9.46 | 12.15 | 11.46 | 2.67 | 4.19 | 2.43 | 8.01 | 7.16 | 5.16 | 7.56 |
| 蔬菜类 Vegetables | 157.40 | 287.96 | 252.04 | 350.40 | 376.86 | 145.62 | 233.04 | 346.47 | 253.60 | 359.84 | 133.84 | 191.95 | 347.27 | 874.64 | 267.81 | 490.58 | 376.86 | 437.59 | 1457.71 | 245.97 | 154.14 | 655.65 | 95.92 | 203.99 | 362.38 |
| 水果类 Fruits | 0.44 | 0.58 | 0.26 | 0.85 | 0.61 | 0.24 | 0.28 | 0.17 | 0.69 | 0.80 | 0.11 | 0.23 | 0.51 | 0.43 | 0.40 | 0.19 | 0.47 | 0.38 | 0.13 | 0.11 | 0.45 | 0.44 | 0.21 | 0.17 | 0.38 |
| 糖类 Sugar | 0.02 | 0.01 | 0.01 | 0.01 | 0.01 | 0.01 | 0.01 | 0.00 | 0.01 | 0.01 | 0.00 | 0.00 | 0.17 | 0.00 | 0.01 | 0.00 | 0.01 | 0.00 | 0.00 | 0.00 | 0.00 | 0.00 | 0.00 | 0.00 | 0.01 |
| 水及饮料类 Water and beverages | 8.56 | 6.97 | 5.43 | 7.75 | 9.11 | 5.22 | 2.42 | 8.35 | 3.62 | 18.03 | 4.33 | 8.27 | 4.92 | 6.06 | 8.27 | 7.06 | 5.50 | 104.53 | 2.00 | 2.20 | 9.12 | 7.43 | 8.35 | 31.24 | 11.86 |
| 酒类 Alcohol beverages | 0.15 | 0.24 | 0.07 | 0.19 | 0.07 | 0.00 | 0.01 | 0.05 | 0.00 | 0.15 | 0.03 | 0.05 | 0.16 | 0.10 | 0.15 | 0.26 | 0.44 | 0.80 | 0.10 | 0.04 | 1.72 | 0.12 | 0.11 | 0.06 | 0.21 |
| 合计 SUM | 281.4 | 448.7 | 380.6 | 469.3 | 491.2 | 243.9 | 392.8 | 437.4 | 402.9 | 520.4 | 233.6 | 375.9 | 494.8 | 1000.0 | 383.2 | 643.6 | 514.6 | 654.3 | 1568.9 | 403.2 | 279.8 | 799.3 | 186.7 | 317.1 | 496.8 |

附表 3-39 第六次中国总膳食研究碘的膳食来源（单位：%）

Annexed Table 3-39 Dietary sources of iodine from the 6th China TDS (Unit: %)

| 膳食类别 Category | 黑龙江 HL | 辽宁 LN | 河北 HE | 北京 BJ | 吉林 JL | 山西 SX | 陕西 SN | 河南 HA | 宁夏 NX | 内蒙古 NM | 青海 QH | 甘肃 GS | 上海 SH | 福建 FJ | 江西 JX | 江苏 JS | 浙江 ZJ | 山东 SD | 湖北 HB | 四川 SC | 广西 GX | 湖南 HN | 广东 GD | 贵州 GZ | 全国平均 AVG |
|---|---|---|---|---|---|---|---|---|---|---|---|---|---|---|---|---|---|---|---|---|---|---|---|---|---|
| 谷类 Cereals | 2.6 | 6.9 | 2.3 | 3.9 | 1.1 | 4.8 | 2.6 | 2.3 | 2.0 | 1.4 | 5.2 | 2.2 | 0.8 | 0.7 | 1.6 | 1.1 | 1.1 | 1.7 | 0.3 | 8.4 | 3.5 | 0.7 | 2.3 | 2.4 | 2.1 |

续表

| 膳食类别 Category | 黑龙江 HL | 辽宁 LN | 河北 HE | 北京 BJ | 吉林 JL | 山西 SX | 陕西 SN | 河南 HA | 宁夏 NX | 内蒙古 NM | 青海 QH | 甘肃 GS | 上海 SH | 福建 FJ | 江西 JX | 江苏 JS | 浙江 ZJ | 山东 SD | 湖北 HB | 四川 SC | 广西 GX | 湖南 HN | 广东 GD | 贵州 GZ | 全国平均 AVG |
|---|---|---|---|---|---|---|---|---|---|---|---|---|---|---|---|---|---|---|---|---|---|---|---|---|---|
| 豆类 Legumes | 3.8 | 8.0 | 3.5 | 1.9 | 3.3 | 4.2 | 9.8 | 1.9 | 2.5 | 2.2 | 0.3 | 4.5 | 2.6 | 0.1 | 4.4 | 3.8 | 2.0 | 1.7 | 1.1 | 4.7 | 2.5 | 1.6 | 2.8 | 5.0 | 2.8 |
| 薯类 Potatoes | 8.4 | 5.3 | 7.8 | 2.9 | 3.9 | 5.9 | 14.0 | 3.7 | 13.9 | 10.2 | 11.6 | 26.0 | 2.5 | 0.7 | 1.5 | 1.7 | 1.3 | 1.7 | 1.6 | 4.8 | 1.9 | 1.7 | 0.9 | 3.2 | 4.7 |
| 肉类 Meats | 10.5 | 4.5 | 6.8 | 5.4 | 4.7 | 14.0 | 6.4 | 5.3 | 12.6 | 8.6 | 12.6 | 6.6 | 7.3 | 3.3 | 12.2 | 8.8 | 11.1 | 5.0 | 1.6 | 16.4 | 18.1 | 7.2 | 19.1 | 10.7 | 7.4 |
| 蛋类 Eggs | 10.1 | 6.6 | 8.6 | 4.7 | 4.2 | 5.1 | 5.1 | 4.3 | 3.5 | 1.5 | 5.9 | 5.5 | 5.4 | 2.1 | 3.2 | 3.6 | 4.0 | 3.6 | 1.0 | 2.4 | 3.4 | 1.5 | 4.3 | 2.5 | 3.6 |
| 水产类 Aquatic foods | 4.2 | 1.0 | 1.2 | 2.3 | 2.4 | 0.6 | 0.5 | 0.4 | 0.2 | 1.0 | 0.7 | 0.7 | 6.4 | 4.2 | 3.5 | 2.2 | 3.6 | 1.5 | 1.1 | 0.7 | 10.6 | 3.2 | 10.9 | 0.3 | 2.4 |
| 乳类 Dairy products | 1.3 | 1.8 | 2.1 | 2.3 | 1.6 | 3.3 | 1.5 | 0.9 | 1.2 | 2.3 | 4.6 | 1.1 | 3.6 | 0.9 | 1.3 | 1.5 | 2.4 | 1.8 | 0.2 | 1.0 | 0.9 | 1.0 | 3.8 | 1.6 | 1.5 |
| 蔬菜类 Vegetables | 55.9 | 64.2 | 66.2 | 74.7 | 76.7 | 59.7 | 59.3 | 79.2 | 62.9 | 69.1 | 57.3 | 51.1 | 70.2 | 87.5 | 69.9 | 76.2 | 73.2 | 66.9 | 92.9 | 61.0 | 55.1 | 82.0 | 51.4 | 64.3 | 72.9 |
| 水果类 Fruits | 0.2 | 0.1 | 0.1 | 0.2 | 0.1 | 0.1 | 0.1 | 0.0 | 0.2 | 0.2 | 0.0 | 0.1 | 0.1 | 0.0 | 0.1 | 0.0 | 0.1 | 0.1 | 0.0 | 0.0 | 0.2 | 0.1 | 0.1 | 0.1 | 0.1 |
| 糖类 Sugar | 0.0 | 0.0 | 0.0 | 0.0 | 0.0 | 0.0 | 0.0 | 0.0 | 0.0 | 0.0 | 0.0 | 0.0 | 0.0 | 0.0 | 0.0 | 0.0 | 0.0 | 0.0 | 0.0 | 0.0 | 0.0 | 0.0 | 0.0 | 0.0 | 0.0 |
| 水及饮料类 Water and beverages | 3.0 | 1.6 | 1.4 | 1.7 | 1.9 | 2.1 | 0.6 | 1.9 | 0.9 | 3.5 | 1.9 | 2.2 | 1.0 | 0.6 | 2.2 | 1.1 | 1.1 | 16.0 | 0.1 | 0.5 | 3.3 | 0.9 | 4.5 | 9.9 | 2.4 |
| 酒类 Alcohol beverages | 0.1 | 0.1 | 0.0 | 0.0 | 0.0 | 0.0 | 0.0 | 0.0 | 0.0 | 0.0 | 0.0 | 0.0 | 0.0 | 0.0 | 0.0 | 0.0 | 0.1 | 0.1 | 0.0 | 0.0 | 0.6 | 0.0 | 0.1 | 0.0 | 0.0 |

附表 3-40 第六次中国总膳食研究膳食样品中铅的含量（单位：μg/kg）

Annexed Table 3-40  Levels of lead in food samples from the 6th China TDS (Unit: μg/kg)

| 膳食类别 Category | 黑龙江 HL | 辽宁 LN | 河北 HE | 北京 BJ | 吉林 JL | 山西 SX | 陕西 SN | 河南 HA | 宁夏 NX | 内蒙古 NM | 青海 QH | 甘肃 GS | 上海 SH | 福建 FJ | 江西 JX | 江苏 JS | 浙江 ZJ | 山东 SD | 湖北 HB | 四川 SC | 广西 GX | 湖南 HN | 广东 GD | 贵州 GZ | 全国平均 AVG |
|---|---|---|---|---|---|---|---|---|---|---|---|---|---|---|---|---|---|---|---|---|---|---|---|---|---|
| 谷类 Cereals | 5.98 | 6.54 | 47.62 | 14.10 | 5.13 | 3.81 | 12.43 | 25.78 | 17.36 | 20.71 | 5.68 | 8.27 | 11.27 | 9.75 | 8.88 | 17.35 | 1.18 | 18.41 | 3.97 | 3.10 | 6.18 | 25.54 | 3.08 | 2.52 | 11.86 |
| 豆类 Legumes | 17.16 | 15.85 | 11.87 | 4.91 | 4.71 | 5.28 | 6.79 | 12.29 | 6.80 | 34.94 | 16.90 | 6.91 | 13.36 | 4.82 | 14.64 | 30.17 | 6.37 | 10.02 | 22.38 | 13.04 | 8.27 | 17.41 | 7.46 | 17.73 | 12.92 |
| 薯类 Potatoes | 6.75 | 11.01 | 18.33 | 11.34 | 5.49 | 6.36 | 3.54 | 12.50 | 19.90 | 18.62 | 18.08 | 0.37 | 7.47 | 11.93 | 11.44 | 35.54 | 14.07 | 6.11 | 1.05 | 2.03 | 7.11 | 2.31 | 13.35 | 23.66 | 11.18 |
| 肉类 Meats | 7.80 | 7.69 | 2.30 | 3.91 | 7.29 | 1.29 | 7.06 | 28.85 | 12.73 | 5.41 | 27.89 | 5.45 | 7.50 | 4.04 | 11.81 | 21.06 | 7.52 | 7.24 | 6.20 | 3.90 | 20.50 | 15.49 | 5.02 | 19.15 | 10.30 |
| 蛋类 Eggs | 5.12 | 9.95 | 11.33 | 1.19 | 5.49 | 4.05 | 13.57 | 11.20 | 25.34 | 18.99 | 9.54 | 10.03 | 10.77 | 5.16 | 22.31 | 15.69 | 13.68 | 9.31 | 5.28 | ND | 9.44 | 7.84 | 2.01 | 5.59 | 9.71 |
| 水产类 Aquatic foods | 7.28 | 10.87 | 26.43 | 13.71 | 7.26 | 3.40 | 2.18 | 8.44 | 11.14 | 9.14 | 37.42 | 3.52 | 5.13 | 33.57 | 10.22 | 20.45 | 21.45 | 20.39 | 16.59 | 9.48 | 18.08 | 3.23 | 10.44 | 29.51 | 14.14 |
| 乳类 Dairy products | 0.86 | 0.32 | 2.09 | 1.56 | 1.69 | 1.58 | 0.23 | 1.70 | 2.17 | 0.50 | 0.86 | 1.45 | 3.12 | 0.32 | 3.28 | 4.69 | 1.98 | 1.80 | 0.29 | 0.26 | 2.30 | ND | 0.48 | 4.79 | 1.60 |
| 蔬菜类 Vegetables | 9.67 | 9.42 | 25.87 | 7.21 | 7.78 | 5.37 | 11.14 | 26.87 | 17.49 | 12.44 | 8.24 | 3.62 | 9.02 | 13.52 | 14.89 | 10.91 | 23.31 | 5.66 | 19.37 | 5.36 | 14.49 | 46.74 | 13.80 | 53.98 | 15.67 |
| 水果类 Fruits | 2.48 | 5.10 | 6.73 | 0.57 | 2.81 | 4.89 | 1.90 | 6.10 | 8.74 | 19.08 | 0.91 | 4.54 | 6.93 | 6.06 | 3.13 | 5.01 | 0.40 | 2.24 | 12.55 | 0.63 | 8.40 | 7.99 | 0.27 | 1.55 | 4.96 |
| 糖类 Sugar | 1.92 | 13.65 | 3.66 | 15.92 | 8.46 | 2.77 | 8.25 | 4.42 | 2.18 | 7.57 | 4.88 | 11.84 | 1.92 | 4.40 | 74.99 | 4.98 | 25.35 | 24.70 | 4.29 | 1.30 | 1.31 | 1.16 | 0.39 | 2.82 | 9.71 |
| 水及饮料类 Water and beverages | 0.23 | 1.04 | 0.75 | 0.74 | 1.37 | 1.52 | 1.18 | 5.67 | 0.43 | 2.82 | 2.19 | 2.75 | 1.11 | 0.77 | 2.30 | 1.34 | 3.43 | 0.92 | 3.67 | 0.67 | 3.23 | 2.05 | 3.93 | 0.44 | 1.86 |

续表

| 膳食类别 Category | 黑龙江 HL | 辽宁 LN | 河北 HE | 北京 BJ | 吉林 JL | 山西 SX | 陕西 SN | 河南 HA | 宁夏 NX | 内蒙古 NM | 青海 QH | 甘肃 GS | 上海 SH | 福建 FJ | 江西 JX | 江苏 JS | 浙江 ZJ | 山东 SD | 湖北 HB | 四川 SC | 广西 GX | 湖南 HN | 广东 GD | 贵州 GZ | 全国平均 AVG |
|---|---|---|---|---|---|---|---|---|---|---|---|---|---|---|---|---|---|---|---|---|---|---|---|---|---|
| 酒类 Alcohol beverages | 0.83 | 1.79 | 3.28 | 1.60 | 1.24 | 0.11 | 0.57 | 3.40 | 0.68 | 7.06 | 0.23 | 0.15 | 0.16 | 0.86 | 1.23 | 2.89 | 0.57 | 1.53 | 2.78 | 0.73 | 5.20 | 3.26 | 3.89 | 1.72 | 1.91 |

注：未检出（ND）按 1/2 检出限（LOD）计
Note: values not detected (ND) were treated as being equal to half of the detection of limit

附表 3-41 第六次中国总膳食研究铅的膳食摄入量（单位：μg/d）
Annexed Table 3-41 Dietary intake of lead from the 6th China TDS (Unit: μg/d)

| 膳食类别 Category | 黑龙江 HL | 辽宁 LN | 河北 HE | 北京 BJ | 吉林 JL | 山西 SX | 陕西 SN | 河南 HA | 宁夏 NX | 内蒙古 NM | 青海 QH | 甘肃 GS | 上海 SH | 福建 FJ | 江西 JX | 江苏 JS | 浙江 ZJ | 山东 SD | 湖北 HB | 四川 SC | 广西 GX | 湖南 HN | 广东 GD | 贵州 GZ | 全国平均 AVG |
|---|---|---|---|---|---|---|---|---|---|---|---|---|---|---|---|---|---|---|---|---|---|---|---|---|---|
| 谷类 Cereals | 3.28 | 4.03 | 35.97 | 11.21 | 3.00 | 3.95 | 9.48 | 23.83 | 11.48 | 14.97 | 4.35 | 5.68 | 5.06 | 6.17 | 5.59 | 13.50 | 0.74 | 18.33 | 2.10 | 3.01 | 5.81 | 14.75 | 1.41 | 1.70 | 8.72 |
| 豆类 Legumes | 0.78 | 1.93 | 0.68 | 0.50 | 0.36 | 0.37 | 0.56 | 0.66 | 0.24 | 1.39 | 0.11 | 0.28 | 1.57 | 0.38 | 1.08 | 2.50 | 0.90 | 0.53 | 1.49 | 0.88 | 0.35 | 1.26 | 0.21 | 1.80 | 0.87 |
| 薯类 Potatoes | 0.52 | 0.79 | 1.12 | 0.66 | 0.66 | 0.75 | 0.41 | 1.00 | 1.99 | 2.28 | 1.83 | 0.05 | 0.27 | 0.50 | 0.37 | 1.19 | 0.52 | 0.28 | 0.09 | 0.13 | 0.09 | 0.12 | 0.33 | 0.81 | 0.70 |
| 肉类 Meats | 0.47 | 0.51 | 0.11 | 0.26 | 0.48 | 0.18 | 0.25 | 1.60 | 0.59 | 0.40 | 1.98 | 0.17 | 0.83 | 0.35 | 1.11 | 1.93 | 0.89 | 0.70 | 0.34 | 0.50 | 3.09 | 2.32 | 0.52 | 2.04 | 0.90 |
| 蛋类 Eggs | 0.21 | 0.41 | 0.36 | 0.05 | 0.22 | 0.09 | 0.30 | 0.33 | 0.33 | 0.56 | 0.13 | 0.22 | 0.42 | 0.10 | 0.46 | 0.44 | 0.33 | 0.41 | 0.13 | 0.00 | 0.13 | 0.18 | 0.05 | 0.09 | 0.25 |
| 水产类 Aquatic foods | 0.20 | 0.17 | 0.25 | 0.23 | 0.08 | 0.02 | 0.01 | 0.04 | 0.03 | 0.09 | 0.13 | 0.01 | 0.35 | 2.16 | 0.45 | 0.80 | 1.08 | 0.46 | 0.68 | 0.08 | 1.75 | 0.21 | 0.53 | 0.10 | 0.41 |
| 乳类 Dairy products | 0.01 | 0.01 | 0.05 | 0.13 | 0.05 | 0.07 | 0.00 | 0.03 | 0.03 | 0.02 | 0.05 | 0.02 | 0.22 | 0.01 | 0.07 | 0.13 | 0.07 | 0.04 | 0.00 | 0.00 | 0.04 | 0.00 | 0.02 | 0.13 | 0.05 |

续表

| 膳食类别<br>Category | 黑龙江<br>HL | 辽宁<br>LN | 河北<br>HE | 北京<br>BJ | 吉林<br>JL | 山西<br>SX | 陕西<br>SN | 河南<br>HA | 宁夏<br>NX | 内蒙古<br>NM | 青海<br>QH | 甘肃<br>GS | 上海<br>SH | 福建<br>FJ | 江西<br>JX | 江苏<br>JS | 浙江<br>ZJ | 山东<br>SD | 湖北<br>HB | 四川<br>SC | 广西<br>GX | 湖南<br>HN | 广东<br>GD | 贵州<br>GZ | 全国平均<br>AVG |
|---|---|---|---|---|---|---|---|---|---|---|---|---|---|---|---|---|---|---|---|---|---|---|---|---|---|
| 蔬菜类 Vegetables | 3.10 | 3.08 | 7.59 | 2.83 | 3.02 | 1.66 | 3.20 | 7.47 | 2.73 | 3.20 | 2.56 | 0.90 | 3.61 | 5.36 | 6.72 | 4.64 | 10.35 | 2.30 | 8.02 | 1.62 | 5.12 | 24.96 | 3.26 | 22.02 | 5.81 |
| 水果类 Fruits | 0.16 | 0.39 | 0.25 | 0.07 | 0.25 | 0.17 | 0.07 | 0.15 | 0.74 | 2.16 | 0.01 | 0.15 | 0.51 | 0.36 | 0.18 | 0.14 | 0.03 | 0.12 | 0.24 | 0.01 | 0.54 | 0.51 | 0.01 | 0.03 | 0.30 |
| 糖类 Sugar | 0.00 | 0.01 | 0.00 | 0.03 | 0.01 | 0.00 | 0.01 | 0.00 | 0.00 | 0.01 | 0.00 | 0.00 | 0.00 | 0.00 | 0.07 | 0.00 | 0.03 | 0.01 | 0.00 | 0.00 | 0.00 | 0.00 | 0.00 | 0.00 | 0.02 |
| 水及饮料类 Water and beverages | 0.28 | 0.51 | 0.58 | 0.82 | 1.79 | 1.13 | 0.41 | 6.76 | 0.22 | 7.26 | 1.35 | 3.25 | 0.78 | 0.67 | 2.72 | 1.35 | 2.70 | 1.66 | 1.05 | 0.21 | 4.21 | 2.18 | 4.69 | 0.55 | 1.96 |
| 酒类 Alcohol beverages | 0.02 | 0.06 | 0.04 | 0.04 | 0.01 | 0.00 | 0.00 | 0.01 | 0.00 | 0.15 | 0.00 | 0.00 | 0.00 | 0.01 | 0.03 | 0.11 | 0.04 | 0.17 | 0.04 | 0.00 | 0.17 | 0.05 | 0.01 | 0.00 | 0.04 |
| 合计 SUM | 9.02 | 11.91 | 47.00 | 16.83 | 9.93 | 8.39 | 15.01 | 41.89 | 18.39 | 32.49 | 12.51 | 10.74 | 13.65 | 16.07 | 18.84 | 26.73 | 17.66 | 25.03 | 14.18 | 6.45 | 21.30 | 46.54 | 11.03 | 29.29 | 20.04 |

附表 3-42 第六次中国总膳食研究铅的膳食来源（单位：%）

Annexed Table 3-42　Dietary sources of lead form the 6$^{th}$ China TDS (Unit: %)

| 膳食类别<br>Category | 黑龙江<br>HL | 辽宁<br>LN | 河北<br>HE | 北京<br>BJ | 吉林<br>JL | 山西<br>SX | 陕西<br>SN | 河南<br>HA | 宁夏<br>NX | 内蒙古<br>NM | 青海<br>QH | 甘肃<br>GS | 上海<br>SH | 福建<br>FJ | 江西<br>JX | 江苏<br>JS | 浙江<br>ZJ | 山东<br>SD | 湖北<br>HB | 四川<br>SC | 广西<br>GX | 湖南<br>HN | 广东<br>GD | 贵州<br>GZ | 全国平均<br>AVG |
|---|---|---|---|---|---|---|---|---|---|---|---|---|---|---|---|---|---|---|---|---|---|---|---|---|---|
| 谷类 Cereals | 36.3 | 33.8 | 76.5 | 66.6 | 30.2 | 47.1 | 63.2 | 56.9 | 62.4 | 46.1 | 34.8 | 52.9 | 37.1 | 38.4 | 29.7 | 50.5 | 4.2 | 73.3 | 14.8 | 46.6 | 27.3 | 31.7 | 12.7 | 5.8 | 43.6 |
| 豆类 Legumes | 8.6 | 16.2 | 1.4 | 3.0 | 3.6 | 4.4 | 3.7 | 1.6 | 1.3 | 4.3 | 0.9 | 2.7 | 11.5 | 2.4 | 5.7 | 9.4 | 5.1 | 2.1 | 10.5 | 13.7 | 1.6 | 2.7 | 1.9 | 6.2 | 4.3 |

续表

| 膳食类别 Category | 黑龙江 HL | 辽宁 LN | 河北 HE | 北京 BJ | 吉林 JL | 山西 SX | 陕西 SN | 河南 HA | 宁夏 NX | 内蒙古 NM | 青海 QH | 甘肃 GS | 上海 SH | 福建 FJ | 江西 JX | 江苏 JS | 浙江 ZJ | 山东 SD | 湖北 HB | 四川 SC | 广西 GX | 湖南 HN | 广东 GD | 贵州 GZ | 全国平均 AVG |
|---|---|---|---|---|---|---|---|---|---|---|---|---|---|---|---|---|---|---|---|---|---|---|---|---|---|
| 薯类 Potatoes | 5.8 | 6.7 | 2.4 | 3.9 | 6.6 | 9.0 | 2.7 | 2.4 | 10.8 | 7.0 | 14.7 | 0.5 | 2.0 | 3.1 | 2.0 | 4.4 | 2.9 | 1.1 | 0.7 | 2.0 | 0.4 | 0.3 | 3.0 | 2.8 | 3.5 |
| 肉类 Meats | 5.2 | 4.3 | 0.2 | 1.6 | 4.9 | 2.1 | 1.7 | 3.8 | 3.2 | 1.2 | 15.8 | 1.6 | 6.1 | 2.2 | 5.9 | 7.2 | 5.0 | 2.8 | 2.4 | 7.8 | 14.5 | 5.0 | 4.7 | 7.0 | 4.5 |
| 蛋类 Eggs | 2.3 | 3.4 | 0.8 | 0.3 | 2.2 | 1.0 | 2.0 | 0.8 | 1.8 | 1.7 | 1.0 | 2.1 | 3.1 | 0.6 | 2.4 | 1.7 | 1.9 | 1.7 | 0.9 | 0.0 | 0.6 | 0.4 | 0.4 | 0.3 | 1.2 |
| 水产类 Aquatic foods | 2.2 | 1.5 | 0.5 | 1.3 | 0.8 | 0.3 | 0.1 | 0.1 | 0.1 | 0.3 | 1.1 | 0.1 | 2.6 | 13.4 | 2.4 | 3.0 | 6.1 | 1.9 | 4.8 | 1.2 | 8.2 | 0.5 | 4.8 | 0.4 | 2.1 |
| 乳类 Dairy products | 0.1 | 0.1 | 0.1 | 0.8 | 0.6 | 0.8 | 0.0 | 0.1 | 0.2 | 0.1 | 0.4 | 0.2 | 1.6 | 0.1 | 0.4 | 0.5 | 0.4 | 0.2 | 0.0 | 0.1 | 0.2 | 0.0 | 0.2 | 0.5 | 0.3 |
| 蔬菜类 Vegetables | 34.4 | 25.8 | 16.2 | 16.8 | 30.4 | 19.8 | 21.3 | 17.8 | 14.9 | 9.9 | 20.5 | 8.4 | 26.5 | 33.4 | 35.7 | 17.4 | 58.6 | 9.2 | 56.6 | 25.2 | 24.0 | 53.6 | 29.6 | 75.2 | 29.0 |
| 水果类 Fruits | 1.7 | 3.3 | 0.5 | 0.4 | 2.5 | 2.0 | 0.5 | 0.4 | 4.0 | 6.6 | 0.1 | 1.4 | 3.7 | 2.3 | 0.9 | 0.5 | 0.2 | 0.5 | 1.7 | 0.1 | 2.5 | 1.1 | 0.1 | 0.1 | 1.5 |
| 糖类 Sugar | 0.0 | 0.1 | 0.0 | 0.2 | 0.1 | 0.0 | 0.0 | 0.0 | 0.0 | 0.0 | 0.0 | 0.0 | 0.1 | 0.0 | 0.4 | 0.0 | 0.2 | 0.0 | 0.0 | 0.0 | 0.0 | 0.0 | 0.0 | 0.0 | 0.0 |
| 水及饮料类 Water and beverages | 3.1 | 4.3 | 1.2 | 4.9 | 18.0 | 13.5 | 2.7 | 16.1 | 1.2 | 22.4 | 10.8 | 30.2 | 5.7 | 4.1 | 14.4 | 5.1 | 15.3 | 6.6 | 7.4 | 3.3 | 19.7 | 4.7 | 42.5 | 1.9 | 9.8 |
| 酒类 Alcohol beverages | 0.2 | 0.5 | 0.1 | 0.3 | 0.1 | 0.0 | 0.0 | 0.0 | 0.0 | 0.5 | 0.0 | 0.0 | 0.0 | 0.1 | 0.1 | 0.4 | 0.2 | 0.7 | 0.3 | 0.1 | 0.8 | 0.1 | 0.0 | 0.0 | 0.2 |

附表 3-43  第六次中国总膳食研究膳食样品中镉的含量（单位：μg/kg）

Annexed Table 3-43  Levels of cadmium in food samples from the 6$^{th}$ China TDS (Unit: μg/kg)

| 膳食类别 Category | 黑龙江 HL | 辽宁 LN | 河北 HE | 北京 BJ | 吉林 JL | 山西 SX | 陕西 SN | 河南 HA | 宁夏 NX | 内蒙古 NM | 青海 QH | 甘肃 GS | 上海 SH | 福建 FJ | 江西 JX | 江苏 JS | 浙江 ZJ | 山东 SD | 湖北 HB | 四川 SC | 广西 GX | 湖南 HN | 广东 GD | 贵州 GZ | 全国平均 AVG |
|---|---|---|---|---|---|---|---|---|---|---|---|---|---|---|---|---|---|---|---|---|---|---|---|---|---|
| 谷类 Cereals | 17.08 | 4.96 | 4.67 | 4.76 | 2.95 | 3.95 | 4.10 | 7.85 | 11.92 | 3.19 | 11.49 | 4.65 | 6.80 | 18.15 | 43.54 | 13.17 | 10.98 | 15.50 | 22.58 | 14.54 | 18.23 | 83.17 | 9.86 | 8.78 | 14.45 |
| 豆类 Legumes | 27.81 | 41.87 | 14.37 | 4.53 | 25.98 | 8.44 | 7.43 | 21.67 | 12.08 | 15.28 | 11.57 | 10.31 | 5.53 | 10.75 | 26.50 | 20.44 | 8.20 | 27.86 | 21.57 | 13.40 | 13.72 | 13.07 | 31.66 | 10.01 | 16.84 |
| 薯类 Potatoes | 11.65 | 26.15 | 11.60 | 5.49 | 20.29 | 4.71 | 2.60 | 3.04 | 4.29 | 30.83 | 2.32 | 3.85 | 8.26 | 4.75 | 12.51 | 11.75 | 5.41 | 12.96 | 15.23 | 11.05 | 12.94 | 15.09 | 14.48 | 14.63 | 11.08 |
| 肉类 Meats | 8.10 | 1.21 | 1.01 | 1.95 | 1.61 | 1.35 | 1.26 | 3.25 | 4.11 | 1.45 | 1.87 | 2.53 | 1.54 | 1.39 | 2.26 | 5.06 | 2.57 | 7.12 | 1.36 | 2.80 | 0.61 | 1.96 | 1.32 | 1.17 | 2.45 |
| 蛋类 Eggs | 6.10 | 0.68 | 0.62 | 0.32 | 0.32 | 0.39 | 0.43 | 0.93 | 1.61 | 0.17 | 0.43 | 0.09 | 0.24 | 1.01 | 0.21 | 0.45 | 0.67 | 8.97 | 0.45 | 0.30 | 0.28 | 0.45 | 0.92 | 0.24 | 1.09 |
| 水产类 Aquatic foods | 7.24 | 83.82 | 4.05 | 22.61 | 3.33 | 3.35 | 1.08 | 26.07 | 1.36 | 2.50 | 5.09 | 3.37 | 7.33 | 70.15 | 0.88 | 3.33 | 52.38 | 48.23 | 1.02 | 1.09 | 19.55 | 5.72 | 29.01 | 3.30 | 16.91 |
| 乳类 Dairy products | 0.94 | ND | ND | ND | ND | ND | 0.08 | 0.05 | 0.31 | 0.07 | 0.05 | 0.08 | 0.08 | ND | ND | 0.05 | ND | 0.89 | ND | 0.08 | ND | ND | 0.27 | ND | 0.14 |
| 蔬菜类 Vegetables | 14.70 | 11.27 | 4.71 | 5.61 | 6.64 | 3.91 | 7.83 | 6.22 | 8.63 | 5.49 | 2.88 | 4.66 | 16.48 | 12.05 | 18.05 | 13.30 | 10.62 | 10.66 | 14.48 | 12.29 | 9.52 | 23.30 | 30.58 | 46.62 | 12.52 |
| 水果类 Fruits | 2.75 | 0.79 | 0.68 | 1.15 | 1.04 | 0.54 | 0.27 | 1.04 | 0.82 | 0.56 | 0.51 | 0.46 | 0.74 | 0.56 | 0.34 | 0.32 | 0.55 | 4.31 | 0.44 | 0.27 | 0.49 | 0.80 | 1.40 | 0.52 | 0.89 |
| 糖类 Sugar | 5.96 | 0.37 | 7.80 | 0.38 | 0.38 | 0.23 | 0.41 | 2.11 | 1.19 | 1.61 | 0.27 | 0.18 | 48.96 | 0.32 | 0.44 | 0.25 | 0.15 | 7.36 | 0.66 | 0.27 | 0.06 | 0.42 | 0.88 | 0.32 | 3.37 |
| 水及饮料类 Water and beverages | 0.53 | 0.07 | ND | ND | ND | ND | 0.06 | ND | 0.14 | ND | 0.08 | ND | 0.07 | 0.10 | ND | 0.07 | ND | 0.92 | ND | 0.16 | ND | 0.09 | 0.16 | ND | 0.11 |

续表

| 膳食类别 Category | 黑龙江 HL | 辽宁 LN | 河北 HE | 北京 BJ | 吉林 JL | 山西 SX | 陕西 SN | 河南 HA | 宁夏 NX | 内蒙古 NM | 青海 QH | 甘肃 GS | 上海 SH | 福建 FJ | 江西 JX | 江苏 JS | 浙江 ZJ | 山东 SD | 湖北 HB | 四川 SC | 广西 GX | 湖南 HN | 广东 GD | 贵州 GZ | 全国平均 AVG |
|---|---|---|---|---|---|---|---|---|---|---|---|---|---|---|---|---|---|---|---|---|---|---|---|---|---|
| 酒类 Alcohol beverages | 0.47 | 0.06 | ND | ND | 0.06 | ND | 0.05 | 0.06 | 0.20 | ND | ND | ND | 1.63 | 0.33 | 0.08 | 0.41 | 0.31 | 0.86 | ND | 0.08 | 0.41 | ND | 2.90 | 0.26 | 0.35 |

注：未检出（ND）按 1/2 检出限（LOD）计

Note: values not detected (ND) were treated as being equal to half of the detection of limit (LOD)

附表 3-44 第六次中国总膳食研究镉的膳食摄入量（单位：μg/d）

Annexed Table 3-44　Dietary intake of cadmium from the 6th China TDS (Unit: μg/d)

| 膳食类别 Category | 黑龙江 HL | 辽宁 LN | 河北 HE | 北京 BJ | 吉林 JL | 山西 SX | 陕西 SN | 河南 HA | 宁夏 NX | 内蒙古 NM | 青海 QH | 甘肃 GS | 上海 SH | 福建 FJ | 江西 JX | 江苏 JS | 浙江 ZJ | 山东 SD | 湖北 HB | 四川 SC | 广西 GX | 湖南 HN | 广东 GD | 贵州 GZ | 全国平均 AVG |
|---|---|---|---|---|---|---|---|---|---|---|---|---|---|---|---|---|---|---|---|---|---|---|---|---|---|
| 谷类 Cereals | 9.36 | 3.05 | 3.53 | 3.79 | 1.73 | 4.10 | 3.13 | 7.26 | 7.89 | 2.30 | 8.81 | 3.19 | 3.05 | 11.47 | 27.43 | 10.25 | 6.95 | 15.43 | 11.93 | 14.10 | 17.15 | 48.02 | 4.50 | 5.93 | 9.76 |
| 豆类 Legumes | 1.26 | 5.11 | 0.82 | 0.46 | 1.96 | 0.59 | 0.62 | 1.17 | 0.42 | 0.61 | 0.08 | 0.42 | 0.65 | 0.84 | 1.95 | 1.70 | 1.16 | 1.46 | 1.44 | 0.91 | 0.58 | 0.95 | 0.88 | 1.02 | 1.13 |
| 薯类 Potatoes | 0.90 | 1.88 | 0.71 | 0.32 | 2.43 | 0.56 | 0.30 | 0.24 | 0.43 | 3.77 | 0.23 | 0.55 | 0.30 | 0.20 | 0.40 | 0.39 | 0.20 | 0.60 | 1.35 | 0.70 | 0.17 | 0.81 | 0.36 | 0.50 | 0.76 |
| 肉类 Meats | 0.49 | 0.08 | 0.05 | 0.13 | 0.11 | 0.19 | 0.05 | 0.18 | 0.19 | 0.11 | 0.13 | 0.08 | 0.17 | 0.12 | 0.21 | 0.46 | 0.30 | 0.69 | 0.07 | 0.36 | 0.09 | 0.29 | 0.14 | 0.12 | 0.20 |
| 蛋类 Eggs | 0.25 | 0.03 | 0.02 | 0.01 | 0.01 | 0.01 | 0.01 | 0.03 | 0.02 | 0.01 | 0.01 | 0.00 | 0.01 | 0.02 | 0.00 | 0.01 | 0.02 | 0.40 | 0.01 | 0.00 | 0.00 | 0.01 | 0.02 | 0.00 | 0.04 |
| 水产类 Aquatic foods | 0.20 | 1.35 | 0.04 | 0.37 | 0.04 | 0.02 | 0.00 | 0.12 | 0.00 | 0.03 | 0.02 | 0.01 | 0.50 | 4.50 | 0.04 | 0.13 | 2.64 | 1.10 | 0.04 | 0.01 | 1.89 | 0.38 | 1.49 | 0.01 | 0.62 |
| 乳类 Dairy products | 0.01 | 0.00 | 0.00 | 0.00 | 0.00 | 0.00 | 0.00 | 0.00 | 0.00 | 0.00 | 0.00 | 0.00 | 0.01 | 0.00 | 0.00 | 0.00 | 0.00 | 0.02 | 0.00 | 0.00 | 0.00 | 0.00 | 0.01 | 0.00 | 0.00 |

续表

| 膳食类别<br>Category | 黑龙江<br>HL | 辽宁<br>LN | 河北<br>HE | 北京<br>BJ | 吉林<br>JL | 山西<br>SX | 陕西<br>SN | 河南<br>HA | 宁夏<br>NX | 内蒙古<br>NM | 青海<br>QH | 甘肃<br>GS | 上海<br>SH | 福建<br>FJ | 江西<br>JX | 江苏<br>JS | 浙江<br>ZJ | 山东<br>SD | 湖北<br>HB | 四川<br>SC | 广西<br>GX | 湖南<br>HN | 广东<br>GD | 贵州<br>GZ | 全国平均<br>AVG |
|---|---|---|---|---|---|---|---|---|---|---|---|---|---|---|---|---|---|---|---|---|---|---|---|---|---|
| 蔬菜类 Vegetables | 4.71 | 3.68 | 1.38 | 2.20 | 2.58 | 1.21 | 2.25 | 1.73 | 1.35 | 1.41 | 0.90 | 1.16 | 6.60 | 4.78 | 8.15 | 5.66 | 4.72 | 4.33 | 5.99 | 3.72 | 3.37 | 12.44 | 7.23 | 19.02 | 4.61 |
| 水果类 Fruits | 0.17 | 0.06 | 0.03 | 0.13 | 0.09 | 0.02 | 0.01 | 0.03 | 0.07 | 0.06 | 0.01 | 0.02 | 0.05 | 0.03 | 0.02 | 0.01 | 0.04 | 0.23 | 0.01 | 0.00 | 0.03 | 0.05 | 0.04 | 0.01 | 0.05 |
| 糖类 Sugar | 0.01 | 0.00 | 0.00 | 0.00 | 0.00 | 0.00 | 0.00 | 0.00 | 0.00 | 0.00 | 0.00 | 0.00 | 0.37 | 0.00 | 0.00 | 0.00 | 0.00 | 0.00 | 0.00 | 0.00 | 0.00 | 0.00 | 0.00 | 0.00 | 0.02 |
| 水及饮料类 Water and beverages | 0.65 | 0.03 | 0.02 | 0.03 | 0.03 | 0.00 | 0.02 | 0.03 | 0.07 | 0.06 | 0.05 | 0.03 | 0.05 | 0.08 | 0.03 | 0.07 | 0.02 | 1.65 | 0.01 | 0.05 | 0.03 | 0.10 | 0.19 | 0.03 | 0.14 |
| 酒类 Alcohol beverages | 0.01 | 0.00 | 0.00 | 0.00 | 0.00 | 0.00 | 0.00 | 0.00 | 0.00 | 0.00 | 0.00 | 0.00 | 0.04 | 0.00 | 0.00 | 0.02 | 0.02 | 0.10 | 0.00 | 0.00 | 0.01 | 0.00 | 0.00 | 0.00 | 0.01 |
| 合计 SUM | 18.02 | 15.28 | 6.60 | 7.44 | 8.98 | 6.70 | 6.38 | 10.79 | 10.45 | 8.36 | 10.23 | 5.46 | 11.80 | 22.06 | 38.24 | 18.70 | 16.05 | 26.02 | 20.86 | 19.85 | 23.32 | 63.05 | 14.86 | 26.65 | 17.34 |

附表 3-45　第六次中国总膳食研究镉的膳食来源（单位：%）

Annexed Table 3-45　Dietary sources of cadmium from the 6$^{th}$ China TDS (Unit: %)

| 膳食类别<br>Category | 黑龙江<br>HL | 辽宁<br>LN | 河北<br>HE | 北京<br>BJ | 吉林<br>JL | 山西<br>SX | 陕西<br>SN | 河南<br>HA | 宁夏<br>NX | 内蒙古<br>NM | 青海<br>QH | 甘肃<br>GS | 上海<br>SH | 福建<br>FJ | 江西<br>JX | 江苏<br>JS | 浙江<br>ZJ | 山东<br>SD | 湖北<br>HB | 四川<br>SC | 广西<br>GX | 湖南<br>HN | 广东<br>GD | 贵州<br>GZ | 全国平均<br>AVG |
|---|---|---|---|---|---|---|---|---|---|---|---|---|---|---|---|---|---|---|---|---|---|---|---|---|---|
| 谷类 Cereals | 51.9 | 20.0 | 53.5 | 50.9 | 19.2 | 61.1 | 48.9 | 67.3 | 75.5 | 27.5 | 86.1 | 58.4 | 25.9 | 52.0 | 71.7 | 54.8 | 43.3 | 59.3 | 57.2 | 71.0 | 73.5 | 76.2 | 30.3 | 22.2 | 56.3 |
| 豆类 Legumes | 7.0 | 33.4 | 12.4 | 6.2 | 21.8 | 8.7 | 9.6 | 10.8 | 4.1 | 7.3 | 0.7 | 7.8 | 5.5 | 3.8 | 5.1 | 9.1 | 7.2 | 5.6 | 6.9 | 4.6 | 2.5 | 1.5 | 5.9 | 3.8 | 6.5 |

续表

| 膳食类别<br>Category | 黑龙江<br>HL | 辽宁<br>LN | 河北<br>HE | 北京<br>BJ | 吉林<br>JL | 山西<br>SX | 陕西<br>SN | 河南<br>HA | 宁夏<br>NX | 内蒙古<br>NM | 青海<br>QH | 甘肃<br>GS | 上海<br>SH | 福建<br>FJ | 江西<br>JX | 江苏<br>JS | 浙江<br>ZJ | 山东<br>SD | 湖北<br>HB | 四川<br>SC | 广西<br>GX | 湖南<br>HN | 广东<br>GD | 贵州<br>GZ | 全国平均<br>AVG |
|---|---|---|---|---|---|---|---|---|---|---|---|---|---|---|---|---|---|---|---|---|---|---|---|---|---|
| 薯类 Potatoes | 5.0 | 12.3 | 10.7 | 4.3 | 27.1 | 8.3 | 4.7 | 2.3 | 4.1 | 45.1 | 2.3 | 10.2 | 2.5 | 0.9 | 1.1 | 2.1 | 1.2 | 2.3 | 6.5 | 3.5 | 0.7 | 1.3 | 2.4 | 1.9 | 4.4 |
| 肉类 Meats | 2.7 | 0.5 | 0.7 | 1.8 | 1.2 | 2.8 | 0.7 | 1.7 | 1.8 | 1.3 | 1.3 | 1.4 | 1.4 | 0.5 | 0.6 | 2.5 | 1.9 | 2.7 | 0.4 | 1.8 | 0.4 | 0.5 | 0.9 | 0.5 | 1.2 |
| 蛋类 Eggs | 1.4 | 0.2 | 0.3 | 0.2 | 0.1 | 0.1 | 0.1 | 0.3 | 0.2 | 0.1 | 0.1 | 0.0 | 0.1 | 0.1 | 0.0 | 0.1 | 0.1 | 1.5 | 0.1 | 0.0 | 0.0 | 0.0 | 0.1 | 0.0 | 0.2 |
| 水产类 Aquatic foods | 1.1 | 8.8 | 0.6 | 5.0 | 0.4 | 0.3 | 0.1 | 1.1 | 0.0 | 0.3 | 0.2 | 0.2 | 4.3 | 20.4 | 0.1 | 0.7 | 16.4 | 4.2 | 0.2 | 0.0 | 8.1 | 0.6 | 10.0 | 0.0 | 3.6 |
| 乳类 Dairy products | 0.1 | 0.0 | 0.0 | 0.0 | 0.0 | 0.0 | 0.0 | 0.0 | 0.0 | 0.0 | 0.0 | 0.0 | 0.1 | 0.0 | 0.0 | 0.0 | 0.0 | 0.1 | 0.0 | 0.0 | 0.0 | 0.0 | 0.1 | 0.0 | 0.0 |
| 蔬菜类 Vegetables | 26.2 | 24.1 | 21.0 | 29.5 | 28.7 | 18.0 | 35.2 | 16.0 | 12.9 | 16.9 | 8.8 | 21.2 | 55.9 | 21.7 | 21.3 | 30.3 | 29.4 | 16.6 | 28.7 | 18.7 | 14.4 | 19.7 | 48.7 | 71.4 | 26.6 |
| 水果类 Fruits | 1.0 | 0.4 | 0.4 | 1.7 | 1.0 | 0.3 | 0.2 | 0.2 | 0.7 | 0.8 | 0.1 | 0.3 | 0.5 | 0.2 | 0.1 | 0.0 | 0.2 | 0.9 | 0.0 | 0.0 | 0.1 | 0.1 | 0.3 | 0.0 | 0.3 |
| 糖类 Sugar | 0.1 | 0.0 | 0.1 | 0.0 | 0.0 | 0.0 | 0.0 | 0.0 | 0.0 | 0.0 | 0.0 | 0.0 | 3.1 | 0.0 | 0.0 | 0.0 | 0.0 | 0.0 | 0.0 | 0.0 | 0.0 | 0.0 | 0.0 | 0.0 | 0.1 |
| 水及饮料类 Water and beverages | 3.6 | 0.2 | 0.3 | 0.4 | 0.4 | 0.3 | 0.3 | 0.3 | 0.7 | 0.8 | 0.5 | 0.5 | 0.4 | 0.4 | 0.1 | 0.4 | 0.1 | 6.3 | 0.0 | 0.3 | 0.1 | 0.2 | 1.3 | 0.1 | 0.8 |
| 酒类 Alcohol beverages | 0.1 | 0.0 | 0.0 | 0.0 | 0.0 | 0.0 | 0.0 | 0.0 | 0.0 | 0.0 | 0.0 | 0.0 | 0.3 | 0.0 | 0.0 | 0.1 | 0.1 | 0.4 | 0.0 | 0.0 | 0.1 | 0.0 | 0.0 | 0.0 | 0.1 |

附表 3-46 第六次中国总膳食研究膳食样品中总汞的含量（单位：μg/kg）

Annexed Table 3-46 Levels of total mercury in food samples from the 6<sup>th</sup> China TDS (Unit: μg/kg)

| 膳食类别 Category | 黑龙江 HL | 辽宁 LN | 河北 HE | 北京 BJ | 吉林 JL | 山西 SX | 陕西 SN | 河南 HA | 宁夏 NX | 内蒙古 NM | 青海 QH | 甘肃 GS | 上海 SH | 福建 FJ | 江西 JX | 江苏 JS | 浙江 ZJ | 山东 SD | 湖北 HB | 四川 SC | 广西 GX | 湖南 HN | 广东 GD | 贵州 GZ | 全国平均 AVG |
|---|---|---|---|---|---|---|---|---|---|---|---|---|---|---|---|---|---|---|---|---|---|---|---|---|---|
| 谷类 Cereals | 0.17 | 1.34 | ND | 0.98 | 0.63 | 0.13 | ND | 0.25 | 1.96 | ND | 2.00 | 0.21 | 0.43 | 1.12 | 2.22 | ND | 0.26 | 0.56 | 0.89 | 1.56 | 1.14 | 0.97 | 0.26 | 0.37 | 0.74 |
| 豆类 Legumes | ND | 1.12 | ND | 0.36 | ND | 0.31 | ND | 0.37 | 0.68 | ND | 0.78 | 0.24 | ND | 0.19 | 0.97 | ND | ND | 0.16 | 0.46 | 0.97 | 0.22 | ND | ND | ND | 0.31 |
| 薯类 Potatoes | ND | 0.83 | ND | 0.22 | ND | 0.38 | ND | ND | 0.54 | ND | 0.95 | 0.29 | ND | 0.22 | 0.62 | ND | ND | 0.85 | 0.46 | 0.68 | 0.58 | ND | ND | ND | 0.30 |
| 肉类 Meats | 0.23 | 1.39 | ND | 0.33 | 0.49 | ND | ND | 0.23 | 0.82 | ND | 0.92 | 0.81 | ND | 0.46 | 0.87 | ND | 0.27 | 0.26 | 0.93 | 0.85 | 0.44 | 0.17 | ND | ND | 0.41 |
| 蛋类 Eggs | 0.30 | 0.63 | ND | 0.24 | 0.23 | 1.17 | ND | 0.24 | 0.77 | ND | 1.51 | 0.22 | 0.19 | 0.52 | 2.21 | 0.28 | 1.85 | 0.51 | 0.47 | 0.65 | 0.29 | 1.67 | ND | ND | 0.59 |
| 水产类 Aquatic foods | 31.43 | 23.82 | 13.44 | 42.84 | 10.80 | 21.66 | 3.64 | 10.01 | 3.88 | 7.30 | 29.17 | 15.84 | 15.89 | 28.05 | 3.80 | 10.26 | 4.92 | 19.31 | 22.69 | 4.08 | 6.28 | 7.34 | 36.13 | 6.33 | 15.79 |
| 乳类 Dairy products | ND | ND | ND | 0.14 | ND | ND | ND | ND | ND | ND | 0.20 | ND | ND | ND | ND | ND | ND | ND | 0.14 | ND | ND | ND | ND | ND | 0.06 |
| 蔬菜类 Vegetables | ND | 0.23 | 0.76 | 0.32 | ND | 0.12 | 0.99 | 0.23 | 0.46 | ND | 0.80 | 0.24 | ND | 1.18 | 0.79 | ND | 0.36 | 0.41 | 0.70 | 0.71 | 0.68 | 0.37 | 0.61 | ND | 0.43 |
| 水果类 Fruits | ND | ND | ND | ND | ND | ND | ND | 0.13 | 0.15 | ND | 0.27 | ND | ND | ND | ND | ND | ND | ND | ND | 0.16 | 0.19 | ND | ND | ND | 0.08 |
| 糖类 Sugar | ND | ND | ND | ND | ND | ND | ND | ND | 0.10 | ND | 0.14 | ND | ND | ND | ND | ND | ND | ND | ND | ND | ND | ND | ND | ND | 0.06 |
| 水及饮料类 Water and beverages | ND | ND | ND | ND | ND | ND | ND | ND | ND | ND | ND | ND | ND | ND | ND | ND | ND | ND | ND | ND | ND | ND | ND | ND | 0.05 |

续表

| 膳食类别 Category | 黑龙江 HL | 辽宁 LN | 河北 HE | 北京 BJ | 吉林 JL | 山西 SX | 陕西 SN | 河南 HA | 宁夏 NX | 内蒙古 NM | 青海 QH | 甘肃 GS | 上海 SH | 福建 FJ | 江西 JX | 江苏 JS | 浙江 ZJ | 山东 SD | 湖北 HB | 四川 SC | 广西 GX | 湖南 HN | 广东 GD | 贵州 GZ | 全国平均 AVG |
|---|---|---|---|---|---|---|---|---|---|---|---|---|---|---|---|---|---|---|---|---|---|---|---|---|---|
| 酒类 Alcohol beverages | 0.10 | 0.12 | ND | ND | ND | ND | ND | ND | ND | ND | ND | ND | ND | ND | ND | ND | ND | ND | ND | ND | ND | ND | ND | ND | 0.06 |

注：未检出（ND）按1/2检出限（LOD）计

Note: values not detected (ND) were treated as being equal to half of the detection of limit (LOD)

附表 3-47 第六次中国总膳食研究总汞的膳食摄入量（单位：μg/d）

Annexed Table 3-47 Dietary intake of total mercury from the 6$^{th}$ China TDS (Unit: μg/d)

| 膳食类别 Category | 黑龙江 HL | 辽宁 LN | 河北 HE | 北京 BJ | 吉林 JL | 山西 SX | 陕西 SN | 河南 HA | 宁夏 NX | 内蒙古 NM | 青海 QH | 甘肃 GS | 上海 SH | 福建 FJ | 江西 JX | 江苏 JS | 浙江 ZJ | 山东 SD | 湖北 HB | 四川 SC | 广西 GX | 湖南 HN | 广东 GD | 贵州 GZ | 全国平均 AVG |
|---|---|---|---|---|---|---|---|---|---|---|---|---|---|---|---|---|---|---|---|---|---|---|---|---|---|
| 谷类 Cereals | 0.10 | 0.83 | 0.06 | 0.78 | 0.37 | 0.13 | 0.07 | 0.23 | 1.30 | 0.05 | 1.53 | 0.14 | 0.19 | 0.71 | 1.40 | 0.05 | 0.17 | 0.56 | 0.47 | 1.51 | 1.07 | 0.56 | 0.12 | 0.25 | 0.53 |
| 豆类 Legumes | 0.00 | 0.14 | 0.00 | 0.04 | 0.01 | 0.02 | 0.00 | 0.02 | 0.02 | 0.00 | 0.01 | 0.01 | 0.01 | 0.01 | 0.07 | 0.00 | 0.01 | 0.01 | 0.03 | 0.07 | 0.01 | 0.00 | 0.00 | 0.01 | 0.02 |
| 薯类 Potatoes | 0.00 | 0.06 | 0.00 | 0.01 | 0.01 | 0.04 | 0.01 | 0.00 | 0.05 | 0.01 | 0.10 | 0.04 | 0.00 | 0.01 | 0.02 | 0.00 | 0.00 | 0.04 | 0.04 | 0.04 | 0.01 | 0.00 | 0.00 | 0.00 | 0.02 |
| 肉类 Meats | 0.01 | 0.09 | 0.00 | 0.02 | 0.03 | 0.01 | 0.00 | 0.01 | 0.04 | 0.00 | 0.07 | 0.02 | 0.01 | 0.04 | 0.08 | 0.00 | 0.03 | 0.02 | 0.05 | 0.11 | 0.07 | 0.03 | 0.01 | 0.01 | 0.03 |
| 蛋类 Eggs | 0.01 | 0.03 | 0.00 | 0.01 | 0.01 | 0.02 | 0.00 | 0.01 | 0.00 | 0.00 | 0.02 | 0.00 | 0.01 | 0.01 | 0.05 | 0.01 | 0.04 | 0.02 | 0.01 | 0.01 | 0.00 | 0.04 | 0.00 | 0.00 | 0.01 |
| 水产类 Aquatic foods | 0.85 | 0.38 | 0.13 | 0.70 | 0.12 | 0.14 | 0.01 | 0.05 | 0.01 | 0.08 | 0.10 | 0.04 | 1.09 | 1.80 | 0.17 | 0.40 | 0.25 | 0.44 | 0.92 | 0.03 | 0.61 | 0.49 | 1.85 | 0.02 | 0.45 |
| 乳类 Dairy products | 0.00 | 0.00 | 0.00 | 0.01 | 0.00 | 0.00 | 0.00 | 0.00 | 0.00 | 0.00 | 0.01 | 0.00 | 0.00 | 0.00 | 0.00 | 0.00 | 0.00 | 0.00 | 0.00 | 0.00 | 0.00 | 0.00 | 0.00 | 0.00 | 0.00 |

续表

| 膳食类别<br>Category | 黑龙江<br>HL | 辽宁<br>LN | 河北<br>HE | 北京<br>BJ | 吉林<br>JL | 山西<br>SX | 陕西<br>SN | 河南<br>HA | 宁夏<br>NX | 内蒙古<br>NM | 青海<br>QH | 甘肃<br>GS | 上海<br>SH | 福建<br>FJ | 江西<br>JX | 江苏<br>JS | 浙江<br>ZJ | 山东<br>SD | 湖北<br>HB | 四川<br>SC | 广西<br>GX | 湖南<br>HN | 广东<br>GD | 贵州<br>GZ | 全国平均<br>AVG |
|---|---|---|---|---|---|---|---|---|---|---|---|---|---|---|---|---|---|---|---|---|---|---|---|---|---|
| 蔬菜类 Vegetables | 0.02 | 0.08 | 0.22 | 0.12 | 0.02 | 0.04 | 0.28 | 0.06 | 0.07 | 0.01 | 0.25 | 0.06 | 0.02 | 0.47 | 0.36 | 0.02 | 0.16 | 0.16 | 0.29 | 0.21 | 0.24 | 0.20 | 0.14 | 0.02 | 0.15 |
| 水果类 Fruits | 0.00 | 0.00 | 0.00 | 0.01 | 0.00 | 0.00 | 0.00 | 0.00 | 0.01 | 0.01 | 0.00 | 0.00 | 0.00 | 0.00 | 0.00 | 0.00 | 0.00 | 0.00 | 0.00 | 0.00 | 0.01 | 0.00 | 0.00 | 0.00 | 0.00 |
| 糖类 Sugar | 0.00 | 0.00 | 0.00 | 0.00 | 0.00 | 0.00 | 0.00 | 0.00 | 0.00 | 0.00 | 0.00 | 0.00 | 0.00 | 0.00 | 0.00 | 0.00 | 0.00 | 0.00 | 0.00 | 0.00 | 0.00 | 0.00 | 0.00 | 0.00 | 0.00 |
| 水及饮料类 Water and beverages | 0.06 | 0.02 | 0.04 | 0.06 | 0.07 | 0.04 | 0.02 | 0.06 | 0.03 | 0.13 | 0.03 | 0.06 | 0.04 | 0.04 | 0.06 | 0.05 | 0.04 | 0.09 | 0.01 | 0.02 | 0.07 | 0.05 | 0.06 | 0.06 | 0.05 |
| 酒类 Alcohol beverages | 0.00 | 0.00 | 0.00 | 0.00 | 0.00 | 0.00 | 0.00 | 0.00 | 0.00 | 0.00 | 0.00 | 0.00 | 0.00 | 0.00 | 0.00 | 0.00 | 0.00 | 0.01 | 0.00 | 0.00 | 0.00 | 0.00 | 0.00 | 0.00 | 0.00 |
| 合计 SUM | 1.07 | 1.63 | 0.47 | 1.77 | 0.63 | 0.45 | 0.41 | 0.45 | 1.54 | 0.29 | 2.12 | 0.39 | 1.37 | 3.10 | 2.20 | 0.55 | 0.71 | 1.36 | 1.83 | 2.01 | 2.08 | 1.37 | 2.19 | 0.37 | 1.26 |

附表 3-48　第六次中国总膳食研究总汞的膳食来源（单位：%）

Annexed Table 3-48　Dietary sources of total mercury from the 6ᵗʰ China TDS (Unit: %)

| 膳食类别<br>Category | 黑龙江<br>HL | 辽宁<br>LN | 河北<br>HE | 北京<br>BJ | 吉林<br>JL | 山西<br>SX | 陕西<br>SN | 河南<br>HA | 宁夏<br>NX | 内蒙古<br>NM | 青海<br>QH | 甘肃<br>GS | 上海<br>SH | 福建<br>FJ | 江西<br>JX | 江苏<br>JS | 浙江<br>ZJ | 山东<br>SD | 湖北<br>HB | 四川<br>SC | 广西<br>GX | 湖南<br>HN | 广东<br>GD | 贵州<br>GZ | 全国平均<br>AVG |
|---|---|---|---|---|---|---|---|---|---|---|---|---|---|---|---|---|---|---|---|---|---|---|---|---|---|
| 谷类 Cereals | 8.9 | 50.6 | 13.4 | 44.3 | 58.4 | 30.0 | 18.1 | 51.8 | 84.0 | 18.1 | 72.3 | 36.2 | 14.2 | 22.8 | 63.4 | 8.9 | 23.6 | 41.0 | 25.7 | 75.3 | 51.3 | 40.6 | 5.5 | 66.8 | 41.7 |
| 豆类 Legumes | 0.3 | 8.3 | 0.7 | 2.1 | 0.8 | 4.7 | 1.1 | 4.4 | 1.6 | 0.7 | 0.2 | 2.5 | 0.5 | 0.5 | 3.3 | 0.9 | 1.1 | 0.6 | 1.7 | 3.3 | 0.5 | 0.3 | 0.1 | 1.6 | 1.7 |

续表

| 膳食类别 Category | 黑龙江 HL | 辽宁 LN | 河北 HE | 北京 BJ | 吉林 JL | 山西 SX | 陕西 SN | 河南 HA | 宁夏 NX | 内蒙古 NM | 青海 QH | 甘肃 GS | 上海 SH | 福建 FJ | 江西 JX | 江苏 JS | 浙江 ZJ | 山东 SD | 湖北 HB | 四川 SC | 广西 GX | 湖南 HN | 广东 GD | 贵州 GZ | 全国平均 AVG |
|---|---|---|---|---|---|---|---|---|---|---|---|---|---|---|---|---|---|---|---|---|---|---|---|---|---|
| 薯类 Potatoes | 0.4 | 3.6 | 0.8 | 0.7 | 0.9 | 10.0 | 1.7 | 1.0 | 3.5 | 2.1 | 4.6 | 10.9 | 0.1 | 0.3 | 0.9 | 0.4 | 0.3 | 2.9 | 2.2 | 2.1 | 0.4 | 0.3 | 0.1 | 0.6 | 1.7 |
| 肉类 Meats | 1.3 | 5.7 | 0.6 | 1.2 | 5.1 | 1.6 | 0.5 | 2.9 | 2.5 | 1.3 | 3.1 | 6.4 | 0.4 | 1.3 | 3.7 | 0.8 | 4.5 | 1.8 | 2.7 | 5.5 | 3.2 | 1.8 | 0.3 | 1.5 | 2.5 |
| 蛋类 Eggs | 1.1 | 1.6 | 0.4 | 0.5 | 1.5 | 5.5 | 0.3 | 1.6 | 0.6 | 0.7 | 0.9 | 1.2 | 0.5 | 0.3 | 2.1 | 1.4 | 6.3 | 1.7 | 0.6 | 0.5 | 0.2 | 2.8 | 0.1 | 0.2 | 1.1 |
| 水产类 Aquatic foods | 79.7 | 23.4 | 27.3 | 39.9 | 18.9 | 30.9 | 3.6 | 10.3 | 0.6 | 25.7 | 4.9 | 11.5 | 79.6 | 58.1 | 7.5 | 73.4 | 35.0 | 32.4 | 50.4 | 1.7 | 29.2 | 35.5 | 84.5 | 6.0 | 35.2 |
| 乳类 Dairy products | 0.1 | 0.1 | 0.3 | 0.7 | 0.3 | 0.5 | 0.2 | 0.2 | 0.0 | 0.6 | 0.5 | 0.2 | 0.3 | 0.1 | 0.0 | 0.3 | 0.2 | 0.1 | 0.1 | 0.0 | 0.0 | 0.1 | 0.1 | 0.4 | 0.2 |
| 蔬菜类 Vegetables | 1.8 | 4.6 | 47.7 | 7.0 | 3.1 | 8.0 | 69.2 | 14.0 | 4.7 | 4.5 | 11.8 | 15.5 | 1.5 | 15.2 | 16.2 | 4.1 | 22.6 | 12.2 | 15.7 | 10.6 | 11.5 | 14.5 | 6.6 | 5.7 | 11.7 |
| 水果类 Fruits | 0.3 | 0.3 | 0.4 | 0.3 | 0.7 | 0.4 | 0.5 | 0.7 | 0.8 | 1.9 | 0.2 | 0.4 | 0.3 | 0.1 | 0.1 | 0.2 | 0.5 | 0.2 | 0.1 | 0.1 | 0.6 | 0.2 | 0.1 | 0.3 | 0.3 |
| 糖类 Sugar | 0.0 | 0.0 | 0.0 | 0.0 | 0.0 | 0.0 | 0.5 | 0.0 | 0.0 | 0.0 | 0.0 | 0.0 | 0.0 | 0.0 | 0.0 | 0.0 | 0.0 | 0.0 | 0.0 | 0.0 | 0.0 | 0.0 | 0.0 | 0.0 | 0.0 |
| 水及饮料类 Water and beverages | 5.7 | 1.5 | 8.3 | 3.1 | 10.3 | 8.3 | 4.2 | 13.2 | 1.7 | 43.9 | 1.5 | 15.2 | 2.6 | 1.4 | 2.7 | 9.3 | 5.6 | 6.6 | 0.8 | 0.8 | 3.1 | 3.9 | 2.7 | 16.9 | 3.9 |
| 酒类 Alcohol beverages | 0.2 | 0.2 | 0.1 | 0.1 | 0.1 | 0.0 | 0.0 | 0.0 | 0.0 | 0.4 | 0.0 | 0.0 | 0.1 | 0.0 | 0.0 | 0.3 | 0.4 | 0.4 | 0.0 | 0.0 | 0.1 | 0.1 | 0.0 | 0.0 | 0.1 |

附表 3-49　第六次中国总膳食研究膳食样品中甲基汞的含量（单位：μg/kg）

Annexed Table 3-49　Levels of methylmercury in food samples from the 6$^{th}$ China TDS (Unit: μg/kg)

| 膳食类别 Category | 黑龙江 HL | 辽宁 LN | 河北 HE | 北京 BJ | 吉林 JL | 山西 SX | 陕西 SN | 河南 HA | 宁夏 NX | 内蒙古 NM | 青海 QH | 甘肃 GS | 上海 SH | 福建 FJ | 江西 JX | 江苏 JS | 浙江 ZJ | 山东 SD | 湖北 HB | 四川 SC | 广西 GX | 湖南 HN | 广东 GD | 贵州 GZ | 全国平均 AVG |
|---|---|---|---|---|---|---|---|---|---|---|---|---|---|---|---|---|---|---|---|---|---|---|---|---|---|
| 水产类 Aquatic foods | 23.43 | 16.18 | 12.13 | 24.57 | 6.16 | 16.71 | 3.20 | 9.69 | ND | 7.10 | 21.57 | 8.60 | 10.60 | 17.29 | ND | 9.71 | 3.30 | 18.35 | 15.46 | ND | 3.84 | 7.10 | 29.48 | 5.61 | 11.44 |

注：未检出（ND）按 1/2 检出限（LOD）计

Note: values not detected (ND) were treated as being equal to half of the detection of limit (LOD)

附表 3-50　第六次中国总膳食研究甲基汞的膳食摄入量（单位：μg/d）

Annexed Table 3-50　Dietary intake of methylmercury from the 6$^{th}$ China TDS (Unit: μg/d)

| 膳食类别 Category | 黑龙江 HL | 辽宁 LN | 河北 HE | 北京 BJ | 吉林 JL | 山西 SX | 陕西 SN | 河南 HA | 宁夏 NX | 内蒙古 NM | 青海 QH | 甘肃 GS | 上海 SH | 福建 FJ | 江西 JX | 江苏 JS | 浙江 ZJ | 山东 SD | 湖北 HB | 四川 SC | 广西 GX | 湖南 HN | 广东 GD | 贵州 GZ | 全国平均 AVG |
|---|---|---|---|---|---|---|---|---|---|---|---|---|---|---|---|---|---|---|---|---|---|---|---|---|---|
| 水产类 Aquatic foods | 0.64 | 0.26 | 0.12 | 0.40 | 0.07 | 0.11 | 0.01 | 0.04 | 0.00 | 0.07 | 0.08 | 0.02 | 0.73 | 1.11 | 0.07 | 0.38 | 0.17 | 0.42 | 0.63 | 0.01 | 0.37 | 0.47 | 1.51 | 0.02 | 0.32 |

附表 3-51　第六次中国总膳食研究膳食样品中总砷的含量（单位：μg/kg）

Annexed Table 3-51　Levels of total arsenic in food samples from the 6$^{th}$ China TDS (Unit: μg/kg)

| 膳食类别 Category | 黑龙江 HL | 辽宁 LN | 河北 HE | 北京 BJ | 吉林 JL | 山西 SX | 陕西 SN | 河南 HA | 宁夏 NX | 内蒙古 NM | 青海 QH | 甘肃 GS | 上海 SH | 福建 FJ | 江西 JX | 江苏 JS | 浙江 ZJ | 山东 SD | 湖北 HB | 四川 SC | 广西 GX | 湖南 HN | 广东 GD | 贵州 GZ | 全国平均 AVG |
|---|---|---|---|---|---|---|---|---|---|---|---|---|---|---|---|---|---|---|---|---|---|---|---|---|---|
| 谷类 Cereals | 15.53 | 12.21 | 12.96 | 10.56 | 18.39 | 5.78 | 10.22 | 12.04 | 10.67 | 6.66 | 9.62 | 11.51 | 22.58 | 21.24 | 30.68 | 20.60 | 28.34 | 6.40 | 20.76 | 8.88 | 32.36 | 31.66 | 24.63 | 22.30 | 16.94 |
| 豆类 Legumes | 3.24 | 4.04 | 4.72 | 3.18 | 2.83 | 1.14 | 6.90 | 6.98 | 6.66 | 3.23 | 1.74 | 7.17 | 4.07 | 1.71 | 8.88 | 5.01 | 1.57 | 3.40 | 4.65 | 4.85 | 3.25 | 0.16 | 5.98 | 7.87 | 4.30 |

续表

| 膳食类别<br>Category | 黑龙江<br>HL | 辽宁<br>LN | 河北<br>HE | 北京<br>BJ | 吉林<br>JL | 山西<br>SX | 陕西<br>SN | 河南<br>HA | 宁夏<br>NX | 内蒙古<br>NM | 青海<br>QH | 甘肃<br>GS | 上海<br>SH | 福建<br>FJ | 江西<br>JX | 江苏<br>JS | 浙江<br>ZJ | 山东<br>SD | 湖北<br>HB | 四川<br>SC | 广西<br>GX | 湖南<br>HN | 广东<br>GD | 贵州<br>GZ | 全国平均<br>AVG |
|---|---|---|---|---|---|---|---|---|---|---|---|---|---|---|---|---|---|---|---|---|---|---|---|---|---|
| 薯类 Potatoes | ND | 1.74 | 3.01 | 7.79 | ND | 2.61 | 4.00 | 3.55 | 4.15 | 1.90 | 0.38 | 6.65 | 4.70 | 1.85 | 5.07 | 3.67 | 1.81 | 3.63 | 1.23 | ND | 6.01 | 1.88 | 4.30 | 1.33 | 2.99 |
| 肉类 Meats | 2.25 | 6.78 | 2.93 | 3.15 | 12.42 | 3.11 | 5.86 | 6.85 | 13.75 | 7.91 | 3.87 | 12.17 | 10.57 | 5.16 | 12.96 | 12.34 | 11.03 | 0.83 | 3.20 | 3.35 | 3.27 | 6.18 | 5.29 | 11.26 | 6.94 |
| 蛋类 Eggs | 0.40 | 2.32 | 2.95 | 1.47 | 5.73 | ND | 1.57 | 2.27 | 6.78 | 1.38 | 1.36 | 5.13 | 4.26 | 3.41 | 9.32 | 14.43 | 7.64 | ND | 1.02 | 0.44 | 3.50 | 2.93 | 5.20 | 2.46 | 3.60 |
| 水产类 Aquatic foods | 188.3 | 749.6 | 239.5 | 1595.2 | 795.2 | 569.3 | 223.8 | 256.5 | 27.4 | 147.0 | 650.8 | 252.3 | 438.5 | 643.3 | 12.9 | 112.0 | 374.5 | 398.9 | 81.5 | 26.0 | 111.3 | 113.7 | 1533.0 | 150.1 | 403.8 |
| 乳类 Dairy products | ND | 0.85 | 0.27 | 0.33 | 0.77 | ND | ND | 0.36 | 2.09 | 0.37 | 0.48 | 0.95 | 0.74 | 0.62 | 2.11 | 0.31 | 0.80 | ND | 1.17 | 0.27 | 0.85 | 0.51 | 0.35 | ND | 0.62 |
| 蔬菜类 Vegetables | 18.49 | 27.72 | 17.77 | 39.35 | 45.77 | 13.49 | 30.82 | 42.84 | 39.44 | 35.94 | 4.89 | 30.19 | 35.72 | 202.97 | 29.96 | 55.63 | 48.55 | 30.97 | 163.11 | 24.14 | 25.24 | 40.01 | 46.10 | 33.01 | 45.09 |
| 水果类 Fruits | ND | 0.83 | 3.32 | 5.46 | 0.72 | 1.90 | 1.55 | 8.85 | 3.68 | 5.78 | 2.23 | 0.68 | 9.90 | 1.64 | 2.26 | 0.31 | 1.37 | ND | 0.32 | 1.14 | 1.78 | 3.23 | 3.06 | 1.09 | 2.56 |
| 糖类 Sugar | ND | 5.85 | 0.52 | 18.50 | 0.80 | ND | 2.00 | 17.68 | 2.30 | 20.65 | ND | 2.54 | 9.59 | 15.52 | 3.72 | 1.15 | 6.93 | 6.02 | 1.38 | 0.97 | 2.22 | 2.70 | 4.35 | 0.66 | 5.27 |
| 水及饮料类 Water and beverages | 0.55 | 0.83 | 1.20 | 1.30 | ND | 0.98 | ND | 0.91 | 0.67 | 0.91 | 1.15 | 1.28 | 0.80 | 1.20 | 0.83 | 1.60 | 0.63 | 0.47 | 0.96 | ND | ND | 1.37 | 1.23 | ND | 0.81 |
| 酒类 Alcohol beverages | 0.70 | 1.39 | 1.55 | 3.49 | 1.61 | 0.61 | 2.26 | 1.99 | 0.50 | 1.24 | 1.41 | 2.62 | 4.48 | 1.56 | 1.52 | 1.50 | 1.95 | 1.12 | 0.83 | 1.88 | 6.51 | 1.48 | 0.98 | 1.55 | 1.86 |

注：未检出（ND）按 1/2 检出限（LOD）计
Note: values not detected (ND) were treated as being equal to half of the detection of limit (LOD)

附表 3-52　第六次中国总膳食研究总砷的膳食摄入量（单位：μg/d）

Annexed Table 3-52　Dietary intake of total arsenic from the 6th China TDS (Unit: μg/d)

| 膳食类别<br>Category | 黑龙江<br>HL | 辽宁<br>LN | 河北<br>HE | 北京<br>BJ | 吉林<br>JL | 山西<br>SX | 陕西<br>SN | 河南<br>HA | 宁夏<br>NX | 内蒙古<br>NM | 青海<br>QH | 甘肃<br>GS | 上海<br>SH | 福建<br>FJ | 江西<br>JX | 江苏<br>JS | 浙江<br>ZJ | 山东<br>SD | 湖北<br>HB | 四川<br>SC | 广西<br>GX | 湖南<br>HN | 广东<br>GD | 贵州<br>GZ | 全国平均<br>AVG |
|---|---|---|---|---|---|---|---|---|---|---|---|---|---|---|---|---|---|---|---|---|---|---|---|---|---|
| 谷类 Cereals | 8.51 | 7.52 | 9.79 | 8.40 | 10.77 | 6.00 | 7.80 | 11.13 | 7.06 | 4.81 | 7.37 | 7.90 | 10.14 | 13.43 | 19.33 | 16.03 | 17.93 | 6.38 | 10.97 | 8.61 | 30.44 | 18.28 | 11.25 | 15.05 | 11.45 |
| 豆类 Legumes | 0.15 | 0.49 | 0.27 | 0.32 | 0.21 | 0.08 | 0.57 | 0.38 | 0.23 | 0.13 | 0.01 | 0.30 | 0.48 | 0.13 | 0.65 | 0.42 | 0.22 | 0.18 | 0.31 | 0.33 | 0.14 | 0.01 | 0.17 | 0.80 | 0.29 |
| 薯类 Potatoes | 0.01 | 0.13 | 0.18 | 0.46 | 0.02 | 0.31 | 0.46 | 0.29 | 0.41 | 0.23 | 0.04 | 0.96 | 0.17 | 0.08 | 0.16 | 0.12 | 0.07 | 0.17 | 0.11 | 0.01 | 0.08 | 0.10 | 0.11 | 0.05 | 0.20 |
| 肉类 Meats | 0.13 | 0.45 | 0.14 | 0.21 | 0.83 | 0.43 | 0.21 | 0.38 | 0.64 | 0.58 | 0.28 | 0.38 | 1.17 | 0.44 | 1.22 | 1.13 | 1.30 | 0.08 | 0.17 | 0.43 | 0.49 | 0.92 | 0.55 | 1.20 | 0.57 |
| 蛋类 Eggs | 0.02 | 0.09 | 0.09 | 0.06 | 0.23 | 0.00 | 0.03 | 0.07 | 0.09 | 0.04 | 0.02 | 0.11 | 0.17 | 0.06 | 0.19 | 0.41 | 0.18 | 0.01 | 0.03 | 0.01 | 0.05 | 0.07 | 0.12 | 0.04 | 0.09 |
| 水产类 Aquatic foods | 5.11 | 12.04 | 2.28 | 26.19 | 8.86 | 3.65 | 0.92 | 1.19 | 0.07 | 1.52 | 2.32 | 0.71 | 30.08 | 41.29 | 0.56 | 4.37 | 18.85 | 9.09 | 3.32 | 0.22 | 10.76 | 7.55 | 78.49 | 0.52 | 11.25 |
| 乳类 Dairy products | 0.00 | 0.04 | 0.01 | 0.03 | 0.02 | 0.01 | 0.00 | 0.01 | 0.03 | 0.01 | 0.03 | 0.01 | 0.05 | 0.02 | 0.05 | 0.01 | 0.03 | 0.00 | 0.01 | 0.00 | 0.02 | 0.01 | 0.01 | 0.00 | 0.02 |
| 蔬菜类 Vegetables | 5.93 | 9.05 | 5.22 | 15.42 | 17.76 | 4.18 | 8.85 | 11.91 | 6.16 | 9.24 | 1.52 | 7.49 | 14.31 | 80.56 | 13.53 | 23.66 | 21.56 | 12.58 | 67.54 | 7.31 | 8.92 | 21.36 | 10.90 | 13.47 | 16.60 |
| 水果类 Fruits | 0.01 | 0.06 | 0.12 | 0.62 | 0.06 | 0.07 | 0.06 | 0.21 | 0.31 | 0.65 | 0.03 | 0.02 | 0.73 | 0.10 | 0.13 | 0.01 | 0.09 | 0.01 | 0.01 | 0.02 | 0.11 | 0.20 | 0.09 | 0.02 | 0.16 |
| 糖类 Sugar | 0.00 | 0.00 | 0.00 | 0.04 | 0.00 | 0.00 | 0.04 | 0.01 | 0.00 | 0.02 | 0.00 | 0.00 | 0.07 | 0.00 | 0.00 | 0.00 | 0.01 | 0.00 | 0.00 | 0.00 | 0.00 | 0.00 | 0.00 | 0.00 | 0.01 |
| 水及饮料类 Water and beverages | 0.68 | 0.41 | 0.93 | 1.44 | 0.16 | 0.73 | 0.04 | 1.08 | 0.35 | 2.35 | 0.71 | 1.51 | 0.56 | 1.04 | 0.98 | 1.62 | 0.50 | 0.84 | 0.27 | 0.04 | 0.16 | 1.46 | 1.47 | 0.16 | 0.81 |

| 膳食类别<br>Category | 黑龙江<br>HL | 辽宁<br>LN | 河北<br>HE | 北京<br>BJ | 吉林<br>JL | 山西<br>SX | 陕西<br>SN | 河南<br>HA | 宁夏<br>NX | 内蒙古<br>NM | 青海<br>QH | 甘肃<br>GS | 上海<br>SH | 福建<br>FJ | 江西<br>JX | 江苏<br>JS | 浙江<br>ZJ | 山东<br>SD | 湖北<br>HB | 四川<br>SC | 广西<br>GX | 湖南<br>HN | 广东<br>GD | 贵州<br>GZ | 全国平均<br>AVG |
|---|---|---|---|---|---|---|---|---|---|---|---|---|---|---|---|---|---|---|---|---|---|---|---|---|---|
| 酒类<br>Alcohol beverages | 0.02 | 0.05 | 0.02 | 0.10 | 0.02 | 0.00 | 0.00 | 0.01 | 0.00 | 0.03 | 0.01 | 0.01 | 0.10 | 0.02 | 0.03 | 0.06 | 0.12 | 0.13 | 0.01 | 0.01 | 0.21 | 0.02 | 0.00 | 0.00 | 0.04 |
| 合计<br>SUM | 20.56 | 30.34 | 19.05 | 53.28 | 38.94 | 15.44 | 19.02 | 26.65 | 15.36 | 19.62 | 12.33 | 19.40 | 58.03 | 137.19 | 36.84 | 47.83 | 60.86 | 29.46 | 82.75 | 16.98 | 51.38 | 49.99 | 103.16 | 31.31 | 41.49 |

注: 未检出 (ND) 按 1/2 检出限 (LOD) 计

Note: values not detected (ND) were treated as being equal to half of the detection of limit (LOD)

附表 3-53　第六次中国总膳食研究总砷的膳食来源（单位: %）

Annexed Table 3-53　Dietary sources of total arsenic form the 6th China TDS (Unit: %)

| 膳食类别<br>Category | 黑龙江<br>HL | 辽宁<br>LN | 河北<br>HE | 北京<br>BJ | 吉林<br>JL | 山西<br>SX | 陕西<br>SN | 河南<br>HA | 宁夏<br>NX | 内蒙古<br>NM | 青海<br>QH | 甘肃<br>GS | 上海<br>SH | 福建<br>FJ | 江西<br>JX | 江苏<br>JS | 浙江<br>ZJ | 山东<br>SD | 湖北<br>HB | 四川<br>SC | 广西<br>GX | 湖南<br>HN | 广东<br>GD | 贵州<br>GZ | 全国平均<br>AVG |
|---|---|---|---|---|---|---|---|---|---|---|---|---|---|---|---|---|---|---|---|---|---|---|---|---|---|
| 谷类<br>Cereals | 41.4 | 24.8 | 51.4 | 15.8 | 27.6 | 38.8 | 41.0 | 41.8 | 46.0 | 24.5 | 59.8 | 40.7 | 17.5 | 9.8 | 52.5 | 33.5 | 29.5 | 21.6 | 13.3 | 50.7 | 59.2 | 36.6 | 10.9 | 48.1 | 27.6 |
| 豆类<br>Legumes | 0.7 | 1.6 | 1.4 | 0.6 | 0.5 | 0.5 | 3.0 | 1.4 | 1.5 | 0.7 | 0.1 | 1.5 | 0.8 | 0.1 | 1.8 | 0.9 | 0.4 | 0.6 | 0.4 | 1.9 | 0.3 | 0.0 | 0.2 | 2.6 | 0.7 |
| 薯类<br>Potatoes | 0.1 | 0.4 | 1.0 | 0.9 | 0.0 | 2.0 | 2.4 | 1.1 | 2.7 | 1.2 | 0.3 | 4.9 | 0.3 | 0.1 | 0.4 | 0.3 | 0.1 | 0.6 | 0.1 | 0.0 | 0.2 | 0.2 | 0.1 | 0.1 | 0.5 |
| 肉类<br>Meats | 0.7 | 1.5 | 0.7 | 0.4 | 2.1 | 2.8 | 1.1 | 1.4 | 4.2 | 3.0 | 2.2 | 1.9 | 2.0 | 0.3 | 3.3 | 2.4 | 2.1 | 0.3 | 0.2 | 2.5 | 1.0 | 1.8 | 0.5 | 3.8 | 1.4 |
| 蛋类<br>Eggs | 0.1 | 0.3 | 0.5 | 0.1 | 0.6 | 0.0 | 0.2 | 0.3 | 0.6 | 0.2 | 0.1 | 0.6 | 0.3 | 0.0 | 0.5 | 0.8 | 0.3 | 0.0 | 0.0 | 0.0 | 0.1 | 0.1 | 0.1 | 0.1 | 0.2 |
| 水产类<br>Aquatic foods | 24.9 | 39.7 | 12.0 | 49.2 | 22.8 | 23.6 | 4.8 | 4.5 | 0.4 | 7.7 | 18.8 | 3.7 | 51.8 | 30.1 | 1.5 | 9.1 | 31.0 | 30.8 | 4.0 | 1.3 | 20.9 | 15.1 | 76.1 | 1.7 | 27.1 |

续表

| 膳食类别 Category | 黑龙江 HL | 辽宁 LN | 河北 HE | 北京 BJ | 吉林 JL | 山西 SX | 陕西 SN | 河南 HA | 宁夏 NX | 内蒙古 NM | 青海 QH | 甘肃 GS | 上海 SH | 福建 FJ | 江西 JX | 江苏 JS | 浙江 ZJ | 山东 SD | 湖北 HB | 四川 SC | 广西 GX | 湖南 HN | 广东 GD | 贵州 GZ | 全国平均 AVG |
|---|---|---|---|---|---|---|---|---|---|---|---|---|---|---|---|---|---|---|---|---|---|---|---|---|---|
| 乳类 Dairy products | 0.0 | 0.1 | 0.0 | 0.1 | 0.1 | 0.0 | 0.0 | 0.0 | 0.2 | 0.1 | 0.2 | 0.1 | 0.1 | 0.0 | 0.1 | 0.0 | 0.0 | 0.0 | 0.0 | 0.0 | 0.0 | 0.0 | 0.0 | 0.0 | 0.0 |
| 蔬菜类 Vegetables | 28.8 | 29.8 | 27.4 | 28.9 | 45.6 | 27.1 | 46.7 | 44.7 | 40.1 | 47.1 | 12.3 | 38.6 | 24.7 | 58.7 | 36.7 | 49.5 | 35.4 | 42.7 | 81.6 | 43.0 | 17.4 | 42.7 | 10.6 | 43.0 | 40.0 |
| 水果类 Fruits | 0.0 | 0.2 | 0.7 | 1.2 | 0.2 | 0.4 | 0.3 | 0.8 | 2.0 | 3.3 | 0.3 | 0.1 | 1.3 | 0.1 | 0.3 | 0.0 | 0.2 | 0.0 | 0.0 | 0.1 | 0.2 | 0.4 | 0.1 | 0.1 | 0.4 |
| 糖类 Sugar | 0.0 | 0.0 | 0.0 | 0.1 | 0.0 | 0.0 | 0.0 | 0.0 | 0.0 | 0.1 | 0.0 | 0.0 | 0.0 | 0.0 | 0.0 | 0.0 | 0.0 | 0.0 | 0.0 | 0.0 | 0.0 | 0.0 | 0.0 | 0.0 | 0.0 |
| 水及饮料类 Water and beverages | 3.3 | 1.4 | 4.9 | 2.7 | 0.4 | 4.7 | 0.2 | 4.1 | 2.2 | 12.0 | 5.8 | 7.8 | 1.0 | 0.8 | 2.7 | 3.4 | 0.8 | 2.8 | 0.3 | 0.2 | 0.3 | 2.9 | 1.4 | 0.5 | 2.0 |
| 酒类 Alcohol beverages | 0.1 | 0.2 | 0.1 | 0.2 | 0.0 | 0.0 | 0.0 | 0.0 | 0.0 | 0.1 | 0.1 | 0.0 | 0.2 | 0.0 | 0.1 | 0.1 | 0.2 | 0.4 | 0.0 | 0.1 | 0.4 | 0.0 | 0.0 | 0.0 | 0.1 |

附表 3-54 第六次中国总膳食研究膳食样品中无机砷的含量（单位：μg/kg）

Annexed Table 3-54 Levels of inorganic arsenic in food samples from the 6$^{th}$ China TDS (Unit: μg/kg)

| 膳食类别 Category | 黑龙江 HL | 辽宁 LN | 河北 HE | 北京 BJ | 吉林 JL | 山西 SX | 陕西 SN | 河南 HA | 宁夏 NX | 内蒙古 NM | 青海 QH | 甘肃 GS | 上海 SH | 福建 FJ | 江西 JX | 江苏 JS | 浙江 ZJ | 山东 SD | 湖北 HB | 四川 SC | 广西 GX | 湖南 HN | 广东 GD | 贵州 GZ | 全国平均 AVG |
|---|---|---|---|---|---|---|---|---|---|---|---|---|---|---|---|---|---|---|---|---|---|---|---|---|---|
| 谷类 Cereals | 9.64 | 9.57 | 6.87 | 8.93 | 10.68 | 3.40 | 7.05 | 7.59 | 8.68 | 4.91 | 5.27 | 8.83 | 5.12 | 11.72 | 20.00 | 6.26 | 19.63 | 5.48 | 15.25 | 7.81 | 25.24 | 25.41 | 12.92 | 17.53 | 10.99 |
| 豆类 Legumes | 2.28 | 2.93 | 2.02 | ND | ND | ND | 3.89 | 2.29 | ND | 1.24 | ND | 3.86 | ND | ND | ND | 3.59 | ND | ND | 1.71 | 2.36 | ND | ND | ND | 6.39 | 1.65 |
| 薯类 Potatoes | ND | 1.49 | ND | 1.57 | ND | 1.31 | ND | 2.21 | ND | ND | ND | 2.28 | 1.03 | ND | ND | 1.41 | ND | 2.57 | ND | ND | ND | 1.48 | ND | 1.28 | 0.96 |

续表

| 膳食类别 Category | 黑龙江 HL | 辽宁 LN | 河北 HE | 北京 BJ | 吉林 JL | 山西 SX | 陕西 SN | 河南 HA | 宁夏 NX | 内蒙古 NM | 青海 QH | 甘肃 GS | 上海 SH | 福建 FJ | 江西 JX | 江苏 JS | 浙江 ZJ | 山东 SD | 湖北 HB | 四川 SC | 广西 GX | 湖南 HN | 广东 GD | 贵州 GZ | 全国平均 AVG |
|---|---|---|---|---|---|---|---|---|---|---|---|---|---|---|---|---|---|---|---|---|---|---|---|---|---|
| 肉类 Meats | ND | ND | ND | 2.05 | ND | ND | ND | ND | ND | ND | ND | 2.49 | ND | 4.27 | 2.03 | 1.48 | 1.65 | ND | ND | ND | 1.02 | ND | ND | 1.58 | 1.05 |
| 蛋类 Eggs | ND | 1.63 | ND | ND | ND | ND | ND | 1.10 | ND | ND | ND | ND | ND | 1.53 | ND | 1.53 | 1.23 | ND | ND | 0.44 | ND | ND | ND | 1.10 | 0.73 |
| 水产类 Aquatic foods | 1.25 | 2.15 | 1.26 | 10.86 | 2.37 | 1.32 | 2.64 | ND | 2.90 | ND | 1.84 | ND | 2.38 | 10.72 | 1.06 | 1.20 | 3.79 | 6.42 | 2.76 | ND | 2.36 | 3.99 | 4.91 | 4.61 | 3.03 |
| 乳类 Dairy products | ND | ND | ND | ND | ND | ND | ND | ND | ND | ND | ND | ND | ND | ND | ND | ND | ND | ND | ND | ND | ND | ND | ND | ND | 0.37 |
| 蔬菜类 Vegetables | 2.34 | 5.43 | 3.13 | 6.34 | 2.38 | 1.36 | 3.97 | 1.46 | 2.56 | 5.09 | 1.86 | 4.39 | 4.06 | 9.52 | 1.63 | 2.70 | 1.87 | 3.58 | 3.14 | 3.93 | 5.61 | 3.58 | 4.46 | 4.86 | 3.72 |
| 水果类 Fruits | ND | ND | ND | 3.45 | ND | 1.22 | ND | ND | ND | 1.04 | ND | ND | 3.95 | 1.01 | 1.73 | ND | ND | ND | 1.22 | ND | ND | ND | ND | ND | 0.84 |
| 糖类 Sugar | ND | 3.80 | ND | 11.40 | ND | ND | 1.68 | 15.53 | ND | 1.26 | ND | 1.99 | 7.87 | 7.34 | 2.23 | 1.06 | ND | 2.87 | ND | ND | 1.56 | 1.75 | ND | ND | 2.73 |
| 水及饮料类 Water and beverages | ND | ND | ND | ND | ND | ND | ND | ND | ND | ND | 1.04 | 1.02 | ND | ND | ND | ND | ND | ND | ND | ND | ND | ND | ND | ND | 0.47 |
| 酒类 Alcohol beverages | ND | ND | ND | 2.29 | ND | ND | 1.17 | 1.69 | ND | ND | 1.16 | 1.47 | 2.26 | 1.51 | ND | ND | ND | ND | ND | ND | 2.75 | 1.12 | ND | 1.14 | 0.98 |

注：未检出（ND）按 1/2 检出限（LOD）计

Note: values not detected (ND) were treated as being equal to half of the detection of limit (LOD)

附表 4-55　第六次中国总膳食研究无机砷的膳食摄入量（单位：μg/d）

Annexed Table 4-55　Dietary intake of inorganic arsenic from the 6<sup>th</sup> China TDS (Unit: μg/d)

| 膳食类别<br>Category | 黑龙江<br>HL | 辽宁<br>LN | 河北<br>HE | 北京<br>BJ | 吉林<br>JL | 山西<br>SX | 陕西<br>SN | 河南<br>HA | 宁夏<br>NX | 内蒙古<br>NM | 青海<br>QH | 甘肃<br>GS | 上海<br>SH | 福建<br>FJ | 江西<br>JX | 江苏<br>JS | 浙江<br>ZJ | 山东<br>SD | 湖北<br>HB | 四川<br>SC | 广西<br>GX | 湖南<br>HN | 广东<br>GD | 贵州<br>GZ | 全国平均<br>AVG |
|---|---|---|---|---|---|---|---|---|---|---|---|---|---|---|---|---|---|---|---|---|---|---|---|---|---|
| 谷类 Cereals | 5.28 | 5.89 | 5.19 | 7.10 | 6.26 | 3.53 | 5.38 | 7.02 | 5.74 | 3.55 | 4.04 | 6.06 | 2.30 | 7.41 | 12.60 | 4.87 | 12.42 | 5.45 | 8.05 | 7.58 | 23.74 | 14.67 | 5.90 | 11.83 | 7.58 |
| 豆类 Legumes | 0.10 | 0.36 | 0.11 | 0.06 | 0.05 | 0.04 | 0.32 | 0.12 | 0.02 | 0.05 | 0.00 | 0.16 | 0.07 | 0.04 | 0.04 | 0.30 | 0.07 | 0.03 | 0.11 | 0.16 | 0.02 | 0.01 | 0.02 | 0.65 | 0.12 |
| 薯类 Potatoes | 0.01 | 0.11 | 0.04 | 0.09 | 0.02 | 0.16 | 0.07 | 0.18 | 0.06 | 0.06 | 0.04 | 0.33 | 0.04 | 0.02 | 0.02 | 0.05 | 0.02 | 0.12 | 0.04 | 0.01 | 0.01 | 0.08 | 0.01 | 0.04 | 0.07 |
| 肉类 Meats | 0.04 | 0.04 | 0.03 | 0.14 | 0.03 | 0.07 | 0.02 | 0.03 | 0.02 | 0.06 | 0.04 | 0.08 | 0.06 | 0.37 | 0.19 | 0.14 | 0.19 | 0.05 | 0.03 | 0.07 | 0.15 | 0.08 | 0.07 | 0.17 | 0.09 |
| 蛋类 Eggs | 0.02 | 0.07 | 0.02 | 0.02 | 0.02 | 0.00 | 0.01 | 0.03 | 0.01 | 0.02 | 0.01 | 0.01 | 0.02 | 0.03 | 0.01 | 0.04 | 0.03 | 0.01 | 0.01 | 0.01 | 0.01 | 0.01 | 0.01 | 0.02 | 0.02 |
| 水产类 Aquatic foods | 0.03 | 0.03 | 0.01 | 0.18 | 0.03 | 0.01 | 0.01 | 0.00 | 0.01 | 0.01 | 0.01 | 0.00 | 0.16 | 0.69 | 0.05 | 0.05 | 0.19 | 0.15 | 0.11 | 0.00 | 0.23 | 0.26 | 0.25 | 0.02 | 0.10 |
| 乳类 Dairy products | 0.00 | 0.02 | 0.01 | 0.03 | 0.02 | 0.01 | 0.00 | 0.01 | 0.01 | 0.01 | 0.03 | 0.01 | 0.04 | 0.02 | 0.01 | 0.01 | 0.02 | 0.00 | 0.00 | 0.00 | 0.01 | 0.01 | 0.01 | 0.00 | 0.01 |
| 蔬菜类 Vegetables | 0.75 | 1.77 | 0.92 | 2.49 | 0.93 | 0.42 | 1.14 | 0.41 | 0.40 | 1.31 | 0.58 | 1.09 | 1.63 | 3.78 | 0.74 | 1.15 | 0.83 | 1.45 | 1.30 | 1.19 | 1.98 | 1.91 | 1.06 | 1.98 | 1.30 |
| 水果类 Fruits | 0.01 | 0.04 | 0.02 | 0.39 | 0.04 | 0.04 | 0.00 | 0.01 | 0.05 | 0.12 | 0.01 | 0.02 | 0.29 | 0.06 | 0.10 | 0.01 | 0.03 | 0.01 | 0.01 | 0.01 | 0.03 | 0.03 | 0.01 | 0.01 | 0.06 |
| 糖类 Sugar | 0.00 | 0.00 | 0.00 | 0.02 | 0.00 | 0.00 | 0.00 | 0.01 | 0.00 | 0.00 | 0.03 | 0.00 | 0.06 | 0.02 | 0.00 | 0.00 | 0.02 | 0.00 | 0.00 | 0.00 | 0.00 | 0.00 | 0.00 | 0.00 | 0.01 |
| 水及饮料类 Water and beverages | 0.61 | 0.25 | 0.39 | 0.55 | 0.16 | 0.37 | 0.04 | 0.60 | 0.26 | 1.29 | 0.64 | 1.20 | 0.35 | 0.43 | 0.59 | 0.50 | 0.39 | 0.84 | 0.14 | 0.04 | 0.16 | 0.53 | 0.60 | 0.16 | 0.46 |

续表

| 膳食类别<br>Category | 黑龙江<br>HL | 辽宁<br>LN | 河北<br>HE | 北京<br>BJ | 吉林<br>JL | 山西<br>SX | 陕西<br>SN | 河南<br>HA | 宁夏<br>NX | 内蒙古<br>NM | 青海<br>QH | 甘肃<br>GS | 上海<br>SH | 福建<br>FJ | 江西<br>JX | 江苏<br>JS | 浙江<br>ZJ | 山东<br>SD | 湖北<br>HB | 四川<br>SC | 广西<br>GX | 湖南<br>HN | 广东<br>GD | 贵州<br>GZ | 全国平均<br>AVG |
|---|---|---|---|---|---|---|---|---|---|---|---|---|---|---|---|---|---|---|---|---|---|---|---|---|---|
| 酒类<br>Alcohol beverages | 0.01 | 0.02 | 0.01 | 0.06 | 0.00 | 0.00 | 0.00 | 0.01 | 0.00 | 0.01 | 0.01 | 0.00 | 0.05 | 0.02 | 0.01 | 0.02 | 0.03 | 0.06 | 0.01 | 0.00 | 0.09 | 0.02 | 0.00 | 0.00 | 0.02 |
| 合计<br>SUM | 6.87 | 8.60 | 6.74 | 11.13 | 7.56 | 4.65 | 7.01 | 8.42 | 6.58 | 6.46 | 5.39 | 8.96 | 5.06 | 12.87 | 14.35 | 7.13 | 14.23 | 8.17 | 9.83 | 9.06 | 26.43 | 17.62 | 7.94 | 14.88 | 9.83 |

注: 计算摄入量时, 表 3-54 中的 ND 原则上按 1/2LOD 代入。无机砷方法检出限 (1.0 μg/kg) 高于总砷方法的检出限 (0.25 μg/kg)。因此样品的无机砷含量不可能大于总砷含量。因此若代入的数值大于总砷含量时, 则用总砷含量代替 ND

Note: values not detected (ND) were treated as being equal to half of the detection of limit (LOD) in principle. The LOD of the inorganic arsenic method (1.0 μg/kg) is higher than that of the total arsenic method (0.25 μg/kg). Because the inorganic arsenic content cannot be higher than the total arsenic content. Therefore, if the substituted value is greater than the total arsenic content, the total arsenic content is used to replace the ND

附表 3-56  第六次中国总膳食研究无机砷的膳食来源（单位: %）

Annexed Table 3-56  Dietary sources of inorganic arsenic form the 6th China TDS (Unit: %)

| 膳食类别<br>Category | 黑龙江<br>HL | 辽宁<br>LN | 河北<br>HE | 北京<br>BJ | 吉林<br>JL | 山西<br>SX | 陕西<br>SN | 河南<br>HA | 宁夏<br>NX | 内蒙古<br>NM | 青海<br>QH | 甘肃<br>GS | 上海<br>SH | 福建<br>FJ | 江西<br>JX | 江苏<br>JS | 浙江<br>ZJ | 山东<br>SD | 湖北<br>HB | 四川<br>SC | 广西<br>GX | 湖南<br>HN | 广东<br>GD | 贵州<br>GZ | 全国平均<br>AVG |
|---|---|---|---|---|---|---|---|---|---|---|---|---|---|---|---|---|---|---|---|---|---|---|---|---|---|
| 谷类<br>Cereals | 76.9 | 68.5 | 77.1 | 63.8 | 82.8 | 75.9 | 76.7 | 83.4 | 87.3 | 54.9 | 74.9 | 67.6 | 45.4 | 57.6 | 87.8 | 68.3 | 87.3 | 66.7 | 82.0 | 83.6 | 89.8 | 83.2 | 74.3 | 79.5 | 77.1% |
| 豆类<br>Legumes | 1.5 | 4.2 | 1.7 | 0.5 | 0.7 | 0.8 | 4.6 | 1.5 | 0.3 | 0.8 | 0.1 | 1.8 | 1.3 | 0.3 | 0.3 | 4.2 | 0.5 | 0.4 | 1.2 | 1.8 | 0.1 | 0.1 | 0.2 | 4.4 | 1.2% |
| 薯类<br>Potatoes | 0.2 | 1.3 | 0.5 | 0.8 | 0.2 | 3.3 | 1.0 | 2.1 | 0.9 | 1.0 | 0.7 | 3.7 | 0.7 | 0.2 | 0.1 | 0.7 | 0.1 | 1.5 | 0.5 | 0.1 | 0.0 | 0.6 | 0.2 | 0.3 | 0.7% |
| 肉类<br>Meats | 0.5 | 0.5 | 0.4 | 1.2 | 0.4 | 1.6 | 0.3 | 0.3 | 0.4 | 0.6 | 0.7 | 0.9 | 1.1 | 2.9 | 1.3 | 1.9 | 1.4 | 0.6 | 0.3 | 0.7 | 0.6 | 0.4 | 0.8 | 1.1 | 0.9% |
| 蛋类<br>Eggs | 0.3 | 0.8 | 0.3 | 0.2 | 0.3 | 0.1 | 0.2 | 0.4 | 0.1 | 0.3 | 0.2 | 0.1 | 0.4 | 0.1 | 0.1 | 0.6 | 0.2 | 0.1 | 0.3 | 0.1 | 0.0 | 0.1 | 0.2 | 0.1 | 0.2% |

续表

| 膳食类别 Category | 黑龙江 HL | 辽宁 LN | 河北 HE | 北京 BJ | 吉林 JL | 山西 SX | 陕西 SN | 河南 HA | 宁夏 NX | 内蒙古 NM | 青海 QH | 甘肃 GS | 上海 SH | 福建 FJ | 江西 JX | 江苏 JS | 浙江 ZJ | 山东 SD | 湖北 HB | 四川 SC | 广西 GX | 湖南 HN | 广东 GD | 贵州 GZ | 全国平均 AVG |
|---|---|---|---|---|---|---|---|---|---|---|---|---|---|---|---|---|---|---|---|---|---|---|---|---|---|
| 水产类 Aquatic foods | 0.5 | 0.4 | 0.2 | 1.6 | 0.3 | 0.2 | 0.2 | 0.0 | 0.1 | 0.1 | 0.1 | 0.0 | 3.2 | 5.3 | 0.3 | 0.7 | 1.3 | 1.8 | 1.1 | 0.0 | 0.9 | 1.5 | 3.2 | 0.1 | 1.1% |
| 乳类 Dairy products | 0.0 | 0.3 | 0.1 | 0.3 | 0.2 | 0.1 | 0.0 | 0.1 | 0.1 | 0.3 | 0.5 | 0.1 | 0.7 | 0.1 | 0.1 | 0.1 | 0.1 | 0.0 | 0.0 | 0.0 | 0.0 | 0.1 | 0.2 | 0.0 | 0.1% |
| 蔬菜类 Vegetables | 10.9 | 20.6 | 13.6 | 22.3 | 12.2 | 9.0 | 16.3 | 4.8 | 6.1 | 20.2 | 10.7 | 12.2 | 32.2 | 29.3 | 5.1 | 16.1 | 5.8 | 17.8 | 13.2 | 13.1 | 7.5 | 10.8 | 13.3 | 13.3 | 13.2% |
| 水果类 Fruits | 0.1 | 0.5 | 0.3 | 3.5 | 0.6 | 0.9 | 0.1 | 0.1 | 0.7 | 1.8 | 0.1 | 0.2 | 5.7 | 0.5 | 0.7 | 0.1 | 0.2 | 0.1 | 0.1 | 0.1 | 0.1 | 0.2 | 0.2 | 0.1 | 0.6% |
| 糖类 Sugar | 0.0 | 0.0 | 0.0 | 0.2 | 0.0 | 0.0 | 0.0 | 0.1 | 0.0 | 0.0 | 0.0 | 0.0 | 1.2 | 0.0 | 0.0 | 0.0 | 0.0 | 0.0 | 0.0 | 0.0 | 0.0 | 0.0 | 0.0 | 0.0 | 0.0% |
| 水及饮料类 Water and beverages | 8.9 | 2.9 | 5.8 | 5.0 | 2.2 | 8.0 | 0.6 | 7.1 | 3.9 | 19.9 | 11.9 | 13.4 | 6.9 | 3.4 | 4.1 | 7.1 | 2.8 | 10.4 | 1.4 | 0.4 | 0.6 | 3.0 | 7.5 | 1.1 | 4.7% |
| 酒类 Alcohol beverages | 0.2 | 0.2 | 0.1 | 0.6 | 0.1 | 0.0 | 0.0 | 0.1 | 0.0 | 0.2 | 0.1 | 0.1 | 1.0 | 0.2 | 0.1 | 0.3 | 0.2 | 0.7 | 0.1 | 0.0 | 0.3 | 0.1 | 0.0 | 0.0 | 0.2% |

附表 3-57 第六次中国总膳食研究膳食样品中铝的含量（单位：mg/kg）

Annexed Table 3-57 Levels of aluminum in food samples from the 6<sup>th</sup> China TDS (Unit: mg/kg)

| 膳食类别 Category | 黑龙江 HL | 辽宁 LN | 河北 HE | 北京 BJ | 吉林 JL | 山西 SX | 陕西 SN | 河南 HA | 宁夏 NX | 内蒙古 NM | 青海 QH | 甘肃 GS | 上海 SH | 福建 FJ | 江西 JX | 江苏 JS | 浙江 ZJ | 山东 SD | 湖北 HB | 四川 SC | 广西 GX | 湖南 HN | 广东 GD | 贵州 GZ | 全国平均 AVG |
|---|---|---|---|---|---|---|---|---|---|---|---|---|---|---|---|---|---|---|---|---|---|---|---|---|---|
| 谷类 Cereals | 31.51 | 12.92 | 13.11 | 9.71 | 19.16 | 5.65 | 7.71 | 5.57 | 6.06 | 3.42 | 1.20 | 1.70 | 1.09 | 2.31 | 2.84 | 1.81 | 0.74 | 7.06 | 1.64 | 1.81 | 0.54 | 0.16 | 0.42 | 2.93 | 5.88 |

续表

| 膳食类别 Category | 黑龙江 HL | 辽宁 LN | 河北 HE | 北京 BJ | 吉林 JL | 山西 SX | 陕西 SN | 河南 HA | 宁夏 NX | 内蒙古 NM | 青海 QH | 甘肃 GS | 上海 SH | 福建 FJ | 江西 JX | 江苏 JS | 浙江 ZJ | 山东 SD | 湖北 HB | 四川 SC | 广西 GX | 湖南 HN | 广东 GD | 贵州 GZ | 全国平均 AVG |
|---|---|---|---|---|---|---|---|---|---|---|---|---|---|---|---|---|---|---|---|---|---|---|---|---|---|
| 豆类 Legumes | 3.07 | 5.35 | 7.48 | 6.60 | 3.40 | 4.74 | 7.56 | 13.28 | 3.19 | 5.48 | 4.11 | 10.33 | 3.53 | 2.53 | 6.77 | 5.38 | 3.17 | 5.42 | 5.13 | 4.93 | 3.15 | 5.64 | 2.42 | 6.44 | 5.38 |
| 薯类 Potatoes | 11.73 | 12.17 | 16.46 | 6.69 | 4.68 | 10.27 | 14.97 | 19.06 | 3.84 | 21.86 | 4.28 | 27.60 | 13.90 | 6.64 | 1.86 | 6.18 | 2.62 | 12.40 | 2.70 | 2.32 | 1.56 | 5.59 | 0.10 | 3.12 | 8.86 |
| 肉类 Meats | 1.13 | 1.36 | 1.14 | 0.90 | 1.21 | 0.35 | 2.69 | 1.87 | 4.12 | 4.35 | 2.48 | 10.66 | 0.53 | 0.43 | 1.57 | 0.19 | 0.59 | 1.41 | 2.18 | 0.82 | 1.07 | 6.79 | ND | 0.71 | 2.02 |
| 蛋类 Eggs | 0.29 | 1.08 | 1.45 | 0.26 | ND | 0.14 | 1.37 | 0.38 | 0.86 | ND | ND | 0.08 | ND | 0.47 | 0.71 | ND | 0.08 | 0.43 | 2.02 | ND | ND | 1.49 | 0.08 | 0.18 | 0.48 |
| 水产类 Aquatic foods | 0.86 | 12.03 | 3.92 | 6.65 | 0.61 | 0.19 | ND | 1.96 | 2.06 | 1.84 | 1.54 | 3.90 | 2.71 | 14.10 | 1.02 | 5.29 | 2.96 | 12.62 | 2.62 | 0.23 | 7.12 | 1.58 | 1.34 | 2.96 | 3.76 |
| 乳类 Dairy products | ND | 0.08 | ND | 0.06 | ND | ND | 0.15 | 0.11 | 0.18 | ND | ND | ND | ND | ND | 0.17 | ND | ND | ND | 0.11 | ND | ND | 0.17 | 0.08 | ND | 0.06 |
| 蔬菜类 Vegetables | 1.81 | 1.66 | 1.47 | 2.54 | 1.42 | 1.18 | 3.20 | 1.98 | 5.61 | 3.35 | 1.25 | 1.77 | 1.16 | 1.58 | 2.85 | 3.74 | 6.17 | 1.72 | 4.87 | 0.27 | 8.15 | 15.05 | 4.09 | 47.21 | 5.17 |
| 水果类 Fruits | 0.18 | 0.41 | ND | 0.40 | ND | ND | 1.29 | 0.13 | 1.33 | 0.24 | ND | 0.15 | 0.35 | 0.13 | ND | 0.18 | ND | 0.31 | 0.48 | ND | ND | ND | ND | 0.10 | 0.25 |
| 糖类 Sugar | ND | 0.16 | 1.58 | 0.82 | 0.26 | ND | 1.54 | 0.92 | 1.10 | 1.58 | ND | 1.43 | 9.81 | ND | 1.24 | ND | 0.29 | 0.52 | ND | 0.49 | ND | 6.30 | ND | 0.27 | 1.19 |
| 水及饮料类 Water and beverages | ND | 0.21 | 0.06 | 0.06 | 0.07 | 0.16 | 1.13 | 0.16 | 0.09 | 0.69 | 4.78 | 0.12 | 1.06 | 0.29 | 0.14 | 0.31 | 0.95 | 0.11 | 0.61 | 0.45 | 0.38 | 3.92 | 0.42 | ND | 0.68 |
| 酒类 Alcohol beverages | 0.40 | 0.06 | 0.14 | 0.12 | 0.27 | ND | 0.17 | 0.32 | 0.17 | 0.20 | 0.08 | 0.05 | 0.48 | 0.11 | 0.12 | 0.62 | 0.26 | 0.14 | 0.31 | 4.33 | 0.44 | 2.84 | 0.24 | 0.67 | 0.52 |

注：未检出（ND）按 1/2 检出限（LOD）计

Note: values not detected (ND) were treated as being equal to half of the detection of limit (LOD)

附表 3-58　第六次中国总膳食研究的铝膳食摄入量（单位：mg/d）

Annexed Table 3-58　Dietary intake of aluminum from the 6$^{th}$ China TDS (Unit: mg/d)

| 膳食类别 Category | 黑龙江 HL | 辽宁 LN | 河北 HE | 北京 BJ | 吉林 JL | 山西 SX | 陕西 SN | 河南 HA | 宁夏 NX | 内蒙古 NM | 青海 QH | 甘肃 GS | 上海 SH | 福建 FJ | 江西 JX | 江苏 JS | 浙江 ZJ | 山东 SD | 湖北 HB | 四川 SC | 广西 GX | 湖南 HN | 广东 GD | 贵州 GZ | 全国平均 AVG |
|---|---|---|---|---|---|---|---|---|---|---|---|---|---|---|---|---|---|---|---|---|---|---|---|---|---|
| 谷类 Cereals | 17.27 | 7.95 | 9.90 | 7.72 | 11.22 | 5.86 | 5.88 | 5.15 | 4.01 | 2.47 | 0.92 | 1.17 | 0.49 | 1.46 | 1.79 | 1.41 | 0.47 | 7.03 | 0.87 | 1.75 | 0.50 | 0.09 | 0.19 | 1.98 | 4.06 |
| 豆类 Legumes | 0.14 | 0.65 | 0.43 | 0.67 | 0.26 | 0.33 | 0.63 | 0.72 | 0.11 | 0.22 | 0.03 | 0.43 | 0.41 | 0.20 | 0.50 | 0.45 | 0.45 | 0.28 | 0.34 | 0.33 | 0.13 | 0.41 | 0.07 | 0.65 | 0.37 |
| 薯类 Potatoes | 0.91 | 0.88 | 1.00 | 0.39 | 0.56 | 1.22 | 1.72 | 1.53 | 0.38 | 2.67 | 0.43 | 3.97 | 0.50 | 0.28 | 0.06 | 0.21 | 0.10 | 0.57 | 0.24 | 0.15 | 0.02 | 0.30 | 0.00 | 0.11 | 0.76 |
| 肉类 Meats | 0.07 | 0.09 | 0.05 | 0.06 | 0.08 | 0.05 | 0.10 | 0.10 | 0.19 | 0.32 | 0.18 | 0.33 | 0.06 | 0.04 | 0.15 | 0.02 | 0.07 | 0.14 | 0.12 | 0.11 | 0.16 | 1.02 | 0.00 | 0.08 | 0.15 |
| 蛋类 Eggs | 0.01 | 0.04 | 0.05 | 0.01 | 0.00 | 0.00 | 0.03 | 0.01 | 0.01 | 0.00 | 0.01 | 0.01 | 0.00 | 0.01 | 0.01 | | 0.00 | 0.02 | 0.05 | 0.00 | 0.00 | 0.03 | 0.00 | 0.00 | 0.01 |
| 水产类 Aquatic foods | 0.02 | 0.19 | 0.04 | 0.11 | 0.01 | 0.00 | 0.00 | 0.01 | 0.00 | 0.02 | 0.01 | 0.00 | 0.19 | 0.91 | 0.04 | 0.21 | 0.15 | 0.29 | 0.11 | 0.00 | 0.69 | 0.10 | 0.07 | 0.01 | 0.13 |
| 乳类 Dairy products | 0.00 | 0.00 | 0.00 | 0.01 | 0.00 | 0.00 | 0.00 | 0.00 | 0.00 | 0.00 | 0.00 | 0.00 | 0.00 | 0.00 | 0.00 | 0.00 | 0.00 | 0.00 | 0.00 | 0.00 | 0.00 | 0.00 | 0.00 | 0.00 | 0.00 |
| 蔬菜类 Vegetables | 0.58 | 0.54 | 0.43 | 1.00 | 0.55 | 0.37 | 0.92 | 0.55 | 0.88 | 0.86 | 0.39 | 0.44 | 0.46 | 0.63 | 1.29 | 1.59 | 2.74 | 0.70 | 2.02 | 0.08 | 2.88 | 8.04 | 0.97 | 19.26 | 2.01 |
| 水果类 Fruits | 0.01 | 0.03 | 0.00 | 0.05 | 0.00 | 0.00 | 0.05 | 0.00 | 0.11 | 0.03 | 0.00 | 0.00 | 0.03 | 0.01 | 0.00 | 0.01 | 0.00 | 0.02 | 0.01 | 0.00 | 0.00 | 0.00 | 0.00 | 0.00 | 0.02 |
| 糖类 Sugar | 0.00 | 0.00 | 0.00 | 0.00 | 0.00 | 0.00 | 0.00 | 0.00 | 0.00 | 0.00 | 0.00 | 0.00 | 0.07 | 0.00 | 0.00 | 0.00 | 0.00 | 0.00 | 0.00 | 0.00 | 0.00 | 0.00 | 0.00 | 0.00 | 0.00 |
| 水及饮料类 Water and beverages | 0.03 | 0.10 | 0.05 | 0.06 | 0.09 | 0.12 | 0.39 | 0.19 | 0.05 | 1.77 | 2.95 | 0.15 | 0.74 | 0.25 | 0.17 | 0.31 | 0.75 | 0.20 | 0.17 | 0.14 | 0.49 | 4.16 | 0.49 | 0.03 | 0.58 |

续表

| 膳食类别<br>Category | 黑龙江<br>HL | 辽宁<br>LN | 河北<br>HE | 北京<br>BJ | 吉林<br>JL | 山西<br>SX | 陕西<br>SN | 河南<br>HA | 宁夏<br>NX | 内蒙古<br>NM | 青海<br>QH | 甘肃<br>GS | 上海<br>SH | 福建<br>FJ | 江西<br>JX | 江苏<br>JS | 浙江<br>ZJ | 山东<br>SD | 湖北<br>HB | 四川<br>SC | 广西<br>GX | 湖南<br>HN | 广东<br>GD | 贵州<br>GZ | 全国平均<br>AVG |
|---|---|---|---|---|---|---|---|---|---|---|---|---|---|---|---|---|---|---|---|---|---|---|---|---|---|
| 酒类<br>Alcohol beverages | 0.01 | 0.00 | 0.00 | 0.00 | 0.00 | 0.00 | 0.00 | 0.00 | 0.00 | 0.00 | 0.00 | 0.00 | 0.01 | 0.00 | 0.00 | 0.02 | 0.02 | 0.02 | 0.00 | 0.02 | 0.01 | 0.05 | 0.00 | 0.00 | 0.01 |
| 合计<br>SUM | 19.05 | 10.50 | 11.95 | 10.08 | 12.77 | 7.95 | 9.71 | 8.26 | 5.75 | 8.37 | 4.91 | 6.50 | 2.97 | 3.78 | 4.02 | 4.22 | 4.74 | 9.27 | 3.93 | 2.59 | 4.90 | 14.21 | 1.80 | 22.12 | 8.10 |

附表 3-59 第六次中国总膳食研究铝的膳食来源（单位：%）

Annexed Table 3-59 Dietary sources of aluminum from the 6th China TDS (Unit: %)

| 膳食类别<br>Category | 黑龙江<br>HL | 辽宁<br>LN | 河北<br>HE | 北京<br>BJ | 吉林<br>JL | 山西<br>SX | 陕西<br>SN | 河南<br>HA | 宁夏<br>NX | 内蒙古<br>NM | 青海<br>QH | 甘肃<br>GS | 上海<br>SH | 福建<br>FJ | 江西<br>JX | 江苏<br>JS | 浙江<br>ZJ | 山东<br>SD | 湖北<br>HB | 四川<br>SC | 广西<br>GX | 湖南<br>HN | 广东<br>GD | 贵州<br>GZ | 全国平均<br>AVG |
|---|---|---|---|---|---|---|---|---|---|---|---|---|---|---|---|---|---|---|---|---|---|---|---|---|---|
| 谷类<br>Cereals | 90.6 | 75.8 | 82.8 | 76.6 | 87.8 | 73.7 | 60.5 | 62.3 | 69.7 | 29.5 | 18.8 | 17.9 | 16.4 | 38.6 | 44.5 | 33.3 | 9.9 | 75.9 | 22.1 | 67.7 | 10.3 | 0.6 | 10.7 | 9.0 | 50.2 |
| 豆类<br>Legumes | 0.7 | 6.2 | 3.6 | 6.7 | 2.0 | 4.1 | 6.4 | 8.7 | 2.0 | 2.6 | 0.5 | 6.6 | 14.0 | 5.3 | 12.4 | 10.6 | 9.4 | 3.1 | 8.7 | 12.9 | 2.7 | 2.9 | 3.7 | 3.0 | 4.5 |
| 薯类<br>Potatoes | 4.8 | 8.4 | 8.4 | 3.9 | 4.4 | 15.3 | 17.7 | 18.5 | 6.7 | 31.9 | 8.8 | 61.1 | 16.8 | 7.4 | 1.5 | 4.9 | 2.0 | 6.2 | 6.1 | 5.7 | 0.4 | 2.1 | 0.1 | 0.5 | 9.4 |
| 肉类<br>Meats | 0.4 | 0.9 | 0.5 | 0.6 | 0.6 | 0.6 | 1.0 | 1.3 | 3.3 | 3.8 | 3.6 | 5.1 | 2.0 | 1.0 | 3.7 | 0.4 | 1.5 | 1.5 | 3.0 | 4.1 | 3.3 | 7.1 | 0.2 | 0.3 | 1.8 |
| 蛋类<br>Eggs | 0.1 | 0.4 | 0.4 | 0.1 | 0.0 | 0.0 | 0.3 | 0.1 | 0.2 | 0.0 | 0.1 | 0.2 | 0.1 | 0.2 | 0.4 | 0.0 | 0.0 | 0.2 | 1.3 | 0.0 | 0.0 | 0.2 | 0.1 | 0.0 | 0.2 |
| 水产类<br>Aquatic foods | 0.1 | 1.8 | 0.3 | 1.1 | 0.1 | 0.0 | 0.0 | 0.1 | 0.1 | 0.2 | 0.0 | 0.2 | 6.3 | 23.9 | 1.1 | 4.9 | 3.1 | 3.1 | 2.7 | 0.1 | 14.1 | 0.7 | 3.8 | 0.0 | 1.6 |
| 乳类<br>Dairy products | 0.0 | 0.0 | 0.0 | 0.0 | 0.0 | 0.0 | 0.0 | 0.0 | 0.0 | 0.0 | 0.0 | 0.0 | 0.1 | 0.0 | 0.1 | 0.0 | 0.0 | 0.0 | 0.0 | 0.0 | 0.0 | 0.0 | 0.2 | 0.0 | 0.0 |

续表

| 膳食类别 Category | 黑龙江 HL | 辽宁 LN | 河北 HE | 北京 BJ | 吉林 JL | 山西 SX | 陕西 SN | 河南 HA | 宁夏 NX | 内蒙古 NM | 青海 QH | 甘肃 GS | 上海 SH | 福建 FJ | 江西 JX | 江苏 JS | 浙江 ZJ | 山东 SD | 湖北 HB | 四川 SC | 广西 GX | 湖南 HN | 广东 GD | 贵州 GZ | 全国平均 AVG |
|---|---|---|---|---|---|---|---|---|---|---|---|---|---|---|---|---|---|---|---|---|---|---|---|---|---|
| 蔬菜类 Vegetables | 3.0 | 5.2 | 3.6 | 9.9 | 4.3 | 4.6 | 9.5 | 6.7 | 15.2 | 10.3 | 7.9 | 6.8 | 15.7 | 16.6 | 32.0 | 37.7 | 57.9 | 7.5 | 51.3 | 3.2 | 58.8 | 56.6 | 53.7 | 87.0 | 24.8 |
| 水果类 Fruits | 0.1 | 0.3 | 0.0 | 0.5 | 0.0 | 0.0 | 0.5 | 0.0 | 2.0 | 0.3 | 0.0 | 0.1 | 0.9 | 0.2 | 0.0 | 0.1 | 0.0 | 0.2 | 0.2 | 0.0 | 0.0 | 0.0 | 0.0 | 0.0 | 0.2 |
| 糖类 Sugar | 0.0 | 0.0 | 0.0 | 0.0 | 0.0 | 0.0 | 0.0 | 0.0 | 0.0 | 0.0 | 0.0 | 0.0 | 2.5 | 0.0 | 0.0 | 0.0 | 0.0 | 0.0 | 0.0 | 0.0 | 0.0 | 0.0 | 0.0 | 0.0 | 0.0 |
| 水及饮料类 Water and beverages | 0.2 | 1.0 | 0.4 | 0.6 | 0.7 | 1.5 | 4.0 | 2.2 | 0.8 | 21.2 | 60.2 | 2.3 | 25.0 | 6.7 | 4.2 | 7.5 | 15.8 | 2.2 | 4.4 | 5.4 | 10.0 | 29.3 | 27.4 | 0.1 | 7.1 |
| 酒类 Alcohol beverages | 0.0 | 0.0 | 0.0 | 0.0 | 0.0 | 0.0 | 0.0 | 0.0 | 0.0 | 0.0 | 0.0 | 0.0 | 0.4 | 0.0 | 0.1 | 0.6 | 0.3 | 0.2 | 0.1 | 0.9 | 0.3 | 0.3 | 0.0 | 0.0 | 0.1 |

# 第四章 附 表
# Annexed Tables of Chapter 4

附表 4-1 第六次中国总膳食研究膳食样品中毒死蜱的含量（单位：μg/kg）

Annexed Table 4-1 Levels of chlorpyrifos in food samples from the 6$^{th}$ China TDS (Unit: μg/kg)

| 膳食类别 Category | 黑龙江 HL | 辽宁 LN | 河北 HE | 北京 BJ | 吉林 JL | 山西 SX | 陕西 SN | 河南 HA | 宁夏 NX | 内蒙古 NM | 青海 QH | 甘肃 GS | 上海 SH | 福建 FJ | 江西 JX | 江苏 JS | 浙江 ZJ | 山东 SD | 湖北 HB | 四川 SC | 广西 GX | 湖南 HN | 广东 GD | 贵州 GZ | 全国平均 AVG |
|---|---|---|---|---|---|---|---|---|---|---|---|---|---|---|---|---|---|---|---|---|---|---|---|---|---|
| 谷类 Cereals | ND | ND | 0.40 | 0.33 | ND | ND | 0.33 | 0.24 | ND | 0.14 | ND | ND | 0.35 | 0.73 | 0.14 | ND | 0.64 | 0.25 | 0.76 | 6.31 | 0.52 | ND | 0.36 | ND | 0.48 |
| 豆类 Legumes | 2.39 | 1.64 | 1.29 | 0.60 | ND | 0.32 | 0.40 | 2.31 | 0.12 | ND | ND | 0.11 | 0.97 | 2.95 | ND | 1.90 | 0.86 | 1.17 | 3.22 | 0.33 | 1.02 | ND | 2.89 | ND | 1.02 |
| 薯类 Potatoes | ND | 0.22 | 2.23 | 2.76 | ND | 0.91 | ND | ND | ND | 0.44 | 0.56 | ND | ND | 4.48 | 0.96 | ND | ND | 1.53 | 3.74 | ND | 2.43 | 1.50 | 1.85 | ND | 0.98 |
| 肉类 Meats | ND | 0.23 | 1.67 | 2.94 | ND | 0.48 | 1.01 | ND | ND | 6.87 | 0.40 | 0.23 | ND | 1.60 | ND | ND | ND | 1.08 | 1.19 | 0.14 | 1.18 | ND | 0.19 | ND | 0.80 |
| 蛋类 Eggs | ND | 0.29 | 2.53 | 4.69 | ND | 0.80 | ND | ND | ND | ND | 0.32 | ND | ND | 11.85 | ND | ND | ND | 0.77 | 3.63 | ND | 2.43 | ND | ND | ND | 1.14 |
| 水产类 Aquatic foods | 0.68 | ND | 0.91 | 4.50 | ND | ND | 0.79 | 0.67 | ND | 4.41 | 0.77 | 1.65 | 0.16 | 10.55 | 0.90 | ND | 0.42 | 1.00 | 2.74 | 3.28 | 3.46 | 2.53 | 2.36 | 1.86 | 1.82 |
| 乳类 Dairy products | ND | ND | ND | ND | ND | ND | ND | ND | ND | ND | ND | ND | ND | ND | ND | ND | ND | ND | ND | ND | ND | ND | ND | ND | 0.00 |
| 蔬菜类 Vegetables | ND | 22.50 | 1.56 | 2.31 | 0.36 | 1.11 | 2.66 | 0.13 | 1.07 | 1.76 | 2.92 | 6.70 | 0.75 | 7.07 | 3.50 | ND | 0.47 | 1.92 | 61.73 | 1.25 | 11.05 | 0.29 | 2.21 | 0.93 | 5.59 |
| 水果类 Fruits | 2.00 | 18.30 | 0.66 | 3.28 | 21.29 | 0.74 | ND | 7.29 | ND | ND | ND | 0.31 | 7.98 | 21.07 | 0.21 | 0.20 | 0.17 | 0.65 | 6.97 | ND | ND | 2.95 | 1.15 | 0.81 | 4.00 |

续表

| 膳食类别<br>Category | 黑龙江<br>HL | 辽宁<br>LN | 河北<br>HE | 北京<br>BJ | 吉林<br>JL | 山西<br>SX | 陕西<br>SN | 河南<br>HA | 宁夏<br>NX | 内蒙古<br>NM | 青海<br>QH | 甘肃<br>GS | 上海<br>SH | 福建<br>FJ | 江西<br>JX | 江苏<br>JS | 浙江<br>ZJ | 山东<br>SD | 湖北<br>HB | 四川<br>SC | 广西<br>GX | 湖南<br>HN | 广东<br>GD | 贵州<br>GZ | 全国平均<br>AVG |
|---|---|---|---|---|---|---|---|---|---|---|---|---|---|---|---|---|---|---|---|---|---|---|---|---|---|
| 糖类 Sugar | ND | ND | ND | ND | ND | ND | ND | ND | ND | ND | ND | ND | 1.13 | ND | ND | ND | ND | ND | ND | ND | ND | ND | ND | ND | 0.05 |
| 水及饮料类 Water and beverages | ND | ND | ND | ND | ND | ND | ND | ND | ND | ND | ND | ND | ND | ND | ND | ND | ND | ND | ND | ND | ND | ND | ND | ND | 0.00 |
| 酒类 Alcohol beverages | ND | ND | ND | ND | ND | ND | ND | ND | ND | ND | ND | ND | ND | ND | ND | ND | ND | ND | ND | ND | ND | ND | ND | ND | 0.00 |

注：未检出（ND）按 0 计

Note: values not detected (ND) were treated as being equal to 0

附表 Table 4-2　第六次中国总膳食研究膳食样品中敌敌畏的含量（单位：μg/kg）

Annexed Table 4-2　Levels of dichlorvos in food samples from the 6$^{th}$ China TDS (Unit: μg/kg)

| 膳食类别<br>Category | 黑龙江<br>HL | 辽宁<br>LN | 河北<br>HE | 北京<br>BJ | 吉林<br>JL | 山西<br>SX | 陕西<br>SN | 河南<br>HA | 宁夏<br>NX | 内蒙古<br>NM | 青海<br>QH | 甘肃<br>GS | 上海<br>SH | 福建<br>FJ | 江西<br>JX | 江苏<br>JS | 浙江<br>ZJ | 山东<br>SD | 湖北<br>HB | 四川<br>SC | 广西<br>GX | 湖南<br>HN | 广东<br>GD | 贵州<br>GZ | 全国平均<br>AVG |
|---|---|---|---|---|---|---|---|---|---|---|---|---|---|---|---|---|---|---|---|---|---|---|---|---|---|
| 谷类 Cereals | 0.17 | 0.95 | 1.27 | 0.12 | ND | ND | ND | ND | ND | ND | ND | 0.10 | ND | ND | ND | ND | ND | 17.26 | 0.19 | ND | ND | ND | ND | ND | 0.84 |
| 豆类 Legumes | 0.38 | ND | 0.12 | ND | ND | ND | ND | 4.31 | 0.68 | ND | ND | ND | ND | ND | ND | ND | ND | 14.70 | 0.07 | ND | ND | ND | ND | ND | 0.84 |
| 薯类 Potatoes | 0.17 | ND | ND | 0.06 | 0.12 | ND | ND | ND | ND | ND | ND | ND | ND | ND | ND | ND | ND | 16.36 | ND | ND | ND | ND | ND | ND | 0.69 |
| 肉类 Meats | ND | ND | ND | ND | ND | ND | ND | ND | ND | ND | ND | ND | ND | ND | ND | ND | ND | 13.49 | ND | ND | ND | ND | ND | ND | 0.57 |
| 蛋类 Eggs | ND | ND | ND | ND | ND | ND | 0.08 | ND | ND | ND | ND | ND | ND | ND | ND | ND | ND | 0.35 | ND | ND | ND | ND | ND | ND | 0.01 |
| 水产类 Aquatic foods | 1.01 | ND | ND | 1.65 | ND | ND | ND | ND | ND | ND | ND | ND | ND | ND | ND | ND | ND | 6.40 | ND | ND | ND | ND | ND | ND | 0.38 |

续表

| 膳食类别 Category | 黑龙江 HL | 辽宁 LN | 河北 HE | 北京 BJ | 吉林 JL | 山西 SX | 陕西 SN | 河南 HA | 宁夏 NX | 内蒙古 NM | 青海 QH | 甘肃 GS | 上海 SH | 福建 FJ | 江西 JX | 江苏 JS | 浙江 ZJ | 山东 SD | 湖北 HB | 四川 SC | 广西 GX | 湖南 HN | 广东 GD | 贵州 GZ | 全国平均 AVG |
|---|---|---|---|---|---|---|---|---|---|---|---|---|---|---|---|---|---|---|---|---|---|---|---|---|---|
| 乳类 Dairy products | 0.09 | ND | 0.18 | ND | ND | 0.10 | ND | 0.18 | ND | 0.06 | ND | ND | ND | ND | ND | 0.30 | ND | 4.79 | ND | ND | ND | ND | ND | 0.06 | 0.24 |
| 蔬菜类 Vegetables | 0.27 | ND | 0.57 | ND | ND | ND | ND | ND | ND | ND | ND | ND | 0.07 | ND | ND | 0.07 | ND | 36.48 | ND | ND | ND | ND | ND | ND | 1.56 |
| 水果类 Fruits | 0.06 | ND | ND | ND | ND | ND | ND | ND | ND | ND | ND | ND | ND | ND | ND | ND | ND | 13.37 | ND | ND | ND | ND | ND | ND | 0.56 |
| 糖类 Sugar | 0.10 | ND | ND | ND | ND | 0.05 | ND | ND | ND | ND | ND | ND | ND | ND | ND | ND | ND | 4.91 | ND | ND | ND | ND | ND | 0.07 | 0.21 |
| 水及饮料类 Water and beverages | 0.08 | ND | ND | ND | ND | ND | ND | ND | ND | 0.06 | ND | ND | ND | ND | ND | ND | ND | 11.42 | ND | ND | ND | 0.12 | ND | ND | 0.49 |
| 酒类 Alcohol beverages | 0.11 | ND | ND | ND | ND | ND | 0.07 | 4.74 | ND | ND | ND | ND | ND | ND | ND | ND | ND | 0.10 | 0.07 | ND | ND | 0.05 | ND | ND | 0.21 |

注：未检出（ND）按 0 计

Note: values not detected (ND) were treated as being equal to 0

附表 4-3 第六次中国总膳食研究膳食样品中乙酰甲胺磷的含量（单位：μg/kg）

Annexed Table 4-3 Levels of acephate in food samples from the 6$^{th}$ China TDS (Unit: μg/kg)

| 膳食类别 Category | 黑龙江 HL | 辽宁 LN | 河北 HE | 北京 BJ | 吉林 JL | 山西 SX | 陕西 SN | 河南 HA | 宁夏 NX | 内蒙古 NM | 青海 QH | 甘肃 GS | 上海 SH | 福建 FJ | 江西 JX | 江苏 JS | 浙江 ZJ | 山东 SD | 湖北 HB | 四川 SC | 广西 GX | 湖南 HN | 广东 GD | 贵州 GZ | 全国平均 AVG |
|---|---|---|---|---|---|---|---|---|---|---|---|---|---|---|---|---|---|---|---|---|---|---|---|---|---|
| 谷类 Cereals | ND | ND | ND | ND | ND | ND | ND | ND | ND | ND | ND | ND | ND | ND | ND | ND | ND | ND | ND | ND | ND | ND | ND | ND | 0.00 |
| 豆类 Legumes | ND | ND | ND | ND | ND | ND | 1.07 | ND | ND | ND | ND | 0.26 | ND | ND | ND | 1.00 | ND | ND | ND | 0.68 | ND | ND | ND | 0.33 | 0.14 |

附录 455

续表

| 膳食类别 Category | 黑龙江 HL | 辽宁 LN | 河北 HE | 北京 BJ | 吉林 JL | 山西 SX | 陕西 SN | 河南 HA | 宁夏 NX | 内蒙古 NM | 青海 QH | 甘肃 GS | 上海 SH | 福建 FJ | 江西 JX | 江苏 JS | 浙江 ZJ | 山东 SD | 湖北 HB | 四川 SC | 广西 GX | 湖南 HN | 广东 GD | 贵州 GZ | 全国平均 AVG |
|---|---|---|---|---|---|---|---|---|---|---|---|---|---|---|---|---|---|---|---|---|---|---|---|---|---|
| 薯类 Potatoes | ND | ND | ND | ND | ND | ND | 1.16 | ND | ND | ND | 0.14 | ND | ND | ND | ND | 2.38 | ND | ND | ND | 2.12 | ND | 0.25 | ND | 0.79 | 0.29 |
| 肉类 Meats | ND | ND | ND | ND | ND | ND | 1.17 | ND | ND | ND | 0.64 | 0.46 | ND | ND | ND | 2.58 | ND | ND | ND | 1.59 | ND | 0.22 | ND | 0.91 | 0.32 |
| 蛋类 Eggs | ND | ND | ND | ND | ND | ND | 1.21 | ND | ND | ND | ND | 0.86 | ND | ND | ND | 2.17 | ND | ND | ND | 1.10 | ND | 0.30 | ND | 0.42 | 0.25 |
| 水产类 Aquatic foods | ND | ND | ND | ND | ND | ND | 1.76 | ND | ND | ND | 0.30 | ND | ND | ND | ND | 0.96 | ND | ND | ND | 0.92 | ND | 0.24 | ND | 0.23 | 0.18 |
| 乳类 Dairy products | ND | ND | ND | ND | ND | ND | ND | ND | ND | ND | ND | ND | ND | ND | ND | ND | ND | ND | ND | ND | ND | ND | ND | ND | 0.00 |
| 蔬菜类 Vegetables | ND | ND | ND | 2.12 | 0.15 | 0.79 | 2.67 | 0.60 | 0.29 | ND | 3.01 | ND | 0.40 | 1.93 | 3.43 | 3.97 | 1.12 | 0.28 | 0.53 | ND | 0.60 | 1.00 | 1.92 | 0.18 | 1.04 |
| 水果类 Fruits | ND | ND | ND | ND | ND | ND | ND | 0.59 | ND | ND | ND | ND | ND | ND | ND | ND | ND | ND | ND | ND | ND | ND | ND | ND | 0.02 |
| 糖类 Sugar | ND | ND | ND | ND | ND | ND | ND | ND | ND | ND | ND | ND | ND | ND | ND | ND | ND | ND | ND | ND | ND | ND | ND | ND | 0.00 |
| 水及饮料类 Water and beverages | ND | ND | ND | ND | ND | ND | ND | ND | ND | ND | ND | ND | ND | ND | ND | ND | ND | ND | ND | ND | ND | ND | ND | ND | 0.00 |
| 酒类 Alcohol beverages | ND | ND | ND | ND | ND | ND | ND | ND | ND | ND | ND | ND | ND | ND | ND | ND | ND | ND | ND | ND | ND | ND | ND | ND | 0.00 |

注：未检出（ND）按 0 计

Note: values not detected (ND) were treated as being equal to 0

附表 4-4　第六次中国总膳食研究膳食样品中三唑磷的含量（单位：μg/kg）

Annexed Table 4-4　Levels of triazophos in food samples from the 6$^{th}$ China TDS (Unit: μg/kg)

| 膳食类别<br>Category | 黑龙江<br>HL | 辽宁<br>LN | 河北<br>HE | 北京<br>BJ | 吉林<br>JL | 山西<br>SX | 陕西<br>SN | 河南<br>HA | 宁夏<br>NX | 内蒙古<br>NM | 青海<br>QH | 甘肃<br>GS | 上海<br>SH | 福建<br>FJ | 江西<br>JX | 江苏<br>JS | 浙江<br>ZJ | 山东<br>SD | 湖北<br>HB | 四川<br>SC | 广西<br>GX | 湖南<br>HN | 广东<br>GD | 贵州<br>GZ | 全国平均<br>AVG |
|---|---|---|---|---|---|---|---|---|---|---|---|---|---|---|---|---|---|---|---|---|---|---|---|---|---|
| 谷类 Cereals | ND | ND | 0.20 | ND | ND | ND | ND | ND | ND | ND | ND | ND | ND | ND | 0.30 | 0.24 | 0.20 | ND | 0.18 | 0.13 | 0.21 | 0.12 | 0.09 | ND | 0.07 |
| 豆类 Legumes | ND | ND | ND | ND | ND | ND | ND | ND | ND | ND | ND | 0.05 | ND | ND | ND | ND | ND | ND | ND | ND | ND | ND | ND | ND | 0.00 |
| 薯类 Potatoes | ND | ND | ND | ND | ND | ND | ND | ND | ND | ND | ND | ND | ND | ND | ND | ND | ND | ND | ND | ND | ND | ND | ND | ND | 0.00 |
| 肉类 Meats | ND | ND | ND | ND | ND | ND | ND | 0.06 | ND | ND | ND | ND | ND | ND | ND | ND | ND | ND | ND | ND | ND | ND | ND | ND | 0.00 |
| 蛋类 Eggs | ND | ND | ND | ND | ND | ND | ND | ND | ND | ND | ND | ND | ND | ND | ND | ND | ND | ND | ND | ND | ND | ND | ND | ND | 0.00 |
| 水产类 Aquatic foods | ND | ND | ND | ND | ND | ND | ND | 0.06 | ND | ND | ND | ND | 0.06 | 0.10 | 0.10 | ND | 0.37 | ND | ND | ND | ND | 0.07 | 0.15 | 0.06 | 0.04 |
| 乳类 Dairy products | ND | ND | ND | ND | ND | ND | ND | ND | ND | ND | ND | ND | ND | ND | ND | ND | ND | ND | ND | ND | ND | ND | ND | ND | 0.00 |
| 蔬菜类 Vegetables | ND | ND | ND | ND | ND | 0.08 | ND | ND | ND | ND | ND | ND | ND | 1.65 | 0.27 | ND | 0.29 | ND | ND | ND | 0.12 | ND | ND | ND | 0.11 |
| 水果类 Fruits | ND | 0.11 | ND | ND | ND | ND | ND | ND | ND | ND | ND | ND | ND | 3.09 | ND | ND | 0.13 | ND | ND | 0.08 | ND | ND | 0.24 | ND | 0.14 |
| 糖类 Sugar | ND | ND | ND | ND | ND | ND | ND | ND | ND | ND | ND | ND | ND | 0.07 | ND | ND | ND | ND | ND | ND | ND | ND | ND | ND | 0.00 |
| 水及饮料类 Water and beverages | ND | ND | ND | ND | ND | ND | ND | ND | ND | ND | ND | ND | ND | ND | ND | ND | ND | ND | ND | ND | ND | ND | ND | ND | 0.00 |

续表

| 膳食类别<br>Category | 黑龙江<br>HL | 辽宁<br>LN | 河北<br>HE | 北京<br>BJ | 吉林<br>JL | 山西<br>SX | 陕西<br>SN | 河南<br>HA | 宁夏<br>NX | 内蒙古<br>NM | 青海<br>QH | 甘肃<br>GS | 上海<br>SH | 福建<br>FJ | 江西<br>JX | 江苏<br>JS | 浙江<br>ZJ | 山东<br>SD | 湖北<br>HB | 四川<br>SC | 广西<br>GX | 湖南<br>HN | 广东<br>GD | 贵州<br>GZ | 全国平均<br>AVG |
|---|---|---|---|---|---|---|---|---|---|---|---|---|---|---|---|---|---|---|---|---|---|---|---|---|---|
| 酒类<br>Alcohol beverages | ND | ND | ND | ND | ND | ND | ND | ND | ND | ND | ND | ND | ND | ND | ND | ND | ND | ND | ND | ND | ND | ND | ND | ND | 0.00 |

注：未检出（ND）按 0 计
Note: values not detected (ND) were treated as being equal to 0

附表 4-5　第六次中国总膳食研究膳食样品中丙溴磷的含量（单位：μg/kg）
Annexed Table 4-5　Levels of profenofos in food samples from the 6th China TDS (Unit: μg/kg)

| 膳食类别<br>Category | 黑龙江<br>HL | 辽宁<br>LN | 河北<br>HE | 北京<br>BJ | 吉林<br>JL | 山西<br>SX | 陕西<br>SN | 河南<br>HA | 宁夏<br>NX | 内蒙古<br>NM | 青海<br>QH | 甘肃<br>GS | 上海<br>SH | 福建<br>FJ | 江西<br>JX | 江苏<br>JS | 浙江<br>ZJ | 山东<br>SD | 湖北<br>HB | 四川<br>SC | 广西<br>GX | 湖南<br>HN | 广东<br>GD | 贵州<br>GZ | 全国平均<br>AVG |
|---|---|---|---|---|---|---|---|---|---|---|---|---|---|---|---|---|---|---|---|---|---|---|---|---|---|
| 谷类<br>Cereals | ND | ND | ND | ND | ND | ND | ND | ND | ND | ND | ND | ND | ND | ND | ND | ND | ND | ND | ND | ND | ND | ND | ND | ND | 0.00 |
| 豆类<br>Legumes | ND | ND | ND | ND | ND | ND | 0.10 | ND | ND | ND | ND | ND | ND | ND | ND | ND | ND | ND | ND | ND | ND | ND | ND | ND | 0.00 |
| 薯类<br>Potatoes | ND | ND | ND | ND | ND | ND | ND | ND | ND | ND | ND | ND | ND | ND | ND | ND | ND | ND | ND | ND | ND | ND | ND | ND | 0.00 |
| 肉类<br>Meats | ND | ND | ND | ND | ND | ND | ND | 0.06 | ND | ND | 0.14 | ND | ND | ND | ND | ND | ND | ND | ND | ND | ND | ND | ND | ND | 0.01 |
| 蛋类<br>Eggs | ND | ND | ND | ND | ND | ND | ND | ND | ND | ND | ND | ND | ND | ND | ND | ND | ND | ND | ND | ND | ND | ND | ND | ND | 0.00 |
| 水产类<br>Aquatic foods | ND | ND | ND | ND | ND | ND | ND | ND | ND | ND | ND | ND | ND | ND | ND | ND | ND | ND | ND | ND | ND | ND | ND | ND | 0.00 |
| 乳类<br>Dairy products | ND | ND | ND | ND | ND | ND | ND | ND | ND | ND | ND | ND | ND | ND | ND | ND | ND | ND | ND | ND | ND | ND | ND | ND | 0.00 |

续表

| 膳食类别<br>Category | 黑龙江<br>HL | 辽宁<br>LN | 河北<br>HE | 北京<br>BJ | 吉林<br>JL | 山西<br>SX | 陕西<br>SN | 河南<br>HA | 宁夏<br>NX | 内蒙古<br>NM | 青海<br>QH | 甘肃<br>GS | 上海<br>SH | 福建<br>FJ | 江西<br>JX | 江苏<br>JS | 浙江<br>ZJ | 山东<br>SD | 湖北<br>HB | 四川<br>SC | 广西<br>GX | 湖南<br>HN | 广东<br>GD | 贵州<br>GZ | 全国平均<br>AVG |
|---|---|---|---|---|---|---|---|---|---|---|---|---|---|---|---|---|---|---|---|---|---|---|---|---|---|
| 蔬菜类<br>Vegetables | ND | ND | 3.00 | ND | ND | 0.47 | 0.09 | 1.00 | ND | ND | 1.40 | 3.62 | 2.74 | 0.15 | 6.55 | ND | ND | ND | 1.62 | ND | 0.55 | 0.54 | 5.73 | ND | 1.14 |
| 水果类<br>Fruits | ND | 0.64 | ND | 0.17 | 0.34 | ND | 0.31 | ND | ND | ND | ND | 15.65 | ND | 0.67 | ND | ND | ND | ND | 0.25 | 0.20 | ND | 0.20 | ND | 0.86 | 0.80 |
| 糖类<br>Sugar | ND | ND | ND | ND | ND | ND | ND | ND | ND | ND | ND | ND | 0.08 | ND | ND | ND | ND | ND | ND | ND | ND | ND | ND | ND | 0.00 |
| 水及饮料类<br>Water and beverages | ND | ND | ND | ND | ND | ND | ND | ND | ND | ND | ND | ND | ND | ND | ND | ND | ND | ND | ND | ND | ND | ND | ND | ND | 0.00 |
| 酒类<br>Alcohol beverages | ND | ND | ND | ND | ND | ND | ND | ND | ND | ND | ND | ND | ND | ND | ND | ND | ND | ND | ND | ND | ND | ND | ND | ND | 0.00 |

注：未检出（ND）按 0 计

Note: values not detected (ND) were treated as being equal to 0

附表 4-6　第六次中国总膳食研究膳食样品中氧乐果的含量（单位：μg/kg）

Annexed Table 4-6　Levels of omethoate in food samples from the 6$^{th}$ China TDS (Unit: μg/kg)

| 膳食类别<br>Category | 黑龙江<br>HL | 辽宁<br>LN | 河北<br>HE | 北京<br>BJ | 吉林<br>JL | 山西<br>SX | 陕西<br>SN | 河南<br>HA | 宁夏<br>NX | 内蒙古<br>NM | 青海<br>QH | 甘肃<br>GS | 上海<br>SH | 福建<br>FJ | 江西<br>JX | 江苏<br>JS | 浙江<br>ZJ | 山东<br>SD | 湖北<br>HB | 四川<br>SC | 广西<br>GX | 湖南<br>HN | 广东<br>GD | 贵州<br>GZ | 全国平均<br>AVG |
|---|---|---|---|---|---|---|---|---|---|---|---|---|---|---|---|---|---|---|---|---|---|---|---|---|---|
| 谷类<br>Cereals | ND | ND | ND | ND | ND | ND | ND | ND | ND | ND | ND | ND | ND | ND | ND | ND | ND | ND | ND | ND | ND | ND | ND | ND | 0.00 |
| 豆类<br>Legumes | ND | ND | ND | ND | ND | ND | ND | ND | ND | ND | ND | ND | ND | ND | ND | ND | ND | ND | ND | ND | ND | ND | ND | ND | 0.00 |
| 薯类<br>Potatoes | ND | ND | ND | ND | ND | ND | ND | ND | ND | ND | ND | ND | ND | ND | ND | ND | ND | ND | 0.10 | ND | ND | ND | ND | ND | 0.00 |

续表

| 膳食类别 Category | 黑龙江 HL | 辽宁 LN | 河北 HE | 北京 BJ | 吉林 JL | 山西 SX | 陕西 SN | 河南 HA | 宁夏 NX | 内蒙古 NM | 青海 QH | 甘肃 GS | 上海 SH | 福建 FJ | 江西 JX | 江苏 JS | 浙江 ZJ | 山东 SD | 湖北 HB | 四川 SC | 广西 GX | 湖南 HN | 广东 GD | 贵州 GZ | 全国平均 AVG |
|---|---|---|---|---|---|---|---|---|---|---|---|---|---|---|---|---|---|---|---|---|---|---|---|---|---|
| 肉类 Meats | ND | ND | ND | ND | ND | ND | ND | ND | ND | ND | ND | ND | ND | ND | ND | ND | ND | ND | ND | ND | ND | ND | ND | ND | 0.00 |
| 蛋类 Eggs | ND | ND | ND | ND | ND | ND | ND | ND | ND | ND | ND | ND | ND | ND | ND | ND | ND | ND | ND | ND | ND | ND | ND | ND | 0.00 |
| 水产类 Aquatic foods | ND | ND | ND | ND | ND | ND | ND | ND | ND | ND | ND | ND | ND | ND | ND | ND | ND | ND | ND | ND | ND | ND | ND | ND | 0.00 |
| 乳类 Dairy products | ND | ND | ND | ND | ND | ND | ND | ND | ND | ND | ND | ND | ND | ND | ND | ND | ND | ND | ND | ND | ND | ND | ND | ND | 0.00 |
| 蔬菜类 Vegetables | ND | 1.68 | ND | ND | 14.45 | ND | ND | ND | ND | ND | ND | ND | 0.23 | ND | ND | ND | ND | ND | 0.58 | ND | ND | 6.96 | 0.11 | ND | 1.00 |
| 水果类 Fruits | ND | 3.15 | ND | ND | ND | ND | 0.19 | ND | ND | ND | ND | ND | ND | ND | ND | ND | ND | ND | 0.14 | ND | 0.31 | ND | ND | ND | 0.16 |
| 糖类 Sugar | ND | ND | ND | ND | ND | ND | ND | ND | ND | ND | ND | ND | ND | ND | ND | ND | ND | ND | ND | ND | ND | ND | ND | ND | 0.00 |
| 水及饮料类 Water and beverages | ND | ND | ND | ND | ND | ND | ND | ND | ND | ND | ND | ND | ND | ND | ND | 0.25 | ND | ND | ND | ND | ND | ND | 0.10 | ND | 0.01 |
| 酒类 Alcohol beverages | ND | ND | ND | ND | ND | ND | ND | ND | ND | ND | ND | ND | ND | ND | ND | ND | ND | ND | ND | ND | ND | ND | ND | ND | 0.00 |

注：未检出（ND）按 0 计

Note: values not detected (ND) were treated as being equal to 0

附表 4-7 第六次中国总膳食研究膳食样品中乐果的含量（单位：μg/kg）

Annexed Table 4-7 Levels of dimethoate in food samples from the 6th China TDS (Unit: μg/kg)

| 膳食类别 Category | 黑龙江 HL | 辽宁 LN | 河北 HE | 北京 BJ | 吉林 JL | 山西 SX | 陕西 SN | 河南 HA | 宁夏 NX | 内蒙古 NM | 青海 QH | 甘肃 GS | 上海 SH | 福建 FJ | 江西 JX | 江苏 JS | 浙江 ZJ | 山东 SD | 湖北 HB | 四川 SC | 广西 GX | 湖南 HN | 广东 GD | 贵州 GZ | 全国平均 AVG |
|---|---|---|---|---|---|---|---|---|---|---|---|---|---|---|---|---|---|---|---|---|---|---|---|---|---|
| 谷类 Cereals | ND | ND | ND | ND | ND | ND | ND | ND | ND | ND | ND | ND | ND | ND | ND | ND | ND | ND | ND | ND | ND | ND | ND | ND | 0.00 |
| 豆类 Legumes | ND | ND | 0.07 | ND | ND | ND | ND | ND | ND | ND | ND | ND | ND | ND | ND | ND | ND | ND | ND | ND | ND | ND | ND | ND | 0.00 |
| 薯类 Potatoes | ND | ND | ND | ND | ND | ND | ND | ND | ND | ND | ND | ND | ND | ND | ND | ND | ND | ND | ND | ND | ND | ND | ND | ND | 0.00 |
| 肉类 Meats | ND | ND | ND | ND | ND | ND | ND | ND | ND | ND | ND | ND | ND | ND | ND | ND | ND | ND | ND | ND | ND | ND | ND | ND | 0.00 |
| 蛋类 Eggs | ND | ND | ND | ND | ND | ND | ND | ND | ND | ND | ND | ND | ND | ND | ND | ND | ND | ND | ND | ND | ND | ND | ND | ND | 0.00 |
| 水产类 Aquatic foods | ND | ND | ND | ND | ND | ND | ND | ND | ND | ND | ND | ND | ND | ND | ND | ND | ND | ND | ND | ND | ND | ND | ND | ND | 0.00 |
| 乳类 Dairy products | ND | ND | ND | ND | ND | ND | ND | ND | ND | ND | ND | ND | ND | ND | ND | ND | ND | ND | ND | ND | ND | ND | ND | ND | 0.00 |
| 蔬菜类 Vegetables | ND | ND | ND | 0.05 | ND | ND | ND | ND | ND | ND | ND | 1.49 | ND | ND | ND | ND | ND | ND | ND | ND | ND | 68.75 | 0.08 | ND | 2.93 |
| 水果类 Fruits | ND | ND | ND | ND | ND | ND | 2.52 | ND | ND | ND | ND | ND | ND | ND | ND | ND | ND | ND | ND | ND | ND | ND | ND | ND | 0.10 |
| 糖类 Sugar | ND | ND | ND | ND | ND | ND | ND | ND | ND | ND | ND | ND | ND | ND | ND | ND | ND | ND | ND | ND | ND | ND | ND | ND | 0.00 |
| 水及饮料类 Water and beverages | ND | ND | ND | ND | 0.04 | ND | ND | ND | ND | ND | ND | ND | 0.05 | ND | ND | 0.11 | ND | ND | ND | ND | ND | ND | ND | ND | 0.01 |

续表

| 膳食类别<br>Category | 黑龙江<br>HL | 辽宁<br>LN | 河北<br>HE | 北京<br>BJ | 吉林<br>JL | 山西<br>SX | 陕西<br>SN | 河南<br>HA | 宁夏<br>NX | 内蒙古<br>NM | 青海<br>QH | 甘肃<br>GS | 上海<br>SH | 福建<br>FJ | 江西<br>JX | 江苏<br>JS | 浙江<br>ZJ | 山东<br>SD | 湖北<br>HB | 四川<br>SC | 广西<br>GX | 湖南<br>HN | 广东<br>GD | 贵州<br>GZ | 全国平均<br>AVG |
|---|---|---|---|---|---|---|---|---|---|---|---|---|---|---|---|---|---|---|---|---|---|---|---|---|---|
| 酒类<br>Alcohol beverages | ND | ND | ND | ND | ND | ND | ND | ND | ND | ND | ND | ND | ND | ND | ND | ND | ND | ND | ND | ND | ND | ND | ND | ND | 0.00 |

注：未检出（ND）按 0 计
Note: values not detected (ND) were treated as being equal to 0

附表 4-8　第六次中国总膳食研究膳食样品中甲胺磷的含量（单位：μg/kg）

Annexed Table 4-8　Levels of methamidophos in food samples from the 6th China TDS (Unit: μg/kg)

| 膳食类别<br>Category | 黑龙江<br>HL | 辽宁<br>LN | 河北<br>HE | 北京<br>BJ | 吉林<br>JL | 山西<br>SX | 陕西<br>SN | 河南<br>HA | 宁夏<br>NX | 内蒙古<br>NM | 青海<br>QH | 甘肃<br>GS | 上海<br>SH | 福建<br>FJ | 江西<br>JX | 江苏<br>JS | 浙江<br>ZJ | 山东<br>SD | 湖北<br>HB | 四川<br>SC | 广西<br>GX | 湖南<br>HN | 广东<br>GD | 贵州<br>GZ | 全国平均<br>AVG |
|---|---|---|---|---|---|---|---|---|---|---|---|---|---|---|---|---|---|---|---|---|---|---|---|---|---|
| 谷类<br>Cereals | ND | ND | ND | ND | ND | ND | ND | ND | ND | ND | ND | ND | ND | ND | ND | ND | ND | ND | ND | ND | ND | ND | ND | ND | 0.00 |
| 豆类<br>Legumes | ND | ND | 0.13 | ND | ND | ND | ND | ND | ND | ND | ND | ND | ND | ND | ND | ND | ND | ND | ND | ND | ND | ND | ND | ND | 0.01 |
| 薯类<br>Potatoes | ND | ND | ND | ND | ND | ND | ND | ND | ND | ND | ND | ND | ND | ND | ND | ND | ND | ND | 0.08 | ND | ND | ND | ND | ND | 0.00 |
| 肉类<br>Meats | ND | ND | ND | ND | ND | ND | ND | ND | ND | ND | ND | ND | ND | ND | ND | ND | ND | ND | ND | ND | ND | ND | ND | ND | 0.00 |
| 蛋类<br>Eggs | ND | ND | ND | ND | ND | ND | ND | ND | ND | ND | ND | ND | ND | ND | ND | ND | ND | ND | ND | ND | ND | ND | ND | ND | 0.00 |
| 水产类<br>Aquatic foods | ND | ND | ND | ND | ND | ND | ND | ND | ND | ND | ND | ND | ND | ND | ND | ND | ND | ND | ND | ND | ND | ND | ND | ND | 0.00 |
| 乳类<br>Dairy products | ND | ND | ND | ND | ND | ND | ND | ND | ND | ND | ND | ND | ND | ND | ND | ND | ND | ND | ND | ND | ND | ND | ND | ND | 0.00 |

续表

| 膳食类别 Category | 黑龙江 HL | 辽宁 LN | 河北 HE | 北京 BJ | 吉林 JL | 山西 SX | 陕西 SN | 河南 HA | 宁夏 NX | 内蒙古 NM | 青海 QH | 甘肃 GS | 上海 SH | 福建 FJ | 江西 JX | 江苏 JS | 浙江 ZJ | 山东 SD | 湖北 HB | 四川 SC | 广西 GX | 湖南 HN | 广东 GD | 贵州 GZ | 全国平均 AVG |
|---|---|---|---|---|---|---|---|---|---|---|---|---|---|---|---|---|---|---|---|---|---|---|---|---|---|
| 蔬菜类 Vegetables | ND | ND | ND | ND | ND | ND | ND | ND | ND | ND | ND | ND | ND | ND | ND | ND | ND | ND | ND | ND | ND | ND | ND | ND | 0.00 |
| 水果类 Fruits | ND | ND | ND | ND | ND | ND | ND | 0.13 | ND | ND | ND | ND | ND | ND | ND | ND | ND | ND | ND | ND | ND | ND | ND | ND | 0.01 |
| 糖类 Sugar | ND | ND | ND | ND | ND | ND | ND | ND | ND | ND | ND | ND | ND | ND | ND | ND | ND | ND | ND | ND | ND | ND | ND | ND | 0.00 |
| 水及饮料类 Water and beverages | ND | ND | ND | ND | ND | ND | ND | ND | ND | ND | ND | ND | ND | ND | ND | ND | ND | ND | ND | ND | ND | ND | ND | ND | 0.00 |
| 酒类 Alcohol beverages | ND | ND | ND | ND | ND | ND | ND | ND | ND | ND | ND | ND | ND | ND | ND | ND | ND | ND | ND | ND | ND | ND | ND | ND | 0.00 |

注：未检出（ND）按 0 计
Note: values not detected (ND) were treated as being equal to 0

附表 4-9　第六次中国总膳食研究膳食样品中二嗪磷的含量（单位：μg/kg）
Annexed Table 4-9　Levels of diazinon in food samples from the 6$^{th}$ China TDS (Unit: μg/kg)

| 膳食类别 Category | 黑龙江 HL | 辽宁 LN | 河北 HE | 北京 BJ | 吉林 JL | 山西 SX | 陕西 SN | 河南 HA | 宁夏 NX | 内蒙古 NM | 青海 QH | 甘肃 GS | 上海 SH | 福建 FJ | 江西 JX | 江苏 JS | 浙江 ZJ | 山东 SD | 湖北 HB | 四川 SC | 广西 GX | 湖南 HN | 广东 GD | 贵州 GZ | 全国平均 AVG |
|---|---|---|---|---|---|---|---|---|---|---|---|---|---|---|---|---|---|---|---|---|---|---|---|---|---|
| 谷类 Cereals | ND | ND | ND | ND | ND | ND | ND | ND | ND | ND | ND | ND | ND | ND | ND | ND | ND | ND | ND | ND | ND | ND | ND | ND | 0.00 |
| 豆类 Legumes | ND | ND | ND | ND | ND | ND | ND | ND | ND | ND | ND | ND | ND | ND | ND | ND | ND | ND | ND | ND | ND | ND | ND | ND | 0.00 |
| 薯类 Potatoes | ND | ND | ND | ND | ND | ND | ND | ND | ND | ND | ND | ND | ND | ND | ND | ND | ND | ND | ND | ND | ND | ND | ND | ND | 0.00 |

续表

| 膳食类别 Category | 黑龙江 HL | 辽宁 LN | 河北 HE | 北京 BJ | 吉林 JL | 山西 SX | 陕西 SN | 河南 HA | 宁夏 NX | 内蒙古 NM | 青海 QH | 甘肃 GS | 上海 SH | 福建 FJ | 江西 JX | 江苏 JS | 浙江 ZJ | 山东 SD | 湖北 HB | 四川 SC | 广西 GX | 湖南 HN | 广东 GD | 贵州 GZ | 全国平均 AVG |
|---|---|---|---|---|---|---|---|---|---|---|---|---|---|---|---|---|---|---|---|---|---|---|---|---|---|
| 肉类 Meats | ND | ND | ND | ND | ND | ND | ND | ND | ND | ND | ND | ND | ND | ND | ND | ND | ND | 0.18 | ND | ND | ND | ND | ND | ND | 0.01 |
| 蛋类 Eggs | ND | ND | ND | ND | ND | ND | ND | ND | ND | ND | ND | ND | ND | ND | ND | ND | ND | ND | ND | ND | ND | ND | ND | ND | 0.00 |
| 水产类 Aquatic foods | ND | ND | ND | ND | ND | ND | 0.07 | ND | ND | ND | ND | ND | ND | ND | ND | ND | ND | ND | ND | ND | ND | ND | ND | ND | 0.00 |
| 乳类 Dairy products | ND | ND | ND | ND | ND | ND | ND | ND | ND | ND | ND | ND | ND | ND | ND | ND | ND | ND | ND | ND | ND | ND | ND | ND | 0.00 |
| 蔬菜类 Vegetables | ND | ND | ND | ND | ND | ND | ND | ND | ND | ND | ND | ND | ND | ND | ND | ND | ND | ND | ND | ND | ND | ND | ND | ND | 0.00 |
| 水果类 Fruits | ND | ND | ND | ND | ND | ND | ND | ND | ND | ND | ND | ND | ND | ND | ND | ND | ND | ND | ND | ND | ND | ND | ND | ND | 0.00 |
| 糖类 Sugar | ND | ND | ND | ND | ND | ND | ND | ND | ND | ND | ND | ND | ND | ND | ND | ND | ND | ND | ND | ND | ND | ND | ND | ND | 0.00 |
| 水及饮料类 Water and beverages | ND | ND | ND | ND | ND | ND | ND | ND | ND | ND | ND | ND | ND | ND | ND | ND | ND | ND | ND | ND | ND | ND | ND | ND | 0.00 |
| 酒类 Alcohol beverages | ND | ND | ND | ND | ND | ND | ND | ND | ND | ND | ND | ND | ND | ND | ND | ND | ND | ND | ND | ND | ND | ND | ND | ND | 0.00 |

注：未检出（ND）按 0 计

Note: values not detected (ND) were treated as being equal to 0

附表 4-10 第六次中国总膳食研究的毒死蜱膳食摄入量 [单位:ng/(kg bw·d)]

Annexed Table 4-10 Dietary intakes of chlorpyrifos from the 6th China TDS [Unit: ng/(kg bw·d)]

| 膳食类别 Category | 黑龙江 HL | 辽宁 LN | 河北 HE | 北京 BJ | 吉林 JL | 山西 SX | 陕西 SN | 河南 HA | 宁夏 NX | 内蒙古 NM | 青海 QH | 甘肃 GS | 上海 SH | 福建 FJ | 江西 JX | 江苏 JS | 浙江 ZJ | 山东 SD | 湖北 HB | 四川 SC | 广西 GX | 湖南 HN | 广东 GD | 贵州 GZ | 全国平均 AVG |
|---|---|---|---|---|---|---|---|---|---|---|---|---|---|---|---|---|---|---|---|---|---|---|---|---|---|
| 谷类 Cereals | 0.000 | 0.000 | 4.768 | 4.164 | 0.000 | 0.000 | 3.955 | 3.461 | 0.000 | 1.620 | 0.000 | 0.000 | 2.521 | 7.339 | 1.436 | 0.000 | 6.473 | 3.881 | 6.366 | 97.180 | 7.804 | 0.000 | 2.597 | 0.000 | 6.399 |
| 豆类 Legumes | 1.723 | 3.181 | 1.165 | 0.965 | 0.000 | 0.352 | 0.532 | 1.982 | 0.065 | 0.000 | 0.000 | 0.072 | 1.803 | 3.679 | 0.000 | 2.509 | 1.930 | 0.977 | 3.411 | 0.357 | 0.687 | 0.000 | 1.280 | 0.000 | 1.111 |
| 薯类 Potatoes | 0.000 | 0.250 | 2.154 | 2.559 | 0.000 | 1.719 | 0.000 | 0.000 | 0.000 | 0.857 | 0.898 | 0.000 | 0.000 | 3.008 | 0.491 | 0.000 | 0.000 | 1.125 | 5.256 | 0.000 | 0.496 | 1.275 | 0.724 | 0.000 | 0.867 |
| 肉类 Meats | 0.000 | 0.241 | 1.253 | 3.139 | 0.000 | 1.038 | 0.580 | 0.000 | 0.000 | 8.012 | 0.446 | 0.113 | 0.000 | 2.187 | 0.000 | 0.000 | 0.000 | 1.674 | 1.021 | 0.295 | 2.833 | 0.000 | 0.311 | 0.000 | 0.964 |
| 蛋类 Eggs | 0.000 | 0.187 | 1.268 | 2.893 | 0.000 | 0.265 | 0.000 | 0.000 | 0.000 | 0.000 | 0.068 | 0.000 | 0.000 | 3.574 | 0.000 | 0.000 | 0.000 | 0.544 | 1.441 | 0.000 | 0.540 | 0.000 | 0.000 | 0.000 | 0.449 |
| 水产类 Aquatic foods | 0.293 | 0.000 | 0.138 | 1.173 | 0.000 | 0.000 | 0.051 | 0.049 | 0.000 | 0.724 | 0.043 | 0.074 | 0.169 | 10.752 | 0.626 | 0.000 | 0.334 | 0.361 | 1.771 | 0.436 | 5.316 | 2.664 | 1.919 | 0.103 | 1.125 |
| 乳类 Dairy products | 0.000 | 0.000 | 0.000 | 0.000 | 0.000 | 0.000 | 0.000 | 0.000 | 0.000 | 0.000 | 0.000 | 0.000 | 0.000 | 0.000 | 0.000 | 0.000 | 0.000 | 0.000 | 0.000 | 0.000 | 0.000 | 0.000 | 0.000 | 0.000 | 0.000 |
| 蔬菜类 Vegetables | 0.000 | 116.600 | 7.259 | 14.370 | 2.224 | 5.436 | 12.140 | 0.589 | 2.642 | 7.164 | 14.370 | 26.370 | 4.788 | 44.570 | 25.110 | 0.000 | 3.280 | 12.390 | 405.800 | 6.025 | 61.980 | 2.426 | 8.308 | 6.000 | 32.910 |
| 水果类 Fruits | 1.994 | 22.320 | 0.393 | 5.909 | 29.680 | 0.408 | 0.000 | 2.796 | 0.000 | 0.000 | 0.000 | 0.161 | 9.300 | 20.014 | 0.186 | 0.085 | 0.185 | 0.564 | 2.125 | 0.000 | 0.000 | 2.970 | 0.537 | 0.268 | 4.162 |
| 糖类 Sugar | 0.000 | 0.000 | 0.000 | 0.000 | 0.000 | 0.000 | 0.000 | 0.000 | 0.000 | 0.000 | 0.000 | 0.000 | 0.137 | 0.000 | 0.000 | 0.000 | 0.000 | 0.000 | 0.000 | 0.000 | 0.000 | 0.000 | 0.000 | 0.000 | 0.006 |
| 水及饮料类 Water and beverages | 0.000 | 0.000 | 0.000 | 0.000 | 0.000 | 0.000 | 0.000 | 0.000 | 0.000 | 0.000 | 0.000 | 0.000 | 0.000 | 0.000 | 0.000 | 0.000 | 0.000 | 0.000 | 0.000 | 0.000 | 0.000 | 0.000 | 0.000 | 0.000 | 0.000 |

续表

| 膳食类别 Category | 黑龙江 HL | 辽宁 LN | 河北 HE | 北京 BJ | 吉林 JL | 山西 SX | 陕西 SN | 河南 HA | 宁夏 NX | 内蒙古 NM | 青海 QH | 甘肃 GS | 上海 SH | 福建 FJ | 江西 JX | 江苏 JS | 浙江 ZJ | 山东 SD | 湖北 HB | 四川 SC | 广西 GX | 湖南 HN | 广东 GD | 贵州 GZ | 全国平均 AVG |
|---|---|---|---|---|---|---|---|---|---|---|---|---|---|---|---|---|---|---|---|---|---|---|---|---|---|
| 酒类 Alcohol beverages | 0.000 | 0.000 | 0.000 | 0.000 | 0.000 | 0.000 | 0.000 | 0.000 | 0.000 | 0.000 | 0.000 | 0.000 | 0.000 | 0.000 | 0.000 | 0.000 | 0.000 | 0.000 | 0.000 | 0.000 | 0.000 | 0.000 | 0.000 | 0.000 | 0.000 |
| 合计 SUM | 4.01 | 142.81 | 18.40 | 35.17 | 31.91 | 9.22 | 17.25 | 8.88 | 2.71 | 18.38 | 15.82 | 26.79 | 18.72 | 95.12 | 27.85 | 2.59 | 12.20 | 21.52 | 427.15 | 104.30 | 79.65 | 9.34 | 15.68 | 6.37 | 47.99 |

附表 4-11 第六次中国总膳食研究的敌敌畏膳食摄入量 [单位: ng/(kg bw·d)]

Annexed Table 4-11 Dietary intakes of dichlorvos from the 6$^{th}$ China TDS [Unit: ng/(kg bw·d)]

| 膳食类别 Category | 黑龙江 HL | 辽宁 LN | 河北 HE | 北京 BJ | 吉林 JL | 山西 SX | 陕西 SN | 河南 HA | 宁夏 NX | 内蒙古 NM | 青海 QH | 甘肃 GS | 上海 SH | 福建 FJ | 江西 JX | 江苏 JS | 浙江 ZJ | 山东 SD | 湖北 HB | 四川 SC | 广西 GX | 湖南 HN | 广东 GD | 贵州 GZ | 全国平均 AVG |
|---|---|---|---|---|---|---|---|---|---|---|---|---|---|---|---|---|---|---|---|---|---|---|---|---|---|
| 谷类 Cereals | 1.498 | 9.320 | 15.210 | 1.461 | 0.000 | 0.000 | 0.000 | 0.000 | 0.000 | 0.000 | 0.000 | 1.139 | 0.000 | 0.000 | 0.000 | 0.000 | 0.000 | 272.800 | 1.618 | 0.000 | 0.000 | 0.000 | 0.000 | 0.000 | 12.63 |
| 豆类 Legumes | 0.274 | 0.000 | 0.104 | 0.000 | 0.000 | 0.000 | 0.000 | 3.689 | 0.378 | 0.000 | 0.000 | 0.000 | 0.000 | 0.000 | 0.000 | 0.000 | 0.000 | 12.250 | 0.069 | 0.000 | 0.000 | 0.000 | 0.000 | 0.000 | 0.698 |
| 薯类 Potatoes | 0.211 | 0.000 | 0.000 | 0.000 | 0.000 | 0.000 | 0.000 | 0.000 | 0.000 | 0.000 | 0.000 | 0.000 | 0.000 | 0.000 | 0.000 | 0.000 | 0.000 | 12.000 | 0.000 | 0.000 | 0.000 | 0.000 | 0.000 | 0.000 | 0.509 |
| 肉类 Meats | 0.000 | 0.000 | 0.000 | 0.069 | 0.126 | 0.000 | 0.000 | 0.000 | 0.000 | 0.000 | 0.000 | 0.000 | 0.000 | 0.000 | 0.000 | 0.000 | 0.000 | 20.830 | 0.000 | 0.000 | 0.000 | 0.000 | 0.000 | 0.000 | 0.876 |
| 蛋类 Eggs | 0.000 | 0.000 | 0.000 | 0.000 | 0.000 | 0.000 | 0.005 | 0.000 | 0.000 | 0.000 | 0.000 | 0.000 | 0.000 | 0.000 | 0.000 | 0.000 | 0.000 | 0.245 | 0.000 | 0.000 | 0.000 | 0.000 | 0.000 | 0.000 | 0.010 |
| 水产类 Aquatic foods | 0.436 | 0.000 | 0.000 | 0.430 | 0.000 | 0.000 | 0.000 | 0.000 | 0.000 | 0.000 | 0.000 | 0.000 | 0.000 | 0.000 | 0.000 | 0.000 | 0.000 | 2.314 | 0.000 | 0.000 | 0.000 | 0.000 | 0.000 | 0.000 | 0.133 |
| 乳类 Dairy products | 0.019 | 0.000 | 0.068 | 0.000 | 0.000 | 0.065 | 0.000 | 0.056 | 0.000 | 0.035 | 0.000 | 0.000 | 0.000 | 0.000 | 0.000 | 0.129 | 0.000 | 1.745 | 0.000 | 0.000 | 0.000 | 0.000 | 0.000 | 0.029 | 0.089 |

续表

| 膳食类别 Category | 黑龙江 HL | 辽宁 LN | 河北 HE | 北京 BJ | 吉林 JL | 山西 SX | 陕西 SN | 河南 HA | 宁夏 NX | 内蒙古 NM | 青海 QH | 甘肃 GS | 上海 SH | 福建 FJ | 江西 JX | 江苏 JS | 浙江 ZJ | 山东 SD | 湖北 HB | 四川 SC | 广西 GX | 湖南 HN | 广东 GD | 贵州 GZ | 全国平均 AVG |
|---|---|---|---|---|---|---|---|---|---|---|---|---|---|---|---|---|---|---|---|---|---|---|---|---|---|
| 蔬菜类 Vegetables | 1.378 | 0.000 | 2.636 | 0.000 | 0.000 | 0.000 | 0.000 | 0.000 | 0.000 | 0.000 | 0.000 | 0.000 | 0.464 | 0.000 | 0.000 | 0.473 | 0.000 | 235.3 | 0.000 | 0.000 | 0.000 | 0.000 | 0.000 | 0.000 | 10.010 |
| 水果类 Fruits | 0.061 | 0.000 | 0.000 | 0.000 | 0.000 | 0.000 | 0.000 | 0.000 | 0.000 | 0.000 | 0.000 | 0.000 | 0.000 | 0.000 | 0.000 | 0.000 | 0.000 | 11.56 | 0.000 | 0.000 | 0.000 | 0.000 | 0.000 | 0.000 | 0.484 |
| 糖类 Sugar | 0.004 | 0.000 | 0.000 | 0.000 | 0.000 | 0.001 | 0.000 | 0.000 | 0.000 | 0.000 | 0.000 | 0.000 | 0.000 | 0.000 | 0.000 | 0.000 | 0.000 | 0.038 | 0.000 | 0.000 | 0.000 | 0.000 | 0.000 | 0.000 | 0.002 |
| 水及饮料类 Water and beverages | 1.626 | 0.000 | 0.000 | 0.000 | 0.000 | 0.000 | 0.000 | 0.000 | 0.000 | 2.279 | 0.000 | 0.000 | 0.000 | 0.000 | 0.000 | 0.000 | 0.000 | 326.5 | 0.000 | 0.000 | 0.000 | 1.990 | 0.000 | 0.000 | 13.850 |
| 酒类 Alcohol beverages | 0.038 | 0.000 | 0.000 | 0.000 | 0.000 | 0.000 | 0.002 | 0.239 | 0.000 | 0.000 | 0.000 | 0.000 | 0.000 | 0.000 | 0.000 | 0.000 | 0.000 | 0.187 | 0.016 | 0.000 | 0.000 | 0.014 | 0.000 | 0.000 | 0.021 |
| 合计 SUM | 5.544 | 9.320 | 18.020 | 1.960 | 0.126 | 0.066 | 0.007 | 3.983 | 0.378 | 2.313 | 0.000 | 1.139 | 0.464 | 0.000 | 0.000 | 0.602 | 0.000 | 895.682 | 1.703 | 0.000 | 0.000 | 2.004 | 0.000 | 0.029 | 39.306 |

附表 4-12 第六次中国总膳食研究的乙酰甲胺磷膳食摄入量 [单位：ng/(kg bw·d)]

Annexed Table 4-12　Dietary intakes of acephate from the 6$^{th}$ China TDS [Unit: ng/(kg bw·d)]

| 膳食类别 Category | 黑龙江 HL | 辽宁 LN | 河北 HE | 北京 BJ | 吉林 JL | 山西 SX | 陕西 SN | 河南 HA | 宁夏 NX | 内蒙古 NM | 青海 QH | 甘肃 GS | 上海 SH | 福建 FJ | 江西 JX | 江苏 JS | 浙江 ZJ | 山东 SD | 湖北 HB | 四川 SC | 广西 GX | 湖南 HN | 广东 GD | 贵州 GZ | 全国平均 AVG |
|---|---|---|---|---|---|---|---|---|---|---|---|---|---|---|---|---|---|---|---|---|---|---|---|---|---|
| 谷类 Cereals | 0.000 | 0.000 | 0.000 | 0.000 | 0.000 | 0.000 | 0.000 | 0.000 | 0.000 | 0.000 | 0.000 | 0.000 | 0.000 | 0.000 | 0.000 | 0.000 | 0.000 | 0.000 | 0.000 | 0.000 | 0.000 | 0.000 | 0.000 | 0.000 | 0.000 |
| 豆类 Legumes | 0.000 | 0.000 | 0.000 | 0.000 | 0.000 | 0.000 | 1.412 | 0.000 | 0.000 | 0.000 | 0.000 | 0.170 | 0.000 | 0.000 | 0.000 | 1.313 | 0.000 | 0.000 | 0.000 | 0.732 | 0.000 | 0.000 | 0.000 | 0.524 | 0.173 |
| 薯类 Potatoes | 0.000 | 0.000 | 0.000 | 0.000 | 0.000 | 0.000 | 2.117 | 0.000 | 0.000 | 0.000 | 0.233 | 0.000 | 0.000 | 0.000 | 0.000 | 1.264 | 0.000 | 0.000 | 0.000 | 2.118 | 0.000 | 0.208 | 0.000 | 0.429 | 0.265 |

续表

| 膳食类别<br>Category | 黑龙江<br>HL | 辽宁<br>LN | 河北<br>HE | 北京<br>BJ | 吉林<br>JL | 山西<br>SX | 陕西<br>SN | 河南<br>HA | 宁夏<br>NX | 内蒙古<br>NM | 青海<br>QH | 甘肃<br>GS | 上海<br>SH | 福建<br>FJ | 江西<br>JX | 江苏<br>JS | 浙江<br>ZJ | 山东<br>SD | 湖北<br>HB | 四川<br>SC | 广西<br>GX | 湖南<br>HN | 广东<br>GD | 贵州<br>GZ | 全国平均<br>AVG |
|---|---|---|---|---|---|---|---|---|---|---|---|---|---|---|---|---|---|---|---|---|---|---|---|---|---|
| 肉类 Meats | 0.000 | 0.000 | 0.000 | 0.000 | 0.000 | 0.000 | 0.670 | 0.000 | 0.000 | 0.000 | 0.723 | 0.227 | 0.000 | 0.000 | 0.000 | 3.753 | 0.000 | 0.000 | 0.000 | 3.260 | 0.000 | 0.520 | 0.000 | 1.535 | 0.445 |
| 蛋类 Eggs | 0.000 | 0.000 | 0.000 | 0.000 | 0.000 | 0.000 | 0.424 | 0.000 | 0.000 | 0.000 | 0.000 | 0.302 | 0.000 | 0.000 | 0.000 | 0.971 | 0.000 | 0.000 | 0.000 | 0.255 | 0.000 | 0.108 | 0.000 | 0.109 | 0.090 |
| 水产类 Aquatic foods | 0.000 | 0.000 | 0.000 | 0.000 | 0.000 | 0.000 | 0.115 | 0.000 | 0.000 | 0.000 | 0.017 | 0.000 | 0.000 | 0.000 | 0.000 | 0.597 | 0.000 | 0.000 | 0.000 | 0.123 | 0.000 | 0.256 | 0.000 | 0.013 | 0.047 |
| 乳类 Dairy products | 0.000 | 0.000 | 0.000 | 0.000 | 0.000 | 0.000 | 0.000 | 0.000 | 0.000 | 0.000 | 0.000 | 0.000 | 0.000 | 0.000 | 0.000 | 0.000 | 0.000 | 0.000 | 0.000 | 0.000 | 0.000 | 0.000 | 0.000 | 0.000 | 0.000 |
| 蔬菜类 Vegetables | 0.000 | 0.000 | 0.000 | 13.180 | 0.946 | 3.867 | 12.160 | 2.649 | 0.725 | 0.000 | 14.840 | 0.000 | 2.554 | 12.130 | 24.620 | 26.830 | 7.927 | 1.833 | 3.502 | 0.000 | 3.361 | 8.468 | 7.198 | 1.139 | 6.164 |
| 水果类 Fruits | 0.000 | 0.000 | 0.000 | 0.000 | 0.000 | 0.000 | 0.000 | 0.227 | 0.000 | 0.000 | 0.000 | 0.000 | 0.000 | 0.000 | 0.000 | 0.000 | 0.000 | 0.000 | 0.000 | 0.000 | 0.000 | 0.000 | 0.000 | 0.000 | 0.009 |
| 糖类 Sugar | 0.000 | 0.000 | 0.000 | 0.000 | 0.000 | 0.000 | 0.000 | 0.000 | 0.000 | 0.000 | 0.000 | 0.000 | 0.000 | 0.000 | 0.000 | 0.000 | 0.000 | 0.000 | 0.000 | 0.000 | 0.000 | 0.000 | 0.000 | 0.000 | 0.000 |
| 水及饮料类 Water and beverages | 0.000 | 0.000 | 0.000 | 0.000 | 0.000 | 0.000 | 0.000 | 0.000 | 0.000 | 0.000 | 0.000 | 0.000 | 0.000 | 0.000 | 0.000 | 0.000 | 0.000 | 0.000 | 0.000 | 0.000 | 0.000 | 0.000 | 0.000 | 0.000 | 0.000 |
| 酒类 Alcohol beverages | 0.000 | 0.000 | 0.000 | 0.000 | 0.000 | 0.000 | 0.000 | 0.000 | 0.000 | 0.000 | 0.000 | 0.000 | 0.000 | 0.000 | 0.000 | 0.000 | 0.000 | 0.000 | 0.000 | 0.000 | 0.000 | 0.000 | 0.000 | 0.000 | 0.000 |
| 合计 SUM | 0.000 | 0.000 | 0.000 | 13.181 | 0.946 | 3.867 | 16.896 | 2.876 | 0.725 | 0.000 | 15.813 | 0.699 | 2.554 | 12.135 | 24.617 | 34.725 | 7.927 | 1.833 | 3.502 | 6.489 | 3.361 | 9.561 | 7.198 | 3.748 | 7.194 |

附表 4-13　第六次中国总膳食研究的三唑磷膳食摄入量 [单位: ng/(kg bw·d)]

Annexed Table 4-13　Dietary intakes of triazophos from the 6th China TDS [Unit: ng/(kg bw·d)]

| 膳食类别 Category | 黑龙江 HL | 辽宁 LN | 河北 HE | 北京 BJ | 吉林 JL | 山西 SX | 陕西 SN | 河南 HA | 宁夏 NX | 内蒙古 NM | 青海 QH | 甘肃 GS | 上海 SH | 福建 FJ | 江西 JX | 江苏 JS | 浙江 ZJ | 山东 SD | 湖北 HB | 四川 SC | 广西 GX | 湖南 HN | 广东 GD | 贵州 GZ | 全国平均 AVG |
|---|---|---|---|---|---|---|---|---|---|---|---|---|---|---|---|---|---|---|---|---|---|---|---|---|---|
| 谷类 Cereals | 0.000 | 0.000 | 2.420 | 0.000 | 0.000 | 0.000 | 0.000 | 0.000 | 0.000 | 0.000 | 0.000 | 0.000 | 0.000 | 0.000 | 2.953 | 2.979 | 2.005 | 0.000 | 1.504 | 1.953 | 3.137 | 1.143 | 0.625 | 0.000 | 0.780 |
| 豆类 Legumes | 0.000 | 0.000 | 0.000 | 0.000 | 0.000 | 0.000 | 0.000 | 0.000 | 0.000 | 0.000 | 0.000 | 0.035 | 0.000 | 0.000 | 0.000 | 0.000 | 0.000 | 0.000 | 0.000 | 0.000 | 0.000 | 0.000 | 0.000 | 0.000 | 0.001 |
| 薯类 Potatoes | 0.000 | 0.000 | 0.000 | 0.000 | 0.000 | 0.000 | 0.000 | 0.000 | 0.000 | 0.000 | 0.000 | 0.000 | 0.000 | 0.000 | 0.000 | 0.000 | 0.000 | 0.000 | 0.000 | 0.000 | 0.000 | 0.000 | 0.000 | 0.000 | 0.000 |
| 肉类 Meats | 0.000 | 0.000 | 0.000 | 0.000 | 0.000 | 0.000 | 0.000 | 0.054 | 0.000 | 0.000 | 0.000 | 0.000 | 0.000 | 0.000 | 0.000 | 0.000 | 0.000 | 0.000 | 0.000 | 0.000 | 0.000 | 0.000 | 0.000 | 0.000 | 0.002 |
| 蛋类 Eggs | 0.000 | 0.000 | 0.000 | 0.000 | 0.000 | 0.000 | 0.000 | 0.004 | 0.000 | 0.000 | 0.000 | 0.000 | 0.000 | 0.000 | 0.000 | 0.000 | 0.000 | 0.000 | 0.000 | 0.000 | 0.000 | 0.000 | 0.000 | 0.000 | 0.000 |
| 水产类 Aquatic foods | 0.000 | 0.000 | 0.000 | 0.000 | 0.000 | 0.000 | 0.000 | 0.000 | 0.000 | 0.000 | 0.000 | 0.000 | 0.067 | 0.101 | 0.070 | 0.000 | 0.294 | 0.000 | 0.000 | 0.000 | 0.000 | 0.075 | 0.118 | 0.004 | 0.031 |
| 乳类 Dairy products | 0.000 | 0.000 | 0.000 | 0.000 | 0.000 | 0.000 | 0.000 | 0.000 | 0.000 | 0.000 | 0.000 | 0.000 | 0.000 | 0.000 | 0.000 | 0.000 | 0.000 | 0.000 | 0.000 | 0.000 | 0.000 | 0.000 | 0.000 | 0.000 | 0.000 |
| 蔬菜类 Vegetables | 0.000 | 0.000 | 0.000 | 0.000 | 0.000 | 0.405 | 0.000 | 0.000 | 0.000 | 0.000 | 0.000 | 0.000 | 0.000 | 10.380 | 1.963 | 0.000 | 2.039 | 0.000 | 0.000 | 0.000 | 0.647 | 0.000 | 0.909 | 0.000 | 0.681 |
| 水果类 Fruits | 0.058 | 0.138 | 0.000 | 0.000 | 0.000 | 0.000 | 0.000 | 0.000 | 0.000 | 0.000 | 0.000 | 0.000 | 0.000 | 2.931 | 0.000 | 0.000 | 0.134 | 0.000 | 0.000 | 0.019 | 0.000 | 0.000 | 0.000 | 0.000 | 0.137 |
| 糖类 Sugar | 0.000 | 0.000 | 0.000 | 0.000 | 0.000 | 0.000 | 0.000 | 0.000 | 0.000 | 0.000 | 0.000 | 0.000 | 0.000 | 0.000 | 0.000 | 0.000 | 0.000 | 0.000 | 0.000 | 0.000 | 0.000 | 0.000 | 0.000 | 0.000 | 0.000 |
| 水及饮料类 Water and beverages | 0.000 | 0.000 | 0.000 | 0.000 | 0.000 | 0.000 | 0.000 | 0.000 | 0.000 | 0.000 | 0.000 | 0.000 | 0.000 | 0.936 | 0.000 | 0.000 | 0.000 | 0.000 | 0.000 | 0.000 | 0.000 | 0.000 | 0.000 | 0.000 | 0.039 |

续表

| 膳食类别 Category | 黑龙江 HL | 辽宁 LN | 河北 HE | 北京 BJ | 吉林 JL | 山西 SX | 陕西 SN | 河南 HA | 宁夏 NX | 内蒙古 NM | 青海 QH | 甘肃 GS | 上海 SH | 福建 FJ | 江西 JX | 江苏 JS | 浙江 ZJ | 山东 SD | 湖北 HB | 四川 SC | 广西 GX | 湖南 HN | 广东 GD | 贵州 GZ | 全国平均 AVG |
|---|---|---|---|---|---|---|---|---|---|---|---|---|---|---|---|---|---|---|---|---|---|---|---|---|---|
| 酒类 Alcohol beverages | 0.000 | 0.000 | 0.000 | 0.000 | 0.000 | 0.000 | 0.000 | 0.000 | 0.000 | 0.000 | 0.000 | 0.000 | 0.000 | 0.000 | 0.000 | 0.000 | 0.000 | 0.000 | 0.000 | 0.000 | 0.000 | 0.000 | 0.000 | 0.000 | 0.000 |
| 合计 SUM | 0.058 | 0.138 | 2.420 | 0.000 | 0.000 | 0.405 | 0.000 | 0.058 | 0.000 | 0.000 | 0.000 | 0.035 | 0.067 | 14.353 | 4.985 | 2.979 | 4.472 | 0.000 | 1.504 | 1.972 | 3.784 | 1.218 | 1.652 | 0.004 | 1.671 |

附表 4-14　第六次中国总膳食研究的丙溴磷膳食摄入量 [ 单位: ng/(kg bw · d)]

Annexed Table 4-14　Dietary intakes of profenofos from the 6$^{th}$ China TDS [Unit: ng/(kg bw · d)]

| 膳食类别 Category | 黑龙江 HL | 辽宁 LN | 河北 HE | 北京 BJ | 吉林 JL | 山西 SX | 陕西 SN | 河南 HA | 宁夏 NX | 内蒙古 NM | 青海 QH | 甘肃 GS | 上海 SH | 福建 FJ | 江西 JX | 江苏 JS | 浙江 ZJ | 山东 SD | 湖北 HB | 四川 SC | 广西 GX | 湖南 HN | 广东 GD | 贵州 GZ | 全国平均 AVG |
|---|---|---|---|---|---|---|---|---|---|---|---|---|---|---|---|---|---|---|---|---|---|---|---|---|---|
| 谷类 Cereals | 0.000 | 0.000 | 0.000 | 0.000 | 0.000 | 0.000 | 0.000 | 0.000 | 0.000 | 0.000 | 0.000 | 0.000 | 0.000 | 0.000 | 0.000 | 0.000 | 0.000 | 0.000 | 0.000 | 0.000 | 0.000 | 0.000 | 0.000 | 0.000 | 0.000 |
| 豆类 Legumes | 0.000 | 0.000 | 0.000 | 0.000 | 0.000 | 0.000 | 0.126 | 0.000 | 0.000 | 0.000 | 0.000 | 0.000 | 0.000 | 0.000 | 0.000 | 0.000 | 0.000 | 0.000 | 0.000 | 0.000 | 0.000 | 0.000 | 0.000 | 0.000 | 0.005 |
| 薯类 Potatoes | 0.000 | 0.000 | 0.000 | 0.000 | 0.000 | 0.000 | 0.000 | 0.000 | 0.000 | 0.000 | 0.162 | 0.000 | 0.000 | 0.000 | 0.000 | 0.000 | 0.000 | 0.000 | 0.000 | 0.000 | 0.000 | 0.000 | 0.000 | 0.000 | 0.000 |
| 肉类 Meats | 0.000 | 0.000 | 0.000 | 0.000 | 0.000 | 0.000 | 0.000 | 0.049 | 0.000 | 0.000 | 0.000 | 0.000 | 0.000 | 0.000 | 0.000 | 0.000 | 0.000 | 0.000 | 0.000 | 0.000 | 0.000 | 0.000 | 0.000 | 0.000 | 0.009 |
| 蛋类 Eggs | 0.000 | 0.000 | 0.000 | 0.000 | 0.000 | 0.000 | 0.000 | 0.000 | 0.000 | 0.000 | 0.000 | 0.000 | 0.000 | 0.000 | 0.000 | 0.000 | 0.000 | 0.000 | 0.000 | 0.000 | 0.000 | 0.000 | 0.000 | 0.000 | 0.000 |
| 水产类 Aquatic foods | 0.000 | 0.000 | 0.000 | 0.000 | 0.000 | 0.000 | 0.000 | 0.000 | 0.000 | 0.000 | 0.000 | 0.000 | 0.000 | 0.000 | 0.000 | 0.000 | 0.000 | 0.000 | 0.000 | 0.000 | 0.000 | 0.000 | 0.000 | 0.000 | 0.000 |
| 乳类 Dairy products | 0.000 | 0.000 | 0.000 | 0.000 | 0.000 | 0.000 | 0.000 | 0.000 | 0.000 | 0.000 | 0.000 | 0.000 | 0.000 | 0.000 | 0.000 | 0.000 | 0.000 | 0.000 | 0.000 | 0.000 | 0.000 | 0.000 | 0.000 | 0.000 | 0.000 |

续表

| 膳食类别<br>Category | 黑龙江<br>HL | 辽宁<br>LN | 河北<br>HE | 北京<br>BJ | 吉林<br>JL | 山西<br>SX | 陕西<br>SN | 河南<br>HA | 宁夏<br>NX | 内蒙古<br>NM | 青海<br>QH | 甘肃<br>GS | 上海<br>SH | 福建<br>FJ | 江西<br>JX | 江苏<br>JS | 浙江<br>ZJ | 山东<br>SD | 湖北<br>HB | 四川<br>SC | 广西<br>GX | 湖南<br>HN | 广东<br>GD | 贵州<br>GZ | 全国平均<br>AVG |
|---|---|---|---|---|---|---|---|---|---|---|---|---|---|---|---|---|---|---|---|---|---|---|---|---|---|
| 蔬菜类<br>Vegetables | 0.000 | 0.000 | 13.98 | 0.000 | 0.000 | 2.319 | 0.421 | 4.392 | 0.000 | 0.000 | 6.920 | 14.25 | 17.45 | 0.925 | 46.97 | 0.000 | 0.000 | 0.000 | 10.62 | 0.000 | 3.113 | 4.570 | 21.51 | 0.000 | 6.143 |
| 水果类<br>Fruits | 0.000 | 0.776 | 0.000 | 0.314 | 0.477 | 0.000 | 0.186 | 0.000 | 0.000 | 0.000 | 0.000 | 8.237 | 0.000 | 0.633 | 0.000 | 0.000 | 0.000 | 0.000 | 0.077 | 0.047 | 0.000 | 0.197 | 0.000 | 0.286 | 0.468 |
| 糖类<br>Sugar | 0.000 | 0.000 | 0.000 | 0.000 | 0.000 | 0.000 | 0.000 | 0.000 | 0.000 | 0.000 | 0.000 | 0.000 | 0.000 | 0.000 | 0.000 | 0.000 | 0.000 | 0.000 | 0.000 | 0.000 | 0.000 | 0.000 | 0.000 | 0.000 | 0.000 |
| 水及饮料类<br>Water and beverages | 0.000 | 0.000 | 0.000 | 0.000 | 0.000 | 0.000 | 0.000 | 0.000 | 0.000 | 0.000 | 0.000 | 0.000 | 0.010 | 0.000 | 0.000 | 0.000 | 0.000 | 0.000 | 0.000 | 0.000 | 0.000 | 0.000 | 0.000 | 0.000 | 0.000 |
| 酒类<br>Alcohol beverages | 0.000 | 0.000 | 0.000 | 0.000 | 0.000 | 0.000 | 0.000 | 0.000 | 0.000 | 0.000 | 0.000 | 0.000 | 0.000 | 0.000 | 0.000 | 0.000 | 0.000 | 0.000 | 0.000 | 0.000 | 0.000 | 0.000 | 0.000 | 0.000 | 0.000 |
| 合计<br>SUM | 0.000 | 0.776 | 13.981 | 0.314 | 0.477 | 2.319 | 0.733 | 4.441 | 0.000 | 0.000 | 7.081 | 22.486 | 17.459 | 1.559 | 46.975 | 0.000 | 0.000 | 0.000 | 10.69 | 0.047 | 3.113 | 4.768 | 21.51 | 0.286 | 6.626 |

附表 4-15 第六次中国总膳食研究的氧乐果膳食摄入量 [单位: ng/(kg bw·d)]
Annexed Table 4-15 Dietary intakes of omethoate from the 6$^{th}$ China TDS [Unit: ng/(kg bw·d)]

| 膳食类别<br>Category | 黑龙江<br>HL | 辽宁<br>LN | 河北<br>HE | 北京<br>BJ | 吉林<br>JL | 山西<br>SX | 陕西<br>SN | 河南<br>HA | 宁夏<br>NX | 内蒙古<br>NM | 青海<br>QH | 甘肃<br>GS | 上海<br>SH | 福建<br>FJ | 江西<br>JX | 江苏<br>JS | 浙江<br>ZJ | 山东<br>SD | 湖北<br>HB | 四川<br>SC | 广西<br>GX | 湖南<br>HN | 广东<br>GD | 贵州<br>GZ | 全国平均<br>AVG |
|---|---|---|---|---|---|---|---|---|---|---|---|---|---|---|---|---|---|---|---|---|---|---|---|---|---|
| 谷类<br>Cereals | 0.000 | 0.000 | 0.000 | 0.000 | 0.000 | 0.000 | 0.000 | 0.000 | 0.000 | 0.000 | 0.000 | 0.000 | 0.000 | 0.000 | 0.000 | 0.000 | 0.000 | 0.000 | 0.000 | 0.000 | 0.000 | 0.000 | 0.000 | 0.000 | 0.000 |
| 豆类<br>Legumes | 0.000 | 0.000 | 0.000 | 0.000 | 0.000 | 0.000 | 0.000 | 0.000 | 0.000 | 0.000 | 0.000 | 0.000 | 0.000 | 0.000 | 0.000 | 0.000 | 0.000 | 0.000 | 0.000 | 0.000 | 0.000 | 0.000 | 0.000 | 0.000 | 0.000 |
| 薯类<br>Potatoes | 0.000 | 0.000 | 0.000 | 0.000 | 0.000 | 0.000 | 0.000 | 0.000 | 0.000 | 0.000 | 0.000 | 0.000 | 0.000 | 0.000 | 0.000 | 0.000 | 0.000 | 0.000 | 0.145 | 0.000 | 0.000 | 0.000 | 0.000 | 0.000 | 0.006 |

续表

| 膳食类别<br>Category | 黑龙江<br>HL | 辽宁<br>LN | 河北<br>HE | 北京<br>BJ | 吉林<br>JL | 山西<br>SX | 陕西<br>SN | 河南<br>HA | 宁夏<br>NX | 内蒙古<br>NM | 青海<br>QH | 甘肃<br>GS | 上海<br>SH | 福建<br>FJ | 江西<br>JX | 江苏<br>JS | 浙江<br>ZJ | 山东<br>SD | 湖北<br>HB | 四川<br>SC | 广西<br>GX | 湖南<br>HN | 广东<br>GD | 贵州<br>GZ | 全国平均<br>AVG |
|---|---|---|---|---|---|---|---|---|---|---|---|---|---|---|---|---|---|---|---|---|---|---|---|---|---|
| 肉类 Meats | 0.000 | 0.000 | 0.000 | 0.000 | 0.000 | 0.000 | 0.000 | 0.000 | 0.000 | 0.000 | 0.000 | 0.000 | 0.000 | 0.000 | 0.000 | 0.000 | 0.000 | 0.000 | 0.000 | 0.000 | 0.000 | 0.000 | 0.000 | 0.000 | 0.000 |
| 蛋类 Eggs | 0.000 | 0.000 | 0.000 | 0.000 | 0.000 | 0.000 | 0.000 | 0.000 | 0.000 | 0.000 | 0.000 | 0.000 | 0.000 | 0.000 | 0.000 | 0.000 | 0.000 | 0.000 | 0.000 | 0.000 | 0.000 | 0.000 | 0.000 | 0.000 | 0.000 |
| 水产类 Aquatic foods | 0.000 | 0.000 | 0.000 | 0.000 | 0.000 | 0.000 | 0.000 | 0.000 | 0.000 | 0.000 | 0.000 | 0.000 | 0.000 | 0.000 | 0.000 | 0.000 | 0.000 | 0.000 | 0.000 | 0.000 | 0.000 | 0.000 | 0.000 | 0.000 | 0.000 |
| 乳类 Dairy products | 0.000 | 0.000 | 0.000 | 0.000 | 0.000 | 0.000 | 0.000 | 0.000 | 0.000 | 0.000 | 0.000 | 0.000 | 0.000 | 0.000 | 0.000 | 0.000 | 0.000 | 0.000 | 0.000 | 0.000 | 0.000 | 0.000 | 0.061 | 0.000 | 0.003 |
| 蔬菜类 Vegetables | 0.000 | 8.731 | 0.000 | 0.000 | 89.020 | 0.000 | 0.000 | 0.000 | 0.000 | 0.000 | 0.000 | 0.000 | 1.449 | 0.000 | 0.000 | 0.000 | 0.000 | 0.000 | 3.817 | 0.000 | 0.000 | 59.000 | 0.000 | 0.000 | 6.751 |
| 水果类 Fruits | 0.000 | 3.844 | 0.000 | 0.000 | 0.000 | 0.000 | 0.117 | 0.000 | 0.000 | 0.000 | 0.000 | 0.000 | 0.000 | 0.000 | 0.000 | 0.000 | 0.000 | 0.000 | 0.043 | 0.000 | 0.320 | 0.000 | 0.000 | 0.000 | 0.180 |
| 糖类 Sugar | 0.000 | 0.000 | 0.000 | 0.000 | 0.000 | 0.000 | 0.000 | 0.000 | 0.000 | 0.000 | 0.000 | 0.000 | 0.000 | 0.000 | 0.000 | 0.000 | 0.000 | 0.000 | 0.000 | 0.000 | 0.000 | 0.000 | 0.000 | 0.000 | 0.000 |
| 水及饮料类 Water and beverages | 0.000 | 0.000 | 0.000 | 0.000 | 0.000 | 0.000 | 0.000 | 0.000 | 0.000 | 0.000 | 0.000 | 0.000 | 0.000 | 0.000 | 0.000 | 3.986 | 0.000 | 0.000 | 0.000 | 0.000 | 0.000 | 0.000 | 0.000 | 0.000 | 0.166 |
| 酒类 Alcohol beverages | 0.000 | 0.000 | 0.000 | 0.000 | 0.000 | 0.000 | 0.000 | 0.000 | 0.000 | 0.000 | 0.000 | 0.000 | 0.000 | 0.000 | 0.000 | 0.000 | 0.000 | 0.000 | 0.000 | 0.000 | 0.000 | 0.000 | 0.000 | 0.000 | 0.000 |
| 合计 SUM | 0.000 | 12.575 | 0.000 | 0.000 | 89.020 | 0.000 | 0.117 | 0.000 | 0.000 | 0.000 | 0.000 | 0.000 | 1.449 | 0.000 | 0.000 | 3.986 | 0.000 | 0.000 | 4.005 | 0.000 | 0.320 | 59.000 | 0.062 | 0.000 | 7.106 |

附表 4-16　第六次中国总膳食研究的乐果膳食摄入量 [单位: ng/(kg bw·d)]

Annexed Table 4-16　Dietary intakes of dimethoate from the 6$^{th}$ China TDS [Unit: ng/(kg bw·d)]

| 膳食类别<br>Category | 黑龙江<br>HL | 辽宁<br>LN | 河北<br>HE | 北京<br>BJ | 吉林<br>JL | 山西<br>SX | 陕西<br>SN | 河南<br>HA | 宁夏<br>NX | 内蒙古<br>NM | 青海<br>QH | 甘肃<br>GS | 上海<br>SH | 福建<br>FJ | 江西<br>JX | 江苏<br>JS | 浙江<br>ZJ | 山东<br>SD | 湖北<br>HB | 四川<br>SC | 广西<br>GX | 湖南<br>HN | 广东<br>GD | 贵州<br>GZ | 全国平均<br>AVG |
|---|---|---|---|---|---|---|---|---|---|---|---|---|---|---|---|---|---|---|---|---|---|---|---|---|---|
| 谷类 Cereals | 0.000 | 0.000 | 0.000 | 0.000 | 0.000 | 0.000 | 0.000 | 0.000 | 0.000 | 0.000 | 0.000 | 0.000 | 0.000 | 0.000 | 0.000 | 0.000 | 0.000 | 0.000 | 0.000 | 0.000 | 0.000 | 0.000 | 0.000 | 0.000 | 0.000 |
| 豆类 Legumes | 0.000 | 0.000 | 0.064 | 0.000 | 0.000 | 0.000 | 0.000 | 0.000 | 0.000 | 0.000 | 0.000 | 0.000 | 0.000 | 0.000 | 0.000 | 0.000 | 0.000 | 0.000 | 0.000 | 0.000 | 0.000 | 0.000 | 0.000 | 0.000 | 0.003 |
| 薯类 Potatoes | 0.000 | 0.000 | 0.000 | 0.000 | 0.000 | 0.000 | 0.000 | 0.000 | 0.000 | 0.000 | 0.000 | 0.000 | 0.000 | 0.000 | 0.000 | 0.000 | 0.000 | 0.000 | 0.000 | 0.000 | 0.000 | 0.000 | 0.000 | 0.000 | 0.000 |
| 肉类 Meats | 0.000 | 0.000 | 0.000 | 0.000 | 0.000 | 0.000 | 0.000 | 0.000 | 0.000 | 0.000 | 0.000 | 0.000 | 0.000 | 0.000 | 0.000 | 0.000 | 0.000 | 0.000 | 0.000 | 0.000 | 0.000 | 0.000 | 0.000 | 0.000 | 0.000 |
| 蛋类 Eggs | 0.000 | 0.000 | 0.000 | 0.000 | 0.000 | 0.000 | 0.000 | 0.000 | 0.000 | 0.000 | 0.000 | 0.000 | 0.000 | 0.000 | 0.000 | 0.000 | 0.000 | 0.000 | 0.000 | 0.000 | 0.000 | 0.000 | 0.000 | 0.000 | 0.000 |
| 水产类 Aquatic foods | 0.000 | 0.000 | 0.000 | 0.000 | 0.000 | 0.000 | 0.000 | 0.000 | 0.000 | 0.000 | 0.000 | 0.000 | 0.000 | 0.000 | 0.000 | 0.000 | 0.000 | 0.000 | 0.000 | 0.000 | 0.000 | 0.000 | 0.000 | 0.000 | 0.000 |
| 乳类 Dairy products | 0.000 | 0.000 | 0.000 | 0.000 | 0.000 | 0.000 | 0.000 | 0.000 | 0.000 | 0.000 | 0.000 | 0.000 | 0.000 | 0.000 | 0.000 | 0.000 | 0.000 | 0.000 | 0.000 | 0.000 | 0.000 | 0.000 | 0.000 | 0.000 | 0.000 |
| 蔬菜类 Vegetables | 0.000 | 0.000 | 0.000 | 0.282 | 0.000 | 0.000 | 0.000 | 0.000 | 0.000 | 0.000 | 0.000 | 5.867 | 0.000 | 0.000 | 0.000 | 0.000 | 0.000 | 0.000 | 0.000 | 0.000 | 0.000 | 582.600 | 0.000 | 0.000 | 24.55 |
| 水果类 Fruits | 0.000 | 0.000 | 0.000 | 0.000 | 0.000 | 0.000 | 1.515 | 0.000 | 0.000 | 0.000 | 0.000 | 0.000 | 0.000 | 0.000 | 0.000 | 0.000 | 0.000 | 0.000 | 0.000 | 0.000 | 0.000 | 0.000 | 0.311 | 0.000 | 0.063 |
| 糖类 Sugar | 0.000 | 0.000 | 0.000 | 0.000 | 0.000 | 0.000 | 0.000 | 0.000 | 0.000 | 0.000 | 0.000 | 0.000 | 0.000 | 0.000 | 0.000 | 0.000 | 0.000 | 0.000 | 0.000 | 0.000 | 0.000 | 0.000 | 0.000 | 0.000 | 0.000 |
| 水及饮料类 Water and beverages | 0.000 | 0.000 | 0.000 | 0.000 | 0.823 | 0.000 | 0.000 | 0.000 | 0.000 | 0.000 | 0.000 | 0.000 | 0.589 | 0.000 | 0.000 | 1.749 | 0.000 | 0.000 | 0.000 | 0.000 | 0.000 | 0.000 | 0.000 | 0.000 | 0.132 |

续表

| 膳食类别<br>Category | 黑龙江<br>HL | 辽宁<br>LN | 河北<br>HE | 北京<br>BJ | 吉林<br>JL | 山西<br>SX | 陕西<br>SN | 河南<br>HA | 宁夏<br>NX | 内蒙古<br>NM | 青海<br>QH | 甘肃<br>GS | 上海<br>SH | 福建<br>FJ | 江西<br>JX | 江苏<br>JS | 浙江<br>ZJ | 山东<br>SD | 湖北<br>HB | 四川<br>SC | 广西<br>GX | 湖南<br>HN | 广东<br>GD | 贵州<br>GZ | 全国平均<br>AVG |
|---|---|---|---|---|---|---|---|---|---|---|---|---|---|---|---|---|---|---|---|---|---|---|---|---|---|
| 酒类 Alcohol beverages | 0.000 | 0.000 | 0.000 | 0.000 | 0.000 | 0.000 | 0.000 | 0.000 | 0.000 | 0.000 | 0.000 | 0.000 | 0.000 | 0.000 | 0.000 | 0.000 | 0.000 | 0.000 | 0.000 | 0.000 | 0.000 | 0.000 | 0.000 | 0.000 | 0.000 |
| 合计 SUM | 0.000 | 0.000 | 0.064 | 0.282 | 0.823 | 0.000 | 1.515 | 0.000 | 0.000 | 0.000 | 0.000 | 5.867 | 5.589 | 0.000 | 0.000 | 1.749 | 0.000 | 0.000 | 0.000 | 0.000 | 0.000 | 582.633 | 0.311 | 0.000 | 24.743 |

附表 4-17　第六次中国总膳食研究的甲胺磷膳食摄入量 [单位：ng/(kg bw·d)]

Annexed Table 4-17　Dietary intakes of methamidophos from the 6th China TDS [Unit: ng/(kg bw·d)]

| 膳食类别<br>Category | 黑龙江<br>HL | 辽宁<br>LN | 河北<br>HE | 北京<br>BJ | 吉林<br>JL | 山西<br>SX | 陕西<br>SN | 河南<br>HA | 宁夏<br>NX | 内蒙古<br>NM | 青海<br>QH | 甘肃<br>GS | 上海<br>SH | 福建<br>FJ | 江西<br>JX | 江苏<br>JS | 浙江<br>ZJ | 山东<br>SD | 湖北<br>HB | 四川<br>SC | 广西<br>GX | 湖南<br>HN | 广东<br>GD | 贵州<br>GZ | 全国平均<br>AVG |
|---|---|---|---|---|---|---|---|---|---|---|---|---|---|---|---|---|---|---|---|---|---|---|---|---|---|
| 谷类 Cereals | 0.000 | 0.000 | 0.000 | 0.000 | 0.000 | 0.000 | 0.000 | 0.000 | 0.000 | 0.000 | 0.000 | 0.000 | 0.000 | 0.000 | 0.000 | 0.000 | 0.000 | 0.000 | 0.000 | 0.000 | 0.000 | 0.000 | 0.000 | 0.000 | 0.000 |
| 豆类 Legumes | 0.000 | 0.000 | 0.120 | 0.000 | 0.000 | 0.000 | 0.000 | 0.000 | 0.000 | 0.000 | 0.000 | 0.000 | 0.000 | 0.000 | 0.000 | 0.000 | 0.000 | 0.000 | 0.000 | 0.000 | 0.000 | 0.000 | 0.000 | 0.000 | 0.005 |
| 薯类 Potatoes | 0.000 | 0.000 | 0.000 | 0.000 | 0.000 | 0.000 | 0.000 | 0.000 | 0.000 | 0.000 | 0.000 | 0.000 | 0.000 | 0.000 | 0.000 | 0.000 | 0.000 | 0.000 | 0.107 | 0.000 | 0.000 | 0.000 | 0.000 | 0.000 | 0.004 |
| 肉类 Meats | 0.000 | 0.000 | 0.000 | 0.000 | 0.000 | 0.000 | 0.000 | 0.000 | 0.000 | 0.000 | 0.000 | 0.000 | 0.000 | 0.000 | 0.000 | 0.000 | 0.000 | 0.000 | 0.000 | 0.000 | 0.000 | 0.000 | 0.000 | 0.000 | 0.000 |
| 蛋类 Eggs | 0.000 | 0.000 | 0.000 | 0.000 | 0.000 | 0.000 | 0.000 | 0.000 | 0.000 | 0.000 | 0.000 | 0.000 | 0.000 | 0.000 | 0.000 | 0.000 | 0.000 | 0.000 | 0.000 | 0.000 | 0.000 | 0.000 | 0.000 | 0.000 | 0.000 |
| 水产类 Aquatic foods | 0.000 | 0.000 | 0.000 | 0.000 | 0.000 | 0.000 | 0.000 | 0.000 | 0.000 | 0.000 | 0.000 | 0.000 | 0.000 | 0.000 | 0.000 | 0.000 | 0.000 | 0.000 | 0.000 | 0.000 | 0.000 | 0.000 | 0.000 | 0.000 | 0.000 |
| 乳类 Dairy products | 0.000 | 0.000 | 0.000 | 0.000 | 0.000 | 0.000 | 0.000 | 0.000 | 0.000 | 0.000 | 0.000 | 0.000 | 0.000 | 0.000 | 0.000 | 0.000 | 0.000 | 0.000 | 0.000 | 0.000 | 0.000 | 0.000 | 0.000 | 0.000 | 0.000 |

续表

| 膳食类别 Category | 黑龙江 HL | 辽宁 LN | 河北 HE | 北京 BJ | 吉林 JL | 山西 SX | 陕西 SN | 河南 HA | 宁夏 NX | 内蒙古 NM | 青海 QH | 甘肃 GS | 上海 SH | 福建 FJ | 江西 JX | 江苏 JS | 浙江 ZJ | 山东 SD | 湖北 HB | 四川 SC | 广西 GX | 湖南 HN | 广东 GD | 贵州 GZ | 全国平均 AVG |
|---|---|---|---|---|---|---|---|---|---|---|---|---|---|---|---|---|---|---|---|---|---|---|---|---|---|
| 蔬菜类 Vegetables | 0.000 | 0.000 | 0.000 | 0.000 | 0.000 | 0.000 | 0.000 | 0.000 | 0.000 | 0.000 | 0.000 | 0.000 | 0.000 | 0.000 | 0.000 | 0.000 | 0.000 | 0.000 | 0.000 | 0.000 | 0.000 | 0.000 | 0.000 | 0.000 | 0.000 |
| 水果类 Fruits | 0.000 | 0.000 | 0.000 | 0.000 | 0.000 | 0.000 | 0.000 | 0.051 | 0.000 | 0.000 | 0.000 | 0.000 | 0.000 | 0.000 | 0.000 | 0.000 | 0.000 | 0.000 | 0.000 | 0.000 | 0.000 | 0.000 | 0.000 | 0.000 | 0.002 |
| 糖类 Sugar | 0.000 | 0.000 | 0.000 | 0.000 | 0.000 | 0.000 | 0.000 | 0.000 | 0.000 | 0.000 | 0.000 | 0.000 | 0.000 | 0.000 | 0.000 | 0.000 | 0.000 | 0.000 | 0.000 | 0.000 | 0.000 | 0.000 | 0.000 | 0.000 | 0.000 |
| 水及饮料类 Water and beverages | 0.000 | 0.000 | 0.000 | 0.000 | 0.000 | 0.000 | 0.000 | 0.000 | 0.000 | 0.000 | 0.000 | 0.000 | 0.000 | 0.000 | 0.000 | 0.000 | 0.000 | 0.000 | 0.000 | 0.000 | 0.000 | 0.000 | 0.000 | 0.000 | 0.000 |
| 酒类 Alcohol beverages | 0.000 | 0.000 | 0.000 | 0.000 | 0.000 | 0.000 | 0.000 | 0.000 | 0.000 | 0.000 | 0.000 | 0.000 | 0.000 | 0.000 | 0.000 | 0.000 | 0.000 | 0.000 | 0.000 | 0.000 | 0.000 | 0.000 | 0.000 | 0.000 | 0.000 |
| 合计 SUM | 0.000 | 0.000 | 0.120 | 0.000 | 0.000 | 0.000 | 0.000 | 0.051 | 0.000 | 0.000 | 0.000 | 0.000 | 0.000 | 0.000 | 0.000 | 0.000 | 0.000 | 0.000 | 0.107 | 0.000 | 0.000 | 0.000 | 0.000 | 0.000 | 0.012 |

附表 4-18 第六次中国总膳食研究的二嗪磷膳食摄入量 [单位: ng/(kg bw·d)]
Annexed Table 4-18　Dietary intakes of diazinon from the 6th China TDS [Unit: ng/(kg bw·d)]

| 膳食类别 Category | 黑龙江 HL | 辽宁 LN | 河北 HE | 北京 BJ | 吉林 JL | 山西 SX | 陕西 SN | 河南 HA | 宁夏 NX | 内蒙古 NM | 青海 QH | 甘肃 GS | 上海 SH | 福建 FJ | 江西 JX | 江苏 JS | 浙江 ZJ | 山东 SD | 湖北 HB | 四川 SC | 广西 GX | 湖南 HN | 广东 GD | 贵州 GZ | 全国平均 AVG |
|---|---|---|---|---|---|---|---|---|---|---|---|---|---|---|---|---|---|---|---|---|---|---|---|---|---|
| 谷类 Cereals | 0.000 | 0.000 | 0.000 | 0.000 | 0.000 | 0.000 | 0.000 | 0.000 | 0.000 | 0.000 | 0.000 | 0.000 | 0.000 | 0.000 | 0.000 | 0.000 | 0.000 | 0.000 | 0.000 | 0.000 | 0.000 | 0.000 | 0.000 | 0.000 | 0.000 |
| 豆类 Legumes | 0.000 | 0.000 | 0.000 | 0.000 | 0.000 | 0.000 | 0.000 | 0.000 | 0.000 | 0.000 | 0.000 | 0.000 | 0.000 | 0.000 | 0.000 | 0.000 | 0.000 | 0.000 | 0.000 | 0.000 | 0.000 | 0.000 | 0.000 | 0.000 | 0.000 |
| 薯类 Potatoes | 0.000 | 0.000 | 0.000 | 0.000 | 0.000 | 0.000 | 0.000 | 0.000 | 0.000 | 0.000 | 0.000 | 0.000 | 0.000 | 0.000 | 0.000 | 0.000 | 0.000 | 0.000 | 0.000 | 0.000 | 0.000 | 0.000 | 0.000 | 0.000 | 0.000 |

续表

| 膳食类别<br>Category | 黑龙江<br>HL | 辽宁<br>LN | 河北<br>HE | 北京<br>BJ | 吉林<br>JL | 山西<br>SX | 陕西<br>SN | 河南<br>HA | 宁夏<br>NX | 内蒙古<br>NM | 青海<br>QH | 甘肃<br>GS | 上海<br>SH | 福建<br>FJ | 江西<br>JX | 江苏<br>JS | 浙江<br>ZJ | 山东<br>SD | 湖北<br>HB | 四川<br>SC | 广西<br>GX | 湖南<br>HN | 广东<br>GD | 贵州<br>GZ | 全国平均<br>AVG |
|---|---|---|---|---|---|---|---|---|---|---|---|---|---|---|---|---|---|---|---|---|---|---|---|---|---|
| 肉类 Meats | 0.000 | 0.000 | 0.000 | 0.000 | 0.000 | 0.000 | 0.000 | 0.000 | 0.000 | 0.000 | 0.000 | 0.000 | 0.000 | 0.000 | 0.000 | 0.000 | 0.000 | 0.286 | 0.000 | 0.000 | 0.000 | 0.000 | 0.000 | 0.000 | 0.012 |
| 蛋类 Eggs | 0.000 | 0.000 | 0.000 | 0.000 | 0.000 | 0.000 | 0.000 | 0.000 | 0.000 | 0.000 | 0.000 | 0.000 | 0.000 | 0.000 | 0.000 | 0.000 | 0.000 | 0.000 | 0.000 | 0.000 | 0.000 | 0.000 | 0.000 | 0.000 | 0.000 |
| 水产类 Aquatic foods | 0.000 | 0.000 | 0.000 | 0.000 | 0.000 | 0.000 | 0.005 | 0.000 | 0.000 | 0.000 | 0.000 | 0.000 | 0.000 | 0.000 | 0.000 | 0.000 | 0.000 | 0.000 | 0.000 | 0.000 | 0.000 | 0.000 | 0.000 | 0.000 | 0.000 |
| 乳类 Dairy products | 0.000 | 0.000 | 0.000 | 0.000 | 0.000 | 0.000 | 0.000 | 0.000 | 0.000 | 0.000 | 0.000 | 0.000 | 0.000 | 0.000 | 0.000 | 0.000 | 0.000 | 0.000 | 0.000 | 0.000 | 0.000 | 0.000 | 0.000 | 0.000 | 0.000 |
| 蔬菜类 Vegetables | 0.000 | 0.000 | 0.000 | 0.000 | 0.000 | 0.000 | 0.000 | 0.000 | 0.000 | 0.000 | 0.000 | 0.000 | 0.000 | 0.000 | 0.000 | 0.000 | 0.000 | 0.000 | 0.000 | 0.000 | 0.000 | 0.000 | 0.000 | 0.000 | 0.000 |
| 水果类 Fruits | 0.000 | 0.000 | 0.000 | 0.000 | 0.000 | 0.000 | 0.000 | 0.000 | 0.000 | 0.000 | 0.000 | 0.000 | 0.000 | 0.000 | 0.000 | 0.000 | 0.000 | 0.000 | 0.000 | 0.000 | 0.000 | 0.000 | 0.000 | 0.000 | 0.000 |
| 糖类 Sugar | 0.000 | 0.000 | 0.000 | 0.000 | 0.000 | 0.000 | 0.000 | 0.000 | 0.000 | 0.000 | 0.000 | 0.000 | 0.000 | 0.000 | 0.000 | 0.000 | 0.000 | 0.000 | 0.000 | 0.000 | 0.000 | 0.000 | 0.000 | 0.000 | 0.000 |
| 水及饮料类 Water and beverages | 0.000 | 0.000 | 0.000 | 0.000 | 0.000 | 0.000 | 0.000 | 0.000 | 0.000 | 0.000 | 0.000 | 0.000 | 0.000 | 0.000 | 0.000 | 0.000 | 0.000 | 0.000 | 0.000 | 0.000 | 0.000 | 0.000 | 0.000 | 0.000 | 0.000 |
| 酒类 Alcohol beverages | 0.000 | 0.000 | 0.000 | 0.000 | 0.000 | 0.000 | 0.000 | 0.000 | 0.000 | 0.000 | 0.000 | 0.000 | 0.000 | 0.000 | 0.000 | 0.000 | 0.000 | 0.000 | 0.000 | 0.000 | 0.000 | 0.000 | 0.000 | 0.000 | 0.000 |
| 合计 SUM | 0.000 | 0.000 | 0.000 | 0.000 | 0.000 | 0.000 | 0.005 | 0.000 | 0.000 | 0.000 | 0.000 | 0.000 | 0.000 | 0.000 | 0.000 | 0.000 | 0.000 | 0.286 | 0.000 | 0.000 | 0.000 | 0.000 | 0.000 | 0.000 | 0.012 |

附表 4-19　第六次中国总膳食研究毒死蜱的膳食来源（单位：%）

Annexed Table 4-19　Dietary sources of chlorpyrifos from the 6$^{th}$ China TDS (Unit: %)

| 膳食类别 Category | 黑龙江 HL | 辽宁 LN | 河北 HE | 北京 BJ | 吉林 JL | 山西 SX | 陕西 SN | 河南 HA | 宁夏 NX | 内蒙古 NM | 青海 QH | 甘肃 GS | 上海 SH | 福建 FJ | 江西 JX | 江苏 JS | 浙江 ZJ | 山东 SD | 湖北 HB | 四川 SC | 广西 GX | 湖南 HN | 广东 GD | 贵州 GZ | 全国平均 AVG |
|---|---|---|---|---|---|---|---|---|---|---|---|---|---|---|---|---|---|---|---|---|---|---|---|---|---|
| 谷类 Cereals | 0.0 | 0.0 | 25.9 | 11.8 | 0.0 | 0.0 | 22.9 | 39.0 | 0.0 | 8.8 | 0.0 | 0.0 | 13.5 | 7.7 | 5.2 | 0.0 | 53.0 | 18.0 | 1.5 | 93.2 | 9.8 | 0.0 | 16.6 | 0.0 | 13.3 |
| 豆类 Legumes | 43.0 | 2.2 | 6.3 | 2.7 | 0.0 | 3.8 | 3.1 | 22.3 | 2.4 | 0.0 | 0.0 | 0.3 | 9.6 | 3.9 | 0.0 | 96.7 | 15.8 | 4.5 | 0.8 | 0.3 | 0.9 | 0.0 | 8.2 | 0.0 | 2.3 |
| 薯类 Potatoes | 0.0 | 0.2 | 11.7 | 7.3 | 0.0 | 18.6 | 0.0 | 0.0 | 0.0 | 4.7 | 5.7 | 0.0 | 0.0 | 3.2 | 1.8 | 0.0 | 0.0 | 5.2 | 1.2 | 0.0 | 0.6 | 13.7 | 4.6 | 0.0 | 1.8 |
| 肉类 Meats | 0.0 | 0.2 | 6.8 | 8.9 | 0.0 | 11.3 | 3.4 | 0.0 | 0.0 | 43.6 | 2.8 | 0.4 | 0.0 | 2.3 | 0.0 | 0.0 | 0.0 | 7.8 | 0.2 | 0.3 | 3.6 | 0.0 | 2.0 | 0.0 | 2.0 |
| 蛋类 Eggs | 0.0 | 0.1 | 6.9 | 8.2 | 0.0 | 2.9 | 0.0 | 0.0 | 0.0 | 0.0 | 0.4 | 0.0 | 0.0 | 3.8 | 0.0 | 0.0 | 0.0 | 2.5 | 0.3 | 0.0 | 0.7 | 0.0 | 0.0 | 0.0 | 0.9 |
| 水产类 Aquatic foods | 7.3 | 0.0 | 0.8 | 3.3 | 0.0 | 0.0 | 0.3 | 0.6 | 0.0 | 3.9 | 0.3 | 0.3 | 0.9 | 11.3 | 2.2 | 0.0 | 2.7 | 1.7 | 0.4 | 0.4 | 6.7 | 28.5 | 12.2 | 1.6 | 2.3 |
| 乳类 Dairy products | 0.0 | 0.0 | 0.0 | 0.0 | 0.0 | 0.0 | 0.0 | 0.0 | 0.0 | 0.0 | 0.0 | 0.0 | 0.0 | 0.0 | 0.0 | 0.0 | 0.0 | 0.0 | 0.0 | 0.0 | 0.0 | 0.0 | 0.0 | 0.0 | 0.0 |
| 蔬菜类 Vegetables | 0.0 | 81.7 | 39.5 | 40.8 | 7.0 | 59.0 | 70.3 | 6.6 | 97.6 | 39.0 | 90.8 | 98.4 | 25.6 | 46.9 | 90.2 | 0.0 | 26.9 | 57.6 | 95.0 | 5.8 | 77.8 | 26.0 | 53.0 | 94.2 | 68.6 |
| 水果类 Fruits | 49.7 | 15.6 | 2.1 | 16.8 | 93.0 | 4.4 | 0.0 | 31.5 | 0.0 | 0.0 | 0.0 | 0.6 | 49.7 | 21.0 | 0.7 | 3.3 | 1.5 | 2.6 | 0.5 | 0.0 | 0.0 | 31.8 | 3.4 | 4.2 | 8.7 |
| 糖类 Sugar | 0.0 | 0.0 | 0.0 | 0.0 | 0.0 | 0.0 | 0.0 | 0.0 | 0.0 | 0.0 | 0.0 | 0.0 | 0.7 | 0.0 | 0.0 | 0.0 | 0.0 | 0.0 | 0.0 | 0.0 | 0.0 | 0.0 | 0.0 | 0.0 | 0.0 |
| 水及饮料类 Water and beverages | 0.0 | 0.0 | 0.0 | 0.0 | 0.0 | 0.0 | 0.0 | 0.0 | 0.0 | 0.0 | 0.0 | 0.0 | 0.0 | 0.0 | 0.0 | 0.0 | 0.0 | 0.0 | 0.0 | 0.0 | 0.0 | 0.0 | 0.0 | 0.0 | 0.0 |

续表

| 膳食类别<br>Category | 黑龙江<br>HL | 辽宁<br>LN | 河北<br>HE | 北京<br>BJ | 吉林<br>JL | 山西<br>SX | 陕西<br>SN | 河南<br>HA | 宁夏<br>NX | 内蒙古<br>NM | 青海<br>QH | 甘肃<br>GS | 上海<br>SH | 福建<br>FJ | 江西<br>JX | 江苏<br>JS | 浙江<br>ZJ | 山东<br>SD | 湖北<br>HB | 四川<br>SC | 广西<br>GX | 湖南<br>HN | 广东<br>GD | 贵州<br>GZ | 全国平均<br>AVG |
|---|---|---|---|---|---|---|---|---|---|---|---|---|---|---|---|---|---|---|---|---|---|---|---|---|---|
| 酒类<br>Alcohol beverages | 0.0 | 0.0 | 0.0 | 0.0 | 0.0 | 0.0 | 0.0 | 0.0 | 0.0 | 0.0 | 0.0 | 0.0 | 0.0 | 0.0 | 0.0 | 0.0 | 0.0 | 0.0 | 0.0 | 0.0 | 0.0 | 0.0 | 0.0 | 0.0 | 0.0 |

附表 4-20 第六次中国总膳食研究敌敌畏的膳食来源（单位：%）
Annexed Table 4-20 Dietary sources of dichlorvos from the 6th China TDS (Unit: %)

| 膳食类别<br>Category | 黑龙江<br>HL | 辽宁<br>LN | 河北<br>HE | 北京<br>BJ | 吉林<br>JL | 山西<br>SX | 陕西<br>SN | 河南<br>HA | 宁夏<br>NX | 内蒙古<br>NM | 青海<br>QH | 甘肃<br>GS | 上海<br>SH | 福建<br>FJ | 江西<br>JX | 江苏<br>JS | 浙江<br>ZJ | 山东<br>SD | 湖北<br>HB | 四川<br>SC | 广西<br>GX | 湖南<br>HN | 广东<br>GD | 贵州<br>GZ | 全国平均<br>AVG |
|---|---|---|---|---|---|---|---|---|---|---|---|---|---|---|---|---|---|---|---|---|---|---|---|---|---|
| 谷类<br>Cereals | 27.0 | 100.0 | 84.4 | 74.5 | 0.0 | 0.0 | 0.0 | 0.0 | 0.0 | 0.0 | 0.0 | 100.0 | 0.0 | 0.0 | 0.0 | 0.0 | 0.0 | 30.5 | 95.0 | 0.0 | 0.0 | 0.0 | 0.0 | 0.0 | 32.1 |
| 豆类<br>Legumes | 4.9 | 0.0 | 0.6 | 0.0 | 0.0 | 0.0 | 0.0 | 92.6 | 100.0 | 0.0 | 0.0 | 0.0 | 0.0 | 0.0 | 0.0 | 0.0 | 0.0 | 1.4 | 4.1 | 0.0 | 0.0 | 0.0 | 0.0 | 0.0 | 1.8 |
| 薯类<br>Potatoes | 3.8 | 0.0 | 0.0 | 0.0 | 0.0 | 0.0 | 0.0 | 0.0 | 0.0 | 0.0 | 0.0 | 0.0 | 0.0 | 0.0 | 0.0 | 0.0 | 0.0 | 1.3 | 0.0 | 0.0 | 0.0 | 0.0 | 0.0 | 0.0 | 1.3 |
| 肉类<br>Meats | 0.0 | 0.0 | 0.0 | 3.5 | 100.0 | 0.0 | 0.0 | 0.0 | 0.0 | 0.0 | 0.0 | 0.0 | 0.0 | 0.0 | 0.0 | 0.0 | 0.0 | 2.3 | 0.0 | 0.0 | 0.0 | 0.0 | 0.0 | 0.0 | 2.2 |
| 蛋类<br>Eggs | 0.0 | 0.0 | 0.0 | 0.0 | 0.0 | 0.0 | 0.0 | 0.0 | 0.0 | 0.0 | 0.0 | 0.0 | 0.0 | 0.0 | 0.0 | 0.0 | 0.0 | 0.0 | 0.0 | 0.0 | 0.0 | 0.0 | 0.0 | 0.0 | 0.0 |
| 水产类<br>Aquatic foods | 7.9 | 0.0 | 0.0 | 22.0 | 0.0 | 0.0 | 75.1 | 0.0 | 0.0 | 1.5 | 0.0 | 0.0 | 0.0 | 0.0 | 0.0 | 0.0 | 0.0 | 0.3 | 0.0 | 0.0 | 0.0 | 0.0 | 0.0 | 0.0 | 0.3 |
| 乳类<br>Dairy products | 0.3 | 0.0 | 0.4 | 0.0 | 0.0 | 98.6 | 0.0 | 1.4 | 0.0 | 0.0 | 0.0 | 0.0 | 0.0 | 0.0 | 0.0 | 21.5 | 0.0 | 0.2 | 0.0 | 0.0 | 0.0 | 0.0 | 0.0 | 99.0 | 0.2 |
| 蔬菜类<br>Vegetables | 24.9 | 0.0 | 14.6 | 0.0 | 0.0 | 0.0 | 0.0 | 0.0 | 0.0 | 0.0 | 0.0 | 0.0 | 100.0 | 0.0 | 0.0 | 78.5 | 0.0 | 26.3 | 0.0 | 0.0 | 0.0 | 0.0 | 0.0 | 0.0 | 25.5 |

续表

| 膳食类别 Category | 黑龙江 HL | 辽宁 LN | 河北 HE | 北京 BJ | 吉林 JL | 山西 SX | 陕西 SN | 河南 HA | 宁夏 NX | 内蒙古 NM | 青海 QH | 甘肃 GS | 上海 SH | 福建 FJ | 江西 JX | 江苏 JS | 浙江 ZJ | 山东 SD | 湖北 HB | 四川 SC | 广西 GX | 湖南 HN | 广东 GD | 贵州 GZ | 全国平均 AVG |
|---|---|---|---|---|---|---|---|---|---|---|---|---|---|---|---|---|---|---|---|---|---|---|---|---|---|
| 水果类 Fruits | 1.1 | 0.0 | 0.0 | 0.0 | 0.0 | 0.0 | 0.0 | 0.0 | 0.0 | 0.0 | 0.0 | 0.0 | 0.0 | 0.0 | 0.0 | 0.0 | 0.0 | 1.3 | 0.0 | 0.0 | 0.0 | 0.0 | 0.0 | 0.0 | 1.2 |
| 糖类 Sugar | 0.1 | 0.0 | 0.0 | 0.0 | 0.0 | 1.4 | 0.0 | 0.0 | 0.0 | 0.0 | 0.0 | 0.0 | 0.0 | 0.0 | 0.0 | 0.0 | 0.0 | 0.0 | 0.0 | 0.0 | 0.0 | 0.0 | 0.0 | 1.0 | 0.0 |
| 水及饮料类 Water and beverages | 29.3 | 0.0 | 0.0 | 0.0 | 0.0 | 0.0 | 0.0 | 0.0 | 0.0 | 98.5 | 0.0 | 0.0 | 0.0 | 0.0 | 0.0 | 0.0 | 0.0 | 36.4 | 0.0 | 0.0 | 0.0 | 99.3 | 0.0 | 0.0 | 35.2 |
| 酒类 Alcohol beverages | 0.7 | 0.0 | 0.0 | 0.0 | 0.0 | 0.0 | 24.9 | 6.0 | 0.0 | 0.0 | 0.0 | 0.0 | 0.0 | 0.0 | 0.0 | 0.0 | 0.0 | 0.0 | 0.9 | 0.0 | 0.0 | 0.7 | 0.0 | 0.0 | 0.1 |

附表 4-21　第六次中国总膳食研究乙酰甲胺磷的膳食来源（单位：%）
Annexed Table 4-21　Dietary sources of acephate from the 6$^{th}$ China TDS (Unit: %)

| 膳食类别 Category | 黑龙江 HL | 辽宁 LN | 河北 HE | 北京 BJ | 吉林 JL | 山西 SX | 陕西 SN | 河南 HA | 宁夏 NX | 内蒙古 NM | 青海 QH | 甘肃 GS | 上海 SH | 福建 FJ | 江西 JX | 江苏 JS | 浙江 ZJ | 山东 SD | 湖北 HB | 四川 SC | 广西 GX | 湖南 HN | 广东 GD | 贵州 GZ | 全国平均 AVG |
|---|---|---|---|---|---|---|---|---|---|---|---|---|---|---|---|---|---|---|---|---|---|---|---|---|---|
| 谷类 Cereals | 0.0 | 0.0 | 0.0 | 0.0 | 0.0 | 0.0 | 0.0 | 0.0 | 0.0 | 0.0 | 0.0 | 0.0 | 0.0 | 0.0 | 0.0 | 0.0 | 0.0 | 0.0 | 0.0 | 0.0 | 0.0 | 0.0 | 0.0 | 0.0 | 0.0 |
| 豆类 Legumes | 0.0 | 0.0 | 0.0 | 0.0 | 0.0 | 0.0 | 8.4 | 0.0 | 0.0 | 0.0 | 0.0 | 24.3 | 0.0 | 0.0 | 0.0 | 3.8 | 0.0 | 0.0 | 0.0 | 11.3 | 0.0 | 0.0 | 0.0 | 14.0 | 2.4 |
| 薯类 Potatoes | 0.0 | 0.0 | 0.0 | 0.0 | 0.0 | 0.0 | 12.5 | 0.0 | 0.0 | 0.0 | 1.5 | 0.0 | 0.0 | 0.0 | 0.0 | 3.6 | 0.0 | 0.0 | 0.0 | 32.6 | 0.0 | 2.2 | 0.0 | 11.4 | 3.7 |
| 肉类 Meats | 0.0 | 0.0 | 0.0 | 0.0 | 0.0 | 0.0 | 4.0 | 0.0 | 0.0 | 0.0 | 4.6 | 32.5 | 0.0 | 0.0 | 0.0 | 10.8 | 0.0 | 0.0 | 0.0 | 50.2 | 0.0 | 5.4 | 0.0 | 40.9 | 6.2 |
| 蛋类 Eggs | 0.0 | 0.0 | 0.0 | 0.0 | 0.0 | 0.0 | 2.5 | 0.0 | 0.0 | 0.0 | 0.0 | 43.2 | 0.0 | 0.0 | 0.0 | 2.8 | 0.0 | 0.0 | 0.0 | 3.9 | 0.0 | 1.1 | 0.0 | 2.9 | 1.3 |

续表

| 膳食类别 Category | 黑龙江 HL | 辽宁 LN | 河北 HE | 北京 BJ | 吉林 JL | 山西 SX | 陕西 SN | 河南 HA | 宁夏 NX | 内蒙古 NM | 青海 QH | 甘肃 GS | 上海 SH | 福建 FJ | 江西 JX | 江苏 JS | 浙江 ZJ | 山东 SD | 湖北 HB | 四川 SC | 广西 GX | 湖南 HN | 广东 GD | 贵州 GZ | 全国平均 AVG |
|---|---|---|---|---|---|---|---|---|---|---|---|---|---|---|---|---|---|---|---|---|---|---|---|---|---|
| 水产类 Aquatic foods | 0.0 | 0.0 | 0.0 | 0.0 | 0.0 | 0.0 | 0.7 | 0.0 | 0.0 | 0.0 | 0.1 | 0.0 | 0.0 | 0.0 | 0.0 | 1.7 | 0.0 | 0.0 | 0.0 | 1.9 | 0.0 | 2.7 | 0.0 | 0.3 | 0.6 |
| 乳类 Dairy products | 0.0 | 0.0 | 0.0 | 0.0 | 0.0 | 0.0 | 0.0 | 0.0 | 0.0 | 0.0 | 0.0 | 0.0 | 0.0 | 0.0 | 0.0 | 0.0 | 0.0 | 0.0 | 0.0 | 0.0 | 0.0 | 0.0 | 0.0 | 0.0 | 0.0 |
| 蔬菜类 Vegetables | 0.0 | 0.0 | 0.0 | 100.0 | 100.0 | 100.0 | 72.0 | 92.1 | 0.0 | 0.0 | 93.8 | 0.0 | 100.0 | 100.0 | 100.0 | 77.3 | 100.0 | 100.0 | 100.0 | 0.0 | 100.0 | 88.6 | 100.0 | 30.4 | 85.7 |
| 水果类 Fruits | 0.0 | 0.0 | 0.0 | 0.0 | 0.0 | 0.0 | 0.0 | 7.9 | 100.0 | 0.0 | 0.0 | 0.0 | 0.0 | 0.0 | 0.0 | 0.0 | 0.0 | 0.0 | 0.0 | 0.0 | 0.0 | 0.0 | 0.0 | 0.0 | 0.1 |
| 糖类 Sugar | 0.0 | 0.0 | 0.0 | 0.0 | 0.0 | 0.0 | 0.0 | 0.0 | 0.0 | 0.0 | 0.0 | 0.0 | 0.0 | 0.0 | 0.0 | 0.0 | 0.0 | 0.0 | 0.0 | 0.0 | 0.0 | 0.0 | 0.0 | 0.0 | 0.0 |
| 水及饮料类 Water and beverages | 0.0 | 0.0 | 0.0 | 0.0 | 0.0 | 0.0 | 0.0 | 0.0 | 0.0 | 0.0 | 0.0 | 0.0 | 0.0 | 0.0 | 0.0 | 0.0 | 0.0 | 0.0 | 0.0 | 0.0 | 0.0 | 0.0 | 0.0 | 0.0 | 0.0 |
| 酒类 Alcohol beverages | 0.0 | 0.0 | 0.0 | 0.0 | 0.0 | 0.0 | 0.0 | 0.0 | 0.0 | 0.0 | 0.0 | 0.0 | 0.0 | 0.0 | 0.0 | 0.0 | 0.0 | 0.0 | 0.0 | 0.0 | 0.0 | 0.0 | 0.0 | 0.0 | 0.0 |

附表 4-22 第六次中国总膳食研究三唑磷的膳食来源（单位：%）

Annexed Table 4-22 Dietary sources of triazophos from the 6$^{th}$ China TDS (Unit: %)

| 膳食类别 Category | 黑龙江 HL | 辽宁 LN | 河北 HE | 北京 BJ | 吉林 JL | 山西 SX | 陕西 SN | 河南 HA | 宁夏 NX | 内蒙古 NM | 青海 QH | 甘肃 GS | 上海 SH | 福建 FJ | 江西 JX | 江苏 JS | 浙江 ZJ | 山东 SD | 湖北 HB | 四川 SC | 广西 GX | 湖南 HN | 广东 GD | 贵州 GZ | 全国平均 AVG |
|---|---|---|---|---|---|---|---|---|---|---|---|---|---|---|---|---|---|---|---|---|---|---|---|---|---|
| 谷类 Cereals | 0.0 | 0.0 | 100.0 | 0.0 | 0.0 | 0.0 | 0.0 | 0.0 | 0.0 | 0.0 | 0.0 | 0.0 | 0.0 | 0.0 | 59.2 | 100.0 | 44.8 | 0.0 | 100.0 | 99.1 | 82.9 | 93.9 | 37.8 | 0.0 | 46.7 |

续表

| 膳食类别<br>Category | 黑龙江<br>HL | 辽宁<br>LN | 河北<br>HE | 北京<br>BJ | 吉林<br>JL | 山西<br>SX | 陕西<br>SN | 河南<br>HA | 宁夏<br>NX | 内蒙古<br>NM | 青海<br>QH | 甘肃<br>GS | 上海<br>SH | 福建<br>FJ | 江西<br>JX | 江苏<br>JS | 浙江<br>ZJ | 山东<br>SD | 湖北<br>HB | 四川<br>SC | 广西<br>GX | 湖南<br>HN | 广东<br>GD | 贵州<br>GZ | 全国平均<br>AVG |
|---|---|---|---|---|---|---|---|---|---|---|---|---|---|---|---|---|---|---|---|---|---|---|---|---|---|
| 豆类 Legumes | 0.0 | 0.0 | 0.0 | 0.0 | 0.0 | 0.0 | 0.0 | 0.0 | 0.0 | 0.0 | 0.0 | 100.0 | 0.0 | 0.0 | 0.0 | 0.0 | 0.0 | 0.0 | 0.0 | 0.0 | 0.0 | 0.0 | 0.0 | 0.0 | 0.1 |
| 薯类 Potatoes | 0.0 | 0.0 | 0.0 | 0.0 | 0.0 | 0.0 | 0.0 | 0.0 | 0.0 | 0.0 | 0.0 | 0.0 | 0.0 | 0.0 | 0.0 | 0.0 | 0.0 | 0.0 | 0.0 | 0.0 | 0.0 | 0.0 | 0.0 | 0.0 | 0.0 |
| 肉类 Meats | 0.0 | 0.0 | 0.0 | 0.0 | 0.0 | 0.0 | 0.0 | 92.3 | 0.0 | 0.0 | 0.0 | 0.0 | 0.0 | 0.0 | 0.0 | 0.0 | 0.0 | 0.0 | 0.0 | 0.0 | 0.0 | 0.0 | 0.0 | 0.0 | 0.1 |
| 蛋类 Eggs | 0.0 | 0.0 | 0.0 | 0.0 | 0.0 | 0.0 | 0.0 | 0.0 | 0.0 | 0.0 | 0.0 | 0.0 | 0.0 | 0.0 | 0.0 | 0.0 | 0.0 | 0.0 | 0.0 | 0.0 | 0.0 | 0.0 | 0.0 | 0.0 | 0.0 |
| 水产类 Aquatic foods | 0.0 | 0.0 | 0.0 | 0.0 | 0.0 | 0.0 | 0.0 | 7.7 | 0.0 | 0.0 | 0.0 | 0.0 | 100.0 | 0.7 | 1.4 | 0.0 | 6.6 | 0.0 | 0.0 | 0.0 | 0.0 | 6.1 | 7.2 | 100.0 | 1.8 |
| 乳类 Dairy products | 0.0 | 0.0 | 0.0 | 0.0 | 0.0 | 0.0 | 0.0 | 0.0 | 0.0 | 0.0 | 0.0 | 0.0 | 0.0 | 0.0 | 0.0 | 0.0 | 0.0 | 0.0 | 0.0 | 0.0 | 0.0 | 0.0 | 0.0 | 0.0 | 0.0 |
| 蔬菜类 Vegetables | 0.0 | 0.0 | 0.0 | 0.0 | 0.0 | 100.0 | 0.0 | 0.0 | 0.0 | 0.0 | 0.0 | 0.0 | 0.0 | 72.4 | 39.4 | 0.0 | 45.6 | 0.0 | 0.0 | 0.0 | 17.1 | 0.0 | 55.0 | 0.0 | 40.8 |
| 水果类 Fruits | 100.0 | 100.0 | 0.0 | 0.0 | 0.0 | 0.0 | 0.0 | 0.0 | 0.0 | 0.0 | 0.0 | 0.0 | 0.0 | 20.4 | 0.0 | 0.0 | 3.0 | 0.0 | 0.0 | 0.9 | 0.0 | 0.0 | 0.0 | 0.0 | 8.2 |
| 糖类 Sugar | 0.0 | 0.0 | 0.0 | 0.0 | 0.0 | 0.0 | 0.0 | 0.0 | 0.0 | 0.0 | 0.0 | 0.0 | 0.0 | 0.0 | 0.0 | 0.0 | 0.0 | 0.0 | 0.0 | 0.0 | 0.0 | 0.0 | 0.0 | 0.0 | 0.0 |
| 水及饮料类 Water and beverages | 0.0 | 0.0 | 0.0 | 0.0 | 0.0 | 0.0 | 0.0 | 0.0 | 0.0 | 0.0 | 0.0 | 0.0 | 0.0 | 6.5 | 0.0 | 0.0 | 0.0 | 0.0 | 0.0 | 0.0 | 0.0 | 0.0 | 0.0 | 0.0 | 2.3 |
| 酒类 Alcohol beverages | 0.0 | 0.0 | 0.0 | 0.0 | 0.0 | 0.0 | 0.0 | 0.0 | 0.0 | 0.0 | 0.0 | 0.0 | 0.0 | 0.0 | 0.0 | 0.0 | 0.0 | 0.0 | 0.0 | 0.0 | 0.0 | 0.0 | 0.0 | 0.0 | 0.0 |

附表 4-23　第六次中国总膳食研究丙溴磷的膳食来源（单位：%）

Annexed Table 4-23　Dietary sources of profenofos from the 6th China TDS (Unit: %)

| 膳食类别<br>Category | 黑龙江<br>HL | 辽宁<br>LN | 河北<br>HE | 北京<br>BJ | 吉林<br>JL | 山西<br>SX | 陕西<br>SN | 河南<br>HA | 宁夏<br>NX | 内蒙古<br>NM | 青海<br>QH | 甘肃<br>GS | 上海<br>SH | 福建<br>FJ | 江西<br>JX | 江苏<br>JS | 浙江<br>ZJ | 山东<br>SD | 湖北<br>HB | 四川<br>SC | 广西<br>GX | 湖南<br>HN | 广东<br>GD | 贵州<br>GZ | 全国平均<br>AVG |
|---|---|---|---|---|---|---|---|---|---|---|---|---|---|---|---|---|---|---|---|---|---|---|---|---|---|
| 谷类 Cereals | 0.0 | 0.0 | 0.0 | 0.0 | 0.0 | 0.0 | 0.0 | 0.0 | 0.0 | 0.0 | 0.0 | 0.0 | 0.0 | 0.0 | 0.0 | 0.0 | 0.0 | 0.0 | 0.0 | 0.0 | 0.0 | 0.0 | 0.0 | 0.0 | 0.0 |
| 豆类 Legumes | 0.0 | 0.0 | 0.0 | 0.0 | 0.0 | 0.0 | 17.2 | 0.0 | 0.0 | 0.0 | 0.0 | 0.0 | 0.0 | 0.0 | 0.0 | 0.0 | 0.0 | 0.0 | 0.0 | 0.0 | 0.0 | 0.0 | 0.0 | 0.0 | 0.1 |
| 薯类 Potatoes | 0.0 | 0.0 | 0.0 | 0.0 | 0.0 | 0.0 | 0.0 | 0.0 | 0.0 | 0.0 | 0.0 | 0.0 | 0.0 | 0.0 | 0.0 | 0.0 | 0.0 | 0.0 | 0.0 | 0.0 | 0.0 | 0.0 | 0.0 | 0.0 | 0.0 |
| 肉类 Meats | 0.0 | 0.0 | 0.0 | 0.0 | 0.0 | 0.0 | 0.0 | 1.1 | 0.0 | 0.0 | 2.3 | 0.0 | 0.0 | 0.0 | 0.0 | 0.0 | 0.0 | 0.0 | 0.0 | 0.0 | 0.0 | 0.0 | 0.0 | 0.0 | 0.1 |
| 蛋类 Eggs | 0.0 | 0.0 | 0.0 | 0.0 | 0.0 | 0.0 | 0.0 | 0.0 | 0.0 | 0.0 | 0.0 | 0.0 | 0.0 | 0.0 | 0.0 | 0.0 | 0.0 | 0.0 | 0.0 | 0.0 | 0.0 | 0.0 | 0.0 | 0.0 | 0.0 |
| 水产类 Aquatic foods | 0.0 | 0.0 | 0.0 | 0.0 | 0.0 | 0.0 | 0.0 | 0.0 | 0.0 | 0.0 | 0.0 | 0.0 | 0.0 | 0.0 | 0.0 | 0.0 | 0.0 | 0.0 | 0.0 | 0.0 | 0.0 | 0.0 | 0.0 | 0.0 | 0.0 |
| 乳类 Dairy products | 0.0 | 0.0 | 0.0 | 0.0 | 0.0 | 0.0 | 0.0 | 0.0 | 0.0 | 0.0 | 0.0 | 0.0 | 0.0 | 0.0 | 0.0 | 0.0 | 0.0 | 0.0 | 0.0 | 0.0 | 0.0 | 0.0 | 0.0 | 0.0 | 0.0 |
| 蔬菜类 Vegetables | 0.0 | 0.0 | 100.0 | 0.0 | 0.0 | 100.0 | 57.5 | 98.9 | 0.0 | 0.0 | 97.7 | 63.4 | 99.9 | 59.4 | 100.0 | 0.0 | 0.0 | 0.0 | 99.3 | 0.0 | 100.0 | 95.9 | 100.0 | 0.0 | 92.7 |
| 水果类 Fruits | 0.0 | 100.0 | 0.0 | 100.0 | 100.0 | 0.0 | 25.4 | 0.0 | 0.0 | 0.0 | 0.0 | 36.6 | 0.0 | 40.6 | 0.0 | 0.0 | 0.0 | 0.0 | 0.7 | 100.0 | 0.0 | 4.1 | 0.0 | 100.0 | 7.1 |
| 糖类 Sugar | 0.0 | 0.0 | 0.0 | 0.0 | 0.0 | 0.0 | 0.0 | 0.0 | 0.0 | 0.0 | 0.0 | 0.0 | 0.1 | 0.0 | 0.0 | 0.0 | 0.0 | 0.0 | 0.0 | 0.0 | 0.0 | 0.0 | 0.0 | 0.0 | 0.0 |
| 水及饮料类 Water and beverages | 0.0 | 0.0 | 0.0 | 0.0 | 0.0 | 0.0 | 0.0 | 0.0 | 0.0 | 0.0 | 0.0 | 0.0 | 0.0 | 0.0 | 0.0 | 0.0 | 0.0 | 0.0 | 0.0 | 0.0 | 0.0 | 0.0 | 0.0 | 0.0 | 0.0 |

续表

| 膳食类别<br>Category | 黑龙江<br>HL | 辽宁<br>LN | 河北<br>HE | 北京<br>BJ | 吉林<br>JL | 山西<br>SX | 陕西<br>SN | 河南<br>HA | 宁夏<br>NX | 内蒙古<br>NM | 青海<br>QH | 甘肃<br>GS | 上海<br>SH | 福建<br>FJ | 江西<br>JX | 江苏<br>JS | 浙江<br>ZJ | 山东<br>SD | 湖北<br>HB | 四川<br>SC | 广西<br>GX | 湖南<br>HN | 广东<br>GD | 贵州<br>GZ | 全国平均<br>AVG |
|---|---|---|---|---|---|---|---|---|---|---|---|---|---|---|---|---|---|---|---|---|---|---|---|---|---|
| 酒类<br>Alcohol beverages | 0.0 | 0.0 | 0.0 | 0.0 | 0.0 | 0.0 | 0.0 | 0.0 | 0.0 | 0.0 | 0.0 | 0.0 | 0.0 | 0.0 | 0.0 | 0.0 | 0.0 | 0.0 | 0.0 | 0.0 | 0.0 | 0.0 | 0.0 | 0.0 | 0.0 |

附表 4-24 第六次中国总膳食研究氧乐果的膳食来源（单位：%）

Annexed Table 4-24 Dietary sources of omethoate from the 6$^{th}$ China TDS (Unit: %)

| 膳食类别<br>Category | 黑龙江<br>HL | 辽宁<br>LN | 河北<br>HE | 北京<br>BJ | 吉林<br>JL | 山西<br>SX | 陕西<br>SN | 河南<br>HA | 宁夏<br>NX | 内蒙古<br>NM | 青海<br>QH | 甘肃<br>GS | 上海<br>SH | 福建<br>FJ | 江西<br>JX | 江苏<br>JS | 浙江<br>ZJ | 山东<br>SD | 湖北<br>HB | 四川<br>SC | 广西<br>GX | 湖南<br>HN | 广东<br>GD | 贵州<br>GZ | 全国平均<br>AVG |
|---|---|---|---|---|---|---|---|---|---|---|---|---|---|---|---|---|---|---|---|---|---|---|---|---|---|
| 谷类<br>Cereals | 0.0 | 0.0 | 0.0 | 0.0 | 0.0 | 0.0 | 0.0 | 0.0 | 0.0 | 0.0 | 0.0 | 0.0 | 0.0 | 0.0 | 0.0 | 0.0 | 0.0 | 0.0 | 0.0 | 0.0 | 0.0 | 0.0 | 0.0 | 0.0 | 0.0 |
| 豆类<br>Legumes | 0.0 | 0.0 | 0.0 | 0.0 | 0.0 | 0.0 | 0.0 | 0.0 | 0.0 | 0.0 | 0.0 | 0.0 | 0.0 | 0.0 | 0.0 | 0.0 | 0.0 | 0.0 | 0.0 | 0.0 | 0.0 | 0.0 | 0.0 | 0.0 | 0.0 |
| 薯类<br>Potatoes | 0.0 | 0.0 | 0.0 | 0.0 | 0.0 | 0.0 | 0.0 | 0.0 | 0.0 | 0.0 | 0.0 | 0.0 | 0.0 | 0.0 | 0.0 | 0.0 | 0.0 | 0.0 | 3.6 | 0.0 | 0.0 | 0.0 | 0.0 | 0.0 | 0.1 |
| 肉类<br>Meats | 0.0 | 0.0 | 0.0 | 0.0 | 0.0 | 0.0 | 0.0 | 0.0 | 0.0 | 0.0 | 0.0 | 0.0 | 0.0 | 0.0 | 0.0 | 0.0 | 0.0 | 0.0 | 0.0 | 0.0 | 0.0 | 0.0 | 0.0 | 0.0 | 0.0 |
| 蛋类<br>Eggs | 0.0 | 0.0 | 0.0 | 0.0 | 0.0 | 0.0 | 0.0 | 0.0 | 0.0 | 0.0 | 0.0 | 0.0 | 0.0 | 0.0 | 0.0 | 0.0 | 0.0 | 0.0 | 0.0 | 0.0 | 0.0 | 0.0 | 0.0 | 0.0 | 0.0 |
| 水产类<br>Aquatic foods | 0.0 | 0.0 | 0.0 | 0.0 | 0.0 | 0.0 | 0.0 | 0.0 | 0.0 | 0.0 | 0.0 | 0.0 | 100.0 | 0.0 | 0.0 | 0.0 | 0.0 | 0.0 | 0.0 | 0.0 | 0.0 | 0.0 | 0.0 | 0.0 | 0.0 |
| 乳类<br>Dairy products | 0.0 | 0.0 | 0.0 | 0.0 | 100.0 | 0.0 | 0.0 | 0.0 | 0.0 | 0.0 | 0.0 | 0.0 | 0.0 | 0.0 | 0.0 | 0.0 | 0.0 | 0.0 | 0.0 | 0.0 | 0.0 | 0.0 | 99.4 | 0.0 | 0.0 |
| 蔬菜类<br>Vegetables | 0.0 | 69.4 | 0.0 | 0.0 | 0.0 | 0.0 | 0.0 | 0.0 | 0.0 | 0.0 | 0.0 | 0.0 | 0.0 | 0.0 | 0.0 | 0.0 | 0.0 | 0.0 | 95.3 | 0.0 | 0.0 | 100.0 | 0.0 | 0.0 | 95.0 |

续表

| 膳食类别 Category | 黑龙江 HL | 辽宁 LN | 河北 HE | 北京 BJ | 吉林 JL | 山西 SX | 陕西 SN | 河南 HA | 宁夏 NX | 内蒙古 NM | 青海 QH | 甘肃 GS | 上海 SH | 福建 FJ | 江西 JX | 江苏 JS | 浙江 ZJ | 山东 SD | 湖北 HB | 四川 SC | 广西 GX | 湖南 HN | 广东 GD | 贵州 GZ | 全国平均 AVG |
|---|---|---|---|---|---|---|---|---|---|---|---|---|---|---|---|---|---|---|---|---|---|---|---|---|---|
| 水果类 Fruits | 0.0 | 30.6 | 0.0 | 0.0 | 0.0 | 0.0 | 100.0 | 0.0 | 0.0 | 0.0 | 0.0 | 0.0 | 0.0 | 0.0 | 0.0 | 0.0 | 0.0 | 0.0 | 1.1 | 0.0 | 100.0 | 0.0 | 0.0 | 0.0 | 2.5 |
| 糖类 Sugar | 0.0 | 0.0 | 0.0 | 0.0 | 0.0 | 0.0 | 0.0 | 0.0 | 0.0 | 0.0 | 0.0 | 0.0 | 0.0 | 0.0 | 0.0 | 0.0 | 0.0 | 0.0 | 0.0 | 0.0 | 0.0 | 0.0 | 0.6 | 0.0 | 0.0 |
| 水及饮料类 Water and beverages | 0.0 | 0.0 | 0.0 | 0.0 | 0.0 | 0.0 | 0.0 | 0.0 | 0.0 | 0.0 | 0.0 | 0.0 | 0.0 | 0.0 | 0.0 | 100.0 | 0.0 | 0.0 | 0.0 | 0.0 | 0.0 | 0.0 | 0.0 | 0.0 | 2.3 |
| 酒类 Alcohol beverages | 0.0 | 0.0 | 0.0 | 0.0 | 0.0 | 0.0 | 0.0 | 0.0 | 0.0 | 0.0 | 0.0 | 0.0 | 0.0 | 0.0 | 0.0 | 0.0 | 0.0 | 0.0 | 0.0 | 0.0 | 0.0 | 0.0 | 0.0 | 0.0 | 0.0 |

附表 4-25 第六次中国总膳食研究乐果的膳食来源（单位：%）

Annexed Table 4-25 Dietary sources of dimethoate from the 6$^{th}$ China TDS (Unit: %)

| 膳食类别 Category | 黑龙江 HL | 辽宁 LN | 河北 HE | 北京 BJ | 吉林 JL | 山西 SX | 陕西 SN | 河南 HA | 宁夏 NX | 内蒙古 NM | 青海 QH | 甘肃 GS | 上海 SH | 福建 FJ | 江西 JX | 江苏 JS | 浙江 ZJ | 山东 SD | 湖北 HB | 四川 SC | 广西 GX | 湖南 HN | 广东 GD | 贵州 GZ | 全国平均 AVG |
|---|---|---|---|---|---|---|---|---|---|---|---|---|---|---|---|---|---|---|---|---|---|---|---|---|---|
| 谷类 Cereals | 0.0 | 0.0 | 0.0 | 0.0 | 0.0 | 0.0 | 0.0 | 0.0 | 0.0 | 0.0 | 0.0 | 0.0 | 0.0 | 0.0 | 0.0 | 0.0 | 0.0 | 0.0 | 0.0 | 0.0 | 0.0 | 0.0 | 0.0 | 0.0 | 0.0 |
| 豆类 Legumes | 0.0 | 0.0 | 100.0 | 0.0 | 0.0 | 0.0 | 0.0 | 0.0 | 0.0 | 0.0 | 0.0 | 0.0 | 0.0 | 0.0 | 0.0 | 0.0 | 0.0 | 0.0 | 0.0 | 0.0 | 0.0 | 0.0 | 0.0 | 0.0 | 0.0 |
| 薯类 Potatoes | 0.0 | 0.0 | 0.0 | 0.0 | 0.0 | 0.0 | 0.0 | 0.0 | 0.0 | 0.0 | 0.0 | 0.0 | 0.0 | 0.0 | 0.0 | 0.0 | 0.0 | 0.0 | 0.0 | 0.0 | 0.0 | 0.0 | 0.0 | 0.0 | 0.0 |
| 肉类 Meats | 0.0 | 0.0 | 0.0 | 0.0 | 0.0 | 0.0 | 0.0 | 0.0 | 0.0 | 0.0 | 0.0 | 0.0 | 0.0 | 0.0 | 0.0 | 0.0 | 0.0 | 0.0 | 0.0 | 0.0 | 0.0 | 0.0 | 0.0 | 0.0 | 0.0 |
| 蛋类 Eggs | 0.0 | 0.0 | 0.0 | 0.0 | 0.0 | 0.0 | 0.0 | 0.0 | 0.0 | 0.0 | 0.0 | 0.0 | 0.0 | 0.0 | 0.0 | 0.0 | 0.0 | 0.0 | 0.0 | 0.0 | 0.0 | 0.0 | 0.0 | 0.0 | 0.0 |

续表

| 膳食类别<br>Category | 黑龙江<br>HL | 辽宁<br>LN | 河北<br>HE | 北京<br>BJ | 吉林<br>JL | 山西<br>SX | 陕西<br>SN | 河南<br>HA | 宁夏<br>NX | 内蒙古<br>NM | 青海<br>QH | 甘肃<br>GS | 上海<br>SH | 福建<br>FJ | 江西<br>JX | 江苏<br>JS | 浙江<br>ZJ | 山东<br>SD | 湖北<br>HB | 四川<br>SC | 广西<br>GX | 湖南<br>HN | 广东<br>GD | 贵州<br>GZ | 全国平均<br>AVG |
|---|---|---|---|---|---|---|---|---|---|---|---|---|---|---|---|---|---|---|---|---|---|---|---|---|---|
| 水产类<br>Aquatic foods | 0.0 | 0.0 | 0.0 | 0.0 | 0.0 | 0.0 | 0.0 | 0.0 | 0.0 | 0.0 | 0.0 | 0.0 | 0.0 | 0.0 | 0.0 | 0.0 | 0.0 | 0.0 | 0.0 | 0.0 | 0.0 | 0.0 | 0.0 | 0.0 | 0.0 |
| 乳类<br>Dairy products | 0.0 | 0.0 | 0.0 | 0.0 | 0.0 | 0.0 | 0.0 | 0.0 | 0.0 | 0.0 | 0.0 | 0.0 | 0.0 | 0.0 | 0.0 | 0.0 | 0.0 | 0.0 | 0.0 | 0.0 | 0.0 | 0.0 | 0.0 | 0.0 | 0.0 |
| 蔬菜类<br>Vegetables | 0.0 | 0.0 | 0.0 | 100.0 | 0.0 | 0.0 | 0.0 | 0.0 | 0.0 | 0.0 | 0.0 | 100.0 | 0.0 | 0.0 | 0.0 | 0.0 | 0.0 | 0.0 | 0.0 | 0.0 | 0.0 | 100.0 | 100.0 | 0.0 | 99.2 |
| 水果类<br>Fruits | 0.0 | 0.0 | 0.0 | 0.0 | 0.0 | 0.0 | 100.0 | 0.0 | 0.0 | 0.0 | 0.0 | 0.0 | 0.0 | 0.0 | 0.0 | 0.0 | 0.0 | 0.0 | 0.0 | 0.0 | 0.0 | 0.0 | 0.0 | 0.0 | 0.3 |
| 糖类<br>Sugar | 0.0 | 0.0 | 0.0 | 0.0 | 0.0 | 0.0 | 0.0 | 0.0 | 0.0 | 0.0 | 0.0 | 0.0 | 0.0 | 0.0 | 0.0 | 0.0 | 0.0 | 0.0 | 0.0 | 0.0 | 0.0 | 0.0 | 0.0 | 0.0 | 0.0 |
| 水及饮料类<br>Water and beverages | 0.0 | 0.0 | 0.0 | 0.0 | 100.0 | 0.0 | 0.0 | 0.0 | 0.0 | 0.0 | 0.0 | 0.0 | 100.0 | 0.0 | 0.0 | 100.0 | 0.0 | 0.0 | 0.0 | 0.0 | 0.0 | 0.0 | 0.0 | 0.0 | 0.5 |
| 酒类<br>Alcohol beverages | 0.0 | 0.0 | 0.0 | 0.0 | 0.0 | 0.0 | 0.0 | 0.0 | 0.0 | 0.0 | 0.0 | 0.0 | 0.0 | 0.0 | 0.0 | 0.0 | 0.0 | 0.0 | 0.0 | 0.0 | 0.0 | 0.0 | 0.0 | 0.0 | 0.0 |

附表 4-26　第六次中国总膳食研究甲胺磷的膳食来源（单位：%）

Annexed Table 4-26　Dietary sources of methamidophos from the 6$^{th}$ China TDS (Unit: %)

| 膳食类别<br>Category | 黑龙江<br>HL | 辽宁<br>LN | 河北<br>HE | 北京<br>BJ | 吉林<br>JL | 山西<br>SX | 陕西<br>SN | 河南<br>HA | 宁夏<br>NX | 内蒙古<br>NM | 青海<br>QH | 甘肃<br>GS | 上海<br>SH | 福建<br>FJ | 江西<br>JX | 江苏<br>JS | 浙江<br>ZJ | 山东<br>SD | 湖北<br>HB | 四川<br>SC | 广西<br>GX | 湖南<br>HN | 广东<br>GD | 贵州<br>GZ | 全国平均<br>AVG |
|---|---|---|---|---|---|---|---|---|---|---|---|---|---|---|---|---|---|---|---|---|---|---|---|---|---|
| 谷类<br>Cereals | 0.0 | 0.0 | 0.0 | 0.0 | 0.0 | 0.0 | 0.0 | 0.0 | 0.0 | 0.0 | 0.0 | 0.0 | 0.0 | 0.0 | 0.0 | 0.0 | 0.0 | 0.0 | 0.0 | 0.0 | 0.0 | 0.0 | 0.0 | 0.0 | 0.0 |

续表

| 膳食类别 Category | 黑龙江 HL | 辽宁 LN | 河北 HE | 北京 BJ | 吉林 JL | 山西 SX | 陕西 SN | 河南 HA | 宁夏 NX | 内蒙古 NM | 青海 QH | 甘肃 GS | 上海 SH | 福建 FJ | 江西 JX | 江苏 JS | 浙江 ZJ | 山东 SD | 湖北 HB | 四川 SC | 广西 GX | 湖南 HN | 广东 GD | 贵州 GZ | 全国平均 AVG |
|---|---|---|---|---|---|---|---|---|---|---|---|---|---|---|---|---|---|---|---|---|---|---|---|---|---|
| 豆类 Legumes | 0.0 | 0.0 | 100.0 | 0.0 | 0.0 | 0.0 | 0.0 | 0.0 | 0.0 | 0.0 | 0.0 | 0.0 | 0.0 | 0.0 | 0.0 | 0.0 | 0.0 | 0.0 | 0.0 | 0.0 | 0.0 | 0.0 | 0.0 | 0.0 | 43.1 |
| 薯类 Potatoes | 0.0 | 0.0 | 0.0 | 0.0 | 0.0 | 0.0 | 0.0 | 0.0 | 0.0 | 0.0 | 0.0 | 0.0 | 0.0 | 0.0 | 0.0 | 0.0 | 0.0 | 0.0 | 100.0 | 0.0 | 0.0 | 0.0 | 0.0 | 0.0 | 38.4 |
| 肉类 Meats | 0.0 | 0.0 | 0.0 | 0.0 | 0.0 | 0.0 | 0.0 | 0.0 | 0.0 | 0.0 | 0.0 | 0.0 | 0.0 | 0.0 | 0.0 | 0.0 | 0.0 | 0.0 | 0.0 | 0.0 | 0.0 | 0.0 | 0.0 | 0.0 | 0.0 |
| 蛋类 Eggs | 0.0 | 0.0 | 0.0 | 0.0 | 0.0 | 0.0 | 0.0 | 0.0 | 0.0 | 0.0 | 0.0 | 0.0 | 0.0 | 0.0 | 0.0 | 0.0 | 0.0 | 0.0 | 0.0 | 0.0 | 0.0 | 0.0 | 0.0 | 0.0 | 0.0 |
| 水产类 Aquatic foods | 0.0 | 0.0 | 0.0 | 0.0 | 0.0 | 0.0 | 0.0 | 0.0 | 0.0 | 0.0 | 0.0 | 0.0 | 0.0 | 0.0 | 0.0 | 0.0 | 0.0 | 0.0 | 0.0 | 0.0 | 0.0 | 0.0 | 0.0 | 0.0 | 0.0 |
| 乳类 Dairy products | 0.0 | 0.0 | 0.0 | 0.0 | 0.0 | 0.0 | 0.0 | 0.0 | 0.0 | 0.0 | 0.0 | 0.0 | 0.0 | 0.0 | 0.0 | 0.0 | 0.0 | 0.0 | 0.0 | 0.0 | 0.0 | 0.0 | 0.0 | 0.0 | 0.0 |
| 蔬菜类 Vegetables | 0.0 | 0.0 | 0.0 | 0.0 | 0.0 | 0.0 | 0.0 | 0.0 | 0.0 | 0.0 | 0.0 | 0.0 | 0.0 | 0.0 | 0.0 | 0.0 | 0.0 | 0.0 | 0.0 | 0.0 | 0.0 | 0.0 | 0.0 | 0.0 | 0.0 |
| 水果类 Fruits | 0.0 | 0.0 | 0.0 | 0.0 | 0.0 | 0.0 | 0.0 | 100.0 | 0.0 | 0.0 | 0.0 | 0.0 | 0.0 | 0.0 | 0.0 | 0.0 | 0.0 | 0.0 | 0.0 | 0.0 | 0.0 | 0.0 | 0.0 | 0.0 | 18.5 |
| 糖类 Sugar | 0.0 | 0.0 | 0.0 | 0.0 | 0.0 | 0.0 | 0.0 | 0.0 | 0.0 | 0.0 | 0.0 | 0.0 | 0.0 | 0.0 | 0.0 | 0.0 | 0.0 | 0.0 | 0.0 | 0.0 | 0.0 | 0.0 | 0.0 | 0.0 | 0.0 |
| 水及饮料类 Water and beverages | 0.0 | 0.0 | 0.0 | 0.0 | 0.0 | 0.0 | 0.0 | 0.0 | 0.0 | 0.0 | 0.0 | 0.0 | 0.0 | 0.0 | 0.0 | 0.0 | 0.0 | 0.0 | 0.0 | 0.0 | 0.0 | 0.0 | 0.0 | 0.0 | 0.0 |
| 酒类 Alcohol beverages | 0.0 | 0.0 | 0.0 | 0.0 | 0.0 | 0.0 | 0.0 | 0.0 | 0.0 | 0.0 | 0.0 | 0.0 | 0.0 | 0.0 | 0.0 | 0.0 | 0.0 | 0.0 | 0.0 | 0.0 | 0.0 | 0.0 | 0.0 | 0.0 | 0.0 |

附表 4-27　第六次中国总膳食研究二嗪磷的膳食来源（单位：%）

Annexed Table 4-27　Dietary sources of diazinon from the 6$^{th}$ China TDS (Unit: %)

| 膳食类别<br>Category | 黑龙江<br>HL | 辽宁<br>LN | 河北<br>HE | 北京<br>BJ | 吉林<br>JL | 山西<br>SX | 陕西<br>SN | 河南<br>HA | 宁夏<br>NX | 内蒙古<br>NM | 青海<br>QH | 甘肃<br>GS | 上海<br>SH | 福建<br>FJ | 江西<br>JX | 江苏<br>JS | 浙江<br>ZJ | 山东<br>SD | 湖北<br>HB | 四川<br>SC | 广西<br>GX | 湖南<br>HN | 广东<br>GD | 贵州<br>GZ | 全国平均<br>AVG |
|---|---|---|---|---|---|---|---|---|---|---|---|---|---|---|---|---|---|---|---|---|---|---|---|---|---|
| 谷类 Cereals | 0.0 | 0.0 | 0.0 | 0.0 | 0.0 | 0.0 | 0.0 | 0.0 | 0.0 | 0.0 | 0.0 | 0.0 | 0.0 | 0.0 | 0.0 | 0.0 | 0.0 | 0.0 | 0.0 | 0.0 | 0.0 | 0.0 | 0.0 | 0.0 | 0.0 |
| 豆类 Legumes | 0.0 | 0.0 | 0.0 | 0.0 | 0.0 | 0.0 | 0.0 | 0.0 | 0.0 | 0.0 | 0.0 | 0.0 | 0.0 | 0.0 | 0.0 | 0.0 | 0.0 | 0.0 | 0.0 | 0.0 | 0.0 | 0.0 | 0.0 | 0.0 | 0.0 |
| 薯类 Potatoes | 0.0 | 0.0 | 0.0 | 0.0 | 0.0 | 0.0 | 0.0 | 0.0 | 0.0 | 0.0 | 0.0 | 0.0 | 0.0 | 0.0 | 0.0 | 0.0 | 0.0 | 0.0 | 0.0 | 0.0 | 0.0 | 0.0 | 0.0 | 0.0 | 0.0 |
| 肉类 Meats | 0.0 | 0.0 | 0.0 | 0.0 | 0.0 | 0.0 | 0.0 | 0.0 | 0.0 | 0.0 | 0.0 | 0.0 | 0.0 | 0.0 | 0.0 | 0.0 | 0.0 | 100.0 | 0.0 | 0.0 | 0.0 | 0.0 | 0.0 | 0.0 | 98.4 |
| 蛋类 Eggs | 0.0 | 0.0 | 0.0 | 0.0 | 0.0 | 0.0 | 0.0 | 0.0 | 0.0 | 0.0 | 0.0 | 0.0 | 0.0 | 0.0 | 0.0 | 0.0 | 0.0 | 0.0 | 0.0 | 0.0 | 0.0 | 0.0 | 0.0 | 0.0 | 0.0 |
| 水产类 Aquatic foods | 0.0 | 0.0 | 0.0 | 0.0 | 0.0 | 0.0 | 100.0 | 0.0 | 0.0 | 0.0 | 0.0 | 0.0 | 0.0 | 0.0 | 0.0 | 0.0 | 0.0 | 0.0 | 0.0 | 0.0 | 0.0 | 0.0 | 0.0 | 0.0 | 1.6 |
| 乳类 Dairy products | 0.0 | 0.0 | 0.0 | 0.0 | 0.0 | 0.0 | 0.0 | 0.0 | 0.0 | 0.0 | 0.0 | 0.0 | 0.0 | 0.0 | 0.0 | 0.0 | 0.0 | 0.0 | 0.0 | 0.0 | 0.0 | 0.0 | 0.0 | 0.0 | 0.0 |
| 蔬菜类 Vegetables | 0.0 | 0.0 | 0.0 | 0.0 | 0.0 | 0.0 | 0.0 | 0.0 | 0.0 | 0.0 | 0.0 | 0.0 | 0.0 | 0.0 | 0.0 | 0.0 | 0.0 | 0.0 | 0.0 | 0.0 | 0.0 | 0.0 | 0.0 | 0.0 | 0.0 |
| 水果类 Fruits | 0.0 | 0.0 | 0.0 | 0.0 | 0.0 | 0.0 | 0.0 | 0.0 | 0.0 | 0.0 | 0.0 | 0.0 | 0.0 | 0.0 | 0.0 | 0.0 | 0.0 | 0.0 | 0.0 | 0.0 | 0.0 | 0.0 | 0.0 | 0.0 | 0.0 |
| 糖类 Sugar | 0.0 | 0.0 | 0.0 | 0.0 | 0.0 | 0.0 | 0.0 | 0.0 | 0.0 | 0.0 | 0.0 | 0.0 | 0.0 | 0.0 | 0.0 | 0.0 | 0.0 | 0.0 | 0.0 | 0.0 | 0.0 | 0.0 | 0.0 | 0.0 | 0.0 |
| 水及饮料类 Water and beverages | 0.0 | 0.0 | 0.0 | 0.0 | 0.0 | 0.0 | 0.0 | 0.0 | 0.0 | 0.0 | 0.0 | 0.0 | 0.0 | 0.0 | 0.0 | 0.0 | 0.0 | 0.0 | 0.0 | 0.0 | 0.0 | 0.0 | 0.0 | 0.0 | 0.0 |

续表

| 膳食类别 Category | 黑龙江 HL | 辽宁 LN | 河北 HE | 北京 BJ | 吉林 JL | 山西 SX | 陕西 SN | 河南 HA | 宁夏 NX | 内蒙古 NM | 青海 QH | 甘肃 GS | 上海 SH | 福建 FJ | 江西 JX | 江苏 JS | 浙江 ZJ | 山东 SD | 湖北 HB | 四川 SC | 广西 GX | 湖南 HN | 广东 GD | 贵州 GZ | 全国平均 AVG |
|---|---|---|---|---|---|---|---|---|---|---|---|---|---|---|---|---|---|---|---|---|---|---|---|---|---|
| 酒类 Alcohol beverages | 0.0 | 0.0 | 0.0 | 0.0 | 0.0 | 0.0 | 0.0 | 0.0 | 0.0 | 0.0 | 0.0 | 0.0 | 0.0 | 0.0 | 0.0 | 0.0 | 0.0 | 0.0 | 0.0 | 0.0 | 0.0 | 0.0 | 0.0 | 0.0 | 0.0 |

附表 4-28　第六次中国总膳食研究膳食样品中吡虫啉的含量（单位：μg/kg）

Annexed Table 4-28　Levels of imidacloprid in food samples from the 6th China TDS (Unit: μg/kg)

| 膳食类别 Category | 黑龙江 HL | 辽宁 LN | 河北 HE | 北京 BJ | 吉林 JL | 山西 SX | 陕西 SN | 河南 HA | 宁夏 NX | 内蒙古 NM | 青海 QH | 甘肃 GS | 上海 SH | 福建 FJ | 江西 JX | 江苏 JS | 浙江 ZJ | 山东 SD | 湖北 HB | 四川 SC | 广西 GX | 湖南 HN | 广东 GD | 贵州 GZ | 全国平均 AVG |
|---|---|---|---|---|---|---|---|---|---|---|---|---|---|---|---|---|---|---|---|---|---|---|---|---|---|
| 谷类 Cereals | 0.06 | ND | 0.48 | ND | ND | ND | ND | 0.45 | ND | 0.31 | 0.03 | ND | 0.45 | 0.44 | 0.06 | 0.11 | 0.11 | ND | 0.24 | 0.03 | 0.14 | 0.17 | 0.13 | 0.08 | 0.14 |
| 豆类 Legumes | ND | 0.42 | 0.84 | 0.18 | ND | 0.02 | 0.32 | 1.00 | 0.02 | ND | 0.03 | 0.06 | 0.06 | 0.08 | 0.25 | 0.20 | 0.22 | 0.08 | 0.12 | 0.94 | 0.08 | 0.06 | 0.20 | 0.08 | 0.22 |
| 薯类 Potatoes | ND | 1.69 | 0.55 | 1.35 | 0.14 | 0.25 | 0.07 | 0.51 | 0.14 | 0.49 | 0.10 | 0.02 | 0.12 | 0.15 | 0.08 | 0.10 | 0.13 | 0.09 | 1.65 | 1.83 | 0.07 | 0.14 | 0.33 | 0.55 | 0.44 |
| 肉类 Meats | ND | 0.28 | 1.80 | 0.21 | ND | ND | 0.01 | 1.73 | 0.16 | 0.02 | 0.14 | 0.07 | 0.04 | 0.12 | 0.01 | 0.03 | 0.10 | ND | 0.28 | 0.62 | ND | 0.03 | 0.34 | 0.05 | 0.25 |
| 蛋类 Eggs | ND | 0.50 | 2.22 | 0.09 | ND | 0.03 | ND | 1.74 | ND | 0.04 | ND | ND | ND | 0.09 | ND | ND | ND | 0.01 | 0.27 | ND | ND | 0.02 | ND | ND | 0.21 |
| 水产类 Aquatic foods | ND | 0.05 | 0.31 | 0.19 | ND | 0.04 | 0.47 | 0.30 | ND | 0.04 | ND | 0.02 | 0.02 | 0.10 | 0.03 | 0.03 | 0.05 | ND | 0.28 | 0.85 | ND | ND | 0.27 | 0.07 | 0.13 |
| 乳类 Dairy products | ND | ND | ND | ND | ND | ND | ND | ND | ND | 0.02 | ND | ND | ND | ND | ND | ND | ND | ND | ND | ND | ND | ND | ND | ND | 0.00 |
| 蔬菜类 Vegetables | 1.72 | 2.89 | 3.14 | 1.61 | 2.14 | 3.28 | 2.53 | 3.14 | 2.34 | 2.26 | 1.02 | 3.94 | 10.13 | 0.86 | 28.05 | 0.82 | 0.90 | 3.10 | 8.68 | 1.03 | 4.24 | 4.19 | 4.88 | 1.07 | 4.08 |

续表

| 膳食类别 Category | 黑龙江 HL | 辽宁 LN | 河北 HE | 北京 BJ | 吉林 JL | 山西 SX | 陕西 SN | 河南 HA | 宁夏 NX | 内蒙古 NM | 青海 QH | 甘肃 GS | 上海 SH | 福建 FJ | 江西 JX | 江苏 JS | 浙江 ZJ | 山东 SD | 湖北 HB | 四川 SC | 广西 GX | 湖南 HN | 广东 GD | 贵州 GZ | 全国平均 AVG |
|---|---|---|---|---|---|---|---|---|---|---|---|---|---|---|---|---|---|---|---|---|---|---|---|---|---|
| 水果类 Fruits | 0.77 | 11.41 | 5.89 | 6.34 | 1.83 | 0.47 | 6.50 | 5.89 | 2.97 | 4.41 | 2.74 | 0.84 | 7.07 | 10.42 | 0.53 | 2.16 | 26.96 | 2.30 | 6.03 | 3.15 | 3.52 | 1.41 | 1.95 | 12.37 | 5.33 |
| 糖类 Sugar | ND | ND | ND | ND | ND | ND | ND | ND | ND | ND | ND | ND | 0.38 | ND | ND | ND | ND | ND | ND | ND | ND | ND | ND | ND | 0.02 |
| 水及饮料类 Water and beverages | ND | 0.02 | ND | ND | 0.03 | ND | 0.05 | ND | ND | 0.12 | 0.72 | ND | 0.28 | 0.03 | ND | 0.33 | 0.13 | ND | 0.23 | 0.34 | 0.05 | 0.18 | 0.41 | ND | 0.12 |
| 酒类 Alcohol beverages | ND | ND | ND | 0.11 | ND | ND | ND | ND | ND | ND | ND | 0.02 | 0.11 | 0.04 | ND | ND | 0.06 | 0.06 | ND | ND | 0.49 | ND | 0.24 | ND | 0.05 |

注：未检出（ND）按 0 计

Note: values not detected (ND) were treated as being equal to 0

附表 4-29　第六次中国总膳食研究膳食样品中啶虫脒的含量（单位：μg/kg）

Annexed Table 4-29　Levels of acetamiprid in food samples from the 6th China TDS (Unit: μg/kg)

| 膳食类别 Category | 黑龙江 HL | 辽宁 LN | 河北 HE | 北京 BJ | 吉林 JL | 山西 SX | 陕西 SN | 河南 HA | 宁夏 NX | 内蒙古 NM | 青海 QH | 甘肃 GS | 上海 SH | 福建 FJ | 江西 JX | 江苏 JS | 浙江 ZJ | 山东 SD | 湖北 HB | 四川 SC | 广西 GX | 湖南 HN | 广东 GD | 贵州 GZ | 全国平均 AVG |
|---|---|---|---|---|---|---|---|---|---|---|---|---|---|---|---|---|---|---|---|---|---|---|---|---|---|
| 谷类 Cereals | 0.03 | ND | ND | ND | ND | ND | 0.74 | ND | ND | ND | 0.11 | ND | 0.32 | 0.16 | 0.21 | 0.05 | 0.22 | 0.01 | 0.77 | ND | 0.31 | 0.12 | 0.02 | 0.05 | 0.13 |
| 豆类 Legumes | ND | 0.25 | 0.12 | 0.12 | 0.12 | 0.04 | 2.23 | 0.15 | 0.01 | 0.04 | 0.17 | 0.09 | 0.03 | ND | 0.12 | ND | 0.01 | ND | 0.04 | 1.82 | ND | 0.04 | 0.06 | ND | 0.23 |
| 薯类 Potatoes | ND | 0.30 | ND | ND | ND | ND | 0.30 | ND | 0.30 | ND | 0.44 | 0.13 | 1.06 | ND | 0.05 | ND | 0.02 | ND | ND | 0.21 | ND | ND | ND | 0.01 | 0.12 |
| 肉类 Meats | 0.02 | 0.31 | 0.04 | 0.51 | 0.10 | 0.02 | ND | 0.04 | 0.54 | ND | 0.66 | 0.24 | 0.02 | ND | 0.07 | 0.02 | 0.13 | ND | 0.10 | 3.20 | ND | 0.51 | 0.04 | 0.03 | 0.28 |
| 蛋类 Eggs | ND | 0.31 | ND | ND | ND | ND | ND | ND | 0.03 | ND | ND | ND | ND | ND | ND | ND | ND | ND | 0.06 | 0.03 | ND | ND | ND | 0.04 | 0.02 |

续表

| 膳食类别<br>Category | 黑龙江<br>HL | 辽宁<br>LN | 河北<br>HE | 北京<br>BJ | 吉林<br>JL | 山西<br>SX | 陕西<br>SN | 河南<br>HA | 宁夏<br>NX | 内蒙古<br>NM | 青海<br>QH | 甘肃<br>GS | 上海<br>SH | 福建<br>FJ | 江西<br>JX | 江苏<br>JS | 浙江<br>ZJ | 山东<br>SD | 湖北<br>HB | 四川<br>SC | 广西<br>GX | 湖南<br>HN | 广东<br>GD | 贵州<br>GZ | 全国平均<br>AVG |
|---|---|---|---|---|---|---|---|---|---|---|---|---|---|---|---|---|---|---|---|---|---|---|---|---|---|
| 水产类<br>Aquatic foods | ND | ND | ND | 0.09 | ND | ND | 2.71 | ND | ND | 0.01 | ND | 0.10 | 0.09 | ND | ND | 0.02 | ND | ND | 0.09 | 2.91 | ND | ND | ND | ND | 0.25 |
| 乳类<br>Dairy products | ND | ND | 0.08 | 0.02 | ND | 0.03 | 0.07 | 0.08 | 0.03 | 0.03 | ND | 0.04 | ND | ND | 0.01 | ND | ND | ND | ND | 0.04 | 0.11 | 0.38 | 0.65 | 2.83 | 0.18 |
| 蔬菜类<br>Vegetables | 1.41 | 12.30 | 6.14 | 8.83 | 1.16 | 4.57 | 7.88 | 6.14 | 41.96 | 0.41 | 6.28 | 7.83 | 185.53 | 8.51 | 9.93 | 34.09 | 51.32 | 1.80 | 41.89 | 2.03 | 8.50 | 15.36 | 65.03 | 0.37 | 22.05 |
| 水果类<br>Fruits | 3.60 | 8.91 | 3.12 | 3.64 | 3.09 | 1.35 | 14.37 | 3.12 | 6.51 | 3.00 | 0.12 | 2.89 | 7.63 | 1.94 | 2.31 | 1.80 | 97.56 | 2.46 | 1.43 | 2.70 | 0.31 | 1.99 | 0.58 | 3.41 | 7.41 |
| 糖类<br>Sugar | ND | ND | ND | ND | ND | ND | ND | ND | ND | ND | ND | ND | 0.11 | ND | ND | ND | ND | ND | ND | ND | ND | ND | ND | ND | 0.00 |
| 水及饮料类<br>Water and beverages | ND | ND | ND | ND | ND | ND | 0.16 | ND | ND | 0.32 | 2.94 | ND | 0.93 | 0.14 | ND | 0.70 | 0.23 | ND | 1.07 | 0.68 | 0.11 | 0.54 | 0.67 | ND | 0.36 |
| 酒类<br>Alcohol beverages | ND | ND | 0.03 | 0.02 | ND | ND | ND | 0.03 | ND | 0.01 | ND | 0.04 | 0.07 | 0.02 | 0.01 | 0.02 | 0.04 | 0.04 | ND | ND | 0.03 | ND | 0.04 | ND | 0.02 |

注：未检出（ND）按 0 计
Note: values not detected (ND) were treated as being equal to 0

附表 4-30　第六次中国总膳食研究膳食样品中噻虫嗪的含量（单位：μg/kg）

Annexed Table 4-30　Levels of thiamethoxam in food samples from the 6th China TDS (Unit: μg/kg)

| 膳食类别<br>Category | 黑龙江<br>HL | 辽宁<br>LN | 河北<br>HE | 北京<br>BJ | 吉林<br>JL | 山西<br>SX | 陕西<br>SN | 河南<br>HA | 宁夏<br>NX | 内蒙古<br>NM | 青海<br>QH | 甘肃<br>GS | 上海<br>SH | 福建<br>FJ | 江西<br>JX | 江苏<br>JS | 浙江<br>ZJ | 山东<br>SD | 湖北<br>HB | 四川<br>SC | 广西<br>GX | 湖南<br>HN | 广东<br>GD | 贵州<br>GZ | 全国平均<br>AVG |
|---|---|---|---|---|---|---|---|---|---|---|---|---|---|---|---|---|---|---|---|---|---|---|---|---|---|
| 谷类<br>Cereals | ND | 0.28 | 0.39 | ND | ND | 0.21 | 0.05 | 0.36 | ND | 0.26 | ND | ND | 0.12 | ND | 0.05 | 0.12 | 0.04 | ND | 0.08 | 0.05 | 0.06 | 0.07 | 0.05 | 0.03 | 0.09 |

续表

| 膳食类别 Category | 黑龙江 HL | 辽宁 LN | 河北 HE | 北京 BJ | 吉林 JL | 山西 SX | 陕西 SN | 河南 HA | 宁夏 NX | 内蒙古 NM | 青海 QH | 甘肃 GS | 上海 SH | 福建 FJ | 江西 JX | 江苏 JS | 浙江 ZJ | 山东 SD | 湖北 HB | 四川 SC | 广西 GX | 湖南 HN | 广东 GD | 贵州 GZ | 全国平均 AVG |
|---|---|---|---|---|---|---|---|---|---|---|---|---|---|---|---|---|---|---|---|---|---|---|---|---|---|
| 豆类 Legumes | ND | ND | 1.82 | 0.62 | 0.24 | ND | 0.38 | 2.18 | 0.05 | ND | ND | 0.16 | ND | ND | ND | 0.05 | ND | 0.04 | 0.18 | 0.35 | 0.02 | ND | 0.10 | ND | 0.26 |
| 薯类 Potatoes | ND | 0.72 | 19.23 | 2.93 | ND | 0.38 | 2.02 | 17.90 | 0.05 | 0.57 | ND | 0.26 | 0.12 | 0.12 | 0.02 | 1.71 | 0.09 | 0.10 | 0.24 | 0.08 | ND | 0.42 | 1.71 | 22.79 | 2.98 |
| 肉类 Meats | ND | 0.47 | 2.54 | 3.12 | ND | 0.06 | 0.40 | 2.43 | 0.08 | 0.39 | ND | 0.35 | 0.03 | 0.02 | ND | 0.04 | 0.04 | 0.10 | 0.32 | 0.38 | ND | 0.08 | 0.04 | ND | 0.45 |
| 蛋类 Eggs | ND | 0.78 | 5.63 | 3.42 | ND | 1.81 | 0.66 | 4.41 | ND | 0.78 | ND | 1.06 | ND | ND | ND | 0.03 | ND | 0.29 | 0.19 | ND | ND | 0.05 | ND | ND | 0.80 |
| 水产类 Aquatic foods | 0.02 | 0.68 | 0.94 | 2.21 | ND | 0.85 | 0.46 | 0.88 | ND | 0.46 | ND | 0.42 | ND | 0.03 | ND | 0.03 | ND | 0.07 | 0.30 | ND | 0.03 | ND | ND | 0.03 | 0.31 |
| 乳类 Dairy products | ND | ND | ND | ND | ND | ND | 0.10 | ND | 0.06 | ND | ND | ND | ND | ND | ND | ND | ND | ND | ND | ND | ND | ND | ND | ND | 0.01 |
| 蔬菜类 Vegetables | 0.31 | 4.09 | 4.53 | 5.30 | 4.03 | 8.64 | 8.52 | 4.54 | 0.58 | 3.93 | 3.60 | 5.54 | 1.50 | 0.76 | 1.64 | 0.51 | 4.40 | 13.97 | 2.16 | 0.41 | 71.31 | 1.03 | 2.17 | 0.28 | 6.41 |
| 水果类 Fruits | 0.82 | 1.32 | 2.28 | 0.30 | 6.13 | 0.53 | 0.24 | 2.28 | 0.58 | 1.22 | 0.24 | 0.84 | 1.29 | 0.87 | 0.06 | 0.48 | 0.21 | 0.49 | 0.22 | 0.22 | ND | 0.17 | 0.96 | 1.28 | 0.96 |
| 糖类 Sugar | ND | ND | ND | ND | ND | ND | ND | ND | ND | ND | ND | ND | 0.07 | ND | ND | ND | ND | ND | ND | ND | 0.02 | ND | ND | ND | 0.00 |
| 水及饮料类 Water and beverages | ND | 0.05 | ND | ND | ND | ND | 0.09 | ND | ND | 0.05 | 0.25 | ND | 0.24 | ND | ND | 0.32 | 0.04 | ND | 0.53 | 0.44 | 0.05 | 0.08 | 0.68 | ND | 0.12 |
| 酒类 Alcohol beverages | ND | 0.02 | ND | ND | ND | ND | ND | ND | ND | 0.02 | ND | ND | ND | ND | ND | ND | ND | ND | 0.09 | ND | ND | ND | ND | ND | 0.01 |

注：未检出（ND）按 0 计

Note: values not detected (ND) were treated as being equal to 0

附表 4-31　第六次中国总膳食研究膳食样品中噻虫胺的含量（单位：μg/kg）

Annexed Table 4-31　Levels of clothianidin in food samples from the 6<sup>th</sup> China TDS (Unit: μg/kg)

| 膳食类别 Category | 黑龙江 HL | 辽宁 LN | 河北 HE | 北京 BJ | 吉林 JL | 山西 SX | 陕西 SN | 河南 HA | 宁夏 NX | 内蒙古 NM | 青海 QH | 甘肃 GS | 上海 SH | 福建 FJ | 江西 JX | 江苏 JS | 浙江 ZJ | 山东 SD | 湖北 HB | 四川 SC | 广西 GX | 湖南 HN | 广东 GD | 贵州 GZ | 全国平均 AVG |
|---|---|---|---|---|---|---|---|---|---|---|---|---|---|---|---|---|---|---|---|---|---|---|---|---|---|
| 谷类 Cereals | ND | ND | 0.08 | ND | ND | 0.06 | 0.07 | 0.07 | ND | 0.13 | ND | ND | 0.07 | 0.06 | 0.31 | 0.13 | 0.06 | 0.05 | 0.24 | 0.06 | 0.25 | 1.11 | 0.09 | 0.15 | 0.13 |
| 豆类 Legumes | 0.08 | 0.14 | 0.40 | ND | 0.04 | ND | 0.09 | 0.48 | 0.04 | ND | ND | ND | ND | ND | ND | 0.07 | ND | ND | 0.04 | 0.20 | ND | ND | 0.05 | ND | 0.07 |
| 薯类 Potatoes | ND | 0.15 | 1.65 | 0.31 | ND | 0.22 | 3.28 | 1.53 | 0.05 | 0.21 | 0.04 | 0.06 | 0.08 | 0.08 | ND | 1.28 | 0.05 | 0.19 | 0.24 | 0.11 | 0.04 | 0.18 | 0.45 | 5.89 | 0.67 |
| 肉类 Meats | 0.12 | 0.11 | 0.83 | 0.33 | ND | ND | 0.07 | 0.79 | 0.06 | 0.15 | 0.05 | 0.05 | ND | ND | ND | ND | 0.13 | 0.04 | 0.05 | 0.16 | ND | ND | ND | ND | 0.12 |
| 蛋类 Eggs | ND | 0.10 | 1.23 | 0.25 | ND | 0.29 | 0.08 | 0.96 | ND | 0.41 | ND | 0.15 | ND | ND | ND | ND | ND | 0.08 | ND | ND | ND | 0.04 | ND | ND | 0.15 |
| 水产类 Aquatic foods | 0.09 | 0.04 | 0.21 | 0.23 | ND | 0.15 | 0.11 | 0.20 | ND | 0.18 | ND | 0.07 | ND | ND | ND | ND | 0.17 | 0.03 | 0.06 | 0.11 | ND | 0.04 | ND | ND | 0.07 |
| 乳类 Dairy products | ND | ND | ND | ND | ND | ND | 0.04 | ND | ND | ND | ND | ND | ND | ND | ND | ND | ND | ND | ND | ND | ND | ND | ND | ND | 0.00 |
| 蔬菜类 Vegetables | 0.06 | 0.16 | 3.59 | 1.93 | 0.16 | 1.61 | 3.47 | 3.59 | 0.35 | 1.91 | 0.48 | 2.75 | 0.24 | 0.53 | 1.04 | 1.02 | 0.51 | 8.61 | 0.34 | 0.08 | 39.01 | 0.65 | 20.57 | 0.07 | 3.86 |
| 水果类 Fruits | 1.43 | 0.80 | 1.76 | 1.05 | 0.82 | 1.78 | 0.10 | 1.76 | 0.39 | 0.17 | 0.06 | 0.55 | 0.60 | 1.02 | 0.20 | 0.50 | 0.13 | 0.26 | 0.92 | 0.26 | ND | 0.67 | 0.64 | 0.61 | 0.69 |
| 糖类 Sugar | ND | ND | ND | ND | ND | ND | 0.03 | ND | 0.03 | ND | 0.03 | ND | 0.07 | ND | 0.04 | ND | ND | 0.04 | 0.04 | ND | 0.10 | 0.06 | ND | ND | 0.02 |
| 水及饮料类 Water and beverages | ND | ND | ND | ND | ND | ND | ND | ND | ND | ND | 0.06 | ND | 0.03 | ND | ND | 0.03 | ND | ND | 0.12 | 0.14 | ND | 0.10 | 0.09 | ND | 0.02 |

续表

| 膳食类别<br>Category | 黑龙江<br>HL | 辽宁<br>LN | 河北<br>HE | 北京<br>BJ | 吉林<br>JL | 山西<br>SX | 陕西<br>SN | 河南<br>HA | 宁夏<br>NX | 内蒙古<br>NM | 青海<br>QH | 甘肃<br>GS | 上海<br>SH | 福建<br>FJ | 江西<br>JX | 江苏<br>JS | 浙江<br>ZJ | 山东<br>SD | 湖北<br>HB | 四川<br>SC | 广西<br>GX | 湖南<br>HN | 广东<br>GD | 贵州<br>GZ | 全国平均<br>AVG |
|---|---|---|---|---|---|---|---|---|---|---|---|---|---|---|---|---|---|---|---|---|---|---|---|---|---|
| 酒类<br>Alcohol beverages | ND | ND | ND | ND | ND | ND | ND | ND | ND | ND | ND | ND | ND | ND | 0.03 | ND | ND | ND | ND | ND | 0.03 | ND | ND | ND | 0.00 |

注：未检出（ND）按 0 计

Note: values not detected (ND) were treated as being equal to 0

附表 4-32　第六次中国总膳食研究膳食样品中 N-脱甲基吡啶虫脒的含量（单位：μg/kg）

Annexed Table 4-32　Levels of acetamiprid-N-desmethyl in food samples from the 6$^{th}$ China TDS (Unit: μg/kg)

| 膳食类别<br>Category | 黑龙江<br>HL | 辽宁<br>LN | 河北<br>HE | 北京<br>BJ | 吉林<br>JL | 山西<br>SX | 陕西<br>SN | 河南<br>HA | 宁夏<br>NX | 内蒙古<br>NM | 青海<br>QH | 甘肃<br>GS | 上海<br>SH | 福建<br>FJ | 江西<br>JX | 江苏<br>JS | 浙江<br>ZJ | 山东<br>SD | 湖北<br>HB | 四川<br>SC | 广西<br>GX | 湖南<br>HN | 广东<br>GD | 贵州<br>GZ | 全国平均<br>AVG |
|---|---|---|---|---|---|---|---|---|---|---|---|---|---|---|---|---|---|---|---|---|---|---|---|---|---|
| 谷类<br>Cereals | ND | ND | ND | ND | ND | ND | 0.05 | ND | ND | ND | ND | ND | 0.02 | ND | 0.02 | ND | ND | ND | 0.09 | ND | ND | ND | ND | ND | 0.01 |
| 豆类<br>Legumes | ND | ND | 0.04 | ND | ND | ND | 0.31 | 0.05 | 0.06 | ND | ND | 0.11 | 0.02 | 0.01 | 0.11 | 0.04 | 0.04 | ND | 0.02 | 0.10 | 0.05 | 0.14 | 0.12 | 0.02 | 0.05 |
| 薯类<br>Potatoes | ND | 0.12 | ND | ND | ND | ND | ND | ND | 0.02 | ND | 0.02 | ND | 0.03 | ND | ND | ND | ND | ND | ND | 0.02 | ND | ND | ND | ND | 0.00 |
| 肉类<br>Meats | 0.04 | 0.04 | 0.04 | ND | ND | ND | ND | 0.03 | 0.32 | ND | 0.06 | 0.03 | 0.02 | ND | ND | 0.02 | 0.06 | ND | 0.03 | 0.12 | 0.01 | 0.03 | ND | 0.03 | 0.04 |
| 蛋类<br>Eggs | 0.05 | 0.12 | ND | ND | ND | ND | ND | ND | 0.04 | ND | ND | 0.04 | 0.01 | ND | ND | ND | 0.06 | ND | ND | 0.02 | ND | ND | ND | 1.51 | 0.08 |
| 水产类<br>Aquatic foods | ND | ND | ND | ND | ND | ND | 0.20 | ND | ND | ND | ND | ND | 0.01 | ND | ND | ND | ND | 0.01 | ND | 0.10 | ND | ND | ND | ND | 0.01 |
| 乳类<br>Dairy products | 0.03 | 0.02 | 0.15 | 0.03 | ND | 0.08 | 0.16 | 0.15 | 0.08 | 0.03 | 0.02 | 0.10 | 0.01 | 0.01 | 0.05 | 0.02 | ND | 0.01 | 0.02 | 0.09 | 0.28 | 0.17 | 1.73 | 7.18 | 0.43 |

续表

附表 4-33 第六次中国总膳食研究膳食样品中呋虫胺的含量（单位：μg/kg）

Annexed Table 4-33 Levels of dinotefuran in food samples from the 6$^{th}$ China TDS (Unit: μg/kg)

| 膳食类别 Category | 黑龙江 HL | 辽宁 LN | 河北 HE | 北京 BJ | 吉林 JL | 山西 SX | 陕西 SN | 河南 HA | 宁夏 NX | 内蒙古 NM | 青海 QH | 甘肃 GS | 上海 SH | 福建 FJ | 江西 JX | 江苏 JS | 浙江 ZJ | 山东 SD | 湖北 HB | 四川 SC | 广西 GX | 湖南 HN | 广东 GD | 贵州 GZ | 全国平均 AVG |
|---|---|---|---|---|---|---|---|---|---|---|---|---|---|---|---|---|---|---|---|---|---|---|---|---|---|
| 蔬菜类 Vegetables | 0.18 | 1.02 | 0.46 | 0.33 | 0.05 | 0.20 | 1.90 | 0.46 | 14.98 | 0.19 | 0.63 | 0.47 | 10.07 | 0.62 | 1.04 | 2.04 | 4.30 | 0.17 | 1.10 | 0.12 | 0.66 | 1.03 | 5.70 | 0.03 | 1.99 |
| 水果类 Fruits | 2.32 | 0.84 | 0.37 | 0.64 | 0.51 | 0.16 | 1.17 | 0.37 | 1.31 | 0.40 | 0.09 | 0.57 | 0.56 | 0.60 | 1.48 | 0.58 | 2.13 | 0.40 | 0.27 | 1.38 | 0.02 | 0.51 | 0.16 | 0.81 | 0.74 |
| 糖类 Sugar | ND | ND | ND | ND | ND | ND | ND | ND | ND | ND | ND | ND | ND | ND | ND | ND | ND | ND | ND | ND | ND | ND | ND | ND | 0.00 |
| 水及饮料类 Water and beverages | ND | ND | ND | ND | ND | ND | ND | ND | ND | 0.01 | 0.17 | ND | 0.03 | ND | ND | 0.03 | ND | ND | 0.03 | 0.02 | ND | 0.02 | 0.03 | ND | 0.01 |
| 酒类 Alcohol beverages | ND | ND | ND | ND | ND | ND | ND | ND | ND | ND | ND | ND | ND | ND | ND | ND | ND | ND | ND | ND | ND | ND | ND | ND | 0.00 |

注：未检出（ND）按 0 计
Note: values not detected (ND) were treated as being equal to 0

| 膳食类别 Category | 黑龙江 HL | 辽宁 LN | 河北 HE | 北京 BJ | 吉林 JL | 山西 SX | 陕西 SN | 河南 HA | 宁夏 NX | 内蒙古 NM | 青海 QH | 甘肃 GS | 上海 SH | 福建 FJ | 江西 JX | 江苏 JS | 浙江 ZJ | 山东 SD | 湖北 HB | 四川 SC | 广西 GX | 湖南 HN | 广东 GD | 贵州 GZ | 全国平均 AVG |
|---|---|---|---|---|---|---|---|---|---|---|---|---|---|---|---|---|---|---|---|---|---|---|---|---|---|
| 谷类 Cereals | ND | ND | ND | ND | ND | ND | ND | ND | ND | ND | ND | ND | ND | ND | 0.07 | ND | ND | ND | ND | ND | ND | ND | ND | ND | 0.00 |
| 豆类 Legumes | ND | ND | ND | ND | ND | ND | ND | ND | ND | ND | ND | ND | ND | ND | ND | ND | ND | ND | ND | ND | ND | ND | ND | ND | 0.00 |
| 薯类 Potatoes | ND | ND | ND | ND | ND | ND | ND | ND | ND | ND | ND | ND | ND | ND | ND | ND | ND | ND | ND | ND | ND | ND | ND | 0.16 | 0.01 |

续表

| 膳食类别<br>Category | 黑龙江<br>HL | 辽宁<br>LN | 河北<br>HE | 北京<br>BJ | 吉林<br>JL | 山西<br>SX | 陕西<br>SN | 河南<br>HA | 宁夏<br>NX | 内蒙古<br>NM | 青海<br>QH | 甘肃<br>GS | 上海<br>SH | 福建<br>FJ | 江西<br>JX | 江苏<br>JS | 浙江<br>ZJ | 山东<br>SD | 湖北<br>HB | 四川<br>SC | 广西<br>GX | 湖南<br>HN | 广东<br>GD | 贵州<br>GZ | 全国平均<br>AVG |
|---|---|---|---|---|---|---|---|---|---|---|---|---|---|---|---|---|---|---|---|---|---|---|---|---|---|
| 肉类 Meats | ND | ND | ND | ND | ND | ND | ND | ND | ND | ND | ND | ND | ND | ND | ND | ND | ND | ND | ND | ND | ND | ND | ND | ND | 0.00 |
| 蛋类 Eggs | ND | ND | ND | ND | ND | ND | ND | ND | ND | ND | ND | ND | ND | ND | ND | ND | ND | ND | ND | ND | ND | ND | ND | ND | 0.00 |
| 水产类 Aquatic foods | ND | ND | ND | ND | ND | ND | ND | ND | ND | ND | ND | ND | ND | ND | ND | ND | ND | ND | ND | ND | ND | ND | ND | ND | 0.00 |
| 乳类 Dairy products | ND | ND | ND | ND | ND | ND | ND | ND | ND | ND | ND | ND | ND | ND | ND | ND | ND | ND | ND | ND | ND | ND | ND | ND | 0.00 |
| 蔬菜类 Vegetables | ND | ND | 0.46 | ND | ND | 0.58 | 0.08 | 0.46 | 0.70 | ND | 1.70 | ND | ND | ND | 0.06 | ND | ND | 0.49 | ND | ND | 0.06 | 0.17 | 0.06 | ND | 0.20 |
| 水果类 Fruits | 0.05 | ND | ND | ND | ND | ND | ND | ND | ND | ND | ND | ND | ND | ND | ND | ND | ND | ND | ND | 0.06 | ND | ND | ND | ND | 0.00 |
| 糖类 Sugar | ND | ND | ND | ND | ND | ND | ND | ND | ND | ND | ND | ND | ND | ND | ND | ND | ND | ND | ND | ND | ND | ND | ND | ND | 0.00 |
| 水及饮料类 Water and beverages | ND | ND | ND | ND | ND | ND | ND | ND | ND | ND | 0.06 | ND | 0.06 | ND | ND | 0.06 | ND | ND | 0.07 | 0.11 | ND | ND | 0.11 | ND | 0.02 |
| 酒类 Alcohol beverages | ND | ND | ND | ND | ND | ND | ND | ND | ND | ND | ND | ND | ND | ND | ND | ND | ND | ND | ND | ND | ND | ND | ND | ND | 0.00 |

注：未检出（ND）按 0 计

Note: values not detected (ND) were treated as being equal to 0

附表 4-34 第六次中国总膳食研究膳食样品中烯啶虫胺的含量（单位：μg/kg）

Annexed Table 4-34　Levels of nitenpyram in food samples from the 6th China TDS (Unit: μg/kg)

| 膳食类别 Category | 黑龙江 HL | 辽宁 LN | 河北 HE | 北京 BJ | 吉林 JL | 山西 SX | 陕西 SN | 河南 HA | 宁夏 NX | 内蒙古 NM | 青海 QH | 甘肃 GS | 上海 SH | 福建 FJ | 江西 JX | 江苏 JS | 浙江 ZJ | 山东 SD | 湖北 HB | 四川 SC | 广西 GX | 湖南 HN | 广东 GD | 贵州 GZ | 全国平均 AVG |
|---|---|---|---|---|---|---|---|---|---|---|---|---|---|---|---|---|---|---|---|---|---|---|---|---|---|
| 谷类 Cereals | ND | ND | ND | ND | ND | ND | 0.03 | ND | ND | ND | ND | ND | ND | ND | ND | ND | ND | ND | ND | ND | 0.01 | ND | ND | ND | 0.00 |
| 豆类 Legumes | ND | ND | ND | ND | ND | ND | ND | ND | ND | ND | ND | ND | ND | ND | ND | ND | ND | ND | ND | ND | ND | ND | ND | ND | 0.00 |
| 薯类 Potatoes | ND | ND | ND | ND | ND | ND | ND | ND | ND | ND | ND | ND | ND | ND | ND | ND | ND | ND | ND | ND | ND | ND | ND | ND | 0.00 |
| 肉类 Meats | ND | ND | ND | ND | ND | ND | ND | ND | ND | ND | ND | ND | ND | ND | ND | ND | ND | ND | ND | ND | ND | ND | ND | ND | 0.00 |
| 蛋类 Eggs | ND | ND | ND | ND | ND | ND | ND | ND | ND | ND | ND | ND | ND | ND | ND | ND | ND | ND | ND | ND | ND | ND | ND | ND | 0.00 |
| 水产类 Aquatic foods | ND | ND | ND | ND | ND | ND | ND | ND | ND | ND | ND | ND | ND | ND | ND | ND | ND | ND | ND | ND | ND | ND | ND | ND | 0.00 |
| 乳类 Dairy products | ND | ND | ND | ND | ND | ND | ND | ND | ND | ND | ND | ND | ND | ND | ND | ND | ND | ND | ND | ND | ND | ND | ND | ND | 0.00 |
| 蔬菜类 Vegetables | ND | ND | 0.38 | 0.42 | ND | 2.34 | 0.25 | 0.38 | 1.17 | ND | 2.18 | 0.29 | ND | 0.12 | 0.16 | 0.15 | ND | 0.47 | ND | ND | ND | 0.08 | 0.24 | ND | 0.36 |
| 水果类 Fruits | ND | ND | 0.16 | ND | ND | ND | ND | 0.16 | 0.24 | ND | ND | ND | 0.07 | ND | ND | ND | ND | ND | ND | ND | ND | ND | ND | ND | 0.03 |
| 糖类 Sugar | ND | ND | ND | ND | ND | ND | ND | ND | ND | ND | ND | ND | ND | ND | ND | ND | ND | ND | ND | ND | ND | ND | ND | ND | 0.00 |
| 水及饮料类 Water and beverages | ND | ND | ND | ND | ND | ND | ND | ND | ND | ND | ND | ND | ND | ND | ND | ND | ND | ND | ND | ND | ND | ND | ND | ND | 0.00 |

续表

| 膳食类别<br>Category | 黑龙江<br>HL | 辽宁<br>LN | 河北<br>HE | 北京<br>BJ | 吉林<br>JL | 山西<br>SX | 陕西<br>SN | 河南<br>HA | 宁夏<br>NX | 内蒙古<br>NM | 青海<br>QH | 甘肃<br>GS | 上海<br>SH | 福建<br>FJ | 江西<br>JX | 江苏<br>JS | 浙江<br>ZJ | 山东<br>SD | 湖北<br>HB | 四川<br>SC | 广西<br>GX | 湖南<br>HN | 广东<br>GD | 贵州<br>GZ | 全国平均<br>AVG |
|---|---|---|---|---|---|---|---|---|---|---|---|---|---|---|---|---|---|---|---|---|---|---|---|---|---|
| 酒类<br>Alcohol beverages | ND | ND | ND | ND | ND | ND | ND | ND | ND | ND | ND | ND | ND | ND | ND | ND | ND | ND | ND | ND | 0.19 | ND | ND | ND | 0.01 |

注：未检出（ND）按 0 计
Note: values not detected (ND) were treated as being equal to 0

附表 4-35　第六次中国总膳食研究膳食样品中噻虫啉的含量（单位：μg/kg）
Annexed Table 4-35　Levels of thiacloprid in food samples from the 6$^{th}$ China TDS (Unit: μg/kg)

| 膳食类别<br>Category | 黑龙江<br>HL | 辽宁<br>LN | 河北<br>HE | 北京<br>BJ | 吉林<br>JL | 山西<br>SX | 陕西<br>SN | 河南<br>HA | 宁夏<br>NX | 内蒙古<br>NM | 青海<br>QH | 甘肃<br>GS | 上海<br>SH | 福建<br>FJ | 江西<br>JX | 江苏<br>JS | 浙江<br>ZJ | 山东<br>SD | 湖北<br>HB | 四川<br>SC | 广西<br>GX | 湖南<br>HN | 广东<br>GD | 贵州<br>GZ | 全国平均<br>AVG |
|---|---|---|---|---|---|---|---|---|---|---|---|---|---|---|---|---|---|---|---|---|---|---|---|---|---|
| 谷类<br>Cereals | ND | ND | ND | ND | ND | ND | ND | ND | ND | ND | ND | ND | ND | ND | ND | ND | ND | ND | ND | ND | ND | ND | ND | ND | 0.00 |
| 豆类<br>Legumes | ND | ND | ND | ND | ND | ND | ND | ND | ND | ND | ND | ND | ND | ND | ND | ND | ND | ND | ND | ND | ND | ND | ND | ND | 0.00 |
| 薯类<br>Potatoes | ND | ND | ND | ND | ND | ND | ND | ND | ND | ND | ND | ND | ND | ND | ND | ND | ND | ND | ND | ND | ND | ND | ND | ND | 0.00 |
| 肉类<br>Meats | ND | ND | ND | ND | ND | ND | ND | ND | ND | ND | ND | ND | ND | ND | ND | ND | ND | ND | ND | ND | ND | ND | ND | ND | 0.00 |
| 蛋类<br>Eggs | ND | ND | ND | ND | ND | ND | ND | ND | ND | ND | ND | ND | ND | ND | ND | ND | ND | ND | ND | ND | ND | ND | ND | ND | 0.00 |
| 水产类<br>Aquatic foods | ND | ND | ND | ND | ND | ND | ND | ND | ND | ND | 0.24 | ND | ND | ND | ND | ND | ND | ND | ND | ND | ND | ND | ND | ND | 0.01 |
| 乳类<br>Dairy products | ND | ND | ND | ND | ND | ND | ND | ND | ND | ND | ND | ND | ND | ND | ND | ND | ND | ND | ND | ND | ND | ND | ND | ND | 0.00 |

续表

| 膳食类别<br>Category | 黑龙江<br>HL | 辽宁<br>LN | 河北<br>HE | 北京<br>BJ | 吉林<br>JL | 山西<br>SX | 陕西<br>SN | 河南<br>HA | 宁夏<br>NX | 内蒙古<br>NM | 青海<br>QH | 甘肃<br>GS | 上海<br>SH | 福建<br>FJ | 江西<br>JX | 江苏<br>JS | 浙江<br>ZJ | 山东<br>SD | 湖北<br>HB | 四川<br>SC | 广西<br>GX | 湖南<br>HN | 广东<br>GD | 贵州<br>GZ | 全国平均<br>AVG |
|---|---|---|---|---|---|---|---|---|---|---|---|---|---|---|---|---|---|---|---|---|---|---|---|---|---|
| 蔬菜类 Vegetables | ND | ND | ND | ND | ND | 1.42 | 0.09 | ND | ND | ND | ND | ND | ND | ND | ND | ND | ND | 0.23 | ND | ND | ND | ND | ND | ND | 0.07 |
| 水果类 Fruits | ND | ND | ND | ND | ND | ND | ND | ND | ND | ND | ND | ND | ND | ND | ND | ND | ND | ND | ND | ND | ND | ND | ND | ND | 0.00 |
| 糖类 Sugar | ND | ND | ND | ND | ND | ND | ND | ND | ND | ND | ND | ND | ND | ND | ND | ND | ND | ND | ND | ND | ND | ND | ND | ND | 0.00 |
| 水及饮料类 Water and beverages | ND | ND | ND | ND | ND | ND | ND | ND | ND | ND | ND | ND | ND | ND | ND | ND | ND | ND | 0.03 | ND | ND | ND | 0.08 | ND | 0.00 |
| 酒类 Alcohol beverages | ND | ND | ND | ND | ND | ND | ND | ND | ND | ND | ND | ND | ND | ND | ND | ND | ND | ND | ND | ND | ND | ND | ND | ND | 0.00 |

注：未检出（ND）按 0 计
Note: values not detected (ND) were treated as being equal to 0

附表 4-36 第六次中国总膳食研究膳食样品中氯噻啉的含量（单位：μg/kg）
Annexed Table 4-36 Levels of imidaclothiz in food samples from the 6<sup>th</sup> China TDS (Unit: μg/kg)

| 膳食类别<br>Category | 黑龙江<br>HL | 辽宁<br>LN | 河北<br>HE | 北京<br>BJ | 吉林<br>JL | 山西<br>SX | 陕西<br>SN | 河南<br>HA | 宁夏<br>NX | 内蒙古<br>NM | 青海<br>QH | 甘肃<br>GS | 上海<br>SH | 福建<br>FJ | 江西<br>JX | 江苏<br>JS | 浙江<br>ZJ | 山东<br>SD | 湖北<br>HB | 四川<br>SC | 广西<br>GX | 湖南<br>HN | 广东<br>GD | 贵州<br>GZ | 全国平均<br>AVG |
|---|---|---|---|---|---|---|---|---|---|---|---|---|---|---|---|---|---|---|---|---|---|---|---|---|---|
| 谷类 Cereals | ND | ND | ND | ND | ND | ND | ND | ND | ND | ND | ND | ND | ND | ND | ND | ND | ND | ND | ND | ND | ND | ND | ND | ND | 0.00 |
| 豆类 Legumes | ND | ND | ND | ND | ND | ND | ND | ND | ND | ND | ND | ND | ND | ND | ND | ND | ND | ND | ND | ND | ND | ND | ND | ND | 0.00 |
| 薯类 Potatoes | ND | ND | ND | ND | ND | ND | ND | ND | ND | ND | ND | ND | ND | ND | ND | ND | ND | ND | ND | ND | ND | ND | ND | ND | 0.00 |

续表

| 膳食类别<br>Category | 黑龙江<br>HL | 辽宁<br>LN | 河北<br>HE | 北京<br>BJ | 吉林<br>JL | 山西<br>SX | 陕西<br>SN | 河南<br>HA | 宁夏<br>NX | 内蒙古<br>NM | 青海<br>QH | 甘肃<br>GS | 上海<br>SH | 福建<br>FJ | 江西<br>JX | 江苏<br>JS | 浙江<br>ZJ | 山东<br>SD | 湖北<br>HB | 四川<br>SC | 广西<br>GX | 湖南<br>HN | 广东<br>GD | 贵州<br>GZ | 全国平均<br>AVG |
|---|---|---|---|---|---|---|---|---|---|---|---|---|---|---|---|---|---|---|---|---|---|---|---|---|---|
| 肉类 Meats | ND | ND | ND | ND | ND | ND | ND | ND | ND | ND | ND | ND | ND | ND | ND | ND | ND | ND | ND | ND | ND | ND | ND | ND | 0.00 |
| 蛋类 Eggs | ND | ND | ND | ND | ND | ND | ND | ND | ND | ND | ND | ND | ND | ND | ND | ND | ND | ND | ND | ND | ND | ND | ND | ND | 0.00 |
| 水产类 Aquatic foods | ND | ND | ND | ND | ND | ND | ND | ND | ND | ND | ND | ND | ND | ND | ND | ND | ND | ND | ND | ND | ND | ND | ND | ND | 0.00 |
| 乳类 Dairy products | ND | ND | ND | ND | ND | ND | ND | ND | ND | ND | ND | ND | ND | ND | ND | ND | ND | ND | ND | ND | ND | ND | ND | ND | 0.00 |
| 蔬菜类 Vegetables | ND | ND | ND | ND | ND | ND | ND | ND | ND | ND | ND | ND | ND | ND | ND | ND | ND | ND | ND | ND | ND | ND | ND | 0.90 | 0.04 |
| 水果类 Fruits | ND | ND | ND | ND | ND | ND | ND | ND | ND | ND | ND | ND | ND | ND | ND | ND | ND | ND | ND | ND | ND | ND | ND | ND | 0.00 |
| 糖类 Sugar | ND | ND | ND | ND | ND | ND | ND | ND | ND | ND | ND | ND | ND | ND | ND | ND | ND | ND | ND | ND | ND | ND | ND | ND | 0.00 |
| 水及饮料类 Water and beverages | ND | ND | ND | ND | ND | ND | ND | ND | ND | ND | ND | ND | ND | ND | ND | ND | ND | ND | ND | ND | ND | ND | ND | ND | 0.00 |
| 酒类 Alcohol beverages | ND | ND | ND | ND | ND | ND | ND | ND | ND | ND | ND | ND | ND | ND | ND | ND | ND | ND | ND | ND | ND | ND | ND | ND | 0.00 |

注：未检出（ND）按 0 计
Note: values not detected (ND) were treated as being equal to 0

附表 4-37　第六次中国总膳食研究的吡虫啉膳食摄入量 [单位：ng/(kg bw·d)]
Annexed Table 4-37　Dietary intakes of imidacloprid from the 6th China TDS [Unit: ng/(kg bw·d)]

| 膳食类别 Category | 黑龙江 HL | 辽宁 LN | 河北 HE | 北京 BJ | 吉林 JL | 山西 SX | 陕西 SN | 河南 HA | 宁夏 NX | 内蒙古 NM | 青海 QH | 甘肃 GS | 上海 SH | 福建 FJ | 江西 JX | 江苏 JS | 浙江 ZJ | 山东 SD | 湖北 HB | 四川 SC | 广西 GX | 湖南 HN | 广东 GD | 贵州 GZ | 全国平均 AVG |
|---|---|---|---|---|---|---|---|---|---|---|---|---|---|---|---|---|---|---|---|---|---|---|---|---|---|
| 谷类 Cereals | 0.492 | 0.000 | 5.737 | 0.000 | 0.000 | 0.000 | 0.000 | 6.621 | 0.000 | 3.577 | 0.312 | 0.000 | 3.224 | 4.443 | 0.596 | 1.312 | 1.152 | 0.000 | 2.019 | 0.400 | 2.151 | 1.551 | 0.973 | 0.813 | 1.474 |
| 豆类 Legumes | 0.000 | 0.811 | 0.759 | 0.290 | 0.000 | 0.019 | 0.419 | 0.860 | 0.012 | 0.000 | 0.003 | 0.041 | 0.121 | 0.095 | 0.289 | 0.264 | 0.497 | 0.070 | 0.125 | 1.004 | 0.051 | 0.071 | 0.088 | 0.127 | 0.251 |
| 薯类 Potatoes | 0.000 | 1.933 | 0.534 | 1.253 | 0.257 | 0.473 | 0.129 | 0.654 | 0.218 | 0.945 | 0.160 | 0.046 | 0.067 | 0.099 | 0.041 | 0.051 | 0.077 | 0.064 | 2.322 | 1.824 | 0.014 | 0.121 | 0.129 | 0.297 | 0.488 |
| 肉类 Meats | 0.000 | 0.293 | 1.354 | 0.224 | 0.000 | 0.000 | 0.006 | 1.517 | 0.116 | 0.020 | 0.162 | 0.035 | 0.065 | 0.164 | 0.021 | 0.043 | 0.183 | 0.000 | 0.237 | 1.269 | 0.000 | 0.078 | 0.570 | 0.091 | 0.269 |
| 蛋类 Eggs | 0.000 | 0.326 | 1.110 | 0.056 | 0.000 | 0.010 | 0.000 | 0.819 | 0.000 | 0.019 | 0.000 | 0.000 | 0.000 | 0.027 | 0.000 | 0.000 | 0.000 | 0.009 | 0.108 | 0.000 | 0.000 | 0.007 | 0.000 | 0.000 | 0.104 |
| 水产类 Aquatic foods | 0.000 | 0.012 | 0.047 | 0.050 | 0.000 | 0.004 | 0.030 | 0.022 | 0.000 | 0.006 | 0.000 | 0.001 | 0.024 | 0.104 | 0.024 | 0.018 | 0.042 | 0.000 | 0.183 | 0.113 | 0.000 | 0.000 | 0.217 | 0.004 | 0.038 |
| 乳类 Dairy products | 0.000 | 0.000 | 0.000 | 0.000 | 0.000 | 0.000 | 0.000 | 0.000 | 0.000 | 0.011 | 0.000 | 0.000 | 0.000 | 0.000 | 0.000 | 0.000 | 0.000 | 0.000 | 0.000 | 0.000 | 0.000 | 0.000 | 0.000 | 0.000 | 0.000 |
| 蔬菜类 Vegetables | 8.745 | 14.96 | 14.63 | 10.01 | 13.20 | 16.09 | 11.55 | 13.86 | 5.792 | 9.221 | 5.050 | 15.50 | 64.42 | 5.448 | 201.0 | 5.549 | 6.344 | 19.99 | 57.05 | 4.959 | 23.76 | 35.54 | 18.33 | 6.915 | 24.50 |
| 水果类 Fruits | 0.763 | 13.92 | 3.522 | 11.43 | 2.554 | 0.261 | 3.910 | 2.259 | 3.989 | 7.914 | 0.678 | 0.443 | 8.233 | 9.896 | 0.474 | 0.935 | 28.81 | 1.989 | 1.836 | 0.747 | 3.598 | 1.420 | 0.906 | 4.110 | 4.775 |
| 糖类 Sugar | 0.000 | 0.000 | 0.000 | 0.000 | 0.000 | 0.000 | 0.000 | 0.000 | 0.000 | 0.000 | 0.000 | 0.000 | 0.045 | 0.000 | 0.000 | 0.000 | 0.000 | 0.000 | 0.000 | 0.000 | 0.000 | 0.000 | 0.000 | 0.000 | 0.002 |
| 水及饮料类 Water and beverages | 0.000 | 0.154 | 0.000 | 0.000 | 0.517 | 0.000 | 0.249 | 0.000 | 0.000 | 5.061 | 7.033 | 0.000 | 3.108 | 0.376 | 0.000 | 5.311 | 1.632 | 0.000 | 1.038 | 1.714 | 1.102 | 2.995 | 7.678 | 0.000 | 1.582 |

续表

| 膳食类别<br>Category | 黑龙江<br>HL | 辽宁<br>LN | 河北<br>HE | 北京<br>BJ | 吉林<br>JL | 山西<br>SX | 陕西<br>SN | 河南<br>HA | 宁夏<br>NX | 内蒙古<br>NM | 青海<br>QH | 甘肃<br>GS | 上海<br>SH | 福建<br>FJ | 江西<br>JX | 江苏<br>JS | 浙江<br>ZJ | 山东<br>SD | 湖北<br>HB | 四川<br>SC | 广西<br>GX | 湖南<br>HN | 广东<br>GD | 贵州<br>GZ | 全国平均<br>AVG |
|---|---|---|---|---|---|---|---|---|---|---|---|---|---|---|---|---|---|---|---|---|---|---|---|---|---|
| 酒类<br>Alcohol beverages | 0.000 | 0.000 | 0.000 | 0.047 | 0.000 | 0.000 | 0.000 | 0.000 | 0.000 | 0.000 | 0.000 | 0.001 | 0.041 | 0.009 | 0.000 | 0.000 | 0.056 | 0.110 | 0.000 | 0.000 | 0.247 | 0.000 | 0.005 | 0.000 | 0.021 |
| 合计<br>SUM | 10.00 | 32.41 | 27.69 | 23.36 | 16.52 | 16.86 | 16.30 | 26.62 | 10.13 | 26.78 | 13.40 | 16.07 | 79.35 | 20.66 | 202.48 | 13.48 | 38.79 | 22.23 | 64.91 | 12.03 | 30.92 | 41.78 | 28.90 | 12.36 | 33.50 |

附表 4-38 第六次中国总膳食研究的啶虫脒膳食摄入量 [单位: ng/(kg bw·d)]

Annexed Table 4-38 Dietary intakes of acetamiprid from the 6$^{th}$ China TDS [Unit: ng/(kg bw·d)]

| 膳食类别<br>Category | 黑龙江<br>HL | 辽宁<br>LN | 河北<br>HE | 北京<br>BJ | 吉林<br>JL | 山西<br>SX | 陕西<br>SN | 河南<br>HA | 宁夏<br>NX | 内蒙古<br>NM | 青海<br>QH | 甘肃<br>GS | 上海<br>SH | 福建<br>FJ | 江西<br>JX | 江苏<br>JS | 浙江<br>ZJ | 山东<br>SD | 湖北<br>HB | 四川<br>SC | 广西<br>GX | 湖南<br>HN | 广东<br>GD | 贵州<br>GZ | 全国平均<br>AVG |
|---|---|---|---|---|---|---|---|---|---|---|---|---|---|---|---|---|---|---|---|---|---|---|---|---|---|
| 谷类<br>Cereals | 0.256 | 0.000 | 0.000 | 0.000 | 0.000 | 0.000 | 8.899 | 0.000 | 0.000 | 0.000 | 1.389 | 0.000 | 2.268 | 1.593 | 2.129 | 0.636 | 2.230 | 0.223 | 6.460 | 0.000 | 4.671 | 1.135 | 0.142 | 0.578 | 1.359 |
| 豆类<br>Legumes | 0.000 | 0.483 | 0.111 | 0.199 | 0.142 | 0.048 | 2.932 | 0.125 | 0.008 | 0.000 | 0.017 | 0.056 | 0.047 | 0.000 | 0.138 | 0.000 | 0.025 | 0.000 | 0.040 | 1.949 | 0.000 | 0.042 | 0.025 | 0.000 | 0.266 |
| 薯类<br>Potatoes | 0.000 | 0.338 | 0.000 | 0.000 | 0.000 | 0.000 | 0.549 | 0.000 | 0.482 | 0.072 | 0.710 | 0.286 | 0.605 | 0.000 | 0.026 | 0.000 | 0.013 | 0.000 | 0.000 | 0.208 | 0.000 | 0.000 | 0.000 | 0.008 | 0.137 |
| 肉类<br>Meats | 0.022 | 0.332 | 0.028 | 0.543 | 0.102 | 0.047 | 0.000 | 0.031 | 0.401 | 0.000 | 0.745 | 0.118 | 0.042 | 0.000 | 0.100 | 0.027 | 0.247 | 0.000 | 0.086 | 6.546 | 0.000 | 1.204 | 0.074 | 0.053 | 0.448 |
| 蛋类<br>Eggs | 0.000 | 0.198 | 0.000 | 0.000 | 0.000 | 0.000 | 0.000 | 0.000 | 0.006 | 0.002 | 0.000 | 0.000 | 0.102 | 0.000 | 0.000 | 0.013 | 0.000 | 0.000 | 0.023 | 0.007 | 0.000 | 0.000 | 0.000 | 0.009 | 0.010 |
| 水产类<br>Aquatic foods | 0.000 | 0.000 | 0.000 | 0.023 | 0.000 | 0.000 | 0.177 | 0.000 | 0.000 | 0.000 | 0.000 | 0.005 | 0.000 | 0.000 | 0.000 | 0.000 | 0.000 | 0.000 | 0.061 | 0.386 | 0.000 | 0.000 | 0.000 | 0.000 | 0.032 |
| 乳类<br>Dairy products | 0.000 | 0.000 | 0.031 | 0.022 | 0.000 | 0.018 | 0.022 | 0.025 | 0.008 | 0.018 | 0.000 | 0.009 | 0.000 | 0.000 | 0.005 | 0.000 | 0.000 | 0.000 | 0.000 | 0.009 | 0.032 | 0.108 | 0.379 | 1.265 | 0.081 |

续表

| 膳食类别 Category | 黑龙江 HL | 辽宁 LN | 河北 HE | 北京 BJ | 吉林 JL | 山西 SX | 陕西 SN | 河南 HA | 宁夏 NX | 内蒙古 NM | 青海 QH | 甘肃 GS | 上海 SH | 福建 FJ | 江西 JX | 江苏 JS | 浙江 ZJ | 山东 SD | 湖北 HB | 四川 SC | 广西 GX | 湖南 HN | 广东 GD | 贵州 GZ | 全国平均 AVG |
|---|---|---|---|---|---|---|---|---|---|---|---|---|---|---|---|---|---|---|---|---|---|---|---|---|---|
| 蔬菜类 Vegetables | 7.159 | 63.77 | 28.60 | 54.90 | 7.116 | 22.46 | 35.93 | 27.11 | 104.08 | 1.683 | 30.98 | 30.85 | 1180 | 53.59 | 71.17 | 230.1 | 361.7 | 11.61 | 275.3 | 9.751 | 47.70 | 130.2 | 244.1 | 2.404 | 126.3 |
| 水果类 Fruits | 3.590 | 10.87 | 1.865 | 6.570 | 4.310 | 0.747 | 8.650 | 1.197 | 8.742 | 5.384 | 0.030 | 1.520 | 8.888 | 1.846 | 2.074 | 0.780 | 104.2 | 2.130 | 0.435 | 0.641 | 0.318 | 2.006 | 0.272 | 1.133 | 7.426 |
| 糖类 Sugar | 0.000 | 0.000 | 0.000 | 0.000 | 0.000 | 0.000 | 0.000 | 0.000 | 0.000 | 0.000 | 0.000 | 0.000 | 0.013 | 0.000 | 0.000 | 0.000 | 0.000 | 0.000 | 0.000 | 0.000 | 0.000 | 0.000 | 0.000 | 0.000 | 0.001 |
| 水及饮料类 Water and beverages | 0.000 | 0.198 | 0.000 | 0.000 | 0.000 | 0.000 | 0.885 | 0.000 | 0.000 | 12.991 | 28.88 | 0.000 | 10.37 | 1.971 | 0.000 | 11.28 | 2.842 | 0.000 | 4.842 | 3.379 | 2.346 | 9.166 | 12.75 | 0.000 | 4.246 |
| 酒类 Alcohol beverages | 0.000 | 0.000 | 0.005 | 0.009 | 0.000 | 0.000 | 0.000 | 0.001 | 0.000 | 0.004 | 0.000 | 0.002 | 0.024 | 0.006 | 0.003 | 0.010 | 0.039 | 0.070 | 0.000 | 0.000 | 0.015 | 0.000 | 0.001 | 0.000 | 0.008 |
| 合计 SUM | 11.03 | 76.19 | 30.64 | 62.27 | 11.67 | 23.32 | 58.04 | 28.49 | 113.73 | 20.15 | 62.75 | 32.84 | 1202.08 | 59.00 | 75.65 | 242.88 | 471.37 | 14.04 | 287.29 | 22.88 | 55.08 | 143.87 | 257.77 | 5.45 | 140.35 |

附表 4-39  第六次中国总膳食研究的噻虫嗪膳食摄入量 [单位：ng/(kg bw · d)]

Annexed Table 4-39  Dietary intakes of thiamethoxam from the 6th China TDS [Unit: ng/(kg bw · d)]

| 膳食类别 Category | 黑龙江 HL | 辽宁 LN | 河北 HE | 北京 BJ | 吉林 JL | 山西 SX | 陕西 SN | 河南 HA | 宁夏 NX | 内蒙古 NM | 青海 QH | 甘肃 GS | 上海 SH | 福建 FJ | 江西 JX | 江苏 JS | 浙江 ZJ | 山东 SD | 湖北 HB | 四川 SC | 广西 GX | 湖南 HN | 广东 GD | 贵州 GZ | 全国平均 AVG |
|---|---|---|---|---|---|---|---|---|---|---|---|---|---|---|---|---|---|---|---|---|---|---|---|---|---|
| 谷类 Cereals | 0.000 | 2.725 | 4.618 | 0.000 | 0.000 | 3.470 | 0.658 | 5.330 | 0.000 | 2.966 | 0.000 | 0.000 | 0.866 | 0.000 | 0.465 | 1.455 | 0.362 | 0.000 | 0.698 | 0.800 | 0.863 | 0.652 | 0.347 | 0.347 | 1.109 |
| 豆类 Legumes | 0.000 | 0.000 | 1.648 | 1.004 | 0.288 | 0.000 | 0.504 | 1.868 | 0.030 | 0.000 | 0.000 | 0.108 | 0.000 | 0.000 | 0.000 | 0.070 | 0.000 | 0.037 | 0.192 | 0.377 | 0.015 | 0.000 | 0.045 | 0.000 | 0.258 |
| 薯类 Potatoes | 0.000 | 0.824 | 18.61 | 2.714 | 0.000 | 0.711 | 3.670 | 22.82 | 0.080 | 1.099 | 0.000 | 0.590 | 0.067 | 0.082 | 0.011 | 0.905 | 0.050 | 0.076 | 0.341 | 0.075 | 0.000 | 0.357 | 0.672 | 12.40 | 2.756 |

续表

| 膳食类别<br>Category | 黑龙江<br>HL | 辽宁<br>LN | 河北<br>HE | 北京<br>BJ | 吉林<br>JL | 山西<br>SX | 陕西<br>SN | 河南<br>HA | 宁夏<br>NX | 内蒙古<br>NM | 青海<br>QH | 甘肃<br>GS | 上海<br>SH | 福建<br>FJ | 江西<br>JX | 江苏<br>JS | 浙江<br>ZJ | 山东<br>SD | 湖北<br>HB | 四川<br>SC | 广西<br>GX | 湖南<br>HN | 广东<br>GD | 贵州<br>GZ | 全国平均<br>AVG |
|---|---|---|---|---|---|---|---|---|---|---|---|---|---|---|---|---|---|---|---|---|---|---|---|---|---|
| 肉类 Meats | 0.000 | 0.503 | 1.908 | 3.338 | 0.000 | 0.126 | 0.228 | 2.137 | 0.059 | 0.458 | 0.000 | 0.170 | 0.058 | 0.030 | 0.000 | 0.061 | 0.071 | 0.152 | 0.278 | 0.784 | 0.000 | 0.199 | 0.067 | 0.000 | 0.443 |
| 蛋类 Eggs | 0.000 | 0.508 | 2.820 | 2.111 | 0.000 | 0.601 | 0.230 | 2.079 | 0.000 | 0.369 | 0.000 | 0.373 | 0.000 | 0.000 | 0.000 | 0.013 | 0.000 | 0.206 | 0.075 | 0.000 | 0.000 | 0.019 | 0.000 | 0.000 | 0.392 |
| 水产类 Aquatic foods | 0.009 | 0.174 | 0.141 | 0.575 | 0.000 | 0.086 | 0.030 | 0.065 | 0.000 | 0.076 | 0.000 | 0.019 | 0.000 | 0.031 | 0.000 | 0.018 | 0.000 | 0.025 | 0.196 | 0.000 | 0.050 | 0.000 | 0.000 | 0.002 | 0.062 |
| 乳类 Dairy products | 0.000 | 0.000 | 0.000 | 0.000 | 0.000 | 0.000 | 0.031 | 0.000 | 0.015 | 0.000 | 0.000 | 0.000 | 0.000 | 0.000 | 0.000 | 0.000 | 0.000 | 0.000 | 0.000 | 0.000 | 0.000 | 0.000 | 0.000 | 0.000 | 0.002 |
| 蔬菜类 Vegetables | 1.589 | 21.220 | 21.120 | 32.970 | 24.800 | 42.460 | 38.820 | 20.010 | 1.432 | 16.030 | 17.720 | 21.830 | 9.525 | 4.775 | 11.780 | 3.476 | 31.030 | 90.100 | 14.170 | 1.968 | 400.000 | 8.740 | 8.140 | 1.804 | 35.230 |
| 水果类 Fruits | 0.815 | 1.606 | 1.361 | 0.542 | 8.541 | 0.296 | 0.146 | 0.873 | 0.782 | 2.193 | 0.060 | 0.440 | 1.506 | 0.828 | 0.052 | 0.209 | 0.223 | 0.426 | 0.066 | 0.052 | 0.000 | 0.175 | 0.448 | 0.426 | 0.919 |
| 糖类 Sugar | 0.000 | 0.000 | 0.000 | 0.000 | 0.000 | 0.000 | 0.000 | 0.000 | 0.000 | 0.000 | 0.000 | 0.000 | 0.009 | 0.000 | 0.000 | 0.000 | 0.000 | 0.000 | 0.000 | 0.000 | 0.000 | 0.000 | 0.000 | 0.000 | 0.000 |
| 水及饮料类 Water and beverages | 0.000 | 0.374 | 0.000 | 0.000 | 0.000 | 0.000 | 0.517 | 0.000 | 0.000 | 1.953 | 2.482 | 0.000 | 2.712 | 0.000 | 0.000 | 5.099 | 0.559 | 0.000 | 2.410 | 2.183 | 1.021 | 1.325 | 12.801 | 0.000 | 1.393 |
| 酒类 Alcohol beverages | 0.000 | 0.013 | 0.000 | 0.000 | 0.000 | 0.000 | 0.000 | 0.000 | 0.000 | 0.008 | 0.000 | 0.000 | 0.000 | 0.000 | 0.000 | 0.000 | 0.000 | 0.000 | 0.020 | 0.000 | 0.000 | 0.000 | 0.000 | 0.000 | 0.002 |
| 合计 SUM | 2.41 | 27.95 | 52.22 | 43.25 | 33.63 | 47.75 | 44.83 | 55.19 | 2.40 | 25.15 | 20.27 | 23.53 | 14.74 | 5.75 | 12.31 | 11.31 | 32.30 | 91.02 | 18.45 | 6.24 | 401.98 | 11.47 | 22.52 | 14.98 | 42.57 |

附表 4-40　第六次中国总膳食研究的噻虫胺膳食摄入量 [单位：ng/(kg bw·d)]

Annexed Table 4-40　Dietary intakes of clothianidin from the 6$^{th}$ China TDS [Unit: ng/(kg bw·d)]

| 膳食类别 Category | 黑龙江 HL | 辽宁 LN | 河北 HE | 北京 BJ | 吉林 JL | 山西 SX | 陕西 SN | 河南 HA | 宁夏 NX | 内蒙古 NM | 青海 QH | 甘肃 GS | 上海 SH | 福建 FJ | 江西 JX | 江苏 JS | 浙江 ZJ | 山东 SD | 湖北 HB | 四川 SC | 广西 GX | 湖南 HN | 广东 GD | 贵州 GZ | 全国平均 AVG |
|---|---|---|---|---|---|---|---|---|---|---|---|---|---|---|---|---|---|---|---|---|---|---|---|---|---|
| 谷类 Cereals | 0.000 | 0.000 | 0.943 | 0.000 | 0.000 | 0.923 | 0.848 | 1.088 | 0.000 | 1.525 | 0.000 | 0.000 | 0.507 | 0.641 | 3.108 | 1.556 | 0.627 | 0.714 | 2.018 | 0.959 | 3.795 | 10.179 | 0.658 | 1.646 | 1.322 |
| 豆类 Legumes | 0.057 | 0.267 | 0.366 | 0.000 | 0.050 | 0.000 | 0.118 | 0.415 | 0.020 | 0.000 | 0.000 | 0.000 | 0.000 | 0.000 | 0.000 | 0.098 | 0.000 | 0.000 | 0.044 | 0.210 | 0.000 | 0.000 | 0.022 | 0.000 | 0.069 |
| 薯类 Potatoes | 0.000 | 0.171 | 1.594 | 0.291 | 0.000 | 0.411 | 5.975 | 1.955 | 0.085 | 0.413 | 0.058 | 0.146 | 0.044 | 0.052 | 0.000 | 0.682 | 0.031 | 0.137 | 0.338 | 0.105 | 0.008 | 0.156 | 0.178 | 3.207 | 0.668 |
| 肉类 Meats | 0.110 | 0.118 | 0.623 | 0.357 | 0.000 | 0.000 | 0.041 | 0.698 | 0.044 | 0.178 | 0.057 | 0.026 | 0.000 | 0.000 | 0.000 | 0.000 | 0.238 | 0.061 | 0.045 | 0.335 | 0.000 | 0.000 | 0.000 | 0.000 | 0.122 |
| 蛋类 Eggs | 0.000 | 0.067 | 0.616 | 0.155 | 0.000 | 0.097 | 0.029 | 0.454 | 0.000 | 0.194 | 0.000 | 0.054 | 0.000 | 0.000 | 0.000 | 0.000 | 0.000 | 0.054 | 0.000 | 0.000 | 0.000 | 0.014 | 0.000 | 0.000 | 0.072 |
| 水产类 Aquatic foods | 0.039 | 0.011 | 0.031 | 0.060 | 0.000 | 0.016 | 0.007 | 0.014 | 0.000 | 0.029 | 0.003 | 0.000 | 0.000 | 0.000 | 0.000 | 0.000 | 0.133 | 0.011 | 0.040 | 0.015 | 0.000 | 0.038 | 0.000 | 0.000 | 0.019 |
| 乳类 Dairy products | 0.000 | 0.000 | 0.000 | 0.000 | 0.000 | 0.000 | 0.011 | 0.000 | 0.000 | 0.000 | 0.000 | 0.054 | 0.000 | 0.000 | 0.000 | 0.000 | 0.000 | 0.000 | 0.000 | 0.000 | 0.000 | 0.000 | 0.000 | 0.000 | 0.000 |
| 蔬菜类 Vegetables | 0.318 | 0.824 | 16.730 | 12.010 | 0.988 | 7.931 | 15.810 | 15.860 | 0.863 | 7.813 | 2.360 | 10.830 | 1.496 | 3.337 | 7.471 | 6.918 | 3.595 | 55.510 | 2.230 | 0.402 | 218.800 | 5.532 | 77.230 | 0.425 | 19.800 |
| 水果类 Fruits | 1.428 | 0.979 | 1.055 | 1.893 | 1.150 | 0.984 | 0.059 | 0.677 | 0.523 | 0.313 | 0.016 | 0.288 | 0.698 | 0.968 | 0.182 | 0.218 | 0.142 | 0.221 | 0.280 | 0.062 | 0.000 | 0.673 | 0.299 | 0.201 | 0.555 |
| 糖类 Sugar | 0.000 | 0.000 | 0.000 | 0.000 | 0.000 | 0.000 | 0.020 | 0.000 | 0.000 | 0.000 | 0.000 | 0.000 | 0.008 | 0.000 | 0.001 | 0.000 | 0.000 | 0.000 | 0.000 | 0.000 | 0.001 | 0.000 | 0.000 | 0.000 | 0.001 |
| 水及饮料类 Water and beverages | 0.000 | 0.000 | 0.000 | 0.000 | 0.000 | 0.000 | 0.000 | 0.000 | 0.000 | 0.000 | 0.548 | 0.333 | 0.000 | 0.000 | 0.000 | 0.481 | 0.000 | 0.000 | 0.543 | 0.709 | 0.000 | 1.666 | 1.610 | 0.000 | 0.245 |

续表

| 膳食类别<br>Category | 黑龙江<br>HL | 辽宁<br>LN | 河北<br>HE | 北京<br>BJ | 吉林<br>JL | 山西<br>SX | 陕西<br>SN | 河南<br>HA | 宁夏<br>NX | 内蒙古<br>NM | 青海<br>QH | 甘肃<br>GS | 上海<br>SH | 福建<br>FJ | 江西<br>JX | 江苏<br>JS | 浙江<br>ZJ | 山东<br>SD | 湖北<br>HB | 四川<br>SC | 广西<br>GX | 湖南<br>HN | 广东<br>GD | 贵州<br>GZ | 全国平均<br>AVG |
|---|---|---|---|---|---|---|---|---|---|---|---|---|---|---|---|---|---|---|---|---|---|---|---|---|---|
| 酒类<br>Alcohol beverages | 0.000 | 0.000 | 0.000 | 0.000 | 0.000 | 0.000 | 0.000 | 0.000 | 0.000 | 0.000 | 0.000 | 0.000 | 0.000 | 0.000 | 0.010 | 0.000 | 0.000 | 0.000 | 0.000 | 0.000 | 0.017 | 0.000 | 0.000 | 0.000 | 0.001 |
| 合计<br>SUM | 1.95 | 2.44 | 21.96 | 14.77 | 2.19 | 10.36 | 22.91 | 21.16 | 1.53 | 10.46 | 3.04 | 11.35 | 3.09 | 5.00 | 10.77 | 9.95 | 4.76 | 56.71 | 5.54 | 2.80 | 222.66 | 18.26 | 79.99 | 5.48 | 22.88 |

附表 4-41  第六次中国总膳食研究的 N-脱甲基吡虫脒膳食摄入量 [单位: ng/(kg bw · d)]

Annexed Table 4-41  Dietary intakes of acetamiprid-N-desmethyl from the 6$^{th}$ China TDS [Unit: ng/(kg bw · d)]

| 膳食类别<br>Category | 黑龙江<br>HL | 辽宁<br>LN | 河北<br>HE | 北京<br>BJ | 吉林<br>JL | 山西<br>SX | 陕西<br>SN | 河南<br>HA | 宁夏<br>NX | 内蒙古<br>NM | 青海<br>QH | 甘肃<br>GS | 上海<br>SH | 福建<br>FJ | 江西<br>JX | 江苏<br>JS | 浙江<br>ZJ | 山东<br>SD | 湖北<br>HB | 四川<br>SC | 广西<br>GX | 湖南<br>HN | 广东<br>GD | 贵州<br>GZ | 全国平均<br>AVG |
|---|---|---|---|---|---|---|---|---|---|---|---|---|---|---|---|---|---|---|---|---|---|---|---|---|---|
| 谷类<br>Cereals | 0.000 | 0.000 | 0.000 | 0.000 | 0.000 | 0.000 | 0.617 | 0.000 | 0.000 | 0.000 | 0.000 | 0.000 | 0.107 | 0.000 | 0.155 | 0.000 | 0.025 | 0.040 | 0.758 | 0.038 | 0.037 | 0.023 | 0.018 | 0.027 | 0.077 |
| 豆类<br>Legumes | 0.000 | 0.000 | 0.039 | 0.000 | 0.000 | 0.000 | 0.408 | 0.044 | 0.032 | 0.000 | 0.000 | 0.069 | 0.046 | 0.013 | 0.132 | 0.054 | 0.085 | 0.002 | 0.020 | 0.102 | 0.031 | 0.163 | 0.051 | 0.028 | 0.055 |
| 薯类<br>Potatoes | 0.000 | 0.000 | 0.000 | 0.000 | 0.000 | 0.000 | 0.000 | 0.000 | 0.032 | 0.000 | 0.037 | 0.000 | 0.020 | 0.000 | 0.000 | 0.000 | 0.001 | 0.002 | 0.004 | 0.023 | 0.001 | 0.002 | 0.001 | 0.001 | 0.005 |
| 肉类<br>Meats | 0.037 | 0.038 | 0.027 | 0.000 | 0.000 | 0.000 | 0.000 | 0.030 | 0.238 | 0.000 | 0.069 | 0.014 | 0.038 | 0.000 | 0.000 | 0.031 | 0.104 | 0.004 | 0.026 | 0.252 | 0.031 | 0.064 | 0.004 | 0.048 | 0.044 |
| 蛋类<br>Eggs | 0.034 | 0.079 | 0.000 | 0.000 | 0.000 | 0.000 | 0.000 | 0.000 | 0.009 | 0.000 | 0.000 | 0.012 | 0.007 | 0.000 | 0.000 | 0.001 | 0.024 | 0.002 | 0.001 | 0.005 | 0.001 | 0.001 | 0.001 | 0.389 | 0.024 |
| 水产类<br>Aquatic foods | 0.000 | 0.000 | 0.000 | 0.000 | 0.000 | 0.000 | 0.013 | 0.000 | 0.018 | 0.014 | 0.017 | 0.023 | 0.015 | 0.008 | 0.016 | 0.007 | 0.002 | 0.001 | 0.002 | 0.014 | 0.004 | 0.003 | 0.002 | 0.000 | 0.002 |
| 乳类<br>Dairy products | 0.007 | 0.011 | 0.056 | 0.036 | 0.000 | 0.051 | 0.049 | 0.045 | 0.018 | 0.000 | 0.017 | 0.023 | 0.015 | 0.008 | 0.016 | 0.007 | 0.001 | 0.005 | 0.002 | 0.017 | 0.081 | 0.050 | 1.004 | 3.214 | 0.198 |

续表

| 膳食类别 Category | 黑龙江 HL | 辽宁 LN | 河北 HE | 北京 BJ | 吉林 JL | 山西 SX | 陕西 SN | 河南 HA | 宁夏 NX | 内蒙古 NM | 青海 QH | 甘肃 GS | 上海 SH | 福建 FJ | 江西 JX | 江苏 JS | 浙江 ZJ | 山东 SD | 湖北 HB | 四川 SC | 广西 GX | 湖南 HN | 广东 GD | 贵州 GZ | 全国平均 AVG |
|---|---|---|---|---|---|---|---|---|---|---|---|---|---|---|---|---|---|---|---|---|---|---|---|---|---|
| 蔬菜类 Vegetables | 0.916 | 5.270 | 2.160 | 2.084 | 0.318 | 0.958 | 8.670 | 2.047 | 37.150 | 0.761 | 3.129 | 1.858 | 64.040 | 3.891 | 7.479 | 13.790 | 30.290 | 1.102 | 7.218 | 0.588 | 3.691 | 8.736 | 21.380 | 0.204 | 9.489 |
| 水果类 Fruits | 2.309 | 1.021 | 0.221 | 1.156 | 0.712 | 0.091 | 0.703 | 0.142 | 1.765 | 0.717 | 0.023 | 0.301 | 0.655 | 0.572 | 1.328 | 0.249 | 2.275 | 0.346 | 0.083 | 0.327 | 0.024 | 0.511 | 0.074 | 0.268 | 0.661 |
| 糖类 Sugar | 0.000 | 0.000 | 0.000 | 0.000 | 0.000 | 0.000 | 0.000 | 0.000 | 0.000 | 0.000 | 0.000 | 0.000 | 0.000 | 0.000 | 0.000 | 0.000 | 0.000 | 0.000 | 0.000 | 0.000 | 0.000 | 0.000 | 0.000 | 0.000 | 0.000 |
| 水及饮料类 Water and beverages | 0.000 | 0.000 | 0.000 | 0.000 | 0.000 | 0.000 | 0.000 | 0.000 | 0.000 | 0.480 | 1.695 | 0.000 | 0.350 | 0.000 | 0.000 | 0.443 | 0.031 | 0.071 | 0.119 | 0.087 | 0.052 | 0.416 | 0.530 | 0.050 | 0.180 |
| 酒类 Alcohol beverages | 0.000 | 0.000 | 0.000 | 0.000 | 0.000 | 0.000 | 0.000 | 0.000 | 0.000 | 0.000 | 0.000 | 0.000 | 0.000 | 0.000 | 0.000 | 0.000 | 0.002 | 0.005 | 0.001 | 0.000 | 0.001 | 0.001 | 0.000 | 0.000 | 0.000 |
| 合计 SUM | 3.303 | 6.419 | 2.503 | 3.276 | 1.030 | 1.099 | 10.460 | 2.308 | 39.244 | 1.972 | 4.970 | 2.278 | 65.277 | 4.485 | 9.110 | 14.574 | 32.846 | 1.578 | 8.232 | 1.454 | 3.954 | 9.969 | 23.068 | 4.229 | 10.735 |

附表 4-42　第六次中国总膳食研究的呋虫胺膳食摄入量 [单位: ng/(kg bw · d)]
Annexed Table 4-42　Dietary intakes of dinotefuran from the 6th China TDS [Unit: ng/(kg bw · d)]

| 膳食类别 Category | 黑龙江 HL | 辽宁 LN | 河北 HE | 北京 BJ | 吉林 JL | 山西 SX | 陕西 SN | 河南 HA | 宁夏 NX | 内蒙古 NM | 青海 QH | 甘肃 GS | 上海 SH | 福建 FJ | 江西 JX | 江苏 JS | 浙江 ZJ | 山东 SD | 湖北 HB | 四川 SC | 广西 GX | 湖南 HN | 广东 GD | 贵州 GZ | 全国平均 AVG |
|---|---|---|---|---|---|---|---|---|---|---|---|---|---|---|---|---|---|---|---|---|---|---|---|---|---|
| 谷类 Cereals | 0.000 | 0.000 | 0.000 | 0.000 | 0.000 | 0.000 | 0.000 | 0.000 | 0.000 | 0.000 | 0.000 | 0.000 | 0.000 | 0.000 | 0.733 | 0.000 | 0.000 | 0.000 | 0.000 | 0.000 | 0.000 | 0.000 | 0.000 | 0.000 | 0.031 |
| 豆类 Legumes | 0.000 | 0.000 | 0.000 | 0.000 | 0.000 | 0.000 | 0.000 | 0.000 | 0.000 | 0.000 | 0.000 | 0.000 | 0.000 | 0.000 | 0.000 | 0.000 | 0.000 | 0.000 | 0.000 | 0.000 | 0.000 | 0.000 | 0.000 | 0.000 | 0.000 |
| 薯类 Potatoes | 0.000 | 0.000 | 0.000 | 0.000 | 0.000 | 0.000 | 0.000 | 0.000 | 0.000 | 0.000 | 0.000 | 0.000 | 0.000 | 0.000 | 0.000 | 0.000 | 0.000 | 0.000 | 0.000 | 0.000 | 0.000 | 0.000 | 0.000 | 0.090 | 0.004 |

续表

| 膳食类别<br>Category | 黑龙江<br>HL | 辽宁<br>LN | 河北<br>HE | 北京<br>BJ | 吉林<br>JL | 山西<br>SX | 陕西<br>SN | 河南<br>HA | 宁夏<br>NX | 内蒙古<br>NM | 青海<br>QH | 甘肃<br>GS | 上海<br>SH | 福建<br>FJ | 江西<br>JX | 江苏<br>JS | 浙江<br>ZJ | 山东<br>SD | 湖北<br>HB | 四川<br>SC | 广西<br>GX | 湖南<br>HN | 广东<br>GD | 贵州<br>GZ | 全国平均<br>AVG |
|---|---|---|---|---|---|---|---|---|---|---|---|---|---|---|---|---|---|---|---|---|---|---|---|---|---|
| 肉类 Meats | 0.000 | 0.000 | 0.000 | 0.000 | 0.000 | 0.000 | 0.000 | 0.000 | 0.000 | 0.000 | 0.000 | 0.000 | 0.000 | 0.000 | 0.000 | 0.000 | 0.000 | 0.000 | 0.000 | 0.000 | 0.000 | 0.000 | 0.000 | 0.000 | 0.000 |
| 蛋类 Eggs | 0.000 | 0.000 | 0.000 | 0.000 | 0.000 | 0.000 | 0.000 | 0.000 | 0.000 | 0.000 | 0.000 | 0.000 | 0.000 | 0.000 | 0.000 | 0.000 | 0.000 | 0.000 | 0.000 | 0.000 | 0.000 | 0.000 | 0.000 | 0.000 | 0.000 |
| 水产类 Aquatic foods | 0.000 | 0.000 | 0.000 | 0.000 | 0.000 | 0.000 | 0.000 | 0.000 | 0.000 | 0.000 | 0.000 | 0.000 | 0.000 | 0.000 | 0.000 | 0.000 | 0.000 | 0.000 | 0.000 | 0.000 | 0.000 | 0.000 | 0.000 | 0.000 | 0.000 |
| 乳类 Dairy products | 0.000 | 0.000 | 0.000 | 0.000 | 0.000 | 0.000 | 0.000 | 0.000 | 0.000 | 0.000 | 0.000 | 0.000 | 0.000 | 0.000 | 0.000 | 0.000 | 0.000 | 0.000 | 0.000 | 0.000 | 0.000 | 0.000 | 0.000 | 0.000 | 0.000 |
| 蔬菜类 Vegetables | 0.000 | 0.000 | 2.132 | 0.000 | 0.000 | 2.865 | 0.364 | 2.021 | 1.738 | 0.000 | 8.366 | 0.000 | 0.000 | 0.000 | 0.395 | 0.000 | 0.000 | 3.190 | 0.000 | 0.000 | 0.348 | 1.472 | 0.229 | 0.000 | 0.963 |
| 水果类 Fruits | 0.053 | 0.000 | 0.000 | 0.000 | 0.000 | 0.000 | 0.000 | 0.000 | 0.000 | 0.000 | 0.000 | 0.000 | 0.000 | 0.000 | 0.000 | 0.000 | 0.000 | 0.000 | 0.000 | 0.014 | 0.000 | 0.000 | 0.000 | 0.000 | 0.003 |
| 糖类 Sugar | 0.000 | 0.000 | 0.000 | 0.000 | 0.000 | 0.000 | 0.000 | 0.000 | 0.000 | 0.000 | 0.000 | 0.000 | 0.000 | 0.000 | 0.000 | 0.000 | 0.000 | 0.000 | 0.000 | 0.000 | 0.000 | 0.000 | 0.000 | 0.000 | 0.000 |
| 水及饮料类 Water and beverages | 0.000 | 0.000 | 0.000 | 0.000 | 0.000 | 0.000 | 0.000 | 0.000 | 0.000 | 0.000 | 0.614 | 0.000 | 0.718 | 0.000 | 0.000 | 0.979 | 0.000 | 0.000 | 0.332 | 0.524 | 0.000 | 0.000 | 2.042 | 0.000 | 0.217 |
| 酒类 Alcohol beverages | 0.000 | 0.000 | 0.000 | 0.000 | 0.000 | 0.000 | 0.000 | 0.000 | 0.000 | 0.000 | 0.000 | 0.000 | 0.000 | 0.000 | 0.000 | 0.000 | 0.000 | 0.000 | 0.000 | 0.000 | 0.000 | 0.000 | 0.000 | 0.000 | 0.000 |
| 合计 SUM | 0.053 | 0.000 | 2.132 | 0.000 | 0.000 | 2.865 | 0.364 | 2.021 | 1.738 | 0.000 | 8.980 | 0.000 | 0.718 | 0.000 | 1.128 | 0.979 | 0.000 | 3.190 | 0.332 | 0.538 | 0.348 | 1.472 | 2.271 | 0.090 | 1.217 |

附表 4-43 第六次中国总膳食研究的烯啶虫胺膳食摄入量 [单位：ng/(kg bw·d)]
Annexed Table 4-43 Dietary intakes of nitenpyram from the 6th China TDS [Unit: ng/(kg bw·d)]

| 膳食类别 Category | 黑龙江 HL | 辽宁 LN | 河北 HE | 北京 BJ | 吉林 JL | 山西 SX | 陕西 SN | 河南 HA | 宁夏 NX | 内蒙古 NM | 青海 QH | 甘肃 GS | 上海 SH | 福建 FJ | 江西 JX | 江苏 JS | 浙江 ZJ | 山东 SD | 湖北 HB | 四川 SC | 广西 GX | 湖南 HN | 广东 GD | 贵州 GZ | 全国平均 AVG |
|---|---|---|---|---|---|---|---|---|---|---|---|---|---|---|---|---|---|---|---|---|---|---|---|---|---|
| 谷类 Cereals | 0.000 | 0.000 | 0.000 | 0.000 | 0.000 | 0.000 | 0.332 | 0.000 | 0.000 | 0.000 | 0.000 | 0.000 | 0.000 | 0.000 | 0.000 | 0.000 | 0.000 | 0.000 | 0.000 | 0.000 | 0.211 | 0.000 | 0.000 | 0.000 | 0.023 |
| 豆类 Legumes | 0.000 | 0.000 | 0.000 | 0.000 | 0.000 | 0.000 | 0.000 | 0.000 | 0.000 | 0.000 | 0.000 | 0.000 | 0.000 | 0.000 | 0.000 | 0.000 | 0.000 | 0.000 | 0.000 | 0.000 | 0.000 | 0.000 | 0.000 | 0.000 | 0.000 |
| 薯类 Potatoes | 0.000 | 0.000 | 0.000 | 0.000 | 0.000 | 0.000 | 0.000 | 0.000 | 0.000 | 0.000 | 0.000 | 0.000 | 0.000 | 0.000 | 0.000 | 0.000 | 0.000 | 0.000 | 0.000 | 0.000 | 0.000 | 0.000 | 0.000 | 0.000 | 0.000 |
| 肉类 Meats | 0.000 | 0.000 | 0.000 | 0.000 | 0.000 | 0.000 | 0.000 | 0.000 | 0.000 | 0.000 | 0.000 | 0.000 | 0.000 | 0.000 | 0.000 | 0.000 | 0.000 | 0.000 | 0.000 | 0.000 | 0.000 | 0.000 | 0.000 | 0.000 | 0.000 |
| 蛋类 Eggs | 0.000 | 0.000 | 0.000 | 0.000 | 0.000 | 0.000 | 0.000 | 0.000 | 0.000 | 0.000 | 0.000 | 0.000 | 0.000 | 0.000 | 0.000 | 0.000 | 0.000 | 0.000 | 0.000 | 0.000 | 0.000 | 0.000 | 0.000 | 0.000 | 0.000 |
| 水产类 Aquatic foods | 0.000 | 0.000 | 0.000 | 0.000 | 0.000 | 0.000 | 0.000 | 0.000 | 0.000 | 0.000 | 0.000 | 0.000 | 0.000 | 0.000 | 0.000 | 0.000 | 0.000 | 0.000 | 0.000 | 0.000 | 0.000 | 0.000 | 0.000 | 0.000 | 0.000 |
| 乳类 Dairy products | 0.000 | 0.000 | 0.000 | 0.000 | 0.000 | 0.000 | 0.000 | 0.000 | 0.000 | 0.000 | 0.000 | 0.000 | 0.000 | 0.000 | 0.000 | 0.000 | 0.000 | 0.000 | 0.000 | 0.000 | 0.000 | 0.000 | 0.000 | 0.000 | 0.000 |
| 蔬菜类 Vegetables | 0.000 | 0.000 | 1.791 | 2.642 | 0.000 | 11.483 | 1.160 | 1.697 | 2.894 | 0.000 | 10.767 | 1.125 | 0.000 | 0.728 | 1.178 | 0.990 | 0.000 | 3.058 | 0.000 | 0.000 | 0.000 | 0.711 | 0.882 | 0.000 | 1.713 |
| 水果类 Fruits | 0.000 | 0.000 | 0.095 | 0.000 | 0.000 | 0.000 | 0.000 | 0.061 | 0.317 | 0.000 | 0.000 | 0.000 | 0.076 | 0.000 | 0.000 | 0.000 | 0.000 | 0.000 | 0.000 | 0.000 | 0.000 | 0.000 | 0.000 | 0.000 | 0.023 |
| 糖类 Sugar | 0.000 | 0.000 | 0.000 | 0.000 | 0.000 | 0.000 | 0.000 | 0.000 | 0.000 | 0.000 | 0.000 | 0.000 | 0.000 | 0.000 | 0.000 | 0.000 | 0.000 | 0.000 | 0.000 | 0.000 | 0.000 | 0.000 | 0.000 | 0.000 | 0.000 |
| 水及饮料类 Water and beverages | 0.000 | 0.000 | 0.000 | 0.000 | 0.000 | 0.000 | 0.000 | 0.000 | 0.000 | 0.000 | 0.000 | 0.000 | 0.000 | 0.000 | 0.000 | 0.000 | 0.000 | 0.000 | 0.000 | 0.000 | 0.000 | 0.000 | 0.000 | 0.000 | 0.000 |

续表

| 膳食类别 Category | 黑龙江 HL | 辽宁 LN | 河北 HE | 北京 BJ | 吉林 JL | 山西 SX | 陕西 SN | 河南 HA | 宁夏 NX | 内蒙古 NM | 青海 QH | 甘肃 GS | 上海 SH | 福建 FJ | 江西 JX | 江苏 JS | 浙江 ZJ | 山东 SD | 湖北 HB | 四川 SC | 广西 GX | 湖南 HN | 广东 GD | 贵州 GZ | 全国平均 AVG |
|---|---|---|---|---|---|---|---|---|---|---|---|---|---|---|---|---|---|---|---|---|---|---|---|---|---|
| 酒类 Alcohol beverages | 0.000 | 0.000 | 0.000 | 0.000 | 0.000 | 0.000 | 0.000 | 0.000 | 0.000 | 0.000 | 0.000 | 0.000 | 0.000 | 0.000 | 0.000 | 0.000 | 0.000 | 0.000 | 0.000 | 0.000 | 0.098 | 0.000 | 0.000 | 0.000 | 0.004 |
| 合计 SUM | 0.000 | 0.000 | 1.885 | 2.642 | 0.000 | 11.483 | 1.493 | 1.758 | 3.211 | 0.000 | 10.767 | 1.125 | 0.076 | 0.728 | 1.178 | 0.990 | 0.000 | 3.058 | 0.000 | 0.000 | 0.309 | 0.711 | 0.882 | 0.000 | 1.762 |

附表 4-44　第六次中国总膳食研究的噻虫啉膳食摄入量 [单位: ng/(kg bw · d)]

Annexed Table 4-44　Dietary intakes of thiacloprid from the 6th China TDS [Unit: ng/(kg bw · d)]

| 膳食类别 Category | 黑龙江 HL | 辽宁 LN | 河北 HE | 北京 BJ | 吉林 JL | 山西 SX | 陕西 SN | 河南 HA | 宁夏 NX | 内蒙古 NM | 青海 QH | 甘肃 GS | 上海 SH | 福建 FJ | 江西 JX | 江苏 JS | 浙江 ZJ | 山东 SD | 湖北 HB | 四川 SC | 广西 GX | 湖南 HN | 广东 GD | 贵州 GZ | 全国平均 AVG |
|---|---|---|---|---|---|---|---|---|---|---|---|---|---|---|---|---|---|---|---|---|---|---|---|---|---|
| 谷类 Cereals | 0.000 | 0.000 | 0.000 | 0.000 | 0.000 | 0.000 | 0.000 | 0.000 | 0.000 | 0.000 | 0.000 | 0.000 | 0.000 | 0.000 | 0.000 | 0.000 | 0.000 | 0.000 | 0.000 | 0.000 | 0.000 | 0.000 | 0.000 | 0.000 | 0.000 |
| 豆类 Legumes | 0.000 | 0.000 | 0.000 | 0.000 | 0.000 | 0.000 | 0.000 | 0.000 | 0.000 | 0.000 | 0.000 | 0.000 | 0.000 | 0.000 | 0.000 | 0.000 | 0.000 | 0.000 | 0.000 | 0.000 | 0.000 | 0.000 | 0.000 | 0.000 | 0.000 |
| 薯类 Potatoes | 0.000 | 0.000 | 0.000 | 0.000 | 0.000 | 0.000 | 0.000 | 0.000 | 0.000 | 0.000 | 0.000 | 0.000 | 0.000 | 0.000 | 0.000 | 0.000 | 0.000 | 0.000 | 0.000 | 0.000 | 0.000 | 0.000 | 0.000 | 0.000 | 0.000 |
| 肉类 Meats | 0.000 | 0.000 | 0.000 | 0.000 | 0.000 | 0.000 | 0.000 | 0.000 | 0.000 | 0.000 | 0.000 | 0.000 | 0.000 | 0.000 | 0.000 | 0.000 | 0.000 | 0.000 | 0.000 | 0.000 | 0.000 | 0.000 | 0.000 | 0.000 | 0.000 |
| 蛋类 Eggs | 0.000 | 0.000 | 0.000 | 0.000 | 0.000 | 0.000 | 0.000 | 0.000 | 0.000 | 0.000 | 0.000 | 0.000 | 0.000 | 0.000 | 0.000 | 0.000 | 0.000 | 0.000 | 0.000 | 0.000 | 0.000 | 0.000 | 0.000 | 0.000 | 0.000 |
| 水产类 Aquatic foods | 0.000 | 0.000 | 0.000 | 0.000 | 0.000 | 0.000 | 0.000 | 0.000 | 0.000 | 0.000 | 0.013 | 0.000 | 0.000 | 0.000 | 0.000 | 0.000 | 0.000 | 0.000 | 0.000 | 0.000 | 0.000 | 0.000 | 0.000 | 0.000 | 0.001 |
| 乳类 Dairy products | 0.000 | 0.000 | 0.000 | 0.000 | 0.000 | 0.000 | 0.000 | 0.000 | 0.000 | 0.000 | 0.000 | 0.000 | 0.000 | 0.000 | 0.000 | 0.000 | 0.000 | 0.000 | 0.000 | 0.000 | 0.000 | 0.000 | 0.000 | 0.000 | 0.000 |

续表

| 膳食类别<br>Category | 黑龙江<br>HL | 辽宁<br>LN | 河北<br>HE | 北京<br>BJ | 吉林<br>JL | 山西<br>SX | 陕西<br>SN | 河南<br>HA | 宁夏<br>NX | 内蒙古<br>NM | 青海<br>QH | 甘肃<br>GS | 上海<br>SH | 福建<br>FJ | 江西<br>JX | 江苏<br>JS | 浙江<br>ZJ | 山东<br>SD | 湖北<br>HB | 四川<br>SC | 广西<br>GX | 湖南<br>HN | 广东<br>GD | 贵州<br>GZ | 全国平均<br>AVG |
|---|---|---|---|---|---|---|---|---|---|---|---|---|---|---|---|---|---|---|---|---|---|---|---|---|---|
| 蔬菜类 Vegetables | 0.000 | 0.000 | 0.000 | 0.000 | 0.000 | 6.982 | 0.427 | 0.000 | 0.000 | 0.000 | 0.000 | 0.000 | 0.000 | 0.000 | 0.000 | 0.000 | 0.000 | 1.465 | 0.000 | 0.000 | 0.000 | 0.000 | 0.000 | 0.000 | 0.370 |
| 水果类 Fruits | 0.000 | 0.000 | 0.000 | 0.000 | 0.000 | 0.000 | 0.000 | 0.000 | 0.000 | 0.000 | 0.000 | 0.000 | 0.000 | 0.000 | 0.000 | 0.000 | 0.000 | 0.000 | 0.000 | 0.000 | 0.000 | 0.000 | 0.000 | 0.000 | 0.000 |
| 糖类 Sugar | 0.000 | 0.000 | 0.000 | 0.000 | 0.000 | 0.000 | 0.000 | 0.000 | 0.000 | 0.000 | 0.000 | 0.000 | 0.000 | 0.000 | 0.000 | 0.000 | 0.000 | 0.000 | 0.000 | 0.000 | 0.000 | 0.000 | 0.000 | 0.000 | 0.000 |
| 水及饮料类 Water and beverages | 0.000 | 0.000 | 0.000 | 0.000 | 0.000 | 0.000 | 0.000 | 0.000 | 0.000 | 0.000 | 0.000 | 0.000 | 0.000 | 0.000 | 0.000 | 0.000 | 0.000 | 0.000 | 0.155 | 0.000 | 0.000 | 0.000 | 1.573 | 0.000 | 0.072 |
| 酒类 Alcohol beverages | 0.000 | 0.000 | 0.000 | 0.000 | 0.000 | 0.000 | 0.000 | 0.000 | 0.000 | 0.000 | 0.000 | 0.000 | 0.000 | 0.000 | 0.000 | 0.000 | 0.000 | 0.000 | 0.000 | 0.000 | 0.000 | 0.000 | 0.000 | 0.000 | 0.000 |
| 合计 SUM | 0.000 | 0.000 | 0.000 | 0.000 | 0.000 | 6.982 | 0.427 | 0.000 | 0.000 | 0.000 | 0.013 | 0.000 | 0.000 | 0.000 | 0.000 | 0.000 | 0.000 | 1.465 | 0.155 | 0.000 | 0.000 | 0.000 | 1.573 | 0.000 | 0.442 |

附表 4-45　第六次中国总膳食研究的氯噻啉膳食摄入量 [单位：ng/(kg bw·d)]
Annexed Table 4-45　Dietary intakes of imidaclothiz from the 6$^{th}$ China TDS [Unit: ng/(kg bw·d)]

| 膳食类别<br>Category | 黑龙江<br>HL | 辽宁<br>LN | 河北<br>HE | 北京<br>BJ | 吉林<br>JL | 山西<br>SX | 陕西<br>SN | 河南<br>HA | 宁夏<br>NX | 内蒙古<br>NM | 青海<br>QH | 甘肃<br>GS | 上海<br>SH | 福建<br>FJ | 江西<br>JX | 江苏<br>JS | 浙江<br>ZJ | 山东<br>SD | 湖北<br>HB | 四川<br>SC | 广西<br>GX | 湖南<br>HN | 广东<br>GD | 贵州<br>GZ | 全国平均<br>AVG |
|---|---|---|---|---|---|---|---|---|---|---|---|---|---|---|---|---|---|---|---|---|---|---|---|---|---|
| 谷类 Cereals | 0.000 | 0.000 | 0.000 | 0.000 | 0.000 | 0.000 | 0.000 | 0.000 | 0.000 | 0.000 | 0.000 | 0.000 | 0.000 | 0.000 | 0.000 | 0.000 | 0.000 | 0.000 | 0.000 | 0.000 | 0.000 | 0.000 | 0.000 | 0.000 | 0.000 |
| 豆类 Legumes | 0.000 | 0.000 | 0.000 | 0.000 | 0.000 | 0.000 | 0.000 | 0.000 | 0.000 | 0.000 | 0.000 | 0.000 | 0.000 | 0.000 | 0.000 | 0.000 | 0.000 | 0.000 | 0.000 | 0.000 | 0.000 | 0.000 | 0.000 | 0.000 | 0.000 |
| 薯类 Potatoes | 0.000 | 0.000 | 0.000 | 0.000 | 0.000 | 0.000 | 0.000 | 0.000 | 0.000 | 0.000 | 0.000 | 0.000 | 0.000 | 0.000 | 0.000 | 0.000 | 0.000 | 0.000 | 0.000 | 0.000 | 0.000 | 0.000 | 0.000 | 0.000 | 0.000 |

续表

| 膳食类别<br>Category | 黑龙江<br>HL | 辽宁<br>LN | 河北<br>HE | 北京<br>BJ | 吉林<br>JL | 山西<br>SX | 陕西<br>SN | 河南<br>HA | 宁夏<br>NX | 内蒙古<br>NM | 青海<br>QH | 甘肃<br>GS | 上海<br>SH | 福建<br>FJ | 江西<br>JX | 江苏<br>JS | 浙江<br>ZJ | 山东<br>SD | 湖北<br>HB | 四川<br>SC | 广西<br>GX | 湖南<br>HN | 广东<br>GD | 贵州<br>GZ | 全国平均<br>AVG |
|---|---|---|---|---|---|---|---|---|---|---|---|---|---|---|---|---|---|---|---|---|---|---|---|---|---|
| 肉类 Meats | 0.000 | 0.000 | 0.000 | 0.000 | 0.000 | 0.000 | 0.000 | 0.000 | 0.000 | 0.000 | 0.000 | 0.000 | 0.000 | 0.000 | 0.000 | 0.000 | 0.000 | 0.000 | 0.000 | 0.000 | 0.000 | 0.000 | 0.000 | 0.000 | 0.000 |
| 蛋类 Eggs | 0.000 | 0.000 | 0.000 | 0.000 | 0.000 | 0.000 | 0.000 | 0.000 | 0.000 | 0.000 | 0.000 | 0.000 | 0.000 | 0.000 | 0.000 | 0.000 | 0.000 | 0.000 | 0.000 | 0.000 | 0.000 | 0.000 | 0.000 | 0.000 | 0.000 |
| 水产类 Aquatic foods | 0.000 | 0.000 | 0.000 | 0.000 | 0.000 | 0.000 | 0.000 | 0.000 | 0.000 | 0.000 | 0.000 | 0.000 | 0.000 | 0.000 | 0.000 | 0.000 | 0.000 | 0.000 | 0.000 | 0.000 | 0.000 | 0.000 | 0.000 | 0.000 | 0.000 |
| 乳类 Dairy products | 0.000 | 0.000 | 0.000 | 0.000 | 0.000 | 0.000 | 0.000 | 0.000 | 0.000 | 0.000 | 0.000 | 0.000 | 0.000 | 0.000 | 0.000 | 0.000 | 0.000 | 0.000 | 0.000 | 0.000 | 0.000 | 0.000 | 0.000 | 0.000 | 0.000 |
| 蔬菜类 Vegetables | 0.000 | 0.000 | 0.000 | 0.000 | 0.000 | 0.000 | 0.000 | 0.000 | 0.000 | 0.000 | 0.000 | 0.000 | 0.000 | 0.000 | 0.000 | 0.000 | 0.000 | 0.000 | 0.000 | 0.000 | 0.000 | 0.000 | 0.000 | 5.809 | 0.242 |
| 水果类 Fruits | 0.000 | 0.000 | 0.000 | 0.000 | 0.000 | 0.000 | 0.000 | 0.000 | 0.000 | 0.000 | 0.000 | 0.000 | 0.000 | 0.000 | 0.000 | 0.000 | 0.000 | 0.000 | 0.000 | 0.000 | 0.000 | 0.000 | 0.000 | 0.000 | 0.000 |
| 糖类 Sugar | 0.000 | 0.000 | 0.000 | 0.000 | 0.000 | 0.000 | 0.000 | 0.000 | 0.000 | 0.000 | 0.000 | 0.000 | 0.000 | 0.000 | 0.000 | 0.000 | 0.000 | 0.000 | 0.000 | 0.000 | 0.000 | 0.000 | 0.000 | 0.000 | 0.000 |
| 水及饮料类 Water and beverages | 0.000 | 0.000 | 0.000 | 0.000 | 0.000 | 0.000 | 0.000 | 0.000 | 0.000 | 0.000 | 0.000 | 0.000 | 0.000 | 0.000 | 0.000 | 0.000 | 0.000 | 0.000 | 0.000 | 0.000 | 0.000 | 0.000 | 0.000 | 0.000 | 0.000 |
| 酒类 Alcohol beverages | 0.000 | 0.000 | 0.000 | 0.000 | 0.000 | 0.000 | 0.000 | 0.000 | 0.000 | 0.000 | 0.000 | 0.000 | 0.000 | 0.000 | 0.000 | 0.000 | 0.000 | 0.000 | 0.000 | 0.000 | 0.000 | 0.000 | 0.000 | 0.000 | 0.000 |
| 合计 SUM | 0.000 | 0.000 | 0.000 | 0.000 | 0.000 | 0.000 | 0.000 | 0.000 | 0.000 | 0.000 | 0.000 | 0.000 | 0.000 | 0.000 | 0.000 | 0.000 | 0.000 | 0.000 | 0.000 | 0.000 | 0.000 | 0.000 | 0.000 | 5.809 | 0.242 |

附表 4-46　第六次中国总膳食研究的总新烟碱膳食摄入量 [单位：ng/(kg bw·d)]
Annexed Table 4-46　Dietary intakes of total neonicotinoids from the 6th China TDS [Unit: ng/(kg bw·d)]

| 膳食类别<br>Category | 黑龙江<br>HL | 辽宁<br>LN | 河北<br>HE | 北京<br>BJ | 吉林<br>JL | 山西<br>SX | 陕西<br>SN | 河南<br>HA | 宁夏<br>NX | 内蒙古<br>NM | 青海<br>QH | 甘肃<br>GS | 上海<br>SH | 福建<br>FJ | 江西<br>JX | 江苏<br>JS | 浙江<br>ZJ | 山东<br>SD | 湖北<br>HB | 四川<br>SC | 广西<br>GX | 湖南<br>HN | 广东<br>GD | 贵州<br>GZ | 全国平均<br>AVG |
|---|---|---|---|---|---|---|---|---|---|---|---|---|---|---|---|---|---|---|---|---|---|---|---|---|---|
| 谷类 Cereals | 1.775 | 0.000 | 55.880 | 0.000 | 0.000 | 39.460 | 19.850 | 66.590 | 0.000 | 41.380 | 2.934 | 0.000 | 16.730 | 10.550 | 27.460 | 25.460 | 10.650 | 6.102 | 26.690 | 14.591 | 37.240 | 68.420 | 8.658 | 14.810 | 20.630 |
| 豆类 Legumes | 0.416 | 15.160 | 18.720 | 10.110 | 3.215 | 0.194 | 8.647 | 17.010 | 0.480 | 0.000 | 0.030 | 1.214 | 0.424 | 0.262 | 0.648 | 1.629 | 0.858 | 0.486 | 2.315 | 7.520 | 0.271 | 0.376 | 0.727 | 0.353 | 3.794 |
| 薯类 Potatoes | 0.000 | 14.170 | 186.600 | 28.790 | 0.501 | 9.745 | 70.300 | 33.850 | 1.974 | 13.970 | 1.269 | 6.870 | 1.491 | 1.228 | 0.203 | 12.653 | 0.775 | 1.628 | 7.624 | 3.397 | 0.086 | 4.471 | 7.575 | 137.0 | 22.760 |
| 肉类 Meats | 0.792 | 11.320 | 23.200 | 34.510 | 0.215 | 1.411 | 2.449 | 37.790 | 1.490 | 5.477 | 1.266 | 1.937 | 0.812 | 0.562 | 0.287 | 0.777 | 2.632 | 1.908 | 3.284 | 16.250 | 0.333 | 3.163 | 1.397 | 0.377 | 6.402 |
| 蛋类 Eggs | 0.110 | 6.773 | 31.520 | 21.050 | 0.000 | 6.304 | 2.376 | 0.000 | 0.037 | 4.683 | 0.000 | 3.885 | 0.085 | 0.066 | 0.000 | 0.160 | 0.068 | 2.327 | 0.865 | 0.038 | 0.000 | 0.288 | 0.000 | 0.352 | 3.375 |
| 水产类 Aquatic foods | 0.340 | 0.665 | 1.581 | 5.897 | 0.000 | 0.922 | 0.512 | 2.691 | 0.000 | 0.906 | 0.195 | 0.205 | 0.240 | 0.484 | 0.113 | 0.250 | 0.906 | 0.327 | 2.362 | 0.533 | 0.604 | 0.345 | 0.321 | 0.023 | 0.851 |
| 乳类 Dairy products | 0.033 | 0.099 | 0.118 | 0.216 | 0.000 | 0.137 | 0.435 | 0.045 | 0.178 | 0.103 | 0.123 | 0.053 | 0.157 | 0.080 | 0.060 | 0.061 | 0.000 | 0.051 | 0.015 | 0.046 | 0.127 | 0.162 | 1.183 | 3.652 | 0.297 |
| 蔬菜类 Vegetables | 32.480 | 141.500 | 345.300 | 441.800 | 260.900 | 603.600 | 516.400 | 584.500 | 145.800 | 209.100 | 249.300 | 313.400 | 1163.000 | 117.440 | 422.100 | 276.000 | 637.300 | 1242.000 | 431.900 | 34.580 | 5139.000 | 267.600 | 759.700 | 34.780 | 598.700 |
| 水果类 Fruits | 21.750 | 54.810 | 24.390 | 35.700 | 94.500 | 9.506 | 13.190 | 13.330 | 23.280 | 35.570 | 1.393 | 7.790 | 34.400 | 25.390 | 4.813 | 5.041 | 117.300 | 9.359 | 4.529 | 2.432 | 3.997 | 9.075 | 7.208 | 10.450 | 23.720 |
| 糖类 Sugar | 0.000 | 0.000 | 0.000 | 0.000 | 0.000 | 0.000 | 0.186 | 0.000 | 0.004 | 0.000 | 0.000 | 0.003 | 0.192 | 0.000 | 0.005 | 0.000 | 0.000 | 0.003 | 0.001 | 0.000 | 0.007 | 0.004 | 0.000 | 0.000 | 0.017 |
| 水及饮料类 Water and beverages | 0.000 | 1.283 | 0.000 | 0.000 | 3.160 | 0.000 | 6.289 | 11.500 | 0.000 | 37.480 | 60.540 | 0.000 | 41.970 | 3.661 | 0.000 | 69.490 | 10.180 | 0.000 | 34.290 | 31.080 | 14.260 | 33.970 | 177.700 | 0.000 | 22.370 |

续表

| 膳食类别<br>Category | 黑龙江<br>HL | 辽宁<br>LN | 河北<br>HE | 北京<br>BJ | 吉林<br>JL | 山西<br>SX | 陕西<br>SN | 河南<br>HA | 宁夏<br>NX | 内蒙古<br>NM | 青海<br>QH | 甘肃<br>GS | 上海<br>SH | 福建<br>FJ | 江西<br>JX | 江苏<br>JS | 浙江<br>ZJ | 山东<br>SD | 湖北<br>HB | 四川<br>SC | 广西<br>GX | 湖南<br>HN | 广东<br>GD | 贵州<br>GZ | 全国平均<br>AVG |
|---|---|---|---|---|---|---|---|---|---|---|---|---|---|---|---|---|---|---|---|---|---|---|---|---|---|
| 酒类<br>Alcohol beverages | 0.000 | 0.000 | 0.025 | 0.108 | 0.000 | 0.000 | 0.000 | 0.011 | 0.000 | 0.102 | 0.000 | 0.009 | 0.105 | 0.042 | 0.100 | 0.083 | 0.210 | 0.390 | 0.207 | 0.000 | 0.511 | 0.000 | 0.008 | 0.000 | 0.080 |
| 合计<br>SUM | 57.7 | 245.8 | 687.4 | 578.2 | 362.4 | 671.2 | 640.6 | 767.3 | 173.2 | 348.8 | 317.1 | 335.4 | 1259.3 | 159.8 | 455.8 | 391.6 | 780.9 | 1264.6 | 514.0 | 110.5 | 5196.8 | 387.8 | 964.5 | 201.8 | 703.0 |

附表 4-47　第六次中国总膳食研究吡虫啉的膳食来源（单位：%）

Annexed Table 4-47　Dietary sources of imidacloprid from the 6ᵗʰ China TDS (Unit: %)

| 膳食类别<br>Category | 黑龙江<br>HL | 辽宁<br>LN | 河北<br>HE | 北京<br>BJ | 吉林<br>JL | 山西<br>SX | 陕西<br>SN | 河南<br>HA | 宁夏<br>NX | 内蒙古<br>NM | 青海<br>QH | 甘肃<br>GS | 上海<br>SH | 福建<br>FJ | 江西<br>JX | 江苏<br>JS | 浙江<br>ZJ | 山东<br>SD | 湖北<br>HB | 四川<br>SC | 广西<br>GX | 湖南<br>HN | 广东<br>GD | 贵州<br>GZ | 全国平均<br>AVG |
|---|---|---|---|---|---|---|---|---|---|---|---|---|---|---|---|---|---|---|---|---|---|---|---|---|---|
| 谷类<br>Cereals | 4.9 | 0.0 | 20.7 | 0.0 | 0.0 | 0.0 | 0.0 | 24.9 | 0.0 | 13.4 | 2.3 | 0.0 | 4.1 | 21.5 | 0.3 | 9.7 | 3.0 | 0.0 | 3.1 | 3.3 | 7.0 | 3.7 | 3.4 | 6.6 | 4.4 |
| 豆类<br>Legumes | 0.0 | 2.5 | 2.7 | 1.2 | 0.0 | 0.1 | 2.6 | 3.2 | 0.1 | 0.0 | 0.0 | 0.3 | 0.2 | 0.5 | 0.1 | 2.0 | 1.3 | 0.3 | 0.2 | 8.3 | 0.2 | 0.2 | 0.3 | 1.0 | 0.7 |
| 薯类<br>Potatoes | 0.0 | 6.0 | 1.9 | 5.4 | 1.6 | 2.8 | 0.8 | 2.5 | 2.2 | 3.5 | 1.2 | 0.3 | 0.1 | 0.5 | 0.0 | 0.4 | 0.2 | 0.3 | 3.6 | 15.2 | 0.0 | 0.3 | 0.4 | 2.4 | 1.5 |
| 肉类<br>Meats | 0.0 | 0.9 | 4.9 | 1.0 | 0.0 | 0.0 | 0.0 | 5.7 | 1.1 | 0.1 | 1.2 | 0.2 | 0.1 | 0.8 | 0.0 | 0.3 | 0.5 | 0.0 | 0.4 | 10.5 | 0.0 | 0.2 | 2.0 | 0.7 | 0.8 |
| 蛋类<br>Eggs | 0.0 | 1.0 | 4.0 | 0.2 | 0.0 | 0.1 | 0.0 | 3.1 | 0.0 | 0.0 | 0.0 | 0.0 | 0.0 | 0.1 | 0.0 | 0.0 | 0.1 | 0.0 | 0.2 | 0.9 | 0.0 | 0.0 | 0.0 | 0.0 | 0.3 |
| 水产类<br>Aquatic foods | 0.0 | 0.0 | 0.2 | 0.2 | 0.0 | 0.0 | 0.2 | 0.1 | 0.0 | 0.0 | 0.0 | 0.0 | 0.0 | 0.5 | 0.0 | 0.1 | 0.1 | 0.0 | 0.3 | 0.0 | 0.0 | 0.0 | 0.8 | 0.0 | 0.1 |
| 乳类<br>Dairy products | 0.0 | 0.0 | 0.0 | 0.0 | 0.0 | 0.0 | 0.0 | 0.0 | 0.0 | 0.0 | 0.0 | 0.0 | 0.0 | 0.0 | 0.0 | 0.0 | 0.0 | 0.0 | 0.0 | 0.0 | 0.0 | 0.0 | 0.0 | 0.0 | 0.0 |

续表

| 膳食类别<br>Category | 黑龙江<br>HL | 辽宁<br>LN | 河北<br>HE | 北京<br>BJ | 吉林<br>JL | 山西<br>SX | 陕西<br>SN | 河南<br>HA | 宁夏<br>NX | 内蒙古<br>NM | 青海<br>QH | 甘肃<br>GS | 上海<br>SH | 福建<br>FJ | 江西<br>JX | 江苏<br>JS | 浙江<br>ZJ | 山东<br>SD | 湖北<br>HB | 四川<br>SC | 广西<br>GX | 湖南<br>HN | 广东<br>GD | 贵州<br>GZ | 全国平均<br>AVG |
|---|---|---|---|---|---|---|---|---|---|---|---|---|---|---|---|---|---|---|---|---|---|---|---|---|---|
| 蔬菜类 Vegetables | 87.5 | 46.1 | 52.8 | 42.9 | 79.9 | 95.5 | 70.9 | 52.1 | 57.2 | 34.4 | 37.7 | 96.5 | 81.2 | 26.4 | 99.3 | 41.2 | 16.4 | 89.9 | 87.9 | 41.2 | 76.8 | 85.1 | 63.4 | 56.0 | 73.1 |
| 水果类 Fruits | 7.6 | 43.0 | 12.7 | 48.9 | 15.5 | 1.5 | 24.0 | 8.5 | 39.4 | 29.6 | 5.1 | 2.8 | 10.4 | 47.9 | 0.2 | 6.9 | 74.3 | 8.9 | 2.8 | 6.2 | 11.6 | 3.4 | 3.1 | 33.3 | 14.3 |
| 糖类 Sugar | 0.0 | 0.0 | 0.0 | 0.0 | 0.0 | 0.0 | 0.0 | 0.0 | 0.0 | 0.0 | 0.0 | 0.0 | 0.1 | 0.0 | 0.0 | 0.0 | 0.0 | 0.0 | 0.0 | 0.0 | 0.0 | 0.0 | 0.0 | 0.0 | 0.0 |
| 水及饮料类 Water and beverages | 0.0 | 0.5 | 0.0 | 0.0 | 3.1 | 0.0 | 1.5 | 0.0 | 0.0 | 18.9 | 52.5 | 0.0 | 3.9 | 1.8 | 0.0 | 39.4 | 4.2 | 0.0 | 1.6 | 14.2 | 3.6 | 7.2 | 26.6 | 0.0 | 4.7 |
| 酒类 Alcohol beverages | 0.0 | 0.0 | 0.0 | 0.2 | 0.0 | 0.0 | 0.0 | 0.0 | 0.0 | 0.0 | 0.0 | 0.0 | 0.1 | 0.0 | 0.0 | 0.0 | 0.1 | 0.5 | 0.0 | 0.0 | 0.8 | 0.0 | 0.0 | 0.0 | 0.1 |

附表 4-48  第六次中国总膳食研究啶虫脒的膳食来源（单位：%）

Annexed Table 4-48  Dietary sources of acetamiprid from the 6th China TDS (Unit: %)

| 膳食类别<br>Category | 黑龙江<br>HL | 辽宁<br>LN | 河北<br>HE | 北京<br>BJ | 吉林<br>JL | 山西<br>SX | 陕西<br>SN | 河南<br>HA | 宁夏<br>NX | 内蒙古<br>NM | 青海<br>QH | 甘肃<br>GS | 上海<br>SH | 福建<br>FJ | 江西<br>JX | 江苏<br>JS | 浙江<br>ZJ | 山东<br>SD | 湖北<br>HB | 四川<br>SC | 广西<br>GX | 湖南<br>HN | 广东<br>GD | 贵州<br>GZ | 全国平均<br>AVG |
|---|---|---|---|---|---|---|---|---|---|---|---|---|---|---|---|---|---|---|---|---|---|---|---|---|---|
| 谷类 Cereals | 2.3 | 0.0 | 0.0 | 0.0 | 0.0 | 0.0 | 15.3 | 0.0 | 0.0 | 0.0 | 2.2 | 0.0 | 0.2 | 2.7 | 2.8 | 0.3 | 0.5 | 1.6 | 2.2 | 0.0 | 8.5 | 0.8 | 0.1 | 10.6 | 1.0 |
| 豆类 Legumes | 0.0 | 0.6 | 0.4 | 0.3 | 1.2 | 0.2 | 5.1 | 0.4 | 0.4 | 0.0 | 0.0 | 0.2 | 0.0 | 0.0 | 0.2 | 0.0 | 0.0 | 0.0 | 0.0 | 8.5 | 0.0 | 0.0 | 0.0 | 0.0 | 0.2 |
| 薯类 Potatoes | 0.0 | 0.4 | 0.0 | 0.0 | 0.0 | 0.0 | 0.9 | 0.0 | 0.0 | 0.4 | 1.1 | 0.9 | 0.1 | 0.0 | 0.0 | 0.0 | 0.1 | 0.0 | 0.0 | 0.9 | 0.0 | 0.0 | 0.0 | 0.0 | 0.1 |
| 肉类 Meats | 0.2 | 0.4 | 0.1 | 0.9 | 0.9 | 0.2 | 0.0 | 0.1 | 0.4 | 0.0 | 1.2 | 0.4 | 0.0 | 0.0 | 0.1 | 0.0 | 0.1 | 0.0 | 0.0 | 28.6 | 0.0 | 0.8 | 0.0 | 1.0 | 0.3 |
| 蛋类 Eggs | 0.0 | 0.3 | 0.0 | 0.0 | 0.0 | 0.0 | 0.0 | 0.0 | 0.0 | 0.0 | 0.0 | 0.0 | 0.0 | 0.0 | 0.0 | 0.0 | 0.0 | 0.0 | 0.0 | 0.0 | 0.0 | 0.0 | 0.0 | 0.2 | 0.0 |

续表

| 膳食类别<br>Category | 黑龙江<br>HL | 辽宁<br>LN | 河北<br>HE | 北京<br>BJ | 吉林<br>JL | 山西<br>SX | 陕西<br>SN | 河南<br>HA | 宁夏<br>NX | 内蒙古<br>NM | 青海<br>QH | 甘肃<br>GS | 上海<br>SH | 福建<br>FJ | 江西<br>JX | 江苏<br>JS | 浙江<br>ZJ | 山东<br>SD | 湖北<br>HB | 四川<br>SC | 广西<br>GX | 湖南<br>HN | 广东<br>GD | 贵州<br>GZ | 全国平均<br>AVG |
|---|---|---|---|---|---|---|---|---|---|---|---|---|---|---|---|---|---|---|---|---|---|---|---|---|---|
| 水产类<br>Aquatic foods | 0.0 | 0.0 | 0.0 | 0.0 | 0.0 | 0.0 | 0.3 | 0.0 | 0.0 | 0.0 | 0.0 | 0.0 | 0.0 | 0.0 | 0.0 | 0.0 | 0.0 | 0.0 | 0.0 | 1.7 | 0.0 | 0.0 | 0.0 | 0.0 | 0.0 |
| 乳类<br>Dairy products | 0.0 | 0.0 | 0.1 | 0.0 | 0.0 | 0.1 | 0.0 | 0.1 | 0.0 | 0.1 | 0.0 | 0.0 | 0.0 | 0.0 | 0.0 | 0.0 | 0.0 | 0.0 | 0.0 | 0.0 | 0.1 | 0.1 | 0.1 | 23.2 | 0.1 |
| 蔬菜类<br>Vegetables | 64.9 | 83.7 | 93.3 | 88.2 | 61.0 | 96.3 | 61.9 | 95.2 | 91.5 | 8.4 | 49.4 | 93.9 | 98.1 | 90.8 | 94.1 | 94.8 | 76.7 | 82.7 | 95.8 | 42.6 | 86.6 | 90.5 | 94.7 | 44.1 | 90.0 |
| 水果类<br>Fruits | 32.6 | 14.3 | 6.1 | 10.6 | 36.9 | 3.2 | 14.9 | 4.2 | 7.7 | 26.7 | 0.0 | 4.6 | 0.7 | 3.1 | 2.7 | 0.3 | 22.1 | 15.2 | 0.2 | 2.8 | 0.6 | 1.4 | 0.1 | 20.8 | 5.3 |
| 糖类<br>Sugar | 0.0 | 0.0 | 0.0 | 0.0 | 0.0 | 0.0 | 0.0 | 0.0 | 0.0 | 0.0 | 0.0 | 0.0 | 0.0 | 0.0 | 0.0 | 0.0 | 0.0 | 0.0 | 0.0 | 0.0 | 0.0 | 0.0 | 0.0 | 0.0 | 0.0 |
| 水及饮料类<br>Water and beverages | 0.0 | 0.3 | 0.0 | 0.0 | 0.0 | 0.0 | 1.5 | 0.0 | 0.0 | 64.5 | 46.0 | 0.0 | 0.9 | 3.3 | 0.0 | 4.6 | 0.6 | 0.0 | 1.7 | 14.8 | 4.3 | 6.4 | 4.9 | 0.0 | 3.0 |
| 酒类<br>Alcohol beverages | 0.0 | 0.0 | 0.0 | 0.0 | 0.0 | 0.0 | 0.0 | 0.0 | 0.0 | 0.0 | 0.0 | 0.0 | 0.0 | 0.0 | 0.0 | 0.0 | 0.0 | 0.5 | 0.0 | 0.0 | 0.0 | 0.0 | 0.0 | 0.0 | 0.0 |

附表 4-49 第六次中国总膳食研究噻虫嗪的膳食来源（单位：%）

Annexed Table 4-49 Dietary sources of thiamethoxam from the 6<sup>th</sup> China TDS (Unit: %)

| 膳食类别<br>Category | 黑龙江<br>HL | 辽宁<br>LN | 河北<br>HE | 北京<br>BJ | 吉林<br>JL | 山西<br>SX | 陕西<br>SN | 河南<br>HA | 宁夏<br>NX | 内蒙古<br>NM | 青海<br>QH | 甘肃<br>GS | 上海<br>SH | 福建<br>FJ | 江西<br>JX | 江苏<br>JS | 浙江<br>ZJ | 山东<br>SD | 湖北<br>HB | 四川<br>SC | 广西<br>GX | 湖南<br>HN | 广东<br>GD | 贵州<br>GZ | 全国平均<br>AVG |
|---|---|---|---|---|---|---|---|---|---|---|---|---|---|---|---|---|---|---|---|---|---|---|---|---|---|
| 谷类<br>Cereals | 0.0 | 9.7 | 8.8 | 0.0 | 0.0 | 7.3 | 1.5 | 9.7 | 0.0 | 11.8 | 0.0 | 0.0 | 5.9 | 0.0 | 3.8 | 12.9 | 1.1 | 0.0 | 3.8 | 12.8 | 0.2 | 5.7 | 1.5 | 2.3 | 2.6 |
| 豆类<br>Legumes | 0.0 | 0.0 | 3.2 | 2.3 | 0.9 | 0.0 | 1.1 | 3.4 | 1.3 | 0.0 | 0.0 | 0.5 | 0.0 | 0.0 | 0.0 | 0.6 | 0.0 | 0.0 | 1.0 | 6.0 | 0.0 | 0.0 | 0.2 | 0.0 | 0.6 |

续表

| 膳食类别<br>Category | 黑龙江<br>HL | 辽宁<br>LN | 河北<br>HE | 北京<br>BJ | 吉林<br>JL | 山西<br>SX | 陕西<br>SN | 河南<br>HA | 宁夏<br>NX | 内蒙古<br>NM | 青海<br>QH | 甘肃<br>GS | 上海<br>SH | 福建<br>FJ | 江西<br>JX | 江苏<br>JS | 浙江<br>ZJ | 山东<br>SD | 湖北<br>HB | 四川<br>SC | 广西<br>GX | 湖南<br>HN | 广东<br>GD | 贵州<br>GZ | 全国平均<br>AVG |
|---|---|---|---|---|---|---|---|---|---|---|---|---|---|---|---|---|---|---|---|---|---|---|---|---|---|
| 薯类 Potatoes | 0.0 | 2.9 | 35.6 | 6.3 | 0.0 | 1.5 | 8.2 | 41.3 | 3.3 | 4.4 | 0.0 | 2.5 | 0.5 | 1.4 | 0.1 | 8.0 | 0.2 | 0.1 | 1.9 | 1.2 | 0.0 | 3.1 | 3.0 | 82.8 | 6.5 |
| 肉类 Meats | 0.0 | 1.8 | 3.7 | 7.7 | 0.0 | 0.3 | 0.5 | 3.9 | 2.5 | 1.8 | 0.0 | 0.7 | 0.4 | 0.5 | 0.0 | 0.5 | 0.2 | 0.2 | 1.5 | 12.6 | 0.0 | 1.7 | 0.3 | 0.0 | 1.0 |
| 蛋类 Eggs | 0.0 | 1.8 | 5.4 | 4.9 | 0.0 | 1.3 | 0.5 | 3.8 | 0.0 | 1.5 | 0.0 | 1.6 | 0.0 | 0.0 | 0.0 | 0.1 | 0.0 | 0.2 | 0.4 | 0.0 | 0.0 | 0.2 | 0.0 | 0.0 | 0.9 |
| 水产类 Aquatic foods | 0.4 | 0.6 | 0.3 | 1.3 | 0.0 | 0.2 | 0.1 | 0.1 | 0.0 | 0.3 | 0.0 | 0.1 | 0.0 | 0.5 | 0.0 | 0.2 | 0.0 | 0.0 | 1.1 | 0.0 | 0.0 | 0.0 | 0.0 | 0.0 | 0.1 |
| 乳类 Dairy products | 0.0 | 0.0 | 0.0 | 0.0 | 0.0 | 0.0 | 0.1 | 0.0 | 0.6 | 0.0 | 0.0 | 0.0 | 0.0 | 0.0 | 0.0 | 0.0 | 0.0 | 0.0 | 0.0 | 0.0 | 0.0 | 0.0 | 0.0 | 0.0 | 0.0 |
| 蔬菜类 Vegetables | 65.9 | 75.9 | 40.4 | 76.2 | 73.7 | 88.9 | 86.6 | 36.3 | 59.7 | 63.7 | 87.5 | 92.8 | 64.6 | 83.1 | 95.7 | 30.7 | 96.1 | 99.0 | 76.8 | 31.5 | 99.5 | 76.2 | 36.1 | 12.0 | 82.8 |
| 水果类 Fruits | 33.8 | 5.7 | 2.6 | 1.3 | 25.4 | 0.6 | 0.3 | 1.6 | 32.6 | 8.7 | 0.3 | 1.9 | 10.2 | 14.4 | 0.4 | 1.8 | 0.7 | 0.5 | 0.4 | 0.8 | 0.0 | 1.5 | 2.0 | 2.8 | 2.2 |
| 糖类 Sugar | 0.0 | 0.0 | 0.0 | 0.0 | 0.0 | 0.0 | 0.0 | 0.0 | 0.0 | 0.0 | 0.0 | 0.0 | 0.1 | 0.0 | 0.0 | 0.0 | 0.0 | 0.0 | 0.0 | 0.0 | 0.0 | 0.0 | 0.0 | 0.0 | 0.0 |
| 水及饮料类 Water and beverages | 0.0 | 1.3 | 0.0 | 0.0 | 0.0 | 0.0 | 1.2 | 0.0 | 0.0 | 7.8 | 12.2 | 0.0 | 18.4 | 0.0 | 0.0 | 45.1 | 1.7 | 0.0 | 13.1 | 35.0 | 0.3 | 11.6 | 56.8 | 0.0 | 3.3 |
| 酒类 Alcohol beverages | 0.0 | 0.0 | 0.0 | 0.0 | 0.0 | 0.0 | 0.0 | 0.0 | 0.0 | 0.0 | 0.0 | 0.0 | 0.0 | 0.0 | 0.0 | 0.0 | 0.0 | 0.0 | 0.1 | 0.0 | 0.0 | 0.0 | 0.0 | 0.0 | 0.0 |

附表 4-50　第六次中国总膳食研究噻虫胺的膳食来源（单位：%）

Annexed Table 4-50　Dietary sources of clothianidin from the 6$^{th}$ China TDS (Unit: %)

| 膳食类别<br>Category | 黑龙江<br>HL | 辽宁<br>LN | 河北<br>HE | 北京<br>BJ | 吉林<br>JL | 山西<br>SX | 陕西<br>SN | 河南<br>HA | 宁夏<br>NX | 内蒙古<br>NM | 青海<br>QH | 甘肃<br>GS | 上海<br>SH | 福建<br>FJ | 江西<br>JX | 江苏<br>JS | 浙江<br>ZJ | 山东<br>SD | 湖北<br>HB | 四川<br>SC | 广西<br>GX | 湖南<br>HN | 广东<br>GD | 贵州<br>GZ | 全国平均<br>AVG |
|---|---|---|---|---|---|---|---|---|---|---|---|---|---|---|---|---|---|---|---|---|---|---|---|---|---|
| 谷类 Cereals | 0.0 | 0.0 | 4.3 | 0.0 | 0.0 | 8.9 | 3.7 | 5.1 | 0.0 | 14.6 | 0.0 | 0.0 | 16.4 | 12.8 | 28.9 | 15.6 | 13.2 | 1.3 | 36.4 | 34.3 | 1.7 | 55.8 | 0.8 | 30.0 | 5.8 |
| 豆类 Legumes | 2.9 | 11.0 | 1.7 | 0.0 | 2.3 | 0.0 | 0.5 | 2.0 | 1.3 | 0.0 | 0.0 | 0.0 | 0.0 | 0.0 | 0.0 | 1.0 | 0.0 | 0.0 | 0.8 | 7.5 | 0.0 | 0.0 | 0.0 | 0.0 | 0.3 |
| 薯类 Potatoes | 0.0 | 7.0 | 7.3 | 2.0 | 0.0 | 4.0 | 26.1 | 9.2 | 5.5 | 3.9 | 1.9 | 1.3 | 1.4 | 1.0 | 0.0 | 6.9 | 0.6 | 0.2 | 6.1 | 3.8 | 0.0 | 0.9 | 0.2 | 58.5 | 2.9 |
| 肉类 Meats | 5.6 | 4.8 | 2.8 | 2.4 | 0.0 | 0.0 | 0.2 | 3.3 | 2.8 | 1.7 | 1.9 | 0.2 | 0.0 | 0.0 | 0.0 | 0.0 | 5.0 | 0.1 | 0.8 | 12.0 | 0.0 | 0.0 | 0.0 | 0.0 | 0.5 |
| 蛋类 Eggs | 0.0 | 2.8 | 2.8 | 1.1 | 0.0 | 0.9 | 0.1 | 2.1 | 0.0 | 1.9 | 0.0 | 0.5 | 0.0 | 0.0 | 0.0 | 0.0 | 0.0 | 0.1 | 0.0 | 0.0 | 0.0 | 0.1 | 0.0 | 0.0 | 0.3 |
| 水产类 Aquatic foods | 2.0 | 0.5 | 0.1 | 0.4 | 0.0 | 0.2 | 0.0 | 0.1 | 0.0 | 0.3 | 0.0 | 0.0 | 0.0 | 0.0 | 0.0 | 0.0 | 2.8 | 0.0 | 0.7 | 0.5 | 0.0 | 0.2 | 0.0 | 0.0 | 0.1 |
| 乳类 Dairy products | 0.0 | 0.0 | 0.0 | 0.0 | 0.0 | 0.0 | 0.0 | 0.0 | 0.0 | 0.0 | 0.0 | 0.0 | 0.0 | 0.0 | 0.0 | 0.0 | 0.0 | 0.0 | 0.0 | 0.0 | 0.0 | 0.0 | 0.0 | 0.0 | 0.0 |
| 蔬菜类 Vegetables | 16.3 | 33.8 | 76.2 | 81.3 | 45.2 | 76.5 | 69.0 | 74.9 | 56.3 | 74.7 | 77.7 | 95.4 | 48.5 | 66.8 | 69.4 | 69.5 | 75.4 | 97.9 | 40.3 | 14.4 | 98.3 | 30.3 | 96.5 | 7.8 | 86.6 |
| 水果类 Fruits | 73.1 | 40.2 | 4.8 | 12.8 | 52.6 | 9.5 | 0.3 | 3.2 | 34.1 | 3.0 | 0.5 | 2.5 | 22.6 | 19.4 | 1.7 | 2.2 | 3.0 | 0.4 | 5.1 | 2.2 | 0.0 | 3.7 | 0.4 | 3.7 | 2.4 |
| 糖类 Sugar | 0.0 | 0.0 | 0.0 | 0.0 | 0.0 | 0.0 | 0.1 | 0.0 | 0.0 | 0.0 | 0.0 | 0.0 | 0.3 | 0.0 | 0.0 | 0.0 | 0.0 | 0.0 | 0.0 | 0.0 | 0.0 | 0.0 | 0.0 | 0.0 | 0.0 |
| 水及饮料类 Water and beverages | 0.0 | 0.0 | 0.0 | 0.0 | 0.0 | 0.0 | 0.0 | 0.0 | 0.0 | 0.0 | 18.0 | 0.0 | 10.8 | 0.0 | 0.0 | 4.8 | 0.0 | 0.0 | 9.8 | 25.4 | 0.0 | 9.1 | 2.0 | 0.0 | 1.1 |

续表

| 膳食类别<br>Category | 黑龙江<br>HL | 辽宁<br>LN | 河北<br>HE | 北京<br>BJ | 吉林<br>JL | 山西<br>SX | 陕西<br>SN | 河南<br>HA | 宁夏<br>NX | 内蒙古<br>NM | 青海<br>QH | 甘肃<br>GS | 上海<br>SH | 福建<br>FJ | 江西<br>JX | 江苏<br>JS | 浙江<br>ZJ | 山东<br>SD | 湖北<br>HB | 四川<br>SC | 广西<br>GX | 湖南<br>HN | 广东<br>GD | 贵州<br>GZ | 全国平均<br>AVG |
|---|---|---|---|---|---|---|---|---|---|---|---|---|---|---|---|---|---|---|---|---|---|---|---|---|---|
| 酒类<br>Alcohol beverages | 0.0 | 0.0 | 0.0 | 0.0 | 0.0 | 0.0 | 0.0 | 0.0 | 0.0 | 0.0 | 0.0 | 0.0 | 0.0 | 0.0 | 0.1 | 0.0 | 0.0 | 0.0 | 0.0 | 0.0 | 0.0 | 0.0 | 0.0 | 0.0 | 0.0 |

附表 4-51　第六次中国总膳食研究 N-脱甲基啶虫脒的膳食来源（单位：%）

Annexed Table 4-51　Dietary sources of acetamiprid-N-desmethyl from the 6th China TDS (Unit: %)

| 膳食类别<br>Category | 黑龙江<br>HL | 辽宁<br>LN | 河北<br>HE | 北京<br>BJ | 吉林<br>JL | 山西<br>SX | 陕西<br>SN | 河南<br>HA | 宁夏<br>NX | 内蒙古<br>NM | 青海<br>QH | 甘肃<br>GS | 上海<br>SH | 福建<br>FJ | 江西<br>JX | 江苏<br>JS | 浙江<br>ZJ | 山东<br>SD | 湖北<br>HB | 四川<br>SC | 广西<br>GX | 湖南<br>HN | 广东<br>GD | 贵州<br>GZ | 全国平均<br>AVG |
|---|---|---|---|---|---|---|---|---|---|---|---|---|---|---|---|---|---|---|---|---|---|---|---|---|---|
| 谷类<br>Cereals | 0.0 | 0.0 | 0.0 | 0.0 | 0.0 | 0.0 | 5.9 | 0.0 | 0.0 | 0.0 | 0.0 | 0.0 | 0.2 | 0.0 | 1.7 | 0.0 | 0.1 | 2.5 | 9.2 | 2.6 | 0.9 | 0.2 | 0.1 | 0.6 | 0.7 |
| 豆类<br>Legumes | 0.0 | 0.6 | 1.5 | 0.0 | 0.0 | 0.0 | 3.9 | 1.9 | 0.1 | 0.0 | 0.0 | 3.1 | 0.1 | 0.3 | 1.4 | 0.4 | 0.3 | 0.1 | 0.2 | 7.0 | 0.8 | 1.6 | 0.2 | 0.7 | 0.5 |
| 薯类<br>Potatoes | 0.0 | 0.0 | 0.0 | 0.0 | 0.0 | 0.0 | 0.0 | 0.0 | 0.1 | 0.0 | 0.7 | 0.0 | 0.0 | 0.0 | 0.0 | 0.0 | 0.0 | 0.0 | 0.0 | 1.6 | 0.0 | 0.0 | 0.0 | 0.0 | 0.0 |
| 肉类<br>Meats | 1.1 | 0.6 | 1.1 | 0.0 | 0.0 | 0.0 | 0.0 | 1.3 | 0.6 | 0.0 | 1.4 | 0.6 | 0.1 | 0.0 | 0.0 | 0.2 | 0.3 | 0.2 | 0.3 | 17.4 | 0.8 | 0.6 | 0.0 | 1.1 | 0.4 |
| 蛋类<br>Eggs | 1.0 | 1.2 | 0.0 | 0.0 | 0.0 | 0.0 | 0.1 | 0.0 | 0.0 | 0.0 | 0.0 | 0.5 | 0.0 | 0.0 | 0.0 | 0.0 | 0.1 | 0.1 | 0.0 | 0.3 | 0.0 | 0.0 | 0.0 | 9.2 | 0.2 |
| 水产类<br>Aquatic foods | 0.0 | 0.0 | 0.0 | 0.0 | 0.0 | 0.0 | 0.0 | 0.0 | 0.0 | 0.0 | 0.0 | 0.0 | 0.0 | 0.0 | 0.0 | 0.0 | 0.0 | 0.1 | 0.0 | 0.9 | 0.0 | 0.0 | 0.0 | 0.0 | 0.0 |
| 乳类<br>Dairy products | 0.2 | 0.2 | 2.3 | 1.1 | 0.0 | 4.6 | 0.5 | 2.0 | 0.0 | 0.7 | 0.3 | 1.0 | 0.0 | 0.2 | 0.2 | 0.0 | 0.0 | 0.3 | 0.0 | 1.2 | 2.0 | 0.5 | 4.4 | 76.0 | 1.8 |
| 蔬菜类<br>Vegetables | 27.7 | 82.1 | 86.3 | 63.6 | 30.9 | 87.2 | 82.9 | 88.7 | 94.7 | 38.6 | 62.9 | 81.6 | 98.1 | 86.8 | 82.1 | 94.6 | 92.2 | 69.8 | 87.7 | 40.4 | 93.4 | 87.6 | 92.7 | 4.8 | 88.4 |

续表

| 膳食类别 Category | 黑龙江 HL | 辽宁 LN | 河北 HE | 北京 BJ | 吉林 JL | 山西 SX | 陕西 SN | 河南 HA | 宁夏 NX | 内蒙古 NM | 青海 QH | 甘肃 GS | 上海 SH | 福建 FJ | 江西 JX | 江苏 JS | 浙江 ZJ | 山东 SD | 湖北 HB | 四川 SC | 广西 GX | 湖南 HN | 广东 GD | 贵州 GZ | 全国平均 AVG |
|---|---|---|---|---|---|---|---|---|---|---|---|---|---|---|---|---|---|---|---|---|---|---|---|---|---|
| 水果类 Fruits | 69.9 | 15.9 | 8.8 | 35.3 | 69.1 | 8.2 | 6.7 | 6.1 | 4.5 | 36.4 | 0.5 | 13.2 | 1.0 | 12.8 | 14.6 | 1.7 | 6.9 | 21.9 | 1.0 | 22.5 | 0.6 | 5.1 | 0.3 | 6.3 | 6.2 |
| 糖类 Sugar | 0.0 | 0.0 | 0.0 | 0.0 | 0.0 | 0.0 | 0.0 | 0.0 | 0.0 | 0.0 | 0.0 | 0.0 | 0.0 | 0.0 | 0.0 | 0.0 | 0.0 | 0.0 | 0.0 | 0.0 | 0.0 | 0.0 | 0.0 | 0.0 | 0.0 |
| 水及饮料类 Water and beverages | 0.0 | 0.0 | 0.0 | 0.0 | 0.0 | 0.0 | 0.0 | 0.0 | 0.0 | 24.4 | 34.1 | 0.0 | 0.5 | 0.0 | 0.0 | 3.0 | 0.1 | 4.5 | 1.4 | 6.0 | 1.3 | 4.2 | 2.3 | 1.2 | 1.7 |
| 酒类 Alcohol beverages | 0.0 | 0.0 | 0.0 | 0.0 | 0.0 | 0.0 | 0.0 | 0.0 | 0.0 | 0.0 | 0.0 | 0.0 | 0.0 | 0.0 | 0.0 | 0.0 | 0.0 | 0.3 | 0.0 | 0.0 | 0.0 | 0.0 | 0.0 | 0.0 | 0.0 |

附表 4-52 第六次中国总膳食研究呋虫胺的膳食来源（单位：%）

Annexed Table 4-52　Dietary sources of dinotefuran from the 6$^{th}$ China TDS (Unit: %)

| 膳食类别 Category | 黑龙江 HL | 辽宁 LN | 河北 HE | 北京 BJ | 吉林 JL | 山西 SX | 陕西 SN | 河南 HA | 宁夏 NX | 内蒙古 NM | 青海 QH | 甘肃 GS | 上海 SH | 福建 FJ | 江西 JX | 江苏 JS | 浙江 ZJ | 山东 SD | 湖北 HB | 四川 SC | 广西 GX | 湖南 HN | 广东 GD | 贵州 GZ | 全国平均 AVG |
|---|---|---|---|---|---|---|---|---|---|---|---|---|---|---|---|---|---|---|---|---|---|---|---|---|---|
| 谷类 Cereals | 0.0 | 0.0 | 0.0 | 0.0 | 0.0 | 0.0 | 0.0 | 0.0 | 0.0 | 0.0 | 0.0 | 0.0 | 0.0 | 0.0 | 65.0 | 0.0 | 0.0 | 0.0 | 0.0 | 0.0 | 0.0 | 0.0 | 0.0 | 0.0 | 2.5 |
| 豆类 Legumes | 0.0 | 0.0 | 0.0 | 0.0 | 0.0 | 0.0 | 0.0 | 0.0 | 0.0 | 0.0 | 0.0 | 0.0 | 0.0 | 0.0 | 0.0 | 0.0 | 0.0 | 0.0 | 0.0 | 0.0 | 0.0 | 0.0 | 0.0 | 0.0 | 0.0 |
| 薯类 Potatoes | 0.0 | 0.0 | 0.0 | 0.0 | 0.0 | 0.0 | 0.0 | 0.0 | 0.0 | 0.0 | 0.0 | 0.0 | 0.0 | 0.0 | 0.0 | 0.0 | 0.0 | 0.0 | 0.0 | 0.0 | 0.0 | 0.0 | 0.0 | 100.0 | 0.3 |
| 肉类 Meats | 0.0 | 0.0 | 0.0 | 0.0 | 0.0 | 0.0 | 0.0 | 0.0 | 0.0 | 0.0 | 0.0 | 0.0 | 0.0 | 0.0 | 0.0 | 0.0 | 0.0 | 0.0 | 0.0 | 0.0 | 0.0 | 0.0 | 0.0 | 0.0 | 0.0 |
| 蛋类 Eggs | 0.0 | 0.0 | 0.0 | 0.0 | 0.0 | 0.0 | 0.0 | 0.0 | 0.0 | 0.0 | 0.0 | 0.0 | 0.0 | 0.0 | 0.0 | 0.0 | 0.0 | 0.0 | 0.0 | 0.0 | 0.0 | 0.0 | 0.0 | 0.0 | 0.0 |

续表

| 膳食类别 Category | 黑龙江 HL | 辽宁 LN | 河北 HE | 北京 BJ | 吉林 JL | 山西 SX | 陕西 SN | 河南 HA | 宁夏 NX | 内蒙古 NM | 青海 QH | 甘肃 GS | 上海 SH | 福建 FJ | 江西 JX | 江苏 JS | 浙江 ZJ | 山东 SD | 湖北 HB | 四川 SC | 广西 GX | 湖南 HN | 广东 GD | 贵州 GZ | 全国平均 AVG |
|---|---|---|---|---|---|---|---|---|---|---|---|---|---|---|---|---|---|---|---|---|---|---|---|---|---|
| 水产类 Aquatic foods | 0.0 | 0.0 | 0.0 | 0.0 | 0.0 | 0.0 | 0.0 | 0.0 | 0.0 | 0.0 | 0.0 | 0.0 | 0.0 | 0.0 | 0.0 | 0.0 | 0.0 | 0.0 | 0.0 | 0.0 | 0.0 | 0.0 | 0.0 | 0.0 | 0.0 |
| 乳类 Dairy products | 0.0 | 0.0 | 0.0 | 0.0 | 0.0 | 0.0 | 0.0 | 0.0 | 0.0 | 0.0 | 0.0 | 0.0 | 0.0 | 0.0 | 0.0 | 0.0 | 0.0 | 0.0 | 0.0 | 0.0 | 0.0 | 0.0 | 0.0 | 0.0 | 0.0 |
| 蔬菜类 Vegetables | 0.0 | 0.0 | 100.0 | 0.0 | 0.0 | 100.0 | 100.0 | 100.0 | 100.0 | 0.0 | 93.2 | 0.0 | 0.0 | 0.0 | 35.0 | 0.0 | 0.0 | 100.0 | 0.0 | 0.0 | 100.0 | 100.0 | 10.1 | 0.0 | 79.1 |
| 水果类 Fruits | 100.0 | 0.0 | 0.0 | 0.0 | 0.0 | 0.0 | 0.0 | 0.0 | 0.0 | 0.0 | 0.0 | 0.0 | 0.0 | 0.0 | 0.0 | 0.0 | 0.0 | 0.0 | 0.0 | 2.6 | 0.0 | 0.0 | 0.0 | 0.0 | 0.2 |
| 糖类 Sugar | 0.0 | 0.0 | 0.0 | 0.0 | 0.0 | 0.0 | 0.0 | 0.0 | 0.0 | 0.0 | 0.0 | 0.0 | 0.0 | 0.0 | 0.0 | 0.0 | 0.0 | 0.0 | 0.0 | 0.0 | 0.0 | 0.0 | 0.0 | 0.0 | 0.0 |
| 水及饮料类 Water and beverages | 0.0 | 0.0 | 0.0 | 0.0 | 0.0 | 0.0 | 0.0 | 0.0 | 0.0 | 0.0 | 6.8 | 0.0 | 100.0 | 0.0 | 0.0 | 100.0 | 0.0 | 0.0 | 100.0 | 97.4 | 0.0 | 0.0 | 89.9 | 0.0 | 17.8 |
| 酒类 Alcohol beverages | 0.0 | 0.0 | 0.0 | 0.0 | 0.0 | 0.0 | 0.0 | 0.0 | 0.0 | 0.0 | 0.0 | 0.0 | 0.0 | 0.0 | 0.0 | 0.0 | 0.0 | 0.0 | 0.0 | 0.0 | 0.0 | 0.0 | 0.0 | 0.0 | 0.0 |

附表 4-53　第六次中国总膳食研究烯啶虫胺的膳食来源（单位：%）

Annexed Table 4-53　Dietary sources of nitenpyram from the 6<sup>th</sup> China TDS (Unit: %)

| 膳食类别 Category | 黑龙江 HL | 辽宁 LN | 河北 HE | 北京 BJ | 吉林 JL | 山西 SX | 陕西 SN | 河南 HA | 宁夏 NX | 内蒙古 NM | 青海 QH | 甘肃 GS | 上海 SH | 福建 FJ | 江西 JX | 江苏 JS | 浙江 ZJ | 山东 SD | 湖北 HB | 四川 SC | 广西 GX | 湖南 HN | 广东 GD | 贵州 GZ | 全国平均 AVG |
|---|---|---|---|---|---|---|---|---|---|---|---|---|---|---|---|---|---|---|---|---|---|---|---|---|---|
| 谷类 Cereals | 0.0 | 0.0 | 0.0 | 0.0 | 0.0 | 0.0 | 22.3 | 0.0 | 0.0 | 0.0 | 0.0 | 0.0 | 0.0 | 0.0 | 0.0 | 0.0 | 0.0 | 0.0 | 0.0 | 0.0 | 68.2 | 0.0 | 0.0 | 0.0 | 1.3 |

续表

| 膳食类别<br>Category | 黑龙江<br>HL | 辽宁<br>LN | 河北<br>HE | 北京<br>BJ | 吉林<br>JL | 山西<br>SX | 陕西<br>SN | 河南<br>HA | 宁夏<br>NX | 内蒙古<br>NM | 青海<br>QH | 甘肃<br>GS | 上海<br>SH | 福建<br>FJ | 江西<br>JX | 江苏<br>JS | 浙江<br>ZJ | 山东<br>SD | 湖北<br>HB | 四川<br>SC | 广西<br>GX | 湖南<br>HN | 广东<br>GD | 贵州<br>GZ | 全国平均<br>AVG |
|---|---|---|---|---|---|---|---|---|---|---|---|---|---|---|---|---|---|---|---|---|---|---|---|---|---|
| 豆类 Legumes | 0.0 | 0.0 | 0.0 | 0.0 | 0.0 | 0.0 | 0.0 | 0.0 | 0.0 | 0.0 | 0.0 | 0.0 | 0.0 | 0.0 | 0.0 | 0.0 | 0.0 | 0.0 | 0.0 | 0.0 | 0.0 | 0.0 | 0.0 | 0.0 | 0.0 |
| 薯类 Potatoes | 0.0 | 0.0 | 0.0 | 0.0 | 0.0 | 0.0 | 0.0 | 0.0 | 0.0 | 0.0 | 0.0 | 0.0 | 0.0 | 0.0 | 0.0 | 0.0 | 0.0 | 0.0 | 0.0 | 0.0 | 0.0 | 0.0 | 0.0 | 0.0 | 0.0 |
| 肉类 Meats | 0.0 | 0.0 | 0.0 | 0.0 | 0.0 | 0.0 | 0.0 | 0.0 | 0.0 | 0.0 | 0.0 | 0.0 | 0.0 | 0.0 | 0.0 | 0.0 | 0.0 | 0.0 | 0.0 | 0.0 | 0.0 | 0.0 | 0.0 | 0.0 | 0.0 |
| 蛋类 Eggs | 0.0 | 0.0 | 0.0 | 0.0 | 0.0 | 0.0 | 0.0 | 0.0 | 0.0 | 0.0 | 0.0 | 0.0 | 0.0 | 0.0 | 0.0 | 0.0 | 0.0 | 0.0 | 0.0 | 0.0 | 0.0 | 0.0 | 0.0 | 0.0 | 0.0 |
| 水产类 Aquatic foods | 0.0 | 0.0 | 0.0 | 0.0 | 0.0 | 0.0 | 0.0 | 0.0 | 0.0 | 0.0 | 0.0 | 0.0 | 0.0 | 0.0 | 0.0 | 0.0 | 0.0 | 0.0 | 0.0 | 0.0 | 0.0 | 0.0 | 0.0 | 0.0 | 0.0 |
| 乳类 Dairy products | 0.0 | 0.0 | 0.0 | 0.0 | 0.0 | 0.0 | 0.0 | 0.0 | 0.0 | 0.0 | 0.0 | 0.0 | 0.0 | 0.0 | 0.0 | 0.0 | 0.0 | 0.0 | 0.0 | 0.0 | 0.0 | 0.0 | 0.0 | 0.0 | 0.0 |
| 蔬菜类 Vegetables | 0.0 | 0.0 | 95.0 | 100.0 | 0.0 | 100.0 | 77.7 | 96.5 | 90.1 | 0.0 | 100.0 | 100.0 | 0.0 | 100.0 | 100.0 | 100.0 | 0.0 | 100.0 | 0.0 | 0.0 | 0.0 | 100.0 | 100.0 | 0.0 | 97.2 |
| 水果类 Fruits | 0.0 | 0.0 | 5.0 | 0.0 | 0.0 | 0.0 | 0.0 | 3.5 | 9.9 | 0.0 | 0.0 | 0.0 | 100.0 | 0.0 | 0.0 | 0.0 | 0.0 | 0.0 | 0.0 | 0.0 | 0.0 | 0.0 | 0.0 | 0.0 | 1.3 |
| 糖类 Sugar | 0.0 | 0.0 | 0.0 | 0.0 | 0.0 | 0.0 | 0.0 | 0.0 | 0.0 | 0.0 | 0.0 | 0.0 | 0.0 | 0.0 | 0.0 | 0.0 | 0.0 | 0.0 | 0.0 | 0.0 | 0.0 | 0.0 | 0.0 | 0.0 | 0.0 |
| 水及饮料类 Water and beverages | 0.0 | 0.0 | 0.0 | 0.0 | 0.0 | 0.0 | 0.0 | 0.0 | 0.0 | 0.0 | 0.0 | 0.0 | 0.0 | 0.0 | 0.0 | 0.0 | 0.0 | 0.0 | 0.0 | 0.0 | 0.0 | 0.0 | 0.0 | 0.0 | 0.0 |
| 酒类 Alcohol beverages | 0.0 | 0.0 | 0.0 | 0.0 | 0.0 | 0.0 | 0.0 | 0.0 | 0.0 | 0.0 | 0.0 | 0.0 | 0.0 | 0.0 | 0.0 | 0.0 | 0.0 | 0.0 | 0.0 | 0.0 | 31.8 | 0.0 | 0.0 | 0.0 | 0.2 |

附表 4-54 第六次中国总膳食研究噻虫啉的膳食来源（单位：%）

Annexed Table 4-54 Dietary sources of thiacloprid from the 6$^{th}$ China TDS (Unit: %)

| 膳食类别<br>Category | 黑龙江<br>HL | 辽宁<br>LN | 河北<br>HE | 北京<br>BJ | 吉林<br>JL | 山西<br>SX | 陕西<br>SN | 河南<br>HA | 宁夏<br>NX | 内蒙古<br>NM | 青海<br>QH | 甘肃<br>GS | 上海<br>SH | 福建<br>FJ | 江西<br>JX | 江苏<br>JS | 浙江<br>ZJ | 山东<br>SD | 湖北<br>HB | 四川<br>SC | 广西<br>GX | 湖南<br>HN | 广东<br>GD | 贵州<br>GZ | 全国平均<br>AVG |
|---|---|---|---|---|---|---|---|---|---|---|---|---|---|---|---|---|---|---|---|---|---|---|---|---|---|
| 谷类 Cereals | 0.0 | 0.0 | 0.0 | 0.0 | 0.0 | 0.0 | 0.0 | 0.0 | 0.0 | 0.0 | 0.0 | 0.0 | 0.0 | 0.0 | 0.0 | 0.0 | 0.0 | 0.0 | 0.0 | 0.0 | 0.0 | 0.0 | 0.0 | 0.0 | 0.0 |
| 豆类 Legumes | 0.0 | 0.0 | 0.0 | 0.0 | 0.0 | 0.0 | 0.0 | 0.0 | 0.0 | 0.0 | 0.0 | 0.0 | 0.0 | 0.0 | 0.0 | 0.0 | 0.0 | 0.0 | 0.0 | 0.0 | 0.0 | 0.0 | 0.0 | 0.0 | 0.0 |
| 薯类 Potatoes | 0.0 | 0.0 | 0.0 | 0.0 | 0.0 | 0.0 | 0.0 | 0.0 | 0.0 | 0.0 | 0.0 | 0.0 | 0.0 | 0.0 | 0.0 | 0.0 | 0.0 | 0.0 | 0.0 | 0.0 | 0.0 | 0.0 | 0.0 | 0.0 | 0.0 |
| 肉类 Meats | 0.0 | 0.0 | 0.0 | 0.0 | 0.0 | 0.0 | 0.0 | 0.0 | 0.0 | 0.0 | 0.0 | 0.0 | 0.0 | 0.0 | 0.0 | 0.0 | 0.0 | 0.0 | 0.0 | 0.0 | 0.0 | 0.0 | 0.0 | 0.0 | 0.0 |
| 蛋类 Eggs | 0.0 | 0.0 | 0.0 | 0.0 | 0.0 | 0.0 | 0.0 | 0.0 | 0.0 | 0.0 | 0.0 | 0.0 | 0.0 | 0.0 | 0.0 | 0.0 | 0.0 | 0.0 | 0.0 | 0.0 | 0.0 | 0.0 | 0.0 | 0.0 | 0.0 |
| 水产类 Aquatic foods | 0.0 | 0.0 | 0.0 | 0.0 | 0.0 | 0.0 | 0.0 | 0.0 | 0.0 | 0.0 | 100.0 | 0.0 | 0.0 | 0.0 | 0.0 | 0.0 | 0.0 | 0.0 | 0.0 | 0.0 | 0.0 | 0.0 | 0.0 | 0.0 | 0.1 |
| 乳类 Dairy products | 0.0 | 0.0 | 0.0 | 0.0 | 0.0 | 0.0 | 0.0 | 0.0 | 0.0 | 0.0 | 0.0 | 0.0 | 0.0 | 0.0 | 0.0 | 0.0 | 0.0 | 0.0 | 0.0 | 0.0 | 0.0 | 0.0 | 0.0 | 0.0 | 0.0 |
| 蔬菜类 Vegetables | 0.0 | 0.0 | 0.0 | 0.0 | 0.0 | 100.0 | 100.0 | 0.0 | 0.0 | 0.0 | 0.0 | 0.0 | 0.0 | 0.0 | 0.0 | 0.0 | 0.0 | 100.0 | 0.0 | 0.0 | 0.0 | 0.0 | 0.0 | 0.0 | 83.6 |
| 水果类 Fruits | 0.0 | 0.0 | 0.0 | 0.0 | 0.0 | 0.0 | 0.0 | 0.0 | 0.0 | 0.0 | 0.0 | 0.0 | 0.0 | 0.0 | 0.0 | 0.0 | 0.0 | 0.0 | 0.0 | 0.0 | 0.0 | 0.0 | 0.0 | 0.0 | 0.0 |
| 糖类 Sugar | 0.0 | 0.0 | 0.0 | 0.0 | 0.0 | 0.0 | 0.0 | 0.0 | 0.0 | 0.0 | 0.0 | 0.0 | 0.0 | 0.0 | 0.0 | 0.0 | 0.0 | 0.0 | 0.0 | 0.0 | 0.0 | 0.0 | 0.0 | 0.0 | 0.0 |
| 水及饮料类 Water and beverages | 0.0 | 0.0 | 0.0 | 0.0 | 0.0 | 0.0 | 0.0 | 0.0 | 0.0 | 0.0 | 0.0 | 0.0 | 0.0 | 0.0 | 0.0 | 0.0 | 0.0 | 0.0 | 100.0 | 0.0 | 0.0 | 0.0 | 100.0 | 0.0 | 16.3 |

续表

| 膳食类别<br>Category | 黑龙江<br>HL | 辽宁<br>LN | 河北<br>HE | 北京<br>BJ | 吉林<br>JL | 山西<br>SX | 陕西<br>SN | 河南<br>HA | 宁夏<br>NX | 内蒙古<br>NM | 青海<br>QH | 甘肃<br>GS | 上海<br>SH | 福建<br>FJ | 江西<br>JX | 江苏<br>JS | 浙江<br>ZJ | 山东<br>SD | 湖北<br>HB | 四川<br>SC | 广西<br>GX | 湖南<br>HN | 广东<br>GD | 贵州<br>GZ | 全国平均<br>AVG |
|---|---|---|---|---|---|---|---|---|---|---|---|---|---|---|---|---|---|---|---|---|---|---|---|---|---|
| 酒类<br>Alcohol beverages | 0.0 | 0.0 | 0.0 | 0.0 | 0.0 | 0.0 | 0.0 | 0.0 | 0.0 | 0.0 | 0.0 | 0.0 | 0.0 | 0.0 | 0.0 | 0.0 | 0.0 | 0.0 | 0.0 | 0.0 | 0.0 | 0.0 | 0.0 | 0.0 | 0.0 |

附表 4-55　第六次中国总膳食研究氯噻啉的膳食来源（单位：%）

Annexed Table 4-55　Dietary sources of imidaclothiz from the 6$^{th}$ China TDS (Unit: %)

| 膳食类别<br>Category | 黑龙江<br>HL | 辽宁<br>LN | 河北<br>HE | 北京<br>BJ | 吉林<br>JL | 山西<br>SX | 陕西<br>SN | 河南<br>HA | 宁夏<br>NX | 内蒙古<br>NM | 青海<br>QH | 甘肃<br>GS | 上海<br>SH | 福建<br>FJ | 江西<br>JX | 江苏<br>JS | 浙江<br>ZJ | 山东<br>SD | 湖北<br>HB | 四川<br>SC | 广西<br>GX | 湖南<br>HN | 广东<br>GD | 贵州<br>GZ | 全国平均<br>AVG |
|---|---|---|---|---|---|---|---|---|---|---|---|---|---|---|---|---|---|---|---|---|---|---|---|---|---|
| 谷类<br>Cereals | 0.0 | 0.0 | 0.0 | 0.0 | 0.0 | 0.0 | 0.0 | 0.0 | 0.0 | 0.0 | 0.0 | 0.0 | 0.0 | 0.0 | 0.0 | 0.0 | 0.0 | 0.0 | 0.0 | 0.0 | 0.0 | 0.0 | 0.0 | 0.0 | 0.0 |
| 豆类<br>Legumes | 0.0 | 0.0 | 0.0 | 0.0 | 0.0 | 0.0 | 0.0 | 0.0 | 0.0 | 0.0 | 0.0 | 0.0 | 0.0 | 0.0 | 0.0 | 0.0 | 0.0 | 0.0 | 0.0 | 0.0 | 0.0 | 0.0 | 0.0 | 0.0 | 0.0 |
| 薯类<br>Potatoes | 0.0 | 0.0 | 0.0 | 0.0 | 0.0 | 0.0 | 0.0 | 0.0 | 0.0 | 0.0 | 0.0 | 0.0 | 0.0 | 0.0 | 0.0 | 0.0 | 0.0 | 0.0 | 0.0 | 0.0 | 0.0 | 0.0 | 0.0 | 0.0 | 0.0 |
| 肉类<br>Meats | 0.0 | 0.0 | 0.0 | 0.0 | 0.0 | 0.0 | 0.0 | 0.0 | 0.0 | 0.0 | 0.0 | 0.0 | 0.0 | 0.0 | 0.0 | 0.0 | 0.0 | 0.0 | 0.0 | 0.0 | 0.0 | 0.0 | 0.0 | 0.0 | 0.0 |
| 蛋类<br>Eggs | 0.0 | 0.0 | 0.0 | 0.0 | 0.0 | 0.0 | 0.0 | 0.0 | 0.0 | 0.0 | 0.0 | 0.0 | 0.0 | 0.0 | 0.0 | 0.0 | 0.0 | 0.0 | 0.0 | 0.0 | 0.0 | 0.0 | 0.0 | 0.0 | 0.0 |
| 水产类<br>Aquatic foods | 0.0 | 0.0 | 0.0 | 0.0 | 0.0 | 0.0 | 0.0 | 0.0 | 0.0 | 0.0 | 0.0 | 0.0 | 0.0 | 0.0 | 0.0 | 0.0 | 0.0 | 0.0 | 0.0 | 0.0 | 0.0 | 0.0 | 0.0 | 0.0 | 0.0 |
| 乳类<br>Dairy products | 0.0 | 0.0 | 0.0 | 0.0 | 0.0 | 0.0 | 0.0 | 0.0 | 0.0 | 0.0 | 0.0 | 0.0 | 0.0 | 0.0 | 0.0 | 0.0 | 0.0 | 0.0 | 0.0 | 0.0 | 0.0 | 0.0 | 0.0 | 0.0 | 0.0 |
| 蔬菜类<br>Vegetables | 0.0 | 0.0 | 0.0 | 0.0 | 0.0 | 0.0 | 0.0 | 0.0 | 0.0 | 0.0 | 0.0 | 0.0 | 0.0 | 0.0 | 0.0 | 0.0 | 0.0 | 0.0 | 0.0 | 0.0 | 0.0 | 0.0 | 0.0 | 100.0 | 100.0 |

续表

| 膳食类别 Category | 黑龙江 HL | 辽宁 LN | 河北 HE | 北京 BJ | 吉林 JL | 山西 SX | 陕西 SN | 河南 HA | 宁夏 NX | 内蒙古 NM | 青海 QH | 甘肃 GS | 上海 SH | 福建 FJ | 江西 JX | 江苏 JS | 浙江 ZJ | 山东 SD | 湖北 HB | 四川 SC | 广西 GX | 湖南 HN | 广东 GD | 贵州 GZ | 全国平均 AVG |
|---|---|---|---|---|---|---|---|---|---|---|---|---|---|---|---|---|---|---|---|---|---|---|---|---|---|
| 水果类 Fruits | 0.0 | 0.0 | 0.0 | 0.0 | 0.0 | 0.0 | 0.0 | 0.0 | 0.0 | 0.0 | 0.0 | 0.0 | 0.0 | 0.0 | 0.0 | 0.0 | 0.0 | 0.0 | 0.0 | 0.0 | 0.0 | 0.0 | 0.0 | 0.0 | 0.0 |
| 糖类 Sugar | 0.0 | 0.0 | 0.0 | 0.0 | 0.0 | 0.0 | 0.0 | 0.0 | 0.0 | 0.0 | 0.0 | 0.0 | 0.0 | 0.0 | 0.0 | 0.0 | 0.0 | 0.0 | 0.0 | 0.0 | 0.0 | 0.0 | 0.0 | 0.0 | 0.0 |
| 水及饮料类 Water and beverages | 0.0 | 0.0 | 0.0 | 0.0 | 0.0 | 0.0 | 0.0 | 0.0 | 0.0 | 0.0 | 0.0 | 0.0 | 0.0 | 0.0 | 0.0 | 0.0 | 0.0 | 0.0 | 0.0 | 0.0 | 0.0 | 0.0 | 0.0 | 0.0 | 0.0 |
| 酒类 Alcohol beverages | 0.0 | 0.0 | 0.0 | 0.0 | 0.0 | 0.0 | 0.0 | 0.0 | 0.0 | 0.0 | 0.0 | 0.0 | 0.0 | 0.0 | 0.0 | 0.0 | 0.0 | 0.0 | 0.0 | 0.0 | 0.0 | 0.0 | 0.0 | 0.0 | 0.0 |

附表 4-56　第六次中国总膳食研究总新烟碱的膳食来源（单位：%）

Annexed Table 4-56　Dietary sources of total neonicotinoids from the 6th China TDS (Unit: %)

| 膳食类别 Category | 黑龙江 HL | 辽宁 LN | 河北 HE | 北京 BJ | 吉林 JL | 山西 SX | 陕西 SN | 河南 HA | 宁夏 NX | 内蒙古 NM | 青海 QH | 甘肃 GS | 上海 SH | 福建 FJ | 江西 JX | 江苏 JS | 浙江 ZJ | 山东 SD | 湖北 HB | 四川 SC | 广西 GX | 湖南 HN | 广东 GD | 贵州 GZ | 全国平均 AVG |
|---|---|---|---|---|---|---|---|---|---|---|---|---|---|---|---|---|---|---|---|---|---|---|---|---|---|
| 谷类 Cereals | 3.1 | 0.0 | 8.1 | 0.0 | 0.0 | 5.9 | 3.1 | 8.7 | 0.0 | 11.9 | 0.9 | 0.0 | 1.3 | 6.6 | 6.0 | 6.5 | 1.4 | 0.5 | 5.2 | 13.2 | 0.7 | 17.6 | 0.9 | 7.3 | 2.9 |
| 豆类 Legumes | 0.7 | 6.2 | 2.7 | 1.7 | 0.9 | 0.0 | 1.3 | 2.2 | 0.3 | 0.0 | 0.0 | 0.4 | 0.0 | 0.2 | 0.1 | 0.4 | 0.1 | 0.0 | 0.5 | 6.8 | 0.0 | 0.1 | 0.1 | 0.2 | 0.5 |
| 薯类 Potatoes | 0.0 | 5.8 | 27.2 | 5.0 | 0.1 | 1.5 | 11.0 | 4.4 | 1.1 | 4.0 | 0.4 | 2.0 | 0.1 | 0.8 | 0.0 | 3.2 | 0.1 | 0.1 | 1.5 | 3.1 | 0.0 | 1.2 | 0.8 | 67.9 | 3.2 |
| 肉类 Meats | 1.4 | 4.6 | 3.4 | 6.0 | 0.1 | 0.2 | 0.4 | 4.9 | 0.9 | 1.6 | 0.4 | 0.6 | 0.1 | 0.4 | 0.1 | 0.2 | 0.3 | 0.2 | 0.6 | 14.7 | 0.0 | 0.8 | 0.1 | 0.2 | 0.9 |
| 蛋类 Eggs | 0.2 | 2.8 | 4.6 | 3.6 | 0.0 | 0.9 | 0.4 | 0.0 | 0.0 | 1.3 | 0.0 | 1.2 | 0.0 | 0.0 | 0.0 | 0.0 | 0.0 | 0.2 | 0.2 | 0.0 | 0.0 | 0.1 | 0.0 | 0.2 | 0.5 |

续表

| 膳食类别<br>Category | 黑龙江<br>HL | 辽宁<br>LN | 河北<br>HE | 北京<br>BJ | 吉林<br>JL | 山西<br>SX | 陕西<br>SN | 河南<br>HA | 宁夏<br>NX | 内蒙古<br>NM | 青海<br>QH | 甘肃<br>GS | 上海<br>SH | 福建<br>FJ | 江西<br>JX | 江苏<br>JS | 浙江<br>ZJ | 山东<br>SD | 湖北<br>HB | 四川<br>SC | 广西<br>GX | 湖南<br>HN | 广东<br>GD | 贵州<br>GZ | 全国平均<br>AVG |
|---|---|---|---|---|---|---|---|---|---|---|---|---|---|---|---|---|---|---|---|---|---|---|---|---|---|
| 水产类 Aquatic foods | 0.6 | 0.3 | 0.2 | 1.0 | 0.0 | 0.1 | 0.1 | 0.4 | 0.0 | 0.3 | 0.1 | 0.1 | 0.0 | 0.3 | 0.0 | 0.1 | 0.1 | 0.0 | 0.5 | 0.5 | 0.0 | 0.1 | 0.0 | 0.0 | 0.1 |
| 乳类 Dairy products | 0.1 | 0.0 | 0.0 | 0.0 | 0.0 | 0.0 | 0.1 | 0.0 | 0.1 | 0.0 | 0.0 | 0.0 | 0.0 | 0.1 | 0.0 | 0.0 | 0.0 | 0.0 | 0.0 | 0.0 | 0.0 | 0.0 | 0.1 | 1.8 | 0.0 |
| 蔬菜类 Vegetables | 56.3 | 57.6 | 50.2 | 76.4 | 72.0 | 89.9 | 80.6 | 76.2 | 84.2 | 60.0 | 78.6 | 93.5 | 92.3 | 73.5 | 92.6 | 70.5 | 81.6 | 98.2 | 84.0 | 31.3 | 98.9 | 69.0 | 78.8 | 17.2 | 85.2 |
| 水果类 Fruits | 37.7 | 22.3 | 3.5 | 6.2 | 26.1 | 1.4 | 2.1 | 1.7 | 13.4 | 10.2 | 0.4 | 2.3 | 2.7 | 15.9 | 1.1 | 1.3 | 15.0 | 0.7 | 0.9 | 2.2 | 0.1 | 2.3 | 0.7 | 5.2 | 3.4 |
| 糖类 Sugar | 0.0 | 0.0 | 0.0 | 0.0 | 0.0 | 0.0 | 0.0 | 0.0 | 0.0 | 0.0 | 0.0 | 0.0 | 0.0 | 0.0 | 0.0 | 0.0 | 0.0 | 0.0 | 0.0 | 0.0 | 0.0 | 0.0 | 0.0 | 0.0 | 0.0 |
| 水及饮料类 Water and beverages | 0.0 | 0.5 | 0.0 | 0.0 | 0.9 | 0.0 | 1.0 | 1.5 | 0.0 | 10.7 | 19.1 | 0.0 | 3.3 | 2.3 | 0.0 | 17.7 | 1.3 | 0.0 | 6.7 | 28.1 | 0.3 | 8.8 | 18.4 | 0.0 | 3.2 |
| 酒类 Alcohol beverages | 0.0 | 0.0 | 0.0 | 0.0 | 0.0 | 0.0 | 0.0 | 0.0 | 0.0 | 0.0 | 0.0 | 0.0 | 0.0 | 0.0 | 0.0 | 0.0 | 0.0 | 0.0 | 0.0 | 0.0 | 0.0 | 0.0 | 0.0 | 0.0 | 0.0 |

附表 4-57　第六次中国总膳食研究膳食样品中氟虫腈的含量（单位：μg/kg）

Annexed Table 4-57　Levels of fipronil in food samples from the 6$^{th}$ China TDS (Unit: μg/kg)

| 膳食类别<br>Category | 黑龙江<br>HL | 辽宁<br>LN | 河北<br>HE | 北京<br>BJ | 吉林<br>JL | 山西<br>SX | 陕西<br>SN | 河南<br>HA | 宁夏<br>NX | 内蒙古<br>NM | 青海<br>QH | 甘肃<br>GS | 上海<br>SH | 福建<br>FJ | 江西<br>JX | 江苏<br>JS | 浙江<br>ZJ | 山东<br>SD | 湖北<br>HB | 四川<br>SC | 广西<br>GX | 湖南<br>HN | 广东<br>GD | 贵州<br>GZ | 全国平均<br>AVG |
|---|---|---|---|---|---|---|---|---|---|---|---|---|---|---|---|---|---|---|---|---|---|---|---|---|---|
| 谷类 Cereals | 0.12 | 0.02 | 0.01 | 0.77 | 0.01 | 0.09 | 0.09 | ND | 0.09 | 0.03 | 0.01 | 0.03 | ND | 0.01 | 0.22 | ND | 0.03 | ND | ND | ND | 0.06 | 0.04 | 0.01 | 0.04 | 0.07 |
| 豆类 Legumes | 0.02 | 0.01 | 0.03 | 0.02 | 0.02 | 0.02 | 0.07 | ND | ND | ND | 0.01 | 0.05 | ND | 0.08 | 0.08 | 0.02 | 0.02 | 0.01 | 0.04 | 0.03 | 0.02 | 0.05 | 0.04 | 0.02 | 0.03 |

续表

| 膳食类别<br>Category | 黑龙江<br>HL | 辽宁<br>LN | 河北<br>HE | 北京<br>BJ | 吉林<br>JL | 山西<br>SX | 陕西<br>SN | 河南<br>HA | 宁夏<br>NX | 内蒙古<br>NM | 青海<br>QH | 甘肃<br>GS | 上海<br>SH | 福建<br>FJ | 江西<br>JX | 江苏<br>JS | 浙江<br>ZJ | 山东<br>SD | 湖北<br>HB | 四川<br>SC | 广西<br>GX | 湖南<br>HN | 广东<br>GD | 贵州<br>GZ | 全国平均<br>AVG |
|---|---|---|---|---|---|---|---|---|---|---|---|---|---|---|---|---|---|---|---|---|---|---|---|---|---|
| 薯类 Potatoes | 0.01 | 0.02 | 0.02 | 0.02 | 0.04 | 0.02 | 0.02 | 0.25 | 0.01 | 0.18 | 0.01 | ND | 0.01 | 0.03 | 0.02 | ND | 0.16 | 0.01 | 0.03 | 0.03 | 0.01 | 0.02 | 0.14 | 0.08 | 0.05 |
| 肉类 Meats | 0.02 | 0.14 | 0.11 | 0.14 | 0.05 | 0.07 | 0.19 | 0.25 | 0.05 | 0.08 | 0.10 | 0.06 | 0.04 | 0.02 | 0.40 | 0.10 | 0.12 | 0.16 | 0.15 | 0.17 | 0.28 | 0.94 | 9.73 | 0.10 | 0.56 |
| 蛋类 Eggs | 0.06 | 42.84 | 0.17 | 18.16 | 0.75 | 0.10 | 0.13 | 0.25 | 0.06 | 52.94 | 0.08 | 383.4 | 0.04 | 0.21 | 0.09 | 1.74 | 0.88 | 5.94 | 0.22 | 0.08 | 0.08 | 0.06 | 3.90 | 0.16 | 21.35 |
| 水产类 Aquatic foods | 0.18 | 0.09 | 0.42 | 0.13 | 0.10 | 0.17 | 0.17 | 0.13 | 0.01 | 0.04 | 0.26 | 0.10 | 0.31 | 0.03 | 4.23 | 0.44 | 0.72 | 0.08 | 0.21 | 0.11 | 0.10 | 1.09 | 0.22 | 0.11 | 0.39 |
| 乳类 Dairy products | 0.01 | 0.01 | 0.03 | 0.04 | 0.01 | 0.07 | 0.03 | 0.07 | 0.02 | 0.01 | 0.02 | 0.01 | 0.08 | 0.05 | 2.77 | 0.17 | 0.03 | 0.05 | 0.03 | ND | 0.07 | 0.02 | 0.07 | 0.02 | 0.15 |
| 蔬菜类 Vegetables | 0.02 | 0.37 | 1.20 | 0.47 | 0.07 | 0.14 | 0.19 | 0.05 | 0.01 | 0.10 | 0.01 | 0.02 | 0.96 | 1.02 | 0.14 | 0.04 | 0.90 | 0.03 | 1.60 | 0.01 | 11.33 | 0.54 | 0.60 | 0.05 | 0.83 |
| 水果类 Fruits | ND | 0.01 | 0.02 | 0.01 | ND | 0.01 | ND | 0.01 | ND | ND | 0.01 | ND | ND | 0.01 | 0.01 | 0.03 | 0.07 | 0.03 | 0.02 | ND | ND | 0.01 | 0.03 | 0.03 | 0.01 |
| 糖类 Sugar | ND | 0.01 | ND | 0.01 | ND | ND | ND | ND | ND | ND | ND | ND | ND | ND | ND | ND | ND | ND | ND | ND | ND | ND | ND | ND | 0.00 |
| 水及饮料类 Water and beverages | ND | ND | ND | ND | ND | ND | ND | ND | ND | ND | ND | ND | ND | ND | 0.02 | ND | 0.02 | ND | ND | 0.01 | ND | ND | ND | ND | 0.00 |
| 酒类 Alcohol beverages | ND | ND | ND | ND | ND | ND | ND | ND | ND | ND | ND | ND | ND | ND | ND | ND | ND | ND | ND | ND | ND | ND | ND | ND | 0.00 |

注：未检出（ND）按 0 计

Note: values not detected (ND) were treated as being equal to 0

附表 4-58　第六次中国总膳食研究的氟虫腈膳食摄入量 [单位: ng/(kg bw · d)]
Annexed Table 4-58　Dietary intakes of fipronil from the 6th China TDS [Unit: ng/(kg bw · d)]

| 膳食类别 Category | 黑龙江 HL | 辽宁 LN | 河北 HE | 北京 BJ | 吉林 JL | 山西 SX | 陕西 SN | 河南 HA | 宁夏 NX | 内蒙古 NM | 青海 QH | 甘肃 GS | 上海 SH | 福建 FJ | 江西 JX | 江苏 JS | 浙江 ZJ | 山东 SD | 湖北 HB | 四川 SC | 广西 GX | 湖南 HN | 广东 GD | 贵州 GZ | 全国平均 AVG |
|---|---|---|---|---|---|---|---|---|---|---|---|---|---|---|---|---|---|---|---|---|---|---|---|---|---|
| 谷类 Cereals | 1.033 | 0.228 | 0.065 | 9.736 | 0.049 | 1.424 | 1.073 | 0.000 | 0.936 | 0.304 | 0.121 | 0.292 | 0.000 | 0.086 | 2.179 | 0.031 | 0.334 | 0.060 | 0.000 | 0.072 | 0.936 | 0.324 | 0.092 | 0.394 | 0.824 |
| 豆类 Legumes | 0.013 | 0.017 | 0.027 | 0.037 | 0.023 | 0.023 | 0.092 | 0.000 | 0.002 | 0.000 | 0.001 | 0.033 | 0.000 | 0.106 | 0.091 | 0.031 | 0.045 | 0.011 | 0.047 | 0.028 | 0.014 | 0.057 | 0.017 | 0.032 | 0.031 |
| 薯类 Potatoes | 0.012 | 0.022 | 0.017 | 0.018 | 0.068 | 0.042 | 0.028 | 0.313 | 0.012 | 0.349 | 0.022 | 0.011 | 0.008 | 0.022 | 0.009 | 0.002 | 0.092 | 0.010 | 0.039 | 0.031 | 0.003 | 0.015 | 0.057 | 0.044 | 0.052 |
| 肉类 Meats | 0.017 | 0.151 | 0.080 | 0.149 | 0.052 | 0.155 | 0.111 | 0.224 | 0.034 | 0.099 | 0.114 | 0.030 | 0.071 | 0.023 | 0.601 | 0.139 | 0.217 | 0.240 | 0.130 | 0.358 | 0.675 | 2.232 | 16.080 | 0.163 | 0.923 |
| 蛋类 Eggs | 0.036 | 27.810 | 0.087 | 11.200 | 0.480 | 0.035 | 0.045 | 0.117 | 0.013 | 24.960 | 0.016 | 135.200 | 0.025 | 0.062 | 0.030 | 0.779 | 0.334 | 4.185 | 0.087 | 0.019 | 0.018 | 0.023 | 1.480 | 0.042 | 8.626 |
| 水产类 Aquatic foods | 0.077 | 0.022 | 0.064 | 0.033 | 0.017 | 0.018 | 0.011 | 0.010 | 0.000 | 0.007 | 0.015 | 0.004 | 0.342 | 0.026 | 2.935 | 0.270 | 0.574 | 0.028 | 0.133 | 0.014 | 0.159 | 1.151 | 0.182 | 0.006 | 0.254 |
| 乳类 Dairy products | 0.001 | 0.007 | 0.010 | 0.060 | 0.007 | 0.046 | 0.010 | 0.020 | 0.004 | 0.004 | 0.013 | 0.003 | 0.091 | 0.028 | 0.960 | 0.075 | 0.014 | 0.017 | 0.003 | 0.001 | 0.021 | 0.006 | 0.039 | 0.009 | 0.060 |
| 蔬菜类 Vegetables | 0.078 | 1.917 | 5.590 | 2.938 | 0.452 | 0.666 | 0.864 | 0.200 | 0.025 | 0.424 | 0.053 | 0.096 | 6.082 | 6.443 | 0.998 | 0.259 | 6.358 | 0.168 | 10.501 | 0.030 | 63.54 | 4.596 | 2.244 | 0.320 | 4.785 |
| 水果类 Fruits | 0.000 | 0.009 | 0.012 | 0.020 | 0.005 | 0.003 | 0.000 | 0.006 | 0.000 | 0.000 | 0.003 | 0.000 | 0.000 | 0.006 | 0.007 | 0.012 | 0.072 | 0.024 | 0.007 | 0.000 | 0.002 | 0.013 | 0.013 | 0.009 | 0.009 |
| 糖类 Sugar | 0.000 | 0.000 | 0.000 | 0.000 | 0.000 | 0.000 | 0.000 | 0.000 | 0.000 | 0.000 | 0.000 | 0.000 | 0.000 | 0.000 | 0.000 | 0.000 | 0.000 | 0.000 | 0.000 | 0.000 | 0.000 | 0.000 | 0.000 | 0.000 | 0.000 |
| 水及饮料类 Water and beverages | 0.000 | 0.000 | 0.000 | 0.000 | 0.034 | 0.000 | 0.000 | 0.025 | 0.000 | 0.149 | 0.000 | 0.050 | 0.000 | 0.000 | 0.290 | 0.000 | 0.187 | 0.000 | 0.000 | 0.048 | 0.000 | 0.000 | 0.089 | 0.000 | 0.036 |

续表

| 膳食类别<br>Category | 黑龙江<br>HL | 辽宁<br>LN | 河北<br>HE | 北京<br>BJ | 吉林<br>JL | 山西<br>SX | 陕西<br>SN | 河南<br>HA | 宁夏<br>NX | 内蒙古<br>NM | 青海<br>QH | 甘肃<br>GS | 上海<br>SH | 福建<br>FJ | 江西<br>JX | 江苏<br>JS | 浙江<br>ZJ | 山东<br>SD | 湖北<br>HB | 四川<br>SC | 广西<br>GX | 湖南<br>HN | 广东<br>GD | 贵州<br>GZ | 全国平均<br>AVG |
|---|---|---|---|---|---|---|---|---|---|---|---|---|---|---|---|---|---|---|---|---|---|---|---|---|---|
| 酒类<br>Alcohol beverages | 0.000 | 0.001 | 0.000 | 0.000 | 0.000 | 0.000 | 0.000 | 0.000 | 0.000 | 0.000 | 0.000 | 0.000 | 0.000 | 0.000 | 0.000 | 0.000 | 0.000 | 0.000 | 0.000 | 0.000 | 0.000 | 0.000 | 0.000 | 0.000 | 0.000 |
| 合计<br>SUM | 1.266 | 30.184 | 5.953 | 24.190 | 1.186 | 2.411 | 2.235 | 0.914 | 1.026 | 26.291 | 0.358 | 135.670 | 6.620 | 6.802 | 8.100 | 1.599 | 8.226 | 4.743 | 10.948 | 0.601 | 65.370 | 8.416 | 20.292 | 1.018 | 15.601 |

附表 4-59 第六次中国总膳食研究氟虫腈的膳食来源（单位：%）

Annexed Table 4-59 Dietary sources of fipronil from the 6th China TDS (Unit: %)

| 膳食类别<br>Category | 黑龙江<br>HL | 辽宁<br>LN | 河北<br>HE | 北京<br>BJ | 吉林<br>JL | 山西<br>SX | 陕西<br>SN | 河南<br>HA | 宁夏<br>NX | 内蒙古<br>NM | 青海<br>QH | 甘肃<br>GS | 上海<br>SH | 福建<br>FJ | 江西<br>JX | 江苏<br>JS | 浙江<br>ZJ | 山东<br>SD | 湖北<br>HB | 四川<br>SC | 广西<br>GX | 湖南<br>HN | 广东<br>GD | 贵州<br>GZ | 全国平均<br>AVG |
|---|---|---|---|---|---|---|---|---|---|---|---|---|---|---|---|---|---|---|---|---|---|---|---|---|---|
| 谷类<br>Cereals | 81.6 | 0.8 | 1.1 | 40.2 | 4.1 | 59.0 | 48.0 | 0.0 | 91.2 | 1.2 | 33.8 | 0.2 | 0.0 | 1.3 | 26.9 | 1.9 | 4.1 | 1.3 | 0.0 | 11.9 | 1.4 | 3.8 | 0.5 | 38.7 | 5.3 |
| 豆类<br>Legumes | 1.0 | 0.1 | 0.5 | 0.2 | 2.0 | 1.0 | 4.1 | 0.0 | 0.2 | 0.0 | 0.2 | 0.0 | 0.0 | 1.6 | 1.1 | 1.9 | 0.5 | 0.2 | 0.4 | 4.7 | 0.0 | 0.7 | 0.1 | 3.1 | 0.2 |
| 薯类<br>Potatoes | 0.9 | 0.1 | 0.3 | 0.1 | 5.7 | 1.7 | 1.2 | 34.2 | 1.2 | 1.3 | 6.1 | 0.0 | 0.1 | 0.3 | 0.1 | 0.1 | 1.1 | 0.2 | 0.4 | 5.2 | 0.0 | 0.2 | 0.3 | 4.3 | 0.3 |
| 肉类<br>Meats | 1.4 | 0.5 | 1.4 | 0.6 | 4.4 | 6.4 | 5.0 | 24.5 | 3.3 | 0.4 | 31.8 | 0.0 | 1.1 | 0.3 | 7.4 | 8.7 | 2.6 | 5.1 | 1.2 | 59.5 | 1.0 | 26.5 | 79.2 | 16.0 | 5.9 |
| 蛋类<br>Eggs | 2.9 | 92.1 | 1.5 | 46.3 | 40.4 | 1.4 | 2.0 | 12.8 | 1.2 | 94.9 | 4.6 | 99.6 | 0.4 | 0.9 | 0.4 | 48.7 | 4.1 | 88.2 | 0.8 | 3.2 | 0.0 | 0.3 | 7.3 | 4.1 | 55.3 |
| 水产类<br>Aquatic foods | 6.0 | 0.1 | 1.1 | 0.1 | 1.5 | 0.7 | 0.5 | 1.1 | 0.0 | 0.0 | 4.2 | 0.0 | 5.2 | 0.4 | 36.2 | 16.9 | 7.0 | 0.6 | 1.2 | 2.3 | 0.2 | 13.7 | 0.9 | 0.6 | 1.6 |
| 乳类<br>Dairy products | 0.1 | 0.0 | 0.2 | 0.2 | 0.6 | 1.9 | 0.5 | 2.2 | 0.4 | 0.0 | 3.6 | 0.0 | 1.4 | 0.4 | 11.9 | 4.7 | 0.2 | 0.4 | 0.0 | 0.1 | 0.0 | 0.1 | 0.2 | 0.9 | 0.4 |

续表

| 膳食类别 Category | 黑龙江 HL | 辽宁 LN | 河北 HE | 北京 BJ | 吉林 JL | 山西 SX | 陕西 SN | 河南 HA | 宁夏 NX | 内蒙古 NM | 青海 QH | 甘肃 GS | 上海 SH | 福建 FJ | 江西 JX | 江苏 JS | 浙江 ZJ | 山东 SD | 湖北 HB | 四川 SC | 广西 GX | 湖南 HN | 广东 GD | 贵州 GZ | 全国平均 AVG |
|---|---|---|---|---|---|---|---|---|---|---|---|---|---|---|---|---|---|---|---|---|---|---|---|---|---|
| 蔬菜类 Vegetables | 6.1 | 6.4 | 93.9 | 12.1 | 38.1 | 27.6 | 38.7 | 21.9 | 2.4 | 1.6 | 14.8 | 0.1 | 91.9 | 94.7 | 12.3 | 16.2 | 77.3 | 3.5 | 95.9 | 4.9 | 97.2 | 54.6 | 11.1 | 31.5 | 30.7 |
| 水果类 Fruits | 0.0 | 0.0 | 0.2 | 0.1 | 0.4 | 0.1 | 0.0 | 0.6 | 0.0 | 0.0 | 0.9 | 0.0 | 0.0 | 0.1 | 0.1 | 0.7 | 0.9 | 0.5 | 0.1 | 0.0 | 0.0 | 0.1 | 0.1 | 0.9 | 0.1 |
| 糖类 Sugar | 0.0 | 0.0 | 0.0 | 0.0 | 0.0 | 0.0 | 0.0 | 0.0 | 0.0 | 0.0 | 0.0 | 0.0 | 0.0 | 0.0 | 0.0 | 0.0 | 0.0 | 0.0 | 0.0 | 0.0 | 0.0 | 0.0 | 0.0 | 0.0 | 0.0 |
| 水及饮料类 Water and beverages | 0.0 | 0.0 | 0.0 | 0.0 | 2.9 | 0.0 | 0.0 | 2.8 | 0.0 | 0.6 | 0.0 | 0.0 | 0.0 | 0.0 | 3.6 | 0.0 | 2.3 | 0.0 | 0.0 | 8.1 | 0.0 | 0.0 | 0.4 | 0.0 | 0.2 |
| 酒类 Alcohol beverages | 0.0 | 0.0 | 0.0 | 0.0 | 0.0 | 0.0 | 0.0 | 0.0 | 0.0 | 0.0 | 0.0 | 0.0 | 0.0 | 0.0 | 0.0 | 0.0 | 0.0 | 0.0 | 0.0 | 0.0 | 0.0 | 0.0 | 0.0 | 0.0 | 0.0 |

附表 4-60　第六次中国总膳食研究膳食样品中克百威的含量（单位：μg/kg）

Annexed Table 4-60　Levels of carbofuran in food samples from the 6$^{th}$ China TDS (Unit: μg/kg)

| 膳食类别 Category | 黑龙江 HL | 辽宁 LN | 河北 HE | 北京 BJ | 吉林 JL | 山西 SX | 陕西 SN | 河南 HA | 宁夏 NX | 内蒙古 NM | 青海 QH | 甘肃 GS | 上海 SH | 福建 FJ | 江西 JX | 江苏 JS | 浙江 ZJ | 山东 SD | 湖北 HB | 四川 SC | 广西 GX | 湖南 HN | 广东 GD | 贵州 GZ | 全国平均 AVG |
|---|---|---|---|---|---|---|---|---|---|---|---|---|---|---|---|---|---|---|---|---|---|---|---|---|---|
| 谷类 Cereals | ND | ND | ND | ND | ND | ND | ND | ND | ND | ND | ND | ND | ND | ND | ND | ND | ND | ND | ND | ND | ND | ND | ND | ND | 0.00 |
| 豆类 Legumes | ND | ND | ND | ND | ND | ND | ND | ND | ND | ND | ND | ND | ND | ND | ND | ND | ND | ND | ND | 0.70 | ND | ND | ND | ND | 0.03 |
| 薯类 Potatoes | ND | ND | ND | ND | ND | ND | 0.15 | ND | ND | ND | ND | ND | ND | ND | ND | ND | ND | ND | ND | ND | ND | ND | ND | ND | 0.01 |
| 肉类 Meats | ND | ND | ND | ND | ND | ND | ND | ND | ND | ND | ND | ND | ND | ND | ND | ND | ND | ND | ND | 0.37 | ND | ND | ND | ND | 0.02 |
| 蛋类 Eggs | ND | ND | ND | ND | ND | ND | ND | ND | ND | ND | ND | ND | ND | ND | ND | ND | ND | ND | ND | ND | ND | ND | ND | ND | 0.00 |

续表

| 膳食类别<br>Category | 黑龙江<br>HL | 辽宁<br>LN | 河北<br>HE | 北京<br>BJ | 吉林<br>JL | 山西<br>SX | 陕西<br>SN | 河南<br>HA | 宁夏<br>NX | 内蒙古<br>NM | 青海<br>QH | 甘肃<br>GS | 上海<br>SH | 福建<br>FJ | 江西<br>JX | 江苏<br>JS | 浙江<br>ZJ | 山东<br>SD | 湖北<br>HB | 四川<br>SC | 广西<br>GX | 湖南<br>HN | 广东<br>GD | 贵州<br>GZ | 全国平均<br>AVG |
|---|---|---|---|---|---|---|---|---|---|---|---|---|---|---|---|---|---|---|---|---|---|---|---|---|---|
| 水产类 Aquatic foods | ND | ND | ND | ND | ND | ND | 1.06 | ND | ND | ND | ND | ND | ND | ND | ND | ND | ND | ND | ND | 0.67 | ND | ND | ND | ND | 0.07 |
| 乳类 Dairy products | ND | ND | ND | ND | ND | ND | ND | ND | ND | ND | ND | ND | ND | ND | ND | ND | ND | ND | ND | ND | ND | ND | ND | ND | 0.00 |
| 蔬菜类 Vegetables | ND | ND | 0.17 | ND | ND | ND | 0.86 | ND | ND | ND | ND | 3.40 | 1.02 | 2.00 | 1.31 | 0.59 | ND | ND | 0.41 | 0.30 | 0.36 | ND | 4.20 | ND | 0.61 |
| 水果类 Fruits | ND | ND | ND | ND | ND | ND | ND | ND | ND | ND | ND | ND | ND | 0.40 | ND | ND | ND | ND | ND | ND | ND | ND | ND | ND | 0.02 |
| 糖类 Sugar | ND | ND | ND | ND | ND | ND | ND | ND | ND | ND | ND | ND | ND | ND | ND | ND | ND | ND | ND | ND | ND | ND | ND | ND | 0.00 |
| 水及饮料类 Water and beverages | ND | ND | ND | ND | ND | ND | ND | ND | ND | ND | ND | ND | ND | ND | ND | ND | ND | ND | ND | ND | ND | ND | ND | ND | 0.00 |
| 酒类 Alcohol beverages | ND | ND | ND | ND | ND | ND | ND | ND | ND | ND | ND | ND | ND | ND | ND | ND | ND | ND | ND | ND | ND | ND | ND | ND | 0.00 |

注：未检出（ND）按 0 计
Note: values not detected (ND) were treated as being equal to 0

附表 4-61　第六次中国总膳食研究膳食样品中茚虫威的含量（单位：μg/kg）
Annexed Table 4-61　Levels of indoxacarb in food samples from the 6$^{th}$ China TDS (Unit: μg/kg)

| 膳食类别<br>Category | 黑龙江<br>HL | 辽宁<br>LN | 河北<br>HE | 北京<br>BJ | 吉林<br>JL | 山西<br>SX | 陕西<br>SN | 河南<br>HA | 宁夏<br>NX | 内蒙古<br>NM | 青海<br>QH | 甘肃<br>GS | 上海<br>SH | 福建<br>FJ | 江西<br>JX | 江苏<br>JS | 浙江<br>ZJ | 山东<br>SD | 湖北<br>HB | 四川<br>SC | 广西<br>GX | 湖南<br>HN | 广东<br>GD | 贵州<br>GZ | 全国平均<br>AVG |
|---|---|---|---|---|---|---|---|---|---|---|---|---|---|---|---|---|---|---|---|---|---|---|---|---|---|
| 谷类 Cereals | ND | ND | ND | ND | ND | ND | ND | ND | ND | ND | ND | ND | ND | ND | ND | ND | ND | ND | ND | ND | ND | ND | ND | ND | 0.00 |

续表

| 膳食类别 Category | 黑龙江 HL | 辽宁 LN | 河北 HE | 北京 BJ | 吉林 JL | 山西 SX | 陕西 SN | 河南 HA | 宁夏 NX | 内蒙古 NM | 青海 QH | 甘肃 GS | 上海 SH | 福建 FJ | 江西 JX | 江苏 JS | 浙江 ZJ | 山东 SD | 湖北 HB | 四川 SC | 广西 GX | 湖南 HN | 广东 GD | 贵州 GZ | 全国平均 AVG |
|---|---|---|---|---|---|---|---|---|---|---|---|---|---|---|---|---|---|---|---|---|---|---|---|---|---|
| 豆类 Legumes | ND | ND | ND | ND | ND | ND | ND | ND | ND | ND | ND | ND | ND | ND | ND | ND | ND | ND | ND | ND | ND | ND | ND | ND | 0.00 |
| 薯类 Potatoes | ND | ND | ND | ND | ND | ND | ND | ND | ND | ND | ND | ND | ND | ND | ND | ND | ND | ND | ND | ND | ND | ND | ND | ND | 0.00 |
| 肉类 Meats | ND | ND | ND | ND | ND | ND | ND | ND | ND | ND | ND | ND | ND | ND | ND | ND | ND | ND | ND | ND | ND | ND | ND | ND | 0.00 |
| 蛋类 Eggs | ND | ND | ND | ND | ND | ND | ND | ND | ND | ND | ND | ND | ND | ND | ND | ND | ND | ND | ND | ND | ND | ND | ND | ND | 0.00 |
| 水产类 Aquatic foods | ND | ND | ND | ND | ND | ND | ND | ND | ND | ND | ND | ND | ND | ND | ND | ND | ND | ND | ND | ND | ND | ND | ND | ND | 0.00 |
| 乳类 Dairy products | ND | ND | ND | ND | ND | ND | ND | ND | ND | ND | ND | ND | ND | ND | 0.27 | ND | ND | ND | ND | ND | ND | ND | ND | ND | 0.01 |
| 蔬菜类 Vegetables | ND | ND | ND | ND | ND | 0.12 | ND | 3.92 | ND | ND | 0.24 | ND | 11.91 | 24.26 | 6.63 | ND | 14.90 | 0.22 | 6.66 | ND | ND | 2.65 | ND | ND | 2.98 |
| 水果类 Fruits | ND | ND | ND | ND | ND | ND | ND | ND | ND | ND | ND | ND | 0.50 | ND | ND | ND | ND | ND | ND | ND | ND | ND | ND | ND | 0.02 |
| 糖类 Sugar | ND | ND | ND | ND | ND | ND | ND | ND | ND | ND | ND | ND | ND | ND | ND | ND | ND | ND | ND | ND | ND | ND | ND | ND | 0.00 |
| 水及饮料类 Water and beverages | ND | ND | ND | ND | ND | ND | ND | ND | ND | ND | ND | ND | ND | ND | ND | ND | ND | ND | ND | ND | ND | ND | ND | ND | 0.00 |
| 酒类 Alcohol beverages | ND | ND | ND | ND | ND | ND | ND | ND | ND | ND | ND | ND | ND | ND | ND | ND | ND | ND | ND | ND | ND | ND | ND | ND | 0.00 |

注：未检出（ND）按0计

Note: values not detected (ND) were treated as being equal to 0

附表 4-62 第六次中国总膳食研究的克百威膳食摄入量 [单位：ng/(kg bw·d)]

Annexed Table 4-62 Dietary intakes of carbofuran from the 6th China TDS [Unit: ng/(kg bw·d)]

| 膳食类别<br>Category | 黑龙江<br>HL | 辽宁<br>LN | 河北<br>HE | 北京<br>BJ | 吉林<br>JL | 山西<br>SX | 陕西<br>SN | 河南<br>HA | 宁夏<br>NX | 内蒙古<br>NM | 青海<br>QH | 甘肃<br>GS | 上海<br>SH | 福建<br>FJ | 江西<br>JX | 江苏<br>JS | 浙江<br>ZJ | 山东<br>SD | 湖北<br>HB | 四川<br>SC | 广西<br>GX | 湖南<br>HN | 广东<br>GD | 贵州<br>GZ | 全国平均<br>AVG |
|---|---|---|---|---|---|---|---|---|---|---|---|---|---|---|---|---|---|---|---|---|---|---|---|---|---|
| 谷类 Cereals | 0.000 | 0.000 | 0.000 | 0.000 | 0.000 | 0.000 | 0.000 | 0.000 | 0.000 | 0.000 | 0.000 | 0.000 | 0.000 | 0.000 | 0.000 | 0.000 | 0.000 | 0.000 | 0.000 | 0.000 | 0.000 | 0.000 | 0.000 | 0.000 | 0.000 |
| 豆类 Legumes | 0.000 | 0.000 | 0.811 | 0.000 | 0.000 | 0.000 | 0.000 | 0.000 | 0.000 | 0.000 | 0.000 | 0.000 | 0.000 | 12.610 | 9.368 | 3.974 | 0.000 | 0.000 | 0.000 | 0.752 | 0.000 | 0.000 | 0.000 | 0.000 | 0.031 |
| 薯类 Potatoes | 0.000 | 0.000 | 0.000 | 0.000 | 0.000 | 0.000 | 0.270 | 0.000 | 0.000 | 0.000 | 0.000 | 0.000 | 0.000 | 0.000 | 0.000 | 0.000 | 0.000 | 0.000 | 0.000 | 0.000 | 0.000 | 0.000 | 0.000 | 0.000 | 0.011 |
| 肉类 Meats | 0.000 | 0.000 | 0.000 | 0.000 | 0.000 | 0.000 | 0.000 | 0.000 | 0.000 | 0.000 | 0.000 | 0.000 | 0.000 | 0.000 | 0.000 | 0.000 | 0.000 | 0.000 | 0.000 | 0.756 | 0.000 | 0.000 | 0.000 | 0.000 | 0.032 |
| 蛋类 Eggs | 0.000 | 0.000 | 0.000 | 0.000 | 0.000 | 0.000 | 0.000 | 0.000 | 0.000 | 0.000 | 0.000 | 0.000 | 0.000 | 0.000 | 0.000 | 0.000 | 0.000 | 0.000 | 0.000 | 0.000 | 0.000 | 0.000 | 0.000 | 0.000 | 0.000 |
| 水产类 Aquatic foods | 0.000 | 0.000 | 0.000 | 0.000 | 0.000 | 0.000 | 0.069 | 0.000 | 0.000 | 0.000 | 0.000 | 0.000 | 0.000 | 0.000 | 0.000 | 0.000 | 0.000 | 0.000 | 0.000 | 0.089 | 0.000 | 0.000 | 0.000 | 0.000 | 0.007 |
| 乳类 Dairy products | 0.000 | 0.000 | 0.000 | 0.000 | 0.000 | 0.000 | 0.000 | 0.000 | 0.000 | 0.000 | 0.000 | 0.000 | 0.000 | 0.000 | 0.000 | 0.000 | 0.000 | 0.000 | 0.000 | 0.000 | 0.000 | 0.000 | 0.000 | 0.000 | 0.000 |
| 蔬菜类 Vegetables | 0.000 | 0.000 | 0.000 | 0.000 | 0.000 | 0.000 | 3.904 | 0.000 | 0.000 | 0.000 | 0.000 | 13.400 | 6.470 | 0.000 | 0.000 | 0.000 | 0.000 | 0.000 | 2.718 | 1.444 | 2.030 | 0.000 | 15.77 | 0.000 | 3.021 |
| 水果类 Fruits | 0.000 | 0.000 | 0.000 | 0.000 | 0.000 | 0.000 | 0.000 | 0.000 | 0.000 | 0.000 | 0.000 | 0.000 | 0.000 | 0.381 | 0.000 | 0.000 | 0.000 | 0.000 | 0.000 | 0.000 | 0.000 | 0.000 | 0.000 | 0.000 | 0.016 |
| 糖类 Sugar | 0.000 | 0.000 | 0.000 | 0.000 | 0.000 | 0.000 | 0.000 | 0.000 | 0.000 | 0.000 | 0.000 | 0.000 | 0.000 | 0.000 | 0.000 | 0.000 | 0.000 | 0.000 | 0.000 | 0.000 | 0.000 | 0.000 | 0.000 | 0.000 | 0.000 |
| 水及饮料类 Water and beverages | 0.000 | 0.000 | 0.000 | 0.000 | 0.000 | 0.000 | 0.000 | 0.000 | 0.000 | 0.000 | 0.000 | 0.000 | 0.000 | 0.000 | 0.000 | 0.000 | 0.000 | 0.000 | 0.000 | 0.000 | 0.000 | 0.000 | 0.000 | 0.000 | 0.000 |

续表

| 膳食类别 Category | 黑龙江 HL | 辽宁 LN | 河北 HE | 北京 BJ | 吉林 JL | 山西 SX | 陕西 SN | 河南 HA | 宁夏 NX | 内蒙古 NM | 青海 QH | 甘肃 GS | 上海 SH | 福建 FJ | 江西 JX | 江苏 JS | 浙江 ZJ | 山东 SD | 湖北 HB | 四川 SC | 广西 GX | 湖南 HN | 广东 GD | 贵州 GZ | 全国平均 AVG |
|---|---|---|---|---|---|---|---|---|---|---|---|---|---|---|---|---|---|---|---|---|---|---|---|---|---|
| 酒类 Alcohol beverages | 0.000 | 0.000 | 0.000 | 0.000 | 0.000 | 0.000 | 0.000 | 0.000 | 0.000 | 0.000 | 0.000 | 0.000 | 0.000 | 0.000 | 0.000 | 0.000 | 0.000 | 0.000 | 0.000 | 0.000 | 0.000 | 0.000 | 0.000 | 0.000 | 0.000 |
| 合计 SUM | 0.000 | 0.000 | 0.811 | 0.000 | 0.000 | 0.000 | 4.243 | 0.000 | 0.000 | 0.000 | 0.000 | 13.399 | 6.470 | 12.989 | 9.368 | 3.974 | 0.000 | 0.000 | 2.718 | 3.041 | 2.030 | 0.000 | 15.767 | 0.000 | 3.117 |

附表 4-63 第六次中国总膳食研究的茚虫威膳食摄入量 [单位: ng/(kg bw·d)]

Annexed Table 4-63 Dietary intakes of indoxacarb from the 6$^{th}$ China TDS [Unit: ng/(kg bw·d)]

| 膳食类别 Category | 黑龙江 HL | 辽宁 LN | 河北 HE | 北京 BJ | 吉林 JL | 山西 SX | 陕西 SN | 河南 HA | 宁夏 NX | 内蒙古 NM | 青海 QH | 甘肃 GS | 上海 SH | 福建 FJ | 江西 JX | 江苏 JS | 浙江 ZJ | 山东 SD | 湖北 HB | 四川 SC | 广西 GX | 湖南 HN | 广东 GD | 贵州 GZ | 全国平均 AVG |
|---|---|---|---|---|---|---|---|---|---|---|---|---|---|---|---|---|---|---|---|---|---|---|---|---|---|
| 谷类 Cereals | 0.000 | 0.000 | 0.000 | 0.000 | 0.000 | 0.000 | 0.000 | 0.000 | 0.000 | 0.000 | 0.000 | 0.000 | 0.000 | 0.000 | 0.000 | 0.000 | 0.000 | 0.000 | 0.000 | 0.000 | 0.000 | 0.000 | 0.000 | 0.000 | 0.000 |
| 豆类 Legumes | 0.000 | 0.000 | 0.000 | 0.000 | 0.000 | 0.000 | 0.000 | 0.000 | 0.000 | 0.000 | 0.000 | 0.000 | 0.000 | 0.000 | 0.000 | 0.000 | 0.000 | 0.000 | 0.000 | 0.000 | 0.000 | 0.000 | 0.000 | 0.000 | 0.000 |
| 薯类 Potatoes | 0.000 | 0.000 | 0.000 | 0.000 | 0.000 | 0.000 | 0.000 | 0.000 | 0.000 | 0.000 | 0.000 | 0.000 | 0.000 | 0.000 | 0.000 | 0.000 | 0.000 | 0.000 | 0.000 | 0.000 | 0.000 | 0.000 | 0.000 | 0.000 | 0.000 |
| 肉类 Meats | 0.000 | 0.000 | 0.000 | 0.000 | 0.000 | 0.000 | 0.000 | 0.000 | 0.000 | 0.000 | 0.000 | 0.000 | 0.000 | 0.000 | 0.000 | 0.000 | 0.000 | 0.000 | 0.000 | 0.000 | 0.000 | 0.000 | 0.000 | 0.000 | 0.000 |
| 蛋类 Eggs | 0.000 | 0.000 | 0.000 | 0.000 | 0.000 | 0.000 | 0.000 | 0.000 | 0.000 | 0.000 | 0.000 | 0.000 | 0.000 | 0.000 | 0.000 | 0.000 | 0.000 | 0.000 | 0.000 | 0.000 | 0.000 | 0.000 | 0.000 | 0.000 | 0.000 |
| 水产类 Aquatic foods | 0.000 | 0.000 | 0.000 | 0.000 | 0.000 | 0.000 | 0.000 | 0.000 | 0.000 | 0.000 | 0.000 | 0.000 | 0.000 | 0.000 | 0.093 | 0.000 | 0.000 | 0.000 | 0.000 | 0.000 | 0.000 | 0.000 | 0.000 | 0.000 | 0.000 |
| 乳类 Dairy products | 0.000 | 0.000 | 0.000 | 0.000 | 0.000 | 0.000 | 0.000 | 0.000 | 0.000 | 0.000 | 0.000 | 0.000 | 0.000 | 0.000 | 0.000 | 0.000 | 0.000 | 0.000 | 0.000 | 0.000 | 0.000 | 0.000 | 0.000 | 0.000 | 0.004 |

续表

| 膳食类别 Category | 黑龙江 HL | 辽宁 LN | 河北 HE | 北京 BJ | 吉林 JL | 山西 SX | 陕西 SN | 河南 HA | 宁夏 NX | 内蒙古 NM | 青海 QH | 甘肃 GS | 上海 SH | 福建 FJ | 江西 JX | 江苏 JS | 浙江 ZJ | 山东 SD | 湖北 HB | 四川 SC | 广西 GX | 湖南 HN | 广东 GD | 贵州 GZ | 全国平均 AVG |
|---|---|---|---|---|---|---|---|---|---|---|---|---|---|---|---|---|---|---|---|---|---|---|---|---|---|
| 蔬菜类 Vegetables | 0.000 | 0.000 | 0.000 | 0.000 | 0.000 | 0.589 | 0.000 | 17.280 | 0.000 | 0.000 | 1.206 | 0.000 | 75.720 | 152.800 | 47.560 | 0.000 | 105.000 | 1.436 | 43.780 | 0.000 | 0.000 | 22.460 | 0.000 | 0.000 | 19.490 |
| 水果类 Fruits | 0.000 | 0.000 | 0.000 | 0.000 | 0.000 | 0.000 | 0.000 | 0.000 | 0.000 | 0.000 | 0.000 | 0.000 | 0.577 | 0.000 | 0.000 | 0.000 | 0.000 | 0.000 | 0.000 | 0.000 | 0.000 | 0.000 | 0.000 | 0.000 | 0.024 |
| 糖类 Sugar | 0.000 | 0.000 | 0.000 | 0.000 | 0.000 | 0.000 | 0.000 | 0.000 | 0.000 | 0.000 | 0.000 | 0.000 | 0.000 | 0.000 | 0.000 | 0.000 | 0.000 | 0.000 | 0.000 | 0.000 | 0.000 | 0.000 | 0.000 | 0.000 | 0.000 |
| 水及饮料类 Water and beverages | 0.000 | 0.000 | 0.000 | 0.000 | 0.000 | 0.000 | 0.000 | 0.000 | 0.000 | 0.000 | 0.000 | 0.000 | 0.000 | 0.000 | 0.000 | 0.000 | 0.000 | 0.000 | 0.000 | 0.000 | 0.000 | 0.000 | 0.000 | 0.000 | 0.000 |
| 酒类 Alcohol beverages | 0.000 | 0.000 | 0.000 | 0.000 | 0.000 | 0.000 | 0.000 | 0.000 | 0.000 | 0.000 | 0.000 | 0.000 | 0.000 | 0.000 | 0.000 | 0.000 | 0.000 | 0.000 | 0.000 | 0.000 | 0.000 | 0.000 | 0.000 | 0.000 | 0.000 |
| 合计 SUM | 0.000 | 0.000 | 0.000 | 0.000 | 0.000 | 0.589 | 0.000 | 17.280 | 0.000 | 0.000 | 1.206 | 0.000 | 76.293 | 152.820 | 47.649 | 0.000 | 105.014 | 1.436 | 43.780 | 0.000 | 0.000 | 22.464 | 0.000 | 0.000 | 19.522 |

附表 4-64　第六次中国总膳食研究克百威的膳食来源（单位：%）

Annexed Table 4-64　Dietary sources of carbofuran from the 6$^{th}$ China TDS (Unit: %)

| 膳食类别 Category | 黑龙江 HL | 辽宁 LN | 河北 HE | 北京 BJ | 吉林 JL | 山西 SX | 陕西 SN | 河南 HA | 宁夏 NX | 内蒙古 NM | 青海 QH | 甘肃 GS | 上海 SH | 福建 FJ | 江西 JX | 江苏 JS | 浙江 ZJ | 山东 SD | 湖北 HB | 四川 SC | 广西 GX | 湖南 HN | 广东 GD | 贵州 GZ | 全国平均 AVG |
|---|---|---|---|---|---|---|---|---|---|---|---|---|---|---|---|---|---|---|---|---|---|---|---|---|---|
| 谷类 Cereals | 0.0 | 0.0 | 0.0 | 0.0 | 0.0 | 0.0 | 0.0 | 0.0 | 0.0 | 0.0 | 0.0 | 0.0 | 0.0 | 0.0 | 0.0 | 0.0 | 0.0 | 0.0 | 0.0 | 0.0 | 0.0 | 0.0 | 0.0 | 0.0 | 0.0 |
| 豆类 Legumes | 0.0 | 0.0 | 0.0 | 0.0 | 0.0 | 0.0 | 0.0 | 0.0 | 0.0 | 0.0 | 0.0 | 0.0 | 0.0 | 0.0 | 0.0 | 0.0 | 0.0 | 0.0 | 0.0 | 24.7 | 0.0 | 0.0 | 0.0 | 0.0 | 1.0 |
| 薯类 Potatoes | 0.0 | 0.0 | 0.0 | 0.0 | 0.0 | 0.0 | 6.4 | 0.0 | 0.0 | 0.0 | 0.0 | 0.0 | 0.0 | 0.0 | 0.0 | 0.0 | 0.0 | 0.0 | 0.0 | 0.0 | 0.0 | 0.0 | 0.0 | 0.0 | 0.4 |
| 肉类 Meats | 0.0 | 0.0 | 0.0 | 0.0 | 0.0 | 0.0 | 0.0 | 0.0 | 0.0 | 0.0 | 0.0 | 0.0 | 0.0 | 0.0 | 0.0 | 0.0 | 0.0 | 0.0 | 0.0 | 24.9 | 0.0 | 0.0 | 0.0 | 0.0 | 1.0 |

续表

| 膳食类别<br>Category | 黑龙江<br>HL | 辽宁<br>LN | 河北<br>HE | 北京<br>BJ | 吉林<br>JL | 山西<br>SX | 陕西<br>SN | 河南<br>HA | 宁夏<br>NX | 内蒙古<br>NM | 青海<br>QH | 甘肃<br>GS | 上海<br>SH | 福建<br>FJ | 江西<br>JX | 江苏<br>JS | 浙江<br>ZJ | 山东<br>SD | 湖北<br>HB | 四川<br>SC | 广西<br>GX | 湖南<br>HN | 广东<br>GD | 贵州<br>GZ | 全国平均<br>AVG |
|---|---|---|---|---|---|---|---|---|---|---|---|---|---|---|---|---|---|---|---|---|---|---|---|---|---|
| 蛋类 Eggs | 0.0 | 0.0 | 0.0 | 0.0 | 0.0 | 0.0 | 0.0 | 0.0 | 0.0 | 0.0 | 0.0 | 0.0 | 0.0 | 0.0 | 0.0 | 0.0 | 0.0 | 0.0 | 0.0 | 0.0 | 0.0 | 0.0 | 0.0 | 0.0 | 0.0 |
| 水产类 Aquatic foods | 0.0 | 0.0 | 0.0 | 0.0 | 0.0 | 0.0 | 1.6 | 0.0 | 0.0 | 0.0 | 0.0 | 0.0 | 0.0 | 0.0 | 0.0 | 0.0 | 0.0 | 0.0 | 0.0 | 2.9 | 0.0 | 0.0 | 0.0 | 0.0 | 0.2 |
| 乳类 Dairy products | 0.0 | 0.0 | 0.0 | 0.0 | 0.0 | 0.0 | 0.0 | 0.0 | 0.0 | 0.0 | 0.0 | 0.0 | 0.0 | 0.0 | 0.0 | 0.0 | 0.0 | 0.0 | 0.0 | 0.0 | 0.0 | 0.0 | 0.0 | 0.0 | 0.0 |
| 蔬菜类 Vegetables | 0.0 | 0.0 | 100.0 | 0.0 | 0.0 | 0.0 | 92.0 | 0.0 | 0.0 | 0.0 | 0.0 | 100.0 | 100.0 | 97.1 | 100.0 | 100.0 | 0.0 | 0.0 | 100.0 | 47.5 | 100.0 | 0.0 | 100.0 | 0.0 | 96.9 |
| 水果类 Fruits | 0.0 | 0.0 | 0.0 | 0.0 | 0.0 | 0.0 | 0.0 | 0.0 | 0.0 | 0.0 | 0.0 | 0.0 | 0.0 | 2.9 | 0.0 | 0.0 | 0.0 | 0.0 | 0.0 | 0.0 | 0.0 | 0.0 | 0.0 | 0.0 | 0.5 |
| 糖类 Sugar | 0.0 | 0.0 | 0.0 | 0.0 | 0.0 | 0.0 | 0.0 | 0.0 | 0.0 | 0.0 | 0.0 | 0.0 | 0.0 | 0.0 | 0.0 | 0.0 | 0.0 | 0.0 | 0.0 | 0.0 | 0.0 | 0.0 | 0.0 | 0.0 | 0.0 |
| 水及饮料类 Water and beverages | 0.0 | 0.0 | 0.0 | 0.0 | 0.0 | 0.0 | 0.0 | 0.0 | 0.0 | 0.0 | 0.0 | 0.0 | 0.0 | 0.0 | 0.0 | 0.0 | 0.0 | 0.0 | 0.0 | 0.0 | 0.0 | 0.0 | 0.0 | 0.0 | 0.0 |
| 酒类 Alcohol beverages | 0.0 | 0.0 | 0.0 | 0.0 | 0.0 | 0.0 | 0.0 | 0.0 | 0.0 | 0.0 | 0.0 | 0.0 | 0.0 | 0.0 | 0.0 | 0.0 | 0.0 | 0.0 | 0.0 | 0.0 | 0.0 | 0.0 | 0.0 | 0.0 | 0.0 |

附表 4-65 第六次中国总膳食研究茚虫威的膳食来源（单位：%）

Annexed Table 4-65 Dietary sources of indoxacarb from the 6$^{th}$ China TDS (Unit: %)

| 膳食类别<br>Category | 黑龙江<br>HL | 辽宁<br>LN | 河北<br>HE | 北京<br>BJ | 吉林<br>JL | 山西<br>SX | 陕西<br>SN | 河南<br>HA | 宁夏<br>NX | 内蒙古<br>NM | 青海<br>QH | 甘肃<br>GS | 上海<br>SH | 福建<br>FJ | 江西<br>JX | 江苏<br>JS | 浙江<br>ZJ | 山东<br>SD | 湖北<br>HB | 四川<br>SC | 广西<br>GX | 湖南<br>HN | 广东<br>GD | 贵州<br>GZ | 全国平均<br>AVG |
|---|---|---|---|---|---|---|---|---|---|---|---|---|---|---|---|---|---|---|---|---|---|---|---|---|---|
| 谷类 Cereals | 0.0 | 0.0 | 0.0 | 0.0 | 0.0 | 0.0 | 0.0 | 0.0 | 0.0 | 0.0 | 0.0 | 0.0 | 0.0 | 0.0 | 0.0 | 0.0 | 0.0 | 0.0 | 0.0 | 0.0 | 0.0 | 0.0 | 0.0 | 0.0 | 0.0 |

续表

| 膳食类别 Category | 黑龙江 HL | 辽宁 LN | 河北 HE | 北京 BJ | 吉林 JL | 山西 SX | 陕西 SN | 河南 HA | 宁夏 NX | 内蒙古 NM | 青海 QH | 甘肃 GS | 上海 SH | 福建 FJ | 江西 JX | 江苏 JS | 浙江 ZJ | 山东 SD | 湖北 HB | 四川 SC | 广西 GX | 湖南 HN | 广东 GD | 贵州 GZ | 全国平均 AVG |
|---|---|---|---|---|---|---|---|---|---|---|---|---|---|---|---|---|---|---|---|---|---|---|---|---|---|
| 豆类 Legumes | 0.0 | 0.0 | 0.0 | 0.0 | 0.0 | 0.0 | 0.0 | 0.0 | 0.0 | 0.0 | 0.0 | 0.0 | 0.0 | 0.0 | 0.0 | 0.0 | 0.0 | 0.0 | 0.0 | 0.0 | 0.0 | 0.0 | 0.0 | 0.0 | 0.0 |
| 薯类 Potatoes | 0.0 | 0.0 | 0.0 | 0.0 | 0.0 | 0.0 | 0.0 | 0.0 | 0.0 | 0.0 | 0.0 | 0.0 | 0.0 | 0.0 | 0.0 | 0.0 | 0.0 | 0.0 | 0.0 | 0.0 | 0.0 | 0.0 | 0.0 | 0.0 | 0.0 |
| 肉类 Meats | 0.0 | 0.0 | 0.0 | 0.0 | 0.0 | 0.0 | 0.0 | 0.0 | 0.0 | 0.0 | 0.0 | 0.0 | 0.0 | 0.0 | 0.0 | 0.0 | 0.0 | 0.0 | 0.0 | 0.0 | 0.0 | 0.0 | 0.0 | 0.0 | 0.0 |
| 蛋类 Eggs | 0.0 | 0.0 | 0.0 | 0.0 | 0.0 | 0.0 | 0.0 | 0.0 | 0.0 | 0.0 | 0.0 | 0.0 | 0.0 | 0.0 | 0.0 | 0.0 | 0.0 | 0.0 | 0.0 | 0.0 | 0.0 | 0.0 | 0.0 | 0.0 | 0.0 |
| 水产类 Aquatic foods | 0.0 | 0.0 | 0.0 | 0.0 | 0.0 | 0.0 | 0.0 | 0.0 | 0.0 | 0.0 | 0.0 | 0.0 | 0.0 | 0.0 | 0.0 | 0.0 | 0.0 | 0.0 | 0.0 | 0.0 | 0.0 | 0.0 | 0.0 | 0.0 | 0.0 |
| 乳类 Dairy products | 0.0 | 0.0 | 0.0 | 0.0 | 0.0 | 0.0 | 0.0 | 0.0 | 0.0 | 0.0 | 0.0 | 0.0 | 0.0 | 0.0 | 0.2 | 0.0 | 0.0 | 0.0 | 0.0 | 0.0 | 0.0 | 0.0 | 0.0 | 0.0 | 0.0 |
| 蔬菜类 Vegetables | 0.0 | 0.0 | 0.0 | 0.0 | 0.0 | 100.0 | 0.0 | 100.0 | 0.0 | 0.0 | 100.0 | 0.0 | 99.2 | 100.0 | 99.8 | 0.0 | 100.0 | 100.0 | 100.0 | 0.0 | 0.0 | 100.0 | 0.0 | 0.0 | 99.9 |
| 水果类 Fruits | 0.0 | 0.0 | 0.0 | 0.0 | 0.0 | 0.0 | 0.0 | 0.0 | 0.0 | 0.0 | 0.0 | 0.0 | 0.8 | 0.0 | 0.0 | 0.0 | 0.0 | 0.0 | 0.0 | 0.0 | 0.0 | 0.0 | 0.0 | 0.0 | 0.1 |
| 糖类 Sugar | 0.0 | 0.0 | 0.0 | 0.0 | 0.0 | 0.0 | 0.0 | 0.0 | 0.0 | 0.0 | 0.0 | 0.0 | 0.0 | 0.0 | 0.0 | 0.0 | 0.0 | 0.0 | 0.0 | 0.0 | 0.0 | 0.0 | 0.0 | 0.0 | 0.0 |
| 水及饮料类 Water and beverages | 0.0 | 0.0 | 0.0 | 0.0 | 0.0 | 0.0 | 0.0 | 0.0 | 0.0 | 0.0 | 0.0 | 0.0 | 0.0 | 0.0 | 0.0 | 0.0 | 0.0 | 0.0 | 0.0 | 0.0 | 0.0 | 0.0 | 0.0 | 0.0 | 0.0 |
| 酒类 Alcohol beverages | 0.0 | 0.0 | 0.0 | 0.0 | 0.0 | 0.0 | 0.0 | 0.0 | 0.0 | 0.0 | 0.0 | 0.0 | 0.0 | 0.0 | 0.0 | 0.0 | 0.0 | 0.0 | 0.0 | 0.0 | 0.0 | 0.0 | 0.0 | 0.0 | 0.0 |

附表 4-66　第六次中国总膳食研究膳食样品中灭蝇胺的含量（单位：μg/kg）

Annexed Table 4-66　Levels of cyromazine in food samples from the 6th China TDS (Unit: μg/kg)

| 膳食类别 Category | 黑龙江 HL | 辽宁 LN | 河北 HE | 北京 BJ | 吉林 JL | 山西 SX | 陕西 SN | 河南 HA | 宁夏 NX | 内蒙古 NM | 青海 QH | 甘肃 GS | 上海 SH | 福建 FJ | 江西 JX | 江苏 JS | 浙江 ZJ | 山东 SD | 湖北 HB | 四川 SC | 广西 GX | 湖南 HN | 广东 GD | 贵州 GZ | 全国平均 AVG |
|---|---|---|---|---|---|---|---|---|---|---|---|---|---|---|---|---|---|---|---|---|---|---|---|---|---|
| 谷类 Cereals | ND | ND | ND | ND | ND | ND | ND | ND | ND | ND | ND | ND | ND | ND | ND | ND | ND | ND | ND | ND | ND | ND | ND | ND | 0.00 |
| 豆类 Legumes | ND | 0.49 | ND | ND | ND | ND | ND | ND | ND | ND | ND | ND | ND | ND | ND | ND | ND | ND | ND | ND | ND | ND | ND | ND | 0.02 |
| 薯类 Potatoes | ND | 0.60 | ND | ND | ND | ND | ND | ND | ND | ND | ND | ND | ND | ND | ND | ND | ND | ND | ND | ND | ND | ND | ND | ND | 0.03 |
| 肉类 Meats | ND | 1.43 | 0.84 | 0.24 | ND | ND | ND | ND | 0.70 | ND | ND | ND | 0.61 | 1.43 | ND | 0.11 | 0.70 | ND | ND | ND | ND | ND | 0.40 | ND | 0.26 |
| 蛋类 Eggs | ND | ND | ND | ND | ND | ND | ND | 2.26 | 1.83 | ND | ND | ND | ND | 1.17 | 0.32 | ND | ND | ND | ND | ND | ND | 3.35 | ND | ND | 0.37 |
| 水产类 Aquatic foods | ND | 0.11 | ND | ND | ND | ND | ND | ND | ND | ND | ND | ND | ND | ND | ND | ND | ND | ND | ND | 0.47 | ND | ND | ND | ND | 0.02 |
| 乳类 Dairy products | ND | ND | ND | ND | ND | ND | ND | ND | ND | ND | 0.61 | ND | ND | 0.08 | ND | ND | ND | ND | ND | ND | ND | ND | ND | ND | 0.03 |
| 蔬菜类 Vegetables | ND | 1.52 | 1.43 | 0.08 | ND | 0.17 | 0.12 | ND | ND | 0.74 | 1.03 | 0.71 | 1.15 | ND | ND | ND | 0.21 | 0.14 | ND | 0.39 | ND | 4.66 | ND | ND | 0.52 |
| 水果类 Fruits | ND | ND | ND | ND | ND | ND | ND | ND | ND | 1.07 | ND | 0.12 | ND | ND | ND | ND | ND | ND | ND | ND | ND | ND | ND | ND | 0.05 |
| 糖类 Sugar | ND | ND | ND | ND | ND | ND | ND | ND | ND | ND | ND | ND | ND | ND | ND | ND | ND | ND | ND | ND | ND | ND | ND | ND | 0.00 |
| 水及饮料类 Water and beverages | ND | ND | ND | ND | ND | ND | ND | ND | ND | ND | ND | ND | ND | ND | ND | ND | ND | ND | ND | ND | ND | ND | ND | ND | 0.00 |

续表

| 膳食类别<br>Category | 黑龙江<br>HL | 辽宁<br>LN | 河北<br>HE | 北京<br>BJ | 吉林<br>JL | 山西<br>SX | 陕西<br>SN | 河南<br>HA | 宁夏<br>NX | 内蒙古<br>NM | 青海<br>QH | 甘肃<br>GS | 上海<br>SH | 福建<br>FJ | 江西<br>JX | 江苏<br>JS | 浙江<br>ZJ | 山东<br>SD | 湖北<br>HB | 四川<br>SC | 广西<br>GX | 湖南<br>HN | 广东<br>GD | 贵州<br>GZ | 全国平均<br>AVG |
|---|---|---|---|---|---|---|---|---|---|---|---|---|---|---|---|---|---|---|---|---|---|---|---|---|---|
| 酒类<br>Alcohol beverages | ND | ND | ND | ND | ND | ND | ND | ND | ND | ND | ND | ND | ND | ND | ND | ND | ND | ND | ND | ND | ND | ND | ND | ND | 0.00 |

注：未检出（ND）按 0 计
Note: values not detected (ND) were treated as being equal to 0

附表 4-67 第六次中国总膳食研究的灭蝇胺膳食摄入量 [单位：ng/(kg bw・d)]
Annexed Table 4-67 Dietary intakes of cyromazine from the 6th China TDS [Unit: ng/(kg bw・d)]

| 膳食类别<br>Category | 黑龙江<br>HL | 辽宁<br>LN | 河北<br>HE | 北京<br>BJ | 吉林<br>JL | 山西<br>SX | 陕西<br>SN | 河南<br>HA | 宁夏<br>NX | 内蒙古<br>NM | 青海<br>QH | 甘肃<br>GS | 上海<br>SH | 福建<br>FJ | 江西<br>JX | 江苏<br>JS | 浙江<br>ZJ | 山东<br>SD | 湖北<br>HB | 四川<br>SC | 广西<br>GX | 湖南<br>HN | 广东<br>GD | 贵州<br>GZ | 全国平均<br>AVG |
|---|---|---|---|---|---|---|---|---|---|---|---|---|---|---|---|---|---|---|---|---|---|---|---|---|---|
| 谷类<br>Cereals | 0.000 | 0.000 | 0.000 | 0.000 | 0.000 | 0.000 | 0.000 | 0.000 | 0.000 | 0.000 | 0.000 | 0.000 | 0.000 | 0.000 | 0.000 | 0.000 | 0.000 | 0.000 | 0.000 | 0.000 | 0.000 | 0.000 | 0.000 | 0.000 | 0.000 |
| 豆类<br>Legumes | 0.000 | 0.952 | 0.000 | 0.000 | 0.000 | 0.000 | 0.000 | 0.000 | 0.000 | 0.000 | 0.000 | 0.000 | 0.000 | 0.000 | 0.000 | 0.000 | 0.000 | 0.000 | 0.000 | 0.000 | 0.000 | 0.000 | 0.000 | 0.000 | 0.040 |
| 薯类<br>Potatoes | 0.000 | 0.684 | 0.000 | 0.000 | 0.000 | 0.000 | 0.000 | 0.000 | 0.000 | 0.000 | 0.000 | 0.000 | 0.000 | 0.000 | 0.000 | 0.057 | 0.000 | 0.000 | 0.000 | 0.000 | 0.000 | 0.000 | 0.000 | 0.000 | 0.031 |
| 肉类<br>Meats | 0.000 | 1.518 | 0.635 | 0.261 | 0.000 | 0.000 | 0.000 | 0.000 | 0.521 | 0.000 | 0.000 | 0.000 | 1.065 | 1.947 | 0.000 | 0.000 | 1.309 | 0.000 | 0.000 | 0.000 | 0.000 | 0.000 | 0.667 | 0.000 | 0.330 |
| 蛋类<br>Eggs | 0.000 | 0.000 | 0.000 | 0.000 | 0.000 | 0.000 | 0.000 | 1.067 | 0.378 | 0.000 | 0.000 | 0.000 | 0.000 | 0.354 | 0.105 | 0.000 | 0.000 | 0.000 | 0.000 | 0.000 | 0.000 | 1.214 | 0.000 | 0.000 | 0.130 |
| 水产类<br>Aquatic foods | 0.000 | 0.029 | 0.000 | 0.000 | 0.000 | 0.000 | 0.000 | 0.000 | 0.000 | 0.000 | 0.000 | 0.000 | 0.000 | 0.000 | 0.000 | 0.000 | 0.000 | 0.000 | 0.000 | 0.000 | 0.000 | 0.000 | 0.382 | 0.000 | 0.017 |
| 乳类<br>Dairy products | 0.000 | 0.000 | 0.000 | 0.000 | 0.000 | 0.000 | 0.000 | 0.000 | 0.000 | 0.000 | 0.519 | 0.000 | 0.000 | 0.043 | 0.000 | 0.000 | 0.000 | 0.000 | 0.000 | 0.000 | 0.000 | 0.000 | 0.000 | 0.000 | 0.023 |

续表

| 膳食类别 Category | 黑龙江 HL | 辽宁 LN | 河北 HE | 北京 BJ | 吉林 JL | 山西 SX | 陕西 SN | 河南 HA | 宁夏 NX | 内蒙古 NM | 青海 QH | 甘肃 GS | 上海 SH | 福建 FJ | 江西 JX | 江苏 JS | 浙江 ZJ | 山东 SD | 湖北 HB | 四川 SC | 广西 GX | 湖南 HN | 广东 GD | 贵州 GZ | 全国平均 AVG |
|---|---|---|---|---|---|---|---|---|---|---|---|---|---|---|---|---|---|---|---|---|---|---|---|---|---|
| 蔬菜类 Vegetables | 0.000 | 7.893 | 6.684 | 0.501 | 0.000 | 0.842 | 0.544 | 0.000 | 0.000 | 3.013 | 5.090 | 2.786 | 7.313 | 0.000 | 0.000 | 0.000 | 1.487 | 0.917 | 0.000 | 1.883 | 0.000 | 39.51 | 0.000 | 0.000 | 3.269 |
| 水果类 Fruits | 0.000 | 0.000 | 0.000 | 0.000 | 0.000 | 0.000 | 0.000 | 0.000 | 0.000 | 1.925 | 0.000 | 0.062 | 0.000 | 0.000 | 0.000 | 0.000 | 0.000 | 0.000 | 0.000 | 0.000 | 0.000 | 0.000 | 0.000 | 0.000 | 0.083 |
| 糖类 Sugar | 0.000 | 0.000 | 0.000 | 0.000 | 0.000 | 0.000 | 0.000 | 0.000 | 0.000 | 0.000 | 0.000 | 0.000 | 0.000 | 0.000 | 0.000 | 0.000 | 0.000 | 0.000 | 0.000 | 0.000 | 0.000 | 0.000 | 0.000 | 0.000 | 0.000 |
| 水及饮料类 Water and beverages | 0.000 | 0.000 | 0.000 | 0.000 | 0.000 | 0.000 | 0.000 | 0.000 | 0.000 | 0.000 | 0.000 | 0.000 | 0.000 | 0.000 | 0.000 | 0.000 | 0.000 | 0.000 | 0.000 | 0.000 | 0.000 | 0.000 | 0.000 | 0.000 | 0.000 |
| 酒类 Alcohol beverages | 0.000 | 0.000 | 0.000 | 0.000 | 0.000 | 0.000 | 0.000 | 0.000 | 0.000 | 0.000 | 0.000 | 0.000 | 0.000 | 0.000 | 0.000 | 0.000 | 0.000 | 0.000 | 0.000 | 0.000 | 0.000 | 0.000 | 0.000 | 0.000 | 0.000 |
| 合计 SUM | 0.000 | 11.076 | 7.318 | 0.762 | 0.000 | 0.842 | 0.544 | 1.067 | 0.899 | 4.938 | 5.609 | 2.848 | 8.378 | 2.344 | 0.105 | 0.057 | 2.796 | 0.917 | 0.000 | 1.883 | 0.000 | 40.724 | 1.049 | 0.000 | 3.923 |

附表 4-68　第六次中国总膳食研究灭蝇胺的膳食来源（单位：%）

Annexed Table 4-68　Dietary sources of cyromazine from the 6$^{th}$ China TDS (Unit: %)

| 膳食类别 Category | 黑龙江 HL | 辽宁 LN | 河北 HE | 北京 BJ | 吉林 JL | 山西 SX | 陕西 SN | 河南 HA | 宁夏 NX | 内蒙古 NM | 青海 QH | 甘肃 GS | 上海 SH | 福建 FJ | 江西 JX | 江苏 JS | 浙江 ZJ | 山东 SD | 湖北 HB | 四川 SC | 广西 GX | 湖南 HN | 广东 GD | 贵州 GZ | 全国平均 AVG |
|---|---|---|---|---|---|---|---|---|---|---|---|---|---|---|---|---|---|---|---|---|---|---|---|---|---|
| 谷类 Cereals | 0.0 | 0.0 | 0.0 | 0.0 | 0.0 | 0.0 | 0.0 | 0.0 | 0.0 | 0.0 | 0.0 | 0.0 | 0.0 | 0.0 | 0.0 | 0.0 | 0.0 | 0.0 | 0.0 | 0.0 | 0.0 | 0.0 | 0.0 | 0.0 | 0.0 |
| 豆类 Legumes | 0.0 | 8.6 | 0.0 | 0.0 | 0.0 | 0.0 | 0.0 | 0.0 | 0.0 | 0.0 | 0.0 | 0.0 | 0.0 | 0.0 | 0.0 | 0.0 | 0.0 | 0.0 | 0.0 | 0.0 | 0.0 | 0.0 | 0.0 | 0.0 | 1.0 |
| 薯类 Potatoes | 0.0 | 6.2 | 0.0 | 0.0 | 0.0 | 0.0 | 0.0 | 0.0 | 57.9 | 0.0 | 0.0 | 0.0 | 12.7 | 0.0 | 0.0 | 100.0 | 46.8 | 0.0 | 0.0 | 0.0 | 0.0 | 0.0 | 0.0 | 0.0 | 0.8 |
| 肉类 Meats | 0.0 | 13.7 | 8.7 | 34.2 | 0.0 | 0.0 | 0.0 | 0.0 | 0.0 | 0.0 | 0.0 | 0.0 | 0.0 | 83.1 | 0.0 | 0.0 | 0.0 | 0.0 | 0.0 | 0.0 | 0.0 | 0.0 | 63.6 | 0.0 | 8.4 |

续表

| 膳食类别 Category | 黑龙江 HL | 辽宁 LN | 河北 HE | 北京 BJ | 吉林 JL | 山西 SX | 陕西 SN | 河南 HA | 宁夏 NX | 内蒙古 NM | 青海 QH | 甘肃 GS | 上海 SH | 福建 FJ | 江西 JX | 江苏 JS | 浙江 ZJ | 山东 SD | 湖北 HB | 四川 SC | 广西 GX | 湖南 HN | 广东 GD | 贵州 GZ | 全国平均 AVG |
|---|---|---|---|---|---|---|---|---|---|---|---|---|---|---|---|---|---|---|---|---|---|---|---|---|---|
| 蛋类 Eggs | 0.0 | 0.0 | 0.0 | 0.0 | 0.0 | 0.0 | 0.0 | 100.0 | 42.1 | 0.0 | 0.0 | 0.0 | 0.0 | 15.1 | 100.0 | 0.0 | 0.0 | 0.0 | 0.0 | 0.0 | 0.0 | 3.0 | 0.0 | 0.0 | 3.3 |
| 水产类 Aquatic foods | 0.0 | 0.3 | 0.0 | 0.0 | 0.0 | 0.0 | 0.0 | 0.0 | 0.0 | 0.0 | 0.0 | 0.0 | 0.0 | 0.0 | 0.0 | 0.0 | 0.0 | 0.0 | 0.0 | 0.0 | 0.0 | 0.0 | 36.4 | 0.0 | 0.4 |
| 乳类 Dairy products | 0.0 | 0.0 | 0.0 | 0.0 | 0.0 | 0.0 | 0.0 | 0.0 | 0.0 | 0.0 | 9.3 | 0.0 | 0.0 | 1.8 | 0.0 | 0.0 | 0.0 | 0.0 | 0.0 | 0.0 | 0.0 | 0.0 | 0.0 | 0.0 | 0.6 |
| 蔬菜类 Vegetables | 0.0 | 71.3 | 91.3 | 65.8 | 0.0 | 100.0 | 100.0 | 0.0 | 0.0 | 61.0 | 90.7 | 97.8 | 87.3 | 0.0 | 0.0 | 0.0 | 53.2 | 100.0 | 0.0 | 100.0 | 0.0 | 97.0 | 0.0 | 0.0 | 83.3 |
| 水果类 Fruits | 0.0 | 0.0 | 0.0 | 0.0 | 0.0 | 0.0 | 0.0 | 0.0 | 0.0 | 39.0 | 0.0 | 2.2 | 0.0 | 0.0 | 0.0 | 0.0 | 0.0 | 0.0 | 0.0 | 0.0 | 0.0 | 0.0 | 0.0 | 0.0 | 2.1 |
| 糖类 Sugar | 0.0 | 0.0 | 0.0 | 0.0 | 0.0 | 0.0 | 0.0 | 0.0 | 0.0 | 0.0 | 0.0 | 0.0 | 0.0 | 0.0 | 0.0 | 0.0 | 0.0 | 0.0 | 0.0 | 0.0 | 0.0 | 0.0 | 0.0 | 0.0 | 0.0 |
| 水及饮料类 Water and beverages | 0.0 | 0.0 | 0.0 | 0.0 | 0.0 | 0.0 | 0.0 | 0.0 | 0.0 | 0.0 | 0.0 | 0.0 | 0.0 | 0.0 | 0.0 | 0.0 | 0.0 | 0.0 | 0.0 | 0.0 | 0.0 | 0.0 | 0.0 | 0.0 | 0.0 |
| 酒类 Alcohol beverages | 0.0 | 0.0 | 0.0 | 0.0 | 0.0 | 0.0 | 0.0 | 0.0 | 0.0 | 0.0 | 0.0 | 0.0 | 0.0 | 0.0 | 0.0 | 0.0 | 0.0 | 0.0 | 0.0 | 0.0 | 0.0 | 0.0 | 0.0 | 0.0 | 0.0 |

附表 4-69 第六次中国总膳食研究膳食样品中甲氧虫酰肼的含量（单位：μg/kg）

Annexed Table 4-69 Levels of methoxyfenozide in food samples from the 6th China TDS (Unit: μg/kg)

| 膳食类别 Category | 黑龙江 HL | 辽宁 LN | 河北 HE | 北京 BJ | 吉林 JL | 山西 SX | 陕西 SN | 河南 HA | 宁夏 NX | 内蒙古 NM | 青海 QH | 甘肃 GS | 上海 SH | 福建 FJ | 江西 JX | 江苏 JS | 浙江 ZJ | 山东 SD | 湖北 HB | 四川 SC | 广西 GX | 湖南 HN | 广东 GD | 贵州 GZ | 全国平均 AVG |
|---|---|---|---|---|---|---|---|---|---|---|---|---|---|---|---|---|---|---|---|---|---|---|---|---|---|
| 谷类 Cereals | ND | ND | ND | ND | ND | ND | ND | ND | ND | ND | ND | ND | ND | ND | ND | ND | ND | ND | ND | ND | ND | ND | ND | ND | 0.00 |

续表

| 膳食类别<br>Category | 黑龙江<br>HL | 辽宁<br>LN | 河北<br>HE | 北京<br>BJ | 吉林<br>JL | 山西<br>SX | 陕西<br>SN | 河南<br>HA | 宁夏<br>NX | 内蒙古<br>NM | 青海<br>QH | 甘肃<br>GS | 上海<br>SH | 福建<br>FJ | 江西<br>JX | 江苏<br>JS | 浙江<br>ZJ | 山东<br>SD | 湖北<br>HB | 四川<br>SC | 广西<br>GX | 湖南<br>HN | 广东<br>GD | 贵州<br>GZ | 全国平均<br>AVG |
|---|---|---|---|---|---|---|---|---|---|---|---|---|---|---|---|---|---|---|---|---|---|---|---|---|---|
| 豆类 Legumes | ND | ND | ND | ND | ND | ND | 0.43 | 0.17 | 1.60 | ND | ND | ND | ND | ND | ND | ND | ND | ND | ND | ND | ND | ND | ND | ND | 0.09 |
| 薯类 Potatoes | ND | ND | ND | ND | ND | ND | ND | ND | ND | ND | ND | ND | ND | ND | ND | ND | ND | ND | ND | ND | ND | ND | ND | ND | 0.00 |
| 肉类 Meats | ND | ND | ND | ND | ND | ND | ND | ND | ND | ND | ND | ND | ND | ND | ND | ND | ND | ND | ND | ND | ND | ND | ND | ND | 0.00 |
| 蛋类 Eggs | ND | ND | ND | ND | 0.16 | ND | ND | ND | ND | ND | ND | ND | ND | ND | ND | ND | ND | ND | ND | ND | ND | ND | ND | ND | 0.01 |
| 水产类 Aquatic foods | ND | ND | ND | ND | ND | ND | ND | ND | ND | ND | ND | ND | ND | ND | ND | ND | ND | ND | ND | ND | ND | ND | ND | ND | 0.00 |
| 乳类 Dairy products | ND | ND | ND | ND | ND | ND | ND | ND | ND | ND | ND | ND | ND | ND | ND | ND | ND | ND | ND | ND | ND | ND | ND | ND | 0.00 |
| 蔬菜类 Vegetables | ND | ND | 0.21 | ND | ND | ND | ND | ND | ND | ND | 0.10 | ND | ND | ND | ND | ND | ND | 0.81 | 38.50 | ND | 0.27 | 0.20 | 0.38 | ND | 1.69 |
| 水果类 Fruits | ND | ND | ND | ND | ND | ND | ND | ND | ND | ND | ND | ND | ND | ND | ND | ND | ND | ND | ND | 0.11 | ND | ND | ND | ND | 0.00 |
| 糖类 Sugar | ND | ND | ND | ND | ND | ND | ND | ND | ND | ND | ND | ND | 0.11 | ND | ND | ND | ND | ND | ND | ND | ND | ND | ND | ND | 0.00 |
| 水及饮料类 Water and beverages | ND | ND | ND | ND | ND | ND | ND | ND | ND | ND | ND | ND | ND | ND | ND | ND | ND | ND | ND | ND | ND | ND | ND | ND | 0.00 |
| 酒类 Alcohol beverages | ND | ND | ND | ND | ND | ND | ND | ND | ND | ND | ND | ND | ND | ND | ND | ND | ND | ND | ND | ND | ND | ND | 0.06 | ND | 0.00 |

注：未检出（ND）按 0 计

Note: values not detected (ND) were treated as being equal to 0

附表 4-70 第六次中国总膳食研究膳食样品中噻嗪酮的含量（单位：μg/kg）

Annexed Table 4-70 Levels of buprofezin in food samples from the 6<sup>th</sup> China TDS (Unit: μg/kg)

| 膳食类别 Category | 黑龙江 HL | 辽宁 LN | 河北 HE | 北京 BJ | 吉林 JL | 山西 SX | 陕西 SN | 河南 HA | 宁夏 NX | 内蒙古 NM | 青海 QH | 甘肃 GS | 上海 SH | 福建 FJ | 江西 JX | 江苏 JS | 浙江 ZJ | 山东 SD | 湖北 HB | 四川 SC | 广西 GX | 湖南 HN | 广东 GD | 贵州 GZ | 全国平均 AVG |
|---|---|---|---|---|---|---|---|---|---|---|---|---|---|---|---|---|---|---|---|---|---|---|---|---|---|
| 谷类 Cereals | ND | ND | ND | ND | ND | ND | ND | ND | ND | ND | ND | ND | 0.10 | ND | 0.27 | ND | 0.27 | ND | ND | ND | 0.19 | 0.11 | ND | ND | 0.04 |
| 豆类 Legumes | ND | ND | ND | ND | ND | ND | ND | ND | ND | ND | ND | ND | ND | ND | ND | ND | ND | ND | ND | ND | ND | ND | ND | ND | 0.00 |
| 薯类 Potatoes | ND | ND | ND | ND | ND | ND | ND | ND | ND | ND | ND | ND | ND | ND | ND | ND | ND | ND | ND | ND | ND | ND | ND | ND | 0.00 |
| 肉类 Meats | ND | ND | ND | ND | ND | ND | 0.29 | ND | ND | ND | ND | ND | ND | ND | ND | ND | ND | ND | ND | ND | ND | ND | ND | ND | 0.01 |
| 蛋类 Eggs | ND | ND | ND | ND | ND | ND | ND | ND | ND | ND | ND | ND | ND | ND | ND | ND | ND | ND | ND | ND | ND | ND | ND | ND | 0.00 |
| 水产类 Aquatic foods | ND | ND | ND | ND | ND | ND | ND | 0.06 | ND | 0.32 | 0.07 | ND | 0.06 | 0.33 | 0.27 | 0.05 | 1.41 | ND | ND | 0.08 | 0.38 | 0.32 | 0.53 | 0.38 | 0.18 |
| 乳类 Dairy products | ND | ND | ND | ND | ND | ND | ND | ND | ND | ND | ND | ND | ND | ND | ND | ND | ND | ND | ND | ND | ND | ND | ND | ND | 0.00 |
| 蔬菜类 Vegetables | ND | ND | ND | 0.08 | ND | 6.70 | ND | 0.11 | 0.15 | ND | 0.18 | ND | 0.07 | ND | 0.31 | 0.08 | 0.09 | ND | ND | ND | 0.08 | ND | ND | ND | 0.34 |
| 水果类 Fruits | 0.11 | 0.10 | 0.26 | 0.13 | 0.05 | ND | ND | ND | ND | ND | ND | 0.07 | ND | 0.35 | ND | ND | 0.07 | ND | 0.23 | ND | ND | 0.10 | 0.20 | ND | 0.07 |
| 糖类 Sugar | ND | ND | ND | ND | ND | ND | ND | ND | ND | ND | ND | ND | ND | ND | ND | ND | ND | ND | ND | ND | ND | ND | 0.13 | ND | 0.00 |
| 水及饮料类 Water and beverages | ND | ND | ND | ND | ND | ND | ND | ND | ND | ND | ND | ND | ND | ND | ND | ND | ND | ND | ND | ND | ND | ND | ND | ND | 0.00 |

续表

| 膳食类别<br>Category | 黑龙江<br>HL | 辽宁<br>LN | 河北<br>HE | 北京<br>BJ | 吉林<br>JL | 山西<br>SX | 陕西<br>SN | 河南<br>HA | 宁夏<br>NX | 内蒙古<br>NM | 青海<br>QH | 甘肃<br>GS | 上海<br>SH | 福建<br>FJ | 江西<br>JX | 江苏<br>JS | 浙江<br>ZJ | 山东<br>SD | 湖北<br>HB | 四川<br>SC | 广西<br>GX | 湖南<br>HN | 广东<br>GD | 贵州<br>GZ | 全国平均<br>AVG |
|---|---|---|---|---|---|---|---|---|---|---|---|---|---|---|---|---|---|---|---|---|---|---|---|---|---|
| 酒类<br>Alcohol beverages | ND | ND | ND | ND | ND | ND | ND | ND | ND | ND | ND | ND | ND | ND | ND | ND | ND | ND | ND | ND | ND | ND | ND | ND | 0.00 |

注: 未检出 (ND) 按 0 计

Note: values not detected (ND) were treated as being equal to 0

附表 4-71 第六次中国总膳食研究膳食样品中吡丙醚的含量（单位：μg/kg）

Annexed Table 4-71 Levels of pyriproxyfen in food samples from the 6th China TDS (Unit: μg/kg)

| 膳食类别<br>Category | 黑龙江<br>HL | 辽宁<br>LN | 河北<br>HE | 北京<br>BJ | 吉林<br>JL | 山西<br>SX | 陕西<br>SN | 河南<br>HA | 宁夏<br>NX | 内蒙古<br>NM | 青海<br>QH | 甘肃<br>GS | 上海<br>SH | 福建<br>FJ | 江西<br>JX | 江苏<br>JS | 浙江<br>ZJ | 山东<br>SD | 湖北<br>HB | 四川<br>SC | 广西<br>GX | 湖南<br>HN | 广东<br>GD | 贵州<br>GZ | 全国平均<br>AVG |
|---|---|---|---|---|---|---|---|---|---|---|---|---|---|---|---|---|---|---|---|---|---|---|---|---|---|
| 谷类<br>Cereals | ND | ND | ND | 0.10 | ND | ND | ND | ND | ND | ND | ND | ND | ND | ND | ND | ND | ND | ND | ND | ND | ND | ND | ND | ND | 0.00 |
| 豆类<br>Legumes | ND | ND | ND | ND | ND | ND | ND | ND | ND | ND | ND | ND | ND | ND | ND | ND | ND | ND | ND | ND | ND | ND | ND | ND | 0.00 |
| 薯类<br>Potatoes | ND | ND | ND | ND | ND | ND | ND | ND | ND | ND | ND | ND | ND | ND | ND | ND | ND | ND | ND | ND | ND | ND | ND | ND | 0.00 |
| 肉类<br>Meats | ND | ND | ND | ND | ND | ND | ND | ND | ND | ND | ND | ND | ND | ND | ND | ND | ND | ND | ND | ND | ND | ND | ND | ND | 0.00 |
| 蛋类<br>Eggs | ND | ND | ND | ND | ND | ND | ND | ND | ND | ND | ND | ND | ND | ND | ND | ND | ND | ND | ND | ND | ND | ND | ND | ND | 0.00 |
| 水产类<br>Aquatic foods | ND | ND | ND | ND | ND | ND | ND | ND | ND | ND | ND | ND | ND | ND | ND | ND | ND | ND | ND | ND | ND | ND | ND | ND | 0.00 |
| 乳类<br>Dairy products | ND | ND | ND | ND | ND | ND | ND | ND | ND | ND | ND | ND | ND | ND | ND | ND | ND | ND | ND | ND | ND | ND | ND | ND | 0.00 |
| 蔬菜类<br>Vegetables | ND | 0.62 | 0.76 | 0.62 | 0.08 | 0.88 | 0.47 | 1.50 | 1.29 | ND | 0.20 | 1.07 | ND | 0.60 | 2.00 | 0.19 | 0.17 | ND | 0.12 | ND | ND | 4.64 | 4.98 | ND | 0.84 |

续表

| 膳食类别<br>Category | 黑龙江<br>HL | 辽宁<br>LN | 河北<br>HE | 北京<br>BJ | 吉林<br>JL | 山西<br>SX | 陕西<br>SN | 河南<br>HA | 宁夏<br>NX | 内蒙古<br>NM | 青海<br>QH | 甘肃<br>GS | 上海<br>SH | 福建<br>FJ | 江西<br>JX | 江苏<br>JS | 浙江<br>ZJ | 山东<br>SD | 湖北<br>HB | 四川<br>SC | 广西<br>GX | 湖南<br>HN | 广东<br>GD | 贵州<br>GZ | 全国平均<br>AVG |
|---|---|---|---|---|---|---|---|---|---|---|---|---|---|---|---|---|---|---|---|---|---|---|---|---|---|
| 水果类 Fruits | 0.13 | ND | ND | 20.34 | ND | ND | ND | ND | ND | ND | ND | ND | ND | ND | ND | ND | ND | ND | ND | ND | ND | ND | ND | ND | 0.85 |
| 糖类 Sugar | ND | ND | ND | ND | ND | ND | ND | ND | ND | ND | ND | ND | ND | ND | ND | ND | ND | ND | ND | ND | ND | ND | ND | ND | 0.00 |
| 水及饮料类 Water and beverages | ND | ND | ND | ND | ND | ND | ND | ND | ND | ND | ND | ND | ND | ND | ND | ND | ND | ND | ND | ND | ND | ND | ND | ND | 0.00 |
| 酒类 Alcohol beverages | ND | ND | ND | ND | ND | ND | ND | ND | ND | ND | ND | ND | ND | ND | ND | ND | ND | ND | ND | ND | ND | ND | ND | ND | 0.00 |

注：未检出（ND）按0计
Note: values not detected (ND) were treated as being equal to 0

附表 4-72 第六次中国总膳食研究的甲氧虫酰肼膳食摄入量 [单位：ng/(kg bw·d)]
Annexed Table 4-72 Dietary intakes of methoxyfenozide from the 6th China TDS [Unit: ng/(kg bw·d)]

| 膳食类别<br>Category | 黑龙江<br>HL | 辽宁<br>LN | 河北<br>HE | 北京<br>BJ | 吉林<br>JL | 山西<br>SX | 陕西<br>SN | 河南<br>HA | 宁夏<br>NX | 内蒙古<br>NM | 青海<br>QH | 甘肃<br>GS | 上海<br>SH | 福建<br>FJ | 江西<br>JX | 江苏<br>JS | 浙江<br>ZJ | 山东<br>SD | 湖北<br>HB | 四川<br>SC | 广西<br>GX | 湖南<br>HN | 广东<br>GD | 贵州<br>GZ | 全国平均<br>AVG |
|---|---|---|---|---|---|---|---|---|---|---|---|---|---|---|---|---|---|---|---|---|---|---|---|---|---|
| 谷类 Cereals | 0.000 | 0.000 | 0.000 | 0.000 | 0.000 | 0.000 | 0.000 | 0.000 | 0.000 | 0.000 | 0.000 | 0.000 | 0.000 | 0.000 | 0.000 | 0.000 | 0.000 | 0.000 | 0.000 | 0.000 | 0.000 | 0.000 | 0.000 | 0.000 | 0.000 |
| 豆类 Legumes | 0.000 | 0.000 | 0.000 | 0.000 | 0.000 | 0.000 | 0.567 | 0.150 | 0.892 | 0.000 | 0.000 | 0.000 | 0.000 | 0.000 | 0.000 | 0.000 | 0.000 | 0.000 | 0.000 | 0.000 | 0.000 | 0.000 | 0.000 | 0.000 | 0.067 |
| 薯类 Potatoes | 0.000 | 0.000 | 0.000 | 0.000 | 0.000 | 0.000 | 0.000 | 0.000 | 0.000 | 0.000 | 0.000 | 0.000 | 0.000 | 0.000 | 0.000 | 0.000 | 0.000 | 0.000 | 0.000 | 0.000 | 0.000 | 0.000 | 0.000 | 0.000 | 0.000 |
| 肉类 Meats | 0.000 | 0.000 | 0.000 | 0.000 | 0.000 | 0.000 | 0.000 | 0.000 | 0.000 | 0.000 | 0.000 | 0.000 | 0.000 | 0.000 | 0.000 | 0.000 | 0.000 | 0.000 | 0.000 | 0.000 | 0.000 | 0.000 | 0.000 | 0.000 | 0.000 |
| 蛋类 Eggs | 0.000 | 0.000 | 0.000 | 0.000 | 0.104 | 0.000 | 0.000 | 0.000 | 0.000 | 0.000 | 0.000 | 0.000 | 0.000 | 0.000 | 0.000 | 0.000 | 0.000 | 0.000 | 0.000 | 0.000 | 0.000 | 0.000 | 0.000 | 0.000 | 0.004 |

续表

| 膳食类别<br>Category | 黑龙江<br>HL | 辽宁<br>LN | 河北<br>HE | 北京<br>BJ | 吉林<br>JL | 山西<br>SX | 陕西<br>SN | 河南<br>HA | 宁夏<br>NX | 内蒙古<br>NM | 青海<br>QH | 甘肃<br>GS | 上海<br>SH | 福建<br>FJ | 江西<br>JX | 江苏<br>JS | 浙江<br>ZJ | 山东<br>SD | 湖北<br>HB | 四川<br>SC | 广西<br>GX | 湖南<br>HN | 广东<br>GD | 贵州<br>GZ | 全国平均<br>AVG |
|---|---|---|---|---|---|---|---|---|---|---|---|---|---|---|---|---|---|---|---|---|---|---|---|---|---|
| 水产类 Aquatic foods | 0.000 | 0.000 | 0.000 | 0.000 | 0.000 | 0.000 | 0.000 | 0.000 | 0.000 | 0.000 | 0.000 | 0.000 | 0.000 | 0.000 | 0.000 | 0.000 | 0.000 | 0.000 | 0.000 | 0.000 | 0.000 | 0.000 | 0.000 | 0.000 | 0.000 |
| 乳类 Dairy products | 0.000 | 0.000 | 0.000 | 0.000 | 0.000 | 0.000 | 0.000 | 0.000 | 0.000 | 0.000 | 0.000 | 0.000 | 0.000 | 0.000 | 0.000 | 0.000 | 0.000 | 0.000 | 0.000 | 0.000 | 0.000 | 0.000 | 0.000 | 0.000 | 0.000 |
| 蔬菜类 Vegetables | 0.000 | 0.000 | 1.001 | 0.000 | 0.000 | 0.000 | 0.000 | 0.000 | 0.000 | 0.000 | 0.510 | 0.000 | 0.000 | 0.000 | 0.000 | 0.000 | 0.000 | 5.196 | 253.100 | 0.000 | 1.524 | 1.734 | 1.430 | 0.000 | 11.020 |
| 水果类 Fruits | 0.000 | 0.000 | 0.000 | 0.000 | 0.000 | 0.000 | 0.000 | 0.000 | 0.000 | 0.000 | 0.000 | 0.000 | 0.000 | 0.000 | 0.000 | 0.000 | 0.000 | 0.000 | 0.000 | 0.027 | 0.000 | 0.000 | 0.000 | 0.000 | 0.001 |
| 糖类 Sugar | 0.000 | 0.000 | 0.000 | 0.000 | 0.000 | 0.000 | 0.000 | 0.000 | 0.000 | 0.000 | 0.000 | 0.000 | 0.014 | 0.000 | 0.000 | 0.000 | 0.000 | 0.000 | 0.000 | 0.000 | 0.000 | 0.000 | 0.000 | 0.000 | 0.001 |
| 水及饮料类 Water and beverages | 0.000 | 0.000 | 0.000 | 0.000 | 0.000 | 0.000 | 0.000 | 0.000 | 0.000 | 0.000 | 0.000 | 0.000 | 0.000 | 0.000 | 0.000 | 0.000 | 0.000 | 0.000 | 0.000 | 0.000 | 0.000 | 0.000 | 0.000 | 0.000 | 0.000 |
| 酒类 Alcohol beverages | 0.000 | 0.000 | 0.000 | 0.000 | 0.000 | 0.000 | 0.000 | 0.000 | 0.000 | 0.000 | 0.000 | 0.000 | 0.000 | 0.000 | 0.000 | 0.000 | 0.000 | 0.000 | 0.000 | 0.000 | 0.000 | 0.000 | 0.001 | 0.000 | 0.000 |
| 合计 SUM | 0.000 | 0.000 | 1.001 | 0.000 | 0.104 | 0.000 | 0.567 | 0.150 | 0.892 | 0.000 | 0.510 | 0.000 | 0.014 | 0.000 | 0.000 | 0.000 | 0.000 | 5.196 | 253.070 | 0.027 | 1.524 | 1.734 | 1.432 | 0.000 | 11.092 |

附表 4-73 第六次中国总膳食研究的噻嗪酮膳食摄入量 [单位: ng/(kg bw·d)]

Annexed Table 4-73 Dietary intakes of buprofezin from the 6<sup>th</sup> China TDS [Unit: ng/(kg bw·d)]

| 膳食类别<br>Category | 黑龙江<br>HL | 辽宁<br>LN | 河北<br>HE | 北京<br>BJ | 吉林<br>JL | 山西<br>SX | 陕西<br>SN | 河南<br>HA | 宁夏<br>NX | 内蒙古<br>NM | 青海<br>QH | 甘肃<br>GS | 上海<br>SH | 福建<br>FJ | 江西<br>JX | 江苏<br>JS | 浙江<br>ZJ | 山东<br>SD | 湖北<br>HB | 四川<br>SC | 广西<br>GX | 湖南<br>HN | 广东<br>GD | 贵州<br>GZ | 全国平均<br>AVG |
|---|---|---|---|---|---|---|---|---|---|---|---|---|---|---|---|---|---|---|---|---|---|---|---|---|---|
| 谷类 Cereals | 0.000 | 0.000 | 0.000 | 0.000 | 0.000 | 0.000 | 0.000 | 0.000 | 0.000 | 0.000 | 0.000 | 0.000 | 0.709 | 0.000 | 2.672 | 0.000 | 2.753 | 0.000 | 0.000 | 0.000 | 2.846 | 0.990 | 0.000 | 0.000 | 0.415 |

续表

| 膳食类别<br>Category | 黑龙江<br>HL | 辽宁<br>LN | 河北<br>HE | 北京<br>BJ | 吉林<br>JL | 山西<br>SX | 陕西<br>SN | 河南<br>HA | 宁夏<br>NX | 内蒙古<br>NM | 青海<br>QH | 甘肃<br>GS | 上海<br>SH | 福建<br>FJ | 江西<br>JX | 江苏<br>JS | 浙江<br>ZJ | 山东<br>SD | 湖北<br>HB | 四川<br>SC | 广西<br>GX | 湖南<br>HN | 广东<br>GD | 贵州<br>GZ | 全国平均<br>AVG |
|---|---|---|---|---|---|---|---|---|---|---|---|---|---|---|---|---|---|---|---|---|---|---|---|---|---|
| 豆类 Legumes | 0.000 | 0.000 | 0.000 | 0.000 | 0.000 | 0.000 | 0.000 | 0.000 | 0.000 | 0.000 | 0.000 | 0.000 | 0.000 | 0.000 | 0.000 | 0.000 | 0.000 | 0.000 | 0.000 | 0.000 | 0.000 | 0.000 | 0.000 | 0.000 | 0.000 |
| 薯类 Potatoes | 0.000 | 0.000 | 0.000 | 0.000 | 0.000 | 0.000 | 0.000 | 0.000 | 0.000 | 0.000 | 0.000 | 0.000 | 0.000 | 0.000 | 0.000 | 0.000 | 0.000 | 0.000 | 0.000 | 0.000 | 0.000 | 0.000 | 0.000 | 0.000 | 0.000 |
| 肉类 Meats | 0.000 | 0.000 | 0.000 | 0.000 | 0.000 | 0.000 | 0.168 | 0.000 | 0.000 | 0.000 | 0.000 | 0.000 | 0.000 | 0.000 | 0.000 | 0.000 | 0.000 | 0.000 | 0.000 | 0.000 | 0.000 | 0.000 | 0.000 | 0.000 | 0.007 |
| 蛋类 Eggs | 0.000 | 0.000 | 0.000 | 0.000 | 0.000 | 0.000 | 0.000 | 0.000 | 0.000 | 0.000 | 0.000 | 0.000 | 0.000 | 0.000 | 0.000 | 0.000 | 0.000 | 0.000 | 0.000 | 0.000 | 0.000 | 0.000 | 0.000 | 0.000 | 0.000 |
| 水产类 Aquatic foods | 0.000 | 0.000 | 0.000 | 0.000 | 0.000 | 0.000 | 0.000 | 0.004 | 0.000 | 0.052 | 0.004 | 0.000 | 0.070 | 0.337 | 0.186 | 0.033 | 1.129 | 0.000 | 0.000 | 0.011 | 0.584 | 0.333 | 0.433 | 0.021 | 0.133 |
| 乳类 Dairy products | 0.000 | 0.000 | 0.000 | 0.000 | 0.000 | 0.000 | 0.000 | 0.000 | 0.000 | 0.000 | 0.000 | 0.000 | 0.000 | 0.000 | 0.000 | 0.000 | 0.000 | 0.000 | 0.000 | 0.000 | 0.000 | 0.000 | 0.000 | 0.000 | 0.000 |
| 蔬菜类 Vegetables | 0.000 | 0.000 | 0.508 | 0.000 | 32.930 | 0.000 | 0.487 | 0.374 | 0.000 | 0.895 | 0.000 | 0.416 | 0.000 | 2.204 | 0.507 | 0.619 | 0.000 | 0.000 | 0.000 | 0.421 | 0.561 | 0.758 | 0.000 | 1.695 |
| 水果类 Fruits | 0.106 | 0.128 | 0.155 | 0.233 | 0.075 | 0.000 | 0.000 | 0.000 | 0.000 | 0.000 | 0.000 | 0.036 | 0.000 | 0.332 | 0.000 | 0.000 | 0.072 | 0.000 | 0.070 | 0.000 | 0.000 | 0.099 | 0.059 | 0.000 | 0.057 |
| 糖类 Sugar | 0.000 | 0.000 | 0.000 | 0.000 | 0.000 | 0.000 | 0.000 | 0.000 | 0.000 | 0.000 | 0.000 | 0.000 | 0.000 | 0.000 | 0.000 | 0.000 | 0.000 | 0.000 | 0.000 | 0.000 | 0.000 | 0.000 | 0.000 | 0.000 | 0.000 |
| 水反饮料类 Water and beverages | 0.000 | 0.000 | 0.000 | 0.000 | 0.000 | 0.000 | 0.000 | 0.000 | 0.000 | 0.000 | 0.000 | 0.000 | 0.000 | 0.000 | 0.000 | 0.000 | 0.000 | 0.000 | 0.000 | 0.000 | 0.000 | 0.000 | 0.000 | 0.000 | 0.000 |
| 酒类 Alcohol beverages | 0.000 | 0.000 | 0.000 | 0.000 | 0.000 | 0.000 | 0.000 | 0.000 | 0.000 | 0.000 | 0.000 | 0.000 | 0.000 | 0.000 | 0.000 | 0.000 | 0.000 | 0.000 | 0.000 | 0.000 | 0.000 | 0.000 | 0.000 | 0.000 | 0.000 |
| 合计 SUM | 0.106 | 0.128 | 0.155 | 0.742 | 0.075 | 32.934 | 0.168 | 0.491 | 0.374 | 0.052 | 0.900 | 0.036 | 1.195 | 0.670 | 5.063 | 0.540 | 4.573 | 0.000 | 0.070 | 0.011 | 3.851 | 1.983 | 1.250 | 0.021 | 2.308 |

附表 4-74 第六次中国总膳食研究的吡丙醚膳食摄入量 [单位: ng/(kg bw·d)]

Annexed Table 4-74 Dietary intakes of pyriproxyfen from the 6th China TDS [Unit: ng/(kg bw·d)]

| 膳食类别<br>Category | 黑龙江<br>HL | 辽宁<br>LN | 河北<br>HE | 北京<br>BJ | 吉林<br>JL | 山西<br>SX | 陕西<br>SN | 河南<br>HA | 宁夏<br>NX | 内蒙古<br>NM | 青海<br>QH | 甘肃<br>GS | 上海<br>SH | 福建<br>FJ | 江西<br>JX | 江苏<br>JS | 浙江<br>ZJ | 山东<br>SD | 湖北<br>HB | 四川<br>SC | 广西<br>GX | 湖南<br>HN | 广东<br>GD | 贵州<br>GZ | 全国平均<br>AVG |
|---|---|---|---|---|---|---|---|---|---|---|---|---|---|---|---|---|---|---|---|---|---|---|---|---|---|
| 谷类 Cereals | 0.000 | 0.000 | 0.000 | 1.265 | 0.000 | 0.000 | 0.000 | 0.000 | 0.000 | 0.000 | 0.000 | 0.000 | 0.000 | 0.000 | 0.000 | 0.000 | 0.000 | 0.000 | 0.000 | 0.000 | 0.000 | 0.000 | 0.000 | 0.000 | 0.053 |
| 豆类 Legumes | 0.000 | 0.000 | 0.000 | 0.000 | 0.000 | 0.000 | 0.000 | 0.000 | 0.000 | 0.000 | 0.000 | 0.000 | 0.000 | 0.000 | 0.000 | 0.000 | 0.000 | 0.000 | 0.000 | 0.000 | 0.000 | 0.000 | 0.000 | 0.000 | 0.000 |
| 薯类 Potatoes | 0.000 | 0.000 | 0.000 | 0.000 | 0.000 | 0.000 | 0.000 | 0.000 | 0.000 | 0.000 | 0.000 | 0.000 | 0.000 | 0.000 | 0.000 | 0.000 | 0.000 | 0.000 | 0.000 | 0.000 | 0.000 | 0.000 | 0.000 | 0.000 | 0.000 |
| 肉类 Meats | 0.000 | 0.000 | 0.000 | 0.000 | 0.000 | 0.000 | 0.000 | 0.000 | 0.000 | 0.000 | 0.000 | 0.000 | 0.000 | 0.000 | 0.000 | 0.000 | 0.000 | 0.000 | 0.000 | 0.000 | 0.000 | 0.000 | 0.000 | 0.000 | 0.000 |
| 蛋类 Eggs | 0.000 | 0.000 | 0.000 | 0.000 | 0.000 | 0.000 | 0.000 | 0.000 | 0.000 | 0.000 | 0.000 | 0.000 | 0.000 | 0.000 | 0.000 | 0.000 | 0.000 | 0.000 | 0.000 | 0.000 | 0.000 | 0.000 | 0.000 | 0.000 | 0.000 |
| 水产类 Aquatic foods | 0.000 | 0.000 | 0.000 | 0.000 | 0.000 | 0.000 | 0.000 | 0.000 | 0.000 | 0.000 | 0.000 | 0.000 | 0.000 | 0.000 | 0.000 | 0.000 | 0.000 | 0.000 | 0.000 | 0.000 | 0.000 | 0.000 | 0.000 | 0.000 | 0.000 |
| 乳类 Dairy products | 0.000 | 0.000 | 0.000 | 0.000 | 0.000 | 0.000 | 0.000 | 0.000 | 0.000 | 0.000 | 0.000 | 0.000 | 0.000 | 0.000 | 0.000 | 0.000 | 0.000 | 0.000 | 0.000 | 0.000 | 0.000 | 0.000 | 0.000 | 0.000 | 0.000 |
| 蔬菜类 Vegetables | 0.000 | 3.206 | 3.537 | 3.834 | 0.467 | 4.334 | 2.143 | 6.619 | 3.199 | 0.000 | 1.000 | 4.232 | 0.000 | 3.760 | 14.30 | 1.303 | 1.225 | 0.000 | 0.796 | 0.000 | 0.000 | 39.36 | 18.700 | 0.000 | 4.667 |
| 水果类 Fruits | 0.132 | 0.000 | 0.000 | 36.68 | 0.000 | 0.000 | 0.000 | 0.000 | 0.000 | 0.000 | 0.000 | 0.000 | 0.000 | 0.000 | 0.000 | 0.000 | 0.000 | 0.000 | 0.000 | 0.000 | 0.000 | 0.000 | 0.000 | 0.000 | 1.534 |
| 糖类 Sugar | 0.000 | 0.000 | 0.000 | 0.000 | 0.000 | 0.000 | 0.000 | 0.000 | 0.000 | 0.000 | 0.000 | 0.000 | 0.000 | 0.000 | 0.000 | 0.000 | 0.000 | 0.000 | 0.000 | 0.000 | 0.000 | 0.000 | 0.000 | 0.000 | 0.000 |
| 水及饮料类 Water and beverages | 0.000 | 0.000 | 0.000 | 0.000 | 0.000 | 0.000 | 0.000 | 0.000 | 0.000 | 0.000 | 0.000 | 0.000 | 0.000 | 0.000 | 0.000 | 0.000 | 0.000 | 0.000 | 0.000 | 0.000 | 0.000 | 0.000 | 0.000 | 0.000 | 0.000 |

续表

| 膳食类别<br>Category | 黑龙江<br>HL | 辽宁<br>LN | 河北<br>HE | 北京<br>BJ | 吉林<br>JL | 山西<br>SX | 陕西<br>SN | 河南<br>HA | 宁夏<br>NX | 内蒙古<br>NM | 青海<br>QH | 甘肃<br>GS | 上海<br>SH | 福建<br>FJ | 江西<br>JX | 江苏<br>JS | 浙江<br>ZJ | 山东<br>SD | 湖北<br>HB | 四川<br>SC | 广西<br>GX | 湖南<br>HN | 广东<br>GD | 贵州<br>GZ | 全国平均<br>AVG |
|---|---|---|---|---|---|---|---|---|---|---|---|---|---|---|---|---|---|---|---|---|---|---|---|---|---|
| 酒类<br>Alcohol beverages | 0.000 | 0.000 | 0.000 | 0.000 | 0.000 | 0.000 | 0.000 | 0.000 | 0.000 | 0.000 | 0.000 | 0.000 | 0.000 | 0.000 | 0.000 | 0.000 | 0.000 | 0.000 | 0.000 | 0.000 | 0.000 | 0.000 | 0.000 | 0.000 | 0.000 |
| 合计<br>SUM | 0.132 | 3.206 | 3.537 | 41.783 | 0.467 | 4.334 | 2.143 | 6.619 | 3.199 | 0.000 | 1.000 | 4.232 | 0.000 | 3.760 | 14.301 | 1.303 | 1.225 | 0.000 | 0.796 | 0.000 | 0.000 | 39.355 | 18.700 | 0.000 | 6.254 |

附表 4-75 第六次中国总膳食研究甲氧虫酰肼的膳食来源（单位：%）

Annexed Table 4-75 Dietary sources of methoxyfenozide from the 6<sup>th</sup> China TDS (Unit: %)

| 膳食类别<br>Category | 黑龙江<br>HL | 辽宁<br>LN | 河北<br>HE | 北京<br>BJ | 吉林<br>JL | 山西<br>SX | 陕西<br>SN | 河南<br>HA | 宁夏<br>NX | 内蒙古<br>NM | 青海<br>QH | 甘肃<br>GS | 上海<br>SH | 福建<br>FJ | 江西<br>JX | 江苏<br>JS | 浙江<br>ZJ | 山东<br>SD | 湖北<br>HB | 四川<br>SC | 广西<br>GX | 湖南<br>HN | 广东<br>GD | 贵州<br>GZ | 全国平均<br>AVG |
|---|---|---|---|---|---|---|---|---|---|---|---|---|---|---|---|---|---|---|---|---|---|---|---|---|---|
| 谷类<br>Cereals | 0.0 | 0.0 | 0.0 | 0.0 | 0.0 | 0.0 | 0.0 | 0.0 | 0.0 | 0.0 | 0.0 | 0.0 | 0.0 | 0.0 | 0.0 | 0.0 | 0.0 | 0.0 | 0.0 | 0.0 | 0.0 | 0.0 | 0.0 | 0.0 | 0.0 |
| 豆类<br>Legumes | 0.0 | 0.0 | 0.0 | 0.0 | 100.0 | 0.0 | 100.0 | 100.0 | 100.0 | 0.0 | 0.0 | 0.0 | 0.0 | 0.0 | 0.0 | 0.0 | 0.0 | 0.0 | 0.0 | 0.0 | 0.0 | 0.0 | 0.0 | 0.0 | 0.6 |
| 薯类<br>Potatoes | 0.0 | 0.0 | 0.0 | 0.0 | 0.0 | 0.0 | 0.0 | 0.0 | 0.0 | 0.0 | 0.0 | 0.0 | 0.0 | 0.0 | 0.0 | 0.0 | 0.0 | 0.0 | 0.0 | 0.0 | 0.0 | 0.0 | 0.0 | 0.0 | 0.0 |
| 肉类<br>Meats | 0.0 | 0.0 | 0.0 | 0.0 | 0.0 | 0.0 | 0.0 | 0.0 | 0.0 | 0.0 | 0.0 | 0.0 | 0.0 | 0.0 | 0.0 | 0.0 | 0.0 | 0.0 | 0.0 | 0.0 | 0.0 | 0.0 | 0.0 | 0.0 | 0.0 |
| 蛋类<br>Eggs | 0.0 | 0.0 | 0.0 | 0.0 | 0.0 | 0.0 | 0.0 | 0.0 | 0.0 | 0.0 | 0.0 | 0.0 | 0.0 | 0.0 | 0.0 | 0.0 | 0.0 | 0.0 | 0.0 | 0.0 | 0.0 | 0.0 | 0.0 | 0.0 | 0.0 |
| 水产类<br>Aquatic foods | 0.0 | 0.0 | 0.0 | 0.0 | 0.0 | 0.0 | 0.0 | 0.0 | 0.0 | 0.0 | 0.0 | 0.0 | 0.0 | 0.0 | 0.0 | 0.0 | 0.0 | 0.0 | 0.0 | 0.0 | 0.0 | 0.0 | 0.0 | 0.0 | 0.0 |
| 乳类<br>Dairy products | 0.0 | 0.0 | 0.0 | 0.0 | 0.0 | 0.0 | 0.0 | 0.0 | 0.0 | 0.0 | 0.0 | 0.0 | 0.0 | 0.0 | 0.0 | 0.0 | 0.0 | 0.0 | 0.0 | 0.0 | 0.0 | 0.0 | 0.0 | 0.0 | 0.0 |

续表

| 膳食类别<br>Category | 黑龙江<br>HL | 辽宁<br>LN | 河北<br>HE | 北京<br>BJ | 吉林<br>JL | 山西<br>SX | 陕西<br>SN | 河南<br>HA | 宁夏<br>NX | 内蒙古<br>NM | 青海<br>QH | 甘肃<br>GS | 上海<br>SH | 福建<br>FJ | 江西<br>JX | 江苏<br>JS | 浙江<br>ZJ | 山东<br>SD | 湖北<br>HB | 四川<br>SC | 广西<br>GX | 湖南<br>HN | 广东<br>GD | 贵州<br>GZ | 全国平均<br>AVG |
|---|---|---|---|---|---|---|---|---|---|---|---|---|---|---|---|---|---|---|---|---|---|---|---|---|---|
| 蔬菜类 Vegetables | 0.0 | 0.0 | 100.0 | 0.0 | 0.0 | 0.0 | 0.0 | 0.0 | 0.0 | 0.0 | 100.0 | 0.0 | 0.0 | 0.0 | 0.0 | 0.0 | 0.0 | 100.0 | 100.0 | 0.0 | 100.0 | 100.0 | 99.9 | 0.0 | 99.3 |
| 水果类 Fruits | 0.0 | 0.0 | 0.0 | 0.0 | 0.0 | 0.0 | 0.0 | 0.0 | 0.0 | 0.0 | 0.0 | 0.0 | 0.0 | 0.0 | 0.0 | 0.0 | 0.0 | 0.0 | 0.0 | 100.0 | 0.0 | 0.0 | 0.0 | 0.0 | 0.0 |
| 糖类 Sugar | 0.0 | 0.0 | 0.0 | 0.0 | 0.0 | 0.0 | 0.0 | 0.0 | 0.0 | 0.0 | 0.0 | 0.0 | 100.0 | 0.0 | 0.0 | 0.0 | 0.0 | 0.0 | 0.0 | 0.0 | 0.0 | 0.0 | 0.0 | 0.0 | 0.0 |
| 水及饮料类 Water and beverages | 0.0 | 0.0 | 0.0 | 0.0 | 0.0 | 0.0 | 0.0 | 0.0 | 0.0 | 0.0 | 0.0 | 0.0 | 0.0 | 0.0 | 0.0 | 0.0 | 0.0 | 0.0 | 0.0 | 0.0 | 0.0 | 0.0 | 0.0 | 0.0 | 0.0 |
| 酒类 Alcohol beverages | 0.0 | 0.0 | 0.0 | 0.0 | 0.0 | 0.0 | 0.0 | 0.0 | 0.0 | 0.0 | 0.0 | 0.0 | 0.0 | 0.0 | 0.0 | 0.0 | 0.0 | 0.0 | 0.0 | 0.0 | 0.0 | 0.0 | 0.1 | 0.0 | 0.0 |

附表 4-76 第六次中国总膳食研究噻嗪酮的膳食来源（单位：%）

Annexed Table 4-76 Dietary sources of buprofezin from the 6$^{th}$ China TDS (Unit: %)

| 膳食类别<br>Category | 黑龙江<br>HL | 辽宁<br>LN | 河北<br>HE | 北京<br>BJ | 吉林<br>JL | 山西<br>SX | 陕西<br>SN | 河南<br>HA | 宁夏<br>NX | 内蒙古<br>NM | 青海<br>QH | 甘肃<br>GS | 上海<br>SH | 福建<br>FJ | 江西<br>JX | 江苏<br>JS | 浙江<br>ZJ | 山东<br>SD | 湖北<br>HB | 四川<br>SC | 广西<br>GX | 湖南<br>HN | 广东<br>GD | 贵州<br>GZ | 全国平均<br>AVG |
|---|---|---|---|---|---|---|---|---|---|---|---|---|---|---|---|---|---|---|---|---|---|---|---|---|---|
| 谷类 Cereals | 0.0 | 0.0 | 0.0 | 0.0 | 0.0 | 0.0 | 0.0 | 0.0 | 0.0 | 0.0 | 0.0 | 0.0 | 59.3 | 0.0 | 52.8 | 0.0 | 60.2 | 0.0 | 0.0 | 0.0 | 73.9 | 49.9 | 0.0 | 0.0 | 18.0 |
| 豆类 Legumes | 0.0 | 0.0 | 0.0 | 0.0 | 0.0 | 0.0 | 0.0 | 0.0 | 0.0 | 0.0 | 0.0 | 0.0 | 0.0 | 0.0 | 0.0 | 0.0 | 0.0 | 0.0 | 0.0 | 0.0 | 0.0 | 0.0 | 0.0 | 0.0 | 0.0 |
| 薯类 Potatoes | 0.0 | 0.0 | 0.0 | 0.0 | 0.0 | 0.0 | 0.0 | 0.0 | 0.0 | 0.0 | 0.0 | 0.0 | 0.0 | 0.0 | 0.0 | 0.0 | 0.0 | 0.0 | 0.0 | 0.0 | 0.0 | 0.0 | 0.0 | 0.0 | 0.0 |
| 肉类 Meats | 0.0 | 0.0 | 0.0 | 0.0 | 0.0 | 0.0 | 100.0 | 0.0 | 0.0 | 0.0 | 0.0 | 0.0 | 0.0 | 0.0 | 0.0 | 0.0 | 0.0 | 0.0 | 0.0 | 0.0 | 0.0 | 0.0 | 0.0 | 0.0 | 0.3 |
| 蛋类 Eggs | 0.0 | 0.0 | 0.0 | 0.0 | 0.0 | 0.0 | 0.0 | 0.0 | 0.0 | 0.0 | 0.0 | 0.0 | 0.0 | 0.0 | 0.0 | 0.0 | 0.0 | 0.0 | 0.0 | 0.0 | 0.0 | 0.0 | 0.0 | 0.0 | 0.0 |

续表

| 膳食类别<br>Category | 黑龙江<br>HL | 辽宁<br>LN | 河北<br>HE | 北京<br>BJ | 吉林<br>JL | 山西<br>SX | 陕西<br>SN | 河南<br>HA | 宁夏<br>NX | 内蒙古<br>NM | 青海<br>QH | 甘肃<br>GS | 上海<br>SH | 福建<br>FJ | 江西<br>JX | 江苏<br>JS | 浙江<br>ZJ | 山东<br>SD | 湖北<br>HB | 四川<br>SC | 广西<br>GX | 湖南<br>HN | 广东<br>GD | 贵州<br>GZ | 全国平均<br>AVG |
|---|---|---|---|---|---|---|---|---|---|---|---|---|---|---|---|---|---|---|---|---|---|---|---|---|---|
| 水产类<br>Aquatic foods | 0.0 | 0.0 | 0.0 | 0.0 | 0.0 | 0.0 | 0.0 | 0.8 | 0.0 | 100.0 | 0.5 | 0.0 | 5.9 | 50.4 | 3.7 | 6.2 | 24.7 | 0.0 | 0.0 | 100.0 | 15.2 | 16.8 | 34.6 | 100.0 | 5.8 |
| 乳类<br>Dairy products | 0.0 | 0.0 | 0.0 | 0.0 | 0.0 | 0.0 | 0.0 | 0.0 | 0.0 | 0.0 | 0.0 | 0.0 | 0.0 | 0.0 | 0.0 | 0.0 | 0.0 | 0.0 | 0.0 | 0.0 | 0.0 | 0.0 | 0.0 | 0.0 | 0.0 |
| 蔬菜类<br>Vegetables | 0.0 | 0.0 | 0.0 | 68.5 | 0.0 | 100.0 | 0.0 | 99.2 | 100.0 | 0.0 | 99.5 | 0.0 | 34.8 | 0.0 | 43.5 | 93.8 | 13.5 | 0.0 | 0.0 | 0.0 | 10.9 | 28.3 | 60.7 | 0.0 | 73.5 |
| 水果类<br>Fruits | 100.0 | 100.0 | 100.0 | 31.5 | 100.0 | 0.0 | 0.0 | 0.0 | 0.0 | 0.0 | 0.0 | 100.0 | 0.0 | 49.6 | 0.0 | 0.0 | 1.6 | 0.0 | 100.0 | 0.0 | 0.0 | 5.0 | 4.7 | 0.0 | 2.5 |
| 糖类<br>Sugar | 0.0 | 0.0 | 0.0 | 0.0 | 0.0 | 0.0 | 0.0 | 0.0 | 0.0 | 0.0 | 0.0 | 0.0 | 0.0 | 0.0 | 0.0 | 0.0 | 0.0 | 0.0 | 0.0 | 0.0 | 0.0 | 0.0 | 0.0 | 0.0 | 0.0 |
| 水及饮料类<br>Water and beverages | 0.0 | 0.0 | 0.0 | 0.0 | 0.0 | 0.0 | 0.0 | 0.0 | 0.0 | 0.0 | 0.0 | 0.0 | 0.0 | 0.0 | 0.0 | 0.0 | 0.0 | 0.0 | 0.0 | 0.0 | 0.0 | 0.0 | 0.0 | 0.0 | 0.0 |
| 酒类<br>Alcohol beverages | 0.0 | 0.0 | 0.0 | 0.0 | 0.0 | 0.0 | 0.0 | 0.0 | 0.0 | 0.0 | 0.0 | 0.0 | 0.0 | 0.0 | 0.0 | 0.0 | 0.0 | 0.0 | 0.0 | 0.0 | 0.0 | 0.0 | 0.0 | 0.0 | 0.0 |

附表 4-77 第六次中国总膳食研究吡丙醚的膳食来源（单位：%）

Annexed Table 4-77 Dietary sources of pyriproxyfen from the 6$^{th}$ China TDS (Unit: %)

| 膳食类别<br>Category | 黑龙江<br>HL | 辽宁<br>LN | 河北<br>HE | 北京<br>BJ | 吉林<br>JL | 山西<br>SX | 陕西<br>SN | 河南<br>HA | 宁夏<br>NX | 内蒙古<br>NM | 青海<br>QH | 甘肃<br>GS | 上海<br>SH | 福建<br>FJ | 江西<br>JX | 江苏<br>JS | 浙江<br>ZJ | 山东<br>SD | 湖北<br>HB | 四川<br>SC | 广西<br>GX | 湖南<br>HN | 广东<br>GD | 贵州<br>GZ | 全国平均<br>AVG |
|---|---|---|---|---|---|---|---|---|---|---|---|---|---|---|---|---|---|---|---|---|---|---|---|---|---|
| 谷类<br>Cereals | 0.0 | 0.0 | 0.0 | 3.0 | 0.0 | 0.0 | 0.0 | 0.0 | 0.0 | 0.0 | 0.0 | 0.0 | 0.0 | 0.0 | 0.0 | 0.0 | 0.0 | 0.0 | 0.0 | 0.0 | 0.0 | 0.0 | 0.0 | 0.0 | 0.8 |

续表

| 膳食类别<br>Category | 黑龙江<br>HL | 辽宁<br>LN | 河北<br>HE | 北京<br>BJ | 吉林<br>JL | 山西<br>SX | 陕西<br>SN | 河南<br>HA | 宁夏<br>NX | 内蒙古<br>NM | 青海<br>QH | 甘肃<br>GS | 上海<br>SH | 福建<br>FJ | 江西<br>JX | 江苏<br>JS | 浙江<br>ZJ | 山东<br>SD | 湖北<br>HB | 四川<br>SC | 广西<br>GX | 湖南<br>HN | 广东<br>GD | 贵州<br>GZ | 全国平均<br>AVG |
|---|---|---|---|---|---|---|---|---|---|---|---|---|---|---|---|---|---|---|---|---|---|---|---|---|---|
| 豆类 Legumes | 0.0 | 0.0 | 0.0 | 0.0 | 0.0 | 0.0 | 0.0 | 0.0 | 0.0 | 0.0 | 0.0 | 0.0 | 0.0 | 0.0 | 0.0 | 0.0 | 0.0 | 0.0 | 0.0 | 0.0 | 0.0 | 0.0 | 0.0 | 0.0 | 0.0 |
| 薯类 Potatoes | 0.0 | 0.0 | 0.0 | 0.0 | 0.0 | 0.0 | 0.0 | 0.0 | 0.0 | 0.0 | 0.0 | 0.0 | 0.0 | 0.0 | 0.0 | 0.0 | 0.0 | 0.0 | 0.0 | 0.0 | 0.0 | 0.0 | 0.0 | 0.0 | 0.0 |
| 肉类 Meats | 0.0 | 0.0 | 0.0 | 0.0 | 0.0 | 0.0 | 0.0 | 0.0 | 0.0 | 0.0 | 0.0 | 0.0 | 0.0 | 0.0 | 0.0 | 0.0 | 0.0 | 0.0 | 0.0 | 0.0 | 0.0 | 0.0 | 0.0 | 0.0 | 0.0 |
| 蛋类 Eggs | 0.0 | 0.0 | 0.0 | 0.0 | 0.0 | 0.0 | 0.0 | 0.0 | 0.0 | 0.0 | 0.0 | 0.0 | 0.0 | 0.0 | 0.0 | 0.0 | 0.0 | 0.0 | 0.0 | 0.0 | 0.0 | 0.0 | 0.0 | 0.0 | 0.0 |
| 水产类 Aquatic foods | 0.0 | 0.0 | 0.0 | 0.0 | 0.0 | 0.0 | 0.0 | 0.0 | 0.0 | 0.0 | 0.0 | 0.0 | 0.0 | 0.0 | 0.0 | 0.0 | 0.0 | 0.0 | 0.0 | 0.0 | 0.0 | 0.0 | 0.0 | 0.0 | 0.0 |
| 乳类 Dairy products | 0.0 | 0.0 | 0.0 | 0.0 | 0.0 | 0.0 | 0.0 | 0.0 | 0.0 | 0.0 | 0.0 | 0.0 | 0.0 | 0.0 | 0.0 | 0.0 | 0.0 | 0.0 | 0.0 | 0.0 | 0.0 | 0.0 | 0.0 | 0.0 | 0.0 |
| 蔬菜类 Vegetables | 0.0 | 100.0 | 100.0 | 9.2 | 100.0 | 100.0 | 100.0 | 100.0 | 100.0 | 0.0 | 100.0 | 100.0 | 0.0 | 100.0 | 100.0 | 100.0 | 100.0 | 0.0 | 100.0 | 0.0 | 0.0 | 100.0 | 100.0 | 0.0 | 74.6 |
| 水果类 Fruits | 100.0 | 0.0 | 0.0 | 87.8 | 0.0 | 0.0 | 0.0 | 0.0 | 0.0 | 0.0 | 0.0 | 0.0 | 0.0 | 0.0 | 0.0 | 0.0 | 0.0 | 0.0 | 0.0 | 0.0 | 0.0 | 0.0 | 0.0 | 0.0 | 24.5 |
| 糖类 Sugar | 0.0 | 0.0 | 0.0 | 0.0 | 0.0 | 0.0 | 0.0 | 0.0 | 0.0 | 0.0 | 0.0 | 0.0 | 0.0 | 0.0 | 0.0 | 0.0 | 0.0 | 0.0 | 0.0 | 0.0 | 0.0 | 0.0 | 0.0 | 0.0 | 0.0 |
| 水及饮料类 Water and beverages | 0.0 | 0.0 | 0.0 | 0.0 | 0.0 | 0.0 | 0.0 | 0.0 | 0.0 | 0.0 | 0.0 | 0.0 | 0.0 | 0.0 | 0.0 | 0.0 | 0.0 | 0.0 | 0.0 | 0.0 | 0.0 | 0.0 | 0.0 | 0.0 | 0.0 |
| 酒类 Alcohol beverages | 0.0 | 0.0 | 0.0 | 0.0 | 0.0 | 0.0 | 0.0 | 0.0 | 0.0 | 0.0 | 0.0 | 0.0 | 0.0 | 0.0 | 0.0 | 0.0 | 0.0 | 0.0 | 0.0 | 0.0 | 0.0 | 0.0 | 0.0 | 0.0 | 0.0 |

附表 4-78 第六次中国总膳食研究膳食样品中粉唑醇的含量（单位：μg/kg）

Annexed Table 4-78 Levels of flutriafol in food samples from the 6$^{th}$ China TDS (Unit: μg/kg)

| 膳食类别 Category | 黑龙江 HL | 辽宁 LN | 河北 HE | 北京 BJ | 吉林 JL | 山西 SX | 陕西 SN | 河南 HA | 宁夏 NX | 内蒙古 NM | 青海 QH | 甘肃 GS | 上海 SH | 福建 FJ | 江西 JX | 江苏 JS | 浙江 ZJ | 山东 SD | 湖北 HB | 四川 SC | 广西 GX | 湖南 HN | 广东 GD | 贵州 GZ | 全国平均 AVG |
|---|---|---|---|---|---|---|---|---|---|---|---|---|---|---|---|---|---|---|---|---|---|---|---|---|---|
| 谷类 Cereals | ND | ND | ND | ND | ND | ND | ND | ND | ND | ND | ND | ND | ND | ND | ND | ND | ND | ND | ND | ND | ND | ND | ND | ND | 0.00 |
| 豆类 Legumes | ND | ND | ND | ND | ND | ND | ND | ND | ND | ND | ND | ND | ND | ND | ND | ND | ND | ND | ND | ND | ND | ND | ND | ND | 0.00 |
| 薯类 Potatoes | ND | ND | ND | ND | 0.12 | ND | ND | ND | ND | ND | ND | ND | ND | ND | ND | ND | ND | ND | ND | ND | ND | ND | ND | ND | 0.01 |
| 肉类 Meats | ND | ND | ND | ND | 0.10 | ND | ND | ND | ND | ND | ND | ND | ND | ND | ND | ND | ND | ND | ND | ND | ND | ND | ND | ND | 0.00 |
| 蛋类 Eggs | ND | ND | ND | ND | ND | ND | ND | ND | ND | ND | ND | ND | ND | ND | ND | ND | ND | ND | ND | ND | ND | ND | ND | ND | 0.00 |
| 水产类 Aquatic foods | ND | ND | ND | ND | 0.08 | ND | ND | ND | ND | ND | ND | ND | ND | ND | ND | ND | ND | ND | ND | ND | ND | ND | ND | ND | 0.00 |
| 乳类 Dairy products | ND | ND | ND | ND | ND | ND | ND | ND | ND | ND | ND | ND | ND | ND | ND | ND | ND | ND | ND | ND | ND | ND | ND | ND | 0.00 |
| 蔬菜类 Vegetables | ND | ND | ND | ND | 0.06 | 0.67 | ND | ND | ND | ND | 0.86 | ND | 0.11 | ND | ND | ND | ND | ND | ND | ND | ND | ND | 0.14 | 0.08 | 0.08 |
| 水果类 Fruits | ND | ND | ND | ND | ND | ND | ND | ND | ND | ND | 0.21 | ND | ND | ND | ND | ND | ND | ND | ND | ND | ND | ND | 0.32 | ND | 0.02 |
| 糖类 Sugar | ND | ND | ND | ND | ND | ND | ND | ND | ND | ND | ND | ND | ND | ND | ND | ND | ND | ND | ND | ND | ND | ND | ND | ND | 0.00 |
| 水及饮料类 Water and beverages | ND | ND | ND | ND | ND | ND | ND | ND | ND | ND | ND | ND | ND | ND | ND | ND | ND | ND | ND | ND | ND | ND | ND | ND | 0.00 |

续表

| 膳食类别<br>Category | 黑龙江<br>HL | 辽宁<br>LN | 河北<br>HE | 北京<br>BJ | 吉林<br>JL | 山西<br>SX | 陕西<br>SN | 河南<br>HA | 宁夏<br>NX | 内蒙古<br>NM | 青海<br>QH | 甘肃<br>GS | 上海<br>SH | 福建<br>FJ | 江西<br>JX | 江苏<br>JS | 浙江<br>ZJ | 山东<br>SD | 湖北<br>HB | 四川<br>SC | 广西<br>GX | 湖南<br>HN | 广东<br>GD | 贵州<br>GZ | 全国平均<br>AVG |
|---|---|---|---|---|---|---|---|---|---|---|---|---|---|---|---|---|---|---|---|---|---|---|---|---|---|
| 酒类<br>Alcohol beverages | ND | ND | ND | ND | ND | ND | ND | ND | ND | ND | ND | ND | ND | ND | ND | ND | ND | ND | ND | ND | ND | ND | ND | ND | 0.00 |

注：未检出（ND）按 0 计

Note: values not detected (ND) were treated as being equal to 0

附表 4-79 第六次中国总膳食研究膳食样品中腈菌唑的含量（单位：μg/kg）

Annexed Table 4-79 Levels of myclobutanil in food samples from the 6th China TDS (Unit: μg/kg)

| 膳食类别<br>Category | 黑龙江<br>HL | 辽宁<br>LN | 河北<br>HE | 北京<br>BJ | 吉林<br>JL | 山西<br>SX | 陕西<br>SN | 河南<br>HA | 宁夏<br>NX | 内蒙古<br>NM | 青海<br>QH | 甘肃<br>GS | 上海<br>SH | 福建<br>FJ | 江西<br>JX | 江苏<br>JS | 浙江<br>ZJ | 山东<br>SD | 湖北<br>HB | 四川<br>SC | 广西<br>GX | 湖南<br>HN | 广东<br>GD | 贵州<br>GZ | 全国平均<br>AVG |
|---|---|---|---|---|---|---|---|---|---|---|---|---|---|---|---|---|---|---|---|---|---|---|---|---|---|
| 谷类<br>Cereals | ND | ND | ND | ND | ND | ND | ND | ND | ND | ND | ND | ND | ND | ND | ND | ND | ND | ND | ND | ND | ND | ND | ND | ND | 0.00 |
| 豆类<br>Legumes | ND | ND | ND | ND | ND | ND | ND | ND | ND | ND | ND | ND | ND | ND | ND | ND | ND | ND | ND | ND | ND | ND | ND | ND | 0.00 |
| 薯类<br>Potatoes | ND | ND | ND | ND | ND | ND | ND | ND | ND | ND | ND | ND | ND | ND | ND | ND | ND | ND | ND | ND | ND | ND | ND | ND | 0.00 |
| 肉类<br>Meats | ND | ND | ND | ND | ND | ND | ND | ND | ND | ND | ND | ND | ND | ND | ND | 0.07 | ND | ND | ND | ND | ND | ND | ND | ND | 0.00 |
| 蛋类<br>Eggs | ND | ND | ND | ND | ND | ND | ND | ND | ND | ND | ND | ND | ND | ND | ND | 0.10 | ND | ND | ND | ND | ND | ND | ND | ND | 0.00 |
| 水产类<br>Aquatic foods | ND | ND | ND | ND | ND | 0.16 | ND | ND | ND | ND | ND | ND | ND | ND | ND | ND | ND | ND | ND | ND | ND | ND | ND | ND | 0.01 |
| 乳类<br>Dairy products | ND | ND | ND | ND | ND | ND | ND | ND | ND | ND | ND | ND | ND | ND | ND | ND | ND | ND | ND | ND | ND | ND | ND | ND | 0.00 |

续表

| 膳食类别 Category | 黑龙江 HL | 辽宁 LN | 河北 HE | 北京 BJ | 吉林 JL | 山西 SX | 陕西 SN | 河南 HA | 宁夏 NX | 内蒙古 NM | 青海 QH | 甘肃 GS | 上海 SH | 福建 FJ | 江西 JX | 江苏 JS | 浙江 ZJ | 山东 SD | 湖北 HB | 四川 SC | 广西 GX | 湖南 HN | 广东 GD | 贵州 GZ | 全国平均 AVG |
|---|---|---|---|---|---|---|---|---|---|---|---|---|---|---|---|---|---|---|---|---|---|---|---|---|---|
| 蔬菜类 Vegetables | ND | ND | 0.06 | ND | 0.33 | 0.50 | 0.13 | 0.11 | 1.38 | 0.11 | 1.10 | 0.21 | ND | ND | ND | 0.09 | ND | ND | 0.14 | ND | 1.35 | 0.38 | 0.15 | ND | 0.25 |
| 水果类 Fruits | ND | 1.74 | ND | ND | 0.45 | ND | ND | ND | ND | 0.20 | ND | ND | 0.33 | 0.19 | 0.05 | ND | ND | ND | ND | ND | ND | ND | 1.52 | ND | 0.19 |
| 糖类 Sugar | ND | ND | ND | ND | ND | ND | ND | ND | ND | ND | ND | ND | ND | ND | ND | ND | ND | ND | ND | ND | ND | ND | ND | ND | 0.00 |
| 水及饮料类 Water and beverages | ND | ND | ND | ND | ND | ND | ND | ND | ND | ND | ND | ND | ND | ND | ND | ND | ND | ND | ND | ND | ND | ND | ND | ND | 0.00 |
| 酒类 Alcohol beverages | ND | 0.09 | ND | ND | ND | ND | ND | ND | ND | ND | ND | ND | ND | ND | ND | ND | ND | ND | ND | ND | 0.11 | ND | ND | ND | 0.01 |

注：未检出（ND）按 0 计

Note: values not detected (ND) were treated as being equal to 0

附表 4-80　第六次中国总膳食研究膳食样品中三唑醇的含量（单位：μg/kg）

Annexed Table 4-80　Levels of triadimenol in food samples from the 6$^{th}$ China TDS (Unit: μg/kg)

| 膳食类别 Category | 黑龙江 HL | 辽宁 LN | 河北 HE | 北京 BJ | 吉林 JL | 山西 SX | 陕西 SN | 河南 HA | 宁夏 NX | 内蒙古 NM | 青海 QH | 甘肃 GS | 上海 SH | 福建 FJ | 江西 JX | 江苏 JS | 浙江 ZJ | 山东 SD | 湖北 HB | 四川 SC | 广西 GX | 湖南 HN | 广东 GD | 贵州 GZ | 全国平均 AVG |
|---|---|---|---|---|---|---|---|---|---|---|---|---|---|---|---|---|---|---|---|---|---|---|---|---|---|
| 谷类 Cereals | ND | ND | ND | ND | ND | ND | ND | ND | ND | ND | ND | ND | 0.30 | ND | 0.14 | 0.52 | 1.36 | ND | ND | ND | ND | ND | 0.82 | 0.41 | 0.15 |
| 豆类 Legumes | ND | ND | ND | ND | ND | ND | ND | ND | ND | ND | ND | ND | ND | ND | ND | ND | ND | ND | ND | ND | ND | ND | ND | ND | 0.00 |
| 薯类 Potatoes | ND | ND | ND | ND | 1.61 | ND | ND | ND | ND | ND | ND | ND | 0.12 | 2.40 | ND | ND | ND | ND | ND | ND | ND | ND | ND | ND | 0.07 |
| 肉类 Meats | ND | ND | ND | ND | ND | ND | ND | ND | ND | ND | ND | ND | ND | ND | ND | ND | ND | ND | 2.18 | ND | ND | ND | 1.56 | ND | 0.26 |

续表

| 膳食类别<br>Category | 黑龙江<br>HL | 辽宁<br>LN | 河北<br>HE | 北京<br>BJ | 吉林<br>JL | 山西<br>SX | 陕西<br>SN | 河南<br>HA | 宁夏<br>NX | 内蒙古<br>NM | 青海<br>QH | 甘肃<br>GS | 上海<br>SH | 福建<br>FJ | 江西<br>JX | 江苏<br>JS | 浙江<br>ZJ | 山东<br>SD | 湖北<br>HB | 四川<br>SC | 广西<br>GX | 湖南<br>HN | 广东<br>GD | 贵州<br>GZ | 全国平均<br>AVG |
|---|---|---|---|---|---|---|---|---|---|---|---|---|---|---|---|---|---|---|---|---|---|---|---|---|---|
| 蛋类 Eggs | ND | ND | ND | ND | ND | ND | ND | ND | ND | ND | ND | ND | ND | ND | ND | ND | ND | ND | 4.17 | ND | ND | ND | ND | ND | 0.17 |
| 水产类 Aquatic foods | ND | ND | ND | ND | ND | ND | ND | ND | ND | 0.11 | ND | ND | 0.13 | ND | ND | ND | ND | ND | 2.83 | ND | ND | ND | ND | 0.23 | 0.14 |
| 乳类 Dairy products | ND | ND | ND | ND | ND | ND | ND | ND | ND | ND | ND | ND | ND | ND | ND | ND | ND | ND | ND | ND | ND | ND | ND | ND | 0.00 |
| 蔬菜类 Vegetables | ND | ND | 3.14 | ND | ND | 7.16 | ND | 1.65 | ND | ND | ND | 0.48 | ND | 0.53 | 2.98 | 0.20 | ND | ND | 6.46 | ND | 0.53 | ND | 10.76 | 0.31 | 1.42 |
| 水果类 Fruits | ND | ND | ND | 1.65 | 0.18 | ND | ND | ND | 0.12 | ND | ND | ND | ND | ND | ND | 0.11 | ND | ND | ND | ND | ND | ND | ND | ND | 0.09 |
| 糖类 Sugar | ND | ND | ND | ND | ND | ND | ND | ND | ND | ND | ND | ND | ND | ND | ND | ND | ND | ND | ND | ND | ND | ND | ND | ND | 0.00 |
| 水及饮料类 Water and beverages | ND | ND | ND | ND | ND | ND | 0.14 | ND | ND | ND | ND | ND | ND | ND | ND | ND | ND | ND | ND | ND | 0.26 | ND | ND | ND | 0.01 |
| 酒类 Alcohol beverages | ND | ND | ND | ND | ND | ND | ND | ND | ND | ND | ND | ND | ND | ND | ND | ND | ND | ND | ND | ND | ND | ND | ND | ND | 0.01 |

注：未检出（ND）按 0 计

Note: values not detected (ND) were treated as being equal to 0

附表 4-81　第六次中国总膳食研究膳食样品中三唑酮的含量（单位：μg/kg）

Annexed Table 4-81　Levels of triadimefon in food samples from the 6th China TDS (Unit: μg/kg)

| 膳食类别<br>Category | 黑龙江<br>HL | 辽宁<br>LN | 河北<br>HE | 北京<br>BJ | 吉林<br>JL | 山西<br>SX | 陕西<br>SN | 河南<br>HA | 宁夏<br>NX | 内蒙古<br>NM | 青海<br>QH | 甘肃<br>GS | 上海<br>SH | 福建<br>FJ | 江西<br>JX | 江苏<br>JS | 浙江<br>ZJ | 山东<br>SD | 湖北<br>HB | 四川<br>SC | 广西<br>GX | 湖南<br>HN | 广东<br>GD | 贵州<br>GZ | 全国平均<br>AVG |
|---|---|---|---|---|---|---|---|---|---|---|---|---|---|---|---|---|---|---|---|---|---|---|---|---|---|
| 谷类 Cereals | ND | ND | ND | ND | ND | ND | ND | ND | ND | ND | ND | ND | 0.38 | ND | 0.14 | 0.52 | 1.66 | ND | ND | ND | ND | ND | 0.82 | 0.41 | 0.16 |

续表

| 膳食类别 Category | 黑龙江 HL | 辽宁 LN | 河北 HE | 北京 BJ | 吉林 JL | 山西 SX | 陕西 SN | 河南 HA | 宁夏 NX | 内蒙古 NM | 青海 QH | 甘肃 GS | 上海 SH | 福建 FJ | 江西 JX | 江苏 JS | 浙江 ZJ | 山东 SD | 湖北 HB | 四川 SC | 广西 GX | 湖南 HN | 广东 GD | 贵州 GZ | 全国平均 AVG |
|---|---|---|---|---|---|---|---|---|---|---|---|---|---|---|---|---|---|---|---|---|---|---|---|---|---|
| 豆类 Legumes | ND | ND | ND | ND | ND | ND | ND | ND | ND | ND | ND | ND | ND | ND | ND | ND | ND | ND | ND | ND | ND | ND | ND | ND | 0.00 |
| 薯类 Potatoes | ND | ND | ND | ND | 1.68 | ND | ND | ND | ND | ND | ND | ND | ND | ND | ND | ND | ND | ND | ND | ND | ND | ND | ND | ND | 0.07 |
| 肉类 Meats | ND | ND | ND | ND | ND | ND | ND | ND | ND | ND | ND | ND | 0.12 | 2.40 | ND | ND | ND | ND | 2.18 | ND | ND | ND | 1.56 | ND | 0.26 |
| 蛋类 Eggs | ND | ND | ND | 1.65 | 0.18 | ND | ND | ND | ND | ND | ND | ND | ND | ND | ND | ND | ND | ND | 4.17 | ND | ND | ND | ND | ND | 0.17 |
| 水产类 Aquatic foods | ND | ND | ND | ND | ND | ND | ND | ND | ND | 0.11 | ND | ND | 0.13 | ND | ND | ND | ND | ND | 2.83 | ND | ND | ND | ND | 0.23 | 0.14 |
| 乳类 Dairy products | ND | ND | ND | ND | ND | ND | ND | ND | ND | ND | ND | ND | ND | ND | ND | ND | ND | ND | ND | ND | ND | ND | ND | ND | 0.00 |
| 蔬菜类 Vegetables | ND | ND | 4.70 | ND | ND | 7.61 | 0.09 | 1.65 | ND | ND | ND | 0.48 | ND | 0.69 | 4.13 | 0.20 | ND | ND | 10.03 | ND | 0.63 | 0.36 | 17.78 | 0.31 | 2.03 |
| 水果类 Fruits | ND | ND | ND | ND | ND | ND | ND | ND | 0.12 | ND | ND | ND | ND | ND | ND | 0.11 | ND | ND | ND | ND | ND | ND | ND | ND | 0.09 |
| 糖类 Sugar | ND | ND | ND | ND | ND | ND | ND | ND | ND | ND | ND | ND | ND | ND | ND | ND | ND | ND | ND | ND | ND | ND | ND | ND | 0.00 |
| 水及饮料类 Water and beverages | ND | ND | ND | ND | ND | ND | 0.14 | ND | ND | ND | ND | ND | ND | ND | ND | ND | ND | ND | ND | ND | ND | ND | ND | ND | 0.01 |
| 酒类 Alcohol beverages | ND | ND | ND | ND | ND | ND | ND | ND | ND | ND | ND | ND | ND | ND | ND | ND | ND | ND | ND | ND | 0.26 | ND | ND | ND | 0.01 |

注：未检出（ND）按 0 计

Note: values not detected (ND) were treated as being equal to 0

附表 4-82  第六次中国总膳食研究膳食样品中四氟醚唑的含量（单位：μg/kg）

Annexed Table 4-82  Levels of tetraconazole in food samples from the 6$^{th}$ China TDS (Unit: μg/kg)

| 膳食类别<br>Category | 黑龙江<br>HL | 辽宁<br>LN | 河北<br>HE | 北京<br>BJ | 吉林<br>JL | 山西<br>SX | 陕西<br>SN | 河南<br>HA | 宁夏<br>NX | 内蒙古<br>NM | 青海<br>QH | 甘肃<br>GS | 上海<br>SH | 福建<br>FJ | 江西<br>JX | 江苏<br>JS | 浙江<br>ZJ | 山东<br>SD | 湖北<br>HB | 四川<br>SC | 广西<br>GX | 湖南<br>HN | 广东<br>GD | 贵州<br>GZ | 全国平均<br>AVG |
|---|---|---|---|---|---|---|---|---|---|---|---|---|---|---|---|---|---|---|---|---|---|---|---|---|---|
| 谷类 Cereals | ND | ND | ND | ND | ND | ND | ND | ND | ND | ND | ND | ND | ND | ND | ND | ND | ND | ND | ND | ND | ND | ND | ND | ND | 0.00 |
| 豆类 Legumes | ND | ND | ND | ND | ND | ND | ND | ND | ND | ND | ND | ND | ND | ND | ND | ND | ND | ND | ND | ND | ND | ND | ND | ND | 0.00 |
| 薯类 Potatoes | ND | ND | ND | ND | ND | ND | ND | ND | ND | ND | ND | ND | ND | ND | ND | ND | ND | ND | ND | ND | ND | ND | ND | ND | 0.00 |
| 肉类 Meats | ND | ND | ND | ND | ND | ND | ND | ND | ND | ND | ND | ND | ND | ND | ND | ND | ND | ND | ND | ND | ND | ND | ND | ND | 0.00 |
| 蛋类 Eggs | ND | ND | ND | ND | ND | ND | ND | ND | ND | ND | ND | ND | ND | ND | ND | ND | ND | ND | ND | ND | ND | ND | ND | ND | 0.00 |
| 水产类 Aquatic foods | ND | ND | ND | ND | ND | ND | ND | ND | ND | ND | ND | ND | ND | ND | ND | ND | ND | ND | ND | ND | ND | ND | ND | ND | 0.00 |
| 乳类 Dairy products | ND | ND | ND | ND | ND | ND | ND | ND | ND | ND | ND | ND | ND | ND | ND | ND | ND | ND | ND | ND | ND | ND | ND | ND | 0.00 |
| 蔬菜类 Vegetables | ND | ND | ND | 0.40 | ND | ND | ND | ND | ND | ND | 0.39 | ND | ND | ND | ND | ND | ND | ND | ND | ND | ND | ND | ND | ND | 0.02 |
| 水果类 Fruits | ND | ND | ND | ND | 0.05 | ND | ND | ND | ND | ND | ND | ND | ND | ND | ND | ND | ND | 0.07 | ND | ND | ND | ND | 0.12 | ND | 0.03 |
| 糖类 Sugar | ND | ND | ND | ND | ND | ND | ND | ND | ND | ND | ND | ND | ND | ND | ND | ND | ND | ND | ND | ND | ND | ND | ND | ND | 0.00 |
| 水及饮料类 Water and beverages | ND | ND | ND | ND | ND | ND | ND | ND | ND | ND | ND | ND | ND | ND | ND | ND | ND | ND | ND | ND | ND | ND | ND | ND | 0.00 |

续表

| 膳食类别<br>Category | 黑龙江<br>HL | 辽宁<br>LN | 河北<br>HE | 北京<br>BJ | 吉林<br>JL | 山西<br>SX | 陕西<br>SN | 河南<br>HA | 宁夏<br>NX | 内蒙古<br>NM | 青海<br>QH | 甘肃<br>GS | 上海<br>SH | 福建<br>FJ | 江西<br>JX | 江苏<br>JS | 浙江<br>ZJ | 山东<br>SD | 湖北<br>HB | 四川<br>SC | 广西<br>GX | 湖南<br>HN | 广东<br>GD | 贵州<br>GZ | 全国平均<br>AVG |
|---|---|---|---|---|---|---|---|---|---|---|---|---|---|---|---|---|---|---|---|---|---|---|---|---|---|
| 酒类<br>Alcohol beverages | ND | ND | ND | ND | ND | ND | ND | ND | ND | ND | ND | ND | ND | ND | ND | ND | ND | ND | ND | ND | ND | ND | ND | ND | 0.00 |

注：未检出（ND）按0计
Note: values not detected (ND) were treated as being equal to 0

附表 Table 4-83　第六次中国总膳食研究膳食样品中氟环唑的含量（单位：μg/kg）
Annexed Table 4-83　Levels of epoxiconazole in food samples from the 6th China TDS (Unit: μg/kg)

| 膳食类别<br>Category | 黑龙江<br>HL | 辽宁<br>LN | 河北<br>HE | 北京<br>BJ | 吉林<br>JL | 山西<br>SX | 陕西<br>SN | 河南<br>HA | 宁夏<br>NX | 内蒙古<br>NM | 青海<br>QH | 甘肃<br>GS | 上海<br>SH | 福建<br>FJ | 江西<br>JX | 江苏<br>JS | 浙江<br>ZJ | 山东<br>SD | 湖北<br>HB | 四川<br>SC | 广西<br>GX | 湖南<br>HN | 广东<br>GD | 贵州<br>GZ | 全国平均<br>AVG |
|---|---|---|---|---|---|---|---|---|---|---|---|---|---|---|---|---|---|---|---|---|---|---|---|---|---|
| 谷类<br>Cereals | 0.10 | ND | ND | ND | ND | ND | ND | ND | ND | ND | ND | ND | ND | 0.08 | 0.10 | ND | ND | ND | ND | ND | ND | ND | ND | ND | 0.01 |
| 豆类<br>Legumes | ND | ND | ND | ND | ND | ND | ND | ND | ND | ND | ND | ND | ND | ND | ND | ND | ND | ND | ND | ND | ND | ND | ND | ND | 0.00 |
| 薯类<br>Potatoes | ND | ND | ND | ND | 0.11 | ND | ND | ND | ND | ND | ND | ND | ND | ND | ND | ND | ND | ND | ND | ND | ND | ND | ND | ND | 0.00 |
| 肉类<br>Meats | ND | ND | ND | ND | ND | ND | ND | ND | ND | ND | ND | ND | ND | ND | ND | ND | ND | ND | ND | ND | ND | ND | ND | ND | 0.00 |
| 蛋类<br>Eggs | ND | ND | ND | ND | 0.11 | ND | ND | ND | ND | ND | ND | ND | ND | ND | ND | ND | ND | ND | ND | ND | ND | ND | ND | ND | 0.00 |
| 水产类<br>Aquatic foods | ND | ND | ND | ND | ND | ND | ND | ND | ND | ND | ND | ND | ND | ND | 0.05 | ND | ND | ND | ND | ND | ND | ND | ND | ND | 0.01 |
| 乳类<br>Dairy products | ND | ND | ND | ND | ND | ND | ND | ND | ND | ND | ND | ND | ND | ND | ND | ND | ND | ND | ND | ND | ND | ND | ND | ND | 0.00 |

续表

| 膳食类别<br>Category | 黑龙江<br>HL | 辽宁<br>LN | 河北<br>HE | 北京<br>BJ | 吉林<br>JL | 山西<br>SX | 陕西<br>SN | 河南<br>HA | 宁夏<br>NX | 内蒙古<br>NM | 青海<br>QH | 甘肃<br>GS | 上海<br>SH | 福建<br>FJ | 江西<br>JX | 江苏<br>JS | 浙江<br>ZJ | 山东<br>SD | 湖北<br>HB | 四川<br>SC | 广西<br>GX | 湖南<br>HN | 广东<br>GD | 贵州<br>GZ | 全国平均<br>AVG |
|---|---|---|---|---|---|---|---|---|---|---|---|---|---|---|---|---|---|---|---|---|---|---|---|---|---|
| 蔬菜类 Vegetables | ND | ND | ND | ND | 0.07 | ND | ND | ND | ND | ND | ND | ND | ND | ND | ND | ND | ND | ND | ND | ND | ND | ND | ND | ND | 0.00 |
| 水果类 Fruits | ND | ND | 0.31 | ND | ND | ND | ND | 0.07 | ND | ND | ND | ND | ND | ND | ND | ND | ND | 1.44 | ND | 0.26 | ND | ND | ND | ND | 0.09 |
| 糖类 Sugar | ND | ND | ND | ND | ND | ND | ND | ND | ND | ND | ND | ND | ND | ND | ND | ND | ND | ND | ND | ND | ND | ND | ND | ND | 0.00 |
| 水及饮料类 Water and beverages | ND | ND | ND | ND | ND | ND | ND | ND | ND | ND | ND | ND | ND | ND | ND | ND | ND | ND | ND | ND | ND | ND | ND | ND | 0.00 |
| 酒类 Alcohol beverages | ND | ND | ND | ND | ND | ND | ND | ND | ND | ND | ND | ND | ND | ND | ND | ND | ND | ND | ND | ND | ND | ND | ND | ND | 0.00 |

注：未检出（ND）按 0 计

Note: values not detected (ND) were treated as being equal to 0

附表 4-84　第六次中国总膳食研究膳食样品中腈苯唑的含量（单位：μg/kg）

Annexed Table 4-84　Levels of fenbuconazole in food samples from the 6$^{th}$ China TDS (Unit: μg/kg)

| 膳食类别<br>Category | 黑龙江<br>HL | 辽宁<br>LN | 河北<br>HE | 北京<br>BJ | 吉林<br>JL | 山西<br>SX | 陕西<br>SN | 河南<br>HA | 宁夏<br>NX | 内蒙古<br>NM | 青海<br>QH | 甘肃<br>GS | 上海<br>SH | 福建<br>FJ | 江西<br>JX | 江苏<br>JS | 浙江<br>ZJ | 山东<br>SD | 湖北<br>HB | 四川<br>SC | 广西<br>GX | 湖南<br>HN | 广东<br>GD | 贵州<br>GZ | 全国平均<br>AVG |
|---|---|---|---|---|---|---|---|---|---|---|---|---|---|---|---|---|---|---|---|---|---|---|---|---|---|
| 谷类 Cereals | ND | ND | ND | ND | ND | ND | ND | ND | ND | ND | ND | ND | ND | ND | ND | ND | ND | ND | ND | ND | 0.08 | ND | ND | ND | 0.00 |
| 豆类 Legumes | 0.29 | 0.42 | ND | ND | ND | ND | ND | ND | ND | ND | ND | ND | 0.87 | ND | ND | ND | ND | ND | 0.81 | ND | 0.28 | ND | ND | 0.55 | 0.13 |
| 薯类 Potatoes | 0.06 | ND | ND | ND | ND | 0.74 | ND | 0.17 | ND | 0.86 | ND | ND | 1.41 | ND | ND | ND | ND | ND | 0.19 | ND | 0.91 | ND | ND | 1.02 | 0.22 |

续表

| 膳食类别 Category | 黑龙江 HL | 辽宁 LN | 河北 HE | 北京 BJ | 吉林 JL | 山西 SX | 陕西 SN | 河南 HA | 宁夏 NX | 内蒙古 NM | 青海 QH | 甘肃 GS | 上海 SH | 福建 FJ | 江西 JX | 江苏 JS | 浙江 ZJ | 山东 SD | 湖北 HB | 四川 SC | 广西 GX | 湖南 HN | 广东 GD | 贵州 GZ | 全国平均 AVG |
|---|---|---|---|---|---|---|---|---|---|---|---|---|---|---|---|---|---|---|---|---|---|---|---|---|---|
| 肉类 Meats | 1.45 | 0.11 | ND | ND | 0.09 | 1.33 | ND | 0.41 | ND | 0.69 | ND | ND | 3.70 | ND | ND | 2.72 | ND | ND | 0.54 | ND | 1.14 | ND | ND | 0.76 | 0.54 |
| 蛋类 Eggs | ND | ND | ND | ND | ND | ND | ND | ND | ND | ND | ND | ND | ND | ND | ND | 0.17 | ND | ND | ND | ND | 1.54 | ND | ND | 0.63 | 0.10 |
| 水产类 Aquatic foods | 0.33 | ND | ND | ND | ND | 0.56 | ND | 0.37 | ND | 7.88 | ND | ND | 2.34 | ND | ND | 0.24 | ND | ND | ND | ND | 0.64 | ND | ND | 1.09 | 0.56 |
| 乳类 Dairy products | ND | 0.10 | ND | ND | ND | ND | ND | ND | ND | ND | ND | ND | ND | ND | ND | ND | ND | ND | ND | ND | ND | ND | ND | ND | 0.00 |
| 蔬菜类 Vegetables | ND | ND | ND | ND | ND | ND | ND | ND | ND | ND | ND | ND | ND | ND | ND | ND | ND | ND | ND | ND | ND | ND | ND | ND | 0.00 |
| 水果类 Fruits | 1.40 | ND | ND | ND | 1.40 | 1.13 | ND | 1.15 | ND | ND | ND | ND | ND | 5.46 | ND | ND | ND | ND | ND | ND | ND | ND | ND | ND | 0.44 |
| 糖类 Sugar | ND | ND | ND | ND | ND | ND | ND | ND | ND | ND | ND | ND | 2.36 | ND | ND | ND | ND | ND | ND | ND | ND | ND | ND | ND | 0.10 |
| 水及饮料类 Water and beverages | ND | ND | ND | ND | ND | ND | ND | ND | ND | 0.24 | ND | ND | ND | ND | 0.09 | 20.05 | ND | ND | ND | ND | ND | ND | ND | ND | 0.00 |
| 酒类 Alcohol beverages | 0.27 | ND | 0.07 | ND | ND | ND | ND | ND | ND | ND | ND | ND | 29.16 | ND | ND | ND | ND | ND | ND | ND | 4.94 | 0.14 | 0.12 | 13.20 | 2.84 |

注：未检出（ND）按 0 计

Note: values not detected (ND) were treated as being equal to 0

附表 4-85　第六次中国总膳食研究膳食样品中氟硅唑的含量（单位：μg/kg）

Annexed Table 4-85　Levels of flusilazole in food samples from the 6<sup>th</sup> China TDS (Unit: μg/kg)

| 膳食类别 Category | 黑龙江 HL | 辽宁 LN | 河北 HE | 北京 BJ | 吉林 JL | 山西 SX | 陕西 SN | 河南 HA | 宁夏 NX | 内蒙古 NM | 青海 QH | 甘肃 GS | 上海 SH | 福建 FJ | 江西 JX | 江苏 JS | 浙江 ZJ | 山东 SD | 湖北 HB | 四川 SC | 广西 GX | 湖南 HN | 广东 GD | 贵州 GZ | 全国平均 AVG |
|---|---|---|---|---|---|---|---|---|---|---|---|---|---|---|---|---|---|---|---|---|---|---|---|---|---|
| 谷类 Cereals | ND | ND | ND | ND | ND | ND | ND | ND | ND | ND | ND | ND | ND | ND | ND | ND | ND | ND | ND | ND | ND | ND | ND | ND | 0.00 |
| 豆类 Legumes | ND | ND | ND | ND | ND | ND | ND | ND | ND | ND | ND | ND | ND | ND | ND | ND | ND | ND | ND | ND | ND | ND | ND | ND | 0.00 |
| 薯类 Potatoes | ND | ND | ND | ND | ND | ND | ND | ND | ND | ND | ND | ND | ND | ND | ND | ND | ND | ND | ND | ND | ND | ND | ND | ND | 0.00 |
| 肉类 Meats | ND | ND | ND | ND | ND | ND | ND | ND | ND | ND | ND | ND | ND | ND | ND | ND | ND | ND | ND | ND | ND | ND | ND | ND | 0.00 |
| 蛋类 Eggs | ND | ND | ND | ND | ND | ND | ND | ND | ND | ND | ND | ND | ND | ND | ND | ND | ND | ND | ND | ND | ND | ND | ND | ND | 0.00 |
| 水产类 Aquatic foods | ND | ND | ND | ND | ND | ND | ND | ND | ND | ND | ND | ND | ND | ND | ND | ND | ND | ND | ND | ND | ND | ND | ND | ND | 0.00 |
| 乳类 Dairy products | ND | ND | ND | ND | ND | ND | ND | ND | ND | ND | ND | ND | ND | ND | ND | ND | ND | ND | ND | ND | ND | ND | ND | ND | 0.00 |
| 蔬菜类 Vegetables | ND | ND | 0.25 | ND | ND | 1.28 | ND | 0.32 | ND | ND | ND | 1.18 | ND | 3.00 | ND | ND | ND | 0.08 | 25.69 | ND | 0.10 | 22.64 | 165.14 | 4.38 | 9.34 |
| 水果类 Fruits | 0.51 | ND | ND | 0.22 | ND | ND | ND | 0.07 | ND | ND | 0.37 | ND | ND | ND | ND | ND | 0.32 | ND | 0.05 | ND | ND | 0.28 | 0.25 | ND | 0.09 |
| 糖类 Sugar | ND | ND | ND | ND | ND | ND | ND | ND | ND | ND | ND | ND | ND | ND | ND | ND | ND | ND | ND | ND | ND | ND | ND | ND | 0.00 |
| 水及饮料类 Water and beverages | ND | ND | ND | ND | ND | ND | ND | ND | ND | ND | ND | ND | ND | ND | ND | ND | ND | ND | ND | ND | ND | ND | ND | ND | 0.00 |

续表

| 膳食类别 Category | 黑龙江 HL | 辽宁 LN | 河北 HE | 北京 BJ | 吉林 JL | 山西 SX | 陕西 SN | 河南 HA | 宁夏 NX | 内蒙古 NM | 青海 QH | 甘肃 GS | 上海 SH | 福建 FJ | 江西 JX | 江苏 JS | 浙江 ZJ | 山东 SD | 湖北 HB | 四川 SC | 广西 GX | 湖南 HN | 广东 GD | 贵州 GZ | 全国平均 AVG |
|---|---|---|---|---|---|---|---|---|---|---|---|---|---|---|---|---|---|---|---|---|---|---|---|---|---|
| 酒类 Alcohol beverages | ND | ND | ND | ND | ND | ND | ND | ND | ND | ND | ND | ND | ND | ND | ND | ND | ND | ND | ND | ND | ND | ND | ND | ND | 0.00 |

注: 未检出 (ND) 按 0 计
Note: values not detected (ND) were treated as being equal to 0

附表 4-86 第六次中国总膳食研究膳食样品中戊唑醇的含量 (单位: μg/kg)
Annexed Table 4-86 Levels of tebuconazole in food samples from the 6th China TDS (Unit: μg/kg)

| 膳食类别 Category | 黑龙江 HL | 辽宁 LN | 河北 HE | 北京 BJ | 吉林 JL | 山西 SX | 陕西 SN | 河南 HA | 宁夏 NX | 内蒙古 NM | 青海 QH | 甘肃 GS | 上海 SH | 福建 FJ | 江西 JX | 江苏 JS | 浙江 ZJ | 山东 SD | 湖北 HB | 四川 SC | 广西 GX | 湖南 HN | 广东 GD | 贵州 GZ | 全国平均 AVG |
|---|---|---|---|---|---|---|---|---|---|---|---|---|---|---|---|---|---|---|---|---|---|---|---|---|---|
| 谷类 Cereals | 0.16 | ND | ND | 0.07 | ND | ND | 0.24 | 0.30 | ND | ND | 0.38 | ND | 0.10 | 0.79 | 1.08 | 0.25 | 0.15 | 0.18 | 0.33 | 0.14 | 0.56 | 0.15 | 0.20 | 0.45 | 0.23 |
| 豆类 Legumes | ND | ND | 0.17 | ND | ND | ND | 0.23 | 0.08 | 0.07 | 0.08 | ND | ND | ND | ND | ND | 0.19 | ND | ND | 0.07 | 0.16 | ND | ND | ND | ND | 0.04 |
| 薯类 Potatoes | ND | ND | ND | ND | 0.13 | ND | 0.95 | ND | ND | ND | 0.05 | ND | ND | ND | ND | ND | ND | 0.23 | ND | 0.09 | ND | ND | ND | ND | 0.07 |
| 肉类 Meats | ND | ND | ND | ND | ND | ND | ND | ND | 0.14 | ND | 0.21 | ND | ND | 0.21 | ND | 0.11 | ND | ND | ND | 0.17 | ND | 0.10 | ND | 0.05 | 0.03 |
| 蛋类 Eggs | ND | ND | ND | ND | 0.10 | ND | 0.39 | ND | ND | ND | 0.13 | ND | ND | 0.07 | ND | 0.08 | ND | ND | ND | 0.11 | ND | 0.10 | ND | ND | 0.01 |
| 水产类 Aquatic foods | ND | ND | ND | ND | ND | ND | ND | ND | ND | ND | ND | ND | ND | ND | ND | 0.11 | ND | ND | ND | ND | ND | ND | ND | 0.06 | 0.04 |
| 乳类 Dairy products | ND | ND | ND | ND | ND | ND | ND | ND | ND | ND | ND | ND | ND | ND | ND | ND | ND | ND | ND | ND | ND | ND | ND | ND | 0.00 |

续表

| 膳食类别 Category | 黑龙江 HL | 辽宁 LN | 河北 HE | 北京 BJ | 吉林 JL | 山西 SX | 陕西 SN | 河南 HA | 宁夏 NX | 内蒙古 NM | 青海 QH | 甘肃 GS | 上海 SH | 福建 FJ | 江西 JX | 江苏 JS | 浙江 ZJ | 山东 SD | 湖北 HB | 四川 SC | 广西 GX | 湖南 HN | 广东 GD | 贵州 GZ | 全国平均 AVG |
|---|---|---|---|---|---|---|---|---|---|---|---|---|---|---|---|---|---|---|---|---|---|---|---|---|---|
| 蔬菜类 Vegetables | 0.09 | 0.22 | 0.13 | 11.01 | ND | 1.26 | 0.45 | 4.77 | 0.19 | 0.08 | 0.91 | 0.28 | 1.28 | 0.33 | 1.19 | 0.22 | 3.75 | 0.09 | 2.20 | 0.12 | 4.72 | 13.75 | 37.21 | 0.38 | 3.53 |
| 水果类 Fruits | 2.33 | 4.25 | 0.76 | 25.59 | 1.15 | 0.16 | 0.35 | 0.66 | 0.14 | ND | 0.11 | 0.09 | 1.25 | 0.53 | 0.35 | 1.27 | 5.52 | 1.33 | 0.20 | 1.36 | 1.01 | 0.13 | 0.73 | 0.44 | 2.07 |
| 糖类 Sugar | ND | ND | ND | ND | ND | ND | ND | ND | ND | ND | ND | ND | ND | ND | ND | ND | ND | ND | ND | ND | ND | ND | ND | ND | 0.00 |
| 水及饮料类 Water and beverages | ND | ND | ND | ND | ND | ND | ND | ND | ND | ND | ND | ND | ND | ND | ND | ND | ND | ND | ND | ND | ND | ND | ND | ND | 0.00 |
| 酒类 Alcohol beverages | ND | ND | ND | ND | ND | ND | ND | ND | ND | ND | ND | ND | ND | ND | ND | ND | ND | ND | ND | ND | ND | ND | 0.04 | ND | 0.00 |

注：未检出（ND）按 0 计
Note: values not detected (ND) were treated as being equal to 0

附表 4-87 第六次中国总膳食研究膳食样品中戊菌唑的含量（单位：μg/kg）
Annexed Table 4-87 Levels of penconazole in food samples from the 6$^{th}$ China TDS (Unit: μg/kg)

| 膳食类别 Category | 黑龙江 HL | 辽宁 LN | 河北 HE | 北京 BJ | 吉林 JL | 山西 SX | 陕西 SN | 河南 HA | 宁夏 NX | 内蒙古 NM | 青海 QH | 甘肃 GS | 上海 SH | 福建 FJ | 江西 JX | 江苏 JS | 浙江 ZJ | 山东 SD | 湖北 HB | 四川 SC | 广西 GX | 湖南 HN | 广东 GD | 贵州 GZ | 全国平均 AVG |
|---|---|---|---|---|---|---|---|---|---|---|---|---|---|---|---|---|---|---|---|---|---|---|---|---|---|
| 谷类 Cereals | ND | ND | ND | ND | ND | ND | ND | ND | ND | ND | ND | ND | ND | ND | ND | ND | ND | ND | ND | ND | ND | ND | ND | ND | 0.00 |
| 豆类 Legumes | ND | ND | ND | ND | ND | ND | ND | ND | ND | ND | ND | ND | ND | ND | ND | ND | ND | ND | ND | ND | ND | ND | ND | ND | 0.00 |
| 薯类 Potatoes | ND | ND | ND | ND | ND | ND | ND | ND | ND | ND | ND | ND | ND | ND | ND | ND | ND | ND | ND | ND | ND | ND | ND | ND | 0.00 |
| 肉类 Meats | ND | ND | ND | ND | ND | ND | ND | ND | ND | ND | ND | ND | ND | ND | ND | ND | ND | ND | ND | ND | ND | ND | ND | ND | 0.00 |

续表

| 膳食类别<br>Category | 黑龙江<br>HL | 辽宁<br>LN | 河北<br>HE | 北京<br>BJ | 吉林<br>JL | 山西<br>SX | 陕西<br>SN | 河南<br>HA | 宁夏<br>NX | 内蒙古<br>NM | 青海<br>QH | 甘肃<br>GS | 上海<br>SH | 福建<br>FJ | 江西<br>JX | 江苏<br>JS | 浙江<br>ZJ | 山东<br>SD | 湖北<br>HB | 四川<br>SC | 广西<br>GX | 湖南<br>HN | 广东<br>GD | 贵州<br>GZ | 全国平均<br>AVG |
|---|---|---|---|---|---|---|---|---|---|---|---|---|---|---|---|---|---|---|---|---|---|---|---|---|---|
| 蛋类 Eggs | ND | ND | ND | ND | ND | ND | ND | ND | ND | 0.11 | ND | ND | ND | ND | ND | ND | ND | ND | ND | ND | ND | ND | ND | ND | 0.00 |
| 水产类 Aquatic foods | ND | ND | ND | ND | ND | ND | ND | ND | ND | ND | ND | ND | ND | ND | ND | ND | ND | ND | ND | ND | ND | ND | ND | ND | 0.00 |
| 乳类 Dairy products | ND | ND | ND | ND | ND | ND | ND | ND | ND | ND | ND | ND | ND | ND | ND | ND | ND | ND | ND | ND | ND | ND | ND | ND | 0.00 |
| 蔬菜类 Vegetables | ND | ND | ND | ND | ND | ND | ND | ND | ND | ND | ND | ND | ND | ND | ND | ND | ND | ND | ND | ND | ND | ND | ND | ND | 0.00 |
| 水果类 Fruits | ND | ND | ND | ND | ND | ND | ND | ND | ND | ND | ND | ND | ND | 0.14 | ND | ND | 1.25 | ND | ND | ND | ND | ND | ND | ND | 0.06 |
| 糖类 Sugar | ND | ND | ND | ND | ND | ND | ND | ND | ND | ND | ND | ND | ND | ND | ND | ND | ND | ND | ND | ND | ND | ND | ND | ND | 0.00 |
| 水及饮料类 Water and beverages | ND | ND | ND | ND | ND | ND | ND | ND | ND | ND | ND | ND | ND | ND | ND | ND | ND | ND | ND | ND | ND | ND | ND | ND | 0.00 |
| 酒类 Alcohol beverages | ND | ND | ND | ND | ND | ND | ND | ND | ND | ND | ND | ND | ND | ND | ND | ND | ND | ND | ND | ND | ND | ND | ND | ND | 0.00 |

注：未检出（ND）按0计
Note: values not detected (ND) were treated as being equal to 0

附表 4-88 第六次中国总膳食研究膳食样品中丙环唑的含量（单位：μg/kg）
Annexed Table 4-88 Levels of propiconazole in food samples from the 6$^{th}$ China TDS (Unit: μg/kg)

| 膳食类别<br>Category | 黑龙江<br>HL | 辽宁<br>LN | 河北<br>HE | 北京<br>BJ | 吉林<br>JL | 山西<br>SX | 陕西<br>SN | 河南<br>HA | 宁夏<br>NX | 内蒙古<br>NM | 青海<br>QH | 甘肃<br>GS | 上海<br>SH | 福建<br>FJ | 江西<br>JX | 江苏<br>JS | 浙江<br>ZJ | 山东<br>SD | 湖北<br>HB | 四川<br>SC | 广西<br>GX | 湖南<br>HN | 广东<br>GD | 贵州<br>GZ | 全国平均<br>AVG |
|---|---|---|---|---|---|---|---|---|---|---|---|---|---|---|---|---|---|---|---|---|---|---|---|---|---|
| 谷类 Cereals | ND | ND | ND | ND | ND | ND | 0.45 | ND | ND | ND | ND | ND | ND | ND | 0.27 | 1.24 | 0.15 | ND | ND | ND | 0.81 | 0.21 | ND | 0.23 | 0.14 |

续表

| 膳食类别<br>Category | 黑龙江<br>HL | 辽宁<br>LN | 河北<br>HE | 北京<br>BJ | 吉林<br>JL | 山西<br>SX | 陕西<br>SN | 河南<br>HA | 宁夏<br>NX | 内蒙古<br>NM | 青海<br>QH | 甘肃<br>GS | 上海<br>SH | 福建<br>FJ | 江西<br>JX | 江苏<br>JS | 浙江<br>ZJ | 山东<br>SD | 湖北<br>HB | 四川<br>SC | 广西<br>GX | 湖南<br>HN | 广东<br>GD | 贵州<br>GZ | 全国平均<br>AVG |
|---|---|---|---|---|---|---|---|---|---|---|---|---|---|---|---|---|---|---|---|---|---|---|---|---|---|
| 豆类 Legumes | ND | ND | ND | ND | ND | ND | ND | ND | ND | ND | ND | ND | ND | ND | ND | 37.00 | ND | ND | ND | ND | ND | ND | ND | ND | 1.54 |
| 薯类 Potatoes | ND | ND | ND | ND | ND | ND | ND | ND | ND | ND | ND | ND | ND | ND | ND | 65.84 | ND | ND | ND | ND | ND | ND | ND | ND | 2.74 |
| 肉类 Meats | ND | ND | ND | ND | ND | ND | ND | ND | ND | ND | ND | ND | ND | ND | ND | 249.10 | ND | ND | ND | ND | ND | ND | ND | ND | 10.38 |
| 蛋类 Eggs | ND | ND | ND | ND | ND | ND | ND | ND | ND | ND | ND | ND | ND | ND | ND | 21.27 | ND | ND | ND | ND | ND | ND | ND | ND | 0.89 |
| 水产类 Aquatic foods | ND | ND | ND | ND | ND | ND | ND | ND | ND | ND | ND | ND | ND | ND | ND | 43.06 | ND | ND | ND | ND | ND | ND | 0.14 | ND | 1.80 |
| 乳类 Dairy products | ND | ND | ND | ND | ND | ND | ND | ND | ND | ND | ND | ND | ND | ND | ND | ND | ND | ND | ND | ND | ND | ND | ND | ND | 0.00 |
| 蔬菜类 Vegetables | ND | ND | 0.17 | ND | 0.12 | 0.91 | 0.34 | ND | 0.26 | ND | ND | 2.70 | ND | ND | 3.09 | 91.88 | ND | ND | 16.59 | ND | 0.09 | 31.44 | 81.27 | 1.61 | 9.60 |
| 水果类 Fruits | ND | ND | ND | 0.23 | ND | ND | ND | ND | ND | ND | ND | ND | ND | 0.19 | ND | 132.20 | ND | ND | ND | ND | ND | ND | 0.11 | ND | 5.53 |
| 糖类 Sugar | ND | ND | ND | ND | ND | ND | ND | ND | ND | ND | ND | ND | ND | ND | ND | 0.18 | ND | ND | ND | ND | ND | ND | ND | ND | 0.00 |
| 水及饮料类 Water and beverages | ND | ND | ND | ND | ND | ND | ND | ND | ND | ND | ND | ND | ND | ND | ND | ND | ND | ND | ND | ND | ND | ND | ND | ND | 0.01 |
| 酒类 Alcohol beverages | ND | ND | ND | ND | ND | ND | ND | ND | ND | ND | ND | ND | ND | ND | ND | ND | ND | ND | ND | ND | ND | ND | ND | ND | 0.00 |

注：未检出（ND）按 0 计

Note: values not detected (ND) were treated as being equal to 0

附表 4-89 第六次中国总膳食研究膳食样品中己唑醇的含量（单位：μg/kg）

Annexed Table 4-89 Levels of hexaconazole in food samples from the 6$^{th}$ China TDS (Unit: μg/kg)

| 膳食类别<br>Category | 黑龙江<br>HL | 辽宁<br>LN | 河北<br>HE | 北京<br>BJ | 吉林<br>JL | 山西<br>SX | 陕西<br>SN | 河南<br>HA | 宁夏<br>NX | 内蒙古<br>NM | 青海<br>QH | 甘肃<br>GS | 上海<br>SH | 福建<br>FJ | 江西<br>JX | 江苏<br>JS | 浙江<br>ZJ | 山东<br>SD | 湖北<br>HB | 四川<br>SC | 广西<br>GX | 湖南<br>HN | 广东<br>GD | 贵州<br>GZ | 全国平均<br>AVG |
|---|---|---|---|---|---|---|---|---|---|---|---|---|---|---|---|---|---|---|---|---|---|---|---|---|---|
| 谷类 Cereals | ND | ND | ND | ND | ND | ND | 0.21 | ND | ND | ND | ND | ND | ND | ND | 0.71 | 0.18 | ND | ND | 0.13 | ND | 0.78 | 0.57 | ND | ND | 0.11 |
| 豆类 Legumes | ND | ND | 0.06 | ND | ND | ND | ND | ND | ND | ND | ND | ND | ND | ND | ND | ND | ND | ND | ND | ND | ND | ND | ND | ND | 0.00 |
| 薯类 Potatoes | ND | ND | ND | ND | ND | ND | ND | ND | ND | ND | ND | ND | ND | ND | ND | ND | ND | ND | 0.10 | ND | ND | ND | ND | ND | 0.00 |
| 肉类 Meats | ND | ND | ND | ND | ND | ND | ND | ND | ND | ND | ND | ND | ND | ND | ND | ND | ND | ND | ND | ND | ND | ND | ND | ND | 0.00 |
| 蛋类 Eggs | ND | ND | ND | ND | ND | ND | ND | ND | ND | ND | ND | ND | ND | ND | ND | ND | ND | ND | ND | ND | ND | ND | ND | ND | 0.00 |
| 水产类 Aquatic foods | ND | ND | ND | ND | ND | ND | ND | ND | ND | ND | ND | ND | ND | ND | 0.13 | ND | ND | ND | ND | ND | ND | 0.11 | ND | ND | 0.01 |
| 乳类 Dairy products | ND | ND | ND | ND | ND | ND | ND | ND | ND | ND | ND | ND | ND | ND | ND | ND | ND | ND | ND | ND | ND | ND | ND | ND | 0.00 |
| 蔬菜类 Vegetables | ND | ND | 0.46 | ND | ND | ND | 0.17 | ND | 0.45 | ND | ND | ND | ND | ND | ND | ND | ND | ND | 0.13 | ND | 40.97 | ND | ND | ND | 1.77 |
| 水果类 Fruits | 0.07 | ND | ND | ND | ND | ND | ND | ND | ND | 0.22 | ND | ND | ND | ND | ND | ND | ND | ND | ND | ND | ND | ND | 0.24 | ND | 0.01 |
| 糖类 Sugar | ND | ND | ND | ND | ND | ND | ND | ND | ND | ND | ND | ND | ND | ND | ND | ND | ND | ND | ND | ND | ND | ND | ND | ND | 0.00 |
| 水及饮料类 Water and beverages | ND | ND | ND | ND | ND | ND | ND | ND | ND | ND | ND | ND | ND | ND | ND | ND | ND | ND | ND | ND | ND | ND | ND | ND | 0.00 |

续表

| 膳食类别<br>Category | 黑龙江<br>HL | 辽宁<br>LN | 河北<br>HE | 北京<br>BJ | 吉林<br>JL | 山西<br>SX | 陕西<br>SN | 河南<br>HA | 宁夏<br>NX | 内蒙古<br>NM | 青海<br>QH | 甘肃<br>GS | 上海<br>SH | 福建<br>FJ | 江西<br>JX | 江苏<br>JS | 浙江<br>ZJ | 山东<br>SD | 湖北<br>HB | 四川<br>SC | 广西<br>GX | 湖南<br>HN | 广东<br>GD | 贵州<br>GZ | 全国平均<br>AVG |
|---|---|---|---|---|---|---|---|---|---|---|---|---|---|---|---|---|---|---|---|---|---|---|---|---|---|
| 酒类<br>Alcohol beverages | ND | ND | ND | ND | ND | ND | ND | ND | ND | ND | ND | ND | ND | ND | ND | ND | ND | ND | ND | ND | ND | ND | ND | ND | 0.00 |

注：未检出（ND）按 0 计
Note: values not detected (ND) were treated as being equal to 0

附表 4-90　第六次中国总膳食研究膳食样品中苯醚甲环唑的含量（单位：μg/kg）
Annexed Table 4-90　Levels of difenoconazole in food samples from the 6th China TDS (Unit: μg/kg)

| 膳食类别<br>Category | 黑龙江<br>HL | 辽宁<br>LN | 河北<br>HE | 北京<br>BJ | 吉林<br>JL | 山西<br>SX | 陕西<br>SN | 河南<br>HA | 宁夏<br>NX | 内蒙古<br>NM | 青海<br>QH | 甘肃<br>GS | 上海<br>SH | 福建<br>FJ | 江西<br>JX | 江苏<br>JS | 浙江<br>ZJ | 山东<br>SD | 湖北<br>HB | 四川<br>SC | 广西<br>GX | 湖南<br>HN | 广东<br>GD | 贵州<br>GZ | 全国平均<br>AVG |
|---|---|---|---|---|---|---|---|---|---|---|---|---|---|---|---|---|---|---|---|---|---|---|---|---|---|
| 谷类<br>Cereals | ND | ND | ND | ND | ND | ND | ND | ND | ND | ND | ND | ND | ND | ND | ND | ND | ND | ND | ND | ND | ND | ND | ND | ND | 0.00 |
| 豆类<br>Legumes | ND | ND | ND | ND | ND | ND | ND | ND | ND | ND | ND | ND | ND | ND | ND | ND | ND | ND | ND | ND | ND | ND | ND | ND | 0.00 |
| 薯类<br>Potatoes | ND | ND | ND | ND | ND | ND | ND | ND | ND | ND | ND | ND | ND | ND | ND | ND | ND | ND | ND | ND | ND | ND | ND | ND | 0.00 |
| 肉类<br>Meats | ND | ND | ND | ND | ND | ND | ND | ND | ND | ND | ND | ND | ND | ND | ND | ND | ND | ND | ND | ND | ND | ND | ND | ND | 0.00 |
| 蛋类<br>Eggs | ND | ND | ND | ND | ND | ND | ND | ND | ND | ND | ND | ND | ND | ND | ND | ND | ND | ND | ND | ND | ND | ND | ND | ND | 0.00 |
| 水产类<br>Aquatic foods | ND | ND | ND | ND | ND | ND | ND | ND | ND | ND | ND | ND | ND | ND | ND | ND | ND | ND | ND | ND | ND | ND | ND | ND | 0.00 |
| 乳类<br>Dairy products | ND | ND | ND | ND | ND | ND | ND | ND | ND | ND | ND | ND | ND | ND | ND | ND | ND | ND | ND | ND | ND | ND | ND | ND | 0.00 |

续表

| 膳食类别<br>Category | 黑龙江<br>HL | 辽宁<br>LN | 河北<br>HE | 北京<br>BJ | 吉林<br>JL | 山西<br>SX | 陕西<br>SN | 河南<br>HA | 宁夏<br>NX | 内蒙古<br>NM | 青海<br>QH | 甘肃<br>GS | 上海<br>SH | 福建<br>FJ | 江西<br>JX | 江苏<br>JS | 浙江<br>ZJ | 山东<br>SD | 湖北<br>HB | 四川<br>SC | 广西<br>GX | 湖南<br>HN | 广东<br>GD | 贵州<br>GZ | 全国平均<br>AVG |
|---|---|---|---|---|---|---|---|---|---|---|---|---|---|---|---|---|---|---|---|---|---|---|---|---|---|
| 蔬菜类<br>Vegetables | 0.09 | ND | 0.09 | ND | 0.99 | 3.65 | 4.25 | 0.31 | 0.06 | 1.54 | 2.23 | 4.34 | 2.23 | 0.95 | 0.87 | 0.18 | 1.75 | 1.65 | 11.24 | ND | 30.00 | 5.84 | 92.07 | 2.64 | 6.96 |
| 水果类<br>Fruits | 0.44 | 2.59 | 1.99 | 2.45 | 0.40 | ND | 1.07 | 11.39 | ND | 0.95 | 0.12 | ND | 0.67 | 1.94 | 0.09 | 4.47 | 0.56 | 5.49 | 1.28 | 3.00 | ND | 0.19 | 0.32 | ND | 1.64 |
| 糖类<br>Sugar | ND | ND | ND | ND | ND | ND | ND | ND | ND | ND | ND | ND | ND | ND | ND | ND | ND | ND | ND | ND | ND | ND | ND | ND | 0.00 |
| 水及饮料类<br>Water and beverages | ND | ND | ND | ND | ND | ND | ND | ND | ND | ND | ND | ND | ND | ND | ND | ND | ND | ND | ND | ND | ND | ND | ND | ND | 0.00 |
| 酒类<br>Alcohol beverages | ND | ND | ND | ND | ND | ND | ND | ND | ND | ND | ND | ND | ND | ND | ND | ND | ND | ND | ND | ND | ND | ND | ND | ND | 0.00 |

注：未检出（ND）按0计
Note: values not detected (ND) were treated as being equal to 0

附表 4-91 第六次中国总膳食研究的粉唑醇膳食摄入量 [单位：ng/(kg bw·d)]
Annexed Table 4-91 Dietary intakes of flutriafol from the 6th China TDS [Unit: ng/(kg bw·d)]

| 膳食类别<br>Category | 黑龙江<br>HL | 辽宁<br>LN | 河北<br>HE | 北京<br>BJ | 吉林<br>JL | 山西<br>SX | 陕西<br>SN | 河南<br>HA | 宁夏<br>NX | 内蒙古<br>NM | 青海<br>QH | 甘肃<br>GS | 上海<br>SH | 福建<br>FJ | 江西<br>JX | 江苏<br>JS | 浙江<br>ZJ | 山东<br>SD | 湖北<br>HB | 四川<br>SC | 广西<br>GX | 湖南<br>HN | 广东<br>GD | 贵州<br>GZ | 全国平均<br>AVG |
|---|---|---|---|---|---|---|---|---|---|---|---|---|---|---|---|---|---|---|---|---|---|---|---|---|---|
| 谷类<br>Cereals | 0.000 | 0.000 | 0.000 | 0.000 | 0.000 | 0.000 | 0.000 | 0.000 | 0.000 | 0.000 | 0.000 | 0.000 | 0.000 | 0.000 | 0.000 | 0.000 | 0.000 | 0.000 | 0.000 | 0.000 | 0.000 | 0.000 | 0.000 | 0.000 | 0.000 |
| 豆类<br>Legumes | 0.000 | 0.000 | 0.000 | 0.000 | 0.000 | 0.000 | 0.000 | 0.000 | 0.000 | 0.000 | 0.000 | 0.000 | 0.000 | 0.000 | 0.000 | 0.000 | 0.000 | 0.000 | 0.000 | 0.000 | 0.000 | 0.000 | 0.000 | 0.000 | 0.000 |
| 薯类<br>Potatoes | 0.000 | 0.000 | 0.000 | 0.000 | 0.235 | 0.000 | 0.000 | 0.000 | 0.000 | 0.000 | 0.000 | 0.000 | 0.000 | 0.000 | 0.000 | 0.000 | 0.000 | 0.000 | 0.000 | 0.000 | 0.000 | 0.000 | 0.000 | 0.000 | 0.010 |

续表

| 膳食类别<br>Category | 黑龙江<br>HL | 辽宁<br>LN | 河北<br>HE | 北京<br>BJ | 吉林<br>JL | 山西<br>SX | 陕西<br>SN | 河南<br>HA | 宁夏<br>NX | 内蒙古<br>NM | 青海<br>QH | 甘肃<br>GS | 上海<br>SH | 福建<br>FJ | 江西<br>JX | 江苏<br>JS | 浙江<br>ZJ | 山东<br>SD | 湖北<br>HB | 四川<br>SC | 广西<br>GX | 湖南<br>HN | 广东<br>GD | 贵州<br>GZ | 全国平均<br>AVG |
|---|---|---|---|---|---|---|---|---|---|---|---|---|---|---|---|---|---|---|---|---|---|---|---|---|---|
| 肉类 Meats | 0.000 | 0.000 | 0.000 | 0.000 | 0.107 | 0.000 | 0.000 | 0.000 | 0.000 | 0.000 | 0.000 | 0.000 | 0.000 | 0.000 | 0.000 | 0.000 | 0.000 | 0.000 | 0.000 | 0.000 | 0.000 | 0.000 | 0.000 | 0.000 | 0.004 |
| 蛋类 Eggs | 0.000 | 0.000 | 0.000 | 0.000 | 0.000 | 0.000 | 0.000 | 0.000 | 0.000 | 0.000 | 0.000 | 0.000 | 0.000 | 0.000 | 0.000 | 0.000 | 0.000 | 0.000 | 0.000 | 0.000 | 0.000 | 0.000 | 0.000 | 0.000 | 0.000 |
| 水产类 Aquatic foods | 0.000 | 0.000 | 0.000 | 0.000 | 0.014 | 0.000 | 0.000 | 0.000 | 0.000 | 0.000 | 0.000 | 0.000 | 0.000 | 0.000 | 0.000 | 0.000 | 0.000 | 0.000 | 0.000 | 0.000 | 0.000 | 0.000 | 0.000 | 0.000 | 0.001 |
| 乳类 Dairy products | 0.000 | 0.000 | 0.000 | 0.000 | 0.000 | 0.000 | 0.000 | 0.000 | 0.000 | 0.000 | 0.000 | 0.000 | 0.000 | 0.000 | 0.000 | 0.000 | 0.000 | 0.000 | 0.000 | 0.000 | 0.000 | 0.000 | 0.000 | 0.000 | 0.000 |
| 蔬菜类 Vegetables | 0.000 | 0.000 | 0.000 | 0.000 | 0.341 | 3.313 | 0.000 | 0.000 | 0.000 | 0.000 | 4.228 | 0.000 | 0.694 | 0.000 | 0.000 | 0.000 | 0.000 | 0.000 | 0.000 | 0.000 | 0.000 | 0.000 | 0.543 | 0.538 | 0.402 |
| 水果类 Fruits | 0.000 | 0.000 | 0.000 | 0.000 | 0.000 | 0.000 | 0.000 | 0.000 | 0.000 | 0.000 | 0.051 | 0.000 | 0.000 | 0.000 | 0.000 | 0.000 | 0.000 | 0.000 | 0.000 | 0.000 | 0.000 | 0.000 | 0.148 | 0.000 | 0.008 |
| 糖类 Sugar | 0.000 | 0.000 | 0.000 | 0.000 | 0.000 | 0.000 | 0.000 | 0.000 | 0.000 | 0.000 | 0.000 | 0.000 | 0.000 | 0.000 | 0.000 | 0.000 | 0.000 | 0.000 | 0.000 | 0.000 | 0.000 | 0.000 | 0.000 | 0.000 | 0.000 |
| 水及饮料类 Water and beverages | 0.000 | 0.000 | 0.000 | 0.000 | 0.000 | 0.000 | 0.000 | 0.000 | 0.000 | 0.000 | 0.000 | 0.000 | 0.000 | 0.000 | 0.000 | 0.000 | 0.000 | 0.000 | 0.000 | 0.000 | 0.000 | 0.000 | 0.000 | 0.000 | 0.000 |
| 酒类 Alcohol beverages | 0.000 | 0.000 | 0.000 | 0.000 | 0.000 | 0.000 | 0.000 | 0.000 | 0.000 | 0.000 | 0.000 | 0.000 | 0.000 | 0.000 | 0.000 | 0.000 | 0.000 | 0.000 | 0.000 | 0.000 | 0.000 | 0.000 | 0.000 | 0.000 | 0.000 |
| 合计 SUM | 0.000 | 0.000 | 0.000 | 0.000 | 0.697 | 3.313 | 0.000 | 0.000 | 0.000 | 0.000 | 4.279 | 0.000 | 0.694 | 0.000 | 0.000 | 0.000 | 0.000 | 0.000 | 0.000 | 0.000 | 0.000 | 0.000 | 0.691 | 0.538 | 0.425 |

附表 4-92  第六次中国总膳食研究的腈菌唑膳食摄入量 [单位：ng/(kg bw·d)]
Annexed Table 4-92  Dietary intakes of myclobutanil from the 6$^{th}$ China TDS [Unit: ng/(kg bw·d)]

| 膳食类别 Category | 黑龙江 HL | 辽宁 LN | 河北 HE | 北京 BJ | 吉林 JL | 山西 SX | 陕西 SN | 河南 HA | 宁夏 NX | 内蒙古 NM | 青海 QH | 甘肃 GS | 上海 SH | 福建 FJ | 江西 JX | 江苏 JS | 浙江 ZJ | 山东 SD | 湖北 HB | 四川 SC | 广西 GX | 湖南 HN | 广东 GD | 贵州 GZ | 全国平均 AVG |
|---|---|---|---|---|---|---|---|---|---|---|---|---|---|---|---|---|---|---|---|---|---|---|---|---|---|
| 谷类 Cereals | 0.000 | 0.000 | 0.000 | 0.000 | 0.000 | 0.000 | 0.000 | 0.000 | 0.000 | 0.000 | 0.000 | 0.000 | 0.000 | 0.000 | 0.000 | 0.000 | 0.000 | 0.000 | 0.000 | 0.000 | 0.000 | 0.000 | 0.000 | 0.000 | 0.000 |
| 豆类 Legumes | 0.000 | 0.000 | 0.000 | 0.000 | 0.000 | 0.000 | 0.000 | 0.000 | 0.000 | 0.000 | 0.000 | 0.000 | 0.000 | 0.000 | 0.000 | 0.000 | 0.000 | 0.000 | 0.000 | 0.000 | 0.000 | 0.000 | 0.000 | 0.000 | 0.000 |
| 薯类 Potatoes | 0.000 | 0.000 | 0.000 | 0.000 | 0.000 | 0.000 | 0.000 | 0.000 | 0.000 | 0.000 | 0.000 | 0.000 | 0.000 | 0.000 | 0.000 | 0.000 | 0.000 | 0.000 | 0.000 | 0.000 | 0.000 | 0.000 | 0.000 | 0.000 | 0.000 |
| 肉类 Meats | 0.000 | 0.000 | 0.000 | 0.000 | 0.000 | 0.000 | 0.000 | 0.000 | 0.000 | 0.000 | 0.000 | 0.000 | 0.000 | 0.000 | 0.000 | 0.098 | 0.000 | 0.000 | 0.000 | 0.000 | 0.000 | 0.000 | 0.000 | 0.000 | 0.004 |
| 蛋类 Eggs | 0.000 | 0.000 | 0.000 | 0.000 | 0.000 | 0.000 | 0.000 | 0.000 | 0.000 | 0.000 | 0.000 | 0.000 | 0.000 | 0.000 | 0.000 | 0.047 | 0.000 | 0.000 | 0.000 | 0.000 | 0.000 | 0.000 | 0.000 | 0.000 | 0.002 |
| 水产类 Aquatic foods | 0.000 | 0.000 | 0.008 | 0.000 | 0.000 | 0.017 | 0.000 | 0.000 | 0.000 | 0.000 | 0.000 | 0.000 | 0.000 | 0.000 | 0.000 | 0.000 | 0.000 | 0.000 | 0.000 | 0.000 | 0.000 | 0.000 | 0.000 | 0.000 | 0.001 |
| 乳类 Dairy products | 0.000 | 0.000 | 0.000 | 0.000 | 0.000 | 0.000 | 0.000 | 0.000 | 0.000 | 0.000 | 0.000 | 0.000 | 0.000 | 0.000 | 0.000 | 0.000 | 0.000 | 0.000 | 0.000 | 0.000 | 0.000 | 0.000 | 0.000 | 0.000 | 0.000 |
| 蔬菜类 Vegetables | 0.000 | 0.000 | 0.286 | 0.000 | 2.046 | 2.433 | 0.600 | 0.487 | 3.415 | 0.431 | 5.421 | 0.822 | 0.000 | 0.000 | 0.000 | 0.632 | 0.000 | 0.000 | 0.908 | 0.000 | 7.568 | 3.236 | 0.548 | 0.000 | 1.201 |
| 水果类 Fruits | 0.000 | 2.128 | 0.000 | 0.000 | 0.626 | 0.000 | 0.000 | 0.000 | 0.000 | 0.354 | 0.000 | 0.000 | 0.385 | 0.184 | 0.046 | 0.000 | 0.000 | 0.000 | 0.000 | 0.000 | 0.000 | 0.000 | 0.707 | 0.000 | 0.185 |
| 糖类 Sugar | 0.000 | 0.000 | 0.000 | 0.000 | 0.000 | 0.000 | 0.000 | 0.000 | 0.000 | 0.000 | 0.000 | 0.000 | 0.000 | 0.000 | 0.000 | 0.000 | 0.000 | 0.000 | 0.000 | 0.000 | 0.000 | 0.000 | 0.000 | 0.000 | 0.000 |
| 水及饮料类 Water and beverages | 0.000 | 0.000 | 0.000 | 0.000 | 0.000 | 0.000 | 0.000 | 0.000 | 0.000 | 0.000 | 0.000 | 0.000 | 0.000 | 0.000 | 0.000 | 0.000 | 0.000 | 0.000 | 0.000 | 0.000 | 0.000 | 0.000 | 0.000 | 0.000 | 0.000 |

| 膳食类别<br>Category | 黑龙江<br>HL | 辽宁<br>LN | 河北<br>HE | 北京<br>BJ | 吉林<br>JL | 山西<br>SX | 陕西<br>SN | 河南<br>HA | 宁夏<br>NX | 内蒙古<br>NM | 青海<br>QH | 甘肃<br>GS | 上海<br>SH | 福建<br>FJ | 江西<br>JX | 江苏<br>JS | 浙江<br>ZJ | 山东<br>SD | 湖北<br>HB | 四川<br>SC | 广西<br>GX | 湖南<br>HN | 广东<br>GD | 贵州<br>GZ | 全国平均<br>AVG |
|---|---|---|---|---|---|---|---|---|---|---|---|---|---|---|---|---|---|---|---|---|---|---|---|---|---|
| 酒类<br>Alcohol beverages | 0.000 | 0.045 | 0.000 | 0.000 | 0.000 | 0.000 | 0.000 | 0.000 | 0.000 | 0.000 | 0.000 | 0.000 | 0.000 | 0.000 | 0.000 | 0.000 | 0.000 | 0.000 | 0.000 | 0.000 | 0.055 | 0.000 | 0.000 | 0.000 | 0.004 |
| 合计<br>SUM | 0.000 | 2.174 | 0.295 | 0.000 | 2.672 | 2.450 | 0.600 | 0.487 | 3.415 | 0.786 | 5.421 | 0.822 | 0.385 | 0.184 | 0.046 | 0.778 | 0.000 | 0.000 | 0.908 | 0.000 | 7.623 | 3.236 | 1.254 | 0.000 | 1.397 |

附表 4-93　第六次中国总膳食研究的三唑醇膳食摄入量 [ 单位：ng/(kg bw · d)]
Annexed Table 4-93　Dietary intakes of triadimenol from the 6th China TDS [Unit: ng/(kg bw · d)]

| 膳食类别<br>Category | 黑龙江<br>HL | 辽宁<br>LN | 河北<br>HE | 北京<br>BJ | 吉林<br>JL | 山西<br>SX | 陕西<br>SN | 河南<br>HA | 宁夏<br>NX | 内蒙古<br>NM | 青海<br>QH | 甘肃<br>GS | 上海<br>SH | 福建<br>FJ | 江西<br>JX | 江苏<br>JS | 浙江<br>ZJ | 山东<br>SD | 湖北<br>HB | 四川<br>SC | 广西<br>GX | 湖南<br>HN | 广东<br>GD | 贵州<br>GZ | 全国平均<br>AVG |
|---|---|---|---|---|---|---|---|---|---|---|---|---|---|---|---|---|---|---|---|---|---|---|---|---|---|
| 谷类<br>Cereals | 0.000 | 0.000 | 0.000 | 0.000 | 0.000 | 0.000 | 0.000 | 0.000 | 0.000 | 0.000 | 0.000 | 0.000 | 2.161 | 0.000 | 1.419 | 6.365 | 13.661 | 0.000 | 0.000 | 0.000 | 0.000 | 0.000 | 5.969 | 4.380 | 1.415 |
| 豆类<br>Legumes | 0.000 | 0.000 | 0.000 | 0.000 | 0.000 | 0.000 | 0.000 | 0.000 | 0.000 | 0.000 | 0.000 | 0.000 | 0.000 | 0.000 | 0.000 | 0.000 | 0.000 | 0.000 | 0.000 | 0.000 | 0.000 | 0.000 | 0.000 | 0.000 | 0.000 |
| 薯类<br>Potatoes | 0.000 | 0.000 | 0.000 | 0.000 | 3.063 | 0.000 | 0.000 | 0.000 | 0.000 | 0.000 | 0.000 | 0.000 | 0.000 | 0.000 | 0.000 | 0.000 | 0.000 | 0.000 | 0.000 | 0.000 | 0.000 | 0.000 | 0.000 | 0.000 | 0.128 |
| 肉类<br>Meats | 0.000 | 0.000 | 0.000 | 0.000 | 0.000 | 0.000 | 0.000 | 0.000 | 0.000 | 0.000 | 0.000 | 0.000 | 0.208 | 3.273 | 0.000 | 0.000 | 0.000 | 0.000 | 1.882 | 0.000 | 0.000 | 0.000 | 2.574 | 0.000 | 0.331 |
| 蛋类<br>Eggs | 0.000 | 0.000 | 0.000 | 0.000 | 0.000 | 0.000 | 0.000 | 0.000 | 0.000 | 0.000 | 0.000 | 0.000 | 0.000 | 0.000 | 0.000 | 0.000 | 0.000 | 0.000 | 1.653 | 0.000 | 0.000 | 0.000 | 0.000 | 0.000 | 0.069 |
| 水产类<br>Aquatic foods | 0.000 | 0.000 | 0.000 | 0.000 | 0.000 | 0.000 | 0.000 | 0.000 | 0.000 | 0.018 | 0.000 | 0.000 | 0.141 | 0.000 | 0.000 | 0.000 | 0.000 | 0.000 | 1.827 | 0.000 | 0.000 | 0.000 | 0.000 | 0.013 | 0.083 |
| 乳类<br>Dairy products | 0.000 | 0.000 | 0.000 | 0.000 | 0.000 | 0.000 | 0.000 | 0.000 | 0.000 | 0.000 | 0.000 | 0.000 | 0.000 | 0.000 | 0.000 | 0.000 | 0.000 | 0.000 | 0.000 | 0.000 | 0.000 | 0.000 | 0.000 | 0.000 | 0.000 |

续表

| 膳食类别 Category | 黑龙江 HL | 辽宁 LN | 河北 HE | 北京 BJ | 吉林 JL | 山西 SX | 陕西 SN | 河南 HA | 宁夏 NX | 内蒙古 NM | 青海 QH | 甘肃 GS | 上海 SH | 福建 FJ | 江西 JX | 江苏 JS | 浙江 ZJ | 山东 SD | 湖北 HB | 四川 SC | 广西 GX | 湖南 HN | 广东 GD | 贵州 GZ | 全国平均 AVG |
|---|---|---|---|---|---|---|---|---|---|---|---|---|---|---|---|---|---|---|---|---|---|---|---|---|---|
| 蔬菜类 Vegetables | 0.000 | 0.000 | 14.627 | 0.000 | 0.000 | 35.184 | 0.000 | 7.270 | 0.000 | 0.000 | 0.000 | 1.881 | 0.000 | 3.329 | 21.376 | 1.334 | 0.000 | 0.000 | 42.441 | 0.000 | 2.994 | 0.000 | 40.377 | 1.978 | 7.200 |
| 水果类 Fruits | 0.000 | 0.000 | 0.000 | 2.976 | 0.245 | 0.000 | 0.000 | 0.000 | 0.163 | 0.000 | 0.000 | 0.000 | 0.000 | 0.000 | 0.000 | 0.047 | 0.000 | 0.000 | 0.000 | 0.000 | 0.000 | 0.000 | 0.000 | 0.000 | 0.143 |
| 糖类 Sugar | 0.000 | 0.000 | 0.000 | 0.000 | 0.000 | 0.000 | 0.000 | 0.000 | 0.000 | 0.000 | 0.000 | 0.000 | 0.000 | 0.000 | 0.000 | 0.000 | 0.000 | 0.000 | 0.000 | 0.000 | 0.000 | 0.000 | 0.000 | 0.000 | 0.000 |
| 水及饮料类 Water and beverages | 0.000 | 0.000 | 0.000 | 0.000 | 0.000 | 0.000 | 0.788 | 0.000 | 0.000 | 0.000 | 0.000 | 0.000 | 0.000 | 0.000 | 0.000 | 0.000 | 0.000 | 0.000 | 0.000 | 0.000 | 0.000 | 0.000 | 0.000 | 0.000 | 0.033 |
| 酒类 Alcohol beverages | 0.000 | 0.000 | 0.000 | 0.000 | 0.000 | 0.000 | 0.000 | 0.000 | 0.000 | 0.018 | 0.000 | 0.000 | 0.000 | 0.000 | 0.000 | 0.000 | 0.000 | 0.000 | 0.000 | 0.000 | 0.130 | 0.000 | 0.000 | 0.000 | 0.005 |
| 合计 SUM | 0.000 | 0.000 | 14.627 | 2.976 | 3.308 | 35.184 | 0.788 | 7.270 | 0.163 | 0.018 | 0.000 | 1.881 | 2.511 | 6.603 | 22.795 | 7.747 | 13.661 | 0.000 | 47.803 | 0.000 | 3.125 | 0.000 | 48.920 | 6.370 | 9.406 |

附表 4-94  第六次中国总膳食研究的三唑酮膳食摄入量 [单位: ng/(kg bw·d)]

Annexed Table 4-94  Dietary intakes of triadimefon from the 6$^{th}$ China TDS [Unit: ng/(kg bw·d)]

| 膳食类别 Category | 黑龙江 HL | 辽宁 LN | 河北 HE | 北京 BJ | 吉林 JL | 山西 SX | 陕西 SN | 河南 HA | 宁夏 NX | 内蒙古 NM | 青海 QH | 甘肃 GS | 上海 SH | 福建 FJ | 江西 JX | 江苏 JS | 浙江 ZJ | 山东 SD | 湖北 HB | 四川 SC | 广西 GX | 湖南 HN | 广东 GD | 贵州 GZ | 全国平均 AVG |
|---|---|---|---|---|---|---|---|---|---|---|---|---|---|---|---|---|---|---|---|---|---|---|---|---|---|
| 谷类 Cereals | 0.000 | 0.000 | 0.000 | 0.000 | 0.000 | 0.000 | 0.000 | 0.000 | 0.000 | 0.000 | 0.000 | 0.000 | 2.678 | 0.000 | 1.419 | 6.365 | 16.630 | 0.000 | 0.000 | 0.000 | 0.000 | 0.000 | 5.969 | 4.380 | 1.560 |
| 豆类 Legumes | 0.000 | 0.000 | 0.000 | 0.000 | 0.000 | 0.000 | 0.000 | 0.000 | 0.000 | 0.000 | 0.000 | 0.000 | 0.000 | 0.000 | 0.000 | 0.000 | 0.000 | 0.000 | 0.000 | 0.000 | 0.000 | 0.000 | 0.000 | 0.000 | 0.000 |
| 薯类 Potatoes | 0.000 | 0.000 | 0.000 | 0.000 | 3.192 | 0.000 | 0.000 | 0.000 | 0.000 | 0.000 | 0.000 | 0.000 | 0.000 | 0.000 | 0.000 | 0.000 | 0.000 | 0.000 | 0.000 | 0.000 | 0.000 | 0.000 | 0.000 | 0.000 | 0.133 |

续表

| 膳食类别<br>Category | 黑龙江<br>HL | 辽宁<br>LN | 河北<br>HE | 北京<br>BJ | 吉林<br>JL | 山西<br>SX | 陕西<br>SN | 河南<br>HA | 宁夏<br>NX | 内蒙古<br>NM | 青海<br>QH | 甘肃<br>GS | 上海<br>SH | 福建<br>FJ | 江西<br>JX | 江苏<br>JS | 浙江<br>ZJ | 山东<br>SD | 湖北<br>HB | 四川<br>SC | 广西<br>GX | 湖南<br>HN | 广东<br>GD | 贵州<br>GZ | 全国平均<br>AVG |
|---|---|---|---|---|---|---|---|---|---|---|---|---|---|---|---|---|---|---|---|---|---|---|---|---|---|
| 肉类 Meats | 0.000 | 0.000 | 0.000 | 0.000 | 0.000 | 0.000 | 0.000 | 0.000 | 0.000 | 0.000 | 0.000 | 0.000 | 0.208 | 3.273 | 0.000 | 0.000 | 0.000 | 0.000 | 1.882 | 0.000 | 0.000 | 0.000 | 2.574 | 0.000 | 0.331 |
| 蛋类 Eggs | 0.000 | 0.000 | 0.000 | 0.000 | 0.000 | 0.000 | 0.000 | 0.000 | 0.000 | 0.000 | 0.000 | 0.000 | 0.000 | 0.000 | 0.000 | 0.000 | 0.000 | 0.000 | 1.653 | 0.000 | 0.000 | 0.000 | 0.000 | 0.000 | 0.069 |
| 水产类 Aquatic foods | 0.000 | 0.000 | 0.000 | 0.000 | 0.000 | 0.000 | 0.000 | 0.000 | 0.000 | 0.018 | 0.000 | 0.000 | 0.141 | 0.000 | 0.000 | 0.000 | 0.000 | 0.000 | 1.827 | 0.000 | 0.000 | 0.000 | 0.000 | 0.013 | 0.083 |
| 乳类 Dairy products | 0.000 | 0.000 | 0.000 | 0.000 | 0.000 | 0.000 | 0.000 | 0.000 | 0.000 | 0.000 | 0.000 | 0.000 | 0.000 | 0.000 | 0.000 | 0.000 | 0.000 | 0.000 | 0.000 | 0.000 | 0.000 | 0.000 | 0.000 | 0.000 | 0.000 |
| 蔬菜类 Vegetables | 0.000 | 0.000 | 21.900 | 0.000 | 0.000 | 37.370 | 0.392 | 7.270 | 0.000 | 0.000 | 0.000 | 1.881 | 0.000 | 4.364 | 29.610 | 1.334 | 0.000 | 0.000 | 65.950 | 0.000 | 3.514 | 3.057 | 66.760 | 1.978 | 10.220 |
| 水果类 Fruits | 0.000 | 0.000 | 0.000 | 2.976 | 0.245 | 0.000 | 0.000 | 0.000 | 0.163 | 0.000 | 0.000 | 0.000 | 0.000 | 0.000 | 0.000 | 0.047 | 0.000 | 0.000 | 0.000 | 0.000 | 0.000 | 0.000 | 0.000 | 0.000 | 0.143 |
| 糖类 Sugar | 0.000 | 0.000 | 0.000 | 0.000 | 0.000 | 0.000 | 0.000 | 0.000 | 0.000 | 0.000 | 0.000 | 0.000 | 0.000 | 0.000 | 0.000 | 0.000 | 0.000 | 0.000 | 0.000 | 0.000 | 0.000 | 0.000 | 0.000 | 0.000 | 0.000 |
| 水及饮料类 Water and beverages | 0.000 | 0.000 | 0.000 | 0.000 | 0.000 | 0.000 | 0.788 | 0.000 | 0.000 | 0.000 | 0.000 | 0.000 | 0.000 | 0.000 | 0.000 | 0.000 | 0.000 | 0.000 | 0.000 | 0.000 | 0.130 | 0.000 | 0.000 | 0.000 | 0.033 |
| 酒类 Alcohol beverages | 0.000 | 0.000 | 0.000 | 0.000 | 0.000 | 0.000 | 0.000 | 0.000 | 0.000 | 0.000 | 0.000 | 0.000 | 0.000 | 0.000 | 0.000 | 0.000 | 0.000 | 0.000 | 0.000 | 0.000 | 0.000 | 0.000 | 0.000 | 0.000 | 0.005 |
| 合计 SUM | 0.000 | 0.000 | 21.901 | 2.976 | 3.437 | 37.367 | 1.179 | 7.270 | 0.163 | 0.018 | 0.000 | 1.881 | 3.028 | 7.638 | 31.025 | 7.747 | 16.626 | 0.000 | 71.312 | 0.000 | 3.644 | 3.057 | 75.304 | 6.370 | 12.581 |

附表 4-95 第六次中国总膳食研究的四氟醚唑膳食摄入量 [单位: ng/(kg bw·d)]
Annexed Table 4-95 Dietary intakes of tetraconazole from the 6th China TDS [Unit: ng/(kg bw·d)]

| 膳食类别 Category | 黑龙江 HL | 辽宁 LN | 河北 HE | 北京 BJ | 吉林 JL | 山西 SX | 陕西 SN | 河南 HA | 宁夏 NX | 内蒙古 NM | 青海 QH | 甘肃 GS | 上海 SH | 福建 FJ | 江西 JX | 江苏 JS | 浙江 ZJ | 山东 SD | 湖北 HB | 四川 SC | 广西 GX | 湖南 HN | 广东 GD | 贵州 GZ | 全国平均 AVG |
|---|---|---|---|---|---|---|---|---|---|---|---|---|---|---|---|---|---|---|---|---|---|---|---|---|---|
| 谷类 Cereals | 0.000 | 0.000 | 0.000 | 0.000 | 0.000 | 0.000 | 0.000 | 0.000 | 0.000 | 0.000 | 0.000 | 0.000 | 0.000 | 0.000 | 0.000 | 0.000 | 0.000 | 0.000 | 0.000 | 0.000 | 0.000 | 0.000 | 0.000 | 0.000 | 0.000 |
| 豆类 Legumes | 0.000 | 0.000 | 0.000 | 0.000 | 0.000 | 0.000 | 0.000 | 0.000 | 0.000 | 0.000 | 0.000 | 0.000 | 0.000 | 0.000 | 0.000 | 0.000 | 0.000 | 0.000 | 0.000 | 0.000 | 0.000 | 0.000 | 0.000 | 0.000 | 0.000 |
| 薯类 Potatoes | 0.000 | 0.000 | 0.000 | 0.000 | 0.000 | 0.000 | 0.000 | 0.000 | 0.000 | 0.000 | 0.000 | 0.000 | 0.000 | 0.000 | 0.000 | 0.000 | 0.000 | 0.000 | 0.000 | 0.000 | 0.000 | 0.000 | 0.000 | 0.000 | 0.000 |
| 肉类 Meats | 0.000 | 0.000 | 0.000 | 0.000 | 0.000 | 0.000 | 0.000 | 0.000 | 0.000 | 0.000 | 0.000 | 0.000 | 0.000 | 0.000 | 0.000 | 0.000 | 0.000 | 0.000 | 0.000 | 0.000 | 0.000 | 0.000 | 0.000 | 0.000 | 0.000 |
| 蛋类 Eggs | 0.000 | 0.000 | 0.000 | 0.000 | 0.000 | 0.000 | 0.000 | 0.000 | 0.000 | 0.000 | 0.000 | 0.000 | 0.000 | 0.000 | 0.000 | 0.000 | 0.000 | 0.000 | 0.000 | 0.000 | 0.000 | 0.000 | 0.000 | 0.000 | 0.000 |
| 水产类 Aquatic foods | 0.000 | 0.000 | 0.000 | 0.000 | 0.000 | 0.000 | 0.000 | 0.000 | 0.000 | 0.000 | 0.000 | 0.000 | 0.000 | 0.000 | 0.000 | 0.000 | 0.000 | 0.000 | 0.000 | 0.000 | 0.000 | 0.000 | 0.000 | 0.000 | 0.000 |
| 乳类 Dairy products | 0.000 | 0.000 | 0.000 | 0.000 | 0.000 | 0.000 | 0.000 | 0.000 | 0.000 | 0.000 | 0.000 | 0.000 | 0.000 | 0.000 | 0.000 | 0.000 | 0.000 | 0.000 | 0.000 | 0.000 | 0.000 | 0.000 | 0.000 | 0.000 | 0.000 |
| 蔬菜类 Vegetables | 0.000 | 0.000 | 0.000 | 0.000 | 0.000 | 0.000 | 0.000 | 0.000 | 0.000 | 0.000 | 1.930 | 0.000 | 0.000 | 0.000 | 0.000 | 0.000 | 0.000 | 0.000 | 0.000 | 0.000 | 0.000 | 0.000 | 0.000 | 0.000 | 0.080 |
| 水果类 Fruits | 0.000 | 0.000 | 0.000 | 0.722 | 0.072 | 0.000 | 0.000 | 0.000 | 0.000 | 0.000 | 0.000 | 0.000 | 0.000 | 0.000 | 0.000 | 0.000 | 0.000 | 0.062 | 0.000 | 0.000 | 0.000 | 0.000 | 0.058 | 0.000 | 0.038 |
| 糖类 Sugar | 0.000 | 0.000 | 0.000 | 0.000 | 0.000 | 0.000 | 0.000 | 0.000 | 0.000 | 0.000 | 0.000 | 0.000 | 0.000 | 0.000 | 0.000 | 0.000 | 0.000 | 0.000 | 0.000 | 0.000 | 0.000 | 0.000 | 0.000 | 0.000 | 0.000 |
| 水及饮料类 Water and beverages | 0.000 | 0.000 | 0.000 | 0.000 | 0.000 | 0.000 | 0.000 | 0.000 | 0.000 | 0.000 | 0.000 | 0.000 | 0.000 | 0.000 | 0.000 | 0.000 | 0.000 | 0.000 | 0.000 | 0.000 | 0.000 | 0.000 | 0.000 | 0.000 | 0.000 |

续表

| 膳食类别<br>Category | 黑龙江<br>HL | 辽宁<br>LN | 河北<br>HE | 北京<br>BJ | 吉林<br>JL | 山西<br>SX | 陕西<br>SN | 河南<br>HA | 宁夏<br>NX | 内蒙古<br>NM | 青海<br>QH | 甘肃<br>GS | 上海<br>SH | 福建<br>FJ | 江西<br>JX | 江苏<br>JS | 浙江<br>ZJ | 山东<br>SD | 湖北<br>HB | 四川<br>SC | 广西<br>GX | 湖南<br>HN | 广东<br>GD | 贵州<br>GZ | 全国平均<br>AVG |
|---|---|---|---|---|---|---|---|---|---|---|---|---|---|---|---|---|---|---|---|---|---|---|---|---|---|
| 酒类<br>Alcohol beverages | 0.000 | 0.000 | 0.000 | 0.000 | 0.000 | 0.000 | 0.000 | 0.000 | 0.000 | 0.000 | 0.000 | 0.000 | 0.000 | 0.000 | 0.000 | 0.000 | 0.000 | 0.000 | 0.000 | 0.000 | 0.000 | 0.000 | 0.000 | 0.000 | 0.000 |
| 合计<br>SUM | 0.000 | 0.000 | 0.000 | 0.722 | 0.072 | 0.000 | 0.000 | 0.000 | 0.000 | 0.000 | 1.930 | 0.000 | 0.000 | 0.000 | 0.000 | 0.000 | 0.000 | 0.062 | 0.000 | 0.000 | 0.000 | 0.000 | 0.058 | 0.000 | 0.119 |

附表 4-96　第六次中国总膳食研究的氟环唑膳食摄入量 [单位: ng/(kg bw · d)]
Annexed Table 4-96　Dietary intakes of epoxiconazole from the 6$^{th}$ China TDS [Unit: ng/(kg bw · d)]

| 膳食类别<br>Category | 黑龙江<br>HL | 辽宁<br>LN | 河北<br>HE | 北京<br>BJ | 吉林<br>JL | 山西<br>SX | 陕西<br>SN | 河南<br>HA | 宁夏<br>NX | 内蒙古<br>NM | 青海<br>QH | 甘肃<br>GS | 上海<br>SH | 福建<br>FJ | 江西<br>JX | 江苏<br>JS | 浙江<br>ZJ | 山东<br>SD | 湖北<br>HB | 四川<br>SC | 广西<br>GX | 湖南<br>HN | 广东<br>GD | 贵州<br>GZ | 全国平均<br>AVG |
|---|---|---|---|---|---|---|---|---|---|---|---|---|---|---|---|---|---|---|---|---|---|---|---|---|---|
| 谷类<br>Cereals | 0.840 | 0.000 | 0.000 | 0.000 | 0.000 | 0.000 | 0.000 | 0.000 | 0.000 | 0.000 | 0.000 | 0.000 | 0.000 | 0.853 | 0.982 | 0.000 | 0.000 | 0.000 | 0.000 | 0.000 | 0.000 | 0.000 | 0.000 | 0.000 | 0.111 |
| 豆类<br>Legumes | 0.000 | 0.000 | 0.000 | 0.000 | 0.000 | 0.000 | 0.000 | 0.000 | 0.000 | 0.000 | 0.000 | 0.000 | 0.000 | 0.000 | 0.000 | 0.000 | 0.000 | 0.000 | 0.000 | 0.000 | 0.000 | 0.000 | 0.000 | 0.000 | 0.000 |
| 薯类<br>Potatoes | 0.000 | 0.000 | 0.000 | 0.000 | 0.204 | 0.000 | 0.000 | 0.000 | 0.000 | 0.000 | 0.000 | 0.000 | 0.000 | 0.000 | 0.000 | 0.000 | 0.000 | 0.000 | 0.000 | 0.000 | 0.000 | 0.000 | 0.000 | 0.000 | 0.009 |
| 肉类<br>Meats | 0.000 | 0.000 | 0.000 | 0.000 | 0.000 | 0.000 | 0.000 | 0.000 | 0.000 | 0.000 | 0.000 | 0.000 | 0.000 | 0.000 | 0.000 | 0.000 | 0.000 | 0.000 | 0.000 | 0.000 | 0.000 | 0.000 | 0.000 | 0.000 | 0.000 |
| 蛋类<br>Eggs | 0.000 | 0.000 | 0.000 | 0.000 | 0.019 | 0.000 | 0.000 | 0.000 | 0.000 | 0.000 | 0.000 | 0.000 | 0.000 | 0.000 | 0.000 | 0.000 | 0.000 | 0.000 | 0.000 | 0.000 | 0.000 | 0.000 | 0.000 | 0.000 | 0.000 |
| 水产类<br>Aquatic foods | 0.000 | 0.000 | 0.000 | 0.000 | 0.000 | 0.000 | 0.000 | 0.000 | 0.000 | 0.000 | 0.000 | 0.000 | 0.000 | 0.000 | 0.035 | 0.000 | 0.000 | 0.000 | 0.000 | 0.000 | 0.000 | 0.000 | 0.000 | 0.000 | 0.002 |
| 乳类<br>Dairy products | 0.000 | 0.000 | 0.000 | 0.000 | 0.000 | 0.000 | 0.000 | 0.000 | 0.000 | 0.000 | 0.000 | 0.000 | 0.000 | 0.000 | 0.000 | 0.000 | 0.000 | 0.000 | 0.000 | 0.000 | 0.000 | 0.000 | 0.000 | 0.000 | 0.000 |

续表

| 膳食类别<br>Category | 黑龙江<br>HL | 辽宁<br>LN | 河北<br>HE | 北京<br>BJ | 吉林<br>JL | 山西<br>SX | 陕西<br>SN | 河南<br>HA | 宁夏<br>NX | 内蒙古<br>NM | 青海<br>QH | 甘肃<br>GS | 上海<br>SH | 福建<br>FJ | 江西<br>JX | 江苏<br>JS | 浙江<br>ZJ | 山东<br>SD | 湖北<br>HB | 四川<br>SC | 广西<br>GX | 湖南<br>HN | 广东<br>GD | 贵州<br>GZ | 全国平均<br>AVG |
|---|---|---|---|---|---|---|---|---|---|---|---|---|---|---|---|---|---|---|---|---|---|---|---|---|---|
| 蔬菜类 Vegetables | 0.000 | 0.000 | 0.000 | 0.000 | 0.400 | 0.000 | 0.000 | 0.000 | 0.000 | 0.000 | 0.000 | 0.000 | 0.000 | 0.000 | 0.000 | 0.000 | 0.000 | 0.000 | 0.000 | 0.000 | 0.000 | 0.000 | 0.000 | 0.000 | 0.017 |
| 水果类 Fruits | 0.000 | 0.000 | 0.187 | 0.000 | 0.000 | 0.000 | 0.000 | 0.027 | 0.000 | 0.000 | 0.000 | 0.000 | 0.000 | 0.000 | 0.000 | 0.000 | 0.000 | 1.244 | 0.000 | 0.063 | 0.000 | 0.000 | 0.000 | 0.000 | 0.063 |
| 糖类 Sugar | 0.000 | 0.000 | 0.000 | 0.000 | 0.000 | 0.000 | 0.000 | 0.000 | 0.000 | 0.000 | 0.000 | 0.000 | 0.000 | 0.000 | 0.000 | 0.000 | 0.000 | 0.000 | 0.000 | 0.000 | 0.000 | 0.000 | 0.000 | 0.000 | 0.000 |
| 水及饮料类 Water and beverages | 0.000 | 0.000 | 0.000 | 0.000 | 0.000 | 0.000 | 0.000 | 0.000 | 0.000 | 0.000 | 0.000 | 0.000 | 0.000 | 0.000 | 0.000 | 0.000 | 0.000 | 0.000 | 0.000 | 0.000 | 0.000 | 0.000 | 0.000 | 0.000 | 0.000 |
| 酒类 Alcohol beverages | 0.000 | 0.000 | 0.000 | 0.000 | 0.000 | 0.000 | 0.000 | 0.000 | 0.000 | 0.000 | 0.000 | 0.000 | 0.000 | 0.853 | 1.017 | 0.000 | 0.000 | 0.000 | 0.000 | 0.000 | 0.000 | 0.000 | 0.000 | 0.000 | 0.000 |
| 合计 SUM | 0.840 | 0.000 | 0.187 | 0.000 | 0.623 | 0.000 | 0.000 | 0.027 | 0.000 | 0.000 | 0.000 | 0.000 | 0.000 | 0.853 | 1.017 | 0.000 | 0.000 | 1.244 | 0.000 | 0.063 | 0.000 | 0.000 | 0.000 | 0.000 | 0.202 |

附表 4-97　第六次中国总膳食研究的腈苯唑膳食摄入量 [单位: ng/(kg bw·d)]

Annexed Table 4-97　Dietary intakes of fenbuconazole from the 6ᵗʰ China TDS [Unit: ng/(kg bw·d)]

| 膳食类别<br>Category | 黑龙江<br>HL | 辽宁<br>LN | 河北<br>HE | 北京<br>BJ | 吉林<br>JL | 山西<br>SX | 陕西<br>SN | 河南<br>HA | 宁夏<br>NX | 内蒙古<br>NM | 青海<br>QH | 甘肃<br>GS | 上海<br>SH | 福建<br>FJ | 江西<br>JX | 江苏<br>JS | 浙江<br>ZJ | 山东<br>SD | 湖北<br>HB | 四川<br>SC | 广西<br>GX | 湖南<br>HN | 广东<br>GD | 贵州<br>GZ | 全国平均<br>AVG |
|---|---|---|---|---|---|---|---|---|---|---|---|---|---|---|---|---|---|---|---|---|---|---|---|---|---|
| 谷类 Cereals | 0.000 | 0.000 | 0.000 | 0.000 | 0.000 | 0.000 | 0.000 | 0.000 | 0.000 | 0.000 | 0.000 | 0.000 | 0.000 | 0.000 | 0.000 | 0.000 | 0.000 | 0.000 | 0.000 | 0.000 | 1.126 | 0.000 | 0.000 | 0.000 | 0.047 |
| 豆类 Legumes | 0.210 | 0.818 | 0.000 | 0.000 | 0.000 | 0.000 | 0.000 | 0.211 | 0.000 | 1.661 | 0.000 | 0.000 | 1.617 | 0.000 | 0.000 | 0.000 | 0.000 | 0.000 | 0.864 | 0.000 | 0.186 | 0.000 | 0.000 | 0.885 | 0.191 |
| 薯类 Potatoes | 0.077 | 0.000 | 0.000 | 0.000 | 0.000 | 1.384 | 0.000 | 0.000 | 0.000 | 0.000 | 0.000 | 0.000 | 0.804 | 0.000 | 0.000 | 0.000 | 0.000 | 0.000 | 0.271 | 0.000 | 0.186 | 0.000 | 0.000 | 0.557 | 0.215 |

续表

| 膳食类别<br>Category | 黑龙江<br>HL | 辽宁<br>LN | 河北<br>HE | 北京<br>BJ | 吉林<br>JL | 山西<br>SX | 陕西<br>SN | 河南<br>HA | 宁夏<br>NX | 内蒙古<br>NM | 青海<br>QH | 甘肃<br>GS | 上海<br>SH | 福建<br>FJ | 江西<br>JX | 江苏<br>JS | 浙江<br>ZJ | 山东<br>SD | 湖北<br>HB | 四川<br>SC | 广西<br>GX | 湖南<br>HN | 广东<br>GD | 贵州<br>GZ | 全国平均<br>AVG |
|---|---|---|---|---|---|---|---|---|---|---|---|---|---|---|---|---|---|---|---|---|---|---|---|---|---|
| 肉类 Meats | 1.375 | 0.116 | 0.000 | 0.000 | 0.099 | 2.898 | 0.000 | 0.359 | 0.000 | 0.808 | 0.000 | 0.000 | 6.494 | 0.000 | 0.000 | 3.956 | 0.000 | 0.000 | 0.462 | 0.000 | 2.731 | 0.000 | 0.000 | 1.289 | 0.858 |
| 蛋类 Eggs | 0.000 | 0.000 | 0.000 | 0.000 | 0.000 | 0.000 | 0.000 | 0.000 | 0.000 | 0.000 | 0.000 | 0.000 | 0.000 | 0.000 | 0.000 | 0.075 | 0.000 | 0.000 | 0.000 | 0.000 | 0.342 | 0.000 | 0.000 | 0.164 | 0.024 |
| 水产类 Aquatic foods | 0.141 | 0.000 | 0.000 | 0.000 | 0.000 | 0.057 | 0.000 | 0.027 | 0.000 | 1.292 | 0.000 | 0.000 | 2.546 | 0.000 | 0.000 | 0.151 | 0.000 | 0.000 | 0.000 | 0.000 | 0.979 | 0.000 | 0.000 | 0.060 | 0.219 |
| 乳类 Dairy products | 0.000 | 0.000 | 0.000 | 0.000 | 0.000 | 0.000 | 0.000 | 0.000 | 0.000 | 0.000 | 0.000 | 0.000 | 0.000 | 0.000 | 0.000 | 0.000 | 0.000 | 0.000 | 0.000 | 0.000 | 0.000 | 0.000 | 0.000 | 0.000 | 0.000 |
| 蔬菜类 Vegetables | 0.000 | 0.531 | 0.000 | 0.000 | 0.000 | 0.000 | 0.000 | 0.000 | 0.000 | 0.000 | 0.000 | 0.000 | 0.000 | 5.184 | 0.000 | 0.000 | 0.000 | 0.000 | 0.000 | 0.000 | 0.000 | 0.000 | 0.000 | 0.000 | 0.022 |
| 水果类 Fruits | 1.394 | 0.000 | 0.000 | 0.000 | 1.956 | 0.627 | 0.000 | 0.442 | 0.000 | 0.000 | 0.000 | 0.000 | 0.000 | 0.000 | 0.000 | 0.000 | 0.000 | 0.000 | 0.000 | 0.000 | 0.000 | 0.000 | 0.000 | 0.000 | 0.400 |
| 糖类 Sugar | 0.000 | 0.000 | 0.000 | 0.000 | 0.000 | 0.000 | 0.000 | 0.000 | 0.000 | 0.000 | 0.000 | 0.000 | 0.285 | 0.000 | 0.000 | 0.000 | 0.000 | 0.000 | 0.000 | 0.000 | 0.000 | 0.000 | 0.000 | 0.000 | 0.012 |
| 水及饮料类 Water and beverages | 0.000 | 0.000 | 0.000 | 0.000 | 0.000 | 0.000 | 0.000 | 0.000 | 0.000 | 0.080 | 0.000 | 0.000 | 0.000 | 0.000 | 0.000 | 0.000 | 0.000 | 0.000 | 0.000 | 0.000 | 0.000 | 0.000 | 0.000 | 0.000 | 0.000 |
| 酒类 Alcohol beverages | 0.093 | 0.000 | 0.012 | 0.000 | 0.000 | 0.000 | 0.000 | 0.000 | 0.000 | 0.000 | 0.000 | 0.000 | 10.430 | 0.000 | 0.030 | 11.930 | 0.000 | 0.000 | 0.000 | 0.000 | 2.509 | 0.038 | 0.002 | 0.457 | 1.066 |
| 合计 SUM | 3.291 | 1.465 | 0.012 | 0.000 | 2.055 | 4.966 | 0.000 | 1.039 | 0.000 | 3.841 | 0.000 | 0.000 | 22.174 | 5.184 | 0.030 | 16.111 | 0.000 | 0.000 | 1.597 | 0.000 | 8.060 | 0.038 | 0.002 | 3.412 | 3.053 |

附表 4-98　第六次中国总膳食研究的氟硅唑膳食摄入量 [单位：ng/(kg bw·d)]

Annexed Table 4-98　Dietary intakes of flusilazole from the 6<sup>th</sup> China TDS [Unit: ng/(kg bw·d)]

| 膳食类别 Category | 黑龙江 HL | 辽宁 LN | 河北 HE | 北京 BJ | 吉林 JL | 山西 SX | 陕西 SN | 河南 HA | 宁夏 NX | 内蒙古 NM | 青海 QH | 甘肃 GS | 上海 SH | 福建 FJ | 江西 JX | 江苏 JS | 浙江 ZJ | 山东 SD | 湖北 HB | 四川 SC | 广西 GX | 湖南 HN | 广东 GD | 贵州 GZ | 全国平均 AVG |
|---|---|---|---|---|---|---|---|---|---|---|---|---|---|---|---|---|---|---|---|---|---|---|---|---|---|
| 谷类 Cereals | 0.000 | 0.000 | 0.000 | 0.000 | 0.000 | 0.000 | 0.000 | 0.000 | 0.000 | 0.000 | 0.000 | 0.000 | 0.000 | 0.000 | 0.000 | 0.000 | 0.000 | 0.000 | 0.000 | 0.000 | 0.000 | 0.000 | 0.000 | 0.000 | 0.000 |
| 豆类 Legumes | 0.000 | 0.000 | 0.000 | 0.000 | 0.000 | 0.000 | 0.000 | 0.000 | 0.000 | 0.000 | 0.000 | 0.000 | 0.000 | 0.000 | 0.000 | 0.000 | 0.000 | 0.000 | 0.000 | 0.000 | 0.000 | 0.000 | 0.000 | 0.000 | 0.000 |
| 薯类 Potatoes | 0.000 | 0.000 | 0.000 | 0.000 | 0.000 | 0.000 | 0.000 | 0.000 | 0.000 | 0.000 | 0.000 | 0.000 | 0.000 | 0.000 | 0.000 | 0.000 | 0.000 | 0.000 | 0.000 | 0.000 | 0.000 | 0.000 | 0.000 | 0.000 | 0.000 |
| 肉类 Meats | 0.000 | 0.000 | 0.000 | 0.000 | 0.000 | 0.000 | 0.000 | 0.000 | 0.000 | 0.000 | 0.000 | 0.000 | 0.000 | 0.000 | 0.000 | 0.000 | 0.000 | 0.000 | 0.000 | 0.000 | 0.000 | 0.000 | 0.000 | 0.000 | 0.000 |
| 蛋类 Eggs | 0.000 | 0.000 | 0.000 | 0.000 | 0.000 | 0.000 | 0.000 | 0.000 | 0.000 | 0.000 | 0.000 | 0.000 | 0.000 | 0.000 | 0.000 | 0.000 | 0.000 | 0.000 | 0.000 | 0.000 | 0.000 | 0.000 | 0.000 | 0.000 | 0.000 |
| 水产类 Aquatic foods | 0.000 | 0.000 | 0.000 | 0.000 | 0.000 | 0.000 | 0.000 | 0.000 | 0.000 | 0.000 | 0.000 | 0.000 | 0.000 | 0.000 | 0.000 | 0.000 | 0.000 | 0.000 | 0.000 | 0.000 | 0.000 | 0.000 | 0.000 | 0.000 | 0.000 |
| 乳类 Dairy products | 0.000 | 0.000 | 0.000 | 0.000 | 0.000 | 0.000 | 0.000 | 0.000 | 0.000 | 0.000 | 0.000 | 0.000 | 0.000 | 0.000 | 0.000 | 0.000 | 0.000 | 0.000 | 0.000 | 0.000 | 0.000 | 0.000 | 0.000 | 0.000 | 0.000 |
| 蔬菜类 Vegetables | 0.000 | 0.000 | 1.149 | 0.000 | 0.000 | 6.312 | 0.000 | 1.415 | 0.000 | 0.000 | 0.000 | 4.655 | 0.000 | 18.930 | 0.000 | 0.000 | 0.000 | 0.504 | 168.800 | 0.000 | 0.547 | 191.900 | 619.900 | 28.390 | 43.440 |
| 水果类 Fruits | 0.506 | 0.000 | 0.000 | 0.394 | 0.000 | 0.000 | 0.000 | 0.026 | 0.000 | 0.000 | 0.091 | 0.000 | 0.000 | 0.000 | 0.000 | 0.000 | 0.343 | 0.000 | 0.016 | 0.000 | 0.000 | 0.286 | 0.115 | 0.000 | 0.074 |
| 糖类 Sugar | 0.000 | 0.000 | 0.000 | 0.000 | 0.000 | 0.000 | 0.000 | 0.000 | 0.000 | 0.000 | 0.000 | 0.000 | 0.000 | 0.000 | 0.000 | 0.000 | 0.000 | 0.000 | 0.000 | 0.000 | 0.000 | 0.000 | 0.000 | 0.000 | 0.000 |
| 水及饮料类 Water and beverages | 0.000 | 0.000 | 0.000 | 0.000 | 0.000 | 0.000 | 0.000 | 0.000 | 0.000 | 0.000 | 0.000 | 0.000 | 0.000 | 0.000 | 0.000 | 0.000 | 0.000 | 0.000 | 0.000 | 0.000 | 0.000 | 0.000 | 0.000 | 0.000 | 0.000 |

续表

| 膳食类别<br>Category | 黑龙江<br>HL | 辽宁<br>LN | 河北<br>HE | 北京<br>BJ | 吉林<br>JL | 山西<br>SX | 陕西<br>SN | 河南<br>HA | 宁夏<br>NX | 内蒙古<br>NM | 青海<br>QH | 甘肃<br>GS | 上海<br>SH | 福建<br>FJ | 江西<br>JX | 江苏<br>JS | 浙江<br>ZJ | 山东<br>SD | 湖北<br>HB | 四川<br>SC | 广西<br>GX | 湖南<br>HN | 广东<br>GD | 贵州<br>GZ | 全国平均<br>AVG |
|---|---|---|---|---|---|---|---|---|---|---|---|---|---|---|---|---|---|---|---|---|---|---|---|---|---|
| 酒类<br>Alcohol beverages | 0.000 | 0.000 | 0.000 | 0.000 | 0.000 | 0.000 | 0.000 | 0.000 | 0.000 | 0.000 | 0.000 | 0.000 | 0.000 | 0.000 | 0.000 | 0.000 | 0.000 | 0.000 | 0.000 | 0.000 | 0.000 | 0.000 | 0.000 | 0.000 | 0.000 |
| 合计<br>SUM | 0.506 | 0.000 | 1.149 | 0.394 | 0.000 | 6.312 | 0.000 | 1.441 | 0.000 | 0.000 | 0.091 | 4.655 | 0.000 | 18.930 | 0.000 | 0.000 | 0.343 | 0.504 | 168.844 | 0.000 | 0.547 | 192.138 | 620.047 | 28.393 | 43.512 |

附表 4-99　第六次中国总膳食研究的戊唑醇膳食摄入量 [单位: ng/(kg bw·d)]

Annexed Table 4-99　Dietary intakes of tebuconazole from the 6th China TDS [Unit: ng/(kg bw·d)]

| 膳食类别<br>Category | 黑龙江<br>HL | 辽宁<br>LN | 河北<br>HE | 北京<br>BJ | 吉林<br>JL | 山西<br>SX | 陕西<br>SN | 河南<br>HA | 宁夏<br>NX | 内蒙古<br>NM | 青海<br>QH | 甘肃<br>GS | 上海<br>SH | 福建<br>FJ | 江西<br>JX | 江苏<br>JS | 浙江<br>ZJ | 山东<br>SD | 湖北<br>HB | 四川<br>SC | 广西<br>GX | 湖南<br>HN | 广东<br>GD | 贵州<br>GZ | 全国平均<br>AVG |
|---|---|---|---|---|---|---|---|---|---|---|---|---|---|---|---|---|---|---|---|---|---|---|---|---|---|
| 谷类<br>Cereals | 1.385 | 0.000 | 0.000 | 0.920 | 0.000 | 0.000 | 2.854 | 4.435 | 0.000 | 0.000 | 4.675 | 0.000 | 0.720 | 7.972 | 10.784 | 3.103 | 1.457 | 2.879 | 2.756 | 2.097 | 8.415 | 1.398 | 1.441 | 4.802 | 2.587 |
| 豆类<br>Legumes | 0.000 | 0.000 | 0.150 | 0.000 | 0.000 | 0.000 | 0.303 | 0.065 | 0.000 | 0.000 | 0.000 | 0.000 | 0.000 | 0.000 | 0.000 | 0.246 | 0.000 | 0.000 | 0.072 | 0.166 | 0.000 | 0.000 | 0.000 | 0.000 | 0.042 |
| 薯类<br>Potatoes | 0.000 | 0.000 | 0.000 | 0.000 | 0.244 | 0.000 | 1.737 | 0.000 | 0.110 | 0.159 | 0.085 | 0.000 | 0.000 | 0.000 | 0.000 | 0.000 | 0.000 | 0.170 | 0.000 | 0.091 | 0.000 | 0.000 | 0.000 | 0.000 | 0.108 |
| 肉类<br>Meats | 0.000 | 0.000 | 0.000 | 0.000 | 0.000 | 0.000 | 0.000 | 0.000 | 0.101 | 0.000 | 0.232 | 0.000 | 0.000 | 0.063 | 0.000 | 0.047 | 0.000 | 0.000 | 0.000 | 0.341 | 0.000 | 0.235 | 0.000 | 0.088 | 0.042 |
| 蛋类<br>Eggs | 0.000 | 0.000 | 0.000 | 0.000 | 0.000 | 0.000 | 0.025 | 0.000 | 0.000 | 0.000 | 0.007 | 0.000 | 0.000 | 0.075 | 0.000 | 0.051 | 0.000 | 0.000 | 0.000 | 0.015 | 0.000 | 0.000 | 0.000 | 0.000 | 0.005 |
| 水产类<br>Aquatic foods | 0.000 | 0.000 | 0.000 | 0.000 | 0.018 | 0.000 | 0.000 | 0.000 | 0.000 | 0.000 | 0.000 | 0.000 | 0.000 | 0.000 | 0.000 | 0.000 | 0.000 | 0.000 | 0.000 | 0.000 | 0.000 | 0.108 | 0.000 | 0.004 | 0.013 |
| 乳类<br>Dairy products | 0.000 | 0.000 | 0.000 | 0.000 | 0.000 | 0.000 | 0.000 | 0.000 | 0.000 | 0.000 | 0.000 | 0.000 | 0.000 | 0.000 | 0.000 | 0.047 | 0.000 | 0.000 | 0.000 | 0.000 | 0.000 | 0.000 | 0.000 | 0.000 | 0.002 |

续表

| 膳食类别<br>Category | 黑龙江<br>HL | 辽宁<br>LN | 河北<br>HE | 北京<br>BJ | 吉林<br>JL | 山西<br>SX | 陕西<br>SN | 河南<br>HA | 宁夏<br>NX | 内蒙古<br>NM | 青海<br>QH | 甘肃<br>GS | 上海<br>SH | 福建<br>FJ | 江西<br>JX | 江苏<br>JS | 浙江<br>ZJ | 山东<br>SD | 湖北<br>HB | 四川<br>SC | 广西<br>GX | 湖南<br>HN | 广东<br>GD | 贵州<br>GZ | 全国平均<br>AVG |
|---|---|---|---|---|---|---|---|---|---|---|---|---|---|---|---|---|---|---|---|---|---|---|---|---|---|
| 蔬菜类 Vegetables | 0.446 | 1.127 | 0.601 | 68.480 | 0.000 | 6.179 | 2.067 | 21.040 | 0.460 | 0.343 | 4.465 | 1.116 | 8.137 | 2.051 | 8.542 | 1.460 | 26.470 | 0.572 | 14.460 | 0.566 | 26.480 | 116.500 | 139.700 | 2.453 | 18.900 |
| 水果类 Fruits | 2.324 | 5.184 | 0.455 | 46.150 | 1.609 | 0.088 | 0.210 | 0.253 | 0.188 | 0.000 | 0.028 | 0.049 | 1.459 | 0.502 | 0.317 | 0.550 | 5.903 | 1.148 | 0.061 | 0.323 | 1.033 | 0.131 | 0.340 | 0.147 | 2.852 |
| 糖类 Sugar | 0.000 | 0.000 | 0.000 | 0.000 | 0.000 | 0.000 | 0.000 | 0.000 | 0.000 | 0.000 | 0.000 | 0.000 | 0.000 | 0.000 | 0.000 | 0.000 | 0.000 | 0.000 | 0.000 | 0.000 | 0.000 | 0.000 | 0.000 | 0.000 | 0.000 |
| 水及饮料类 Water and beverages | 0.000 | 0.000 | 0.000 | 0.000 | 0.000 | 0.000 | 0.000 | 0.000 | 0.000 | 0.000 | 0.000 | 0.000 | 0.000 | 0.000 | 0.000 | 0.000 | 0.000 | 0.000 | 0.000 | 0.000 | 0.000 | 0.000 | 0.000 | 0.000 | 0.000 |
| 酒类 Alcohol beverages | 0.000 | 0.000 | 0.000 | 0.000 | 0.000 | 0.000 | 0.000 | 0.000 | 0.000 | 0.000 | 0.000 | 0.000 | 0.000 | 0.000 | 0.000 | 0.000 | 0.000 | 0.000 | 0.000 | 0.000 | 0.000 | 0.000 | 0.001 | 0.000 | 0.000 |
| 合计 SUM | 4.155 | 6.311 | 1.206 | 115.545 | 1.871 | 6.266 | 7.197 | 25.787 | 0.859 | 0.502 | 9.492 | 1.165 | 10.315 | 10.664 | 19.643 | 5.504 | 33.827 | 4.769 | 17.350 | 3.600 | 35.932 | 118.367 | 141.461 | 7.494 | 24.553 |

附表 4-100 第六次中国总膳食研究的戊菌唑膳食摄入量 [ 单位：ng/(kg bw·d)]

Annexed Table 4-100 Dietary intakes of penconazole from the 6<sup>th</sup> China TDS [Unit: ng/(kg bw·d)]

| 膳食类别<br>Category | 黑龙江<br>HL | 辽宁<br>LN | 河北<br>HE | 北京<br>BJ | 吉林<br>JL | 山西<br>SX | 陕西<br>SN | 河南<br>HA | 宁夏<br>NX | 内蒙古<br>NM | 青海<br>QH | 甘肃<br>GS | 上海<br>SH | 福建<br>FJ | 江西<br>JX | 江苏<br>JS | 浙江<br>ZJ | 山东<br>SD | 湖北<br>HB | 四川<br>SC | 广西<br>GX | 湖南<br>HN | 广东<br>GD | 贵州<br>GZ | 全国平均<br>AVG |
|---|---|---|---|---|---|---|---|---|---|---|---|---|---|---|---|---|---|---|---|---|---|---|---|---|---|
| 谷类 Cereals | 0.000 | 0.000 | 0.000 | 0.000 | 0.000 | 0.000 | 0.000 | 0.000 | 0.000 | 0.000 | 0.000 | 0.000 | 0.000 | 0.000 | 0.000 | 0.000 | 0.000 | 0.000 | 0.000 | 0.000 | 0.000 | 0.000 | 0.000 | 0.000 | 0.000 |
| 豆类 Legumes | 0.000 | 0.000 | 0.000 | 0.000 | 0.000 | 0.000 | 0.000 | 0.000 | 0.000 | 0.000 | 0.000 | 0.000 | 0.000 | 0.000 | 0.000 | 0.000 | 0.000 | 0.000 | 0.000 | 0.000 | 0.000 | 0.000 | 0.000 | 0.000 | 0.000 |
| 薯类 Potatoes | 0.000 | 0.000 | 0.000 | 0.000 | 0.000 | 0.000 | 0.000 | 0.000 | 0.000 | 0.000 | 0.000 | 0.000 | 0.000 | 0.000 | 0.000 | 0.000 | 0.000 | 0.000 | 0.000 | 0.000 | 0.000 | 0.000 | 0.000 | 0.000 | 0.000 |

续表

| 膳食类别<br>Category | 黑龙江<br>HL | 辽宁<br>LN | 河北<br>HE | 北京<br>BJ | 吉林<br>JL | 山西<br>SX | 陕西<br>SN | 河南<br>HA | 宁夏<br>NX | 内蒙古<br>NM | 青海<br>QH | 甘肃<br>GS | 上海<br>SH | 福建<br>FJ | 江西<br>JX | 江苏<br>JS | 浙江<br>ZJ | 山东<br>SD | 湖北<br>HB | 四川<br>SC | 广西<br>GX | 湖南<br>HN | 广东<br>GD | 贵州<br>GZ | 全国平均<br>AVG |
|---|---|---|---|---|---|---|---|---|---|---|---|---|---|---|---|---|---|---|---|---|---|---|---|---|---|
| 肉类 Meats | 0.000 | 0.000 | 0.000 | 0.000 | 0.000 | 0.000 | 0.000 | 0.000 | 0.000 | 0.000 | 0.000 | 0.000 | 0.000 | 0.000 | 0.000 | 0.000 | 0.000 | 0.000 | 0.000 | 0.000 | 0.000 | 0.000 | 0.000 | 0.000 | 0.000 |
| 蛋类 Eggs | 0.000 | 0.000 | 0.000 | 0.000 | 0.000 | 0.000 | 0.000 | 0.000 | 0.000 | 0.053 | 0.000 | 0.000 | 0.000 | 0.000 | 0.000 | 0.000 | 0.000 | 0.000 | 0.000 | 0.000 | 0.000 | 0.000 | 0.000 | 0.000 | 0.002 |
| 水产类 Aquatic foods | 0.000 | 0.000 | 0.000 | 0.000 | 0.000 | 0.000 | 0.000 | 0.000 | 0.000 | 0.000 | 0.000 | 0.000 | 0.000 | 0.000 | 0.000 | 0.000 | 0.000 | 0.000 | 0.000 | 0.000 | 0.000 | 0.000 | 0.000 | 0.000 | 0.000 |
| 乳类 Dairy products | 0.000 | 0.000 | 0.000 | 0.000 | 0.000 | 0.000 | 0.000 | 0.000 | 0.000 | 0.000 | 0.000 | 0.000 | 0.000 | 0.000 | 0.000 | 0.000 | 0.000 | 0.000 | 0.000 | 0.000 | 0.000 | 0.000 | 0.000 | 0.000 | 0.000 |
| 蔬菜类 Vegetables | 0.000 | 0.000 | 0.000 | 0.000 | 0.000 | 0.000 | 0.000 | 0.000 | 0.000 | 0.000 | 0.000 | 0.000 | 0.000 | 0.000 | 0.000 | 0.000 | 0.000 | 0.000 | 0.000 | 0.000 | 0.000 | 0.000 | 0.000 | 0.000 | 0.000 |
| 水果类 Fruits | 0.000 | 0.000 | 0.000 | 0.000 | 0.000 | 0.000 | 0.000 | 0.000 | 0.000 | 0.000 | 0.000 | 0.000 | 0.000 | 0.135 | 0.000 | 0.000 | 1.337 | 0.000 | 0.000 | 0.000 | 0.000 | 0.000 | 0.000 | 0.000 | 0.061 |
| 糖类 Sugar | 0.000 | 0.000 | 0.000 | 0.000 | 0.000 | 0.000 | 0.000 | 0.000 | 0.000 | 0.000 | 0.000 | 0.000 | 0.000 | 0.000 | 0.000 | 0.000 | 0.000 | 0.000 | 0.000 | 0.000 | 0.000 | 0.000 | 0.000 | 0.000 | 0.000 |
| 水及饮料类 Water and beverages | 0.000 | 0.000 | 0.000 | 0.000 | 0.000 | 0.000 | 0.000 | 0.000 | 0.000 | 0.000 | 0.000 | 0.000 | 0.000 | 0.000 | 0.000 | 0.000 | 0.000 | 0.000 | 0.000 | 0.000 | 0.000 | 0.000 | 0.000 | 0.000 | 0.000 |
| 酒类 Alcohol beverages | 0.000 | 0.000 | 0.000 | 0.000 | 0.000 | 0.000 | 0.000 | 0.000 | 0.000 | 0.000 | 0.000 | 0.000 | 0.000 | 0.000 | 0.000 | 0.000 | 0.000 | 0.000 | 0.000 | 0.000 | 0.000 | 0.000 | 0.000 | 0.000 | 0.000 |
| 合计 SUM | 0.000 | 0.000 | 0.000 | 0.000 | 0.000 | 0.000 | 0.000 | 0.000 | 0.000 | 0.053 | 0.000 | 0.000 | 0.000 | 0.135 | 0.000 | 0.000 | 1.337 | 0.000 | 0.000 | 0.000 | 0.000 | 0.000 | 0.000 | 0.000 | 0.064 |

附表 4-101 第六次中国总膳食研究的丙环唑膳食摄入量 [单位: ng/(kg bw·d)]
Annexed Table 4-101 Dietary intakes of propiconazole from the 6th China TDS [Unit: ng/(kg bw·d)]

| 膳食类别 Category | 黑龙江 HL | 辽宁 LN | 河北 HE | 北京 BJ | 吉林 JL | 山西 SX | 陕西 SN | 河南 HA | 宁夏 NX | 内蒙古 NM | 青海 QH | 甘肃 GS | 上海 SH | 福建 FJ | 江西 JX | 江苏 JS | 浙江 ZJ | 山东 SD | 湖北 HB | 四川 SC | 广西 GX | 湖南 HN | 广东 GD | 贵州 GZ | 全国平均 AVG |
|---|---|---|---|---|---|---|---|---|---|---|---|---|---|---|---|---|---|---|---|---|---|---|---|---|---|
| 谷类 Cereals | 0.000 | 0.000 | 0.000 | 0.000 | 0.000 | 0.000 | 5.409 | 0.000 | 0.000 | 0.000 | 0.000 | 0.000 | 0.000 | 0.000 | 2.657 | 15.315 | 1.483 | 0.000 | 0.000 | 0.000 | 12.100 | 1.887 | 0.000 | 2.476 | 1.722 |
| 豆类 Legumes | 0.000 | 0.000 | 0.000 | 0.000 | 0.000 | 0.000 | 0.000 | 0.000 | 0.000 | 0.000 | 0.000 | 0.000 | 0.000 | 0.000 | 0.000 | 48.740 | 0.000 | 0.000 | 0.000 | 0.000 | 0.000 | 0.000 | 0.000 | 0.000 | 2.031 |
| 薯类 Potatoes | 0.000 | 0.000 | 0.000 | 0.000 | 0.000 | 0.000 | 0.000 | 0.000 | 0.000 | 0.000 | 0.000 | 0.000 | 0.000 | 0.000 | 0.000 | 34.960 | 0.000 | 0.000 | 0.000 | 0.000 | 0.000 | 0.000 | 0.000 | 0.000 | 1.457 |
| 肉类 Meats | 0.000 | 0.000 | 0.000 | 0.000 | 0.000 | 0.000 | 0.000 | 0.000 | 0.000 | 0.000 | 0.000 | 0.000 | 0.000 | 0.000 | 0.000 | 362.900 | 0.000 | 0.000 | 0.000 | 0.000 | 0.000 | 0.000 | 0.000 | 0.000 | 15.120 |
| 蛋类 Eggs | 0.000 | 0.000 | 0.000 | 0.000 | 0.000 | 0.000 | 0.000 | 0.000 | 0.000 | 0.000 | 0.000 | 0.000 | 0.000 | 0.000 | 0.000 | 9.502 | 0.000 | 0.000 | 0.000 | 0.000 | 0.000 | 0.000 | 0.000 | 0.000 | 0.396 |
| 水产类 Aquatic foods | 0.000 | 0.000 | 0.000 | 0.000 | 0.000 | 0.000 | 0.000 | 0.000 | 0.000 | 0.000 | 0.000 | 0.000 | 0.000 | 0.000 | 0.000 | 26.660 | 0.000 | 0.000 | 0.000 | 0.000 | 0.000 | 0.000 | 0.116 | 0.000 | 1.116 |
| 乳类 Dairy products | 0.000 | 0.000 | 0.000 | 0.000 | 0.000 | 0.000 | 0.000 | 0.000 | 0.000 | 0.000 | 0.000 | 0.000 | 0.000 | 0.000 | 0.000 | 0.000 | 0.000 | 0.000 | 0.000 | 0.000 | 0.000 | 0.000 | 0.000 | 0.000 | 0.000 |
| 蔬菜类 Vegetables | 0.000 | 0.000 | 0.791 | 0.000 | 0.761 | 4.447 | 1.571 | 0.000 | 0.649 | 0.000 | 0.000 | 10.640 | 0.000 | 0.000 | 22.150 | 620.300 | 0.000 | 0.000 | 109.100 | 0.000 | 0.525 | 266.500 | 305.100 | 10.460 | 56.370 |
| 水果类 Fruits | 0.000 | 0.000 | 0.000 | 0.416 | 0.000 | 0.000 | 0.000 | 0.000 | 0.000 | 0.000 | 0.000 | 0.000 | 0.000 | 0.176 | 0.000 | 57.140 | 0.000 | 0.000 | 0.000 | 0.000 | 0.000 | 0.000 | 0.052 | 0.000 | 2.408 |
| 糖类 Sugar | 0.000 | 0.000 | 0.000 | 0.000 | 0.000 | 0.000 | 0.000 | 0.000 | 0.000 | 0.000 | 0.000 | 0.000 | 0.000 | 0.000 | 0.000 | 0.000 | 0.000 | 0.000 | 0.000 | 0.000 | 0.000 | 0.000 | 0.000 | 0.000 | 0.000 |
| 水及饮料类 Water and beverages | 0.000 | 0.000 | 0.000 | 0.000 | 0.000 | 0.000 | 0.000 | 0.000 | 0.000 | 0.000 | 0.000 | 0.000 | 0.000 | 0.000 | 0.000 | 2.823 | 0.000 | 0.000 | 0.000 | 0.000 | 0.000 | 0.000 | 0.000 | 0.000 | 0.118 |

续表

| 膳食类别<br>Category | 黑龙江<br>HL | 辽宁<br>LN | 河北<br>HE | 北京<br>BJ | 吉林<br>JL | 山西<br>SX | 陕西<br>SN | 河南<br>HA | 宁夏<br>NX | 内蒙古<br>NM | 青海<br>QH | 甘肃<br>GS | 上海<br>SH | 福建<br>FJ | 江西<br>JX | 江苏<br>JS | 浙江<br>ZJ | 山东<br>SD | 湖北<br>HB | 四川<br>SC | 广西<br>GX | 湖南<br>HN | 广东<br>GD | 贵州<br>GZ | 全国平均<br>AVG |
|---|---|---|---|---|---|---|---|---|---|---|---|---|---|---|---|---|---|---|---|---|---|---|---|---|---|
| 酒类 Alcohol beverages | 0.000 | 0.000 | 0.000 | 0.000 | 0.000 | 0.000 | 0.000 | 0.000 | 0.000 | 0.000 | 0.000 | 0.000 | 0.000 | 0.000 | 0.000 | 0.000 | 0.000 | 0.000 | 0.000 | 0.000 | 0.000 | 0.000 | 0.000 | 0.000 | 0.000 |
| 合计 SUM | 0.000 | 0.000 | 0.791 | 0.416 | 0.761 | 4.447 | 6.980 | 0.000 | 0.649 | 0.000 | 0.000 | 10.641 | 0.000 | 0.176 | 24.807 | 1178.343 | 1.483 | 0.000 | 109.068 | 0.000 | 12.627 | 268.351 | 305.252 | 12.932 | 80.739 |

附表 4-102　第六次中国总膳食研究的己唑醇膳食摄入量 [单位: ng/(kg bw · d)]

Annexed Table 4-102　Dietary intakes of hexaconazole from the 6th China TDS [Unit: ng/(kg bw · d)]

| 膳食类别<br>Category | 黑龙江<br>HL | 辽宁<br>LN | 河北<br>HE | 北京<br>BJ | 吉林<br>JL | 山西<br>SX | 陕西<br>SN | 河南<br>HA | 宁夏<br>NX | 内蒙古<br>NM | 青海<br>QH | 甘肃<br>GS | 上海<br>SH | 福建<br>FJ | 江西<br>JX | 江苏<br>JS | 浙江<br>ZJ | 山东<br>SD | 湖北<br>HB | 四川<br>SC | 广西<br>GX | 湖南<br>HN | 广东<br>GD | 贵州<br>GZ | 全国平均<br>AVG |
|---|---|---|---|---|---|---|---|---|---|---|---|---|---|---|---|---|---|---|---|---|---|---|---|---|---|
| 谷类 Cereals | 0.000 | 0.000 | 0.000 | 0.000 | 0.000 | 0.000 | 2.597 | 0.000 | 0.000 | 0.000 | 0.000 | 0.000 | 0.000 | 0.000 | 7.132 | 2.202 | 0.000 | 0.000 | 1.062 | 0.000 | 11.617 | 5.215 | 0.000 | 0.000 | 1.243 |
| 豆类 Legumes | 0.000 | 0.000 | 0.058 | 0.000 | 0.000 | 0.000 | 0.000 | 0.000 | 0.000 | 0.000 | 0.000 | 0.000 | 0.000 | 0.000 | 0.000 | 0.000 | 0.000 | 0.000 | 0.000 | 0.000 | 0.000 | 0.000 | 0.000 | 0.000 | 0.002 |
| 薯类 Potatoes | 0.000 | 0.000 | 0.000 | 0.000 | 0.000 | 0.000 | 0.000 | 0.000 | 0.000 | 0.000 | 0.000 | 0.000 | 0.000 | 0.000 | 0.000 | 0.000 | 0.000 | 0.000 | 0.146 | 0.000 | 0.000 | 0.000 | 0.000 | 0.000 | 0.006 |
| 肉类 Meats | 0.000 | 0.000 | 0.000 | 0.000 | 0.000 | 0.000 | 0.000 | 0.000 | 0.000 | 0.000 | 0.000 | 0.000 | 0.000 | 0.000 | 0.000 | 0.000 | 0.000 | 0.000 | 0.000 | 0.000 | 0.000 | 0.000 | 0.000 | 0.000 | 0.000 |
| 蛋类 Eggs | 0.000 | 0.000 | 0.000 | 0.000 | 0.000 | 0.000 | 0.000 | 0.000 | 0.000 | 0.000 | 0.000 | 0.000 | 0.000 | 0.000 | 0.000 | 0.000 | 0.000 | 0.000 | 0.000 | 0.000 | 0.000 | 0.000 | 0.000 | 0.000 | 0.000 |
| 水产类 Aquatic foods | 0.000 | 0.000 | 0.000 | 0.000 | 0.000 | 0.000 | 0.000 | 0.000 | 0.000 | 0.000 | 0.000 | 0.000 | 0.000 | 0.000 | 0.087 | 0.000 | 0.000 | 0.000 | 0.000 | 0.000 | 0.000 | 0.119 | 0.000 | 0.000 | 0.009 |
| 乳类 Dairy products | 0.000 | 0.000 | 0.000 | 0.000 | 0.000 | 0.000 | 0.000 | 0.000 | 0.000 | 0.000 | 0.000 | 0.000 | 0.000 | 0.000 | 0.000 | 0.000 | 0.000 | 0.000 | 0.000 | 0.000 | 0.000 | 0.000 | 0.000 | 0.000 | 0.000 |

续表

| 膳食类别 Category | 黑龙江 HL | 辽宁 LN | 河北 HE | 北京 BJ | 吉林 JL | 山西 SX | 陕西 SN | 河南 HA | 宁夏 NX | 内蒙古 NM | 青海 QH | 甘肃 GS | 上海 SH | 福建 FJ | 江西 JX | 江苏 JS | 浙江 ZJ | 山东 SD | 湖北 HB | 四川 SC | 广西 GX | 湖南 HN | 广东 GD | 贵州 GZ | 全国平均 AVG |
|---|---|---|---|---|---|---|---|---|---|---|---|---|---|---|---|---|---|---|---|---|---|---|---|---|---|
| 蔬菜类 Vegetables | 0.000 | 0.000 | 2.138 | 0.000 | 0.000 | 0.000 | 0.775 | 0.000 | 1.108 | 0.000 | 0.000 | 0.000 | 0.000 | 0.000 | 0.000 | 0.000 | 0.000 | 0.000 | 0.839 | 0.000 | 229.800 | 0.000 | 0.908 | 0.000 | 9.816 |
| 水果类 Fruits | 0.072 | 0.000 | 0.000 | 0.000 | 0.000 | 0.000 | 0.000 | 0.000 | 0.000 | 0.395 | 0.000 | 0.000 | 0.000 | 0.000 | 0.000 | 0.000 | 0.000 | 0.000 | 0.000 | 0.000 | 0.000 | 0.000 | 0.000 | 0.000 | 0.019 |
| 糖类 Sugar | 0.000 | 0.000 | 0.000 | 0.000 | 0.000 | 0.000 | 0.000 | 0.000 | 0.000 | 0.000 | 0.000 | 0.000 | 0.000 | 0.000 | 0.000 | 0.000 | 0.000 | 0.000 | 0.000 | 0.000 | 0.000 | 0.000 | 0.000 | 0.000 | 0.000 |
| 水及饮料类 Water and beverages | 0.000 | 0.000 | 0.000 | 0.000 | 0.000 | 0.000 | 0.000 | 0.000 | 0.000 | 0.000 | 0.000 | 0.000 | 0.000 | 0.000 | 0.000 | 0.000 | 0.000 | 0.000 | 0.000 | 0.000 | 0.000 | 0.000 | 0.000 | 0.000 | 0.000 |
| 酒类 Alcohol beverages | 0.000 | 0.000 | 0.000 | 0.000 | 0.000 | 0.000 | 0.000 | 0.000 | 0.000 | 0.000 | 0.000 | 0.000 | 0.000 | 0.000 | 0.000 | 0.000 | 0.000 | 0.000 | 0.000 | 0.000 | 0.000 | 0.000 | 0.000 | 0.000 | 0.000 |
| 合计 SUM | 0.072 | 0.000 | 2.195 | 0.000 | 0.000 | 0.000 | 3.372 | 0.000 | 1.108 | 0.395 | 0.000 | 0.000 | 0.000 | 0.000 | 7.219 | 2.202 | 0.000 | 0.000 | 2.048 | 0.000 | 241.425 | 5.335 | 0.908 | 0.000 | 11.095 |

附表 4-103 第六次中国总膳食研究的苯醚甲环唑膳食摄入量 [单位：ng/(kg bw·d)]

Annexed Table 4-103　Dietary intakes of difenoconazole from the 6$^{th}$ China TDS [Unit: ng/(kg bw · d)]

| 膳食类别 Category | 黑龙江 HL | 辽宁 LN | 河北 HE | 北京 BJ | 吉林 JL | 山西 SX | 陕西 SN | 河南 HA | 宁夏 NX | 内蒙古 NM | 青海 QH | 甘肃 GS | 上海 SH | 福建 FJ | 江西 JX | 江苏 JS | 浙江 ZJ | 山东 SD | 湖北 HB | 四川 SC | 广西 GX | 湖南 HN | 广东 GD | 贵州 GZ | 全国平均 AVG |
|---|---|---|---|---|---|---|---|---|---|---|---|---|---|---|---|---|---|---|---|---|---|---|---|---|---|
| 谷类 Cereals | 0.000 | 0.000 | 0.000 | 0.000 | 0.000 | 0.000 | 0.000 | 0.000 | 0.000 | 0.000 | 0.000 | 0.000 | 0.000 | 0.000 | 0.000 | 0.000 | 0.000 | 0.000 | 0.000 | 0.000 | 0.000 | 0.000 | 0.000 | 0.000 | 0.000 |
| 豆类 Legumes | 0.000 | 0.000 | 0.000 | 0.000 | 0.000 | 0.000 | 0.000 | 0.000 | 0.000 | 0.000 | 0.000 | 0.000 | 0.000 | 0.000 | 0.000 | 0.000 | 0.000 | 0.000 | 0.000 | 0.000 | 0.000 | 0.000 | 0.000 | 0.000 | 0.000 |
| 薯类 Potatoes | 0.000 | 0.000 | 0.000 | 0.000 | 0.000 | 0.000 | 0.000 | 0.000 | 0.000 | 0.000 | 0.000 | 0.000 | 0.000 | 0.000 | 0.000 | 0.000 | 0.000 | 0.000 | 0.000 | 0.000 | 0.000 | 0.000 | 0.000 | 0.000 | 0.000 |

续表

| 膳食类别 Category | 黑龙江 HL | 辽宁 LN | 河北 HE | 北京 BJ | 吉林 JL | 山西 SX | 陕西 SN | 河南 HA | 宁夏 NX | 内蒙古 NM | 青海 QH | 甘肃 GS | 上海 SH | 福建 FJ | 江西 JX | 江苏 JS | 浙江 ZJ | 山东 SD | 湖北 HB | 四川 SC | 广西 GX | 湖南 HN | 广东 GD | 贵州 GZ | 全国平均 AVG |
|---|---|---|---|---|---|---|---|---|---|---|---|---|---|---|---|---|---|---|---|---|---|---|---|---|---|
| 肉类 Meats | 0.000 | 0.000 | 0.000 | 0.000 | 0.000 | 0.000 | 0.000 | 0.000 | 0.000 | 0.000 | 0.000 | 0.000 | 0.000 | 0.000 | 0.000 | 0.000 | 0.000 | 0.000 | 0.000 | 0.000 | 0.000 | 0.000 | 0.000 | 0.000 | 0.000 |
| 蛋类 Eggs | 0.000 | 0.000 | 0.000 | 0.000 | 0.000 | 0.000 | 0.000 | 0.000 | 0.000 | 0.000 | 0.000 | 0.000 | 0.000 | 0.000 | 0.000 | 0.000 | 0.000 | 0.000 | 0.000 | 0.000 | 0.000 | 0.000 | 0.000 | 0.000 | 0.000 |
| 水产类 Aquatic foods | 0.000 | 0.000 | 0.000 | 0.000 | 0.000 | 0.000 | 0.000 | 0.000 | 0.000 | 0.000 | 0.000 | 0.000 | 0.000 | 0.000 | 0.000 | 0.000 | 0.000 | 0.000 | 0.000 | 0.000 | 0.000 | 0.000 | 0.000 | 0.000 | 0.000 |
| 乳类 Dairy products | 0.000 | 0.000 | 0.000 | 0.000 | 0.000 | 0.000 | 0.000 | 0.000 | 0.000 | 0.000 | 0.000 | 0.000 | 0.000 | 0.000 | 0.000 | 0.000 | 0.000 | 0.000 | 0.000 | 0.000 | 0.000 | 0.000 | 0.000 | 0.000 | 0.000 |
| 蔬菜类 Vegetables | 0.469 | 0.000 | 0.423 | 0.000 | 6.097 | 17.930 | 19.360 | 1.363 | 0.152 | 6.276 | 11.010 | 17.090 | 14.160 | 5.995 | 6.225 | 1.213 | 12.300 | 10.660 | 73.860 | 0.000 | 168.300 | 49.480 | 345.600 | 17.090 | 32.710 |
| 水果类 Fruits | 0.442 | 3.157 | 1.187 | 4.426 | 0.554 | 0.000 | 0.642 | 4.370 | 0.000 | 1.704 | 0.030 | 0.000 | 0.783 | 1.840 | 0.080 | 1.933 | 0.594 | 4.743 | 0.391 | 0.712 | 0.000 | 0.189 | 0.150 | 0.000 | 1.164 |
| 糖类 Sugar | 0.000 | 0.000 | 0.000 | 0.000 | 0.000 | 0.000 | 0.000 | 0.000 | 0.000 | 0.000 | 0.000 | 0.000 | 0.000 | 0.000 | 0.000 | 0.000 | 0.000 | 0.000 | 0.000 | 0.000 | 0.000 | 0.000 | 0.000 | 0.000 | 0.000 |
| 水及饮料类 Water and beverages | 0.000 | 0.000 | 0.000 | 0.000 | 0.000 | 0.000 | 0.000 | 0.000 | 0.000 | 0.000 | 0.000 | 0.000 | 0.000 | 0.000 | 0.000 | 0.000 | 0.000 | 0.000 | 0.000 | 0.000 | 0.000 | 0.000 | 0.000 | 0.000 | 0.000 |
| 酒类 Alcohol beverages | 0.000 | 0.000 | 0.000 | 0.000 | 0.000 | 0.000 | 0.000 | 0.000 | 0.000 | 0.000 | 0.000 | 0.000 | 0.000 | 0.000 | 0.000 | 0.000 | 0.000 | 0.000 | 0.000 | 0.000 | 0.000 | 0.000 | 0.000 | 0.000 | 0.000 |
| 合计 SUM | 0.912 | 3.157 | 1.610 | 4.426 | 6.651 | 17.932 | 20.006 | 5.734 | 0.152 | 7.980 | 11.037 | 17.089 | 14.946 | 7.835 | 6.304 | 3.146 | 12.897 | 15.407 | 74.253 | 0.712 | 168.283 | 49.670 | 345.782 | 17.094 | 33.876 |

附表 4-104  第六次中国总膳食研究粉唑醇的膳食来源（单位：%）
Annexed Table 4-104  Dietary sources of flutriafol from the 6$^{th}$ China TDS (Unit: %)

| 膳食类别 Category | 黑龙江 HL | 辽宁 LN | 河北 HE | 北京 BJ | 吉林 JL | 山西 SX | 陕西 SN | 河南 HA | 宁夏 NX | 内蒙古 NM | 青海 QH | 甘肃 GS | 上海 SH | 福建 FJ | 江西 JX | 江苏 JS | 浙江 ZJ | 山东 SD | 湖北 HB | 四川 SC | 广西 GX | 湖南 HN | 广东 GD | 贵州 GZ | 全国平均 AVG |
|---|---|---|---|---|---|---|---|---|---|---|---|---|---|---|---|---|---|---|---|---|---|---|---|---|---|
| 谷类 Cereals | 0.0 | 0.0 | 0.0 | 0.0 | 0.0 | 0.0 | 0.0 | 0.0 | 0.0 | 0.0 | 0.0 | 0.0 | 0.0 | 0.0 | 0.0 | 0.0 | 0.0 | 0.0 | 0.0 | 0.0 | 0.0 | 0.0 | 0.0 | 0.0 | 0.0 |
| 豆类 Legumes | 0.0 | 0.0 | 0.0 | 0.0 | 0.0 | 0.0 | 0.0 | 0.0 | 0.0 | 0.0 | 0.0 | 0.0 | 0.0 | 0.0 | 0.0 | 0.0 | 0.0 | 0.0 | 0.0 | 0.0 | 0.0 | 0.0 | 0.0 | 0.0 | 0.0 |
| 薯类 Potatoes | 0.0 | 0.0 | 0.0 | 0.0 | 33.7 | 0.0 | 0.0 | 0.0 | 0.0 | 0.0 | 0.0 | 0.0 | 0.0 | 0.0 | 0.0 | 0.0 | 0.0 | 0.0 | 0.0 | 0.0 | 0.0 | 0.0 | 0.0 | 0.0 | 2.3 |
| 肉类 Meats | 0.0 | 0.0 | 0.0 | 0.0 | 15.3 | 0.0 | 0.0 | 0.0 | 0.0 | 0.0 | 0.0 | 0.0 | 0.0 | 0.0 | 0.0 | 0.0 | 0.0 | 0.0 | 0.0 | 0.0 | 0.0 | 0.0 | 0.0 | 0.0 | 1.0 |
| 蛋类 Eggs | 0.0 | 0.0 | 0.0 | 0.0 | 0.0 | 0.0 | 0.0 | 0.0 | 0.0 | 0.0 | 0.0 | 0.0 | 0.0 | 0.0 | 0.0 | 0.0 | 0.0 | 0.0 | 0.0 | 0.0 | 0.0 | 0.0 | 0.0 | 0.0 | 0.0 |
| 水产类 Aquatic foods | 0.0 | 0.0 | 0.0 | 0.0 | 2.0 | 0.0 | 0.0 | 0.0 | 0.0 | 0.0 | 0.0 | 0.0 | 0.0 | 0.0 | 0.0 | 0.0 | 0.0 | 0.0 | 0.0 | 0.0 | 0.0 | 0.0 | 0.0 | 0.0 | 0.1 |
| 乳类 Dairy products | 0.0 | 0.0 | 0.0 | 0.0 | 0.0 | 0.0 | 0.0 | 0.0 | 0.0 | 0.0 | 0.0 | 0.0 | 0.0 | 0.0 | 0.0 | 0.0 | 0.0 | 0.0 | 0.0 | 0.0 | 0.0 | 0.0 | 0.0 | 0.0 | 0.0 |
| 蔬菜类 Vegetables | 0.0 | 0.0 | 0.0 | 0.0 | 49.0 | 100.0 | 0.0 | 0.0 | 0.0 | 0.0 | 98.8 | 0.0 | 100.0 | 0.0 | 0.0 | 0.0 | 0.0 | 0.0 | 0.0 | 0.0 | 0.0 | 0.0 | 78.6 | 100.0 | 94.6 |
| 水果类 Fruits | 0.0 | 0.0 | 0.0 | 0.0 | 0.0 | 0.0 | 0.0 | 0.0 | 0.0 | 0.0 | 1.2 | 0.0 | 0.0 | 0.0 | 0.0 | 0.0 | 0.0 | 0.0 | 0.0 | 0.0 | 0.0 | 0.0 | 21.4 | 0.0 | 1.9 |
| 糖类 Sugar | 0.0 | 0.0 | 0.0 | 0.0 | 0.0 | 0.0 | 0.0 | 0.0 | 0.0 | 0.0 | 0.0 | 0.0 | 0.0 | 0.0 | 0.0 | 0.0 | 0.0 | 0.0 | 0.0 | 0.0 | 0.0 | 0.0 | 0.0 | 0.0 | 0.0 |
| 水及饮料类 Water and beverages | 0.0 | 0.0 | 0.0 | 0.0 | 0.0 | 0.0 | 0.0 | 0.0 | 0.0 | 0.0 | 0.0 | 0.0 | 0.0 | 0.0 | 0.0 | 0.0 | 0.0 | 0.0 | 0.0 | 0.0 | 0.0 | 0.0 | 0.0 | 0.0 | 0.0 |

续表

| 膳食类别<br>Category | 黑龙江<br>HL | 辽宁<br>LN | 河北<br>HE | 北京<br>BJ | 吉林<br>JL | 山西<br>SX | 陕西<br>SN | 河南<br>HA | 宁夏<br>NX | 内蒙古<br>NM | 青海<br>QH | 甘肃<br>GS | 上海<br>SH | 福建<br>FJ | 江西<br>JX | 江苏<br>JS | 浙江<br>ZJ | 山东<br>SD | 湖北<br>HB | 四川<br>SC | 广西<br>GX | 湖南<br>HN | 广东<br>GD | 贵州<br>GZ | 全国平均<br>AVG |
|---|---|---|---|---|---|---|---|---|---|---|---|---|---|---|---|---|---|---|---|---|---|---|---|---|---|
| 酒类<br>Alcohol beverages | 0.0 | 0.0 | 0.0 | 0.0 | 0.0 | 0.0 | 0.0 | 0.0 | 0.0 | 0.0 | 0.0 | 0.0 | 0.0 | 0.0 | 0.0 | 0.0 | 0.0 | 0.0 | 0.0 | 0.0 | 0.0 | 0.0 | 0.0 | 0.0 | 0.0 |

附表 4-105 第六次中国总膳食研究腈菌唑的膳食来源（单位：%）

Annexed Table 4-105　Dietary sources of myclobutanil from the 6$^{th}$ China TDS (Unit: %)

| 膳食类别<br>Category | 黑龙江<br>HL | 辽宁<br>LN | 河北<br>HE | 北京<br>BJ | 吉林<br>JL | 山西<br>SX | 陕西<br>SN | 河南<br>HA | 宁夏<br>NX | 内蒙古<br>NM | 青海<br>QH | 甘肃<br>GS | 上海<br>SH | 福建<br>FJ | 江西<br>JX | 江苏<br>JS | 浙江<br>ZJ | 山东<br>SD | 湖北<br>HB | 四川<br>SC | 广西<br>GX | 湖南<br>HN | 广东<br>GD | 贵州<br>GZ | 全国平均<br>AVG |
|---|---|---|---|---|---|---|---|---|---|---|---|---|---|---|---|---|---|---|---|---|---|---|---|---|---|
| 谷类<br>Cereals | 0.0 | 0.0 | 0.0 | 0.0 | 0.0 | 0.0 | 0.0 | 0.0 | 0.0 | 0.0 | 0.0 | 0.0 | 0.0 | 0.0 | 0.0 | 0.0 | 0.0 | 0.0 | 0.0 | 0.0 | 0.0 | 0.0 | 0.0 | 0.0 | 0.0 |
| 豆类<br>Legumes | 0.0 | 0.0 | 0.0 | 0.0 | 0.0 | 0.0 | 0.0 | 0.0 | 0.0 | 0.0 | 0.0 | 0.0 | 0.0 | 0.0 | 0.0 | 0.0 | 0.0 | 0.0 | 0.0 | 0.0 | 0.0 | 0.0 | 0.0 | 0.0 | 0.0 |
| 薯类<br>Potatoes | 0.0 | 0.0 | 0.0 | 0.0 | 0.0 | 0.0 | 0.0 | 0.0 | 0.0 | 0.0 | 0.0 | 0.0 | 0.0 | 0.0 | 0.0 | 0.0 | 0.0 | 0.0 | 0.0 | 0.0 | 0.0 | 0.0 | 0.0 | 0.0 | 0.0 |
| 肉类<br>Meats | 0.0 | 0.0 | 0.0 | 0.0 | 0.0 | 0.0 | 0.0 | 0.0 | 0.0 | 0.0 | 0.0 | 0.0 | 0.0 | 0.0 | 0.0 | 12.6 | 0.0 | 0.0 | 0.0 | 0.0 | 0.0 | 0.0 | 0.0 | 0.0 | 0.3 |
| 蛋类<br>Eggs | 0.0 | 0.0 | 0.0 | 0.0 | 0.0 | 0.0 | 0.0 | 0.0 | 0.0 | 0.0 | 0.0 | 0.0 | 0.0 | 0.0 | 0.0 | 6.0 | 0.0 | 0.0 | 0.0 | 0.0 | 0.0 | 0.0 | 0.0 | 0.0 | 0.1 |
| 水产类<br>Aquatic foods | 0.0 | 0.0 | 2.9 | 0.0 | 0.0 | 0.7 | 0.0 | 0.0 | 0.0 | 0.0 | 0.0 | 0.0 | 0.0 | 0.0 | 0.0 | 0.0 | 0.0 | 0.0 | 0.0 | 0.0 | 0.0 | 0.0 | 0.0 | 0.0 | 0.1 |
| 乳类<br>Dairy products | 0.0 | 0.0 | 0.0 | 0.0 | 0.0 | 0.0 | 0.0 | 0.0 | 0.0 | 0.0 | 0.0 | 0.0 | 0.0 | 0.0 | 0.0 | 0.0 | 0.0 | 0.0 | 0.0 | 0.0 | 0.0 | 0.0 | 0.0 | 0.0 | 0.0 |
| 蔬菜类<br>Vegetables | 0.0 | 0.0 | 97.1 | 0.0 | 76.6 | 99.3 | 100.0 | 100.0 | 100.0 | 54.9 | 100.0 | 100.0 | 0.0 | 0.0 | 0.0 | 81.3 | 0.0 | 0.0 | 100.0 | 0.0 | 99.3 | 100.0 | 43.7 | 0.0 | 86.0 |

续表

| 膳食类别 Category | 黑龙江 HL | 辽宁 LN | 河北 HE | 北京 BJ | 吉林 JL | 山西 SX | 陕西 SN | 河南 HA | 宁夏 NX | 内蒙古 NM | 青海 QH | 甘肃 GS | 上海 SH | 福建 FJ | 江西 JX | 江苏 JS | 浙江 ZJ | 山东 SD | 湖北 HB | 四川 SC | 广西 GX | 湖南 HN | 广东 GD | 贵州 GZ | 全国平均 AVG |
|---|---|---|---|---|---|---|---|---|---|---|---|---|---|---|---|---|---|---|---|---|---|---|---|---|---|
| 水果类 Fruits | 0.0 | 97.9 | 0.0 | 0.0 | 23.4 | 0.0 | 0.0 | 0.0 | 0.0 | 45.1 | 0.0 | 0.0 | 100.0 | 100.0 | 100.0 | 0.0 | 0.0 | 0.0 | 0.0 | 0.0 | 0.0 | 0.0 | 56.3 | 0.0 | 13.2 |
| 糖类 Sugar | 0.0 | 0.0 | 0.0 | 0.0 | 0.0 | 0.0 | 0.0 | 0.0 | 0.0 | 0.0 | 0.0 | 0.0 | 0.0 | 0.0 | 0.0 | 0.0 | 0.0 | 0.0 | 0.0 | 0.0 | 0.0 | 0.0 | 0.0 | 0.0 | 0.0 |
| 水及饮料类 Water and beverages | 0.0 | 0.0 | 0.0 | 0.0 | 0.0 | 0.0 | 0.0 | 0.0 | 0.0 | 0.0 | 0.0 | 0.0 | 0.0 | 0.0 | 0.0 | 0.0 | 0.0 | 0.0 | 0.0 | 0.0 | 0.0 | 0.0 | 0.0 | 0.0 | 0.0 |
| 酒类 Alcohol beverages | 0.0 | 2.1 | 0.0 | 0.0 | 0.0 | 0.0 | 0.0 | 0.0 | 0.0 | 0.0 | 0.0 | 0.0 | 0.0 | 0.0 | 0.0 | 0.0 | 0.0 | 0.0 | 0.0 | 0.0 | 0.7 | 0.0 | 0.0 | 0.0 | 0.3 |

附表 4-106　第六次中国总膳食研究三唑醇的膳食来源（单位：%）

Annexed Table 4-106　Dietary sources of triadimenol from the 6$^{th}$ China TDS (Unit: %)

| 膳食类别 Category | 黑龙江 HL | 辽宁 LN | 河北 HE | 北京 BJ | 吉林 JL | 山西 SX | 陕西 SN | 河南 HA | 宁夏 NX | 内蒙古 NM | 青海 QH | 甘肃 GS | 上海 SH | 福建 FJ | 江西 JX | 江苏 JS | 浙江 ZJ | 山东 SD | 湖北 HB | 四川 SC | 广西 GX | 湖南 HN | 广东 GD | 贵州 GZ | 全国平均 AVG |
|---|---|---|---|---|---|---|---|---|---|---|---|---|---|---|---|---|---|---|---|---|---|---|---|---|---|
| 谷类 Cereals | 0.0 | 0.0 | 0.0 | 0.0 | 0.0 | 0.0 | 0.0 | 0.0 | 0.0 | 0.0 | 0.0 | 0.0 | 0.0 | 0.0 | 0.0 | 0.0 | 0.0 | 0.0 | 0.0 | 0.0 | 0.0 | 0.0 | 0.0 | 0.0 | 0.0 |
| 豆类 Legumes | 0.0 | 0.0 | 0.0 | 0.0 | 0.0 | 0.0 | 0.0 | 0.0 | 0.0 | 0.0 | 0.0 | 0.0 | 0.0 | 0.0 | 0.0 | 0.0 | 0.0 | 0.0 | 0.0 | 0.0 | 0.0 | 0.0 | 0.0 | 0.0 | 0.0 |
| 薯类 Potatoes | 0.0 | 0.0 | 0.0 | 0.0 | 0.0 | 0.0 | 0.0 | 0.0 | 0.0 | 0.0 | 0.0 | 0.0 | 0.0 | 0.0 | 0.0 | 0.0 | 0.0 | 0.0 | 0.0 | 0.0 | 0.0 | 0.0 | 0.0 | 0.0 | 0.0 |
| 肉类 Meats | 0.0 | 0.0 | 0.0 | 0.0 | 0.0 | 0.0 | 0.0 | 0.0 | 0.0 | 0.0 | 0.0 | 0.0 | 0.0 | 0.0 | 0.0 | 12.6 | 0.0 | 0.0 | 0.0 | 0.0 | 0.0 | 0.0 | 0.0 | 0.0 | 0.3 |
| 蛋类 Eggs | 0.0 | 0.0 | 0.0 | 0.0 | 0.0 | 0.0 | 0.0 | 0.0 | 0.0 | 0.0 | 0.0 | 0.0 | 0.0 | 0.0 | 0.0 | 6.0 | 0.0 | 0.0 | 0.0 | 0.0 | 0.0 | 0.0 | 0.0 | 0.0 | 0.1 |

续表

| 膳食类别<br>Category | 黑龙江<br>HL | 辽宁<br>LN | 河北<br>HE | 北京<br>BJ | 吉林<br>JL | 山西<br>SX | 陕西<br>SN | 河南<br>HA | 宁夏<br>NX | 内蒙古<br>NM | 青海<br>QH | 甘肃<br>GS | 上海<br>SH | 福建<br>FJ | 江西<br>JX | 江苏<br>JS | 浙江<br>ZJ | 山东<br>SD | 湖北<br>HB | 四川<br>SC | 广西<br>GX | 湖南<br>HN | 广东<br>GD | 贵州<br>GZ | 全国平均<br>AVG |
|---|---|---|---|---|---|---|---|---|---|---|---|---|---|---|---|---|---|---|---|---|---|---|---|---|---|
| 水产类 Aquatic foods | 0.0 | 0.0 | 2.9 | 0.0 | 0.0 | 0.7 | 0.0 | 0.0 | 0.0 | 0.0 | 0.0 | 0.0 | 0.0 | 0.0 | 0.0 | 0.0 | 0.0 | 0.0 | 0.0 | 0.0 | 0.0 | 0.0 | 0.0 | 0.0 | 0.1 |
| 乳类 Dairy products | 0.0 | 0.0 | 0.0 | 0.0 | 0.0 | 0.0 | 0.0 | 0.0 | 0.0 | 0.0 | 0.0 | 0.0 | 0.0 | 0.0 | 0.0 | 0.0 | 0.0 | 0.0 | 0.0 | 0.0 | 0.0 | 0.0 | 0.0 | 0.0 | 0.0 |
| 蔬菜类 Vegetables | 0.0 | 0.0 | 97.1 | 0.0 | 76.6 | 99.3 | 100.0 | 100.0 | 100.0 | 54.9 | 100.0 | 100.0 | 0.0 | 0.0 | 0.0 | 81.3 | 0.0 | 0.0 | 100.0 | 0.0 | 99.3 | 100.0 | 43.7 | 0.0 | 86.0 |
| 水果类 Fruits | 0.0 | 97.9 | 0.0 | 0.0 | 23.4 | 0.0 | 0.0 | 0.0 | 0.0 | 45.1 | 0.0 | 0.0 | 0.0 | 0.0 | 100.0 | 0.0 | 0.0 | 0.0 | 0.0 | 0.0 | 0.0 | 0.0 | 56.3 | 0.0 | 13.2 |
| 糖类 Sugar | 0.0 | 0.0 | 0.0 | 0.0 | 0.0 | 0.0 | 0.0 | 0.0 | 0.0 | 0.0 | 0.0 | 0.0 | 100.0 | 100.0 | 0.0 | 0.0 | 0.0 | 0.0 | 0.0 | 0.0 | 0.0 | 0.0 | 0.0 | 0.0 | 0.0 |
| 水及饮料类 Water and beverages | 0.0 | 0.0 | 0.0 | 0.0 | 0.0 | 0.0 | 0.0 | 0.0 | 0.0 | 0.0 | 0.0 | 0.0 | 0.0 | 0.0 | 0.0 | 0.0 | 0.0 | 0.0 | 0.0 | 0.0 | 0.0 | 0.0 | 0.0 | 0.0 | 0.0 |
| 酒类 Alcohol beverages | 0.0 | 2.1 | 0.0 | 0.0 | 0.0 | 0.0 | 0.0 | 0.0 | 0.0 | 0.0 | 0.0 | 0.0 | 0.0 | 0.0 | 0.0 | 0.0 | 0.0 | 0.0 | 0.0 | 0.0 | 0.7 | 0.0 | 0.0 | 0.0 | 0.3 |

附表 4-107　第六次中国总膳食研究三唑酮的膳食来源（单位：%）

Annexed Table 4-107　Dietary sources of triadimefon from the 6$^{th}$ China TDS (Unit: %)

| 膳食类别<br>Category | 黑龙江<br>HL | 辽宁<br>LN | 河北<br>HE | 北京<br>BJ | 吉林<br>JL | 山西<br>SX | 陕西<br>SN | 河南<br>HA | 宁夏<br>NX | 内蒙古<br>NM | 青海<br>QH | 甘肃<br>GS | 上海<br>SH | 福建<br>FJ | 江西<br>JX | 江苏<br>JS | 浙江<br>ZJ | 山东<br>SD | 湖北<br>HB | 四川<br>SC | 广西<br>GX | 湖南<br>HN | 广东<br>GD | 贵州<br>GZ | 全国平均<br>AVG |
|---|---|---|---|---|---|---|---|---|---|---|---|---|---|---|---|---|---|---|---|---|---|---|---|---|---|
| 谷类 Cereals | 0.0 | 0.0 | 0.0 | 0.0 | 0.0 | 0.0 | 0.0 | 0.0 | 0.0 | 0.0 | 0.0 | 0.0 | 88.4 | 0.0 | 4.6 | 82.2 | 100.0 | 0.0 | 0.0 | 0.0 | 0.0 | 0.0 | 7.9 | 68.8 | 12.4 |

续表

| 膳食类别 Category | 黑龙江 HL | 辽宁 LN | 河北 HE | 北京 BJ | 吉林 JL | 山西 SX | 陕西 SN | 河南 HA | 宁夏 NX | 内蒙古 NM | 青海 QH | 甘肃 GS | 上海 SH | 福建 FJ | 江西 JX | 江苏 JS | 浙江 ZJ | 山东 SD | 湖北 HB | 四川 SC | 广西 GX | 湖南 HN | 广东 GD | 贵州 GZ | 全国平均 AVG |
|---|---|---|---|---|---|---|---|---|---|---|---|---|---|---|---|---|---|---|---|---|---|---|---|---|---|
| 豆类 Legumes | 0.0 | 0.0 | 0.0 | 0.0 | 0.0 | 0.0 | 0.0 | 0.0 | 0.0 | 0.0 | 0.0 | 0.0 | 0.0 | 0.0 | 0.0 | 0.0 | 0.0 | 0.0 | 0.0 | 0.0 | 0.0 | 0.0 | 0.0 | 0.0 | 0.0 |
| 薯类 Potatoes | 0.0 | 0.0 | 0.0 | 0.0 | 92.9 | 0.0 | 0.0 | 0.0 | 0.0 | 0.0 | 0.0 | 0.0 | 0.0 | 0.0 | 0.0 | 0.0 | 0.0 | 0.0 | 0.0 | 0.0 | 0.0 | 0.0 | 0.0 | 0.0 | 1.1 |
| 肉类 Meats | 0.0 | 0.0 | 0.0 | 0.0 | 0.0 | 0.0 | 0.0 | 0.0 | 0.0 | 0.0 | 0.0 | 0.0 | 6.9 | 42.9 | 0.0 | 0.0 | 0.0 | 0.0 | 2.6 | 0.0 | 0.0 | 0.0 | 3.4 | 0.0 | 2.6 |
| 蛋类 Eggs | 0.0 | 0.0 | 0.0 | 0.0 | 0.0 | 0.0 | 0.0 | 0.0 | 0.0 | 0.0 | 0.0 | 0.0 | 0.0 | 0.0 | 0.0 | 0.0 | 0.0 | 0.0 | 2.3 | 0.0 | 0.0 | 0.0 | 0.0 | 0.0 | 0.5 |
| 水产类 Aquatic foods | 0.0 | 0.0 | 0.0 | 0.0 | 0.0 | 0.0 | 0.0 | 0.0 | 0.0 | 100.0 | 0.0 | 0.0 | 4.7 | 0.0 | 0.0 | 0.0 | 0.0 | 0.0 | 2.6 | 0.0 | 0.0 | 0.0 | 0.0 | 0.2 | 0.7 |
| 乳类 Dairy products | 0.0 | 0.0 | 0.0 | 0.0 | 0.0 | 0.0 | 0.0 | 0.0 | 100.0 | 0.0 | 0.0 | 0.0 | 0.0 | 0.0 | 0.0 | 0.0 | 0.0 | 0.0 | 0.0 | 0.0 | 0.0 | 0.0 | 0.0 | 0.0 | 0.0 |
| 蔬菜类 Vegetables | 0.0 | 0.0 | 100.0 | 0.0 | 0.0 | 100.0 | 33.2 | 100.0 | 0.0 | 0.0 | 0.0 | 100.0 | 0.0 | 57.1 | 95.4 | 17.2 | 0.0 | 0.0 | 92.5 | 0.0 | 96.4 | 100.0 | 88.7 | 31.0 | 81.3 |
| 水果类 Fruits | 0.0 | 0.0 | 0.0 | 100.0 | 7.1 | 0.0 | 0.0 | 0.0 | 0.0 | 0.0 | 0.0 | 0.0 | 0.0 | 0.0 | 0.0 | 0.6 | 0.0 | 0.0 | 0.0 | 0.0 | 0.0 | 0.0 | 0.0 | 0.0 | 1.1 |
| 糖类 Sugar | 0.0 | 0.0 | 0.0 | 0.0 | 0.0 | 0.0 | 0.0 | 0.0 | 0.0 | 0.0 | 0.0 | 0.0 | 0.0 | 0.0 | 0.0 | 0.0 | 0.0 | 0.0 | 0.0 | 0.0 | 0.0 | 0.0 | 0.0 | 0.0 | 0.0 |
| 水及饮料类 Water and beverages | 0.0 | 0.0 | 0.0 | 0.0 | 0.0 | 0.0 | 66.8 | 0.0 | 0.0 | 0.0 | 0.0 | 0.0 | 0.0 | 0.0 | 0.0 | 0.0 | 0.0 | 0.0 | 0.0 | 0.0 | 0.0 | 0.0 | 0.0 | 0.0 | 0.3 |
| 酒类 Alcohol beverages | 0.0 | 0.0 | 0.0 | 0.0 | 0.0 | 0.0 | 0.0 | 0.0 | 0.0 | 0.0 | 0.0 | 0.0 | 0.0 | 0.0 | 0.0 | 0.0 | 0.0 | 0.0 | 0.0 | 0.0 | 3.6 | 0.0 | 0.0 | 0.0 | 0.0 |

附表 4-108 第六次中国总膳食研究四氟醚唑的膳食来源（单位：%）

Annexed Table 4-108 Dietary sources of tetraconazole from the 6$^{th}$ China TDS (Unit: %)

| 膳食类别 Category | 黑龙江 HL | 辽宁 LN | 河北 HE | 北京 BJ | 吉林 JL | 山西 SX | 陕西 SN | 河南 HA | 宁夏 NX | 内蒙古 NM | 青海 QH | 甘肃 GS | 上海 SH | 福建 FJ | 江西 JX | 江苏 JS | 浙江 ZJ | 山东 SD | 湖北 HB | 四川 SC | 广西 GX | 湖南 HN | 广东 GD | 贵州 GZ | 全国平均 AVG |
|---|---|---|---|---|---|---|---|---|---|---|---|---|---|---|---|---|---|---|---|---|---|---|---|---|---|
| 谷类 Cereals | 0.0 | 0.0 | 0.0 | 0.0 | 0.0 | 0.0 | 0.0 | 0.0 | 0.0 | 0.0 | 0.0 | 0.0 | 0.0 | 0.0 | 0.0 | 0.0 | 0.0 | 0.0 | 0.0 | 0.0 | 0.0 | 0.0 | 0.0 | 0.0 | 0.0 |
| 豆类 Legumes | 0.0 | 0.0 | 0.0 | 0.0 | 0.0 | 0.0 | 0.0 | 0.0 | 0.0 | 0.0 | 0.0 | 0.0 | 0.0 | 0.0 | 0.0 | 0.0 | 0.0 | 0.0 | 0.0 | 0.0 | 0.0 | 0.0 | 0.0 | 0.0 | 0.0 |
| 薯类 Potatoes | 0.0 | 0.0 | 0.0 | 0.0 | 0.0 | 0.0 | 0.0 | 0.0 | 0.0 | 0.0 | 0.0 | 0.0 | 0.0 | 0.0 | 0.0 | 0.0 | 0.0 | 0.0 | 0.0 | 0.0 | 0.0 | 0.0 | 0.0 | 0.0 | 0.0 |
| 肉类 Meats | 0.0 | 0.0 | 0.0 | 0.0 | 0.0 | 0.0 | 0.0 | 0.0 | 0.0 | 0.0 | 0.0 | 0.0 | 0.0 | 0.0 | 0.0 | 0.0 | 0.0 | 0.0 | 0.0 | 0.0 | 0.0 | 0.0 | 0.0 | 0.0 | 0.0 |
| 蛋类 Eggs | 0.0 | 0.0 | 0.0 | 0.0 | 0.0 | 0.0 | 0.0 | 0.0 | 0.0 | 0.0 | 0.0 | 0.0 | 0.0 | 0.0 | 0.0 | 0.0 | 0.0 | 0.0 | 0.0 | 0.0 | 0.0 | 0.0 | 0.0 | 0.0 | 0.0 |
| 水产类 Aquatic foods | 0.0 | 0.0 | 0.0 | 0.0 | 0.0 | 0.0 | 0.0 | 0.0 | 0.0 | 0.0 | 100.0 | 0.0 | 0.0 | 0.0 | 0.0 | 0.0 | 0.0 | 0.0 | 0.0 | 0.0 | 0.0 | 0.0 | 0.0 | 0.0 | 0.0 |
| 乳类 Dairy products | 0.0 | 0.0 | 0.0 | 0.0 | 0.0 | 0.0 | 0.0 | 0.0 | 0.0 | 0.0 | 0.0 | 0.0 | 0.0 | 0.0 | 0.0 | 0.0 | 0.0 | 0.0 | 0.0 | 0.0 | 0.0 | 0.0 | 0.0 | 0.0 | 0.0 |
| 蔬菜类 Vegetables | 0.0 | 0.0 | 0.0 | 100.0 | 100.0 | 0.0 | 0.0 | 0.0 | 0.0 | 0.0 | 0.0 | 0.0 | 0.0 | 0.0 | 0.0 | 0.0 | 0.0 | 0.0 | 0.0 | 0.0 | 0.0 | 0.0 | 0.0 | 0.0 | 67.9 |
| 水果类 Fruits | 0.0 | 0.0 | 0.0 | 0.0 | 0.0 | 0.0 | 0.0 | 0.0 | 0.0 | 0.0 | 0.0 | 0.0 | 0.0 | 0.0 | 0.0 | 0.0 | 0.0 | 100.0 | 0.0 | 0.0 | 0.0 | 0.0 | 100.0 | 0.0 | 32.1 |
| 糖类 Sugar | 0.0 | 0.0 | 0.0 | 0.0 | 0.0 | 0.0 | 0.0 | 0.0 | 0.0 | 0.0 | 0.0 | 0.0 | 0.0 | 0.0 | 0.0 | 0.0 | 0.0 | 0.0 | 0.0 | 0.0 | 0.0 | 0.0 | 0.0 | 0.0 | 0.0 |
| 水及饮料类 Water and beverages | 0.0 | 0.0 | 0.0 | 0.0 | 0.0 | 0.0 | 0.0 | 0.0 | 0.0 | 0.0 | 0.0 | 0.0 | 0.0 | 0.0 | 0.0 | 0.0 | 0.0 | 0.0 | 0.0 | 0.0 | 0.0 | 0.0 | 0.0 | 0.0 | 0.0 |

续表

| 膳食类别<br>Category | 黑龙江<br>HL | 辽宁<br>LN | 河北<br>HE | 北京<br>BJ | 吉林<br>JL | 山西<br>SX | 陕西<br>SN | 河南<br>HA | 宁夏<br>NX | 内蒙古<br>NM | 青海<br>QH | 甘肃<br>GS | 上海<br>SH | 福建<br>FJ | 江西<br>JX | 江苏<br>JS | 浙江<br>ZJ | 山东<br>SD | 湖北<br>HB | 四川<br>SC | 广西<br>GX | 湖南<br>HN | 广东<br>GD | 贵州<br>GZ | 全国平均<br>AVG |
|---|---|---|---|---|---|---|---|---|---|---|---|---|---|---|---|---|---|---|---|---|---|---|---|---|---|
| 酒类<br>Alcohol beverages | 0.0 | 0.0 | 0.0 | 0.0 | 0.0 | 0.0 | 0.0 | 0.0 | 0.0 | 0.0 | 0.0 | 0.0 | 0.0 | 0.0 | 0.0 | 0.0 | 0.0 | 0.0 | 0.0 | 0.0 | 0.0 | 0.0 | 0.0 | 0.0 | 0.0 |

附表 4-109　第六次中国总膳食研究氟环唑的膳食来源（单位：%）

Annexed Table 4-109　Dietary sources of epoxiconazole from the 6th China TDS (Unit: %)

| 膳食类别<br>Category | 黑龙江<br>HL | 辽宁<br>LN | 河北<br>HE | 北京<br>BJ | 吉林<br>JL | 山西<br>SX | 陕西<br>SN | 河南<br>HA | 宁夏<br>NX | 内蒙古<br>NM | 青海<br>QH | 甘肃<br>GS | 上海<br>SH | 福建<br>FJ | 江西<br>JX | 江苏<br>JS | 浙江<br>ZJ | 山东<br>SD | 湖北<br>HB | 四川<br>SC | 广西<br>GX | 湖南<br>HN | 广东<br>GD | 贵州<br>GZ | 全国平均<br>AVG |
|---|---|---|---|---|---|---|---|---|---|---|---|---|---|---|---|---|---|---|---|---|---|---|---|---|---|
| 谷类<br>Cereals | 100.0 | 0.0 | 0.0 | 0.0 | 0.0 | 0.0 | 0.0 | 0.0 | 0.0 | 0.0 | 0.0 | 0.0 | 0.0 | 100.0 | 96.5 | 0.0 | 0.0 | 0.0 | 0.0 | 0.0 | 0.0 | 0.0 | 0.0 | 0.0 | 55.1 |
| 豆类<br>Legumes | 0.0 | 0.0 | 0.0 | 0.0 | 0.0 | 0.0 | 0.0 | 0.0 | 0.0 | 0.0 | 0.0 | 0.0 | 0.0 | 0.0 | 0.0 | 0.0 | 0.0 | 0.0 | 0.0 | 0.0 | 0.0 | 0.0 | 0.0 | 0.0 | 0.0 |
| 薯类<br>Potatoes | 0.0 | 0.0 | 0.0 | 0.0 | 32.7 | 0.0 | 0.0 | 0.0 | 0.0 | 0.0 | 0.0 | 0.0 | 0.0 | 0.0 | 0.0 | 0.0 | 0.0 | 0.0 | 0.0 | 0.0 | 0.0 | 0.0 | 0.0 | 0.0 | 4.2 |
| 肉类<br>Meats | 0.0 | 0.0 | 0.0 | 0.0 | 0.0 | 0.0 | 0.0 | 0.0 | 0.0 | 0.0 | 0.0 | 0.0 | 0.0 | 0.0 | 0.0 | 0.0 | 0.0 | 0.0 | 0.0 | 0.0 | 0.0 | 0.0 | 0.0 | 0.0 | 0.0 |
| 蛋类<br>Eggs | 0.0 | 0.0 | 0.0 | 0.0 | 0.0 | 0.0 | 0.0 | 0.0 | 0.0 | 0.0 | 0.0 | 0.0 | 0.0 | 0.0 | 0.0 | 0.0 | 0.0 | 0.0 | 0.0 | 0.0 | 0.0 | 0.0 | 0.0 | 0.0 | 0.0 |
| 水产类<br>Aquatic foods | 0.0 | 0.0 | 0.0 | 0.0 | 3.0 | 0.0 | 0.0 | 0.0 | 0.0 | 0.0 | 0.0 | 0.0 | 0.0 | 0.0 | 3.5 | 0.0 | 0.0 | 0.0 | 0.0 | 0.0 | 0.0 | 0.0 | 0.0 | 0.0 | 1.1 |
| 乳类<br>Dairy products | 0.0 | 0.0 | 0.0 | 0.0 | 0.0 | 0.0 | 0.0 | 0.0 | 0.0 | 0.0 | 0.0 | 0.0 | 0.0 | 0.0 | 0.0 | 0.0 | 0.0 | 0.0 | 0.0 | 0.0 | 0.0 | 0.0 | 0.0 | 0.0 | 0.0 |
| 蔬菜类<br>Vegetables | 0.0 | 0.0 | 0.0 | 0.0 | 64.3 | 0.0 | 0.0 | 0.0 | 0.0 | 0.0 | 0.0 | 0.0 | 0.0 | 0.0 | 0.0 | 0.0 | 0.0 | 0.0 | 0.0 | 0.0 | 0.0 | 0.0 | 0.0 | 0.0 | 8.2 |

续表

| 膳食类别<br>Category | 黑龙江<br>HL | 辽宁<br>LN | 河北<br>HE | 北京<br>BJ | 吉林<br>JL | 山西<br>SX | 陕西<br>SN | 河南<br>HA | 宁夏<br>NX | 内蒙古<br>NM | 青海<br>QH | 甘肃<br>GS | 上海<br>SH | 福建<br>FJ | 江西<br>JX | 江苏<br>JS | 浙江<br>ZJ | 山东<br>SD | 湖北<br>HB | 四川<br>SC | 广西<br>GX | 湖南<br>HN | 广东<br>GD | 贵州<br>GZ | 全国平均<br>AVG |
|---|---|---|---|---|---|---|---|---|---|---|---|---|---|---|---|---|---|---|---|---|---|---|---|---|---|
| 水果类 Fruits | 0.0 | 0.0 | 100.0 | 0.0 | 0.0 | 0.0 | 0.0 | 100.0 | 0.0 | 0.0 | 0.0 | 0.0 | 0.0 | 0.0 | 0.0 | 0.0 | 0.0 | 100.0 | 0.0 | 100.0 | 0.0 | 0.0 | 0.0 | 0.0 | 31.3 |
| 糖类 Sugar | 0.0 | 0.0 | 0.0 | 0.0 | 0.0 | 0.0 | 0.0 | 0.0 | 0.0 | 0.0 | 0.0 | 0.0 | 0.0 | 0.0 | 0.0 | 0.0 | 0.0 | 0.0 | 0.0 | 0.0 | 0.0 | 0.0 | 0.0 | 0.0 | 0.0 |
| 水及饮料类 Water and beverages | 0.0 | 0.0 | 0.0 | 0.0 | 0.0 | 0.0 | 0.0 | 0.0 | 0.0 | 0.0 | 0.0 | 0.0 | 0.0 | 0.0 | 0.0 | 0.0 | 0.0 | 0.0 | 0.0 | 0.0 | 0.0 | 0.0 | 0.0 | 0.0 | 0.0 |
| 酒类 Alcohol beverages | 0.0 | 0.0 | 0.0 | 0.0 | 0.0 | 0.0 | 0.0 | 0.0 | 0.0 | 0.0 | 0.0 | 0.0 | 0.0 | 0.0 | 0.0 | 0.0 | 0.0 | 0.0 | 0.0 | 0.0 | 0.0 | 0.0 | 0.0 | 0.0 | 0.0 |

附表 4-110　第六次中国总膳食研究腈苯唑的膳食来源（单位：%）

Annexed Table 4-110　Dietary sources of fenbuconazole from the 6$^{th}$ China TDS (Unit: %)

| 膳食类别<br>Category | 黑龙江<br>HL | 辽宁<br>LN | 河北<br>HE | 北京<br>BJ | 吉林<br>JL | 山西<br>SX | 陕西<br>SN | 河南<br>HA | 宁夏<br>NX | 内蒙古<br>NM | 青海<br>QH | 甘肃<br>GS | 上海<br>SH | 福建<br>FJ | 江西<br>JX | 江苏<br>JS | 浙江<br>ZJ | 山东<br>SD | 湖北<br>HB | 四川<br>SC | 广西<br>GX | 湖南<br>HN | 广东<br>GD | 贵州<br>GZ | 全国平均<br>AVG |
|---|---|---|---|---|---|---|---|---|---|---|---|---|---|---|---|---|---|---|---|---|---|---|---|---|---|
| 谷类 Cereals | 0.0 | 0.0 | 0.0 | 0.0 | 0.0 | 0.0 | 0.0 | 0.0 | 0.0 | 0.0 | 0.0 | 0.0 | 0.0 | 0.0 | 0.0 | 0.0 | 0.0 | 0.0 | 0.0 | 0.0 | 14.0 | 0.0 | 0.0 | 0.0 | 1.5 |
| 豆类 Legumes | 6.4 | 55.8 | 0.0 | 0.0 | 0.0 | 0.0 | 0.0 | 0.0 | 0.0 | 0.0 | 0.0 | 0.0 | 7.3 | 0.0 | 0.0 | 0.0 | 0.0 | 0.0 | 54.1 | 0.0 | 2.3 | 0.0 | 0.0 | 25.9 | 6.3 |
| 薯类 Potatoes | 2.3 | 0.0 | 0.0 | 0.0 | 0.0 | 27.9 | 0.0 | 20.4 | 0.0 | 43.2 | 0.0 | 0.0 | 3.6 | 0.0 | 0.0 | 0.0 | 0.0 | 0.0 | 17.0 | 0.0 | 2.3 | 0.0 | 0.0 | 16.3 | 7.0 |
| 肉类 Meats | 41.8 | 7.9 | 0.0 | 0.0 | 4.8 | 58.4 | 0.0 | 34.5 | 0.0 | 21.0 | 0.0 | 0.0 | 29.3 | 0.0 | 0.0 | 24.6 | 0.0 | 0.0 | 28.9 | 0.0 | 33.9 | 0.0 | 0.0 | 37.8 | 28.1 |
| 蛋类 Eggs | 0.0 | 0.0 | 0.0 | 0.0 | 0.0 | 0.0 | 0.0 | 0.0 | 0.0 | 0.0 | 0.0 | 0.0 | 0.0 | 0.0 | 0.0 | 0.5 | 0.0 | 0.0 | 0.0 | 0.0 | 4.2 | 0.0 | 0.0 | 4.8 | 0.8 |

续表

| 膳食类别<br>Category | 黑龙江<br>HL | 辽宁<br>LN | 河北<br>HE | 北京<br>BJ | 吉林<br>JL | 山西<br>SX | 陕西<br>SN | 河南<br>HA | 宁夏<br>NX | 内蒙古<br>NM | 青海<br>QH | 甘肃<br>GS | 上海<br>SH | 福建<br>FJ | 江西<br>JX | 江苏<br>JS | 浙江<br>ZJ | 山东<br>SD | 湖北<br>HB | 四川<br>SC | 广西<br>GX | 湖南<br>HN | 广东<br>GD | 贵州<br>GZ | 全国平均<br>AVG |
|---|---|---|---|---|---|---|---|---|---|---|---|---|---|---|---|---|---|---|---|---|---|---|---|---|---|
| 水产类<br>Aquatic foods | 4.3 | 0.0 | 0.0 | 0.0 | 0.0 | 1.1 | 0.0 | 2.6 | 0.0 | 33.6 | 0.0 | 0.0 | 11.5 | 0.0 | 0.0 | 0.9 | 0.0 | 0.0 | 0.0 | 0.0 | 12.2 | 0.0 | 0.0 | 1.8 | 7.2 |
| 乳类<br>Dairy products | 0.0 | 0.0 | 0.0 | 0.0 | 0.0 | 0.0 | 0.0 | 0.0 | 0.0 | 0.0 | 0.0 | 0.0 | 0.0 | 0.0 | 0.0 | 0.0 | 0.0 | 0.0 | 0.0 | 0.0 | 0.0 | 0.0 | 0.0 | 0.0 | 0.0 |
| 蔬菜类<br>Vegetables | 0.0 | 36.3 | 0.0 | 0.0 | 0.0 | 0.0 | 0.0 | 0.0 | 0.0 | 0.0 | 0.0 | 0.0 | 0.0 | 100.0 | 0.0 | 0.0 | 0.0 | 0.0 | 0.0 | 0.0 | 0.0 | 0.0 | 0.0 | 0.0 | 0.7 |
| 水果类<br>Fruits | 42.4 | 0.0 | 0.0 | 0.0 | 95.2 | 12.6 | 0.0 | 42.5 | 0.0 | 0.0 | 0.0 | 0.0 | 0.0 | 0.0 | 0.0 | 0.0 | 0.0 | 0.0 | 0.0 | 0.0 | 0.0 | 0.0 | 0.0 | 0.0 | 13.1 |
| 糖类<br>Sugar | 0.0 | 0.0 | 0.0 | 0.0 | 0.0 | 0.0 | 0.0 | 0.0 | 0.0 | 0.0 | 0.0 | 0.0 | 1.3 | 0.0 | 0.0 | 0.0 | 0.0 | 0.0 | 0.0 | 0.0 | 0.0 | 0.0 | 0.0 | 0.0 | 0.4 |
| 水及饮料类<br>Water and beverages | 0.0 | 0.0 | 100.0 | 0.0 | 0.0 | 0.0 | 0.0 | 0.0 | 0.0 | 0.0 | 0.0 | 0.0 | 0.0 | 0.0 | 0.0 | 0.0 | 0.0 | 0.0 | 0.0 | 0.0 | 0.0 | 0.0 | 0.0 | 0.0 | 0.0 |
| 酒类<br>Alcohol beverages | 2.8 | 0.0 | 0.0 | 0.0 | 0.0 | 0.0 | 0.0 | 0.0 | 0.0 | 2.1 | 0.0 | 0.0 | 47.0 | 0.0 | 100.0 | 74.0 | 0.0 | 0.0 | 0.0 | 0.0 | 31.1 | 100.0 | 100.0 | 13.4 | 34.9 |

附表 4-111 第六次中国总膳食研究氟硅唑的膳食来源（单位：%）

Annexed Table 4-111 Dietary sources of flusilazole from the 6th China TDS (Unit: %)

| 膳食类别<br>Category | 黑龙江<br>HL | 辽宁<br>LN | 河北<br>HE | 北京<br>BJ | 吉林<br>JL | 山西<br>SX | 陕西<br>SN | 河南<br>HA | 宁夏<br>NX | 内蒙古<br>NM | 青海<br>QH | 甘肃<br>GS | 上海<br>SH | 福建<br>FJ | 江西<br>JX | 江苏<br>JS | 浙江<br>ZJ | 山东<br>SD | 湖北<br>HB | 四川<br>SC | 广西<br>GX | 湖南<br>HN | 广东<br>GD | 贵州<br>GZ | 全国平均<br>AVG |
|---|---|---|---|---|---|---|---|---|---|---|---|---|---|---|---|---|---|---|---|---|---|---|---|---|---|
| 谷类<br>Cereals | 0.0 | 0.0 | 0.0 | 0.0 | 0.0 | 0.0 | 0.0 | 0.0 | 0.0 | 0.0 | 0.0 | 0.0 | 0.0 | 0.0 | 0.0 | 0.0 | 0.0 | 0.0 | 0.0 | 0.0 | 0.0 | 0.0 | 0.0 | 0.0 | 0.0 |
| 豆类<br>Legumes | 0.0 | 0.0 | 0.0 | 0.0 | 0.0 | 0.0 | 0.0 | 0.0 | 0.0 | 0.0 | 0.0 | 0.0 | 0.0 | 0.0 | 0.0 | 0.0 | 0.0 | 0.0 | 0.0 | 0.0 | 0.0 | 0.0 | 0.0 | 0.0 | 0.0 |

续表

| 膳食类别 Category | 黑龙江 HL | 辽宁 LN | 河北 HE | 北京 BJ | 吉林 JL | 山西 SX | 陕西 SN | 河南 HA | 宁夏 NX | 内蒙古 NM | 青海 QH | 甘肃 GS | 上海 SH | 福建 FJ | 江西 JX | 江苏 JS | 浙江 ZJ | 山东 SD | 湖北 HB | 四川 SC | 广西 GX | 湖南 HN | 广东 GD | 贵州 GZ | 全国平均 AVG |
|---|---|---|---|---|---|---|---|---|---|---|---|---|---|---|---|---|---|---|---|---|---|---|---|---|---|
| 薯类 Potatoes | 0.0 | 0.0 | 0.0 | 0.0 | 0.0 | 0.0 | 0.0 | 0.0 | 0.0 | 0.0 | 0.0 | 0.0 | 0.0 | 0.0 | 0.0 | 0.0 | 0.0 | 0.0 | 0.0 | 0.0 | 0.0 | 0.0 | 0.0 | 0.0 | 0.0 |
| 肉类 Meats | 0.0 | 0.0 | 0.0 | 0.0 | 0.0 | 0.0 | 0.0 | 0.0 | 0.0 | 0.0 | 0.0 | 0.0 | 0.0 | 0.0 | 0.0 | 0.0 | 0.0 | 0.0 | 0.0 | 0.0 | 0.0 | 0.0 | 0.0 | 0.0 | 0.0 |
| 蛋类 Eggs | 0.0 | 0.0 | 0.0 | 0.0 | 0.0 | 0.0 | 0.0 | 0.0 | 0.0 | 0.0 | 0.0 | 0.0 | 0.0 | 0.0 | 0.0 | 0.0 | 0.0 | 0.0 | 0.0 | 0.0 | 0.0 | 0.0 | 0.0 | 0.0 | 0.0 |
| 水产类 Aquatic foods | 0.0 | 0.0 | 0.0 | 0.0 | 0.0 | 0.0 | 0.0 | 0.0 | 0.0 | 0.0 | 0.0 | 0.0 | 0.0 | 0.0 | 0.0 | 0.0 | 0.0 | 0.0 | 0.0 | 0.0 | 0.0 | 0.0 | 0.0 | 0.0 | 0.0 |
| 乳类 Dairy products | 0.0 | 0.0 | 0.0 | 0.0 | 0.0 | 0.0 | 0.0 | 0.0 | 0.0 | 0.0 | 0.0 | 100.0 | 0.0 | 0.0 | 0.0 | 0.0 | 0.0 | 0.0 | 0.0 | 0.0 | 0.0 | 0.0 | 0.0 | 0.0 | 0.0 |
| 蔬菜类 Vegetables | 0.0 | 0.0 | 100.0 | 100.0 | 0.0 | 100.0 | 0.0 | 98.2 | 0.0 | 0.0 | 0.0 | 0.0 | 0.0 | 100.0 | 0.0 | 0.0 | 0.0 | 100.0 | 100.0 | 0.0 | 100.0 | 99.9 | 100.0 | 100.0 | 99.8 |
| 水果类 Fruits | 100.0 | 0.0 | 0.0 | 0.0 | 0.0 | 0.0 | 0.0 | 1.8 | 0.0 | 0.0 | 100.0 | 0.0 | 0.0 | 0.0 | 0.0 | 0.0 | 100.0 | 0.0 | 0.0 | 0.0 | 0.0 | 0.1 | 0.0 | 0.0 | 0.2 |
| 糖类 Sugar | 0.0 | 0.0 | 0.0 | 0.0 | 0.0 | 0.0 | 0.0 | 0.0 | 0.0 | 0.0 | 0.0 | 0.0 | 0.0 | 0.0 | 0.0 | 0.0 | 0.0 | 0.0 | 0.0 | 0.0 | 0.0 | 0.0 | 0.0 | 0.0 | 0.0 |
| 水及饮料类 Water and beverages | 0.0 | 0.0 | 0.0 | 0.0 | 0.0 | 0.0 | 0.0 | 0.0 | 0.0 | 0.0 | 0.0 | 0.0 | 0.0 | 0.0 | 0.0 | 0.0 | 0.0 | 0.0 | 0.0 | 0.0 | 0.0 | 0.0 | 0.0 | 0.0 | 0.0 |
| 酒类 Alcohol beverages | 0.0 | 0.0 | 0.0 | 0.0 | 0.0 | 0.0 | 0.0 | 0.0 | 0.0 | 0.0 | 0.0 | 0.0 | 0.0 | 0.0 | 0.0 | 0.0 | 0.0 | 0.0 | 0.0 | 0.0 | 0.0 | 0.0 | 0.0 | 0.0 | 0.0 |

附表 4-112　第六次中国总膳食研究戊唑醇的膳食来源（单位：%）

Annexed Table 4-112　Dietary sources of tebuconazole from the 6th China TDS (Unit: %)

| 膳食类别 Category | 黑龙江 HL | 辽宁 LN | 河北 HE | 北京 BJ | 吉林 JL | 山西 SX | 陕西 SN | 河南 HA | 宁夏 NX | 内蒙古 NM | 青海 QH | 甘肃 GS | 上海 SH | 福建 FJ | 江西 JX | 江苏 JS | 浙江 ZJ | 山东 SD | 湖北 HB | 四川 SC | 广西 GX | 湖南 HN | 广东 GD | 贵州 GZ | 全国平均 AVG |
|---|---|---|---|---|---|---|---|---|---|---|---|---|---|---|---|---|---|---|---|---|---|---|---|---|---|
| 谷类 Cereals | 33.3 | 0.0 | 0.0 | 0.8 | 0.0 | 0.0 | 39.7 | 17.2 | 0.0 | 0.0 | 49.3 | 0.0 | 7.0 | 74.8 | 54.9 | 56.4 | 4.3 | 60.4 | 15.9 | 58.3 | 23.4 | 1.2 | 1.0 | 64.1 | 10.5 |
| 豆类 Legumes | 0.0 | 0.0 | 12.4 | 0.0 | 0.0 | 0.0 | 4.2 | 0.3 | 0.0 | 0.0 | 0.0 | 0.0 | 0.0 | 0.0 | 0.0 | 4.5 | 0.0 | 0.0 | 0.4 | 4.6 | 0.0 | 0.0 | 0.0 | 0.0 | 0.2 |
| 薯类 Potatoes | 0.0 | 0.0 | 0.0 | 0.0 | 13.0 | 0.0 | 24.1 | 0.0 | 12.8 | 31.7 | 0.9 | 0.0 | 0.0 | 0.0 | 0.0 | 0.0 | 0.0 | 3.6 | 0.0 | 2.5 | 0.0 | 0.0 | 0.0 | 0.0 | 0.4 |
| 肉类 Meats | 0.0 | 0.0 | 0.0 | 0.0 | 0.0 | 0.0 | 0.0 | 0.0 | 11.7 | 0.0 | 2.4 | 0.0 | 0.0 | 0.0 | 0.0 | 0.0 | 0.0 | 0.0 | 0.0 | 9.5 | 0.0 | 0.2 | 0.0 | 1.2 | 0.2 |
| 蛋类 Eggs | 0.0 | 0.0 | 0.0 | 0.0 | 1.0 | 0.0 | 0.0 | 0.0 | 0.0 | 0.0 | 0.0 | 0.0 | 0.0 | 0.6 | 0.0 | 0.9 | 0.0 | 0.0 | 0.0 | 0.0 | 0.0 | 0.0 | 0.0 | 0.0 | 0.0 |
| 水产类 Aquatic foods | 0.0 | 0.0 | 0.0 | 0.0 | 0.0 | 0.0 | 0.4 | 0.0 | 0.0 | 0.0 | 0.1 | 0.0 | 0.0 | 0.7 | 0.0 | 0.9 | 0.0 | 0.0 | 0.0 | 0.4 | 0.0 | 0.1 | 0.0 | 0.0 | 0.1 |
| 乳类 Dairy products | 0.0 | 0.0 | 0.0 | 0.0 | 0.0 | 0.0 | 0.0 | 0.0 | 0.0 | 0.0 | 0.0 | 0.0 | 0.0 | 0.0 | 0.0 | 0.9 | 0.0 | 0.0 | 0.0 | 0.0 | 0.0 | 0.0 | 0.0 | 0.0 | 0.0 |
| 蔬菜类 Vegetables | 10.7 | 17.9 | 49.8 | 59.3 | 0.0 | 98.6 | 28.7 | 81.6 | 53.6 | 68.3 | 47.0 | 95.8 | 78.9 | 19.2 | 43.5 | 26.5 | 78.2 | 12.0 | 83.4 | 15.7 | 73.7 | 98.4 | 98.7 | 32.7 | 77.0 |
| 水果类 Fruits | 55.9 | 82.1 | 37.7 | 39.9 | 86.0 | 1.4 | 2.9 | 1.0 | 21.9 | 0.0 | 0.3 | 4.2 | 14.1 | 4.7 | 1.6 | 10.0 | 17.5 | 24.1 | 0.4 | 9.0 | 2.9 | 0.1 | 0.2 | 2.0 | 11.6 |
| 糖类 Sugar | 0.0 | 0.0 | 0.0 | 0.0 | 0.0 | 0.0 | 0.0 | 0.0 | 0.0 | 0.0 | 0.0 | 0.0 | 0.0 | 0.0 | 0.0 | 0.0 | 0.0 | 0.0 | 0.0 | 0.0 | 0.0 | 0.0 | 0.0 | 0.0 | 0.0 |
| 水及饮料类 Water and beverages | 0.0 | 0.0 | 0.0 | 0.0 | 0.0 | 0.0 | 0.0 | 0.0 | 0.0 | 0.0 | 0.0 | 0.0 | 0.0 | 0.0 | 0.0 | 0.0 | 0.0 | 0.0 | 0.0 | 0.0 | 0.0 | 0.0 | 0.0 | 0.0 | 0.0 |

续表

| 膳食类别 Category | 黑龙江 HL | 辽宁 LN | 河北 HE | 北京 BJ | 吉林 JL | 山西 SX | 陕西 SN | 河南 HA | 宁夏 NX | 内蒙古 NM | 青海 QH | 甘肃 GS | 上海 SH | 福建 FJ | 江西 JX | 江苏 JS | 浙江 ZJ | 山东 SD | 湖北 HB | 四川 SC | 广西 GX | 湖南 HN | 广东 GD | 贵州 GZ | 全国平均 AVG |
|---|---|---|---|---|---|---|---|---|---|---|---|---|---|---|---|---|---|---|---|---|---|---|---|---|---|
| 酒类 Alcohol beverages | 0.0 | 0.0 | 0.0 | 0.0 | 0.0 | 0.0 | 0.0 | 0.0 | 0.0 | 0.0 | 0.0 | 0.0 | 0.0 | 0.0 | 0.0 | 0.0 | 0.0 | 0.0 | 0.0 | 0.0 | 0.0 | 0.0 | 0.0 | 0.0 | 0.0 |

附表 4-113 第六次中国总膳食研究戊菌唑的膳食来源（单位：%）

Annexed Table 4-113 Dietary sources of penconazole from the 6$^{th}$ China TDS (Unit: %)

| 膳食类别 Category | 黑龙江 HL | 辽宁 LN | 河北 HE | 北京 BJ | 吉林 JL | 山西 SX | 陕西 SN | 河南 HA | 宁夏 NX | 内蒙古 NM | 青海 QH | 甘肃 GS | 上海 SH | 福建 FJ | 江西 JX | 江苏 JS | 浙江 ZJ | 山东 SD | 湖北 HB | 四川 SC | 广西 GX | 湖南 HN | 广东 GD | 贵州 GZ | 全国平均 AVG |
|---|---|---|---|---|---|---|---|---|---|---|---|---|---|---|---|---|---|---|---|---|---|---|---|---|---|
| 谷类 Cereals | 0.0 | 0.0 | 0.0 | 0.0 | 0.0 | 0.0 | 0.0 | 0.0 | 0.0 | 0.0 | 0.0 | 0.0 | 0.0 | 0.0 | 0.0 | 0.0 | 0.0 | 0.0 | 0.0 | 0.0 | 0.0 | 0.0 | 0.0 | 0.0 | 0.0 |
| 豆类 Legumes | 0.0 | 0.0 | 0.0 | 0.0 | 0.0 | 0.0 | 0.0 | 0.0 | 0.0 | 0.0 | 0.0 | 0.0 | 0.0 | 0.0 | 0.0 | 0.0 | 0.0 | 0.0 | 0.0 | 0.0 | 0.0 | 0.0 | 0.0 | 0.0 | 0.0 |
| 薯类 Potatoes | 0.0 | 0.0 | 0.0 | 0.0 | 0.0 | 0.0 | 0.0 | 0.0 | 0.0 | 0.0 | 0.0 | 0.0 | 0.0 | 0.0 | 0.0 | 0.0 | 0.0 | 0.0 | 0.0 | 0.0 | 0.0 | 0.0 | 0.0 | 0.0 | 0.0 |
| 肉类 Meats | 0.0 | 0.0 | 0.0 | 0.0 | 0.0 | 0.0 | 0.0 | 0.0 | 0.0 | 0.0 | 0.0 | 0.0 | 0.0 | 0.0 | 0.0 | 0.0 | 0.0 | 0.0 | 0.0 | 0.0 | 0.0 | 0.0 | 0.0 | 0.0 | 0.0 |
| 蛋类 Eggs | 0.0 | 0.0 | 0.0 | 0.0 | 0.0 | 0.0 | 0.0 | 0.0 | 0.0 | 100.0 | 0.0 | 0.0 | 0.0 | 0.0 | 0.0 | 0.0 | 0.0 | 0.0 | 0.0 | 0.0 | 0.0 | 0.0 | 0.0 | 0.0 | 3.5 |
| 水产类 Aquatic foods | 0.0 | 0.0 | 0.0 | 0.0 | 0.0 | 0.0 | 0.0 | 0.0 | 0.0 | 0.0 | 0.0 | 0.0 | 0.0 | 0.0 | 0.0 | 0.0 | 0.0 | 0.0 | 0.0 | 0.0 | 0.0 | 0.0 | 0.0 | 0.0 | 0.0 |
| 乳类 Dairy products | 0.0 | 0.0 | 0.0 | 0.0 | 0.0 | 0.0 | 0.0 | 0.0 | 0.0 | 0.0 | 0.0 | 0.0 | 0.0 | 0.0 | 0.0 | 0.0 | 0.0 | 0.0 | 0.0 | 0.0 | 0.0 | 0.0 | 0.0 | 0.0 | 0.0 |
| 蔬菜类 Vegetables | 0.0 | 0.0 | 0.0 | 0.0 | 0.0 | 0.0 | 0.0 | 0.0 | 0.0 | 0.0 | 0.0 | 0.0 | 0.0 | 0.0 | 0.0 | 0.0 | 0.0 | 0.0 | 0.0 | 0.0 | 0.0 | 0.0 | 0.0 | 0.0 | 0.0 |

续表

| 膳食类别<br>Category | 黑龙江<br>HL | 辽宁<br>LN | 河北<br>HE | 北京<br>BJ | 吉林<br>JL | 山西<br>SX | 陕西<br>SN | 河南<br>HA | 宁夏<br>NX | 内蒙古<br>NM | 青海<br>QH | 甘肃<br>GS | 上海<br>SH | 福建<br>FJ | 江西<br>JX | 江苏<br>JS | 浙江<br>ZJ | 山东<br>SD | 湖北<br>HB | 四川<br>SC | 广西<br>GX | 湖南<br>HN | 广东<br>GD | 贵州<br>GZ | 全国平均<br>AVG |
|---|---|---|---|---|---|---|---|---|---|---|---|---|---|---|---|---|---|---|---|---|---|---|---|---|---|
| 水果类 Fruits | 0.0 | 0.0 | 0.0 | 0.0 | 0.0 | 0.0 | 0.0 | 0.0 | 0.0 | 0.0 | 0.0 | 0.0 | 0.0 | 100.0 | 0.0 | 0.0 | 100.0 | 0.0 | 0.0 | 0.0 | 0.0 | 0.0 | 0.0 | 0.0 | 96.5 |
| 糖类 Sugar | 0.0 | 0.0 | 0.0 | 0.0 | 0.0 | 0.0 | 0.0 | 0.0 | 0.0 | 0.0 | 0.0 | 0.0 | 0.0 | 0.0 | 0.0 | 0.0 | 0.0 | 0.0 | 0.0 | 0.0 | 0.0 | 0.0 | 0.0 | 0.0 | 0.0 |
| 水及饮料类 Water and beverages | 0.0 | 0.0 | 0.0 | 0.0 | 0.0 | 0.0 | 0.0 | 0.0 | 0.0 | 0.0 | 0.0 | 0.0 | 0.0 | 0.0 | 0.0 | 0.0 | 0.0 | 0.0 | 0.0 | 0.0 | 0.0 | 0.0 | 0.0 | 0.0 | 0.0 |
| 酒类 Alcohol beverages | 0.0 | 0.0 | 0.0 | 0.0 | 0.0 | 0.0 | 0.0 | 0.0 | 0.0 | 0.0 | 0.0 | 0.0 | 0.0 | 0.0 | 0.0 | 0.0 | 0.0 | 0.0 | 0.0 | 0.0 | 0.0 | 0.0 | 0.0 | 0.0 | 0.0 |

附表 4-114 第六次中国总膳食研究丙环唑的膳食来源（单位：%）

Annexed Table 4-114  Dietary sources of propiconazole from the 6$^{th}$ China TDS (Unit: %)

| 膳食类别<br>Category | 黑龙江<br>HL | 辽宁<br>LN | 河北<br>HE | 北京<br>BJ | 吉林<br>JL | 山西<br>SX | 陕西<br>SN | 河南<br>HA | 宁夏<br>NX | 内蒙古<br>NM | 青海<br>QH | 甘肃<br>GS | 上海<br>SH | 福建<br>FJ | 江西<br>JX | 江苏<br>JS | 浙江<br>ZJ | 山东<br>SD | 湖北<br>HB | 四川<br>SC | 广西<br>GX | 湖南<br>HN | 广东<br>GD | 贵州<br>GZ | 全国平均<br>AVG |
|---|---|---|---|---|---|---|---|---|---|---|---|---|---|---|---|---|---|---|---|---|---|---|---|---|---|
| 谷类 Cereals | 0.0 | 0.0 | 0.0 | 0.0 | 0.0 | 0.0 | 77.5 | 0.0 | 0.0 | 0.0 | 0.0 | 0.0 | 0.0 | 0.0 | 10.7 | 1.3 | 100.0 | 0.0 | 0.0 | 0.0 | 95.8 | 0.7 | 0.0 | 19.1 | 2.1 |
| 豆类 Legumes | 0.0 | 0.0 | 0.0 | 0.0 | 0.0 | 0.0 | 0.0 | 0.0 | 0.0 | 0.0 | 0.0 | 0.0 | 0.0 | 0.0 | 0.0 | 4.1 | 0.0 | 0.0 | 0.0 | 0.0 | 0.0 | 0.0 | 0.0 | 0.0 | 2.5 |
| 薯类 Potatoes | 0.0 | 0.0 | 0.0 | 0.0 | 0.0 | 0.0 | 0.0 | 0.0 | 0.0 | 0.0 | 0.0 | 0.0 | 0.0 | 0.0 | 0.0 | 3.0 | 0.0 | 0.0 | 0.0 | 0.0 | 0.0 | 0.0 | 0.0 | 0.0 | 1.8 |
| 肉类 Meats | 0.0 | 0.0 | 0.0 | 0.0 | 0.0 | 0.0 | 0.0 | 0.0 | 0.0 | 0.0 | 0.0 | 0.0 | 0.0 | 0.0 | 0.0 | 30.8 | 0.0 | 0.0 | 0.0 | 0.0 | 0.0 | 0.0 | 0.0 | 0.0 | 18.7 |
| 蛋类 Eggs | 0.0 | 0.0 | 0.0 | 0.0 | 0.0 | 0.0 | 0.0 | 0.0 | 0.0 | 0.0 | 0.0 | 0.0 | 0.0 | 0.0 | 0.0 | 0.8 | 0.0 | 0.0 | 0.0 | 0.0 | 0.0 | 0.0 | 0.0 | 0.0 | 0.5 |

续表

| 膳食类别 Category | 黑龙江 HL | 辽宁 LN | 河北 HE | 北京 BJ | 吉林 JL | 山西 SX | 陕西 SN | 河南 HA | 宁夏 NX | 内蒙古 NM | 青海 QH | 甘肃 GS | 上海 SH | 福建 FJ | 江西 JX | 江苏 JS | 浙江 ZJ | 山东 SD | 湖北 HB | 四川 SC | 广西 GX | 湖南 HN | 广东 GD | 贵州 GZ | 全国平均 AVG |
|---|---|---|---|---|---|---|---|---|---|---|---|---|---|---|---|---|---|---|---|---|---|---|---|---|---|
| 水产类 Aquatic foods | 0.0 | 0.0 | 0.0 | 0.0 | 0.0 | 0.0 | 0.0 | 0.0 | 0.0 | 0.0 | 0.0 | 0.0 | 0.0 | 0.0 | 0.0 | 2.3 | 0.0 | 0.0 | 0.0 | 0.0 | 0.0 | 0.0 | 0.0 | 0.0 | 1.4 |
| 乳类 Dairy products | 0.0 | 0.0 | 0.0 | 100.0 | 0.0 | 0.0 | 0.0 | 0.0 | 0.0 | 0.0 | 0.0 | 0.0 | 0.0 | 0.0 | 0.0 | 0.0 | 0.0 | 0.0 | 0.0 | 0.0 | 0.0 | 0.0 | 0.0 | 0.0 | 0.0 |
| 蔬菜类 Vegetables | 0.0 | 0.0 | 100.0 | 0.0 | 100.0 | 100.0 | 22.5 | 0.0 | 100.0 | 0.0 | 0.0 | 100.0 | 0.0 | 0.0 | 89.3 | 52.6 | 0.0 | 0.0 | 100.0 | 0.0 | 4.2 | 99.3 | 99.9 | 80.9 | 69.8 |
| 水果类 Fruits | 0.0 | 0.0 | 0.0 | 0.0 | 0.0 | 0.0 | 0.0 | 0.0 | 0.0 | 0.0 | 0.0 | 0.0 | 0.0 | 100.0 | 0.0 | 4.8 | 0.0 | 0.0 | 0.0 | 0.0 | 0.0 | 0.0 | 0.0 | 0.0 | 3.0 |
| 糖类 Sugar | 0.0 | 0.0 | 0.0 | 0.0 | 0.0 | 0.0 | 0.0 | 0.0 | 0.0 | 0.0 | 0.0 | 0.0 | 0.0 | 0.0 | 0.0 | 0.0 | 0.0 | 0.0 | 0.0 | 0.0 | 0.0 | 0.0 | 0.0 | 0.0 | 0.0 |
| 水及饮料类 Water and beverages | 0.0 | 0.0 | 0.0 | 0.0 | 0.0 | 0.0 | 0.0 | 0.0 | 0.0 | 0.0 | 0.0 | 0.0 | 0.0 | 0.0 | 0.0 | 0.2 | 0.0 | 0.0 | 0.0 | 0.0 | 0.0 | 0.0 | 0.0 | 0.0 | 0.1 |
| 酒类 Alcohol beverages | 0.0 | 0.0 | 0.0 | 0.0 | 0.0 | 0.0 | 0.0 | 0.0 | 0.0 | 0.0 | 0.0 | 0.0 | 0.0 | 0.0 | 0.0 | 0.0 | 0.0 | 0.0 | 0.0 | 0.0 | 0.0 | 0.0 | 0.0 | 0.0 | 0.0 |

附表 4-115　第六次中国总膳食研究己唑醇的膳食来源（单位：%）

Annexed Table 4-115　Dietary sources of hexaconazole from the 6$^{th}$ China TDS (Unit: %)

| 膳食类别 Category | 黑龙江 HL | 辽宁 LN | 河北 HE | 北京 BJ | 吉林 JL | 山西 SX | 陕西 SN | 河南 HA | 宁夏 NX | 内蒙古 NM | 青海 QH | 甘肃 GS | 上海 SH | 福建 FJ | 江西 JX | 江苏 JS | 浙江 ZJ | 山东 SD | 湖北 HB | 四川 SC | 广西 GX | 湖南 HN | 广东 GD | 贵州 GZ | 全国平均 AVG |
|---|---|---|---|---|---|---|---|---|---|---|---|---|---|---|---|---|---|---|---|---|---|---|---|---|---|
| 谷类 Cereals | 0.0 | 0.0 | 0.0 | 0.0 | 0.0 | 0.0 | 77.0 | 0.0 | 0.0 | 0.0 | 0.0 | 0.0 | 0.0 | 0.0 | 98.8 | 100.0 | 0.0 | 0.0 | 51.9 | 0.0 | 4.8 | 97.8 | 0.0 | 0.0 | 11.2 |

续表

| 膳食类别 Category | 黑龙江 HL | 辽宁 LN | 河北 HE | 北京 BJ | 吉林 JL | 山西 SX | 陕西 SN | 河南 HA | 宁夏 NX | 内蒙古 NM | 青海 QH | 甘肃 GS | 上海 SH | 福建 FJ | 江西 JX | 江苏 JS | 浙江 ZJ | 山东 SD | 湖北 HB | 四川 SC | 广西 GX | 湖南 HN | 广东 GD | 贵州 GZ | 全国平均 AVG |
|---|---|---|---|---|---|---|---|---|---|---|---|---|---|---|---|---|---|---|---|---|---|---|---|---|---|
| 豆类 Legumes | 0.0 | 0.0 | 2.6 | 0.0 | 0.0 | 0.0 | 0.0 | 0.0 | 0.0 | 0.0 | 0.0 | 0.0 | 0.0 | 0.0 | 0.0 | 0.0 | 0.0 | 0.0 | 0.0 | 0.0 | 0.0 | 0.0 | 0.0 | 0.0 | 0.0 |
| 薯类 Potatoes | 0.0 | 0.0 | 0.0 | 0.0 | 0.0 | 0.0 | 0.0 | 0.0 | 0.0 | 0.0 | 0.0 | 0.0 | 0.0 | 0.0 | 0.0 | 0.0 | 0.0 | 0.0 | 7.1 | 0.0 | 0.0 | 0.0 | 0.0 | 0.0 | 0.1 |
| 肉类 Meats | 0.0 | 0.0 | 0.0 | 0.0 | 0.0 | 0.0 | 0.0 | 0.0 | 0.0 | 0.0 | 0.0 | 0.0 | 0.0 | 0.0 | 0.0 | 0.0 | 0.0 | 0.0 | 0.0 | 0.0 | 0.0 | 0.0 | 0.0 | 0.0 | 0.0 |
| 蛋类 Eggs | 0.0 | 0.0 | 0.0 | 0.0 | 0.0 | 0.0 | 0.0 | 0.0 | 0.0 | 0.0 | 0.0 | 0.0 | 0.0 | 0.0 | 0.0 | 0.0 | 0.0 | 0.0 | 0.0 | 0.0 | 0.0 | 0.0 | 0.0 | 0.0 | 0.0 |
| 水产类 Aquatic foods | 0.0 | 0.0 | 0.0 | 0.0 | 0.0 | 0.0 | 0.0 | 0.0 | 0.0 | 0.0 | 0.0 | 0.0 | 0.0 | 0.0 | 1.2 | 0.0 | 0.0 | 0.0 | 0.0 | 0.0 | 0.0 | 2.2 | 0.0 | 0.0 | 0.1 |
| 乳类 Dairy products | 0.0 | 0.0 | 0.0 | 0.0 | 0.0 | 0.0 | 0.0 | 0.0 | 0.0 | 0.0 | 0.0 | 0.0 | 0.0 | 0.0 | 0.0 | 0.0 | 0.0 | 0.0 | 0.0 | 0.0 | 0.0 | 0.0 | 0.0 | 0.0 | 0.0 |
| 蔬菜类 Vegetables | 0.0 | 0.0 | 97.4 | 0.0 | 0.0 | 0.0 | 23.0 | 0.0 | 100.0 | 0.0 | 0.0 | 0.0 | 0.0 | 0.0 | 0.0 | 0.0 | 0.0 | 0.0 | 41.0 | 0.0 | 95.2 | 0.0 | 100.0 | 0.0 | 88.5 |
| 水果类 Fruits | 100.0 | 0.0 | 0.0 | 0.0 | 0.0 | 0.0 | 0.0 | 0.0 | 0.0 | 100.0 | 0.0 | 0.0 | 0.0 | 0.0 | 0.0 | 0.0 | 0.0 | 0.0 | 0.0 | 0.0 | 0.0 | 0.0 | 0.0 | 0.0 | 0.2 |
| 糖类 Sugar | 0.0 | 0.0 | 0.0 | 0.0 | 0.0 | 0.0 | 0.0 | 0.0 | 0.0 | 0.0 | 0.0 | 0.0 | 0.0 | 0.0 | 0.0 | 0.0 | 0.0 | 0.0 | 0.0 | 0.0 | 0.0 | 0.0 | 0.0 | 0.0 | 0.0 |
| 水及饮料类 Water and beverages | 0.0 | 0.0 | 0.0 | 0.0 | 0.0 | 0.0 | 0.0 | 0.0 | 0.0 | 0.0 | 0.0 | 0.0 | 0.0 | 0.0 | 0.0 | 0.0 | 0.0 | 0.0 | 0.0 | 0.0 | 0.0 | 0.0 | 0.0 | 0.0 | 0.0 |
| 酒类 Alcohol beverages | 0.0 | 0.0 | 0.0 | 0.0 | 0.0 | 0.0 | 0.0 | 0.0 | 0.0 | 0.0 | 0.0 | 0.0 | 0.0 | 0.0 | 0.0 | 0.0 | 0.0 | 0.0 | 0.0 | 0.0 | 0.0 | 0.0 | 0.0 | 0.0 | 0.0 |

附表 4-116　第六次中国总膳食研究苯醚甲环唑的膳食来源（单位：%）

Annexed Table 4-116　Dietary sources of difenoconazole from the 6$^{th}$ China TDS (Unit: %)

| 膳食类别<br>Category | 黑龙江<br>HL | 辽宁<br>LN | 河北<br>HE | 北京<br>BJ | 吉林<br>JL | 山西<br>SX | 陕西<br>SN | 河南<br>HA | 宁夏<br>NX | 内蒙古<br>NM | 青海<br>QH | 甘肃<br>GS | 上海<br>SH | 福建<br>FJ | 江西<br>JX | 江苏<br>JS | 浙江<br>ZJ | 山东<br>SD | 湖北<br>HB | 四川<br>SC | 广西<br>GX | 湖南<br>HN | 广东<br>GD | 贵州<br>GZ | 全国平均<br>AVG |
|---|---|---|---|---|---|---|---|---|---|---|---|---|---|---|---|---|---|---|---|---|---|---|---|---|---|
| 谷类 Cereals | 0.0 | 0.0 | 0.0 | 0.0 | 0.0 | 0.0 | 0.0 | 0.0 | 0.0 | 0.0 | 0.0 | 0.0 | 0.0 | 0.0 | 0.0 | 0.0 | 0.0 | 0.0 | 0.0 | 0.0 | 0.0 | 0.0 | 0.0 | 0.0 | 0.0 |
| 豆类 Legumes | 0.0 | 0.0 | 0.0 | 0.0 | 0.0 | 0.0 | 0.0 | 0.0 | 0.0 | 0.0 | 0.0 | 0.0 | 0.0 | 0.0 | 0.0 | 0.0 | 0.0 | 0.0 | 0.0 | 0.0 | 0.0 | 0.0 | 0.0 | 0.0 | 0.0 |
| 薯类 Potatoes | 0.0 | 0.0 | 0.0 | 0.0 | 0.0 | 0.0 | 0.0 | 0.0 | 0.0 | 0.0 | 0.0 | 0.0 | 0.0 | 0.0 | 0.0 | 0.0 | 0.0 | 0.0 | 0.0 | 0.0 | 0.0 | 0.0 | 0.0 | 0.0 | 0.0 |
| 肉类 Meats | 0.0 | 0.0 | 0.0 | 0.0 | 0.0 | 0.0 | 0.0 | 0.0 | 0.0 | 0.0 | 0.0 | 0.0 | 0.0 | 0.0 | 0.0 | 0.0 | 0.0 | 0.0 | 0.0 | 0.0 | 0.0 | 0.0 | 0.0 | 0.0 | 0.0 |
| 蛋类 Eggs | 0.0 | 0.0 | 0.0 | 0.0 | 0.0 | 0.0 | 0.0 | 0.0 | 0.0 | 0.0 | 0.0 | 0.0 | 0.0 | 0.0 | 0.0 | 0.0 | 0.0 | 0.0 | 0.0 | 0.0 | 0.0 | 0.0 | 0.0 | 0.0 | 0.0 |
| 水产类 Aquatic foods | 0.0 | 0.0 | 0.0 | 0.0 | 0.0 | 0.0 | 0.0 | 0.0 | 0.0 | 0.0 | 0.0 | 0.0 | 0.0 | 0.0 | 0.0 | 0.0 | 0.0 | 0.0 | 0.0 | 0.0 | 0.0 | 0.0 | 0.0 | 0.0 | 0.0 |
| 乳类 Dairy products | 0.0 | 0.0 | 0.0 | 0.0 | 0.0 | 0.0 | 0.0 | 0.0 | 0.0 | 0.0 | 0.0 | 0.0 | 0.0 | 0.0 | 0.0 | 0.0 | 0.0 | 0.0 | 0.0 | 0.0 | 0.0 | 0.0 | 0.0 | 0.0 | 0.0 |
| 蔬菜类 Vegetables | 51.5 | 0.0 | 26.3 | 0.0 | 91.7 | 100.0 | 96.8 | 23.8 | 100.0 | 78.7 | 99.7 | 100.0 | 94.8 | 76.5 | 98.7 | 38.6 | 95.4 | 69.2 | 99.5 | 0.0 | 100.0 | 99.6 | 100.0 | 100.0 | 96.6 |
| 水果类 Fruits | 48.5 | 100.0 | 73.7 | 100.0 | 8.3 | 0.0 | 3.2 | 76.2 | 0.0 | 21.3 | 0.3 | 0.0 | 5.2 | 23.5 | 1.3 | 61.4 | 4.6 | 30.8 | 0.5 | 100.0 | 0.0 | 0.4 | 0.0 | 0.0 | 3.4 |
| 糖类 Sugar | 0.0 | 0.0 | 0.0 | 0.0 | 0.0 | 0.0 | 0.0 | 0.0 | 0.0 | 0.0 | 0.0 | 0.0 | 0.0 | 0.0 | 0.0 | 0.0 | 0.0 | 0.0 | 0.0 | 0.0 | 0.0 | 0.0 | 0.0 | 0.0 | 0.0 |
| 水及饮料类 Water and beverages | 0.0 | 0.0 | 0.0 | 0.0 | 0.0 | 0.0 | 0.0 | 0.0 | 0.0 | 0.0 | 0.0 | 0.0 | 0.0 | 0.0 | 0.0 | 0.0 | 0.0 | 0.0 | 0.0 | 0.0 | 0.0 | 0.0 | 0.0 | 0.0 | 0.0 |

续表

| 膳食类别 Category | 黑龙江 HL | 辽宁 LN | 河北 HE | 北京 BJ | 吉林 JL | 山西 SX | 陕西 SN | 河南 HA | 宁夏 NX | 内蒙古 NM | 青海 QH | 甘肃 GS | 上海 SH | 福建 FJ | 江西 JX | 江苏 JS | 浙江 ZJ | 山东 SD | 湖北 HB | 四川 SC | 广西 GX | 湖南 HN | 广东 GD | 贵州 GZ | 全国平均 AVG |
|---|---|---|---|---|---|---|---|---|---|---|---|---|---|---|---|---|---|---|---|---|---|---|---|---|---|
| 酒类 Alcohol beverages | 0.0 | 0.0 | 0.0 | 0.0 | 0.0 | 0.0 | 0.0 | 0.0 | 0.0 | 0.0 | 0.0 | 0.0 | 0.0 | 0.0 | 0.0 | 0.0 | 0.0 | 0.0 | 0.0 | 0.0 | 0.0 | 0.0 | 0.0 | 0.0 | 0.0 |

附表 4-117 第六次中国总膳食研究膳食样品中多菌灵的含量（单位：μg/kg）

Annexed Table 4-117 Levels of carbendazim in food samples from the 6$^{th}$ China TDS (Unit: μg/kg)

| 膳食类别 Category | 黑龙江 HL | 辽宁 LN | 河北 HE | 北京 BJ | 吉林 JL | 山西 SX | 陕西 SN | 河南 HA | 宁夏 NX | 内蒙古 NM | 青海 QH | 甘肃 GS | 上海 SH | 福建 FJ | 江西 JX | 江苏 JS | 浙江 ZJ | 山东 SD | 湖北 HB | 四川 SC | 广西 GX | 湖南 HN | 广东 GD | 贵州 GZ | 全国平均 AVG |
|---|---|---|---|---|---|---|---|---|---|---|---|---|---|---|---|---|---|---|---|---|---|---|---|---|---|
| 谷类 Cereals | ND | ND | 0.10 | ND | ND | ND | 0.33 | ND | ND | ND | ND | ND | ND | ND | 0.16 | ND | ND | ND | ND | 2.72 | 0.39 | ND | ND | ND | 0.15 |
| 豆类 Legumes | ND | ND | ND | ND | 0.06 | ND | ND | ND | ND | ND | ND | ND | ND | 0.05 | ND | ND | ND | ND | ND | 0.04 | ND | ND | ND | ND | 0.01 |
| 薯类 Potatoes | ND | ND | ND | ND | 0.14 | 0.04 | 0.35 | 0.54 | ND | 0.16 | 0.11 | ND | ND | ND | ND | ND | ND | ND | ND | 0.06 | 0.32 | ND | ND | 0.11 | 0.08 |
| 肉类 Meats | ND | ND | ND | 0.23 | 0.10 | ND | ND | 0.03 | ND | 0.11 | ND | ND | ND | ND | ND | ND | ND | ND | ND | ND | ND | ND | ND | 0.05 | 0.02 |
| 蛋类 Eggs | ND | ND | ND | ND | 0.05 | ND | ND | ND | ND | ND | ND | ND | ND | ND | ND | ND | ND | ND | 1.49 | ND | ND | 0.09 | ND | ND | 0.06 |
| 水产类 Aquatic foods | ND | ND | ND | ND | 0.13 | 0.41 | ND | ND | ND | ND | 0.07 | ND | ND | ND | 0.07 | 0.06 | ND | ND | 0.04 | ND | ND | ND | ND | ND | 0.04 |
| 乳类 Dairy products | ND | ND | ND | ND | ND | ND | ND | ND | ND | ND | ND | ND | ND | ND | ND | ND | ND | ND | ND | ND | ND | ND | ND | ND | 0.00 |
| 蔬菜类 Vegetables | 0.28 | ND | 0.90 | 4.77 | 0.86 | 6.31 | 2.69 | 0.17 | 0.03 | 0.44 | 19.77 | 2.65 | 0.45 | 11.27 | 0.13 | 0.60 | 0.28 | 1.10 | 0.67 | 0.44 | 3.26 | 0.27 | 2.59 | 6.43 | 2.77 |

续表

| 膳食类别 Category | 黑龙江 HL | 辽宁 LN | 河北 HE | 北京 BJ | 吉林 JL | 山西 SX | 陕西 SN | 河南 HA | 宁夏 NX | 内蒙古 NM | 青海 QH | 甘肃 GS | 上海 SH | 福建 FJ | 江西 JX | 江苏 JS | 浙江 ZJ | 山东 SD | 湖北 HB | 四川 SC | 广西 GX | 湖南 HN | 广东 GD | 贵州 GZ | 全国平均 AVG |
|---|---|---|---|---|---|---|---|---|---|---|---|---|---|---|---|---|---|---|---|---|---|---|---|---|---|
| 水果类 Fruits | 2.41 | 3.97 | 0.49 | 1.60 | 0.36 | ND | 1.27 | 24.39 | ND | 1.26 | ND | 2.24 | 0.14 | 3.05 | 2.67 | 1.33 | 8.48 | 1.22 | 1.51 | 4.46 | 0.15 | 0.53 | 3.14 | ND | 2.69 |
| 糖类 Sugar | ND | ND | ND | ND | ND | ND | ND | ND | ND | ND | ND | ND | ND | ND | ND | ND | ND | ND | ND | ND | ND | ND | ND | ND | 0.00 |
| 水及饮料类 Water and beverages | ND | ND | ND | ND | ND | ND | ND | ND | ND | ND | ND | ND | ND | ND | ND | ND | ND | ND | ND | 0.06 | ND | ND | ND | ND | 0.00 |
| 酒类 Alcohol beverages | ND | 0.07 | ND | 0.05 | 0.07 | ND | 0.06 | ND | ND | ND | ND | ND | ND | 0.10 | ND | ND | 0.10 | 0.17 | ND | ND | 0.87 | ND | ND | ND | 0.06 |

注：未检出（ND）按 0 计

Note: values not detected (ND) were treated as being equal to 0

**附表 4-118　第六次中国总膳食研究膳食样品中噻菌灵的含量（单位：μg/kg）**

**Annexed Table 4-118　Levels of thiabendazole in food samples from the 6th China TDS (Unit: μg/kg)**

| 膳食类别 Category | 黑龙江 HL | 辽宁 LN | 河北 HE | 北京 BJ | 吉林 JL | 山西 SX | 陕西 SN | 河南 HA | 宁夏 NX | 内蒙古 NM | 青海 QH | 甘肃 GS | 上海 SH | 福建 FJ | 江西 JX | 江苏 JS | 浙江 ZJ | 山东 SD | 湖北 HB | 四川 SC | 广西 GX | 湖南 HN | 广东 GD | 贵州 GZ | 全国平均 AVG |
|---|---|---|---|---|---|---|---|---|---|---|---|---|---|---|---|---|---|---|---|---|---|---|---|---|---|
| 谷类 Cereals | ND | ND | ND | 0.08 | ND | ND | ND | ND | ND | ND | ND | ND | 0.12 | ND | ND | ND | ND | ND | ND | ND | ND | ND | ND | ND | 0.01 |
| 豆类 Legumes | 0.34 | ND | ND | ND | ND | ND | ND | ND | ND | ND | ND | ND | ND | ND | ND | ND | ND | ND | ND | ND | ND | ND | ND | ND | 0.01 |
| 薯类 Potatoes | ND | ND | ND | ND | ND | ND | ND | ND | ND | 0.06 | ND | 0.51 | ND | ND | ND | ND | ND | 0.08 | ND | ND | ND | ND | ND | ND | 0.03 |
| 肉类 Meats | ND | ND | 0.07 | ND | ND | ND | ND | ND | 0.07 | ND | ND | ND | ND | ND | ND | ND | ND | ND | ND | ND | ND | ND | 0.74 | ND | 0.04 |
| 蛋类 Eggs | ND | ND | ND | ND | ND | ND | ND | ND | ND | ND | ND | ND | ND | ND | ND | ND | ND | ND | ND | ND | ND | ND | ND | ND | 0.00 |

续表

| 膳食类别<br>Category | 黑龙江<br>HL | 辽宁<br>LN | 河北<br>HE | 北京<br>BJ | 吉林<br>JL | 山西<br>SX | 陕西<br>SN | 河南<br>HA | 宁夏<br>NX | 内蒙古<br>NM | 青海<br>QH | 甘肃<br>GS | 上海<br>SH | 福建<br>FJ | 江西<br>JX | 江苏<br>JS | 浙江<br>ZJ | 山东<br>SD | 湖北<br>HB | 四川<br>SC | 广西<br>GX | 湖南<br>HN | 广东<br>GD | 贵州<br>GZ | 全国平均<br>AVG |
|---|---|---|---|---|---|---|---|---|---|---|---|---|---|---|---|---|---|---|---|---|---|---|---|---|---|
| 水产类 Aquatic foods | ND | ND | ND | ND | ND | ND | ND | ND | ND | ND | ND | ND | ND | ND | ND | ND | ND | ND | ND | ND | ND | ND | ND | ND | 0.00 |
| 乳类 Dairy products | ND | 0.08 | ND | ND | ND | ND | ND | ND | ND | ND | ND | ND | ND | ND | ND | ND | ND | ND | ND | ND | ND | ND | ND | ND | 0.00 |
| 蔬菜类 Vegetables | ND | ND | ND | ND | ND | ND | ND | ND | 0.09 | ND | ND | ND | ND | ND | ND | ND | ND | ND | 0.06 | 0.38 | ND | ND | ND | ND | 0.02 |
| 水果类 Fruits | ND | 7.88 | 6.53 | ND | ND | ND | ND | ND | ND | ND | ND | 0.08 | 47.29 | 17.73 | ND | 1.06 | 41.74 | 4.36 | 11.48 | ND | ND | ND | ND | ND | 5.76 |
| 糖类 Sugar | ND | ND | ND | ND | ND | ND | ND | ND | 0.09 | ND | ND | ND | ND | 0.05 | ND | ND | ND | ND | ND | 0.08 | ND | ND | ND | ND | 0.01 |
| 水反饮料类 Water and beverages | ND | ND | ND | ND | ND | ND | ND | ND | ND | ND | ND | ND | ND | ND | ND | 0.06 | ND | ND | ND | ND | 0.09 | ND | ND | ND | 0.01 |
| 酒类 Alcohol beverages | ND | ND | ND | ND | ND | ND | ND | ND | ND | ND | ND | ND | ND | ND | ND | ND | ND | ND | ND | 0.06 | ND | ND | ND | ND | 0.00 |

注：未检出（ND）按 0 计

Note: values not detected (ND) were treated as being equal to 0

附表 4-119　第六次中国总膳食研究膳食样品中抑霉唑的含量（单位：μg/kg）

Annexed Table 4-119　Levels of imazalil in food samples from the 6th China TDS (Unit: μg/kg)

| 膳食类别<br>Category | 黑龙江<br>HL | 辽宁<br>LN | 河北<br>HE | 北京<br>BJ | 吉林<br>JL | 山西<br>SX | 陕西<br>SN | 河南<br>HA | 宁夏<br>NX | 内蒙古<br>NM | 青海<br>QH | 甘肃<br>GS | 上海<br>SH | 福建<br>FJ | 江西<br>JX | 江苏<br>JS | 浙江<br>ZJ | 山东<br>SD | 湖北<br>HB | 四川<br>SC | 广西<br>GX | 湖南<br>HN | 广东<br>GD | 贵州<br>GZ | 全国平均<br>AVG |
|---|---|---|---|---|---|---|---|---|---|---|---|---|---|---|---|---|---|---|---|---|---|---|---|---|---|
| 谷类 Cereals | ND | ND | ND | ND | ND | 0.14 | ND | ND | ND | ND | ND | ND | ND | ND | ND | ND | ND | 0.13 | ND | 0.12 | ND | ND | ND | ND | 0.02 |

续表

| 膳食类别 Category | 黑龙江 HL | 辽宁 LN | 河北 HE | 北京 BJ | 吉林 JL | 山西 SX | 陕西 SN | 河南 HA | 宁夏 NX | 内蒙古 NM | 青海 QH | 甘肃 GS | 上海 SH | 福建 FJ | 江西 JX | 江苏 JS | 浙江 ZJ | 山东 SD | 湖北 HB | 四川 SC | 广西 GX | 湖南 HN | 广东 GD | 贵州 GZ | 全国平均 AVG |
|---|---|---|---|---|---|---|---|---|---|---|---|---|---|---|---|---|---|---|---|---|---|---|---|---|---|
| 豆类 Legumes | 0.18 | ND | ND | ND | ND | ND | ND | 0.16 | ND | ND | ND | ND | ND | ND | ND | ND | 0.13 | ND | ND | ND | ND | ND | ND | ND | 0.02 |
| 薯类 Potatoes | ND | ND | ND | ND | ND | 0.11 | ND | 0.15 | 0.19 | 0.16 | ND | 0.51 | ND | ND | ND | ND | ND | ND | ND | ND | ND | ND | ND | ND | 0.05 |
| 肉类 Meats | ND | ND | 0.13 | ND | ND | ND | ND | 0.14 | 0.31 | ND | 0.09 | ND | ND | ND | ND | ND | ND | ND | ND | ND | ND | ND | 0.31 | ND | 0.04 |
| 蛋类 Eggs | ND | ND | 0.10 | ND | ND | ND | 0.23 | ND | ND | ND | ND | ND | ND | ND | ND | ND | ND | ND | ND | ND | ND | ND | ND | ND | 0.01 |
| 水产类 Aquatic foods | ND | ND | ND | 0.08 | ND | ND | ND | ND | ND | 0.09 | 0.10 | ND | ND | ND | ND | ND | ND | ND | ND | ND | ND | ND | ND | ND | 0.01 |
| 乳类 Dairy products | ND | 0.09 | ND | ND | ND | ND | ND | ND | ND | ND | ND | ND | ND | ND | 0.08 | ND | ND | ND | ND | ND | ND | ND | ND | ND | 0.01 |
| 蔬菜类 Vegetables | ND | ND | ND | ND | ND | ND | ND | 0.13 | 0.14 | ND | ND | ND | ND | ND | ND | ND | ND | ND | 0.08 | 0.25 | ND | ND | ND | ND | 0.03 |
| 水果类 Fruits | 0.08 | 5.93 | 5.88 | ND | 0.78 | 1.53 | 1.53 | 0.78 | ND | 0.22 | ND | 0.08 | 15.91 | 12.73 | 0.32 | 0.84 | 29.35 | 1.33 | 33.46 | 1.30 | ND | ND | 0.35 | 0.12 | 4.69 |
| 糖类 Sugar | ND | ND | ND | ND | ND | ND | ND | ND | 0.10 | ND | ND | ND | ND | ND | ND | ND | ND | ND | ND | ND | ND | ND | ND | ND | 0.00 |
| 水及饮料类 Water and beverages | ND | ND | ND | ND | ND | ND | ND | ND | ND | ND | ND | 0.07 | ND | ND | ND | 0.12 | ND | ND | ND | 0.13 | 0.25 | ND | ND | ND | 0.02 |
| 酒类 Alcohol beverages | ND | ND | ND | ND | ND | ND | ND | ND | ND | ND | ND | ND | ND | ND | ND | ND | ND | ND | ND | 0.09 | 0.29 | ND | ND | ND | 0.02 |

注：未检出（ND）按0计

Note: values not detected (ND) were treated as being equal to 0

附表 4-120 第六次中国总膳食研究膳食样品中咪鲜胺的含量（单位：µg/kg）

Annexed Table 4-120 Levels of prochloraz in food samples from the 6$^{th}$ China TDS (Unit: µg/kg)

| 膳食类别 Category | 黑龙江 HL | 辽宁 LN | 河北 HE | 北京 BJ | 吉林 JL | 山西 SX | 陕西 SN | 河南 HA | 宁夏 NX | 内蒙古 NM | 青海 QH | 甘肃 GS | 上海 SH | 福建 FJ | 江西 JX | 江苏 JS | 浙江 ZJ | 山东 SD | 湖北 HB | 四川 SC | 广西 GX | 湖南 HN | 广东 GD | 贵州 GZ | 全国平均 AVG |
|---|---|---|---|---|---|---|---|---|---|---|---|---|---|---|---|---|---|---|---|---|---|---|---|---|---|
| 谷类 Cereals | ND | 0.34 | ND | 0.08 | 0.21 | 0.29 | ND | ND | 0.12 | ND | ND | ND | 0.12 | ND | ND | ND | ND | ND | ND | 2.70 | ND | ND | ND | ND | 0.16 |
| 豆类 Legumes | 0.10 | ND | ND | ND | 0.45 | ND | 0.08 | 2.91 | ND | ND | ND | ND | ND | ND | ND | ND | ND | ND | ND | ND | ND | ND | ND | ND | 0.15 |
| 薯类 Potatoes | 0.07 | ND | ND | ND | 0.26 | 2.09 | ND | 0.98 | 0.16 | 0.08 | 0.12 | ND | 0.40 | ND | ND | ND | ND | 1.16 | ND | 0.16 | ND | ND | ND | ND | 0.23 |
| 肉类 Meats | ND | ND | ND | ND | ND | ND | ND | 0.19 | 0.23 | ND | 0.14 | ND | ND | ND | ND | ND | ND | 0.10 | ND | 0.10 | ND | 0.08 | ND | ND | 0.03 |
| 蛋类 Eggs | ND | ND | ND | ND | ND | ND | ND | ND | ND | ND | ND | ND | 0.16 | ND | ND | ND | ND | ND | ND | ND | ND | ND | ND | ND | 0.01 |
| 水产类 Aquatic foods | ND | ND | ND | 0.16 | ND | 0.23 | 0.07 | ND | ND | ND | 0.07 | ND | ND | ND | ND | ND | ND | ND | ND | ND | ND | 0.06 | ND | ND | 0.02 |
| 乳类 Dairy products | ND | ND | ND | ND | ND | ND | ND | ND | ND | ND | ND | ND | ND | ND | ND | 0.08 | ND | ND | ND | ND | ND | ND | ND | ND | 0.00 |
| 蔬菜类 Vegetables | ND | 1.49 | 0.69 | 0.87 | 0.14 | 0.59 | 2.50 | 0.33 | 2.61 | 0.13 | ND | 0.07 | ND | 0.23 | 0.29 | 0.18 | 1.30 | 0.06 | 0.64 | 0.24 | 0.69 | 1.68 | 28.54 | 0.64 | 1.83 |
| 水果类 Fruits | 0.20 | 0.45 | 0.51 | 0.85 | 1.45 | 1.02 | 1.12 | 0.65 | 0.31 | 0.09 | ND | 0.09 | 0.21 | 4.68 | ND | 0.77 | 0.66 | 1.75 | 1.22 | 19.73 | 0.59 | 0.90 | 0.07 | 0.77 | 1.59 |
| 糖类 Sugar | ND | ND | ND | ND | ND | ND | ND | ND | ND | ND | ND | ND | ND | ND | ND | ND | ND | ND | ND | ND | ND | ND | ND | ND | 0.00 |
| 水及饮料类 Water and beverages | ND | ND | ND | ND | ND | ND | ND | ND | ND | ND | ND | ND | ND | ND | ND | ND | ND | ND | ND | 0.39 | ND | ND | ND | ND | 0.02 |

续表

| 膳食类别 Category | 黑龙江 HL | 辽宁 LN | 河北 HE | 北京 BJ | 吉林 JL | 山西 SX | 陕西 SN | 河南 HA | 宁夏 NX | 内蒙古 NM | 青海 QH | 甘肃 GS | 上海 SH | 福建 FJ | 江西 JX | 江苏 JS | 浙江 ZJ | 山东 SD | 湖北 HB | 四川 SC | 广西 GX | 湖南 HN | 广东 GD | 贵州 GZ | 全国平均 AVG |
|---|---|---|---|---|---|---|---|---|---|---|---|---|---|---|---|---|---|---|---|---|---|---|---|---|---|
| 酒类 Alcohol beverages | ND | ND | ND | ND | ND | ND | ND | 0.43 | ND | ND | ND | ND | ND | ND | ND | ND | ND | ND | ND | ND | ND | ND | ND | ND | 0.02 |

注：未检出（ND）按 0 计

Note: values not detected (ND) were treated as being equal to 0

附表 4-121　第六次中国总膳食研究的多菌灵膳食摄入量 [ 单位：ng/(kg bw・d)]

Annexed Table 4-121　Dietary intakes of carbendazim from the 6th China TDS [Unit: ng/(kg bw・d)]

| 膳食类别 Category | 黑龙江 HL | 辽宁 LN | 河北 HE | 北京 BJ | 吉林 JL | 山西 SX | 陕西 SN | 河南 HA | 宁夏 NX | 内蒙古 NM | 青海 QH | 甘肃 GS | 上海 SH | 福建 FJ | 江西 JX | 江苏 JS | 浙江 ZJ | 山东 SD | 湖北 HB | 四川 SC | 广西 GX | 湖南 HN | 广东 GD | 贵州 GZ | 全国平均 AVG |
|---|---|---|---|---|---|---|---|---|---|---|---|---|---|---|---|---|---|---|---|---|---|---|---|---|---|
| 谷类 Cereals | 4.397 | 21.010 | 4.702 | 3.865 | 3.955 | 5.607 | 4.870 | 13.840 | 4.351 | 16.000 | 3.985 | 4.570 | 7.865 | 5.841 | 2.278 | 10.910 | 9.512 | 8.378 | 2.799 | 10.020 | 3.127 | 2.232 | 2.506 | 0.000 | 6.526 |
| 豆类 Legumes | 0.480 | 0.000 | 0.416 | 0.000 | 0.190 | 0.319 | 0.454 | 1.827 | 0.000 | 0.000 | 0.020 | 0.212 | 0.302 | 0.215 | 0.261 | 0.000 | 0.448 | 1.298 | 0.377 | 3.749 | 0.094 | 0.369 | 0.146 | 0.000 | 0.466 |
| 薯类 Potatoes | 0.000 | 0.437 | 0.216 | 0.215 | 0.000 | 20.540 | 0.591 | 1.437 | 0.654 | 0.820 | 0.442 | 0.715 | 0.153 | 0.101 | 0.107 | 0.178 | 0.110 | 8.519 | 0.469 | 0.490 | 0.000 | 0.345 | 0.104 | 0.238 | 1.537 |
| 肉类 Meats | 0.000 | 0.688 | 0.000 | 0.000 | 0.000 | 0.000 | 0.000 | 0.000 | 0.000 | 0.000 | 0.000 | 0.000 | 0.000 | 0.000 | 0.000 | 0.000 | 0.000 | 0.000 | 3.805 | 0.000 | 0.000 | 0.000 | 1.075 | 0.000 | 0.232 |
| 蛋类 Eggs | 0.000 | 0.337 | 0.203 | 0.000 | 0.000 | 0.000 | 0.000 | 0.000 | 0.000 | 0.000 | 0.000 | 0.000 | 0.000 | 0.000 | 0.000 | 0.000 | 0.000 | 0.000 | 0.837 | 0.000 | 0.000 | 0.198 | 0.000 | 0.000 | 0.057 |
| 水产类 Aquatic foods | 0.000 | 0.000 | 0.000 | 0.000 | 0.000 | 0.000 | 0.000 | 0.000 | 0.000 | 0.000 | 0.000 | 0.000 | 0.000 | 0.000 | 0.000 | 0.000 | 0.209 | 0.000 | 1.996 | 0.330 | 0.000 | 0.597 | 0.251 | 0.000 | 0.149 |
| 乳类 Dairy products | 0.000 | 0.000 | 0.000 | 0.000 | 0.000 | 0.202 | 0.000 | 0.000 | 0.000 | 0.000 | 0.000 | 0.000 | 0.000 | 0.000 | 0.000 | 0.000 | 0.000 | 0.000 | 0.000 | 0.000 | 0.000 | 0.000 | 0.000 | 0.000 | 0.008 |

续表

| 膳食类别<br>Category | 黑龙江<br>HL | 辽宁<br>LN | 河北<br>HE | 北京<br>BJ | 吉林<br>JL | 山西<br>SX | 陕西<br>SN | 河南<br>HA | 宁夏<br>NX | 内蒙古<br>NM | 青海<br>QH | 甘肃<br>GS | 上海<br>SH | 福建<br>FJ | 江西<br>JX | 江苏<br>JS | 浙江<br>ZJ | 山东<br>SD | 湖北<br>HB | 四川<br>SC | 广西<br>GX | 湖南<br>HN | 广东<br>GD | 贵州<br>GZ | 全国平均<br>AVG |
|---|---|---|---|---|---|---|---|---|---|---|---|---|---|---|---|---|---|---|---|---|---|---|---|---|---|
| 蔬菜类 Vegetables | 4.99 | 20.88 | 180.90 | 126.70 | 6.18 | 64.90 | 5.79 | 13.47 | 23.65 | 2.99 | 57.14 | 96.38 | 34.66 | 14.07 | 50.31 | 14.38 | 133.10 | 140.20 | 49.70 | 35.31 | 14.36 | 25.22 | 12.94 | 59.80 | 49.50 |
| 水果类 Fruits | 13.60 | 76.29 | 10.50 | 114.80 | 32.57 | 6.15 | 10.24 | 18.07 | 23.88 | 11.49 | 0.405 | 0.77 | 39.42 | 36.96 | 29.20 | 7.93 | 18.46 | 49.42 | 4.93 | 2.26 | 4.79 | 13.28 | 5.08 | 5.09 | 22.32 |
| 糖类 Sugar | 0.000 | 0.000 | 0.000 | 0.000 | 0.000 | 0.000 | 0.000 | 0.000 | 0.000 | 0.000 | 0.000 | 0.003 | 0.079 | 0.000 | 0.000 | 0.000 | 0.000 | 0.000 | 0.000 | 0.000 | 0.000 | 0.000 | 0.000 | 0.000 | 0.003 |
| 水及饮料类 Water and beverages | 0.000 | 0.000 | 0.000 | 0.000 | 1.989 | 0.000 | 0.000 | 0.000 | 0.000 | 0.000 | 4.551 | 0.000 | 6.758 | 3.130 | 0.000 | 2.519 | 2.951 | 0.000 | 0.876 | 0.000 | 5.203 | 3.807 | 15.160 | 0.000 | 1.739 |
| 酒类 Alcohol beverages | 0.000 | 0.000 | 0.000 | 0.358 | 0.067 | 0.000 | 0.000 | 0.000 | 0.000 | 0.065 | 0.000 | 0.000 | 0.686 | 0.065 | 0.000 | 0.197 | 0.819 | 6.768 | 0.000 | 0.000 | 0.000 | 0.000 | 0.023 | 0.000 | 0.594 |
| 合计 SUM | 23.47 | 119.64 | 197.98 | 246.98 | 44.95 | 97.72 | 21.94 | 48.63 | 52.53 | 31.36 | 66.54 | 102.65 | 89.92 | 60.39 | 82.15 | 36.12 | 165.57 | 214.54 | 65.79 | 52.16 | 27.57 | 46.05 | 37.29 | 65.13 | 83.13 |

附表 4-122　第六次中国总膳食研究的噻菌灵膳食摄入量 [单位: ng/(kg bw·d)]

Annexed Table 4-122　Dietary intakes of thiabendazole from the 6$^{th}$ China TDS [Unit: ng/(kg bw·d)]

| 膳食类别<br>Category | 黑龙江<br>HL | 辽宁<br>LN | 河北<br>HE | 北京<br>BJ | 吉林<br>JL | 山西<br>SX | 陕西<br>SN | 河南<br>HA | 宁夏<br>NX | 内蒙古<br>NM | 青海<br>QH | 甘肃<br>GS | 上海<br>SH | 福建<br>FJ | 江西<br>JX | 江苏<br>JS | 浙江<br>ZJ | 山东<br>SD | 湖北<br>HB | 四川<br>SC | 广西<br>GX | 湖南<br>HN | 广东<br>GD | 贵州<br>GZ | 全国平均<br>AVG |
|---|---|---|---|---|---|---|---|---|---|---|---|---|---|---|---|---|---|---|---|---|---|---|---|---|---|
| 谷类 Cereals | 0.000 | 0.000 | 0.000 | 1.043 | 0.000 | 0.000 | 0.000 | 0.000 | 0.000 | 0.000 | 0.000 | 0.000 | 0.826 | 0.000 | 0.000 | 0.000 | 0.000 | 0.000 | 0.000 | 0.000 | 0.000 | 0.000 | 0.000 | 0.000 | 0.078 |
| 豆类 Legumes | 0.242 | 0.000 | 0.000 | 0.000 | 0.000 | 0.000 | 0.000 | 0.000 | 0.000 | 0.000 | 0.000 | 0.000 | 0.000 | 0.000 | 0.000 | 0.000 | 0.000 | 0.058 | 0.000 | 0.000 | 0.000 | 0.000 | 0.000 | 0.000 | 0.010 |
| 薯类 Potatoes | 0.000 | 0.000 | 0.000 | 0.000 | 0.000 | 0.000 | 0.000 | 0.000 | 0.000 | 0.118 | 0.000 | 1.163 | 0.000 | 0.000 | 0.000 | 0.000 | 0.000 | 0.000 | 0.000 | 0.000 | 0.000 | 0.000 | 0.000 | 0.000 | 0.056 |

续表

| 膳食类别<br>Category | 黑龙江<br>HL | 辽宁<br>LN | 河北<br>HE | 北京<br>BJ | 吉林<br>JL | 山西<br>SX | 陕西<br>SN | 河南<br>HA | 宁夏<br>NX | 内蒙古<br>NM | 青海<br>QH | 甘肃<br>GS | 上海<br>SH | 福建<br>FJ | 江西<br>JX | 江苏<br>JS | 浙江<br>ZJ | 山东<br>SD | 湖北<br>HB | 四川<br>SC | 广西<br>GX | 湖南<br>HN | 广东<br>GD | 贵州<br>GZ | 全国平均<br>AVG |
|---|---|---|---|---|---|---|---|---|---|---|---|---|---|---|---|---|---|---|---|---|---|---|---|---|---|
| 肉类 Meats | 0.000 | 0.000 | 0.052 | 0.000 | 0.000 | 0.000 | 0.000 | 0.000 | 0.052 | 0.000 | 0.000 | 0.000 | 0.000 | 0.000 | 0.000 | 0.000 | 0.000 | 0.000 | 0.000 | 0.000 | 0.000 | 0.000 | 1.222 | 0.000 | 0.055 |
| 蛋类 Eggs | 0.000 | 0.000 | 0.000 | 0.000 | 0.000 | 0.000 | 0.000 | 0.000 | 0.000 | 0.000 | 0.000 | 0.000 | 0.000 | 0.000 | 0.000 | 0.000 | 0.000 | 0.000 | 0.000 | 0.000 | 0.000 | 0.000 | 0.000 | 0.000 | 0.000 |
| 水产类 Aquatic foods | 0.000 | 0.000 | 0.000 | 0.000 | 0.000 | 0.000 | 0.000 | 0.000 | 0.000 | 0.000 | 0.000 | 0.000 | 0.000 | 0.000 | 0.000 | 0.000 | 0.000 | 0.000 | 0.000 | 0.000 | 0.000 | 0.000 | 0.000 | 0.000 | 0.000 |
| 乳类 Dairy products | 0.000 | 0.053 | 0.000 | 0.000 | 0.000 | 0.000 | 0.000 | 0.000 | 0.000 | 0.000 | 0.000 | 0.000 | 0.000 | 0.000 | 0.000 | 0.000 | 0.000 | 0.000 | 0.000 | 0.000 | 0.000 | 0.000 | 0.000 | 0.000 | 0.002 |
| 蔬菜类 Vegetables | 0.000 | 0.000 | 0.000 | 0.000 | 0.000 | 0.000 | 0.000 | 0.000 | 0.216 | 0.000 | 0.000 | 0.040 | 0.000 | 0.000 | 0.000 | 0.000 | 0.000 | 0.000 | 0.381 | 1.843 | 0.000 | 0.000 | 0.000 | 0.000 | 0.102 |
| 水果类 Fruits | 0.000 | 9.615 | 3.903 | 0.000 | 0.000 | 0.000 | 0.000 | 0.000 | 0.000 | 0.000 | 0.000 | 0.000 | 55.110 | 16.840 | 0.000 | 0.457 | 44.600 | 3.767 | 3.499 | 0.000 | 0.000 | 0.000 | 0.000 | 0.000 | 5.742 |
| 糖类 Sugar | 0.000 | 0.000 | 0.000 | 0.000 | 0.000 | 0.000 | 0.000 | 0.000 | 0.000 | 0.000 | 0.000 | 0.000 | 0.000 | 0.000 | 0.000 | 0.000 | 0.000 | 0.000 | 0.000 | 0.000 | 0.000 | 0.000 | 0.000 | 0.000 | 0.000 |
| 水及饮料类 Water and beverages | 0.000 | 0.000 | 0.000 | 0.000 | 0.000 | 0.000 | 0.000 | 0.000 | 0.000 | 0.000 | 0.000 | 0.000 | 0.000 | 0.000 | 0.000 | 0.988 | 0.000 | 0.000 | 0.000 | 0.000 | 1.894 | 0.000 | 0.000 | 0.000 | 0.120 |
| 酒类 Alcohol beverages | 0.000 | 0.000 | 0.000 | 0.000 | 0.000 | 0.000 | 0.000 | 0.000 | 0.001 | 0.000 | 0.000 | 0.000 | 0.000 | 0.000 | 0.000 | 0.000 | 0.000 | 0.000 | 0.000 | 0.005 | 0.000 | 0.000 | 0.000 | 0.000 | 0.000 |
| 合计 SUM | 0.242 | 9.668 | 3.955 | 1.043 | 0.000 | 0.000 | 0.000 | 0.000 | 0.269 | 0.118 | 0.000 | 1.203 | 55.932 | 16.837 | 0.000 | 1.445 | 44.596 | 3.825 | 3.880 | 1.848 | 1.894 | 0.000 | 1.222 | 0.000 | 6.166 |

附表 4-123　第六次中国总膳食研究的抑霉唑膳食摄入量 [单位：ng/(kg bw·d)]
Annexed Table 4-123　Dietary intakes of imazalil from the 6th China TDS [Unit: ng/(kg bw·d)]

| 膳食类别 Category | 黑龙江 HL | 辽宁 LN | 河北 HE | 北京 BJ | 吉林 JL | 山西 SX | 陕西 SN | 河南 HA | 宁夏 NX | 内蒙古 NM | 青海 QH | 甘肃 GS | 上海 SH | 福建 FJ | 江西 JX | 江苏 JS | 浙江 ZJ | 山东 SD | 湖北 HB | 四川 SC | 广西 GX | 湖南 HN | 广东 GD | 贵州 GZ | 全国平均 AVG |
|---|---|---|---|---|---|---|---|---|---|---|---|---|---|---|---|---|---|---|---|---|---|---|---|---|---|
| 谷类 Cereals | 0.000 | 0.000 | 0.000 | 0.000 | 0.000 | 2.326 | 0.000 | 0.000 | 0.000 | 0.000 | 0.000 | 0.000 | 0.000 | 0.000 | 0.000 | 0.000 | 0.000 | 1.978 | 0.000 | 1.838 | 0.000 | 0.000 | 0.000 | 0.000 | 0.256 |
| 豆类 Legumes | 0.127 | 0.000 | 0.000 | 0.000 | 0.000 | 0.000 | 0.000 | 0.134 | 0.000 | 0.000 | 0.000 | 0.000 | 0.000 | 0.000 | 0.000 | 0.000 | 0.280 | 0.000 | 0.000 | 0.000 | 0.000 | 0.000 | 0.000 | 0.000 | 0.023 |
| 薯类 Potatoes | 0.000 | 0.000 | 0.000 | 0.000 | 0.000 | 0.212 | 0.000 | 0.188 | 0.294 | 0.304 | 0.000 | 1.164 | 0.000 | 0.000 | 0.000 | 0.000 | 0.000 | 0.000 | 0.000 | 0.000 | 0.000 | 0.000 | 0.000 | 0.000 | 0.090 |
| 肉类 Meats | 0.000 | 0.000 | 0.099 | 0.000 | 0.000 | 0.000 | 0.000 | 0.126 | 0.230 | 0.000 | 0.097 | 0.000 | 0.000 | 0.000 | 0.000 | 0.000 | 0.000 | 0.000 | 0.000 | 0.000 | 0.000 | 0.000 | 0.506 | 0.000 | 0.044 |
| 蛋类 Eggs | 0.000 | 0.000 | 0.049 | 0.021 | 0.000 | 0.000 | 0.079 | 0.000 | 0.000 | 0.000 | 0.000 | 0.000 | 0.000 | 0.000 | 0.000 | 0.000 | 0.000 | 0.000 | 0.000 | 0.000 | 0.000 | 0.000 | 0.000 | 0.000 | 0.005 |
| 水产类 Aquatic foods | 0.000 | 0.065 | 0.000 | 0.000 | 0.000 | 0.000 | 0.000 | 0.000 | 0.000 | 0.015 | 0.005 | 0.000 | 0.000 | 0.000 | 0.000 | 0.000 | 0.000 | 0.000 | 0.000 | 0.000 | 0.000 | 0.000 | 0.000 | 0.000 | 0.002 |
| 乳类 Dairy products | 0.000 | 0.000 | 0.000 | 0.000 | 0.000 | 0.000 | 0.000 | 0.000 | 0.000 | 0.000 | 0.000 | 0.000 | 0.000 | 0.000 | 0.026 | 0.000 | 0.000 | 0.000 | 0.000 | 0.000 | 0.000 | 0.000 | 0.000 | 0.000 | 0.004 |
| 蔬菜类 Vegetables | 0.000 | 0.000 | 0.000 | 0.000 | 0.000 | 0.000 | 0.000 | 0.578 | 0.359 | 0.450 | 0.000 | 0.043 | 0.000 | 0.000 | 0.000 | 0.000 | 0.000 | 0.000 | 0.523 | 1.216 | 0.000 | 0.000 | 0.000 | 0.000 | 0.130 |
| 水果类 Fruits | 0.080 | 7.240 | 3.519 | 0.000 | 1.086 | 0.848 | 0.924 | 0.300 | 0.000 | 0.400 | 0.000 | 0.000 | 18.540 | 12.090 | 0.289 | 0.362 | 31.354 | 1.151 | 10.200 | 0.310 | 0.000 | 0.000 | 0.165 | 0.039 | 3.706 |
| 糖类 Sugar | 0.000 | 0.000 | 0.000 | 0.000 | 0.000 | 0.000 | 0.000 | 0.000 | 0.001 | 0.000 | 0.000 | 0.000 | 0.000 | 0.000 | 0.000 | 0.000 | 0.000 | 0.000 | 0.000 | 0.000 | 0.000 | 0.000 | 0.000 | 0.000 | 0.000 |
| 水及饮料类 Water and beverages | 0.000 | 0.000 | 0.000 | 0.000 | 0.000 | 0.000 | 0.000 | 0.000 | 0.000 | 0.000 | 0.000 | 1.323 | 0.000 | 0.000 | 0.000 | 1.929 | 0.000 | 0.000 | 0.000 | 0.657 | 5.261 | 0.000 | 0.000 | 0.000 | 0.382 |

续表

| 膳食类别<br>Category | 黑龙江<br>HL | 辽宁<br>LN | 河北<br>HE | 北京<br>BJ | 吉林<br>JL | 山西<br>SX | 陕西<br>SN | 河南<br>HA | 宁夏<br>NX | 内蒙古<br>NM | 青海<br>QH | 甘肃<br>GS | 上海<br>SH | 福建<br>FJ | 江西<br>JX | 江苏<br>JS | 浙江<br>ZJ | 山东<br>SD | 湖北<br>HB | 四川<br>SC | 广西<br>GX | 湖南<br>HN | 广东<br>GD | 贵州<br>GZ | 全国平均<br>AVG |
|---|---|---|---|---|---|---|---|---|---|---|---|---|---|---|---|---|---|---|---|---|---|---|---|---|---|
| 酒类<br>Alcohol beverages | 0.000 | 0.000 | 0.000 | 0.000 | 0.000 | 0.000 | 0.000 | 0.000 | 0.000 | 0.000 | 0.000 | 0.000 | 0.000 | 0.000 | 0.000 | 0.000 | 0.000 | 0.000 | 0.000 | 0.000 | 0.145 | 0.000 | 0.000 | 0.000 | 0.006 |
| 合计<br>SUM | 0.207 | 7.304 | 3.666 | 0.021 | 1.086 | 3.386 | 1.003 | 1.326 | 0.884 | 1.169 | 0.103 | 2.530 | 18.542 | 12.095 | 0.315 | 2.292 | 31.634 | 3.129 | 10.721 | 4.028 | 5.406 | 0.000 | 0.671 | 0.039 | 4.648 |

附表 4-124 第六次中国总膳食研究的咪鲜胺膳食摄入量 [单位: ng/(kg bw · d)]

Annexed Table 4-124 Dietary intakes of prochloraz from the 6<sup>th</sup> China TDS [Unit: ng/(kg bw · d)]

| 膳食类别<br>Category | 黑龙江<br>HL | 辽宁<br>LN | 河北<br>HE | 北京<br>BJ | 吉林<br>JL | 山西<br>SX | 陕西<br>SN | 河南<br>HA | 宁夏<br>NX | 内蒙古<br>NM | 青海<br>QH | 甘肃<br>GS | 上海<br>SH | 福建<br>FJ | 江西<br>JX | 江苏<br>JS | 浙江<br>ZJ | 山东<br>SD | 湖北<br>HB | 四川<br>SC | 广西<br>GX | 湖南<br>HN | 广东<br>GD | 贵州<br>GZ | 全国平均<br>AVG |
|---|---|---|---|---|---|---|---|---|---|---|---|---|---|---|---|---|---|---|---|---|---|---|---|---|---|
| 谷类<br>Cereals | 0.000 | 3.334 | 0.000 | 0.997 | 1.984 | 4.821 | 0.000 | 0.000 | 1.273 | 0.000 | 0.000 | 0.000 | 0.887 | 0.000 | 0.000 | 0.000 | 0.000 | 0.000 | 0.000 | 41.630 | 0.000 | 0.000 | 0.000 | 0.000 | 2.289 |
| 豆类<br>Legumes | 0.075 | 0.000 | 0.000 | 0.000 | 0.537 | 0.000 | 0.111 | 2.491 | 0.000 | 0.163 | 0.185 | 0.000 | 0.000 | 0.000 | 0.000 | 0.000 | 0.000 | 0.000 | 0.000 | 0.000 | 0.000 | 0.000 | 0.000 | 0.000 | 0.134 |
| 薯类<br>Potatoes | 0.085 | 0.000 | 0.000 | 0.000 | 0.503 | 3.943 | 0.000 | 1.253 | 0.247 | 0.000 | 0.152 | 0.000 | 0.226 | 0.000 | 0.000 | 0.000 | 0.000 | 0.849 | 0.000 | 0.156 | 0.000 | 0.000 | 0.000 | 0.000 | 0.317 |
| 肉类<br>Meats | 0.000 | 0.000 | 0.000 | 0.000 | 0.000 | 0.000 | 0.000 | 0.163 | 0.172 | 0.000 | 0.152 | 0.000 | 0.000 | 0.000 | 0.000 | 0.000 | 0.000 | 0.147 | 0.000 | 0.212 | 0.000 | 0.195 | 0.000 | 0.000 | 0.043 |
| 蛋类<br>Eggs | 0.000 | 0.000 | 0.000 | 0.042 | 0.000 | 0.023 | 0.004 | 0.000 | 0.000 | 0.000 | 0.004 | 0.000 | 0.100 | 0.000 | 0.000 | 0.000 | 0.000 | 0.000 | 0.000 | 0.024 | 0.000 | 0.000 | 0.000 | 0.021 | 0.006 |
| 水产类<br>Aquatic foods | 0.000 | 0.000 | 0.000 | 0.000 | 0.000 | 0.000 | 0.004 | 0.000 | 0.000 | 0.000 | 0.000 | 0.000 | 0.000 | 0.000 | 0.000 | 0.034 | 0.000 | 0.000 | 0.000 | 0.000 | 0.000 | 0.058 | 0.000 | 0.000 | 0.005 |
| 乳类<br>Dairy products | 0.000 | 0.000 | 0.000 | 0.000 | 0.000 | 0.000 | 0.000 | 0.000 | 0.000 | 0.000 | 0.000 | 0.000 | 0.000 | 0.000 | 0.000 | 0.000 | 0.000 | 0.000 | 0.000 | 0.000 | 0.000 | 0.000 | 0.000 | 0.000 | 0.001 |

续表

| 膳食类别 Category | 黑龙江 HL | 辽宁 LN | 河北 HE | 北京 BJ | 吉林 JL | 山西 SX | 陕西 SN | 河南 HA | 宁夏 NX | 内蒙古 NM | 青海 QH | 甘肃 GS | 上海 SH | 福建 FJ | 江西 JX | 江苏 JS | 浙江 ZJ | 山东 SD | 湖北 HB | 四川 SC | 广西 GX | 湖南 HN | 广东 GD | 贵州 GZ | 全国平均 AVG |
|---|---|---|---|---|---|---|---|---|---|---|---|---|---|---|---|---|---|---|---|---|---|---|---|---|---|
| 蔬菜类 Vegetables | 0.000 | 7.706 | 3.202 | 5.443 | 0.845 | 2.891 | 11.370 | 1.446 | 6.465 | 0.513 | 0.000 | 0.268 | 0.000 | 1.449 | 2.066 | 1.189 | 9.165 | 0.360 | 4.220 | 1.159 | 3.863 | 14.220 | 107.200 | 4.127 | 7.880 |
| 水果类 Fruits | 0.197 | 0.552 | 0.306 | 1.530 | 2.016 | 0.565 | 0.674 | 0.248 | 0.420 | 0.163 | 0.000 | 0.047 | 0.243 | 4.445 | 0.000 | 0.332 | 0.701 | 1.511 | 0.373 | 4.681 | 0.608 | 0.909 | 0.034 | 0.255 | 0.867 |
| 糖类 Sugar | 0.000 | 0.000 | 0.000 | 0.000 | 0.000 | 0.000 | 0.000 | 0.000 | 0.000 | 0.000 | 0.000 | 0.000 | 0.000 | 0.000 | 0.000 | 0.000 | 0.000 | 0.000 | 0.000 | 0.000 | 0.000 | 0.000 | 0.000 | 0.000 | 0.000 |
| 水及饮料类 Water and beverages | 0.000 | 0.000 | 0.000 | 0.000 | 0.000 | 0.000 | 0.000 | 0.000 | 0.000 | 0.000 | 0.000 | 0.000 | 0.000 | 0.000 | 0.000 | 0.000 | 0.000 | 0.000 | 0.000 | 1.953 | 0.000 | 0.000 | 0.000 | 0.000 | 0.081 |
| 酒类 Alcohol beverages | 0.000 | 0.000 | 0.000 | 0.000 | 0.000 | 0.000 | 0.000 | 0.022 | 0.000 | 0.000 | 0.000 | 0.000 | 0.000 | 0.000 | 0.000 | 0.000 | 0.000 | 0.000 | 0.000 | 0.000 | 0.000 | 0.000 | 0.000 | 0.000 | 0.001 |
| 合计 SUM | 0.357 | 11.592 | 3.508 | 8.012 | 5.885 | 12.244 | 12.162 | 5.623 | 8.578 | 0.839 | 0.341 | 0.314 | 1.455 | 5.893 | 2.066 | 1.555 | 9.866 | 2.867 | 4.594 | 49.814 | 4.471 | 15.386 | 107.188 | 4.404 | 11.626 |

附表 4-125　第六次中国总膳食研究多菌灵的膳食来源（单位：%）

Annexed Table 4-125　Dietary sources of carbendazim from the 6<sup>th</sup> China TDS (Unit: %)

| 膳食类别 Category | 黑龙江 HL | 辽宁 LN | 河北 HE | 北京 BJ | 吉林 JL | 山西 SX | 陕西 SN | 河南 HA | 宁夏 NX | 内蒙古 NM | 青海 QH | 甘肃 GS | 上海 SH | 福建 FJ | 江西 JX | 江苏 JS | 浙江 ZJ | 山东 SD | 湖北 HB | 四川 SC | 广西 GX | 湖南 HN | 广东 GD | 贵州 GZ | 全国平均 AVG |
|---|---|---|---|---|---|---|---|---|---|---|---|---|---|---|---|---|---|---|---|---|---|---|---|---|---|
| 谷类 Cereals | 0.51 | 2.15 | 0.39 | 0.31 | 0.43 | 0.34 | 0.40 | 0.94 | 0.41 | 1.39 | 0.33 | 0.42 | 1.10 | 0.58 | 0.23 | 0.88 | 0.95 | 0.53 | 0.33 | 0.65 | 0.21 | 0.24 | 0.35 | 0.00 | 0.59 |
| 豆类 Legumes | 0.67 | 0.00 | 0.46 | 0.00 | 0.16 | 0.29 | 0.35 | 2.13 | 0.00 | 0.00 | 0.20 | 0.32 | 0.16 | 0.17 | 0.22 | 0.00 | 0.20 | 1.56 | 0.36 | 3.49 | 0.14 | 0.32 | 0.33 | 0.00 | 0.48 |
| 薯类 Potatoes | 0.00 | 0.38 | 0.22 | 0.23 | 0.00 | 10.91 | 0.32 | 1.13 | 0.41 | 0.42 | 0.27 | 0.31 | 0.27 | 0.15 | 0.21 | 0.34 | 0.19 | 11.61 | 0.33 | 0.49 | 0.00 | 0.41 | 0.27 | 0.44 | 1.22 |
| 肉类 Meats | 0.00 | 0.65 | 0.00 | 0.00 | 0.00 | 0.00 | 0.00 | 0.00 | 0.00 | 0.00 | 0.00 | 0.00 | 0.00 | 0.00 | 0.00 | 0.00 | 0.00 | 0.00 | 4.42 | 0.00 | 0.00 | 0.00 | 0.65 | 0.00 | 0.24 |

续表

| 膳食类别 Category | 黑龙江 HL | 辽宁 LN | 河北 HE | 北京 BJ | 吉林 JL | 山西 SX | 陕西 SN | 河南 HA | 宁夏 NX | 内蒙古 NM | 青海 QH | 甘肃 GS | 上海 SH | 福建 FJ | 江西 JX | 江苏 JS | 浙江 ZJ | 山东 SD | 湖北 HB | 四川 SC | 广西 GX | 湖南 HN | 广东 GD | 贵州 GZ | 全国平均 AVG |
|---|---|---|---|---|---|---|---|---|---|---|---|---|---|---|---|---|---|---|---|---|---|---|---|---|---|
| 蛋类 Eggs | 0.00 | 0.52 | 0.00 | 0.00 | 0.00 | 0.00 | 0.00 | 0.00 | 0.00 | 0.00 | 0.00 | 0.00 | 0.00 | 0.00 | 0.00 | 0.00 | 0.00 | 0.00 | 2.11 | 0.00 | 0.00 | 0.55 | 0.00 | 0.00 | 0.13 |
| 水产类 Aquatic foods | 0.00 | 0.00 | 1.34 | 0.00 | 0.00 | 0.00 | 0.00 | 0.00 | 0.00 | 0.00 | 0.00 | 0.00 | 0.00 | 0.00 | 0.00 | 0.00 | 0.26 | 0.00 | 3.09 | 2.49 | 0.00 | 0.57 | 0.31 | 0.00 | 0.34 |
| 乳类 Dairy products | 0.00 | 0.00 | 0.00 | 0.00 | 0.00 | 0.31 | 0.00 | 0.00 | 0.00 | 0.00 | 0.00 | 0.00 | 0.00 | 0.00 | 0.00 | 0.00 | 0.00 | 0.00 | 0.00 | 0.00 | 0.00 | 0.00 | 0.00 | 0.00 | 0.01 |
| 蔬菜类 Vegetables | 0.98 | 4.03 | 38.83 | 20.37 | 1.00 | 13.21 | 1.27 | 3.05 | 9.54 | 0.73 | 11.59 | 24.48 | 5.45 | 2.23 | 7.02 | 2.13 | 18.88 | 21.73 | 7.56 | 7.35 | 2.56 | 2.98 | 3.45 | 9.24 | 9.15 |
| 水果类 Fruits | 13.65 | 62.53 | 17.57 | 63.66 | 23.36 | 11.10 | 17.00 | 47.09 | 17.78 | 6.41 | 1.64 | 1.47 | 33.83 | 38.92 | 32.47 | 18.36 | 17.28 | 57.18 | 16.19 | 9.53 | 4.68 | 13.20 | 10.93 | 15.32 | 22.96 |
| 糖类 Sugar | 0.00 | 0.00 | 0.00 | 0.00 | 0.00 | 0.00 | 0.00 | 0.00 | 0.00 | 0.00 | 0.00 | 0.52 | 0.66 | 0.00 | 0.00 | 0.09 | 0.00 | 0.00 | 0.00 | 0.00 | 0.00 | 0.00 | 0.00 | 0.00 | 0.05 |
| 水及饮料类 Water and beverages | 0.00 | 0.00 | 0.00 | 0.00 | 0.10 | 0.00 | 0.00 | 0.00 | 0.00 | 0.00 | 0.46 | 0.00 | 0.61 | 0.23 | 0.00 | 0.16 | 0.24 | 0.00 | 0.19 | 0.00 | 0.00 | 0.23 | 0.80 | 0.00 | 0.13 |
| 酒类 Alcohol beverages | 0.00 | 0.00 | 0.00 | 0.82 | 0.44 | 0.00 | 0.00 | 0.00 | 0.20 | 0.00 | 0.00 | 0.00 | 1.92 | 0.29 | 0.00 | 0.33 | 0.82 | 3.75 | 0.00 | 0.00 | 10.24 | 0.00 | 1.10 | 0.00 | 0.83 |

附表 4-126　第六次中国总膳食研究噻菌灵的膳食来源（单位：%）

Annexed Table 4-126　Dietary sources of thiabendazole from the 6$^{th}$ China TDS (Unit: %)

| 膳食类别 Category | 黑龙江 HL | 辽宁 LN | 河北 HE | 北京 BJ | 吉林 JL | 山西 SX | 陕西 SN | 河南 HA | 宁夏 NX | 内蒙古 NM | 青海 QH | 甘肃 GS | 上海 SH | 福建 FJ | 江西 JX | 江苏 JS | 浙江 ZJ | 山东 SD | 湖北 HB | 四川 SC | 广西 GX | 湖南 HN | 广东 GD | 贵州 GZ | 全国平均 AVG |
|---|---|---|---|---|---|---|---|---|---|---|---|---|---|---|---|---|---|---|---|---|---|---|---|---|---|
| 谷类 Cereals | 0.0 | 0.0 | 0.0 | 100.0 | 0.0 | 0.0 | 0.0 | 0.0 | 0.0 | 0.0 | 0.0 | 0.0 | 1.5 | 0.0 | 0.0 | 0.0 | 0.0 | 0.0 | 0.0 | 0.0 | 0.0 | 0.0 | 0.0 | 0.0 | 1.3 |

续表

| 膳食类别 Category | 黑龙江 HL | 辽宁 LN | 河北 HE | 北京 BJ | 吉林 JL | 山西 SX | 陕西 SN | 河南 HA | 宁夏 NX | 内蒙古 NM | 青海 QH | 甘肃 GS | 上海 SH | 福建 FJ | 江西 JX | 江苏 JS | 浙江 ZJ | 山东 SD | 湖北 HB | 四川 SC | 广西 GX | 湖南 HN | 广东 GD | 贵州 GZ | 全国平均 AVG |
|---|---|---|---|---|---|---|---|---|---|---|---|---|---|---|---|---|---|---|---|---|---|---|---|---|---|
| 豆类 Legumes | 100.0 | 0.0 | 0.0 | 0.0 | 0.0 | 0.0 | 0.0 | 0.0 | 0.0 | 0.0 | 0.0 | 0.0 | 0.0 | 0.0 | 0.0 | 0.0 | 0.0 | 0.0 | 0.0 | 0.0 | 0.0 | 0.0 | 0.0 | 0.0 | 0.2 |
| 薯类 Potatoes | 0.0 | 0.0 | 0.0 | 0.0 | 0.0 | 0.0 | 0.0 | 0.0 | 0.0 | 100.0 | 0.0 | 96.7 | 0.0 | 0.0 | 0.0 | 0.0 | 0.0 | 1.5 | 0.0 | 0.0 | 0.0 | 0.0 | 0.0 | 0.0 | 0.9 |
| 肉类 Meats | 0.0 | 0.0 | 1.3 | 0.0 | 0.0 | 0.0 | 0.0 | 0.0 | 19.2 | 0.0 | 0.0 | 0.0 | 0.0 | 0.0 | 0.0 | 0.0 | 0.0 | 0.0 | 0.0 | 0.0 | 0.0 | 0.0 | 100.0 | 0.0 | 0.9 |
| 蛋类 Eggs | 0.0 | 0.0 | 0.0 | 0.0 | 0.0 | 0.0 | 0.0 | 0.0 | 0.0 | 0.0 | 0.0 | 0.0 | 0.0 | 0.0 | 0.0 | 0.0 | 0.0 | 0.0 | 0.0 | 0.0 | 0.0 | 0.0 | 0.0 | 0.0 | 0.0 |
| 水产类 Aquatic foods | 0.0 | 0.0 | 0.0 | 0.0 | 0.0 | 0.0 | 0.0 | 0.0 | 0.0 | 0.0 | 0.0 | 0.0 | 0.0 | 0.0 | 0.0 | 0.0 | 0.0 | 0.0 | 0.0 | 0.0 | 0.0 | 0.0 | 0.0 | 0.0 | 0.0 |
| 乳类 Dairy products | 0.0 | 0.5 | 0.0 | 0.0 | 0.0 | 0.0 | 0.0 | 0.0 | 0.0 | 0.0 | 0.0 | 0.0 | 0.0 | 0.0 | 0.0 | 0.0 | 0.0 | 0.0 | 0.0 | 0.0 | 0.0 | 0.0 | 0.0 | 0.0 | 0.0 |
| 蔬菜类 Vegetables | 0.0 | 0.0 | 0.0 | 0.0 | 0.0 | 0.0 | 0.0 | 0.0 | 80.4 | 0.0 | 0.0 | 3.3 | 98.5 | 100.0 | 0.0 | 31.6 | 100.0 | 98.5 | 9.8 | 99.7 | 0.0 | 0.0 | 0.0 | 0.0 | 1.6 |
| 水果类 Fruits | 0.0 | 99.5 | 98.7 | 0.0 | 0.0 | 0.0 | 0.0 | 0.0 | 0.0 | 0.0 | 0.0 | 0.0 | 0.0 | 0.0 | 0.0 | 0.0 | 0.0 | 0.0 | 90.2 | 0.0 | 0.0 | 0.0 | 0.0 | 0.0 | 93.1 |
| 糖类 Sugar | 0.0 | 0.0 | 0.0 | 0.0 | 0.0 | 0.0 | 0.0 | 0.0 | 0.4 | 0.0 | 0.0 | 0.0 | 0.0 | 0.0 | 0.0 | 0.0 | 0.0 | 0.0 | 0.0 | 0.0 | 0.0 | 0.0 | 0.0 | 0.0 | 0.0 |
| 水及饮料类 Water and beverages | 0.0 | 0.0 | 0.0 | 0.0 | 0.0 | 0.0 | 0.0 | 0.0 | 0.0 | 0.0 | 0.0 | 0.0 | 0.0 | 0.0 | 0.0 | 68.4 | 0.0 | 0.0 | 0.0 | 0.0 | 100.0 | 0.0 | 0.0 | 0.0 | 1.9 |
| 酒类 Alcohol beverages | 0.0 | 0.0 | 0.0 | 0.0 | 0.0 | 0.0 | 0.0 | 0.0 | 0.0 | 0.0 | 0.0 | 0.0 | 0.0 | 0.0 | 0.0 | 0.0 | 0.0 | 0.0 | 0.0 | 0.3 | 0.0 | 0.0 | 0.0 | 0.0 | 0.0 |

附表 4-127　第六次中国总膳食研究抑霉唑的膳食来源（单位：%）
Annexed Table 4-127　Dietary sources of imazalil from the 6th China TDS (Unit: %)

| 膳食类别<br>Category | 黑龙江<br>HL | 辽宁<br>LN | 河北<br>HE | 北京<br>BJ | 吉林<br>JL | 山西<br>SX | 陕西<br>SN | 河南<br>HA | 宁夏<br>NX | 内蒙古<br>NM | 青海<br>QH | 甘肃<br>GS | 上海<br>SH | 福建<br>FJ | 江西<br>JX | 江苏<br>JS | 浙江<br>ZJ | 山东<br>SD | 湖北<br>HB | 四川<br>SC | 广西<br>GX | 湖南<br>HN | 广东<br>GD | 贵州<br>GZ | 全国平均<br>AVG |
|---|---|---|---|---|---|---|---|---|---|---|---|---|---|---|---|---|---|---|---|---|---|---|---|---|---|
| 谷类 Cereals | 0.0 | 0.0 | 0.0 | 0.0 | 0.0 | 68.7 | 0.0 | 0.0 | 0.0 | 0.0 | 0.0 | 0.0 | 0.0 | 0.0 | 0.0 | 0.0 | 0.0 | 63.2 | 0.0 | 45.6 | 0.0 | 0.0 | 0.0 | 0.0 | 5.5 |
| 豆类 Legumes | 61.3 | 0.0 | 0.0 | 0.0 | 0.0 | 0.0 | 0.0 | 10.1 | 33.3 | 0.0 | 0.0 | 0.0 | 0.0 | 0.0 | 0.0 | 0.0 | 0.9 | 0.0 | 0.0 | 0.0 | 0.0 | 0.0 | 0.0 | 0.0 | 0.5 |
| 薯类 Potatoes | 0.0 | 0.0 | 0.0 | 0.0 | 0.0 | 6.3 | 0.0 | 14.2 | 26.0 | 26.0 | 0.0 | 46.0 | 0.0 | 0.0 | 0.0 | 0.0 | 0.0 | 0.0 | 0.0 | 0.0 | 0.0 | 0.0 | 0.0 | 0.0 | 1.9 |
| 肉类 Meats | 0.0 | 0.0 | 2.7 | 100.0 | 0.0 | 0.0 | 0.0 | 9.5 | 26.0 | 0.0 | 94.7 | 0.0 | 0.0 | 0.0 | 0.0 | 0.0 | 0.0 | 0.0 | 0.0 | 0.0 | 0.0 | 0.0 | 75.4 | 0.0 | 0.9 |
| 蛋类 Eggs | 0.0 | 0.0 | 1.3 | 0.0 | 0.0 | 0.0 | 7.9 | 0.0 | 0.0 | 0.0 | 0.0 | 0.0 | 0.0 | 0.0 | 0.0 | 0.0 | 0.0 | 0.0 | 0.0 | 0.0 | 0.0 | 0.0 | 0.0 | 0.0 | 0.1 |
| 水产类 Aquatic foods | 0.0 | 0.0 | 0.0 | 0.0 | 0.0 | 0.0 | 0.0 | 0.0 | 0.0 | 1.3 | 5.3 | 0.0 | 0.0 | 0.0 | 8.3 | 0.0 | 0.0 | 0.0 | 0.0 | 0.0 | 0.0 | 0.0 | 0.0 | 0.0 | 0.0 |
| 乳类 Dairy products | 0.0 | 0.9 | 0.0 | 0.0 | 0.0 | 0.0 | 0.0 | 0.0 | 0.0 | 0.0 | 0.0 | 0.0 | 0.0 | 0.0 | 0.0 | 0.0 | 0.0 | 0.0 | 0.0 | 0.0 | 0.0 | 0.0 | 0.0 | 0.0 | 0.1 |
| 蔬菜类 Vegetables | 0.0 | 0.0 | 0.0 | 0.0 | 0.0 | 0.0 | 0.0 | 43.6 | 40.6 | 38.5 | 0.0 | 0.0 | 0.0 | 0.0 | 0.0 | 0.0 | 0.0 | 0.0 | 4.9 | 30.2 | 0.0 | 0.0 | 0.0 | 0.0 | 2.8 |
| 水果类 Fruits | 38.7 | 99.1 | 96.0 | 0.0 | 100.0 | 25.1 | 92.1 | 22.6 | 0.0 | 34.2 | 0.0 | 1.7 | 100.0 | 100.0 | 91.7 | 15.8 | 99.1 | 36.8 | 95.1 | 7.7 | 0.0 | 0.0 | 24.6 | 100.0 | 79.7 |
| 糖类 Sugar | 0.0 | 0.0 | 0.0 | 0.0 | 0.0 | 0.0 | 0.0 | 0.0 | 0.1 | 0.0 | 0.0 | 0.0 | 0.0 | 0.0 | 0.0 | 0.0 | 0.0 | 0.0 | 0.0 | 0.0 | 0.0 | 0.0 | 0.0 | 0.0 | 0.0 |
| 水及饮料类 Water and beverages | 0.0 | 0.0 | 0.0 | 0.0 | 0.0 | 0.0 | 0.0 | 0.0 | 0.0 | 0.0 | 0.0 | 52.3 | 0.0 | 0.0 | 0.0 | 84.2 | 0.0 | 0.0 | 0.0 | 16.3 | 97.3 | 0.0 | 0.0 | 0.0 | 8.2 |

续表

| 膳食类别 Category | 黑龙江 HL | 辽宁 LN | 河北 HE | 北京 BJ | 吉林 JL | 山西 SX | 陕西 SN | 河南 HA | 宁夏 NX | 内蒙古 NM | 青海 QH | 甘肃 GS | 上海 SH | 福建 FJ | 江西 JX | 江苏 JS | 浙江 ZJ | 山东 SD | 湖北 HB | 四川 SC | 广西 GX | 湖南 HN | 广东 GD | 贵州 GZ | 全国平均 AVG |
|---|---|---|---|---|---|---|---|---|---|---|---|---|---|---|---|---|---|---|---|---|---|---|---|---|---|
| 酒类 Alcohol beverages | 0.0 | 0.0 | 0.0 | 0.0 | 0.0 | 0.0 | 0.0 | 0.0 | 0.0 | 0.0 | 0.0 | 0.0 | 0.0 | 0.0 | 0.0 | 0.0 | 0.0 | 0.0 | 0.0 | 0.2 | 2.7 | 0.0 | 0.0 | 0.0 | 0.1 |

附表 4-128　第六次中国总膳食研究咪鲜胺的膳食来源（单位：%）

Annexed Table 4-128　Dietary sources of prochloraz from the 6th China TDS (Unit: %)

| 膳食类别 Category | 黑龙江 HL | 辽宁 LN | 河北 HE | 北京 BJ | 吉林 JL | 山西 SX | 陕西 SN | 河南 HA | 宁夏 NX | 内蒙古 NM | 青海 QH | 甘肃 GS | 上海 SH | 福建 FJ | 江西 JX | 江苏 JS | 浙江 ZJ | 山东 SD | 湖北 HB | 四川 SC | 广西 GX | 湖南 HN | 广东 GD | 贵州 GZ | 全国平均 AVG |
|---|---|---|---|---|---|---|---|---|---|---|---|---|---|---|---|---|---|---|---|---|---|---|---|---|---|
| 谷类 Cereals | 0.0 | 28.8 | 0.0 | 12.4 | 33.7 | 39.4 | 0.0 | 0.0 | 14.8 | 0.0 | 0.0 | 0.0 | 60.9 | 0.0 | 0.0 | 0.0 | 0.0 | 0.0 | 0.0 | 83.6 | 0.0 | 0.0 | 0.0 | 0.0 | 19.7 |
| 豆类 Legumes | 20.9 | 0.0 | 0.0 | 0.0 | 9.1 | 0.0 | 0.9 | 44.3 | 0.0 | 0.0 | 0.0 | 0.0 | 0.0 | 0.0 | 0.0 | 0.0 | 0.0 | 0.0 | 0.0 | 0.0 | 0.0 | 0.0 | 0.0 | 0.0 | 1.2 |
| 薯类 Potatoes | 23.7 | 0.0 | 0.0 | 0.0 | 8.5 | 32.2 | 0.0 | 22.3 | 2.9 | 19.4 | 54.2 | 0.0 | 15.5 | 0.0 | 0.0 | 0.0 | 0.0 | 29.6 | 0.0 | 0.3 | 0.0 | 0.0 | 0.0 | 0.0 | 2.7 |
| 肉类 Meats | 0.0 | 0.0 | 0.0 | 0.0 | 0.0 | 0.0 | 0.0 | 2.9 | 2.0 | 0.0 | 44.6 | 0.0 | 0.0 | 0.0 | 0.0 | 0.0 | 0.0 | 5.1 | 0.0 | 0.4 | 0.0 | 1.3 | 0.0 | 0.0 | 0.4 |
| 蛋类 Eggs | 0.0 | 0.0 | 0.0 | 0.5 | 0.0 | 0.2 | 0.0 | 0.0 | 0.0 | 0.0 | 1.2 | 0.0 | 6.9 | 0.0 | 0.0 | 0.0 | 0.0 | 0.0 | 0.0 | 0.4 | 0.0 | 0.0 | 0.0 | 0.5 | 0.1 |
| 水产类 Aquatic foods | 0.0 | 0.0 | 0.0 | 0.0 | 0.0 | 0.0 | 0.0 | 0.0 | | 0.0 | 0.0 | 0.0 | 0.0 | 0.0 | 0.0 | 0.0 | 0.0 | 0.0 | 0.0 | 0.0 | 0.0 | 0.4 | 0.0 | 0.0 | 0.0 |
| 乳类 Dairy products | 0.0 | 0.0 | 0.0 | 0.0 | 0.0 | 0.0 | 0.0 | 0.0 | 0.0 | 0.0 | 0.0 | 0.0 | 0.0 | 0.0 | 0.0 | 2.2 | 0.0 | 0.0 | 0.0 | 0.0 | 0.0 | 0.0 | 0.0 | 0.0 | 0.0 |
| 蔬菜类 Vegetables | 0.0 | 66.5 | 91.3 | 67.9 | 14.4 | 23.6 | 93.5 | 25.7 | 75.4 | 61.1 | 0.0 | 85.1 | 0.0 | 24.6 | 100.0 | 76.5 | 92.9 | 12.6 | 91.9 | 2.3 | 86.4 | 92.4 | 100.0 | 93.7 | 67.8 |

续表

| 膳食类别 Category | 黑龙江 HL | 辽宁 LN | 河北 HE | 北京 BJ | 吉林 JL | 山西 SX | 陕西 SN | 河南 HA | 宁夏 NX | 内蒙古 NM | 青海 QH | 甘肃 GS | 上海 SH | 福建 FJ | 江西 JX | 江苏 JS | 浙江 ZJ | 山东 SD | 湖北 HB | 四川 SC | 广西 GX | 湖南 HN | 广东 GD | 贵州 GZ | 全国平均 AVG |
|---|---|---|---|---|---|---|---|---|---|---|---|---|---|---|---|---|---|---|---|---|---|---|---|---|---|
| 水果类 Fruits | 55.4 | 4.8 | 8.7 | 19.1 | 34.3 | 4.6 | 5.5 | 4.4 | 4.9 | 19.4 | 0.0 | 14.9 | 16.7 | 75.4 | 0.0 | 21.3 | 7.1 | 52.7 | 8.1 | 9.4 | 13.6 | 5.9 | 0.0 | 5.8 | 7.5 |
| 糖类 Sugar | 0.0 | 0.0 | 0.0 | 0.0 | 0.0 | 0.0 | 0.0 | 0.0 | 0.0 | 0.0 | 0.0 | 0.0 | 0.0 | 0.0 | 0.0 | 0.0 | 0.0 | 0.0 | 0.0 | 0.0 | 0.0 | 0.0 | 0.0 | 0.0 | 0.0 |
| 水及饮料类 Water and beverages | 0.0 | 0.0 | 0.0 | 0.0 | 0.0 | 0.0 | 0.0 | 0.0 | 0.0 | 0.0 | 0.0 | 0.0 | 0.0 | 0.0 | 0.0 | 0.0 | 0.0 | 0.0 | 0.0 | 3.9 | 0.0 | 0.0 | 0.0 | 0.0 | 0.7 |
| 酒类 Alcohol beverages | 0.0 | 0.0 | 0.0 | 0.0 | 0.0 | 0.0 | 0.0 | 0.4 | 0.0 | 0.0 | 0.0 | 0.0 | 0.0 | 0.0 | 0.0 | 0.0 | 0.0 | 0.0 | 0.0 | 0.0 | 0.0 | 0.0 | 0.0 | 0.0 | 0.0 |

附表 4-129 第六次中国总膳食研究膳食样品中嘧菌酯的含量（单位：μg/kg）

Annexed Table 4-129 Levels of azoxystrobin in food samples from the 6$^{th}$ China TDS (Unit: μg/kg)

| 膳食类别 Category | 黑龙江 HL | 辽宁 LN | 河北 HE | 北京 BJ | 吉林 JL | 山西 SX | 陕西 SN | 河南 HA | 宁夏 NX | 内蒙古 NM | 青海 QH | 甘肃 GS | 上海 SH | 福建 FJ | 江西 JX | 江苏 JS | 浙江 ZJ | 山东 SD | 湖北 HB | 四川 SC | 广西 GX | 湖南 HN | 广东 GD | 贵州 GZ | 全国平均 AVG |
|---|---|---|---|---|---|---|---|---|---|---|---|---|---|---|---|---|---|---|---|---|---|---|---|---|---|
| 谷类 Cereals | ND | ND | 0.10 | ND | ND | ND | 0.33 | ND | ND | ND | ND | ND | ND | ND | 0.16 | ND | ND | ND | ND | 2.72 | 0.39 | ND | ND | ND | 0.15 |
| 豆类 Legumes | ND | ND | ND | ND | 0.06 | ND | ND | ND | ND | ND | ND | ND | ND | 0.05 | ND | ND | ND | ND | ND | 0.04 | ND | ND | ND | ND | 0.01 |
| 薯类 Potatoes | ND | ND | ND | ND | 0.14 | 0.04 | 0.35 | 0.54 | ND | 0.16 | 0.11 | ND | ND | ND | ND | ND | ND | ND | ND | 0.06 | 0.32 | ND | ND | 0.11 | 0.08 |
| 肉类 Meats | ND | ND | ND | 0.23 | 0.10 | ND | ND | 0.03 | ND | 0.11 | ND | ND | ND | ND | ND | ND | ND | ND | ND | ND | ND | ND | ND | 0.05 | 0.02 |
| 蛋类 Eggs | ND | ND | ND | ND | 0.05 | ND | ND | ND | ND | ND | ND | ND | ND | ND | ND | ND | ND | ND | 1.49 | ND | ND | ND | ND | ND | 0.06 |

续表

| 膳食类别 Category | 黑龙江 HL | 辽宁 LN | 河北 HE | 北京 BJ | 吉林 JL | 山西 SX | 陕西 SN | 河南 HA | 宁夏 NX | 内蒙古 NM | 青海 QH | 甘肃 GS | 上海 SH | 福建 FJ | 江西 JX | 江苏 JS | 浙江 ZJ | 山东 SD | 湖北 HB | 四川 SC | 广西 GX | 湖南 HN | 广东 GD | 贵州 GZ | 全国平均 AVG |
|---|---|---|---|---|---|---|---|---|---|---|---|---|---|---|---|---|---|---|---|---|---|---|---|---|---|
| 水产类 Aquatic foods | ND | ND | ND | ND | 0.13 | 0.41 | ND | ND | ND | ND | 0.07 | ND | ND | ND | 0.07 | 0.06 | ND | ND | 0.04 | ND | ND | 0.09 | ND | ND | 0.04 |
| 乳类 Dairy products | ND | ND | ND | ND | ND | ND | ND | ND | ND | ND | ND | ND | ND | ND | ND | ND | ND | ND | ND | ND | ND | ND | ND | ND | 0.00 |
| 蔬菜类 Vegetables | 0.28 | ND | 0.90 | 4.77 | 0.86 | 6.31 | 2.69 | 0.17 | 0.03 | 0.44 | 19.77 | 2.65 | 0.45 | 11.27 | 0.13 | 0.60 | 0.28 | 1.10 | 0.67 | 0.44 | 3.26 | 0.27 | 2.59 | 6.43 | 2.77 |
| 水果类 Fruits | 2.41 | 3.97 | 0.49 | 1.60 | 0.36 | ND | 1.27 | 24.39 | ND | 1.26 | ND | 2.24 | 0.14 | 3.05 | 2.67 | 1.33 | 8.48 | 1.22 | 1.51 | 4.46 | 0.15 | 0.53 | 3.14 | ND | 2.69 |
| 糖类 Sugar | ND | ND | ND | ND | ND | ND | ND | ND | ND | ND | ND | ND | ND | ND | ND | ND | ND | ND | ND | ND | ND | ND | ND | ND | 0.00 |
| 水及饮料类 Water and beverages | ND | ND | ND | ND | ND | ND | ND | ND | ND | ND | ND | ND | ND | ND | ND | ND | ND | ND | ND | 0.06 | 0.87 | ND | ND | ND | 0.00 |
| 酒类 Alcohol beverages | ND | 0.07 | ND | 0.05 | 0.07 | ND | 0.06 | ND | ND | ND | ND | ND | ND | 0.10 | ND | ND | 0.10 | 0.17 | ND | ND | ND | ND | ND | ND | 0.06 |

注：未检出（ND）按 0 计
Note: values not detected (ND) were treated as being equal to 0

附表 4-130 第六次中国总膳食研究膳食样品中吡唑醚菌酯的含量（单位：μg/kg）
Annexed Table 4-130 Levels of pyraclostrobin in food samples from the 6th China TDS (Unit: μg/kg)

| 膳食类别 Category | 黑龙江 HL | 辽宁 LN | 河北 HE | 北京 BJ | 吉林 JL | 山西 SX | 陕西 SN | 河南 HA | 宁夏 NX | 内蒙古 NM | 青海 QH | 甘肃 GS | 上海 SH | 福建 FJ | 江西 JX | 江苏 JS | 浙江 ZJ | 山东 SD | 湖北 HB | 四川 SC | 广西 GX | 湖南 HN | 广东 GD | 贵州 GZ | 全国平均 AVG |
|---|---|---|---|---|---|---|---|---|---|---|---|---|---|---|---|---|---|---|---|---|---|---|---|---|---|
| 谷类 Cereals | 0.20 | ND | ND | ND | ND | ND | 0.41 | 0.09 | ND | 0.36 | ND | ND | ND | ND | ND | ND | ND | ND | ND | 0.11 | ND | 0.11 | ND | ND | 0.05 |

续表

| 膳食类别<br>Category | 黑龙江<br>HL | 辽宁<br>LN | 河北<br>HE | 北京<br>BJ | 吉林<br>JL | 山西<br>SX | 陕西<br>SN | 河南<br>HA | 宁夏<br>NX | 内蒙古<br>NM | 青海<br>QH | 甘肃<br>GS | 上海<br>SH | 福建<br>FJ | 江西<br>JX | 江苏<br>JS | 浙江<br>ZJ | 山东<br>SD | 湖北<br>HB | 四川<br>SC | 广西<br>GX | 湖南<br>HN | 广东<br>GD | 贵州<br>GZ | 全国平均<br>AVG |
|---|---|---|---|---|---|---|---|---|---|---|---|---|---|---|---|---|---|---|---|---|---|---|---|---|---|
| 豆类<br>Legumes | ND | ND | ND | ND | ND | ND | 0.32 | 0.09 | ND | ND | ND | ND | ND | ND | ND | ND | ND | ND | ND | 0.12 | ND | ND | ND | ND | 0.02 |
| 薯类<br>Potatoes | ND | ND | ND | ND | 0.12 | ND | 0.12 | ND | ND | ND | 0.09 | ND | 0.14 | ND | 0.06 | ND | ND | ND | 0.05 | 0.08 | ND | ND | 0.20 | ND | 0.04 |
| 肉类<br>Meats | ND | ND | ND | ND | ND | ND | 0.05 | ND | 0.06 | 0.06 | 0.10 | ND | ND | ND | ND | 0.06 | ND | ND | ND | 0.14 | ND | 0.08 | ND | 0.22 | 0.03 |
| 蛋类<br>Eggs | ND | ND | ND | ND | 0.09 | ND | ND | ND | ND | ND | ND | ND | ND | ND | ND | 0.09 | ND | 0.06 | ND | ND | ND | ND | ND | ND | 0.01 |
| 水产类<br>Aquatic foods | ND | ND | ND | ND | 0.14 | ND | 0.19 | ND | ND | ND | 0.09 | ND | ND | ND | ND | 0.06 | ND | ND | ND | ND | 0.12 | 0.06 | 0.10 | ND | 0.03 |
| 乳类<br>Dairy products | ND | ND | ND | ND | ND | 0.05 | ND | ND | ND | ND | ND | ND | ND | ND | ND | ND | ND | ND | ND | ND | ND | ND | ND | ND | 0.00 |
| 蔬菜类<br>Vegetables | 0.10 | 0.10 | 0.13 | 0.34 | 0.15 | 1.12 | 10.38 | 0.07 | 0.11 | 0.74 | 4.79 | 0.16 | 13.61 | 7.03 | 21.27 | 0.17 | 4.24 | 2.82 | 12.00 | 0.86 | 26.52 | 2.74 | 47.10 | 0.46 | 6.54 |
| 水果类<br>Fruits | 0.17 | 4.02 | 1.01 | 0.60 | 0.05 | 0.06 | 0.44 | 3.64 | 0.57 | 0.23 | 0.10 | 0.16 | 5.76 | 2.78 | 0.84 | 1.76 | 0.41 | 5.64 | 0.46 | 0.98 | ND | 0.67 | 0.59 | 0.25 | 1.30 |
| 糖类<br>Sugar | ND | ND | ND | ND | ND | ND | ND | ND | ND | ND | ND | ND | ND | ND | ND | ND | ND | ND | ND | ND | ND | ND | ND | ND | 0.00 |
| 水及饮料类<br>Water and beverages | ND | ND | ND | ND | ND | ND | ND | ND | ND | ND | ND | ND | ND | ND | ND | ND | ND | ND | ND | ND | ND | ND | ND | ND | 0.00 |
| 酒类<br>Alcohol beverages | ND | ND | ND | ND | ND | ND | ND | ND | ND | ND | ND | ND | ND | ND | ND | ND | ND | ND | ND | ND | ND | ND | ND | ND | 0.00 |

注：未检出（ND）按0计

Note: values not detected (ND) were treated as being equal to 0

附表 4-131　第六次中国总膳食研究膳食样品中肟菌酯的含量（单位：μg/kg）

Annexed Table 4-131　Levels of trifloxystrobin in food samples from the 6$^{th}$ China TDS (Unit: μg/kg)

| 膳食类别<br>Category | 黑龙江<br>HL | 辽宁<br>LN | 河北<br>HE | 北京<br>BJ | 吉林<br>JL | 山西<br>SX | 陕西<br>SN | 河南<br>HA | 宁夏<br>NX | 内蒙古<br>NM | 青海<br>QH | 甘肃<br>GS | 上海<br>SH | 福建<br>FJ | 江西<br>JX | 江苏<br>JS | 浙江<br>ZJ | 山东<br>SD | 湖北<br>HB | 四川<br>SC | 广西<br>GX | 湖南<br>HN | 广东<br>GD | 贵州<br>GZ | 全国平均<br>AVG |
|---|---|---|---|---|---|---|---|---|---|---|---|---|---|---|---|---|---|---|---|---|---|---|---|---|---|
| 谷类 Cereals | ND | 0.07 | ND | ND | ND | ND | ND | ND | ND | ND | ND | ND | ND | ND | ND | ND | ND | ND | ND | ND | ND | ND | ND | ND | 0.00 |
| 豆类 Legumes | ND | ND | ND | ND | ND | ND | ND | ND | ND | ND | ND | ND | ND | ND | ND | ND | ND | ND | ND | ND | ND | ND | ND | ND | 0.00 |
| 薯类 Potatoes | ND | ND | ND | ND | 0.15 | ND | ND | ND | ND | ND | ND | ND | ND | ND | ND | ND | ND | ND | ND | ND | ND | ND | ND | ND | 0.01 |
| 肉类 Meats | ND | ND | ND | ND | 0.08 | ND | ND | 0.09 | ND | ND | ND | ND | ND | ND | ND | ND | ND | ND | ND | ND | ND | ND | ND | ND | 0.01 |
| 蛋类 Eggs | ND | ND | ND | ND | 0.07 | ND | ND | ND | ND | ND | ND | ND | ND | ND | ND | ND | ND | ND | ND | ND | ND | ND | ND | ND | 0.00 |
| 水产类 Aquatic foods | ND | ND | ND | ND | 0.19 | ND | ND | ND | ND | ND | ND | ND | ND | ND | 0.12 | ND | ND | ND | ND | ND | ND | ND | ND | ND | 0.01 |
| 乳类 Dairy products | ND | ND | ND | ND | ND | ND | ND | ND | ND | ND | ND | ND | ND | ND | ND | ND | ND | ND | ND | ND | ND | ND | ND | ND | 0.00 |
| 蔬菜类 Vegetables | 0.64 | ND | 1.72 | ND | 0.14 | ND | 0.43 | 0.13 | 3.80 | 0.50 | 0.27 | ND | 0.29 | 0.07 | ND | ND | 0.07 | 0.14 | ND | ND | 0.59 | ND | ND | ND | 0.37 |
| 水果类 Fruits | ND | ND | 0.27 | 19.46 | ND | ND | ND | ND | ND | ND | ND | ND | 0.67 | ND | ND | ND | 0.12 | 0.24 | 0.12 | ND | ND | 0.39 | ND | ND | 0.89 |
| 糖类 Sugar | ND | ND | ND | ND | ND | ND | ND | ND | ND | ND | ND | ND | ND | ND | ND | ND | ND | ND | ND | ND | ND | ND | ND | ND | 0.00 |
| 水及饮料类 Water and beverages | ND | ND | ND | ND | ND | ND | ND | ND | ND | ND | ND | ND | ND | ND | ND | ND | ND | ND | ND | ND | ND | ND | ND | ND | 0.00 |

续表

| 膳食类别 Category | 黑龙江 HL | 辽宁 LN | 河北 HE | 北京 BJ | 吉林 JL | 山西 SX | 陕西 SN | 河南 HA | 宁夏 NX | 内蒙古 NM | 青海 QH | 甘肃 GS | 上海 SH | 福建 FJ | 江西 JX | 江苏 JS | 浙江 ZJ | 山东 SD | 湖北 HB | 四川 SC | 广西 GX | 湖南 HN | 广东 GD | 贵州 GZ | 全国平均 AVG |
|---|---|---|---|---|---|---|---|---|---|---|---|---|---|---|---|---|---|---|---|---|---|---|---|---|---|
| 酒类 Alcohol beverages | ND | ND | ND | ND | ND | ND | ND | ND | ND | ND | ND | ND | ND | ND | ND | ND | ND | ND | ND | ND | ND | ND | ND | ND | 0.00 |

注：未检出（ND）按 0 计
Note: values not detected (ND) were treated as being equal to 0

附表 4-132　第六次中国总膳食研究的嘧菌酯膳食摄入量 [单位：ng/(kg bw·d)]
Annexed Table 4-132　Dietary intakes of azoxystrobin from the 6th China TDS [Unit: ng/(kg bw·d)]

| 膳食类别 Category | 黑龙江 HL | 辽宁 LN | 河北 HE | 北京 BJ | 吉林 JL | 山西 SX | 陕西 SN | 河南 HA | 宁夏 NX | 内蒙古 NM | 青海 QH | 甘肃 GS | 上海 SH | 福建 FJ | 江西 JX | 江苏 JS | 浙江 ZJ | 山东 SD | 湖北 HB | 四川 SC | 广西 GX | 湖南 HN | 广东 GD | 贵州 GZ | 全国平均 AVG |
|---|---|---|---|---|---|---|---|---|---|---|---|---|---|---|---|---|---|---|---|---|---|---|---|---|---|
| 谷类 Cereals | 0.000 | 0.000 | 1.185 | 0.000 | 0.000 | 0.000 | 3.946 | 0.000 | 0.000 | 0.000 | 0.000 | 0.000 | 0.000 | 0.000 | 1.626 | 0.000 | 0.000 | 0.000 | 0.000 | 41.800 | 5.805 | 0.000 | 0.000 | 0.000 | 2.265 |
| 豆类 Legumes | 0.000 | 0.000 | 0.000 | 0.000 | 0.075 | 0.000 | 0.000 | 0.000 | 0.000 | 0.000 | 0.000 | 0.000 | 0.000 | 0.069 | 0.000 | 0.000 | 0.000 | 0.000 | 0.000 | 0.042 | 0.000 | 0.000 | 0.000 | 0.000 | 0.008 |
| 薯类 Potatoes | 0.000 | 0.000 | 0.000 | 0.000 | 0.261 | 0.074 | 0.641 | 0.694 | 0.000 | 0.313 | 0.174 | 0.000 | 0.000 | 0.000 | 0.000 | 0.000 | 0.000 | 0.000 | 0.000 | 0.063 | 0.065 | 0.000 | 0.000 | 0.058 | 0.098 |
| 肉类 Meats | 0.000 | 0.000 | 0.000 | 0.243 | 0.102 | 0.000 | 0.000 | 0.029 | 0.000 | 0.125 | 0.000 | 0.000 | 0.000 | 0.000 | 0.000 | 0.000 | 0.000 | 0.000 | 0.592 | 0.000 | 0.000 | 0.000 | 0.000 | 0.088 | 0.024 |
| 蛋类 Eggs | 0.000 | 0.000 | 0.000 | 0.000 | 0.030 | 0.000 | 0.000 | 0.000 | 0.000 | 0.000 | 0.004 | 0.000 | 0.000 | 0.000 | 0.000 | 0.000 | 0.000 | 0.000 | 0.026 | 0.000 | 0.000 | 0.091 | 0.000 | 0.000 | 0.026 |
| 水产类 Aquatic foods | 0.000 | 0.000 | 0.000 | 0.000 | 0.023 | 0.042 | 0.000 | 0.000 | 0.000 | 0.000 | 0.000 | 0.000 | 0.000 | 0.000 | 0.050 | 0.035 | 0.000 | 0.000 | 0.000 | 0.000 | 0.000 | 0.000 | 0.000 | 0.000 | 0.011 |
| 乳类 Dairy products | 0.000 | 0.000 | 0.000 | 0.000 | 0.000 | 0.000 | 0.000 | 0.000 | 0.000 | 0.000 | 0.000 | 0.000 | 0.000 | 0.000 | 0.000 | 0.000 | 0.000 | 0.000 | 0.000 | 0.000 | 0.000 | 0.000 | 0.000 | 0.000 | 0.000 |

续表

| 膳食类别<br>Category | 黑龙江<br>HL | 辽宁<br>LN | 河北<br>HE | 北京<br>BJ | 吉林<br>JL | 山西<br>SX | 陕西<br>SN | 河南<br>HA | 宁夏<br>NX | 内蒙古<br>NM | 青海<br>QH | 甘肃<br>GS | 上海<br>SH | 福建<br>FJ | 江西<br>JX | 江苏<br>JS | 浙江<br>ZJ | 山东<br>SD | 湖北<br>HB | 四川<br>SC | 广西<br>GX | 湖南<br>HN | 广东<br>GD | 贵州<br>GZ | 全国平均<br>AVG |
|---|---|---|---|---|---|---|---|---|---|---|---|---|---|---|---|---|---|---|---|---|---|---|---|---|---|
| 蔬菜类<br>Vegetables | 1.445 | 0.000 | 4.203 | 29.700 | 5.285 | 30.990 | 12.280 | 0.769 | 0.082 | 1.813 | 97.440 | 10.440 | 2.856 | 70.980 | 0.927 | 4.045 | 1.999 | 7.076 | 4.436 | 2.130 | 18.270 | 2.318 | 9.741 | 41.630 | 15.040 |
| 水果类<br>Fruits | 2.400 | 4.844 | 0.295 | 2.878 | 0.497 | 0.000 | 0.762 | 9.356 | 0.000 | 2.257 | 0.000 | 1.181 | 0.163 | 2.893 | 2.403 | 0.576 | 9.056 | 1.050 | 0.460 | 1.057 | 0.154 | 0.531 | 1.458 | 0.000 | 1.845 |
| 糖类<br>Sugar | 0.000 | 0.000 | 0.000 | 0.000 | 0.000 | 0.000 | 0.000 | 0.000 | 0.000 | 0.000 | 0.000 | 0.000 | 0.000 | 0.000 | 0.000 | 0.000 | 0.000 | 0.000 | 0.000 | 0.000 | 0.000 | 0.000 | 0.000 | 0.000 | 0.000 |
| 水及饮料类<br>Water and beverages | 0.000 | 0.000 | 0.000 | 0.000 | 0.000 | 0.000 | 0.000 | 0.000 | 0.000 | 0.000 | 0.000 | 0.000 | 0.000 | 0.000 | 0.000 | 0.000 | 0.000 | 0.000 | 0.000 | 0.301 | 0.000 | 0.000 | 0.000 | 0.000 | 0.013 |
| 酒类<br>Alcohol beverages | 0.000 | 0.040 | 0.000 | 0.020 | 0.010 | 0.000 | 0.002 | 0.000 | 0.000 | 0.000 | 0.000 | 0.000 | 0.000 | 0.023 | 0.000 | 0.000 | 0.095 | 0.306 | 0.000 | 0.000 | 0.444 | 0.000 | 0.000 | 0.000 | 0.039 |
| 合计<br>SUM | 3.845 | 4.884 | 5.683 | 32.835 | 6.283 | 31.110 | 17.627 | 10.848 | 0.082 | 4.508 | 97.620 | 11.616 | 3.019 | 73.965 | 5.007 | 4.656 | 11.149 | 8.432 | 5.515 | 45.391 | 24.735 | 2.940 | 11.199 | 41.776 | 19.364 |

附表 4-133　第六次中国总膳食研究的吡唑醚菌酯膳食摄入量 [单位: ng/(kg bw·d)]

Annexed Table 4-133　Dietary intakes of pyraclostrobin from the 6$^{th}$ China TDS [Unit: ng/(kg bw·d)]

| 膳食类别<br>Category | 黑龙江<br>HL | 辽宁<br>LN | 河北<br>HE | 北京<br>BJ | 吉林<br>JL | 山西<br>SX | 陕西<br>SN | 河南<br>HA | 宁夏<br>NX | 内蒙古<br>NM | 青海<br>QH | 甘肃<br>GS | 上海<br>SH | 福建<br>FJ | 江西<br>JX | 江苏<br>JS | 浙江<br>ZJ | 山东<br>SD | 湖北<br>HB | 四川<br>SC | 广西<br>GX | 湖南<br>HN | 广东<br>GD | 贵州<br>GZ | 全国平均<br>AVG |
|---|---|---|---|---|---|---|---|---|---|---|---|---|---|---|---|---|---|---|---|---|---|---|---|---|---|
| 谷类<br>Cereals | 1.698 | 0.000 | 0.000 | 0.000 | 0.000 | 0.000 | 4.978 | 1.294 | 0.000 | 4.074 | 0.000 | 0.000 | 0.000 | 0.000 | 0.000 | 0.000 | 0.000 | 0.000 | 0.000 | 1.650 | 0.000 | 0.977 | 0.000 | 0.000 | 0.611 |
| 豆类<br>Legumes | 0.000 | 0.000 | 0.000 | 0.000 | 0.000 | 0.000 | 0.415 | 0.080 | 0.000 | 0.000 | 0.150 | 0.000 | 0.000 | 0.000 | 0.029 | 0.000 | 0.000 | 0.000 | 0.000 | 0.126 | 0.000 | 0.000 | 0.000 | 0.000 | 0.026 |
| 薯类<br>Potatoes | 0.000 | 0.000 | 0.000 | 0.000 | 0.236 | 0.000 | 0.213 | 0.000 | 0.000 | 0.000 | 0.000 | 0.000 | 0.081 | 0.000 | 0.000 | 0.000 | 0.000 | 0.000 | 0.071 | 0.076 | 0.000 | 0.000 | 0.078 | 0.000 | 0.039 |

续表

| 膳食类别<br>Category | 黑龙江<br>HL | 辽宁<br>LN | 河北<br>HE | 北京<br>BJ | 吉林<br>JL | 山西<br>SX | 陕西<br>SN | 河南<br>HA | 宁夏<br>NX | 内蒙古<br>NM | 青海<br>QH | 甘肃<br>GS | 上海<br>SH | 福建<br>FJ | 江西<br>JX | 江苏<br>JS | 浙江<br>ZJ | 山东<br>SD | 湖北<br>HB | 四川<br>SC | 广西<br>GX | 湖南<br>HN | 广东<br>GD | 贵州<br>GZ | 全国平均<br>AVG |
|---|---|---|---|---|---|---|---|---|---|---|---|---|---|---|---|---|---|---|---|---|---|---|---|---|---|
| 肉类 Meats | 0.000 | 0.000 | 0.000 | 0.000 | 0.000 | 0.000 | 0.030 | 0.000 | 0.042 | 0.070 | 0.108 | 0.000 | 0.000 | 0.000 | 0.000 | 0.086 | 0.000 | 0.000 | 0.000 | 0.290 | 0.000 | 0.181 | 0.000 | 0.378 | 0.049 |
| 蛋类 Eggs | 0.000 | 0.000 | 0.000 | 0.000 | 0.059 | 0.000 | 0.000 | 0.000 | 0.000 | 0.000 | 0.000 | 0.000 | 0.000 | 0.000 | 0.000 | 0.040 | 0.000 | 0.045 | 0.000 | 0.000 | 0.000 | 0.000 | 0.000 | 0.000 | 0.006 |
| 水产类 Aquatic foods | 0.000 | 0.000 | 0.000 | 0.000 | 0.025 | 0.000 | 0.013 | 0.000 | 0.000 | 0.000 | 0.005 | 0.000 | 0.000 | 0.000 | 0.000 | 0.035 | 0.000 | 0.000 | 0.000 | 0.000 | 0.189 | 0.066 | 0.085 | 0.000 | 0.017 |
| 乳类 Dairy products | 0.000 | 0.000 | 0.000 | 0.000 | 0.000 | 0.033 | 0.000 | 0.000 | 0.000 | 0.000 | 0.000 | 0.000 | 0.000 | 0.000 | 0.000 | 0.000 | 0.000 | 0.000 | 0.000 | 0.000 | 0.000 | 0.000 | 0.000 | 0.000 | 0.001 |
| 蔬菜类 Vegetables | 0.498 | 0.493 | 0.627 | 2.086 | 0.912 | 5.484 | 47.300 | 0.328 | 0.263 | 3.011 | 23.620 | 0.624 | 86.560 | 44.270 | 152.500 | 1.169 | 29.870 | 18.160 | 78.870 | 4.147 | 148.800 | 23.250 | 176.800 | 2.973 | 35.520 |
| 水果类 Fruits | 0.172 | 4.909 | 0.602 | 1.081 | 0.073 | 0.034 | 0.267 | 1.398 | 0.762 | 0.407 | 0.025 | 0.086 | 6.708 | 2.643 | 0.757 | 0.761 | 0.443 | 4.876 | 0.139 | 0.233 | 0.000 | 0.675 | 0.272 | 0.083 | 1.142 |
| 糖类 Sugar | 0.000 | 0.000 | 0.000 | 0.000 | 0.000 | 0.000 | 0.000 | 0.000 | 0.000 | 0.000 | 0.000 | 0.000 | 0.000 | 0.000 | 0.000 | 0.000 | 0.000 | 0.000 | 0.000 | 0.000 | 0.000 | 0.000 | 0.000 | 0.000 | 0.000 |
| 水及饮料类 Water and beverages | 0.000 | 0.000 | 0.000 | 0.000 | 0.000 | 0.000 | 0.000 | 0.000 | 0.000 | 0.000 | 0.000 | 0.000 | 0.000 | 0.000 | 0.000 | 0.000 | 0.000 | 0.000 | 0.000 | 0.000 | 0.000 | 0.000 | 0.000 | 0.000 | 0.000 |
| 酒类 Alcohol beverages | 0.000 | 0.000 | 0.000 | 0.000 | 0.000 | 0.000 | 0.000 | 0.000 | 0.000 | 0.000 | 0.000 | 0.000 | 0.000 | 0.000 | 0.000 | 0.000 | 0.000 | 0.000 | 0.000 | 0.000 | 0.000 | 0.000 | 0.000 | 0.000 | 0.000 |
| 合计 SUM | 2.368 | 5.402 | 1.229 | 3.167 | 1.305 | 5.551 | 53.214 | 3.100 | 1.067 | 7.563 | 23.905 | 0.710 | 93.346 | 46.914 | 153.263 | 2.091 | 30.314 | 23.081 | 79.080 | 6.523 | 149.982 | 25.148 | 177.245 | 3.434 | 37.417 |

附表 4-134　第六次中国总膳食研究的肟菌酯膳食摄入量 [单位：ng/(kg bw·d)]

Annexed Table 4-134　Dietary intakes of trifloxystrobin from the 6th China TDS [Unit: ng/(kg bw·d)]

| 膳食类别 Category | 黑龙江 HL | 辽宁 LN | 河北 HE | 北京 BJ | 吉林 JL | 山西 SX | 陕西 SN | 河南 HA | 宁夏 NX | 内蒙古 NM | 青海 QH | 甘肃 GS | 上海 SH | 福建 FJ | 江西 JX | 江苏 JS | 浙江 ZJ | 山东 SD | 湖北 HB | 四川 SC | 广西 GX | 湖南 HN | 广东 GD | 贵州 GZ | 全国平均 AVG |
|---|---|---|---|---|---|---|---|---|---|---|---|---|---|---|---|---|---|---|---|---|---|---|---|---|---|
| 谷类 Cereals | 0.000 | 0.000 | 0.000 | 0.000 | 0.000 | 0.000 | 0.000 | 0.000 | 0.000 | 0.000 | 0.000 | 0.000 | 0.000 | 0.000 | 0.000 | 0.000 | 0.000 | 0.000 | 0.000 | 0.000 | 0.000 | 0.000 | 0.000 | 0.000 | 0.000 |
| 豆类 Legumes | 0.000 | 0.000 | 0.000 | 0.000 | 0.000 | 0.000 | 0.000 | 0.000 | 0.000 | 0.000 | 0.000 | 0.000 | 0.000 | 0.000 | 0.000 | 0.000 | 0.000 | 0.000 | 0.000 | 0.000 | 0.000 | 0.000 | 0.000 | 0.000 | 0.000 |
| 薯类 Potatoes | 0.000 | 0.000 | 0.000 | 0.000 | 0.288 | 0.000 | 0.000 | 0.000 | 0.000 | 0.000 | 0.000 | 0.000 | 0.000 | 0.000 | 0.000 | 0.000 | 0.000 | 0.000 | 0.000 | 0.000 | 0.000 | 0.000 | 0.000 | 0.000 | 0.012 |
| 肉类 Meats | 0.000 | 0.000 | 0.000 | 0.000 | 0.086 | 0.000 | 0.000 | 0.077 | 0.000 | 0.000 | 0.000 | 0.000 | 0.000 | 0.000 | 0.000 | 0.000 | 0.000 | 0.000 | 0.000 | 0.000 | 0.000 | 0.000 | 0.000 | 0.000 | 0.007 |
| 蛋类 Eggs | 0.000 | 0.000 | 0.000 | 0.000 | 0.043 | 0.000 | 0.000 | 0.000 | 0.000 | 0.000 | 0.000 | 0.000 | 0.000 | 0.000 | 0.000 | 0.000 | 0.000 | 0.000 | 0.000 | 0.000 | 0.000 | 0.000 | 0.000 | 0.000 | 0.002 |
| 水产类 Aquatic foods | 0.000 | 0.000 | 0.000 | 0.000 | 0.033 | 0.000 | 0.000 | 0.000 | 0.000 | 0.000 | 0.000 | 0.000 | 0.000 | 0.000 | 0.085 | 0.000 | 0.000 | 0.000 | 0.000 | 0.000 | 0.000 | 0.000 | 0.000 | 0.000 | 0.005 |
| 乳类 Dairy products | 0.000 | 0.000 | 0.000 | 0.000 | 0.000 | 0.000 | 0.000 | 0.000 | 0.000 | 0.000 | 0.000 | 0.000 | 0.000 | 0.000 | 0.000 | 0.000 | 0.000 | 0.000 | 0.000 | 0.000 | 0.000 | 0.000 | 0.000 | 0.000 | 0.000 |
| 蔬菜类 Vegetables | 3.249 | 0.355 | 8.038 | 0.000 | 0.883 | 0.000 | 1.968 | 0.570 | 9.424 | 2.041 | 1.323 | 0.000 | 1.831 | 0.439 | 0.000 | 0.000 | 0.471 | 0.933 | 0.000 | 0.000 | 3.287 | 0.000 | 0.000 | 0.000 | 1.451 |
| 水果类 Fruits | 0.000 | 0.000 | 0.164 | 35.100 | 0.000 | 0.000 | 0.000 | 0.000 | 0.000 | 0.000 | 0.000 | 0.000 | 0.784 | 0.000 | 0.000 | 0.000 | 0.133 | 0.204 | 0.037 | 0.000 | 0.000 | 0.394 | 0.000 | 0.000 | 1.534 |
| 糖类 Sugar | 0.000 | 0.000 | 0.000 | 0.000 | 0.000 | 0.000 | 0.000 | 0.000 | 0.000 | 0.000 | 0.000 | 0.000 | 0.000 | 0.000 | 0.000 | 0.000 | 0.000 | 0.000 | 0.000 | 0.000 | 0.000 | 0.000 | 0.000 | 0.000 | 0.000 |
| 水及饮料类 Water and beverages | 0.000 | 0.000 | 0.000 | 0.000 | 0.000 | 0.000 | 0.000 | 0.000 | 0.000 | 0.000 | 0.000 | 0.000 | 0.000 | 0.000 | 0.000 | 0.000 | 0.000 | 0.000 | 0.000 | 0.000 | 0.000 | 0.000 | 0.000 | 0.000 | 0.000 |

续表

| 膳食类别<br>Category | 黑龙江<br>HL | 辽宁<br>LN | 河北<br>HE | 北京<br>BJ | 吉林<br>JL | 山西<br>SX | 陕西<br>SN | 河南<br>HA | 宁夏<br>NX | 内蒙古<br>NM | 青海<br>QH | 甘肃<br>GS | 上海<br>SH | 福建<br>FJ | 江西<br>JX | 江苏<br>JS | 浙江<br>ZJ | 山东<br>SD | 湖北<br>HB | 四川<br>SC | 广西<br>GX | 湖南<br>HN | 广东<br>GD | 贵州<br>GZ | 全国平均<br>AVG |
|---|---|---|---|---|---|---|---|---|---|---|---|---|---|---|---|---|---|---|---|---|---|---|---|---|---|
| 酒类<br>Alcohol beverages | 0.000 | 0.000 | 0.000 | 0.000 | 0.000 | 0.000 | 0.000 | 0.000 | 0.000 | 0.000 | 0.000 | 0.000 | 0.000 | 0.000 | 0.000 | 0.000 | 0.000 | 0.000 | 0.000 | 0.000 | 0.000 | 0.000 | 0.000 | 0.000 | 0.000 |
| 合计<br>SUM | 3.249 | 0.355 | 8.202 | 35.100 | 1.333 | 0.000 | 1.968 | 0.647 | 9.424 | 2.041 | 1.323 | 0.000 | 2.616 | 0.439 | 0.085 | 0.000 | 0.604 | 1.138 | 0.037 | 0.000 | 3.287 | 0.394 | 0.000 | 0.000 | 3.010 |

附表 4-135 第六次中国总膳食研究嘧菌酯的膳食来源（单位：%）
Annexed Table 4-135 Dietary sources of azoxystrobin from the 6$^{th}$ China TDS (Unit: %)

| 膳食类别<br>Category | 黑龙江<br>HL | 辽宁<br>LN | 河北<br>HE | 北京<br>BJ | 吉林<br>JL | 山西<br>SX | 陕西<br>SN | 河南<br>HA | 宁夏<br>NX | 内蒙古<br>NM | 青海<br>QH | 甘肃<br>GS | 上海<br>SH | 福建<br>FJ | 江西<br>JX | 江苏<br>JS | 浙江<br>ZJ | 山东<br>SD | 湖北<br>HB | 四川<br>SC | 广西<br>GX | 湖南<br>HN | 广东<br>GD | 贵州<br>GZ | 全国平均<br>AVG |
|---|---|---|---|---|---|---|---|---|---|---|---|---|---|---|---|---|---|---|---|---|---|---|---|---|---|
| 谷类<br>Cereals | 0.0 | 0.0 | 20.9 | 0.0 | 0.0 | 0.0 | 22.4 | 0.0 | 0.0 | 0.0 | 0.0 | 0.0 | 0.0 | 0.0 | 32.5 | 0.0 | 0.0 | 0.0 | 0.0 | 92.1 | 23.5 | 0.0 | 0.0 | 0.0 | 11.7 |
| 豆类<br>Legumes | 0.0 | 0.0 | 0.0 | 0.0 | 1.2 | 0.0 | 0.0 | 0.0 | 0.0 | 0.0 | 0.0 | 0.0 | 0.0 | 0.1 | 0.0 | 0.0 | 0.0 | 0.0 | 0.0 | 0.1 | 0.0 | 0.0 | 0.0 | 0.0 | 0.0 |
| 薯类<br>Potatoes | 0.0 | 0.0 | 0.0 | 0.0 | 4.1 | 0.2 | 3.6 | 6.4 | 0.0 | 6.9 | 0.2 | 0.0 | 0.0 | 0.0 | 0.0 | 0.0 | 0.0 | 0.0 | 0.0 | 0.1 | 0.3 | 0.0 | 0.0 | 0.1 | 0.5 |
| 肉类<br>Meats | 0.0 | 0.0 | 0.0 | 0.7 | 1.6 | 0.0 | 0.0 | 0.3 | 0.0 | 2.8 | 0.0 | 0.0 | 0.0 | 0.0 | 0.0 | 0.0 | 0.0 | 0.0 | 0.0 | 0.0 | 0.0 | 0.0 | 0.0 | 0.2 | 0.1 |
| 蛋类<br>Eggs | 0.0 | 0.0 | 0.0 | 0.0 | 0.5 | 0.1 | 0.0 | 0.0 | 0.0 | 0.0 | 0.0 | 0.0 | 0.0 | 0.0 | 0.0 | 0.7 | 0.0 | 0.0 | 10.7 | 0.0 | 0.0 | 0.0 | 0.0 | 0.0 | 0.1 |
| 水产类<br>Aquatic foods | 0.0 | 0.0 | 0.0 | 0.0 | 0.4 | 0.0 | 0.0 | 0.0 | 0.0 | 0.0 | 0.0 | 0.0 | 0.0 | 0.0 | 1.0 | 0.0 | 0.0 | 0.0 | 0.5 | 0.0 | 0.0 | 3.1 | 0.0 | 0.0 | 0.1 |
| 乳类<br>Dairy products | 0.0 | 0.0 | 0.0 | 0.0 | 0.0 | 0.0 | 0.0 | 0.0 | 0.0 | 0.0 | 0.0 | 0.0 | 0.0 | 0.0 | 0.0 | 0.0 | 0.0 | 0.0 | 0.0 | 0.0 | 0.0 | 0.0 | 0.0 | 0.0 | 0.0 |

续表

| 膳食类别<br>Category | 黑龙江<br>HL | 辽宁<br>LN | 河北<br>HE | 北京<br>BJ | 吉林<br>JL | 山西<br>SX | 陕西<br>SN | 河南<br>HA | 宁夏<br>NX | 内蒙古<br>NM | 青海<br>QH | 甘肃<br>GS | 上海<br>SH | 福建<br>FJ | 江西<br>JX | 江苏<br>JS | 浙江<br>ZJ | 山东<br>SD | 湖北<br>HB | 四川<br>SC | 广西<br>GX | 湖南<br>HN | 广东<br>GD | 贵州<br>GZ | 全国平均<br>AVG |
|---|---|---|---|---|---|---|---|---|---|---|---|---|---|---|---|---|---|---|---|---|---|---|---|---|---|
| 蔬菜类 Vegetables | 37.6 | 0.0 | 74.0 | 90.4 | 84.1 | 99.6 | 69.6 | 7.1 | 100.0 | 40.2 | 99.8 | 89.8 | 94.6 | 96.0 | 18.5 | 86.9 | 17.9 | 83.9 | 80.4 | 4.7 | 73.9 | 78.8 | 87.0 | 99.7 | 77.6 |
| 水果类 Fruits | 62.4 | 99.2 | 5.2 | 8.8 | 7.9 | 0.0 | 4.3 | 86.2 | 0.0 | 50.1 | 0.0 | 10.2 | 5.4 | 3.9 | 48.0 | 12.4 | 81.2 | 12.5 | 8.3 | 2.3 | 0.6 | 18.1 | 13.0 | 0.0 | 9.5 |
| 糖类 Sugar | 0.0 | 0.0 | 0.0 | 0.0 | 0.0 | 0.0 | 0.0 | 0.0 | 0.0 | 0.0 | 0.0 | 0.0 | 0.0 | 0.0 | 0.0 | 0.0 | 0.0 | 0.0 | 0.0 | 0.0 | 0.0 | 0.0 | 0.0 | 0.0 | 0.0 |
| 水及饮料类 Water and beverages | 0.0 | 0.0 | 0.0 | 0.0 | 0.0 | 0.0 | 0.0 | 0.0 | 0.0 | 0.0 | 0.0 | 0.0 | 0.0 | 0.0 | 0.0 | 0.0 | 0.0 | 0.0 | 0.0 | 0.7 | 0.0 | 0.0 | 0.0 | 0.0 | 0.1 |
| 酒类 Alcohol beverages | 0.0 | 0.8 | 0.0 | 0.1 | 0.2 | 0.0 | 0.0 | 0.0 | 0.0 | 0.0 | 0.0 | 0.0 | 0.0 | 0.0 | 0.0 | 0.0 | 0.8 | 3.6 | 0.0 | 0.0 | 1.8 | 0.0 | 0.0 | 0.0 | 0.2 |

附表 4-136 第六次中国总膳食研究吡唑醚菌酯的膳食来源（单位：%）
Annexed Table 4-136 Dietary sources of pyraclostrobin from the 6th China TDS (Unit: %)

| 膳食类别<br>Category | 黑龙江<br>HL | 辽宁<br>LN | 河北<br>HE | 北京<br>BJ | 吉林<br>JL | 山西<br>SX | 陕西<br>SN | 河南<br>HA | 宁夏<br>NX | 内蒙古<br>NM | 青海<br>QH | 甘肃<br>GS | 上海<br>SH | 福建<br>FJ | 江西<br>JX | 江苏<br>JS | 浙江<br>ZJ | 山东<br>SD | 湖北<br>HB | 四川<br>SC | 广西<br>GX | 湖南<br>HN | 广东<br>GD | 贵州<br>GZ | 全国平均<br>AVG |
|---|---|---|---|---|---|---|---|---|---|---|---|---|---|---|---|---|---|---|---|---|---|---|---|---|---|
| 谷类 Cereals | 71.7 | 0.0 | 0.0 | 0.0 | 0.0 | 0.0 | 9.4 | 41.7 | 0.0 | 53.9 | 0.0 | 0.0 | 0.0 | 0.0 | 0.0 | 0.0 | 0.0 | 0.0 | 0.0 | 25.3 | 0.0 | 3.9 | 0.0 | 0.0 | 1.6 |
| 豆类 Legumes | 0.0 | 0.0 | 0.0 | 0.0 | 0.0 | 0.0 | 0.8 | 2.6 | 0.0 | 0.0 | 0.0 | 0.0 | 0.0 | 0.0 | 0.0 | 0.0 | 0.0 | 0.0 | 0.0 | 1.9 | 0.0 | 0.0 | 0.0 | 0.0 | 0.1 |
| 薯类 Potatoes | 0.0 | 0.0 | 0.0 | 0.0 | 18.1 | 0.0 | 0.4 | 0.0 | 4.0 | 0.0 | 0.6 | 0.0 | 0.1 | 0.0 | 0.0 | 4.1 | 0.0 | 0.0 | 0.1 | 1.2 | 0.0 | 0.0 | 0.0 | 0.0 | 0.1 |
| 肉类 Meats | 0.0 | 0.0 | 0.0 | 0.0 | 0.0 | 0.0 | 0.1 | 0.0 | 0.0 | 0.9 | 0.5 | 0.0 | 0.0 | 0.0 | 0.0 | 1.9 | 0.0 | 0.0 | 0.0 | 4.5 | 0.0 | 0.7 | 0.0 | 11.0 | 0.1 |
| 蛋类 Eggs | 0.0 | 0.0 | 0.0 | 0.0 | 4.5 | 0.0 | 0.0 | 0.0 | 0.0 | 0.0 | 0.0 | 0.0 | 0.0 | 0.0 | 0.0 | 0.0 | 0.0 | 0.2 | 0.0 | 0.0 | 0.0 | 0.0 | 0.0 | 0.0 | 0.0 |

续表

| 膳食类别<br>Category | 黑龙江<br>HL | 辽宁<br>LN | 河北<br>HE | 北京<br>BJ | 吉林<br>JL | 山西<br>SX | 陕西<br>SN | 河南<br>HA | 宁夏<br>NX | 内蒙古<br>NM | 青海<br>QH | 甘肃<br>GS | 上海<br>SH | 福建<br>FJ | 江西<br>JX | 江苏<br>JS | 浙江<br>ZJ | 山东<br>SD | 湖北<br>HB | 四川<br>SC | 广西<br>GX | 湖南<br>HN | 广东<br>GD | 贵州<br>GZ | 全国平均<br>AVG |
|---|---|---|---|---|---|---|---|---|---|---|---|---|---|---|---|---|---|---|---|---|---|---|---|---|---|
| 水产类<br>Aquatic foods | 0.0 | 0.0 | 0.0 | 0.0 | 1.9 | 0.0 | 0.0 | 0.0 | 0.0 | 0.0 | 0.0 | 0.0 | 0.0 | 0.0 | 0.0 | 1.7 | 0.0 | 0.0 | 0.0 | 0.0 | 0.1 | 0.3 | 0.0 | 0.0 | 0.0 |
| 乳类<br>Dairy products | 0.0 | 0.0 | 0.0 | 0.0 | 0.0 | 0.6 | 0.0 | 0.0 | 0.0 | 0.0 | 0.0 | 0.0 | 0.0 | 0.0 | 0.0 | 0.0 | 0.0 | 0.0 | 0.0 | 0.0 | 0.0 | 0.0 | 0.0 | 0.0 | 0.0 |
| 蔬菜类<br>Vegetables | 21.0 | 9.1 | 51.0 | 65.9 | 69.9 | 98.8 | 88.9 | 10.6 | 24.7 | 39.8 | 98.8 | 87.9 | 92.7 | 94.4 | 99.5 | 55.9 | 98.5 | 78.7 | 99.7 | 63.6 | 99.9 | 92.4 | 99.8 | 86.6 | 94.9 |
| 水果类<br>Fruits | 7.3 | 90.9 | 49.0 | 34.1 | 5.6 | 0.6 | 0.5 | 45.1 | 71.4 | 5.4 | 0.1 | 12.1 | 7.2 | 5.6 | 0.5 | 36.4 | 1.5 | 21.1 | 0.2 | 3.6 | 0.0 | 2.7 | 0.2 | 2.4 | 3.1 |
| 糖类<br>Sugar | 0.0 | 0.0 | 0.0 | 0.0 | 0.0 | 0.0 | 0.0 | 0.0 | 0.0 | 0.0 | 0.0 | 0.0 | 0.0 | 0.0 | 0.0 | 0.0 | 0.0 | 0.0 | 0.0 | 0.0 | 0.0 | 0.0 | 0.0 | 0.0 | 0.0 |
| 水及饮料类<br>Water and beverages | 0.0 | 0.0 | 0.0 | 0.0 | 0.0 | 0.0 | 0.0 | 0.0 | 0.0 | 0.0 | 0.0 | 0.0 | 0.0 | 0.0 | 0.0 | 0.0 | 0.0 | 0.0 | 0.0 | 0.0 | 0.0 | 0.0 | 0.0 | 0.0 | 0.0 |
| 酒类<br>Alcohol beverages | 0.0 | 0.0 | 0.0 | 0.0 | 0.0 | 0.0 | 0.0 | 0.0 | 0.0 | 0.0 | 0.0 | 0.0 | 0.0 | 0.0 | 0.0 | 0.0 | 0.0 | 0.0 | 0.0 | 0.0 | 0.0 | 0.0 | 0.0 | 0.0 | 0.0 |

附表 4-137　第六次中国总膳食研究肟菌酯的膳食来源（单位：%）

Annexed Table 4-137　Dietary sources of trifloxystrobin from the 6$^{th}$ China TDS (Unit: %)

| 膳食类别<br>Category | 黑龙江<br>HL | 辽宁<br>LN | 河北<br>HE | 北京<br>BJ | 吉林<br>JL | 山西<br>SX | 陕西<br>SN | 河南<br>HA | 宁夏<br>NX | 内蒙古<br>NM | 青海<br>QH | 甘肃<br>GS | 上海<br>SH | 福建<br>FJ | 江西<br>JX | 江苏<br>JS | 浙江<br>ZJ | 山东<br>SD | 湖北<br>HB | 四川<br>SC | 广西<br>GX | 湖南<br>HN | 广东<br>GD | 贵州<br>GZ | 全国平均<br>AVG |
|---|---|---|---|---|---|---|---|---|---|---|---|---|---|---|---|---|---|---|---|---|---|---|---|---|---|
| 谷类<br>Cereals | 0.0 | 0.0 | 0.0 | 0.0 | 0.0 | 0.0 | 0.0 | 0.0 | 0.0 | 0.0 | 0.0 | 0.0 | 0.0 | 0.0 | 0.0 | 0.0 | 0.0 | 0.0 | 0.0 | 0.0 | 0.0 | 0.0 | 0.0 | 0.0 | 0.0 |
| 豆类<br>Legumes | 0.0 | 0.0 | 0.0 | 0.0 | 0.0 | 0.0 | 0.0 | 0.0 | 0.0 | 0.0 | 0.0 | 0.0 | 0.0 | 0.0 | 0.0 | 0.0 | 0.0 | 0.0 | 0.0 | 0.0 | 0.0 | 0.0 | 0.0 | 0.0 | 0.0 |

续表

| 膳食类别 Category | 黑龙江 HL | 辽宁 LN | 河北 HE | 北京 BJ | 吉林 JL | 山西 SX | 陕西 SN | 河南 HA | 宁夏 NX | 内蒙古 NM | 青海 QH | 甘肃 GS | 上海 SH | 福建 FJ | 江西 JX | 江苏 JS | 浙江 ZJ | 山东 SD | 湖北 HB | 四川 SC | 广西 GX | 湖南 HN | 广东 GD | 贵州 GZ | 全国平均 AVG |
|---|---|---|---|---|---|---|---|---|---|---|---|---|---|---|---|---|---|---|---|---|---|---|---|---|---|
| 薯类 Potatoes | 0.0 | 0.0 | 0.0 | 0.0 | 21.6 | 0.0 | 0.0 | 0.0 | 0.0 | 0.0 | 0.0 | 0.0 | 0.0 | 0.0 | 0.0 | 0.0 | 0.0 | 0.0 | 0.0 | 0.0 | 0.0 | 0.0 | 0.0 | 0.0 | 0.4 |
| 肉类 Meats | 0.0 | 0.0 | 0.0 | 0.0 | 6.4 | 0.0 | 0.0 | 11.9 | 0.0 | 0.0 | 0.0 | 0.0 | 0.0 | 0.0 | 0.0 | 0.0 | 0.0 | 0.0 | 0.0 | 0.0 | 0.0 | 0.0 | 0.0 | 0.0 | 0.2 |
| 蛋类 Eggs | 0.0 | 0.0 | 0.0 | 0.0 | 3.3 | 0.0 | 0.0 | 0.0 | 0.0 | 0.0 | 0.0 | 0.0 | 0.0 | 0.0 | 0.0 | 0.0 | 0.0 | 0.0 | 0.0 | 0.0 | 0.0 | 0.0 | 0.0 | 0.0 | 0.1 |
| 水产类 Aquatic foods | 0.0 | 0.0 | 0.0 | 0.0 | 2.5 | 0.0 | 0.0 | 0.0 | 0.0 | 0.0 | 0.0 | 0.0 | 0.0 | 0.0 | 100.0 | 0.0 | 0.0 | 0.0 | 0.0 | 0.0 | 0.0 | 0.0 | 0.0 | 0.0 | 0.2 |
| 乳类 Dairy products | 0.0 | 0.0 | 0.0 | 0.0 | 0.0 | 0.0 | 0.0 | 0.0 | 0.0 | 0.0 | 0.0 | 0.0 | 0.0 | 0.0 | 0.0 | 0.0 | 0.0 | 0.0 | 0.0 | 0.0 | 0.0 | 0.0 | 0.0 | 0.0 | 0.0 |
| 蔬菜类 Vegetables | 100.0 | 100.0 | 98.0 | 0.0 | 66.2 | 0.0 | 100.0 | 88.1 | 100.0 | 100.0 | 100.0 | 0.0 | 70.0 | 100.0 | 0.0 | 0.0 | 77.9 | 82.0 | 0.0 | 0.0 | 100.0 | 0.0 | 0.0 | 0.0 | 48.2 |
| 水果类 Fruits | 0.0 | 0.0 | 2.0 | 100.0 | 0.0 | 0.0 | 0.0 | 0.0 | 0.0 | 0.0 | 0.0 | 0.0 | 30.0 | 0.0 | 0.0 | 0.0 | 22.1 | 18.0 | 100.0 | 0.0 | 0.0 | 100.0 | 0.0 | 0.0 | 51.0 |
| 糖类 Sugar | 0.0 | 0.0 | 0.0 | 0.0 | 0.0 | 0.0 | 0.0 | 0.0 | 0.0 | 0.0 | 0.0 | 0.0 | 0.0 | 0.0 | 0.0 | 0.0 | 0.0 | 0.0 | 0.0 | 0.0 | 0.0 | 0.0 | 0.0 | 0.0 | 0.0 |
| 水及饮料类 Water and beverages | 0.0 | 0.0 | 0.0 | 0.0 | 0.0 | 0.0 | 0.0 | 0.0 | 0.0 | 0.0 | 0.0 | 0.0 | 0.0 | 0.0 | 0.0 | 0.0 | 0.0 | 0.0 | 0.0 | 0.0 | 0.0 | 0.0 | 0.0 | 0.0 | 0.0 |
| 酒类 Alcohol beverages | 0.0 | 0.0 | 0.0 | 0.0 | 0.0 | 0.0 | 0.0 | 0.0 | 0.0 | 0.0 | 0.0 | 0.0 | 0.0 | 0.0 | 0.0 | 0.0 | 0.0 | 0.0 | 0.0 | 0.0 | 0.0 | 0.0 | 0.0 | 0.0 | 0.0 |

附表 4-138 第六次中国总膳食研究膳食样品中甲霜灵的含量（单位：μg/kg）

Annexed Table 4-138 Levels of metalaxyl in food samples from the 6$^{th}$ China TDS (Unit: μg/kg)

| 膳食类别 Category | 黑龙江 HL | 辽宁 LN | 河北 HE | 北京 BJ | 吉林 JL | 山西 SX | 陕西 SN | 河南 HA | 宁夏 NX | 内蒙古 NM | 青海 QH | 甘肃 GS | 上海 SH | 福建 FJ | 江西 JX | 江苏 JS | 浙江 ZJ | 山东 SD | 湖北 HB | 四川 SC | 广西 GX | 湖南 HN | 广东 GD | 贵州 GZ | 全国平均 AVG |
|---|---|---|---|---|---|---|---|---|---|---|---|---|---|---|---|---|---|---|---|---|---|---|---|---|---|
| 谷类 Cereals | ND | ND | ND | ND | ND | ND | ND | ND | ND | ND | ND | ND | ND | ND | ND | ND | ND | ND | ND | ND | ND | ND | ND | ND | 0.00 |
| 豆类 Legumes | ND | ND | ND | ND | ND | ND | ND | ND | ND | ND | ND | ND | ND | ND | ND | ND | 0.14 | ND | ND | ND | ND | ND | ND | ND | 0.01 |
| 薯类 Potatoes | ND | ND | ND | ND | ND | ND | 0.42 | ND | ND | 0.15 | 0.19 | ND | ND | ND | ND | 2.69 | ND | 0.47 | 0.50 | ND | ND | ND | ND | 0.12 | 0.17 |
| 肉类 Meats | ND | ND | ND | ND | ND | 0.41 | ND | ND | ND | ND | ND | ND | ND | ND | ND | 0.08 | 0.37 | ND | ND | 0.11 | ND | ND | ND | ND | 0.06 |
| 蛋类 Eggs | ND | ND | ND | ND | ND | ND | ND | ND | ND | 0.09 | ND | ND | ND | ND | ND | ND | ND | ND | 0.51 | ND | ND | ND | ND | ND | 0.03 |
| 水产类 Aquatic foods | ND | ND | ND | 0.16 | ND | 0.11 | ND | ND | ND | ND | ND | ND | ND | ND | ND | ND | 0.27 | ND | 0.53 | 0.08 | ND | ND | ND | ND | 0.05 |
| 乳类 Dairy products | ND | ND | ND | ND | ND | ND | ND | ND | ND | ND | ND | ND | ND | ND | ND | ND | ND | ND | ND | ND | ND | ND | ND | ND | 0.00 |
| 蔬菜类 Vegetables | 1.45 | ND | 0.34 | 1.86 | 1.25 | 0.66 | 0.26 | 1.18 | 0.12 | 0.55 | 1.51 | 9.12 | 4.59 | 0.20 | 1.53 | 10.63 | 0.35 | 0.52 | 1.27 | 0.85 | 6.76 | 10.91 | 25.50 | 3.69 | 3.56 |
| 水果类 Fruits | ND | 0.21 | ND | 0.15 | ND | ND | 0.73 | ND | ND | 0.11 | ND | ND | ND | 1.71 | ND | ND | ND | 0.34 | 0.08 | ND | 0.21 | ND | 1.72 | 0.08 | 0.21 |
| 糖类 Sugar | ND | ND | ND | ND | ND | ND | ND | ND | ND | ND | ND | ND | 0.52 | ND | ND | ND | ND | ND | ND | ND | ND | ND | ND | ND | 0.02 |
| 水及饮料类 Water and beverages | ND | ND | ND | ND | ND | ND | ND | ND | ND | ND | ND | ND | ND | ND | ND | ND | ND | ND | ND | ND | ND | ND | ND | ND | 0.00 |

续表

| 膳食类别<br>Category | 黑龙江<br>HL | 辽宁<br>LN | 河北<br>HE | 北京<br>BJ | 吉林<br>JL | 山西<br>SX | 陕西<br>SN | 河南<br>HA | 宁夏<br>NX | 内蒙古<br>NM | 青海<br>QH | 甘肃<br>GS | 上海<br>SH | 福建<br>FJ | 江西<br>JX | 江苏<br>JS | 浙江<br>ZJ | 山东<br>SD | 湖北<br>HB | 四川<br>SC | 广西<br>GX | 湖南<br>HN | 广东<br>GD | 贵州<br>GZ | 全国平均<br>AVG |
|---|---|---|---|---|---|---|---|---|---|---|---|---|---|---|---|---|---|---|---|---|---|---|---|---|---|
| 酒类<br>Alcohol beverages | ND | ND | ND | 0.16 | ND | ND | ND | ND | ND | ND | ND | ND | 0.22 | ND | ND | 0.06 | 0.25 | 0.29 | ND | ND | 2.75 | ND | 0.14 | ND | 0.16 |

注：未检出（ND）按 0 计
Note: values not detected (ND) were treated as being equal to 0

附表 4-139 第六次中国总膳食研究膳食样品中环酰菌胺的含量（单位：μg/kg）
Annexed Table 4-139 Levels of fenhexamid in food samples from the 6$^{th}$ China TDS (Unit: μg/kg)

| 膳食类别<br>Category | 黑龙江<br>HL | 辽宁<br>LN | 河北<br>HE | 北京<br>BJ | 吉林<br>JL | 山西<br>SX | 陕西<br>SN | 河南<br>HA | 宁夏<br>NX | 内蒙古<br>NM | 青海<br>QH | 甘肃<br>GS | 上海<br>SH | 福建<br>FJ | 江西<br>JX | 江苏<br>JS | 浙江<br>ZJ | 山东<br>SD | 湖北<br>HB | 四川<br>SC | 广西<br>GX | 湖南<br>HN | 广东<br>GD | 贵州<br>GZ | 全国平均<br>AVG |
|---|---|---|---|---|---|---|---|---|---|---|---|---|---|---|---|---|---|---|---|---|---|---|---|---|---|
| 谷类<br>Cereals | ND | ND | ND | ND | ND | ND | ND | ND | ND | ND | ND | ND | ND | ND | ND | ND | ND | ND | ND | ND | ND | ND | ND | ND | 0.00 |
| 豆类<br>Legumes | ND | ND | ND | ND | ND | ND | ND | ND | ND | ND | ND | ND | ND | ND | ND | ND | ND | ND | ND | ND | ND | ND | ND | ND | 0.00 |
| 薯类<br>Potatoes | ND | ND | ND | ND | ND | ND | ND | ND | ND | ND | ND | ND | ND | ND | ND | ND | ND | ND | ND | ND | ND | ND | ND | ND | 0.00 |
| 肉类<br>Meats | ND | ND | ND | ND | ND | ND | ND | ND | ND | ND | ND | ND | ND | ND | ND | ND | ND | ND | ND | ND | ND | ND | ND | ND | 0.00 |
| 蛋类<br>Eggs | ND | ND | ND | ND | ND | ND | ND | ND | ND | ND | ND | ND | ND | ND | ND | ND | ND | ND | ND | ND | ND | ND | ND | ND | 0.00 |
| 水产类<br>Aquatic foods | ND | ND | ND | ND | ND | ND | ND | ND | ND | ND | ND | ND | ND | ND | ND | ND | ND | ND | ND | ND | ND | ND | ND | ND | 0.00 |
| 乳类<br>Dairy products | ND | ND | ND | ND | ND | ND | ND | ND | ND | ND | ND | ND | ND | ND | ND | ND | ND | ND | ND | ND | ND | ND | ND | ND | 0.00 |

续表

| 膳食类别<br>Category | 黑龙江<br>HL | 辽宁<br>LN | 河北<br>HE | 北京<br>BJ | 吉林<br>JL | 山西<br>SX | 陕西<br>SN | 河南<br>HA | 宁夏<br>NX | 内蒙古<br>NM | 青海<br>QH | 甘肃<br>GS | 上海<br>SH | 福建<br>FJ | 江西<br>JX | 江苏<br>JS | 浙江<br>ZJ | 山东<br>SD | 湖北<br>HB | 四川<br>SC | 广西<br>GX | 湖南<br>HN | 广东<br>GD | 贵州<br>GZ | 全国平均<br>AVG |
|---|---|---|---|---|---|---|---|---|---|---|---|---|---|---|---|---|---|---|---|---|---|---|---|---|---|
| 蔬菜类 Vegetables | ND | ND | ND | ND | ND | ND | ND | ND | ND | ND | ND | ND | ND | ND | ND | ND | ND | ND | ND | ND | ND | ND | ND | ND | 0.00 |
| 水果类 Fruits | ND | ND | ND | ND | ND | ND | ND | ND | ND | ND | ND | ND | 0.47 | ND | ND | ND | ND | ND | ND | ND | ND | ND | ND | ND | 0.02 |
| 糖类 Sugar | ND | ND | ND | ND | ND | ND | ND | ND | ND | ND | ND | ND | ND | ND | ND | ND | ND | ND | ND | ND | ND | ND | ND | ND | 0.00 |
| 水及饮料类 Water and beverages | ND | ND | ND | ND | ND | ND | ND | ND | ND | ND | ND | ND | ND | ND | ND | ND | ND | ND | ND | ND | ND | ND | ND | ND | 0.00 |
| 酒类 Alcohol beverages | ND | ND | ND | ND | ND | ND | ND | ND | ND | ND | ND | ND | ND | ND | ND | ND | ND | ND | ND | ND | ND | ND | ND | ND | 0.00 |

注：未检出（ND）按 0 计
Note: values not detected (ND) were treated as being equal to 0

附表 4-140　第六次中国总膳食研究膳食样品中嘧霉胺的含量（单位：μg/kg）
Annexed Table 4-140　Levels of pyrimethanil in food samples from the 6$^{th}$ China TDS (Unit: μg/kg)

| 膳食类别<br>Category | 黑龙江<br>HL | 辽宁<br>LN | 河北<br>HE | 北京<br>BJ | 吉林<br>JL | 山西<br>SX | 陕西<br>SN | 河南<br>HA | 宁夏<br>NX | 内蒙古<br>NM | 青海<br>QH | 甘肃<br>GS | 上海<br>SH | 福建<br>FJ | 江西<br>JX | 江苏<br>JS | 浙江<br>ZJ | 山东<br>SD | 湖北<br>HB | 四川<br>SC | 广西<br>GX | 湖南<br>HN | 广东<br>GD | 贵州<br>GZ | 全国平均<br>AVG |
|---|---|---|---|---|---|---|---|---|---|---|---|---|---|---|---|---|---|---|---|---|---|---|---|---|---|
| 谷类 Cereals | ND | 0.30 | ND | ND | ND | ND | ND | ND | ND | ND | ND | ND | ND | ND | ND | ND | ND | ND | ND | ND | ND | ND | ND | ND | 0.01 |
| 豆类 Legumes | ND | ND | ND | ND | ND | ND | ND | ND | ND | ND | ND | ND | ND | ND | ND | ND | ND | ND | ND | ND | ND | ND | ND | ND | 0.00 |
| 薯类 Potatoes | ND | ND | 0.14 | ND | ND | ND | ND | ND | ND | ND | ND | ND | 0.19 | ND | ND | ND | ND | ND | ND | ND | ND | ND | ND | ND | 0.01 |

续表

| 膳食类别<br>Category | 黑龙江<br>HL | 辽宁<br>LN | 河北<br>HE | 北京<br>BJ | 吉林<br>JL | 山西<br>SX | 陕西<br>SN | 河南<br>HA | 宁夏<br>NX | 内蒙古<br>NM | 青海<br>QH | 甘肃<br>GS | 上海<br>SH | 福建<br>FJ | 江西<br>JX | 江苏<br>JS | 浙江<br>ZJ | 山东<br>SD | 湖北<br>HB | 四川<br>SC | 广西<br>GX | 湖南<br>HN | 广东<br>GD | 贵州<br>GZ | 全国平均<br>AVG |
|---|---|---|---|---|---|---|---|---|---|---|---|---|---|---|---|---|---|---|---|---|---|---|---|---|---|
| 肉类 Meats | ND | ND | ND | ND | ND | ND | ND | ND | ND | ND | ND | ND | ND | ND | ND | ND | ND | ND | ND | ND | ND | ND | 0.04 | ND | 0.00 |
| 蛋类 Eggs | ND | ND | ND | ND | ND | ND | ND | ND | ND | ND | ND | ND | ND | ND | ND | ND | ND | ND | ND | ND | ND | ND | ND | ND | 0.00 |
| 水产类 Aquatic foods | ND | 0.17 | ND | ND | ND | ND | ND | ND | ND | ND | ND | 0.41 | ND | ND | ND | 0.17 | 0.08 | ND | ND | ND | ND | ND | 0.10 | ND | 0.04 |
| 乳类 Dairy products | ND | ND | ND | ND | ND | ND | ND | ND | ND | ND | ND | ND | ND | ND | ND | 0.05 | ND | ND | ND | ND | ND | ND | ND | ND | 0.00 |
| 蔬菜类 Vegetables | ND | ND | 0.75 | 0.96 | 0.14 | 0.40 | 1.15 | 0.10 | 0.24 | 0.10 | 0.79 | 130.61 | 1.03 | 0.21 | 0.18 | 0.24 | 0.09 | 4.21 | 1.25 | 2.61 | 0.24 | 12.12 | 8.80 | 0.17 | 6.93 |
| 水果类 Fruits | 0.27 | 4.56 | 2.14 | 0.17 | 4.91 | ND | ND | 0.91 | 0.08 | 0.35 | 0.78 | 0.06 | 4.91 | 11.91 | ND | 0.19 | 14.60 | 0.04 | 8.94 | 7.25 | ND | ND | 3.17 | ND | 2.72 |
| 糖类 Sugar | ND | ND | ND | ND | ND | ND | ND | ND | ND | ND | ND | ND | ND | ND | ND | ND | ND | ND | ND | ND | ND | ND | ND | ND | 0.00 |
| 水及饮料类 Water and beverages | ND | ND | ND | ND | ND | ND | ND | 0.96 | ND | ND | ND | ND | 0.12 | ND | ND | ND | ND | ND | ND | ND | ND | ND | ND | ND | 0.00 |
| 酒类 Alcohol beverages | ND | ND | ND | ND | ND | ND | ND | ND | ND | ND | ND | ND | ND | ND | ND | ND | ND | ND | ND | ND | 1.04 | ND | 0.03 | ND | 0.09 |

注：未检出（ND）按 0 计

Note: values not detected (ND) were treated as being equal to 0

附表 4-141　第六次中国总膳食研究膳食样品中乙嘧酚磺酸酯的含量（单位：μg/kg）

Annexed Table 4-141　Levels of bupirimate in food samples from the 6th China TDS (Unit: μg/kg)

| 膳食类别 Category | 黑龙江 HL | 辽宁 LN | 河北 HE | 北京 BJ | 吉林 JL | 山西 SX | 陕西 SN | 河南 HA | 宁夏 NX | 内蒙古 NM | 青海 QH | 甘肃 GS | 上海 SH | 福建 FJ | 江西 JX | 江苏 JS | 浙江 ZJ | 山东 SD | 湖北 HB | 四川 SC | 广西 GX | 湖南 HN | 广东 GD | 贵州 GZ | 全国平均 AVG |
|---|---|---|---|---|---|---|---|---|---|---|---|---|---|---|---|---|---|---|---|---|---|---|---|---|---|
| 谷类 Cereals | ND | ND | ND | ND | ND | ND | ND | ND | ND | ND | ND | ND | ND | ND | ND | ND | ND | ND | ND | ND | ND | ND | ND | ND | 0.00 |
| 豆类 Legumes | ND | ND | ND | ND | ND | ND | ND | ND | ND | ND | ND | ND | ND | ND | ND | ND | ND | ND | ND | ND | ND | ND | ND | ND | 0.00 |
| 薯类 Potatoes | ND | ND | ND | ND | ND | ND | ND | ND | ND | ND | ND | ND | ND | ND | ND | ND | 0.08 | ND | ND | ND | ND | ND | ND | ND | 0.00 |
| 肉类 Meats | ND | ND | ND | ND | ND | ND | ND | ND | ND | ND | ND | ND | ND | ND | ND | ND | ND | ND | ND | ND | ND | ND | ND | ND | 0.00 |
| 蛋类 Eggs | ND | ND | ND | ND | ND | ND | ND | ND | ND | ND | ND | ND | ND | ND | ND | ND | ND | ND | ND | ND | ND | ND | ND | ND | 0.00 |
| 水产类 Aquatic foods | ND | ND | ND | ND | ND | ND | ND | ND | ND | ND | 0.11 | ND | ND | ND | ND | ND | ND | ND | ND | ND | ND | ND | ND | ND | 0.00 |
| 乳类 Dairy products | ND | ND | ND | ND | ND | ND | ND | ND | ND | ND | ND | ND | ND | ND | ND | ND | ND | ND | ND | ND | ND | ND | ND | ND | 0.00 |
| 蔬菜类 Vegetables | ND | ND | ND | ND | 0.42 | ND | ND | ND | ND | ND | 1.78 | ND | ND | ND | ND | ND | ND | ND | ND | ND | ND | ND | ND | ND | 0.09 |
| 水果类 Fruits | ND | ND | ND | ND | ND | ND | ND | ND | ND | ND | ND | ND | ND | ND | ND | ND | ND | 0.11 | ND | ND | ND | ND | ND | ND | 0.00 |
| 糖类 Sugar | ND | ND | ND | ND | ND | ND | ND | ND | ND | ND | ND | ND | ND | ND | ND | ND | ND | ND | ND | ND | ND | ND | ND | ND | 0.00 |
| 水及饮料类 Water and beverages | ND | ND | ND | ND | ND | ND | ND | ND | ND | ND | ND | ND | ND | ND | ND | ND | ND | ND | ND | ND | ND | ND | ND | ND | 0.00 |

续表

| 膳食类别<br>Category | 黑龙江<br>HL | 辽宁<br>LN | 河北<br>HE | 北京<br>BJ | 吉林<br>JL | 山西<br>SX | 陕西<br>SN | 河南<br>HA | 宁夏<br>NX | 内蒙古<br>NM | 青海<br>QH | 甘肃<br>GS | 上海<br>SH | 福建<br>FJ | 江西<br>JX | 江苏<br>JS | 浙江<br>ZJ | 山东<br>SD | 湖北<br>HB | 四川<br>SC | 广西<br>GX | 湖南<br>HN | 广东<br>GD | 贵州<br>GZ | 全国平均<br>AVG |
|---|---|---|---|---|---|---|---|---|---|---|---|---|---|---|---|---|---|---|---|---|---|---|---|---|---|
| 酒类<br>Alcohol beverages | ND | ND | ND | ND | ND | ND | ND | ND | ND | ND | ND | ND | ND | ND | ND | ND | ND | ND | ND | ND | ND | ND | ND | ND | 0.00 |

注：未检出（ND）按 0 计

Note: values not detected (ND) were treated as being equal to 0

附表 4-142　第六次中国总膳食研究膳食样品中嘧菌环胺的含量（单位：μg/kg）

Annexed Table 4-142　Levels of cyprodinil in food samples from the 6<sup>th</sup> China TDS (Unit: μg/kg)

| 膳食类别<br>Category | 黑龙江<br>HL | 辽宁<br>LN | 河北<br>HE | 北京<br>BJ | 吉林<br>JL | 山西<br>SX | 陕西<br>SN | 河南<br>HA | 宁夏<br>NX | 内蒙古<br>NM | 青海<br>QH | 甘肃<br>GS | 上海<br>SH | 福建<br>FJ | 江西<br>JX | 江苏<br>JS | 浙江<br>ZJ | 山东<br>SD | 湖北<br>HB | 四川<br>SC | 广西<br>GX | 湖南<br>HN | 广东<br>GD | 贵州<br>GZ | 全国平均<br>AVG |
|---|---|---|---|---|---|---|---|---|---|---|---|---|---|---|---|---|---|---|---|---|---|---|---|---|---|
| 谷类<br>Cereals | ND | ND | ND | ND | ND | ND | ND | ND | ND | ND | ND | ND | ND | ND | ND | ND | ND | ND | ND | ND | ND | ND | ND | ND | 0.00 |
| 豆类<br>Legumes | ND | ND | ND | ND | ND | ND | ND | ND | ND | ND | ND | ND | ND | ND | ND | ND | ND | ND | ND | ND | ND | ND | ND | ND | 0.00 |
| 薯类<br>Potatoes | ND | ND | ND | ND | ND | ND | ND | ND | ND | ND | ND | ND | ND | ND | ND | ND | ND | ND | ND | ND | ND | ND | ND | ND | 0.00 |
| 肉类<br>Meats | ND | ND | 0.08 | ND | ND | ND | ND | ND | ND | ND | ND | ND | ND | ND | ND | ND | ND | ND | ND | ND | ND | ND | ND | ND | 0.00 |
| 蛋类<br>Eggs | ND | ND | ND | ND | ND | ND | ND | ND | ND | ND | ND | ND | ND | ND | ND | ND | ND | ND | ND | ND | ND | ND | ND | ND | 0.00 |
| 水产类<br>Aquatic foods | ND | ND | ND | ND | ND | ND | ND | ND | ND | ND | ND | ND | ND | ND | ND | ND | ND | ND | ND | ND | ND | ND | ND | ND | 0.00 |
| 乳类<br>Dairy products | ND | ND | ND | ND | ND | ND | ND | ND | ND | ND | ND | ND | ND | ND | ND | ND | ND | ND | ND | ND | ND | ND | ND | ND | 0.00 |

续表

| 膳食类别<br>Category | 黑龙江<br>HL | 辽宁<br>LN | 河北<br>HE | 北京<br>BJ | 吉林<br>JL | 山西<br>SX | 陕西<br>SN | 河南<br>HA | 宁夏<br>NX | 内蒙古<br>NM | 青海<br>QH | 甘肃<br>GS | 上海<br>SH | 福建<br>FJ | 江西<br>JX | 江苏<br>JS | 浙江<br>ZJ | 山东<br>SD | 湖北<br>HB | 四川<br>SC | 广西<br>GX | 湖南<br>HN | 广东<br>GD | 贵州<br>GZ | 全国平均<br>AVG |
|---|---|---|---|---|---|---|---|---|---|---|---|---|---|---|---|---|---|---|---|---|---|---|---|---|---|
| 蔬菜类<br>Vegetables | ND | ND | ND | 0.08 | ND | ND | ND | 0.31 | 0.24 | ND | ND | ND | ND | ND | ND | ND | ND | ND | ND | ND | ND | ND | 0.41 | ND | 0.04 |
| 水果类<br>Fruits | ND | ND | 4.10 | ND | ND | ND | ND | ND | ND | ND | ND | ND | 34.03 | 2.59 | ND | ND | ND | 0.71 | ND | ND | ND | ND | ND | ND | 1.73 |
| 糖类<br>Sugar | ND | ND | ND | ND | ND | ND | ND | ND | ND | ND | ND | ND | ND | ND | ND | ND | ND | ND | ND | ND | ND | ND | ND | ND | 0.00 |
| 水及饮料类<br>Water and beverages | ND | ND | ND | ND | ND | ND | ND | ND | ND | ND | ND | ND | ND | ND | ND | ND | ND | ND | ND | ND | ND | ND | ND | ND | 0.00 |
| 酒类<br>Alcohol beverages | ND | ND | ND | ND | ND | ND | ND | ND | ND | ND | ND | ND | ND | ND | ND | ND | ND | ND | ND | ND | ND | ND | ND | ND | 0.00 |

注：未检出（ND）按 0 计
Note: values not detected (ND) were treated as being equal to 0

附表 4-143　第六次中国总膳食研究膳食样品中氟吡菌胺的含量（单位：μg/kg）
Annexed Table 4-143　Levels of fluopicolide in food samples from the 6<sup>th</sup> China TDS (Unit: μg/kg)

| 膳食类别<br>Category | 黑龙江<br>HL | 辽宁<br>LN | 河北<br>HE | 北京<br>BJ | 吉林<br>JL | 山西<br>SX | 陕西<br>SN | 河南<br>HA | 宁夏<br>NX | 内蒙古<br>NM | 青海<br>QH | 甘肃<br>GS | 上海<br>SH | 福建<br>FJ | 江西<br>JX | 江苏<br>JS | 浙江<br>ZJ | 山东<br>SD | 湖北<br>HB | 四川<br>SC | 广西<br>GX | 湖南<br>HN | 广东<br>GD | 贵州<br>GZ | 全国平均<br>AVG |
|---|---|---|---|---|---|---|---|---|---|---|---|---|---|---|---|---|---|---|---|---|---|---|---|---|---|
| 谷类<br>Cereals | ND | ND | ND | ND | ND | ND | ND | ND | ND | ND | ND | ND | ND | ND | ND | ND | ND | ND | ND | ND | ND | ND | ND | ND | 0.00 |
| 豆类<br>Legumes | ND | ND | 0.12 | ND | ND | ND | ND | ND | ND | ND | ND | ND | ND | ND | ND | ND | ND | ND | ND | ND | ND | ND | ND | ND | 0.00 |
| 薯类<br>Potatoes | ND | ND | ND | ND | 0.26 | ND | ND | 0.13 | ND | ND | ND | ND | ND | ND | ND | ND | ND | ND | ND | ND | ND | ND | ND | ND | 0.02 |

续表

| 膳食类别<br>Category | 黑龙江<br>HL | 辽宁<br>LN | 河北<br>HE | 北京<br>BJ | 吉林<br>JL | 山西<br>SX | 陕西<br>SN | 河南<br>HA | 宁夏<br>NX | 内蒙古<br>NM | 青海<br>QH | 甘肃<br>GS | 上海<br>SH | 福建<br>FJ | 江西<br>JX | 江苏<br>JS | 浙江<br>ZJ | 山东<br>SD | 湖北<br>HB | 四川<br>SC | 广西<br>GX | 湖南<br>HN | 广东<br>GD | 贵州<br>GZ | 全国平均<br>AVG |
|---|---|---|---|---|---|---|---|---|---|---|---|---|---|---|---|---|---|---|---|---|---|---|---|---|---|
| 肉类 Meats | ND | ND | ND | ND | ND | ND | ND | ND | ND | ND | ND | ND | ND | ND | ND | ND | ND | ND | ND | ND | ND | ND | ND | ND | 0.00 |
| 蛋类 Eggs | ND | ND | ND | ND | ND | ND | ND | ND | ND | ND | ND | ND | ND | ND | ND | ND | ND | ND | ND | ND | ND | ND | ND | ND | 0.00 |
| 水产类 Aquatic foods | ND | ND | ND | ND | ND | ND | ND | ND | ND | ND | ND | ND | ND | ND | ND | ND | ND | ND | ND | ND | ND | ND | ND | ND | 0.00 |
| 乳类 Dairy products | ND | ND | ND | ND | ND | 0.06 | ND | ND | ND | ND | ND | ND | ND | ND | ND | ND | ND | ND | ND | ND | ND | ND | ND | ND | 0.00 |
| 蔬菜类 Vegetables | ND | ND | 0.36 | 0.64 | ND | 1.48 | ND | ND | ND | ND | ND | 0.34 | 0.17 | 0.04 | 1.27 | ND | 0.24 | 0.05 | 0.16 | 2.39 | ND | 0.06 | 1.48 | 0.62 | 0.39 |
| 水果类 Fruits | ND | ND | ND | ND | 1.40 | ND | ND | ND | ND | ND | ND | ND | ND | ND | ND | ND | ND | 0.08 | ND | 0.73 | ND | ND | 0.05 | ND | 0.09 |
| 糖类 Sugar | ND | ND | ND | ND | ND | ND | ND | ND | ND | ND | ND | ND | ND | ND | ND | ND | ND | ND | ND | ND | ND | ND | ND | ND | 0.00 |
| 水及饮料类 Water and beverages | ND | ND | ND | ND | ND | ND | ND | ND | ND | ND | ND | ND | ND | ND | ND | ND | ND | ND | ND | ND | ND | ND | ND | ND | 0.00 |
| 酒类 Alcohol beverages | ND | ND | ND | ND | ND | ND | ND | ND | ND | ND | ND | ND | ND | ND | ND | ND | ND | ND | ND | ND | ND | ND | ND | ND | 0.00 |

注：未检出（ND）按0计

Note: values not detected (ND) were treated as being equal to 0

附表 4-144 第六次中国总膳食研究膳食样品中烯酰吗啉的含量（单位：μg/kg）

Annexed Table 4-144 Levels of dimethomorph in food samples from the 6th China TDS (Unit: μg/kg)

| 膳食类别 Category | 黑龙江 HL | 辽宁 LN | 河北 HE | 北京 BJ | 吉林 JL | 山西 SX | 陕西 SN | 河南 HA | 宁夏 NX | 内蒙古 NM | 青海 QH | 甘肃 GS | 上海 SH | 福建 FJ | 江西 JX | 江苏 JS | 浙江 ZJ | 山东 SD | 湖北 HB | 四川 SC | 广西 GX | 湖南 HN | 广东 GD | 贵州 GZ | 全国平均 AVG |
|---|---|---|---|---|---|---|---|---|---|---|---|---|---|---|---|---|---|---|---|---|---|---|---|---|---|
| 谷类 Cereals | ND | ND | 0.09 | 0.08 | ND | ND | ND | 0.12 | ND | ND | ND | ND | ND | ND | 0.12 | ND | ND | ND | ND | ND | ND | ND | ND | ND | 0.02 |
| 豆类 Legumes | ND | ND | 0.12 | ND | ND | ND | ND | 0.08 | ND | ND | ND | ND | ND | ND | ND | ND | ND | ND | ND | ND | ND | ND | ND | 0.07 | 0.01 |
| 薯类 Potatoes | ND | ND | 1.14 | ND | 0.34 | 0.11 | 2.04 | 0.20 | ND | 0.21 | ND | 0.19 | 1.63 | 0.07 | ND | ND | 0.06 | 0.07 | ND | 0.12 | 0.56 | ND | 0.80 | 0.12 | 0.32 |
| 肉类 Meats | ND | ND | 0.23 | 0.15 | ND | 0.38 | ND | 0.06 | ND | 0.32 | ND | ND | ND | ND | ND | 0.07 | ND | ND | 0.07 | ND | 0.06 | 0.07 | ND | 0.20 | 0.06 |
| 蛋类 Eggs | ND | ND | 0.11 | 0.21 | ND | ND | ND | ND | ND | ND | ND | ND | ND | ND | ND | ND | ND | ND | ND | ND | ND | ND | ND | ND | 0.01 |
| 水产类 Aquatic foods | ND | ND | 0.11 | 0.15 | 0.10 | 0.08 | ND | 0.06 | ND | ND | ND | 0.30 | ND | 0.09 | ND | ND | ND | ND | ND | ND | 0.06 | ND | 0.13 | 0.08 | 0.05 |
| 乳类 Dairy products | ND | ND | ND | ND | ND | 0.14 | ND | ND | ND | ND | ND | ND | ND | ND | ND | ND | ND | ND | ND | ND | ND | ND | ND | ND | 0.01 |
| 蔬菜类 Vegetables | 0.34 | 0.09 | 10.45 | 0.72 | 0.09 | 6.61 | 2.11 | 1.15 | 1.74 | 0.85 | 28.05 | 85.67 | 91.37 | 29.24 | 38.95 | 88.76 | 1.77 | 1.91 | 180.63 | 10.12 | 6.74 | 180.62 | 516.98 | 118.55 | 58.48 |
| 水果类 Fruits | 1.91 | 4.00 | 0.07 | 1.67 | 3.21 | ND | 0.11 | 18.90 | ND | 1.15 | 0.85 | ND | 0.06 | 1.37 | 0.38 | ND | 4.52 | 0.13 | 0.60 | 4.02 | 2.41 | ND | 6.31 | ND | 2.15 |
| 糖类 Sugar | ND | ND | ND | ND | ND | ND | ND | ND | ND | ND | ND | ND | ND | ND | ND | ND | ND | ND | ND | ND | ND | ND | ND | ND | 0.00 |
| 水及饮料类 Water and beverages | ND | ND | ND | ND | ND | ND | ND | ND | ND | ND | ND | ND | ND | ND | ND | ND | ND | ND | ND | ND | ND | ND | ND | ND | 0.00 |

续表

| 膳食类别 Category | 黑龙江 HL | 辽宁 LN | 河北 HE | 北京 BJ | 吉林 JL | 山西 SX | 陕西 SN | 河南 HA | 宁夏 NX | 内蒙古 NM | 青海 QH | 甘肃 GS | 上海 SH | 福建 FJ | 江西 JX | 江苏 JS | 浙江 ZJ | 山东 SD | 湖北 HB | 四川 SC | 广西 GX | 湖南 HN | 广东 GD | 贵州 GZ | 全国平均 AVG |
|---|---|---|---|---|---|---|---|---|---|---|---|---|---|---|---|---|---|---|---|---|---|---|---|---|---|
| 酒类 Alcohol beverages | 0.09 | 0.25 | 0.13 | 0.34 | 0.12 | ND | ND | 0.30 | ND | ND | 0.11 | ND | 0.42 | 0.14 | ND | 0.25 | 0.44 | 1.42 | ND | 0.14 | 17.01 | 0.07 | 0.32 | 0.14 | 0.90 |

注：未检出（ND）按 0 计
Note: values not detected (ND) were treated as being equal to 0

附表 4-145　第六次中国总膳食研究膳食样品中咯菌腈的含量（单位：μg/kg）
Annexed Table 4-145　Levels of fludioxonil in food samples from the 6<sup>th</sup> China TDS (Unit: μg/kg)

| 膳食类别 Category | 黑龙江 HL | 辽宁 LN | 河北 HE | 北京 BJ | 吉林 JL | 山西 SX | 陕西 SN | 河南 HA | 宁夏 NX | 内蒙古 NM | 青海 QH | 甘肃 GS | 上海 SH | 福建 FJ | 江西 JX | 江苏 JS | 浙江 ZJ | 山东 SD | 湖北 HB | 四川 SC | 广西 GX | 湖南 HN | 广东 GD | 贵州 GZ | 全国平均 AVG |
|---|---|---|---|---|---|---|---|---|---|---|---|---|---|---|---|---|---|---|---|---|---|---|---|---|---|
| 谷类 Cereals | ND | ND | ND | ND | ND | ND | ND | ND | ND | ND | ND | ND | ND | ND | ND | ND | ND | ND | ND | ND | ND | ND | ND | ND | 0.00 |
| 豆类 Legumes | ND | ND | ND | ND | ND | ND | ND | ND | ND | ND | ND | ND | ND | ND | ND | ND | ND | ND | ND | ND | ND | ND | ND | ND | 0.00 |
| 薯类 Potatoes | ND | ND | ND | ND | ND | ND | ND | ND | ND | ND | ND | ND | ND | ND | ND | ND | ND | ND | ND | ND | ND | ND | ND | ND | 0.00 |
| 肉类 Meats | ND | ND | ND | ND | ND | ND | ND | ND | ND | ND | ND | ND | ND | ND | ND | ND | ND | ND | ND | ND | ND | ND | ND | ND | 0.00 |
| 蛋类 Eggs | ND | ND | ND | ND | ND | ND | ND | ND | ND | ND | ND | ND | ND | ND | ND | ND | ND | ND | ND | ND | ND | ND | ND | ND | 0.00 |
| 水产类 Aquatic foods | ND | ND | ND | ND | ND | ND | ND | ND | ND | ND | ND | ND | ND | ND | ND | ND | ND | ND | ND | ND | ND | ND | ND | ND | 0.00 |
| 乳类 Dairy products | ND | ND | ND | ND | ND | ND | ND | ND | ND | ND | ND | ND | ND | ND | ND | ND | ND | ND | ND | ND | ND | ND | ND | ND | 0.00 |

续表

| 膳食类别<br>Category | 黑龙江<br>HL | 辽宁<br>LN | 河北<br>HE | 北京<br>BJ | 吉林<br>JL | 山西<br>SX | 陕西<br>SN | 河南<br>HA | 宁夏<br>NX | 内蒙古<br>NM | 青海<br>QH | 甘肃<br>GS | 上海<br>SH | 福建<br>FJ | 江西<br>JX | 江苏<br>JS | 浙江<br>ZJ | 山东<br>SD | 湖北<br>HB | 四川<br>SC | 广西<br>GX | 湖南<br>HN | 广东<br>GD | 贵州<br>GZ | 全国平均<br>AVG |
|---|---|---|---|---|---|---|---|---|---|---|---|---|---|---|---|---|---|---|---|---|---|---|---|---|---|
| 蔬菜类 Vegetables | ND | ND | ND | ND | ND | ND | ND | ND | ND | ND | ND | ND | ND | ND | ND | ND | ND | ND | ND | ND | ND | ND | ND | ND | 0.00 |
| 水果类 Fruits | ND | ND | 0.38 | ND | ND | ND | ND | 0.06 | ND | ND | ND | ND | 1.80 | ND | ND | ND | ND | ND | ND | ND | ND | ND | ND | ND | 0.09 |
| 糖类 Sugar | ND | ND | ND | ND | ND | ND | ND | ND | ND | ND | ND | ND | ND | ND | ND | ND | ND | ND | ND | ND | ND | ND | ND | ND | 0.00 |
| 水及饮料类 Water and beverages | ND | ND | ND | ND | ND | ND | ND | ND | ND | ND | ND | ND | ND | ND | ND | ND | ND | ND | ND | ND | ND | ND | ND | ND | 0.00 |
| 酒类 Alcohol beverages | ND | ND | ND | ND | ND | ND | ND | ND | ND | ND | ND | ND | ND | ND | ND | ND | ND | ND | ND | ND | ND | ND | ND | ND | 0.00 |

注：未检出（ND）按 0 计

Note: values not detected (ND) were treated as being equal to 0

附表 4-146　第六次中国总膳食研究的甲霜灵膳食摄入量 [单位：ng/(kg bw・d)]

Annexed Table 4-146　Dietary intakes of metalaxyl from the 6$^{th}$ China TDS [Unit: ng/(kg bw・d)]

| 膳食类别<br>Category | 黑龙江<br>HL | 辽宁<br>LN | 河北<br>HE | 北京<br>BJ | 吉林<br>JL | 山西<br>SX | 陕西<br>SN | 河南<br>HA | 宁夏<br>NX | 内蒙古<br>NM | 青海<br>QH | 甘肃<br>GS | 上海<br>SH | 福建<br>FJ | 江西<br>JX | 江苏<br>JS | 浙江<br>ZJ | 山东<br>SD | 湖北<br>HB | 四川<br>SC | 广西<br>GX | 湖南<br>HN | 广东<br>GD | 贵州<br>GZ | 全国平均<br>AVG |
|---|---|---|---|---|---|---|---|---|---|---|---|---|---|---|---|---|---|---|---|---|---|---|---|---|---|
| 谷类 Cereals | 0.000 | 0.000 | 0.000 | 0.000 | 0.000 | 0.000 | 0.000 | 0.000 | 0.000 | 0.000 | 0.000 | 0.000 | 0.000 | 0.000 | 0.000 | 0.000 | 0.000 | 0.000 | 0.000 | 0.000 | 0.000 | 0.000 | 0.000 | 0.000 | 0.000 |
| 豆类 Legumes | 0.000 | 0.000 | 0.000 | 0.000 | 0.000 | 0.000 | 0.757 | 0.000 | 0.000 | 0.285 | 0.307 | 0.000 | 0.000 | 0.000 | 0.000 | 1.427 | 0.313 | 0.000 | 0.000 | 0.000 | 0.000 | 0.000 | 0.000 | 0.000 | 0.013 |
| 薯类 Potatoes | 0.000 | 0.000 | 0.000 | 0.000 | 0.000 | 0.000 | 0.000 | 0.000 | 0.000 | 0.000 | 0.000 | 0.000 | 0.000 | 0.000 | 0.000 | 0.000 | 0.000 | 0.346 | 0.000 | 0.000 | 0.000 | 0.000 | 0.000 | 0.065 | 0.133 |

续表

| 膳食类别 Category | 黑龙江 HL | 辽宁 LN | 河北 HE | 北京 BJ | 吉林 JL | 山西 SX | 陕西 SN | 河南 HA | 宁夏 NX | 内蒙古 NM | 青海 QH | 甘肃 GS | 上海 SH | 福建 FJ | 江西 JX | 江苏 JS | 浙江 ZJ | 山东 SD | 湖北 HB | 四川 SC | 广西 GX | 湖南 HN | 广东 GD | 贵州 GZ | 全国平均 AVG |
|---|---|---|---|---|---|---|---|---|---|---|---|---|---|---|---|---|---|---|---|---|---|---|---|---|---|
| 肉类 Meats | 0.000 | 0.000 | 0.000 | 0.000 | 0.000 | 0.887 | 0.000 | 0.000 | 0.000 | 0.000 | 0.000 | 0.000 | 0.000 | 0.000 | 0.000 | 0.122 | 0.704 | 0.000 | 0.429 | 0.235 | 0.000 | 0.000 | 0.000 | 0.000 | 0.099 |
| 蛋类 Eggs | 0.000 | 0.000 | 0.000 | 0.000 | 0.000 | 0.000 | 0.000 | 0.000 | 0.000 | 0.044 | 0.000 | 0.000 | 0.000 | 0.000 | 0.000 | 0.000 | 0.000 | 0.000 | 0.202 | 0.000 | 0.000 | 0.000 | 0.000 | 0.000 | 0.010 |
| 水产类 Aquatic foods | 0.021 | 0.000 | 0.000 | 0.042 | 0.000 | 0.011 | 0.000 | 0.000 | 0.000 | 0.000 | 0.000 | 0.000 | 0.000 | 0.000 | 0.000 | 0.000 | 0.213 | 0.000 | 0.340 | 0.010 | 0.000 | 0.000 | 0.000 | 0.000 | 0.027 |
| 乳类 Dairy products | 0.000 | 0.000 | 0.000 | 0.000 | 0.000 | 0.000 | 0.000 | 0.000 | 0.000 | 0.000 | 0.000 | 0.000 | 0.000 | 0.000 | 0.000 | 0.000 | 0.000 | 0.000 | 0.000 | 0.000 | 0.000 | 0.000 | 0.000 | 0.000 | 0.000 |
| 蔬菜类 Vegetables | 7.382 | 1.109 | 1.603 | 11.550 | 7.707 | 3.253 | 1.201 | 5.220 | 0.296 | 2.243 | 7.434 | 35.890 | 29.220 | 1.287 | 10.990 | 71.790 | 2.476 | 3.378 | 8.328 | 4.066 | 37.910 | 92.490 | 95.730 | 23.880 | 19.440 |
| 水果类 Fruits | 0.000 | 0.000 | 0.000 | 0.274 | 0.000 | 0.000 | 0.438 | 0.000 | 0.000 | 0.196 | 0.000 | 0.000 | 0.000 | 1.623 | 0.000 | 0.000 | 0.000 | 0.293 | 0.025 | 0.000 | 0.210 | 0.000 | 0.801 | 0.028 | 0.162 |
| 糖类 Sugar | 0.000 | 0.000 | 0.000 | 0.000 | 0.000 | 0.000 | 0.000 | 0.000 | 0.000 | 0.000 | 0.000 | 0.000 | 0.063 | 0.000 | 0.000 | 0.000 | 0.000 | 0.000 | 0.000 | 0.000 | 0.000 | 0.000 | 0.000 | 0.000 | 0.003 |
| 水及饮料类 Water and beverages | 0.000 | 0.000 | 0.000 | 0.000 | 0.000 | 0.000 | 0.000 | 0.000 | 0.000 | 0.000 | 0.000 | 0.000 | 0.000 | 0.000 | 0.000 | 0.000 | 0.000 | 0.000 | 0.000 | 0.000 | 0.000 | 0.000 | 0.000 | 0.000 | 0.000 |
| 酒类 Alcohol beverages | 0.000 | 0.000 | 0.000 | 0.069 | 0.000 | 0.000 | 0.000 | 0.000 | 0.000 | 0.000 | 0.000 | 0.000 | 0.080 | 0.000 | 0.000 | 0.036 | 0.245 | 0.514 | 0.000 | 0.000 | 1.398 | 0.000 | 0.003 | 0.000 | 0.098 |
| 合计 SUM | 7.403 | 1.109 | 1.603 | 11.939 | 7.707 | 4.151 | 2.396 | 5.220 | 0.296 | 2.768 | 7.740 | 35.894 | 29.360 | 2.910 | 10.992 | 73.379 | 3.951 | 4.530 | 9.324 | 4.311 | 39.523 | 92.492 | 96.532 | 23.972 | 19.979 |

附表 4-147 第六次中国总膳食研究的环酰菌胺膳食摄入量 [单位: ng/(kg bw·d)]
Annexed Table 4-147 Dietary intakes of fenhexamid from the 6$^{th}$ China TDS [Unit: ng/(kg bw·d)]

| 膳食类别<br>Category | 黑龙江<br>HL | 辽宁<br>LN | 河北<br>HE | 北京<br>BJ | 吉林<br>JL | 山西<br>SX | 陕西<br>SN | 河南<br>HA | 宁夏<br>NX | 内蒙古<br>NM | 青海<br>QH | 甘肃<br>GS | 上海<br>SH | 福建<br>FJ | 江西<br>JX | 江苏<br>JS | 浙江<br>ZJ | 山东<br>SD | 湖北<br>HB | 四川<br>SC | 广西<br>GX | 湖南<br>HN | 广东<br>GD | 贵州<br>GZ | 全国平均<br>AVG |
|---|---|---|---|---|---|---|---|---|---|---|---|---|---|---|---|---|---|---|---|---|---|---|---|---|---|
| 谷类 Cereals | 0.000 | 0.000 | 0.000 | 0.000 | 0.000 | 0.000 | 0.000 | 0.000 | 0.000 | 0.000 | 0.000 | 0.000 | 0.000 | 0.000 | 0.000 | 0.000 | 0.000 | 0.000 | 0.000 | 0.000 | 0.000 | 0.000 | 0.000 | 0.000 | 0.000 |
| 豆类 Legumes | 0.000 | 0.000 | 0.000 | 0.000 | 0.000 | 0.000 | 0.000 | 0.000 | 0.000 | 0.000 | 0.000 | 0.000 | 0.000 | 0.000 | 0.000 | 0.000 | 0.000 | 0.000 | 0.000 | 0.000 | 0.000 | 0.000 | 0.000 | 0.000 | 0.000 |
| 薯类 Potatoes | 0.000 | 0.000 | 0.000 | 0.000 | 0.000 | 0.000 | 0.000 | 0.000 | 0.000 | 0.000 | 0.000 | 0.000 | 0.000 | 0.000 | 0.000 | 0.000 | 0.000 | 0.000 | 0.000 | 0.000 | 0.000 | 0.000 | 0.000 | 0.000 | 0.000 |
| 肉类 Meats | 0.000 | 0.000 | 0.000 | 0.000 | 0.000 | 0.000 | 0.000 | 0.000 | 0.000 | 0.000 | 0.000 | 0.000 | 0.000 | 0.000 | 0.000 | 0.000 | 0.000 | 0.000 | 0.000 | 0.000 | 0.000 | 0.000 | 0.000 | 0.000 | 0.000 |
| 蛋类 Eggs | 0.000 | 0.000 | 0.000 | 0.000 | 0.000 | 0.000 | 0.000 | 0.000 | 0.000 | 0.000 | 0.000 | 0.000 | 0.000 | 0.000 | 0.000 | 0.000 | 0.000 | 0.000 | 0.000 | 0.000 | 0.000 | 0.000 | 0.000 | 0.000 | 0.000 |
| 水产类 Aquatic foods | 0.000 | 0.000 | 0.000 | 0.000 | 0.000 | 0.000 | 0.000 | 0.000 | 0.000 | 0.000 | 0.000 | 0.000 | 0.000 | 0.000 | 0.000 | 0.000 | 0.000 | 0.000 | 0.000 | 0.000 | 0.000 | 0.000 | 0.000 | 0.000 | 0.000 |
| 乳类 Dairy products | 0.000 | 0.000 | 0.000 | 0.000 | 0.000 | 0.000 | 0.000 | 0.000 | 0.000 | 0.000 | 0.000 | 0.000 | 0.000 | 0.000 | 0.000 | 0.000 | 0.000 | 0.000 | 0.000 | 0.000 | 0.000 | 0.000 | 0.000 | 0.000 | 0.000 |
| 蔬菜类 Vegetables | 0.000 | 0.000 | 0.000 | 0.000 | 0.000 | 0.000 | 0.000 | 0.000 | 0.000 | 0.000 | 0.000 | 0.000 | 0.000 | 0.000 | 0.000 | 0.000 | 0.000 | 0.000 | 0.000 | 0.000 | 0.000 | 0.000 | 0.000 | 0.000 | 0.000 |
| 水果类 Fruits | 0.000 | 0.000 | 0.000 | 0.000 | 0.000 | 0.000 | 0.000 | 0.000 | 0.000 | 0.000 | 0.000 | 0.000 | 0.548 | 0.000 | 0.000 | 0.000 | 0.000 | 0.000 | 0.000 | 0.000 | 0.000 | 0.000 | 0.000 | 0.000 | 0.023 |
| 糖类 Sugar | 0.000 | 0.000 | 0.000 | 0.000 | 0.000 | 0.000 | 0.000 | 0.000 | 0.000 | 0.000 | 0.000 | 0.000 | 0.000 | 0.000 | 0.000 | 0.000 | 0.000 | 0.000 | 0.000 | 0.000 | 0.000 | 0.000 | 0.000 | 0.000 | 0.000 |
| 水及饮料类 Water and beverages | 0.000 | 0.000 | 0.000 | 0.000 | 0.000 | 0.000 | 0.000 | 0.000 | 0.000 | 0.000 | 0.000 | 0.000 | 0.000 | 0.000 | 0.000 | 0.000 | 0.000 | 0.000 | 0.000 | 0.000 | 0.000 | 0.000 | 0.000 | 0.000 | 0.000 |

续表

| 膳食类别 Category | 黑龙江 HL | 辽宁 LN | 河北 HE | 北京 BJ | 吉林 JL | 山西 SX | 陕西 SN | 河南 HA | 宁夏 NX | 内蒙古 NM | 青海 QH | 甘肃 GS | 上海 SH | 福建 FJ | 江西 JX | 江苏 JS | 浙江 ZJ | 山东 SD | 湖北 HB | 四川 SC | 广西 GX | 湖南 HN | 广东 GD | 贵州 GZ | 全国平均 AVG |
|---|---|---|---|---|---|---|---|---|---|---|---|---|---|---|---|---|---|---|---|---|---|---|---|---|---|
| 酒类 Alcohol beverages | 0.000 | 0.000 | 0.000 | 0.000 | 0.000 | 0.000 | 0.000 | 0.000 | 0.000 | 0.000 | 0.000 | 0.000 | 0.000 | 0.000 | 0.000 | 0.000 | 0.000 | 0.000 | 0.000 | 0.000 | 0.000 | 0.000 | 0.000 | 0.000 | 0.000 |
| 合计 SUM | 0.000 | 0.000 | 0.000 | 0.000 | 0.000 | 0.000 | 0.000 | 0.000 | 0.000 | 0.000 | 0.000 | 0.000 | 0.548 | 0.000 | 0.000 | 0.000 | 0.000 | 0.000 | 0.000 | 0.000 | 0.000 | 0.000 | 0.000 | 0.000 | 0.023 |

附表 4-148 第六次中国总膳食研究的嘧霉胺膳食摄入量 [单位: ng/(kg bw · d)]

Annexed Table 4-148 Dietary intakes of pyrimethanil from the 6$^{th}$ China TDS [Unit: ng/(kg bw · d)]

| 膳食类别 Category | 黑龙江 HL | 辽宁 LN | 河北 HE | 北京 BJ | 吉林 JL | 山西 SX | 陕西 SN | 河南 HA | 宁夏 NX | 内蒙古 NM | 青海 QH | 甘肃 GS | 上海 SH | 福建 FJ | 江西 JX | 江苏 JS | 浙江 ZJ | 山东 SD | 湖北 HB | 四川 SC | 广西 GX | 湖南 HN | 广东 GD | 贵州 GZ | 全国平均 AVG |
|---|---|---|---|---|---|---|---|---|---|---|---|---|---|---|---|---|---|---|---|---|---|---|---|---|---|
| 谷类 Cereals | 0.000 | 2.948 | 0.000 | 0.000 | 0.000 | 0.000 | 0.000 | 0.000 | 0.000 | 0.000 | 0.000 | 0.000 | 0.000 | 0.000 | 0.000 | 0.000 | 0.000 | 0.000 | 0.000 | 0.000 | 0.000 | 0.000 | 0.000 | 0.000 | 0.123 |
| 豆类 Legumes | 0.000 | 0.000 | 0.000 | 0.000 | 0.000 | 0.000 | 0.000 | 0.000 | 0.000 | 0.000 | 0.000 | 0.000 | 0.000 | 0.000 | 0.000 | 0.000 | 0.000 | 0.000 | 0.000 | 0.000 | 0.000 | 0.000 | 0.000 | 0.000 | 0.000 |
| 薯类 Potatoes | 0.000 | 0.000 | 0.131 | 0.000 | 0.000 | 0.000 | 0.000 | 0.000 | 0.000 | 0.000 | 0.000 | 0.000 | 0.106 | 0.000 | 0.000 | 0.000 | 0.000 | 0.000 | 0.000 | 0.000 | 0.000 | 0.000 | 0.000 | 0.000 | 0.010 |
| 肉类 Meats | 0.000 | 0.000 | 0.000 | 0.000 | 0.000 | 0.000 | 0.000 | 0.000 | 0.000 | 0.000 | 0.000 | 0.000 | 0.000 | 0.000 | 0.000 | 0.000 | 0.000 | 0.000 | 0.000 | 0.000 | 0.000 | 0.000 | 0.071 | 0.000 | 0.003 |
| 蛋类 Eggs | 0.000 | 0.000 | 0.000 | 0.000 | 0.000 | 0.000 | 0.000 | 0.000 | 0.000 | 0.000 | 0.000 | 0.018 | 0.000 | 0.000 | 0.000 | 0.000 | 0.000 | 0.000 | 0.000 | 0.000 | 0.000 | 0.000 | 0.000 | 0.000 | 0.000 |
| 水产类 Aquatic foods | 0.000 | 0.043 | 0.000 | 0.000 | 0.000 | 0.000 | 0.000 | 0.000 | 0.000 | 0.000 | 0.000 | 0.000 | 0.000 | 0.000 | 0.000 | 0.103 | 0.060 | 0.000 | 0.000 | 0.000 | 0.000 | 0.000 | 0.079 | 0.000 | 0.013 |
| 乳类 Dairy products | 0.000 | 0.000 | 0.000 | 0.000 | 0.000 | 0.000 | 0.000 | 0.000 | 0.000 | 0.000 | 0.000 | 0.000 | 0.000 | 0.000 | 0.000 | 0.022 | 0.000 | 0.000 | 0.000 | 0.000 | 0.000 | 0.000 | 0.000 | 0.000 | 0.001 |

续表

| 膳食类别<br>Category | 黑龙江<br>HL | 辽宁<br>LN | 河北<br>HE | 北京<br>BJ | 吉林<br>JL | 山西<br>SX | 陕西<br>SN | 河南<br>HA | 宁夏<br>NX | 内蒙古<br>NM | 青海<br>QH | 甘肃<br>GS | 上海<br>SH | 福建<br>FJ | 江西<br>JX | 江苏<br>JS | 浙江<br>ZJ | 山东<br>SD | 湖北<br>HB | 四川<br>SC | 广西<br>GX | 湖南<br>HN | 广东<br>GD | 贵州<br>GZ | 全国平均<br>AVG |
|---|---|---|---|---|---|---|---|---|---|---|---|---|---|---|---|---|---|---|---|---|---|---|---|---|---|
| 蔬菜类 Vegetables | 0.000 | 0.000 | 3.503 | 5.994 | 0.850 | 1.951 | 5.237 | 0.440 | 0.593 | 0.422 | 3.902 | 514.200 | 6.544 | 1.343 | 1.255 | 1.625 | 0.607 | 27.120 | 8.241 | 12.560 | 1.324 | 102.700 | 33.020 | 1.126 | 30.610 |
| 水果类 Fruits | 0.267 | 5.565 | 1.279 | 0.299 | 6.842 | 0.000 | 0.000 | 0.351 | 0.108 | 0.623 | 0.194 | 0.032 | 5.716 | 11.310 | 0.000 | 0.082 | 15.600 | 0.036 | 2.725 | 1.721 | 0.000 | 0.000 | 1.474 | 0.000 | 2.259 |
| 糖类 Sugar | 0.000 | 0.000 | 0.000 | 0.000 | 0.000 | 0.000 | 0.000 | 0.000 | 0.000 | 0.000 | 0.000 | 0.000 | 0.000 | 0.000 | 0.000 | 0.000 | 0.000 | 0.000 | 0.000 | 0.000 | 0.000 | 0.000 | 0.000 | 0.000 | 0.000 |
| 水及饮料类 Water and beverages | 0.000 | 0.000 | 0.000 | 0.000 | 0.000 | 0.000 | 0.000 | 0.048 | 0.000 | 0.000 | 0.000 | 0.000 | 0.044 | 0.000 | 0.000 | 0.000 | 0.000 | 0.000 | 0.000 | 0.000 | 0.528 | 0.000 | 0.001 | 0.000 | 0.026 |
| 酒类 Alcohol beverages | 0.000 | 0.000 | 0.000 | 0.000 | 0.000 | 0.000 | 0.000 | 0.048 | 0.000 | 0.000 | 0.000 | 0.000 | 0.044 | 0.000 | 0.000 | 0.000 | 0.000 | 0.000 | 0.000 | 0.000 | 0.528 | 0.000 | 0.001 | 0.000 | 0.026 |
| 合计 SUM | 0.267 | 8.556 | 4.913 | 6.293 | 7.692 | 1.951 | 5.237 | 0.839 | 0.701 | 1.045 | 4.097 | 514.299 | 12.410 | 12.656 | 1.255 | 1.831 | 16.269 | 27.159 | 10.966 | 14.277 | 1.853 | 102.695 | 34.649 | 1.126 | 33.043 |

附表 4-149 第六次中国总膳食研究的乙嘧酚磺酸酯膳食摄入量 [单位：ng/(kg bw·d)]
Annexed Table 4-149 Dietary intakes of bupirimate from the 6$^{th}$ China TDS [Unit: ng/(kg bw·d)]

| 膳食类别<br>Category | 黑龙江<br>HL | 辽宁<br>LN | 河北<br>HE | 北京<br>BJ | 吉林<br>JL | 山西<br>SX | 陕西<br>SN | 河南<br>HA | 宁夏<br>NX | 内蒙古<br>NM | 青海<br>QH | 甘肃<br>GS | 上海<br>SH | 福建<br>FJ | 江西<br>JX | 江苏<br>JS | 浙江<br>ZJ | 山东<br>SD | 湖北<br>HB | 四川<br>SC | 广西<br>GX | 湖南<br>HN | 广东<br>GD | 贵州<br>GZ | 全国平均<br>AVG |
|---|---|---|---|---|---|---|---|---|---|---|---|---|---|---|---|---|---|---|---|---|---|---|---|---|---|
| 谷类 Cereals | 0.000 | 0.000 | 0.000 | 0.000 | 0.000 | 0.000 | 0.000 | 0.000 | 0.000 | 0.000 | 0.000 | 0.000 | 0.000 | 0.000 | 0.000 | 0.000 | 0.000 | 0.000 | 0.000 | 0.000 | 0.000 | 0.000 | 0.000 | 0.000 | 0.000 |
| 豆类 Legumes | 0.000 | 0.000 | 0.000 | 0.000 | 0.000 | 0.000 | 0.000 | 0.000 | 0.000 | 0.000 | 0.000 | 0.000 | 0.000 | 0.000 | 0.000 | 0.000 | 0.000 | 0.000 | 0.000 | 0.000 | 0.000 | 0.000 | 0.000 | 0.000 | 0.000 |
| 薯类 Potatoes | 0.000 | 0.000 | 0.000 | 0.000 | 0.000 | 0.000 | 0.000 | 0.000 | 0.000 | 0.000 | 0.000 | 0.000 | 0.000 | 0.000 | 0.000 | 0.000 | 0.045 | 0.000 | 0.000 | 0.000 | 0.000 | 0.000 | 0.000 | 0.000 | 0.002 |

续表

| 膳食类别<br>Category | 黑龙江<br>HL | 辽宁<br>LN | 河北<br>HE | 北京<br>BJ | 吉林<br>JL | 山西<br>SX | 陕西<br>SN | 河南<br>HA | 宁夏<br>NX | 内蒙古<br>NM | 青海<br>QH | 甘肃<br>GS | 上海<br>SH | 福建<br>FJ | 江西<br>JX | 江苏<br>JS | 浙江<br>ZJ | 山东<br>SD | 湖北<br>HB | 四川<br>SC | 广西<br>GX | 湖南<br>HN | 广东<br>GD | 贵州<br>GZ | 全国平均<br>AVG |
|---|---|---|---|---|---|---|---|---|---|---|---|---|---|---|---|---|---|---|---|---|---|---|---|---|---|
| 肉类 Meats | 0.000 | 0.000 | 0.000 | 0.000 | 0.000 | 0.000 | 0.000 | 0.000 | 0.000 | 0.000 | 0.000 | 0.000 | 0.000 | 0.000 | 0.000 | 0.000 | 0.000 | 0.000 | 0.000 | 0.000 | 0.000 | 0.000 | 0.000 | 0.000 | 0.000 |
| 蛋类 Eggs | 0.000 | 0.000 | 0.000 | 0.000 | 0.000 | 0.000 | 0.000 | 0.000 | 0.000 | 0.000 | 0.000 | 0.000 | 0.000 | 0.000 | 0.000 | 0.000 | 0.000 | 0.000 | 0.000 | 0.000 | 0.000 | 0.000 | 0.000 | 0.000 | 0.000 |
| 水产类 Aquatic foods | 0.000 | 0.000 | 0.000 | 0.000 | 0.000 | 0.000 | 0.000 | 0.000 | 0.000 | 0.000 | 0.006 | 0.000 | 0.000 | 0.000 | 0.000 | 0.000 | 0.000 | 0.000 | 0.000 | 0.000 | 0.000 | 0.000 | 0.000 | 0.000 | 0.000 |
| 乳类 Dairy products | 0.000 | 0.000 | 0.000 | 0.000 | 0.000 | 0.000 | 0.000 | 0.000 | 0.000 | 0.000 | 0.000 | 0.000 | 0.000 | 0.000 | 0.000 | 0.000 | 0.000 | 0.000 | 0.000 | 0.000 | 0.000 | 0.000 | 0.000 | 0.000 | 0.000 |
| 蔬菜类 Vegetables | 0.000 | 0.000 | 0.000 | 0.000 | 2.617 | 0.000 | 0.000 | 0.000 | 0.000 | 0.000 | 8.797 | 0.000 | 0.000 | 0.000 | 0.000 | 0.000 | 0.000 | 0.000 | 0.000 | 0.000 | 0.000 | 0.000 | 0.000 | 0.000 | 0.476 |
| 水果类 Fruits | 0.000 | 0.000 | 0.000 | 0.000 | 0.000 | 0.000 | 0.000 | 0.000 | 0.000 | 0.000 | 0.000 | 0.000 | 0.000 | 0.000 | 0.000 | 0.000 | 0.000 | 0.099 | 0.000 | 0.000 | 0.000 | 0.000 | 0.000 | 0.000 | 0.004 |
| 糖类 Sugar | 0.000 | 0.000 | 0.000 | 0.000 | 0.000 | 0.000 | 0.000 | 0.000 | 0.000 | 0.000 | 0.000 | 0.000 | 0.000 | 0.000 | 0.000 | 0.000 | 0.000 | 0.000 | 0.000 | 0.000 | 0.000 | 0.000 | 0.000 | 0.000 | 0.000 |
| 水及饮料类 Water and beverages | 0.000 | 0.000 | 0.000 | 0.000 | 0.000 | 0.000 | 0.000 | 0.000 | 0.000 | 0.000 | 0.000 | 0.000 | 0.000 | 0.000 | 0.000 | 0.000 | 0.000 | 0.000 | 0.000 | 0.000 | 0.000 | 0.000 | 0.000 | 0.000 | 0.000 |
| 酒类 Alcohol beverages | 0.000 | 0.000 | 0.000 | 0.000 | 0.000 | 0.000 | 0.000 | 0.000 | 0.000 | 0.000 | 0.000 | 0.000 | 0.000 | 0.000 | 0.000 | 0.000 | 0.000 | 0.000 | 0.000 | 0.000 | 0.000 | 0.000 | 0.000 | 0.000 | 0.000 |
| 合计 SUM | 0.000 | 0.000 | 0.000 | 0.000 | 2.617 | 0.000 | 0.000 | 0.000 | 0.000 | 0.000 | 8.803 | 0.000 | 0.000 | 0.000 | 0.000 | 0.000 | 0.045 | 0.099 | 0.000 | 0.000 | 0.000 | 0.000 | 0.000 | 0.000 | 0.482 |

附表 4-150 第六次中国总膳食研究的嘧菌环胺膳食摄入量 [单位：ng/(kg bw·d)]

Annexed Table 4-150　Dietary intakes of cyprodinil from the 6<sup>th</sup> China TDS [Unit: ng/(kg bw·d)]

| 膳食类别 Category | 黑龙江 HL | 辽宁 LN | 河北 HE | 北京 BJ | 吉林 JL | 山西 SX | 陕西 SN | 河南 HA | 宁夏 NX | 内蒙古 NM | 青海 QH | 甘肃 GS | 上海 SH | 福建 FJ | 江西 JX | 江苏 JS | 浙江 ZJ | 山东 SD | 湖北 HB | 四川 SC | 广西 GX | 湖南 HN | 广东 GD | 贵州 GZ | 全国平均 AVG |
|---|---|---|---|---|---|---|---|---|---|---|---|---|---|---|---|---|---|---|---|---|---|---|---|---|---|
| 谷类 Cereals | 0.000 | 0.000 | 0.000 | 0.000 | 0.000 | 0.000 | 0.000 | 0.000 | 0.000 | 0.000 | 0.000 | 0.000 | 0.000 | 0.000 | 0.000 | 0.000 | 0.000 | 0.000 | 0.000 | 0.000 | 0.000 | 0.000 | 0.000 | 0.000 | 0.000 |
| 豆类 Legumes | 0.000 | 0.000 | 0.000 | 0.000 | 0.000 | 0.000 | 0.000 | 0.000 | 0.000 | 0.000 | 0.000 | 0.000 | 0.000 | 0.000 | 0.000 | 0.000 | 0.000 | 0.000 | 0.000 | 0.000 | 0.000 | 0.000 | 0.000 | 0.000 | 0.000 |
| 薯类 Potatoes | 0.000 | 0.000 | 0.000 | 0.000 | 0.000 | 0.000 | 0.000 | 0.000 | 0.000 | 0.000 | 0.000 | 0.000 | 0.000 | 0.000 | 0.000 | 0.000 | 0.000 | 0.000 | 0.000 | 0.000 | 0.000 | 0.000 | 0.000 | 0.000 | 0.000 |
| 肉类 Meats | 0.000 | 0.000 | 0.062 | 0.000 | 0.000 | 0.000 | 0.000 | 0.000 | 0.000 | 0.000 | 0.000 | 0.000 | 0.000 | 0.000 | 0.000 | 0.000 | 0.000 | 0.000 | 0.000 | 0.000 | 0.000 | 0.000 | 0.000 | 0.000 | 0.003 |
| 蛋类 Eggs | 0.000 | 0.000 | 0.000 | 0.000 | 0.000 | 0.000 | 0.000 | 0.000 | 0.000 | 0.000 | 0.000 | 0.000 | 0.000 | 0.000 | 0.000 | 0.000 | 0.000 | 0.000 | 0.000 | 0.000 | 0.000 | 0.000 | 0.000 | 0.000 | 0.000 |
| 水产类 Aquatic foods | 0.000 | 0.000 | 0.000 | 0.000 | 0.000 | 0.000 | 0.000 | 0.000 | 0.000 | 0.000 | 0.000 | 0.000 | 0.000 | 0.000 | 0.000 | 0.000 | 0.000 | 0.000 | 0.000 | 0.000 | 0.000 | 0.000 | 0.000 | 0.000 | 0.000 |
| 乳类 Dairy products | 0.000 | 0.000 | 0.000 | 0.000 | 0.000 | 0.000 | 0.000 | 0.000 | 0.000 | 0.000 | 0.000 | 0.000 | 0.000 | 0.000 | 0.000 | 0.000 | 0.000 | 0.000 | 0.000 | 0.000 | 0.000 | 0.000 | 0.000 | 0.000 | 0.000 |
| 蔬菜类 Vegetables | 0.000 | 0.000 | 0.000 | 0.508 | 0.000 | 0.000 | 0.000 | 1.372 | 0.585 | 0.000 | 0.000 | 0.000 | 0.000 | 0.000 | 0.000 | 0.000 | 0.000 | 0.000 | 0.000 | 0.000 | 0.000 | 0.000 | 1.540 | 0.000 | 0.167 |
| 水果类 Fruits | 0.000 | 0.000 | 2.452 | 0.000 | 0.000 | 0.000 | 0.000 | 0.000 | 0.000 | 0.000 | 0.000 | 0.000 | 39.650 | 2.458 | 0.000 | 0.000 | 0.000 | 0.615 | 0.000 | 0.000 | 0.000 | 0.000 | 0.000 | 0.000 | 1.882 |
| 糖类 Sugar | 0.000 | 0.000 | 0.000 | 0.000 | 0.000 | 0.000 | 0.000 | 0.000 | 0.000 | 0.000 | 0.000 | 0.000 | 0.000 | 0.000 | 0.000 | 0.000 | 0.000 | 0.000 | 0.000 | 0.000 | 0.000 | 0.000 | 0.000 | 0.000 | 0.000 |
| 水及饮料类 Water and beverages | 0.000 | 0.000 | 0.000 | 0.000 | 0.000 | 0.000 | 0.000 | 0.000 | 0.000 | 0.000 | 0.000 | 0.000 | 0.000 | 0.000 | 0.000 | 0.000 | 0.000 | 0.000 | 0.000 | 0.000 | 0.000 | 0.000 | 0.000 | 0.000 | 0.000 |

续表

| 膳食类别 Category | 黑龙江 HL | 辽宁 LN | 河北 HE | 北京 BJ | 吉林 JL | 山西 SX | 陕西 SN | 河南 HA | 宁夏 NX | 内蒙古 NM | 青海 QH | 甘肃 GS | 上海 SH | 福建 FJ | 江西 JX | 江苏 JS | 浙江 ZJ | 山东 SD | 湖北 HB | 四川 SC | 广西 GX | 湖南 HN | 广东 GD | 贵州 GZ | 全国平均 AVG |
|---|---|---|---|---|---|---|---|---|---|---|---|---|---|---|---|---|---|---|---|---|---|---|---|---|---|
| 酒类 Alcohol beverages | 0.000 | 0.000 | 0.000 | 0.000 | 0.000 | 0.000 | 0.000 | 0.000 | 0.000 | 0.000 | 0.000 | 0.000 | 0.000 | 0.000 | 0.000 | 0.000 | 0.000 | 0.000 | 0.000 | 0.000 | 0.000 | 0.000 | 0.000 | 0.000 | 0.000 |
| 合计 SUM | 0.000 | 0.000 | 2.514 | 0.508 | 0.000 | 0.000 | 0.000 | 1.372 | 0.585 | 0.000 | 0.000 | 0.000 | 39.653 | 2.458 | 0.000 | 0.000 | 0.000 | 0.615 | 0.000 | 0.000 | 0.000 | 0.000 | 1.540 | 0.000 | 2.052 |

附表 4-151　第六次中国总膳食研究的氟吡菌胺膳食摄入量 [单位：ng/(kg bw·d)]
Annexed Table 4-151　Dietary intakes of fluopicolide from the 6th China TDS [Unit: ng/(kg bw·d)]

| 膳食类别 Category | 黑龙江 HL | 辽宁 LN | 河北 HE | 北京 BJ | 吉林 JL | 山西 SX | 陕西 SN | 河南 HA | 宁夏 NX | 内蒙古 NM | 青海 QH | 甘肃 GS | 上海 SH | 福建 FJ | 江西 JX | 江苏 JS | 浙江 ZJ | 山东 SD | 湖北 HB | 四川 SC | 广西 GX | 湖南 HN | 广东 GD | 贵州 GZ | 全国平均 AVG |
|---|---|---|---|---|---|---|---|---|---|---|---|---|---|---|---|---|---|---|---|---|---|---|---|---|---|
| 谷类 Cereals | 0.000 | 0.000 | 0.000 | 0.000 | 0.000 | 0.000 | 0.000 | 0.000 | 0.000 | 0.000 | 0.000 | 0.000 | 0.000 | 0.000 | 0.000 | 0.000 | 0.000 | 0.000 | 0.000 | 0.000 | 0.000 | 0.000 | 0.000 | 0.000 | 0.000 |
| 豆类 Legumes | 0.000 | 0.000 | 0.000 | 0.000 | 0.000 | 0.000 | 0.000 | 0.000 | 0.000 | 0.000 | 0.000 | 0.000 | 0.000 | 0.000 | 0.000 | 0.000 | 0.000 | 0.000 | 0.000 | 0.000 | 0.000 | 0.000 | 0.000 | 0.000 | 0.000 |
| 薯类 Potatoes | 0.000 | 0.000 | 0.118 | 0.000 | 0.504 | 0.000 | 0.000 | 0.171 | 0.000 | 0.000 | 0.000 | 0.000 | 0.000 | 0.000 | 0.000 | 0.000 | 0.000 | 0.000 | 0.000 | 0.000 | 0.000 | 0.000 | 0.000 | 0.000 | 0.033 |
| 肉类 Meats | 0.000 | 0.000 | 0.000 | 0.000 | 0.000 | 0.000 | 0.000 | 0.000 | 0.000 | 0.000 | 0.000 | 0.000 | 0.000 | 0.000 | 0.000 | 0.000 | 0.000 | 0.000 | 0.000 | 0.000 | 0.000 | 0.000 | 0.000 | 0.000 | 0.000 |
| 蛋类 Eggs | 0.000 | 0.000 | 0.000 | 0.000 | 0.000 | 0.000 | 0.000 | 0.000 | 0.000 | 0.000 | 0.000 | 0.000 | 0.000 | 0.000 | 0.000 | 0.000 | 0.000 | 0.000 | 0.000 | 0.000 | 0.000 | 0.000 | 0.000 | 0.000 | 0.000 |
| 水产类 Aquatic foods | 0.000 | 0.000 | 0.000 | 0.000 | 0.000 | 0.000 | 0.000 | 0.000 | 0.000 | 0.000 | 0.000 | 0.000 | 0.000 | 0.000 | 0.000 | 0.000 | 0.000 | 0.000 | 0.000 | 0.000 | 0.000 | 0.000 | 0.000 | 0.000 | 0.000 |
| 乳类 Dairy products | 0.000 | 0.000 | 0.000 | 0.000 | 0.000 | 0.042 | 0.000 | 0.000 | 0.000 | 0.000 | 0.000 | 0.000 | 0.000 | 0.000 | 0.000 | 0.000 | 0.000 | 0.000 | 0.000 | 0.000 | 0.000 | 0.000 | 0.000 | 0.000 | 0.002 |

续表

| 膳食类别 Category | 黑龙江 HL | 辽宁 LN | 河北 HE | 北京 BJ | 吉林 JL | 山西 SX | 陕西 SN | 河南 HA | 宁夏 NX | 内蒙古 NM | 青海 QH | 甘肃 GS | 上海 SH | 福建 FJ | 江西 JX | 江苏 JS | 浙江 ZJ | 山东 SD | 湖北 HB | 四川 SC | 广西 GX | 湖南 HN | 广东 GD | 贵州 GZ | 全国平均 AVG |
|---|---|---|---|---|---|---|---|---|---|---|---|---|---|---|---|---|---|---|---|---|---|---|---|---|---|
| 蔬菜类 Vegetables | 0.000 | 0.000 | 1.658 | 3.962 | 0.000 | 7.252 | 0.000 | 0.000 | 0.000 | 0.000 | 0.000 | 1.341 | 1.076 | 0.246 | 9.137 | 0.000 | 1.718 | 0.299 | 1.056 | 11.460 | 0.000 | 0.534 | 5.542 | 3.984 | 2.053 |
| 水果类 Fruits | 0.000 | 0.000 | 0.000 | 0.000 | 1.945 | 0.000 | 0.000 | 0.000 | 0.000 | 0.000 | 0.000 | 0.000 | 0.000 | 0.000 | 0.000 | 0.000 | 0.000 | 0.070 | 0.000 | 0.173 | 0.000 | 0.000 | 0.025 | 0.000 | 0.092 |
| 糖类 Sugar | 0.000 | 0.000 | 0.000 | 0.000 | 0.000 | 0.000 | 0.000 | 0.000 | 0.000 | 0.000 | 0.000 | 0.000 | 0.000 | 0.000 | 0.000 | 0.000 | 0.000 | 0.000 | 0.000 | 0.000 | 0.000 | 0.000 | 0.000 | 0.000 | 0.000 |
| 水及饮料类 Water and beverages | 0.000 | 0.000 | 0.000 | 0.000 | 0.000 | 0.000 | 0.000 | 0.000 | 0.000 | 0.000 | 0.000 | 0.000 | 0.000 | 0.000 | 0.000 | 0.000 | 0.000 | 0.000 | 0.000 | 0.000 | 0.000 | 0.000 | 0.000 | 0.000 | 0.000 |
| 酒类 Alcohol beverages | 0.000 | 0.000 | 0.000 | 0.000 | 0.000 | 0.000 | 0.000 | 0.000 | 0.000 | 0.000 | 0.000 | 0.000 | 0.000 | 0.000 | 0.000 | 0.000 | 0.000 | 0.000 | 0.000 | 0.000 | 0.000 | 0.000 | 0.000 | 0.000 | 0.000 |
| 合计 SUM | 0.000 | 0.000 | 1.776 | 3.962 | 2.449 | 7.294 | 0.000 | 0.171 | 0.000 | 0.000 | 0.000 | 1.341 | 1.076 | 0.246 | 9.137 | 0.000 | 1.718 | 0.369 | 1.056 | 11.635 | 0.000 | 0.534 | 5.566 | 3.984 | 2.180 |

附表 4-152　第六次中国总膳食研究的烯酰吗啉膳食摄入量 [单位：ng/(kg bw·d)]

Annexed Table 4-152　Dietary intakes of dimethomorph from the 6$^{th}$ China TDS [Unit: ng/(kg bw·d)]

| 膳食类别 Category | 黑龙江 HL | 辽宁 LN | 河北 HE | 北京 BJ | 吉林 JL | 山西 SX | 陕西 SN | 河南 HA | 宁夏 NX | 内蒙古 NM | 青海 QH | 甘肃 GS | 上海 SH | 福建 FJ | 江西 JX | 江苏 JS | 浙江 ZJ | 山东 SD | 湖北 HB | 四川 SC | 广西 GX | 湖南 HN | 广东 GD | 贵州 GZ | 全国平均 AVG |
|---|---|---|---|---|---|---|---|---|---|---|---|---|---|---|---|---|---|---|---|---|---|---|---|---|---|
| 谷类 Cereals | 0.000 | 0.000 | 1.118 | 0.954 | 0.000 | 0.000 | 0.000 | 1.750 | 0.000 | 0.000 | 0.000 | 0.000 | 0.000 | 0.000 | 1.179 | 0.000 | 0.000 | 0.000 | 0.094 | 0.120 | 0.000 | 0.000 | 0.000 | 0.000 | 0.208 |
| 豆类 Legumes | 0.000 | 0.000 | 0.111 | 0.000 | 0.000 | 0.000 | 0.000 | 0.070 | 0.000 | 0.000 | 0.000 | 0.430 | 0.929 | 0.046 | 0.000 | 0.000 | 0.034 | 0.051 | 0.000 | 0.000 | 0.115 | 0.000 | 0.000 | 0.110 | 0.012 |
| 薯类 Potatoes | 0.000 | 0.000 | 1.107 | 0.000 | 0.653 | 0.216 | 3.705 | 0.252 | 0.000 | 0.416 | 0.000 | 0.000 | 0.000 | 0.000 | 0.000 | 0.000 | 0.000 | 0.000 | 0.000 | 0.000 | 0.000 | 0.000 | 0.315 | 0.064 | 0.356 |

续表

| 膳食类别 Category | 黑龙江 HL | 辽宁 LN | 河北 HE | 北京 BJ | 吉林 JL | 山西 SX | 陕西 SN | 河南 HA | 宁夏 NX | 内蒙古 NM | 青海 QH | 甘肃 GS | 上海 SH | 福建 FJ | 江西 JX | 江苏 JS | 浙江 ZJ | 山东 SD | 湖北 HB | 四川 SC | 广西 GX | 湖南 HN | 广东 GD | 贵州 GZ | 全国平均 AVG |
|---|---|---|---|---|---|---|---|---|---|---|---|---|---|---|---|---|---|---|---|---|---|---|---|---|---|
| 肉类 Meats | 0.000 | 0.000 | 0.175 | 0.161 | 0.000 | 0.825 | 0.000 | 0.052 | 0.000 | 0.378 | 0.000 | 0.000 | 0.000 | 0.000 | 0.000 | 0.107 | 0.000 | 0.000 | 0.000 | 0.000 | 0.134 | 0.162 | 0.000 | 0.335 | 0.097 |
| 蛋类 Eggs | 0.000 | 0.000 | 0.053 | 0.130 | 0.000 | 0.000 | 0.000 | 0.000 | 0.000 | 0.000 | 0.000 | 0.000 | 0.000 | 0.000 | 0.000 | 0.000 | 0.000 | 0.000 | 0.000 | 0.000 | 0.000 | 0.000 | 0.000 | 0.000 | 0.008 |
| 水产类 Aquatic foods | 0.000 | 0.000 | 0.016 | 0.039 | 0.018 | 0.008 | 0.000 | 0.004 | 0.000 | 0.000 | 0.000 | 0.013 | 0.000 | 0.092 | 0.000 | 0.000 | 0.000 | 0.000 | 0.000 | 0.000 | 0.090 | 0.000 | 0.107 | 0.004 | 0.016 |
| 乳类 Dairy products | 0.000 | 0.000 | 0.000 | 0.000 | 0.000 | 0.089 | 0.000 | 0.000 | 0.000 | 0.000 | 0.000 | 0.000 | 0.000 | 0.000 | 0.000 | 0.000 | 0.000 | 0.000 | 0.000 | 0.000 | 0.000 | 0.000 | 0.000 | 0.000 | 0.004 |
| 蔬菜类 Vegetables | 1.752 | 0.443 | 48.680 | 4.509 | 0.572 | 32.480 | 9.598 | 5.072 | 4.315 | 3.473 | 138.300 | 337.300 | 581.000 | 184.200 | 279.200 | 599.200 | 12.490 | 12.290 | 1187.000 | 48.640 | 37.830 | 1531.000 | 1941.000 | 767.600 | 323.700 |
| 水果类 Fruits | 1.904 | 4.875 | 0.039 | 3.005 | 4.478 | 0.000 | 0.065 | 7.252 | 0.000 | 2.055 | 0.211 | 0.000 | 0.070 | 1.300 | 0.346 | 0.000 | 4.829 | 0.116 | 0.184 | 0.954 | 2.467 | 0.000 | 2.934 | 0.000 | 1.545 |
| 糖类 Sugar | 0.000 | 0.000 | 0.000 | 0.000 | 0.000 | 0.000 | 0.000 | 0.000 | 0.000 | 0.000 | 0.000 | 0.000 | 0.000 | 0.000 | 0.000 | 0.000 | 0.000 | 0.000 | 0.000 | 0.000 | 0.000 | 0.000 | 0.000 | 0.000 | 0.000 |
| 水及饮料类 Water and beverages | 0.000 | 0.000 | 0.000 | 0.000 | 0.000 | 0.000 | 0.000 | 0.000 | 0.000 | 0.000 | 0.000 | 0.000 | 0.000 | 0.000 | 0.000 | 0.000 | 0.000 | 0.000 | 0.000 | 0.000 | 0.000 | 0.000 | 0.000 | 0.000 | 0.000 |
| 酒类 Alcohol beverages | 0.031 | 0.132 | 0.023 | 0.149 | 0.018 | 0.000 | 0.000 | 0.015 | 0.000 | 0.000 | 0.008 | 0.000 | 0.149 | 0.031 | 0.000 | 0.147 | 0.434 | 2.562 | 0.000 | 0.012 | 8.645 | 0.018 | 0.007 | 0.005 | 0.516 |
| 合计 SUM | 3.69 | 5.45 | 51.33 | 8.95 | 5.74 | 33.62 | 13.37 | 14.47 | 4.32 | 6.32 | 138.50 | 337.74 | 582.11 | 185.70 | 280.73 | 599.50 | 17.79 | 15.02 | 1187.53 | 49.73 | 49.28 | 1530.90 | 1944.08 | 768.15 | 326.42 |

附表 4-153　第六次中国总膳食研究的咯菌腈膳食摄入量 [单位: ng/(kg bw·d)]
Annexed Table 4-153　Dietary intakes of fludioxonil from the 6th China TDS [Unit: ng/(kg bw·d)]

| 膳食类别<br>Category | 黑龙江<br>HL | 辽宁<br>LN | 河北<br>HE | 北京<br>BJ | 吉林<br>JL | 山西<br>SX | 陕西<br>SN | 河南<br>HA | 宁夏<br>NX | 内蒙古<br>NM | 青海<br>QH | 甘肃<br>GS | 上海<br>SH | 福建<br>FJ | 江西<br>JX | 江苏<br>JS | 浙江<br>ZJ | 山东<br>SD | 湖北<br>HB | 四川<br>SC | 广西<br>GX | 湖南<br>HN | 广东<br>GD | 贵州<br>GZ | 全国平均<br>AVG |
|---|---|---|---|---|---|---|---|---|---|---|---|---|---|---|---|---|---|---|---|---|---|---|---|---|---|
| 谷类 Cereals | 0.000 | 0.000 | 0.000 | 0.000 | 0.000 | 0.000 | 0.000 | 0.000 | 0.000 | 0.000 | 0.000 | 0.000 | 0.000 | 0.000 | 0.000 | 0.000 | 0.000 | 0.000 | 0.000 | 0.000 | 0.000 | 0.000 | 0.000 | 0.000 | 0.000 |
| 豆类 Legumes | 0.000 | 0.000 | 0.000 | 0.000 | 0.000 | 0.000 | 0.000 | 0.000 | 0.000 | 0.000 | 0.000 | 0.000 | 0.000 | 0.000 | 0.000 | 0.000 | 0.000 | 0.000 | 0.000 | 0.000 | 0.000 | 0.000 | 0.000 | 0.000 | 0.000 |
| 薯类 Potatoes | 0.000 | 0.000 | 0.000 | 0.000 | 0.000 | 0.000 | 0.000 | 0.000 | 0.000 | 0.000 | 0.000 | 0.000 | 0.000 | 0.000 | 0.000 | 0.000 | 0.000 | 0.000 | 0.000 | 0.000 | 0.000 | 0.000 | 0.000 | 0.000 | 0.000 |
| 肉类 Meats | 0.000 | 0.000 | 0.000 | 0.000 | 0.000 | 0.000 | 0.000 | 0.000 | 0.000 | 0.000 | 0.000 | 0.000 | 0.000 | 0.000 | 0.000 | 0.000 | 0.000 | 0.000 | 0.000 | 0.000 | 0.000 | 0.000 | 0.000 | 0.000 | 0.000 |
| 蛋类 Eggs | 0.000 | 0.000 | 0.000 | 0.000 | 0.000 | 0.000 | 0.000 | 0.000 | 0.000 | 0.000 | 0.000 | 0.000 | 0.000 | 0.000 | 0.000 | 0.000 | 0.000 | 0.000 | 0.000 | 0.000 | 0.000 | 0.000 | 0.000 | 0.000 | 0.000 |
| 水产类 Aquatic foods | 0.000 | 0.000 | 0.000 | 0.000 | 0.000 | 0.000 | 0.000 | 0.000 | 0.000 | 0.000 | 0.000 | 0.000 | 0.000 | 0.000 | 0.000 | 0.000 | 0.000 | 0.000 | 0.000 | 0.000 | 0.000 | 0.000 | 0.000 | 0.000 | 0.000 |
| 乳类 Dairy products | 0.000 | 0.000 | 0.000 | 0.000 | 0.000 | 0.000 | 0.000 | 0.000 | 0.000 | 0.000 | 0.000 | 0.000 | 0.000 | 0.000 | 0.000 | 0.000 | 0.000 | 0.000 | 0.000 | 0.000 | 0.000 | 0.000 | 0.000 | 0.000 | 0.000 |
| 蔬菜类 Vegetables | 0.000 | 0.000 | 0.000 | 0.000 | 0.000 | 0.000 | 0.000 | 0.000 | 0.000 | 0.000 | 0.000 | 0.000 | 0.000 | 0.000 | 0.000 | 0.000 | 0.000 | 0.000 | 0.000 | 0.000 | 0.000 | 0.000 | 0.000 | 0.000 | 0.000 |
| 水果类 Fruits | 0.000 | 0.000 | 0.227 | 0.000 | 0.000 | 0.000 | 0.000 | 0.025 | 0.000 | 0.000 | 0.000 | 0.000 | 2.099 | 0.000 | 0.000 | 0.000 | 0.000 | 0.000 | 0.000 | 0.000 | 0.000 | 0.000 | 0.000 | 0.000 | 0.098 |
| 糖类 Sugar | 0.000 | 0.000 | 0.000 | 0.000 | 0.000 | 0.000 | 0.000 | 0.000 | 0.000 | 0.000 | 0.000 | 0.000 | 0.000 | 0.000 | 0.000 | 0.000 | 0.000 | 0.000 | 0.000 | 0.000 | 0.000 | 0.000 | 0.000 | 0.000 | 0.000 |
| 水及饮料类 Water and beverages | 0.000 | 0.000 | 0.000 | 0.000 | 0.000 | 0.000 | 0.000 | 0.000 | 0.000 | 0.000 | 0.000 | 0.000 | 0.000 | 0.000 | 0.000 | 0.000 | 0.000 | 0.000 | 0.000 | 0.000 | 0.000 | 0.000 | 0.000 | 0.000 | 0.000 |

续表

| 膳食类别<br>Category | 黑龙江<br>HL | 辽宁<br>LN | 河北<br>HE | 北京<br>BJ | 吉林<br>JL | 山西<br>SX | 陕西<br>SN | 河南<br>HA | 宁夏<br>NX | 内蒙古<br>NM | 青海<br>QH | 甘肃<br>GS | 上海<br>SH | 福建<br>FJ | 江西<br>JX | 江苏<br>JS | 浙江<br>ZJ | 山东<br>SD | 湖北<br>HB | 四川<br>SC | 广西<br>GX | 湖南<br>HN | 广东<br>GD | 贵州<br>GZ | 全国平均<br>AVG |
|---|---|---|---|---|---|---|---|---|---|---|---|---|---|---|---|---|---|---|---|---|---|---|---|---|---|
| 酒类<br>Alcohol beverages | 0.000 | 0.000 | 0.000 | 0.000 | 0.000 | 0.000 | 0.000 | 0.000 | 0.000 | 0.000 | 0.000 | 0.000 | 0.000 | 0.000 | 0.000 | 0.000 | 0.000 | 0.000 | 0.000 | 0.000 | 0.000 | 0.000 | 0.000 | 0.000 | 0.000 |
| 合计<br>SUM | 0.000 | 0.000 | 0.227 | 0.000 | 0.000 | 0.000 | 0.000 | 0.025 | 0.000 | 0.000 | 0.000 | 0.000 | 2.099 | 0.000 | 0.000 | 0.000 | 0.000 | 0.000 | 0.000 | 0.000 | 0.000 | 0.000 | 0.000 | 0.000 | 0.098 |

附表 4-154　第六次中国总膳食研究甲霜灵的膳食来源（单位：%）

Annexed Table 4-154　Dietary sources of metalaxyl from the 6$^{th}$ China TDS (Unit: %)

| 膳食类别<br>Category | 黑龙江<br>HL | 辽宁<br>LN | 河北<br>HE | 北京<br>BJ | 吉林<br>JL | 山西<br>SX | 陕西<br>SN | 河南<br>HA | 宁夏<br>NX | 内蒙古<br>NM | 青海<br>QH | 甘肃<br>GS | 上海<br>SH | 福建<br>FJ | 江西<br>JX | 江苏<br>JS | 浙江<br>ZJ | 山东<br>SD | 湖北<br>HB | 四川<br>SC | 广西<br>GX | 湖南<br>HN | 广东<br>GD | 贵州<br>GZ | 全国平均<br>AVG |
|---|---|---|---|---|---|---|---|---|---|---|---|---|---|---|---|---|---|---|---|---|---|---|---|---|---|
| 谷类<br>Cereals | 0.0 | 0.0 | 0.0 | 0.0 | 0.0 | 0.0 | 0.0 | 0.0 | 0.0 | 0.0 | 0.0 | 0.0 | 0.0 | 0.0 | 0.0 | 0.0 | 0.0 | 0.0 | 0.0 | 0.0 | 0.0 | 0.0 | 0.0 | 0.0 | 0.0 |
| 豆类<br>Legumes | 0.0 | 0.0 | 0.0 | 0.0 | 0.0 | 0.0 | 0.0 | 0.0 | 0.0 | 0.0 | 0.0 | 0.0 | 0.0 | 0.0 | 0.0 | 0.0 | 7.9 | 0.0 | 0.0 | 0.0 | 0.0 | 0.0 | 0.0 | 0.0 | 0.1 |
| 薯类<br>Potatoes | 0.0 | 0.0 | 0.0 | 0.0 | 0.0 | 0.0 | 31.6 | 0.0 | 0.0 | 10.3 | 4.0 | 0.0 | 0.0 | 0.0 | 0.0 | 1.9 | 0.0 | 7.6 | 0.0 | 0.0 | 0.0 | 0.0 | 0.0 | 0.3 | 0.7 |
| 肉类<br>Meats | 0.0 | 0.0 | 0.0 | 0.0 | 0.0 | 21.4 | 0.0 | 0.0 | 0.0 | 0.0 | 0.0 | 0.0 | 0.0 | 0.0 | 0.0 | 0.2 | 17.8 | 0.0 | 4.6 | 5.4 | 0.0 | 0.0 | 0.0 | 0.0 | 0.5 |
| 蛋类<br>Eggs | 0.0 | 0.0 | 0.0 | 0.0 | 0.0 | 0.0 | 0.0 | 0.0 | 0.0 | 1.6 | 0.0 | 0.0 | 0.0 | 0.0 | 0.0 | 0.0 | 0.0 | 0.0 | 2.2 | 0.0 | 0.0 | 0.0 | 0.0 | 0.0 | 0.1 |
| 水产类<br>Aquatic foods | 0.3 | 0.0 | 0.0 | 0.4 | 0.0 | 0.3 | 0.0 | 0.0 | 0.0 | 0.0 | 0.0 | 0.0 | 0.0 | 0.0 | 0.0 | 0.0 | 5.4 | 0.0 | 3.6 | 0.2 | 0.0 | 0.0 | 0.0 | 0.0 | 0.1 |
| 乳类<br>Dairy products | 0.0 | 0.0 | 0.0 | 0.0 | 0.0 | 0.0 | 0.0 | 0.0 | 0.0 | 0.0 | 0.0 | 0.0 | 0.0 | 0.0 | 0.0 | 0.0 | 0.0 | 0.0 | 0.0 | 0.0 | 0.0 | 0.0 | 0.0 | 0.0 | 0.0 |

续表

| 膳食类别<br>Category | 黑龙江<br>HL | 辽宁<br>LN | 河北<br>HE | 北京<br>BJ | 吉林<br>JL | 山西<br>SX | 陕西<br>SN | 河南<br>HA | 宁夏<br>NX | 内蒙古<br>NM | 青海<br>QH | 甘肃<br>GS | 上海<br>SH | 福建<br>FJ | 江西<br>JX | 江苏<br>JS | 浙江<br>ZJ | 山东<br>SD | 湖北<br>HB | 四川<br>SC | 广西<br>GX | 湖南<br>HN | 广东<br>GD | 贵州<br>GZ | 全国平均<br>AVG |
|---|---|---|---|---|---|---|---|---|---|---|---|---|---|---|---|---|---|---|---|---|---|---|---|---|---|
| 蔬菜类<br>Vegetables | 99.7 | 100.0 | 100.0 | 96.8 | 100.0 | 78.4 | 50.1 | 100.0 | 100.0 | 81.0 | 96.0 | 100.0 | 99.5 | 44.2 | 100.0 | 97.8 | 62.7 | 74.6 | 89.3 | 94.3 | 95.9 | 100.0 | 99.2 | 99.6 | 97.3 |
| 水果类<br>Fruits | 0.0 | 0.0 | 0.0 | 2.3 | 0.0 | 0.0 | 18.3 | 0.0 | 0.0 | 7.1 | 0.0 | 0.0 | 0.0 | 55.8 | 0.0 | 0.0 | 0.0 | 6.5 | 0.3 | 0.0 | 0.5 | 0.0 | 0.8 | 0.1 | 0.8 |
| 糖类<br>Sugar | 0.0 | 0.0 | 0.0 | 0.0 | 0.0 | 0.0 | 0.0 | 0.0 | 0.0 | 0.0 | 0.0 | 0.0 | 0.2 | 0.0 | 0.0 | 0.0 | 0.0 | 0.0 | 0.0 | 0.0 | 0.0 | 0.0 | 0.0 | 0.0 | 0.0 |
| 水及饮料类<br>Water and beverages | 0.0 | 0.0 | 0.0 | 0.0 | 0.0 | 0.0 | 0.0 | 0.0 | 0.0 | 0.0 | 0.0 | 0.0 | 0.0 | 0.0 | 0.0 | 0.0 | 0.0 | 0.0 | 0.0 | 0.0 | 0.0 | 0.0 | 0.0 | 0.0 | 0.0 |
| 酒类<br>Alcohol beverages | 0.0 | 0.0 | 0.0 | 0.6 | 0.0 | 0.0 | 0.0 | 0.0 | 0.0 | 0.0 | 0.0 | 0.0 | 0.3 | 0.0 | 0.0 | 0.0 | 6.2 | 11.3 | 0.0 | 0.0 | 3.5 | 0.0 | 0.0 | 0.0 | 0.5 |

附表 4-155　第六次中国总膳食研究环己酰菌胺的膳食来源（单位：%）
Annexed Table 4-155　Dietary sources of fenhexamid from the 6$^{th}$ China TDS (Unit: %)

| 膳食类别<br>Category | 黑龙江<br>HL | 辽宁<br>LN | 河北<br>HE | 北京<br>BJ | 吉林<br>JL | 山西<br>SX | 陕西<br>SN | 河南<br>HA | 宁夏<br>NX | 内蒙古<br>NM | 青海<br>QH | 甘肃<br>GS | 上海<br>SH | 福建<br>FJ | 江西<br>JX | 江苏<br>JS | 浙江<br>ZJ | 山东<br>SD | 湖北<br>HB | 四川<br>SC | 广西<br>GX | 湖南<br>HN | 广东<br>GD | 贵州<br>GZ | 全国平均<br>AVG |
|---|---|---|---|---|---|---|---|---|---|---|---|---|---|---|---|---|---|---|---|---|---|---|---|---|---|
| 谷类<br>Cereals | 0.0 | 0.0 | 0.0 | 0.0 | 0.0 | 0.0 | 0.0 | 0.0 | 0.0 | 0.0 | 0.0 | 0.0 | 0.0 | 0.0 | 0.0 | 0.0 | 0.0 | 0.0 | 0.0 | 0.0 | 0.0 | 0.0 | 0.0 | 0.0 | 0.0 |
| 豆类<br>Legumes | 0.0 | 0.0 | 0.0 | 0.0 | 0.0 | 0.0 | 0.0 | 0.0 | 0.0 | 0.0 | 0.0 | 0.0 | 0.0 | 0.0 | 0.0 | 0.0 | 0.0 | 0.0 | 0.0 | 0.0 | 0.0 | 0.0 | 0.0 | 0.0 | 0.0 |
| 薯类<br>Potatoes | 0.0 | 0.0 | 0.0 | 0.0 | 0.0 | 0.0 | 0.0 | 0.0 | 0.0 | 0.0 | 0.0 | 0.0 | 0.0 | 0.0 | 0.0 | 0.0 | 0.0 | 0.0 | 0.0 | 0.0 | 0.0 | 0.0 | 0.0 | 0.0 | 0.0 |
| 肉类<br>Meats | 0.0 | 0.0 | 0.0 | 0.0 | 0.0 | 0.0 | 0.0 | 0.0 | 0.0 | 0.0 | 0.0 | 0.0 | 0.0 | 0.0 | 0.0 | 0.0 | 0.0 | 0.0 | 0.0 | 0.0 | 0.0 | 0.0 | 0.0 | 0.0 | 0.0 |
| 蛋类<br>Eggs | 0.0 | 0.0 | 0.0 | 0.0 | 0.0 | 0.0 | 0.0 | 0.0 | 0.0 | 0.0 | 0.0 | 0.0 | 0.0 | 0.0 | 0.0 | 0.0 | 0.0 | 0.0 | 0.0 | 0.0 | 0.0 | 0.0 | 0.0 | 0.0 | 0.0 |

续表

| 膳食类别<br>Category | 黑龙江<br>HL | 辽宁<br>LN | 河北<br>HE | 北京<br>BJ | 吉林<br>JL | 山西<br>SX | 陕西<br>SN | 河南<br>HA | 宁夏<br>NX | 内蒙古<br>NM | 青海<br>QH | 甘肃<br>GS | 上海<br>SH | 福建<br>FJ | 江西<br>JX | 江苏<br>JS | 浙江<br>ZJ | 山东<br>SD | 湖北<br>HB | 四川<br>SC | 广西<br>GX | 湖南<br>HN | 广东<br>GD | 贵州<br>GZ | 全国平均<br>AVG |
|---|---|---|---|---|---|---|---|---|---|---|---|---|---|---|---|---|---|---|---|---|---|---|---|---|---|
| 水产类<br>Aquatic foods | 0.0 | 0.0 | 0.0 | 0.0 | 0.0 | 0.0 | 0.0 | 0.0 | 0.0 | 0.0 | 0.0 | 0.0 | 0.0 | 0.0 | 0.0 | 0.0 | 0.0 | 0.0 | 0.0 | 0.0 | 0.0 | 0.0 | 0.0 | 0.0 | 0.0 |
| 乳类<br>Dairy products | 0.0 | 0.0 | 0.0 | 0.0 | 0.0 | 0.0 | 0.0 | 0.0 | 0.0 | 0.0 | 0.0 | 0.0 | 0.0 | 0.0 | 0.0 | 0.0 | 0.0 | 0.0 | 0.0 | 0.0 | 0.0 | 0.0 | 0.0 | 0.0 | 0.0 |
| 蔬菜类<br>Vegetables | 0.0 | 0.0 | 0.0 | 0.0 | 0.0 | 0.0 | 0.0 | 0.0 | 0.0 | 0.0 | 0.0 | 0.0 | 0.0 | 0.0 | 0.0 | 0.0 | 0.0 | 0.0 | 0.0 | 0.0 | 0.0 | 0.0 | 0.0 | 0.0 | 0.0 |
| 水果类<br>Fruits | 0.0 | 0.0 | 0.0 | 0.0 | 0.0 | 0.0 | 0.0 | 0.0 | 0.0 | 0.0 | 0.0 | 0.0 | 100.0 | 0.0 | 0.0 | 0.0 | 0.0 | 0.0 | 0.0 | 0.0 | 0.0 | 0.0 | 0.0 | 0.0 | 100.0 |
| 糖类<br>Sugar | 0.0 | 0.0 | 0.0 | 0.0 | 0.0 | 0.0 | 0.0 | 0.0 | 0.0 | 0.0 | 0.0 | 0.0 | 0.0 | 0.0 | 0.0 | 0.0 | 0.0 | 0.0 | 0.0 | 0.0 | 0.0 | 0.0 | 0.0 | 0.0 | 0.0 |
| 水及饮料类<br>Water and beverages | 0.0 | 0.0 | 0.0 | 0.0 | 0.0 | 0.0 | 0.0 | 0.0 | 0.0 | 0.0 | 0.0 | 0.0 | 0.0 | 0.0 | 0.0 | 0.0 | 0.0 | 0.0 | 0.0 | 0.0 | 0.0 | 0.0 | 0.0 | 0.0 | 0.0 |
| 酒类<br>Alcohol beverages | 0.0 | 0.0 | 0.0 | 0.0 | 0.0 | 0.0 | 0.0 | 0.0 | 0.0 | 0.0 | 0.0 | 0.0 | 0.0 | 0.0 | 0.0 | 0.0 | 0.0 | 0.0 | 0.0 | 0.0 | 0.0 | 0.0 | 0.0 | 0.0 | 0.0 |

附表 4-156　第六次中国总膳食研究嘧霉胺的膳食来源（单位：%）

Annexed Table 4-156　Dietary sources of pyrimethanil from the 6$^{th}$ China TDS (Unit: %)

| 膳食类别<br>Category | 黑龙江<br>HL | 辽宁<br>LN | 河北<br>HE | 北京<br>BJ | 吉林<br>JL | 山西<br>SX | 陕西<br>SN | 河南<br>HA | 宁夏<br>NX | 内蒙古<br>NM | 青海<br>QH | 甘肃<br>GS | 上海<br>SH | 福建<br>FJ | 江西<br>JX | 江苏<br>JS | 浙江<br>ZJ | 山东<br>SD | 湖北<br>HB | 四川<br>SC | 广西<br>GX | 湖南<br>HN | 广东<br>GD | 贵州<br>GZ | 全国平均<br>AVG |
|---|---|---|---|---|---|---|---|---|---|---|---|---|---|---|---|---|---|---|---|---|---|---|---|---|---|
| 谷类<br>Cereals | 0.0 | 34.5 | 0.0 | 0.0 | 0.0 | 0.4 | 0.0 | 0.0 | 0.0 | 0.0 | 0.0 | 0.0 | 0.0 | 0.0 | 0.0 | 0.0 | 0.0 | 0.0 | 0.0 | 0.0 | 0.0 | 0.0 | 0.0 | 0.0 | 0.4 |
| 豆类<br>Legumes | 0.0 | 0.0 | 0.0 | 0.0 | 0.0 | 0.0 | 0.0 | 0.0 | 0.0 | 0.0 | 0.0 | 0.0 | 0.0 | 0.0 | 0.0 | 0.0 | 0.0 | 0.0 | 0.0 | 0.0 | 0.0 | 0.0 | 0.0 | 0.0 | 0.0 |

续表

| 膳食类别<br>Category | 黑龙江<br>HL | 辽宁<br>LN | 河北<br>HE | 北京<br>BJ | 吉林<br>JL | 山西<br>SX | 陕西<br>SN | 河南<br>HA | 宁夏<br>NX | 内蒙古<br>NM | 青海<br>QH | 甘肃<br>GS | 上海<br>SH | 福建<br>FJ | 江西<br>JX | 江苏<br>JS | 浙江<br>ZJ | 山东<br>SD | 湖北<br>HB | 四川<br>SC | 广西<br>GX | 湖南<br>HN | 广东<br>GD | 贵州<br>GZ | 全国平均<br>AVG |
|---|---|---|---|---|---|---|---|---|---|---|---|---|---|---|---|---|---|---|---|---|---|---|---|---|---|
| 薯类 Potatoes | 0.0 | 0.0 | 2.7 | 0.0 | 0.0 | 0.0 | 0.0 | 0.0 | 0.0 | 0.0 | 0.0 | 0.0 | 0.9 | 0.0 | 0.0 | 0.0 | 0.0 | 0.0 | 0.0 | 0.0 | 0.0 | 0.0 | 0.0 | 0.0 | 0.0 |
| 肉类 Meats | 0.0 | 0.0 | 0.0 | 0.0 | 0.0 | 0.0 | 0.0 | 0.0 | 0.0 | 0.0 | 0.0 | 0.0 | 0.0 | 0.0 | 0.0 | 0.0 | 0.0 | 0.0 | 0.0 | 0.0 | 0.0 | 0.0 | 0.2 | 0.0 | 0.0 |
| 蛋类 Eggs | 0.0 | 0.0 | 0.0 | 0.0 | 0.0 | 0.0 | 0.0 | 0.0 | 0.0 | 0.0 | 0.0 | 0.0 | 0.0 | 0.0 | 0.0 | 0.0 | 0.0 | 0.0 | 0.0 | 0.0 | 0.0 | 0.0 | 0.0 | 0.0 | 0.0 |
| 水产类 Aquatic foods | 0.0 | 0.5 | 0.0 | 0.0 | 0.0 | 0.0 | 0.0 | 0.0 | 0.0 | 0.0 | 0.0 | 0.0 | 0.0 | 0.0 | 0.0 | 5.6 | 0.4 | 0.0 | 0.0 | 0.0 | 0.0 | 0.0 | 0.2 | 0.0 | 0.0 |
| 乳类 Dairy products | 0.0 | 0.0 | 0.0 | 0.0 | 0.0 | 0.0 | 0.0 | 0.0 | 0.0 | 0.0 | 0.0 | 0.0 | 0.0 | 0.0 | 0.0 | 1.2 | 0.0 | 0.0 | 0.0 | 0.0 | 0.0 | 0.0 | 0.0 | 0.0 | 0.0 |
| 蔬菜类 Vegetables | 0.0 | 0.0 | 71.3 | 95.2 | 11.0 | 100.0 | 100.0 | 52.4 | 84.6 | 40.4 | 95.3 | 100.0 | 52.7 | 10.6 | 100.0 | 88.8 | 3.7 | 99.9 | 75.2 | 87.9 | 71.5 | 100.0 | 95.3 | 100.0 | 92.6 |
| 水果类 Fruits | 100.0 | 65.0 | 26.0 | 4.8 | 89.0 | 0.0 | 0.0 | 41.8 | 15.4 | 59.6 | 4.7 | 0.0 | 46.1 | 89.4 | 0.0 | 4.5 | 95.9 | 0.1 | 24.8 | 12.1 | 0.0 | 0.0 | 4.3 | 0.0 | 6.8 |
| 糖类 Sugar | 0.0 | 0.0 | 0.0 | 0.0 | 0.0 | 0.0 | 0.0 | 0.0 | 0.0 | 0.0 | 0.0 | 0.0 | 0.0 | 0.0 | 0.0 | 0.0 | 0.0 | 0.0 | 0.0 | 0.0 | 0.0 | 0.0 | 0.0 | 0.0 | 0.0 |
| 水及饮料类 Water and beverages | 0.0 | 0.0 | 0.0 | 0.0 | 0.0 | 0.0 | 0.0 | 5.7 | 0.0 | 0.0 | 0.0 | 0.0 | 0.4 | 0.0 | 0.0 | 0.0 | 0.0 | 0.0 | 0.0 | 0.0 | 0.0 | 0.0 | 0.0 | 0.0 | 0.0 |
| 酒类 Alcohol beverages | 0.0 | 0.0 | 0.0 | 0.0 | 0.0 | 0.0 | 0.0 | 0.0 | 0.0 | 0.0 | 0.0 | 0.0 | 0.0 | 0.0 | 0.0 | 0.0 | 0.0 | 0.0 | 0.0 | 0.0 | 28.5 | 0.0 | 0.0 | 0.0 | 0.1 |

附表 4-157　第六次中国总膳食研究乙嘧酚磺酸酯的膳食来源（单位：%）

Annexed Table 4-157　Dietary sources of bupirimate from the 6<sup>th</sup> China TDS (Unit: %)

| 膳食类别<br>Category | 黑龙江<br>HL | 辽宁<br>LN | 河北<br>HE | 北京<br>BJ | 吉林<br>JL | 山西<br>SX | 陕西<br>SN | 河南<br>HA | 宁夏<br>NX | 内蒙古<br>NM | 青海<br>QH | 甘肃<br>GS | 上海<br>SH | 福建<br>FJ | 江西<br>JX | 江苏<br>JS | 浙江<br>ZJ | 山东<br>SD | 湖北<br>HB | 四川<br>SC | 广西<br>GX | 湖南<br>HN | 广东<br>GD | 贵州<br>GZ | 全国平均<br>AVG |
|---|---|---|---|---|---|---|---|---|---|---|---|---|---|---|---|---|---|---|---|---|---|---|---|---|---|
| 谷类 Cereals | 0.0 | 0.0 | 0.0 | 0.0 | 0.0 | 0.0 | 0.0 | 0.0 | 0.0 | 0.0 | 0.0 | 0.0 | 0.0 | 0.0 | 0.0 | 0.0 | 0.0 | 0.0 | 0.0 | 0.0 | 0.0 | 0.0 | 0.0 | 0.0 | 0.0 |
| 豆类 Legumes | 0.0 | 0.0 | 0.0 | 0.0 | 0.0 | 0.0 | 0.0 | 0.0 | 0.0 | 0.0 | 0.0 | 0.0 | 0.0 | 0.0 | 0.0 | 0.0 | 0.0 | 0.0 | 0.0 | 0.0 | 0.0 | 0.0 | 0.0 | 0.0 | 0.0 |
| 薯类 Potatoes | 0.0 | 0.0 | 0.0 | 0.0 | 0.0 | 0.0 | 0.0 | 0.0 | 0.0 | 0.0 | 0.0 | 0.0 | 0.0 | 0.0 | 0.0 | 0.0 | 100.0 | 0.0 | 0.0 | 0.0 | 0.0 | 0.0 | 0.0 | 0.0 | 0.4 |
| 肉类 Meats | 0.0 | 0.0 | 0.0 | 0.0 | 0.0 | 0.0 | 0.0 | 0.0 | 0.0 | 0.0 | 0.0 | 0.0 | 0.0 | 0.0 | 0.0 | 0.0 | 0.0 | 0.0 | 0.0 | 0.0 | 0.0 | 0.0 | 0.0 | 0.0 | 0.0 |
| 蛋类 Eggs | 0.0 | 0.0 | 0.0 | 0.0 | 0.0 | 0.0 | 0.0 | 0.0 | 0.0 | 0.0 | 0.0 | 0.0 | 0.0 | 0.0 | 0.0 | 0.0 | 0.0 | 0.0 | 0.0 | 0.0 | 0.0 | 0.0 | 0.0 | 0.0 | 0.0 |
| 水产类 Aquatic foods | 0.0 | 0.0 | 0.0 | 0.0 | 0.0 | 0.0 | 0.0 | 0.0 | 0.0 | 0.0 | 0.1 | 0.0 | 0.0 | 0.0 | 0.0 | 0.0 | 0.0 | 0.0 | 0.0 | 0.0 | 0.0 | 0.0 | 0.0 | 0.0 | 0.1 |
| 乳类 Dairy products | 0.0 | 0.0 | 0.0 | 0.0 | 0.0 | 0.0 | 0.0 | 0.0 | 0.0 | 0.0 | 0.0 | 0.0 | 0.0 | 0.0 | 0.0 | 0.0 | 0.0 | 0.0 | 0.0 | 0.0 | 0.0 | 0.0 | 0.0 | 0.0 | 0.0 |
| 蔬菜类 Vegetables | 0.0 | 0.0 | 0.0 | 0.0 | 100.0 | 0.0 | 0.0 | 0.0 | 0.0 | 0.0 | 99.9 | 0.0 | 0.0 | 0.0 | 0.0 | 0.0 | 0.0 | 0.0 | 0.0 | 0.0 | 0.0 | 0.0 | 0.0 | 0.0 | 98.7 |
| 水果类 Fruits | 0.0 | 0.0 | 0.0 | 0.0 | 0.0 | 0.0 | 0.0 | 0.0 | 0.0 | 0.0 | 0.0 | 0.0 | 0.0 | 0.0 | 0.0 | 0.0 | 0.0 | 100.0 | 0.0 | 0.0 | 0.0 | 0.0 | 0.0 | 0.0 | 0.9 |
| 糖类 Sugar | 0.0 | 0.0 | 0.0 | 0.0 | 0.0 | 0.0 | 0.0 | 0.0 | 0.0 | 0.0 | 0.0 | 0.0 | 0.0 | 0.0 | 0.0 | 0.0 | 0.0 | 0.0 | 0.0 | 0.0 | 0.0 | 0.0 | 0.0 | 0.0 | 0.0 |
| 水及饮料类 Water and beverages | 0.0 | 0.0 | 0.0 | 0.0 | 0.0 | 0.0 | 0.0 | 0.0 | 0.0 | 0.0 | 0.0 | 0.0 | 0.0 | 0.0 | 0.0 | 0.0 | 0.0 | 0.0 | 0.0 | 0.0 | 0.0 | 0.0 | 0.0 | 0.0 | 0.0 |

续表

| 膳食类别 Category | 黑龙江 HL | 辽宁 LN | 河北 HE | 北京 BJ | 吉林 JL | 山西 SX | 陕西 SN | 河南 HA | 宁夏 NX | 内蒙古 NM | 青海 QH | 甘肃 GS | 上海 SH | 福建 FJ | 江西 JX | 江苏 JS | 浙江 ZJ | 山东 SD | 湖北 HB | 四川 SC | 广西 GX | 湖南 HN | 广东 GD | 贵州 GZ | 全国平均 AVG |
|---|---|---|---|---|---|---|---|---|---|---|---|---|---|---|---|---|---|---|---|---|---|---|---|---|---|
| 酒类 Alcohol beverages | 0.0 | 0.0 | 0.0 | 0.0 | 0.0 | 0.0 | 0.0 | 0.0 | 0.0 | 0.0 | 0.0 | 0.0 | 0.0 | 0.0 | 0.0 | 0.0 | 0.0 | 0.0 | 0.0 | 0.0 | 0.0 | 0.0 | 0.0 | 0.0 | 0.0 |

附表 4-158 第六次中国总膳食研究嘧菌环胺的膳食来源（单位：%）

Annexed Table 4-158 Dietary sources of cyprodinil from the 6th China TDS (Unit: %)

| 膳食类别 Category | 黑龙江 HL | 辽宁 LN | 河北 HE | 北京 BJ | 吉林 JL | 山西 SX | 陕西 SN | 河南 HA | 宁夏 NX | 内蒙古 NM | 青海 QH | 甘肃 GS | 上海 SH | 福建 FJ | 江西 JX | 江苏 JS | 浙江 ZJ | 山东 SD | 湖北 HB | 四川 SC | 广西 GX | 湖南 HN | 广东 GD | 贵州 GZ | 全国平均 AVG |
|---|---|---|---|---|---|---|---|---|---|---|---|---|---|---|---|---|---|---|---|---|---|---|---|---|---|
| 谷类 Cereals | 0.0 | 0.0 | 0.0 | 0.0 | 0.0 | 0.0 | 0.0 | 0.0 | 0.0 | 0.0 | 0.0 | 0.0 | 0.0 | 0.0 | 0.0 | 0.0 | 0.0 | 0.0 | 0.0 | 0.0 | 0.0 | 0.0 | 0.0 | 0.0 | 0.0 |
| 豆类 Legumes | 0.0 | 0.0 | 0.0 | 0.0 | 0.0 | 0.0 | 0.0 | 0.0 | 0.0 | 0.0 | 0.0 | 0.0 | 0.0 | 0.0 | 0.0 | 0.0 | 0.0 | 0.0 | 0.0 | 0.0 | 0.0 | 0.0 | 0.0 | 0.0 | 0.0 |
| 薯类 Potatoes | 0.0 | 0.0 | 0.0 | 0.0 | 0.0 | 0.0 | 0.0 | 0.0 | 0.0 | 0.0 | 0.0 | 0.0 | 0.0 | 0.0 | 0.0 | 0.0 | 0.0 | 0.0 | 0.0 | 0.0 | 0.0 | 0.0 | 0.0 | 0.0 | 0.0 |
| 肉类 Meats | 0.0 | 0.0 | 2.5 | 0.0 | 0.0 | 0.0 | 0.0 | 0.0 | 0.0 | 0.0 | 0.0 | 0.0 | 0.0 | 0.0 | 0.0 | 0.0 | 0.0 | 0.0 | 0.0 | 0.0 | 0.0 | 0.0 | 0.0 | 0.0 | 0.1 |
| 蛋类 Eggs | 0.0 | 0.0 | 0.0 | 0.0 | 0.0 | 0.0 | 0.0 | 0.0 | 0.0 | 0.0 | 0.0 | 0.0 | 0.0 | 0.0 | 0.0 | 0.0 | 0.0 | 0.0 | 0.0 | 0.0 | 0.0 | 0.0 | 0.0 | 0.0 | 0.0 |
| 水产类 Aquatic foods | 0.0 | 0.0 | 0.0 | 0.0 | 0.0 | 0.0 | 0.0 | 0.0 | 0.0 | 0.0 | 0.0 | 0.0 | 0.0 | 0.0 | 0.0 | 0.0 | 0.0 | 0.0 | 0.0 | 0.0 | 0.0 | 0.0 | 0.0 | 0.0 | 0.0 |
| 乳类 Dairy products | 0.0 | 0.0 | 0.0 | 100.0 | 0.0 | 0.0 | 0.0 | 0.0 | 0.0 | 0.0 | 0.0 | 0.0 | 0.0 | 0.0 | 0.0 | 0.0 | 0.0 | 0.0 | 0.0 | 0.0 | 0.0 | 0.0 | 0.0 | 0.0 | 0.0 |
| 蔬菜类 Vegetables | 0.0 | 0.0 | 0.0 | 0.0 | 0.0 | 8.1 | 0.0 | 100.0 | 100.0 | 0.0 | 0.0 | 0.0 | 0.0 | 0.0 | 0.0 | 0.0 | 0.0 | 0.0 | 0.0 | 0.0 | 0.0 | 0.0 | 100.0 | 0.0 | 8.1 |

续表

| 膳食类别<br>Category | 黑龙江<br>HL | 辽宁<br>LN | 河北<br>HE | 北京<br>BJ | 吉林<br>JL | 山西<br>SX | 陕西<br>SN | 河南<br>HA | 宁夏<br>NX | 内蒙古<br>NM | 青海<br>QH | 甘肃<br>GS | 上海<br>SH | 福建<br>FJ | 江西<br>JX | 江苏<br>JS | 浙江<br>ZJ | 山东<br>SD | 湖北<br>HB | 四川<br>SC | 广西<br>GX | 湖南<br>HN | 广东<br>GD | 贵州<br>GZ | 全国平均<br>AVG |
|---|---|---|---|---|---|---|---|---|---|---|---|---|---|---|---|---|---|---|---|---|---|---|---|---|---|
| 水果类 Fruits | 0.0 | 0.0 | 97.5 | 0.0 | 0.0 | 0.0 | 0.0 | 0.0 | 0.0 | 0.0 | 0.0 | 0.0 | 100.0 | 100.0 | 0.0 | 0.0 | 0.0 | 100.0 | 0.0 | 0.0 | 0.0 | 0.0 | 0.0 | 0.0 | 91.7 |
| 糖类 Sugar | 0.0 | 0.0 | 0.0 | 0.0 | 0.0 | 0.0 | 0.0 | 0.0 | 0.0 | 0.0 | 0.0 | 0.0 | 0.0 | 0.0 | 0.0 | 0.0 | 0.0 | 0.0 | 0.0 | 0.0 | 0.0 | 0.0 | 0.0 | 0.0 | 0.0 |
| 水及饮料类 Water and beverages | 0.0 | 0.0 | 0.0 | 0.0 | 0.0 | 0.0 | 0.0 | 0.0 | 0.0 | 0.0 | 0.0 | 0.0 | 0.0 | 0.0 | 0.0 | 0.0 | 0.0 | 0.0 | 0.0 | 0.0 | 0.0 | 0.0 | 0.0 | 0.0 | 0.0 |
| 酒类 Alcohol beverages | 0.0 | 0.0 | 0.0 | 0.0 | 0.0 | 0.0 | 0.0 | 0.0 | 0.0 | 0.0 | 0.0 | 0.0 | 0.0 | 0.0 | 0.0 | 0.0 | 0.0 | 0.0 | 0.0 | 0.0 | 0.0 | 0.0 | 0.0 | 0.0 | 0.0 |

附表 4-159 第六次中国总膳食研究氟吡菌胺的膳食来源（单位：%）
Annexed Table 4-159 Dietary sources of fluopicolide from the 6th China TDS (Unit: %)

| 膳食类别<br>Category | 黑龙江<br>HL | 辽宁<br>LN | 河北<br>HE | 北京<br>BJ | 吉林<br>JL | 山西<br>SX | 陕西<br>SN | 河南<br>HA | 宁夏<br>NX | 内蒙古<br>NM | 青海<br>QH | 甘肃<br>GS | 上海<br>SH | 福建<br>FJ | 江西<br>JX | 江苏<br>JS | 浙江<br>ZJ | 山东<br>SD | 湖北<br>HB | 四川<br>SC | 广西<br>GX | 湖南<br>HN | 广东<br>GD | 贵州<br>GZ | 全国平均<br>AVG |
|---|---|---|---|---|---|---|---|---|---|---|---|---|---|---|---|---|---|---|---|---|---|---|---|---|---|
| 谷类 Cereals | 0.0 | 0.0 | 0.0 | 0.0 | 0.0 | 0.0 | 0.0 | 0.0 | 0.0 | 0.0 | 0.0 | 0.0 | 0.0 | 0.0 | 0.0 | 0.0 | 0.0 | 0.0 | 0.0 | 0.0 | 0.0 | 0.0 | 0.0 | 0.0 | 0.0 |
| 豆类 Legumes | 0.0 | 0.0 | 0.0 | 0.0 | 0.0 | 0.0 | 0.0 | 0.0 | 0.0 | 0.0 | 0.0 | 0.0 | 0.0 | 0.0 | 0.0 | 0.0 | 0.0 | 0.0 | 0.0 | 0.0 | 0.0 | 0.0 | 0.0 | 0.0 | 0.0 |
| 薯类 Potatoes | 0.0 | 0.0 | 6.6 | 0.0 | 20.6 | 0.0 | 0.0 | 100.0 | 0.0 | 0.0 | 0.0 | 0.0 | 0.0 | 0.0 | 0.0 | 0.0 | 0.0 | 0.0 | 0.0 | 0.0 | 0.0 | 0.0 | 0.0 | 0.0 | 1.5 |
| 肉类 Meats | 0.0 | 0.0 | 0.0 | 0.0 | 0.0 | 0.0 | 0.0 | 0.0 | 0.0 | 0.0 | 0.0 | 0.0 | 0.0 | 0.0 | 0.0 | 0.0 | 0.0 | 0.0 | 0.0 | 0.0 | 0.0 | 0.0 | 0.0 | 0.0 | 0.0 |
| 蛋类 Eggs | 0.0 | 0.0 | 0.0 | 0.0 | 0.0 | 0.0 | 0.0 | 0.0 | 0.0 | 0.0 | 0.0 | 0.0 | 0.0 | 0.0 | 0.0 | 0.0 | 0.0 | 0.0 | 0.0 | 0.0 | 0.0 | 0.0 | 0.0 | 0.0 | 0.0 |

续表

| 膳食类别 Category | 黑龙江 HL | 辽宁 LN | 河北 HE | 北京 BJ | 吉林 JL | 山西 SX | 陕西 SN | 河南 HA | 宁夏 NX | 内蒙古 NM | 青海 QH | 甘肃 GS | 上海 SH | 福建 FJ | 江西 JX | 江苏 JS | 浙江 ZJ | 山东 SD | 湖北 HB | 四川 SC | 广西 GX | 湖南 HN | 广东 GD | 贵州 GZ | 全国平均 AVG |
|---|---|---|---|---|---|---|---|---|---|---|---|---|---|---|---|---|---|---|---|---|---|---|---|---|---|
| 水产类 Aquatic foods | 0.0 | 0.0 | 0.0 | 0.0 | 0.0 | 0.0 | 0.0 | 0.0 | 0.0 | 0.0 | 0.0 | 0.0 | 0.0 | 0.0 | 0.0 | 0.0 | 0.0 | 0.0 | 0.0 | 0.0 | 0.0 | 0.0 | 0.0 | 0.0 | 0.0 |
| 乳类 Dairy products | 0.0 | 0.0 | 0.0 | 0.0 | 0.0 | 0.6 | 0.0 | 0.0 | 0.0 | 0.0 | 0.0 | 0.0 | 0.0 | 0.0 | 0.0 | 0.0 | 0.0 | 0.0 | 0.0 | 0.0 | 0.0 | 0.0 | 0.0 | 0.0 | 0.1 |
| 蔬菜类 Vegetables | 0.0 | 0.0 | 93.4 | 100.0 | 0.0 | 99.4 | 0.0 | 0.0 | 0.0 | 0.0 | 0.0 | 100.0 | 100.0 | 100.0 | 100.0 | 0.0 | 100.0 | 81.1 | 100.0 | 98.5 | 0.0 | 100.0 | 99.6 | 100.0 | 94.2 |
| 水果类 Fruits | 0.0 | 0.0 | 0.0 | 0.0 | 79.4 | 0.0 | 0.0 | 0.0 | 0.0 | 0.0 | 0.0 | 0.0 | 0.0 | 0.0 | 0.0 | 0.0 | 0.0 | 18.9 | 0.0 | 1.5 | 0.0 | 0.0 | 0.4 | 0.0 | 4.2 |
| 糖类 Sugar | 0.0 | 0.0 | 0.0 | 0.0 | 0.0 | 0.0 | 0.0 | 0.0 | 0.0 | 0.0 | 0.0 | 0.0 | 0.0 | 0.0 | 0.0 | 0.0 | 0.0 | 0.0 | 0.0 | 0.0 | 0.0 | 0.0 | 0.0 | 0.0 | 0.0 |
| 水及饮料类 Water and beverages | 0.0 | 0.0 | 0.0 | 0.0 | 0.0 | 0.0 | 0.0 | 0.0 | 0.0 | 0.0 | 0.0 | 0.0 | 0.0 | 0.0 | 0.0 | 0.0 | 0.0 | 0.0 | 0.0 | 0.0 | 0.0 | 0.0 | 0.0 | 0.0 | 0.0 |
| 酒类 Alcohol beverages | 0.0 | 0.0 | 0.0 | 0.0 | 0.0 | 0.0 | 0.0 | 0.0 | 0.0 | 0.0 | 0.0 | 0.0 | 0.0 | 0.0 | 0.0 | 0.0 | 0.0 | 0.0 | 0.0 | 0.0 | 0.0 | 0.0 | 0.0 | 0.0 | 0.0 |

附表 4-160　第六次中国总膳食研究烯酰吗啉的膳食来源（单位：%）

Annexed Table 4-160　Dietary sources of dimethomorph from the 6$^{th}$ China TDS (Unit: %)

| 膳食类别 Category | 黑龙江 HL | 辽宁 LN | 河北 HE | 北京 BJ | 吉林 JL | 山西 SX | 陕西 SN | 河南 HA | 宁夏 NX | 内蒙古 NM | 青海 QH | 甘肃 GS | 上海 SH | 福建 FJ | 江西 JX | 江苏 JS | 浙江 ZJ | 山东 SD | 湖北 HB | 四川 SC | 广西 GX | 湖南 HN | 广东 GD | 贵州 GZ | 全国平均 AVG |
|---|---|---|---|---|---|---|---|---|---|---|---|---|---|---|---|---|---|---|---|---|---|---|---|---|---|
| 谷类 Cereals | 0.0 | 0.0 | 2.2 | 10.7 | 0.0 | 0.0 | 0.0 | 12.1 | 0.0 | 0.0 | 0.0 | 0.0 | 0.0 | 0.0 | 0.4 | 0.0 | 0.0 | 0.0 | 0.0 | 0.0 | 0.0 | 0.0 | 0.0 | 0.0 | 0.1 |
| 豆类 Legumes | 0.0 | 0.0 | 0.2 | 0.0 | 0.0 | 0.0 | 0.0 | 0.5 | 0.0 | 0.0 | 0.0 | 0.0 | 0.0 | 0.0 | 0.0 | 0.0 | 0.0 | 0.0 | 0.0 | 0.0 | 0.0 | 0.0 | 0.0 | 0.0 | 0.0 |

续表

| 膳食类别<br>Category | 黑龙江<br>HL | 辽宁<br>LN | 河北<br>HE | 北京<br>BJ | 吉林<br>JL | 山西<br>SX | 陕西<br>SN | 河南<br>HA | 宁夏<br>NX | 内蒙古<br>NM | 青海<br>QH | 甘肃<br>GS | 上海<br>SH | 福建<br>FJ | 江西<br>JX | 江苏<br>JS | 浙江<br>ZJ | 山东<br>SD | 湖北<br>HB | 四川<br>SC | 广西<br>GX | 湖南<br>HN | 广东<br>GD | 贵州<br>GZ | 全国平均<br>AVG |
|---|---|---|---|---|---|---|---|---|---|---|---|---|---|---|---|---|---|---|---|---|---|---|---|---|---|
| 薯类<br>Potatoes | 0.0 | 0.0 | 2.2 | 0.0 | 11.4 | 0.6 | 27.7 | 1.7 | 0.0 | 6.6 | 0.0 | 0.1 | 0.2 | 0.0 | 0.0 | 0.0 | 0.2 | 0.3 | 0.0 | 0.2 | 0.2 | 0.0 | 0.0 | 0.0 | 0.1 |
| 肉类<br>Meats | 0.0 | 0.0 | 0.3 | 1.8 | 0.0 | 2.5 | 0.0 | 0.4 | 0.0 | 6.0 | 0.0 | 0.0 | 0.0 | 0.0 | 0.0 | 0.0 | 0.0 | 0.0 | 0.0 | 0.0 | 0.3 | 0.0 | 0.0 | 0.0 | 0.0 |
| 蛋类<br>Eggs | 0.0 | 0.0 | 0.1 | 1.5 | 0.0 | 0.0 | 0.0 | 0.0 | 0.0 | 0.0 | 0.0 | 0.0 | 0.0 | 0.0 | 0.0 | 0.0 | 0.0 | 0.0 | 0.0 | 0.0 | 0.0 | 0.0 | 0.0 | 0.0 | 0.0 |
| 水产类<br>Aquatic foods | 0.0 | 0.0 | 0.0 | 0.4 | 0.3 | 0.0 | 0.0 | 0.0 | 0.0 | 0.0 | 0.0 | 0.0 | 0.0 | 0.0 | 0.0 | 0.0 | 0.0 | 0.0 | 0.0 | 0.0 | 0.2 | 0.0 | 0.0 | 0.0 | 0.0 |
| 乳类<br>Dairy products | 0.0 | 0.0 | 0.0 | 0.0 | 0.0 | 0.3 | 0.0 | 0.0 | 0.0 | 0.0 | 0.0 | 0.0 | 0.0 | 0.0 | 0.0 | 0.0 | 0.0 | 0.0 | 0.0 | 0.0 | 0.0 | 0.0 | 0.0 | 0.0 | 0.0 |
| 蔬菜类<br>Vegetables | 47.5 | 8.1 | 94.9 | 50.4 | 10.0 | 96.6 | 71.8 | 35.1 | 100.0 | 54.9 | 99.8 | 99.9 | 99.8 | 99.2 | 99.5 | 100.0 | 70.2 | 81.8 | 100.0 | 97.8 | 76.8 | 100.0 | 99.8 | 99.9 | 99.2 |
| 水果类<br>Fruits | 51.7 | 89.5 | 0.1 | 33.6 | 78.0 | 0.0 | 0.5 | 50.1 | 0.0 | 32.5 | 0.2 | 0.0 | 0.0 | 0.7 | 0.1 | 0.0 | 27.1 | 0.8 | 0.0 | 1.9 | 5.0 | 0.0 | 0.2 | 0.0 | 0.5 |
| 糖类<br>Sugar | 0.0 | 0.0 | 0.0 | 0.0 | 0.0 | 0.0 | 0.0 | 0.0 | 0.0 | 0.0 | 0.0 | 0.0 | 0.0 | 0.0 | 0.0 | 0.0 | 0.0 | 0.0 | 0.0 | 0.0 | 0.0 | 0.0 | 0.0 | 0.0 | 0.0 |
| 水及饮料类<br>Water and beverages | 0.0 | 0.0 | 0.0 | 0.0 | 0.0 | 0.0 | 0.0 | 0.1 | 0.0 | 0.0 | 0.0 | 0.0 | 0.0 | 0.0 | 0.0 | 0.0 | 0.0 | 0.0 | 0.0 | 0.0 | 0.0 | 0.0 | 0.0 | 0.0 | 0.0 |
| 酒类<br>Alcohol beverages | 0.8 | 2.4 | 0.0 | 1.7 | 0.3 | 0.0 | 0.0 | 0.0 | 0.0 | 0.0 | 0.0 | 0.0 | 0.0 | 0.0 | 0.0 | 0.0 | 2.4 | 17.1 | 0.0 | 0.0 | 17.5 | 0.0 | 0.0 | 0.0 | 0.2 |

附表 4-161 第六次中国总膳食研究略菌腈的膳食来源（单位：%）

Annexed Table 4-161 Dietary sources of fludioxonil from the 6$^{th}$ China TDS (Unit: %)

| 膳食类别 Category | 黑龙江 HL | 辽宁 LN | 河北 HE | 北京 BJ | 吉林 JL | 山西 SX | 陕西 SN | 河南 HA | 宁夏 NX | 内蒙古 NM | 青海 QH | 甘肃 GS | 上海 SH | 福建 FJ | 江西 JX | 江苏 JS | 浙江 ZJ | 山东 SD | 湖北 HB | 四川 SC | 广西 GX | 湖南 HN | 广东 GD | 贵州 GZ | 全国平均 AVG |
|---|---|---|---|---|---|---|---|---|---|---|---|---|---|---|---|---|---|---|---|---|---|---|---|---|---|
| 谷类 Cereals | 0.0 | 0.0 | 0.0 | 0.0 | 0.0 | 0.0 | 0.0 | 0.0 | 0.0 | 0.0 | 0.0 | 0.0 | 0.0 | 0.0 | 0.0 | 0.0 | 0.0 | 0.0 | 0.0 | 0.0 | 0.0 | 0.0 | 0.0 | 0.0 | 0.0 |
| 豆类 Legumes | 0.0 | 0.0 | 0.0 | 0.0 | 0.0 | 0.0 | 0.0 | 0.0 | 0.0 | 0.0 | 0.0 | 0.0 | 0.0 | 0.0 | 0.0 | 0.0 | 0.0 | 0.0 | 0.0 | 0.0 | 0.0 | 0.0 | 0.0 | 0.0 | 0.0 |
| 薯类 Potatoes | 0.0 | 0.0 | 0.0 | 0.0 | 0.0 | 0.0 | 0.0 | 0.0 | 0.0 | 0.0 | 0.0 | 0.0 | 0.0 | 0.0 | 0.0 | 0.0 | 0.0 | 0.0 | 0.0 | 0.0 | 0.0 | 0.0 | 0.0 | 0.0 | 0.0 |
| 肉类 Meats | 0.0 | 0.0 | 0.0 | 0.0 | 0.0 | 0.0 | 0.0 | 0.0 | 0.0 | 0.0 | 0.0 | 0.0 | 0.0 | 0.0 | 0.0 | 0.0 | 0.0 | 0.0 | 0.0 | 0.0 | 0.0 | 0.0 | 0.0 | 0.0 | 0.0 |
| 蛋类 Eggs | 0.0 | 0.0 | 0.0 | 0.0 | 0.0 | 0.0 | 0.0 | 0.0 | 0.0 | 0.0 | 0.0 | 0.0 | 0.0 | 0.0 | 0.0 | 0.0 | 0.0 | 0.0 | 0.0 | 0.0 | 0.0 | 0.0 | 0.0 | 0.0 | 0.0 |
| 水产类 Aquatic foods | 0.0 | 0.0 | 0.0 | 0.0 | 0.0 | 0.0 | 0.0 | 0.0 | 0.0 | 0.0 | 0.0 | 0.0 | 0.0 | 0.0 | 0.0 | 0.0 | 0.0 | 0.0 | 0.0 | 0.0 | 0.0 | 0.0 | 0.0 | 0.0 | 0.0 |
| 乳类 Dairy products | 0.0 | 0.0 | 0.0 | 0.0 | 0.0 | 0.0 | 0.0 | 0.0 | 0.0 | 0.0 | 0.0 | 0.0 | 0.0 | 0.0 | 0.0 | 0.0 | 0.0 | 0.0 | 0.0 | 0.0 | 0.0 | 0.0 | 0.0 | 0.0 | 0.0 |
| 蔬菜类 Vegetables | 0.0 | 0.0 | 100.0 | 0.0 | 0.0 | 0.0 | 0.0 | 100.0 | 0.0 | 0.0 | 0.0 | 0.0 | 0.0 | 0.0 | 0.0 | 0.0 | 0.0 | 0.0 | 0.0 | 0.0 | 0.0 | 0.0 | 0.0 | 0.0 | 0.0 |
| 水果类 Fruits | 0.0 | 0.0 | 0.0 | 0.0 | 0.0 | 0.0 | 0.0 | 0.0 | 0.0 | 0.0 | 0.0 | 0.0 | 100.0 | 0.0 | 0.0 | 0.0 | 0.0 | 0.0 | 0.0 | 0.0 | 0.0 | 0.0 | 0.0 | 0.0 | 100.0 |
| 糖类 Sugar | 0.0 | 0.0 | 0.0 | 0.0 | 0.0 | 0.0 | 0.0 | 0.0 | 0.0 | 0.0 | 0.0 | 0.0 | 0.0 | 0.0 | 0.0 | 0.0 | 0.0 | 0.0 | 0.0 | 0.0 | 0.0 | 0.0 | 0.0 | 0.0 | 0.0 |
| 水及饮料类 Water and beverages | 0.0 | 0.0 | 0.0 | 0.0 | 0.0 | 0.0 | 0.0 | 0.0 | 0.0 | 0.0 | 0.0 | 0.0 | 0.0 | 0.0 | 0.0 | 0.0 | 0.0 | 0.0 | 0.0 | 0.0 | 0.0 | 0.0 | 0.0 | 0.0 | 0.0 |

续表

| 膳食类别 Category | 黑龙江 HL | 辽宁 LN | 河北 HE | 北京 BJ | 吉林 JL | 山西 SX | 陕西 SN | 河南 HA | 宁夏 NX | 内蒙古 NM | 青海 QH | 甘肃 GS | 上海 SH | 福建 FJ | 江西 JX | 江苏 JS | 浙江 ZJ | 山东 SD | 湖北 HB | 四川 SC | 广西 GX | 湖南 HN | 广东 GD | 贵州 GZ | 全国平均 AVG |
|---|---|---|---|---|---|---|---|---|---|---|---|---|---|---|---|---|---|---|---|---|---|---|---|---|---|
| 酒类 Alcohol beverages | 0.0 | 0.0 | 0.0 | 0.0 | 0.0 | 0.0 | 0.0 | 0.0 | 0.0 | 0.0 | 0.0 | 0.0 | 0.0 | 0.0 | 0.0 | 0.0 | 0.0 | 0.0 | 0.0 | 0.0 | 0.0 | 0.0 | 0.0 | 0.0 | 0.0 |

附表 4-162　第六次中国总膳食研究膳食样品中哒螨特的含量（单位：μg/kg）

Annexed Table 4-162　Levels of propargite in food samples from the 6$^{th}$ China TDS (Unit: μg/kg)

| 膳食类别 Category | 黑龙江 HL | 辽宁 LN | 河北 HE | 北京 BJ | 吉林 JL | 山西 SX | 陕西 SN | 河南 HA | 宁夏 NX | 内蒙古 NM | 青海 QH | 甘肃 GS | 上海 SH | 福建 FJ | 江西 JX | 江苏 JS | 浙江 ZJ | 山东 SD | 湖北 HB | 四川 SC | 广西 GX | 湖南 HN | 广东 GD | 贵州 GZ | 全国平均 AVG |
|---|---|---|---|---|---|---|---|---|---|---|---|---|---|---|---|---|---|---|---|---|---|---|---|---|---|
| 谷类 Cereals | ND | ND | ND | ND | ND | ND | ND | ND | ND | ND | ND | ND | ND | ND | ND | 0.20 | ND | ND | ND | ND | ND | ND | ND | ND | 0.01 |
| 豆类 Legumes | ND | ND | ND | ND | ND | ND | ND | ND | ND | ND | ND | ND | ND | ND | ND | ND | ND | ND | ND | ND | ND | ND | ND | ND | 0.00 |
| 薯类 Potatoes | ND | ND | ND | ND | ND | ND | ND | ND | ND | 0.30 | 0.12 | 0.12 | ND | ND | ND | ND | ND | ND | ND | ND | ND | ND | ND | ND | 0.02 |
| 肉类 Meats | ND | ND | ND | ND | ND | ND | ND | 0.07 | ND | ND | 0.16 | 0.16 | ND | ND | ND | ND | ND | ND | ND | 0.35 | ND | ND | ND | ND | 0.03 |
| 蛋类 Eggs | ND | ND | ND | ND | ND | ND | ND | ND | ND | ND | ND | ND | ND | ND | ND | ND | ND | ND | ND | ND | ND | ND | ND | ND | 0.00 |
| 水产类 Aquatic foods | ND | ND | ND | ND | ND | ND | ND | ND | ND | 0.15 | 0.09 | ND | ND | ND | ND | ND | ND | ND | ND | 0.28 | ND | ND | ND | ND | 0.02 |
| 乳类 Dairy products | ND | ND | ND | ND | ND | ND | ND | ND | ND | ND | ND | ND | ND | ND | ND | ND | ND | ND | ND | ND | ND | ND | ND | ND | 0.00 |
| 蔬菜类 Vegetables | ND | ND | 0.07 | ND | 0.16 | ND | ND | 0.11 | ND | 0.17 | ND | 0.74 | ND | 0.11 | ND | ND | ND | ND | 0.12 | 0.07 | ND | 0.83 | ND | ND | 0.10 |

续表

| 膳食类别 Category | 黑龙江 HL | 辽宁 LN | 河北 HE | 北京 BJ | 吉林 JL | 山西 SX | 陕西 SN | 河南 HA | 宁夏 NX | 内蒙古 NM | 青海 QH | 甘肃 GS | 上海 SH | 福建 FJ | 江西 JX | 江苏 JS | 浙江 ZJ | 山东 SD | 湖北 HB | 四川 SC | 广西 GX | 湖南 HN | 广东 GD | 贵州 GZ | 全国平均 AVG |
|---|---|---|---|---|---|---|---|---|---|---|---|---|---|---|---|---|---|---|---|---|---|---|---|---|---|
| 水果类 Fruits | ND | 15.23 | ND | ND | ND | ND | ND | ND | ND | ND | ND | ND | 0.23 | 1.03 | ND | ND | ND | ND | 0.44 | ND | ND | ND | ND | ND | 0.71 |
| 糖类 Sugar | ND | ND | ND | ND | ND | ND | ND | ND | ND | ND | ND | ND | ND | ND | ND | ND | ND | ND | ND | ND | ND | ND | ND | ND | 0.00 |
| 水及饮料类 Water and beverages | ND | ND | ND | ND | ND | ND | ND | ND | ND | ND | ND | ND | ND | ND | ND | ND | ND | ND | ND | ND | ND | ND | ND | ND | 0.00 |
| 酒类 Alcohol beverages | ND | ND | ND | ND | ND | ND | ND | 0.09 | ND | ND | ND | ND | ND | ND | ND | ND | ND | ND | ND | ND | ND | ND | ND | ND | 0.00 |

注：未检出（ND）按0计

Note: values not detected (ND) were treated as being equal to 0

附表 4-163　第六次中国总膳食研究膳食样品中螺螨酯的含量（单位：μg/kg）

Annexed Table 4-163　Levels of spirodiclofen in food samples from the 6<sup>th</sup> China TDS (Unit: μg/kg)

| 膳食类别 Category | 黑龙江 HL | 辽宁 LN | 河北 HE | 北京 BJ | 吉林 JL | 山西 SX | 陕西 SN | 河南 HA | 宁夏 NX | 内蒙古 NM | 青海 QH | 甘肃 GS | 上海 SH | 福建 FJ | 江西 JX | 江苏 JS | 浙江 ZJ | 山东 SD | 湖北 HB | 四川 SC | 广西 GX | 湖南 HN | 广东 GD | 贵州 GZ | 全国平均 AVG |
|---|---|---|---|---|---|---|---|---|---|---|---|---|---|---|---|---|---|---|---|---|---|---|---|---|---|
| 谷类 Cereals | ND | ND | ND | ND | ND | ND | ND | ND | ND | ND | ND | ND | ND | ND | ND | ND | ND | ND | ND | ND | ND | ND | ND | ND | 0.00 |
| 豆类 Legumes | ND | ND | ND | ND | ND | ND | ND | ND | ND | ND | ND | ND | ND | ND | ND | ND | ND | ND | ND | ND | ND | ND | ND | ND | 0.00 |
| 薯类 Potatoes | ND | ND | ND | ND | ND | ND | ND | ND | ND | ND | ND | ND | ND | ND | ND | ND | ND | ND | ND | ND | ND | ND | ND | ND | 0.00 |
| 肉类 Meats | ND | ND | ND | ND | ND | ND | ND | ND | ND | ND | ND | ND | ND | ND | ND | ND | ND | ND | ND | ND | ND | ND | ND | ND | 0.00 |
| 蛋类 Eggs | ND | ND | ND | ND | ND | ND | ND | ND | ND | ND | ND | ND | ND | ND | ND | ND | ND | ND | ND | ND | ND | ND | ND | ND | 0.00 |

续表

| 膳食类别 Category | 黑龙江 HL | 辽宁 LN | 河北 HE | 北京 BJ | 吉林 JL | 山西 SX | 陕西 SN | 河南 HA | 宁夏 NX | 内蒙古 NM | 青海 QH | 甘肃 GS | 上海 SH | 福建 FJ | 江西 JX | 江苏 JS | 浙江 ZJ | 山东 SD | 湖北 HB | 四川 SC | 广西 GX | 湖南 HN | 广东 GD | 贵州 GZ | 全国平均 AVG |
|---|---|---|---|---|---|---|---|---|---|---|---|---|---|---|---|---|---|---|---|---|---|---|---|---|---|
| 水产类 Aquatic foods | ND | ND | ND | ND | ND | ND | ND | ND | ND | ND | ND | ND | ND | ND | ND | ND | ND | ND | ND | ND | ND | ND | ND | ND | 0.00 |
| 乳类 Dairy products | ND | ND | ND | ND | ND | ND | ND | ND | ND | ND | ND | ND | ND | ND | ND | ND | ND | ND | ND | ND | ND | ND | ND | ND | 0.00 |
| 蔬菜类 Vegetables | ND | ND | 0.10 | ND | ND | 0.19 | ND | 0.63 | ND | ND | 1.13 | 0.36 | 0.50 | ND | 4.62 | ND | ND | 0.24 | 0.30 | ND | ND | ND | ND | ND | 0.34 |
| 水果类 Fruits | 0.99 | ND | 0.10 | ND | ND | ND | ND | 0.24 | 0.29 | ND | 0.14 | ND | 0.54 | ND | ND | 0.12 | ND | ND | ND | ND | ND | 0.15 | 1.22 | ND | 0.16 |
| 糖类 Sugar | ND | ND | ND | ND | ND | ND | ND | ND | ND | ND | ND | ND | ND | ND | ND | ND | ND | ND | ND | ND | ND | ND | ND | ND | 0.00 |
| 水及饮料类 Water and beverages | ND | ND | ND | ND | ND | ND | ND | ND | ND | ND | ND | ND | ND | ND | ND | ND | ND | ND | ND | ND | ND | ND | ND | ND | 0.00 |
| 酒类 Alcohol beverages | ND | ND | ND | ND | ND | ND | ND | ND | ND | ND | ND | ND | ND | ND | ND | ND | ND | ND | ND | ND | ND | ND | ND | ND | 0.00 |

注：未检出（ND）按 0 计

Note: values not detected (ND) were treated as being equal to 0

附表 4-164　第六次中国总膳食研究膳食样品中哒螨灵的含量（单位：μg/kg）

Annexed Table 4-164　Levels of pyridaben in food samples from the 6th China TDS (Unit: μg/kg)

| 膳食类别 Category | 黑龙江 HL | 辽宁 LN | 河北 HE | 北京 BJ | 吉林 JL | 山西 SX | 陕西 SN | 河南 HA | 宁夏 NX | 内蒙古 NM | 青海 QH | 甘肃 GS | 上海 SH | 福建 FJ | 江西 JX | 江苏 JS | 浙江 ZJ | 山东 SD | 湖北 HB | 四川 SC | 广西 GX | 湖南 HN | 广东 GD | 贵州 GZ | 全国平均 AVG |
|---|---|---|---|---|---|---|---|---|---|---|---|---|---|---|---|---|---|---|---|---|---|---|---|---|---|
| 谷类 Cereals | ND | ND | ND | ND | ND | ND | ND | ND | ND | ND | ND | ND | ND | ND | ND | ND | ND | ND | ND | ND | ND | ND | ND | ND | 0.00 |

续表

| 膳食类别<br>Category | 黑龙江<br>HL | 辽宁<br>LN | 河北<br>HE | 北京<br>BJ | 吉林<br>JL | 山西<br>SX | 陕西<br>SN | 河南<br>HA | 宁夏<br>NX | 内蒙古<br>NM | 青海<br>QH | 甘肃<br>GS | 上海<br>SH | 福建<br>FJ | 江西<br>JX | 江苏<br>JS | 浙江<br>ZJ | 山东<br>SD | 湖北<br>HB | 四川<br>SC | 广西<br>GX | 湖南<br>HN | 广东<br>GD | 贵州<br>GZ | 全国平均<br>AVG |
|---|---|---|---|---|---|---|---|---|---|---|---|---|---|---|---|---|---|---|---|---|---|---|---|---|---|
| 豆类 Legumes | ND | ND | ND | ND | ND | ND | ND | ND | ND | ND | ND | ND | ND | ND | ND | ND | ND | ND | ND | ND | ND | ND | ND | ND | 0.00 |
| 薯类 Potatoes | ND | ND | 0.82 | 0.07 | ND | ND | ND | ND | ND | ND | ND | ND | 0.46 | ND | ND | ND | ND | ND | 0.13 | ND | ND | ND | ND | ND | 0.02 |
| 肉类 Meats | ND | 0.10 | 0.10 | ND | ND | ND | ND | ND | ND | ND | ND | ND | ND | ND | ND | ND | 0.11 | ND | ND | ND | ND | ND | ND | ND | 0.01 |
| 蛋类 Eggs | ND | ND | ND | ND | ND | ND | ND | ND | ND | ND | ND | ND | ND | ND | ND | ND | ND | ND | ND | ND | ND | ND | ND | ND | 0.00 |
| 水产类 Aquatic foods | ND | ND | ND | ND | ND | 0.12 | ND | ND | ND | ND | ND | ND | ND | ND | ND | ND | ND | ND | ND | ND | ND | ND | ND | ND | 0.01 |
| 乳类 Dairy products | ND | ND | ND | ND | ND | ND | ND | ND | ND | ND | ND | ND | ND | ND | ND | ND | ND | ND | ND | ND | ND | ND | ND | ND | 0.00 |
| 蔬菜类 Vegetables | 0.23 | 0.09 | 0.82 | 0.07 | 0.18 | 6.25 | 0.23 | 0.16 | 0.25 | ND | 0.75 | 1.27 | 28.85 | 13.62 | 2.14 | 24.11 | 60.42 | 0.35 | 16.40 | ND | 7.11 | 7.11 | 4.25 | 0.82 | 7.31 |
| 水果类 Fruits | ND | 3.93 | 0.10 | ND | ND | ND | 0.06 | ND | ND | ND | ND | ND | ND | 0.11 | ND | 0.14 | ND | 0.11 | 0.06 | ND | ND | ND | ND | ND | 0.19 |
| 糖类 Sugar | ND | ND | ND | ND | ND | ND | ND | ND | ND | ND | ND | ND | ND | ND | ND | ND | ND | ND | ND | ND | ND | ND | ND | ND | 0.00 |
| 水及饮料类 Water and beverages | ND | ND | ND | ND | ND | ND | ND | ND | ND | ND | ND | ND | ND | ND | ND | ND | ND | ND | ND | ND | ND | ND | ND | ND | 0.00 |
| 酒类 Alcohol beverages | ND | ND | ND | ND | ND | ND | ND | ND | ND | ND | ND | ND | ND | ND | ND | ND | ND | ND | ND | ND | ND | ND | ND | ND | 0.00 |

注：未检出（ND）按 0 计

Note: values not detected (ND) were treated as being equal to 0

附表 4-165　第六次中国总膳食研究的炔螨特膳食摄入量 [单位：ng/(kg bw·d)]
Annexed Table 4-165　Dietary intakes of propargite from the 6th China TDS [Unit: ng/(kg bw·d)]

| 膳食类别 Category | 黑龙江 HL | 辽宁 LN | 河北 HE | 北京 BJ | 吉林 JL | 山西 SX | 陕西 SN | 河南 HA | 宁夏 NX | 内蒙古 NM | 青海 QH | 甘肃 GS | 上海 SH | 福建 FJ | 江西 JX | 江苏 JS | 浙江 ZJ | 山东 SD | 湖北 HB | 四川 SC | 广西 GX | 湖南 HN | 广东 GD | 贵州 GZ | 全国平均 AVG |
|---|---|---|---|---|---|---|---|---|---|---|---|---|---|---|---|---|---|---|---|---|---|---|---|---|---|
| 谷类 Cereals | 0.000 | 0.000 | 0.000 | 0.000 | 0.000 | 0.000 | 0.000 | 0.000 | 0.000 | 0.000 | 0.000 | 0.000 | 0.000 | 0.000 | 0.000 | 2.528 | 0.000 | 0.000 | 0.000 | 0.000 | 0.000 | 0.000 | 0.000 | 0.000 | 0.105 |
| 豆类 Legumes | 0.000 | 0.000 | 0.000 | 0.000 | 0.000 | 0.000 | 0.000 | 0.000 | 0.000 | 0.000 | 0.000 | 0.000 | 0.000 | 0.000 | 0.000 | 0.000 | 0.000 | 0.000 | 0.000 | 0.000 | 0.000 | 0.000 | 0.000 | 0.000 | 0.000 |
| 薯类 Potatoes | 0.000 | 0.000 | 0.000 | 0.000 | 0.000 | 0.000 | 0.000 | 0.000 | 0.000 | 0.591 | 0.196 | 0.280 | 0.000 | 0.000 | 0.000 | 0.000 | 0.000 | 0.000 | 0.000 | 0.000 | 0.000 | 0.000 | 0.000 | 0.000 | 0.044 |
| 肉类 Meats | 0.000 | 0.000 | 0.000 | 0.000 | 0.000 | 0.000 | 0.000 | 0.065 | 0.000 | 0.000 | 0.184 | 0.080 | 0.000 | 0.000 | 0.000 | 0.000 | 0.000 | 0.000 | 0.000 | 0.719 | 0.000 | 0.000 | 0.000 | 0.000 | 0.044 |
| 蛋类 Eggs | 0.000 | 0.000 | 0.000 | 0.000 | 0.000 | 0.000 | 0.000 | 0.000 | 0.000 | 0.000 | 0.000 | 0.000 | 0.000 | 0.000 | 0.000 | 0.000 | 0.000 | 0.000 | 0.000 | 0.000 | 0.000 | 0.000 | 0.000 | 0.000 | 0.000 |
| 水产类 Aquatic foods | 0.000 | 0.000 | 0.000 | 0.000 | 0.000 | 0.000 | 0.000 | 0.000 | 0.000 | 0.025 | 0.005 | 0.000 | 0.000 | 0.000 | 0.000 | 0.000 | 0.000 | 0.000 | 0.000 | 0.037 | 0.000 | 0.000 | 0.000 | 0.000 | 0.003 |
| 乳类 Dairy products | 0.000 | 0.000 | 0.000 | 0.000 | 0.000 | 0.000 | 0.000 | 0.000 | 0.000 | 0.000 | 0.000 | 0.000 | 0.000 | 0.000 | 0.000 | 0.000 | 0.000 | 0.000 | 0.000 | 0.000 | 0.000 | 0.000 | 0.000 | 0.000 | 0.000 |
| 蔬菜类 Vegetables | 0.000 | 0.000 | 0.332 | 0.000 | 1.001 | 0.000 | 0.000 | 0.495 | 0.000 | 0.678 | 0.000 | 2.896 | 0.000 | 0.681 | 0.000 | 0.000 | 0.000 | 0.000 | 0.757 | 0.320 | 0.000 | 0.000 | 0.000 | 0.000 | 0.592 |
| 水果类 Fruits | 0.000 | 18.580 | 0.000 | 0.000 | 0.000 | 0.000 | 0.000 | 0.000 | 0.000 | 0.000 | 0.000 | 0.000 | 0.271 | 0.978 | 0.000 | 0.000 | 0.000 | 0.000 | 0.134 | 0.000 | 0.000 | 0.000 | 0.000 | 0.000 | 0.832 |
| 糖类 Sugar | 0.000 | 0.000 | 0.000 | 0.000 | 0.000 | 0.000 | 0.000 | 0.000 | 0.000 | 0.000 | 0.000 | 0.000 | 0.000 | 0.000 | 0.000 | 0.000 | 0.000 | 0.000 | 0.000 | 0.000 | 0.000 | 0.000 | 0.000 | 0.000 | 0.000 |
| 水及饮料类 Water and beverages | 0.000 | 0.000 | 0.000 | 0.000 | 0.000 | 0.000 | 0.000 | 0.000 | 0.000 | 0.000 | 0.000 | 0.000 | 0.000 | 0.000 | 0.000 | 0.000 | 0.000 | 0.000 | 0.000 | 0.000 | 0.000 | 0.000 | 0.000 | 0.000 | 0.000 |

续表

| 膳食类别<br>Category | 黑龙江<br>HL | 辽宁<br>LN | 河北<br>HE | 北京<br>BJ | 吉林<br>JL | 山西<br>SX | 陕西<br>SN | 河南<br>HA | 宁夏<br>NX | 内蒙古<br>NM | 青海<br>QH | 甘肃<br>GS | 上海<br>SH | 福建<br>FJ | 江西<br>JX | 江苏<br>JS | 浙江<br>ZJ | 山东<br>SD | 湖北<br>HB | 四川<br>SC | 广西<br>GX | 湖南<br>HN | 广东<br>GD | 贵州<br>GZ | 全国平均<br>AVG |
|---|---|---|---|---|---|---|---|---|---|---|---|---|---|---|---|---|---|---|---|---|---|---|---|---|---|
| 酒类<br>Alcohol beverages | 0.000 | 0.000 | 0.000 | 0.000 | 0.000 | 0.000 | 0.000 | 0.005 | 0.000 | 0.000 | 0.000 | 0.000 | 0.000 | 0.000 | 0.000 | 0.000 | 0.000 | 0.000 | 0.000 | 0.000 | 0.000 | 0.000 | 0.000 | 0.000 | 0.000 |
| 合计<br>SUM | 0.000 | 18.585 | 0.332 | 0.000 | 1.001 | 0.000 | 0.000 | 0.565 | 0.000 | 1.294 | 0.385 | 3.256 | 0.271 | 1.659 | 0.000 | 2.528 | 0.000 | 0.000 | 0.890 | 1.076 | 0.000 | 7.041 | 0.000 | 0.000 | 1.620 |

附表 4-166 第六次中国总膳食研究的螺螨酯膳食摄入量 [单位：ng/(kg bw·d)]

Annexed Table 4-166 Dietary intakes of spirodiclofen from the 6$^{th}$ China TDS [Unit: ng/(kg bw · d)]

| 膳食类别<br>Category | 黑龙江<br>HL | 辽宁<br>LN | 河北<br>HE | 北京<br>BJ | 吉林<br>JL | 山西<br>SX | 陕西<br>SN | 河南<br>HA | 宁夏<br>NX | 内蒙古<br>NM | 青海<br>QH | 甘肃<br>GS | 上海<br>SH | 福建<br>FJ | 江西<br>JX | 江苏<br>JS | 浙江<br>ZJ | 山东<br>SD | 湖北<br>HB | 四川<br>SC | 广西<br>GX | 湖南<br>HN | 广东<br>GD | 贵州<br>GZ | 全国平均<br>AVG |
|---|---|---|---|---|---|---|---|---|---|---|---|---|---|---|---|---|---|---|---|---|---|---|---|---|---|
| 谷类<br>Cereals | 0.000 | 0.000 | 0.000 | 0.000 | 0.000 | 0.000 | 0.000 | 0.000 | 0.000 | 0.000 | 0.000 | 0.000 | 0.000 | 0.000 | 0.000 | 0.000 | 0.000 | 0.000 | 0.000 | 0.000 | 0.000 | 0.000 | 0.000 | 0.000 | 0.000 |
| 豆类<br>Legumes | 0.000 | 0.000 | 0.000 | 0.000 | 0.000 | 0.000 | 0.000 | 0.000 | 0.000 | 0.000 | 0.000 | 0.000 | 0.000 | 0.000 | 0.000 | 0.000 | 0.000 | 0.000 | 0.000 | 0.000 | 0.000 | 0.000 | 0.000 | 0.000 | 0.000 |
| 薯类<br>Potatoes | 0.000 | 0.000 | 0.000 | 0.000 | 0.000 | 0.000 | 0.000 | 0.000 | 0.000 | 0.000 | 0.000 | 0.000 | 0.000 | 0.000 | 0.000 | 0.000 | 0.000 | 0.000 | 0.000 | 0.000 | 0.000 | 0.000 | 0.000 | 0.000 | 0.000 |
| 肉类<br>Meats | 0.000 | 0.000 | 0.000 | 0.000 | 0.000 | 0.000 | 0.000 | 0.000 | 0.000 | 0.000 | 0.000 | 0.000 | 0.000 | 0.000 | 0.000 | 0.000 | 0.000 | 0.000 | 0.000 | 0.000 | 0.000 | 0.000 | 0.000 | 0.000 | 0.000 |
| 蛋类<br>Eggs | 0.000 | 0.000 | 0.000 | 0.000 | 0.000 | 0.000 | 0.000 | 0.000 | 0.000 | 0.000 | 0.000 | 0.000 | 0.000 | 0.000 | 0.000 | 0.000 | 0.000 | 0.000 | 0.000 | 0.000 | 0.000 | 0.000 | 0.000 | 0.000 | 0.000 |
| 水产类<br>Aquatic foods | 0.000 | 0.000 | 0.000 | 0.000 | 0.000 | 0.000 | 0.000 | 0.000 | 0.000 | 0.000 | 0.000 | 0.000 | 0.000 | 0.000 | 0.000 | 0.000 | 0.000 | 0.000 | 0.000 | 0.000 | 0.000 | 0.000 | 0.000 | 0.000 | 0.000 |
| 乳类<br>Dairy products | 0.000 | 0.000 | 0.000 | 0.000 | 0.000 | 0.000 | 0.000 | 0.000 | 0.000 | 0.000 | 0.000 | 0.000 | 0.000 | 0.000 | 0.000 | 0.000 | 0.000 | 0.000 | 0.000 | 0.000 | 0.000 | 0.000 | 0.000 | 0.000 | 0.000 |

续表

附表 4-167 第六次中国总膳食研究的哒螨灵膳食摄入量 [单位: ng/(kg bw·d)]
Annexed Table 4-167 Dietary intakes of pyridaben from the 6th China TDS [Unit: ng/(kg bw·d)]

| 膳食类别<br>Category | 黑龙江<br>HL | 辽宁<br>LN | 河北<br>HE | 北京<br>BJ | 吉林<br>JL | 山西<br>SX | 陕西<br>SN | 河南<br>HA | 宁夏<br>NX | 内蒙古<br>NM | 青海<br>QH | 甘肃<br>GS | 上海<br>SH | 福建<br>FJ | 江西<br>JX | 江苏<br>JS | 浙江<br>ZJ | 山东<br>SD | 湖北<br>HB | 四川<br>SC | 广西<br>GX | 湖南<br>HN | 广东<br>GD | 贵州<br>GZ | 全国平均<br>AVG |
|---|---|---|---|---|---|---|---|---|---|---|---|---|---|---|---|---|---|---|---|---|---|---|---|---|---|
| 蔬菜类 Vegetables | 0.000 | 0.000 | 0.479 | 0.000 | 0.000 | 0.941 | 0.000 | 2.762 | 0.000 | 0.000 | 5.557 | 1.418 | 3.185 | 0.000 | 33.120 | 0.000 | 0.000 | 1.561 | 1.988 | 0.000 | 0.000 | 0.000 | 0.000 | 0.000 | 2.125 |
| 水果类 Fruits | 0.985 | 0.000 | 0.062 | 0.000 | 0.000 | 0.000 | 0.000 | 0.092 | 0.386 | 0.000 | 0.034 | 0.000 | 0.626 | 0.000 | 0.000 | 0.053 | 0.000 | 0.000 | 0.000 | 0.000 | 0.000 | 0.155 | 0.569 | 0.000 | 0.123 |
| 糖类 Sugar | 0.000 | 0.000 | 0.000 | 0.000 | 0.000 | 0.000 | 0.000 | 0.000 | 0.000 | 0.000 | 0.000 | 0.000 | 0.000 | 0.000 | 0.000 | 0.000 | 0.000 | 0.000 | 0.000 | 0.000 | 0.000 | 0.000 | 0.000 | 0.000 | 0.000 |
| 水及饮料类 Water and beverages | 0.000 | 0.000 | 0.000 | 0.000 | 0.000 | 0.000 | 0.000 | 0.000 | 0.000 | 0.000 | 0.000 | 0.000 | 0.000 | 0.000 | 0.000 | 0.000 | 0.000 | 0.000 | 0.000 | 0.000 | 0.000 | 0.000 | 0.000 | 0.000 | 0.000 |
| 酒类 Alcohol beverages | 0.000 | 0.000 | 0.000 | 0.000 | 0.000 | 0.000 | 0.000 | 0.000 | 0.000 | 0.000 | 0.000 | 0.000 | 0.000 | 0.000 | 0.000 | 0.000 | 0.000 | 0.000 | 0.000 | 0.000 | 0.000 | 0.000 | 0.000 | 0.000 | 0.000 |
| 合计 SUM | 0.985 | 0.000 | 0.541 | 0.000 | 0.000 | 0.941 | 0.000 | 2.855 | 0.386 | 0.000 | 5.591 | 1.418 | 3.811 | 0.000 | 33.119 | 0.053 | 0.000 | 1.561 | 1.988 | 0.000 | 0.000 | 0.155 | 0.569 | 0.000 | 2.249 |

| 膳食类别<br>Category | 黑龙江<br>HL | 辽宁<br>LN | 河北<br>HE | 北京<br>BJ | 吉林<br>JL | 山西<br>SX | 陕西<br>SN | 河南<br>HA | 宁夏<br>NX | 内蒙古<br>NM | 青海<br>QH | 甘肃<br>GS | 上海<br>SH | 福建<br>FJ | 江西<br>JX | 江苏<br>JS | 浙江<br>ZJ | 山东<br>SD | 湖北<br>HB | 四川<br>SC | 广西<br>GX | 湖南<br>HN | 广东<br>GD | 贵州<br>GZ | 全国平均<br>AVG |
|---|---|---|---|---|---|---|---|---|---|---|---|---|---|---|---|---|---|---|---|---|---|---|---|---|---|
| 谷类 Cereals | 0.000 | 0.000 | 0.000 | 0.000 | 0.000 | 0.000 | 0.000 | 0.000 | 0.000 | 0.000 | 0.000 | 0.000 | 0.000 | 0.000 | 0.000 | 0.000 | 0.000 | 0.000 | 0.000 | 0.000 | 0.000 | 0.000 | 0.000 | 0.000 | 0.000 |
| 豆类 Legumes | 0.000 | 0.000 | 0.000 | 0.000 | 0.000 | 0.000 | 0.000 | 0.000 | 0.000 | 0.000 | 0.000 | 0.000 | 0.264 | 0.000 | 0.000 | 0.000 | 0.000 | 0.000 | 0.000 | 0.000 | 0.000 | 0.000 | 0.000 | 0.000 | 0.000 |
| 薯类 Potatoes | 0.000 | 0.000 | 0.000 | 0.000 | 0.000 | 0.000 | 0.000 | 0.000 | 0.000 | 0.000 | 0.000 | 0.000 | 0.000 | 0.000 | 0.000 | 0.000 | 0.000 | 0.000 | 0.185 | 0.000 | 0.000 | 0.000 | 0.000 | 0.000 | 0.019 |

续表

| 膳食类别 Category | 黑龙江 HL | 辽宁 LN | 河北 HE | 北京 BJ | 吉林 JL | 山西 SX | 陕西 SN | 河南 HA | 宁夏 NX | 内蒙古 NM | 青海 QH | 甘肃 GS | 上海 SH | 福建 FJ | 江西 JX | 江苏 JS | 浙江 ZJ | 山东 SD | 湖北 HB | 四川 SC | 广西 GX | 湖南 HN | 广东 GD | 贵州 GZ | 全国平均 AVG |
|---|---|---|---|---|---|---|---|---|---|---|---|---|---|---|---|---|---|---|---|---|---|---|---|---|---|
| 肉类 Meats | 0.000 | 0.102 | 0.000 | 0.000 | 0.000 | 0.000 | 0.000 | 0.000 | 0.000 | 0.000 | 0.000 | 0.000 | 0.000 | 0.000 | 0.000 | 0.000 | 0.203 | 0.000 | 0.000 | 0.000 | 0.000 | 0.000 | 0.000 | 0.000 | 0.013 |
| 蛋类 Eggs | 0.000 | 0.000 | 0.000 | 0.000 | 0.000 | 0.000 | 0.000 | 0.000 | 0.000 | 0.000 | 0.000 | 0.000 | 0.000 | 0.000 | 0.000 | 0.000 | 0.000 | 0.000 | 0.000 | 0.000 | 0.000 | 0.000 | 0.000 | 0.000 | 0.000 |
| 水产类 Aquatic foods | 0.000 | 0.000 | 0.000 | 0.000 | 0.000 | 0.012 | 0.000 | 0.000 | 0.000 | 0.000 | 0.000 | 0.000 | 0.000 | 0.000 | 0.000 | 0.000 | 0.000 | 0.000 | 0.000 | 0.000 | 0.000 | 0.000 | 0.000 | 0.000 | 0.001 |
| 乳类 Dairy products | 0.000 | 0.000 | 0.000 | 0.000 | 0.000 | 0.000 | 0.000 | 0.000 | 0.000 | 0.000 | 0.000 | 0.000 | 0.000 | 0.000 | 0.000 | 0.000 | 0.000 | 0.000 | 0.000 | 0.000 | 0.000 | 0.000 | 0.000 | 0.000 | 0.000 |
| 蔬菜类 Vegetables | 1.155 | 0.461 | 3.823 | 0.455 | 1.133 | 30.720 | 1.045 | 0.685 | 0.632 | 0.000 | 3.696 | 5.017 | 183.500 | 85.820 | 15.310 | 162.800 | 425.900 | 2.274 | 107.800 | 0.000 | 39.870 | 60.260 | 15.940 | 5.336 | 48.070 |
| 水果类 Fruits | 0.000 | 4.794 | 0.063 | 0.000 | 0.000 | 0.000 | 0.037 | 0.000 | 0.000 | 0.000 | 0.000 | 0.000 | 0.000 | 0.103 | 0.000 | 0.059 | 0.000 | 0.095 | 0.019 | 0.000 | 0.000 | 0.000 | 0.000 | 0.000 | 0.215 |
| 糖类 Sugar | 0.000 | 0.000 | 0.000 | 0.000 | 0.000 | 0.000 | 0.000 | 0.000 | 0.000 | 0.000 | 0.000 | 0.000 | 0.000 | 0.000 | 0.000 | 0.000 | 0.000 | 0.000 | 0.000 | 0.000 | 0.000 | 0.000 | 0.000 | 0.000 | 0.000 |
| 水及饮料类 Water and beverages | 0.000 | 0.000 | 0.000 | 0.000 | 0.000 | 0.000 | 0.000 | 0.000 | 0.000 | 0.000 | 0.000 | 0.000 | 0.000 | 0.000 | 0.000 | 0.000 | 0.000 | 0.000 | 0.000 | 0.000 | 0.000 | 0.000 | 0.000 | 0.000 | 0.000 |
| 酒类 Alcohol beverages | 0.000 | 0.000 | 0.000 | 0.000 | 0.000 | 0.000 | 0.000 | 0.000 | 0.000 | 0.000 | 0.000 | 0.000 | 0.000 | 0.000 | 0.000 | 0.000 | 0.000 | 0.000 | 0.000 | 0.000 | 0.000 | 0.000 | 0.000 | 0.000 | 0.000 |
| 合计 SUM | 1.155 | 5.358 | 3.886 | 0.455 | 1.133 | 30.736 | 1.082 | 0.685 | 0.632 | 0.000 | 3.696 | 5.017 | 183.723 | 85.922 | 15.314 | 162.813 | 426.142 | 2.369 | 108.004 | 0.000 | 39.871 | 60.256 | 15.937 | 5.336 | 48.313 |

附表 4-168　第六次中国总膳食研究炔螨特的膳食来源（单位：%）

Annexed Table 4-168　Dietary sources of propargite from the 6th China TDS (Unit: %)

| 膳食类别 Category | 黑龙江 HL | 辽宁 LN | 河北 HE | 北京 BJ | 吉林 JL | 山西 SX | 陕西 SN | 河南 HA | 宁夏 NX | 内蒙古 NM | 青海 QH | 甘肃 GS | 上海 SH | 福建 FJ | 江西 JX | 江苏 JS | 浙江 ZJ | 山东 SD | 湖北 HB | 四川 SC | 广西 GX | 湖南 HN | 广东 GD | 贵州 GZ | 全国平均 AVG |
|---|---|---|---|---|---|---|---|---|---|---|---|---|---|---|---|---|---|---|---|---|---|---|---|---|---|
| 谷类 Cereals | 0.0 | 0.0 | 0.0 | 0.0 | 0.0 | 0.0 | 0.0 | 0.0 | 0.0 | 0.0 | 0.0 | 0.0 | 0.0 | 0.0 | 0.0 | 100.0 | 0.0 | 0.0 | 0.0 | 0.0 | 0.0 | 0.0 | 0.0 | 0.0 | 6.5 |
| 豆类 Legumes | 0.0 | 0.0 | 0.0 | 0.0 | 0.0 | 0.0 | 0.0 | 0.0 | 0.0 | 0.0 | 0.0 | 0.0 | 0.0 | 0.0 | 0.0 | 0.0 | 0.0 | 0.0 | 0.0 | 0.0 | 0.0 | 0.0 | 0.0 | 0.0 | 0.0 |
| 薯类 Potatoes | 0.0 | 0.0 | 0.0 | 0.0 | 0.0 | 0.0 | 0.0 | 0.0 | 0.0 | 45.7 | 50.9 | 8.6 | 0.0 | 0.0 | 0.0 | 0.0 | 0.0 | 0.0 | 0.0 | 0.0 | 0.0 | 0.0 | 0.0 | 0.0 | 2.7 |
| 肉类 Meats | 0.0 | 0.0 | 0.0 | 0.0 | 0.0 | 0.0 | 0.0 | 11.5 | 0.0 | 0.0 | 47.7 | 2.5 | 0.0 | 0.0 | 0.0 | 0.0 | 0.0 | 0.0 | 0.0 | 66.8 | 0.0 | 0.0 | 0.0 | 0.0 | 2.7 |
| 蛋类 Eggs | 0.0 | 0.0 | 0.0 | 0.0 | 0.0 | 0.0 | 0.0 | 0.0 | 0.0 | 0.0 | 0.0 | 0.0 | 0.0 | 0.0 | 0.0 | 0.0 | 0.0 | 0.0 | 0.0 | 0.0 | 0.0 | 0.0 | 0.0 | 0.0 | 0.0 |
| 水产类 Aquatic foods | 0.0 | 0.0 | 0.0 | 0.0 | 0.0 | 0.0 | 0.0 | 0.0 | 0.0 | 2.0 | 1.4 | 0.0 | 0.0 | 0.0 | 0.0 | 0.0 | 0.0 | 0.0 | 0.0 | 3.4 | 0.0 | 0.0 | 0.0 | 0.0 | 0.2 |
| 乳类 Dairy products | 0.0 | 0.0 | 0.0 | 0.0 | 0.0 | 0.0 | 0.0 | 0.0 | 0.0 | 0.0 | 0.0 | 0.0 | 0.0 | 0.0 | 0.0 | 0.0 | 0.0 | 0.0 | 0.0 | 0.0 | 0.0 | 0.0 | 0.0 | 0.0 | 0.0 |
| 蔬菜类 Vegetables | 0.0 | 0.0 | 100.0 | 0.0 | 100.0 | 0.0 | 0.0 | 87.7 | 0.0 | 52.4 | 0.0 | 89.0 | 0.0 | 41.0 | 0.0 | 0.0 | 0.0 | 0.0 | 85.0 | 29.8 | 0.0 | 100.0 | 0.0 | 0.0 | 36.5 |
| 水果类 Fruits | 0.0 | 100.0 | 0.0 | 0.0 | 0.0 | 0.0 | 0.0 | 0.0 | 0.0 | 0.0 | 0.0 | 0.0 | 100.0 | 59.0 | 0.0 | 0.0 | 0.0 | 0.0 | 15.0 | 0.0 | 0.0 | 0.0 | 0.0 | 0.0 | 51.4 |
| 糖类 Sugar | 0.0 | 0.0 | 0.0 | 0.0 | 0.0 | 0.0 | 0.0 | 0.0 | 0.0 | 0.0 | 0.0 | 0.0 | 0.0 | 0.0 | 0.0 | 0.0 | 0.0 | 0.0 | 0.0 | 0.0 | 0.0 | 0.0 | 0.0 | 0.0 | 0.0 |
| 水及饮料类 Water and beverages | 0.0 | 0.0 | 0.0 | 0.0 | 0.0 | 0.0 | 0.0 | 0.0 | 0.0 | 0.0 | 0.0 | 0.0 | 0.0 | 0.0 | 0.0 | 0.0 | 0.0 | 0.0 | 0.0 | 0.0 | 0.0 | 0.0 | 0.0 | 0.0 | 0.0 |

续表

| 膳食类别<br>Category | 黑龙江<br>HL | 辽宁<br>LN | 河北<br>HE | 北京<br>BJ | 吉林<br>JL | 山西<br>SX | 陕西<br>SN | 河南<br>HA | 宁夏<br>NX | 内蒙古<br>NM | 青海<br>QH | 甘肃<br>GS | 上海<br>SH | 福建<br>FJ | 江西<br>JX | 江苏<br>JS | 浙江<br>ZJ | 山东<br>SD | 湖北<br>HB | 四川<br>SC | 广西<br>GX | 湖南<br>HN | 广东<br>GD | 贵州<br>GZ | 全国平均<br>AVG |
|---|---|---|---|---|---|---|---|---|---|---|---|---|---|---|---|---|---|---|---|---|---|---|---|---|---|
| 酒类<br>Alcohol beverages | 0.0 | 0.0 | 0.0 | 0.0 | 0.0 | 0.0 | 0.0 | 0.8 | 0.0 | 0.0 | 0.0 | 0.0 | 0.0 | 0.0 | 0.0 | 0.0 | 0.0 | 0.0 | 0.0 | 0.0 | 0.0 | 0.0 | 0.0 | 0.0 | 0.0 |

附表 4-169 第六次中国总膳食研究螺螨酯的膳食来源（单位：%）

Annexed Table 4-169 Dietary sources of spirodiclofen from the 6<sup>th</sup> China TDS (Unit: %)

| 膳食类别<br>Category | 黑龙江<br>HL | 辽宁<br>LN | 河北<br>HE | 北京<br>BJ | 吉林<br>JL | 山西<br>SX | 陕西<br>SN | 河南<br>HA | 宁夏<br>NX | 内蒙古<br>NM | 青海<br>QH | 甘肃<br>GS | 上海<br>SH | 福建<br>FJ | 江西<br>JX | 江苏<br>JS | 浙江<br>ZJ | 山东<br>SD | 湖北<br>HB | 四川<br>SC | 广西<br>GX | 湖南<br>HN | 广东<br>GD | 贵州<br>GZ | 全国平均<br>AVG |
|---|---|---|---|---|---|---|---|---|---|---|---|---|---|---|---|---|---|---|---|---|---|---|---|---|---|
| 谷类<br>Cereals | 0.0 | 0.0 | 0.0 | 0.0 | 0.0 | 0.0 | 0.0 | 0.0 | 0.0 | 0.0 | 0.0 | 0.0 | 0.0 | 0.0 | 0.0 | 0.0 | 0.0 | 0.0 | 0.0 | 0.0 | 0.0 | 0.0 | 0.0 | 0.0 | 0.0 |
| 豆类<br>Legumes | 0.0 | 0.0 | 0.0 | 0.0 | 0.0 | 0.0 | 0.0 | 0.0 | 0.0 | 0.0 | 0.0 | 0.0 | 0.0 | 0.0 | 0.0 | 0.0 | 0.0 | 0.0 | 0.0 | 0.0 | 0.0 | 0.0 | 0.0 | 0.0 | 0.0 |
| 薯类<br>Potatoes | 0.0 | 0.0 | 0.0 | 0.0 | 0.0 | 0.0 | 0.0 | 0.0 | 0.0 | 0.0 | 0.0 | 0.0 | 0.0 | 0.0 | 0.0 | 0.0 | 0.0 | 0.0 | 0.0 | 0.0 | 0.0 | 0.0 | 0.0 | 0.0 | 0.0 |
| 肉类<br>Meats | 0.0 | 0.0 | 0.0 | 0.0 | 0.0 | 0.0 | 0.0 | 0.0 | 0.0 | 0.0 | 0.0 | 0.0 | 0.0 | 0.0 | 0.0 | 0.0 | 0.0 | 0.0 | 0.0 | 0.0 | 0.0 | 0.0 | 0.0 | 0.0 | 0.0 |
| 蛋类<br>Eggs | 0.0 | 0.0 | 0.0 | 0.0 | 0.0 | 0.0 | 0.0 | 0.0 | 0.0 | 0.0 | 0.0 | 0.0 | 0.0 | 0.0 | 0.0 | 0.0 | 0.0 | 0.0 | 0.0 | 0.0 | 0.0 | 0.0 | 0.0 | 0.0 | 0.0 |
| 水产类<br>Aquatic foods | 0.0 | 0.0 | 0.0 | 0.0 | 0.0 | 0.0 | 0.0 | 0.0 | 0.0 | 0.0 | 0.0 | 0.0 | 83.6 | 0.0 | 0.0 | 0.0 | 0.0 | 0.0 | 0.0 | 0.0 | 0.0 | 0.0 | 0.0 | 0.0 | 0.0 |
| 乳类<br>Dairy products | 0.0 | 0.0 | 0.0 | 0.0 | 0.0 | 0.0 | 0.0 | 0.0 | 0.0 | 0.0 | 99.4 | 100.0 | 0.0 | 0.0 | 100.0 | 0.0 | 0.0 | 100.0 | 100.0 | 0.0 | 0.0 | 0.0 | 0.0 | 0.0 | 0.0 |
| 蔬菜类<br>Vegetables | 0.0 | 0.0 | 88.6 | 0.0 | 0.0 | 100.0 | 0.0 | 96.8 | 0.0 | 0.0 | 0.0 | 0.0 | 0.0 | 0.0 | 0.0 | 0.0 | 0.0 | 0.0 | 0.0 | 0.0 | 0.0 | 0.0 | 0.0 | 0.0 | 94.5 |

续表

| 膳食类别<br>Category | 黑龙江<br>HL | 辽宁<br>LN | 河北<br>HE | 北京<br>BJ | 吉林<br>JL | 山西<br>SX | 陕西<br>SN | 河南<br>HA | 宁夏<br>NX | 内蒙古<br>NM | 青海<br>QH | 甘肃<br>GS | 上海<br>SH | 福建<br>FJ | 江西<br>JX | 江苏<br>JS | 浙江<br>ZJ | 山东<br>SD | 湖北<br>HB | 四川<br>SC | 广西<br>GX | 湖南<br>HN | 广东<br>GD | 贵州<br>GZ | 全国平均<br>AVG |
|---|---|---|---|---|---|---|---|---|---|---|---|---|---|---|---|---|---|---|---|---|---|---|---|---|---|
| 水果类 Fruits | 100.0 | 0.0 | 11.4 | 0.0 | 0.0 | 0.0 | 0.0 | 3.2 | 100.0 | 0.0 | 0.6 | 0.0 | 16.4 | 0.0 | 0.0 | 100.0 | 0.0 | 0.0 | 0.0 | 0.0 | 0.0 | 100.0 | 100.0 | 0.0 | 5.5 |
| 糖类 Sugar | 0.0 | 0.0 | 0.0 | 0.0 | 0.0 | 0.0 | 0.0 | 0.0 | 0.0 | 0.0 | 0.0 | 0.0 | 0.0 | 0.0 | 0.0 | 0.0 | 0.0 | 0.0 | 0.0 | 0.0 | 0.0 | 0.0 | 0.0 | 0.0 | 0.0 |
| 水及饮料类 Water and beverages | 0.0 | 0.0 | 0.0 | 0.0 | 0.0 | 0.0 | 0.0 | 0.0 | 0.0 | 0.0 | 0.0 | 0.0 | 0.0 | 0.0 | 0.0 | 0.0 | 0.0 | 0.0 | 0.0 | 0.0 | 0.0 | 0.0 | 0.0 | 0.0 | 0.0 |
| 酒类 Alcohol beverages | 0.0 | 0.0 | 0.0 | 0.0 | 0.0 | 0.0 | 0.0 | 0.0 | 0.0 | 0.0 | 0.0 | 0.0 | 0.0 | 0.0 | 0.0 | 0.0 | 0.0 | 0.0 | 0.0 | 0.0 | 0.0 | 0.0 | 0.0 | 0.0 | 0.0 |

附表 4-170　第六次中国总膳食研究哒螨灵的膳食来源（单位：%）

Annexed Table 4-170　Dietary sources of pyridaben from the 6$^{th}$ China TDS (Unit: %)

| 膳食类别<br>Category | 黑龙江<br>HL | 辽宁<br>LN | 河北<br>HE | 北京<br>BJ | 吉林<br>JL | 山西<br>SX | 陕西<br>SN | 河南<br>HA | 宁夏<br>NX | 内蒙古<br>NM | 青海<br>QH | 甘肃<br>GS | 上海<br>SH | 福建<br>FJ | 江西<br>JX | 江苏<br>JS | 浙江<br>ZJ | 山东<br>SD | 湖北<br>HB | 四川<br>SC | 广西<br>GX | 湖南<br>HN | 广东<br>GD | 贵州<br>GZ | 全国平均<br>AVG |
|---|---|---|---|---|---|---|---|---|---|---|---|---|---|---|---|---|---|---|---|---|---|---|---|---|---|
| 谷类 Cereals | 0.0 | 0.0 | 0.0 | 0.0 | 0.0 | 0.0 | 0.0 | 0.0 | 0.0 | 0.0 | 0.0 | 0.0 | 0.0 | 0.0 | 0.0 | 0.0 | 0.0 | 0.0 | 0.0 | 0.0 | 0.0 | 0.0 | 0.0 | 0.0 | 0.0 |
| 豆类 Legumes | 0.0 | 0.0 | 0.0 | 0.0 | 0.0 | 0.0 | 0.0 | 0.0 | 0.0 | 0.0 | 0.0 | 0.0 | 0.0 | 0.0 | 0.0 | 0.0 | 0.0 | 0.0 | 0.0 | 0.0 | 0.0 | 0.0 | 0.0 | 0.0 | 0.0 |
| 薯类 Potatoes | 0.0 | 0.0 | 0.0 | 0.0 | 0.0 | 0.0 | 0.0 | 0.0 | 0.0 | 0.0 | 0.0 | 0.0 | 0.1 | 0.0 | 0.0 | 0.0 | 0.0 | 0.0 | 0.2 | 0.0 | 0.0 | 0.0 | 0.0 | 0.0 | 0.0 |
| 肉类 Meats | 0.0 | 1.9 | 0.0 | 0.0 | 0.0 | 0.0 | 0.0 | 0.0 | 0.0 | 0.0 | 0.0 | 0.0 | 0.0 | 0.0 | 0.0 | 0.0 | 0.0 | 0.0 | 0.0 | 0.0 | 0.0 | 0.0 | 0.0 | 0.0 | 0.0 |
| 蛋类 Eggs | 0.0 | 0.0 | 0.0 | 0.0 | 0.0 | 0.0 | 0.0 | 0.0 | 0.0 | 0.0 | 0.0 | 0.0 | 0.0 | 0.0 | 0.0 | 0.0 | 0.0 | 0.0 | 0.0 | 0.0 | 0.0 | 0.0 | 0.0 | 0.0 | 0.0 |

续表

| 膳食类别<br>Category | 黑龙江<br>HL | 辽宁<br>LN | 河北<br>HE | 北京<br>BJ | 吉林<br>JL | 山西<br>SX | 陕西<br>SN | 河南<br>HA | 宁夏<br>NX | 内蒙古<br>NM | 青海<br>QH | 甘肃<br>GS | 上海<br>SH | 福建<br>FJ | 江西<br>JX | 江苏<br>JS | 浙江<br>ZJ | 山东<br>SD | 湖北<br>HB | 四川<br>SC | 广西<br>GX | 湖南<br>HN | 广东<br>GD | 贵州<br>GZ | 全国平均<br>AVG |
|---|---|---|---|---|---|---|---|---|---|---|---|---|---|---|---|---|---|---|---|---|---|---|---|---|---|
| 水产类<br>Aquatic foods | 0.0 | 0.0 | 0.0 | 0.0 | 0.0 | 0.0 | 0.0 | 0.0 | 0.0 | 0.0 | 0.0 | 0.0 | 0.0 | 0.0 | 0.0 | 0.0 | 0.0 | 0.0 | 0.0 | 0.0 | 0.0 | 0.0 | 0.0 | 0.0 | 0.0 |
| 乳类<br>Dairy products | 0.0 | 0.0 | 0.0 | 0.0 | 0.0 | 0.0 | 0.0 | 0.0 | 0.0 | 0.0 | 0.0 | 0.0 | 0.0 | 0.0 | 0.0 | 0.0 | 0.0 | 0.0 | 0.0 | 0.0 | 0.0 | 0.0 | 0.0 | 0.0 | 0.0 |
| 蔬菜类<br>Vegetables | 100.0 | 8.6 | 98.4 | 100.0 | 100.0 | 100.0 | 96.6 | 100.0 | 100.0 | 0.0 | 100.0 | 100.0 | 99.9 | 99.9 | 100.0 | 100.0 | 100.0 | 96.0 | 99.8 | 0.0 | 100.0 | 100.0 | 100.0 | 100.0 | 99.5 |
| 水果类<br>Fruits | 0.0 | 89.5 | 1.6 | 0.0 | 0.0 | 0.0 | 3.4 | 0.0 | 0.0 | 0.0 | 0.0 | 0.0 | 0.0 | 0.1 | 0.0 | 0.0 | 0.0 | 4.0 | 0.0 | 0.0 | 0.0 | 0.0 | 0.0 | 0.0 | 0.4 |
| 糖类<br>Sugar | 0.0 | 0.0 | 0.0 | 0.0 | 0.0 | 0.0 | 0.0 | 0.0 | 0.0 | 0.0 | 0.0 | 0.0 | 0.0 | 0.0 | 0.0 | 0.0 | 0.0 | 0.0 | 0.0 | 0.0 | 0.0 | 0.0 | 0.0 | 0.0 | 0.0 |
| 水及饮料类<br>Water and beverages | 0.0 | 0.0 | 0.0 | 0.0 | 0.0 | 0.0 | 0.0 | 0.0 | 0.0 | 0.0 | 0.0 | 0.0 | 0.0 | 0.0 | 0.0 | 0.0 | 0.0 | 0.0 | 0.0 | 0.0 | 0.0 | 0.0 | 0.0 | 0.0 | 0.0 |
| 酒类<br>Alcohol beverages | 0.0 | 0.0 | 0.0 | 0.0 | 0.0 | 0.0 | 0.0 | 0.0 | 0.0 | 0.0 | 0.0 | 0.0 | 0.0 | 0.0 | 0.0 | 0.0 | 0.0 | 0.0 | 0.0 | 0.0 | 0.0 | 0.0 | 0.0 | 0.0 | 0.0 |

附表 4-171 第六次中国总膳食研究膳食样品中莠去津的含量（单位：μg/kg）

Annexed Table 4-171 Levels of atrazine in food samples from the 6$^{th}$ China TDS (Unit: μg/kg)

| 膳食类别<br>Category | 黑龙江<br>HL | 辽宁<br>LN | 河北<br>HE | 北京<br>BJ | 吉林<br>JL | 山西<br>SX | 陕西<br>SN | 河南<br>HA | 宁夏<br>NX | 内蒙古<br>NM | 青海<br>QH | 甘肃<br>GS | 上海<br>SH | 福建<br>FJ | 江西<br>JX | 江苏<br>JS | 浙江<br>ZJ | 山东<br>SD | 湖北<br>HB | 四川<br>SC | 广西<br>GX | 湖南<br>HN | 广东<br>GD | 贵州<br>GZ | 全国平均<br>AVG |
|---|---|---|---|---|---|---|---|---|---|---|---|---|---|---|---|---|---|---|---|---|---|---|---|---|---|
| 谷类<br>Cereals | 0.14 | ND | ND | ND | 0.21 | ND | ND | ND | ND | ND | ND | ND | ND | ND | ND | ND | ND | ND | 0.10 | ND | ND | ND | 0.09 | 0.11 | 0.03 |
| 豆类<br>Legumes | 0.13 | ND | ND | ND | 0.52 | ND | ND | ND | ND | ND | ND | ND | ND | ND | ND | 0.60 | ND | ND | ND | ND | ND | ND | 0.08 | ND | 0.06 |

附录 671

续表

| 膳食类别 Category | 黑龙江 HL | 辽宁 LN | 河北 HE | 北京 BJ | 吉林 JL | 山西 SX | 陕西 SN | 河南 HA | 宁夏 NX | 内蒙古 NM | 青海 QH | 甘肃 GS | 上海 SH | 福建 FJ | 江西 JX | 江苏 JS | 浙江 ZJ | 山东 SD | 湖北 HB | 四川 SC | 广西 GX | 湖南 HN | 广东 GD | 贵州 GZ | 全国平均 AVG |
|---|---|---|---|---|---|---|---|---|---|---|---|---|---|---|---|---|---|---|---|---|---|---|---|---|---|
| 薯类 Potatoes | 0.11 | ND | ND | ND | 0.22 | ND | ND | ND | ND | ND | 0.09 | ND | ND | 0.08 | ND | ND | ND | ND | ND | ND | ND | ND | ND | ND | 0.02 |
| 肉类 Meats | 0.12 | 0.09 | ND | ND | 0.20 | ND | ND | ND | ND | ND | 0.32 | 0.08 | ND | 0.07 | ND | ND | ND | 0.26 | ND | ND | ND | ND | 0.09 | ND | 0.05 |
| 蛋类 Eggs | ND | ND | ND | ND | 0.63 | ND | ND | ND | ND | ND | ND | ND | ND | 0.10 | ND | ND | ND | 0.16 | ND | ND | ND | ND | ND | ND | 0.04 |
| 水产类 Aquatic foods | 0.28 | 0.12 | ND | 0.07 | 1.11 | ND | ND | 0.20 | 0.22 | ND | 0.35 | 0.07 | ND | 0.09 | 0.16 | 0.14 | 0.06 | 0.09 | ND | 0.13 | 0.17 | 0.12 | ND | ND | 0.14 |
| 乳类 Dairy products | 0.28 | ND | ND | ND | ND | ND | ND | ND | ND | ND | ND | ND | ND | ND | ND | ND | ND | ND | ND | ND | ND | ND | ND | ND | 0.01 |
| 蔬菜类 Vegetables | 0.61 | ND | ND | 0.13 | 1.12 | ND | ND | 0.07 | ND | 0.29 | ND | ND | ND | 0.09 | 0.13 | ND | 0.09 | 0.08 | 0.16 | ND | 0.10 | 0.10 | 0.14 | ND | 0.11 |
| 水果类 Fruits | 0.09 | ND | ND | 0.06 | ND | ND | ND | 0.08 | ND | ND | ND | ND | ND | ND | ND | 0.06 | ND | ND | ND | ND | ND | ND | ND | ND | 0.02 |
| 糖类 Sugar | ND | ND | ND | ND | ND | ND | ND | ND | ND | ND | ND | ND | ND | ND | ND | ND | ND | ND | ND | ND | ND | ND | ND | ND | 0.00 |
| 水及饮料类 Water and beverages | 0.06 | 0.07 | ND | ND | 0.25 | ND | ND | ND | ND | ND | ND | ND | ND | ND | ND | ND | ND | ND | ND | ND | ND | ND | ND | 0.07 | 0.02 |
| 酒类 Alcohol beverages | ND | ND | ND | ND | ND | ND | ND | ND | ND | ND | ND | ND | ND | ND | ND | ND | ND | ND | ND | ND | ND | ND | ND | ND | 0.00 |

注：未检出（ND）按 0 计

Note: values not detected (ND) were treated as being equal to 0

附表 4-172　第六次中国总膳食研究膳食样品中多效唑的含量（单位：μg/kg）

Annexed Table 4-172　Levels of paclobutrazol in food samples from the 6$^{th}$ China TDS (Unit: μg/kg)

| 膳食类别<br>Category | 黑龙江<br>HL | 辽宁<br>LN | 河北<br>HE | 北京<br>BJ | 吉林<br>JL | 山西<br>SX | 陕西<br>SN | 河南<br>HA | 宁夏<br>NX | 内蒙古<br>NM | 青海<br>QH | 甘肃<br>GS | 上海<br>SH | 福建<br>FJ | 江西<br>JX | 江苏<br>JS | 浙江<br>ZJ | 山东<br>SD | 湖北<br>HB | 四川<br>SC | 广西<br>GX | 湖南<br>HN | 广东<br>GD | 贵州<br>GZ | 全国平均<br>AVG |
|---|---|---|---|---|---|---|---|---|---|---|---|---|---|---|---|---|---|---|---|---|---|---|---|---|---|
| 谷类 Cereals | ND | ND | ND | ND | ND | ND | ND | ND | ND | ND | ND | ND | ND | ND | ND | ND | ND | ND | ND | ND | ND | ND | ND | ND | 0.00 |
| 豆类 Legumes | ND | ND | ND | ND | ND | ND | ND | ND | ND | ND | ND | ND | ND | ND | ND | ND | ND | ND | 0.12 | ND | 0.10 | ND | ND | ND | 0.01 |
| 薯类 Potatoes | ND | ND | ND | 0.31 | ND | ND | ND | ND | ND | ND | ND | ND | ND | ND | ND | ND | ND | ND | ND | ND | 0.33 | ND | 2.70 | ND | 0.14 |
| 肉类 Meats | ND | ND | ND | ND | ND | ND | ND | ND | ND | ND | ND | ND | ND | ND | ND | ND | ND | ND | ND | ND | ND | ND | ND | ND | 0.00 |
| 蛋类 Eggs | ND | ND | ND | ND | ND | ND | ND | ND | ND | ND | ND | ND | ND | ND | ND | ND | ND | ND | ND | ND | ND | ND | ND | ND | 0.00 |
| 水产类 Aquatic foods | ND | ND | ND | ND | ND | ND | ND | ND | ND | ND | 0.24 | ND | ND | ND | ND | ND | ND | ND | ND | ND | ND | ND | ND | ND | 0.00 |
| 乳类 Dairy products | ND | ND | ND | ND | ND | ND | ND | ND | ND | ND | ND | ND | ND | ND | ND | ND | ND | ND | ND | ND | ND | ND | ND | ND | 0.00 |
| 蔬菜类 Vegetables | ND | ND | ND | ND | ND | ND | ND | ND | ND | ND | ND | ND | ND | ND | ND | ND | ND | ND | 0.12 | ND | ND | ND | ND | ND | 0.01 |
| 水果类 Fruits | 0.26 | ND | 1.75 | ND | ND | ND | ND | ND | ND | ND | ND | ND | ND | 1.58 | ND | ND | ND | ND | 0.57 | ND | ND | ND | ND | ND | 0.17 |
| 糖类 Sugar | ND | ND | ND | ND | ND | ND | ND | ND | ND | ND | ND | ND | ND | ND | ND | ND | ND | ND | ND | ND | ND | ND | ND | ND | 0.00 |
| 水及饮料类 Water and beverages | ND | ND | ND | ND | ND | ND | ND | ND | ND | ND | ND | ND | ND | ND | ND | ND | ND | ND | ND | ND | ND | ND | ND | ND | 0.00 |

续表

| 膳食类别 Category | 黑龙江 HL | 辽宁 LN | 河北 HE | 北京 BJ | 吉林 JL | 山西 SX | 陕西 SN | 河南 HA | 宁夏 NX | 内蒙古 NM | 青海 QH | 甘肃 GS | 上海 SH | 福建 FJ | 江西 JX | 江苏 JS | 浙江 ZJ | 山东 SD | 湖北 HB | 四川 SC | 广西 GX | 湖南 HN | 广东 GD | 贵州 GZ | 全国平均 AVG |
|---|---|---|---|---|---|---|---|---|---|---|---|---|---|---|---|---|---|---|---|---|---|---|---|---|---|
| 酒类 Alcohol beverages | ND | ND | ND | ND | ND | ND | ND | ND | ND | ND | ND | ND | ND | ND | ND | ND | ND | ND | ND | ND | ND | ND | ND | ND | 0.00 |

注：未检出（ND）按 0 计
Note: values not detected (ND) were treated as being equal to 0

附表 4-173　第六次中国总膳食研究的莠去津膳食摄入量 [ 单位：ng/(kg bw · d]
Annexed Table 4-173　Dietary intakes of atrazine from the 6th China TDS [Unit: ng/(kg bw · d)]

| 膳食类别 Category | 黑龙江 HL | 辽宁 LN | 河北 HE | 北京 BJ | 吉林 JL | 山西 SX | 陕西 SN | 河南 HA | 宁夏 NX | 内蒙古 NM | 青海 QH | 甘肃 GS | 上海 SH | 福建 FJ | 江西 JX | 江苏 JS | 浙江 ZJ | 山东 SD | 湖北 HB | 四川 SC | 广西 GX | 湖南 HN | 广东 GD | 贵州 GZ | 全国平均 AVG |
|---|---|---|---|---|---|---|---|---|---|---|---|---|---|---|---|---|---|---|---|---|---|---|---|---|---|
| 谷类 Cereals | 1.179 | 0.000 | 0.000 | 0.000 | 1.956 | 0.000 | 0.000 | 0.000 | 0.000 | 0.000 | 0.000 | 0.000 | 0.000 | 0.000 | 0.000 | 0.000 | 0.000 | 0.000 | 0.804 | 0.000 | 0.000 | 0.000 | 0.686 | 1.209 | 0.243 |
| 豆类 Legumes | 0.094 | 0.000 | 0.000 | 0.000 | 0.618 | 0.000 | 0.000 | 0.000 | 0.000 | 0.000 | 0.000 | 0.000 | 0.000 | 0.000 | 0.000 | 0.797 | 0.000 | 0.000 | 0.000 | 0.000 | 0.000 | 0.000 | 0.035 | 0.000 | 0.064 |
| 薯类 Potatoes | 0.132 | 0.000 | 0.000 | 0.000 | 0.424 | 0.000 | 0.000 | 0.000 | 0.000 | 0.000 | 0.150 | 0.000 | 0.000 | 0.052 | 0.000 | 0.000 | 0.000 | 0.000 | 0.000 | 0.000 | 0.000 | 0.000 | 0.000 | 0.000 | 0.032 |
| 肉类 Meats | 0.112 | 0.092 | 0.000 | 0.000 | 0.209 | 0.000 | 0.000 | 0.000 | 0.000 | 0.000 | 0.358 | 0.039 | 0.000 | 0.091 | 0.000 | 0.000 | 0.000 | 0.399 | 0.000 | 0.000 | 0.000 | 0.000 | 0.000 | 0.000 | 0.060 |
| 蛋类 Eggs | 0.000 | 0.000 | 0.000 | 0.000 | 0.404 | 0.000 | 0.000 | 0.000 | 0.000 | 0.000 | 0.000 | 0.003 | 0.000 | 0.029 | 0.000 | 0.000 | 0.000 | 0.115 | 0.000 | 0.000 | 0.000 | 0.000 | 0.146 | 0.000 | 0.023 |
| 水产类 Aquatic foods | 0.120 | 0.030 | 0.000 | 0.019 | 0.197 | 0.000 | 0.000 | 0.015 | 0.008 | 0.000 | 0.020 | 0.000 | 0.000 | 0.092 | 0.111 | 0.088 | 0.050 | 0.032 | 0.000 | 0.017 | 0.263 | 0.128 | 0.000 | 0.000 | 0.050 |
| 乳类 Dairy products | 0.059 | 0.000 | 0.000 | 0.000 | 0.000 | 0.000 | 0.000 | 0.000 | 0.000 | 0.000 | 0.000 | 0.000 | 0.000 | 0.000 | 0.000 | 0.000 | 0.000 | 0.000 | 0.000 | 0.000 | 0.000 | 0.000 | 0.000 | 0.000 | 0.002 |

续表

| 膳食类别<br>Category | 黑龙江<br>HL | 辽宁<br>LN | 河北<br>HE | 北京<br>BJ | 吉林<br>JL | 山西<br>SX | 陕西<br>SN | 河南<br>HA | 宁夏<br>NX | 内蒙古<br>NM | 青海<br>QH | 甘肃<br>GS | 上海<br>SH | 福建<br>FJ | 江西<br>JX | 江苏<br>JS | 浙江<br>ZJ | 山东<br>SD | 湖北<br>HB | 四川<br>SC | 广西<br>GX | 湖南<br>HN | 广东<br>GD | 贵州<br>GZ | 全国平均<br>AVG |
|---|---|---|---|---|---|---|---|---|---|---|---|---|---|---|---|---|---|---|---|---|---|---|---|---|---|
| 蔬菜类 Vegetables | 3.083 | 0.000 | 0.000 | 0.817 | 6.924 | 0.000 | 0.000 | 0.000 | 0.000 | 0.000 | 0.000 | 0.000 | 0.000 | 0.550 | 0.932 | 0.000 | 0.602 | 0.497 | 1.052 | 0.000 | 0.572 | 0.874 | 0.542 | 0.000 | 0.685 |
| 水果类 Fruits | 0.086 | 0.000 | 0.000 | 0.114 | 0.000 | 0.000 | 0.000 | 0.027 | 0.000 | 0.525 | 0.000 | 0.000 | 0.000 | 0.000 | 0.000 | 0.000 | 0.000 | 0.000 | 0.000 | 0.000 | 0.000 | 0.000 | 0.000 | 0.000 | 0.031 |
| 糖类 Sugar | 0.000 | 0.000 | 0.000 | 0.000 | 0.000 | 0.000 | 0.000 | 0.000 | 0.000 | 0.000 | 0.000 | 0.000 | 0.000 | 0.000 | 0.000 | 0.000 | 0.000 | 0.000 | 0.000 | 0.000 | 0.000 | 0.000 | 0.000 | 0.000 | 0.000 |
| 水及饮料类 Water and beverages | 1.164 | 0.548 | 0.000 | 0.000 | 5.165 | 0.000 | 0.000 | 1.514 | 0.000 | 0.000 | 0.000 | 0.000 | 0.000 | 0.000 | 0.000 | 0.961 | 0.000 | 0.000 | 0.000 | 0.000 | 0.000 | 0.000 | 0.000 | 1.392 | 0.448 |
| 酒类 Alcohol beverages | 0.000 | 0.000 | 0.000 | 0.000 | 0.000 | 0.000 | 0.000 | 0.000 | 0.000 | 0.000 | 0.000 | 0.000 | 0.000 | 0.000 | 0.000 | 0.000 | 0.000 | 0.000 | 0.000 | 0.000 | 0.000 | 0.000 | 0.000 | 0.000 | 0.000 |
| 合计 SUM | 6.030 | 0.670 | 0.000 | 0.951 | 15.895 | 0.000 | 0.000 | 1.556 | 0.008 | 0.525 | 0.528 | 0.042 | 0.000 | 0.814 | 1.043 | 1.846 | 0.652 | 1.043 | 1.856 | 0.017 | 0.836 | 1.001 | 1.409 | 2.601 | 1.638 |

附表 4-174　第六次中国总膳食研究的多效唑膳食摄入量 [单位: ng/(kg bw·d)]
Annexed Table 4-174　Dietary intakes of paclobutrazol from the 6th China TDS [Unit: ng/(kg bw·d)]

| 膳食类别<br>Category | 黑龙江<br>HL | 辽宁<br>LN | 河北<br>HE | 北京<br>BJ | 吉林<br>JL | 山西<br>SX | 陕西<br>SN | 河南<br>HA | 宁夏<br>NX | 内蒙古<br>NM | 青海<br>QH | 甘肃<br>GS | 上海<br>SH | 福建<br>FJ | 江西<br>JX | 江苏<br>JS | 浙江<br>ZJ | 山东<br>SD | 湖北<br>HB | 四川<br>SC | 广西<br>GX | 湖南<br>HN | 广东<br>GD | 贵州<br>GZ | 全国平均<br>AVG |
|---|---|---|---|---|---|---|---|---|---|---|---|---|---|---|---|---|---|---|---|---|---|---|---|---|---|
| 谷类 Cereals | 0.000 | 0.000 | 0.000 | 0.000 | 0.000 | 0.000 | 0.000 | 0.000 | 0.000 | 0.000 | 0.000 | 0.000 | 0.000 | 0.000 | 0.000 | 0.000 | 0.000 | 0.000 | 0.000 | 0.000 | 0.000 | 0.000 | 0.000 | 0.000 | 0.000 |
| 豆类 Legumes | 0.000 | 0.000 | 0.000 | 0.000 | 0.000 | 0.000 | 0.000 | 0.000 | 0.000 | 0.000 | 0.000 | 0.000 | 0.000 | 0.000 | 0.000 | 0.000 | 0.000 | 0.000 | 0.131 | 0.000 | 0.065 | 0.000 | 0.000 | 0.000 | 0.008 |
| 薯类 Potatoes | 0.000 | 0.000 | 0.000 | 0.291 | 0.000 | 0.000 | 0.000 | 0.000 | 0.000 | 0.000 | 0.000 | 0.000 | 0.000 | 0.000 | 0.000 | 0.000 | 0.000 | 0.000 | 0.000 | 0.000 | 0.067 | 0.000 | 1.058 | 0.000 | 0.059 |

续表

| 膳食类别 Category | 黑龙江 HL | 辽宁 LN | 河北 HE | 北京 BJ | 吉林 JL | 山西 SX | 陕西 SN | 河南 HA | 宁夏 NX | 内蒙古 NM | 青海 QH | 甘肃 GS | 上海 SH | 福建 FJ | 江西 JX | 江苏 JS | 浙江 ZJ | 山东 SD | 湖北 HB | 四川 SC | 广西 GX | 湖南 HN | 广东 GD | 贵州 GZ | 全国平均 AVG |
|---|---|---|---|---|---|---|---|---|---|---|---|---|---|---|---|---|---|---|---|---|---|---|---|---|---|
| 肉类 Meats | 0.000 | 0.000 | 0.000 | 0.000 | 0.000 | 0.000 | 0.000 | 0.000 | 0.000 | 0.000 | 0.000 | 0.000 | 0.000 | 0.000 | 0.000 | 0.000 | 0.000 | 0.000 | 0.000 | 0.000 | 0.000 | 0.000 | 0.000 | 0.000 | 0.000 |
| 蛋类 Eggs | 0.000 | 0.000 | 0.000 | 0.000 | 0.000 | 0.000 | 0.000 | 0.000 | 0.000 | 0.000 | 0.000 | 0.000 | 0.000 | 0.000 | 0.000 | 0.000 | 0.000 | 0.000 | 0.000 | 0.000 | 0.000 | 0.000 | 0.000 | 0.000 | 0.000 |
| 水产类 Aquatic foods | 0.000 | 0.000 | 0.000 | 0.000 | 0.000 | 0.000 | 0.000 | 0.000 | 0.000 | 0.000 | 0.000 | 0.000 | 0.000 | 0.000 | 0.000 | 0.000 | 0.000 | 0.000 | 0.000 | 0.000 | 0.000 | 0.000 | 0.000 | 0.000 | 0.000 |
| 乳类 Dairy products | 0.000 | 0.000 | 0.000 | 0.000 | 0.000 | 0.000 | 0.000 | 0.000 | 0.000 | 0.000 | 0.000 | 0.000 | 0.000 | 0.000 | 0.000 | 0.000 | 0.000 | 0.000 | 0.000 | 0.000 | 0.000 | 0.000 | 0.000 | 0.000 | 0.000 |
| 蔬菜类 Vegetables | 0.000 | 0.000 | 0.000 | 0.000 | 0.000 | 0.000 | 0.000 | 0.000 | 0.000 | 0.000 | 1.182 | 0.000 | 0.000 | 0.000 | 0.000 | 0.000 | 0.000 | 0.000 | 0.770 | 0.000 | 0.000 | 0.000 | 0.000 | 0.000 | 0.081 |
| 水果类 Fruits | 0.258 | 0.000 | 1.046 | 0.000 | 0.000 | 0.000 | 0.000 | 0.000 | 0.000 | 0.000 | 0.000 | 0.000 | 0.000 | 1.498 | 0.000 | 0.000 | 0.000 | 0.000 | 0.174 | 0.000 | 0.000 | 0.000 | 0.000 | 0.000 | 0.124 |
| 糖类 Sugar | 0.000 | 0.000 | 0.000 | 0.000 | 0.000 | 0.000 | 0.000 | 0.000 | 0.000 | 0.000 | 0.000 | 0.000 | 0.000 | 0.000 | 0.000 | 0.000 | 0.000 | 0.000 | 0.000 | 0.000 | 0.000 | 0.000 | 0.000 | 0.000 | 0.000 |
| 水及饮料类 Water and beverages | 0.000 | 0.000 | 0.000 | 0.000 | 0.000 | 0.000 | 0.000 | 0.000 | 0.000 | 0.000 | 0.000 | 0.000 | 0.000 | 0.000 | 0.000 | 0.000 | 0.000 | 0.000 | 0.000 | 0.000 | 0.000 | 0.000 | 0.000 | 0.000 | 0.000 |
| 酒类 Alcohol beverages | 0.000 | 0.000 | 0.000 | 0.291 | 0.000 | 0.000 | 0.000 | 0.000 | 0.000 | 0.000 | 0.000 | 0.000 | 0.000 | 0.000 | 0.000 | 0.000 | 0.000 | 0.000 | 0.000 | 0.000 | 0.132 | 0.000 | 1.058 | 0.000 | 0.000 |
| 合计 SUM | 0.258 | 0.000 | 1.046 | 0.291 | 0.000 | 0.000 | 0.000 | 0.000 | 0.000 | 0.000 | 1.182 | 0.000 | 0.000 | 1.498 | 0.000 | 0.000 | 0.000 | 0.000 | 1.075 | 0.000 | 0.132 | 0.000 | 1.058 | 0.000 | 0.273 |

附表 4-175　第六次中国总膳食研究莠去津的膳食来源（单位：%）

Annexed Table 4-175　Dietary sources of atrazine from the 6th China TDS (Unit: %)

| 膳食类别<br>Category | 黑龙江<br>HL | 辽宁<br>LN | 河北<br>HE | 北京<br>BJ | 吉林<br>JL | 山西<br>SX | 陕西<br>SN | 河南<br>HA | 宁夏<br>NX | 内蒙古<br>NM | 青海<br>QH | 甘肃<br>GS | 上海<br>SH | 福建<br>FJ | 江西<br>JX | 江苏<br>JS | 浙江<br>ZJ | 山东<br>SD | 湖北<br>HB | 四川<br>SC | 广西<br>GX | 湖南<br>HN | 广东<br>GD | 贵州<br>GZ | 全国平均<br>AVG |
|---|---|---|---|---|---|---|---|---|---|---|---|---|---|---|---|---|---|---|---|---|---|---|---|---|---|
| 谷类 Cereals | 19.5 | 0.0 | 0.0 | 0.0 | 12.3 | 0.0 | 0.0 | 0.0 | 0.0 | 0.0 | 0.0 | 0.0 | 0.0 | 0.0 | 0.0 | 0.0 | 0.0 | 0.0 | 43.3 | 0.0 | 0.0 | 0.0 | 48.7 | 46.5 | 14.8 |
| 豆类 Legumes | 1.6 | 0.0 | 0.0 | 0.0 | 3.9 | 0.0 | 0.0 | 0.0 | 0.0 | 0.0 | 0.0 | 0.0 | 0.0 | 0.0 | 0.0 | 43.1 | 0.0 | 0.0 | 0.0 | 0.0 | 0.0 | 0.0 | 2.5 | 0.0 | 3.9 |
| 薯类 Potatoes | 2.2 | 0.0 | 0.0 | 0.0 | 2.7 | 0.0 | 0.0 | 0.0 | 0.0 | 0.0 | 28.4 | 0.0 | 0.0 | 6.4 | 0.0 | 0.0 | 0.0 | 0.0 | 0.0 | 0.0 | 0.0 | 0.0 | 0.0 | 0.0 | 1.9 |
| 肉类 Meats | 1.9 | 13.7 | 0.0 | 0.0 | 1.3 | 0.0 | 0.0 | 0.0 | 0.0 | 0.0 | 67.8 | 92.5 | 0.0 | 11.2 | 0.0 | 0.0 | 0.0 | 38.2 | 0.0 | 0.0 | 0.0 | 0.0 | 10.4 | 0.0 | 3.7 |
| 蛋类 Eggs | 0.0 | 0.0 | 0.0 | 0.0 | 2.5 | 0.0 | 0.0 | 0.0 | 0.0 | 0.0 | 0.0 | 0.0 | 0.0 | 3.5 | 0.0 | 0.0 | 0.0 | 11.0 | 0.0 | 0.0 | 0.0 | 0.0 | 0.0 | 0.0 | 1.4 |
| 水产类 Aquatic foods | 2.0 | 4.5 | 0.0 | 2.0 | 1.2 | 0.0 | 0.0 | 0.9 | 100.0 | 0.0 | 3.8 | 7.5 | 0.0 | 11.3 | 10.6 | 4.8 | 7.7 | 3.1 | 0.0 | 100.0 | 31.5 | 12.8 | 0.0 | 0.0 | 3.0 |
| 乳类 Dairy products | 1.0 | 0.0 | 0.0 | 0.0 | 0.0 | 0.0 | 0.0 | 0.0 | 0.0 | 0.0 | 0.0 | 0.0 | 0.0 | 0.0 | 0.0 | 0.0 | 0.0 | 0.0 | 0.0 | 0.0 | 0.0 | 0.0 | 0.0 | 0.0 | 0.2 |
| 蔬菜类 Vegetables | 51.1 | 0.0 | 0.0 | 85.9 | 43.6 | 0.0 | 0.0 | 0.0 | 0.0 | 100.0 | 0.0 | 0.0 | 0.0 | 67.5 | 89.4 | 0.0 | 92.3 | 47.7 | 56.7 | 0.0 | 68.5 | 87.2 | 38.5 | 0.0 | 41.8 |
| 水果类 Fruits | 1.4 | 0.0 | 0.0 | 12.0 | 0.0 | 0.0 | 0.0 | 1.7 | 0.0 | 0.0 | 0.0 | 0.0 | 0.0 | 0.0 | 0.0 | 0.0 | 0.0 | 0.0 | 0.0 | 0.0 | 0.0 | 0.0 | 0.0 | 0.0 | 1.9 |
| 糖类 Sugar | 0.0 | 0.0 | 0.0 | 0.0 | 0.0 | 0.0 | 0.0 | 0.0 | 0.0 | 0.0 | 0.0 | 0.0 | 0.0 | 0.0 | 0.0 | 0.0 | 0.0 | 0.0 | 0.0 | 0.0 | 0.0 | 0.0 | 0.0 | 0.0 | 0.0 |

续表

| 膳食类别<br>Category | 黑龙江<br>HL | 辽宁<br>LN | 河北<br>HE | 北京<br>BJ | 吉林<br>JL | 山西<br>SX | 陕西<br>SN | 河南<br>HA | 宁夏<br>NX | 内蒙古<br>NM | 青海<br>QH | 甘肃<br>GS | 上海<br>SH | 福建<br>FJ | 江西<br>JX | 江苏<br>JS | 浙江<br>ZJ | 山东<br>SD | 湖北<br>HB | 四川<br>SC | 广西<br>GX | 湖南<br>HN | 广东<br>GD | 贵州<br>GZ | 全国平均<br>AVG |
|---|---|---|---|---|---|---|---|---|---|---|---|---|---|---|---|---|---|---|---|---|---|---|---|---|---|
| 水及饮料类<br>Water and beverages | 19.3 | 81.9 | 0.0 | 0.0 | 32.5 | 0.0 | 0.0 | 97.3 | 0.0 | 0.0 | 0.0 | 0.0 | 0.0 | 0.0 | 0.0 | 52.1 | 0.0 | 0.0 | 0.0 | 0.0 | 0.0 | 0.0 | 0.0 | 53.5 | 27.3 |
| 酒类<br>Alcohol beverages | 0.0 | 0.0 | 0.0 | 0.0 | 0.0 | 0.0 | 0.0 | 0.0 | 0.0 | 0.0 | 0.0 | 0.0 | 0.0 | 0.0 | 0.0 | 0.0 | 0.0 | 0.0 | 0.0 | 0.0 | 0.0 | 0.0 | 0.0 | 0.0 | 0.0 |

附表 4-176　第六次中国总膳食研究多效唑的膳食来源（单位：%）

Annexed Table 4-176　Dietary sources of paclobutrazol from the 6$^{th}$ China TDS (Unit: %)

| 膳食类别<br>Category | 黑龙江<br>HL | 辽宁<br>LN | 河北<br>HE | 北京<br>BJ | 吉林<br>JL | 山西<br>SX | 陕西<br>SN | 河南<br>HA | 宁夏<br>NX | 内蒙古<br>NM | 青海<br>QH | 甘肃<br>GS | 上海<br>SH | 福建<br>FJ | 江西<br>JX | 江苏<br>JS | 浙江<br>ZJ | 山东<br>SD | 湖北<br>HB | 四川<br>SC | 广西<br>GX | 湖南<br>HN | 广东<br>GD | 贵州<br>GZ | 全国平均<br>AVG |
|---|---|---|---|---|---|---|---|---|---|---|---|---|---|---|---|---|---|---|---|---|---|---|---|---|---|
| 谷类<br>Cereals | 0.0 | 0.0 | 0.0 | 0.0 | 0.0 | 0.0 | 0.0 | 0.0 | 0.0 | 0.0 | 0.0 | 0.0 | 0.0 | 0.0 | 0.0 | 0.0 | 0.0 | 0.0 | 0.0 | 0.0 | 0.0 | 0.0 | 0.0 | 0.0 | 0.0 |
| 豆类<br>Legumes | 0.0 | 0.0 | 0.0 | 0.0 | 0.0 | 0.0 | 0.0 | 0.0 | 0.0 | 0.0 | 0.0 | 0.0 | 0.0 | 0.0 | 0.0 | 0.0 | 0.0 | 0.0 | 12.2 | 0.0 | 49.4 | 0.0 | 0.0 | 0.0 | 3.0 |
| 薯类<br>Potatoes | 0.0 | 0.0 | 0.0 | 100.0 | 0.0 | 0.0 | 0.0 | 0.0 | 0.0 | 0.0 | 0.0 | 0.0 | 0.0 | 0.0 | 0.0 | 0.0 | 0.0 | 0.0 | 0.0 | 0.0 | 50.6 | 0.0 | 100.0 | 0.0 | 21.7 |
| 肉类<br>Meats | 0.0 | 0.0 | 0.0 | 0.0 | 0.0 | 0.0 | 0.0 | 0.0 | 0.0 | 0.0 | 0.0 | 0.0 | 0.0 | 0.0 | 0.0 | 0.0 | 0.0 | 0.0 | 0.0 | 0.0 | 0.0 | 0.0 | 0.0 | 0.0 | 0.0 |
| 蛋类<br>Eggs | 0.0 | 0.0 | 0.0 | 0.0 | 0.0 | 0.0 | 0.0 | 0.0 | 0.0 | 0.0 | 0.0 | 0.0 | 0.0 | 0.0 | 0.0 | 0.0 | 0.0 | 0.0 | 0.0 | 0.0 | 0.0 | 0.0 | 0.0 | 0.0 | 0.0 |
| 水产类<br>Aquatic foods | 0.0 | 0.0 | 0.0 | 0.0 | 0.0 | 0.0 | 0.0 | 0.0 | 0.0 | 0.0 | 0.0 | 0.0 | 0.0 | 0.0 | 0.0 | 0.0 | 0.0 | 0.0 | 0.0 | 0.0 | 0.0 | 0.0 | 0.0 | 0.0 | 0.0 |

续表

| 膳食类别 Category | 黑龙江 HL | 辽宁 LN | 河北 HE | 北京 BJ | 吉林 JL | 山西 SX | 陕西 SN | 河南 HA | 宁夏 NX | 内蒙古 NM | 青海 QH | 甘肃 GS | 上海 SH | 福建 FJ | 江西 JX | 江苏 JS | 浙江 ZJ | 山东 SD | 湖北 HB | 四川 SC | 广西 GX | 湖南 HN | 广东 GD | 贵州 GZ | 全国平均 AVG |
|---|---|---|---|---|---|---|---|---|---|---|---|---|---|---|---|---|---|---|---|---|---|---|---|---|---|
| 乳类 Dairy products | 0.0 | 0.0 | 0.0 | 0.0 | 0.0 | 0.0 | 0.0 | 0.0 | 0.0 | 0.0 | 0.0 | 0.0 | 0.0 | 0.0 | 0.0 | 0.0 | 0.0 | 0.0 | 0.0 | 0.0 | 0.0 | 0.0 | 0.0 | 0.0 | 0.0 |
| 蔬菜类 Vegetables | 0.0 | 0.0 | 0.0 | 0.0 | 0.0 | 0.0 | 0.0 | 0.0 | 0.0 | 0.0 | 100.0 | 0.0 | 0.0 | 0.0 | 0.0 | 0.0 | 0.0 | 0.0 | 71.6 | 0.0 | 0.0 | 0.0 | 0.0 | 0.0 | 29.8 |
| 水果类 Fruits | 100.0 | 0.0 | 100.0 | 0.0 | 0.0 | 0.0 | 0.0 | 0.0 | 0.0 | 0.0 | 0.0 | 0.0 | 0.0 | 100.0 | 0.0 | 0.0 | 0.0 | 0.0 | 16.2 | 0.0 | 0.0 | 0.0 | 0.0 | 0.0 | 45.5 |
| 糖类 Sugar | 0.0 | 0.0 | 0.0 | 0.0 | 0.0 | 0.0 | 0.0 | 0.0 | 0.0 | 0.0 | 0.0 | 0.0 | 0.0 | 0.0 | 0.0 | 0.0 | 0.0 | 0.0 | 0.0 | 0.0 | 0.0 | 0.0 | 0.0 | 0.0 | 0.0 |
| 水及饮料类 Water and beverages | 0.0 | 0.0 | 0.0 | 0.0 | 0.0 | 0.0 | 0.0 | 0.0 | 0.0 | 0.0 | 0.0 | 0.0 | 0.0 | 0.0 | 0.0 | 0.0 | 0.0 | 0.0 | 0.0 | 0.0 | 0.0 | 0.0 | 0.0 | 0.0 | 0.0 |
| 酒类 Alcohol beverages | 0.0 | 0.0 | 0.0 | 0.0 | 0.0 | 0.0 | 0.0 | 0.0 | 0.0 | 0.0 | 0.0 | 0.0 | 0.0 | 0.0 | 0.0 | 0.0 | 0.0 | 0.0 | 0.0 | 0.0 | 0.0 | 0.0 | 0.0 | 0.0 | 0.0 |

# 第五章 附 表
# Annexed Tables of Chapter 5

附表 5-1 第六次中国总膳食研究膳食样品中甲氧苄啶的含量（单位：μg/kg）

Annexed Table 5-1 Levels of trimethoprim in food samples from the 6<sup>th</sup> China TDS (Unit: μg/kg)

| 膳食类别<br>Category | 黑龙江<br>HL | 辽宁<br>LN | 河北<br>HE | 北京<br>BJ | 吉林<br>JL | 山西<br>SX | 陕西<br>SN | 河南<br>HA | 宁夏<br>NX | 内蒙古<br>NM | 青海<br>QH | 甘肃<br>GS | 上海<br>SH | 福建<br>FJ | 江西<br>JX | 江苏<br>JS | 浙江<br>ZJ | 山东<br>SD | 湖北<br>HB | 四川<br>SC | 广西<br>GX | 湖南<br>HN | 广东<br>GD | 贵州<br>GZ | 全国平均<br>AVG |
|---|---|---|---|---|---|---|---|---|---|---|---|---|---|---|---|---|---|---|---|---|---|---|---|---|---|
| 肉类 Meats | 1.42 | 0.06 | ND | 2.14 | 0.78 | 0.14 | ND | 0.18 | 1.05 | ND | 0.06 | 0.05 | 0.21 | ND | 0.25 | 0.71 | 13.67 | 0.14 | 0.04 | 0.07 | 0.39 | 13.30 | 0.53 | 0.47 | 1.49 |
| 蛋类 Eggs | 7.60 | 0.23 | 0.39 | 0.31 | 13.40 | 0.08 | ND | ND | ND | ND | 0.06 | 0.33 | 0.17 | 0.12 | 0.11 | 0.98 | 0.25 | 173.15 | 0.13 | 0.13 | 0.05 | ND | 0.15 | 3.98 | 8.40 |
| 水产类 Aquatic foods | ND | ND | 0.05 | ND | ND | ND | 0.14 | ND | 0.03 | ND | 0.07 | ND | ND | ND | ND | ND | 0.10 | ND | 0.09 | ND | ND | 0.22 | ND | ND | 0.03 |
| 乳类 Dairy products | ND | 0.06 | ND | ND | ND | ND | ND | ND | ND | ND | 0.10 | 0.05 | 0.08 | ND | ND | ND | ND | 0.04 | ND | ND | ND | ND | 0.11 | ND | 0.02 |

注：未检出（ND）按 0 计
Note: values not detected (ND) were treated as being equal to 0

附表 5-2 第六次中国总膳食研究的甲氧苄啶膳食摄入量 [单位：ng/(kg bw·d)]

Annexed Table 5-2 Dietary intakes of trimethoprim from the 6<sup>th</sup> China TDS [Unit: ng/(kg bw·d)]

| 膳食类别<br>Category | 黑龙江<br>HL | 辽宁<br>LN | 河北<br>HE | 北京<br>BJ | 吉林<br>JL | 山西<br>SX | 陕西<br>SN | 河南<br>HA | 宁夏<br>NX | 内蒙古<br>NM | 青海<br>QH | 甘肃<br>GS | 上海<br>SH | 福建<br>FJ | 江西<br>JX | 江苏<br>JS | 浙江<br>ZJ | 山东<br>SD | 湖北<br>HB | 四川<br>SC | 广西<br>GX | 湖南<br>HN | 广东<br>GD | 贵州<br>GZ | 全国平均<br>AVG |
|---|---|---|---|---|---|---|---|---|---|---|---|---|---|---|---|---|---|---|---|---|---|---|---|---|---|
| 肉类 Meats | 1.354 | 0.067 | 0.000 | 2.281 | 0.822 | 0.303 | 0.000 | 0.158 | 0.777 | 0.000 | 0.065 | 0.027 | 0.375 | 0.000 | 0.377 | 1.030 | 25.668 | 0.217 | 0.038 | 0.143 | 0.942 | 31.568 | 0.872 | 0.800 | 2.828 |

续表

| 膳食类别<br>Category | 黑龙江<br>HL | 辽宁<br>LN | 河北<br>HE | 北京<br>BJ | 吉林<br>JL | 山西<br>SX | 陕西<br>SN | 河南<br>HA | 宁夏<br>NX | 内蒙古<br>NM | 青海<br>QH | 甘肃<br>GS | 上海<br>SH | 福建<br>FJ | 江西<br>JX | 江苏<br>JS | 浙江<br>ZJ | 山东<br>SD | 湖北<br>HB | 四川<br>SC | 广西<br>GX | 湖南<br>HN | 广东<br>GD | 贵州<br>GZ | 全国平均<br>AVG |
|---|---|---|---|---|---|---|---|---|---|---|---|---|---|---|---|---|---|---|---|---|---|---|---|---|---|
| 蛋类<br>Eggs | 4.884 | 0.151 | 0.193 | 0.189 | 8.546 | 0.026 | 0.000 | 0.000 | 0.000 | 0.000 | 0.012 | 0.116 | 0.105 | 0.036 | 0.037 | 0.437 | 0.093 | 122.085 | 0.050 | 0.029 | 0.011 | 0.000 | 0.059 | 1.027 | 5.754 |
| 水产类<br>Aquatic foods | 0.000 | 0.000 | 0.007 | 0.000 | 0.000 | 0.000 | 0.009 | 0.000 | 0.001 | 0.000 | 0.004 | 0.000 | 0.000 | 0.000 | 0.000 | 0.000 | 0.082 | 0.000 | 0.057 | 0.000 | 0.000 | 0.230 | 0.000 | 0.000 | 0.016 |
| 乳类<br>Dairy products | 0.000 | 0.045 | 0.000 | 0.000 | 0.000 | 0.000 | 0.000 | 0.000 | 0.000 | 0.000 | 0.085 | 0.011 | 0.094 | 0.000 | 0.000 | 0.000 | 0.000 | 0.014 | 0.000 | 0.000 | 0.000 | 0.000 | 0.066 | 0.000 | 0.013 |
| 合计<br>SUM | 6.237 | 0.262 | 0.200 | 2.470 | 9.368 | 0.329 | 0.009 | 0.158 | 0.778 | 0.000 | 0.166 | 0.153 | 0.573 | 0.036 | 0.413 | 1.467 | 25.843 | 122.317 | 0.145 | 0.172 | 0.953 | 31.798 | 0.996 | 1.827 | 8.611 |

附表 5-3 第六次中国总膳食研究甲氧苄啶的膳食来源（单位：%）

Annexed Table 5-3 Dietary sources of trimethoprim from the 6th China TDS (Unit: %)

| 膳食类别<br>Category | 黑龙江<br>HL | 辽宁<br>LN | 河北<br>HE | 北京<br>BJ | 吉林<br>JL | 山西<br>SX | 陕西<br>SN | 河南<br>HA | 宁夏<br>NX | 内蒙古<br>NM | 青海<br>QH | 甘肃<br>GS | 上海<br>SH | 福建<br>FJ | 江西<br>JX | 江苏<br>JS | 浙江<br>ZJ | 山东<br>SD | 湖北<br>HB | 四川<br>SC | 广西<br>GX | 湖南<br>HN | 广东<br>GD | 贵州<br>GZ | 全国平均<br>AVG |
|---|---|---|---|---|---|---|---|---|---|---|---|---|---|---|---|---|---|---|---|---|---|---|---|---|---|
| 肉类<br>Meats | 21.7 | 25.5 | 0.0 | 92.4 | 8.8 | 92.1 | 0.0 | 100.0 | 99.8 | 0.0 | 39.5 | 17.4 | 65.4 | 0.0 | 91.1 | 70.2 | 99.3 | 0.2 | 26.3 | 82.9 | 98.8 | 99.3 | 87.5 | 43.8 | 32.8 |
| 蛋类<br>Eggs | 78.3 | 57.5 | 96.5 | 7.6 | 91.2 | 7.9 | 0.0 | 0.0 | 0.0 | 0.0 | 7.1 | 75.7 | 18.2 | 100.0 | 8.9 | 29.8 | 0.4 | 99.8 | 34.5 | 17.1 | 1.2 | 0.0 | 5.9 | 56.2 | 66.8 |
| 水产类<br>Aquatic foods | 0.0 | 0.0 | 0.0 | 0.0 | 0.0 | 0.0 | 100.0 | 0.0 | 0.2 | 0.0 | 2.2 | 0.0 | 0.0 | 0.0 | 0.0 | 0.0 | 0.3 | 0.0 | 39.2 | 0.0 | 0.0 | 0.7 | 0.0 | 0.0 | 0.2 |
| 乳类<br>Dairy products | 0.0 | 17.0 | 0.0 | 0.0 | 0.0 | 0.0 | 0.0 | 0.0 | 0.0 | 0.0 | 51.2 | 6.9 | 16.4 | 0.0 | 0.0 | 0.0 | 0.0 | 0.0 | 0.0 | 0.0 | 0.0 | 0.0 | 6.6 | 0.0 | 0.2 |

附表 5-4　第六次中国总膳食研究膳食样品中麻保沙星的含量（单位：µg/kg）

Annexed Table 5-4　Levels of marbofloxacin in food samples from the 6$^{th}$ China TDS (Unit: µg/kg)

| 膳食类别 Category | 黑龙江 HL | 辽宁 LN | 河北 HE | 北京 BJ | 吉林 JL | 山西 SX | 陕西 SN | 河南 HA | 宁夏 NX | 内蒙古 NM | 青海 QH | 甘肃 GS | 上海 SH | 福建 FJ | 江西 JX | 江苏 JS | 浙江 ZJ | 山东 SD | 湖北 HB | 四川 SC | 广西 GX | 湖南 HN | 广东 GD | 贵州 GZ | 全国平均 AVG |
|---|---|---|---|---|---|---|---|---|---|---|---|---|---|---|---|---|---|---|---|---|---|---|---|---|---|
| 肉类 Meats | ND | ND | ND | ND | ND | ND | ND | ND | ND | ND | ND | ND | ND | ND | ND | ND | ND | ND | ND | ND | ND | ND | ND | ND | 0.00 |
| 蛋类 Eggs | ND | ND | ND | ND | ND | ND | ND | ND | ND | ND | ND | ND | ND | ND | ND | ND | ND | ND | ND | ND | ND | ND | ND | ND | 0.00 |
| 水产类 Aquatic foods | ND | ND | ND | ND | ND | ND | ND | ND | ND | ND | ND | ND | ND | ND | ND | ND | ND | ND | ND | ND | ND | ND | ND | ND | 0.00 |
| 乳类 Dairy products | ND | 0.17 | ND | ND | ND | 0.03 | ND | ND | ND | ND | ND | ND | ND | ND | ND | ND | ND | ND | 0.24 | ND | ND | 0.38 | ND | ND | 0.03 |

注：未检出（ND）按 0 计

Note: values not detected (ND) were treated as being equal to 0

附表 5-5　第六次中国总膳食研究的麻保沙星膳食摄入量 [单位：ng/(kg bw·d)]

Annexed Table 5-5　Dietary intakes of marbofloxacin from the 6$^{th}$ China TDS [Unit: ng/(kg bw·d)]

| 膳食类别 Category | 黑龙江 HL | 辽宁 LN | 河北 HE | 北京 BJ | 吉林 JL | 山西 SX | 陕西 SN | 河南 HA | 宁夏 NX | 内蒙古 NM | 青海 QH | 甘肃 GS | 上海 SH | 福建 FJ | 江西 JX | 江苏 JS | 浙江 ZJ | 山东 SD | 湖北 HB | 四川 SC | 广西 GX | 湖南 HN | 广东 GD | 贵州 GZ | 全国平均 AVG |
|---|---|---|---|---|---|---|---|---|---|---|---|---|---|---|---|---|---|---|---|---|---|---|---|---|---|
| 肉类 Meats | 0.000 | 0.000 | 0.000 | 0.000 | 0.000 | 0.000 | 0.000 | 0.000 | 0.000 | 0.000 | 0.000 | 0.000 | 0.000 | 0.000 | 0.000 | 0.000 | 0.000 | 0.000 | 0.000 | 0.000 | 0.000 | 0.000 | 0.000 | 0.000 | 0.000 |
| 蛋类 Eggs | 0.000 | 0.000 | 0.000 | 0.000 | 0.000 | 0.000 | 0.000 | 0.000 | 0.000 | 0.000 | 0.000 | 0.000 | 0.000 | 0.000 | 0.000 | 0.000 | 0.000 | 0.000 | 0.000 | 0.000 | 0.000 | 0.000 | 0.000 | 0.000 | 0.000 |
| 水产类 Aquatic foods | 0.000 | 0.000 | 0.000 | 0.000 | 0.000 | 0.000 | 0.000 | 0.000 | 0.000 | 0.000 | 0.000 | 0.000 | 0.000 | 0.000 | 0.000 | 0.000 | 0.000 | 0.000 | 0.000 | 0.000 | 0.000 | 0.000 | 0.000 | 0.000 | 0.000 |

续表

| 膳食类别<br>Category | 黑龙江<br>HL | 辽宁<br>LN | 河北<br>HE | 北京<br>BJ | 吉林<br>JL | 山西<br>SX | 陕西<br>SN | 河南<br>HA | 宁夏<br>NX | 内蒙古<br>NM | 青海<br>QH | 甘肃<br>GS | 上海<br>SH | 福建<br>FJ | 江西<br>JX | 江苏<br>JS | 浙江<br>ZJ | 山东<br>SD | 湖北<br>HB | 四川<br>SC | 广西<br>GX | 湖南<br>HN | 广东<br>GD | 贵州<br>GZ | 全国平均<br>AVG |
|---|---|---|---|---|---|---|---|---|---|---|---|---|---|---|---|---|---|---|---|---|---|---|---|---|---|
| 乳类 Dairy products | 0.000 | 0.123 | 0.000 | 0.000 | 0.000 | 0.018 | 0.000 | 0.000 | 0.000 | 0.000 | 0.000 | 0.000 | 0.000 | 0.000 | 0.000 | 0.000 | 0.000 | 0.000 | 0.025 | 0.000 | 0.000 | 0.108 | 0.000 | 0.000 | 0.011 |
| 合计 SUM | 0.000 | 0.123 | 0.000 | 0.000 | 0.000 | 0.018 | 0.000 | 0.000 | 0.000 | 0.000 | 0.000 | 0.000 | 0.000 | 0.000 | 0.000 | 0.000 | 0.000 | 0.000 | 0.025 | 0.000 | 0.000 | 0.108 | 0.000 | 0.000 | 0.011 |

附表 5-6 第六次中国总膳食研究麻保沙星的膳食来源（单位：%）
Annexed Table 5-6　Dietary sources of marbofloxacin from the 6$^{th}$ China TDS (Unit: %)

| 膳食类别<br>Category | 黑龙江<br>HL | 辽宁<br>LN | 河北<br>HE | 北京<br>BJ | 吉林<br>JL | 山西<br>SX | 陕西<br>SN | 河南<br>HA | 宁夏<br>NX | 内蒙古<br>NM | 青海<br>QH | 甘肃<br>GS | 上海<br>SH | 福建<br>FJ | 江西<br>JX | 江苏<br>JS | 浙江<br>ZJ | 山东<br>SD | 湖北<br>HB | 四川<br>SC | 广西<br>GX | 湖南<br>HN | 广东<br>GD | 贵州<br>GZ | 全国平均<br>AVG |
|---|---|---|---|---|---|---|---|---|---|---|---|---|---|---|---|---|---|---|---|---|---|---|---|---|---|
| 肉类 Meats | 0.0 | 0.0 | 0.0 | 0.0 | 0.0 | 0.0 | 0.0 | 0.0 | 0.0 | 0.0 | 0.0 | 0.0 | 0.0 | 0.0 | 0.0 | 0.0 | 0.0 | 0.0 | 0.0 | 0.0 | 0.0 | 0.0 | 0.0 | 0.0 | 0.0 |
| 蛋类 Eggs | 0.0 | 0.0 | 0.0 | 0.0 | 0.0 | 0.0 | 0.0 | 0.0 | 0.0 | 0.0 | 0.0 | 0.0 | 0.0 | 0.0 | 0.0 | 0.0 | 0.0 | 0.0 | 0.0 | 0.0 | 0.0 | 0.0 | 0.0 | 0.0 | 0.0 |
| 水产类 Aquatic foods | 0.0 | 0.0 | 0.0 | 0.0 | 0.0 | 0.0 | 0.0 | 0.0 | 0.0 | 0.0 | 0.0 | 0.0 | 0.0 | 0.0 | 0.0 | 0.0 | 0.0 | 0.0 | 0.0 | 0.0 | 0.0 | 0.0 | 0.0 | 0.0 | 0.0 |
| 乳类 Dairy products | 0.0 | 100.0 | 0.0 | 0.0 | 0.0 | 100.0 | 0.0 | 0.0 | 0.0 | 0.0 | 0.0 | 0.0 | 0.0 | 0.0 | 0.0 | 0.0 | 0.0 | 0.0 | 100.0 | 0.0 | 0.0 | 100.0 | 0.0 | 0.0 | 100.0 |

附表 5-7 第六次中国总膳食研究膳食样品中氧氟沙星的含量（单位：μg/kg）
Annexed Table 5-7　Levels of ofloxacin in food samples from the 6$^{th}$ China TDS (Unit: μg/kg)

| 膳食类别<br>Category | 黑龙江<br>HL | 辽宁<br>LN | 河北<br>HE | 北京<br>BJ | 吉林<br>JL | 山西<br>SX | 陕西<br>SN | 河南<br>HA | 宁夏<br>NX | 内蒙古<br>NM | 青海<br>QH | 甘肃<br>GS | 上海<br>SH | 福建<br>FJ | 江西<br>JX | 江苏<br>JS | 浙江<br>ZJ | 山东<br>SD | 湖北<br>HB | 四川<br>SC | 广西<br>GX | 湖南<br>HN | 广东<br>GD | 贵州<br>GZ | 全国平均<br>AVG |
|---|---|---|---|---|---|---|---|---|---|---|---|---|---|---|---|---|---|---|---|---|---|---|---|---|---|
| 肉类 Meats | 0.36 | ND | ND | 4.10 | ND | ND | ND | ND | 0.02 | ND | ND | 0.02 | 0.08 | 0.09 | ND | 0.58 | ND | 0.03 | ND | ND | 0.33 | ND | ND | 0.91 | 0.27 |

续表

| 膳食类别 Category | 黑龙江 HL | 辽宁 LN | 河北 HE | 北京 BJ | 吉林 JL | 山西 SX | 陕西 SN | 河南 HA | 宁夏 NX | 内蒙古 NM | 青海 QH | 甘肃 GS | 上海 SH | 福建 FJ | 江西 JX | 江苏 JS | 浙江 ZJ | 山东 SD | 湖北 HB | 四川 SC | 广西 GX | 湖南 HN | 广东 GD | 贵州 GZ | 全国平均 AVG |
|---|---|---|---|---|---|---|---|---|---|---|---|---|---|---|---|---|---|---|---|---|---|---|---|---|---|
| 蛋类 Eggs | ND | 0.21 | ND | 0.99 | ND | ND | 0.26 | ND | ND | ND | ND | 0.32 | ND | ND | ND | ND | 0.13 | ND | ND | ND | ND | ND | ND | ND | 0.08 |
| 水产类 Aquatic foods | ND | ND | ND | ND | ND | ND | ND | ND | ND | ND | ND | ND | ND | ND | ND | ND | ND | ND | ND | ND | ND | ND | ND | ND | 0.00 |
| 乳类 Dairy products | ND | ND | ND | ND | 0.04 | ND | ND | 0.48 | ND | ND | ND | 0.09 | 3.21 | ND | ND | ND | ND | ND | 0.19 | ND | ND | ND | ND | ND | 0.17 |

注：未检出（ND）按 0 计

Note: values not detected (ND) were treated as being equal to 0

附表 5-8 第六次中国总膳食研究的氧氟沙星膳食摄入量 [单位: ng/(kg bw·d)]

Annexed Table 5-8 Dietary intakes of ofloxacin from the 6$^{th}$ China TDS [Unit: ng/(kg bw·d)]

| 膳食类别 Category | 黑龙江 HL | 辽宁 LN | 河北 HE | 北京 BJ | 吉林 JL | 山西 SX | 陕西 SN | 河南 HA | 宁夏 NX | 内蒙古 NM | 青海 QH | 甘肃 GS | 上海 SH | 福建 FJ | 江西 JX | 江苏 JS | 浙江 ZJ | 山东 SD | 湖北 HB | 四川 SC | 广西 GX | 湖南 HN | 广东 GD | 贵州 GZ | 全国平均 AVG |
|---|---|---|---|---|---|---|---|---|---|---|---|---|---|---|---|---|---|---|---|---|---|---|---|---|---|
| 肉类 Meats | 0.345 | 0.000 | 0.000 | 4.381 | 0.000 | 0.000 | 0.000 | 0.000 | 0.018 | 0.000 | 0.000 | 0.008 | 0.140 | 0.122 | 0.000 | 0.844 | 0.000 | 0.041 | 0.000 | 0.000 | 0.793 | 0.000 | 0.000 | 1.538 | 0.343 |
| 蛋类 Eggs | 0.000 | 0.136 | 0.000 | 0.611 | 0.000 | 0.000 | 0.091 | 0.000 | 0.000 | 0.000 | 0.000 | 0.114 | 0.000 | 0.000 | 0.000 | 0.000 | 0.050 | 0.000 | 0.000 | 0.000 | 0.000 | 0.000 | 0.000 | 0.000 | 0.042 |
| 水产类 Aquatic foods | 0.000 | 0.000 | 0.000 | 0.000 | 0.000 | 0.000 | 0.000 | 0.000 | 0.000 | 0.000 | 0.000 | 0.000 | 0.000 | 0.000 | 0.000 | 0.000 | 0.000 | 0.000 | 0.000 | 0.000 | 0.000 | 0.000 | 0.000 | 0.000 | 0.000 |
| 乳类 Dairy products | 0.000 | 0.000 | 0.000 | 0.000 | 0.020 | 0.000 | 0.000 | 0.149 | 0.000 | 0.000 | 0.000 | 0.019 | 3.636 | 0.000 | 0.000 | 0.000 | 0.000 | 0.000 | 0.020 | 0.000 | 0.000 | 0.000 | 0.000 | 0.000 | 0.160 |
| 合计 SUM | 0.345 | 0.136 | 0.000 | 4.992 | 0.020 | 0.000 | 0.091 | 0.149 | 0.018 | 0.000 | 0.000 | 0.141 | 3.776 | 0.122 | 0.000 | 0.844 | 0.050 | 0.041 | 0.020 | 0.000 | 0.793 | 0.000 | 0.000 | 1.538 | 0.545 |

附表 5-9　第六次中国总膳食研究氧氟沙星的膳食来源（单位：%）
Annexed Table 5-9　Dietary sources of ofloxacin from the 6th China TDS (Unit: %)

| 膳食类别<br>Category | 黑龙江<br>HL | 辽宁<br>LN | 河北<br>HE | 北京<br>BJ | 吉林<br>JL | 山西<br>SX | 陕西<br>SN | 河南<br>HA | 宁夏<br>NX | 内蒙古<br>NM | 青海<br>QH | 甘肃<br>GS | 上海<br>SH | 福建<br>FJ | 江西<br>JX | 江苏<br>JS | 浙江<br>ZJ | 山东<br>SD | 湖北<br>HB | 四川<br>SC | 广西<br>GX | 湖南<br>HN | 广东<br>GD | 贵州<br>GZ | 全国平均<br>AVG |
|---|---|---|---|---|---|---|---|---|---|---|---|---|---|---|---|---|---|---|---|---|---|---|---|---|---|
| 肉类 Meats | 100.0 | 0.0 | 0.0 | 87.8 | 0.0 | 0.0 | 0.0 | 0.0 | 100.0 | 0.0 | 0.0 | 5.7 | 3.7 | 100.0 | 0.0 | 100.0 | 0.0 | 100.0 | 0.0 | 0.0 | 100.0 | 0.0 | 0.0 | 100.0 | 62.9 |
| 蛋类 Eggs | 0.0 | 100.0 | 0.0 | 12.2 | 0.0 | 0.0 | 100.0 | 0.0 | 0.0 | 0.0 | 0.0 | 80.7 | 0.0 | 0.0 | 0.0 | 0.0 | 100.0 | 0.0 | 0.0 | 0.0 | 0.0 | 0.0 | 0.0 | 0.0 | 7.7 |
| 水产类 Aquatic foods | 0.0 | 0.0 | 0.0 | 0.0 | 0.0 | 0.0 | 0.0 | 0.0 | 0.0 | 0.0 | 0.0 | 0.0 | 0.0 | 0.0 | 0.0 | 0.0 | 0.0 | 0.0 | 0.0 | 0.0 | 0.0 | 0.0 | 0.0 | 0.0 | 0.0 |
| 乳类 Dairy products | 0.0 | 0.0 | 0.0 | 0.0 | 100.0 | 0.0 | 0.0 | 100.0 | 0.0 | 0.0 | 0.0 | 13.5 | 96.3 | 0.0 | 0.0 | 0.0 | 0.0 | 0.0 | 100.0 | 0.0 | 0.0 | 0.0 | 0.0 | 0.0 | 29.4 |

附表 5-10　第六次中国总膳食研究膳食样品中培氟沙星的含量（单位：μg/kg）
Annexed Table 5-10　Levels of pefloxacin in food samples from the 6th China TDS (Unit: μg/kg)

| 膳食类别<br>Category | 黑龙江<br>HL | 辽宁<br>LN | 河北<br>HE | 北京<br>BJ | 吉林<br>JL | 山西<br>SX | 陕西<br>SN | 河南<br>HA | 宁夏<br>NX | 内蒙古<br>NM | 青海<br>QH | 甘肃<br>GS | 上海<br>SH | 福建<br>FJ | 江西<br>JX | 江苏<br>JS | 浙江<br>ZJ | 山东<br>SD | 湖北<br>HB | 四川<br>SC | 广西<br>GX | 湖南<br>HN | 广东<br>GD | 贵州<br>GZ | 全国平均<br>AVG |
|---|---|---|---|---|---|---|---|---|---|---|---|---|---|---|---|---|---|---|---|---|---|---|---|---|---|
| 肉类 Meats | 0.14 | ND | 0.08 | ND | 0.05 | ND | ND | 0.08 | ND | ND | ND | ND | ND | ND | ND | 0.27 | 0.04 | ND | ND | ND | ND | ND | ND | ND | 0.03 |
| 蛋类 Eggs | ND | ND | ND | ND | 0.10 | ND | ND | ND | ND | ND | ND | ND | ND | ND | ND | ND | ND | ND | ND | ND | ND | ND | 0.08 | ND | 0.01 |
| 水产类 Aquatic foods | ND | ND | ND | ND | ND | ND | ND | ND | ND | ND | ND | ND | ND | ND | ND | ND | ND | ND | ND | ND | ND | ND | ND | ND | 0.00 |
| 乳类 Dairy products | ND | ND | ND | ND | 0.06 | ND | ND | ND | ND | ND | ND | ND | ND | ND | ND | ND | ND | ND | ND | ND | ND | ND | ND | ND | 0.00 |

注：未检出（ND）按 0 计
Note: values not detected (ND) were treated as being equal to 0

附表 5-11 第六次中国总膳食研究的培氟沙星膳食摄入量 [单位: ng/(kg bw·d)]
Annexed Table 5-11  Dietary intakes of pefloxacin from the 6th China TDS [Unit: ng/(kg bw·d)]

| 膳食类别 Category | 黑龙江 HL | 辽宁 LN | 河北 HE | 北京 BJ | 吉林 JL | 山西 SX | 陕西 SN | 河南 HA | 宁夏 NX | 内蒙古 NM | 青海 QH | 甘肃 GS | 上海 SH | 福建 FJ | 江西 JX | 江苏 JS | 浙江 ZJ | 山东 SD | 湖北 HB | 四川 SC | 广西 GX | 湖南 HN | 广东 GD | 贵州 GZ | 全国平均 AVG |
|---|---|---|---|---|---|---|---|---|---|---|---|---|---|---|---|---|---|---|---|---|---|---|---|---|---|
| 肉类 Meats | 0.131 | 0.000 | 0.057 | 0.000 | 0.058 | 0.000 | 0.000 | 0.072 | 0.000 | 0.000 | 0.000 | 0.000 | 0.000 | 0.000 | 0.000 | 0.397 | 0.078 | 0.000 | 0.000 | 0.000 | 0.000 | 0.000 | 0.000 | 0.000 | 0.033 |
| 蛋类 Eggs | 0.000 | 0.000 | 0.000 | 0.000 | 0.065 | 0.000 | 0.000 | 0.000 | 0.000 | 0.000 | 0.000 | 0.000 | 0.000 | 0.000 | 0.000 | 0.000 | 0.000 | 0.000 | 0.000 | 0.000 | 0.000 | 0.000 | 0.031 | 0.000 | 0.004 |
| 水产类 Aquatic foods | 0.000 | 0.000 | 0.000 | 0.000 | 0.000 | 0.000 | 0.000 | 0.000 | 0.000 | 0.000 | 0.000 | 0.000 | 0.000 | 0.000 | 0.000 | 0.000 | 0.000 | 0.000 | 0.000 | 0.000 | 0.000 | 0.000 | 0.000 | 0.000 | 0.000 |
| 乳类 Dairy products | 0.000 | 0.000 | 0.000 | 0.000 | 0.031 | 0.000 | 0.000 | 0.000 | 0.000 | 0.000 | 0.000 | 0.000 | 0.000 | 0.000 | 0.000 | 0.000 | 0.000 | 0.000 | 0.000 | 0.000 | 0.000 | 0.000 | 0.000 | 0.000 | 0.001 |
| 合计 SUM | 0.131 | 0.000 | 0.057 | 0.000 | 0.153 | 0.000 | 0.000 | 0.072 | 0.000 | 0.000 | 0.000 | 0.000 | 0.000 | 0.000 | 0.000 | 0.397 | 0.078 | 0.000 | 0.000 | 0.000 | 0.000 | 0.000 | 0.031 | 0.000 | 0.038 |

附表 5-12 第六次中国总膳食研究培氟沙星的膳食来源（单位：%）
Annexed Table 5-12  Dietary sources of pefloxacin from the 6th China TDS (Unit: %)

| 膳食类别 Category | 黑龙江 HL | 辽宁 LN | 河北 HE | 北京 BJ | 吉林 JL | 山西 SX | 陕西 SN | 河南 HA | 宁夏 NX | 内蒙古 NM | 青海 QH | 甘肃 GS | 上海 SH | 福建 FJ | 江西 JX | 江苏 JS | 浙江 ZJ | 山东 SD | 湖北 HB | 四川 SC | 广西 GX | 湖南 HN | 广东 GD | 贵州 GZ | 全国平均 AVG |
|---|---|---|---|---|---|---|---|---|---|---|---|---|---|---|---|---|---|---|---|---|---|---|---|---|---|
| 肉类 Meats | 100.0 | 0.0 | 100.0 | 0.0 | 37.6 | 0.0 | 0.0 | 100.0 | 0.0 | 0.0 | 0.0 | 0.0 | 0.0 | 0.0 | 0.0 | 100.0 | 100.0 | 0.0 | 0.0 | 0.0 | 0.0 | 0.0 | 0.0 | 0.0 | 86.2 |
| 蛋类 Eggs | 0.0 | 0.0 | 0.0 | 0.0 | 42.2 | 0.0 | 0.0 | 0.0 | 0.0 | 0.0 | 0.0 | 0.0 | 0.0 | 0.0 | 0.0 | 0.0 | 0.0 | 0.0 | 0.0 | 0.0 | 0.0 | 0.0 | 100.0 | 0.0 | 10.5 |
| 水产类 Aquatic foods | 0.0 | 0.0 | 0.0 | 0.0 | 0.0 | 0.0 | 0.0 | 0.0 | 0.0 | 0.0 | 0.0 | 0.0 | 0.0 | 0.0 | 0.0 | 0.0 | 0.0 | 0.0 | 0.0 | 0.0 | 0.0 | 0.0 | 0.0 | 0.0 | 0.0 |
| 乳类 Dairy products | 0.0 | 0.0 | 0.0 | 0.0 | 20.2 | 0.0 | 0.0 | 0.0 | 0.0 | 0.0 | 0.0 | 0.0 | 0.0 | 0.0 | 0.0 | 0.0 | 0.0 | 0.0 | 0.0 | 0.0 | 0.0 | 0.0 | 0.0 | 0.0 | 3.4 |

附表 5-13 第六次中国总膳食研究膳食样品中诺氟沙星的含量（单位：μg/kg）

Annexed Table 5-13　Levels of norfloxacin in food samples from the 6th China TDS (Unit: μg/kg)

| 膳食类别<br>Category | 黑龙江<br>HL | 辽宁<br>LN | 河北<br>HE | 北京<br>BJ | 吉林<br>JL | 山西<br>SX | 陕西<br>SN | 河南<br>HA | 宁夏<br>NX | 内蒙古<br>NM | 青海<br>QH | 甘肃<br>GS | 上海<br>SH | 福建<br>FJ | 江西<br>JX | 江苏<br>JS | 浙江<br>ZJ | 山东<br>SD | 湖北<br>HB | 四川<br>SC | 广西<br>GX | 湖南<br>HN | 广东<br>GD | 贵州<br>GZ | 全国平均<br>AVG |
|---|---|---|---|---|---|---|---|---|---|---|---|---|---|---|---|---|---|---|---|---|---|---|---|---|---|
| 肉类 Meats | ND | ND | ND | ND | ND | ND | ND | ND | ND | ND | ND | ND | ND | ND | ND | ND | ND | ND | ND | ND | ND | ND | ND | ND | 0.00 |
| 蛋类 Eggs | ND | ND | ND | ND | ND | ND | ND | ND | ND | ND | ND | ND | ND | ND | ND | ND | ND | ND | ND | ND | ND | ND | ND | ND | 0.00 |
| 水产类 Aquatic foods | ND | ND | ND | ND | ND | ND | ND | ND | ND | ND | ND | ND | ND | ND | ND | ND | ND | ND | ND | ND | ND | ND | ND | ND | 0.00 |
| 乳类 Dairy products | ND | ND | ND | ND | 0.32 | ND | ND | ND | ND | ND | ND | ND | ND | ND | ND | ND | ND | ND | ND | ND | ND | ND | ND | ND | 0.01 |

注：未检出（ND）按 0 计
Note: values not detected (ND) were treated as being equal to 0

附表 5-14 第六次中国总膳食研究的诺氟沙星膳食摄入量 [单位：ng/(kg bw·d)]

Annexed Table 5-14　Dietary intakes of norfloxacin from the 6th China TDS [Unit: ng/(kg bw·d)]

| 膳食类别<br>Category | 黑龙江<br>HL | 辽宁<br>LN | 河北<br>HE | 北京<br>BJ | 吉林<br>JL | 山西<br>SX | 陕西<br>SN | 河南<br>HA | 宁夏<br>NX | 内蒙古<br>NM | 青海<br>QH | 甘肃<br>GS | 上海<br>SH | 福建<br>FJ | 江西<br>JX | 江苏<br>JS | 浙江<br>ZJ | 山东<br>SD | 湖北<br>HB | 四川<br>SC | 广西<br>GX | 湖南<br>HN | 广东<br>GD | 贵州<br>GZ | 全国平均<br>AVG |
|---|---|---|---|---|---|---|---|---|---|---|---|---|---|---|---|---|---|---|---|---|---|---|---|---|---|
| 肉类 Meats | 0.000 | 0.000 | 0.000 | 0.000 | 0.000 | 0.000 | 0.000 | 0.000 | 0.000 | 0.000 | 0.000 | 0.000 | 0.000 | 0.000 | 0.000 | 0.000 | 0.000 | 0.000 | 0.000 | 0.000 | 0.000 | 0.000 | 0.000 | 0.000 | 0.000 |
| 蛋类 Eggs | 0.000 | 0.000 | 0.000 | 0.000 | 0.000 | 0.000 | 0.000 | 0.000 | 0.000 | 0.000 | 0.000 | 0.000 | 0.000 | 0.000 | 0.000 | 0.000 | 0.000 | 0.000 | 0.000 | 0.000 | 0.000 | 0.000 | 0.000 | 0.000 | 0.000 |
| 水产类 Aquatic foods | 0.000 | 0.000 | 0.000 | 0.000 | 0.000 | 0.000 | 0.000 | 0.000 | 0.000 | 0.000 | 0.000 | 0.000 | 0.000 | 0.000 | 0.000 | 0.000 | 0.000 | 0.000 | 0.000 | 0.000 | 0.000 | 0.000 | 0.000 | 0.000 | 0.000 |
| 乳类 Dairy products | 0.000 | 0.000 | 0.000 | 0.000 | 0.163 | 0.000 | 0.000 | 0.000 | 0.000 | 0.000 | 0.000 | 0.000 | 0.000 | 0.000 | 0.000 | 0.000 | 0.000 | 0.000 | 0.000 | 0.000 | 0.000 | 0.000 | 0.000 | 0.000 | 0.007 |

续表

| 膳食类别 Category | 黑龙江 HL | 辽宁 LN | 河北 HE | 北京 BJ | 吉林 JL | 山西 SX | 陕西 SN | 河南 HA | 宁夏 NX | 内蒙古 NM | 青海 QH | 甘肃 GS | 上海 SH | 福建 FJ | 江西 JX | 江苏 JS | 浙江 ZJ | 山东 SD | 湖北 HB | 四川 SC | 广西 GX | 湖南 HN | 广东 GD | 贵州 GZ | 全国平均 AVG |
|---|---|---|---|---|---|---|---|---|---|---|---|---|---|---|---|---|---|---|---|---|---|---|---|---|---|
| 合计 SUM | 0.000 | 0.000 | 0.000 | 0.000 | 0.163 | 0.000 | 0.000 | 0.000 | 0.000 | 0.000 | 0.000 | 0.000 | 0.000 | 0.000 | 0.000 | 0.000 | 0.000 | 0.000 | 0.000 | 0.000 | 0.000 | 0.000 | 0.000 | 0.000 | 0.007 |

附表 5-15　第六次中国总膳食研究诺氟沙星的膳食来源（单位：%）

Annexed Table 5-15　Dietary sources of norfloxacin from the 6th China TDS (Unit: %)

| 膳食类别 Category | 黑龙江 HL | 辽宁 LN | 河北 HE | 北京 BJ | 吉林 JL | 山西 SX | 陕西 SN | 河南 HA | 宁夏 NX | 内蒙古 NM | 青海 QH | 甘肃 GS | 上海 SH | 福建 FJ | 江西 JX | 江苏 JS | 浙江 ZJ | 山东 SD | 湖北 HB | 四川 SC | 广西 GX | 湖南 HN | 广东 GD | 贵州 GZ | 全国平均 AVG |
|---|---|---|---|---|---|---|---|---|---|---|---|---|---|---|---|---|---|---|---|---|---|---|---|---|---|
| 肉类 Meats | 0.0 | 0.0 | 0.0 | 0.0 | 0.0 | 0.0 | 0.0 | 0.0 | 0.0 | 0.0 | 0.0 | 0.0 | 0.0 | 0.0 | 0.0 | 0.0 | 0.0 | 0.0 | 0.0 | 0.0 | 0.0 | 0.0 | 0.0 | 0.0 | 0.0 |
| 蛋类 Eggs | 0.0 | 0.0 | 0.0 | 0.0 | 0.0 | 0.0 | 0.0 | 0.0 | 0.0 | 0.0 | 0.0 | 0.0 | 0.0 | 0.0 | 0.0 | 0.0 | 0.0 | 0.0 | 0.0 | 0.0 | 0.0 | 0.0 | 0.0 | 0.0 | 0.0 |
| 水产类 Aquatic foods | 0.0 | 0.0 | 0.0 | 0.0 | 0.0 | 0.0 | 0.0 | 0.0 | 0.0 | 0.0 | 0.0 | 0.0 | 0.0 | 0.0 | 0.0 | 0.0 | 0.0 | 0.0 | 0.0 | 0.0 | 0.0 | 0.0 | 0.0 | 0.0 | 0.0 |
| 乳类 Dairy products | 0.0 | 0.0 | 0.0 | 0.0 | 100.0 | 0.0 | 0.0 | 0.0 | 0.0 | 0.0 | 0.0 | 0.0 | 0.0 | 0.0 | 0.0 | 0.0 | 0.0 | 0.0 | 0.0 | 0.0 | 0.0 | 0.0 | 0.0 | 0.0 | 100.0 |

附表 5-16　第六次中国总膳食研究膳食样品中恩诺沙星的含量（单位：μg/kg）

Annexed Table 5-16　Levels of enrofloxacin in food samples from the 6th China TDS (Unit: μg/kg)

| 膳食类别 Category | 黑龙江 HL | 辽宁 LN | 河北 HE | 北京 BJ | 吉林 JL | 山西 SX | 陕西 SN | 河南 HA | 宁夏 NX | 内蒙古 NM | 青海 QH | 甘肃 GS | 上海 SH | 福建 FJ | 江西 JX | 江苏 JS | 浙江 ZJ | 山东 SD | 湖北 HB | 四川 SC | 广西 GX | 湖南 HN | 广东 GD | 贵州 GZ | 全国平均 AVG |
|---|---|---|---|---|---|---|---|---|---|---|---|---|---|---|---|---|---|---|---|---|---|---|---|---|---|
| 肉类 Meats | 0.08 | ND | 117.81 | 475.10 | 2.27 | ND | ND | 0.13 | 46.55 | ND | 84.41 | 0.05 | 0.25 | 0.10 | 0.49 | 6.82 | 0.02 | 0.01 | 0.59 | ND | 0.27 | 2.34 | 0.18 | 0.26 | 30.74 |

续表

| 膳食类别 Category | 黑龙江 HL | 辽宁 LN | 河北 HE | 北京 BJ | 吉林 JL | 山西 SX | 陕西 SN | 河南 HA | 宁夏 NX | 内蒙古 NM | 青海 QH | 甘肃 GS | 上海 SH | 福建 FJ | 江西 JX | 江苏 JS | 浙江 ZJ | 山东 SD | 湖北 HB | 四川 SC | 广西 GX | 湖南 HN | 广东 GD | 贵州 GZ | 全国平均 AVG |
|---|---|---|---|---|---|---|---|---|---|---|---|---|---|---|---|---|---|---|---|---|---|---|---|---|---|
| 蛋类 Eggs | 2.79 | ND | ND | 0.20 | ND | ND | 0.02 | ND | ND | ND | 3.76 | ND | 0.17 | ND | ND | 0.17 | 0.08 | 0.15 | ND | 0.16 | 0.07 | 12.64 | 0.86 | ND | 0.88 |
| 水产类 Aquatic foods | 3.31 | 15.11 | 4.95 | 0.91 | 11.43 | 18.87 | 6.13 | 7.64 | 2.49 | 3.28 | 5.29 | 3.38 | 19.38 | 0.29 | 1.21 | 16.02 | 28.42 | 0.71 | 19.43 | 1.60 | 1.67 | 8.75 | 1.42 | 1.14 | 7.62 |
| 乳类 Dairy products | ND | ND | ND | ND | ND | ND | ND | 0.05 | ND | 0.02 | ND | 0.10 | ND | ND | 0.03 | 0.01 | ND | 0.02 | 0.10 | ND | 0.19 | ND | ND | ND | 0.02 |

注：未检出（ND）按 0 计
Note: values not detected (ND) were treated as being equal to 0

附表 5-17　第六次中国总膳食研究的恩诺沙星膳食摄入量 [单位：ng/(kg bw・d)]
Annexed Table 5-17　Dietary intakes of enrofloxacin from the 6<sup>th</sup> China TDS [Unit: ng/(kg bw・d)]

| 膳食类别 Category | 黑龙江 HL | 辽宁 LN | 河北 HE | 北京 BJ | 吉林 JL | 山西 SX | 陕西 SN | 河南 HA | 宁夏 NX | 内蒙古 NM | 青海 QH | 甘肃 GS | 上海 SH | 福建 FJ | 江西 JX | 江苏 JS | 浙江 ZJ | 山东 SD | 湖北 HB | 四川 SC | 广西 GX | 湖南 HN | 广东 GD | 贵州 GZ | 全国平均 AVG |
|---|---|---|---|---|---|---|---|---|---|---|---|---|---|---|---|---|---|---|---|---|---|---|---|---|---|
| 肉类 Meats | 0.079 | 0.000 | 88.609 | 507.528 | 2.400 | 0.000 | 0.000 | 0.114 | 34.479 | 0.000 | 95.131 | 0.022 | 0.431 | 0.137 | 0.727 | 9.937 | 0.039 | 0.021 | 0.510 | 0.000 | 0.639 | 5.544 | 0.303 | 0.433 | 31.128 |
| 蛋类 Eggs | 1.793 | 0.000 | 0.000 | 0.126 | 0.000 | 0.000 | 0.009 | 0.000 | 0.000 | 0.000 | 0.784 | 0.000 | 0.107 | 0.000 | 0.000 | 0.074 | 0.032 | 0.106 | 0.000 | 0.037 | 0.015 | 4.573 | 0.325 | 0.000 | 0.333 |
| 水产类 Aquatic foods | 1.428 | 3.851 | 0.747 | 0.238 | 2.020 | 1.919 | 0.399 | 0.561 | 0.096 | 0.538 | 0.299 | 0.151 | 21.098 | 0.298 | 0.839 | 9.921 | 22.696 | 0.257 | 12.553 | 0.213 | 2.570 | 9.218 | 1.153 | 0.063 | 3.880 |
| 乳类 Dairy products | 0.000 | 0.000 | 0.000 | 0.000 | 0.000 | 0.000 | 0.000 | 0.016 | 0.000 | 0.012 | 0.000 | 0.021 | 0.000 | 0.000 | 0.009 | 0.006 | 0.000 | 0.009 | 0.011 | 0.000 | 0.054 | 0.000 | 0.000 | 0.000 | 0.006 |
| 合计 SUM | 3.300 | 3.851 | 89.356 | 507.892 | 4.420 | 1.919 | 0.408 | 0.691 | 34.575 | 0.551 | 96.214 | 0.195 | 21.636 | 0.435 | 1.576 | 19.938 | 22.767 | 0.393 | 13.074 | 0.249 | 3.277 | 19.335 | 1.782 | 0.496 | 35.350 |

附表 5-18　第六次中国总膳食研究恩诺沙星的膳食来源（单位：%）
Annexed Table 5-18　Dietary sources of enrofloxacin from the 6th China TDS (Unit: %)

| 膳食类别<br>Category | 黑龙江<br>HL | 辽宁<br>LN | 河北<br>HE | 北京<br>BJ | 吉林<br>JL | 山西<br>SX | 陕西<br>SN | 河南<br>HA | 宁夏<br>NX | 内蒙古<br>NM | 青海<br>QH | 甘肃<br>GS | 上海<br>SH | 福建<br>FJ | 江西<br>JX | 江苏<br>JS | 浙江<br>ZJ | 山东<br>SD | 湖北<br>HB | 四川<br>SC | 广西<br>GX | 湖南<br>HN | 广东<br>GD | 贵州<br>GZ | 全国平均<br>AVG |
|---|---|---|---|---|---|---|---|---|---|---|---|---|---|---|---|---|---|---|---|---|---|---|---|---|---|
| 肉类 Meats | 2.4 | 0.0 | 99.2 | 99.9 | 54.3 | 0.0 | 0.0 | 16.5 | 99.7 | 0.0 | 98.9 | 11.4 | 2.0 | 31.6 | 46.2 | 49.8 | 0.2 | 5.3 | 3.9 | 0.0 | 19.5 | 28.7 | 17.0 | 87.3 | 88.1 |
| 蛋类 Eggs | 54.3 | 0.0 | 0.0 | 0.0 | 0.0 | 0.0 | 2.1 | 0.0 | 0.0 | 0.0 | 0.8 | 0.0 | 0.5 | 0.0 | 0.0 | 0.4 | 0.1 | 27.1 | 0.0 | 14.7 | 0.5 | 23.7 | 18.3 | 0.0 | 0.9 |
| 水产类 Aquatic foods | 43.3 | 100.0 | 0.8 | 0.0 | 45.7 | 100.0 | 97.9 | 81.2 | 0.3 | 97.8 | 0.3 | 77.6 | 97.5 | 68.4 | 53.3 | 49.8 | 99.7 | 65.4 | 96.0 | 85.3 | 78.4 | 47.7 | 64.7 | 12.7 | 11.0 |
| 乳类 Dairy products | 0.0 | 0.0 | 0.0 | 0.0 | 0.0 | 0.0 | 0.0 | 2.3 | 0.0 | 2.2 | 0.0 | 11.0 | 0.0 | 0.0 | 0.6 | 0.0 | 0.0 | 2.2 | 0.1 | 0.0 | 1.6 | 0.0 | 0.0 | 0.0 | 0.0 |

附表 5-19　第六次中国总膳食研究膳食样品中达氟沙星的含量（单位：μg/kg）
Annexed Table 5-19　Levels of danofloxacin in food samples from the 6th China TDS (Unit: μg/kg)

| 膳食类别<br>Category | 黑龙江<br>HL | 辽宁<br>LN | 河北<br>HE | 北京<br>BJ | 吉林<br>JL | 山西<br>SX | 陕西<br>SN | 河南<br>HA | 宁夏<br>NX | 内蒙古<br>NM | 青海<br>QH | 甘肃<br>GS | 上海<br>SH | 福建<br>FJ | 江西<br>JX | 江苏<br>JS | 浙江<br>ZJ | 山东<br>SD | 湖北<br>HB | 四川<br>SC | 广西<br>GX | 湖南<br>HN | 广东<br>GD | 贵州<br>GZ | 全国平均<br>AVG |
|---|---|---|---|---|---|---|---|---|---|---|---|---|---|---|---|---|---|---|---|---|---|---|---|---|---|
| 肉类 Meats | ND | ND | ND | ND | ND | ND | ND | ND | ND | ND | ND | ND | ND | ND | ND | ND | ND | ND | ND | ND | ND | ND | ND | ND | 0.00 |
| 蛋类 Eggs | ND | ND | ND | ND | ND | ND | ND | ND | ND | ND | ND | 0.04 | ND | ND | ND | ND | ND | ND | ND | ND | ND | ND | ND | ND | 0.00 |
| 水产类 Aquatic foods | ND | ND | ND | ND | 0.13 | ND | ND | ND | ND | ND | ND | ND | ND | ND | ND | ND | ND | ND | ND | ND | ND | ND | ND | ND | 0.01 |
| 乳类 Dairy products | ND | ND | ND | ND | ND | ND | ND | ND | ND | ND | ND | ND | ND | ND | ND | ND | ND | ND | ND | ND | ND | ND | ND | ND | 0.00 |

注：未检出（ND）按 0 计
Note: values not detected (ND) were treated as being equal to 0

附表 5-20　第六次中国总膳食研究的达氟沙星膳食摄入量 [ 单位：ng/(kg bw・d)]
Annexed Table 5-20　Dietary intakes of danofloxacin from the 6th China TDS [Unit: ng/(kg bw・d)]

| 膳食类别<br>Category | 黑龙江<br>HL | 辽宁<br>LN | 河北<br>HE | 北京<br>BJ | 吉林<br>JL | 山西<br>SX | 陕西<br>SN | 河南<br>HA | 宁夏<br>NX | 内蒙古<br>NM | 青海<br>QH | 甘肃<br>GS | 上海<br>SH | 福建<br>FJ | 江西<br>JX | 江苏<br>JS | 浙江<br>ZJ | 山东<br>SD | 湖北<br>HB | 四川<br>SC | 广西<br>GX | 湖南<br>HN | 广东<br>GD | 贵州<br>GZ | 全国平均<br>AVG |
|---|---|---|---|---|---|---|---|---|---|---|---|---|---|---|---|---|---|---|---|---|---|---|---|---|---|
| 肉类 Meats | 0.000 | 0.000 | 0.000 | 0.000 | 0.000 | 0.000 | 0.000 | 0.000 | 0.000 | 0.000 | 0.000 | 0.000 | 0.000 | 0.000 | 0.000 | 0.000 | 0.000 | 0.000 | 0.000 | 0.000 | 0.000 | 0.000 | 0.000 | 0.000 | 0.000 |
| 蛋类 Eggs | 0.000 | 0.000 | 0.000 | 0.000 | 0.000 | 0.000 | 0.000 | 0.000 | 0.000 | 0.000 | 0.000 | 0.000 | 0.000 | 0.000 | 0.000 | 0.000 | 0.000 | 0.000 | 0.000 | 0.000 | 0.000 | 0.000 | 0.000 | 0.000 | 0.000 |
| 水产类 Aquatic foods | 0.000 | 0.000 | 0.000 | 0.000 | 0.023 | 0.000 | 0.000 | 0.000 | 0.000 | 0.000 | 0.000 | 0.002 | 0.000 | 0.000 | 0.000 | 0.000 | 0.000 | 0.000 | 0.000 | 0.000 | 0.000 | 0.000 | 0.000 | 0.000 | 0.001 |
| 乳类 Dairy products | 0.000 | 0.000 | 0.000 | 0.000 | 0.000 | 0.000 | 0.000 | 0.000 | 0.000 | 0.000 | 0.000 | 0.000 | 0.000 | 0.000 | 0.000 | 0.000 | 0.000 | 0.000 | 0.000 | 0.000 | 0.000 | 0.000 | 0.000 | 0.000 | 0.000 |
| 合计 SUM | 0.000 | 0.000 | 0.000 | 0.000 | 0.023 | 0.000 | 0.000 | 0.000 | 0.000 | 0.000 | 0.000 | 0.002 | 0.000 | 0.000 | 0.000 | 0.000 | 0.000 | 0.000 | 0.000 | 0.000 | 0.000 | 0.000 | 0.000 | 0.000 | 0.001 |

附表 5-21　第六次中国总膳食研究达氟沙星的膳食来源（单位：%）
Annexed Table 5-21　Dietary sources of danofloxacin from the 6th China TDS (Unit: %)

| 膳食类别<br>Category | 黑龙江<br>HL | 辽宁<br>LN | 河北<br>HE | 北京<br>BJ | 吉林<br>JL | 山西<br>SX | 陕西<br>SN | 河南<br>HA | 宁夏<br>NX | 内蒙古<br>NM | 青海<br>QH | 甘肃<br>GS | 上海<br>SH | 福建<br>FJ | 江西<br>JX | 江苏<br>JS | 浙江<br>ZJ | 山东<br>SD | 湖北<br>HB | 四川<br>SC | 广西<br>GX | 湖南<br>HN | 广东<br>GD | 贵州<br>GZ | 全国平均<br>AVG |
|---|---|---|---|---|---|---|---|---|---|---|---|---|---|---|---|---|---|---|---|---|---|---|---|---|---|
| 肉类 Meats | 0.0 | 0.0 | 0.0 | 0.0 | 0.0 | 0.0 | 0.0 | 0.0 | 0.0 | 0.0 | 0.0 | 0.0 | 0.0 | 0.0 | 0.0 | 0.0 | 0.0 | 0.0 | 0.0 | 0.0 | 0.0 | 0.0 | 0.0 | 0.0 | 0.0 |
| 蛋类 Eggs | 0.0 | 0.0 | 0.0 | 0.0 | 0.0 | 0.0 | 0.0 | 0.0 | 0.0 | 0.0 | 0.0 | 0.0 | 0.0 | 0.0 | 0.0 | 0.0 | 0.0 | 0.0 | 0.0 | 0.0 | 0.0 | 0.0 | 0.0 | 0.0 | 0.0 |
| 水产类 Aquatic foods | 0.0 | 0.0 | 0.0 | 0.0 | 100.0 | 0.0 | 0.0 | 0.0 | 0.0 | 0.0 | 0.0 | 100.0 | 0.0 | 0.0 | 0.0 | 0.0 | 0.0 | 0.0 | 0.0 | 0.0 | 0.0 | 0.0 | 0.0 | 0.0 | 100.0 |
| 乳类 Dairy products | 0.0 | 0.0 | 0.0 | 0.0 | 0.0 | 0.0 | 0.0 | 0.0 | 0.0 | 0.0 | 0.0 | 0.0 | 0.0 | 0.0 | 0.0 | 0.0 | 0.0 | 0.0 | 0.0 | 0.0 | 0.0 | 0.0 | 0.0 | 0.0 | 0.0 |

附表 5-22　第六次中国总膳食研究膳食样品中洛美沙星的含量（单位：μg/kg）

Annexed Table 5-22　Levels of lomefloxacin in food samples from the 6th China TDS (Unit: μg/kg)

| 膳食类别<br>Category | 黑龙江<br>HL | 辽宁<br>LN | 河北<br>HE | 北京<br>BJ | 吉林<br>JL | 山西<br>SX | 陕西<br>SN | 河南<br>HA | 宁夏<br>NX | 内蒙古<br>NM | 青海<br>QH | 甘肃<br>GS | 上海<br>SH | 福建<br>FJ | 江西<br>JX | 江苏<br>JS | 浙江<br>ZJ | 山东<br>SD | 湖北<br>HB | 四川<br>SC | 广西<br>GX | 湖南<br>HN | 广东<br>GD | 贵州<br>GZ | 全国平均<br>AVG |
|---|---|---|---|---|---|---|---|---|---|---|---|---|---|---|---|---|---|---|---|---|---|---|---|---|---|
| 肉类 Meats | ND | ND | ND | ND | ND | ND | ND | ND | ND | ND | ND | ND | ND | ND | ND | ND | ND | ND | ND | ND | ND | ND | ND | ND | 0.00 |
| 蛋类 Eggs | ND | ND | ND | ND | ND | ND | ND | ND | ND | ND | ND | ND | ND | ND | ND | ND | ND | ND | ND | ND | ND | ND | ND | ND | 0.00 |
| 水产类 Aquatic foods | ND | ND | 0.05 | ND | ND | ND | ND | ND | ND | ND | ND | ND | ND | ND | ND | ND | 0.02 | ND | ND | ND | ND | ND | ND | ND | 0.00 |
| 乳类 Dairy products | ND | ND | ND | ND | ND | ND | ND | ND | ND | ND | ND | ND | ND | ND | ND | ND | ND | ND | ND | ND | ND | ND | ND | ND | 0.00 |

注：未检出（ND）按 0 计

Note: values not detected (ND) were treated as being equal to 0

附表 5-23　第六次中国总膳食研究的洛美沙星膳食摄入量 [单位：ng/(kg bw·d)]

Annexed Table 5-23　Dietary intakes of lomefloxacin from the 6th China TDS [Unit: ng/(kg bw·d)]

| 膳食类别<br>Category | 黑龙江<br>HL | 辽宁<br>LN | 河北<br>HE | 北京<br>BJ | 吉林<br>JL | 山西<br>SX | 陕西<br>SN | 河南<br>HA | 宁夏<br>NX | 内蒙古<br>NM | 青海<br>QH | 甘肃<br>GS | 上海<br>SH | 福建<br>FJ | 江西<br>JX | 江苏<br>JS | 浙江<br>ZJ | 山东<br>SD | 湖北<br>HB | 四川<br>SC | 广西<br>GX | 湖南<br>HN | 广东<br>GD | 贵州<br>GZ | 全国平均<br>AVG |
|---|---|---|---|---|---|---|---|---|---|---|---|---|---|---|---|---|---|---|---|---|---|---|---|---|---|
| 肉类 Meats | 0.000 | 0.000 | 0.000 | 0.000 | 0.000 | 0.000 | 0.000 | 0.000 | 0.000 | 0.000 | 0.000 | 0.000 | 0.000 | 0.000 | 0.000 | 0.000 | 0.000 | 0.000 | 0.000 | 0.000 | 0.000 | 0.000 | 0.000 | 0.000 | 0.000 |
| 蛋类 Eggs | 0.000 | 0.000 | 0.000 | 0.000 | 0.000 | 0.000 | 0.000 | 0.000 | 0.000 | 0.000 | 0.000 | 0.000 | 0.000 | 0.000 | 0.000 | 0.000 | 0.000 | 0.000 | 0.000 | 0.000 | 0.000 | 0.000 | 0.000 | 0.000 | 0.000 |
| 水产类 Aquatic foods | 0.000 | 0.000 | 0.007 | 0.000 | 0.000 | 0.000 | 0.000 | 0.000 | 0.000 | 0.000 | 0.000 | 0.000 | 0.000 | 0.000 | 0.000 | 0.000 | 0.009 | 0.000 | 0.000 | 0.000 | 0.000 | 0.000 | 0.000 | 0.000 | 0.000 |
| 乳类 Dairy products | 0.000 | 0.000 | 0.000 | 0.000 | 0.000 | 0.000 | 0.000 | 0.000 | 0.000 | 0.000 | 0.000 | 0.000 | 0.000 | 0.000 | 0.000 | 0.000 | 0.000 | 0.000 | 0.000 | 0.000 | 0.000 | 0.000 | 0.000 | 0.000 | 0.000 |

续表

| 膳食类别<br>Category | 黑龙江<br>HL | 辽宁<br>LN | 河北<br>HE | 北京<br>BJ | 吉林<br>JL | 山西<br>SX | 陕西<br>SN | 河南<br>HA | 宁夏<br>NX | 内蒙古<br>NM | 青海<br>QH | 甘肃<br>GS | 上海<br>SH | 福建<br>FJ | 江西<br>JX | 江苏<br>JS | 浙江<br>ZJ | 山东<br>SD | 湖北<br>HB | 四川<br>SC | 广西<br>GX | 湖南<br>HN | 广东<br>GD | 贵州<br>GZ | 全国平均<br>AVG |
|---|---|---|---|---|---|---|---|---|---|---|---|---|---|---|---|---|---|---|---|---|---|---|---|---|---|
| 合计<br>SUM | 0.000 | 0.000 | 0.007 | 0.000 | 0.000 | 0.000 | 0.000 | 0.000 | 0.000 | 0.000 | 0.000 | 0.000 | 0.000 | 0.000 | 0.000 | 0.000 | 0.009 | 0.000 | 0.000 | 0.000 | 0.000 | 0.000 | 0.000 | 0.000 | 0.001 |

附表 5-24 第六次中国总膳食研究洛美沙星的膳食来源（单位：%）

Annexed Table 5-24　Dietary sources of lomefloxacin from the 6th China TDS (Unit: %)

| 膳食类别<br>Category | 黑龙江<br>HL | 辽宁<br>LN | 河北<br>HE | 北京<br>BJ | 吉林<br>JL | 山西<br>SX | 陕西<br>SN | 河南<br>HA | 宁夏<br>NX | 内蒙古<br>NM | 青海<br>QH | 甘肃<br>GS | 上海<br>SH | 福建<br>FJ | 江西<br>JX | 江苏<br>JS | 浙江<br>ZJ | 山东<br>SD | 湖北<br>HB | 四川<br>SC | 广西<br>GX | 湖南<br>HN | 广东<br>GD | 贵州<br>GZ | 全国平均<br>AVG |
|---|---|---|---|---|---|---|---|---|---|---|---|---|---|---|---|---|---|---|---|---|---|---|---|---|---|
| 肉类<br>Meats | 0.0 | 0.0 | 0.0 | 0.0 | 0.0 | 0.0 | 0.0 | 0.0 | 0.0 | 0.0 | 0.0 | 0.0 | 0.0 | 0.0 | 0.0 | 0.0 | 0.0 | 0.0 | 0.0 | 0.0 | 0.0 | 0.0 | 0.0 | 0.0 | 0.0 |
| 蛋类<br>Eggs | 0.0 | 0.0 | 0.0 | 0.0 | 0.0 | 0.0 | 0.0 | 0.0 | 0.0 | 0.0 | 0.0 | 0.0 | 0.0 | 0.0 | 0.0 | 0.0 | 100.0 | 0.0 | 0.0 | 0.0 | 0.0 | 0.0 | 0.0 | 0.0 | 56.7 |
| 水产类<br>Aquatic foods | 0.0 | 0.0 | 100.0 | 0.0 | 0.0 | 0.0 | 0.0 | 0.0 | 0.0 | 0.0 | 0.0 | 0.0 | 0.0 | 0.0 | 0.0 | 0.0 | 0.0 | 0.0 | 0.0 | 0.0 | 0.0 | 0.0 | 0.0 | 0.0 | 43.3 |
| 乳类<br>Dairy products | 0.0 | 0.0 | 0.0 | 0.0 | 0.0 | 0.0 | 0.0 | 0.0 | 0.0 | 0.0 | 0.0 | 0.0 | 0.0 | 0.0 | 0.0 | 0.0 | 0.0 | 0.0 | 0.0 | 0.0 | 0.0 | 0.0 | 0.0 | 0.0 | 0.0 |

附表 5-25 第六次中国总膳食研究膳食样品中奥比沙星的含量（单位：μg/kg）

Annexed Table 5-25　Levels of orbifloxacin in food samples from the 6th China TDS (Unit: μg/kg)

| 膳食类别<br>Category | 黑龙江<br>HL | 辽宁<br>LN | 河北<br>HE | 北京<br>BJ | 吉林<br>JL | 山西<br>SX | 陕西<br>SN | 河南<br>HA | 宁夏<br>NX | 内蒙古<br>NM | 青海<br>QH | 甘肃<br>GS | 上海<br>SH | 福建<br>FJ | 江西<br>JX | 江苏<br>JS | 浙江<br>ZJ | 山东<br>SD | 湖北<br>HB | 四川<br>SC | 广西<br>GX | 湖南<br>HN | 广东<br>GD | 贵州<br>GZ | 全国平均<br>AVG |
|---|---|---|---|---|---|---|---|---|---|---|---|---|---|---|---|---|---|---|---|---|---|---|---|---|---|
| 肉类<br>Meats | ND | ND | ND | ND | ND | ND | ND | ND | ND | ND | ND | ND | ND | ND | ND | ND | ND | ND | ND | ND | ND | ND | ND | ND | 0.00 |

续表

| 膳食类别 Category | 黑龙江 HL | 辽宁 LN | 河北 HE | 北京 BJ | 吉林 JL | 山西 SX | 陕西 SN | 河南 HA | 宁夏 NX | 内蒙古 NM | 青海 QH | 甘肃 GS | 上海 SH | 福建 FJ | 江西 JX | 江苏 JS | 浙江 ZJ | 山东 SD | 湖北 HB | 四川 SC | 广西 GX | 湖南 HN | 广东 GD | 贵州 GZ | 全国平均 AVG |
|---|---|---|---|---|---|---|---|---|---|---|---|---|---|---|---|---|---|---|---|---|---|---|---|---|---|
| 蛋类 Eggs | ND | ND | ND | ND | ND | ND | ND | ND | ND | ND | ND | ND | ND | ND | ND | ND | ND | ND | ND | ND | ND | ND | ND | ND | 0.00 |
| 水产类 Aquatic foods | ND | ND | ND | ND | ND | ND | ND | ND | ND | ND | ND | ND | ND | ND | ND | ND | ND | ND | ND | ND | ND | ND | ND | ND | 0.00 |
| 乳类 Dairy products | ND | ND | ND | ND | ND | ND | ND | ND | ND | ND | ND | ND | ND | ND | ND | ND | ND | ND | ND | ND | 2.43 | ND | ND | ND | 0.10 |

注：未检出（ND）按 0 计
Note: values not detected (ND) were treated as being equal to 0

附表 5-26　第六次中国总膳食研究的奥比沙星膳食摄入量 [单位：ng/(kg bw·d)]
Annexed Table 5-26　Dietary intakes of orbifloxacin from the 6th China TDS [Unit: ng/(kg bw·d)]

| 膳食类别 Category | 黑龙江 HL | 辽宁 LN | 河北 HE | 北京 BJ | 吉林 JL | 山西 SX | 陕西 SN | 河南 HA | 宁夏 NX | 内蒙古 NM | 青海 QH | 甘肃 GS | 上海 SH | 福建 FJ | 江西 JX | 江苏 JS | 浙江 ZJ | 山东 SD | 湖北 HB | 四川 SC | 广西 GX | 湖南 HN | 广东 GD | 贵州 GZ | 全国平均 AVG |
|---|---|---|---|---|---|---|---|---|---|---|---|---|---|---|---|---|---|---|---|---|---|---|---|---|---|
| 肉类 Meats | 0.000 | 0.000 | 0.000 | 0.000 | 0.000 | 0.000 | 0.000 | 0.000 | 0.000 | 0.000 | 0.000 | 0.000 | 0.000 | 0.000 | 0.000 | 0.000 | 0.000 | 0.000 | 0.000 | 0.000 | 0.000 | 0.000 | 0.000 | 0.000 | 0.000 |
| 蛋类 Eggs | 0.000 | 0.000 | 0.000 | 0.000 | 0.000 | 0.000 | 0.000 | 0.000 | 0.000 | 0.000 | 0.000 | 0.000 | 0.000 | 0.000 | 0.000 | 0.000 | 0.000 | 0.000 | 0.000 | 0.000 | 0.000 | 0.000 | 0.000 | 0.000 | 0.000 |
| 水产类 Aquatic foods | 0.000 | 0.000 | 0.000 | 0.000 | 0.000 | 0.000 | 0.000 | 0.000 | 0.000 | 0.000 | 0.000 | 0.000 | 0.000 | 0.000 | 0.000 | 0.000 | 0.000 | 0.000 | 0.000 | 0.000 | 0.000 | 0.000 | 0.000 | 0.000 | 0.000 |
| 乳类 Dairy products | 0.000 | 0.000 | 0.000 | 0.000 | 0.000 | 0.000 | 0.000 | 0.000 | 0.000 | 0.000 | 0.000 | 0.000 | 0.000 | 0.000 | 0.000 | 0.000 | 0.000 | 0.000 | 0.000 | 0.000 | 0.698 | 0.000 | 0.000 | 0.000 | 0.029 |
| 合计 SUM | 0.000 | 0.000 | 0.000 | 0.000 | 0.000 | 0.000 | 0.000 | 0.000 | 0.000 | 0.000 | 0.000 | 0.000 | 0.000 | 0.000 | 0.000 | 0.000 | 0.000 | 0.000 | 0.000 | 0.000 | 0.698 | 0.000 | 0.000 | 0.000 | 0.029 |

附表 5-27 第六次中国总膳食研究奥比沙星奥比沙星的膳食来源（单位：%）
Annexed Table 5-27 Dietary sources of orbifloxacin from the 6th China TDS (Unit: %)

| 膳食类别 Category | 黑龙江 HL | 辽宁 LN | 河北 HE | 北京 BJ | 吉林 JL | 山西 SX | 陕西 SN | 河南 HA | 宁夏 NX | 内蒙古 NM | 青海 QH | 甘肃 GS | 上海 SH | 福建 FJ | 江西 JX | 江苏 JS | 浙江 ZJ | 山东 SD | 湖北 HB | 四川 SC | 广西 GX | 湖南 HN | 广东 GD | 贵州 GZ | 全国平均 AVG |
|---|---|---|---|---|---|---|---|---|---|---|---|---|---|---|---|---|---|---|---|---|---|---|---|---|---|
| 肉类 Meats | 0.0 | 0.0 | 0.0 | 0.0 | 0.0 | 0.0 | 0.0 | 0.0 | 0.0 | 0.0 | 0.0 | 0.0 | 0.0 | 0.0 | 0.0 | 0.0 | 0.0 | 0.0 | 0.0 | 0.0 | 0.0 | 0.0 | 0.0 | 0.0 | 0.0 |
| 蛋类 Eggs | 0.0 | 0.0 | 0.0 | 0.0 | 0.0 | 0.0 | 0.0 | 0.0 | 0.0 | 0.0 | 0.0 | 0.0 | 0.0 | 0.0 | 0.0 | 0.0 | 0.0 | 0.0 | 0.0 | 0.0 | 0.0 | 0.0 | 0.0 | 0.0 | 0.0 |
| 水产类 Aquatic foods | 0.0 | 0.0 | 0.0 | 0.0 | 0.0 | 0.0 | 0.0 | 0.0 | 0.0 | 0.0 | 0.0 | 0.0 | 0.0 | 0.0 | 0.0 | 0.0 | 0.0 | 0.0 | 0.0 | 0.0 | 0.0 | 0.0 | 0.0 | 0.0 | 0.0 |
| 乳类 Dairy products | 0.0 | 0.0 | 0.0 | 0.0 | 0.0 | 0.0 | 0.0 | 0.0 | 0.0 | 0.0 | 0.0 | 0.0 | 0.0 | 0.0 | 0.0 | 0.0 | 0.0 | 0.0 | 0.0 | 0.0 | 100.0 | 0.0 | 0.0 | 0.0 | 100.0 |

附表 5-28 第六次中国总膳食研究膳食样品中沙拉沙星的含量（单位：μg/kg）
Annexed Table 5-28 Levels of sarafloxacin in food samples from the 6th China TDS (Unit: μg/kg)

| 膳食类别 Category | 黑龙江 HL | 辽宁 LN | 河北 HE | 北京 BJ | 吉林 JL | 山西 SX | 陕西 SN | 河南 HA | 宁夏 NX | 内蒙古 NM | 青海 QH | 甘肃 GS | 上海 SH | 福建 FJ | 江西 JX | 江苏 JS | 浙江 ZJ | 山东 SD | 湖北 HB | 四川 SC | 广西 GX | 湖南 HN | 广东 GD | 贵州 GZ | 全国平均 AVG |
|---|---|---|---|---|---|---|---|---|---|---|---|---|---|---|---|---|---|---|---|---|---|---|---|---|---|
| 肉类 Meats | ND | ND | ND | ND | ND | ND | ND | ND | ND | ND | ND | ND | ND | ND | ND | ND | ND | ND | ND | 0.04 | ND | ND | ND | ND | 0.00 |
| 蛋类 Eggs | ND | ND | ND | ND | ND | ND | ND | ND | ND | ND | ND | 6.78 | ND | ND | ND | ND | 0.02 | ND | ND | ND | ND | ND | 0.03 | ND | 0.28 |
| 水产类 Aquatic foods | ND | ND | ND | ND | ND | ND | ND | ND | ND | ND | ND | ND | ND | ND | ND | ND | ND | ND | ND | 0.06 | ND | ND | ND | ND | 0.00 |
| 乳类 Dairy products | ND | ND | ND | ND | ND | ND | ND | ND | ND | ND | ND | ND | ND | ND | ND | ND | ND | ND | ND | ND | ND | ND | ND | ND | 0.00 |

注：未检出（ND）按 0 计
Note: values not detected (ND) were treated as being equal to 0

附表 5-29　第六次中国总膳食研究的沙拉沙星膳食摄入量 [单位: ng/(kg bw·d)]
Annexed Table 5-29　Dietary intakes of sarafloxacin from the 6$^{th}$ China TDS [Unit: ng/(kg bw·d)]

| 膳食类别<br>Category | 黑龙江<br>HL | 辽宁<br>LN | 河北<br>HE | 北京<br>BJ | 吉林<br>JL | 山西<br>SX | 陕西<br>SN | 河南<br>HA | 宁夏<br>NX | 内蒙古<br>NM | 青海<br>QH | 甘肃<br>GS | 上海<br>SH | 福建<br>FJ | 江西<br>JX | 江苏<br>JS | 浙江<br>ZJ | 山东<br>SD | 湖北<br>HB | 四川<br>SC | 广西<br>GX | 湖南<br>HN | 广东<br>GD | 贵州<br>GZ | 全国平均<br>AVG |
|---|---|---|---|---|---|---|---|---|---|---|---|---|---|---|---|---|---|---|---|---|---|---|---|---|---|
| 肉类<br>Meats | 0.000 | 0.000 | 0.000 | 0.000 | 0.000 | 0.000 | 0.000 | 0.000 | 0.000 | 0.000 | 0.000 | 0.000 | 0.000 | 0.000 | 0.000 | 0.000 | 0.000 | 0.000 | 0.000 | 0.088 | 0.000 | 0.000 | 0.000 | 0.000 | 0.004 |
| 蛋类<br>Eggs | 0.000 | 0.000 | 0.000 | 0.000 | 0.000 | 0.000 | 0.000 | 0.000 | 0.000 | 0.000 | 0.000 | 2.391 | 0.000 | 0.000 | 0.000 | 0.000 | 0.006 | 0.000 | 0.000 | 0.000 | 0.000 | 0.000 | 0.012 | 0.000 | 0.100 |
| 水产类<br>Aquatic foods | 0.000 | 0.000 | 0.000 | 0.000 | 0.000 | 0.000 | 0.000 | 0.000 | 0.000 | 0.000 | 0.000 | 0.000 | 0.000 | 0.000 | 0.000 | 0.000 | 0.000 | 0.000 | 0.000 | 0.008 | 0.000 | 0.000 | 0.000 | 0.000 | 0.000 |
| 乳类<br>Dairy products | 0.000 | 0.000 | 0.000 | 0.000 | 0.000 | 0.000 | 0.000 | 0.000 | 0.000 | 0.000 | 0.000 | 0.000 | 0.000 | 0.000 | 0.000 | 0.000 | 0.000 | 0.000 | 0.000 | 0.000 | 0.000 | 0.000 | 0.000 | 0.000 | 0.000 |
| 合计<br>SUM | 0.000 | 0.000 | 0.000 | 0.000 | 0.000 | 0.000 | 0.000 | 0.000 | 0.000 | 0.000 | 0.000 | 2.391 | 0.000 | 0.000 | 0.000 | 0.000 | 0.006 | 0.000 | 0.000 | 0.096 | 0.000 | 0.000 | 0.012 | 0.000 | 0.104 |

附表 5-30　第六次中国总膳食研究沙拉沙星的膳食来源（单位：%）
Annexed Table 5-30　Dietary sources of sarafloxacin from the 6$^{th}$ China TDS (Unit: %)

| 膳食类别<br>Category | 黑龙江<br>HL | 辽宁<br>LN | 河北<br>HE | 北京<br>BJ | 吉林<br>JL | 山西<br>SX | 陕西<br>SN | 河南<br>HA | 宁夏<br>NX | 内蒙古<br>NM | 青海<br>QH | 甘肃<br>GS | 上海<br>SH | 福建<br>FJ | 江西<br>JX | 江苏<br>JS | 浙江<br>ZJ | 山东<br>SD | 湖北<br>HB | 四川<br>SC | 广西<br>GX | 湖南<br>HN | 广东<br>GD | 贵州<br>GZ | 全国平均<br>AVG |
|---|---|---|---|---|---|---|---|---|---|---|---|---|---|---|---|---|---|---|---|---|---|---|---|---|---|
| 肉类<br>Meats | 0.0 | 0.0 | 0.0 | 0.0 | 0.0 | 0.0 | 0.0 | 0.0 | 0.0 | 0.0 | 0.0 | 0.0 | 0.0 | 0.0 | 0.0 | 0.0 | 0.0 | 0.0 | 0.0 | 92.1 | 0.0 | 0.0 | 0.0 | 0.0 | 3.5 |
| 蛋类<br>Eggs | 0.0 | 0.0 | 0.0 | 0.0 | 0.0 | 0.0 | 0.0 | 0.0 | 0.0 | 0.0 | 0.0 | 100.0 | 0.0 | 0.0 | 0.0 | 0.0 | 100.0 | 0.0 | 0.0 | 0.0 | 0.0 | 0.0 | 100.0 | 0.0 | 96.2 |
| 水产类<br>Aquatic foods | 0.0 | 0.0 | 0.0 | 0.0 | 0.0 | 0.0 | 0.0 | 0.0 | 0.0 | 0.0 | 0.0 | 0.0 | 0.0 | 0.0 | 0.0 | 0.0 | 0.0 | 0.0 | 0.0 | 7.9 | 0.0 | 0.0 | 0.0 | 0.0 | 0.3 |
| 乳类<br>Dairy products | 0.0 | 0.0 | 0.0 | 0.0 | 0.0 | 0.0 | 0.0 | 0.0 | 0.0 | 0.0 | 0.0 | 0.0 | 0.0 | 0.0 | 0.0 | 0.0 | 0.0 | 0.0 | 0.0 | 0.0 | 0.0 | 0.0 | 0.0 | 0.0 | 0.0 |

附表 5-31　第六次中国总膳食研究膳食样品中氟甲喹的含量（单位：μg/kg）
Annexed Table 5-31　Levels of flumequine in food samples from the 6$^{th}$ China TDS (Unit: μg/kg)

| 膳食类别<br>Category | 黑龙江<br>HL | 辽宁<br>LN | 河北<br>HE | 北京<br>BJ | 吉林<br>JL | 山西<br>SX | 陕西<br>SN | 河南<br>HA | 宁夏<br>NX | 内蒙古<br>NM | 青海<br>QH | 甘肃<br>GS | 上海<br>SH | 福建<br>FJ | 江西<br>JX | 江苏<br>JS | 浙江<br>ZJ | 山东<br>SD | 湖北<br>HB | 四川<br>SC | 广西<br>GX | 湖南<br>HN | 广东<br>GD | 贵州<br>GZ | 全国平均<br>AVG |
|---|---|---|---|---|---|---|---|---|---|---|---|---|---|---|---|---|---|---|---|---|---|---|---|---|---|
| 肉类 Meats | ND | ND | ND | 0.02 | ND | ND | ND | ND | ND | ND | ND | ND | ND | ND | ND | ND | ND | ND | ND | ND | ND | ND | ND | ND | 0.00 |
| 蛋类 Eggs | ND | ND | ND | ND | ND | 0.03 | 0.02 | 0.03 | ND | ND | ND | ND | ND | ND | ND | ND | 0.06 | ND | ND | ND | ND | ND | ND | ND | 0.01 |
| 水产类 Aquatic foods | ND | ND | 0.03 | ND | ND | ND | ND | ND | ND | ND | ND | ND | ND | ND | ND | ND | ND | ND | ND | ND | ND | ND | ND | ND | 0.00 |
| 乳类 Dairy products | ND | ND | ND | ND | ND | ND | ND | ND | ND | ND | ND | ND | ND | ND | ND | ND | ND | ND | ND | ND | ND | ND | ND | ND | 0.00 |

注：未检出（ND）按 0 计
Note: values not detected (ND) were treated as being equal to 0

附表 5-32　第六次中国总膳食研究的氟甲喹膳食摄入量 [单位：ng/(kg bw·d)]
Annexed Table 5-32　Dietary intakes of flumequine from the 6$^{th}$ China TDS [Unit: ng/(kg bw·d)]

| 膳食类别<br>Category | 黑龙江<br>HL | 辽宁<br>LN | 河北<br>HE | 北京<br>BJ | 吉林<br>JL | 山西<br>SX | 陕西<br>SN | 河南<br>HA | 宁夏<br>NX | 内蒙古<br>NM | 青海<br>QH | 甘肃<br>GS | 上海<br>SH | 福建<br>FJ | 江西<br>JX | 江苏<br>JS | 浙江<br>ZJ | 山东<br>SD | 湖北<br>HB | 四川<br>SC | 广西<br>GX | 湖南<br>HN | 广东<br>GD | 贵州<br>GZ | 全国平均<br>AVG |
|---|---|---|---|---|---|---|---|---|---|---|---|---|---|---|---|---|---|---|---|---|---|---|---|---|---|
| 肉类 Meats | 0.000 | 0.000 | 0.000 | 0.022 | 0.000 | 0.000 | 0.000 | 0.000 | 0.000 | 0.000 | 0.000 | 0.000 | 0.000 | 0.000 | 0.000 | 0.000 | 0.000 | 0.000 | 0.000 | 0.000 | 0.000 | 0.000 | 0.000 | 0.000 | 0.001 |
| 蛋类 Eggs | 0.000 | 0.000 | 0.000 | 0.000 | 0.000 | 0.009 | 0.006 | 0.016 | 0.000 | 0.000 | 0.000 | 0.000 | 0.000 | 0.000 | 0.000 | 0.000 | 0.023 | 0.000 | 0.000 | 0.000 | 0.000 | 0.000 | 0.000 | 0.000 | 0.002 |
| 水产类 Aquatic foods | 0.000 | 0.000 | 0.005 | 0.000 | 0.000 | 0.000 | 0.000 | 0.000 | 0.000 | 0.000 | 0.000 | 0.000 | 0.000 | 0.000 | 0.000 | 0.000 | 0.000 | 0.000 | 0.000 | 0.000 | 0.000 | 0.000 | 0.000 | 0.000 | 0.000 |
| 乳类 Dairy products | 0.000 | 0.000 | 0.000 | 0.000 | 0.000 | 0.000 | 0.000 | 0.000 | 0.000 | 0.000 | 0.000 | 0.000 | 0.000 | 0.000 | 0.000 | 0.000 | 0.000 | 0.000 | 0.000 | 0.000 | 0.000 | 0.000 | 0.000 | 0.000 | 0.000 |

续表

| 膳食类别<br>Category | 黑龙江<br>HL | 辽宁<br>LN | 河北<br>HE | 北京<br>BJ | 吉林<br>JL | 山西<br>SX | 陕西<br>SN | 河南<br>HA | 宁夏<br>NX | 内蒙古<br>NM | 青海<br>QH | 甘肃<br>GS | 上海<br>SH | 福建<br>FJ | 江西<br>JX | 江苏<br>JS | 浙江<br>ZJ | 山东<br>SD | 湖北<br>HB | 四川<br>SC | 广西<br>GX | 湖南<br>HN | 广东<br>GD | 贵州<br>GZ | 全国平均<br>AVG |
|---|---|---|---|---|---|---|---|---|---|---|---|---|---|---|---|---|---|---|---|---|---|---|---|---|---|
| 合计<br>SUM | 0.000 | 0.000 | 0.005 | 0.022 | 0.000 | 0.009 | 0.006 | 0.016 | 0.000 | 0.000 | 0.000 | 0.000 | 0.000 | 0.000 | 0.000 | 0.000 | 0.023 | 0.000 | 0.000 | 0.000 | 0.000 | 0.000 | 0.000 | 0.000 | 0.003 |

附表 5-33　第六次中国总膳食研究氟甲喹的膳食来源（单位：%）

Annexed Table 5-33　Dietary sources of flumequine from the 6$^{th}$ China TDS (Unit: %)

| 膳食类别<br>Category | 黑龙江<br>HL | 辽宁<br>LN | 河北<br>HE | 北京<br>BJ | 吉林<br>JL | 山西<br>SX | 陕西<br>SN | 河南<br>HA | 宁夏<br>NX | 内蒙古<br>NM | 青海<br>QH | 甘肃<br>GS | 上海<br>SH | 福建<br>FJ | 江西<br>JX | 江苏<br>JS | 浙江<br>ZJ | 山东<br>SD | 湖北<br>HB | 四川<br>SC | 广西<br>GX | 湖南<br>HN | 广东<br>GD | 贵州<br>GZ | 全国平均<br>AVG |
|---|---|---|---|---|---|---|---|---|---|---|---|---|---|---|---|---|---|---|---|---|---|---|---|---|---|
| 肉类<br>Meats | 0.0 | 0.0 | 0.0 | 100.0 | 0.0 | 0.0 | 100.0 | 0.0 | 0.0 | 0.0 | 0.0 | 0.0 | 0.0 | 0.0 | 0.0 | 0.0 | 0.0 | 0.0 | 0.0 | 0.0 | 0.0 | 0.0 | 0.0 | 0.0 | 27.3 |
| 蛋类<br>Eggs | 0.0 | 0.0 | 0.0 | 0.0 | 0.0 | 100.0 | 100.0 | 100.0 | 0.0 | 0.0 | 0.0 | 0.0 | 0.0 | 0.0 | 0.0 | 0.0 | 100.0 | 0.0 | 0.0 | 0.0 | 0.0 | 0.0 | 0.0 | 0.0 | 67.0 |
| 水产类<br>Aquatic foods | 0.0 | 0.0 | 100.0 | 0.0 | 0.0 | 0.0 | 0.0 | 0.0 | 0.0 | 0.0 | 0.0 | 0.0 | 0.0 | 0.0 | 0.0 | 0.0 | 0.0 | 0.0 | 0.0 | 0.0 | 0.0 | 0.0 | 0.0 | 0.0 | 5.7 |
| 乳类<br>Dairy products | 0.0 | 0.0 | 0.0 | 0.0 | 0.0 | 0.0 | 0.0 | 0.0 | 0.0 | 0.0 | 0.0 | 0.0 | 0.0 | 0.0 | 0.0 | 0.0 | 0.0 | 0.0 | 0.0 | 0.0 | 0.0 | 0.0 | 0.0 | 0.0 | 0.0 |

附表 5-34　第六次中国总膳食研究食样品中磺胺二甲嘧啶的含量（单位：μg/kg）

Annexed Table 5-34　Levels of sulfamethazine in food samples from the 6$^{th}$ China TDS (Unit: μg/kg)

| 膳食类别<br>Category | 黑龙江<br>HL | 辽宁<br>LN | 河北<br>HE | 北京<br>BJ | 吉林<br>JL | 山西<br>SX | 陕西<br>SN | 河南<br>HA | 宁夏<br>NX | 内蒙古<br>NM | 青海<br>QH | 甘肃<br>GS | 上海<br>SH | 福建<br>FJ | 江西<br>JX | 江苏<br>JS | 浙江<br>ZJ | 山东<br>SD | 湖北<br>HB | 四川<br>SC | 广西<br>GX | 湖南<br>HN | 广东<br>GD | 贵州<br>GZ | 全国平均<br>AVG |
|---|---|---|---|---|---|---|---|---|---|---|---|---|---|---|---|---|---|---|---|---|---|---|---|---|---|
| 肉类<br>Meats | ND | ND | 0.04 | 0.08 | ND | ND | ND | ND | 2.37 | ND | ND | ND | 0.75 | 0.02 | ND | 0.06 | 0.87 | 0.12 | ND | 0.08 | ND | 0.76 | 3.11 | 0.02 | 0.34 |

续表

| 膳食类别 Category | 黑龙江 HL | 辽宁 LN | 河北 HE | 北京 BJ | 吉林 JL | 山西 SX | 陕西 SN | 河南 HA | 宁夏 NX | 内蒙古 NM | 青海 QH | 甘肃 GS | 上海 SH | 福建 FJ | 江西 JX | 江苏 JS | 浙江 ZJ | 山东 SD | 湖北 HB | 四川 SC | 广西 GX | 湖南 HN | 广东 GD | 贵州 GZ | 全国平均 AVG |
|---|---|---|---|---|---|---|---|---|---|---|---|---|---|---|---|---|---|---|---|---|---|---|---|---|---|
| 蛋类 Eggs | ND | ND | ND | ND | ND | ND | ND | ND | ND | ND | ND | 0.05 | ND | ND | ND | ND | ND | ND | ND | ND | ND | ND | 0.02 | ND | 0.00 |
| 水产类 Aquatic foods | ND | ND | ND | ND | ND | ND | ND | ND | ND | ND | ND | ND | ND | ND | ND | ND | ND | ND | ND | ND | ND | ND | ND | ND | 0.00 |
| 乳类 Dairy products | ND | ND | ND | ND | ND | ND | ND | ND | ND | ND | ND | ND | ND | ND | ND | ND | ND | ND | ND | ND | ND | ND | ND | ND | 0.00 |

注：未检出（ND）按 0 计

Note: values not detected (ND) were treated as being equal to 0

附表 5-35 第六次中国总膳食研究的磺胺二甲嘧啶膳食摄入量 [单位：ng/(kg bw·d)]

Annexed Table 5-35　Dietary intakes of sulfamethazine from the 6th China TDS [Unit: ng/(kg bw·d)]

| 膳食类别 Category | 黑龙江 HL | 辽宁 LN | 河北 HE | 北京 BJ | 吉林 JL | 山西 SX | 陕西 SN | 河南 HA | 宁夏 NX | 内蒙古 NM | 青海 QH | 甘肃 GS | 上海 SH | 福建 FJ | 江西 JX | 江苏 JS | 浙江 ZJ | 山东 SD | 湖北 HB | 四川 SC | 广西 GX | 湖南 HN | 广东 GD | 贵州 GZ | 全国平均 AVG |
|---|---|---|---|---|---|---|---|---|---|---|---|---|---|---|---|---|---|---|---|---|---|---|---|---|---|
| 肉类 Meats | 0.000 | 0.000 | 0.031 | 0.080 | 0.000 | 0.000 | 0.000 | 0.000 | 1.758 | 0.000 | 0.000 | 0.000 | 1.321 | 0.021 | 0.000 | 0.088 | 1.627 | 0.182 | 0.000 | 0.166 | 0.000 | 1.802 | 5.135 | 0.031 | 0.510 |
| 蛋类 Eggs | 0.000 | 0.000 | 0.000 | 0.000 | 0.000 | 0.000 | 0.000 | 0.000 | 0.000 | 0.000 | 0.000 | 0.017 | 0.000 | 0.000 | 0.000 | 0.000 | 0.000 | 0.000 | 0.000 | 0.000 | 0.000 | 0.000 | 0.008 | 0.000 | 0.001 |
| 水产类 Aquatic foods | 0.000 | 0.000 | 0.000 | 0.000 | 0.000 | 0.000 | 0.000 | 0.000 | | 0.000 | 0.000 | 0.000 | 0.000 | 0.000 | 0.000 | 0.000 | 0.000 | 0.000 | 0.000 | 0.000 | 0.000 | 0.000 | 0.000 | 0.000 | 0.000 |
| 乳类 Dairy products | 0.000 | 0.000 | 0.000 | 0.000 | 0.000 | 0.000 | 0.000 | 0.000 | | 0.000 | 0.000 | 0.000 | 0.000 | 0.000 | 0.000 | 0.000 | 0.000 | 0.000 | 0.000 | 0.000 | 0.000 | 0.000 | 0.000 | 0.000 | 0.000 |
| 合计 SUM | 0.000 | 0.000 | 0.031 | 0.080 | 0.000 | 0.000 | 0.000 | 0.000 | 1.758 | 0.000 | 0.000 | 0.017 | 1.321 | 0.021 | 0.000 | 0.088 | 1.627 | 0.182 | 0.000 | 0.166 | 0.000 | 1.802 | 5.144 | 0.031 | 0.511 |

附表 5-36 第六次中国总膳食研究的磺胺噻唑膳食摄入量 [单位: ng/(kg bw·d)]
Annexed Table 5-36 Dietary intakes of sulfathiazole from the 6th China TDS [Unit: ng/(kg bw·d)]

| 膳食类别 Category | 黑龙江 HL | 辽宁 LN | 河北 HE | 北京 BJ | 吉林 JL | 山西 SX | 陕西 SN | 河南 HA | 宁夏 NX | 内蒙古 NM | 青海 QH | 甘肃 GS | 上海 SH | 福建 FJ | 江西 JX | 江苏 JS | 浙江 ZJ | 山东 SD | 湖北 HB | 四川 SC | 广西 GX | 湖南 HN | 广东 GD | 贵州 GZ | 全国平均 AVG |
|---|---|---|---|---|---|---|---|---|---|---|---|---|---|---|---|---|---|---|---|---|---|---|---|---|---|
| 肉类 Meats | 0.000 | 0.000 | 0.000 | 0.000 | 0.000 | 0.000 | 0.000 | 0.000 | 0.000 | 0.000 | 0.000 | 0.000 | 0.000 | 0.000 | 0.000 | 0.000 | 0.000 | 0.000 | 0.000 | 0.000 | 0.000 | 0.000 | 0.000 | 0.000 | 0.000 |
| 蛋类 Eggs | 0.000 | 0.000 | 0.000 | 0.000 | 0.000 | 0.000 | 0.000 | 0.000 | 0.000 | 0.000 | 0.000 | 0.000 | 0.000 | 0.000 | 0.000 | 0.000 | 0.000 | 0.000 | 0.000 | 0.000 | 0.000 | 0.000 | 0.000 | 0.000 | 0.000 |
| 水产类 Aquatic foods | 0.000 | 0.000 | 0.000 | 0.000 | 0.000 | 0.000 | 0.000 | 0.000 | 0.000 | 0.000 | 0.000 | 0.000 | 0.000 | 0.000 | 0.000 | 0.000 | 0.000 | 0.000 | 0.000 | 0.000 | 0.000 | 0.000 | 0.000 | 0.000 | 0.000 |
| 乳类 Dairy products | 0.000 | 0.015 | 0.000 | 0.000 | 0.000 | 0.000 | 0.005 | 0.000 | 0.005 | 0.010 | 0.000 | 0.000 | 0.000 | 0.009 | 0.000 | 0.009 | 0.000 | 0.014 | 0.000 | 0.000 | 0.000 | 0.000 | 0.000 | 0.000 | 0.003 |
| 合计 SUM | 0.000 | 0.015 | 0.000 | 0.000 | 0.000 | 0.000 | 0.005 | 0.000 | 0.005 | 0.010 | 0.000 | 0.000 | 0.000 | 0.009 | 0.000 | 0.009 | 0.000 | 0.014 | 0.000 | 0.000 | 0.000 | 0.000 | 0.000 | 0.000 | 0.003 |

附表 5-37 第六次中国总膳食研究的磺胺甲噁唑膳食摄入量 [单位: ng/(kg bw·d)]
Annexed Table 5-37 Dietary intakes of sulfamethoxazole from the 6th China TDS [Unit: ng/(kg bw·d)]

| 膳食类别 Category | 黑龙江 HL | 辽宁 LN | 河北 HE | 北京 BJ | 吉林 JL | 山西 SX | 陕西 SN | 河南 HA | 宁夏 NX | 内蒙古 NM | 青海 QH | 甘肃 GS | 上海 SH | 福建 FJ | 江西 JX | 江苏 JS | 浙江 ZJ | 山东 SD | 湖北 HB | 四川 SC | 广西 GX | 湖南 HN | 广东 GD | 贵州 GZ | 全国平均 AVG |
|---|---|---|---|---|---|---|---|---|---|---|---|---|---|---|---|---|---|---|---|---|---|---|---|---|---|
| 肉类 Meats | 0.000 | 0.000 | 0.000 | 0.109 | 0.000 | 0.000 | 0.000 | 0.000 | 0.127 | 0.000 | 0.000 | 0.000 | 0.000 | 0.000 | 0.084 | 0.000 | 0.000 | 0.000 | 0.010 | 0.010 | 0.000 | 0.000 | 0.281 | 0.000 | 0.025 |
| 蛋类 Eggs | 0.000 | 0.009 | 0.019 | 0.056 | 0.032 | 0.004 | 0.004 | 0.000 | 0.000 | 0.009 | 0.000 | 0.000 | 0.010 | 0.004 | 0.006 | 0.093 | 0.040 | 263.047 | 0.012 | 0.000 | 0.000 | 0.006 | 0.000 | 0.056 | 10.976 |
| 水产类 Aquatic foods | 0.000 | 0.000 | 0.000 | 0.000 | 0.000 | 0.000 | 0.000 | 0.000 | 0.000 | 0.000 | 0.000 | 0.000 | 0.000 | 0.000 | 0.000 | 0.000 | 0.029 | 0.000 | 0.000 | 0.000 | 0.033 | 0.000 | 0.000 | 0.000 | 0.003 |
| 乳类 Dairy products | 0.000 | 0.026 | 0.000 | 0.000 | 0.000 | 0.000 | 0.000 | 0.000 | 0.000 | 0.013 | 0.024 | 0.000 | 0.027 | 0.000 | 0.000 | 0.000 | 0.000 | 0.000 | 0.000 | 0.002 | 0.000 | 0.000 | 0.029 | 0.000 | 0.005 |

续表

| 膳食类别<br>Category | 黑龙江<br>HL | 辽宁<br>LN | 河北<br>HE | 北京<br>BJ | 吉林<br>JL | 山西<br>SX | 陕西<br>SN | 河南<br>HA | 宁夏<br>NX | 内蒙古<br>NM | 青海<br>QH | 甘肃<br>GS | 上海<br>SH | 福建<br>FJ | 江西<br>JX | 江苏<br>JS | 浙江<br>ZJ | 山东<br>SD | 湖北<br>HB | 四川<br>SC | 广西<br>GX | 湖南<br>HN | 广东<br>GD | 贵州<br>GZ | 全国平均<br>AVG |
|---|---|---|---|---|---|---|---|---|---|---|---|---|---|---|---|---|---|---|---|---|---|---|---|---|---|
| 合计<br>SUM | 0.000 | 0.035 | 0.019 | 0.165 | 0.032 | 0.004 | 0.004 | 0.000 | 0.127 | 0.022 | 0.024 | 0.000 | 0.037 | 0.004 | 0.089 | 0.093 | 0.068 | 263.047 | 0.022 | 0.012 | 0.033 | 0.006 | 0.311 | 0.056 | 11.01 |

附表 5-38　第六次中国总膳食研究的磺胺间甲氧嘧啶膳食摄入量 [单位: ng/(kg bw·d)]

Annexed Table 5-38　Dietary intakes of sulfamonomethoxine from the 6$^{th}$ China TDS [Unit: ng/(kg bw·d)]

| 膳食类别<br>Category | 黑龙江<br>HL | 辽宁<br>LN | 河北<br>HE | 北京<br>BJ | 吉林<br>JL | 山西<br>SX | 陕西<br>SN | 河南<br>HA | 宁夏<br>NX | 内蒙古<br>NM | 青海<br>QH | 甘肃<br>GS | 上海<br>SH | 福建<br>FJ | 江西<br>JX | 江苏<br>JS | 浙江<br>ZJ | 山东<br>SD | 湖北<br>HB | 四川<br>SC | 广西<br>GX | 湖南<br>HN | 广东<br>GD | 贵州<br>GZ | 全国平均<br>AVG |
|---|---|---|---|---|---|---|---|---|---|---|---|---|---|---|---|---|---|---|---|---|---|---|---|---|---|
| 肉类<br>Meats | 16.569 | 0.000 | 0.122 | 17.780 | 0.171 | 0.000 | 0.000 | 0.057 | 1.395 | 0.000 | 0.000 | 0.000 | 0.324 | 0.000 | 0.000 | 1.033 | 0.000 | 0.000 | 0.000 | 0.000 | 0.000 | 0.000 | 0.000 | 0.000 | 1.560 |
| 蛋类<br>Eggs | 55.997 | 0.000 | 0.000 | 0.000 | 3.888 | 0.000 | 0.000 | 0.000 | 0.000 | 0.000 | 0.000 | 0.000 | 0.000 | 0.000 | 0.000 | 0.000 | 0.000 | 0.715 | 0.000 | 0.000 | 0.000 | 0.000 | 0.000 | 3.853 | 2.686 |
| 水产类<br>Aquatic foods | 0.000 | 0.000 | 0.000 | 0.000 | 0.000 | 0.000 | 0.000 | 0.000 | 0.000 | 0.000 | 0.000 | 0.000 | 0.000 | 0.000 | 0.000 | 0.000 | 0.000 | 0.000 | 0.000 | 0.000 | 0.000 | 0.000 | 0.000 | 0.000 | 0.000 |
| 乳类<br>Dairy products | 0.000 | 0.000 | 0.000 | 0.000 | 0.000 | 0.000 | 0.000 | 0.000 | 0.000 | 0.000 | 0.000 | 0.000 | 0.000 | 0.000 | 0.000 | 0.000 | 0.000 | 0.000 | 0.000 | 0.000 | 0.000 | 0.000 | 0.000 | 0.000 | 0.000 |
| 合计<br>SUM | 72.565 | 0.000 | 0.122 | 17.780 | 4.059 | 0.000 | 0.000 | 0.057 | 1.395 | 0.000 | 0.000 | 0.000 | 0.324 | 0.000 | 0.000 | 1.033 | 0.000 | 0.715 | 0.000 | 0.000 | 0.000 | 0.000 | 0.000 | 3.853 | 4.246 |

附表 5-39　第六次中国总膳食研究膳食样品中磺胺噻唑的含量（单位：μg/kg）

Annexed Table 5-39　Levels of sulfathiazole in food samples from the 6$^{th}$ China TDS (Unit: μg/kg)

| 膳食类别<br>Category | 黑龙江<br>HL | 辽宁<br>LN | 河北<br>HE | 北京<br>BJ | 吉林<br>JL | 山西<br>SX | 陕西<br>SN | 河南<br>HA | 宁夏<br>NX | 内蒙古<br>NM | 青海<br>QH | 甘肃<br>GS | 上海<br>SH | 福建<br>FJ | 江西<br>JX | 江苏<br>JS | 浙江<br>ZJ | 山东<br>SD | 湖北<br>HB | 四川<br>SC | 广西<br>GX | 湖南<br>HN | 广东<br>GD | 贵州<br>GZ | 全国平均<br>AVG |
|---|---|---|---|---|---|---|---|---|---|---|---|---|---|---|---|---|---|---|---|---|---|---|---|---|---|
| 肉类<br>Meats | ND | ND | ND | ND | ND | ND | ND | ND | ND | ND | ND | ND | ND | ND | ND | ND | ND | ND | ND | ND | ND | ND | ND | ND | 0.00 |

续表

| 膳食类别 Category | 黑龙江 HL | 辽宁 LN | 河北 HE | 北京 BJ | 吉林 JL | 山西 SX | 陕西 SN | 河南 HA | 宁夏 NX | 内蒙古 NM | 青海 QH | 甘肃 GS | 上海 SH | 福建 FJ | 江西 JX | 江苏 JS | 浙江 ZJ | 山东 SD | 湖北 HB | 四川 SC | 广西 GX | 湖南 HN | 广东 GD | 贵州 GZ | 全国平均 AVG |
|---|---|---|---|---|---|---|---|---|---|---|---|---|---|---|---|---|---|---|---|---|---|---|---|---|---|
| 蛋类 Eggs | ND | ND | ND | ND | ND | ND | ND | ND | ND | ND | ND | ND | ND | ND | ND | ND | ND | ND | ND | ND | ND | ND | ND | ND | 0.00 |
| 水产类 Aquatic foods | ND | ND | ND | ND | ND | ND | ND | ND | ND | ND | ND | ND | ND | ND | ND | ND | ND | ND | ND | ND | ND | ND | ND | ND | 0.00 |
| 乳类 Dairy products | ND | 0.02 | ND | ND | ND | ND | 0.02 | ND | 0.02 | 0.02 | ND | ND | ND | 0.02 | ND | 0.02 | ND | 0.04 | ND | ND | ND | ND | ND | ND | 0.01 |

注：未检出（ND）按 0 计

Note: values not detected (ND) were treated as being equal to 0

附表 5-40 第六次中国总膳食研究膳食样品中磺胺甲噁唑的含量（单位：μg/kg）

Annexed Table 5-40 Levels of sulfamethoxazole in food samples from the 6th China TDS (Unit: μg/kg)

| 膳食类别 Category | 黑龙江 HL | 辽宁 LN | 河北 HE | 北京 BJ | 吉林 JL | 山西 SX | 陕西 SN | 河南 HA | 宁夏 NX | 内蒙古 NM | 青海 QH | 甘肃 GS | 上海 SH | 福建 FJ | 江西 JX | 江苏 JS | 浙江 ZJ | 山东 SD | 湖北 HB | 四川 SC | 广西 GX | 湖南 HN | 广东 GD | 贵州 GZ | 全国平均 AVG |
|---|---|---|---|---|---|---|---|---|---|---|---|---|---|---|---|---|---|---|---|---|---|---|---|---|---|
| 肉类 Meats | ND | ND | ND | 0.10 | ND | ND | ND | ND | 0.17 | ND | ND | ND | ND | ND | 0.06 | ND | ND | ND | 0.01 | ND | ND | ND | 0.17 | ND | 0.02 |
| 蛋类 Eggs | ND | 0.01 | 0.04 | 0.09 | 0.05 | 0.01 | 0.01 | ND | ND | 0.02 | ND | ND | 0.02 | 0.01 | 0.02 | 0.21 | 0.10 | 373.07 | 0.03 | 0.04 | 0.02 | 0.02 | ND | 0.22 | 15.58 |
| 水产类 Aquatic foods | ND | ND | ND | ND | ND | ND | ND | ND | ND | ND | ND | ND | ND | ND | ND | ND | 0.04 | ND | ND | ND | ND | ND | ND | ND | 0.00 |
| 乳类 Dairy products | ND | 0.04 | ND | ND | ND | ND | ND | ND | ND | 0.02 | 0.03 | ND | 0.02 | ND | ND | ND | ND | ND | ND | 0.01 | ND | ND | 0.05 | ND | 0.01 |

注：未检出（ND）按 0 计

Note: values not detected (ND) were treated as being equal to 0

附表 5-41  第六次中国总膳食研究膳食样品中磺胺间甲氧嘧啶的含量（单位：μg/kg）

Annexed Table 5-41  Levels of sulfamonomethoxine in food samples from the 6th China TDS (Unit: μg/kg)

| 膳食类别 Category | 黑龙江 HL | 辽宁 LN | 河北 HE | 北京 BJ | 吉林 JL | 山西 SX | 陕西 SN | 河南 HA | 宁夏 NX | 内蒙古 NM | 青海 QH | 甘肃 GS | 上海 SH | 福建 FJ | 江西 JX | 江苏 JS | 浙江 ZJ | 山东 SD | 湖北 HB | 四川 SC | 广西 GX | 湖南 HN | 广东 GD | 贵州 GZ | 全国平均 AVG |
|---|---|---|---|---|---|---|---|---|---|---|---|---|---|---|---|---|---|---|---|---|---|---|---|---|---|
| 肉类 Meats | 17.43 | ND | 0.16 | 16.64 | 0.16 | ND | ND | 0.06 | 1.88 | ND | ND | ND | 0.18 | ND | ND | 0.71 | ND | ND | ND | ND | ND | ND | ND | ND | 1.55 |
| 蛋类 Eggs | 87.20 | ND | ND | ND | 6.09 | ND | ND | ND | ND | ND | ND | ND | ND | ND | ND | ND | ND | 1.01 | ND | ND | ND | ND | ND | 14.93 | 4.55 |
| 水产类 Aquatic foods | ND | ND | ND | ND | ND | ND | ND | ND | ND | ND | ND | ND | ND | ND | ND | ND | ND | ND | ND | ND | ND | ND | ND | ND | 0.00 |
| 乳类 Dairy products | ND | ND | ND | ND | ND | ND | ND | ND | ND | ND | ND | ND | ND | ND | ND | ND | ND | ND | ND | ND | ND | ND | ND | ND | 0.00 |

注：未检出（ND）按 0 计
Note: values not detected (ND) were treated as being equal to 0

附表 5-42  第六次中国总膳食研究膳食样品中总磺胺的含量（单位：μg/kg）

Annexed Table 5-42  Levels of total sulfonamides in food samples from the 6th China TDS (Unit: μg/kg)

| 膳食类别 Category | 黑龙江 HL | 辽宁 LN | 河北 HE | 北京 BJ | 吉林 JL | 山西 SX | 陕西 SN | 河南 HA | 宁夏 NX | 内蒙古 NM | 青海 QH | 甘肃 GS | 上海 SH | 福建 FJ | 江西 JX | 江苏 JS | 浙江 ZJ | 山东 SD | 湖北 HB | 四川 SC | 广西 GX | 湖南 HN | 广东 GD | 贵州 GZ | 全国平均 AVG |
|---|---|---|---|---|---|---|---|---|---|---|---|---|---|---|---|---|---|---|---|---|---|---|---|---|---|
| 肉类 Meats | 17.43 | ND | 0.20 | 16.82 | 0.16 | ND | ND | 0.06 | 4.43 | ND | ND | ND | 0.94 | 0.02 | 0.06 | 0.77 | 0.87 | 0.12 | 0.01 | 0.08 | ND | 0.76 | 3.28 | 0.02 | 1.92 |
| 蛋类 Eggs | 87.20 | 0.01 | 0.04 | 0.09 | 6.15 | 0.01 | 0.01 | ND | ND | 0.02 | 0.05 | 0.05 | 0.02 | 0.01 | 0.02 | 0.21 | 0.10 | 374.09 | 0.03 | 0.04 | ND | 0.02 | 0.02 | 15.15 | 20.14 |
| 水产类 Aquatic foods | ND | ND | ND | ND | ND | ND | ND | ND | ND | ND | ND | ND | ND | ND | ND | ND | 0.04 | ND | ND | ND | 0.02 | ND | ND | ND | 0.00 |

续表

| 膳食类别<br>Category | 黑龙江<br>HL | 辽宁<br>LN | 河北<br>HE | 北京<br>BJ | 吉林<br>JL | 山西<br>SX | 陕西<br>SN | 河南<br>HA | 宁夏<br>NX | 内蒙古<br>NM | 青海<br>QH | 甘肃<br>GS | 上海<br>SH | 福建<br>FJ | 江西<br>JX | 江苏<br>JS | 浙江<br>ZJ | 山东<br>SD | 湖北<br>HB | 四川<br>SC | 广西<br>GX | 湖南<br>HN | 广东<br>GD | 贵州<br>GZ | 全国平均<br>AVG |
|---|---|---|---|---|---|---|---|---|---|---|---|---|---|---|---|---|---|---|---|---|---|---|---|---|---|
| 乳类<br>Dairy products | ND | 0.06 | ND | ND | ND | ND | 0.02 | ND | 0.02 | 0.04 | 0.03 | ND | 0.02 | 0.02 | ND | 0.02 | ND | 0.04 | ND | 0.01 | ND | ND | 0.05 | ND | 0.01 |

注：未检出（ND）按0计

Note: values not detected (ND) were treated as being equal to 0

附表 5-43　第六次中国总膳食研究的总磺胺膳食摄入量 [单位: ng/(kg bw·d)]

Annexed Table 5-43　Dietary intakes of total sulfonamides from the 6th China TDS [Unit: ng/(kg bw·d)]

| 膳食类别<br>Category | 黑龙江<br>HL | 辽宁<br>LN | 河北<br>HE | 北京<br>BJ | 吉林<br>JL | 山西<br>SX | 陕西<br>SN | 河南<br>HA | 宁夏<br>NX | 内蒙古<br>NM | 青海<br>QH | 甘肃<br>GS | 上海<br>SH | 福建<br>FJ | 江西<br>JX | 江苏<br>JS | 浙江<br>ZJ | 山东<br>SD | 湖北<br>HB | 四川<br>SC | 广西<br>GX | 湖南<br>HN | 广东<br>GD | 贵州<br>GZ | 全国平均<br>AVG |
|---|---|---|---|---|---|---|---|---|---|---|---|---|---|---|---|---|---|---|---|---|---|---|---|---|---|
| 肉类<br>Meats | 16.569 | 0.000 | 0.153 | 17.969 | 0.171 | 0.000 | 0.000 | 0.057 | 3.280 | 0.000 | 0.000 | 0.000 | 1.645 | 0.021 | 0.084 | 1.121 | 1.627 | 0.182 | 0.010 | 0.166 | 0.000 | 1.802 | 5.416 | 0.031 | 2.096 |
| 蛋类<br>Eggs | 55.997 | 0.009 | 0.019 | 0.056 | 3.920 | 0.004 | 0.004 | 0.000 | 0.000 | 0.009 | 0.000 | 0.017 | 0.010 | 0.004 | 0.006 | 0.093 | 0.040 | 263.762 | 0.012 | 0.010 | 0.000 | 0.006 | 0.008 | 3.909 | 13.662 |
| 水产类<br>Aquatic foods | 0.000 | 0.000 | 0.000 | 0.000 | 0.000 | 0.000 | 0.000 | 0.000 | 0.000 | 0.000 | 0.000 | 0.000 | 0.000 | 0.000 | 0.000 | 0.000 | 0.029 | 0.000 | 0.000 | 0.000 | 0.033 | 0.000 | 0.000 | 0.000 | 0.003 |
| 乳类<br>Dairy products | 0.000 | 0.041 | 0.000 | 0.000 | 0.000 | 0.000 | 0.005 | 0.000 | 0.005 | 0.023 | 0.024 | 0.000 | 0.027 | 0.009 | 0.000 | 0.009 | 0.000 | 0.014 | 0.000 | 0.002 | 0.000 | 0.000 | 0.029 | 0.000 | 0.008 |
| 合计<br>SUM | 72.565 | 0.050 | 0.173 | 18.025 | 4.091 | 0.004 | 0.010 | 0.057 | 3.285 | 0.032 | 0.024 | 0.017 | 1.682 | 0.035 | 0.089 | 1.223 | 1.695 | 263.958 | 0.022 | 0.178 | 0.033 | 1.807 | 5.454 | 3.941 | 15.769 |

附表 5-44 第六次中国总膳食研究总磺胺的膳食来源（单位：%）

Annexed Table 5-44 Dietary sources of total sulfonamides from the 6th China TDS (Unit: %)

| 膳食类别<br>Category | 黑龙江<br>HL | 辽宁<br>LN | 河北<br>HE | 北京<br>BJ | 吉林<br>JL | 山西<br>SX | 陕西<br>SN | 河南<br>HA | 宁夏<br>NX | 内蒙古<br>NM | 青海<br>QH | 甘肃<br>GS | 上海<br>SH | 福建<br>FJ | 江西<br>JX | 江苏<br>JS | 浙江<br>ZJ | 山东<br>SD | 湖北<br>HB | 四川<br>SC | 广西<br>GX | 湖南<br>HN | 广东<br>GD | 贵州<br>GZ | 全国平均<br>AVG |
|---|---|---|---|---|---|---|---|---|---|---|---|---|---|---|---|---|---|---|---|---|---|---|---|---|---|
| 肉类 Meats | 22.8 | 0.0 | 88.8 | 99.7 | 4.2 | 0.0 | 0.0 | 100.0 | 99.9 | 0.0 | 0.0 | 0.0 | 97.8 | 61.5 | 93.5 | 91.7 | 96.0 | 0.1 | 46.4 | 93.2 | 0.0 | 99.7 | 99.3 | 0.8 | 13.3 |
| 蛋类 Eggs | 77.2 | 18.7 | 11.2 | 0.3 | 95.8 | 100.0 | 45.2 | 0.0 | 0.0 | 29.3 | 0.0 | 100.0 | 0.6 | 11.6 | 6.5 | 7.6 | 2.3 | 99.9 | 53.6 | 5.8 | 0.0 | 0.3 | 0.2 | 99.2 | 86.6 |
| 水产类 Aquatic foods | 0.0 | 0.0 | 0.0 | 0.0 | 0.0 | 0.0 | 0.0 | 0.0 | 0.0 | 0.0 | 0.0 | 0.0 | 0.0 | 0.0 | 0.0 | 0.0 | 1.7 | 0.0 | 0.0 | 0.0 | 100.0 | 0.0 | 0.0 | 0.0 | 0.0 |
| 乳类 Dairy products | 0.0 | 81.3 | 0.0 | 0.0 | 0.0 | 0.0 | 54.8 | 0.0 | 0.1 | 70.7 | 100.0 | 0.0 | 1.6 | 27.0 | 0.0 | 0.7 | 0.0 | 0.0 | 0.0 | 1.0 | 0.0 | 0.0 | 0.5 | 0.0 | 0.0 |

附表 5-45 第六次中国总膳食研究膳食样品中结晶紫的含量（单位：μg/kg）

Annexed Table 5-45 Levels of crystal violet in food samples from the 6th China TDS (Unit: μg/kg)

| 膳食类别<br>Category | 黑龙江<br>HL | 辽宁<br>LN | 河北<br>HE | 北京<br>BJ | 吉林<br>JL | 山西<br>SX | 陕西<br>SN | 河南<br>HA | 宁夏<br>NX | 内蒙古<br>NM | 青海<br>QH | 甘肃<br>GS | 上海<br>SH | 福建<br>FJ | 江西<br>JX | 江苏<br>JS | 浙江<br>ZJ | 山东<br>SD | 湖北<br>HB | 四川<br>SC | 广西<br>GX | 湖南<br>HN | 广东<br>GD | 贵州<br>GZ | 全国平均<br>AVG |
|---|---|---|---|---|---|---|---|---|---|---|---|---|---|---|---|---|---|---|---|---|---|---|---|---|---|
| 肉类 Meats | 1.95 | 0.79 | 1.97 | 3.56 | 11.45 | 6.74 | 2.33 | 6.62 | 2.60 | 4.26 | 2.69 | 0.77 | 1.88 | 6.34 | 11.73 | 9.61 | 0.48 | 2.14 | 7.86 | 21.32 | 0.69 | 1.78 | 16.51 | 10.82 | 5.70 |
| 蛋类 Eggs | 0.80 | 24.21 | 0.93 | 3.93 | 11.32 | 6.65 | 19.39 | 2.07 | 2.57 | 5.69 | 39.42 | 0.89 | 3.98 | 0.43 | 26.48 | 1.10 | 22.03 | 0.75 | 0.52 | 0.76 | 47.51 | 3.31 | 0.38 | 0.58 | 9.40 |
| 水产类 Aquatic foods | 0.48 | 0.21 | 0.42 | 0.09 | 0.59 | 0.73 | 0.39 | 0.40 | 1.73 | 0.58 | 0.37 | 7.72 | 0.31 | 0.25 | 0.47 | 0.13 | 0.34 | 0.92 | 0.13 | 0.17 | 45.43 | 0.29 | 0.48 | 1.07 | 2.65 |
| 乳类 Dairy products | 0.14 | 1.66 | 0.19 | 0.24 | 9.26 | 0.15 | 0.51 | 0.73 | 0.70 | 0.28 | 7.10 | 1.83 | 0.21 | 1.51 | 0.23 | 3.41 | 0.38 | 0.32 | 0.64 | 1.34 | 0.31 | 1.88 | 30.62 | 0.19 | 2.66 |

附表 5-46 第六次中国总膳食研究的结晶紫膳食摄入量 [单位：ng/(kg bw·d)]
Annexed Table 5-46 Dietary intakes of crystal violet from the 6th China TDS [Unit: ng/(kg bw·d)]

| 膳食类别<br>Category | 黑龙江<br>HL | 辽宁<br>LN | 河北<br>HE | 北京<br>BJ | 吉林<br>JL | 山西<br>SX | 陕西<br>SN | 河南<br>HA | 宁夏<br>NX | 内蒙古<br>NM | 青海<br>QH | 甘肃<br>GS | 上海<br>SH | 福建<br>FJ | 江西<br>JX | 江苏<br>JS | 浙江<br>ZJ | 山东<br>SD | 湖北<br>HB | 四川<br>SC | 广西<br>GX | 湖南<br>HN | 广东<br>GD | 贵州<br>GZ | 全国平均<br>AVG |
|---|---|---|---|---|---|---|---|---|---|---|---|---|---|---|---|---|---|---|---|---|---|---|---|---|---|
| 肉类 Meats | 1.852 | 0.839 | 1.479 | 3.799 | 12.095 | 14.680 | 1.333 | 5.813 | 1.929 | 4.970 | 3.036 | 0.379 | 3.309 | 8.656 | 17.478 | 14.003 | 0.905 | 3.310 | 6.773 | 43.620 | 1.646 | 4.225 | 27.279 | 18.292 | 8.404 |
| 蛋类 Eggs | 0.517 | 15.714 | 0.467 | 2.422 | 7.224 | 2.212 | 6.763 | 0.977 | 0.532 | 2.684 | 8.221 | 0.313 | 2.461 | 0.130 | 8.616 | 0.491 | 8.364 | 0.527 | 0.205 | 0.177 | 10.565 | 1.200 | 0.146 | 0.150 | 3.378 |
| 水产类 Aquatic foods | 0.206 | 0.053 | 0.064 | 0.023 | 0.105 | 0.074 | 0.025 | 0.030 | 0.066 | 0.095 | 0.021 | 0.346 | 0.341 | 0.259 | 0.324 | 0.082 | 0.271 | 0.332 | 0.083 | 0.023 | 69.709 | 0.305 | 0.389 | 0.059 | 3.053 |
| 乳类 Dairy products | 0.029 | 1.170 | 0.071 | 0.320 | 4.758 | 0.101 | 0.158 | 0.228 | 0.170 | 0.153 | 6.027 | 0.409 | 0.239 | 0.864 | 0.079 | 1.488 | 0.203 | 0.117 | 0.068 | 0.267 | 0.089 | 0.537 | 17.740 | 0.086 | 1.474 |
| 合计 SUM | 2.604 | 17.776 | 2.082 | 6.564 | 24.182 | 17.067 | 8.279 | 7.047 | 2.697 | 7.902 | 17.305 | 1.446 | 6.351 | 9.909 | 26.497 | 16.064 | 9.743 | 4.285 | 7.129 | 44.087 | 82.009 | 6.267 | 45.555 | 18.587 | 16.310 |

附表 5-47 第六次中国总膳食研究结晶紫的膳食来源（单位：%）
Annexed Table 5-47 Dietary sources of crystal violet from the 6th China TDS (Unit: %)

| 膳食类别<br>Category | 黑龙江<br>HL | 辽宁<br>LN | 河北<br>HE | 北京<br>BJ | 吉林<br>JL | 山西<br>SX | 陕西<br>SN | 河南<br>HA | 宁夏<br>NX | 内蒙古<br>NM | 青海<br>QH | 甘肃<br>GS | 上海<br>SH | 福建<br>FJ | 江西<br>JX | 江苏<br>JS | 浙江<br>ZJ | 山东<br>SD | 湖北<br>HB | 四川<br>SC | 广西<br>GX | 湖南<br>HN | 广东<br>GD | 贵州<br>GZ | 全国平均<br>AVG |
|---|---|---|---|---|---|---|---|---|---|---|---|---|---|---|---|---|---|---|---|---|---|---|---|---|---|
| 肉类 Meats | 71.1 | 4.7 | 71.1 | 57.9 | 50.0 | 86.0 | 16.1 | 82.5 | 71.5 | 62.9 | 17.5 | 26.2 | 52.1 | 87.4 | 66.0 | 87.2 | 9.3 | 77.2 | 95.0 | 98.9 | 2.0 | 67.4 | 59.9 | 98.4 | 51.5 |
| 蛋类 Eggs | 19.8 | 88.4 | 22.4 | 36.9 | 29.9 | 13.0 | 81.7 | 13.9 | 19.7 | 34.0 | 47.5 | 21.6 | 38.8 | 1.3 | 32.5 | 3.1 | 85.8 | 12.3 | 2.9 | 0.4 | 12.9 | 19.1 | 0.3 | 0.8 | 20.7 |
| 水产类 Aquatic foods | 7.9 | 0.3 | 3.1 | 0.4 | 0.4 | 0.4 | 0.3 | 0.4 | 2.5 | 1.2 | 0.1 | 23.9 | 5.4 | 2.6 | 1.2 | 0.5 | 2.8 | 7.7 | 1.2 | 0.1 | 85.0 | 4.9 | 0.9 | 0.3 | 18.7 |
| 乳类 Dairy products | 1.1 | 6.6 | 3.4 | 4.9 | 19.7 | 0.6 | 1.9 | 3.2 | 6.3 | 1.9 | 34.8 | 28.3 | 3.8 | 8.7 | 0.3 | 9.3 | 2.1 | 2.7 | 1.0 | 0.6 | 0.1 | 8.6 | 38.9 | 0.5 | 9.0 |

附表 5-48　第六次中国总膳食研究膳食样品中甲硝唑的含量（单位：µg/kg）
Annexed Table 5-48　Levels of metronidazole in food samples from the 6<sup>th</sup> China TDS (Unit: µg/kg)

| 膳食类别<br>Category | 黑龙江<br>HL | 辽宁<br>LN | 河北<br>HE | 北京<br>BJ | 吉林<br>JL | 山西<br>SX | 陕西<br>SN | 河南<br>HA | 宁夏<br>NX | 内蒙古<br>NM | 青海<br>QH | 甘肃<br>GS | 上海<br>SH | 福建<br>FJ | 江西<br>JX | 江苏<br>JS | 浙江<br>ZJ | 山东<br>SD | 湖北<br>HB | 四川<br>SC | 广西<br>GX | 湖南<br>HN | 广东<br>GD | 贵州<br>GZ | 全国平均<br>AVG |
|---|---|---|---|---|---|---|---|---|---|---|---|---|---|---|---|---|---|---|---|---|---|---|---|---|---|
| 肉类 Meats | ND | ND | ND | ND | 0.18 | ND | ND | ND | ND | ND | ND | ND | ND | 9.96 | ND | ND | ND | ND | ND | ND | ND | ND | ND | ND | 0.42 |
| 蛋类 Eggs | ND | ND | 4.26 | ND | 21.06 | 0.24 | 10.98 | 0.20 | ND | 0.20 | ND | 0.83 | 2.23 | 0.84 | ND | 0.04 | 0.42 | 0.13 | 0.06 | ND | 0.18 | 602.90 | 0.18 | 0.14 | 26.87 |
| 水产类 Aquatic foods | ND | ND | ND | ND | ND | ND | ND | ND | ND | ND | ND | ND | ND | ND | ND | ND | ND | ND | ND | ND | ND | ND | ND | ND | 0.00 |
| 乳类 Dairy products | ND | ND | ND | ND | ND | ND | ND | ND | ND | ND | 0.04 | ND | ND | ND | ND | ND | ND | ND | ND | ND | ND | ND | ND | ND | 0.00 |

注：未检出（ND）按 0 计
Note: values not detected (ND) were treated as being equal to 0

附表 5-49　第六次中国总膳食研究的甲硝唑膳食摄入量 [单位：ng/(kg bw · d)]
Annexed Table 5-49　Dietary intakes of metronidazole from the 6<sup>th</sup> China TDS [Unit: ng/(kg bw · d)]

| 膳食类别<br>Category | 黑龙江<br>HL | 辽宁<br>LN | 河北<br>HE | 北京<br>BJ | 吉林<br>JL | 山西<br>SX | 陕西<br>SN | 河南<br>HA | 宁夏<br>NX | 内蒙古<br>NM | 青海<br>QH | 甘肃<br>GS | 上海<br>SH | 福建<br>FJ | 江西<br>JX | 江苏<br>JS | 浙江<br>ZJ | 山东<br>SD | 湖北<br>HB | 四川<br>SC | 广西<br>GX | 湖南<br>HN | 广东<br>GD | 贵州<br>GZ | 全国平均<br>AVG |
|---|---|---|---|---|---|---|---|---|---|---|---|---|---|---|---|---|---|---|---|---|---|---|---|---|---|
| 肉类 Meats | 0.000 | 0.000 | 0.000 | 0.000 | 0.185 | 0.000 | 0.000 | 0.000 | 0.000 | 0.000 | 0.000 | 0.000 | 0.000 | 13.594 | 0.000 | 0.000 | 0.000 | 0.000 | 0.000 | 0.000 | 0.000 | 0.000 | 0.000 | 0.000 | 0.574 |
| 蛋类 Eggs | 0.000 | 0.000 | 2.136 | 0.000 | 13.434 | 0.079 | 3.832 | 0.095 | 0.000 | 0.093 | 0.000 | 0.291 | 1.378 | 0.254 | 0.000 | 0.017 | 0.161 | 0.091 | 0.025 | 0.000 | 0.040 | 218.191 | 0.068 | 0.036 | 10.009 |
| 水产类 Aquatic foods | 0.000 | 0.000 | 0.000 | 0.000 | 0.000 | 0.000 | 0.000 | 0.000 | 0.000 | 0.000 | 0.033 | 0.000 | 0.000 | 0.000 | 0.000 | 0.000 | 0.000 | 0.000 | 0.000 | 0.000 | 0.000 | 0.000 | 0.000 | 0.000 | 0.000 |
| 乳类 Dairy products | 0.000 | 0.000 | 0.000 | 0.000 | 0.000 | 0.000 | 0.000 | 0.000 | 0.000 | 0.000 | 0.000 | 0.000 | 0.000 | 0.000 | 0.000 | 0.000 | 0.000 | 0.000 | 0.000 | 0.000 | 0.000 | 0.000 | 0.000 | 0.000 | 0.001 |

续表

| 膳食类别<br>Category | 黑龙江<br>HL | 辽宁<br>LN | 河北<br>HE | 北京<br>BJ | 吉林<br>JL | 山西<br>SX | 陕西<br>SN | 河南<br>HA | 宁夏<br>NX | 内蒙古<br>NM | 青海<br>QH | 甘肃<br>GS | 上海<br>SH | 福建<br>FJ | 江西<br>JX | 江苏<br>JS | 浙江<br>ZJ | 山东<br>SD | 湖北<br>HB | 四川<br>SC | 广西<br>GX | 湖南<br>HN | 广东<br>GD | 贵州<br>GZ | 全国平均<br>AVG |
|---|---|---|---|---|---|---|---|---|---|---|---|---|---|---|---|---|---|---|---|---|---|---|---|---|---|
| 合计 SUM | 0.000 | 0.000 | 2.136 | 0.000 | 13.619 | 0.079 | 3.832 | 0.095 | 0.000 | 0.093 | 0.033 | 0.291 | 1.378 | 13.849 | 0.000 | 0.017 | 0.161 | 0.091 | 0.025 | 0.000 | 0.040 | 218.191 | 0.068 | 0.036 | 10.585 |

附表 5-50 第六次中国总膳食研究甲硝唑的膳食来源（单位：%）
Annexed Table 5-50 Dietary sources of metronidazole from the 6$^{th}$ China TDS (Unit: %)

| 膳食类别<br>Category | 黑龙江<br>HL | 辽宁<br>LN | 河北<br>HE | 北京<br>BJ | 吉林<br>JL | 山西<br>SX | 陕西<br>SN | 河南<br>HA | 宁夏<br>NX | 内蒙古<br>NM | 青海<br>QH | 甘肃<br>GS | 上海<br>SH | 福建<br>FJ | 江西<br>JX | 江苏<br>JS | 浙江<br>ZJ | 山东<br>SD | 湖北<br>HB | 四川<br>SC | 广西<br>GX | 湖南<br>HN | 广东<br>GD | 贵州<br>GZ | 全国平均<br>AVG |
|---|---|---|---|---|---|---|---|---|---|---|---|---|---|---|---|---|---|---|---|---|---|---|---|---|---|
| 肉类 Meats | 0.0 | 0.0 | 0.0 | 0.0 | 1.4 | 0.0 | 0.0 | 0.0 | 0.0 | 0.0 | 0.0 | 0.0 | 0.0 | 98.2 | 0.0 | 0.0 | 0.0 | 0.0 | 0.0 | 0.0 | 0.0 | 0.0 | 0.0 | 0.0 | 5.4 |
| 蛋类 Eggs | 0.0 | 0.0 | 100.0 | 0.0 | 98.6 | 100.0 | 100.0 | 100.0 | 0.0 | 100.0 | 0.0 | 100.0 | 100.0 | 1.8 | 0.0 | 100.0 | 100.0 | 100.0 | 100.0 | 0.0 | 100.0 | 100.0 | 100.0 | 100.0 | 94.6 |
| 水产类 Aquatic foods | 0.0 | 0.0 | 0.0 | 0.0 | 0.0 | 0.0 | 0.0 | 0.0 | 0.0 | 0.0 | 0.0 | 0.0 | 0.0 | 0.0 | 0.0 | 0.0 | 0.0 | 0.0 | 0.0 | 0.0 | 0.0 | 0.0 | 0.0 | 0.0 | 0.0 |
| 乳类 Dairy products | 0.0 | 0.0 | 0.0 | 0.0 | 0.0 | 0.0 | 0.0 | 0.0 | 0.0 | 0.0 | 100.0 | 0.0 | 0.0 | 0.0 | 0.0 | 0.0 | 0.0 | 0.0 | 0.0 | 0.0 | 0.0 | 0.0 | 0.0 | 0.0 | 0.0 |

附表 5-51 第六次中国总膳食研究膳食样品中地美硝唑的含量（单位：μg/kg）
Annexed Table 5-51 Levels of dimetridazole in food samples from the 6$^{th}$ China TDS (Unit: μg/kg)

| 膳食类别<br>Category | 黑龙江<br>HL | 辽宁<br>LN | 河北<br>HE | 北京<br>BJ | 吉林<br>JL | 山西<br>SX | 陕西<br>SN | 河南<br>HA | 宁夏<br>NX | 内蒙古<br>NM | 青海<br>QH | 甘肃<br>GS | 上海<br>SH | 福建<br>FJ | 江西<br>JX | 江苏<br>JS | 浙江<br>ZJ | 山东<br>SD | 湖北<br>HB | 四川<br>SC | 广西<br>GX | 湖南<br>HN | 广东<br>GD | 贵州<br>GZ | 全国平均<br>AVG |
|---|---|---|---|---|---|---|---|---|---|---|---|---|---|---|---|---|---|---|---|---|---|---|---|---|---|
| 肉类 Meats | ND | ND | ND | ND | ND | ND | ND | ND | ND | ND | ND | ND | ND | ND | ND | ND | ND | ND | ND | ND | ND | ND | ND | ND | 0.00 |

续表

| 膳食类别<br>Category | 黑龙江<br>HL | 辽宁<br>LN | 河北<br>HE | 北京<br>BJ | 吉林<br>JL | 山西<br>SX | 陕西<br>SN | 河南<br>HA | 宁夏<br>NX | 内蒙古<br>NM | 青海<br>QH | 甘肃<br>GS | 上海<br>SH | 福建<br>FJ | 江西<br>JX | 江苏<br>JS | 浙江<br>ZJ | 山东<br>SD | 湖北<br>HB | 四川<br>SC | 广西<br>GX | 湖南<br>HN | 广东<br>GD | 贵州<br>GZ | 全国平均<br>AVG |
|---|---|---|---|---|---|---|---|---|---|---|---|---|---|---|---|---|---|---|---|---|---|---|---|---|---|
| 蛋类 Eggs | ND | ND | ND | ND | ND | ND | ND | ND | ND | 51.41 | ND | ND | 169.22 | ND | ND | ND | ND | ND | ND | ND | ND | ND | ND | ND | 9.19 |
| 水产类 Aquatic foods | ND | ND | ND | ND | ND | ND | ND | ND | ND | ND | ND | ND | ND | ND | ND | ND | ND | ND | ND | ND | ND | ND | ND | ND | 0.00 |
| 乳类 Dairy products | ND | ND | ND | ND | ND | ND | ND | ND | ND | ND | ND | ND | ND | ND | ND | ND | ND | ND | ND | ND | ND | ND | ND | ND | 0.00 |

注：未检出（ND）按 0 计

Note: values not detected (ND) were treated as being equal to 0

附表 5-52　第六次中国总膳食研究的地美硝唑膳食摄入量［单位：ng/(kg bw·d)］

Annexed Table 5-52　Dietary intakes of dimetridazole from the 6$^{th}$ China TDS [Unit: ng/(kg bw·d)]

| 膳食类别<br>Category | 黑龙江<br>HL | 辽宁<br>LN | 河北<br>HE | 北京<br>BJ | 吉林<br>JL | 山西<br>SX | 陕西<br>SN | 河南<br>HA | 宁夏<br>NX | 内蒙古<br>NM | 青海<br>QH | 甘肃<br>GS | 上海<br>SH | 福建<br>FJ | 江西<br>JX | 江苏<br>JS | 浙江<br>ZJ | 山东<br>SD | 湖北<br>HB | 四川<br>SC | 广西<br>GX | 湖南<br>HN | 广东<br>GD | 贵州<br>GZ | 全国平均<br>AVG |
|---|---|---|---|---|---|---|---|---|---|---|---|---|---|---|---|---|---|---|---|---|---|---|---|---|---|
| 肉类 Meats | 0.000 | 0.000 | 0.000 | 0.000 | 0.000 | 0.000 | 0.000 | 0.000 | 0.000 | 0.000 | 0.000 | 0.000 | 0.000 | 0.000 | 0.000 | 0.000 | 0.000 | 0.000 | 0.000 | 0.000 | 0.000 | 0.000 | 0.000 | 0.000 | 0.000 |
| 蛋类 Eggs | 0.000 | 0.000 | 0.000 | 0.000 | 0.000 | 0.000 | 0.000 | 0.000 | 0.000 | 24.234 | 0.000 | 0.000 | 104.780 | 0.000 | 0.000 | 0.000 | 0.000 | 0.000 | 0.000 | 0.000 | 0.000 | 0.000 | 0.000 | 0.000 | 5.376 |
| 水产类 Aquatic foods | 0.000 | 0.000 | 0.000 | 0.000 | 0.000 | 0.000 | 0.000 | 0.000 | 0.000 | 0.000 | 0.000 | 0.000 | 0.000 | 0.000 | 0.000 | 0.000 | 0.000 | 0.000 | 0.000 | 0.000 | 0.000 | 0.000 | 0.000 | 0.000 | 0.000 |
| 乳类 Dairy products | 0.000 | 0.000 | 0.000 | 0.000 | 0.000 | 0.000 | 0.000 | 0.000 | 0.000 | 0.000 | 0.000 | 0.000 | 0.000 | 0.000 | 0.000 | 0.000 | 0.000 | 0.000 | 0.000 | 0.000 | 0.000 | 0.000 | 0.000 | 0.000 | 0.000 |
| 合计 SUM | 0.000 | 0.000 | 0.000 | 0.000 | 0.000 | 0.000 | 0.000 | 0.000 | 0.000 | 24.234 | 0.000 | 0.000 | 104.780 | 0.000 | 0.000 | 0.000 | 0.000 | 0.000 | 0.000 | 0.000 | 0.000 | 0.000 | 0.000 | 0.000 | 5.376 |

附表 5-53 第六次中国总膳食研究地美硝唑的膳食来源（单位：%）
Annexed Table 5-53 Dietary sources of dimetridazole from the 6th China TDS (Unit: %)

| 膳食类别<br>Category | 黑龙江<br>HL | 辽宁<br>LN | 河北<br>HE | 北京<br>BJ | 吉林<br>JL | 山西<br>SX | 陕西<br>SN | 河南<br>HA | 宁夏<br>NX | 内蒙古<br>NM | 青海<br>QH | 甘肃<br>GS | 上海<br>SH | 福建<br>FJ | 江西<br>JX | 江苏<br>JS | 浙江<br>ZJ | 山东<br>SD | 湖北<br>HB | 四川<br>SC | 广西<br>GX | 湖南<br>HN | 广东<br>GD | 贵州<br>GZ | 全国平均<br>AVG |
|---|---|---|---|---|---|---|---|---|---|---|---|---|---|---|---|---|---|---|---|---|---|---|---|---|---|
| 肉类 Meats | 0.0 | 0.0 | 0.0 | 0.0 | 0.0 | 0.0 | 0.0 | 0.0 | 0.0 | 0.0 | 0.0 | 0.0 | 0.0 | 0.0 | 0.0 | 0.0 | 0.0 | 0.0 | 0.0 | 0.0 | 0.0 | 0.0 | 0.0 | 0.0 | 0.0 |
| 蛋类 Eggs | 0.0 | 0.0 | 0.0 | 0.0 | 0.0 | 0.0 | 0.0 | 0.0 | 0.0 | 100.0 | 0.0 | 0.0 | 100.0 | 0.0 | 0.0 | 0.0 | 0.0 | 0.0 | 0.0 | 0.0 | 0.0 | 0.0 | 0.0 | 0.0 | 100.0 |
| 水产类 Aquatic foods | 0.0 | 0.0 | 0.0 | 0.0 | 0.0 | 0.0 | 0.0 | 0.0 | 0.0 | 0.0 | 0.0 | 0.0 | 0.0 | 0.0 | 0.0 | 0.0 | 0.0 | 0.0 | 0.0 | 0.0 | 0.0 | 0.0 | 0.0 | 0.0 | 0.0 |
| 乳类 Dairy products | 0.0 | 0.0 | 0.0 | 0.0 | 0.0 | 0.0 | 0.0 | 0.0 | 0.0 | 0.0 | 0.0 | 0.0 | 0.0 | 0.0 | 0.0 | 0.0 | 0.0 | 0.0 | 0.0 | 0.0 | 0.0 | 0.0 | 0.0 | 0.0 | 0.0 |

附表 5-54 第六次中国总膳食研究膳食样品中左旋咪唑的含量（单位：μg/kg）
Annexed Table 5-54 Levels of levamisole in food samples from the 6th China TDS (Unit: μg/kg)

| 膳食类别<br>Category | 黑龙江<br>HL | 辽宁<br>LN | 河北<br>HE | 北京<br>BJ | 吉林<br>JL | 山西<br>SX | 陕西<br>SN | 河南<br>HA | 宁夏<br>NX | 内蒙古<br>NM | 青海<br>QH | 甘肃<br>GS | 上海<br>SH | 福建<br>FJ | 江西<br>JX | 江苏<br>JS | 浙江<br>ZJ | 山东<br>SD | 湖北<br>HB | 四川<br>SC | 广西<br>GX | 湖南<br>HN | 广东<br>GD | 贵州<br>GZ | 全国平均<br>AVG |
|---|---|---|---|---|---|---|---|---|---|---|---|---|---|---|---|---|---|---|---|---|---|---|---|---|---|
| 肉类 Meats | ND | ND | ND | ND | ND | ND | ND | ND | ND | ND | ND | ND | ND | ND | ND | ND | ND | ND | ND | ND | ND | ND | ND | ND | 0.00 |
| 蛋类 Eggs | ND | ND | ND | ND | ND | ND | ND | ND | ND | ND | ND | ND | ND | ND | 2.25 | ND | ND | ND | ND | ND | ND | ND | ND | ND | 0.00 |
| 水产类 Aquatic foods | ND | ND | ND | ND | ND | ND | ND | ND | ND | ND | ND | ND | 2.25 | ND | ND | ND | ND | ND | ND | ND | ND | ND | ND | ND | 0.00 |
| 乳类 Dairy products | ND | ND | ND | ND | ND | ND | ND | ND | ND | ND | ND | ND | ND | ND | ND | ND | ND | ND | ND | ND | ND | ND | ND | ND | 0.19 |

注：未检出（ND）按 0 计
Note: values not detected (ND) were treated as being equal to 0

附表 5-55 第六次中国总膳食研究的左旋咪唑膳食摄入量 [单位: ng/(kg bw・d)]
Annexed Table 5-55 Dietary intakes of levamisole from the 6th China TDS [Unit: ng/(kg bw・d)]

| 膳食类别 Category | 黑龙江 HL | 辽宁 LN | 河北 HE | 北京 BJ | 吉林 JL | 山西 SX | 陕西 SN | 河南 HA | 宁夏 NX | 内蒙古 NM | 青海 QH | 甘肃 GS | 上海 SH | 福建 FJ | 江西 JX | 江苏 JS | 浙江 ZJ | 山东 SD | 湖北 HB | 四川 SC | 广西 GX | 湖南 HN | 广东 GD | 贵州 GZ | 全国平均 AVG |
|---|---|---|---|---|---|---|---|---|---|---|---|---|---|---|---|---|---|---|---|---|---|---|---|---|---|
| 肉类 Meats | 0.000 | 0.000 | 0.000 | 0.000 | 0.000 | 0.000 | 0.000 | 0.000 | 0.000 | 0.000 | 0.000 | 0.000 | 0.000 | 0.000 | 0.000 | 0.000 | 0.000 | 0.000 | 0.000 | 0.000 | 0.000 | 0.000 | 0.000 | 0.000 | 0.000 |
| 蛋类 Eggs | 0.000 | 0.000 | 0.000 | 0.000 | 0.000 | 0.000 | 0.000 | 0.000 | 0.000 | 0.000 | 0.000 | 0.000 | 0.000 | 0.000 | 0.000 | 0.000 | 0.000 | 0.000 | 0.000 | 0.000 | 0.000 | 0.000 | 0.000 | 0.000 | 0.000 |
| 水产类 Aquatic foods | 0.000 | 0.000 | 0.000 | 0.000 | 0.000 | 0.000 | 0.000 | 0.000 | 0.000 | 0.000 | 0.000 | 0.000 | 0.000 | 0.000 | 0.000 | 0.000 | 0.000 | 0.000 | 0.000 | 0.000 | 0.000 | 0.000 | 0.000 | 0.000 | 0.000 |
| 乳类 Dairy products | 0.000 | 0.000 | 0.000 | 0.000 | 0.000 | 0.000 | 0.000 | 0.000 | 0.000 | 0.000 | 0.000 | 0.000 | 2.549 | 0.000 | 0.781 | 0.000 | 0.000 | 0.000 | 0.000 | 0.000 | 0.000 | 0.000 | 0.000 | 0.000 | 0.139 |
| 合计 SUM | 0.000 | 0.000 | 0.000 | 0.000 | 0.000 | 0.000 | 0.000 | 0.000 | 0.000 | 0.000 | 0.000 | 0.000 | 2.549 | 0.000 | 0.781 | 0.000 | 0.000 | 0.000 | 0.000 | 0.000 | 0.000 | 0.000 | 0.000 | 0.000 | 0.139 |

附表 5-56 第六次中国总膳食研究左旋咪唑的膳食来源（单位：%）
Annexed Table 5-56 Dietary sources of levamisole from the 6th China TDS (Unit: %)

| 膳食类别 Category | 黑龙江 HL | 辽宁 LN | 河北 HE | 北京 BJ | 吉林 JL | 山西 SX | 陕西 SN | 河南 HA | 宁夏 NX | 内蒙古 NM | 青海 QH | 甘肃 GS | 上海 SH | 福建 FJ | 江西 JX | 江苏 JS | 浙江 ZJ | 山东 SD | 湖北 HB | 四川 SC | 广西 GX | 湖南 HN | 广东 GD | 贵州 GZ | 全国平均 AVG |
|---|---|---|---|---|---|---|---|---|---|---|---|---|---|---|---|---|---|---|---|---|---|---|---|---|---|
| 肉类 Meats | 0.0 | 0.0 | 0.0 | 0.0 | 0.0 | 0.0 | 0.0 | 0.0 | 0.0 | 0.0 | 0.0 | 0.0 | 0.0 | 0.0 | 0.0 | 0.0 | 0.0 | 0.0 | 0.0 | 0.0 | 0.0 | 0.0 | 0.0 | 0.0 | 0.0 |
| 蛋类 Eggs | 0.0 | 0.0 | 0.0 | 0.0 | 0.0 | 0.0 | 0.0 | 0.0 | 0.0 | 0.0 | 0.0 | 0.0 | 0.0 | 0.0 | 0.0 | 0.0 | 0.0 | 0.0 | 0.0 | 0.0 | 0.0 | 0.0 | 0.0 | 0.0 | 0.0 |
| 水产类 Aquatic foods | 0.0 | 0.0 | 0.0 | 0.0 | 0.0 | 0.0 | 0.0 | 0.0 | 0.0 | 0.0 | 0.0 | 0.0 | 0.0 | 0.0 | 0.0 | 0.0 | 0.0 | 0.0 | 0.0 | 0.0 | 0.0 | 0.0 | 0.0 | 0.0 | 0.0 |
| 乳类 Dairy products | 0.0 | 0.0 | 0.0 | 0.0 | 0.0 | 0.0 | 0.0 | 0.0 | 0.0 | 0.0 | 0.0 | 0.0 | 100.0 | 0.0 | 100.0 | 0.0 | 0.0 | 0.0 | 0.0 | 0.0 | 0.0 | 0.0 | 0.0 | 0.0 | 100.0 |

附表 5-57 第六次中国总膳食研究膳食样品中阿苯达唑的含量（单位：μg/kg）

Annexed Table 5-57 Levels of albendazole in food samples from the 6th China TDS (Unit: μg/kg)

| 膳食类别 Category | 黑龙江 HL | 辽宁 LN | 河北 HE | 北京 BJ | 吉林 JL | 山西 SX | 陕西 SN | 河南 HA | 宁夏 NX | 内蒙古 NM | 青海 QH | 甘肃 GS | 上海 SH | 福建 FJ | 江西 JX | 江苏 JS | 浙江 ZJ | 山东 SD | 湖北 HB | 四川 SC | 广西 GX | 湖南 HN | 广东 GD | 贵州 GZ | 全国平均 AVG |
|---|---|---|---|---|---|---|---|---|---|---|---|---|---|---|---|---|---|---|---|---|---|---|---|---|---|
| 肉类 Meats | ND | 0.06 | 4.29 | 0.05 | ND | ND | 0.31 | 0.18 | ND | 0.09 | 0.24 | 0.19 | ND | ND | 0.02 | 0.03 | ND | ND | ND | ND | ND | ND | ND | 0.07 | 0.23 |
| 蛋类 Eggs | ND | ND | 0.38 | ND | ND | 0.65 | ND | 0.05 | 0.88 | ND | ND | ND | ND | 0.18 | ND | 0.96 | ND | ND | ND | ND | ND | ND | ND | ND | 0.13 |
| 水产类 Aquatic foods | ND | ND | ND | ND | ND | ND | ND | 0.04 | ND | ND | ND | 0.03 | 0.17 | ND | ND | ND | ND | ND | ND | ND | ND | ND | ND | ND | 0.01 |
| 乳类 Dairy products | ND | ND | ND | ND | 0.04 | ND | ND | ND | ND | ND | ND | ND | ND | ND | ND | ND | ND | ND | ND | ND | ND | ND | ND | ND | 0.00 |

注：未检出（ND）按 0 计

Note: values not detected (ND) were treated as being equal to 0

附表 5-58 第六次中国总膳食研究的阿苯达唑膳食摄入量 [单位：ng/(kg bw·d)]

Annexed Table 5-58 Dietary intakes of albendazole from the 6th China TDS [Unit: ng/(kg bw·d)]

| 膳食类别 Category | 黑龙江 HL | 辽宁 LN | 河北 HE | 北京 BJ | 吉林 JL | 山西 SX | 陕西 SN | 河南 HA | 宁夏 NX | 内蒙古 NM | 青海 QH | 甘肃 GS | 上海 SH | 福建 FJ | 江西 JX | 江苏 JS | 浙江 ZJ | 山东 SD | 湖北 HB | 四川 SC | 广西 GX | 湖南 HN | 广东 GD | 贵州 GZ | 全国平均 AVG |
|---|---|---|---|---|---|---|---|---|---|---|---|---|---|---|---|---|---|---|---|---|---|---|---|---|---|
| 肉类 Meats | 0.000 | 0.064 | 3.229 | 0.052 | 0.000 | 0.000 | 0.179 | 0.160 | 0.000 | 0.101 | 0.273 | 0.094 | 0.000 | 0.000 | 0.024 | 0.044 | 0.000 | 0.000 | 0.000 | 0.000 | 0.000 | 0.000 | 0.000 | 0.125 | 0.181 |
| 蛋类 Eggs | 0.000 | 0.000 | 0.193 | 0.000 | 0.000 | 0.217 | 0.000 | 0.022 | 0.181 | 0.000 | 0.000 | 0.000 | 0.000 | 0.055 | 0.000 | 0.430 | 0.000 | 0.000 | 0.000 | 0.000 | 0.000 | 0.000 | 0.000 | 0.000 | 0.046 |
| 水产类 Aquatic foods | 0.000 | 0.000 | 0.000 | 0.000 | 0.000 | 0.000 | 0.000 | 0.003 | 0.000 | 0.000 | 0.000 | 0.002 | 0.180 | 0.000 | 0.000 | 0.000 | 0.000 | 0.000 | 0.000 | 0.000 | 0.000 | 0.000 | 0.000 | 0.000 | 0.008 |
| 乳类 Dairy products | 0.000 | 0.000 | 0.000 | 0.000 | 0.022 | 0.000 | 0.000 | 0.000 | 0.000 | 0.000 | 0.000 | 0.000 | 0.000 | 0.000 | 0.000 | 0.000 | 0.000 | 0.000 | 0.000 | 0.000 | 0.000 | 0.000 | 0.000 | 0.000 | 0.001 |

续表

| 膳食类别<br>Category | 黑龙江<br>HL | 辽宁<br>LN | 河北<br>HE | 北京<br>BJ | 吉林<br>JL | 山西<br>SX | 陕西<br>SN | 河南<br>HA | 宁夏<br>NX | 内蒙古<br>NM | 青海<br>QH | 甘肃<br>GS | 上海<br>SH | 福建<br>FJ | 江西<br>JX | 江苏<br>JS | 浙江<br>ZJ | 山东<br>SD | 湖北<br>HB | 四川<br>SC | 广西<br>GX | 湖南<br>HN | 广东<br>GD | 贵州<br>GZ | 全国平均<br>AVG |
|---|---|---|---|---|---|---|---|---|---|---|---|---|---|---|---|---|---|---|---|---|---|---|---|---|---|
| 合计<br>SUM | 0.000 | 0.064 | 3.422 | 0.052 | 0.022 | 0.217 | 0.179 | 0.185 | 0.181 | 0.101 | 0.273 | 0.096 | 0.180 | 0.055 | 0.024 | 0.474 | 0.000 | 0.000 | 0.000 | 0.000 | 0.000 | 0.000 | 0.000 | 0.125 | 0.235 |

附表 5-59　第六次中国总膳食研究阿苯达唑的膳食来源（单位：%）

Annexed Table 5-59　Dietary sources of albendazole from the 6th China TDS (Unit: %)

| 膳食类别<br>Category | 黑龙江<br>HL | 辽宁<br>LN | 河北<br>HE | 北京<br>BJ | 吉林<br>JL | 山西<br>SX | 陕西<br>SN | 河南<br>HA | 宁夏<br>NX | 内蒙古<br>NM | 青海<br>QH | 甘肃<br>GS | 上海<br>SH | 福建<br>FJ | 江西<br>JX | 江苏<br>JS | 浙江<br>ZJ | 山东<br>SD | 湖北<br>HB | 四川<br>SC | 广西<br>GX | 湖南<br>HN | 广东<br>GD | 贵州<br>GZ | 全国平均<br>AVG |
|---|---|---|---|---|---|---|---|---|---|---|---|---|---|---|---|---|---|---|---|---|---|---|---|---|---|
| 肉类<br>Meats | 0.0 | 100.0 | 94.4 | 100.0 | 0.0 | 0.0 | 100.0 | 86.4 | 0.0 | 100.0 | 100.0 | 98.4 | 0.0 | 0.0 | 100.0 | 9.3 | 0.0 | 0.0 | 0.0 | 0.0 | 0.0 | 0.0 | 0.0 | 100.0 | 76.9 |
| 蛋类<br>Eggs | 0.0 | 0.0 | 5.6 | 0.0 | 0.0 | 100.0 | 0.0 | 12.0 | 100.0 | 0.0 | 0.0 | 0.0 | 0.0 | 100.0 | 0.0 | 90.7 | 0.0 | 0.0 | 0.0 | 0.0 | 0.0 | 0.0 | 0.0 | 0.0 | 19.4 |
| 水产类<br>Aquatic foods | 0.0 | 0.0 | 0.0 | 0.0 | 0.0 | 0.0 | 0.0 | 1.5 | 0.0 | 0.0 | 0.0 | 1.6 | 100.0 | 0.0 | 0.0 | 0.0 | 0.0 | 0.0 | 0.0 | 0.0 | 0.0 | 0.0 | 0.0 | 0.0 | 3.3 |
| 乳类<br>Dairy products | 0.0 | 0.0 | 0.0 | 0.0 | 100.0 | 0.0 | 0.0 | 0.0 | 0.0 | 0.0 | 0.0 | 0.0 | 0.0 | 0.0 | 0.0 | 0.0 | 0.0 | 0.0 | 0.0 | 0.0 | 0.0 | 0.0 | 0.0 | 0.0 | 0.4 |

附表 5-60　第六次中国总膳食研究膳食样品中芬苯达唑的含量（单位：μg/kg）

Annexed Table 5-60　Levels of fenbendazole in food samples from the 6th China TDS (Unit: μg/kg)

| 膳食类别<br>Category | 黑龙江<br>HL | 辽宁<br>LN | 河北<br>HE | 北京<br>BJ | 吉林<br>JL | 山西<br>SX | 陕西<br>SN | 河南<br>HA | 宁夏<br>NX | 内蒙古<br>NM | 青海<br>QH | 甘肃<br>GS | 上海<br>SH | 福建<br>FJ | 江西<br>JX | 江苏<br>JS | 浙江<br>ZJ | 山东<br>SD | 湖北<br>HB | 四川<br>SC | 广西<br>GX | 湖南<br>HN | 广东<br>GD | 贵州<br>GZ | 全国平均<br>AVG |
|---|---|---|---|---|---|---|---|---|---|---|---|---|---|---|---|---|---|---|---|---|---|---|---|---|---|
| 肉类<br>Meats | 0.05 | 0.05 | 0.08 | 0.10 | 0.07 | 0.06 | 0.08 | 0.08 | 0.06 | 0.05 | 0.07 | 0.05 | 0.52 | 0.10 | 0.09 | 0.07 | 0.09 | 0.07 | 0.02 | 0.06 | 0.08 | 0.08 | 0.06 | 0.08 | 0.09 |

续表

| 膳食类别<br>Category | 黑龙江<br>HL | 辽宁<br>LN | 河北<br>HE | 北京<br>BJ | 吉林<br>JL | 山西<br>SX | 陕西<br>SN | 河南<br>HA | 宁夏<br>NX | 内蒙古<br>NM | 青海<br>QH | 甘肃<br>GS | 上海<br>SH | 福建<br>FJ | 江西<br>JX | 江苏<br>JS | 浙江<br>ZJ | 山东<br>SD | 湖北<br>HB | 四川<br>SC | 广西<br>GX | 湖南<br>HN | 广东<br>GD | 贵州<br>GZ | 全国平均<br>AVG |
|---|---|---|---|---|---|---|---|---|---|---|---|---|---|---|---|---|---|---|---|---|---|---|---|---|---|
| 蛋类 Eggs | 0.07 | 0.09 | 0.09 | 0.08 | 0.08 | 0.10 | 0.09 | 0.08 | 0.09 | 0.09 | 0.10 | 0.10 | 0.08 | 0.10 | 0.13 | 0.10 | 0.08 | 0.09 | 0.07 | 0.10 | 0.07 | 0.07 | 0.08 | 0.07 | 0.09 |
| 水产类 Aquatic foods | 0.00 | 0.18 | ND | ND | ND | ND | ND | ND | ND | ND | ND | ND | ND | ND | ND | ND | ND | ND | ND | ND | ND | ND | ND | ND | 0.01 |
| 乳类 Dairy products | 0.07 | 0.09 | 0.08 | 0.08 | 0.03 | 0.08 | 0.07 | 0.10 | 0.03 | 0.09 | 0.09 | 0.08 | 0.09 | 0.08 | 0.07 | 0.09 | 0.09 | 0.08 | 0.13 | 0.09 | 0.09 | 0.10 | 0.08 | 0.08 | 0.08 |

注：未检出（ND）按 0 计

Note: values not detected (ND) were treated as being equal to 0

附表 5-61 第六次中国总膳食研究的芬苯达唑膳食摄入量 [单位：ng/(kg bw·d)]

Annexed Table 5-61 Dietary intakes of fenbendazole from the 6th China TDS [Unit: ng/(kg bw·d)]

| 膳食类别<br>Category | 黑龙江<br>HL | 辽宁<br>LN | 河北<br>HE | 北京<br>BJ | 吉林<br>JL | 山西<br>SX | 陕西<br>SN | 河南<br>HA | 宁夏<br>NX | 内蒙古<br>NM | 青海<br>QH | 甘肃<br>GS | 上海<br>SH | 福建<br>FJ | 江西<br>JX | 江苏<br>JS | 浙江<br>ZJ | 山东<br>SD | 湖北<br>HB | 四川<br>SC | 广西<br>GX | 湖南<br>HN | 广东<br>GD | 贵州<br>GZ | 全国平均<br>AVG |
|---|---|---|---|---|---|---|---|---|---|---|---|---|---|---|---|---|---|---|---|---|---|---|---|---|---|
| 肉类 Meats | 0.051 | 0.054 | 0.059 | 0.104 | 0.073 | 0.128 | 0.046 | 0.069 | 0.047 | 0.055 | 0.080 | 0.024 | 0.918 | 0.136 | 0.132 | 0.104 | 0.164 | 0.112 | 0.016 | 0.116 | 0.193 | 0.184 | 0.102 | 0.130 | 0.129 |
| 蛋类 Eggs | 0.046 | 0.059 | 0.044 | 0.048 | 0.049 | 0.033 | 0.030 | 0.037 | 0.019 | 0.041 | 0.020 | 0.035 | 0.050 | 0.029 | 0.041 | 0.043 | 0.031 | 0.066 | 0.026 | 0.023 | 0.016 | 0.025 | 0.029 | 0.017 | 0.036 |
| 水产类 Aquatic foods | 0.000 | 0.047 | 0.000 | 0.000 | 0.000 | 0.000 | 0.000 | 0.000 | 0.000 | 0.000 | 0.000 | 0.000 | 0.000 | 0.000 | 0.000 | 0.000 | 0.000 | 0.000 | 0.000 | 0.000 | 0.000 | 0.000 | 0.000 | 0.000 | 0.002 |
| 乳类 Dairy products | 0.016 | 0.060 | 0.031 | 0.112 | 0.018 | 0.053 | 0.022 | 0.030 | 0.008 | 0.046 | 0.077 | 0.018 | 0.100 | 0.046 | 0.025 | 0.040 | 0.046 | 0.031 | 0.014 | 0.018 | 0.026 | 0.028 | 0.049 | 0.036 | 0.040 |
| 合计 SUM | 0.113 | 0.220 | 0.134 | 0.264 | 0.141 | 0.213 | 0.097 | 0.136 | 0.074 | 0.143 | 0.177 | 0.077 | 1.067 | 0.211 | 0.198 | 0.187 | 0.241 | 0.209 | 0.056 | 0.157 | 0.235 | 0.237 | 0.180 | 0.184 | 0.206 |

附表 5-62 第六次中国总膳食研究芬苯达唑的膳食来源（单位：%）
Annexed Table 5-62　Dietary sources of fenbendazole from the 6th China TDS (Unit: %)

| 膳食类别 Category | 黑龙江 HL | 辽宁 LN | 河北 HE | 北京 BJ | 吉林 JL | 山西 SX | 陕西 SN | 河南 HA | 宁夏 NX | 内蒙古 NM | 青海 QH | 甘肃 GS | 上海 SH | 福建 FJ | 江西 JX | 江苏 JS | 浙江 ZJ | 山东 SD | 湖北 HB | 四川 SC | 广西 GX | 湖南 HN | 广东 GD | 贵州 GZ | 全国平均 AVG |
|---|---|---|---|---|---|---|---|---|---|---|---|---|---|---|---|---|---|---|---|---|---|---|---|---|---|
| 肉类 Meats | 45.2 | 24.4 | 44.3 | 39.6 | 52.2 | 60.1 | 47.0 | 50.8 | 63.1 | 38.5 | 45.1 | 30.8 | 86.0 | 64.4 | 66.7 | 55.6 | 68.1 | 53.8 | 28.8 | 73.8 | 82.2 | 77.6 | 56.9 | 70.8 | 62.6 |
| 蛋类 Eggs | 40.9 | 26.7 | 32.8 | 18.1 | 35.1 | 15.3 | 30.6 | 26.9 | 25.6 | 29.0 | 11.2 | 45.6 | 4.7 | 13.7 | 20.6 | 23.0 | 12.9 | 31.6 | 46.7 | 14.6 | 6.8 | 10.5 | 15.9 | 9.4 | 17.3 |
| 水产类 Aquatic foods | 0.0 | 21.4 | 0.0 | 0.0 | 0.0 | 0.0 | 0.0 | 0.0 | 0.0 | 0.0 | 0.0 | 0.0 | 0.0 | 0.0 | 0.0 | 0.0 | 0.0 | 0.0 | 0.0 | 0.0 | 0.0 | 0.0 | 0.0 | 0.0 | 0.9 |
| 乳类 Dairy products | 13.9 | 27.5 | 22.8 | 42.3 | 12.7 | 24.6 | 22.4 | 22.3 | 11.3 | 32.5 | 43.6 | 23.6 | 9.4 | 21.9 | 12.7 | 21.4 | 19.0 | 14.6 | 24.4 | 11.6 | 11.1 | 11.9 | 27.2 | 19.8 | 19.2 |

附表 5-63 第六次中国总膳食研究膳食样品中氟苯达唑的含量（单位：μg/kg）
Annexed Table 5-63　Levels of flubendazole in food samples from the 6th China TDS (Unit: μg/kg)

| 膳食类别 Category | 黑龙江 HL | 辽宁 LN | 河北 HE | 北京 BJ | 吉林 JL | 山西 SX | 陕西 SN | 河南 HA | 宁夏 NX | 内蒙古 NM | 青海 QH | 甘肃 GS | 上海 SH | 福建 FJ | 江西 JX | 江苏 JS | 浙江 ZJ | 山东 SD | 湖北 HB | 四川 SC | 广西 GX | 湖南 HN | 广东 GD | 贵州 GZ | 全国平均 AVG |
|---|---|---|---|---|---|---|---|---|---|---|---|---|---|---|---|---|---|---|---|---|---|---|---|---|---|
| 肉类 Meats | 0.11 | 0.01 | 0.03 | 0.03 | 0.08 | 0.01 | 0.01 | 0.07 | 0.02 | ND | 0.01 | 0.01 | 0.02 | 0.01 | 0.06 | 0.02 | 0.01 | 0.04 | 0.01 | 0.01 | 0.11 | ND | 0.12 | 0.03 | 0.03 |
| 蛋类 Eggs | 0.06 | 0.04 | 0.04 | 0.03 | 0.03 | ND | 0.03 | 0.03 | 0.03 | 0.03 | 0.05 | ND | 0.03 | 0.03 | 0.06 | 0.03 | 0.04 | 0.04 | 0.02 | 0.02 | 0.02 | 0.02 | 0.03 | 0.03 | 0.03 |
| 水产类 Aquatic foods | ND | ND | ND | ND | ND | ND | 0.01 | ND | ND | ND | ND | ND | ND | ND | ND | ND | ND | 0.01 | ND | ND | ND | 0.01 | 0.02 | ND | 0.00 |
| 乳类 Dairy products | 0.04 | 0.03 | 0.04 | 0.04 | 0.01 | 0.03 | 0.04 | 0.03 | 0.02 | 0.04 | 0.04 | 0.04 | 0.04 | 0.04 | 0.03 | 0.04 | 0.04 | 0.04 | 0.07 | 0.04 | 0.04 | 0.04 | 0.03 | 0.04 | 0.04 |

注：未检出（ND）按 0 计
Note: values not detected (ND) were treated as being equal to 0

附表 5-64　第六次中国总膳食研究的氟苯达唑膳食摄入量［单位：ng/(kg bw·d)］
Annexed Table 5-64　Dietary intakes of flubendazole from the 6th China TDS [Unit: ng/(kg bw·d)]

| 膳食类别 Category | 黑龙江 HL | 辽宁 LN | 河北 HE | 北京 BJ | 吉林 JL | 山西 SX | 陕西 SN | 河南 HA | 宁夏 NX | 内蒙古 NM | 青海 QH | 甘肃 GS | 上海 SH | 福建 FJ | 江西 JX | 江苏 JS | 浙江 ZJ | 山东 SD | 湖北 HB | 四川 SC | 广西 GX | 湖南 HN | 广东 GD | 贵州 GZ | 全国平均 AVG |
|---|---|---|---|---|---|---|---|---|---|---|---|---|---|---|---|---|---|---|---|---|---|---|---|---|---|
| 肉类 Meats | 0.105 | 0.006 | 0.021 | 0.037 | 0.080 | 0.017 | 0.008 | 0.059 | 0.016 | 0.000 | 0.016 | 0.004 | 0.029 | 0.017 | 0.095 | 0.031 | 0.023 | 0.055 | 0.005 | 0.014 | 0.256 | 0.000 | 0.194 | 0.044 | 0.047 |
| 蛋类 Eggs | 0.037 | 0.024 | 0.019 | 0.017 | 0.019 | 0.008 | 0.010 | 0.015 | 0.006 | 0.015 | 0.010 | 0.015 | 0.019 | 0.009 | 0.020 | 0.014 | 0.014 | 0.029 | 0.007 | 0.004 | 0.005 | 0.009 | 0.010 | 0.007 | 0.014 |
| 水产类 Aquatic foods | 0.000 | 0.000 | 0.000 | 0.000 | 0.000 | 0.000 | 0.000 | 0.000 | 0.000 | 0.000 | 0.000 | 0.000 | 0.000 | 0.000 | 0.000 | 0.002 | 0.000 | 0.002 | 0.000 | 0.000 | 0.006 | 0.011 | 0.016 | 0.000 | 0.002 |
| 乳类 Dairy products | 0.008 | 0.025 | 0.015 | 0.051 | 0.007 | 0.023 | 0.012 | 0.011 | 0.004 | 0.019 | 0.031 | 0.008 | 0.042 | 0.022 | 0.011 | 0.017 | 0.022 | 0.014 | 0.008 | 0.008 | 0.011 | 0.013 | 0.019 | 0.016 | 0.017 |
| 合计 SUM | 0.150 | 0.054 | 0.056 | 0.105 | 0.107 | 0.048 | 0.029 | 0.085 | 0.026 | 0.035 | 0.058 | 0.027 | 0.090 | 0.049 | 0.127 | 0.064 | 0.058 | 0.100 | 0.019 | 0.026 | 0.278 | 0.032 | 0.239 | 0.067 | 0.080 |

附表 5-65　第六次中国总膳食研究氟苯达唑的膳食来源（单位：%）
Annexed Table 5-65　Dietary sources of flubendazole from the 6th China TDS (Unit: %)

| 膳食类别 Category | 黑龙江 HL | 辽宁 LN | 河北 HE | 北京 BJ | 吉林 JL | 山西 SX | 陕西 SN | 河南 HA | 宁夏 NX | 内蒙古 NM | 青海 QH | 甘肃 GS | 上海 SH | 福建 FJ | 江西 JX | 江苏 JS | 浙江 ZJ | 山东 SD | 湖北 HB | 四川 SC | 广西 GX | 湖南 HN | 广东 GD | 贵州 GZ | 全国平均 AVG |
|---|---|---|---|---|---|---|---|---|---|---|---|---|---|---|---|---|---|---|---|---|---|---|---|---|---|
| 肉类 Meats | 70.0 | 10.6 | 37.5 | 35.2 | 74.9 | 34.9 | 26.4 | 69.0 | 60.5 | 0.0 | 28.7 | 14.1 | 31.9 | 36.0 | 75.2 | 47.7 | 39.9 | 54.7 | 24.0 | 54.4 | 92.0 | 0.0 | 81.2 | 64.7 | 58.6 |
| 蛋类 Eggs | 24.5 | 44.3 | 35.0 | 15.8 | 18.2 | 17.6 | 32.9 | 18.0 | 22.2 | 44.7 | 16.9 | 56.1 | 21.0 | 18.3 | 16.2 | 21.7 | 23.2 | 29.3 | 35.0 | 13.9 | 2.0 | 27.2 | 4.0 | 10.9 | 17.8 |
| 水产类 Aquatic foods | 0.0 | 0.0 | 0.0 | 0.0 | 0.0 | 0.0 | 1.3 | 0.4 | 0.0 | 0.0 | 0.0 | 0.7 | 0.0 | 0.0 | 0.0 | 3.5 | 0.0 | 2.3 | 0.0 | 0.0 | 2.2 | 33.2 | 6.9 | 0.0 | 2.0 |
| 乳类 Dairy products | 5.6 | 45.1 | 27.5 | 48.9 | 6.9 | 47.4 | 39.5 | 12.6 | 17.3 | 55.3 | 54.5 | 29.1 | 47.0 | 45.6 | 8.6 | 27.1 | 36.9 | 13.7 | 41.0 | 31.7 | 3.9 | 39.6 | 7.9 | 24.4 | 21.7 |

附表 5-66　第六次中国总膳食研究膳食样品中甲苯达唑的含量（单位：μg/kg）
Annexed Table 5-66　Levels of mebendazole in food samples from the 6th China TDS (Unit: μg/kg)

| 膳食类别<br>Category | 黑龙江<br>HL | 辽宁<br>LN | 河北<br>HE | 北京<br>BJ | 吉林<br>JL | 山西<br>SX | 陕西<br>SN | 河南<br>HA | 宁夏<br>NX | 内蒙古<br>NM | 青海<br>QH | 甘肃<br>GS | 上海<br>SH | 福建<br>FJ | 江西<br>JX | 江苏<br>JS | 浙江<br>ZJ | 山东<br>SD | 湖北<br>HB | 四川<br>SC | 广西<br>GX | 湖南<br>HN | 广东<br>GD | 贵州<br>GZ | 全国平均<br>AVG |
|---|---|---|---|---|---|---|---|---|---|---|---|---|---|---|---|---|---|---|---|---|---|---|---|---|---|
| 肉类 Meats | 0.01 | 0.01 | 0.01 | 0.02 | 0.01 | 0.04 | ND | 0.02 | 0.02 | 0.03 | ND | 0.01 | ND | 0.01 | 0.02 | 0.01 | 0.01 | 0.02 | ND | ND | ND | 0.02 | 0.02 | 0.01 | 0.01 |
| 蛋类 Eggs | 0.02 | 0.02 | 0.02 | 0.02 | 0.05 | 0.01 | 0.02 | 0.03 | 0.03 | 0.03 | 0.03 | 0.03 | 0.01 | 0.02 | 0.03 | ND | ND | ND | 0.01 | 0.03 | 0.01 | 0.01 | 0.02 | 0.02 | 0.02 |
| 水产类 Aquatic foods | ND | ND | ND | ND | ND | ND | ND | ND | ND | ND | ND | ND | ND | ND | ND | ND | ND | ND | ND | ND | ND | ND | ND | ND | 0.00 |
| 乳类 Dairy products | 0.01 | 0.03 | 0.03 | 0.02 | 0.02 | 0.02 | 0.01 | 0.03 | 0.01 | 0.03 | 0.04 | 0.01 | 0.03 | 0.03 | 0.04 | 0.03 | 0.03 | 0.03 | 0.05 | 0.04 | 0.02 | 0.02 | 0.04 | 0.03 | 0.03 |

注：未检出（ND）按 0 计
Note: values not detected (ND) were treated as being equal to 0

附表 5-67　第六次中国总膳食研究的甲苯达唑膳食摄入量 [单位：ng/(kg bw·d)]
Annexed Table 5-67　Dietary intakes of mebendazole from the 6th China TDS [Unit: ng/(kg bw·d)]

| 膳食类别<br>Category | 黑龙江<br>HL | 辽宁<br>LN | 河北<br>HE | 北京<br>BJ | 吉林<br>JL | 山西<br>SX | 陕西<br>SN | 河南<br>HA | 宁夏<br>NX | 内蒙古<br>NM | 青海<br>QH | 甘肃<br>GS | 上海<br>SH | 福建<br>FJ | 江西<br>JX | 江苏<br>JS | 浙江<br>ZJ | 山东<br>SD | 湖北<br>HB | 四川<br>SC | 广西<br>GX | 湖南<br>HN | 广东<br>GD | 贵州<br>GZ | 全国平均<br>AVG |
|---|---|---|---|---|---|---|---|---|---|---|---|---|---|---|---|---|---|---|---|---|---|---|---|---|---|
| 肉类 Meats | 0.007 | 0.008 | 0.004 | 0.021 | 0.013 | 0.078 | 0.000 | 0.015 | 0.018 | 0.031 | 0.000 | 0.004 | 0.000 | 0.014 | 0.032 | 0.020 | 0.016 | 0.026 | 0.000 | 0.000 | 0.000 | 0.043 | 0.037 | 0.014 | 0.017 |
| 蛋类 Eggs | 0.012 | 0.016 | 0.011 | 0.015 | 0.031 | 0.004 | 0.006 | 0.013 | 0.006 | 0.016 | 0.006 | 0.011 | 0.009 | 0.006 | 0.009 | 0.008 | 0.005 | 0.006 | 0.003 | 0.006 | 0.003 | 0.004 | 0.007 | 0.006 | 0.009 |
| 水产类 Aquatic foods | 0.000 | 0.000 | 0.000 | 0.000 | 0.000 | 0.000 | 0.000 | 0.000 | 0.000 | 0.000 | 0.000 | 0.000 | 0.000 | 0.000 | 0.000 | 0.000 | 0.000 | 0.000 | 0.000 | 0.000 | 0.000 | 0.000 | 0.000 | 0.000 | 0.000 |
| 乳类 Dairy products | 0.003 | 0.023 | 0.011 | 0.026 | 0.010 | 0.013 | 0.004 | 0.010 | 0.003 | 0.018 | 0.032 | 0.003 | 0.038 | 0.016 | 0.013 | 0.014 | 0.017 | 0.011 | 0.005 | 0.007 | 0.007 | 0.005 | 0.021 | 0.013 | 0.013 |

续表

| 膳食类别<br>Category | 黑龙江<br>HL | 辽宁<br>LN | 河北<br>HE | 北京<br>BJ | 吉林<br>JL | 山西<br>SX | 陕西<br>SN | 河南<br>HA | 宁夏<br>NX | 内蒙古<br>NM | 青海<br>QH | 甘肃<br>GS | 上海<br>SH | 福建<br>FJ | 江西<br>JX | 江苏<br>JS | 浙江<br>ZJ | 山东<br>SD | 湖北<br>HB | 四川<br>SC | 广西<br>GX | 湖南<br>HN | 广东<br>GD | 贵州<br>GZ | 全国<br>平均<br>AVG |
|---|---|---|---|---|---|---|---|---|---|---|---|---|---|---|---|---|---|---|---|---|---|---|---|---|---|
| 合计<br>SUM | 0.023 | 0.047 | 0.026 | 0.062 | 0.054 | 0.094 | 0.010 | 0.038 | 0.027 | 0.065 | 0.038 | 0.018 | 0.047 | 0.036 | 0.054 | 0.041 | 0.038 | 0.044 | 0.009 | 0.013 | 0.010 | 0.051 | 0.066 | 0.033 | 0.039 |

附表 5-68 第六次中国总膳食研究甲苯达唑的膳食来源（单位：%）
Annexed Table 5-68 Dietary sources of mebendazole from the 6th China TDS (Unit: %)

| 膳食类别<br>Category | 黑龙江<br>HL | 辽宁<br>LN | 河北<br>HE | 北京<br>BJ | 吉林<br>JL | 山西<br>SX | 陕西<br>SN | 河南<br>HA | 宁夏<br>NX | 内蒙古<br>NM | 青海<br>QH | 甘肃<br>GS | 上海<br>SH | 福建<br>FJ | 江西<br>JX | 江苏<br>JS | 浙江<br>ZJ | 山东<br>SD | 湖北<br>HB | 四川<br>SC | 广西<br>GX | 湖南<br>HN | 广东<br>GD | 贵州<br>GZ | 全国<br>平均<br>AVG |
|---|---|---|---|---|---|---|---|---|---|---|---|---|---|---|---|---|---|---|---|---|---|---|---|---|---|
| 肉类<br>Meats | 32.5 | 17.9 | 16.6 | 33.8 | 24.1 | 82.2 | 0.0 | 39.3 | 67.4 | 47.4 | 0.0 | 23.6 | 0.0 | 40.2 | 59.5 | 48.4 | 42.6 | 60.7 | 0.0 | 0.0 | 0.0 | 83.4 | 56.5 | 43.5 | 42.7 |
| 蛋类<br>Eggs | 54.4 | 33.7 | 40.8 | 23.9 | 57.7 | 4.0 | 60.4 | 34.2 | 21.6 | 25.3 | 14.8 | 59.2 | 19.1 | 16.0 | 17.3 | 18.2 | 13.0 | 14.0 | 35.9 | 45.6 | 31.4 | 7.6 | 11.4 | 18.3 | 23.2 |
| 水产类<br>Aquatic foods | 0.0 | 0.0 | 0.0 | 0.0 | 0.0 | 0.0 | 0.0 | 0.0 | 0.0 | 0.0 | 0.0 | 0.0 | 0.0 | 0.0 | 0.0 | 0.0 | 0.0 | 0.0 | 0.0 | 0.0 | 0.0 | 0.0 | 0.0 | 0.0 | 0.0 |
| 乳类<br>Dairy products | 13.1 | 48.4 | 42.5 | 42.2 | 18.2 | 13.9 | 39.6 | 26.5 | 11.0 | 27.3 | 85.2 | 17.2 | 80.9 | 43.8 | 23.2 | 33.3 | 44.4 | 25.3 | 64.1 | 54.4 | 68.6 | 9.0 | 32.2 | 38.2 | 34.1 |

附表 5-69 第六次中国总膳食研究膳食样品中氟苯尼考的含量（单位：μg/kg）
Annexed Table 5-69 Levels of florfenicol in food samples from the 6th China TDS (Unit: μg/kg)

| 膳食类别<br>Category | 黑龙江<br>HL | 辽宁<br>LN | 河北<br>HE | 北京<br>BJ | 吉林<br>JL | 山西<br>SX | 陕西<br>SN | 河南<br>HA | 宁夏<br>NX | 内蒙古<br>NM | 青海<br>QH | 甘肃<br>GS | 上海<br>SH | 福建<br>FJ | 江西<br>JX | 江苏<br>JS | 浙江<br>ZJ | 山东<br>SD | 湖北<br>HB | 四川<br>SC | 广西<br>GX | 湖南<br>HN | 广东<br>GD | 贵州<br>GZ | 全国<br>平均<br>AVG |
|---|---|---|---|---|---|---|---|---|---|---|---|---|---|---|---|---|---|---|---|---|---|---|---|---|---|
| 肉类<br>Meats | 48.28 | 0.06 | 0.06 | 0.32 | 0.12 | 0.26 | 0.16 | 0.06 | 0.13 | ND | 0.03 | 0.05 | ND | 0.16 | ND | 4.00 | 0.34 | ND | 49.85 | ND | ND | 0.33 | 1.09 | ND | 4.39 |

续表

| 膳食类别<br>Category | 黑龙江<br>HL | 辽宁<br>LN | 河北<br>HE | 北京<br>BJ | 吉林<br>JL | 山西<br>SX | 陕西<br>SN | 河南<br>HA | 宁夏<br>NX | 内蒙古<br>NM | 青海<br>QH | 甘肃<br>GS | 上海<br>SH | 福建<br>FJ | 江西<br>JX | 江苏<br>JS | 浙江<br>ZJ | 山东<br>SD | 湖北<br>HB | 四川<br>SC | 广西<br>GX | 湖南<br>HN | 广东<br>GD | 贵州<br>GZ | 全国平均<br>AVG |
|---|---|---|---|---|---|---|---|---|---|---|---|---|---|---|---|---|---|---|---|---|---|---|---|---|---|
| 蛋类 Eggs | 0.05 | ND | 0.24 | ND | 0.79 | 0.13 | 0.08 | 0.51 | ND | 0.05 | 0.04 | ND | 1.15 | 7.93 | 0.05 | ND | 0.29 | ND | 0.05 | 0.07 | ND | 1.85 | 2.46 | ND | 0.66 |
| 水产类 Aquatic foods | ND | ND | ND | ND | ND | ND | ND | ND | ND | ND | ND | ND | 0.19 | ND | ND | ND | ND | ND | ND | ND | ND | ND | 0.23 | ND | 0.02 |
| 乳类 Dairy products | ND | 0.06 | ND | ND | ND | ND | ND | ND | ND | ND | ND | ND | ND | ND | 0.16 | ND | ND | ND | ND | ND | ND | ND | ND | ND | 0.01 |

注：未检出（ND）按 0 计

Note: values not detected (ND) were treated as being equal to 0

附表 5-70　第六次中国总膳食研究的氟苯尼考膳食摄入量 [单位：ng/(kg bw·d)]

Annexed Table 5-70　Dietary intakes of florfenicol from the 6th China TDS [Unit: ng/(kg bw·d)]

| 膳食类别<br>Category | 黑龙江<br>HL | 辽宁<br>LN | 河北<br>HE | 北京<br>BJ | 吉林<br>JL | 山西<br>SX | 陕西<br>SN | 河南<br>HA | 宁夏<br>NX | 内蒙古<br>NM | 青海<br>QH | 甘肃<br>GS | 上海<br>SH | 福建<br>FJ | 江西<br>JX | 江苏<br>JS | 浙江<br>ZJ | 山东<br>SD | 湖北<br>HB | 四川<br>SC | 广西<br>GX | 湖南<br>HN | 广东<br>GD | 贵州<br>GZ | 全国平均<br>AVG |
|---|---|---|---|---|---|---|---|---|---|---|---|---|---|---|---|---|---|---|---|---|---|---|---|---|---|
| 肉类 Meats | 45.895 | 0.068 | 0.042 | 0.344 | 0.125 | 0.567 | 0.090 | 0.050 | 0.094 | 0.000 | 0.038 | 0.025 | 0.000 | 0.221 | 0.000 | 5.829 | 0.645 | 0.000 | 42.963 | 0.000 | 0.000 | 0.772 | 1.801 | 0.000 | 4.149 |
| 蛋类 Eggs | 0.029 | 0.000 | 0.121 | 0.000 | 0.506 | 0.042 | 0.027 | 0.243 | 0.000 | 0.025 | 0.009 | 0.000 | 0.710 | 2.390 | 0.015 | 0.000 | 0.110 | 0.000 | 0.018 | 0.016 | 0.000 | 0.670 | 0.932 | 0.000 | 0.244 |
| 水产类 Aquatic foods | 0.000 | 0.000 | 0.000 | 0.000 | 0.000 | 0.000 | 0.000 | 0.000 | 0.000 | 0.000 | 0.000 | 0.000 | 0.202 | 0.000 | 0.000 | 0.000 | 0.000 | 0.000 | 0.000 | 0.000 | 0.000 | 0.000 | 0.184 | 0.000 | 0.016 |
| 乳类 Dairy products | 0.000 | 0.040 | 0.000 | 0.000 | 0.000 | 0.000 | 0.000 | 0.000 | 0.000 | 0.000 | 0.000 | 0.000 | 0.000 | 0.000 | 0.057 | 0.000 | 0.000 | 0.000 | 0.000 | 0.000 | 0.000 | 0.000 | 0.000 | 0.000 | 0.004 |

续表

| 膳食类别 Category | 黑龙江 HL | 辽宁 LN | 河北 HE | 北京 BJ | 吉林 JL | 山西 SX | 陕西 SN | 河南 HA | 宁夏 NX | 内蒙古 NM | 青海 QH | 甘肃 GS | 上海 SH | 福建 FJ | 江西 JX | 江苏 JS | 浙江 ZJ | 山东 SD | 湖北 HB | 四川 SC | 广西 GX | 湖南 HN | 广东 GD | 贵州 GZ | 全国平均 AVG |
|---|---|---|---|---|---|---|---|---|---|---|---|---|---|---|---|---|---|---|---|---|---|---|---|---|---|
| 合计 SUM | 45.924 | 0.107 | 0.163 | 0.344 | 0.631 | 0.609 | 0.117 | 0.293 | 0.094 | 0.025 | 0.047 | 0.025 | 0.911 | 2.611 | 0.071 | 5.829 | 0.755 | 0.000 | 42.982 | 0.016 | 0.000 | 1.443 | 2.918 | 0.000 | 4.413 |

附表 5-71 第六次中国总膳食研究氟苯尼考的膳食来源（单位：%）

Annexed Table 5-71 Dietary sources of florfenicol from the 6th China TDS (Unit: %)

| 膳食类别 Category | 黑龙江 HL | 辽宁 LN | 河北 HE | 北京 BJ | 吉林 JL | 山西 SX | 陕西 SN | 河南 HA | 宁夏 NX | 内蒙古 NM | 青海 QH | 甘肃 GS | 上海 SH | 福建 FJ | 江西 JX | 江苏 JS | 浙江 ZJ | 山东 SD | 湖北 HB | 四川 SC | 广西 GX | 湖南 HN | 广东 GD | 贵州 GZ | 全国平均 AVG |
|---|---|---|---|---|---|---|---|---|---|---|---|---|---|---|---|---|---|---|---|---|---|---|---|---|---|
| 肉类 Meats | 99.9 | 63.0 | 25.8 | 100.0 | 19.7 | 93.1 | 77.3 | 17.1 | 100.0 | 0.0 | 81.5 | 100.0 | 0.0 | 8.5 | 0.0 | 100.0 | 85.5 | 0.0 | 100.0 | 0.0 | 0.0 | 53.5 | 61.7 | 0.0 | 94.0 |
| 蛋类 Eggs | 0.1 | 0.0 | 74.2 | 0.0 | 80.3 | 6.9 | 22.7 | 82.9 | 0.0 | 100.0 | 18.5 | 0.0 | 77.9 | 91.5 | 20.6 | 0.0 | 14.5 | 0.0 | 0.0 | 100.0 | 0.0 | 46.5 | 31.9 | 0.0 | 5.5 |
| 水产类 Aquatic foods | 0.0 | 0.0 | 0.0 | 0.0 | 0.0 | 0.0 | 0.0 | 0.0 | 0.0 | 0.0 | 0.0 | 0.0 | 22.1 | 0.0 | 79.4 | 0.0 | 0.0 | 0.0 | 0.0 | 0.0 | 0.0 | 0.0 | 6.3 | 0.0 | 0.4 |
| 乳类 Dairy products | 0.0 | 37.0 | 0.0 | 0.0 | 0.0 | 0.0 | 0.0 | 0.0 | 0.0 | 0.0 | 0.0 | 0.0 | 0.0 | 0.0 | 0.0 | 0.0 | 0.0 | 0.0 | 0.0 | 0.0 | 0.0 | 0.0 | 0.0 | 0.0 | 0.1 |

附表 5-72 第六次中国总膳食研究膳食样品中氯霉素的含量（单位：μg/kg）

Annexed Table 5-72 Levels of chloramphenicol in food samples from the 6th China TDS (Unit: μg/kg)

| 膳食类别 Category | 黑龙江 HL | 辽宁 LN | 河北 HE | 北京 BJ | 吉林 JL | 山西 SX | 陕西 SN | 河南 HA | 宁夏 NX | 内蒙古 NM | 青海 QH | 甘肃 GS | 上海 SH | 福建 FJ | 江西 JX | 江苏 JS | 浙江 ZJ | 山东 SD | 湖北 HB | 四川 SC | 广西 GX | 湖南 HN | 广东 GD | 贵州 GZ | 全国平均 AVG |
|---|---|---|---|---|---|---|---|---|---|---|---|---|---|---|---|---|---|---|---|---|---|---|---|---|---|
| 肉类 Meats | ND | ND | ND | ND | ND | ND | ND | ND | ND | ND | ND | ND | ND | ND | ND | ND | ND | ND | ND | ND | ND | ND | 0.23 | ND | 0.01 |
| 蛋类 Eggs | ND | ND | ND | ND | ND | ND | ND | ND | ND | ND | ND | ND | ND | ND | ND | ND | ND | ND | ND | ND | ND | ND | ND | ND | 0.00 |

续表

| 膳食类别 Category | 黑龙江 HL | 辽宁 LN | 河北 HE | 北京 BJ | 吉林 JL | 山西 SX | 陕西 SN | 河南 HA | 宁夏 NX | 内蒙古 NM | 青海 QH | 甘肃 GS | 上海 SH | 福建 FJ | 江西 JX | 江苏 JS | 浙江 ZJ | 山东 SD | 湖北 HB | 四川 SC | 广西 GX | 湖南 HN | 广东 GD | 贵州 GZ | 全国平均 AVG |
|---|---|---|---|---|---|---|---|---|---|---|---|---|---|---|---|---|---|---|---|---|---|---|---|---|---|
| 水产类 Aquatic foods | ND | ND | ND | ND | ND | ND | ND | ND | ND | ND | ND | ND | ND | ND | ND | 0.03 | ND | 0.08 | ND | ND | 0.03 | ND | ND | ND | 0.01 |
| 乳类 Dairy products | ND | ND | ND | ND | ND | ND | ND | ND | ND | ND | ND | ND | ND | ND | ND | ND | ND | ND | ND | ND | ND | ND | ND | ND | 0.00 |

注：未检出（ND）按 0 计

Note: values not detected (ND) were treated as being equal to 0

附表 5-73　第六次中国总膳食研究的氯霉素膳食摄入量 [单位：ng/(kg bw·d)]

Annexed Table 5-73　Dietary intakes of chloramphenicol from the 6th China TDS [Unit: ng/(kg bw·d)]

| 膳食类别 Category | 黑龙江 HL | 辽宁 LN | 河北 HE | 北京 BJ | 吉林 JL | 山西 SX | 陕西 SN | 河南 HA | 宁夏 NX | 内蒙古 NM | 青海 QH | 甘肃 GS | 上海 SH | 福建 FJ | 江西 JX | 江苏 JS | 浙江 ZJ | 山东 SD | 湖北 HB | 四川 SC | 广西 GX | 湖南 HN | 广东 GD | 贵州 GZ | 全国平均 AVG |
|---|---|---|---|---|---|---|---|---|---|---|---|---|---|---|---|---|---|---|---|---|---|---|---|---|---|
| 肉类 Meats | 0.000 | 0.000 | 0.000 | 0.000 | 0.000 | 0.000 | 0.000 | 0.000 | 0.000 | 0.000 | 0.000 | 0.000 | 0.000 | 0.000 | 0.000 | 0.000 | 0.000 | 0.000 | 0.000 | 0.000 | 0.000 | 0.000 | 0.374 | 0.000 | 0.016 |
| 蛋类 Eggs | 0.000 | 0.000 | 0.000 | 0.000 | 0.000 | 0.000 | 0.000 | 0.000 | 0.000 | 0.000 | 0.000 | 0.000 | 0.000 | 0.000 | 0.000 | 0.000 | 0.000 | 0.000 | 0.000 | 0.000 | 0.000 | 0.000 | 0.000 | 0.000 | 0.000 |
| 水产类 Aquatic foods | 0.000 | 0.000 | 0.000 | 0.000 | 0.000 | 0.000 | 0.000 | 0.000 | 0.000 | 0.000 | 0.000 | 0.000 | 0.000 | 0.000 | 0.000 | 0.021 | 0.000 | 0.028 | 0.000 | 0.000 | 0.045 | 0.000 | 0.000 | 0.000 | 0.004 |
| 乳类 Dairy products | 0.000 | 0.000 | 0.000 | 0.000 | 0.000 | 0.000 | 0.000 | 0.000 | 0.000 | 0.000 | 0.000 | 0.000 | 0.000 | 0.000 | 0.000 | 0.000 | 0.000 | 0.000 | 0.000 | 0.000 | 0.000 | 0.000 | 0.000 | 0.000 | 0.000 |
| 合计 SUM | 0.000 | 0.000 | 0.000 | 0.000 | 0.000 | 0.000 | 0.000 | 0.000 | 0.000 | 0.000 | 0.000 | 0.000 | 0.000 | 0.000 | 0.000 | 0.021 | 0.000 | 0.028 | 0.000 | 0.000 | 0.045 | 0.000 | 0.374 | 0.000 | 0.019 |

附表 5-74　第六次中国总膳食研究氯霉素的膳食来源（单位：%）

Annexed Table 5-74　Dietary sources of chloramphenicol from the 6$^{th}$ China TDS (Unit: %)

| 膳食类别<br>Category | 黑龙江<br>HL | 辽宁<br>LN | 河北<br>HE | 北京<br>BJ | 吉林<br>JL | 山西<br>SX | 陕西<br>SN | 河南<br>HA | 宁夏<br>NX | 内蒙古<br>NM | 青海<br>QH | 甘肃<br>GS | 上海<br>SH | 福建<br>FJ | 江西<br>JX | 江苏<br>JS | 浙江<br>ZJ | 山东<br>SD | 湖北<br>HB | 四川<br>SC | 广西<br>GX | 湖南<br>HN | 广东<br>GD | 贵州<br>GZ | 全国平均<br>AVG |
|---|---|---|---|---|---|---|---|---|---|---|---|---|---|---|---|---|---|---|---|---|---|---|---|---|---|
| 肉类 Meats | 0.0 | 0.0 | 0.0 | 0.0 | 0.0 | 0.0 | 0.0 | 0.0 | 0.0 | 0.0 | 0.0 | 0.0 | 0.0 | 0.0 | 0.0 | 0.0 | 0.0 | 0.0 | 0.0 | 0.0 | 0.0 | 0.0 | 100.0 | 0.0 | 80.0 |
| 蛋类 Eggs | 0.0 | 0.0 | 0.0 | 0.0 | 0.0 | 0.0 | 0.0 | 0.0 | 0.0 | 0.0 | 0.0 | 0.0 | 0.0 | 0.0 | 0.0 | 0.0 | 0.0 | 0.0 | 0.0 | 0.0 | 0.0 | 0.0 | 0.0 | 0.0 | 0.0 |
| 水产类 Aquatic foods | 0.0 | 0.0 | 0.0 | 0.0 | 0.0 | 0.0 | 0.0 | 0.0 | 0.0 | 0.0 | 0.0 | 0.0 | 0.0 | 0.0 | 0.0 | 100.0 | 0.0 | 100.0 | 0.0 | 0.0 | 100.0 | 0.0 | 0.0 | 0.0 | 20.0 |
| 乳类 Dairy products | 0.0 | 0.0 | 0.0 | 0.0 | 0.0 | 0.0 | 0.0 | 0.0 | 0.0 | 0.0 | 0.0 | 0.0 | 0.0 | 0.0 | 0.0 | 0.0 | 0.0 | 0.0 | 0.0 | 0.0 | 0.0 | 0.0 | 0.0 | 0.0 | 0.0 |

附表 5-75　第六次中国总膳食研究膳食样品中甲砜霉素的含量（单位：μg/kg）

Annexed Table 5-75　Levels of thiamphenicol in food samples from the 6$^{th}$ China TDS (Unit: μg/kg)

| 膳食类别<br>Category | 黑龙江<br>HL | 辽宁<br>LN | 河北<br>HE | 北京<br>BJ | 吉林<br>JL | 山西<br>SX | 陕西<br>SN | 河南<br>HA | 宁夏<br>NX | 内蒙古<br>NM | 青海<br>QH | 甘肃<br>GS | 上海<br>SH | 福建<br>FJ | 江西<br>JX | 江苏<br>JS | 浙江<br>ZJ | 山东<br>SD | 湖北<br>HB | 四川<br>SC | 广西<br>GX | 湖南<br>HN | 广东<br>GD | 贵州<br>GZ | 全国平均<br>AVG |
|---|---|---|---|---|---|---|---|---|---|---|---|---|---|---|---|---|---|---|---|---|---|---|---|---|---|
| 肉类 Meats | 0.27 | ND | ND | ND | ND | ND | ND | ND | ND | ND | ND | ND | ND | ND | ND | 0.06 | ND | ND | 0.06 | ND | ND | ND | ND | ND | 0.02 |
| 蛋类 Eggs | ND | ND | ND | ND | ND | ND | ND | ND | ND | ND | ND | ND | ND | 0.12 | ND | ND | ND | ND | ND | ND | ND | ND | ND | ND | 0.00 |
| 水产类 Aquatic foods | ND | ND | ND | ND | ND | ND | ND | ND | ND | ND | ND | ND | ND | ND | ND | ND | ND | ND | ND | ND | ND | ND | ND | ND | 0.00 |
| 乳类 Dairy products | ND | ND | ND | ND | ND | ND | ND | ND | ND | ND | ND | ND | ND | ND | ND | ND | ND | ND | ND | ND | ND | ND | ND | ND | 0.00 |

注：未检出（ND）按 0 计

Note: values not detected (ND) were treated as being equal to 0

附表 5-76 第六次中国总膳食研究的甲砜霉素膳食摄入量 [单位: ng/(kg bw · d)]
Annexed Table 5-76 Dietary intakes of thiamphenicol from the 6th China TDS [Unit: ng/(kg bw · d)]

| 膳食类别<br>Category | 黑龙江<br>HL | 辽宁<br>LN | 河北<br>HE | 北京<br>BJ | 吉林<br>JL | 山西<br>SX | 陕西<br>SN | 河南<br>HA | 宁夏<br>NX | 内蒙古<br>NM | 青海<br>QH | 甘肃<br>GS | 上海<br>SH | 福建<br>FJ | 江西<br>JX | 江苏<br>JS | 浙江<br>ZJ | 山东<br>SD | 湖北<br>HB | 四川<br>SC | 广西<br>GX | 湖南<br>HN | 广东<br>GD | 贵州<br>GZ | 全国平均<br>AVG |
|---|---|---|---|---|---|---|---|---|---|---|---|---|---|---|---|---|---|---|---|---|---|---|---|---|---|
| 肉类 Meats | 0.252 | 0.000 | 0.000 | 0.000 | 0.000 | 0.000 | 0.000 | 0.000 | 0.000 | 0.000 | 0.000 | 0.000 | 0.000 | 0.000 | 0.000 | 0.084 | 0.000 | 0.000 | 0.049 | 0.000 | 0.000 | 0.000 | 0.000 | 0.000 | 0.016 |
| 蛋类 Eggs | 0.000 | 0.000 | 0.000 | 0.000 | 0.000 | 0.000 | 0.000 | 0.000 | 0.000 | 0.000 | 0.000 | 0.000 | 0.000 | 0.035 | 0.000 | 0.000 | 0.000 | 0.000 | 0.000 | 0.000 | 0.000 | 0.000 | 0.000 | 0.000 | 0.001 |
| 水产类 Aquatic foods | 0.000 | 0.000 | 0.000 | 0.000 | 0.000 | 0.000 | 0.000 | 0.000 | 0.000 | 0.000 | 0.000 | 0.000 | 0.000 | 0.000 | 0.000 | 0.000 | 0.000 | 0.000 | 0.000 | 0.000 | 0.000 | 0.000 | 0.000 | 0.000 | 0.000 |
| 乳类 Dairy products | 0.000 | 0.000 | 0.000 | 0.000 | 0.000 | 0.000 | 0.000 | 0.000 | 0.000 | 0.000 | 0.000 | 0.000 | 0.000 | 0.000 | 0.000 | 0.000 | 0.000 | 0.000 | 0.000 | 0.000 | 0.000 | 0.000 | 0.000 | 0.000 | 0.000 |
| 合计 SUM | 0.252 | 0.000 | 0.000 | 0.000 | 0.000 | 0.000 | 0.000 | 0.000 | 0.000 | 0.000 | 0.000 | 0.000 | 0.000 | 0.035 | 0.000 | 0.084 | 0.000 | 0.000 | 0.049 | 0.000 | 0.000 | 0.000 | 0.000 | 0.000 | 0.017 |

附表 5-77 第六次中国总膳食研究甲砜霉素的膳食来源（单位: %）
Annexed Table 5-77 Dietary sources of thiamphenicol from the 6th China TDS (Unit: %)

| 膳食类别<br>Category | 黑龙江<br>HL | 辽宁<br>LN | 河北<br>HE | 北京<br>BJ | 吉林<br>JL | 山西<br>SX | 陕西<br>SN | 河南<br>HA | 宁夏<br>NX | 内蒙古<br>NM | 青海<br>QH | 甘肃<br>GS | 上海<br>SH | 福建<br>FJ | 江西<br>JX | 江苏<br>JS | 浙江<br>ZJ | 山东<br>SD | 湖北<br>HB | 四川<br>SC | 广西<br>GX | 湖南<br>HN | 广东<br>GD | 贵州<br>GZ | 全国平均<br>AVG |
|---|---|---|---|---|---|---|---|---|---|---|---|---|---|---|---|---|---|---|---|---|---|---|---|---|---|
| 肉类 Meats | 100.0 | 0.0 | 0.0 | 0.0 | 0.0 | 0.0 | 0.0 | 0.0 | 0.0 | 0.0 | 0.0 | 0.0 | 0.0 | 0.0 | 0.0 | 100.0 | 0.0 | 0.0 | 100.0 | 0.0 | 0.0 | 0.0 | 0.0 | 0.0 | 91.7 |
| 蛋类 Eggs | 0.0 | 0.0 | 0.0 | 0.0 | 0.0 | 0.0 | 0.0 | 0.0 | 0.0 | 0.0 | 0.0 | 0.0 | 0.0 | 100.0 | 0.0 | 0.0 | 0.0 | 0.0 | 0.0 | 0.0 | 0.0 | 0.0 | 0.0 | 0.0 | 8.3 |
| 水产类 Aquatic foods | 0.0 | 0.0 | 0.0 | 0.0 | 0.0 | 0.0 | 0.0 | 0.0 | 0.0 | 0.0 | 0.0 | 0.0 | 0.0 | 0.0 | 0.0 | 0.0 | 0.0 | 0.0 | 0.0 | 0.0 | 0.0 | 0.0 | 0.0 | 0.0 | 0.0 |
| 乳类 Dairy products | 0.0 | 0.0 | 0.0 | 0.0 | 0.0 | 0.0 | 0.0 | 0.0 | 0.0 | 0.0 | 0.0 | 0.0 | 0.0 | 0.0 | 0.0 | 0.0 | 0.0 | 0.0 | 0.0 | 0.0 | 0.0 | 0.0 | 0.0 | 0.0 | 0.0 |

# 第六章 附 表
# Annexed Tables of Chapter 6

附表 6-1 第六次中国总膳食研究膳食样品中 3-MCPD 的含量（单位：μg/kg）

Annexed Table 6-1 Levels of 3-MCPD in food samples from the 6<sup>th</sup> China TDS (Unit: μg/kg)

| 膳食类别 Category | 黑龙江 HL | 辽宁 LN | 河北 HE | 北京 BJ | 吉林 JL | 山西 SX | 陕西 SN | 河南 HA | 宁夏 NX | 内蒙古 NM | 青海 QH | 甘肃 GS | 上海 SH | 福建 FJ | 江西 JX | 江苏 JS | 浙江 ZJ | 山东 SD | 湖北 HB | 四川 SC | 广西 GX | 湖南 HN | 广东 GD | 贵州 GZ | 全国平均 AVG |
|---|---|---|---|---|---|---|---|---|---|---|---|---|---|---|---|---|---|---|---|---|---|---|---|---|---|
| 谷类 Cereals | ND | ND | ND | 4.8 | ND | ND | 2.5 | ND | ND | ND | ND | 3.0 | ND | ND | ND | ND | ND | ND | ND | ND | ND | ND | ND | ND | 1.3 |
| 豆类 Legumes | ND | 6.3 | ND | 3.7 | ND | ND | 3.3 | 9.6 | ND | ND | 5.0 | 14.6 | ND | 5.0 | 2.7 | 5.3 | ND | 3.5 | ND | 6.1 | ND | ND | ND | 3.1 | 3.2 |
| 薯类 Potatoes | ND | ND | ND | 6.4 | 2.6 | 2.9 | 4.3 | 21.7 | 3.1 | 13.1 | 5.7 | 6.0 | 2.8 | ND | 28.5 | 12.4 | ND | ND | 3.3 | 11.0 | ND | 8.4 | ND | ND | 6.1 |
| 肉类 Meats | 2.6 | 3.0 | ND | 3.9 | ND | 2.8 | 14.5 | ND | ND | 2.7 | ND | 2.6 | ND | ND | ND | ND | ND | ND | 5.5 | 23.0 | ND | 6.4 | 5.2 | 12.0 | 4.0 |
| 蛋类 Eggs | ND | ND | 4.8 | 2.9 | 13.6 | ND | ND | 4.2 | ND | ND | ND | ND | ND | ND | 3.5 | ND | ND | ND | ND | 60.7 | ND | ND | ND | 8.2 | 4.8 |
| 水产类 Aquatic foods | ND | ND | ND | 6.8 | 9.4 | ND | ND | ND | 9.4 | ND | 9.3 | ND | ND | ND | ND | ND | 6.4 | 5.9 | ND | 3.0 | ND | ND | ND | ND | 2.8 |
| 乳类 Dairy products | ND | ND | ND | ND | ND | ND | ND | ND | ND | ND | ND | ND | ND | ND | ND | ND | ND | ND | ND | ND | ND | ND | ND | ND | ND |
| 蔬菜类 Vegetables | 7.4 | ND | 38.6 | 3.9 | 37.3 | 4.8 | 12.0 | 26.8 | 33.4 | ND | 9.1 | ND | 10.7 | 7.2 | 16.5 | 6.8 | 4.4 | 19.7 | 6.1 | 33.1 | 5.1 | 27.5 | 14.5 | 88.9 | 17.4 |
| 水果类 Fruits | ND | ND | ND | ND | ND | ND | ND | ND | ND | ND | ND | ND | ND | ND | ND | ND | ND | ND | ND | ND | ND | ND | ND | ND | ND |

续表

| 膳食类别<br>Category | 黑龙江<br>HL | 辽宁<br>LN | 河北<br>HE | 北京<br>BJ | 吉林<br>JL | 山西<br>SX | 陕西<br>SN | 河南<br>HA | 宁夏<br>NX | 内蒙古<br>NM | 青海<br>QH | 甘肃<br>GS | 上海<br>SH | 福建<br>FJ | 江西<br>JX | 江苏<br>JS | 浙江<br>ZJ | 山东<br>SD | 湖北<br>HB | 四川<br>SC | 广西<br>GX | 湖南<br>HN | 广东<br>GD | 贵州<br>GZ | 全国平均<br>AVG |
|---|---|---|---|---|---|---|---|---|---|---|---|---|---|---|---|---|---|---|---|---|---|---|---|---|---|
| 糖类<br>Sugar | ND | ND | ND | ND | ND | ND | ND | ND | ND | ND | ND | ND | ND | ND | ND | ND | ND | ND | ND | ND | ND | ND | ND | ND | ND |
| 水及饮料类<br>Water and beverages | ND | ND | ND | ND | ND | ND | ND | ND | ND | ND | ND | ND | ND | ND | ND | ND | ND | ND | ND | ND | ND | ND | ND | ND | ND |
| 酒类<br>Alcohol beverages | ND | 3.1 | ND | 3.3 | 4.2 | ND | ND | 4.1 | ND | ND | ND | 3.2 | 2.9 | 3.7 | ND | 2.9 | ND | ND | ND | ND | 2.7 | 2.6 | 4.0 | ND | 2.1 |

注: 未检出 (ND) 按 1/2 检出限 (LOD) 计

Note: values not detected (ND) were treated as being equal to half of the detection of limit (LOD)

附表 Table 6-2 第六次中国总膳食研究膳食样品中 2-MCPD 的含量 (单位: µg/kg)

Annexed Table 6-2  Levels of 2-MCPD in food samples from the 6$^{th}$ China TDS (Unit: µg/kg)

| 膳食类别<br>Category | 黑龙江<br>HL | 辽宁<br>LN | 河北<br>HE | 北京<br>BJ | 吉林<br>JL | 山西<br>SX | 陕西<br>SN | 河南<br>HA | 宁夏<br>NX | 内蒙古<br>NM | 青海<br>QH | 甘肃<br>GS | 上海<br>SH | 福建<br>FJ | 江西<br>JX | 江苏<br>JS | 浙江<br>ZJ | 山东<br>SD | 湖北<br>HB | 四川<br>SC | 广西<br>GX | 湖南<br>HN | 广东<br>GD | 贵州<br>GZ | 全国平均<br>AVG |
|---|---|---|---|---|---|---|---|---|---|---|---|---|---|---|---|---|---|---|---|---|---|---|---|---|---|
| 谷类<br>Cereals | ND | ND | ND | ND | ND | ND | ND | ND | ND | ND | ND | ND | ND | ND | ND | ND | ND | ND | ND | ND | ND | ND | ND | ND | ND |
| 豆类<br>Legumes | ND | ND | ND | ND | ND | ND | ND | ND | ND | ND | ND | ND | ND | ND | ND | ND | ND | ND | ND | ND | ND | ND | ND | ND | ND |
| 薯类<br>Potatoes | ND | ND | ND | ND | ND | ND | ND | ND | ND | ND | ND | ND | ND | ND | 5.0 | ND | ND | ND | ND | 2.2 | ND | ND | ND | ND | 1.2 |
| 肉类<br>Meats | ND | ND | ND | ND | ND | ND | ND | ND | ND | ND | ND | ND | ND | ND | ND | ND | ND | ND | ND | ND | ND | ND | ND | ND | 1.1 |
| 蛋类<br>Eggs | ND | ND | ND | ND | ND | ND | ND | ND | ND | ND | ND | ND | ND | ND | ND | ND | ND | ND | ND | 19.2 | ND | ND | ND | ND | 1.8 |

续表

| 膳食类别 Category | 黑龙江 HL | 辽宁 LN | 河北 HE | 北京 BJ | 吉林 JL | 山西 SX | 陕西 SN | 河南 HA | 宁夏 NX | 内蒙古 NM | 青海 QH | 甘肃 GS | 上海 SH | 福建 FJ | 江西 JX | 江苏 JS | 浙江 ZJ | 山东 SD | 湖北 HB | 四川 SC | 广西 GX | 湖南 HN | 广东 GD | 贵州 GZ | 全国平均 AVG |
|---|---|---|---|---|---|---|---|---|---|---|---|---|---|---|---|---|---|---|---|---|---|---|---|---|---|
| 水产类 Aquatic foods | ND | ND | ND | ND | ND | ND | ND | ND | ND | ND | ND | ND | ND | ND | ND | ND | ND | ND | ND | ND | ND | ND | ND | ND | ND |
| 乳类 Dairy products | ND | ND | ND | ND | ND | ND | ND | ND | ND | ND | ND | ND | ND | ND | ND | ND | ND | ND | ND | ND | ND | ND | ND | ND | ND |
| 蔬菜类 Vegetables | ND | ND | ND | ND | ND | ND | ND | ND | ND | ND | ND | ND | ND | ND | ND | ND | ND | 2.0 | ND | ND | ND | ND | ND | 3.4 | 1.1 |
| 水果类 Fruits | ND | ND | ND | ND | ND | ND | ND | ND | ND | ND | ND | ND | ND | ND | ND | ND | ND | ND | ND | ND | ND | ND | ND | ND | ND |
| 糖类 Sugar | ND | ND | ND | ND | ND | ND | ND | ND | ND | ND | ND | ND | ND | ND | ND | ND | ND | ND | ND | ND | ND | ND | ND | ND | ND |
| 水及饮料类 Water and beverages | ND | ND | ND | ND | ND | ND | ND | ND | ND | ND | ND | ND | ND | ND | ND | ND | ND | ND | ND | ND | ND | ND | ND | ND | ND |
| 酒类 Alcohol beverages | ND | ND | ND | ND | ND | ND | ND | ND | ND | ND | ND | ND | ND | ND | ND | ND | ND | ND | ND | ND | ND | ND | ND | ND | ND |

注：未检出（ND）按 1/2 检出限（LOD）计

Note: values not detected (ND) were treated as being equal to half of the detection of limit (LOD)

附表 6-3 第六次中国总膳食研究 3-MCPD 的膳食摄入量 [单位：μg/(kg bw·d)]

Annexed Table 6-3 Dietary intakes of 3-MCPD from the 6$^{th}$ China TDS [Unit: μg/(kg bw·d)]

| 膳食类别 Category | 黑龙江 HL | 辽宁 LN | 河北 HE | 北京 BJ | 吉林 JL | 山西 SX | 陕西 SN | 河南 HA | 宁夏 NX | 内蒙古 NM | 青海 QH | 甘肃 GS | 上海 SH | 福建 FJ | 江西 JX | 江苏 JS | 浙江 ZJ | 山东 SD | 湖北 HB | 四川 SC | 广西 GX | 湖南 HN | 广东 GD | 贵州 GZ | 全国平均 AVG |
|---|---|---|---|---|---|---|---|---|---|---|---|---|---|---|---|---|---|---|---|---|---|---|---|---|---|
| 谷类 Cereals | 0.017 | 0.016 | 0.020 | 0.085 | 0.012 | 0.027 | 0.059 | 0.023 | 0.019 | 0.017 | 0.028 | 0.055 | 0.009 | 0.015 | 0.014 | 0.015 | 0.013 | 0.025 | 0.011 | 0.024 | 0.022 | 0.013 | 0.010 | 0.017 | 0.024 |

续表

| 膳食类别<br>Category | 黑龙江<br>HL | 辽宁<br>LN | 河北<br>HE | 北京<br>BJ | 吉林<br>JL | 山西<br>SX | 陕西<br>SN | 河南<br>HA | 宁夏<br>NX | 内蒙古<br>NM | 青海<br>QH | 甘肃<br>GS | 上海<br>SH | 福建<br>FJ | 江西<br>JX | 江苏<br>JS | 浙江<br>ZJ | 山东<br>SD | 湖北<br>HB | 四川<br>SC | 广西<br>GX | 湖南<br>HN | 广东<br>GD | 贵州<br>GZ | 全国平均<br>AVG |
|---|---|---|---|---|---|---|---|---|---|---|---|---|---|---|---|---|---|---|---|---|---|---|---|---|---|
| 豆类 Legumes | 0.001 | 0.017 | 0.001 | 0.006 | 0.002 | 0.001 | 0.005 | 0.012 | 0.001 | 0.001 | 0.001 | 0.010 | 0.002 | 0.001 | 0.004 | 0.008 | 0.002 | 0.004 | 0.001 | 0.008 | 0.001 | 0.001 | 0.001 | 0.006 | 0.004 |
| 薯类 Potatoes | 0.001 | 0.001 | 0.001 | 0.007 | 0.005 | 0.007 | 0.010 | 0.030 | 0.006 | 0.026 | 0.010 | 0.014 | 0.002 | 0.004 | 0.015 | 0.008 | 0.001 | 0.001 | 0.005 | 0.011 | <0.001 | 0.010 | <0.001 | 0.001 | 0.007 |
| 肉类 Meats | 0.003 | 0.004 | 0.001 | 0.005 | 0.001 | 0.006 | 0.009 | 0.001 | 0.001 | 0.003 | 0.001 | 0.001 | 0.002 | 0.001 | 0.002 | 0.001 | 0.002 | 0.002 | 0.005 | 0.047 | 0.002 | 0.015 | 0.011 | 0.021 | 0.006 |
| 蛋类 Eggs | 0.001 | 0.001 | 0.003 | 0.002 | 0.010 | <0.001 | <0.001 | 0.002 | <0.001 | 0.001 | <0.001 | <0.001 | 0.001 | <0.001 | 0.001 | <0.001 | <0.001 | 0.001 | <0.001 | 0.016 | <0.001 | <0.001 | <0.001 | 0.002 | 0.002 |
| 水产类 Aquatic foods | <0.001 | <0.001 | <0.001 | 0.002 | 0.002 | <0.001 | <0.001 | <0.001 | <0.001 | <0.001 | 0.001 | <0.001 | 0.001 | 0.001 | 0.001 | 0.001 | 0.005 | 0.003 | 0.001 | <0.001 | 0.002 | 0.001 | <0.001 | <0.001 | 0.001 |
| 乳类 Dairy products | <0.001 | <0.001 | <0.001 | <0.001 | <0.001 | <0.001 | <0.001 | <0.001 | <0.001 | <0.001 | <0.001 | <0.001 | <0.001 | <0.001 | <0.001 | <0.001 | <0.001 | <0.001 | <0.001 | <0.001 | <0.001 | <0.001 | <0.001 | <0.001 | <0.001 |
| 蔬菜类 Vegetables | 0.046 | 0.006 | 0.182 | 0.025 | 0.232 | 0.024 | 0.056 | 0.119 | 0.083 | 0.004 | 0.045 | 0.004 | 0.068 | 0.046 | 0.118 | 0.048 | 0.038 | 0.128 | 0.040 | 0.160 | 0.029 | 0.240 | 0.056 | 0.593 | 0.100 |
| 水果类 Fruits | <0.001 | <0.001 | <0.001 | <0.001 | <0.001 | <0.001 | <0.001 | <0.001 | <0.001 | <0.001 | <0.001 | <0.001 | <0.001 | <0.001 | <0.001 | <0.001 | <0.001 | <0.001 | <0.001 | <0.001 | <0.001 | <0.001 | <0.001 | <0.001 | <0.001 |
| 糖类 Sugar | <0.001 | <0.001 | <0.001 | <0.001 | <0.001 | <0.001 | <0.001 | <0.001 | <0.001 | <0.001 | <0.001 | <0.001 | <0.001 | <0.001 | <0.001 | <0.001 | <0.001 | <0.001 | <0.001 | <0.001 | <0.001 | <0.001 | <0.001 | <0.001 | <0.001 |
| 水及饮料类 Water and beverages | <0.001 | <0.001 | <0.001 | 0.001 | 0.001 | <0.001 | <0.001 | <0.001 | <0.001 | <0.001 | <0.001 | <0.001 | 0.001 | 0.001 | 0.001 | 0.002 | 0.001 | 0.002 | <0.001 | <0.001 | 0.001 | 0.001 | 0.001 | <0.001 | 0.001 |
| 酒类 Alcohol beverages | <0.001 | 0.002 | <0.001 | <0.001 | <0.001 | <0.001 | <0.001 | <0.001 | <0.001 | <0.001 | <0.001 | <0.001 | <0.001 | <0.001 | <0.001 | <0.001 | <0.001 | 0.002 | <0.001 | <0.001 | <0.001 | <0.001 | <0.001 | <0.001 | 0.001 |
| 合计 SUM | 0.070 | 0.046 | 0.208 | 0.134 | 0.264 | 0.066 | 0.139 | 0.187 | 0.109 | 0.052 | 0.085 | 0.085 | 0.086 | 0.069 | 0.154 | 0.084 | 0.063 | 0.165 | 0.064 | 0.267 | 0.058 | 0.282 | 0.079 | 0.640 | 0.144 |

注：摄入量合计时，摄入量<0.001 的结果按 0 计
Note: values <0.001 were treated as 0

附表 6-4 第六次中国总膳食研究 2-MCPD 的膳食摄入量 [单位: μg/(kg bw·d)]

Annexed Table 6-4 Dietary intakes of 2-MCPD from the 6th China TDS [Unit: μg/(kg bw·d)]

| 膳食类别<br>Category | 黑龙江<br>HL | 辽宁<br>LN | 河北<br>HE | 北京<br>BJ | 吉林<br>JL | 山西<br>SX | 陕西<br>SN | 河南<br>HA | 宁夏<br>NX | 内蒙古<br>NM | 青海<br>QH | 甘肃<br>GS | 上海<br>SH | 福建<br>FJ | 江西<br>JX | 江苏<br>JS | 浙江<br>ZJ | 山东<br>SD | 湖北<br>HB | 四川<br>SC | 广西<br>GX | 湖南<br>HN | 广东<br>GD | 贵州<br>GZ | 全国平均<br>AVG |
|---|---|---|---|---|---|---|---|---|---|---|---|---|---|---|---|---|---|---|---|---|---|---|---|---|---|
| 谷类 Cereals | <0.001 | 0.001 | <0.001 | <0.001 | <0.001 | <0.001 | <0.001 | <0.001 | <0.001 | <0.001 | <0.001 | <0.001 | <0.001 | <0.001 | <0.001 | <0.001 | <0.001 | <0.001 | <0.001 | <0.001 | <0.001 | <0.001 | <0.001 | <0.001 | <0.001 |
| 豆类 Legumes | <0.001 | <0.001 | <0.001 | <0.001 | <0.001 | <0.001 | <0.001 | <0.001 | <0.001 | <0.001 | <0.001 | <0.001 | <0.001 | <0.001 | <0.001 | <0.001 | <0.001 | <0.001 | <0.001 | <0.001 | <0.001 | <0.001 | <0.001 | <0.001 | <0.001 |
| 薯类 Potatoes | 0.001 | 0.001 | 0.001 | 0.001 | 0.002 | 0.002 | 0.002 | 0.001 | 0.002 | 0.002 | 0.002 | 0.002 | 0.001 | 0.001 | 0.003 | 0.001 | 0.001 | <0.001 | 0.001 | 0.001 | <0.001 | 0.001 | <0.001 | 0.001 | 0.001 |
| 肉类 Meats | 0.001 | 0.001 | 0.001 | 0.001 | 0.001 | 0.002 | 0.001 | <0.001 | 0.001 | 0.001 | 0.001 | 0.001 | 0.002 | 0.001 | 0.002 | 0.001 | 0.002 | 0.002 | 0.001 | 0.005 | 0.002 | 0.002 | 0.002 | 0.002 | 0.002 |
| 蛋类 Eggs | 0.001 | <0.001 | 0.001 | 0.001 | 0.001 | <0.001 | <0.001 | <0.001 | <0.001 | <0.001 | <0.001 | <0.001 | 0.001 | <0.001 | <0.001 | <0.001 | <0.001 | 0.001 | <0.001 | 0.005 | <0.001 | <0.001 | <0.001 | 0.001 | 0.001 |
| 水产类 Aquatic foods | <0.001 | <0.001 | <0.001 | <0.001 | <0.001 | <0.001 | <0.001 | <0.001 | <0.001 | <0.001 | <0.001 | <0.001 | <0.001 | <0.001 | <0.001 | <0.001 | <0.001 | <0.001 | <0.001 | <0.001 | <0.001 | <0.001 | <0.001 | <0.001 | <0.001 |
| 乳类 Dairy products | <0.001 | <0.001 | <0.001 | <0.001 | <0.001 | <0.001 | <0.001 | <0.001 | <0.001 | <0.001 | <0.001 | <0.001 | <0.001 | <0.001 | <0.001 | <0.001 | <0.001 | <0.001 | <0.001 | <0.001 | <0.001 | <0.001 | <0.001 | <0.001 | <0.001 |
| 蔬菜类 Vegetables | 0.006 | 0.006 | 0.005 | 0.006 | 0.006 | 0.005 | 0.005 | 0.004 | 0.002 | 0.004 | 0.005 | 0.004 | 0.006 | 0.006 | 0.007 | 0.007 | 0.009 | 0.013 | 0.007 | 0.005 | 0.006 | 0.009 | 0.004 | 0.023 | 0.007 |
| 水果类 Fruits | <0.001 | <0.001 | <0.001 | <0.001 | <0.001 | <0.001 | <0.001 | <0.001 | <0.001 | <0.001 | <0.001 | <0.001 | <0.001 | <0.001 | <0.001 | <0.001 | <0.001 | <0.001 | <0.001 | <0.001 | <0.001 | <0.001 | <0.001 | <0.001 | <0.001 |
| 糖类 Sugar | <0.001 | <0.001 | <0.001 | <0.001 | <0.001 | <0.001 | <0.001 | <0.001 | <0.001 | <0.001 | <0.001 | <0.001 | <0.001 | <0.001 | <0.001 | <0.001 | <0.001 | <0.001 | <0.001 | <0.001 | <0.001 | <0.001 | <0.001 | <0.001 | <0.001 |
| 水及饮料类 Water and beverages | <0.001 | <0.001 | <0.001 | <0.001 | <0.001 | <0.001 | <0.001 | <0.001 | <0.001 | <0.001 | <0.001 | <0.001 | <0.001 | <0.001 | <0.001 | <0.001 | <0.001 | <0.001 | <0.001 | <0.001 | <0.001 | <0.001 | <0.001 | <0.001 | <0.001 |

续表

| 膳食类别 Category | 黑龙江 HL | 辽宁 LN | 河北 HE | 北京 BJ | 吉林 JL | 山西 SX | 陕西 SN | 河南 HA | 宁夏 NX | 内蒙古 NM | 青海 QH | 甘肃 GS | 上海 SH | 福建 FJ | 江西 JX | 江苏 JS | 浙江 ZJ | 山东 SD | 湖北 HB | 四川 SC | 广西 GX | 湖南 HN | 广东 GD | 贵州 GZ | 全国平均 AVG |
|---|---|---|---|---|---|---|---|---|---|---|---|---|---|---|---|---|---|---|---|---|---|---|---|---|---|
| 酒类 Alcohol beverages | <0.001 | <0.001 | <0.001 | <0.001 | <0.001 | <0.001 | <0.001 | <0.001 | <0.001 | <0.001 | <0.001 | <0.001 | <0.001 | <0.001 | <0.001 | <0.001 | <0.001 | <0.001 | <0.001 | <0.001 | <0.001 | <0.001 | <0.001 | <0.001 | <0.001 |
| 合计 SUM | 0.010 | 0.009 | 0.007 | 0.009 | 0.010 | 0.010 | 0.008 | 0.007 | 0.005 | 0.008 | 0.008 | 0.007 | 0.009 | 0.009 | 0.012 | 0.010 | 0.012 | 0.016 | 0.009 | 0.015 | 0.009 | 0.013 | 0.007 | 0.025 | 0.010 |

注：摄入量合计时，摄入量<0.001 的结果按 0 计
Note: values <0.001 were treated as 0

附表 6-5 第六次中国总膳研究 3-MCPD 的膳食来源（单位：%）
Annexed Table 6-5 Dietary sources of 3-MCPD from the 6th China TDS (Unit: %)

| 膳食类别 Category | 黑龙江 HL | 辽宁 LN | 河北 HE | 北京 BJ | 吉林 JL | 山西 SX | 陕西 SN | 河南 HA | 宁夏 NX | 内蒙古 NM | 青海 QH | 甘肃 GS | 上海 SH | 福建 FJ | 江西 JX | 江苏 JS | 浙江 ZJ | 山东 SD | 湖北 HB | 四川 SC | 广西 GX | 湖南 HN | 广东 GD | 贵州 GZ | 全国平均 AVG |
|---|---|---|---|---|---|---|---|---|---|---|---|---|---|---|---|---|---|---|---|---|---|---|---|---|---|
| 谷类 Cereals | 24.0 | 33.7 | 9.6 | 63.7 | 4.6 | 40.5 | 42.3 | 12.2 | 17.1 | 32.4 | 32.6 | 64.9 | 10.8 | 21.3 | 8.9 | 18.5 | 21.2 | 15.2 | 18.0 | 9.1 | 38.1 | 4.8 | 12.4 | 2.7 | 16.4 |
| 豆类 Legumes | 1.5 | 36.3 | 0.5 | 4.9 | 0.6 | 1.9 | 3.5 | 6.3 | 0.6 | 1.3 | 0.7 | 11.5 | 2.5 | 1.8 | 2.3 | 9.7 | 3.8 | 2.2 | 1.8 | 2.8 | 1.2 | 0.5 | 0.6 | 0.9 | 2.7 |
| 薯类 Potatoes | 2.1 | 3.2 | 0.5 | 5.2 | 1.9 | 10.4 | 7.0 | 16.0 | 5.1 | 49.9 | 11.3 | 16.6 | 1.9 | 5.3 | 9.4 | 9.5 | 1.0 | 0.5 | 7.4 | 4.3 | 0.5 | 3.4 | 0.5 | 0.1 | 5.0 |
| 肉类 Meats | 4.2 | 8.5 | 0.4 | 3.9 | 0.4 | 9.8 | 6.4 | 0.5 | 0.7 | 6.2 | 1.3 | 1.7 | 2.1 | 2.0 | 1.0 | 1.8 | 3.2 | 1.0 | 7.7 | 17.8 | 4.2 | 5.4 | 13.8 | 3.3 | 4.3 |
| 蛋类 Eggs | 0.9 | 1.9 | 1.5 | 1.6 | 3.8 | 0.7 | 0.3 | 1.1 | 0.3 | 1.2 | 0.3 | 0.5 | 0.8 | 0.6 | 0.9 | 0.6 | 0.7 | 0.5 | 0.7 | 6.0 | 0.4 | 0.1 | 0.5 | 0.3 | 1.3 |
| 水产类 Aquatic foods | 0.6 | 0.8 | 0.1 | 1.4 | 0.6 | 0.2 | 0.0 | 0.0 | 0.3 | 0.3 | 0.7 | 0.1 | 1.3 | 1.5 | 0.5 | 0.8 | 8.5 | 1.5 | 1.0 | 0.1 | 2.7 | 0.4 | 1.1 | 0.0 | 0.6 |
| 乳类 Dairy products | 0.0 | 0.0 | 0.0 | 0.0 | 0.0 | 0.0 | 0.0 | 0.0 | 0.0 | 0.0 | 0.0 | 0.0 | 0.0 | 0.0 | 0.0 | 0.0 | 0.0 | 0.0 | 0.0 | 0.0 | 0.0 | 0.0 | 0.0 | 0.0 | 0.0 |

续表

| 膳食类别 Category | 黑龙江 HL | 辽宁 LN | 河北 HE | 北京 BJ | 吉林 JL | 山西 SX | 陕西 SN | 河南 HA | 宁夏 NX | 内蒙古 NM | 青海 QH | 甘肃 GS | 上海 SH | 福建 FJ | 江西 JX | 江苏 JS | 浙江 ZJ | 山东 SD | 湖北 HB | 四川 SC | 广西 GX | 湖南 HN | 广东 GD | 贵州 GZ | 全国平均 AVG |
|---|---|---|---|---|---|---|---|---|---|---|---|---|---|---|---|---|---|---|---|---|---|---|---|---|---|
| 蔬菜类 Vegetables | 66.2 | 12.1 | 87.4 | 18.3 | 87.8 | 36.6 | 40.5 | 63.8 | 75.8 | 8.1 | 52.9 | 4.6 | 79.5 | 66.2 | 76.8 | 57.2 | 60.0 | 77.9 | 62.9 | 59.9 | 50.6 | 85.1 | 71.0 | 92.7 | 69.2 |
| 水果类 Fruits | 0.0 | 0.0 | 0.0 | 0.0 | 0.0 | 0.0 | 0.0 | 0.0 | 0.0 | 0.0 | 0.0 | 0.0 | 0.0 | 0.0 | 0.0 | 0.0 | 0.0 | 0.0 | 0.0 | 0.0 | 0.0 | 0.0 | 0.0 | 0.0 | 0.0 |
| 糖类 Sugar | 0.0 | 0.0 | 0.0 | 0.0 | 0.0 | 0.0 | 0.0 | 0.0 | 0.0 | 0.0 | 0.0 | 0.0 | 0.0 | 0.0 | 0.0 | 0.0 | 0.0 | 0.0 | 0.0 | 0.0 | 0.0 | 0.0 | 0.0 | 0.0 | 0.0 |
| 水及饮料类 Water and beverages | 0.0 | 0.0 | 0.0 | 0.0 | 0.0 | 0.0 | 0.0 | 0.1 | 0.0 | 0.6 | 0.1 | 0.2 | 1.2 | 1.2 | 0.2 | 2.1 | 1.6 | 1.1 | 0.4 | 0.0 | 2.4 | 0.2 | 0.1 | 0.0 | 0.4 |
| 酒类 Alcohol beverages | 0.5 | 3.6 | 0.1 | 1.1 | 0.2 | 0.0 | 0.0 | 0.1 | 0.0 | 0.6 | 0.1 | 0.2 | 1.2 | 1.2 | 0.2 | 2.1 | 1.6 | 1.1 | 0.4 | 0.0 | 2.4 | 0.2 | 0.1 | 0.0 | 0.4 |

附表 6-6 第六次中国总膳食研究膳食样品中 3-MCPD 酯的含量（单位：μg/kg）

Annexed Table 6-6 Levels of 3-MCPD esters in food samples from the 6$^{th}$ China TDS (Unit: μg/kg)

| 膳食类别 Category | 黑龙江 HL | 辽宁 LN | 河北 HE | 北京 BJ | 吉林 JL | 山西 SX | 陕西 SN | 河南 HA | 宁夏 NX | 内蒙古 NM | 青海 QH | 甘肃 GS | 上海 SH | 福建 FJ | 江西 JX | 江苏 JS | 浙江 ZJ | 山东 SD | 湖北 HB | 四川 SC | 广西 GX | 湖南 HN | 广东 GD | 贵州 GZ | 全国平均 AVG |
|---|---|---|---|---|---|---|---|---|---|---|---|---|---|---|---|---|---|---|---|---|---|---|---|---|---|
| 谷类 Cereals | 8 | 15 | 14 | 12 | 9 | 5 | 7 | 6 | 6 | 24 | 7 | 4 | 10 | 11 | 17 | 19 | 6 | 9 | 9 | 5 | 4 | ND | 9 | 11 | 9.5 |
| 豆类 Legumes | 13 | 14 | 15 | 9 | 21 | 19 | 46 | 28 | 53 | 23 | 54 | 65 | 19 | 75 | 28 | 28 | 16 | 10 | 18 | 35 | 18 | 19 | 34 | 33 | 28.9 |
| 薯类 Potatoes | 15 | 6 | 55 | 42 | 9 | 9 | 100 | 38 | 237 | 34 | 226 | 189 | 48 | 46 | 13 | 30 | 30 | 12 | 35 | 37 | 19 | 13 | 7 | 163 | 58.9 |
| 肉类 Meats | 25 | 16 | 40 | 39 | 40 | 17 | 145 | 37 | 317 | 114 | 188 | 193 | 46 | 100 | 64 | 54 | 47 | 29 | 48 | 119 | 57 | 59 | 24 | 121 | 80.8 |
| 蛋类 Eggs | 52 | 14 | 150 | 59 | 258 | 21 | 113 | 56 | 432 | 98 | 160 | 168 | 69 | 88 | 82 | 67 | 4390 | 45 | 20 | 67 | 18 | 44 | 11 | 224 | 279.4 |

续表

| 膳食类别<br>Category | 黑龙江<br>HL | 辽宁<br>LN | 河北<br>HE | 北京<br>BJ | 吉林<br>JL | 山西<br>SX | 陕西<br>SN | 河南<br>HA | 宁夏<br>NX | 内蒙古<br>NM | 青海<br>QH | 甘肃<br>GS | 上海<br>SH | 福建<br>FJ | 江西<br>JX | 江苏<br>JS | 浙江<br>ZJ | 山东<br>SD | 湖北<br>HB | 四川<br>SC | 广西<br>GX | 湖南<br>HN | 广东<br>GD | 贵州<br>GZ | 全国平均<br>AVG |
|---|---|---|---|---|---|---|---|---|---|---|---|---|---|---|---|---|---|---|---|---|---|---|---|---|---|
| 水产类 Aquatic foods | 11 | 4 | 16 | 23 | 152 | 11 | 60 | 16 | 99 | 13 | 106 | 231 | 33 | 249 | 37 | 33 | 37 | 25 | 16 | 42 | 22 | 41 | 28 | 91 | 58.2 |
| 乳类 Dairy products | ND | 4 | ND | ND | 4 | ND | 5 | 4 | 4 | 5 | ND | ND | ND | ND | ND | ND | ND | ND | ND | ND | ND | ND | ND | ND | 2.6 |
| 蔬菜类 Vegetables | 31 | 13 | 93 | 20 | 85 | 22 | 141 | 49 | 208 | 54 | 181 | 137 | 64 | 230 | 85 | 59 | 126 | 44 | 34 | 83 | 30 | 38 | 52 | 162 | 85.0 |
| 水果类 Fruits | 6 | 5 | 6 | 4 | ND | ND | 5 | 5 | ND | 4 | 4 | ND | 5 | 5 | 9 | 5 | ND | ND | 6 | 6 | 4 | 4 | 4 | 4 | 4.3 |
| 糖类 Sugar | 13 | 10 | 14 | 27 | 23 | 10 | 10 | 12 | 13 | 11 | 13 | 11 | 20 | 10 | 9 | 11 | 15 | 9 | 15 | 18 | 12 | 15 | 9 | 13 | 13.5 |
| 水及饮料类 Water and beverages | 6 | ND | 7 | ND | ND | ND | ND | 5 | 5 | ND | ND | ND | 7 | 5 | 10 | ND | 7 | 4 | 9 | 5 | ND | ND | ND | 5 | 4.1 |
| 酒类 Alcohol beverages | 13 | 8 | 8 | 8 | 7 | 7 | 13 | 10 | 4 | 13 | 8 | 7 | 7 | 11 | 7 | 14 | 19 | 9 | 13 | 18 | 14 | 9 | 8 | 6 | 10.0 |

注：未检出（ND）按 1/2 检出限（LOD）计

Note: values not detected (ND) were treated as being equal to half of the detection of limit (LOD)

附表 6-7 第六次中国总膳食研究膳食样品中 2-MCPD 酯的含量（单位：μg/kg）

Annexed Table 6-7　Levels of 2-MCPD esters in food samples from the 6$^{th}$ China TDS (Unit: μg/kg)

| 膳食类别<br>Category | 黑龙江<br>HL | 辽宁<br>LN | 河北<br>HE | 北京<br>BJ | 吉林<br>JL | 山西<br>SX | 陕西<br>SN | 河南<br>HA | 宁夏<br>NX | 内蒙古<br>NM | 青海<br>QH | 甘肃<br>GS | 上海<br>SH | 福建<br>FJ | 江西<br>JX | 江苏<br>JS | 浙江<br>ZJ | 山东<br>SD | 湖北<br>HB | 四川<br>SC | 广西<br>GX | 湖南<br>HN | 广东<br>GD | 贵州<br>GZ | 全国平均<br>AVG |
|---|---|---|---|---|---|---|---|---|---|---|---|---|---|---|---|---|---|---|---|---|---|---|---|---|---|
| 谷类 Cereals | ND | ND | ND | ND | ND | ND | ND | ND | ND | 8 | ND | ND | ND | ND | ND | 4 | ND | ND | ND | ND | ND | ND | ND | ND | 2.3 |

续表

| 膳食类别<br>Category | 黑龙江<br>HL | 辽宁<br>LN | 河北<br>HE | 北京<br>BJ | 吉林<br>JL | 山西<br>SX | 陕西<br>SN | 河南<br>HA | 宁夏<br>NX | 内蒙古<br>NM | 青海<br>QH | 甘肃<br>GS | 上海<br>SH | 福建<br>FJ | 江西<br>JX | 江苏<br>JS | 浙江<br>ZJ | 山东<br>SD | 湖北<br>HB | 四川<br>SC | 广西<br>GX | 湖南<br>HN | 广东<br>GD | 贵州<br>GZ | 全国平均<br>AVG |
|---|---|---|---|---|---|---|---|---|---|---|---|---|---|---|---|---|---|---|---|---|---|---|---|---|---|
| 豆类 Legumes | ND | ND | ND | ND | ND | ND | 16 | 5 | 11 | ND | 14 | 19 | 4 | 29 | 8 | 10 | ND | ND | 4 | 9 | 7 | 4 | 13 | 11 | 7.6 |
| 薯类 Potatoes | ND | ND | 15 | 8 | ND | ND | 39 | 4 | 47 | 5 | 74 | 60 | 15 | 15 | ND | 11 | 5 | 5 | 9 | 13 | 6 | ND | ND | 32 | 15.6 |
| 肉类 Meats | ND | ND | 11 | 7 | 7 | ND | 46 | 6 | 40 | 8 | 47 | 56 | 12 | 24 | 10 | 21 | 12 | 5 | 8 | 23 | 13 | 12 | 8 | 20 | 16.8 |
| 蛋类 Eggs | 4 | ND | 34 | 15 | 72 | 4 | 37 | 11 | 89 | 29 | 22 | 47 | 16 | 43 | 20 | 21 | 837 | 7 | ND | 19 | 4 | 10 | ND | 65 | 58.8 |
| 水产类 Aquatic foods | ND | ND | 4 | 6 | 29 | ND | 23 | ND | 21 | 4 | 25 | 53 | 10 | 114 | 11 | 12 | 12 | 7 | ND | 12 | 7 | 9 | 11 | 19 | 16.6 |
| 乳类 Dairy products | ND | ND | ND | ND | ND | ND | ND | ND | ND | ND | ND | ND | ND | ND | ND | ND | ND | ND | ND | ND | ND | ND | ND | ND | ND |
| 蔬菜类 Vegetables | 5 | ND | 20 | 5 | 14 | 4 | 51 | 6 | 50 | 10 | 39 | 51 | 17 | 102 | 21 | 24 | 23 | 10 | 9 | 27 | 11 | 9 | 18 | 32 | 23.3 |
| 水果类 Fruits | ND | ND | ND | ND | ND | ND | ND | ND | ND | ND | ND | ND | ND | ND | ND | ND | ND | ND | ND | ND | ND | ND | ND | ND | ND |
| 糖类 Sugar | ND | ND | ND | ND | 4 | ND | ND | ND | ND | ND | ND | ND | 4 | ND | ND | ND | ND | ND | ND | ND | ND | ND | ND | ND | 2.2 |
| 水及饮料类 Water and beverages | ND | ND | ND | ND | ND | ND | ND | ND | ND | ND | ND | ND | ND | ND | ND | ND | ND | ND | ND | ND | ND | ND | ND | ND | ND |
| 酒类 Alcohol beverages | ND | ND | ND | ND | ND | ND | ND | ND | ND | ND | ND | ND | ND | ND | ND | ND | ND | ND | ND | ND | ND | ND | ND | ND | ND |

注：未检出（ND）按 1/2 检出限（LOD）计

Note: values not detected (ND) were treated as being equal to half of the detection of limit (LOD)

附表 6-8 第六次中国总膳食研究 3-MCPD 酯的膳食摄入量 [单位: μg/(kg bw·d)]

Annexed Table 6-8 Dietary intakes of 3-MCPD esters from the 6<sup>th</sup> China TDS [Unit: μg/(kg bw·d)]

| 膳食类别 Category | 黑龙江 HL | 辽宁 LN | 河北 HE | 北京 BJ | 吉林 JL | 山西 SX | 陕西 SN | 河南 HA | 宁夏 NX | 内蒙古 NM | 青海 QH | 甘肃 GS | 上海 SH | 福建 FJ | 江西 JX | 江苏 JS | 浙江 ZJ | 山东 SD | 湖北 HB | 四川 SC | 广西 GX | 湖南 HN | 广东 GD | 贵州 GZ | 全国平均 AVG |
|---|---|---|---|---|---|---|---|---|---|---|---|---|---|---|---|---|---|---|---|---|---|---|---|---|---|
| 谷类 Cereals | 0.135 | 0.233 | 0.278 | 0.213 | 0.110 | 0.133 | 0.165 | 0.138 | 0.112 | 0.405 | 0.193 | 0.074 | 0.093 | 0.162 | 0.233 | 0.293 | 0.080 | 0.226 | 0.103 | 0.122 | 0.088 | 0.027 | 0.088 | 0.190 | 0.162 |
| 豆类 Legumes | 0.014 | 0.037 | 0.016 | 0.016 | 0.034 | 0.023 | 0.068 | 0.034 | 0.035 | 0.016 | 0.006 | 0.044 | 0.041 | 0.095 | 0.037 | 0.043 | 0.038 | 0.010 | 0.021 | 0.043 | 0.012 | 0.028 | 0.017 | 0.063 | 0.033 |
| 薯类 Potatoes | 0.022 | 0.009 | 0.062 | 0.045 | 0.017 | 0.021 | 0.225 | 0.053 | 0.429 | 0.067 | 0.379 | 0.445 | 0.027 | 0.034 | 0.007 | 0.019 | 0.018 | 0.009 | 0.050 | 0.038 | 0.005 | 0.015 | 0.003 | 0.108 | 0.088 |
| 肉类 Meats | 0.028 | 0.021 | 0.033 | 0.052 | 0.043 | 0.039 | 0.089 | 0.034 | 0.245 | 0.136 | 0.214 | 0.107 | 0.081 | 0.141 | 0.096 | 0.079 | 0.095 | 0.048 | 0.043 | 0.246 | 0.137 | 0.141 | 0.050 | 0.211 | 0.100 |
| 蛋类 Eggs | 0.034 | 0.012 | 0.096 | 0.043 | 0.189 | 0.010 | 0.046 | 0.026 | 0.131 | 0.061 | 0.046 | 0.069 | 0.046 | 0.034 | 0.031 | 0.032 | 2.058 | 0.039 | 0.009 | 0.018 | 0.004 | 0.016 | 0.004 | 0.058 | 0.130 |
| 水产类 Aquatic foods | 0.005 | 0.001 | 0.003 | 0.006 | 0.027 | 0.001 | 0.004 | 0.001 | 0.004 | 0.002 | 0.007 | 0.010 | 0.036 | 0.264 | 0.026 | 0.021 | 0.031 | 0.011 | 0.010 | 0.006 | 0.034 | 0.044 | 0.024 | 0.006 | 0.024 |
| 乳类 Dairy products | <0.001 | 0.003 | 0.001 | 0.003 | 0.002 | 0.001 | 0.002 | 0.001 | 0.001 | 0.003 | 0.002 | <0.001 | 0.002 | 0.001 | 0.001 | 0.001 | 0.001 | 0.001 | <0.001 | <0.001 | 0.001 | 0.001 | 0.001 | 0.001 | 0.001 |
| 蔬菜类 Vegetables | 0.194 | 0.072 | 0.437 | 0.126 | 0.529 | 0.110 | 0.663 | 0.218 | 0.516 | 0.227 | 0.892 | 0.539 | 0.407 | 1.464 | 0.609 | 0.415 | 1.083 | 0.287 | 0.223 | 0.402 | 0.172 | 0.332 | 0.201 | 1.081 | 0.467 |
| 水果类 Fruits | 0.006 | 0.007 | 0.004 | 0.008 | 0.003 | 0.001 | 0.003 | 0.002 | 0.003 | 0.007 | 0.001 | 0.001 | 0.006 | 0.005 | 0.008 | 0.002 | 0.002 | 0.002 | 0.002 | 0.002 | 0.004 | 0.004 | 0.002 | 0.002 | 0.004 |
| 糖类 Sugar | <0.001 | <0.001 | <0.001 | 0.001 | <0.001 | <0.001 | <0.001 | <0.001 | <0.001 | <0.001 | <0.001 | <0.001 | 0.002 | <0.001 | <0.001 | <0.001 | <0.001 | <0.001 | <0.001 | <0.001 | <0.001 | <0.001 | <0.001 | <0.001 | 0.001 |
| 水及饮料类 Water and beverages | 0.116 | 0.016 | 0.086 | 0.035 | 0.041 | 0.024 | 0.011 | 0.095 | 0.041 | 0.082 | 0.020 | 0.037 | 0.078 | 0.069 | 0.188 | 0.032 | 0.087 | 0.114 | 0.041 | 0.025 | 0.041 | 0.034 | 0.038 | 0.099 | 0.060 |

续表

| 膳食类别 Category | 黑龙江 HL | 辽宁 LN | 河北 HE | 北京 BJ | 吉林 JL | 山西 SX | 陕西 SN | 河南 HA | 宁夏 NX | 内蒙古 NM | 青海 QH | 甘肃 GS | 上海 SH | 福建 FJ | 江西 JX | 江苏 JS | 浙江 ZJ | 山东 SD | 湖北 HB | 四川 SC | 广西 GX | 湖南 HN | 广东 GD | 贵州 GZ | 全国平均 AVG |
|---|---|---|---|---|---|---|---|---|---|---|---|---|---|---|---|---|---|---|---|---|---|---|---|---|---|
| 酒类 Alcohol beverages | 0.005 | 0.004 | 0.001 | 0.003 | 0.001 | <0.001 | <0.001 | 0.001 | <0.001 | 0.004 | 0.001 | <0.001 | 0.003 | 0.002 | 0.002 | 0.008 | 0.019 | 0.016 | 0.003 | 0.001 | 0.007 | 0.002 | <0.001 | <0.001 | 0.004 |
| 合计 SUM | 0.559 | 0.415 | 1.017 | 0.551 | 0.996 | 0.364 | 1.283 | 0.603 | 1.517 | 1.010 | 1.761 | 1.328 | 0.822 | 2.272 | 1.238 | 0.946 | 3.513 | 0.763 | 0.506 | 0.902 | 0.505 | 0.644 | 0.429 | 1.820 | 1.074 |

注：摄入量合计时，摄入量<0.001 的结果按 0 计
Note: values <0.001 were treated as 0

附表 6-9　第六次中国总膳食研究 2-MCPD 酯的膳食摄入量 [单位：μg/(kg bw·d)]
Annexed Table 6-9　Dietary intakes of 2-MCPD esters from the 6th China TDS [Unit: μg/(kg bw·d)]

| 膳食类别 Category | 黑龙江 HL | 辽宁 LN | 河北 HE | 北京 BJ | 吉林 JL | 山西 SX | 陕西 SN | 河南 HA | 宁夏 NX | 内蒙古 NM | 青海 QH | 甘肃 GS | 上海 SH | 福建 FJ | 江西 JX | 江苏 JS | 浙江 ZJ | 山东 SD | 湖北 HB | 四川 SC | 广西 GX | 湖南 HN | 广东 GD | 贵州 GZ | 全国平均 AVG |
|---|---|---|---|---|---|---|---|---|---|---|---|---|---|---|---|---|---|---|---|---|---|---|---|---|---|
| 谷类 Cereals | 0.034 | 0.031 | 0.040 | 0.036 | 0.024 | 0.053 | 0.047 | 0.046 | 0.037 | 0.135 | 0.055 | 0.037 | 0.019 | 0.030 | 0.027 | 0.062 | 0.027 | 0.050 | 0.023 | 0.049 | 0.044 | 0.027 | 0.020 | 0.035 | 0.041 |
| 豆类 Legumes | 0.002 | 0.005 | 0.002 | 0.004 | 0.003 | 0.002 | 0.024 | 0.006 | 0.007 | 0.001 | 0.002 | 0.013 | 0.009 | 0.037 | 0.011 | 0.015 | 0.005 | 0.002 | 0.005 | 0.011 | 0.005 | 0.006 | 0.007 | 0.021 | 0.009 |
| 薯类 Potatoes | 0.003 | 0.003 | 0.017 | 0.009 | 0.004 | 0.005 | 0.088 | 0.006 | 0.085 | 0.010 | 0.124 | 0.141 | 0.009 | 0.011 | 0.001 | 0.007 | 0.003 | 0.002 | 0.013 | 0.013 | 0.002 | 0.002 | 0.001 | 0.021 | 0.024 |
| 肉类 Meats | 0.002 | 0.003 | 0.009 | 0.009 | 0.007 | 0.005 | 0.028 | 0.005 | 0.031 | 0.010 | 0.054 | 0.031 | 0.021 | 0.034 | 0.015 | 0.031 | 0.024 | 0.008 | 0.007 | 0.047 | 0.031 | 0.029 | 0.017 | 0.035 | 0.021 |
| 蛋类 Eggs | 0.003 | 0.002 | 0.022 | 0.011 | 0.053 | 0.002 | 0.015 | 0.005 | 0.027 | 0.018 | 0.006 | 0.019 | 0.011 | 0.017 | 0.008 | 0.010 | 0.392 | 0.006 | 0.001 | 0.005 | 0.001 | 0.004 | 0.001 | 0.017 | 0.027 |
| 水产类 Aquatic foods | 0.001 | 0.001 | 0.001 | 0.002 | 0.005 | 0.000 | 0.001 | 0.005 | 0.001 | 0.001 | 0.002 | 0.002 | 0.011 | 0.121 | 0.008 | 0.008 | 0.010 | 0.003 | 0.001 | 0.002 | 0.011 | 0.010 | 0.009 | 0.001 | 0.009 |
| 乳类 Dairy products | <0.001 | <0.001 | <0.001 | <0.001 | <0.001 | <0.001 | <0.001 | <0.001 | <0.001 | <0.001 | <0.001 | <0.001 | <0.001 | <0.001 | <0.001 | <0.001 | <0.001 | <0.001 | <0.001 | <0.001 | <0.001 | <0.001 | <0.001 | <0.001 | <0.001 |

续表

| 膳食类别 Category | 黑龙江 HL | 辽宁 LN | 河北 HE | 北京 BJ | 吉林 JL | 山西 SX | 陕西 SN | 河南 HA | 宁夏 NX | 内蒙古 NM | 青海 QH | 甘肃 GS | 上海 SH | 福建 FJ | 江西 JX | 江苏 JS | 浙江 ZJ | 山东 SD | 湖北 HB | 四川 SC | 广西 GX | 湖南 HN | 广东 GD | 贵州 GZ | 全国平均 AVG |
|---|---|---|---|---|---|---|---|---|---|---|---|---|---|---|---|---|---|---|---|---|---|---|---|---|---|
| 蔬菜类 Vegetables | 0.031 | 0.011 | 0.094 | 0.031 | 0.087 | 0.020 | 0.240 | 0.027 | 0.124 | 0.042 | 0.192 | 0.201 | 0.108 | 0.649 | 0.151 | 0.169 | 0.198 | 0.065 | 0.059 | 0.131 | 0.063 | 0.079 | 0.070 | 0.214 | 0.127 |
| 水果类 Fruits | <0.001 | <0.001 | <0.001 | <0.001 | <0.001 | <0.001 | <0.001 | <0.001 | <0.001 | <0.001 | <0.001 | <0.001 | <0.001 | <0.001 | <0.001 | <0.001 | <0.001 | <0.001 | <0.001 | <0.001 | <0.001 | <0.001 | <0.001 | <0.001 | <0.001 |
| 糖类 Sugar | <0.001 | <0.001 | <0.001 | <0.001 | <0.001 | <0.001 | 0.001 | <0.001 | <0.001 | <0.001 | <0.001 | <0.001 | <0.001 | <0.001 | <0.001 | <0.001 | <0.001 | <0.001 | <0.001 | <0.001 | <0.001 | <0.001 | <0.001 | <0.001 | <0.001 |
| 水及饮料类 Water and beverages | <0.001 | <0.001 | <0.001 | <0.001 | <0.001 | <0.001 | <0.001 | <0.001 | <0.001 | <0.001 | <0.001 | <0.001 | <0.001 | <0.001 | <0.001 | <0.001 | <0.001 | <0.001 | <0.001 | <0.001 | <0.001 | <0.001 | <0.001 | <0.001 | <0.001 |
| 酒类 Alcohol beverages | <0.001 | <0.001 | <0.001 | <0.001 | <0.001 | <0.001 | <0.001 | <0.001 | <0.001 | <0.001 | <0.001 | <0.001 | <0.001 | <0.001 | <0.001 | <0.001 | <0.001 | <0.001 | <0.001 | <0.001 | <0.001 | <0.001 | <0.001 | <0.001 | <0.001 |
| 合计 SUM | 0.076 | 0.056 | 0.184 | 0.101 | 0.184 | 0.087 | 0.445 | 0.095 | 0.312 | 0.217 | 0.435 | 0.444 | 0.187 | 0.898 | 0.220 | 0.301 | 0.659 | 0.136 | 0.109 | 0.258 | 0.156 | 0.156 | 0.123 | 0.343 | 0.258 |

注：摄入量合计时，摄入量<0.001 的结果按 0 计

Note: values <0.001 were treated as 0

附表 6-10 第六次中国总膳食研究 3-MCPD 酯的膳食来源（单位：%）

Annexed Table 6-10　Dietary sources of 3-MCPD esters from the 6$^{th}$ China TDS (Unit: %)

| 膳食类别 Category | 黑龙江 HL | 辽宁 LN | 河北 HE | 北京 BJ | 吉林 JL | 山西 SX | 陕西 SN | 河南 HA | 宁夏 NX | 内蒙古 NM | 青海 QH | 甘肃 GS | 上海 SH | 福建 FJ | 江西 JX | 江苏 JS | 浙江 ZJ | 山东 SD | 湖北 HB | 四川 SC | 广西 GX | 湖南 HN | 广东 GD | 贵州 GZ | 全国平均 AVG |
|---|---|---|---|---|---|---|---|---|---|---|---|---|---|---|---|---|---|---|---|---|---|---|---|---|---|
| 谷类 Cereals | 24.1 | 56.1 | 27.3 | 38.7 | 11.0 | 36.5 | 12.9 | 22.8 | 7.4 | 40.1 | 11.0 | 5.6 | 11.3 | 7.1 | 18.8 | 31.0 | 2.3 | 29.6 | 20.4 | 13.5 | 17.4 | 4.2 | 20.6 | 10.4 | 15.1 |
| 豆类 Legumes | 2.4 | 8.9 | 1.6 | 2.9 | 3.4 | 6.4 | 5.3 | 5.7 | 2.3 | 1.5 | 0.4 | 3.3 | 5.0 | 4.2 | 3.0 | 4.5 | 1.1 | 1.3 | 4.2 | 4.8 | 2.4 | 4.4 | 4.0 | 3.5 | 3.1 |

续表

| 膳食类别 Category | 黑龙江 HL | 辽宁 LN | 河北 HE | 北京 BJ | 吉林 JL | 山西 SX | 陕西 SN | 河南 HA | 宁夏 NX | 内蒙古 NM | 青海 QH | 甘肃 GS | 上海 SH | 福建 FJ | 江西 JX | 江苏 JS | 浙江 ZJ | 山东 SD | 湖北 HB | 四川 SC | 广西 GX | 湖南 HN | 广东 GD | 贵州 GZ | 全国平均 AVG |
|---|---|---|---|---|---|---|---|---|---|---|---|---|---|---|---|---|---|---|---|---|---|---|---|---|---|
| 薯类 Potatoes | 3.9 | 2.1 | 6.1 | 8.2 | 1.7 | 5.8 | 17.6 | 8.7 | 28.3 | 6.7 | 21.5 | 33.5 | 3.3 | 1.5 | 0.5 | 2.0 | 0.5 | 1.2 | 9.8 | 4.2 | 1.0 | 2.3 | 0.7 | 5.9 | 8.2 |
| 肉类 Meats | 5.0 | 5.0 | 3.2 | 9.4 | 4.3 | 10.7 | 6.9 | 5.6 | 16.2 | 13.4 | 12.2 | 8.0 | 9.8 | 6.2 | 7.8 | 8.4 | 2.7 | 6.3 | 8.5 | 27.2 | 27.0 | 21.9 | 11.7 | 11.6 | 9.3 |
| 蛋类 Eggs | 6.0 | 2.9 | 9.4 | 7.8 | 19.0 | 2.6 | 3.6 | 4.4 | 8.6 | 6.0 | 2.6 | 5.2 | 5.6 | 1.5 | 2.5 | 3.4 | 58.6 | 5.1 | 1.8 | 2.0 | 0.9 | 2.5 | 1.0 | 3.2 | 12.1 |
| 水产类 Aquatic foods | 0.8 | 0.4 | 0.3 | 1.2 | 2.7 | 0.4 | 0.3 | 0.2 | 0.3 | 0.2 | 0.4 | 0.8 | 4.4 | 11.6 | 2.1 | 2.2 | 0.9 | 1.4 | 2.0 | 0.6 | 6.7 | 6.8 | 5.5 | 0.3 | 2.3 |
| 乳类 Dairy products | 0.1 | 0.7 | 0.1 | 0.5 | 0.2 | 0.4 | 0.1 | 0.2 | 0.1 | 0.3 | 0.1 | 0.0 | 0.3 | 0.1 | 0.1 | 0.1 | 0.0 | 0.1 | 0.0 | 0.0 | 0.1 | 0.1 | 0.3 | 0.0 | 0.1 |
| 蔬菜类 Vegetables | 34.8 | 17.5 | 43.0 | 22.8 | 53.1 | 30.3 | 51.7 | 36.2 | 34.0 | 22.5 | 50.7 | 40.6 | 49.5 | 64.4 | 49.2 | 43.9 | 30.8 | 37.6 | 44.1 | 44.5 | 34.0 | 51.5 | 47.0 | 59.4 | 43.5 |
| 水果类 Fruits | 1.1 | 1.6 | 0.4 | 1.4 | 0.3 | 0.3 | 0.2 | 0.3 | 0.2 | 0.7 | 0.1 | 0.1 | 0.7 | 0.2 | 0.7 | 0.2 | 0.1 | 0.2 | 0.4 | 0.2 | 0.8 | 0.6 | 0.4 | 0.1 | 0.3 |
| 糖类 Sugar | 0.1 | 0.0 | 0.0 | 0.2 | 0.0 | 0.0 | 0.5 | 0.0 | 0.0 | 0.0 | 0.0 | 0.0 | 0.3 | 0.0 | 0.0 | 0.0 | 0.0 | 0.0 | 0.0 | 0.0 | 0.0 | 0.0 | 0.0 | 0.0 | 0.0 |
| 水及饮料类 Water and beverages | 20.8 | 3.8 | 8.5 | 6.4 | 4.1 | 6.5 | 0.9 | 15.7 | 2.7 | 8.1 | 1.1 | 2.8 | 9.5 | 3.0 | 15.1 | 3.4 | 2.5 | 15.0 | 8.0 | 2.8 | 8.2 | 5.2 | 8.8 | 5.5 | 5.6 |
| 酒类 Alcohol beverages | 0.8 | 1.0 | 0.1 | 0.6 | 0.1 | 0.0 | 0.0 | 0.1 | 0.0 | 0.4 | 0.0 | 0.0 | 0.3 | 0.1 | 0.2 | 0.9 | 0.5 | 2.1 | 0.6 | 0.2 | 1.4 | 0.4 | 0.0 | 0.0 | 0.3 |

附表 6-11 第六次中国总膳食研究 2-MCPD 酯的膳食来源（单位：%）

Annexed Table 6-11 Dietary sources of 2-MCPD esters from the 6th China TDS (Unit: %)

| 膳食类别 Category | 黑龙江 HL | 辽宁 LN | 河北 HE | 北京 BJ | 吉林 JL | 山西 SX | 陕西 SN | 河南 HA | 宁夏 NX | 内蒙古 NM | 青海 QH | 甘肃 GS | 上海 SH | 福建 FJ | 江西 JX | 江苏 JS | 浙江 ZJ | 山东 SD | 湖北 HB | 四川 SC | 广西 GX | 湖南 HN | 广东 GD | 贵州 GZ | 全国平均 AVG |
|---|---|---|---|---|---|---|---|---|---|---|---|---|---|---|---|---|---|---|---|---|---|---|---|---|---|
| 谷类 Cereals | 44.4 | 55.8 | 21.5 | 35.2 | 13.3 | 61.1 | 10.6 | 48.2 | 12.0 | 62.3 | 12.7 | 8.3 | 9.9 | 3.3 | 12.5 | 20.5 | 4.1 | 36.8 | 21.1 | 18.9 | 28.1 | 17.3 | 15.9 | 10.1 | 15.9 |
| 豆类 Legumes | 2.8 | 9.5 | 1.2 | 3.5 | 1.8 | 2.8 | 5.3 | 6.4 | 2.3 | 0.6 | 0.4 | 2.9 | 4.6 | 4.1 | 4.8 | 5.1 | 0.7 | 1.5 | 4.3 | 4.3 | 3.1 | 3.8 | 5.3 | 6.2 | 3.3 |
| 薯类 Potatoes | 3.9 | 5.4 | 9.2 | 8.5 | 2.1 | 5.4 | 19.8 | 5.8 | 27.2 | 4.6 | 28.5 | 31.8 | 4.6 | 1.2 | 0.5 | 2.3 | 0.5 | 1.1 | 11.7 | 5.2 | 1.0 | 1.5 | 0.7 | 6.2 | 9.4 |
| 肉类 Meats | 3.0 | 4.7 | 4.9 | 9.2 | 4.1 | 5.3 | 6.3 | 5.8 | 9.9 | 4.4 | 12.3 | 7.0 | 11.3 | 3.8 | 6.8 | 10.3 | 3.7 | 6.1 | 6.6 | 18.4 | 19.9 | 18.4 | 13.6 | 10.1 | 8.0 |
| 蛋类 Eggs | 3.4 | 3.1 | 11.8 | 10.8 | 28.7 | 2.1 | 3.4 | 5.5 | 8.6 | 8.3 | 1.5 | 4.3 | 5.8 | 1.9 | 3.5 | 3.3 | 59.5 | 4.5 | 0.9 | 1.9 | 0.6 | 2.4 | 0.6 | 4.9 | 10.6 |
| 水产类 Aquatic foods | 1.1 | 1.4 | 0.4 | 1.6 | 2.8 | 0.3 | 0.3 | 0.2 | 0.3 | 0.3 | 0.4 | 0.5 | 5.8 | 13.5 | 3.5 | 2.5 | 1.5 | 2.2 | 1.2 | 0.6 | 6.9 | 6.1 | 7.5 | 0.4 | 3.4 |
| 乳类 Dairy products | 0.0 | 0.0 | 0.0 | 0.0 | 0.0 | 0.0 | 0.0 | 0.0 | 0.0 | 0.0 | 0.0 | 0.0 | 0.3 | 0.0 | 0.0 | 0.0 | 0.0 | 0.0 | 0.0 | 0.0 | 0.0 | 0.0 | 0.0 | 0.0 | 0.0 |
| 蔬菜类 Vegetables | 41.3 | 20.1 | 51.0 | 31.1 | 47.3 | 23.0 | 54.0 | 28.1 | 39.7 | 19.4 | 44.2 | 45.2 | 57.8 | 72.3 | 68.4 | 56.0 | 30.0 | 47.8 | 54.3 | 50.7 | 40.3 | 50.4 | 56.4 | 62.2 | 49.4 |
| 水果类 Fruits | 0.0 | 0.0 | 0.0 | 0.0 | 0.0 | 0.0 | 0.0 | 0.0 | 0.0 | 0.0 | 0.0 | 0.0 | 0.0 | 0.0 | 0.0 | 0.0 | 0.0 | 0.0 | 0.0 | 0.0 | 0.0 | 0.0 | 0.0 | 0.0 | 0.0 |
| 糖类 Sugar | 0.1 | 0.0 | 0.0 | 0.1 | 0.0 | 0.0 | 0.3 | 0.0 | 0.0 | 0.0 | 0.0 | 0.0 | 0.0 | 0.0 | 0.0 | 0.0 | 0.0 | 0.0 | 0.0 | 0.0 | 0.0 | 0.0 | 0.0 | 0.0 | 0.0 |
| 水及饮料类 Water and beverages | 0.0 | 0.0 | 0.0 | 0.0 | 0.0 | 0.0 | 0.0 | 0.0 | 0.0 | 0.0 | 0.0 | 0.0 | 0.0 | 0.0 | 0.0 | 0.0 | 0.0 | 0.0 | 0.0 | 0.0 | 0.0 | 0.0 | 0.0 | 0.0 | 0.0 |
| 酒类 Alcohol beverages | 0.0 | 0.0 | 0.0 | 0.0 | 0.0 | 0.0 | 0.0 | 0.0 | 0.0 | 0.0 | 0.0 | 0.0 | 0.0 | 0.0 | 0.0 | 0.0 | 0.0 | 0.0 | 0.0 | 0.0 | 0.0 | 0.0 | 0.0 | 0.0 | 0.0 |

附表 6-12 第六次中国总膳食研究混合膳食样品中缩水甘油酯的含量（单位：μg/kg）

Annexed Table 6-12 Levels of glycidyl fatty acid esters in food samples from the 6th China TDS (Unit: μg/kg)

| 膳食类别 Category | 黑龙江 HL | 辽宁 LN | 河北 HE | 北京 BJ | 吉林 JL | 山西 SX | 陕西 SN | 河南 HA | 宁夏 NX | 内蒙古 NM | 青海 QH | 甘肃 GS | 上海 SH | 福建 FJ | 江西 JX | 江苏 JS | 浙江 ZJ | 山东 SD | 湖北 HB | 四川 SC | 广西 GX | 湖南 HN | 广东 GD | 贵州 GZ | 全国平均 AVG |
|---|---|---|---|---|---|---|---|---|---|---|---|---|---|---|---|---|---|---|---|---|---|---|---|---|---|
| 谷类 Cereals | 4 | ND | 10 | 4 | 5 | ND | 4 | 5 | 5 | 16 | ND | ND | 4 | ND | 5 | 5 | ND | ND | 4 | ND | ND | ND | ND | 9 | 4.3 |
| 豆类 Legumes | 9 | 19 | 14 | 5 | 9 | 41 | 106 | 14 | 42 | 16 | 30 | 80 | 20 | 30 | 27 | 32 | 10 | 23 | 18 | 28 | 9 | 14 | 29 | 18 | 26.8 |
| 薯类 Potatoes | 18 | 7 | 31 | 18 | 6 | 8 | 152 | 15 | 134 | 12 | 92 | 146 | 59 | 19 | 7 | 19 | 14 | 16 | 15 | 33 | 10 | 4 | ND | 65 | 37.6 |
| 肉类 Meats | 60 | 22 | 48 | 35 | 55 | 22 | 196 | 32 | 107 | 60 | 81 | 145 | 64 | 117 | 117 | 57 | 64 | 46 | 53 | 82 | 70 | 72 | 22 | 78 | 71.0 |
| 蛋类 Eggs | 28 | 8 | 64 | 26 | 87 | 12 | 115 | 35 | 202 | 51 | 61 | 107 | 42 | 36 | 43 | 47 | 1294 | 31 | 21 | 30 | 20 | 32 | 5 | 77 | 103.1 |
| 水产类 Aquatic foods | 20 | 7 | 14 | 12 | 51 | 9 | 114 | 22 | 35 | 19 | 61 | 59 | 46 | 111 | 47 | 34 | 42 | 27 | 19 | 40 | 16 | 40 | 38 | 42 | 38.5 |
| 乳类 Dairy products | ND | ND | 4 | 5 | ND | ND | ND | 5 | ND | ND | ND | 6 | ND | 4 | ND | ND | ND | 4 | ND | ND | 5 | ND | 4 | 5 | 2.9 |
| 蔬菜类 Vegetables | 38 | 20 | 157 | 17 | 74 | 14 | 267 | 137 | 198 | 27 | 93 | 161 | 88 | 81 | 60 | 54 | 67 | 104 | 19 | 67 | 20 | 14 | 52 | 60 | 78.7 |
| 水果类 Fruits | ND | ND | ND | ND | ND | ND | ND | ND | ND | ND | ND | ND | ND | ND | ND | ND | ND | ND | ND | ND | ND | ND | ND | ND | ND |
| 糖类 Sugar | 5 | 5 | 6 | 13 | 44 | ND | ND | 5 | ND | 6 | 5 | 6 | 14 | 4 | ND | 5 | 16 | 7 | 17 | 19 | 4 | 11 | 4 | 4 | 9.0 |
| 水及饮料类 Water and beverages | 6 | ND | 8 | ND | ND | ND | ND | ND | 6 | ND | ND | ND | ND | 4 | 6 | 6 | ND | ND | 6 | ND | ND | ND | ND | 10 | 3.3 |
| 酒类 Alcohol beverages | 6 | 4 | 5 | 5 | 5 | 4 | 15 | 5 | ND | 12 | ND | 4 | 4 | 5 | 4 | 6 | 16 | 4 | 6 | 30 | 9 | 4 | 4 | ND | 6.8 |

注：未检出（ND）按 1/2 检出限（LOD）计

Note: values not detected (ND) were treated as being equal to half of the detection of limit (LOD)

附表 6-13 第六次中国总膳食研究缩水甘油酯的膳食摄入量 [单位: μg/(kg bw·d)]

Annexed Table 6-13 Dietary intakes of glycidyl fatty acid esters from the 6th China TDS [Unit: μg/(kg bw·d)]

| 膳食类别 Category | 黑龙江 HL | 辽宁 LN | 河北 HE | 北京 BJ | 吉林 JL | 山西 SX | 陕西 SN | 河南 HA | 宁夏 NX | 内蒙古 NM | 青海 QH | 甘肃 GS | 上海 SH | 福建 FJ | 江西 JX | 江苏 JS | 浙江 ZJ | 山东 SD | 湖北 HB | 四川 SC | 广西 GX | 湖南 HN | 广东 GD | 贵州 GZ | 全国平均 AVG |
|---|---|---|---|---|---|---|---|---|---|---|---|---|---|---|---|---|---|---|---|---|---|---|---|---|---|
| 谷类 Cereals | 0.067 | 0.031 | 0.199 | 0.071 | 0.061 | 0.053 | 0.094 | 0.115 | 0.094 | 0.270 | 0.055 | 0.037 | 0.037 | 0.030 | 0.068 | 0.077 | 0.027 | 0.050 | 0.046 | 0.049 | 0.044 | 0.027 | 0.020 | 0.156 | 0.074 |
| 豆类 Legumes | 0.009 | 0.050 | 0.015 | 0.009 | 0.015 | 0.050 | 0.157 | 0.017 | 0.028 | 0.011 | 0.004 | 0.054 | 0.043 | 0.038 | 0.036 | 0.049 | 0.024 | 0.024 | 0.021 | 0.034 | 0.006 | 0.021 | 0.015 | 0.035 | 0.032 |
| 薯类 Potatoes | 0.026 | 0.010 | 0.035 | 0.019 | 0.011 | 0.019 | 0.343 | 0.021 | 0.243 | 0.024 | 0.154 | 0.344 | 0.034 | 0.014 | 0.004 | 0.012 | 0.008 | 0.012 | 0.021 | 0.034 | 0.003 | 0.005 | 0.001 | 0.043 | 0.060 |
| 肉类 Meats | 0.067 | 0.029 | 0.039 | 0.047 | 0.059 | 0.050 | 0.120 | 0.029 | 0.083 | 0.071 | 0.092 | 0.080 | 0.112 | 0.165 | 0.176 | 0.084 | 0.129 | 0.076 | 0.048 | 0.169 | 0.168 | 0.173 | 0.046 | 0.136 | 0.094 |
| 蛋类 Eggs | 0.018 | 0.007 | 0.041 | 0.019 | 0.064 | 0.005 | 0.047 | 0.017 | 0.061 | 0.032 | 0.018 | 0.044 | 0.028 | 0.014 | 0.016 | 0.022 | 0.607 | 0.027 | 0.010 | 0.008 | 0.005 | 0.012 | 0.002 | 0.020 | 0.048 |
| 水产类 Aquatic foods | 0.009 | 0.003 | 0.002 | 0.003 | 0.009 | 0.001 | 0.007 | 0.002 | 0.001 | 0.003 | 0.004 | 0.003 | 0.050 | 0.118 | 0.033 | 0.021 | 0.035 | 0.011 | 0.012 | 0.005 | 0.025 | 0.043 | 0.032 | 0.003 | 0.018 |
| 乳类 Dairy products | <0.001 | 0.001 | 0.002 | 0.007 | 0.001 | 0.001 | 0.001 | 0.002 | <0.001 | 0.001 | 0.002 | 0.001 | 0.002 | 0.001 | 0.001 | 0.001 | 0.001 | 0.001 | <0.001 | <0.001 | <0.001 | 0.001 | 0.002 | 0.002 | 0.001 |
| 蔬菜类 Vegetables | 0.238 | 0.111 | 0.738 | 0.107 | 0.460 | 0.070 | 1.256 | 0.611 | 0.491 | 0.114 | 0.458 | 0.634 | 0.560 | 0.515 | 0.430 | 0.380 | 0.576 | 0.678 | 0.125 | 0.324 | 0.114 | 0.122 | 0.201 | 0.401 | 0.405 |
| 水果类 Fruits | <0.001 | <0.001 | <0.001 | <0.001 | <0.001 | <0.001 | <0.001 | <0.001 | <0.001 | <0.001 | <0.001 | <0.001 | <0.001 | <0.001 | <0.001 | <0.001 | <0.001 | <0.001 | <0.001 | <0.001 | <0.001 | <0.001 | <0.001 | <0.001 | <0.001 |
| 糖类 Sugar | <0.001 | <0.001 | <0.001 | <0.001 | <0.001 | <0.001 | <0.001 | <0.001 | <0.001 | <0.001 | <0.001 | <0.001 | 0.002 | <0.001 | <0.001 | <0.001 | <0.001 | <0.001 | <0.001 | <0.001 | <0.001 | <0.001 | <0.001 | <0.001 | <0.001 |
| 水及饮料类 Water and beverages | 0.116 | 0.016 | 0.098 | 0.035 | 0.041 | 0.024 | 0.011 | 0.038 | 0.049 | 0.082 | 0.020 | 0.037 | 0.022 | 0.055 | 0.113 | 0.096 | 0.025 | 0.057 | 0.009 | 0.010 | 0.041 | 0.034 | 0.038 | 0.199 | 0.053 |

续表

| 膳食类别 Category | 黑龙江 HL | 辽宁 LN | 河北 HE | 北京 BJ | 吉林 JL | 山西 SX | 陕西 SN | 河南 HA | 宁夏 NX | 内蒙古 NM | 青海 QH | 甘肃 GS | 上海 SH | 福建 FJ | 江西 JX | 江苏 JS | 浙江 ZJ | 山东 SD | 湖北 HB | 四川 SC | 广西 GX | 湖南 HN | 广东 GD | 贵州 GZ | 全国平均 AVG |
|---|---|---|---|---|---|---|---|---|---|---|---|---|---|---|---|---|---|---|---|---|---|---|---|---|---|
| 酒类 Alcohol beverages | 0.002 | 0.002 | 0.001 | 0.002 | 0.001 | <0.001 | <0.001 | <0.001 | <0.001 | 0.004 | <0.001 | <0.001 | 0.001 | 0.001 | 0.001 | 0.004 | 0.016 | 0.007 | 0.001 | 0.002 | 0.005 | 0.001 | <0.001 | <0.001 | 0.002 |
| 合计 SUM | 0.555 | 0.261 | 1.171 | 0.320 | 0.723 | 0.274 | 2.039 | 0.850 | 1.050 | 0.611 | 0.807 | 1.234 | 0.892 | 0.951 | 0.878 | 0.746 | 1.448 | 0.945 | 0.294 | 0.637 | 0.412 | 0.437 | 0.357 | 0.993 | 0.787 |

注：摄入量合计时，摄入量<0.001的结果按0计

Note: values <0.001 were treated as 0

附表 6-14 第六次中国总膳食研究缩水甘油酯的膳食来源（单位：%）

Annexed Table 6-14 Dietary sources of glycidyl fatty acid esters from the 6$^{th}$ China TDS (Unit: %)

| 膳食类别 Category | 黑龙江 HL | 辽宁 LN | 河北 HE | 北京 BJ | 吉林 JL | 山西 SX | 陕西 SN | 河南 HA | 宁夏 NX | 内蒙古 NM | 青海 QH | 甘肃 GS | 上海 SH | 福建 FJ | 江西 JX | 江苏 JS | 浙江 ZJ | 山东 SD | 湖北 HB | 四川 SC | 广西 GX | 湖南 HN | 广东 GD | 贵州 GZ | 全国平均 AVG |
|---|---|---|---|---|---|---|---|---|---|---|---|---|---|---|---|---|---|---|---|---|---|---|---|---|---|
| 谷类 Cereals | 12.1 | 11.8 | 16.9 | 22.0 | 8.4 | 19.3 | 4.6 | 13.5 | 8.9 | 43.9 | 6.8 | 3.0 | 4.1 | 3.1 | 7.8 | 10.3 | 1.8 | 5.3 | 15.6 | 7.6 | 10.6 | 6.1 | 5.5 | 15.6 | 9.4 |
| 豆类 Legumes | 1.7 | 19.1 | 1.3 | 2.7 | 2.0 | 18.2 | 7.7 | 2.0 | 2.6 | 1.8 | 0.4 | 4.4 | 4.8 | 4.0 | 4.1 | 6.6 | 1.6 | 2.5 | 7.2 | 5.4 | 1.5 | 4.8 | 4.1 | 3.5 | 4.0 |
| 薯类 Potatoes | 4.7 | 3.9 | 3.0 | 6.0 | 1.6 | 6.8 | 16.8 | 2.4 | 23.0 | 3.9 | 19.1 | 27.8 | 3.8 | 1.5 | 0.4 | 1.6 | 0.6 | 1.3 | 7.2 | 5.3 | 0.6 | 1.0 | 0.2 | 4.3 | 7.6 |
| 肉类 Meats | 12.1 | 10.9 | 3.3 | 14.4 | 8.1 | 18.3 | 5.9 | 3.4 | 7.9 | 11.6 | 11.4 | 6.5 | 12.6 | 17.3 | 20.0 | 11.2 | 8.9 | 8.1 | 16.2 | 26.6 | 40.5 | 39.3 | 12.9 | 13.7 | 11.9 |
| 蛋类 Eggs | 3.3 | 2.6 | 3.5 | 5.8 | 8.8 | 2.0 | 2.3 | 1.9 | 5.8 | 5.1 | 2.2 | 3.6 | 3.2 | 1.5 | 1.9 | 3.0 | 41.8 | 2.9 | 3.3 | 1.2 | 1.2 | 2.7 | 0.5 | 2.0 | 6.1 |
| 水产类 Aquatic foods | 1.5 | 1.0 | 0.2 | 1.0 | 1.2 | 0.4 | 0.4 | 0.2 | 0.1 | 0.5 | 0.5 | 0.2 | 5.6 | 12.4 | 3.7 | 2.9 | 2.4 | 1.2 | 4.2 | 0.8 | 6.0 | 9.7 | 9.0 | 0.3 | 2.3 |
| 乳类 Dairy products | 0.1 | 0.5 | 0.1 | 2.1 | 0.1 | 0.5 | 0.0 | 0.2 | 0.0 | 0.2 | 0.2 | 0.1 | 0.3 | 0.1 | 0.1 | 0.1 | 0.1 | 0.2 | 0.1 | 0.1 | 0.3 | 0.1 | 0.6 | 0.2 | 0.2 |

续表

| 膳食类别 Category | 黑龙江 HL | 辽宁 LN | 河北 HE | 北京 BJ | 吉林 JL | 山西 SX | 陕西 SN | 河南 HA | 宁夏 NX | 内蒙古 NM | 青海 QH | 甘肃 GS | 上海 SH | 福建 FJ | 江西 JX | 江苏 JS | 浙江 ZJ | 山东 SD | 湖北 HB | 四川 SC | 广西 GX | 湖南 HN | 广东 GD | 贵州 GZ | 全国平均 AVG |
|---|---|---|---|---|---|---|---|---|---|---|---|---|---|---|---|---|---|---|---|---|---|---|---|---|---|
| 蔬菜类 Vegetables | 42.8 | 42.3 | 63.0 | 33.0 | 63.5 | 25.5 | 61.6 | 71.7 | 46.6 | 18.5 | 56.8 | 51.3 | 62.6 | 54.1 | 48.9 | 50.8 | 39.7 | 71.6 | 42.4 | 50.9 | 27.6 | 27.8 | 56.3 | 40.3 | 51.4 |
| 水果类 Fruits | 0.0 | 0.0 | 0.0 | 0.0 | 0.0 | 0.0 | 0.0 | 0.0 | 0.0 | 0.0 | 0.0 | 0.0 | 0.0 | 0.0 | 0.0 | 0.0 | 0.0 | 0.0 | 0.0 | 0.0 | 0.0 | 0.0 | 0.0 | 0.0 | 0.0 |
| 糖类 Sugar | 0.0 | 0.0 | 0.0 | 0.1 | 0.0 | 0.0 | 0.0 | 0.0 | 0.0 | 0.0 | 0.0 | 0.0 | 0.2 | 0.0 | 0.0 | 0.0 | 0.0 | 0.0 | 0.0 | 0.0 | 0.0 | 0.0 | 0.0 | 0.0 | 0.0 |
| 水及饮料类 Water and beverages | 20.9 | 5.9 | 8.4 | 10.9 | 5.7 | 8.6 | 0.5 | 4.4 | 4.7 | 13.3 | 2.4 | 3.0 | 2.5 | 5.8 | 12.8 | 12.9 | 1.7 | 6.0 | 3.1 | 1.6 | 10.0 | 7.7 | 10.6 | 20.0 | 6.7 |
| 酒类 Alcohol beverages | 0.4 | 0.8 | 0.1 | 0.7 | 0.1 | 0.0 | 0.0 | 0.0 | 0.0 | 0.6 | 0.0 | 0.0 | 0.2 | 0.1 | 0.2 | 0.5 | 1.1 | 0.8 | 0.5 | 0.4 | 1.1 | 0.2 | 0.0 | 0.0 | 0.3 |

附表 6-15 第六次中国总膳食研究膳食样品中丙烯酰胺的含量 （单位：μg/kg）

Annexed Table 6-15 Levels of acrylamide in food samples from the 6th China TDS (Unit: μg/kg)

| 膳食类别 Category | 黑龙江 HL | 辽宁 LN | 河北 HE | 北京 BJ | 吉林 JL | 山西 SX | 陕西 SN | 河南 HA | 宁夏 NX | 内蒙古 NM | 青海 QH | 甘肃 GS | 上海 SH | 福建 FJ | 江西 JX | 江苏 JS | 浙江 ZJ | 山东 SD | 湖北 HB | 四川 SC | 广西 GX | 湖南 HN | 广东 GD | 贵州 GZ | 全国平均 AVG |
|---|---|---|---|---|---|---|---|---|---|---|---|---|---|---|---|---|---|---|---|---|---|---|---|---|---|
| 谷类 Cereals | 5.69 | 1.93 | 3.21 | 2.78 | 6.38 | 2.14 | 3.00 | 2.52 | 2.57 | 7.39 | 2.58 | ND | 2.28 | 1.77 | 7.76 | 2.26 | ND | 3.15 | 1.79 | 2.25 | 2.27 | 2.64 | 1.82 | 2.47 | 2.95 |
| 豆类 Legumes | 3.11 | 10.62 | 7.32 | 3.10 | 2.44 | 6.49 | 3.12 | 11.98 | 4.56 | 3.84 | 1.89 | 14.20 | 6.54 | 4.19 | 6.37 | 28.14 | 3.44 | 11.56 | 13.74 | 9.84 | 2.83 | 10.08 | 1.75 | 3.51 | 7.28 |
| 薯类 Potatoes | 2.04 | 5.36 | 3.52 | 16.51 | 33.90 | 2.91 | 6.83 | 40.22 | 10.42 | 30.20 | 7.75 | 14.53 | 6.08 | 8.34 | 176.90 | 3.75 | 18.96 | 10.48 | 5.15 | 2.42 | 7.25 | 5.57 | ND | 6.68 | 17.74 |
| 肉类 Meats | 2.84 | ND | 3.01 | 2.36 | 1.57 | 2.69 | ND | 2.08 | 3.23 | 3.73 | 4.85 | 3.82 | 2.87 | 2.91 | 2.41 | ND | 3.30 | ND | 14.70 | 4.91 | 0.08 | 3.76 | ND | 4.13 | 2.90 |
| 蛋类 Eggs | ND | ND | 2.53 | 1.21 | ND | ND | 1.86 | 1.83 | 2.92 | 3.32 | 4.00 | 1.24 | 1.64 | 1.98 | 4.21 | 2.58 | 2.03 | 2.34 | 7.23 | 2.52 | 1.79 | 4.52 | 1.09 | 2.05 | 2.22 |

续表

| 膳食类别 Category | 黑龙江 HL | 辽宁 LN | 河北 HE | 北京 BJ | 吉林 JL | 山西 SX | 陕西 SN | 河南 HA | 宁夏 NX | 内蒙古 NM | 青海 QH | 甘肃 GS | 上海 SH | 福建 FJ | 江西 JX | 江苏 JS | 浙江 ZJ | 山东 SD | 湖北 HB | 四川 SC | 广西 GX | 湖南 HN | 广东 GD | 贵州 GZ | 全国平均 AVG |
|---|---|---|---|---|---|---|---|---|---|---|---|---|---|---|---|---|---|---|---|---|---|---|---|---|---|
| 水产类 Aquatic foods | 4.53 | ND | 1.63 | 1.09 | 3.09 | 2.96 | 5.10 | 2.26 | ND | 2.83 | 8.67 | 4.47 | 1.31 | 1.17 | 2.25 | ND | 2.85 | 3.58 | 3.23 | 3.90 | ND | 3.91 | 1.56 | 2.45 | 2.63 |
| 乳类 Dairy products | 3.50 | ND | 3.60 | 1.28 | 1.48 | 1.46 | ND | 1.06 | 2.21 | ND | 1.63 | ND | 2.02 | ND | 2.61 | 1.59 | 3.52 | 1.21 | 1.22 | 1.37 | ND | 1.50 | 2.22 | 1.89 | 1.49 |
| 蔬菜类 Vegetables | 21.57 | 11.29 | 20.26 | 7.01 | 34.24 | 4.90 | 3.31 | 35.15 | 29.30 | 11.66 | 10.29 | 5.56 | 4.53 | 6.38 | 10.06 | 1.86 | 10.98 | 15.69 | 4.23 | 12.52 | 3.28 | 3.69 | 22.06 | 154.85 | 18.53 |
| 水果类 Fruits | 1.30 | 1.13 | ND | 1.28 | ND | 1.46 | ND | ND | ND | ND | ND | ND | ND | 1.16 | ND | ND | ND | ND | 1.00 | 1.41 | ND | 1.40 | ND | 1.51 | 0.54 |
| 糖类 Sugar | ND | 4.02 | 129.31 | 9.30 | 4.03 | 1.21 | 7.27 | 19.44 | 11.28 | 14.43 | ND | 1.06 | 19.62 | 4.02 | 9.24 | 3.34 | 7.45 | 61.24 | 7.20 | 9.30 | 7.27 | 8.71 | 5.17 | 6.23 | 14.60 |
| 水及饮料类 Water and beverages | ND | 2.66 | ND | ND | ND | ND | ND | ND | ND | ND | ND | ND | 1.65 | 6.09 | ND | ND | ND | ND | ND | ND | ND | ND | ND | ND | 0.50 |
| 酒类 Alcohol beverages | ND | ND | ND | 1.13 | 1.73 | ND | 6.29 | 8.10 | ND | ND | ND | 1.36 | ND | 4.88 | ND | ND | 5.88 | ND | ND | ND | 6.29 | ND | ND | ND | 1.54 |

注：未检出（ND）按 1/2 检出限（LOD）计

Note: values not detected (ND) were treated as being equal to half of the detection of limit (LOD)

附表 6-16 第六次中国总膳食研究的丙烯酰胺膳食摄入量［单位：ng/(kg bw · d)］

Annexed Table 6-16　Dietary intakes of acrylamide from the 6th China TDS [Unit: ng/(kg bw · d)]

| 膳食类别 Category | 黑龙江 HL | 辽宁 LN | 河北 HE | 北京 BJ | 吉林 JL | 山西 SX | 陕西 SN | 河南 HA | 宁夏 NX | 内蒙古 NM | 青海 QH | 甘肃 GS | 上海 SH | 福建 FJ | 江西 JX | 江苏 JS | 浙江 ZJ | 山东 SD | 湖北 HB | 四川 SC | 广西 GX | 湖南 HN | 广东 GD | 贵州 GZ | 全国平均 AVG |
|---|---|---|---|---|---|---|---|---|---|---|---|---|---|---|---|---|---|---|---|---|---|---|---|---|---|
| 谷类 Cereals | 49.534 | 18.904 | 38.530 | 35.095 | 59.296 | 35.194 | 36.363 | 36.991 | 26.951 | 84.811 | 31.417 | 1.477 | 16.243 | 17.780 | 77.592 | 27.915 | 1.071 | 49.742 | 15.037 | 34.590 | 33.861 | 24.197 | 13.182 | 26.459 | 33.010 |

续表

| 膳食类别 Category | 黑龙江 HL | 辽宁 LN | 河北 HE | 北京 BJ | 吉林 JL | 山西 SX | 陕西 SN | 河南 HA | 宁夏 NX | 内蒙古 NM | 青海 QH | 甘肃 GS | 上海 SH | 福建 FJ | 江西 JX | 江苏 JS | 浙江 ZJ | 山东 SD | 湖北 HB | 四川 SC | 广西 GX | 湖南 HN | 广东 GD | 贵州 GZ | 全国平均 AVG |
|---|---|---|---|---|---|---|---|---|---|---|---|---|---|---|---|---|---|---|---|---|---|---|---|---|---|
| 豆类 Legumes | 2.242 | 20.557 | 6.630 | 5.003 | 2.917 | 7.144 | 4.102 | 10.259 | 2.546 | 2.427 | 0.194 | 9.290 | 12.202 | 5.225 | 7.458 | 37.068 | 7.702 | 9.627 | 14.572 | 10.561 | 1.902 | 11.618 | 0.775 | 5.660 | 8.237 |
| 薯类 Potatoes | 2.502 | 6.130 | 3.408 | 15.317 | 64.571 | 5.474 | 12.423 | 51.261 | 16.517 | 58.639 | 12.466 | 33.194 | 3.464 | 5.601 | 90.303 | 1.990 | 11.038 | 7.691 | 7.240 | 2.413 | 1.479 | 4.743 | 0.033 | 3.632 | 17.564 |
| 肉类 Meats | 2.704 | 0.105 | 2.264 | 2.526 | 1.661 | 5.854 | 0.049 | 1.829 | 2.394 | 4.349 | 5.462 | 1.878 | 5.038 | 3.969 | 3.588 | 0.118 | 6.201 | 0.133 | 12.667 | 10.039 | 0.192 | 8.931 | 0.167 | 6.984 | 3.713 |
| 蛋类 Eggs | 0.052 | 0.068 | 1.269 | 0.745 | 0.059 | 0.036 | 0.649 | 0.865 | 0.604 | 1.567 | 0.834 | 0.438 | 1.018 | 0.596 | 1.369 | 1.153 | 0.771 | 1.647 | 2.868 | 0.585 | 0.398 | 1.636 | 0.413 | 0.529 | 0.840 |
| 水产类 Aquatic foods | 1.952 | 0.030 | 0.245 | 0.284 | 0.547 | 0.301 | 0.332 | 0.166 | 0.003 | 0.464 | 0.490 | 0.200 | 1.426 | 1.196 | 1.561 | 0.051 | 2.274 | 1.294 | 2.085 | 0.518 | 0.124 | 4.123 | 1.268 | 0.135 | 0.878 |
| 乳类 Dairy products | 0.743 | 0.056 | 1.385 | 1.737 | 0.759 | 0.960 | 0.025 | 0.330 | 0.534 | 0.044 | 1.386 | 0.018 | 2.288 | 0.046 | 0.904 | 0.694 | 1.871 | 0.443 | 0.130 | 0.273 | 0.023 | 0.428 | 1.284 | 0.844 | 0.717 |
| 蔬菜类 Vegetables | 109.745 | 58.522 | 94.417 | 43.580 | 210.912 | 224.088 | 15.105 | 155.119 | 72.678 | 47.589 | 50.715 | 21.895 | 28.835 | 40.181 | 72.121 | 12.547 | 77.428 | 101.180 | 27.798 | 60.173 | 18.383 | 31.233 | 82.820 | 100.636 | 102.487 |
| 水果类 Fruits | 1.291 | 1.375 | 0.048 | 2.303 | 0.112 | 0.809 | 0.051 | 0.031 | 0.125 | 0.145 | 0.020 | 0.042 | 0.093 | 1.101 | 0.072 | 0.035 | 0.085 | 0.069 | 0.305 | 0.335 | 0.082 | 1.406 | 0.037 | 0.503 | 0.436 |
| 糖类 Sugar | 0.003 | 0.047 | 1.006 | 0.291 | 0.061 | 0.021 | 4.378 | 0.120 | 0.143 | 0.238 | 0.001 | 0.007 | 2.364 | 0.019 | 0.141 | 0.014 | 0.125 | 0.476 | 0.021 | 0.060 | 0.054 | 0.069 | 0.019 | 0.029 | 0.404 |
| 水及饮料类 Water and beverages | 1.552 | 20.827 | 0.985 | 1.407 | 1.653 | 0.947 | 0.439 | 1.514 | 0.657 | 3.270 | 0.785 | 1.500 | 18.414 | 83.638 | 1.500 | 1.281 | 0.999 | 2.287 | 0.362 | 0.399 | 1.654 | 1.349 | 1.515 | 1.590 | 6.272 |
| 酒类 Alcohol beverages | 0.028 | 0.043 | 0.014 | 0.490 | 0.263 | 0.000 | 0.166 | 0.407 | 0.001 | 0.026 | 0.006 | 0.071 | 0.029 | 1.104 | 0.027 | 0.048 | 5.858 | 0.144 | 0.018 | 0.007 | 3.196 | 0.021 | 0.002 | 0.003 | 0.499 |
| 合计 SUM | 172.348 | 126.664 | 150.200 | 108.778 | 342.811 | 80.827 | 74.080 | 258.893 | 123.152 | 203.569 | 103.777 | 70.010 | 91.413 | 160.457 | 256.637 | 82.913 | 115.424 | 174.733 | 83.103 | 119.954 | 61.348 | 89.755 | 101.514 | 1049.005 | 175.057 |

附表 6-17　第六次中国总膳食研究丙烯酰胺的膳食来源（单位：%）

Annexed Table 6-17　Dietary sources of acrylamide from the 6<sup>th</sup> China TDS (Unit: %)

| 膳食类别<br>Category | 黑龙江<br>HL | 辽宁<br>LN | 河北<br>HE | 北京<br>BJ | 吉林<br>JL | 山西<br>SX | 陕西<br>SN | 河南<br>HA | 宁夏<br>NX | 内蒙古<br>NM | 青海<br>QH | 甘肃<br>GS | 上海<br>SH | 福建<br>FJ | 江西<br>JX | 江苏<br>JS | 浙江<br>ZJ | 山东<br>SD | 湖北<br>HB | 四川<br>SC | 广西<br>GX | 湖南<br>HN | 广东<br>GD | 贵州<br>GZ | 全国平均<br>AVG |
|---|---|---|---|---|---|---|---|---|---|---|---|---|---|---|---|---|---|---|---|---|---|---|---|---|---|
| 谷类 Cereals | 29.0 | 15.0 | 25.8 | 32.7 | 17.4 | 44.1 | 49.5 | 14.4 | 22.0 | 42.4 | 30.5 | 0.0 | 17.8 | 11.1 | 30.4 | 34.3 | 0.0 | 28.9 | 18.2 | 28.9 | 57.1 | 27.4 | 13.2 | 2.5 | 18.9 |
| 豆类 Legumes | 1.3 | 16.3 | 4.4 | 4.7 | 0.9 | 8.9 | 5.6 | 4.0 | 2.1 | 1.2 | 0.2 | 13.9 | 13.4 | 3.3 | 2.9 | 45.5 | 6.8 | 5.6 | 17.6 | 8.8 | 3.2 | 13.1 | 0.8 | 0.5 | 4.7 |
| 薯类 Potatoes | 1.5 | 4.9 | 2.3 | 14.3 | 18.9 | 6.9 | 16.9 | 19.9 | 13.5 | 29.3 | 12.1 | 49.6 | 3.8 | 3.5 | 35.4 | 2.4 | 9.7 | 4.5 | 8.8 | 2.0 | 2.5 | 5.4 | 0.0 | 0.3 | 10.1 |
| 肉类 Meats | 1.6 | 0.0 | 1.5 | 2.4 | 0.5 | 7.3 | 0.0 | 0.7 | 2.0 | 2.2 | 5.3 | 2.8 | 5.5 | 2.5 | 1.4 | 0.0 | 5.5 | 0.0 | 15.3 | 8.4 | 0.0 | 10.1 | 0.0 | 0.7 | 2.1 |
| 蛋类 Eggs | 0.0 | 0.0 | 0.9 | 0.7 | 0.0 | 0.0 | 0.9 | 0.3 | 0.5 | 0.8 | 0.8 | 0.7 | 1.1 | 0.4 | 0.5 | 1.4 | 0.7 | 1.0 | 3.5 | 0.5 | 0.7 | 1.9 | 0.4 | 0.1 | 0.5 |
| 水产类 Aquatic foods | 1.1 | 0.0 | 0.2 | 0.3 | 0.2 | 0.4 | 0.5 | 0.1 | 0.0 | 0.2 | 0.5 | 0.3 | 1.6 | 0.7 | 0.6 | 0.0 | 2.0 | 0.8 | 2.5 | 0.4 | 0.0 | 4.7 | 1.3 | 0.0 | 0.5 |
| 乳类 Dairy products | 0.4 | 0.0 | 0.9 | 1.6 | 0.2 | 1.2 | 0.0 | 0.1 | 0.4 | 0.0 | 1.3 | 0.0 | 2.5 | 0.0 | 0.4 | 0.9 | 1.7 | 0.3 | 0.2 | 0.2 | 0.0 | 0.5 | 1.3 | 0.1 | 0.4 |
| 蔬菜类 Vegetables | 64.3 | 46.3 | 63.3 | 40.6 | 61.9 | 30.2 | 20.5 | 60.3 | 59.4 | 23.8 | 49.3 | 32.7 | 31.6 | 25.0 | 28.3 | 15.4 | 68.4 | 58.8 | 33.6 | 50.3 | 31.0 | 35.3 | 83.0 | 95.7 | 59.0 |
| 水果类 Fruits | 0.8 | 1.1 | 0.0 | 2.1 | 0.0 | 1.0 | 0.0 | 0.0 | 0.0 | 0.0 | 0.0 | 0.0 | 0.0 | 0.7 | 0.0 | 0.0 | 0.0 | 0.0 | 0.4 | 0.3 | 0.0 | 1.6 | 0.0 | 0.0 | 0.2 |
| 糖类 Sugar | 0.0 | 0.0 | 0.7 | 0.3 | 0.0 | 0.0 | 6.0 | 0.1 | 0.1 | 0.1 | 0.0 | 0.0 | 2.6 | 0.0 | 0.1 | 0.0 | 0.1 | 0.3 | 0.0 | 0.1 | 0.1 | 0.1 | 0.0 | 0.0 | 0.2 |
| 水及饮料类 Water and beverages | 0.0 | 16.5 | 0.0 | 0.0 | 0.0 | 0.0 | 0.0 | 0.2 | 0.0 | 0.0 | 0.0 | 0.1 | 20.2 | 52.1 | 0.0 | 0.0 | 0.0 | 0.0 | 0.0 | 0.0 | 0.0 | 0.0 | 0.0 | 0.0 | 2.9 |
| 酒类 Alcohol beverages | 0.0 | 0.0 | 0.0 | 0.5 | 0.1 | 0.0 | 0.2 | 0.2 | 0.0 | 0.0 | 0.0 | 0.1 | 0.0 | 0.7 | 0.0 | 0.0 | 5.2 | 0.0 | 0.0 | 0.0 | 5.4 | 0.0 | 0.0 | 0.0 | 0.3 |

附表 6-18 第六次中国总膳食研究膳食样品中苯并 [a] 芘的含量（单位：μg/kg）

Annexed Table 6-18 Levels of benzo [a] pyrene in food samples from the 6$^{th}$ China TDS (Unit: μg/kg)

| 膳食类别 Category | 黑龙江 HL | 辽宁 LN | 河北 HE | 北京 BJ | 吉林 JL | 山西 SX | 陕西 SN | 河南 HA | 宁夏 NX | 内蒙古 NM | 青海 QH | 甘肃 GS | 上海 SH | 福建 FJ | 江西 JX | 江苏 JS | 浙江 ZJ | 山东 SD | 湖北 HB | 四川 SC | 广西 GX | 湖南 HN | 广东 GD | 贵州 GZ | 全国平均 AVG |
|---|---|---|---|---|---|---|---|---|---|---|---|---|---|---|---|---|---|---|---|---|---|---|---|---|---|
| 谷类 Cereals | 0.07 | 0.03 | 0.05 | ND | ND | 0.05 | 0.03 | 0.10 | ND | 0.09 | 0.04 | 0.04 | 0.02 | ND | 0.03 | 0.02 | 0.02 | 0.02 | 0.04 | 0.04 | ND | ND | 0.03 | 0.03 | 0.03 |
| 豆类 Legumes | 0.08 | 0.11 | 0.11 | 0.16 | 0.19 | 0.55 | 0.25 | 0.16 | 0.34 | 0.58 | 0.33 | 0.49 | 0.07 | 0.09 | 0.14 | 0.17 | 0.11 | 0.14 | 0.40 | 0.09 | 0.16 | 0.59 | 0.08 | 0.73 | 0.25 |
| 薯类 Potatoes | 0.12 | 0.04 | 0.15 | 0.20 | 0.05 | 0.13 | 0.12 | 0.03 | 0.61 | 0.13 | 0.42 | 0.23 | 0.13 | 0.04 | 0.02 | 0.06 | 0.04 | 0.05 | 0.17 | 0.06 | 0.06 | 0.07 | ND | 0.18 | 0.13 |
| 肉类 Meats | 0.22 | 0.06 | 0.16 | 0.18 | 0.11 | 0.21 | 0.36 | 0.07 | 0.50 | 0.12 | 2.24 | 0.23 | 1.02 | ND | ND | 0.19 | 0.13 | 0.19 | 0.46 | 0.13 | 0.12 | 0.22 | 0.06 | 0.71 | 0.32 |
| 蛋类 Eggs | 0.14 | 0.03 | 0.18 | 0.22 | 0.08 | 0.24 | 0.19 | ND | 0.48 | 0.12 | 0.38 | 0.26 | 0.12 | 0.07 | 0.04 | 0.12 | 0.08 | 0.20 | 0.29 | 0.10 | 0.09 | 0.14 | ND | 0.21 | 0.16 |
| 水产类 Aquatic foods | 0.12 | 0.06 | 0.05 | 0.24 | 0.18 | 0.07 | 0.15 | 0.06 | 0.14 | 0.10 | 0.56 | 0.07 | 0.18 | 0.09 | 0.03 | 0.07 | 0.28 | 0.14 | 0.39 | 0.07 | 0.12 | 0.17 | 0.07 | 0.15 | 0.15 |
| 乳类 Dairy products | ND | ND | ND | ND | ND | ND | ND | ND | ND | ND | ND | ND | ND | ND | 0.03 | ND | ND | 0.01 | ND | 0.03 | 0.02 | ND | ND | ND | 0.01 |
| 蔬菜类 Vegetables | 0.12 | 0.08 | 0.30 | 0.26 | 0.08 | 0.23 | 0.20 | 0.06 | 0.74 | 0.10 | 0.45 | 0.29 | 0.35 | 0.10 | 0.06 | 0.14 | 0.12 | 0.19 | 0.28 | 0.10 | 0.16 | 0.17 | 0.14 | 1.36 | 0.25 |
| 水果类 Fruits | ND | 0.01 | ND | ND | 0.01 | ND | ND | ND | ND | ND | 0.02 | ND | ND | ND | ND | ND | ND | 0.02 | ND | 0.04 | ND | ND | ND | 0.01 | 0.01 |
| 糖类 Sugar | ND | ND | 0.01 | 0.04 | ND | 0.05 | ND | 0.02 | ND | 0.02 | 0.02 | ND | 0.10 | ND | ND | ND | 0.05 | 0.06 | ND | 0.01 | ND | ND | ND | ND | 0.02 |
| 水及饮料类 Water and beverages | ND | ND | ND | ND | ND | ND | ND | ND | ND | ND | 0.03 | ND | ND | ND | ND | ND | ND | ND | ND | ND | 0.01 | ND | ND | ND | 0.01 |

续表

| 膳食类别 Category | 黑龙江 HL | 辽宁 LN | 河北 HE | 北京 BJ | 吉林 JL | 山西 SX | 陕西 SN | 河南 HA | 宁夏 NX | 内蒙古 NM | 青海 QH | 甘肃 GS | 上海 SH | 福建 FJ | 江西 JX | 江苏 JS | 浙江 ZJ | 山东 SD | 湖北 HB | 四川 SC | 广西 GX | 湖南 HN | 广东 GD | 贵州 GZ | 全国平均 AVG |
|---|---|---|---|---|---|---|---|---|---|---|---|---|---|---|---|---|---|---|---|---|---|---|---|---|---|
| 酒类 Alcohol beverages | ND | ND | ND | ND | ND | ND | ND | ND | ND | ND | ND | ND | ND | ND | ND | ND | ND | ND | ND | ND | ND | ND | ND | 0.01 | 0.01 |
| 合计 SUM | 0.90 | 0.44 | 1.02 | 1.33 | 0.73 | 1.55 | 1.33 | 0.53 | 2.83 | 1.28 | 4.50 | 1.64 | 2.01 | 0.43 | 0.36 | 0.80 | 0.85 | 1.02 | 2.06 | 0.68 | 0.76 | 1.39 | 0.42 | 3.42 | 1.35 |

注: 未检出 (ND) 按 1/2 检出限 (LOD) 计

Note: values not detected (ND) were treated as being equal to half of the detection of limit (LOD)

附表 6-19 第六次中国总膳食研究膳食样品中䓛的含量 (单位: μg/kg)

Annexed Table 6-19 Levels of chrysene in food samples from the 6$^{th}$ China TDS (Unit: μg/kg)

| 膳食类别 Category | 黑龙江 HL | 辽宁 LN | 河北 HE | 北京 BJ | 吉林 JL | 山西 SX | 陕西 SN | 河南 HA | 宁夏 NX | 内蒙古 NM | 青海 QH | 甘肃 GS | 上海 SH | 福建 FJ | 江西 JX | 江苏 JS | 浙江 ZJ | 山东 SD | 湖北 HB | 四川 SC | 广西 GX | 湖南 HN | 广东 GD | 贵州 GZ | 全国平均 AVG |
|---|---|---|---|---|---|---|---|---|---|---|---|---|---|---|---|---|---|---|---|---|---|---|---|---|---|
| 谷类 Cereals | 0.19 | 0.05 | 0.17 | 0.01 | 0.09 | 0.13 | 0.07 | 0.41 | 0.10 | 0.22 | 0.09 | 0.13 | 0.09 | 0.05 | 0.06 | 0.08 | 0.06 | 0.14 | 0.11 | 0.09 | 0.06 | 0.07 | 0.09 | 0.07 | 0.11 |
| 豆类 Legumes | 0.23 | 0.21 | 0.34 | 0.32 | 0.29 | 0.83 | 0.64 | 0.54 | 0.63 | 2.17 | 0.39 | 1.43 | 0.14 | 0.17 | 0.31 | 0.50 | 0.22 | 0.32 | 0.83 | 0.21 | 0.43 | 1.85 | 0.33 | 2.15 | 0.65 |
| 薯类 Potatoes | 0.34 | 0.09 | 0.30 | 0.34 | 0.17 | 0.28 | 0.16 | 0.09 | 0.86 | 0.26 | 0.52 | 0.59 | 0.18 | 0.09 | 0.05 | 0.12 | 0.08 | 0.15 | 0.34 | 0.10 | 0.13 | 0.14 | 0.02 | 0.36 | 0.24 |
| 肉类 Meats | 0.56 | 0.15 | 0.30 | 0.32 | 0.39 | 0.43 | 0.38 | 0.22 | 0.81 | 0.29 | 1.77 | 0.60 | 0.74 | 0.12 | 0.07 | 0.36 | 0.22 | 0.24 | 0.68 | 0.25 | 0.31 | 0.56 | 0.27 | 1.09 | 0.46 |
| 蛋类 Eggs | 0.37 | 0.11 | 0.37 | 0.44 | 0.23 | 0.49 | 0.22 | 0.11 | 0.77 | 0.22 | 0.61 | 0.59 | 0.16 | 0.15 | 0.08 | 0.26 | 0.08 | 0.35 | 0.61 | 0.11 | 0.20 | 0.30 | ND | 0.41 | 0.30 |
| 水产类 Aquatic foods | 0.42 | 0.14 | 0.20 | 0.52 | 0.66 | 0.18 | 0.25 | 0.21 | 0.39 | 0.26 | 0.77 | 0.24 | 0.28 | 0.26 | 0.10 | 0.23 | 0.48 | 0.25 | 0.82 | 0.17 | 0.31 | 0.46 | 0.25 | 0.34 | 0.34 |
| 乳类 Dairy products | 0.03 | 0.02 | ND | 0.02 | 0.04 | 0.07 | 0.05 | 0.03 | 0.06 | ND | ND | ND | 0.03 | 0.03 | 0.10 | 0.04 | ND | ND | 0.08 | 0.03 | 0.07 | ND | 0.04 | ND | 0.03 |

续表

| 膳食类别 Category | 黑龙江 HL | 辽宁 LN | 河北 HE | 北京 BJ | 吉林 JL | 山西 SX | 陕西 SN | 河南 HA | 宁夏 NX | 内蒙古 NM | 青海 QH | 甘肃 GS | 上海 SH | 福建 FJ | 江西 JX | 江苏 JS | 浙江 ZJ | 山东 SD | 湖北 HB | 四川 SC | 广西 GX | 湖南 HN | 广东 GD | 贵州 GZ | 全国平均 AVG |
|---|---|---|---|---|---|---|---|---|---|---|---|---|---|---|---|---|---|---|---|---|---|---|---|---|---|
| 蔬菜类 Vegetables | 0.34 | 0.19 | 0.54 | 0.64 | 0.31 | 0.55 | 0.36 | 0.21 | 1.10 | 0.21 | 0.62 | 0.73 | 0.39 | 0.30 | 0.35 | 0.30 | 0.28 | 0.30 | 0.63 | 0.24 | 0.47 | 0.45 | 0.58 | 0.99 | 0.46 |
| 水果类 Fruits | ND | 0.03 | 0.01 | 0.02 | ND | 0.05 | ND | ND | ND | 0.03 | 0.04 | 0.02 | 0.08 | ND | ND | 0.03 | ND | ND | ND | 0.01 | ND | ND | ND | ND | 0.02 |
| 糖类 Sugar | ND | ND | 0.01 | 0.04 | ND | 0.06 | ND | 0.04 | 0.02 | 0.04 | ND | 0.05 | 0.32 | ND | ND | 0.02 | 0.08 | 0.02 | ND | 0.03 | ND | ND | ND | ND | 0.03 |
| 水及饮料类 Water and beverages | ND | ND | 0.04 | ND | ND | ND | ND | ND | ND | ND | ND | ND | ND | ND | ND | ND | ND | ND | ND | ND | ND | ND | ND | ND | 0.01 |
| 酒类 Alcohol beverages | ND | ND | ND | ND | ND | ND | ND | ND | ND | ND | ND | ND | ND | ND | ND | ND | ND | ND | ND | ND | ND | ND | ND | 0.02 | 0.01 |
| 合计 SUM | 2.50 | 1.01 | 2.28 | 2.67 | 2.20 | 3.08 | 2.15 | 1.87 | 4.76 | 3.72 | 4.82 | 4.40 | 2.42 | 1.19 | 1.13 | 1.95 | 1.52 | 1.80 | 4.12 | 1.25 | 1.99 | 3.86 | 1.61 | 5.46 | 2.66 |

注: 未检出 (ND) 按 1/2 检出限 (LOD) 计
Note: values not detected (ND) were treated as being equal to half of the detection of limit (LOD)

附表 6-20 第六次中国总膳食研究膳食样品中苯并 [a] 蒽的含量（单位：μg/kg）

Annexed Table 6-20 Levels of benzo [a] anthracene in food samples from the 6$^{th}$ China TDS (Unit: μg/kg)

| 膳食类别 Category | 黑龙江 HL | 辽宁 LN | 河北 HE | 北京 BJ | 吉林 JL | 山西 SX | 陕西 SN | 河南 HA | 宁夏 NX | 内蒙古 NM | 青海 QH | 甘肃 GS | 上海 SH | 福建 FJ | 江西 JX | 江苏 JS | 浙江 ZJ | 山东 SD | 湖北 HB | 四川 SC | 广西 GX | 湖南 HN | 广东 GD | 贵州 GZ | 全国平均 AVG |
|---|---|---|---|---|---|---|---|---|---|---|---|---|---|---|---|---|---|---|---|---|---|---|---|---|---|
| 谷类 Cereals | 0.14 | 0.05 | 0.13 | 0.01 | 0.07 | 0.11 | 0.05 | 0.35 | 0.09 | 0.16 | 0.09 | 0.10 | 0.07 | 0.04 | 0.07 | 0.06 | 0.05 | 0.09 | 0.08 | 0.07 | 0.05 | 0.06 | 0.07 | 0.07 | 0.09 |
| 豆类 Legumes | 0.19 | 0.17 | 0.29 | 0.32 | 0.29 | 0.81 | 0.53 | 0.52 | 0.61 | 2.41 | 0.40 | 1.22 | 0.12 | 0.14 | 0.31 | 0.41 | 0.21 | 0.26 | 0.82 | 0.18 | 0.27 | 1.89 | 0.29 | 2.08 | 0.61 |
| 薯类 Potatoes | 0.25 | 0.07 | 0.24 | 0.30 | 0.12 | 0.24 | 0.12 | 0.08 | 0.70 | 0.22 | 0.51 | 0.46 | 0.16 | 0.06 | 0.07 | 0.09 | 0.04 | 0.11 | 0.27 | 0.06 | 0.11 | 0.10 | 0.01 | 0.32 | 0.20 |

续表

| 膳食类别<br>Category | 黑龙江<br>HL | 辽宁<br>LN | 河北<br>HE | 北京<br>BJ | 吉林<br>JL | 山西<br>SX | 陕西<br>SN | 河南<br>HA | 宁夏<br>NX | 内蒙古<br>NM | 青海<br>QH | 甘肃<br>GS | 上海<br>SH | 福建<br>FJ | 江西<br>JX | 江苏<br>JS | 浙江<br>ZJ | 山东<br>SD | 湖北<br>HB | 四川<br>SC | 广西<br>GX | 湖南<br>HN | 广东<br>GD | 贵州<br>GZ | 全国平均<br>AVG |
|---|---|---|---|---|---|---|---|---|---|---|---|---|---|---|---|---|---|---|---|---|---|---|---|---|---|
| 肉类 Meats | 0.23 | 0.13 | 0.26 | 0.28 | 0.25 | 0.40 | 0.56 | 0.18 | 0.87 | 0.20 | 1.87 | 0.49 | 0.82 | 0.06 | 0.28 | 0.25 | 0.15 | 0.18 | 0.54 | 0.24 | 0.20 | 0.39 | 0.16 | 1.08 | 0.42 |
| 蛋类 Eggs | 0.28 | 0.09 | 0.31 | 0.43 | 0.17 | 0.43 | 0.20 | 0.09 | 0.64 | 0.17 | 0.64 | 0.47 | 0.12 | 0.11 | 0.09 | 0.29 | 0.07 | 0.27 | 0.53 | 0.10 | 0.16 | 0.20 | ND | 0.37 | 0.26 |
| 水产类 Aquatic foods | 0.26 | 0.06 | 0.09 | 0.41 | 0.42 | 0.13 | 0.14 | 0.10 | 0.21 | 0.16 | 0.74 | 0.15 | 0.16 | 0.16 | 0.12 | 0.13 | 0.27 | 0.08 | 0.62 | 0.07 | 0.16 | 0.25 | 0.12 | 0.28 | 0.22 |
| 乳类 Dairy products | ND | ND | ND | 0.03 | 0.02 | 0.07 | ND | ND | ND | 0.04 | ND | ND | 0.02 | 0.01 | 0.10 | 0.03 | ND | ND | 0.05 | 0.03 | 0.01 | ND | 0.02 | 0.04 | 0.02 |
| 蔬菜类 Vegetables | 0.26 | 0.11 | 0.50 | 0.38 | 0.19 | 0.41 | 0.23 | 0.17 | 0.90 | 0.14 | 0.59 | 0.47 | 0.31 | 0.19 | 0.10 | 0.21 | 0.15 | 0.20 | 0.46 | 0.12 | 0.30 | 0.25 | 0.32 | 1.05 | 0.33 |
| 水果类 Fruits | ND | 0.04 | 0.03 | ND | ND | 0.03 | ND | ND | ND | ND | 0.05 | ND | 0.04 | ND | 0.02 | 0.02 | 0.05 | ND | ND | 0.01 | ND | ND | ND | ND | 0.02 |
| 糖类 Sugar | ND | ND | 0.02 | 0.03 | ND | 0.06 | ND | 0.04 | 0.04 | 0.03 | 0.05 | 0.05 | 0.27 | ND | 0.03 | ND | 0.06 | 0.06 | ND | 0.02 | ND | ND | ND | ND | 0.03 |
| 水及饮料类 Water and beverages | ND | ND | 0.03 | ND | ND | 0.05 | ND | ND | ND | ND | ND | ND | 0.04 | ND | 0.01 | ND | 0.04 | ND | ND | ND | ND | ND | ND | ND | 0.01 |
| 酒类 Alcohol beverages | ND | ND | ND | ND | ND | 0.06 | ND | ND | ND | ND | ND | ND | ND | ND | ND | ND | 0.03 | ND | ND | ND | ND | ND | ND | 0.03 | 0.01 |
| 合计 SUM | 1.64 | 0.74 | 1.92 | 2.20 | 1.55 | 2.80 | 1.86 | 1.55 | 4.06 | 3.54 | 4.94 | 3.43 | 2.14 | 0.79 | 1.20 | 1.51 | 1.12 | 1.26 | 3.39 | 0.89 | 1.29 | 3.17 | 1.02 | 5.34 | 2.22 |

注: 未检出 (ND) 按 1/2 检出限 (LOD) 计

Note: values not detected (ND) were treated as being equal to half of the detection of limit (LOD)

附表 6-21 第六次中国总膳食研究膳食样品中苯并[b]荧蒽的含量（单位：μg/kg）

Annexed Table 6-21 Levels of benzo[b]fluoranthene in food samples from the 6$^{th}$ China TDS (Unit: μg/kg)

| 膳食类别 Category | 黑龙江 HL | 辽宁 LN | 河北 HE | 北京 BJ | 吉林 JL | 山西 SX | 陕西 SN | 河南 HA | 宁夏 NX | 内蒙古 NM | 青海 QH | 甘肃 GS | 上海 SH | 福建 FJ | 江西 JX | 江苏 JS | 浙江 ZJ | 山东 SD | 湖北 HB | 四川 SC | 广西 GX | 湖南 HN | 广东 GD | 贵州 GZ | 全国平均 AVG |
|---|---|---|---|---|---|---|---|---|---|---|---|---|---|---|---|---|---|---|---|---|---|---|---|---|---|
| 谷类 Cereals | 0.11 | 0.03 | 0.09 | ND | 0.04 | 0.07 | 0.08 | 0.18 | 0.06 | 0.12 | 0.06 | 0.07 | 0.04 | 0.03 | 0.03 | 0.04 | 0.03 | 0.06 | 0.05 | 0.05 | 0.02 | 0.02 | 0.05 | 0.03 | 0.06 |
| 豆类 Legumes | 0.14 | 0.12 | 0.16 | 0.17 | 0.14 | 0.67 | 0.37 | 0.25 | 0.34 | 0.80 | 0.47 | 0.60 | 0.10 | 0.11 | 0.14 | 0.23 | 0.14 | 0.19 | 0.50 | 0.10 | 0.26 | 0.81 | 0.13 | 0.78 | 0.32 |
| 薯类 Potatoes | 0.19 | 0.05 | 0.20 | 0.23 | 0.07 | 0.18 | 0.19 | 0.05 | 0.51 | 0.18 | 0.36 | 0.36 | 0.16 | 0.05 | 0.02 | 0.07 | 0.05 | 0.07 | 0.23 | 0.07 | 0.08 | 0.10 | 0.01 | 0.20 | 0.15 |
| 肉类 Meats | 0.31 | 0.08 | 0.20 | 0.23 | 0.18 | 0.28 | 0.44 | 0.22 | 0.54 | 0.19 | 1.23 | 0.36 | 0.56 | 0.07 | ND | 0.22 | 0.14 | 0.20 | 0.41 | 0.14 | 0.16 | 0.32 | 0.11 | 0.48 | 0.29 |
| 蛋类 Eggs | 0.23 | 0.06 | 0.22 | 0.30 | 0.09 | 0.32 | 0.22 | 0.06 | 0.49 | 0.16 | 0.46 | 0.37 | 0.16 | 0.09 | 0.04 | 0.15 | 0.07 | 0.21 | 0.30 | 0.09 | 0.12 | 0.20 | ND | 0.23 | 0.19 |
| 水产类 Aquatic foods | 0.20 | 0.06 | 0.08 | 0.30 | 0.26 | 0.10 | 0.18 | 0.10 | 0.15 | 0.15 | 0.55 | 0.12 | 0.18 | 0.14 | 0.03 | 0.10 | 0.25 | 0.17 | 0.34 | 0.08 | 0.13 | 0.25 | 0.12 | 0.17 | 0.18 |
| 乳类 Dairy products | ND | ND | ND | ND | ND | 0.02 | ND | ND | ND | ND | ND | ND | ND | 0.01 | 0.04 | ND | 0.04 | 0.02 | 0.03 | ND | 0.02 | ND | 0.01 | ND | 0.01 |
| 蔬菜类 Vegetables | 0.23 | 0.08 | 0.37 | 0.32 | 0.12 | 0.31 | 0.32 | 0.14 | 0.65 | 0.14 | 0.44 | 0.44 | 0.29 | 0.16 | 0.11 | 0.19 | 0.18 | 0.27 | 0.39 | 0.14 | 0.27 | 0.28 | 0.24 | 0.63 | 0.28 |
| 水果类 Fruits | ND | 0.01 | ND | ND | 0.02 | 0.02 | ND | ND | ND | ND | 0.02 | ND | 0.02 | ND | ND | 0.02 | ND | 0.01 | ND | 0.02 | 0.02 | ND | ND | ND | 0.01 |
| 糖类 Sugar | ND | ND | ND | 0.08 | 0.02 | 0.05 | ND | 0.03 | ND | 0.03 | ND | ND | 0.15 | ND | ND | 0.01 | 0.05 | 0.06 | ND | ND | ND | ND | ND | ND | 0.03 |
| 水及饮料类 Water and beverages | ND | ND | 0.02 | ND | ND | ND | ND | ND | ND | ND | ND | ND | ND | ND | ND | ND | ND | ND | ND | ND | ND | ND | ND | ND | 0.01 |

续表

| 膳食类别<br>Category | 黑龙江<br>HL | 辽宁<br>LN | 河北<br>HE | 北京<br>BJ | 吉林<br>JL | 山西<br>SX | 陕西<br>SN | 河南<br>HA | 宁夏<br>NX | 内蒙古<br>NM | 青海<br>QH | 甘肃<br>GS | 上海<br>SH | 福建<br>FJ | 江西<br>JX | 江苏<br>JS | 浙江<br>ZJ | 山东<br>SD | 湖北<br>HB | 四川<br>SC | 广西<br>GX | 湖南<br>HN | 广东<br>GD | 贵州<br>GZ | 全国平均<br>AVG |
|---|---|---|---|---|---|---|---|---|---|---|---|---|---|---|---|---|---|---|---|---|---|---|---|---|---|
| 酒类<br>Alcohol beverages | ND | ND | ND | ND | ND | ND | ND | ND | ND | ND | ND | ND | ND | ND | ND | ND | ND | ND | ND | ND | ND | ND | ND | ND | 0.01 |
| 合计<br>SUM | 1.44 | 0.51 | 1.34 | 1.66 | 0.96 | 2.03 | 1.83 | 1.05 | 2.75 | 1.79 | 3.61 | 2.35 | 1.68 | 0.68 | 0.44 | 1.05 | 0.97 | 1.26 | 2.27 | 0.71 | 1.10 | 2.01 | 0.70 | 2.54 | 1.53 |

注：未检出（ND）按 1/2 检出限（LOD）计
Note: values not detected (ND) were treated as being equal to half of the detection of limit (LOD)

附表 6-22　第六次中国总膳食研究膳食样品中苯并 [k] 荧蒽的含量　（单位：μg/kg）
Annexed Table 6-22　Levels of benzo [k] fluoranthene in food samples from the 6$^{th}$ China TDS (Unit: μg/kg)

| 膳食类别<br>Category | 黑龙江<br>HL | 辽宁<br>LN | 河北<br>HE | 北京<br>BJ | 吉林<br>JL | 山西<br>SX | 陕西<br>SN | 河南<br>HA | 宁夏<br>NX | 内蒙古<br>NM | 青海<br>QH | 甘肃<br>GS | 上海<br>SH | 福建<br>FJ | 江西<br>JX | 江苏<br>JS | 浙江<br>ZJ | 山东<br>SD | 湖北<br>HB | 四川<br>SC | 广西<br>GX | 湖南<br>HN | 广东<br>GD | 贵州<br>GZ | 全国平均<br>AVG |
|---|---|---|---|---|---|---|---|---|---|---|---|---|---|---|---|---|---|---|---|---|---|---|---|---|---|
| 谷类<br>Cereals | 0.05 | 0.01 | 0.04 | ND | 0.02 | 0.03 | 0.04 | 0.90 | 0.03 | 0.05 | 0.03 | 0.04 | 0.01 | 0.03 | ND | 0.02 | 0.01 | 0.04 | 0.02 | 0.04 | 0.01 | ND | 0.02 | ND | 0.06 |
| 豆类<br>Legumes | 0.06 | 0.05 | 0.07 | 0.08 | 0.07 | 0.34 | 0.15 | 0.13 | 0.16 | 0.43 | 0.27 | 0.28 | 0.04 | 0.09 | 0.06 | 0.11 | 0.06 | 0.07 | 0.24 | 0.07 | 0.10 | 0.34 | 0.05 | 0.52 | 0.16 |
| 薯类<br>Potatoes | 0.09 | 0.02 | 0.10 | 0.10 | 0.03 | 0.09 | 0.07 | 0.02 | 0.25 | 0.10 | 0.24 | 0.19 | 0.07 | 0.04 | 0.01 | 0.04 | 0.02 | 0.10 | 0.10 | 0.05 | 0.03 | 0.04 | ND | 0.12 | 0.08 |
| 肉类<br>Meats | 0.13 | 0.02 | 0.09 | 0.10 | 0.07 | 0.14 | 0.15 | 0.03 | 0.36 | 0.08 | 0.90 | 0.17 | 0.32 | 0.04 | ND | 0.08 | 0.06 | 0.10 | 0.26 | 0.08 | 0.07 | 0.12 | 0.04 | 0.31 | 0.16 |
| 蛋类<br>Eggs | 0.10 | ND | 0.09 | 0.14 | 0.04 | 0.17 | 0.09 | 0.02 | 0.35 | 0.08 | 0.26 | 0.10 | 0.07 | 0.06 | ND | 0.07 | 0.03 | 0.08 | 0.32 | 0.05 | 0.06 | 0.07 | ND | 0.11 | 0.10 |
| 水产类<br>Aquatic foods | 0.09 | 0.02 | 0.03 | 0.14 | 0.12 | 0.05 | 0.08 | 0.04 | 0.06 | 0.06 | 0.31 | 0.03 | 0.08 | 0.09 | 0.02 | 0.05 | 0.10 | 0.07 | 0.22 | 0.05 | 0.10 | 0.08 | 0.05 | 0.10 | 0.08 |
| 乳类<br>Dairy products | ND | ND | ND | ND | ND | 0.01 | ND | ND | ND | ND | ND | ND | ND | ND | 0.02 | ND | ND | ND | 0.01 | 0.02 | ND | ND | ND | ND | 0.01 |

续表

| 膳食类别 Category | 黑龙江 HL | 辽宁 LN | 河北 HE | 北京 BJ | 吉林 JL | 山西 SX | 陕西 SN | 河南 HA | 宁夏 NX | 内蒙古 NM | 青海 QH | 甘肃 GS | 上海 SH | 福建 FJ | 江西 JX | 江苏 JS | 浙江 ZJ | 山东 SD | 湖北 HB | 四川 SC | 广西 GX | 湖南 HN | 广东 GD | 贵州 GZ | 全国平均 AVG |
|---|---|---|---|---|---|---|---|---|---|---|---|---|---|---|---|---|---|---|---|---|---|---|---|---|---|
| 蔬菜类 Vegetables | 0.09 | 0.03 | 0.16 | 0.20 | 0.05 | 0.15 | 0.11 | 0.05 | 0.52 | 0.06 | 0.26 | 0.17 | 0.14 | 0.11 | 0.05 | 0.10 | 0.07 | 0.13 | 0.17 | 0.09 | 0.24 | 0.10 | 0.09 | 0.43 | 0.15 |
| 水果类 Fruits | ND | ND | ND | ND | ND | ND | ND | ND | ND | ND | 0.01 | ND | 0.01 | ND | ND | ND | ND | ND | ND | ND | ND | ND | ND | ND | 0.01 |
| 糖类 Sugar | ND | ND | ND | 0.02 | ND | 0.02 | ND | 0.01 | ND | 0.01 | ND | ND | 0.05 | ND | ND | ND | 0.02 | 0.02 | ND | 0.02 | ND | ND | ND | ND | 0.01 |
| 水及饮料类 Water and beverages | ND | ND | 0.01 | ND | ND | ND | ND | ND | ND | ND | 0.01 | ND | ND | ND | ND | ND | ND | ND | ND | ND | ND | ND | ND | ND | 0.01 |
| 酒类 Alcohol beverages | ND | ND | ND | ND | ND | ND | ND | ND | ND | ND | ND | ND | ND | ND | ND | ND | ND | ND | ND | ND | ND | ND | ND | ND | 0.01 |
| 合计 SUM | 0.64 | 0.18 | 0.60 | 0.81 | 0.43 | 1.02 | 0.72 | 1.22 | 1.75 | 0.89 | 2.30 | 1.01 | 0.81 | 0.49 | 0.19 | 0.50 | 0.39 | 0.53 | 1.36 | 0.48 | 0.62 | 0.78 | 0.29 | 1.61 | 0.82 |

注：未检出（ND）按 1/2 检出限（LOD）计  
Note: values not detected (ND) were treated as being equal to half of the detection of limit (LOD)

附表 6-23　第六次中国总膳食研究膳食样品中二苯并[a,h]蒽的含量（单位：μg/kg）

Annexed Table 6-23　Levels of dibenzo [a,h] anthracene in food samples from the 6$^{th}$ China TDS (Unit: μg/kg)

| 膳食类别 Category | 黑龙江 HL | 辽宁 LN | 河北 HE | 北京 BJ | 吉林 JL | 山西 SX | 陕西 SN | 河南 HA | 宁夏 NX | 内蒙古 NM | 青海 QH | 甘肃 GS | 上海 SH | 福建 FJ | 江西 JX | 江苏 JS | 浙江 ZJ | 山东 SD | 湖北 HB | 四川 SC | 广西 GX | 湖南 HN | 广东 GD | 贵州 GZ | 全国平均 AVG |
|---|---|---|---|---|---|---|---|---|---|---|---|---|---|---|---|---|---|---|---|---|---|---|---|---|---|
| 谷类 Cereals | ND | ND | ND | ND | ND | ND | ND | ND | ND | ND | ND | ND | ND | ND | ND | ND | ND | ND | ND | 0.02 | ND | ND | ND | ND | 0.01 |
| 豆类 Legumes | ND | ND | ND | ND | ND | ND | 0.03 | ND | 0.08 | ND | ND | 0.04 | ND | ND | 0.08 | ND | ND | ND | ND | 0.02 | ND | ND | ND | 0.05 | 0.01 |
| 薯类 Potatoes | ND | ND | 0.02 | ND | ND | ND | 0.01 | ND | ND | ND | 0.04 | 0.03 | 0.02 | ND | ND | ND | ND | ND | ND | ND | ND | ND | ND | ND | 0.02 |

续表

| 膳食类别<br>Category | 黑龙江<br>HL | 辽宁<br>LN | 河北<br>HE | 北京<br>BJ | 吉林<br>JL | 山西<br>SX | 陕西<br>SN | 河南<br>HA | 宁夏<br>NX | 内蒙古<br>NM | 青海<br>QH | 甘肃<br>GS | 上海<br>SH | 福建<br>FJ | 江西<br>JX | 江苏<br>JS | 浙江<br>ZJ | 山东<br>SD | 湖北<br>HB | 四川<br>SC | 广西<br>GX | 湖南<br>HN | 广东<br>GD | 贵州<br>GZ | 全国平均<br>AVG |
|---|---|---|---|---|---|---|---|---|---|---|---|---|---|---|---|---|---|---|---|---|---|---|---|---|---|
| 肉类 Meats | ND | ND | ND | ND | ND | ND | ND | ND | ND | ND | ND | ND | 0.06 | ND | ND | ND | ND | ND | ND | ND | ND | ND | ND | ND | 0.01 |
| 蛋类 Eggs | ND | ND | ND | ND | ND | ND | 0.04 | ND | ND | ND | ND | ND | ND | ND | ND | ND | ND | ND | ND | ND | ND | ND | ND | ND | 0.01 |
| 水产类 Aquatic foods | ND | ND | ND | ND | ND | ND | 0.03 | ND | ND | ND | 0.08 | ND | ND | ND | ND | ND | ND | ND | ND | ND | ND | ND | ND | ND | 0.01 |
| 乳类 Dairy products | ND | ND | ND | ND | ND | ND | ND | ND | ND | ND | ND | ND | ND | ND | ND | ND | ND | ND | ND | ND | ND | ND | ND | ND | 0.01 |
| 蔬菜类 Vegetables | ND | ND | ND | ND | ND | ND | 0.02 | ND | 0.07 | ND | 0.07 | ND | ND | ND | ND | ND | ND | ND | ND | ND | ND | ND | ND | 0.03 | 0.01 |
| 水果类 Fruits | ND | ND | ND | ND | ND | ND | ND | ND | ND | ND | ND | ND | ND | ND | ND | ND | ND | ND | ND | ND | ND | ND | ND | ND | 0.01 |
| 糖类 Sugar | ND | ND | ND | ND | ND | ND | ND | ND | ND | ND | ND | ND | ND | ND | ND | ND | ND | ND | ND | ND | ND | ND | ND | ND | 0.01 |
| 水及饮料类 Water and beverages | ND | ND | ND | ND | ND | ND | ND | ND | ND | ND | ND | ND | ND | ND | ND | ND | ND | ND | ND | ND | ND | ND | ND | ND | 0.01 |
| 酒类 Alcohol beverages | ND | ND | ND | ND | ND | ND | ND | ND | ND | ND | ND | ND | ND | ND | ND | ND | ND | ND | ND | ND | ND | ND | ND | ND | 0.01 |
| 合计 SUM | 0.06 | 0.06 | 0.07 | 0.06 | 0.06 | 0.06 | 0.17 | 0.06 | 0.20 | 0.06 | 0.23 | 0.12 | 0.13 | 0.06 | 0.14 | 0.06 | 0.06 | 0.06 | 0.06 | 0.09 | 0.06 | 0.06 | 0.06 | 0.13 | 0.09 |

注：未检出（ND）按 1/2 检出限（LOD）计

Note: values not detected (ND) were treated as being equal to half of the detection of limit (LOD)

附表 6-24　第六次中国总膳食研究膳食样品中苯并[g,h,i]芘的含量（单位：μg/kg）

Annexed Table 6-24　Levels of benzo [g,h,i] perylene in food samples from the 6th China TDS (Unit: μg/kg)

| 膳食类别 Category | 黑龙江 HL | 辽宁 LN | 河北 HE | 北京 BJ | 吉林 JL | 山西 SX | 陕西 SN | 河南 HA | 宁夏 NX | 内蒙古 NM | 青海 QH | 甘肃 GS | 上海 SH | 福建 FJ | 江西 JX | 江苏 JS | 浙江 ZJ | 山东 SD | 湖北 HB | 四川 SC | 广西 GX | 湖南 HN | 广东 GD | 贵州 GZ | 全国平均 AVG |
|---|---|---|---|---|---|---|---|---|---|---|---|---|---|---|---|---|---|---|---|---|---|---|---|---|---|
| 谷类 Cereals | 0.08 | 0.02 | 0.05 | ND | ND | 0.05 | 0.03 | 0.07 | ND | 0.14 | 0.04 | 0.03 | ND | ND | 0.06 | 0.01 | 0.03 | 0.01 | 0.08 | 0.05 | ND | 0.08 | 0.03 | 0.04 | 0.04 |
| 豆类 Legumes | 0.09 | 0.08 | 0.09 | 0.16 | 0.18 | 1.07 | 0.36 | 0.08 | 0.33 | 0.16 | 0.14 | 0.23 | 0.08 | 0.05 | 0.16 | 0.09 | 0.09 | 0.13 | 0.27 | 0.07 | 0.10 | 0.23 | 0.10 | 0.27 | 0.19 |
| 薯类 Potatoes | 0.10 | 0.04 | 0.14 | 0.22 | 0.10 | 0.19 | 0.13 | 0.03 | 0.76 | 0.14 | 0.43 | 0.21 | 0.15 | 0.03 | ND | 0.06 | 0.05 | 0.08 | 0.20 | 0.06 | 0.04 | 0.07 | 0.04 | 0.13 | 0.14 |
| 肉类 Meats | 0.20 | 0.06 | 0.15 | 0.23 | 0.14 | 0.29 | 0.47 | 0.09 | 0.52 | 0.16 | 2.36 | 0.21 | 1.04 | ND | 0.10 | 0.32 | 0.23 | 0.33 | 0.61 | 0.12 | 0.17 | 0.24 | 0.13 | 0.63 | 0.37 |
| 蛋类 Eggs | 0.13 | 0.05 | 0.17 | 0.21 | 0.12 | 0.35 | 0.19 | ND | 1.05 | ND | 0.34 | 0.24 | 0.15 | 0.06 | 0.08 | 0.11 | 0.30 | 0.32 | 0.35 | 0.08 | 0.09 | 0.15 | ND | 0.17 | 0.20 |
| 水产类 Aquatic foods | 0.12 | 0.03 | 0.07 | 0.47 | 0.29 | 0.09 | 0.15 | 0.07 | 0.19 | 0.11 | 0.58 | 0.07 | 0.20 | 0.08 | 0.06 | 0.08 | 0.32 | 0.16 | 0.52 | 0.08 | 0.08 | 0.17 | 0.08 | 0.14 | 0.18 |
| 乳类 Dairy products | 0.03 | ND | ND | ND | ND | ND | ND | ND | ND | ND | ND | ND | ND | ND | 0.04 | ND | ND | ND | ND | 0.04 | 0.01 | ND | 0.04 | ND | 0.01 |
| 蔬菜类 Vegetables | 0.12 | 0.05 | 0.12 | 0.23 | 0.12 | 0.28 | 0.20 | 0.06 | 0.72 | 0.12 | 0.45 | 0.26 | 0.34 | 0.08 | 0.08 | 0.14 | 0.12 | 0.22 | 0.35 | 0.11 | 0.12 | 0.17 | 0.13 | 1.28 | 0.24 |
| 水果类 Fruits | ND | 0.02 | 0.02 | 0.02 | ND | ND | ND | ND | ND | 0.02 | 0.02 | ND | ND | ND | ND | ND | ND | ND | ND | 0.02 | ND | ND | ND | ND | 0.01 |
| 糖类 Sugar | ND | ND | 0.02 | 0.04 | ND | ND | ND | 0.02 | ND | 0.03 | ND | ND | 0.12 | ND | ND | ND | 0.10 | 0.05 | ND | ND | ND | ND | ND | ND | 0.03 |
| 水及饮料类 Water and beverages | ND | ND | 0.02 | ND | ND | ND | ND | ND | ND | ND | ND | ND | ND | ND | 0.03 | ND | ND | 0.02 | ND | ND | ND | ND | ND | ND | 0.01 |

续表

| 膳食类别<br>Category | 黑龙江<br>HL | 辽宁<br>LN | 河北<br>HE | 北京<br>BJ | 吉林<br>JL | 山西<br>SX | 陕西<br>SN | 河南<br>HA | 宁夏<br>NX | 内蒙古<br>NM | 青海<br>QH | 甘肃<br>GS | 上海<br>SH | 福建<br>FJ | 江西<br>JX | 江苏<br>JS | 浙江<br>ZJ | 山东<br>SD | 湖北<br>HB | 四川<br>SC | 广西<br>GX | 湖南<br>HN | 广东<br>GD | 贵州<br>GZ | 全国平均<br>AVG |
|---|---|---|---|---|---|---|---|---|---|---|---|---|---|---|---|---|---|---|---|---|---|---|---|---|---|
| 酒类<br>Alcohol beverages | ND | ND | ND | ND | ND | ND | ND | ND | ND | ND | ND | ND | ND | ND | ND | ND | ND | 0.01 | ND | ND | ND | ND | ND | ND | 0.01 |
| 合计<br>SUM | 0.89 | 0.37 | 0.86 | 1.60 | 0.98 | 2.35 | 1.56 | 0.44 | 3.59 | 0.90 | 4.38 | 1.28 | 2.11 | 0.34 | 0.63 | 0.84 | 1.26 | 1.34 | 2.44 | 0.65 | 0.63 | 1.14 | 0.58 | 2.69 | 1.42 |

注：未检出（ND）按 1/2 检出限（LOD）计

Note: values not detected (ND) were treated as being equal to half of the detection of limit (LOD)

附表 6-25　第六次中国总膳食研究膳食样品中茚并 [1,2,3-cd] 芘的含量（单位：μg/kg）

Annexed Table 6-25　Levels of indeno [1,2,3-cd] pyrene in food samples from the 6$^{th}$ China TDS (Unit: μg/kg)

| 膳食类别<br>Category | 黑龙江<br>HL | 辽宁<br>LN | 河北<br>HE | 北京<br>BJ | 吉林<br>JL | 山西<br>SX | 陕西<br>SN | 河南<br>HA | 宁夏<br>NX | 内蒙古<br>NM | 青海<br>QH | 甘肃<br>GS | 上海<br>SH | 福建<br>FJ | 江西<br>JX | 江苏<br>JS | 浙江<br>ZJ | 山东<br>SD | 湖北<br>HB | 四川<br>SC | 广西<br>GX | 湖南<br>HN | 广东<br>GD | 贵州<br>GZ | 全国平均<br>AVG |
|---|---|---|---|---|---|---|---|---|---|---|---|---|---|---|---|---|---|---|---|---|---|---|---|---|---|
| 谷类<br>Cereals | 0.07 | ND | 0.03 | ND | ND | ND | 0.02 | ND | ND | 0.07 | 0.04 | 0.03 | 0.01 | ND | ND | ND | ND | 0.02 | ND | 0.04 | ND | ND | 0.01 | ND | 0.02 |
| 豆类<br>Legumes | 0.08 | 0.07 | 0.06 | 0.10 | 0.10 | 0.35 | 0.15 | 0.08 | 0.27 | 0.14 | 0.13 | 0.20 | 0.04 | 0.04 | 0.09 | 0.08 | 0.05 | 0.04 | 0.19 | 0.06 | 0.10 | 0.19 | 0.03 | 0.20 | 0.12 |
| 薯类<br>Potatoes | 0.11 | ND | 0.10 | 0.13 | 0.02 | 0.12 | 0.09 | ND | 0.53 | 0.10 | 0.34 | 0.15 | 0.09 | 0.03 | ND | 0.04 | 0.03 | ND | 0.13 | 0.05 | 0.05 | 0.06 | ND | 0.09 | 0.09 |
| 肉类<br>Meats | 0.21 | 0.12 | 0.12 | 0.14 | 0.06 | ND | 0.23 | ND | 0.31 | 0.11 | 1.78 | 0.14 | 0.65 | 0.01 | ND | 0.13 | ND | 0.16 | 0.31 | 0.09 | 0.09 | 0.21 | 0.03 | 0.42 | 0.22 |
| 蛋类<br>Eggs | 0.11 | 0.07 | 0.14 | 0.18 | 0.03 | 0.25 | 0.14 | 0.05 | 0.33 | ND | 0.31 | 1.90 | 0.09 | 0.04 | ND | 0.09 | 0.06 | 0.66 | 0.12 | 0.07 | 0.09 | 0.12 | ND | 0.10 | 0.21 |
| 水产类<br>Aquatic foods | 0.12 | ND | 0.04 | 0.17 | 0.10 | 0.06 | 0.11 | 0.07 | 0.14 | 0.08 | 0.45 | 0.05 | 0.12 | 0.05 | 0.03 | 0.05 | 0.17 | 0.12 | 0.14 | 0.05 | 0.10 | 0.14 | 0.04 | 0.09 | 0.10 |
| 乳类<br>Dairy products | ND | ND | ND | ND | ND | ND | ND | ND | ND | ND | ND | ND | ND | ND | 0.01 | ND | ND | ND | ND | ND | ND | ND | ND | ND | 0.01 |

续表

| 膳食类别<br>Category | 黑龙江<br>HL | 辽宁<br>LN | 河北<br>HE | 北京<br>BJ | 吉林<br>JL | 山西<br>SX | 陕西<br>SN | 河南<br>HA | 宁夏<br>NX | 内蒙古<br>NM | 青海<br>QH | 甘肃<br>GS | 上海<br>SH | 福建<br>FJ | 江西<br>JX | 江苏<br>JS | 浙江<br>ZJ | 山东<br>SD | 湖北<br>HB | 四川<br>SC | 广西<br>GX | 湖南<br>HN | 广东<br>GD | 贵州<br>GZ | 全国平均<br>AVG |
|---|---|---|---|---|---|---|---|---|---|---|---|---|---|---|---|---|---|---|---|---|---|---|---|---|---|
| 蔬菜类 Vegetables | 0.12 | ND | 0.08 | 0.16 | 0.04 | 0.19 | 0.16 | 0.06 | 0.47 | 0.08 | 0.35 | 0.20 | 0.21 | 0.06 | 0.06 | 0.10 | 0.08 | 0.08 | 0.22 | 0.09 | 0.14 | 0.14 | 0.09 | 0.76 | 0.16 |
| 水果类 Fruits | ND | 0.01 | ND | ND | ND | ND | ND | ND | ND | ND | ND | ND | ND | ND | ND | ND | ND | ND | ND | ND | ND | ND | ND | ND | 0.01 |
| 糖类 Sugar | ND | ND | ND | 0.02 | ND | ND | ND | ND | ND | 0.02 | ND | ND | 0.06 | ND | ND | ND | 0.03 | 0.05 | ND | ND | ND | ND | ND | ND | 0.01 |
| 水及饮料类 Water and beverages | ND | ND | ND | ND | ND | ND | ND | ND | ND | ND | ND | ND | ND | ND | ND | ND | ND | ND | ND | ND | ND | ND | ND | ND | 0.01 |
| 酒类 Alcohol beverages | ND | ND | ND | ND | ND | ND | ND | ND | ND | ND | ND | ND | ND | ND | ND | ND | ND | ND | ND | ND | ND | ND | ND | ND | 0.01 |
| 合计 SUM | 0.85 | 0.20 | 0.60 | 0.92 | 0.38 | 1.01 | 0.93 | 0.30 | 2.07 | 0.62 | 3.42 | 2.70 | 1.29 | 0.26 | 0.23 | 0.52 | 0.45 | 1.16 | 1.14 | 0.46 | 0.60 | 0.89 | 0.24 | 1.69 | 0.96 |

注：未检出（ND）按 1/2 检出限（LOD）计

Note: values not detected (ND) were treated as being equal to half of the detection of limit (LOD)

附表 6-26 第六次中国总膳食研究膳食样品中苯并[j]荧蒽的含量（单位：μg/kg）

Annexed Table 6-26 Levels of benzo [j] fluoranthene in food samples from the 6$^{th}$ China TDS (Unit: μg/kg)

| 膳食类别<br>Category | 黑龙江<br>HL | 辽宁<br>LN | 河北<br>HE | 北京<br>BJ | 吉林<br>JL | 山西<br>SX | 陕西<br>SN | 河南<br>HA | 宁夏<br>NX | 内蒙古<br>NM | 青海<br>QH | 甘肃<br>GS | 上海<br>SH | 福建<br>FJ | 江西<br>JX | 江苏<br>JS | 浙江<br>ZJ | 山东<br>SD | 湖北<br>HB | 四川<br>SC | 广西<br>GX | 湖南<br>HN | 广东<br>GD | 贵州<br>GZ | 全国平均<br>AVG |
|---|---|---|---|---|---|---|---|---|---|---|---|---|---|---|---|---|---|---|---|---|---|---|---|---|---|
| 谷类 Cereals | 0.05 | 0.02 | 0.03 | ND | 0.02 | 0.04 | 0.02 | 0.09 | ND | 0.05 | 0.02 | 0.04 | 0.01 | ND | ND | 0.01 | 0.01 | 0.03 | 0.02 | 0.06 | 0.01 | ND | 0.02 | ND | 0.02 |
| 豆类 Legumes | 0.06 | 0.06 | 0.07 | 0.09 | 0.10 | 0.37 | 0.17 | 0.13 | 0.21 | 0.43 | 0.24 | 0.28 | 0.05 | 0.06 | 0.07 | 0.12 | 0.07 | 0.07 | 0.24 | 0.07 | 0.11 | 0.40 | 0.06 | 0.34 | 0.16 |
| 薯类 Potatoes | 0.09 | 0.02 | 0.05 | 0.13 | 0.03 | 0.10 | 0.07 | 0.01 | 0.33 | 0.11 | 0.24 | 0.18 | 0.04 | 0.03 | 0.01 | 0.04 | 0.03 | 0.01 | 0.11 | 0.05 | 0.04 | 0.04 | ND | 0.10 | 0.08 |

续表

| 膳食类别 Category | 黑龙江 HL | 辽宁 LN | 河北 HE | 北京 BJ | 吉林 JL | 山西 SX | 陕西 SN | 河南 HA | 宁夏 NX | 内蒙古 NM | 青海 QH | 甘肃 GS | 上海 SH | 福建 FJ | 江西 JX | 江苏 JS | 浙江 ZJ | 山东 SD | 湖北 HB | 四川 SC | 广西 GX | 湖南 HN | 广东 GD | 贵州 GZ | 全国平均 AVG |
|---|---|---|---|---|---|---|---|---|---|---|---|---|---|---|---|---|---|---|---|---|---|---|---|---|---|
| 肉类 Meats | 0.16 | 0.04 | 0.08 | 0.04 | 0.09 | 0.12 | 0.21 | 0.03 | 0.23 | 0.06 | 1.18 | 0.19 | 0.54 | 0.02 | ND | 0.11 | 0.08 | 0.06 | 0.26 | 0.12 | 0.07 | 0.12 | 0.05 | 0.31 | 0.17 |
| 蛋类 Eggs | 0.10 | 0.02 | 0.07 | 0.15 | 0.05 | 0.17 | 0.10 | 0.02 | 0.22 | 0.08 | 0.25 | 0.17 | 0.05 | 0.03 | ND | 0.08 | 0.03 | 0.06 | 0.20 | 0.05 | 0.06 | 0.08 | ND | 0.10 | 0.09 |
| 水产类 Aquatic foods | 0.06 | 0.03 | 0.02 | 0.18 | 0.13 | 0.05 | 0.08 | 0.05 | 0.07 | 0.07 | 0.30 | 0.06 | 0.10 | 0.06 | 0.02 | 0.05 | 0.17 | 0.09 | 0.26 | 0.07 | 0.04 | 0.10 | 0.05 | 0.10 | 0.09 |
| 乳类 Dairy products | ND | ND | ND | 0.04 | ND | ND | ND | ND | ND | ND | ND | ND | ND | ND | 0.03 | ND | ND | ND | 0.01 | ND | ND | ND | ND | ND | 0.01 |
| 蔬菜类 Vegetables | 0.10 | 0.04 | 0.19 | 0.20 | 0.06 | 0.16 | 0.13 | ND | 0.38 | 0.07 | 0.27 | 0.22 | 0.13 | 0.09 | 0.06 | 0.11 | 0.10 | 0.14 | 0.19 | 0.14 | 0.14 | 0.07 | 0.13 | 0.67 | 0.16 |
| 水果类 Fruits | ND | ND | ND | ND | ND | ND | ND | 0.01 | ND | ND | ND | ND | 0.01 | ND | ND | ND | ND | ND | ND | ND | ND | ND | ND | ND | 0.01 |
| 糖类 Sugar | ND | ND | ND | 0.03 | ND | 0.02 | ND | ND | ND | 0.02 | ND | ND | 0.12 | ND | ND | ND | 0.02 | 0.02 | ND | 0.02 | ND | ND | ND | ND | 0.02 |
| 水及饮料类 Water and beverages | ND | ND | 0.01 | ND | ND | ND | ND | ND | ND | ND | ND | ND | ND | ND | ND | ND | ND | ND | ND | ND | ND | ND | ND | ND | 0.01 |
| 酒类 Alcohol beverages | ND | ND | ND | ND | ND | ND | ND | ND | ND | ND | ND | ND | ND | ND | ND | ND | ND | ND | ND | ND | ND | ND | ND | ND | 0.01 |
| 合计 SUM | 0.65 | 0.26 | 0.53 | 0.88 | 0.51 | 1.05 | 0.81 | 0.41 | 1.46 | 0.91 | 2.52 | 1.17 | 1.07 | 0.32 | 0.22 | 0.55 | 0.53 | 0.50 | 1.31 | 0.59 | 0.49 | 0.84 | 0.35 | 1.65 | 0.82 |

注：未检出（ND）按1/2检出限（LOD）计

Note: values not detected (ND) were treated as being equal to half of the detection of limit (LOD)

附表 6-27　第六次中国总膳食研究膳食样品中环戊井[c,d]芘的含量（单位：μg/kg）

Annexed Table 6-27　Levels of cyclopenta [c,d] pyrene in food samples from the 6$^{th}$ China TDS (Unit: μg/kg)

| 膳食类别 Category | 黑龙江 HL | 辽宁 LN | 河北 HE | 北京 BJ | 吉林 JL | 山西 SX | 陕西 SN | 河南 HA | 宁夏 NX | 内蒙古 NM | 青海 QH | 甘肃 GS | 上海 SH | 福建 FJ | 江西 JX | 江苏 JS | 浙江 ZJ | 山东 SD | 湖北 HB | 四川 SC | 广西 GX | 湖南 HN | 广东 GD | 贵州 GZ | 全国平均 AVG |
|---|---|---|---|---|---|---|---|---|---|---|---|---|---|---|---|---|---|---|---|---|---|---|---|---|---|
| 谷类 Cereals | ND | ND | ND | ND | ND | ND | ND | ND | ND | ND | ND | ND | ND | ND | ND | ND | ND | ND | ND | 0.03 | ND | ND | ND | 0.03 | 0.01 |
| 豆类 Legumes | ND | 0.04 | ND | ND | 0.57 | ND | ND | ND | 0.21 | ND | 0.07 | ND | 0.09 | ND | 0.23 | ND | ND | ND | ND | 0.02 | ND | ND | ND | 0.96 | 0.09 |
| 薯类 Potatoes | ND | ND | ND | ND | ND | ND | ND | ND | 0.33 | ND | 0.56 | ND | ND | ND | ND | ND | 0.04 | ND | ND | 0.01 | ND | ND | ND | 0.16 | 0.05 |
| 肉类 Meats | 0.06 | ND | 0.01 | 0.12 | ND | ND | 0.27 | ND | ND | ND | 4.48 | ND | 0.47 | ND | ND | ND | 0.41 | ND | 0.98 | 0.05 | ND | ND | ND | 1.31 | 0.34 |
| 蛋类 Eggs | ND | ND | ND | ND | ND | ND | ND | ND | 0.37 | ND | ND | ND | ND | ND | ND | ND | 0.27 | ND | ND | ND | 0.05 | ND | ND | 0.19 | 0.05 |
| 水产类 Aquatic foods | ND | ND | ND | ND | ND | ND | ND | ND | ND | ND | 0.55 | ND | 0.25 | ND | ND | ND | 0.81 | ND | 0.22 | 0.03 | ND | ND | ND | 0.15 | 0.09 |
| 乳类 Dairy products | ND | ND | ND | ND | ND | ND | ND | ND | ND | ND | ND | ND | ND | ND | ND | ND | ND | ND | ND | ND | ND | ND | ND | ND | 0.01 |
| 蔬菜类 Vegetables | ND | ND | 0.09 | ND | ND | 0.06 | ND | ND | 0.71 | ND | 0.42 | ND | 1.05 | ND | 0.03 | ND | ND | 0.02 | 0.01 | 0.04 | ND | ND | ND | 2.87 | 0.22 |
| 水果类 Fruits | ND | ND | ND | ND | ND | ND | ND | ND | ND | ND | ND | ND | ND | ND | ND | ND | ND | ND | ND | ND | ND | ND | ND | ND | 0.01 |
| 糖类 Sugar | ND | ND | ND | 0.02 | ND | ND | ND | ND | ND | ND | ND | ND | 0.06 | ND | ND | ND | ND | ND | ND | ND | 0.01 | ND | ND | 0.04 | 0.01 |
| 水及饮料类 Water and beverages | ND | ND | ND | ND | ND | ND | ND | ND | ND | ND | ND | ND | ND | ND | ND | ND | ND | ND | ND | ND | ND | ND | ND | ND | 0.01 |

续表

| 膳食类别<br>Category | 黑龙江<br>HL | 辽宁<br>LN | 河北<br>HE | 北京<br>BJ | 吉林<br>JL | 山西<br>SX | 陕西<br>SN | 河南<br>HA | 宁夏<br>NX | 内蒙古<br>NM | 青海<br>QH | 甘肃<br>GS | 上海<br>SH | 福建<br>FJ | 江西<br>JX | 江苏<br>JS | 浙江<br>ZJ | 山东<br>SD | 湖北<br>HB | 四川<br>SC | 广西<br>GX | 湖南<br>HN | 广东<br>GD | 贵州<br>GZ | 全国平均<br>AVG |
|---|---|---|---|---|---|---|---|---|---|---|---|---|---|---|---|---|---|---|---|---|---|---|---|---|---|
| 酒类<br>Alcohol beverages | ND | ND | ND | ND | ND | ND | ND | ND | ND | ND | ND | ND | ND | ND | ND | ND | ND | ND | ND | ND | ND | ND | ND | ND | 0.01 |
| 合计<br>SUM | 0.12 | 0.10 | 0.15 | 0.19 | 0.63 | 0.12 | 0.33 | 0.06 | 1.65 | 0.06 | 6.11 | 0.06 | 1.96 | 0.06 | 0.30 | 0.06 | 1.57 | 0.07 | 1.26 | 0.20 | 0.11 | 0.06 | 0.06 | 5.73 | 0.87 |

注: 未检出 (ND) 按 1/2 检出限 (LOD) 计
Note: values not detected (ND) were treated as being equal to half of the detection of limit (LOD)

附表 6-28 第六次中国总膳食研究膳食样品中 PAH4 的含量 (单位: μg/kg)
Annexed Table 6-28 Levels of PAH4 in food samples from the 6th China TDS (Unit: μg/kg)

| 膳食类别<br>Category | 黑龙江<br>HL | 辽宁<br>LN | 河北<br>HE | 北京<br>BJ | 吉林<br>JL | 山西<br>SX | 陕西<br>SN | 河南<br>HA | 宁夏<br>NX | 内蒙古<br>NM | 青海<br>QH | 甘肃<br>GS | 上海<br>SH | 福建<br>FJ | 江西<br>JX | 江苏<br>JS | 浙江<br>ZJ | 山东<br>SD | 湖北<br>HB | 四川<br>SC | 广西<br>GX | 湖南<br>HN | 广东<br>GD | 贵州<br>GZ | 全国平均<br>AVG |
|---|---|---|---|---|---|---|---|---|---|---|---|---|---|---|---|---|---|---|---|---|---|---|---|---|---|
| 谷类<br>Cereals | 0.51 | 0.16 | 0.44 | 0.03 | 0.21 | 0.36 | 0.23 | 1.04 | 0.26 | 0.59 | 0.27 | 0.34 | 0.22 | 0.13 | 0.19 | 0.20 | 0.16 | 0.30 | 0.28 | 0.25 | 0.14 | 0.16 | 0.24 | 0.21 | 0.29 |
| 豆类<br>Legumes | 0.64 | 0.61 | 0.90 | 0.97 | 0.91 | 2.86 | 1.79 | 1.47 | 1.93 | 5.96 | 1.59 | 3.74 | 0.43 | 0.51 | 0.89 | 1.31 | 0.68 | 0.90 | 2.55 | 0.58 | 1.12 | 5.14 | 0.83 | 5.75 | 1.84 |
| 薯类<br>Potatoes | 0.90 | 0.25 | 0.90 | 1.07 | 0.41 | 0.83 | 0.59 | 0.25 | 2.68 | 0.79 | 1.81 | 1.64 | 0.63 | 0.24 | 0.15 | 0.34 | 0.21 | 0.38 | 1.01 | 0.29 | 0.37 | 0.41 | 0.05 | 1.05 | 0.72 |
| 肉类<br>Meats | 1.32 | 0.42 | 0.91 | 1.01 | 0.93 | 1.32 | 1.74 | 0.69 | 2.71 | 0.80 | 7.11 | 1.68 | 3.14 | 0.26 | 0.36 | 1.02 | 0.64 | 0.82 | 2.09 | 0.76 | 0.80 | 1.49 | 0.60 | 3.36 | 1.50 |
| 蛋类<br>Eggs | 1.02 | 0.29 | 1.08 | 1.39 | 0.57 | 1.48 | 0.83 | 0.27 | 2.37 | 0.67 | 2.09 | 1.69 | 0.56 | 0.42 | 0.25 | 0.82 | 0.30 | 1.03 | 1.73 | 0.40 | 0.57 | 0.84 | 0.02 | 1.23 | 0.91 |
| 水产类<br>Aquatic foods | 1.00 | 0.32 | 0.41 | 1.46 | 1.52 | 0.48 | 0.72 | 0.47 | 0.90 | 0.67 | 2.61 | 0.58 | 0.80 | 0.65 | 0.28 | 0.53 | 1.28 | 0.63 | 2.17 | 0.38 | 0.73 | 1.13 | 0.56 | 0.94 | 0.88 |
| 乳类<br>Dairy products | 0.05 | 0.04 | 0.02 | 0.06 | 0.07 | 0.17 | 0.07 | 0.05 | 0.08 | 0.06 | 0.02 | 0.02 | 0.06 | 0.06 | 0.27 | 0.08 | 0.06 | 0.04 | 0.17 | 0.09 | 0.12 | 0.02 | 0.08 | 0.06 | 0.07 |

续表

| 膳食类别<br>Category | 黑龙江<br>HL | 辽宁<br>LN | 河北<br>HE | 北京<br>BJ | 吉林<br>JL | 山西<br>SX | 陕西<br>SN | 河南<br>HA | 宁夏<br>NX | 内蒙古<br>NM | 青海<br>QH | 甘肃<br>GS | 上海<br>SH | 福建<br>FJ | 江西<br>JX | 江苏<br>JS | 浙江<br>ZJ | 山东<br>SD | 湖北<br>HB | 四川<br>SC | 广西<br>GX | 湖南<br>HN | 广东<br>GD | 贵州<br>GZ | 全国平均<br>AVG |
|---|---|---|---|---|---|---|---|---|---|---|---|---|---|---|---|---|---|---|---|---|---|---|---|---|---|
| 蔬菜类 Vegetables | 0.95 | 0.46 | 1.71 | 1.59 | 0.70 | 1.50 | 1.11 | 0.58 | 3.38 | 0.59 | 2.09 | 1.93 | 1.34 | 0.75 | 0.62 | 0.84 | 0.73 | 0.96 | 1.76 | 0.60 | 1.20 | 1.15 | 1.28 | 4.03 | 1.33 |
| 水果类 Fruits | 0.02 | 0.09 | 0.05 | 0.04 | 0.04 | 0.11 | 0.02 | 0.02 | ND | 0.05 | 0.13 | 0.04 | 0.15 | 0.02 | 0.04 | 0.08 | 0.07 | 0.04 | 0.02 | 0.08 | 0.02 | 0.02 | 0.02 | 0.03 | 0.05 |
| 糖类 Sugar | 0.02 | 0.02 | 0.04 | 0.19 | 0.04 | 0.22 | 0.02 | 0.13 | 0.07 | 0.13 | 0.08 | 0.11 | 0.84 | 0.02 | 0.05 | 0.04 | 0.23 | 0.19 | 0.02 | 0.08 | 0.03 | 0.02 | 0.02 | 0.02 | 0.12 |
| 水及饮料类 Water and beverages | 0.02 | 0.02 | 0.10 | 0.02 | 0.02 | 0.07 | 0.02 | 0.02 | 0.02 | 0.02 | 0.04 | 0.02 | 0.06 | 0.02 | 0.02 | 0.02 | 0.06 | 0.02 | 0.02 | 0.02 | 0.03 | 0.02 | 0.02 | 0.02 | 0.03 |
| 酒类 Alcohol beverages | 0.02 | 0.02 | ND | 0.02 | 0.02 | 0.08 | 0.02 | 0.02 | 0.02 | 0.02 | 0.02 | 0.02 | 0.02 | 0.02 | 0.03 | 0.02 | 0.05 | 0.02 | 0.02 | 0.02 | 0.02 | 0.02 | 0.02 | 0.06 | 0.03 |
| 合计 SUM | 6.47 | 2.70 | 6.55 | 7.85 | 5.43 | 9.46 | 7.16 | 5.00 | 14.4 | 10.3 | 17.9 | 11.8 | 8.24 | 3.09 | 3.13 | 5.30 | 4.45 | 5.34 | 11.8 | 3.54 | 5.15 | 10.4 | 3.73 | 16.8 | 7.76 |

注：未检出（ND）按 1/2 检出限（LOD）计
Note: values not detected (ND) were treated as being equal to half of the detection of limit (LOD)

附表 6-29 第六次中国总膳食研究膳食样品中 PAH16 的含量（单位：μg/kg）
Annexed Table 6-29 Levels of PAH16 in food samples from the 6$^{th}$ China TDS (Unit: μg/kg)

| 膳食类别<br>Category | 黑龙江<br>HL | 辽宁<br>LN | 河北<br>HE | 北京<br>BJ | 吉林<br>JL | 山西<br>SX | 陕西<br>SN | 河南<br>HA | 宁夏<br>NX | 内蒙古<br>NM | 青海<br>QH | 甘肃<br>GS | 上海<br>SH | 福建<br>FJ | 江西<br>JX | 江苏<br>JS | 浙江<br>ZJ | 山东<br>SD | 湖北<br>HB | 四川<br>SC | 广西<br>GX | 湖南<br>HN | 广东<br>GD | 贵州<br>GZ | 全国平均<br>AVG |
|---|---|---|---|---|---|---|---|---|---|---|---|---|---|---|---|---|---|---|---|---|---|---|---|---|---|
| 谷类 Cereals | 0.80 | 0.26 | 0.63 | 0.09 | 0.30 | 0.53 | 0.38 | 2.15 | 0.34 | 0.94 | 0.43 | 0.52 | 0.30 | 0.21 | 0.30 | 0.29 | 0.26 | 0.44 | 0.45 | 0.51 | 0.21 | 0.29 | 0.36 | 0.32 | 0.47 |
| 豆类 Legumes | 0.97 | 0.95 | 1.24 | 1.44 | 1.97 | 5.03 | 2.69 | 1.93 | 3.14 | 7.16 | 2.48 | 4.81 | 0.77 | 0.79 | 1.53 | 1.75 | 0.99 | 1.26 | 3.53 | 0.92 | 1.56 | 6.34 | 1.11 | 8.13 | 2.60 |
| 薯类 Potatoes | 1.33 | 0.38 | 1.34 | 1.69 | 0.63 | 1.37 | 1.00 | 0.36 | 4.99 | 1.28 | 3.68 | 2.44 | 1.04 | 0.41 | 0.30 | 0.56 | 0.42 | 0.53 | 1.59 | 0.54 | 0.58 | 0.66 | 0.14 | 1.69 | 1.20 |

续表

| 膳食类别<br>Category | 黑龙江<br>HL | 辽宁<br>LN | 河北<br>HE | 北京<br>BJ | 吉林<br>JL | 山西<br>SX | 陕西<br>SN | 河南<br>HA | 宁夏<br>NX | 内蒙古<br>NM | 青海<br>QH | 甘肃<br>GS | 上海<br>SH | 福建<br>FJ | 江西<br>JX | 江苏<br>JS | 浙江<br>ZJ | 山东<br>SD | 湖北<br>HB | 四川<br>SC | 广西<br>GX | 湖南<br>HN | 广东<br>GD | 贵州<br>GZ | 全国平均<br>AVG |
|---|---|---|---|---|---|---|---|---|---|---|---|---|---|---|---|---|---|---|---|---|---|---|---|---|---|
| 肉类 Meats | 2.12 | 0.59 | 1.40 | 1.56 | 1.33 | 1.92 | 3.11 | 0.89 | 4.17 | 1.25 | 17.84 | 2.43 | 6.25 | 0.37 | 0.51 | 1.70 | 1.46 | 1.50 | 4.55 | 1.25 | 1.23 | 2.22 | 0.89 | 6.37 | 2.79 |
| 蛋类 Eggs | 1.50 | 0.48 | 1.59 | 2.22 | 0.85 | 2.46 | 1.43 | 0.40 | 4.72 | 0.88 | 3.29 | 4.14 | 0.96 | 0.65 | 0.38 | 1.21 | 1.03 | 2.19 | 2.76 | 0.68 | 0.94 | 1.30 | 0.08 | 1.94 | 1.59 |
| 水产类 Aquatic foods | 1.43 | 0.45 | 0.61 | 2.46 | 2.20 | 0.77 | 1.21 | 0.74 | 1.39 | 1.03 | 4.91 | 0.83 | 1.59 | 0.97 | 0.44 | 0.80 | 2.89 | 1.10 | 3.57 | 0.69 | 1.09 | 1.66 | 0.82 | 1.54 | 1.47 |
| 乳类 Dairy products | 0.13 | 0.10 | 0.08 | 0.15 | 0.13 | 0.23 | 0.13 | 0.11 | 0.14 | 0.12 | 0.08 | 0.08 | 0.12 | 0.12 | 0.41 | 0.14 | 0.12 | 0.10 | 0.27 | 0.21 | 0.19 | 0.08 | 0.17 | 0.12 | 0.15 |
| 蔬菜类 Vegetables | 1.42 | 0.63 | 2.39 | 2.42 | 1.01 | 2.38 | 1.77 | 0.84 | 6.28 | 0.96 | 3.93 | 2.82 | 3.25 | 1.13 | 0.93 | 1.33 | 1.14 | 1.57 | 2.74 | 1.10 | 1.88 | 1.67 | 1.76 | 10.1 | 2.31 |
| 水果类 Fruits | 0.08 | 0.17 | 0.12 | 0.11 | 0.10 | 0.17 | 0.08 | 0.08 | ND | 0.12 | 0.21 | 0.10 | 0.22 | 0.08 | 0.10 | 0.14 | 0.13 | 0.10 | 0.08 | 0.14 | 0.08 | 0.08 | 0.08 | 0.09 | 0.11 |
| 糖类 Sugar | 0.08 | 0.08 | 0.12 | 0.35 | 0.10 | 0.31 | 0.08 | 0.21 | 0.13 | 0.24 | 0.14 | 0.17 | 1.29 | 0.08 | 0.11 | 0.10 | 0.44 | 0.38 | 0.08 | 0.19 | 0.10 | 0.08 | 0.08 | 0.12 | 0.23 |
| 水及饮料类 Water and beverages | 0.08 | 0.08 | 0.18 | 0.08 | 0.08 | 0.13 | 0.08 | 0.08 | 0.08 | 0.08 | 0.11 | 0.08 | 0.12 | 0.08 | 0.11 | 0.08 | 0.12 | 0.09 | 0.08 | 0.08 | 0.09 | 0.08 | 0.08 | 0.08 | 0.09 |
| 酒类 Alcohol beverages | 0.08 | 0.08 | ND | 0.08 | 0.08 | 0.14 | 0.08 | 0.08 | 0.08 | 0.08 | 0.08 | 0.08 | 0.08 | 0.08 | 0.09 | 0.08 | 0.11 | 0.09 | 0.08 | 0.08 | 0.08 | 0.08 | 0.08 | 0.12 | 0.09 |
| 合计 SUM | 10.02 | 4.21 | 9.69 | 12.66 | 8.77 | 15.41 | 12.01 | 7.85 | 25.45 | 14.14 | 37.18 | 18.49 | 15.95 | 4.97 | 5.19 | 8.17 | 9.07 | 9.35 | 19.76 | 6.38 | 8.02 | 14.54 | 5.65 | 30.61 | 13.10 |

注：未检出（ND）按 1/2 检出限（LOD）计

Note: values not detected (ND) were treated as being equal to half of the detection of limit (LOD)

附表 6-30  第六次中国总膳食研究苯并[a]芘膳食摄入量 [单位：ng/(kg bw·d)]
Annexed Table 6-30  Dietary intakes of benzo[a] pyrene from the 6$^{th}$ China TDS[Unit: ng/(kg bw·d)]

| 膳食类别<br>Category | 黑龙江<br>HL | 辽宁<br>LN | 河北<br>HE | 北京<br>BJ | 吉林<br>JL | 山西<br>SX | 陕西<br>SN | 河南<br>HA | 宁夏<br>NX | 内蒙古<br>NM | 青海<br>QH | 甘肃<br>GS | 上海<br>SH | 福建<br>FJ | 江西<br>JX | 江苏<br>JS | 浙江<br>ZJ | 山东<br>SD | 湖北<br>HB | 四川<br>SC | 广西<br>GX | 湖南<br>HN | 广东<br>GD | 贵州<br>GZ | 全国平均<br>AVG |
|---|---|---|---|---|---|---|---|---|---|---|---|---|---|---|---|---|---|---|---|---|---|---|---|---|---|
| 谷类 Cereals | 0.61 | 0.29 | 0.61 | 0.06 | 0.05 | 0.82 | 0.36 | 1.47 | 0.05 | 1.03 | 0.47 | 0.44 | 0.14 | 0.05 | 0.26 | 0.25 | 0.20 | 0.27 | 0.34 | 0.58 | 0.07 | 0.05 | 0.22 | 0.35 | 0.37 |
| 豆类 Legumes | 0.06 | 0.21 | 0.10 | 0.26 | 0.23 | 0.61 | 0.33 | 0.14 | 0.19 | 0.37 | 0.03 | 0.32 | 0.13 | 0.11 | 0.16 | 0.22 | 0.25 | 0.11 | 0.42 | 0.10 | 0.10 | 0.68 | 0.04 | 1.18 | 0.28 |
| 薯类 Potatoes | 0.15 | 0.05 | 0.15 | 0.19 | 0.10 | 0.24 | 0.22 | 0.04 | 0.97 | 0.25 | 0.67 | 0.53 | 0.07 | 0.03 | 0.01 | 0.03 | 0.02 | 0.03 | 0.24 | 0.06 | 0.01 | 0.06 | 0.00 | 0.10 | 0.14 |
| 肉类 Meats | 0.21 | 0.06 | 0.12 | 0.19 | 0.12 | 0.46 | 0.21 | 0.06 | 0.37 | 0.14 | 2.53 | 0.11 | 1.79 | 0.01 | 0.01 | 0.28 | 0.24 | 0.29 | 0.40 | 0.27 | 0.29 | 0.52 | 0.10 | 1.21 | 0.44 |
| 蛋类 Eggs | 0.09 | 0.02 | 0.09 | 0.14 | 0.05 | 0.08 | 0.07 | 0.00 | 0.10 | 0.06 | 0.08 | 0.09 | 0.07 | 0.02 | 0.01 | 0.05 | 0.03 | 0.14 | 0.12 | 0.02 | 0.02 | 0.05 | 0.00 | 0.05 | 0.07 |
| 水产类 Aquatic foods | 0.05 | 0.02 | 0.01 | 0.06 | 0.03 | 0.01 | 0.01 | 0.00 | 0.01 | 0.02 | 0.03 | 0.00 | 0.20 | 0.09 | 0.02 | 0.04 | 0.22 | 0.05 | 0.25 | 0.01 | 0.19 | 0.18 | 0.06 | 0.01 | 0.07 |
| 乳类 Dairy products | 0.00 | 0.00 | 0.00 | 0.01 | 0.00 | 0.00 | 0.00 | 0.00 | 0.00 | 0.00 | 0.00 | 0.00 | 0.01 | 0.00 | 0.01 | 0.00 | 0.00 | 0.01 | 0.00 | 0.01 | 0.01 | 0.00 | 0.00 | 0.00 | 0.00 |
| 蔬菜类 Vegetables | 0.61 | 0.41 | 1.40 | 1.62 | 0.49 | 1.13 | 0.91 | 0.26 | 1.83 | 0.41 | 2.22 | 1.14 | 2.23 | 0.63 | 0.40 | 0.95 | 0.85 | 1.24 | 1.84 | 0.49 | 0.91 | 1.44 | 0.53 | 8.81 | 1.40 |
| 水果类 Fruits | 0.00 | 0.01 | 0.00 | 0.01 | 0.01 | 0.00 | 0.00 | 0.00 | ND | 0.01 | 0.01 | 0.00 | 0.01 | 0.00 | 0.00 | 0.00 | 0.01 | 0.02 | 0.00 | 0.01 | 0.01 | 0.01 | 0.00 | 0.00 | 0.01 |
| 糖类 Sugar | 0.00 | 0.00 | 0.00 | 0.00 | 0.00 | 0.00 | 0.00 | 0.00 | 0.00 | 0.00 | 0.00 | 0.00 | 0.01 | 0.00 | 0.00 | 0.00 | 0.00 | 0.00 | 0.00 | 0.00 | 0.00 | 0.00 | 0.00 | 0.00 | 0.00 |
| 水及饮料类 Water and beverages | 0.10 | 0.04 | 0.06 | 0.09 | 0.10 | 0.06 | 0.03 | 0.09 | 0.04 | 0.20 | 0.27 | 0.09 | 0.06 | 0.07 | 0.09 | 0.08 | 0.06 | 0.14 | 0.02 | 0.02 | 0.21 | 0.08 | 0.09 | 0.10 | 0.10 |

续表

| 膳食类别<br>Category | 黑龙江<br>HL | 辽宁<br>LN | 河北<br>HE | 北京<br>BJ | 吉林<br>JL | 山西<br>SX | 陕西<br>SN | 河南<br>HA | 宁夏<br>NX | 内蒙古<br>NM | 青海<br>QH | 甘肃<br>GS | 上海<br>SH | 福建<br>FJ | 江西<br>JX | 江苏<br>JS | 浙江<br>ZJ | 山东<br>SD | 湖北<br>HB | 四川<br>SC | 广西<br>GX | 湖南<br>HN | 广东<br>GD | 贵州<br>GZ | 全国平均<br>AVG |
|---|---|---|---|---|---|---|---|---|---|---|---|---|---|---|---|---|---|---|---|---|---|---|---|---|---|
| 酒类<br>Alcohol beverages | 0.00 | 0.00 | ND | 0.00 | 0.00 | 0.00 | 0.00 | 0.00 | 0.00 | 0.00 | 0.00 | 0.00 | 0.00 | 0.00 | 0.00 | 0.00 | 0.00 | 0.01 | 0.00 | 0.00 | 0.00 | 0.00 | 0.00 | 0.00 | 0.00 |
| 合计<br>SUM | 1.88 | 1.11 | 2.54 | 2.63 | 1.18 | 3.41 | 2.14 | 2.06 | 3.56 | 2.49 | 6.31 | 2.72 | 4.72 | 1.01 | 0.97 | 1.90 | 1.88 | 2.31 | 3.63 | 1.57 | 1.82 | 3.07 | 1.04 | 11.81 | 2.82 |

附表 6-31　第六次中国总膳食研究 PAH4 膳食摄入量 [单位：ng/(kg bw · d)]

Annexed Table 6-31　Dietary intakes of PAH4 from the 6th China TDS[Unit: ng/(kg bw · d)]

| 膳食类别<br>Category | 黑龙江<br>HL | 辽宁<br>LN | 河北<br>HE | 北京<br>BJ | 吉林<br>JL | 山西<br>SX | 陕西<br>SN | 河南<br>HA | 宁夏<br>NX | 内蒙古<br>NM | 青海<br>QH | 甘肃<br>GS | 上海<br>SH | 福建<br>FJ | 江西<br>JX | 江苏<br>JS | 浙江<br>ZJ | 山东<br>SD | 湖北<br>HB | 四川<br>SC | 广西<br>GX | 湖南<br>HN | 广东<br>GD | 贵州<br>GZ | 全国平均<br>AVG |
|---|---|---|---|---|---|---|---|---|---|---|---|---|---|---|---|---|---|---|---|---|---|---|---|---|---|
| 谷类<br>Cereals | 4.44 | 1.56 | 5.22 | 0.39 | 1.91 | 5.93 | 2.78 | 15.26 | 2.68 | 6.77 | 3.32 | 3.70 | 1.57 | 1.25 | 1.89 | 2.47 | 1.61 | 4.69 | 2.35 | 3.82 | 2.02 | 1.42 | 1.74 | 2.23 | 3.25 |
| 豆类<br>Legumes | 0.46 | 1.18 | 0.82 | 1.57 | 1.09 | 3.15 | 2.35 | 1.26 | 1.08 | 3.77 | 0.16 | 2.45 | 0.80 | 0.64 | 1.04 | 1.73 | 1.52 | 0.75 | 2.70 | 0.63 | 0.75 | 5.92 | 0.37 | 9.28 | 2.01 |
| 薯类<br>Potatoes | 1.11 | 0.29 | 0.87 | 0.99 | 0.78 | 1.56 | 1.07 | 0.32 | 4.25 | 1.53 | 2.91 | 3.75 | 0.36 | 0.16 | 0.08 | 0.18 | 0.12 | 0.28 | 1.42 | 0.29 | 0.08 | 0.35 | 0.02 | 0.57 | 0.80 |
| 肉类<br>Meats | 1.25 | 0.45 | 0.69 | 1.08 | 0.98 | 2.87 | 1.00 | 0.61 | 2.01 | 0.93 | 8.01 | 0.83 | 5.52 | 0.35 | 0.53 | 1.49 | 1.20 | 1.26 | 1.80 | 1.54 | 1.90 | 3.54 | 0.99 | 5.67 | 2.03 |
| 蛋类<br>Eggs | 0.66 | 0.19 | 0.54 | 0.85 | 0.36 | 0.49 | 0.29 | 0.13 | 0.49 | 0.32 | 0.43 | 0.60 | 0.35 | 0.13 | 0.08 | 0.37 | 0.11 | 0.73 | 0.69 | 0.09 | 0.13 | 0.30 | 0.01 | 0.32 | 0.38 |
| 水产类<br>Aquatic foods | 0.43 | 0.08 | 0.06 | 0.38 | 0.27 | 0.05 | 0.05 | 0.03 | 0.03 | 0.11 | 0.15 | 0.03 | 0.87 | 0.66 | 0.19 | 0.33 | 1.02 | 0.23 | 1.40 | 0.05 | 1.13 | 1.19 | 0.46 | 0.05 | 0.39 |
| 乳类<br>Dairy products | 0.01 | 0.02 | 0.01 | 0.08 | 0.04 | 0.11 | 0.02 | 0.01 | 0.02 | 0.03 | 0.02 | 0.00 | 0.07 | 0.03 | 0.09 | 0.03 | 0.03 | 0.02 | 0.02 | 0.02 | 0.03 | 0.01 | 0.04 | 0.03 | 0.04 |

续表

| 膳食类别 Category | 黑龙江 HL | 辽宁 LN | 河北 HE | 北京 BJ | 吉林 JL | 山西 SX | 陕西 SN | 河南 HA | 宁夏 NX | 内蒙古 NM | 青海 QH | 甘肃 GS | 上海 SH | 福建 FJ | 江西 JX | 江苏 JS | 浙江 ZJ | 山东 SD | 湖北 HB | 四川 SC | 广西 GX | 湖南 HN | 广东 GD | 贵州 GZ | 全国平均 AVG |
|---|---|---|---|---|---|---|---|---|---|---|---|---|---|---|---|---|---|---|---|---|---|---|---|---|---|
| 蔬菜类 Vegetables | 4.83 | 2.38 | 7.97 | 9.91 | 4.31 | 7.37 | 5.06 | 2.56 | 8.38 | 2.41 | 10.30 | 7.60 | 8.52 | 4.73 | 4.41 | 5.67 | 5.15 | 6.22 | 11.57 | 2.89 | 6.74 | 9.75 | 4.81 | 26.11 | 7.32 |
| 水果类 Fruits | 0.02 | 0.11 | 0.03 | 0.06 | 0.06 | 0.06 | 0.01 | 0.01 | 0.00 | 0.08 | 0.03 | 0.02 | 0.17 | 0.02 | 0.03 | 0.03 | 0.07 | 0.04 | 0.01 | 0.02 | 0.02 | 0.02 | 0.01 | 0.01 | 0.04 |
| 糖类 Sugar | 0.00 | 0.00 | 0.00 | 0.01 | 0.00 | 0.00 | 0.01 | 0.00 | ND | 0.00 | 0.00 | 0.00 | 0.10 | 0.00 | 0.00 | 0.00 | 0.00 | 0.00 | 0.00 | 0.00 | 0.00 | 0.00 | 0.00 | 0.00 | 0.00 |
| 水及饮料类 Water and beverages | 0.39 | 0.16 | 1.17 | 0.35 | 0.41 | 0.77 | 0.11 | 0.38 | 0.16 | 0.82 | 0.42 | 0.37 | 0.61 | 0.27 | 0.38 | 0.32 | 0.69 | 0.57 | 0.09 | 0.10 | 0.52 | 0.34 | 0.38 | 0.40 | 0.46 |
| 酒类 Alcohol beverages | 0.01 | 0.01 | ND | 0.01 | 0.00 | 0.00 | 0.00 | 0.00 | 0.00 | 0.01 | 0.00 | 0.00 | 0.01 | 0.00 | 0.01 | 0.01 | 0.04 | 0.04 | 0.00 | 0.00 | 0.01 | 0.01 | 0.00 | 0.00 | 0.01 |
| 合计 SUM | 13.61 | 6.43 | 17.38 | 15.68 | 10.21 | 22.36 | 12.75 | 20.57 | 19.10 | 16.78 | 25.75 | 19.35 | 18.95 | 8.24 | 8.73 | 12.63 | 11.56 | 14.83 | 22.05 | 9.45 | 13.33 | 22.85 | 8.82 | 44.67 | 16.50 |

附表 6-32　第六次中国总膳食研究 PAH16 膳食摄入量 [单位: ng/(kg bw·d)]

Annexed Table 6-32　Dietary intakes of PAH16 from the 6th China TDS [Unit: ng/(kg bw·d)]

| 膳食类别 Category | 黑龙江 HL | 辽宁 LN | 河北 HE | 北京 BJ | 吉林 JL | 山西 SX | 陕西 SN | 河南 HA | 宁夏 NX | 内蒙古 NM | 青海 QH | 甘肃 GS | 上海 SH | 福建 FJ | 江西 JX | 江苏 JS | 浙江 ZJ | 山东 SD | 湖北 HB | 四川 SC | 广西 GX | 湖南 HN | 广东 GD | 贵州 GZ | 全国平均 AVG |
|---|---|---|---|---|---|---|---|---|---|---|---|---|---|---|---|---|---|---|---|---|---|---|---|---|---|
| 谷类 Cereals | 6.96 | 2.49 | 7.51 | 1.15 | 2.74 | 8.65 | 4.60 | 31.47 | 3.55 | 10.79 | 5.25 | 5.66 | 2.10 | 2.11 | 3.02 | 3.52 | 2.56 | 6.97 | 3.73 | 7.84 | 3.06 | 2.66 | 2.61 | 3.46 | 5.60 |
| 豆类 Legumes | 0.70 | 1.83 | 1.12 | 2.33 | 2.35 | 5.54 | 3.53 | 1.65 | 1.75 | 4.53 | 0.25 | 3.14 | 1.43 | 0.99 | 1.79 | 2.31 | 2.21 | 1.05 | 3.74 | 0.99 | 1.05 | 7.31 | 0.49 | 13.12 | 2.72 |
| 薯类 Potatoes | 1.63 | 0.43 | 1.29 | 1.57 | 1.20 | 2.58 | 1.81 | 0.45 | 7.91 | 2.49 | 5.93 | 5.56 | 0.59 | 0.28 | 0.15 | 0.30 | 0.24 | 0.39 | 2.24 | 0.54 | 0.12 | 0.56 | 0.05 | 0.92 | 1.63 |

续表

| 膳食类别<br>Category | 黑龙江<br>HL | 辽宁<br>LN | 河北<br>HE | 北京<br>BJ | 吉林<br>JL | 山西<br>SX | 陕西<br>SN | 河南<br>HA | 宁夏<br>NX | 内蒙古<br>NM | 青海<br>QH | 甘肃<br>GS | 上海<br>SH | 福建<br>FJ | 江西<br>JX | 江苏<br>JS | 浙江<br>ZJ | 山东<br>SD | 湖北<br>HB | 四川<br>SC | 广西<br>GX | 湖南<br>HN | 广东<br>GD | 贵州<br>GZ | 全国平均<br>AVG |
|---|---|---|---|---|---|---|---|---|---|---|---|---|---|---|---|---|---|---|---|---|---|---|---|---|---|
| 肉类 Meats | 2.01 | 0.62 | 1.05 | 1.67 | 1.40 | 4.17 | 1.78 | 0.78 | 3.09 | 1.46 | 20.11 | 1.20 | 10.99 | 0.51 | 0.76 | 2.48 | 2.74 | 2.32 | 3.92 | 2.55 | 2.95 | 5.27 | 1.47 | 10.76 | 3.59 |
| 蛋类 Eggs | 0.96 | 0.31 | 0.80 | 1.37 | 0.54 | 0.82 | 0.50 | 0.19 | 0.98 | 0.41 | 0.69 | 1.46 | 0.59 | 0.20 | 0.12 | 0.54 | 0.39 | 1.54 | 1.10 | 0.16 | 0.21 | 0.47 | 0.03 | 0.50 | 0.62 |
| 水产类 Aquatic foods | 0.62 | 0.11 | 0.09 | 0.64 | 0.39 | 0.08 | 0.08 | 0.05 | 0.05 | 0.17 | 0.28 | 0.04 | 1.73 | 0.99 | 0.30 | 0.50 | 2.30 | 0.40 | 2.30 | 0.09 | 1.67 | 1.75 | 0.67 | 0.09 | 0.64 |
| 乳类 Dairy products | 0.03 | 0.07 | 0.03 | 0.20 | 0.07 | 0.15 | 0.04 | 0.03 | 0.03 | 0.06 | 0.07 | 0.02 | 0.14 | 0.07 | 0.14 | 0.06 | 0.06 | 0.04 | 0.03 | 0.04 | 0.05 | 0.02 | 0.10 | 0.05 | 0.07 |
| 蔬菜类 Vegetables | 7.23 | 3.24 | 11.11 | 15.07 | 6.22 | 11.67 | 8.04 | 3.71 | 15.57 | 3.92 | 19.35 | 11.10 | 20.63 | 7.12 | 6.64 | 8.98 | 8.04 | 10.15 | 17.98 | 5.29 | 10.56 | 14.15 | 6.61 | 65.40 | 12.41 |
| 水果类 Fruits | 0.08 | 0.21 | 0.07 | 0.20 | 0.14 | 0.09 | 0.05 | 0.03 | 0.00 | 0.22 | 0.05 | 0.05 | 0.25 | 0.08 | 0.09 | 0.06 | 0.13 | 0.09 | 0.02 | 0.03 | 0.08 | 0.08 | 0.04 | 0.03 | 0.09 |
| 糖类 Sugar | 0.00 | 0.00 | 0.00 | 0.01 | 0.00 | 0.01 | 0.05 | 0.00 | 0.00 | 0.00 | 0.00 | 0.00 | 0.15 | 0.00 | 0.00 | 0.00 | 0.01 | 0.00 | 0.00 | 0.00 | 0.00 | 0.00 | 0.00 | 0.00 | 0.01 |
| 水及饮料类 Water and beverages | 1.55 | 0.63 | 2.22 | 1.41 | 1.65 | 1.48 | 0.44 | 1.51 | 0.66 | 3.27 | 1.09 | 1.50 | 1.28 | 1.10 | 2.04 | 1.28 | 1.44 | 2.63 | 0.36 | 0.40 | 1.76 | 1.35 | 1.51 | 1.59 | 1.42 |
| 酒类 Alcohol beverages | 0.03 | 0.04 | 0.00 | 0.03 | 0.01 | 0.00 | 0.00 | 0.00 | 0.00 | 0.03 | 0.01 | 0.00 | 0.03 | 0.02 | 0.03 | 0.05 | 0.10 | 0.16 | 0.02 | 0.01 | 0.04 | 0.02 | 0.00 | 0.00 | 0.03 |
| 合计 SUM | 21.80 | 9.98 | 25.29 | 25.64 | 16.72 | 35.23 | 20.91 | 39.88 | 33.59 | 27.34 | 53.07 | 29.74 | 39.91 | 13.44 | 15.09 | 20.06 | 20.23 | 25.73 | 35.44 | 17.94 | 21.55 | 33.64 | 13.58 | 95.92 | 28.82 |

附表 6-33 第六次中国总膳食研究膳食样品中氨基甲酸乙酯的含量（单位：μg/kg）

Annexed Table 6-33 Levels of ethyl carbamate in food samples from the 6$^{th}$ China TDS (Unit: μg/kg)

| 膳食类别<br>Category | 黑龙江<br>HL | 辽宁<br>LN | 河北<br>HE | 北京<br>BJ | 吉林<br>JL | 山西<br>SX | 陕西<br>SN | 河南<br>HA | 宁夏<br>NX | 内蒙古<br>NM | 青海<br>QH | 甘肃<br>GS | 上海<br>SH | 福建<br>FJ | 江西<br>JX | 江苏<br>JS | 浙江<br>ZJ | 山东<br>SD | 湖北<br>HB | 四川<br>SC | 广西<br>GX | 湖南<br>HN | 广东<br>GD | 贵州<br>GZ | 全国平均<br>AVG |
|---|---|---|---|---|---|---|---|---|---|---|---|---|---|---|---|---|---|---|---|---|---|---|---|---|---|
| 谷类 Cereals | ND | ND | ND | ND | ND | ND | ND | ND | ND | ND | ND | ND | ND | ND | ND | ND | ND | ND | ND | ND | ND | ND | ND | ND | ND |
| 豆类 Legumes | ND | ND | ND | ND | ND | ND | ND | ND | ND | ND | ND | ND | ND | ND | ND | ND | ND | ND | ND | ND | ND | ND | ND | ND | ND |
| 薯类 Potatoes | ND | ND | ND | ND | ND | ND | ND | ND | ND | ND | ND | ND | ND | ND | ND | ND | ND | ND | ND | ND | ND | ND | ND | ND | ND |
| 肉类 Meats | 94.61 | 12.59 | 35.41 | 13.45 | 8.96 | 8.74 | 124.41 | 58.36 | ND | 33.84 | 27.05 | 10.12 | ND | 64.57 | ND | ND | 8.73 | 21.72 | ND | 8.36 | ND | 39.29 | ND | 15.34 | 24.40 |
| 蛋类 Eggs | ND | ND | ND | ND | ND | ND | ND | ND | ND | ND | ND | ND | ND | ND | ND | ND | ND | ND | ND | ND | ND | ND | ND | ND | ND |
| 水产类 Aquatic foods | 30.10 | 145.16 | 35.32 | 16.51 | ND | ND | 50.36 | 105.26 | 14.55 | 47.69 | 7.37 | ND | ND | 7.19 | 10.01 | ND | 17.91 | 7.82 | ND | ND | 45.63 | ND | ND | 9.39 | 22.93 |
| 乳类 Dairy products | ND | ND | ND | ND | ND | ND | ND | ND | ND | ND | ND | ND | ND | ND | ND | ND | ND | ND | ND | ND | ND | ND | ND | ND | ND |
| 蔬菜类 Vegetables | ND | 15.05 | ND | 3.42 | ND | 3.47 | ND | 3.45 | 2.92 | 8.70 | 10.89 | ND | ND | ND | ND | ND | 8.38 | ND | ND | ND | ND | ND | ND | 1.70 | 2.42 |
| 水果类 Fruits | ND | ND | ND | ND | ND | ND | ND | ND | ND | ND | ND | ND | ND | ND | ND | ND | ND | ND | ND | ND | ND | ND | ND | ND | ND |
| 糖类 Sugar | ND | ND | ND | ND | ND | ND | ND | ND | ND | ND | ND | ND | ND | ND | ND | ND | ND | ND | ND | ND | ND | ND | ND | ND | ND |
| 水及饮料类 Water and beverages | ND | ND | ND | ND | ND | ND | ND | ND | ND | ND | ND | ND | ND | ND | ND | ND | ND | ND | ND | ND | ND | ND | ND | ND | ND |
| 酒类 Alcohol beverages | 5.10 | 12.06 | 5.40 | ND | 4.58 | 9.16 | 16.57 | 6.79 | 24.21 | 3.72 | 4.93 | ND | ND | 6.54 | 17.33 | 11.56 | 24.66 | 6.06 | 12.13 | 18.93 | 4.10 | 14.06 | 4.08 | 33.75 | 10.24 |

注：未检出（ND）按 1/2 检出限（LOD）计

Note: values not detected (ND) were treated as being equal to half of the detection of limit (LOD)

附表 6-34 第六次中国总膳食研究的氨基甲酸乙酯膳食摄入量 [单位：μg/(kg bw·d)]
Annexed Table 6-34 Dietary intakes of ethyl carbamate from the 6$^{th}$ China TDS [Unit: μg/(kg bw·d)]

| 膳食类别 Category | 黑龙江 HL | 辽宁 LN | 河北 HE | 北京 BJ | 吉林 JL | 山西 SX | 陕西 SN | 河南 HA | 宁夏 NX | 内蒙古 NM | 青海 QH | 甘肃 GS | 上海 SH | 福建 FJ | 江西 JX | 江苏 JS | 浙江 ZJ | 山东 SD | 湖北 HB | 四川 SC | 广西 GX | 湖南 HN | 广东 GD | 贵州 GZ | 全国平均 AVG |
|---|---|---|---|---|---|---|---|---|---|---|---|---|---|---|---|---|---|---|---|---|---|---|---|---|---|
| 谷类 Cereals | 0 | 0 | 0 | 0 | 0 | 0 | 0 | 0 | 0 | 0 | 0 | 0 | 0 | 0 | 0 | 0 | 0 | 0 | 0 | 0 | 0 | 0 | 0 | 0 | 0 |
| 豆类 Legumes | 0 | 0 | 0 | 0 | 0 | 0 | 0 | 0 | 0 | 0 | 0 | 0 | 0 | 0 | 0 | 0 | 0 | 0 | 0 | 0 | 0 | 0 | 0 | 0 | 0 |
| 薯类 Potatoes | 0 | 0 | 0 | 0 | 0 | 0 | 0 | 0 | 0 | 0 | 0 | 0 | 0 | 0 | 0 | 0 | 0 | 0 | 0 | 0 | 0 | 0 | 0 | 0 | 0 |
| 肉类 Meats | 0.090 | 0.013 | 0.027 | 0.014 | 0.009 | 0.019 | 0.071 | 0.051 | 0.000 | 0.039 | 0.030 | 0.005 | 0.000 | 0.088 | 0.000 | 0.000 | 0.016 | 0.034 | 0.000 | 0.017 | 0.000 | 0.093 | 0.000 | 0.026 | 0.027 |
| 蛋类 Eggs | 0 | 0 | 0 | 0 | 0 | 0 | 0 | 0 | 0 | 0 | 0 | 0 | 0 | 0 | 0 | 0 | 0 | 0 | 0 | 0 | 0 | 0 | 0 | 0 | 0 |
| 水产类 Aquatic foods | 0.013 | 0.037 | 0.005 | 0.004 | 0.000 | 0.000 | 0.003 | 0.008 | 0.001 | 0.008 | 0.000 | 0.000 | 0.000 | 0.007 | 0.007 | 0.000 | 0.014 | 0.003 | 0.000 | 0.000 | 0.070 | 0.000 | 0.000 | 0.001 | 0.008 |
| 乳类 Dairy products | 0 | 0 | 0 | 0 | 0 | 0 | 0 | 0 | 0 | 0 | 0 | 0 | 0 | 0 | 0 | 0 | 0 | 0 | 0 | 0 | 0 | 0 | 0 | 0 | 0 |
| 蔬菜类 Vegetables | 0.000 | 0.078 | 0.000 | 0.021 | 0.000 | 0.017 | 0.000 | 0.015 | 0.007 | 0.036 | 0.054 | 0.000 | 0.000 | 0.000 | 0.000 | 0.000 | 0.059 | 0.000 | 0.000 | 0.000 | 0.000 | 0.000 | 0.000 | 0.011 | 0.012 |
| 水果类 Fruits | 0 | 0 | 0 | 0 | 0 | 0 | 0 | 0 | 0 | 0 | 0 | 0 | 0 | 0 | 0 | 0 | 0 | 0 | 0 | 0 | 0 | 0 | 0 | 0 | 0 |
| 糖类 Sugar | 0 | 0 | 0 | 0 | 0 | 0 | 0 | 0 | 0 | 0 | 0 | 0 | 0 | 0 | 0 | 0 | 0 | 0 | 0 | 0 | 0 | 0 | 0 | 0 | 0 |
| 水及饮料类 Water and beverages | 0 | 0 | 0 | 0 | 0 | 0 | 0 | 0 | 0 | 0 | 0 | 0 | 0 | 0 | 0 | 0 | 0 | 0 | 0 | 0 | 0 | 0 | 0 | 0 | 0 |

续表

| 膳食类别 Category | 黑龙江 HL | 辽宁 LN | 河北 HE | 北京 BJ | 吉林 JL | 山西 SX | 陕西 SN | 河南 HA | 宁夏 NX | 内蒙古 NM | 青海 QH | 甘肃 GS | 上海 SH | 福建 FJ | 江西 JX | 江苏 JS | 浙江 ZJ | 山东 SD | 湖北 HB | 四川 SC | 广西 GX | 湖南 HN | 广东 GD | 贵州 GZ | 全国平均 AVG |
|---|---|---|---|---|---|---|---|---|---|---|---|---|---|---|---|---|---|---|---|---|---|---|---|---|---|
| 酒类 Alcohol beverages | 0.002 | 0.006 | 0.001 | 0.000 | 0.001 | 0.000 | 0.000 | 0.000 | 0.000 | 0.001 | 0.000 | 0.000 | 0.000 | 0.001 | 0.006 | 0.007 | 0.025 | 0.011 | 0.003 | 0.002 | 0.002 | 0.004 | 0.000 | 0.001 | 0.003 |
| 合计 SUM | 0.105 | 0.135 | 0.033 | 0.040 | 0.010 | 0.036 | 0.075 | 0.075 | 0.008 | 0.084 | 0.085 | 0.005 | 0.000 | 0.097 | 0.013 | 0.007 | 0.114 | 0.047 | 0.003 | 0.019 | 0.072 | 0.097 | 0.000 | 0.039 | 0.050 |

附表 6-35 第六次中国总膳食研究氨基甲酸乙酯的膳食来源（单位：%）

Annexed Table 6-35 Dietary sources of ethyl carbamate from the 6$^{th}$ China TDS (Unit: %)

| 膳食类别 Category | 黑龙江 HL | 辽宁 LN | 河北 HE | 北京 BJ | 吉林 JL | 山西 SX | 陕西 SN | 河南 HA | 宁夏 NX | 内蒙古 NM | 青海 QH | 甘肃 GS | 上海 SH | 福建 FJ | 江西 JX | 江苏 JS | 浙江 ZJ | 山东 SD | 湖北 HB | 四川 SC | 广西 GX | 湖南 HN | 广东 GD | 贵州 GZ | 全国平均 AVG |
|---|---|---|---|---|---|---|---|---|---|---|---|---|---|---|---|---|---|---|---|---|---|---|---|---|---|
| 谷类 Cereals | 0 | 0 | 0 | 0 | 0 | 0 | 0 | 0 | 0 | 0 | 0 | 0 | 0 | 0 | 0 | 0 | 0 | 0 | 0 | 0 | 0 | 0 | 0 | 0 | 0 |
| 豆类 Legumes | 0 | 0 | 0 | 0 | 0 | 0 | 0 | 0 | 0 | 0 | 0 | 0 | 0 | 0 | 0 | 0 | 0 | 0 | 0 | 0 | 0 | 0 | 0 | 0 | 0 |
| 薯类 Potatoes | 0 | 0 | 0 | 0 | 0 | 0 | 0 | 0 | 0 | 0 | 0 | 0 | 0 | 0 | 0 | 0 | 0 | 0 | 0 | 0 | 0 | 0 | 0 | 0 | 0 |
| 肉类 Meats | 85.91 | 9.90 | 81.00 | 35.94 | 93.16 | 52.65 | 95.04 | 68.74 | 0.00 | 46.97 | 35.89 | 100.00 | 0.00 | 90.92 | 0.00 | 0.00 | 14.34 | 70.92 | 0.00 | 91.71 | 0.00 | 96.16 | 0.00 | 67.12 | 53.82 |
| 蛋类 Eggs | 0 | 0 | 0 | 0 | 0 | 0 | 0 | 0 | 0 | 0 | 0 | 0 | 0 | 0 | 0 | 0 | 0 | 0 | 0 | 0 | 0 | 0 | 0 | 0 | 0 |
| 水产类 Aquatic foods | 12.39 | 27.45 | 16.22 | 10.77 | 0.00 | 0.00 | 4.37 | 10.37 | 7.02 | 9.31 | 0.49 | 0.00 | 0.00 | 7.55 | 53.94 | 0.00 | 12.51 | 5.98 | 0.00 | 0.00 | 97.11 | 0.00 | 0.00 | 1.34 | 15.14 |
| 乳类 Dairy products | 0 | 0 | 0 | 0 | 0 | 0 | 0 | 0 | 0 | 0 | 0 | 0 | 0 | 0 | 0 | 0 | 0 | 0 | 0 | 0 | 0 | 0 | 0 | 0 | 0 |

续表

| 膳食类别 Category | 黑龙江 HL | 辽宁 LN | 河北 HE | 北京 BJ | 吉林 JL | 山西 SX | 陕西 SN | 河南 HA | 宁夏 NX | 内蒙古 NM | 青海 QH | 甘肃 GS | 上海 SH | 福建 FJ | 江西 JX | 江苏 JS | 浙江 ZJ | 山东 SD | 湖北 HB | 四川 SC | 广西 GX | 湖南 HN | 广东 GD | 贵州 GZ | 全国平均 AVG |
|---|---|---|---|---|---|---|---|---|---|---|---|---|---|---|---|---|---|---|---|---|---|---|---|---|---|
| 蔬菜类 Vegetables | 0.00 | 57.87 | 0.00 | 53.29 | 0.00 | 47.23 | 0.00 | 20.44 | 90.78 | 42.27 | 63.19 | 0.00 | 0.00 | 0.00 | 0.00 | 0.00 | 51.66 | 0.00 | 0.00 | 0.00 | 0.00 | 0.00 | 0.00 | 28.52 | 24.90 |
| 水果类 Fruits | 0 | 0 | 0 | 0 | 0 | 0 | 0 | 0 | 0 | 0 | 0 | 0 | 0 | 0 | 0 | 0 | 0 | 0 | 0 | 0 | 0 | 0 | 0 | 0 | 0 |
| 糖类 Sugar | 0 | 0 | 0 | 0 | 0 | 0 | 0 | 0 | 0 | 0 | 0 | 0 | 0 | 0 | 0 | 0 | 0 | 0 | 0 | 0 | 0 | 0 | 0 | 0 | 0 |
| 水及饮料类 Water and beverages | 0 | 0 | 0 | 0 | 0 | 0 | 0 | 0 | 0 | 0 | 0 | 0 | 0 | 0 | 0 | 0 | 0 | 0 | 0 | 0 | 0 | 0 | 0 | 0 | 0 |
| 酒类 Alcohol beverages | 1.70 | 4.78 | 2.78 | 0.00 | 6.84 | 0.12 | 0.58 | 0.46 | 2.20 | 1.46 | 0.43 | 0.00 | 0.00 | 1.53 | 46.06 | 100.00 | 21.48 | 23.10 | 100.00 | 8.29 | 2.89 | 3.84 | 100.00 | 3.02 | 6.14 |

附表 6-36 第六次中国总膳食研究膳食样品中 DBP 的含量（单位：µg/kg）

Annexed Table 6-36　Levels of DBP in food samples from the 6$^{th}$ China TDS (Unit: µg/kg)

| 膳食类别 Category | 黑龙江 HL | 辽宁 LN | 河北 HE | 北京 BJ | 吉林 JL | 山西 SX | 陕西 SN | 河南 HA | 宁夏 NX | 内蒙古 NM | 青海 QH | 甘肃 GS | 上海 SH | 福建 FJ | 江西 JX | 江苏 JS | 浙江 ZJ | 山东 SD | 湖北 HB | 四川 SC | 广西 GX | 湖南 HN | 广东 GD | 贵州 GZ | 全国平均 AVG |
|---|---|---|---|---|---|---|---|---|---|---|---|---|---|---|---|---|---|---|---|---|---|---|---|---|---|
| 谷类 Cereals | 51.50 | 29.21 | 10.10 | 126.90 | 23.68 | 17.90 | 10.71 | 44.53 | 19.43 | 29.26 | 20.23 | 37.63 | 23.12 | 53.09 | 18.08 | 11.75 | 16.53 | 12.06 | 24.38 | 17.87 | 16.62 | 28.24 | 34.86 | 28.23 | 29.41 |
| 豆类 Legumes | 28.40 | 51.78 | 21.24 | 11.41 | ND | 16.33 | 34.46 | 60.43 | 59.29 | 27.53 | 19.89 | 83.92 | 43.68 | 23.67 | 44.32 | 44.07 | 26.28 | 17.78 | 38.56 | 34.56 | 34.29 | 82.34 | 37.16 | 33.10 | 36.52 |
| 薯类 Potatoes | ND | 22.60 | 11.32 | 56.63 | 119.50 | 17.00 | 8.79 | 21.09 | 43.63 | 16.73 | 32.71 | 8.45 | 48.20 | 53.30 | 43.70 | 42.41 | 15.63 | 13.62 | 20.61 | 30.82 | 20.13 | ND | 15.21 | 40.73 | 29.44 |

续表

| 膳食类别 Category | 黑龙江 HL | 辽宁 LN | 河北 HE | 北京 BJ | 吉林 JL | 山西 SX | 陕西 SN | 河南 HA | 宁夏 NX | 内蒙古 NM | 青海 QH | 甘肃 GS | 上海 SH | 福建 FJ | 江西 JX | 江苏 JS | 浙江 ZJ | 山东 SD | 湖北 HB | 四川 SC | 广西 GX | 湖南 HN | 广东 GD | 贵州 GZ | 全国平均 AVG |
|---|---|---|---|---|---|---|---|---|---|---|---|---|---|---|---|---|---|---|---|---|---|---|---|---|---|
| 肉类 Meats | 29.80 | 22.22 | 14.02 | 112.13 | 201.41 | 14.63 | 23.89 | 34.48 | 51.84 | 11.22 | 37.47 | 48.31 | 49.10 | ND | 24.24 | 14.04 | 29.03 | 13.55 | 33.13 | 32.59 | 31.80 | 25.15 | 31.14 | 35.67 | 38.43 |
| 蛋类 Eggs | ND | 42.63 | 21.72 | 111.76 | ND | 24.11 | 19.61 | 15.00 | 45.01 | 48.55 | 54.03 | 48.60 | 50.54 | 48.44 | ND | 38.51 | 38.52 | 10.62 | 21.53 | 26.99 | 18.43 | 45.31 | 22.02 | 28.00 | 32.71 |
| 水产类 Aquatic foods | 23.43 | 34.26 | 17.30 | 93.09 | 440.10 | 13.76 | 8.60 | 23.65 | 17.90 | 22.80 | 36.07 | ND | 46.90 | 30.94 | 40.00 | 31.33 | 23.65 | 25.65 | 25.30 | 29.90 | 24.65 | 24.55 | 23.13 | 55.42 | 46.41 |
| 乳类 Dairy products | 13.00 | ND | 40.10 | 38.10 | 16.00 | 14.90 | 19.80 | 23.80 | 40.40 | 18.50 | 15.80 | ND | 105.50 | 17.10 | 1.50 | 18.80 | 21.20 | 26.30 | 17.30 | 17.70 | 15.90 | 20.60 | 21.00 | 33.10 | 23.31 |
| 蔬菜类 Vegetables | ND | 37.63 | 18.87 | 53.74 | 204.04 | 11.72 | 17.13 | 35.35 | 39.60 | 24.12 | 35.10 | 37.80 | 51.90 | 24.04 | 25.90 | 51.77 | 25.49 | 15.56 | 34.80 | ND | 29.59 | 42.16 | 26.80 | 30.52 | 36.54 |
| 水果类 Fruits | ND | ND | 5.40 | 64.79 | 11.00 | 9.80 | 8.40 | 14.50 | 21.10 | 14.44 | 6.70 | 15.40 | 41.70 | 23.30 | ND | 14.40 | 13.50 | 7.40 | 14.10 | 6.00 | 12.70 | 13.80 | 14.70 | 20.34 | 14.92 |
| 糖类 Sugar | 9.20 | 14.90 | 6.50 | 70.80 | 10.20 | 21.20 | 6.10 | 14.90 | 7.30 | 13.40 | 7.90 | 28.90 | 57.30 | 16.10 | 19.50 | 14.00 | 13.50 | 7.40 | 14.60 | 6.00 | 14.20 | 63.20 | 12.60 | 16.60 | 19.43 |
| 水及饮料类 Water and beverages | 8.00 | 15.40 | 8.20 | 62.60 | 12.40 | 35.30 | 8.70 | 17.70 | 9.50 | 4.90 | ND | 26.80 | 35.60 | 16.50 | 21.80 | 12.40 | 11.00 | 7.50 | 15.50 | 8.20 | 12.80 | 20.30 | 11.60 | 17.30 | 16.73 |
| 酒类 Alcohol beverages | 23.90 | 29.50 | 11.40 | 56.80 | 127.80 | 12.20 | 9.10 | 22.30 | 17.20 | 19.20 | 9.90 | ND | 61.70 | 18.20 | 25.40 | 28.60 | 17.30 | ND | 18.50 | 44.80 | 29.30 | 41.20 | 18.00 | 235.60 | 36.70 |

注：未检出（ND）按 1/2 检出限（LOD）计

Note: values not detected (ND) were treated as being equal to half of the limit of detection (LOD)

附表 6-37 第六次中国总膳食研究膳食样品中 DiBP 的含量（单位：μg/kg）

Annexed Table 6-37  Levels of DiBP in food samples from the 6$^{th}$ China TDS (Unit: μg/kg)

| 膳食类别 Category | 黑龙江 HL | 辽宁 LN | 河北 HE | 北京 BJ | 吉林 JL | 山西 SX | 陕西 SN | 河南 HA | 宁夏 NX | 内蒙古 NM | 青海 QH | 甘肃 GS | 上海 SH | 福建 FJ | 江西 JX | 江苏 JS | 浙江 ZJ | 山东 SD | 湖北 HB | 四川 SC | 广西 GX | 湖南 HN | 广东 GD | 贵州 GZ | 全国平均 AVG |
|---|---|---|---|---|---|---|---|---|---|---|---|---|---|---|---|---|---|---|---|---|---|---|---|---|---|
| 谷类 Cereals | 8.52 | 36.03 | 7.29 | 38.73 | 15.92 | 5.81 | 6.62 | 21.09 | 11.76 | 6.47 | 13.86 | 44.24 | 22.86 | 130.74 | 14.79 | 8.25 | 23.20 | 6.51 | 13.01 | 5.54 | 11.03 | 18.09 | 45.81 | 28.23 | 29.41 |
| 豆类 Legumes | 10.58 | 31.78 | 7.52 | 27.93 | ND | 6.00 | 4.62 | 36.00 | 6.23 | 6.77 | 3.45 | 20.41 | 20.23 | 21.33 | 25.45 | 19.77 | 11.28 | 8.02 | 18.22 | 9.41 | 14.80 | 35.97 | 27.50 | 33.10 | 36.52 |
| 薯类 Potatoes | 4.88 | 27.40 | 6.30 | 28.84 | 13.00 | 7.50 | ND | 24.35 | 19.87 | 5.51 | 9.06 | 13.92 | 34.90 | 78.57 | 16.20 | 12.17 | 20.83 | 5.74 | 10.30 | 5.48 | 18.82 | 28.92 | 26.15 | 40.73 | 29.44 |
| 肉类 Meats | 7.69 | 25.43 | 7.61 | 41.50 | 21.72 | 7.37 | 11.57 | 22.71 | 32.30 | 7.14 | 7.07 | 48.31 | 26.60 | 16.29 | 31.92 | 1.52 | 31.83 | 5.81 | 11.98 | 7.27 | 15.20 | 16.36 | 31.14 | 35.67 | 38.43 |
| 蛋类 Eggs | ND | 65.53 | 12.01 | 41.06 | ND | 10.41 | 14.71 | 16.90 | 12.42 | 12.37 | 13.89 | 27.33 | 25.33 | 29.09 | ND | 26.17 | 149.01 | ND | 13.18 | 8.05 | 13.48 | 66.12 | 42.63 | 28.00 | 32.71 |
| 水产类 Aquatic foods | 6.21 | 40.00 | 8.81 | 37.66 | 47.90 | 6.94 | 3.50 | 15.00 | 12.70 | 8.00 | 7.75 | ND | 26.70 | 29.06 | 25.20 | 10.71 | 30.73 | 12.94 | 10.40 | 5.60 | 12.12 | 18.48 | 29.06 | 55.42 | 46.41 |
| 乳类 Dairy products | ND | ND | 14.70 | 20.90 | 26.80 | 7.30 | 13.90 | 36.80 | 14.70 | 14.70 | 4.60 | ND | 42.50 | 11.00 | ND | 9.40 | 12.30 | 4.70 | 11.10 | 11.80 | 9.20 | 34.40 | 60.20 | 33.10 | 23.31 |
| 蔬菜类 Vegetables | ND | 33.33 | 6.86 | 24.55 | 18.69 | 5.91 | 6.91 | 31.31 | 19.80 | 7.01 | 5.20 | 22.00 | 29.20 | 31.52 | 21.60 | 15.83 | 45.37 | 6.26 | 23.60 | ND | 13.57 | 27.22 | 7.22 | 30.52 | 36.54 |
| 水果类 Fruits | ND | 26.09 | 3.30 | 9.04 | 10.30 | 4.80 | 4.20 | 8.30 | 21.91 | 3.33 | 4.23 | 12.60 | 30.40 | 23.09 | ND | 20.70 | 17.80 | 3.40 | 20.50 | 1.64 | 16.40 | 14.10 | 28.50 | 20.34 | 14.92 |
| 糖类 Sugar | 6.00 | 15.90 | 4.90 | 30.70 | 13.30 | 8.20 | ND | 16.40 | 3.40 | 4.90 | 3.50 | 18.20 | 63.50 | 13.60 | 12.80 | 18.30 | 16.10 | 3.90 | 6.40 | 3.80 | 8.30 | 13.90 | 19.10 | 16.60 | 19.43 |
| 水及饮料类 Water and beverages | 3.30 | 18.60 | 5.30 | 46.50 | 32.90 | 7.00 | 45.50 | 15.80 | 6.00 | 5.30 | 115.10 | 14.50 | 71.50 | 17.60 | 22.20 | 25.40 | 19.90 | 3.10 | 19.60 | 23.50 | 17.20 | 52.30 | 34.30 | 17.30 | 16.73 |

续表

| 膳食类别<br>Category | 黑龙江<br>HL | 辽宁<br>LN | 河北<br>HE | 北京<br>BJ | 吉林<br>JL | 山西<br>SX | 陕西<br>SN | 河南<br>HA | 宁夏<br>NX | 内蒙古<br>NM | 青海<br>QH | 甘肃<br>GS | 上海<br>SH | 福建<br>FJ | 江西<br>JX | 江苏<br>JS | 浙江<br>ZJ | 山东<br>SD | 湖北<br>HB | 四川<br>SC | 广西<br>GX | 湖南<br>HN | 广东<br>GD | 贵州<br>GZ | 全国平均<br>AVG |
|---|---|---|---|---|---|---|---|---|---|---|---|---|---|---|---|---|---|---|---|---|---|---|---|---|---|
| 酒类<br>Alcohol beverages | 23.00 | 15.60 | 7.20 | 25.80 | 45.90 | 6.50 | 6.90 | 12.40 | 423.20 | 7.20 | 4.40 | ND | 27.70 | 10.60 | 14.10 | 42.50 | 12.90 | ND | 11.00 | 60.10 | 13.40 | 57.40 | 18.50 | 235.60 | 36.70 |

注：未检出（ND）按 1/2 检出限（LOD）计
Note: values not detected (ND) were treated as being equal to half of the limit of detection (LOD)

附表 Table 6-38　第六次中国总膳食研究膳食样品中 DEHP 的含量（单位：μg/kg）
Annexed Table 6-38　Levels of DEHP in food samples from the 6$^{th}$ China TDS (Unit: μg/kg)

| 膳食类别<br>Category | 黑龙江<br>HL | 辽宁<br>LN | 河北<br>HE | 北京<br>BJ | 吉林<br>JL | 山西<br>SX | 陕西<br>SN | 河南<br>HA | 宁夏<br>NX | 内蒙古<br>NM | 青海<br>QH | 甘肃<br>GS | 上海<br>SH | 福建<br>FJ | 江西<br>JX | 江苏<br>JS | 浙江<br>ZJ | 山东<br>SD | 湖北<br>HB | 四川<br>SC | 广西<br>GX | 湖南<br>HN | 广东<br>GD | 贵州<br>GZ | 全国平均<br>AVG |
|---|---|---|---|---|---|---|---|---|---|---|---|---|---|---|---|---|---|---|---|---|---|---|---|---|---|
| 谷类<br>Cereals | 43.76 | 19.68 | 20.54 | 45.49 | 16.84 | 28.23 | 15.00 | 111.09 | 24.06 | 365.88 | 38.41 | 19.66 | 12.86 | 10.59 | 8.77 | 1.88 | 12.80 | 21.43 | 17.40 | 27.52 | 17.35 | 13.24 | 25.54 | 14.03 | 38.83 |
| 豆类<br>Legumes | 41.73 | 36.58 | 28.04 | 11.30 | 2.03 | 10.67 | 7.88 | 25.14 | 22.82 | 39.78 | 7.36 | 35.05 | 21.72 | 22.96 | 18.07 | 25.58 | 8.72 | 12.22 | 25.56 | 25.26 | 26.43 | 18.83 | 29.32 | 31.31 | 22.27 |
| 薯类<br>Potatoes | 28.80 | 21.69 | 38.18 | 28.26 | 6.90 | 22.63 | 8.92 | 7.83 | 20.10 | 138.57 | 17.40 | 62.68 | 21.30 | 12.75 | 9.80 | 18.07 | 13.13 | 13.83 | 38.38 | 22.86 | 24.61 | 16.35 | 6.46 | 61.34 | 27.53 |
| 肉类<br>Meats | 53.09 | 53.33 | 46.17 | 50.13 | 39.29 | 43.26 | 24.32 | 42.29 | 35.75 | 6.94 | 32.22 | 63.26 | 55.90 | 40.62 | 30.71 | 51.92 | 37.74 | 26.24 | 65.83 | 74.67 | 64.30 | 46.67 | 91.39 | 55.77 | 47.16 |
| 蛋类<br>Eggs | ND | 23.29 | 48.04 | 45.41 | ND | 52.19 | 13.07 | 12.60 | 16.66 | 33.42 | 24.44 | 30.93 | 23.48 | 43.64 | ND | 20.21 | 16.05 | 23.46 | 46.94 | 21.89 | 31.80 | 60.61 | 5.45 | 33.20 | 26.32 |
| 水产类<br>Aquatic foods | 23.43 | 32.21 | 61.91 | 50.11 | 39.60 | 14.59 | 10.10 | 17.40 | 75.10 | 27.10 | 80.00 | ND | 37.20 | 71.77 | 21.40 | 24.49 | 22.60 | 117.06 | 53.00 | 40.40 | 40.10 | 15.35 | 76.04 | 81.93 | 43.10 |
| 乳类<br>Dairy products | 7.50 | 4.00 | 8.40 | 8.20 | 11.80 | ND | 18.70 | 7.30 | 45.70 | 9.20 | 10.50 | ND | 12.20 | 6.10 | ND | ND | 4.60 | 3.70 | ND | 9.20 | ND | 6.90 | 4.50 | 9.50 | 8.21 |

续表

| 膳食类别 Category | 黑龙江 HL | 辽宁 LN | 河北 HE | 北京 BJ | 吉林 JL | 山西 SX | 陕西 SN | 河南 HA | 宁夏 NX | 内蒙古 NM | 青海 QH | 甘肃 GS | 上海 SH | 福建 FJ | 江西 JX | 江苏 JS | 浙江 ZJ | 山东 SD | 湖北 HB | 四川 SC | 广西 GX | 湖南 HN | 广东 GD | 贵州 GZ | 全国平均 AVG |
|---|---|---|---|---|---|---|---|---|---|---|---|---|---|---|---|---|---|---|---|---|---|---|---|---|---|
| 蔬菜类 Vegetables | ND | 40.11 | 51.68 | 24.65 | 24.85 | 30.88 | 53.87 | 30.20 | 22.10 | 793.09 | 21.70 | 109.10 | 26.50 | 45.25 | 29.40 | 28.23 | 50.49 | 42.93 | 114.10 | ND | 53.27 | 32.06 | 68.35 | 82.16 | 74.10 |
| 水果类 Fruits | ND | 11.74 | 6.40 | 16.49 | ND | 14.50 | 17.43 | 62.00 | 6.03 | 9.49 | ND | ND | 11.40 | 8.04 | ND | 9.90 | 6.90 | 36.60 | 7.30 | 13.19 | 9.30 | 8.13 | ND | 6.59 | 11.27 |
| 糖类 Sugar | 9.20 | 14.90 | 6.50 | 70.80 | 10.20 | 21.20 | 6.10 | 14.90 | 7.30 | 13.40 | 7.90 | 28.90 | 57.30 | 16.10 | 19.50 | 14.00 | 13.50 | 7.40 | 14.60 | 6.00 | 14.20 | 63.20 | 12.60 | 16.60 | 19.43 |
| 水及饮料类 Water and beverages | 8.00 | 15.40 | 8.20 | 62.60 | 12.40 | 35.30 | 8.70 | 17.70 | 9.50 | 4.90 | ND | 26.80 | 35.60 | 16.50 | 21.80 | 12.40 | 11.00 | 7.50 | 15.50 | 8.20 | 12.80 | 20.30 | 11.60 | 17.30 | 16.73 |
| 酒类 Alcohol beverages | 23.90 | 29.50 | 11.40 | 56.80 | 127.80 | 12.20 | 9.10 | 22.30 | 17.20 | 19.20 | 9.90 | ND | 61.70 | 18.20 | 25.40 | 28.60 | 17.30 | ND | 18.50 | 44.80 | 29.30 | 41.20 | 18.00 | 235.60 | 36.70 |

注：未检出（ND）按 1/2 检出限（LOD）计

Note: values not detected (ND) were treated as being equal to half of the limit of detection (LOD)

附表 6-39  第六次中国总膳食研究的 DBP 膳食摄入量 [单位：μg/(kg bw · d)]

Annexed Table 6-39  Dietary intakes of DBP from the 6th China TDS [Unit: μg/(kg bw · d)]

| 膳食类别 Category | 黑龙江 HL | 辽宁 LN | 河北 HE | 北京 BJ | 吉林 JL | 山西 SX | 陕西 SN | 河南 HA | 宁夏 NX | 内蒙古 NM | 青海 QH | 甘肃 GS | 上海 SH | 福建 FJ | 江西 JX | 江苏 JS | 浙江 ZJ | 山东 SD | 湖北 HB | 四川 SC | 广西 GX | 湖南 HN | 广东 GD | 贵州 GZ | 全国平均 AVG |
|---|---|---|---|---|---|---|---|---|---|---|---|---|---|---|---|---|---|---|---|---|---|---|---|---|---|
| 谷类 Cereals | 0.45 | 0.29 | 0.12 | 1.60 | 0.22 | 0.29 | 0.13 | 0.65 | 0.20 | 0.34 | 0.25 | 0.41 | 0.16 | 0.53 | 0.18 | 0.15 | 0.17 | 0.19 | 0.20 | 0.28 | 0.25 | 0.26 | 0.25 | 0.30 | 0.33 |
| 豆类 Legumes | 0.02 | 0.10 | 0.02 | 0.02 | 0.00 | 0.02 | 0.05 | 0.05 | 0.03 | 0.02 | 0.00 | 0.05 | 0.08 | 0.03 | 0.05 | 0.06 | 0.06 | 0.01 | 0.04 | 0.04 | 0.02 | 0.09 | 0.02 | 0.05 | 0.04 |
| 薯类 Potatoes | 0.00 | 0.03 | 0.01 | 0.05 | 0.23 | 0.03 | 0.02 | 0.03 | 0.07 | 0.03 | 0.05 | 0.02 | 0.03 | 0.04 | 0.02 | 0.02 | 0.01 | 0.01 | 0.03 | 0.03 | 0.00 | 0.00 | 0.01 | 0.02 | 0.03 |

续表

| 膳食类别<br>Category | 黑龙江<br>HL | 辽宁<br>LN | 河北<br>HE | 北京<br>BJ | 吉林<br>JL | 山西<br>SX | 陕西<br>SN | 河南<br>HA | 宁夏<br>NX | 内蒙古<br>NM | 青海<br>QH | 甘肃<br>GS | 上海<br>SH | 福建<br>FJ | 江西<br>JX | 江苏<br>JS | 浙江<br>ZJ | 山东<br>SD | 湖北<br>HB | 四川<br>SC | 广西<br>GX | 湖南<br>HN | 广东<br>GD | 贵州<br>GZ | 全国平均<br>AVG |
|---|---|---|---|---|---|---|---|---|---|---|---|---|---|---|---|---|---|---|---|---|---|---|---|---|---|
| 肉类 Meats | 0.03 | 0.02 | 0.01 | 0.12 | 0.21 | 0.03 | 0.01 | 0.03 | 0.04 | 0.01 | 0.04 | 0.02 | 0.09 | 0.00 | 0.04 | 0.02 | 0.05 | 0.02 | 0.03 | 0.07 | 0.08 | 0.06 | 0.05 | 0.06 | 0.05 |
| 蛋类 Eggs | 0.00 | 0.03 | 0.01 | 0.07 | 0.00 | 0.01 | 0.01 | 0.01 | 0.01 | 0.02 | 0.01 | 0.02 | 0.03 | 0.01 | 0.00 | 0.02 | 0.01 | 0.01 | 0.01 | 0.01 | 0.00 | 0.02 | 0.01 | 0.01 | 0.01 |
| 水产类 Aquatic foods | 0.01 | 0.01 | 0.00 | 0.02 | 0.08 | 0.00 | 0.00 | 0.00 | 0.00 | 0.00 | 0.00 | 0.00 | 0.05 | 0.03 | 0.03 | 0.02 | 0.02 | 0.01 | 0.02 | 0.00 | 0.04 | 0.03 | 0.02 | 0.00 | 0.02 |
| 乳类 Dairy products | 0.00 | 0.00 | 0.02 | 0.05 | 0.01 | 0.01 | 0.01 | 0.01 | 0.01 | 0.01 | 0.01 | 0.00 | 0.12 | 0.01 | 0.00 | 0.01 | 0.01 | 0.01 | 0.00 | 0.00 | 0.00 | 0.01 | 0.01 | 0.01 | 0.01 |
| 蔬菜类 Vegetables | 0.01 | 0.20 | 0.09 | 0.33 | 1.26 | 0.06 | 0.08 | 0.16 | 0.10 | 0.10 | 0.17 | 0.15 | 0.33 | 0.15 | 0.19 | 0.35 | 0.18 | 0.10 | 0.23 | 0.01 | 0.17 | 0.36 | 0.10 | 0.20 | 0.21 |
| 水果类 Fruits | 0.00 | 0.00 | 0.00 | 0.12 | 0.02 | 0.01 | 0.01 | 0.01 | 0.03 | 0.03 | 0.00 | 0.01 | 0.05 | 0.02 | 0.00 | 0.01 | 0.01 | 0.01 | 0.00 | 0.00 | 0.01 | 0.01 | 0.01 | 0.01 | 0.02 |
| 糖类 Sugar | 0.00 | 0.00 | 0.00 | 0.00 | 0.00 | 0.00 | 0.00 | 0.00 | 0.00 | 0.00 | 0.00 | 0.00 | 0.01 | 0.00 | 0.00 | 0.00 | 0.00 | 0.00 | 0.00 | 0.00 | 0.00 | 0.00 | 0.00 | 0.00 | 0.00 |
| 水及饮料类 Water and beverages | 0.16 | 0.12 | 0.10 | 1.10 | 0.26 | 0.42 | 0.05 | 0.34 | 0.08 | 0.20 | 0.01 | 0.50 | 0.40 | 0.23 | 0.41 | 0.20 | 0.14 | 0.21 | 0.07 | 0.04 | 0.26 | 0.34 | 0.22 | 0.34 | 0.26 |
| 酒类 Alcohol beverages | 0.01 | 0.02 | 0.00 | 0.02 | 0.02 | 0.00 | 0.00 | 0.00 | 0.00 | 0.01 | 0.00 | 0.00 | 0.02 | 0.00 | 0.01 | 0.02 | 0.02 | 0.00 | 0.00 | 0.00 | 0.01 | 0.01 | 0.00 | 0.01 | 0.01 |
| 合计 SUM | 0.69 | 0.81 | 0.38 | 3.52 | 2.30 | 0.88 | 0.35 | 1.28 | 0.57 | 0.77 | 0.56 | 1.18 | 1.37 | 1.06 | 0.92 | 0.86 | 0.68 | 0.59 | 0.64 | 0.48 | 0.86 | 1.19 | 0.69 | 1.02 | 0.99 |

附录 773

附表 6-40 第六次中国总膳食研究的 DiBP 膳食摄入量 [单位: μg/(kg bw·d)]
Annexed Table 6-40 Dietary intakes of DiBP from the 6<sup>th</sup> China TDS [Unit: μg/(kg bw·d)]

| 膳食类别 Category | 黑龙江 HL | 辽宁 LN | 河北 HE | 北京 BJ | 吉林 JL | 山西 SX | 陕西 SN | 河南 HA | 宁夏 NX | 内蒙古 NM | 青海 QH | 甘肃 GS | 上海 SH | 福建 FJ | 江西 JX | 江苏 JS | 浙江 ZJ | 山东 SD | 湖北 HB | 四川 SC | 广西 GX | 湖南 HN | 广东 GD | 贵州 GZ | 全国平均 AVG |
|---|---|---|---|---|---|---|---|---|---|---|---|---|---|---|---|---|---|---|---|---|---|---|---|---|---|
| 谷类 Cereals | 0.07 | 0.35 | 0.09 | 0.49 | 0.15 | 0.10 | 0.08 | 0.31 | 0.12 | 0.07 | 0.17 | 0.48 | 0.16 | 1.31 | 0.15 | 0.10 | 0.23 | 0.10 | 0.11 | 0.09 | 0.16 | 0.17 | 0.33 | 0.17 | 0.23 |
| 豆类 Legumes | 0.01 | 0.06 | 0.01 | 0.05 | 0.00 | 0.01 | 0.01 | 0.03 | 0.00 | 0.00 | 0.00 | 0.01 | 0.04 | 0.03 | 0.03 | 0.03 | 0.03 | 0.01 | 0.02 | 0.01 | 0.01 | 0.04 | 0.01 | 0.04 | 0.02 |
| 薯类 Potatoes | 0.01 | 0.03 | 0.01 | 0.03 | 0.02 | 0.01 | 0.00 | 0.03 | 0.03 | 0.01 | 0.01 | 0.03 | 0.02 | 0.05 | 0.01 | 0.00 | 0.01 | 0.00 | 0.01 | 0.01 | 0.00 | 0.02 | 0.01 | 0.02 | 0.02 |
| 肉类 Meats | 0.01 | 0.03 | 0.01 | 0.04 | 0.02 | 0.02 | 0.01 | 0.02 | 0.02 | 0.01 | 0.01 | 0.02 | 0.05 | 0.02 | 0.05 | 0.00 | 0.06 | 0.01 | 0.01 | 0.01 | 0.04 | 0.04 | 0.05 | 0.03 | 0.02 |
| 蛋类 Eggs | 0.00 | 0.04 | 0.01 | 0.03 | 0.00 | 0.00 | 0.01 | 0.01 | 0.00 | 0.01 | 0.00 | 0.01 | 0.02 | 0.03 | 0.00 | 0.01 | 0.06 | 0.00 | 0.01 | 0.00 | 0.00 | 0.02 | 0.02 | 0.00 | 0.01 |
| 水产类 Aquatic foods | 0.00 | 0.01 | 0.00 | 0.01 | 0.01 | 0.00 | 0.00 | 0.00 | 0.00 | 0.00 | 0.00 | 0.00 | 0.03 | 0.01 | 0.02 | 0.01 | 0.02 | 0.00 | 0.01 | 0.00 | 0.02 | 0.02 | 0.02 | 0.00 | 0.01 |
| 乳类 Dairy products | 0.00 | 0.00 | 0.01 | 0.03 | 0.01 | 0.00 | 0.00 | 0.01 | 0.00 | 0.01 | 0.00 | 0.00 | 0.05 | 0.03 | 0.00 | 0.01 | 0.01 | 0.00 | 0.00 | 0.00 | 0.00 | 0.01 | 0.03 | 0.02 | 0.01 |
| 蔬菜类 Vegetables | 0.01 | 0.17 | 0.03 | 0.15 | 0.12 | 0.03 | 0.03 | 0.14 | 0.05 | 0.03 | 0.03 | 0.09 | 0.19 | 0.20 | 0.15 | 0.11 | 0.32 | 0.04 | 0.16 | 0.01 | 0.08 | 0.23 | 0.03 | 0.09 | 0.10 |
| 水果类 Fruits | 0.00 | 0.03 | 0.00 | 0.02 | 0.01 | 0.00 | 0.00 | 0.00 | 0.03 | 0.01 | 0.00 | 0.01 | 0.04 | 0.02 | 0.00 | 0.01 | 0.02 | 0.00 | 0.01 | 0.00 | 0.02 | 0.01 | 0.01 | 0.00 | 0.01 |
| 糖类 Sugar | 0.00 | 0.00 | 0.00 | 0.00 | 0.00 | 0.00 | 0.00 | 0.01 | 0.00 | 0.00 | 0.00 | 0.00 | 0.01 | 0.00 | 0.00 | 0.00 | 0.00 | 0.00 | 0.00 | 0.00 | 0.00 | 0.00 | 0.00 | 0.00 | 0.00 |
| 水及饮料类 Water and beverages | 0.06 | 0.15 | 0.07 | 0.82 | 0.68 | 0.08 | 0.25 | 0.30 | 0.05 | 0.22 | 1.13 | 0.27 | 0.80 | 0.24 | 0.42 | 0.41 | 0.25 | 0.09 | 0.09 | 0.12 | 0.36 | 0.88 | 0.65 | 0.17 | 0.36 |

续表

| 膳食类别 Category | 黑龙江 HL | 辽宁 LN | 河北 HE | 北京 BJ | 吉林 JL | 山西 SX | 陕西 SN | 河南 HA | 宁夏 NX | 内蒙古 NM | 青海 QH | 甘肃 GS | 上海 SH | 福建 FJ | 江西 JX | 江苏 JS | 浙江 ZJ | 山东 SD | 湖北 HB | 四川 SC | 广西 GX | 湖南 HN | 广东 GD | 贵州 GZ | 全国平均 AVG |
|---|---|---|---|---|---|---|---|---|---|---|---|---|---|---|---|---|---|---|---|---|---|---|---|---|---|
| 酒类 Alcohol beverages | 0.01 | 0.01 | 0.00 | 0.01 | 0.01 | 0.00 | 0.00 | 0.00 | 0.00 | 0.00 | 0.00 | 0.00 | 0.01 | 0.00 | 0.00 | 0.03 | 0.01 | 0.00 | 0.00 | 0.00 | 0.01 | 0.02 | 0.00 | 0.00 | 0.01 |
| 合计 SUM | 0.18 | 0.88 | 0.22 | 1.67 | 1.04 | 0.26 | 0.39 | 0.85 | 0.32 | 0.37 | 1.36 | 0.93 | 1.40 | 1.92 | 0.83 | 0.71 | 1.02 | 0.27 | 0.42 | 0.25 | 0.69 | 1.47 | 1.17 | 0.54 | 0.80 |

附表 6-41 第六次中国总膳食研究的 DEHP 膳食摄入量 [单位: μg/(kg bw · d)]
Annexed Table 6-41 Dietary intakes of DEHP from the 6th China TDS [Unit: μg/(kg bw · d)]

| 膳食类别 Category | 黑龙江 HL | 辽宁 LN | 河北 HE | 北京 BJ | 吉林 JL | 山西 SX | 陕西 SN | 河南 HA | 宁夏 NX | 内蒙古 NM | 青海 QH | 甘肃 GS | 上海 SH | 福建 FJ | 江西 JX | 江苏 JS | 浙江 ZJ | 山东 SD | 湖北 HB | 四川 SC | 广西 GX | 湖南 HN | 广东 GD | 贵州 GZ | 全国平均 AVG |
|---|---|---|---|---|---|---|---|---|---|---|---|---|---|---|---|---|---|---|---|---|---|---|---|---|---|
| 谷类 Cereals | 0.38 | 0.19 | 0.25 | 0.57 | 0.16 | 0.46 | 0.18 | 1.63 | 0.25 | 4.20 | 0.47 | 0.21 | 0.09 | 0.11 | 0.09 | 0.02 | 0.13 | 0.34 | 0.15 | 0.42 | 0.26 | 0.12 | 0.19 | 0.15 | 0.46 |
| 豆类 Legumes | 0.03 | 0.07 | 0.03 | 0.02 | 0.00 | 0.01 | 0.01 | 0.02 | 0.01 | 0.03 | 0.00 | 0.02 | 0.04 | 0.03 | 0.02 | 0.03 | 0.02 | 0.01 | 0.03 | 0.03 | 0.02 | 0.02 | 0.01 | 0.05 | 0.02 |
| 薯类 Potatoes | 0.04 | 0.02 | 0.04 | 0.03 | 0.01 | 0.04 | 0.02 | 0.01 | 0.03 | 0.27 | 0.03 | 0.14 | 0.01 | 0.01 | 0.01 | 0.01 | 0.01 | 0.01 | 0.05 | 0.02 | 0.01 | 0.01 | 0.00 | 0.03 | 0.04 |
| 肉类 Meats | 0.05 | 0.06 | 0.03 | 0.05 | 0.04 | 0.09 | 0.01 | 0.04 | 0.03 | 0.01 | 0.04 | 0.03 | 0.10 | 0.06 | 0.05 | 0.08 | 0.07 | 0.04 | 0.06 | 0.15 | 0.15 | 0.11 | 0.15 | 0.09 | 0.07 |
| 蛋类 Eggs | 0.00 | 0.02 | 0.02 | 0.03 | 0.00 | 0.02 | 0.00 | 0.01 | 0.00 | 0.02 | 0.00 | 0.01 | 0.01 | 0.01 | 0.00 | 0.01 | 0.01 | 0.02 | 0.02 | 0.01 | 0.01 | 0.02 | 0.00 | 0.01 | 0.01 |
| 水产类 Aquatic foods | 0.01 | 0.01 | 0.01 | 0.01 | 0.01 | 0.00 | 0.00 | 0.01 | 0.01 | 0.00 | 0.00 | 0.00 | 0.04 | 0.07 | 0.01 | 0.02 | 0.02 | 0.04 | 0.03 | 0.01 | 0.06 | 0.02 | 0.06 | 0.00 | 0.02 |
| 乳类 Dairy products | 0.00 | 0.00 | 0.00 | 0.01 | 0.01 | 0.00 | 0.01 | 0.00 | 0.01 | 0.01 | 0.01 | 0.00 | 0.01 | 0.00 | 0.00 | 0.00 | 0.00 | 0.00 | 0.00 | 0.00 | 0.00 | 0.00 | 0.00 | 0.00 | 0.00 |

续表

| 膳食类别 Category | 黑龙江 HL | 辽宁 LN | 河北 HE | 北京 BJ | 吉林 JL | 山西 SX | 陕西 SN | 河南 HA | 宁夏 NX | 内蒙古 NM | 青海 QH | 甘肃 GS | 上海 SH | 福建 FJ | 江西 JX | 江苏 JS | 浙江 ZJ | 山东 SD | 湖北 HB | 四川 SC | 广西 GX | 湖南 HN | 广东 GD | 贵州 GZ | 全国平均 AVG |
|---|---|---|---|---|---|---|---|---|---|---|---|---|---|---|---|---|---|---|---|---|---|---|---|---|---|
| 蔬菜类 Vegetables | 0.01 | 0.21 | 0.24 | 0.15 | 0.15 | 0.15 | 0.25 | 0.13 | 0.05 | 3.24 | 0.11 | 0.43 | 0.17 | 0.29 | 0.21 | 0.19 | 0.36 | 0.28 | 0.75 | 0.01 | 0.30 | 0.27 | 0.26 | 0.53 | 0.36 |
| 水果类 Fruits | 0.00 | 0.01 | 0.00 | 0.03 | 0.00 | 0.01 | 0.01 | 0.02 | 0.01 | 0.00 | 0.00 | 0.00 | 0.01 | 0.01 | 0.00 | 0.00 | 0.01 | 0.03 | 0.00 | 0.00 | 0.00 | 0.01 | 0.00 | 0.00 | 0.01 |
| 糖类 Sugar | 0.00 | 0.00 | 0.00 | 0.00 | 0.00 | 0.00 | 0.01 | 0.00 | 0.00 | 0.00 | 0.00 | 0.00 | 0.01 | 0.00 | 0.00 | 0.00 | 0.00 | 0.00 | 0.00 | 0.00 | 0.00 | 0.00 | 0.00 | 0.00 | 0.00 |
| 水及饮料类 Water and beverages | 0.26 | 0.02 | 0.02 | 0.30 | 0.07 | 0.36 | 0.02 | 0.05 | 0.01 | 0.18 | 0.03 | 1.49 | 0.14 | 0.02 | 0.18 | 0.02 | 0.02 | 0.10 | 0.43 | 0.02 | 0.10 | 0.06 | 0.08 | 0.05 | 0.17 |
| 酒类 Alcohol beverages | 0.00 | 0.00 | 0.00 | 0.00 | 0.00 | 0.00 | 0.00 | 0.00 | 0.00 | 0.00 | 0.00 | 0.00 | 0.00 | 0.00 | 0.00 | 0.00 | 0.00 | 0.00 | 0.01 | 0.00 | 0.00 | 0.00 | 0.00 | 0.00 | 0.00 |
| 合计 SUM | 0.78 | 0.62 | 0.64 | 1.21 | 0.45 | 1.15 | 0.52 | 1.91 | 0.42 | 7.97 | 0.69 | 2.34 | 0.64 | 0.60 | 0.57 | 0.39 | 0.64 | 0.87 | 1.52 | 0.67 | 0.91 | 0.65 | 0.75 | 0.93 | 1.16 |

附表 6-42　第六次中国总膳食研究 DBP 的膳食来源（单位：%）

Annexed Table 6-42　Dietary sources of DBP from the 6$^{th}$ China TDS (Unit: %)

| 膳食类别 Category | 黑龙江 HL | 辽宁 LN | 河北 HE | 北京 BJ | 吉林 JL | 山西 SX | 陕西 SN | 河南 HA | 宁夏 NX | 内蒙古 NM | 青海 QH | 甘肃 GS | 上海 SH | 福建 FJ | 江西 JX | 江苏 JS | 浙江 ZJ | 山东 SD | 湖北 HB | 四川 SC | 广西 GX | 湖南 HN | 广东 GD | 贵州 GZ | 全国平均 AVG |
|---|---|---|---|---|---|---|---|---|---|---|---|---|---|---|---|---|---|---|---|---|---|---|---|---|---|
| 谷类 Cereals | 65.15 | 35.40 | 31.48 | 45.55 | 9.58 | 33.62 | 36.75 | 51.19 | 35.84 | 43.80 | 43.94 | 34.59 | 12.06 | 50.24 | 19.55 | 16.83 | 24.34 | 32.50 | 32.10 | 57.71 | 28.97 | 21.78 | 36.44 | 29.65 | 34.54 |
| 豆类 Legumes | 2.98 | 12.44 | 5.00 | 0.52 | 0.11 | 2.05 | 12.83 | 4.06 | 5.81 | 2.27 | 0.37 | 4.63 | 5.97 | 2.78 | 5.61 | 6.73 | 8.62 | 2.52 | 6.42 | 7.78 | 2.69 | 7.99 | 2.37 | 5.24 | 4.91 |
| 薯类 Potatoes | 0.32 | 3.21 | 2.85 | 1.49 | 9.91 | 3.65 | 4.54 | 2.11 | 12.15 | 4.24 | 9.40 | 1.63 | 2.01 | 3.37 | 2.41 | 2.61 | 1.33 | 1.70 | 4.55 | 6.46 | 0.48 | 0.15 | 0.86 | 2.17 | 3.48 |

续表

| 膳食类别 Category | 黑龙江 HL | 辽宁 LN | 河北 HE | 北京 BJ | 吉林 JL | 山西 SX | 陕西 SN | 河南 HA | 宁夏 NX | 内蒙古 NM | 青海 QH | 甘肃 GS | 上海 SH | 福建 FJ | 江西 JX | 江苏 JS | 浙江 ZJ | 山东 SD | 湖北 HB | 四川 SC | 广西 GX | 湖南 HN | 广东 GD | 贵州 GZ | 全国平均 AVG |
|---|---|---|---|---|---|---|---|---|---|---|---|---|---|---|---|---|---|---|---|---|---|---|---|---|---|
| 肉类 Meats | 4.12 | 2.92 | 2.74 | 3.41 | 9.26 | 3.63 | 3.88 | 2.37 | 6.75 | 1.71 | 7.54 | 2.01 | 6.31 | 0.20 | 3.91 | 2.37 | 7.99 | 3.57 | 4.48 | 13.99 | 8.89 | 5.02 | 7.42 | 5.91 | 5.02 |
| 蛋类 Eggs | 0.14 | 3.43 | 2.83 | 1.96 | 0.05 | 0.92 | 1.94 | 0.55 | 1.63 | 2.99 | 2.01 | 1.45 | 2.29 | 1.38 | 0.06 | 1.99 | 2.14 | 1.28 | 1.34 | 1.32 | 0.48 | 1.38 | 1.20 | 0.71 | 1.48 |
| 水产类 Aquatic foods | 1.47 | 1.08 | 0.68 | 0.69 | 3.39 | 0.16 | 0.16 | 0.14 | 0.12 | 0.49 | 0.36 | 0.01 | 3.74 | 2.97 | 3.00 | 2.25 | 2.77 | 1.58 | 2.57 | 0.83 | 4.42 | 2.18 | 2.71 | 0.30 | 1.59 |
| 乳类 Dairy products | 0.40 | 0.13 | 4.01 | 1.47 | 0.36 | 1.12 | 1.72 | 0.58 | 1.72 | 1.32 | 2.39 | 0.03 | 8.75 | 0.92 | 0.06 | 0.95 | 1.65 | 1.63 | 0.29 | 0.74 | 0.53 | 0.50 | 1.75 | 1.45 | 1.44 |
| 蔬菜类 Vegetables | 1.37 | 24.20 | 22.85 | 9.51 | 54.69 | 6.56 | 22.13 | 12.23 | 17.26 | 12.84 | 30.90 | 12.56 | 24.15 | 14.28 | 20.08 | 40.53 | 26.34 | 17.10 | 35.91 | 1.52 | 19.38 | 30.08 | 14.51 | 19.38 | 20.43 |
| 水果类 Fruits | 0.22 | 0.25 | 0.84 | 3.32 | 0.67 | 0.62 | 1.43 | 0.44 | 4.98 | 3.38 | 0.30 | 0.68 | 3.56 | 2.09 | 0.15 | 0.72 | 2.11 | 1.09 | 0.67 | 0.30 | 1.52 | 1.17 | 0.99 | 0.66 | 1.34 |
| 糖类 Sugar | 0.05 | 0.02 | 0.01 | 0.06 | 0.01 | 0.04 | 1.04 | 0.01 | 0.02 | 0.03 | 0.01 | 0.02 | 0.51 | 0.01 | 0.03 | 0.01 | 0.03 | 0.01 | 0.01 | 0.01 | 0.01 | 0.04 | 0.01 | 0.01 | 0.08 |
| 水及饮料类 Water and beverages | 22.58 | 14.97 | 26.22 | 31.30 | 11.15 | 47.62 | 13.52 | 26.25 | 13.70 | 26.12 | 2.63 | 42.40 | 29.05 | 21.37 | 44.21 | 23.03 | 20.13 | 36.54 | 11.01 | 8.57 | 30.89 | 28.80 | 31.67 | 33.73 | 24.89 |
| 酒类 Alcohol beverages | 1.22 | 1.96 | 0.50 | 0.70 | 0.84 | 0.01 | 0.07 | 0.09 | 0.02 | 0.83 | 0.13 | 0.01 | 1.61 | 0.39 | 0.94 | 1.97 | 2.53 | 0.46 | 0.66 | 0.77 | 1.74 | 0.92 | 0.05 | 0.80 | 0.80 |

附表 6-43　第六次中国总膳食研究 DiBP 的膳食来源（单位：%）

Annexed Table 6-43　Dietary sources of DiBP from the 6th China TDS (Unit: %)

| 膳食类别<br>Category | 黑龙江<br>HL | 辽宁<br>LN | 河北<br>HE | 北京<br>BJ | 吉林<br>JL | 山西<br>SX | 陕西<br>SN | 河南<br>HA | 宁夏<br>NX | 内蒙古<br>NM | 青海<br>QH | 甘肃<br>GS | 上海<br>SH | 福建<br>FJ | 江西<br>JX | 江苏<br>JS | 浙江<br>ZJ | 山东<br>SD | 湖北<br>HB | 四川<br>SC | 广西<br>GX | 湖南<br>HN | 广东<br>GD | 贵州<br>GZ | 全国平均<br>AVG |
|---|---|---|---|---|---|---|---|---|---|---|---|---|---|---|---|---|---|---|---|---|---|---|---|---|---|
| 谷类 Cereals | 40.67 | 39.80 | 39.82 | 29.32 | 14.26 | 37.34 | 20.53 | 36.28 | 38.61 | 20.27 | 12.44 | 52.03 | 11.67 | 68.23 | 17.83 | 14.41 | 22.88 | 38.80 | 26.05 | 34.04 | 23.71 | 11.31 | 28.36 | 31.13 | 29.57 |
| 豆类 Legumes | 4.19 | 6.96 | 3.10 | 2.71 | 0.23 | 2.58 | 1.55 | 3.62 | 1.09 | 1.17 | 0.03 | 1.44 | 2.70 | 1.38 | 3.59 | 3.68 | 2.48 | 2.52 | 4.61 | 4.04 | 1.43 | 2.83 | 1.04 | 6.53 | 2.73 |
| 薯类 Potatoes | 3.29 | 3.54 | 2.78 | 1.60 | 2.39 | 5.51 | 0.87 | 3.64 | 9.85 | 2.92 | 1.08 | 3.43 | 1.43 | 2.74 | 1.00 | 0.91 | 1.19 | 1.59 | 3.46 | 2.19 | 0.55 | 1.68 | 0.88 | 2.88 | 2.56 |
| 肉类 Meats | 4.01 | 3.05 | 2.61 | 2.66 | 2.21 | 6.27 | 1.70 | 2.34 | 7.48 | 2.27 | 0.59 | 2.57 | 3.35 | 1.16 | 5.73 | 0.31 | 5.87 | 3.38 | 2.46 | 5.94 | 5.24 | 2.65 | 4.40 | 5.86 | 3.50 |
| 蛋类 Eggs | 0.54 | 4.81 | 2.74 | 1.52 | 0.11 | 1.35 | 1.31 | 0.93 | 0.80 | 1.59 | 0.21 | 1.04 | 1.12 | 0.46 | 0.07 | 1.65 | 5.56 | 0.49 | 1.25 | 0.75 | 0.43 | 1.63 | 1.38 | 0.92 | 1.36 |
| 水产类 Aquatic foods | 1.47 | 1.15 | 0.61 | 0.59 | 0.82 | 0.28 | 0.06 | 0.13 | 0.15 | 0.36 | 0.03 | 0.01 | 2.08 | 1.54 | 2.11 | 0.94 | 2.41 | 1.77 | 1.60 | 0.30 | 2.68 | 1.33 | 2.02 | 0.21 | 1.03 |
| 乳类 Dairy products | 0.18 | 0.12 | 2.58 | 1.71 | 1.33 | 1.88 | 1.09 | 1.34 | 1.11 | 2.19 | 0.29 | 0.04 | 3.45 | 0.33 | 0.06 | 0.58 | 0.64 | 0.65 | 0.28 | 0.94 | 0.38 | 0.67 | 2.98 | 3.34 | 1.17 |
| 蔬菜类 Vegetables | 5.16 | 19.53 | 14.57 | 9.16 | 11.09 | 11.34 | 8.07 | 16.20 | 15.35 | 7.81 | 1.89 | 9.35 | 13.30 | 10.32 | 18.66 | 15.12 | 31.41 | 15.24 | 37.03 | 2.90 | 10.96 | 15.74 | 2.31 | 17.48 | 13.33 |
| 水果类 Fruits | 0.82 | 3.60 | 0.90 | 0.98 | 1.38 | 1.04 | 0.65 | 0.37 | 9.20 | 1.63 | 0.08 | 0.72 | 2.54 | 1.14 | 0.16 | 1.27 | 1.87 | 1.11 | 1.49 | 0.16 | 2.41 | 0.97 | 1.13 | 0.55 | 1.51 |
| 糖类 Sugar | 0.12 | 0.02 | 0.02 | 0.06 | 0.02 | 0.06 | 0.23 | 0.01 | 0.01 | 0.02 | 0.00 | 0.01 | 0.55 | 0.00 | 0.02 | 0.01 | 0.03 | 0.01 | 0.00 | 0.01 | 0.01 | 0.01 | 0.01 | 0.01 | 0.05 |
| 水及饮料类 Water and beverages | 35.15 | 16.47 | 29.72 | 49.04 | 65.50 | 32.34 | 63.89 | 35.06 | 15.39 | 59.12 | 83.34 | 29.35 | 57.11 | 12.57 | 50.18 | 57.54 | 24.40 | 33.42 | 21.16 | 46.79 | 51.20 | 60.15 | 55.47 | 31.02 | 42.31 |
| 酒类 Alcohol beverages | 4.41 | 0.94 | 0.56 | 0.67 | 0.67 | 0.01 | 0.05 | 0.07 | 0.96 | 0.65 | 0.02 | 0.01 | 0.71 | 0.12 | 0.58 | 3.58 | 1.26 | 1.02 | 0.60 | 1.96 | 0.98 | 1.04 | 0.03 | 0.07 | 0.87 |

附表 6-44　第六次中国总膳食研究 DEHP 的膳食来源（单位：%）

Annexed Table 6-44　Dietary sources of DEHP from the 6th China TDS (Unit: %)

| 膳食类别 Category | 黑龙江 HL | 辽宁 LN | 河北 HE | 北京 BJ | 吉林 JL | 山西 SX | 陕西 SN | 河南 HA | 宁夏 NX | 内蒙古 NM | 青海 QH | 甘肃 GS | 上海 SH | 福建 FJ | 江西 JX | 江苏 JS | 浙江 ZJ | 山东 SD | 湖北 HB | 四川 SC | 广西 GX | 湖南 HN | 广东 GD | 贵州 GZ | 全国平均 AVG |
|---|---|---|---|---|---|---|---|---|---|---|---|---|---|---|---|---|---|---|---|---|---|---|---|---|---|
| 谷类 Cereals | 48.61 | 31.15 | 38.23 | 47.38 | 34.78 | 40.37 | 35.03 | 85.12 | 60.65 | 52.71 | 67.61 | 9.15 | 14.34 | 17.64 | 15.50 | 5.96 | 20.19 | 38.88 | 9.57 | 63.29 | 28.40 | 18.78 | 24.60 | 16.17 | 34.34 |
| 豆类 Legumes | 3.84 | 11.47 | 3.94 | 1.51 | 0.54 | 1.02 | 2.00 | 1.13 | 3.06 | 0.32 | 0.11 | 0.98 | 6.34 | 4.75 | 3.74 | 8.67 | 3.06 | 1.17 | 1.78 | 4.05 | 1.95 | 3.36 | 1.73 | 5.43 | 3.16 |
| 薯类 Potatoes | 4.52 | 4.02 | 5.74 | 2.16 | 2.92 | 3.70 | 3.13 | 0.52 | 7.65 | 3.38 | 4.05 | 6.11 | 1.90 | 1.42 | 0.88 | 2.47 | 1.20 | 1.16 | 3.54 | 3.41 | 0.55 | 2.15 | 0.34 | 3.59 | 2.94 |
| 肉类 Meats | 6.45 | 9.16 | 5.39 | 4.42 | 9.22 | 8.18 | 2.69 | 1.94 | 6.36 | 0.10 | 5.26 | 1.33 | 15.37 | 9.20 | 8.09 | 19.46 | 11.13 | 4.65 | 3.72 | 22.83 | 16.88 | 17.14 | 20.07 | 10.14 | 9.13 |
| 蛋类 Eggs | 0.12 | 2.45 | 3.73 | 2.31 | 0.24 | 1.51 | 0.88 | 0.31 | 0.83 | 0.20 | 0.74 | 0.47 | 2.27 | 2.18 | 0.10 | 2.32 | 0.96 | 1.90 | 1.22 | 0.76 | 0.78 | 3.40 | 0.28 | 0.92 | 1.29 |
| 水产类 Aquatic foods | 1.29 | 1.33 | 1.45 | 1.08 | 1.56 | 0.13 | 0.13 | 0.07 | 0.69 | 0.06 | 0.65 | 0.00 | 6.34 | 12.13 | 2.62 | 3.90 | 2.84 | 4.86 | 2.25 | 0.80 | 6.75 | 2.51 | 8.21 | 0.49 | 2.59 |
| 乳类 Dairy products | 0.20 | 0.46 | 0.50 | 0.92 | 1.35 | 0.09 | 1.11 | 0.12 | 2.66 | 0.06 | 1.29 | 0.01 | 2.16 | 0.58 | 0.09 | 0.17 | 0.38 | 0.15 | 0.01 | 0.27 | 0.05 | 0.31 | 0.35 | 0.46 | 0.57 |
| 蔬菜类 Vegetables | 1.20 | 33.68 | 37.39 | 12.65 | 34.01 | 13.17 | 47.37 | 6.96 | 13.16 | 40.64 | 15.48 | 18.34 | 26.36 | 47.31 | 37.26 | 49.02 | 55.89 | 31.78 | 49.20 | 1.08 | 32.76 | 42.06 | 34.10 | 57.22 | 30.75 |
| 水果类 Fruits | 0.19 | 2.32 | 0.59 | 2.45 | 0.46 | 0.70 | 2.02 | 1.24 | 1.94 | 0.21 | 0.06 | 0.03 | 2.08 | 1.27 | 0.24 | 1.10 | 1.16 | 3.63 | 0.15 | 0.47 | 1.04 | 1.27 | 0.09 | 0.24 | 1.04 |
| 糖类 Sugar | 0.01 | 0.01 | 0.01 | 0.04 | 0.01 | 0.04 | 2.14 | 0.00 | 0.03 | 0.00 | 0.01 | 0.00 | 0.97 | 0.00 | 0.01 | 0.00 | 0.02 | 0.02 | 0.00 | 0.01 | 0.00 | 0.00 | 0.00 | 0.00 | 0.14 |
| 水及饮料类 Water and beverages | 32.96 | 3.68 | 2.87 | 24.96 | 14.69 | 31.03 | 3.49 | 2.57 | 2.96 | 2.31 | 4.69 | 63.56 | 21.63 | 3.42 | 31.17 | 6.18 | 2.94 | 11.48 | 27.90 | 2.98 | 10.65 | 8.87 | 10.22 | 5.35 | 13.86 |
| 酒类 Alcohol beverages | 0.60 | 0.29 | 0.16 | 0.11 | 0.22 | 0.07 | 0.02 | 0.02 | 0.01 | 0.02 | 0.06 | 0.00 | 0.23 | 0.10 | 0.30 | 0.75 | 0.23 | 0.31 | 0.67 | 0.05 | 0.20 | 0.16 | 0.01 | 0.01 | 0.19 |

# 第七章 附 表
# Annexed Tables of Chapter 7

附表 7-1 第六次中国总膳食研究混合膳食样品中二噁英及其类似物的含量（单位：pg TEQ/g）

Annexed Table 7-1  Levels of PCDD/Fs and dl-PCBs in food samples from the 6$^{th}$ China TDS (Unit: pg TEQ/g)

| 膳食类别<br>Category | 黑龙江<br>HL | 辽宁<br>LN | 河北<br>HE | 北京<br>BJ | 吉林<br>JL | 山西<br>SX | 陕西<br>SN | 河南<br>HA | 宁夏<br>NX | 内蒙古<br>NM | 青海<br>QH | 甘肃<br>GS | 上海<br>SH | 福建<br>FJ | 江西<br>JX | 江苏<br>JS | 浙江<br>ZJ | 山东<br>SD | 四川<br>SC | 广西<br>GX | 湖南<br>HN | 广东<br>GD | 贵州<br>GZ | 全国平均<br>AVG |
|---|---|---|---|---|---|---|---|---|---|---|---|---|---|---|---|---|---|---|---|---|---|---|---|---|
| 肉类<br>Meats | 0.06 | 0.15 | 0.08 | 0.11 | 0.11 | 0.05 | 0.10 | 0.08 | 0.06 | 0.10 | 0.05 | 0.18 | 0.07 | 0.05 | 0.08 | 0.05 | 0.15 | 0.03 | 0.05 | 0.21 | 0.14 | 0.05 | 0.06 | 0.09 |
| 蛋类<br>Eggs | 0.04 | 0.13 | 0.14 | 0.13 | 0.10 | 0.02 | 0.03 | 0.03 | 0.03 | 0.07 | 0.02 | 0.04 | 0.10 | 0.13 | 0.08 | 0.07 | 0.16 | 0.01 | 0.01 | 0.03 | 0.09 | 0.02 | 0.03 | 0.07 |
| 水产类<br>Aquatic foods | 0.08 | 0.22 | 0.12 | 0.19 | 0.13 | 0.10 | 0.07 | 0.13 | 0.03 | 0.10 | 0.09 | 0.11 | 0.25 | 0.16 | 0.21 | 0.33 | 0.20 | 0.15 | 0.16 | 0.16 | 0.16 | 0.32 | 0.12 | 0.16 |
| 乳类<br>Dairy products | 0.004 | 0.03 | 0.04 | 0.04 | 0.08 | 0.02 | 0.02 | 0.03 | 0.02 | 0.10 | 0.02 | 0.02 | 0.04 | 0.02 | 0.05 | 0.04 | 0.04 | 0.03 | 0.01 | 0.01 | 0.04 | 0.03 | 0.01 | 0.03 |

注：未检出（ND）按检出限（LOD）计

Note: values not detected (ND) were treated as being equal to the detection of limit (LOD)

附表 7-2 第六次中国总膳食研究二噁英及其类似物的膳食摄入量 [单位：pg TEQ/(kg bw·月)]

Annexed Table 7-2  Dietary intakes of PCDD/Fs and dl-PCBs from the 6$^{th}$ China TDS [Unit: pg TEQ/(kg bw·month)]

| 膳食类别<br>Category | 黑龙江<br>HL | 辽宁<br>LN | 河北<br>HE | 北京<br>BJ | 吉林<br>JL | 山西<br>SX | 陕西<br>SN | 河南<br>HA | 宁夏<br>NX | 内蒙古<br>NM | 青海<br>QH | 甘肃<br>GS | 上海<br>SH | 福建<br>FJ | 江西<br>JX | 江苏<br>JS | 浙江<br>ZJ | 山东<br>SD | 四川<br>SC | 广西<br>GX | 湖南<br>HN | 广东<br>GD | 贵州<br>GZ | 全国平均<br>AVG |
|---|---|---|---|---|---|---|---|---|---|---|---|---|---|---|---|---|---|---|---|---|---|---|---|---|
| 肉类<br>Meats | 1.7 | 4.7 | 1.9 | 3.6 | 3.6 | 3.1 | 1.8 | 2.2 | 1.3 | 3.4 | 1.7 | 2.7 | 3.9 | 2.0 | 3.5 | 2.4 | 8.5 | 1.4 | 2.9 | 15.1 | 9.9 | 2.6 | 2.9 | 3.8 |
| 蛋类<br>Eggs | 0.8 | 2.5 | 2.1 | 2.4 | 2.0 | 0.2 | 0.3 | 0.5 | 0.2 | 1.0 | 0.1 | 0.4 | 1.8 | 1.2 | 0.8 | 0.9 | 1.8 | 0.3 | 0.1 | 0.2 | 1.0 | 0.3 | 0.2 | 0.9 |
| 水产类<br>Aquatic foods | 1.0 | 1.6 | 0.5 | 1.5 | 0.7 | 0.3 | 0.1 | 0.3 | 0.0 | 0.5 | 0.2 | 0.1 | 8.3 | 4.8 | 4.5 | 6.2 | 4.9 | 1.6 | 0.6 | 7.2 | 5.0 | 7.7 | 0.2 | 2.5 |

续表

| 膳食类别<br>Category | 黑龙江<br>HL | 辽宁<br>LN | 河北<br>HE | 北京<br>BJ | 吉林<br>JL | 山西<br>SX | 陕西<br>SN | 河南<br>HA | 宁夏<br>NX | 内蒙古<br>NM | 青海<br>QH | 甘肃<br>GS | 上海<br>SH | 福建<br>FJ | 江西<br>JX | 江苏<br>JS | 浙江<br>ZJ | 山东<br>SD | 四川<br>SC | 广西<br>GX | 湖南<br>HN | 广东<br>GD | 贵州<br>GZ | 全国平均<br>AVG |
|---|---|---|---|---|---|---|---|---|---|---|---|---|---|---|---|---|---|---|---|---|---|---|---|---|
| 乳类<br>Dairy products | 0.0 | 0.6 | 0.5 | 1.7 | 1.3 | 0.4 | 0.2 | 0.2 | 0.2 | 1.6 | 0.6 | 0.2 | 1.3 | 0.4 | 0.5 | 0.5 | 0.6 | 0.3 | 0.1 | 0.1 | 0.3 | 0.5 | 0.2 | 0.5 |
| 合计<br>SUM | 3.5 | 9.5 | 5.0 | 9.2 | 7.5 | 4.0 | 2.4 | 3.2 | 1.7 | 6.6 | 2.6 | 3.3 | 15.2 | 8.4 | 9.2 | 10.0 | 15.8 | 3.6 | 3.7 | 22.6 | 16.2 | 11.1 | 3.5 | 7.7 |

附表 7-3　第六次中国总膳食研究二噁英及其类似物的膳食来源（单位：%）
Annexed Table 7-3　Dietary sources of PCDD/Fs and dl-PCBs from the 6th China TDS (Unit: %)

| 膳食类别<br>Category | 黑龙江<br>HL | 辽宁<br>LN | 河北<br>HE | 北京<br>BJ | 吉林<br>JL | 山西<br>SX | 陕西<br>SN | 河南<br>HA | 宁夏<br>NX | 内蒙古<br>NM | 青海<br>QH | 甘肃<br>GS | 上海<br>SH | 福建<br>FJ | 江西<br>JX | 江苏<br>JS | 浙江<br>ZJ | 山东<br>SD | 四川<br>SC | 广西<br>GX | 湖南<br>HN | 广东<br>GD | 贵州<br>GZ | 全国平均<br>AVG |
|---|---|---|---|---|---|---|---|---|---|---|---|---|---|---|---|---|---|---|---|---|---|---|---|---|
| 肉类<br>Meats | 47.3 | 49.7 | 38.4 | 38.9 | 47.6 | 76.7 | 72.8 | 68.6 | 76.3 | 52.2 | 65.9 | 79.6 | 25.4 | 23.7 | 37.7 | 23.9 | 54.0 | 39.4 | 79.5 | 66.8 | 61.1 | 23.5 | 82.4 | 48.7 |
| 蛋类<br>Eggs | 23.7 | 26.2 | 41.9 | 26.0 | 26.2 | 5.1 | 12.9 | 14.6 | 11.0 | 15.5 | 5.2 | 11.3 | 11.8 | 14.4 | 8.4 | 8.8 | 11.3 | 7.9 | 2.1 | 0.8 | 6.1 | 2.3 | 7.1 | 11.8 |
| 水产类<br>Aquatic foods | 28.1 | 17.3 | 10.6 | 16.3 | 9.4 | 7.8 | 6.0 | 9.2 | 2.3 | 7.7 | 5.9 | 4.3 | 54.3 | 57.3 | 48.3 | 62.2 | 30.8 | 44.6 | 16.8 | 32.0 | 31.0 | 70.0 | 5.6 | 32.6 |
| 乳类<br>Dairy products | 0.9 | 6.8 | 9.1 | 18.8 | 16.9 | 10.4 | 8.2 | 7.7 | 10.5 | 24.6 | 23.1 | 4.9 | 8.5 | 4.6 | 5.6 | 5.1 | 3.9 | 8.1 | 1.6 | 0.4 | 1.9 | 4.2 | 4.8 | 6.9 |

附表 7-4　第六次中国总膳食研究混合膳食样品中指示性 PCB 的含量（单位：pg/g）
Annexed Table 7-4　Levels of indicator PCBs in food samples from the 6th China TDS (Unit: pg/g)

| 膳食类别<br>Category | 黑龙江<br>HL | 辽宁<br>LN | 河北<br>HE | 北京<br>BJ | 吉林<br>JL | 山西<br>SX | 陕西<br>SN | 河南<br>HA | 宁夏<br>NX | 内蒙古<br>NM | 青海<br>QH | 甘肃<br>GS | 上海<br>SH | 福建<br>FJ | 江西<br>JX | 江苏<br>JS | 浙江<br>ZJ | 山东<br>SD | 湖北<br>HB | 四川<br>SC | 广西<br>GX | 湖南<br>HN | 广东<br>GD | 贵州<br>GZ | 全国平均<br>AVG |
|---|---|---|---|---|---|---|---|---|---|---|---|---|---|---|---|---|---|---|---|---|---|---|---|---|---|
| 谷类<br>Cereals | 8.5 | 0.3 | 4.5 | 2.4 | 3.8 | 9.0 | 0.1 | 4.2 | 0.1 | 10.5 | 0.6 | 15.7 | 3.7 | 1.7 | 0.9 | 2.9 | 2.3 | 7.0 | 7.7 | 3.9 | 29.6 | 5.0 | 3.0 | 5.6 | 5.5 |
| 豆类<br>Legumes | 16.0 | 11.7 | 3.5 | 4.8 | 8.4 | 28.6 | 4.2 | 9.8 | 3.6 | 22.0 | 2.3 | 13.0 | 9.1 | 3.4 | 3.8 | 9.8 | 4.0 | 17.0 | 29.7 | 9.9 | 19.3 | 9.4 | 13.4 | 9.1 | 11.1 |

续表

| 膳食类别 Category | 黑龙江 HL | 辽宁 LN | 河北 HE | 北京 BJ | 吉林 JL | 山西 SX | 陕西 SN | 河南 HA | 宁夏 NX | 内蒙古 NM | 青海 QH | 甘肃 GS | 上海 SH | 福建 FJ | 江西 JX | 江苏 JS | 浙江 ZJ | 山东 SD | 湖北 HB | 四川 SC | 广西 GX | 湖南 HN | 广东 GD | 贵州 GZ | 全国平均 AVG |
|---|---|---|---|---|---|---|---|---|---|---|---|---|---|---|---|---|---|---|---|---|---|---|---|---|---|
| 薯类 Potatoes | 6.1 | 6.1 | 31.8 | 2.5 | 3.0 | 11.1 | 1.3 | 0.7 | 2.9 | 15.5 | 4.5 | 13.1 | 7.8 | 5.2 | 5.6 | 8.2 | 3.1 | 7.3 | 16.7 | 8.0 | 12.2 | 8.0 | 1.1 | 8.7 | 7.9 |
| 肉类 Meats | 41.4 | 55.0 | 56.5 | 24.2 | 37.9 | 32.7 | 23.0 | 39.1 | 54.7 | 30.1 | 21.4 | 40.8 | 41.7 | 21.2 | 27.4 | 28.1 | 135.5 | 24.3 | 42.3 | 30.1 | 1319.7 | 31.0 | 235.9 | 22.0 | 100.7 |
| 蛋类 Eggs | 15.0 | 52.8 | 32.6 | 130.1 | 48.0 | 62.2 | 13.9 | 24.0 | 19.4 | 37.6 | 34.2 | 21.0 | 25.1 | 56.8 | 42.3 | 23.9 | 31.2 | 11.6 | 20.6 | 17.7 | 65.4 | 21.6 | 11.2 | 14.1 | 34.7 |
| 水产类 Aquatic foods | 165.6 | 498.2 | 138.6 | 168.7 | 131.0 | 138.0 | 105.8 | 127.4 | 21.0 | 12.6 | 147.5 | 153.0 | 212.2 | 127.2 | 74.7 | 122.1 | 139.2 | 151.2 | 123.2 | 86.2 | 72.1 | 99.9 | 705.0 | 70.6 | 158.0 |
| 乳类 Dairy products | 3.1 | 13.3 | 3.0 | 4.7 | 27.3 | 12.5 | 23.7 | 12.3 | 1.7 | 223.3 | 12.1 | 16.2 | 6.3 | 10.2 | 5.7 | 9.9 | 4.8 | 15.0 | 24.6 | 12.3 | 35.2 | 10.1 | 17.0 | 9.4 | 21.4 |
| 蔬菜类 Vegetables | 5.9 | 7.3 | 4.5 | 5.6 | 4.5 | 12.4 | 1.8 | 9.6 | 2.0 | 8.7 | 3.1 | 6.3 | 8.5 | 5.4 | 5.2 | 9.9 | 11.0 | 7.2 | 9.9 | 8.5 | 9.1 | 12.7 | 16.3 | 8.4 | 7.7 |

注：未检出（ND）按检出限（LOD）计

Note: values not detected (ND) were treated as being equal to the detection of limit (LOD)

附表 7-5 第六次中国总膳食研究指示性 PCB 膳食摄入量 [单位：pg/(kg bw·d)]

Annexed Table 7-5 Dietary intakes of indicator PCBs from the 6$^{th}$ China TDS [Unit: pg/(kg bw·d)]

| 膳食类别 Category | 黑龙江 HL | 辽宁 LN | 河北 HE | 北京 BJ | 吉林 JL | 山西 SX | 陕西 SN | 河南 HA | 宁夏 NX | 内蒙古 NM | 青海 QH | 甘肃 GS | 上海 SH | 福建 FJ | 江西 JX | 江苏 JS | 浙江 ZJ | 山东 SD | 湖北 HB | 四川 SC | 广西 GX | 湖南 HN | 广东 GD | 贵州 GZ | 全国平均 AVG |
|---|---|---|---|---|---|---|---|---|---|---|---|---|---|---|---|---|---|---|---|---|---|---|---|---|---|
| 谷类 Cereals | 74.3 | 3.1 | 53.6 | 29.7 | 35.0 | 148.4 | 1.6 | 62.0 | 0.8 | 120.3 | 7.3 | 171.5 | 26.7 | 17.0 | 8.8 | 36.3 | 22.9 | 110.3 | 65.0 | 59.8 | 442.0 | 45.5 | 21.9 | 60.5 | 67.7 |
| 豆类 Legumes | 11.6 | 22.7 | 3.1 | 7.7 | 10.0 | 31.5 | 5.5 | 8.4 | 2.0 | 13.9 | 0.2 | 8.5 | 17.0 | 4.3 | 4.4 | 13.0 | 9.0 | 14.1 | 31.4 | 10.6 | 13.0 | 10.8 | 5.9 | 14.7 | 11.4 |
| 薯类 Potatoes | 7.4 | 7.0 | 30.7 | 2.3 | 5.6 | 20.9 | 2.4 | 1.0 | 4.6 | 30.0 | 7.2 | 29.9 | 4.5 | 3.5 | 2.8 | 4.4 | 1.8 | 5.3 | 23.5 | 7.9 | 2.5 | 6.8 | 0.4 | 4.7 | 9.0 |

续表

| 膳食类别 Category | 黑龙江 HL | 辽宁 LN | 河北 HE | 北京 BJ | 吉林 JL | 山西 SX | 陕西 SN | 河南 HA | 宁夏 NX | 内蒙古 NM | 青海 QH | 甘肃 GS | 上海 SH | 福建 FJ | 江西 JX | 江苏 JS | 浙江 ZJ | 山东 SD | 湖北 HB | 四川 SC | 广西 GX | 湖南 HN | 广东 GD | 贵州 GZ | 全国平均 AVG |
|---|---|---|---|---|---|---|---|---|---|---|---|---|---|---|---|---|---|---|---|---|---|---|---|---|---|
| 肉类 Meats | 39.4 | 58.3 | 42.5 | 25.9 | 40.1 | 71.2 | 13.2 | 34.3 | 40.5 | 35.1 | 24.1 | 20.1 | 73.2 | 28.9 | 40.8 | 40.9 | 254.3 | 37.4 | 36.5 | 61.6 | 3161.0 | 73.6 | 389.8 | 37.2 | 195.0 |
| 蛋类 Eggs | 9.6 | 34.3 | 16.3 | 80.2 | 30.7 | 20.7 | 4.8 | 11.3 | 4.0 | 17.7 | 7.1 | 7.4 | 15.5 | 17.1 | 13.8 | 10.7 | 11.8 | 8.2 | 8.2 | 4.1 | 14.5 | 7.8 | 4.2 | 3.6 | 15.2 |
| 水产类 Aquatic foods | 71.4 | 127.0 | 20.9 | 44.0 | 23.2 | 14.0 | 6.9 | 9.4 | 0.8 | 2.1 | 8.3 | 6.8 | 231.0 | 129.6 | 51.8 | 75.6 | 111.2 | 54.7 | 79.6 | 11.5 | 110.7 | 105.3 | 573.0 | 3.9 | 78.0 |
| 乳类 Dairy products | 0.7 | 9.4 | 1.2 | 6.4 | 14.0 | 8.2 | 7.3 | 3.8 | 0.4 | 121.7 | 10.3 | 3.6 | 7.1 | 5.8 | 2.0 | 4.3 | 2.6 | 5.5 | 2.6 | 2.5 | 10.1 | 2.9 | 9.8 | 4.2 | 10.3 |
| 蔬菜类 Vegetables | 29.9 | 37.9 | 20.9 | 34.8 | 28.0 | 60.7 | 8.3 | 42.3 | 4.8 | 35.7 | 15.2 | 24.9 | 54.1 | 34.1 | 37.6 | 66.9 | 77.4 | 46.5 | 65.2 | 40.9 | 51.0 | 107.7 | 61.3 | 54.6 | 43.4 |
| 合计 SUM | 244.2 | 299.7 | 189.4 | 230.9 | 186.5 | 375.7 | 50.0 | 172.5 | 57.9 | 376.5 | 79.8 | 272.8 | 429.1 | 240.2 | 162.0 | 252.0 | 491.1 | 282.0 | 311.9 | 198.9 | 3804.7 | 360.3 | 1066.3 | 183.5 | 429.9 |

附表 7-6  第六次中国总膳食研究指示性 PCB 的膳食来源（单位：%）

Annexed Table 7-6  Dietary sources of indicator PCBs from the 6th China TDS (Unit: %)

| 膳食类别 Category | 黑龙江 HL | 辽宁 LN | 河北 HE | 北京 BJ | 吉林 JL | 山西 SX | 陕西 SN | 河南 HA | 宁夏 NX | 内蒙古 NM | 青海 QH | 甘肃 GS | 上海 SH | 福建 FJ | 江西 JX | 江苏 JS | 浙江 ZJ | 山东 SD | 湖北 HB | 四川 SC | 广西 GX | 湖南 HN | 广东 GD | 贵州 GZ | 全国平均 AVG |
|---|---|---|---|---|---|---|---|---|---|---|---|---|---|---|---|---|---|---|---|---|---|---|---|---|---|
| 谷类 Cereals | 30.4 | 1.0 | 28.3 | 12.9 | 18.7 | 39.5 | 3.2 | 35.9 | 1.3 | 31.9 | 9.2 | 62.9 | 6.2 | 7.1 | 5.4 | 14.4 | 4.7 | 39.1 | 20.8 | 30.1 | 11.6 | 12.6 | 2.0 | 33.0 | 19.3 |
| 豆类 Legumes | 4.7 | 7.6 | 1.7 | 3.3 | 5.4 | 8.4 | 11.0 | 4.9 | 3.5 | 3.7 | 0.3 | 3.1 | 4.0 | 1.8 | 2.7 | 5.1 | 1.8 | 5.0 | 10.1 | 5.3 | 0.3 | 3.0 | 0.6 | 8.0 | 4.4 |
| 薯类 Potatoes | 3.0 | 2.3 | 16.2 | 1.0 | 3.0 | 5.6 | 4.8 | 0.6 | 7.9 | 8.0 | 9.0 | 11.0 | 1.0 | 1.4 | 1.8 | 1.7 | 0.4 | 1.9 | 7.5 | 4.0 | 0.1 | 1.9 | 0.0 | 2.6 | 4.0 |
| 肉类 Meats | 16.1 | 19.4 | 22.4 | 11.2 | 21.5 | 19.0 | 26.4 | 19.9 | 69.9 | 9.3 | 30.2 | 7.4 | 17.1 | 12.0 | 25.2 | 16.2 | 51.8 | 13.3 | 11.7 | 31.0 | 83.1 | 20.4 | 36.6 | 20.3 | 25.5 |

续表

| 膳食类别 Category | 黑龙江 HL | 辽宁 LN | 河北 HE | 北京 BJ | 吉林 JL | 山西 SX | 陕西 SN | 河南 HA | 宁夏 NX | 内蒙古 NM | 青海 QH | 甘肃 GS | 上海 SH | 福建 FJ | 江西 JX | 江苏 JS | 浙江 ZJ | 山东 SD | 湖北 HB | 四川 SC | 广西 GX | 湖南 HN | 广东 GD | 贵州 GZ | 全国平均 AVG |
|---|---|---|---|---|---|---|---|---|---|---|---|---|---|---|---|---|---|---|---|---|---|---|---|---|---|
| 蛋类 Eggs | 3.9 | 11.4 | 8.6 | 34.7 | 16.4 | 5.5 | 9.7 | 6.6 | 6.9 | 4.7 | 8.9 | 2.7 | 3.6 | 7.1 | 8.5 | 4.2 | 2.4 | 2.9 | 2.6 | 2.1 | 0.4 | 2.2 | 0.4 | 2.0 | 6.6 |
| 水产类 Aquatic foods | 29.2 | 42.4 | 11.1 | 19.0 | 12.4 | 3.7 | 13.8 | 5.4 | 1.4 | 0.5 | 10.4 | 2.5 | 53.8 | 53.9 | 32.0 | 30.0 | 22.6 | 19.4 | 25.5 | 5.8 | 2.9 | 29.2 | 53.7 | 2.1 | 20.1 |
| 乳类 Dairy products | 0.3 | 3.1 | 0.6 | 2.8 | 7.5 | 2.2 | 14.5 | 2.2 | 0.7 | 32.3 | 12.9 | 1.3 | 1.7 | 2.4 | 1.2 | 1.7 | 0.5 | 1.9 | 0.8 | 1.2 | 0.3 | 0.8 | 0.9 | 2.3 | 4.0 |
| 蔬菜类 Vegetables | 12.2 | 12.6 | 11.0 | 15.1 | 15.0 | 16.2 | 16.7 | 24.5 | 8.4 | 9.5 | 19.0 | 9.1 | 12.6 | 14.2 | 23.2 | 26.5 | 15.8 | 16.5 | 20.9 | 20.6 | 1.3 | 29.9 | 5.7 | 29.8 | 16.1 |

附表 7-7 第六次中国总膳食研究混合膳食样品中多溴二苯醚的含量（单位：pg/g）

Annexed Table 7-7 Levels of PBDEs in food samples from the 6$^{th}$ China TDS (Unit: pg/g)

| 膳食类别 Category | 黑龙江 HL | 辽宁 LN | 河北 HE | 北京 BJ | 吉林 JL | 山西 SX | 陕西 SN | 河南 HA | 宁夏 NX | 内蒙古 NM | 青海 QH | 甘肃 GS | 上海 SH | 福建 FJ | 江西 JX | 江苏 JS | 浙江 ZJ | 山东 SD | 湖北 HB | 四川 SC | 广西 GX | 湖南 HN | 广东 GD | 贵州 GZ | 全国平均 AVG |
|---|---|---|---|---|---|---|---|---|---|---|---|---|---|---|---|---|---|---|---|---|---|---|---|---|---|
| 谷类 Cereals | 1.1 | 3.6 | 0.6 | 1.8 | 12.1 | 1.5 | 0.1 | 0.1 | 0.1 | 4.1 | 0.4 | 5.8 | 4.0 | 8.6 | 0.6 | 2.2 | 77.1 | 0.4 | 1.1 | 1.3 | 4.7 | 0.4 | 0.4 | 2.3 | 5.6 |
| 豆类 Legumes | 1.6 | 9.4 | 1.0 | 9.8 | 5.8 | 1.8 | 0.7 | 1.5 | 0.7 | 10.1 | 1.3 | 39.7 | 4.1 | 7.2 | 7.1 | 4.7 | 42.2 | 0.8 | 2.2 | 4.6 | 3.2 | 0.7 | 1.2 | 8.3 | 7.1 |
| 薯类 Potatoes | 1.0 | 6.1 | 3.7 | 5.5 | 4.8 | 0.9 | 1.4 | 1.6 | 1.3 | 4.3 | 5.9 | 6.2 | 3.2 | 9.2 | 2.9 | 1.5 | 122.9 | 1.5 | 4.4 | 4.5 | 3.3 | 2.0 | 0.3 | 20.5 | 9.1 |
| 肉类 Meats | 7.6 | 30.1 | 14.9 | 21.4 | 21.1 | 11.6 | 4.4 | 14.8 | 11.1 | 19.4 | 7.8 | 28.4 | 19.4 | 31.1 | 6.1 | 16.4 | 153.6 | 12.2 | 14.9 | 76.9 | 87.6 | 35.3 | 20.3 | 47.7 | 29.8 |
| 蛋类 Eggs | 3.8 | 25.7 | 8.2 | 30.0 | 9.6 | 5.0 | 4.9 | 6.2 | 4.0 | 22.2 | 17.7 | 18.2 | 17.7 | 36.4 | 9.0 | 10.4 | 167.4 | 4.6 | 7.1 | 35.1 | 10.9 | 31.6 | 22.2 | 24.6 | 22.2 |
| 水产类 Aquatic foods | 18.3 | 41.0 | 17.2 | 26.9 | 28.7 | 13.2 | 9.5 | 29.6 | 11.0 | 3.0 | 27.6 | 43.6 | 87.0 | 48.5 | 20.7 | 32.3 | 108.2 | 33.7 | 38.7 | 39.8 | 26.8 | 43.6 | 157.3 | 50.5 | 39.9 |

续表

| 膳食类别 Category | 黑龙江 HL | 辽宁 LN | 河北 HE | 北京 BJ | 吉林 JL | 山西 SX | 陕西 SN | 河南 HA | 宁夏 NX | 内蒙古 NM | 青海 QH | 甘肃 GS | 上海 SH | 福建 FJ | 江西 JX | 江苏 JS | 浙江 ZJ | 山东 SD | 湖北 HB | 四川 SC | 广西 GX | 湖南 HN | 广东 GD | 贵州 GZ | 全国平均 AVG |
|---|---|---|---|---|---|---|---|---|---|---|---|---|---|---|---|---|---|---|---|---|---|---|---|---|---|
| 乳类 Dairy products | 2.8 | 3.3 | 0.4 | 1.3 | 6.5 | 1.7 | 8.7 | 1.7 | 0.8 | 31.6 | 2.4 | 1.9 | 3.8 | 2.1 | 2.0 | 2.2 | 3.3 | 2.1 | 3.6 | 0.4 | 8.5 | 3.9 | 1.0 | 4.0 | 4.2 |
| 蔬菜类 Vegetables | 0.4 | 10.0 | 0.1 | 9.7 | 8.5 | 2.3 | 0.7 | 0.9 | 1.6 | 59.1 | 11.0 | 6.6 | 3.3 | 16.1 | 7.4 | 5.5 | 31.7 | 2.4 | 3.1 | 7.6 | 2.8 | 4.8 | 3.5 | 15.4 | 8.9 |

注：未检出（ND）按检出限（LOD）计

Note: values not detected (ND) were treated as being equal to the detection of limit (LOD)

附表 7-8 第六次中国总膳食研究多溴二苯醚膳食摄入量 [单位：pg/(kg bw·d)]

Annexed Table 7-8  Dietary intakes of PBDEs from the 6th China TDS [Unit: pg/(kg bw·d)]

| 膳食类别 Category | 黑龙江 HL | 辽宁 LN | 河北 HE | 北京 BJ | 吉林 JL | 山西 SX | 陕西 SN | 河南 HA | 宁夏 NX | 内蒙古 NM | 青海 QH | 甘肃 GS | 上海 SH | 福建 FJ | 江西 JX | 江苏 JS | 浙江 ZJ | 山东 SD | 湖北 HB | 四川 SC | 广西 GX | 湖南 HN | 广东 GD | 贵州 GZ | 全国平均 AVG |
|---|---|---|---|---|---|---|---|---|---|---|---|---|---|---|---|---|---|---|---|---|---|---|---|---|---|
| 谷类 Cereals | 18.9 | 55.8 | 11.3 | 32.4 | 148.2 | 39.8 | 1.9 | 1.9 | 2.5 | 69.4 | 10.9 | 107.3 | 36.9 | 126.5 | 8.5 | 33.8 | 1031.9 | 10.0 | 12.9 | 32.3 | 102.3 | 5.6 | 3.8 | 39.0 | 81.0 |
| 豆类 Legumes | 1.7 | 25.0 | 1.1 | 17.2 | 9.3 | 2.2 | 1.0 | 1.8 | 0.4 | 6.9 | 0.1 | 26.8 | 8.8 | 9.1 | 9.4 | 7.3 | 100.3 | 0.9 | 2.6 | 5.6 | 2.2 | 1.0 | 0.6 | 16.0 | 10.7 |
| 薯类 Potatoes | 1.5 | 9.1 | 4.1 | 5.9 | 9.2 | 2.1 | 3.2 | 2.1 | 2.4 | 8.4 | 9.9 | 14.7 | 1.8 | 6.8 | 1.5 | 1.0 | 74.5 | 1.2 | 6.3 | 4.6 | 0.9 | 2.3 | 0.1 | 13.6 | 7.8 |
| 肉类 Meats | 8.6 | 39.3 | 12.2 | 28.6 | 22.5 | 26.7 | 2.7 | 13.5 | 8.6 | 23.0 | 8.9 | 15.7 | 34.2 | 43.8 | 9.2 | 24.1 | 310.1 | 20.2 | 13.4 | 158.7 | 209.8 | 84.7 | 42.4 | 83.1 | 51.8 |
| 蛋类 Eggs | 2.5 | 22.0 | 5.3 | 21.8 | 7.1 | 2.3 | 2.0 | 2.9 | 1.2 | 13.8 | 5.1 | 7.5 | 11.9 | 14.3 | 3.5 | 5.0 | 78.5 | 4.0 | 3.3 | 9.2 | 2.7 | 11.7 | 8.5 | 6.3 | 10.5 |
| 水产类 Aquatic foods | 7.9 | 15.4 | 2.9 | 7.4 | 5.1 | 1.6 | 0.6 | 2.3 | 0.4 | 0.5 | 1.8 | 2.0 | 94.7 | 51.5 | 14.3 | 20.4 | 90.0 | 14.3 | 25.0 | 5.3 | 41.5 | 46.5 | 133.1 | 3.4 | 24.5 |
| 乳类 Dairy products | 0.6 | 2.3 | 0.2 | 1.8 | 3.3 | 1.1 | 2.7 | 0.5 | 0.2 | 17.2 | 2.0 | 0.4 | 4.3 | 1.2 | 0.7 | 1.0 | 1.7 | 0.8 | 0.4 | 0.1 | 2.5 | 1.1 | 0.6 | 1.8 | 2.0 |

续表

| 膳食类别 Category | 黑龙江 HL | 辽宁 LN | 河北 HE | 北京 BJ | 吉林 JL | 山西 SX | 陕西 SN | 河南 HA | 宁夏 NX | 内蒙古 NM | 青海 QH | 甘肃 GS | 上海 SH | 福建 FJ | 江西 JX | 江苏 JS | 浙江 ZJ | 山东 SD | 湖北 HB | 四川 SC | 广西 GX | 湖南 HN | 广东 GD | 贵州 GZ | 全国平均 AVG |
|---|---|---|---|---|---|---|---|---|---|---|---|---|---|---|---|---|---|---|---|---|---|---|---|---|---|
| 蔬菜类 Vegetables | 2.4 | 55.8 | 0.4 | 61.1 | 52.9 | 11.6 | 3.3 | 4.1 | 4.0 | 248.8 | 54.0 | 26.1 | 20.9 | 102.5 | 53.2 | 38.4 | 272.9 | 15.7 | 20.5 | 36.7 | 16.3 | 42.3 | 13.7 | 102.8 | 52.5 |
| 合计 SUM | 44.0 | 224.7 | 37.3 | 176.2 | 257.7 | 87.4 | 17.4 | 29.2 | 19.7 | 388.0 | 92.8 | 200.5 | 213.5 | 355.6 | 100.2 | 130.9 | 1959.9 | 67.0 | 84.3 | 252.5 | 378.2 | 195.2 | 202.7 | 266.0 | 240.9 |

附表 7-9 第六次中国总膳食研究多溴二苯醚的膳食来源（单位：%）

Annexed Table 7-9 Dietary sources of PBDEs from the 6$^{th}$ China TDS (Unit: %)

| 膳食类别 Category | 黑龙江 HL | 辽宁 LN | 河北 HE | 北京 BJ | 吉林 JL | 山西 SX | 陕西 SN | 河南 HA | 宁夏 NX | 内蒙古 NM | 青海 QH | 甘肃 GS | 上海 SH | 福建 FJ | 江西 JX | 江苏 JS | 浙江 ZJ | 山东 SD | 湖北 HB | 四川 SC | 广西 GX | 湖南 HN | 广东 GD | 贵州 GZ | 全国平均 AVG |
|---|---|---|---|---|---|---|---|---|---|---|---|---|---|---|---|---|---|---|---|---|---|---|---|---|---|
| 谷类 Cereals | 43.0 | 24.8 | 30.2 | 18.4 | 57.5 | 45.6 | 10.8 | 6.5 | 12.6 | 17.9 | 11.8 | 53.5 | 17.3 | 35.6 | 8.5 | 25.8 | 52.6 | 14.9 | 15.3 | 12.8 | 27.0 | 2.8 | 1.9 | 14.7 | 23.4 |
| 豆类 Legumes | 3.8 | 11.1 | 2.9 | 9.8 | 3.6 | 2.5 | 5.9 | 6.3 | 2.2 | 1.8 | 0.2 | 13.4 | 4.1 | 2.6 | 9.4 | 5.5 | 5.1 | 1.3 | 3.1 | 2.2 | 0.6 | 0.5 | 0.3 | 6.0 | 4.3 |
| 薯类 Potatoes | 3.5 | 4.1 | 11.1 | 3.4 | 3.6 | 2.4 | 18.2 | 7.4 | 11.9 | 2.2 | 10.7 | 7.3 | 0.8 | 1.9 | 1.5 | 0.7 | 3.8 | 1.8 | 7.4 | 1.8 | 0.2 | 1.2 | 0.1 | 5.1 | 4.7 |
| 肉类 Meats | 19.5 | 17.5 | 32.6 | 16.2 | 8.7 | 30.6 | 15.5 | 46.3 | 43.4 | 5.9 | 9.6 | 7.8 | 16.0 | 12.3 | 9.2 | 18.4 | 15.8 | 30.1 | 15.9 | 62.8 | 55.5 | 43.4 | 20.9 | 31.2 | 24.4 |
| 蛋类 Eggs | 5.6 | 9.8 | 14.1 | 12.3 | 2.7 | 2.6 | 11.4 | 10.0 | 6.1 | 3.5 | 5.5 | 3.7 | 5.6 | 4.0 | 3.4 | 3.8 | 4.0 | 6.0 | 3.9 | 3.7 | 0.7 | 6.0 | 4.2 | 2.4 | 5.6 |
| 水产类 Aquatic foods | 17.9 | 6.8 | 7.7 | 4.2 | 2.0 | 1.8 | 3.5 | 7.8 | 2.1 | 0.1 | 1.9 | 1.0 | 44.4 | 14.5 | 14.3 | 15.6 | 4.6 | 21.4 | 29.6 | 2.1 | 11.0 | 23.8 | 65.7 | 1.3 | 12.7 |
| 乳类 Dairy products | 1.4 | 1.0 | 0.4 | 1.0 | 1.3 | 1.3 | 15.4 | 1.8 | 1.0 | 4.4 | 2.2 | 0.2 | 2.0 | 0.3 | 0.7 | 0.7 | 0.1 | 1.1 | 0.5 | 0.0 | 0.6 | 0.6 | 0.3 | 0.7 | 1.6 |
| 蔬菜类 Vegetables | 5.4 | 24.8 | 1.1 | 34.7 | 20.5 | 13.2 | 19.3 | 14.0 | 20.5 | 64.1 | 58.2 | 13.0 | 9.8 | 28.8 | 53.1 | 29.3 | 13.9 | 23.4 | 24.3 | 14.5 | 4.3 | 21.7 | 6.7 | 38.6 | 23.2 |

附表 7-10 第六次中国总膳食研究膳食样品中六溴环十二烷的含量（单位：pg/g）

Annexed Table 7-10　Levels of HBCD in food samples from the 6<sup>th</sup> China TDS (Unit: pg/g)

| 膳食类别 Category | 黑龙江 HL | 辽宁 LN | 河北 HE | 北京 BJ | 吉林 JL | 山西 SX | 陕西 SN | 河南 HA | 宁夏 NX | 内蒙古 NM | 青海 QH | 甘肃 GS | 上海 SH | 福建 FJ | 江西 JX | 江苏 JS | 浙江 ZJ | 山东 SD | 湖北 HB | 四川 SC | 广西 GX | 湖南 HN | 广东 GD | 贵州 GZ | 全国平均 AVG |
|---|---|---|---|---|---|---|---|---|---|---|---|---|---|---|---|---|---|---|---|---|---|---|---|---|---|
| 肉类 Meats | 300.4 | 14013.0 | 1720.1 | 8225.1 | 11185.6 | 666.8 | 235.9 | 366.7 | 264.6 | 3397.2 | 342.4 | 392.8 | 1808.2 | 38.3 | 60.8 | 823.7 | 1400.7 | 814.7 | 410.1 | 6152.9 | 268.2 | 841.8 | 116.6 | 314.2 | 1840.0 |
| 蛋类 Eggs | 100.6 | 51.5 | 47.2 | 277.6 | 44.2 | 57.6 | 22.0 | 29.1 | 70.0 | 840.7 | 55.2 | 146.7 | 71.3 | 29.7 | 16.0 | 17.1 | 22.8 | 51.6 | 67.4 | 61.1 | 38.0 | 99.5 | 14.7 | 17.9 | 93.7 |
| 水产类 Aquatic foods | 294.0 | 103.5 | 866.3 | 292.3 | 291.5 | 81.4 | 103.7 | 498.8 | 481.8 | 288.0 | 127.2 | 324.2 | 258.8 | 4476.2 | 91.3 | 92.2 | 75.3 | 407.5 | 190.3 | 202.7 | 596.1 | 137.9 | 118.2 | 187.4 | 441.1 |
| 乳类 Dairy products | 61.3 | 30.6 | 143.7 | 42.6 | 68.7 | 43.7 | 99.8 | 19.5 | 36.1 | 150.5 | 12.0 | 8.1 | 14.1 | 62.9 | 26.6 | 9.0 | 31.3 | 34.8 | 36.2 | 18.1 | 6.3 | 23.8 | 22.5 | 3.6 | 41.9 |

注：未检出（ND）按 1/2 检出限（LOD）计

Note: values not detected (ND) were treated as being equal to half of the detection of limit (LOD)

附表 7-11 第六次中国总膳食研究六溴环十二烷的膳食摄入量 [单位：pg/(kg bw·d)]

Annexed Table 7-11　Dietary intakes of HBCD from the 6<sup>th</sup> China TDS [Unit: pg/(kg bw·d)]

| 膳食类别 Category | 黑龙江 HL | 辽宁 LN | 河北 HE | 北京 BJ | 吉林 JL | 山西 SX | 陕西 SN | 河南 HA | 宁夏 NX | 内蒙古 NM | 青海 QH | 甘肃 GS | 上海 SH | 福建 FJ | 江西 JX | 江苏 JS | 浙江 ZJ | 山东 SD | 湖北 HB | 四川 SC | 广西 GX | 湖南 HN | 广东 GD | 贵州 GZ | 全国平均 AVG |
|---|---|---|---|---|---|---|---|---|---|---|---|---|---|---|---|---|---|---|---|---|---|---|---|---|---|
| 肉类 Meats | 337.7 | 18335.2 | 1405.5 | 10983.2 | 1264.7 | 1528.5 | 144.7 | 335.6 | 204.8 | 4043.2 | 389.7 | 217.2 | 3178.1 | 53.9 | 91.5 | 1212.2 | 2828.2 | 1352.9 | 368.2 | 12702.6 | 642.4 | 2017.8 | 244.0 | 547.4 | 2684.5 |
| 蛋类 Eggs | 65.4 | 44.0 | 30.2 | 201.3 | 32.4 | 26.3 | 8.9 | 13.7 | 21.1 | 521.5 | 16.0 | 60.1 | 48.0 | 11.6 | 6.1 | 8.1 | 10.7 | 44.9 | 31.4 | 16.1 | 9.5 | 36.8 | 5.6 | 4.6 | 53.1 |
| 水产类 Aquatic foods | 126.8 | 38.8 | 144.0 | 81.1 | 51.5 | 9.7 | 6.8 | 38.2 | 18.6 | 47.2 | 8.1 | 14.5 | 281.8 | 4750.8 | 63.3 | 58.2 | 62.6 | 173.3 | 123.0 | 26.9 | 924.0 | 146.8 | 100.1 | 12.5 | 304.5 |
| 乳类 Dairy products | 13.0 | 21.5 | 55.3 | 58.0 | 35.3 | 28.8 | 30.6 | 6.1 | 8.7 | 82.0 | 10.2 | 1.8 | 15.9 | 35.9 | 9.2 | 3.9 | 16.6 | 12.7 | 3.9 | 3.6 | 1.8 | 6.8 | 13.1 | 1.6 | 19.8 |
| 合计 SUM | 543.0 | 18439.6 | 1635.0 | 11323.6 | 1383.9 | 1593.3 | 191.0 | 393.6 | 253.3 | 4694.0 | 424.0 | 293.7 | 3523.7 | 4852.2 | 170.2 | 1282.5 | 2918.1 | 1583.9 | 526.5 | 12749.2 | 1577.7 | 2208.1 | 362.7 | 566.1 | 3062.0 |

附表 7-12　第六次中国总膳食研究膳食样品中六氯苯的含量（单位：μg/kg）

Annexed Table 7-12　Levels of HCB in food samples from the 6th China TDS (Unit: μg/kg)

| 膳食类别<br>Category | 黑龙江<br>HL | 辽宁<br>LN | 河北<br>HE | 北京<br>BJ | 吉林<br>JL | 山西<br>SX | 陕西<br>SN | 河南<br>HA | 宁夏<br>NX | 内蒙古<br>NM | 青海<br>QH | 甘肃<br>GS | 上海<br>SH | 福建<br>FJ | 江西<br>JX | 江苏<br>JS | 浙江<br>ZJ | 山东<br>SD | 湖北<br>HB | 四川<br>SC | 广西<br>GX | 湖南<br>HN | 广东<br>GD | 贵州<br>GZ | 全国平均<br>AVG |
|---|---|---|---|---|---|---|---|---|---|---|---|---|---|---|---|---|---|---|---|---|---|---|---|---|---|
| 谷类 Cereals | ND | ND | ND | ND | ND | ND | ND | 0.07 | ND | ND | ND | ND | ND | ND | ND | 0.05 | ND | ND | ND | ND | ND | ND | ND | ND | 0.01 |
| 豆类 Legumes | ND | ND | ND | ND | ND | 0.45 | ND | 0.11 | 0.06 | ND | 0.07 | ND | ND | ND | ND | 0.05 | ND | ND | 0.08 | 0.08 | ND | ND | ND | ND | 0.04 |
| 薯类 Potatoes | 0.09 | ND | ND | ND | ND | ND | ND | ND | ND | 0.05 | ND | ND | ND | ND | ND | 0.10 | ND | ND | 0.07 | 0.11 | 0.07 | ND | ND | ND | 0.02 |
| 肉类 Meats | 0.10 | ND | 0.34 | 0.13 | ND | ND | ND | 0.39 | 1.27 | ND | 0.07 | ND | 0.27 | 0.07 | ND | 0.09 | 0.07 | 0.08 | ND | 0.11 | 0.39 | 0.11 | ND | 0.06 | 0.15 |
| 蛋类 Eggs | 0.14 | ND | 0.39 | ND | 0.07 | 0.27 | 0.09 | ND | ND | 0.06 | ND | ND | 0.15 | 0.18 | ND | 0.19 | 0.10 | 0.09 | 0.42 | 0.14 | 0.07 | 0.15 | 0.05 | 0.06 | 0.11 |
| 水产类 Aquatic foods | 0.17 | ND | 0.18 | 0.06 | ND | ND | 0.16 | 0.07 | 0.19 | ND | 0.12 | 0.09 | 0.23 | 0.19 | 0.62 | 0.10 | 0.10 | ND | 0.20 | 0.11 | 0.06 | 2.78 | 0.09 | 0.31 | 0.24 |
| 乳类 Dairy products | 0.06 | ND | 0.05 | ND | ND | 0.04 | 0.05 | ND | 0.05 | ND | 0.04 | 0.08 | ND | ND | 0.05 | 0.05 | ND | 0.06 | ND | 0.06 | ND | ND | ND | ND | 0.03 |
| 蔬菜类 Vegetables | ND | ND | 0.11 | ND | 0.06 | ND | ND | ND | ND | ND | ND | 0.16 | 0.12 | ND | ND | 0.06 | ND | ND | ND | 0.10 | 0.05 | 0.07 | ND | ND | 0.03 |
| 水果类 Fruits | ND | ND | ND | ND | ND | ND | ND | ND | ND | ND | ND | ND | ND | ND | ND | ND | ND | ND | ND | ND | ND | ND | ND | ND | 0.00 |

注：未检出（ND）按 0 计

Note: values not detected (ND) were treated as 0

附表 7-13　第六次中国总膳食研究膳食样品中滴滴涕的含量（单位：μg/kg）

Annexed Table 7-13　Levels of DDT in food samples from the 6th China TDS (Unit: μg/kg)

| 膳食类别 Category | 黑龙江 HL | 辽宁 LN | 河北 HE | 北京 BJ | 吉林 JL | 山西 SX | 陕西 SN | 河南 HA | 宁夏 NX | 内蒙古 NM | 青海 QH | 甘肃 GS | 上海 SH | 福建 FJ | 江西 JX | 江苏 JS | 浙江 ZJ | 山东 SD | 湖北 HB | 四川 SC | 广西 GX | 湖南 HN | 广东 GD | 贵州 GZ | 全国平均 AVG |
|---|---|---|---|---|---|---|---|---|---|---|---|---|---|---|---|---|---|---|---|---|---|---|---|---|---|
| 谷类 Cereals | ND | ND | ND | 0.03 | ND | ND | 0.01 | 0.03 | 0.05 | ND | ND | ND | ND | ND | ND | 0.03 | ND | ND | 0.06 | ND | ND | ND | ND | ND | 0.01 |
| 豆类 Legumes | 0.09 | ND | ND | ND | ND | ND | ND | 0.07 | ND | ND | ND | 0.34 | 0.04 | ND | ND | 0.06 | ND | ND | 0.09 | ND | ND | ND | ND | ND | 0.03 |
| 薯类 Potatoes | ND | ND | ND | ND | ND | 0.01 | ND | ND | ND | ND | ND | 0.23 | ND | ND | ND | ND | ND | ND | ND | ND | ND | ND | ND | ND | 0.01 |
| 肉类 Meats | 0.07 | 0.84 | 0.41 | 1.52 | 0.25 | 0.06 | 0.03 | 0.93 | 0.12 | 0.03 | 0.22 | 0.90 | 0.78 | 1.26 | 1.29 | 0.15 | 1.31 | ND | 0.75 | 0.08 | 0.29 | 1.45 | 0.08 | 0.81 | 0.57 |
| 蛋类 Eggs | 0.07 | 0.23 | 1.90 | 0.67 | 0.22 | ND | 0.02 | 0.04 | 0.02 | 0.36 | 0.01 | 0.28 | 1.38 | 1.81 | 1.35 | 0.18 | 1.15 | 0.05 | 2.08 | ND | 1.66 | ND | 0.07 | 0.15 | 0.57 |
| 水产类 Aquatic foods | 0.34 | 0.92 | 0.49 | 1.49 | 1.93 | 0.55 | 1.20 | 4.05 | 0.16 | 1.03 | 0.33 | 1.19 | 9.83 | 1.46 | 4.02 | 2.29 | 2.96 | 1.09 | 5.45 | 1.27 | 2.00 | 3.89 | 2.43 | 3.67 | 2.25 |
| 乳类 Dairy products | 0.06 | 0.44 | 0.15 | 0.50 | 0.10 | 0.05 | 0.58 | 0.23 | ND | 0.06 | 0.05 | 0.59 | 0.17 | 1.04 | 0.85 | 0.12 | 0.15 | 0.11 | 1.01 | 0.02 | 0.90 | 0.07 | 0.22 | 0.78 | 0.34 |
| 蔬菜类 Vegetables | ND | 0.03 | 0.16 | 0.04 | ND | ND | ND | ND | ND | ND | ND | ND | 0.04 | 0.07 | ND | ND | ND | ND | 0.21 | ND | ND | ND | ND | ND | 0.02 |
| 水果类 Fruits | ND | ND | ND | ND | ND | ND | ND | ND | ND | ND | ND | ND | ND | ND | ND | ND | ND | ND | ND | ND | ND | ND | ND | ND | 0.00 |

注：未检出（ND）按 0 计

Note: values not detected (ND) were treated as 0

附表 7-14 第六次中国总膳食研究膳食样品中六六六的含量（单位：μg/kg）

Annexed Table 7-14　Levels of HCH in food samples from the 6th China TDS (Unit: μg/kg)

| 膳食类别 Category | 黑龙江 HL | 辽宁 LN | 河北 HE | 北京 BJ | 吉林 JL | 山西 SX | 陕西 SN | 河南 HA | 宁夏 NX | 内蒙古 NM | 青海 QH | 甘肃 GS | 上海 SH | 福建 FJ | 江西 JX | 江苏 JS | 浙江 ZJ | 山东 SD | 湖北 HB | 四川 SC | 广西 GX | 湖南 HN | 广东 GD | 贵州 GZ | 全国平均 AVG |
|---|---|---|---|---|---|---|---|---|---|---|---|---|---|---|---|---|---|---|---|---|---|---|---|---|---|
| 谷类 Cereals | ND | ND | 0.26 | ND | ND | ND | ND | ND | ND | ND | ND | ND | ND | ND | ND | ND | ND | ND | ND | ND | ND | ND | ND | ND | 0.01 |
| 豆类 Legumes | 0.12 | 0.20 | 0.20 | ND | 0.42 | ND | ND | ND | 0.19 | ND | ND | 0.07 | ND | ND | ND | ND | ND | ND | ND | ND | ND | ND | 0.04 | ND | 0.05 |
| 薯类 Potatoes | ND | ND | 0.15 | 0.07 | ND | ND | ND | ND | ND | ND | ND | 0.32 | ND | ND | ND | ND | ND | 0.14 | ND | ND | ND | ND | ND | ND | 0.04 |
| 肉类 Meats | 0.40 | 0.40 | 0.41 | 0.24 | 0.18 | 0.31 | 0.09 | 0.17 | 3.56 | 0.09 | 0.11 | 0.61 | 0.06 | 0.21 | ND | 0.17 | 0.10 | 0.14 | 0.07 | 0.13 | 0.19 | 0.12 | ND | 0.11 | 0.33 |
| 蛋类 Eggs | 0.18 | ND | 0.44 | 0.24 | 0.12 | 0.28 | 0.03 | 0.09 | 0.05 | 0.68 | 0.07 | 0.05 | 0.05 | 0.14 | 0.27 | 0.08 | ND | 0.14 | 0.37 | 0.09 | 0.08 | 0.15 | 0.05 | 0.04 | 0.15 |
| 水产类 Aquatic foods | 6.62 | 0.19 | 0.93 | 0.59 | 4.27 | 0.41 | 0.32 | 0.72 | 0.43 | 0.18 | 0.44 | 0.26 | 0.79 | 0.44 | 0.42 | 0.51 | 1.04 | 0.43 | 0.66 | 0.77 | 0.21 | 0.22 | 0.20 | 0.29 | 0.89 |
| 乳类 Dairy products | 0.12 | 0.12 | 0.13 | 0.13 | 0.14 | 0.11 | 0.09 | 0.14 | 0.20 | 0.06 | 0.20 | 0.24 | 0.08 | 0.07 | 0.24 | 0.10 | 0.12 | 0.15 | 0.08 | ND | 0.04 | 0.18 | 0.07 | 0.03 | 0.12 |
| 蔬菜类 Vegetables | ND | 0.09 | 0.23 | 0.08 | ND | ND | 0.12 | ND | ND | 0.27 | ND | ND | ND | ND | ND | ND | ND | 0.19 | 0.11 | ND | ND | 0.07 | ND | 0.08 | 0.05 |
| 水果类 Fruits | ND | ND | ND | ND | ND | ND | ND | ND | ND | ND | ND | ND | ND | ND | ND | ND | ND | ND | ND | ND | ND | ND | ND | ND | 0.00 |

注：未检出（ND）按 0 计

Note: values not detected (ND) were treated as 0

附表 7-15 第六次中国总膳食研究膳食样品中硫丹的含量（单位：μg/kg）

Annexed Table 7-15 Levels of endosulfans in food samples from the 6$^{th}$ China TDS (Unit: μg/kg)

| 膳食类别<br>Category | 黑龙江<br>HL | 辽宁<br>LN | 河北<br>HE | 北京<br>BJ | 吉林<br>JL | 山西<br>SX | 陕西<br>SN | 河南<br>HA | 宁夏<br>NX | 内蒙古<br>NM | 青海<br>QH | 甘肃<br>GS | 上海<br>SH | 福建<br>FJ | 江西<br>JX | 江苏<br>JS | 浙江<br>ZJ | 山东<br>SD | 湖北<br>HB | 四川<br>SC | 广西<br>GX | 湖南<br>HN | 广东<br>GD | 贵州<br>GZ | 全国平均<br>AVG |
|---|---|---|---|---|---|---|---|---|---|---|---|---|---|---|---|---|---|---|---|---|---|---|---|---|---|
| 谷类 Cereals | ND | ND | ND | ND | ND | ND | ND | ND | ND | ND | ND | ND | ND | ND | ND | ND | ND | ND | ND | ND | ND | ND | ND | ND | 0.00 |
| 豆类 Legumes | ND | ND | ND | ND | ND | ND | ND | ND | ND | ND | ND | ND | ND | ND | ND | ND | ND | ND | ND | ND | ND | ND | ND | ND | 0.00 |
| 薯类 Potatoes | ND | ND | ND | 0.86 | ND | ND | ND | ND | ND | ND | ND | ND | ND | ND | ND | ND | ND | ND | 1.68 | ND | ND | ND | ND | ND | 0.07 |
| 肉类 Meats | ND | 2.06 | ND | ND | ND | ND | ND | ND | ND | ND | ND | ND | 0.97 | ND | ND | 1.72 | 0.91 | ND | ND | ND | ND | ND | ND | ND | 0.27 |
| 蛋类 Eggs | ND | 3.12 | ND | 1.31 | ND | ND | ND | ND | ND | ND | ND | ND | 0.30 | 3.22 | ND | ND | ND | ND | ND | ND | ND | 0.96 | ND | ND | 0.32 |
| 水产类 Aquatic foods | ND | 1.33 | ND | ND | ND | ND | ND | 8.19 | ND | ND | ND | ND | 3.19 | 1.12 | ND | 2.80 | 2.76 | ND | 2.73 | ND | ND | 2.13 | 2.25 | ND | 1.16 |
| 乳类 Dairy products | ND | 2.09 | ND | 0.67 | ND | ND | ND | 1.37 | ND | ND | ND | 1.01 | ND | 0.65 | 0.74 | 1.44 | 0.60 | ND | 0.86 | ND | ND | 1.66 | 2.34 | ND | 0.56 |
| 蔬菜类 Vegetables | ND | ND | ND | 1.61 | ND | ND | ND | ND | ND | ND | ND | ND | ND | ND | ND | ND | ND | ND | ND | ND | ND | 1.08 | 1.88 | ND | 0.19 |
| 水果类 Fruits | ND | ND | ND | ND | ND | ND | ND | 0.75 | ND | 0.50 | ND | ND | ND | ND | ND | ND | ND | ND | ND | ND | ND | ND | ND | ND | 0.05 |

注：未检出（ND）按 0 计

Note: values not detected (ND) were treated as 0

附表 7-16 第六次中国总膳食研究膳食样品中五氯苯的含量（单位：μg/kg）

Annexed Table 7-16 Levels of pentachlorobenzene in food samples from the 6th China TDS (Unit: μg/kg)

| 膳食类别 Category | 黑龙江 HL | 辽宁 LN | 河北 HE | 北京 BJ | 吉林 JL | 山西 SX | 陕西 SN | 河南 HA | 宁夏 NX | 内蒙古 NM | 青海 QH | 甘肃 GS | 上海 SH | 福建 FJ | 江西 JX | 江苏 JS | 浙江 ZJ | 山东 SD | 湖北 HB | 四川 SC | 广西 GX | 湖南 HN | 广东 GD | 贵州 GZ | 全国平均 AVG |
|---|---|---|---|---|---|---|---|---|---|---|---|---|---|---|---|---|---|---|---|---|---|---|---|---|---|
| 谷类 Cereals | 0.18 | 0.10 | 0.13 | 0.11 | 0.09 | 0.11 | 0.20 | 0.20 | 0.13 | 0.08 | 0.14 | 0.12 | 0.12 | 0.08 | 0.13 | 0.15 | 0.07 | 0.11 | 0.09 | 0.11 | 0.13 | 0.10 | 0.09 | 0.18 | 0.12 |
| 豆类 Legumes | 0.16 | 0.09 | 0.10 | 0.08 | 0.10 | 0.13 | 0.19 | 0.23 | 0.13 | 0.09 | 0.12 | 0.23 | 0.07 | 0.07 | 0.06 | 0.12 | 0.05 | 0.09 | 0.11 | 0.17 | 0.05 | 0.09 | 0.07 | 0.16 | 0.12 |
| 薯类 Potatoes | 0.11 | 0.06 | 0.23 | 0.09 | 0.05 | 0.31 | 0.08 | 0.11 | 0.08 | 0.09 | 0.12 | 0.08 | 0.05 | 0.05 | 0.06 | 0.21 | 0.07 | 0.07 | 0.08 | 0.14 | 0.09 | 0.10 | 0.15 | 0.11 | 0.11 |
| 肉类 Meats | 0.14 | 0.14 | 0.34 | 0.08 | 0.14 | 0.06 | 0.13 | 0.37 | 0.43 | 0.08 | 0.15 | 0.14 | 0.22 | 0.20 | 0.20 | 0.14 | 0.13 | 0.12 | 0.07 | 0.16 | 0.52 | 0.15 | 0.08 | 0.14 | 0.18 |
| 蛋类 Eggs | 0.27 | 0.11 | 0.42 | 0.11 | 0.11 | 0.27 | 0.21 | 0.13 | 0.09 | 0.12 | 0.09 | 0.10 | 0.12 | 0.25 | 0.08 | 0.21 | 0.10 | 0.16 | 0.22 | 0.19 | 0.14 | 0.24 | 0.10 | 0.27 | 0.17 |
| 水产类 Aquatic foods | 0.26 | 0.11 | 0.22 | 0.13 | 0.33 | 0.12 | 0.27 | 0.17 | ND | 0.07 | 0.17 | 0.10 | 0.34 | 0.23 | 0.44 | 0.19 | 0.15 | 0.11 | 0.23 | 0.27 | 0.11 | 1.06 | 0.12 | 0.26 | 0.23 |
| 乳类 Dairy products | 0.12 | 0.05 | 0.07 | ND | 0.06 | 0.07 | 0.07 | 0.08 | 0.07 | 0.06 | 0.07 | 0.12 | 0.06 | 0.06 | | 0.08 | 0.08 | 0.11 | 0.05 | 0.19 | 0.06 | 0.06 | 0.08 | 0.12 | 0.08 |
| 蔬菜类 Vegetables | 0.09 | 0.06 | 0.21 | 0.06 | 0.10 | 0.06 | 0.09 | 0.09 | 0.13 | 0.07 | 0.09 | 0.18 | 0.10 | 0.09 | 0.13 | 0.11 | 0.09 | 0.09 | 0.19 | 0.17 | 0.09 | 0.12 | 0.06 | 0.09 | 0.11 |
| 水果类 Fruits | 0.13 | 0.11 | ND | 0.05 | 0.07 | ND | 0.10 | 0.06 | ND | 0.11 | 0.05 | 0.06 | 0.09 | 0.09 | 0.07 | 0.10 | 0.06 | 0.08 | 0.07 | 0.05 | 0.09 | 0.07 | 0.06 | 0.13 | 0.07 |

注：未检出（ND）按 0 计

Note: values not detected (ND) were treated as 0

附表 7-17  第六次中国总膳食研究膳食样品中艾氏剂和狄氏剂的含量（单位：μg/kg）

Annexed Table 7-17  Levels of aldrin and dieldrin in food samples from the 6$^{th}$ China TDS (Unit: μg/kg)

| 膳食类别<br>Category | 黑龙江<br>HL | 辽宁<br>LN | 河北<br>HE | 北京<br>BJ | 吉林<br>JL | 山西<br>SX | 陕西<br>SN | 河南<br>HA | 宁夏<br>NX | 内蒙古<br>NM | 青海<br>QH | 甘肃<br>GS | 上海<br>SH | 福建<br>FJ | 江西<br>JX | 江苏<br>JS | 浙江<br>ZJ | 山东<br>SD | 湖北<br>HB | 四川<br>SC | 广西<br>GX | 湖南<br>HN | 广东<br>GD | 贵州<br>GZ | 全国平均<br>AVG |
|---|---|---|---|---|---|---|---|---|---|---|---|---|---|---|---|---|---|---|---|---|---|---|---|---|---|
| 谷类 Cereals | ND | ND | ND | ND | ND | ND | ND | ND | ND | ND | ND | ND | ND | ND | ND | ND | ND | ND | ND | ND | ND | ND | ND | ND | 0.00 |
| 豆类 Legumes | ND | ND | ND | ND | ND | ND | ND | ND | ND | ND | ND | ND | ND | ND | ND | ND | ND | ND | ND | ND | ND | ND | ND | ND | 0.00 |
| 薯类 Potatoes | ND | ND | ND | ND | ND | ND | ND | ND | ND | ND | ND | ND | ND | ND | ND | ND | ND | ND | ND | ND | ND | ND | ND | ND | 0.00 |
| 肉类 Meats | ND | 0.09 | ND | ND | ND | ND | ND | ND | ND | ND | ND | ND | ND | 0.17 | ND | 0.07 | 0.08 | ND | ND | ND | ND | ND | 0.09 | ND | 0.02 |
| 蛋类 Eggs | ND | ND | ND | ND | ND | ND | ND | ND | ND | ND | ND | ND | ND | ND | ND | 0.12 | 0.07 | ND | ND | ND | ND | ND | ND | ND | 0.01 |
| 水产类 Aquatic foods | ND | ND | ND | ND | ND | ND | ND | ND | ND | ND | ND | ND | ND | ND | 0.06 | 0.10 | ND | ND | ND | ND | ND | ND | ND | ND | 0.01 |
| 乳类 Dairy products | ND | 0.07 | ND | ND | 0.08 | ND | ND | ND | ND | ND | ND | ND | ND | 0.11 | ND | ND | 0.07 | ND | ND | ND | ND | ND | ND | ND | 0.01 |
| 蔬菜类 Vegetables | ND | ND | ND | ND | ND | ND | ND | ND | ND | ND | ND | ND | ND | ND | ND | ND | ND | ND | ND | ND | ND | ND | ND | ND | 0.00 |
| 水果类 Fruits | ND | ND | ND | ND | ND | ND | ND | ND | ND | ND | ND | ND | ND | ND | ND | ND | ND | ND | ND | ND | ND | ND | ND | ND | 0.00 |

注：未检出（ND）按 0 计

Note: values not detected (ND) were treated as 0

附表 7-18　第六次中国总膳食研究膳食样品中氯丹的含量（单位：μg/kg）

Annexed Table 7-18　Levels of CHLs in food samples from the 6$^{th}$ China TDS (Unit: μg/kg)

| 膳食类别 Category | 黑龙江 HL | 辽宁 LN | 河北 HE | 北京 BJ | 吉林 JL | 山西 SX | 陕西 SN | 河南 HA | 宁夏 NX | 内蒙古 NM | 青海 QH | 甘肃 GS | 上海 SH | 福建 FJ | 江西 JX | 江苏 JS | 浙江 ZJ | 山东 SD | 湖北 HB | 四川 SC | 广西 GX | 湖南 HN | 广东 GD | 贵州 GZ | 全国平均 AVG |
|---|---|---|---|---|---|---|---|---|---|---|---|---|---|---|---|---|---|---|---|---|---|---|---|---|---|
| 谷类 Cereals | ND | ND | ND | ND | ND | ND | ND | ND | ND | ND | ND | ND | ND | ND | ND | ND | ND | ND | ND | ND | ND | ND | ND | ND | 0.000 |
| 豆类 Legumes | ND | ND | ND | ND | ND | ND | ND | ND | ND | ND | ND | ND | ND | ND | ND | ND | ND | ND | ND | ND | ND | ND | ND | ND | 0.000 |
| 薯类 Potatoes | ND | ND | ND | ND | ND | ND | ND | ND | ND | ND | ND | ND | ND | ND | ND | ND | ND | ND | ND | ND | ND | ND | ND | ND | 0.000 |
| 肉类 Meats | ND | ND | ND | ND | ND | ND | ND | ND | ND | ND | ND | ND | 0.02 | ND | ND | ND | ND | ND | ND | ND | ND | ND | ND | ND | 0.001 |
| 蛋类 Eggs | ND | 0.03 | ND | ND | ND | ND | ND | ND | ND | ND | ND | 0.04 | ND | ND | ND | ND | ND | ND | ND | ND | ND | ND | ND | ND | 0.003 |
| 水产类 Aquatic foods | ND | ND | ND | ND | 0.04 | ND | ND | ND | ND | ND | ND | ND | 0.08 | ND | ND | ND | ND | ND | ND | ND | ND | ND | ND | ND | 0.005 |
| 乳类 Dairy products | ND | ND | ND | ND | 0.01 | ND | ND | ND | ND | ND | ND | ND | 0.03 | ND | ND | ND | 0.03 | ND | ND | ND | ND | ND | ND | ND | 0.003 |
| 蔬菜类 Vegetables | ND | ND | ND | ND | ND | ND | ND | ND | ND | ND | ND | ND | ND | ND | ND | ND | ND | ND | ND | ND | ND | ND | ND | ND | 0.000 |
| 水果类 Fruits | ND | ND | ND | ND | ND | ND | ND | ND | ND | ND | ND | ND | ND | ND | ND | ND | ND | ND | ND | ND | ND | ND | ND | ND | 0.000 |

注：未检出（ND）按 0 计

Note: values not detected (ND) were treated as 0

附表 7-19 第六次中国总膳食研究膳食样品中七氯的含量（单位：μg/kg）

Annexed Table 7-19 Levels of heptachlor in food samples from the 6th China TDS (Unit: μg/kg)

| 膳食类别<br>Category | 黑龙江<br>HL | 辽宁<br>LN | 河北<br>HE | 北京<br>BJ | 吉林<br>JL | 山西<br>SX | 陕西<br>SN | 河南<br>HA | 宁夏<br>NX | 内蒙古<br>NM | 青海<br>QH | 甘肃<br>GS | 上海<br>SH | 福建<br>FJ | 江西<br>JX | 江苏<br>JS | 浙江<br>ZJ | 山东<br>SD | 湖北<br>HB | 四川<br>SC | 广西<br>GX | 湖南<br>HN | 广东<br>GD | 贵州<br>GZ | 全国平均<br>AVG |
|---|---|---|---|---|---|---|---|---|---|---|---|---|---|---|---|---|---|---|---|---|---|---|---|---|---|
| 谷类 Cereals | ND | ND | ND | ND | ND | ND | ND | ND | ND | ND | ND | ND | ND | ND | ND | ND | ND | ND | ND | ND | ND | ND | ND | ND | 0.00 |
| 豆类 Legumes | ND | ND | ND | ND | ND | ND | ND | ND | ND | ND | ND | ND | ND | ND | ND | ND | ND | ND | ND | ND | ND | ND | ND | ND | 0.00 |
| 薯类 Potatoes | ND | ND | ND | ND | ND | 0.07 | ND | ND | ND | ND | ND | ND | ND | 0.06 | ND | ND | ND | ND | ND | ND | ND | ND | ND | ND | 0.01 |
| 肉类 Meats | ND | ND | ND | ND | ND | ND | ND | ND | ND | ND | ND | ND | ND | ND | ND | ND | ND | ND | ND | ND | ND | ND | ND | ND | 0.00 |
| 蛋类 Eggs | ND | ND | ND | 0.06 | ND | ND | ND | ND | ND | ND | ND | ND | ND | 0.08 | ND | ND | ND | ND | ND | ND | ND | ND | ND | ND | 0.01 |
| 水产类 Aquatic foods | ND | ND | ND | ND | ND | ND | ND | ND | ND | ND | ND | ND | ND | 0.09 | ND | ND | ND | ND | ND | ND | ND | ND | ND | ND | 0.00 |
| 乳类 Dairy products | ND | ND | ND | ND | ND | ND | ND | ND | ND | ND | ND | ND | ND | 0.06 | ND | ND | ND | ND | ND | ND | ND | ND | ND | ND | 0.00 |
| 蔬菜类 Vegetables | ND | ND | ND | ND | ND | ND | ND | ND | ND | ND | ND | ND | ND | ND | ND | ND | ND | ND | ND | ND | ND | ND | ND | ND | 0.00 |
| 水果类 Fruits | ND | ND | ND | ND | ND | ND | ND | ND | ND | ND | ND | ND | ND | ND | ND | ND | ND | ND | ND | ND | ND | ND | ND | ND | 0.00 |

注：未检出（ND）按 0 计

Note: values not detected (ND) were treated as 0

附表 7-20　第六次中国总膳食研究的滴滴涕膳食摄入量 [单位：ng/(kg bw·d)]

Annexed Table 7-20　Dietary intakes of DDTs from the 6th China TDS [Unit: ng/(kg bw·d)]

| 膳食类别<br>Category | 黑龙江<br>HL | 辽宁<br>LN | 河北<br>HE | 北京<br>BJ | 吉林<br>JL | 山西<br>SX | 陕西<br>SN | 河南<br>HA | 宁夏<br>NX | 内蒙古<br>NM | 青海<br>QH | 甘肃<br>GS | 上海<br>SH | 福建<br>FJ | 江西<br>JX | 江苏<br>JS | 浙江<br>ZJ | 山东<br>SD | 湖北<br>HB | 四川<br>SC | 广西<br>GX | 湖南<br>HN | 广东<br>GD | 贵州<br>GZ | 全国平均<br>AVG |
|---|---|---|---|---|---|---|---|---|---|---|---|---|---|---|---|---|---|---|---|---|---|---|---|---|---|
| 谷类 Cereals | 0.000 | 0.000 | 0.000 | 0.379 | 0.000 | 0.000 | 0.121 | 0.440 | 0.525 | 0.000 | 0.000 | 0.000 | 0.000 | 0.000 | 0.000 | 0.370 | 0.000 | 0.000 | 0.503 | 0.000 | 0.000 | 0.000 | 0.000 | 0.000 | 0.097 |
| 豆类 Legumes | 0.065 | 0.000 | 0.000 | 0.000 | 0.000 | 0.000 | 0.000 | 0.060 | 0.000 | 0.000 | 0.000 | 0.222 | 0.075 | 0.000 | 0.000 | 0.079 | 0.000 | 0.000 | 0.095 | 0.000 | 0.000 | 0.000 | 0.000 | 0.000 | 0.025 |
| 薯类 Potatoes | 0.000 | 0.000 | 0.000 | 0.000 | 0.000 | 0.019 | 0.000 | 0.000 | 0.000 | 0.000 | 0.000 | 0.525 | 0.000 | 0.000 | 0.000 | 0.000 | 0.000 | 0.000 | 0.000 | 0.000 | 0.000 | 0.000 | 0.000 | 0.000 | 0.023 |
| 肉类 Meats | 0.067 | 0.890 | 0.308 | 1.624 | 0.264 | 0.131 | 0.017 | 0.817 | 0.089 | 0.035 | 0.248 | 0.443 | 1.371 | 1.720 | 1.923 | 0.219 | 2.460 | 0.000 | 0.646 | 0.164 | 0.695 | 3.441 | 0.132 | 1.369 | 0.795 |
| 蛋类 Eggs | 0.045 | 0.149 | 0.951 | 0.413 | 0.140 | 0.000 | 0.007 | 0.019 | 0.004 | 0.170 | 0.002 | 0.099 | 0.855 | 0.546 | 0.439 | 0.080 | 0.437 | 0.035 | 0.825 | 0.000 | 0.369 | 0.000 | 0.027 | 0.039 | 0.235 |
| 水产类 Aquatic foods | 0.147 | 0.235 | 0.074 | 0.388 | 0.341 | 0.056 | 0.078 | 0.298 | 0.006 | 0.169 | 0.019 | 0.053 | 10.704 | 1.488 | 2.788 | 1.418 | 2.364 | 0.394 | 3.521 | 0.169 | 3.069 | 4.100 | 1.975 | 0.203 | 1.419 |
| 乳类 Dairy products | 0.013 | 0.310 | 0.058 | 0.680 | 0.051 | 0.033 | 0.178 | 0.071 | 0.000 | 0.033 | 0.042 | 0.132 | 0.193 | 0.594 | 0.295 | 0.052 | 0.080 | 0.040 | 0.107 | 0.004 | 0.258 | 0.020 | 0.127 | 0.349 | 0.155 |
| 蔬菜类 Vegetables | 0.000 | 0.156 | 0.746 | 0.249 | 0.000 | 0.000 | 0.000 | 0.000 | 0.000 | 0.000 | 0.000 | 0.000 | 0.254 | 0.441 | 0.000 | 0.000 | 0.000 | 0.000 | 1.380 | 0.000 | 0.000 | 0.000 | 0.000 | 0.000 | 0.134 |
| 水果类 Fruits | 0.000 | 0.000 | 0.000 | 0.000 | 0.000 | 0.000 | 0.000 | 0.000 | 0.000 | 0.000 | 0.000 | 0.000 | 0.000 | 0.000 | 0.000 | 0.000 | 0.000 | 0.000 | 0.000 | 0.000 | 0.000 | 0.000 | 0.000 | 0.000 | 0.000 |
| 合计 SUM | 0.336 | 1.740 | 2.137 | 3.733 | 0.797 | 0.238 | 0.401 | 1.705 | 0.624 | 0.406 | 0.311 | 1.475 | 13.451 | 4.788 | 5.445 | 2.219 | 5.341 | 0.469 | 7.079 | 0.336 | 4.391 | 7.561 | 2.261 | 1.959 | 2.883 |

附表 7-21 第六次中国总膳食研究的六六膳食摄入量 [单位: ng/(kg bw·d)]

Annexed Table 7-21 Dietary intakes of HCHs from the 6th China TDS [Unit: ng/(kg bw·d)]

| 膳食类别<br>Category | 黑龙江<br>HL | 辽宁<br>LN | 河北<br>HE | 北京<br>BJ | 吉林<br>JL | 山西<br>SX | 陕西<br>SN | 河南<br>HA | 宁夏<br>NX | 内蒙古<br>NM | 青海<br>QH | 甘肃<br>GS | 上海<br>SH | 福建<br>FJ | 江西<br>JX | 江苏<br>JS | 浙江<br>ZJ | 山东<br>SD | 湖北<br>HB | 四川<br>SC | 广西<br>GX | 湖南<br>HN | 广东<br>GD | 贵州<br>GZ | 全国平均<br>AVG |
|---|---|---|---|---|---|---|---|---|---|---|---|---|---|---|---|---|---|---|---|---|---|---|---|---|---|
| 谷类 Cereals | 0.000 | 0.000 | 3.117 | 0.000 | 0.000 | 0.000 | 0.000 | 0.000 | 0.000 | 0.000 | 0.000 | 0.000 | 0.000 | 0.000 | 0.000 | 0.000 | 0.000 | 0.000 | 0.000 | 0.000 | 0.000 | 0.000 | 0.000 | 0.000 | 0.130 |
| 豆类 Legumes | 0.087 | 0.387 | 0.181 | 0.000 | 0.503 | 0.000 | 0.000 | 0.000 | 0.106 | 0.000 | 0.000 | 0.046 | 0.000 | 0.000 | 0.000 | 0.000 | 0.000 | 0.000 | 0.000 | 0.000 | 0.000 | 0.000 | 0.018 | 0.000 | 0.055 |
| 薯类 Potatoes | 0.000 | 0.000 | 0.145 | 0.065 | 0.000 | 0.000 | 0.000 | 0.000 | 0.270 | 0.388 | 0.000 | 0.731 | 0.000 | 0.000 | 0.000 | 0.000 | 0.000 | 0.103 | 0.000 | 0.000 | 0.000 | 0.000 | 0.000 | 0.000 | 0.071 |
| 肉类 Meats | 0.380 | 0.424 | 0.308 | 0.256 | 0.190 | 0.675 | 0.052 | 0.149 | 2.637 | 0.105 | 0.124 | 0.300 | 0.105 | 0.287 | 0.000 | 0.248 | 0.188 | 0.216 | 0.060 | 0.266 | 0.455 | 0.285 | 0.000 | 0.186 | 0.329 |
| 蛋类 Eggs | 0.116 | 0.000 | 0.220 | 0.148 | 0.077 | 0.093 | 0.010 | 0.042 | 0.010 | 0.321 | 0.015 | 0.018 | 0.031 | 0.042 | 0.088 | 0.036 | 0.000 | 0.099 | 0.147 | 0.021 | 0.018 | 0.054 | 0.019 | 0.010 | 0.068 |
| 水产类 Aquatic foods | 2.853 | 0.048 | 0.140 | 0.154 | 0.755 | 0.042 | 0.021 | 0.053 | 0.017 | 0.030 | 0.025 | 0.012 | 0.860 | 0.448 | 0.291 | 0.316 | 0.831 | 0.155 | 0.426 | 0.102 | 0.322 | 0.232 | 0.163 | 0.016 | 0.346 |
| 乳类 Dairy products | 0.026 | 0.085 | 0.050 | 0.177 | 0.072 | 0.072 | 0.028 | 0.043 | 0.048 | 0.033 | 0.170 | 0.054 | 0.091 | 0.040 | 0.083 | 0.044 | 0.064 | 0.055 | 0.009 | 0.000 | 0.011 | 0.051 | 0.041 | 0.013 | 0.057 |
| 蔬菜类 Vegetables | 0.000 | 0.467 | 1.072 | 0.498 | 0.000 | 0.000 | 0.547 | 0.000 | 0.000 | 1.102 | 0.000 | 0.000 | 0.000 | 0.000 | 0.000 | 0.000 | 0.000 | 1.225 | 0.723 | 0.000 | 0.000 | 0.593 | 0.000 | 0.518 | 0.281 |
| 水果类 Fruits | 0.000 | 0.000 | 0.000 | 0.000 | 0.000 | 0.000 | 0.000 | 0.000 | 0.000 | 0.000 | 0.000 | 0.000 | 0.000 | 0.000 | 0.000 | 0.000 | 0.000 | 0.000 | 0.000 | 0.000 | 0.000 | 0.000 | 0.000 | 0.000 | 0.000 |
| 合计 SUM | 3.461 | 1.411 | 5.234 | 1.298 | 1.596 | 0.882 | 0.657 | 0.288 | 3.088 | 1.978 | 0.333 | 1.160 | 1.087 | 0.817 | 0.462 | 0.643 | 1.082 | 1.853 | 1.365 | 0.389 | 0.807 | 1.216 | 0.240 | 0.744 | 1.337 |

附表 7-22　第六次中国总膳食研究的硫丹膳食摄入量 [单位：ng/(kg bw·d)]

Annexed Table 7-22　Dietary intakes of endosulfans from the 6th China TDS [Unit: ng/(kg bw·d)]

| 膳食类别<br>Category | 黑龙江<br>HL | 辽宁<br>LN | 河北<br>HE | 北京<br>BJ | 吉林<br>JL | 山西<br>SX | 陕西<br>SN | 河南<br>HA | 宁夏<br>NX | 内蒙古<br>NM | 青海<br>QH | 甘肃<br>GS | 上海<br>SH | 福建<br>FJ | 江西<br>JX | 江苏<br>JS | 浙江<br>ZJ | 山东<br>SD | 湖北<br>HB | 四川<br>SC | 广西<br>GX | 湖南<br>HN | 广东<br>GD | 贵州<br>GZ | 全国平均<br>AVG |
|---|---|---|---|---|---|---|---|---|---|---|---|---|---|---|---|---|---|---|---|---|---|---|---|---|---|
| 谷类 Cereals | 0.000 | 0.000 | 0.000 | 0.000 | 0.000 | 0.000 | 0.000 | 0.000 | 0.000 | 0.000 | 0.000 | 0.000 | 0.000 | 0.000 | 0.000 | 0.000 | 0.000 | 0.000 | 0.000 | 0.000 | 0.000 | 0.000 | 0.000 | 0.000 | 0.000 |
| 豆类 Legumes | 0.000 | 0.000 | 0.000 | 0.000 | 0.000 | 0.000 | 0.000 | 0.000 | 0.000 | 0.000 | 0.000 | 0.000 | 0.000 | 0.000 | 0.000 | 0.000 | 0.000 | 0.000 | 0.000 | 0.000 | 0.000 | 0.000 | 0.000 | 0.000 | 0.000 |
| 薯类 Potatoes | 0.000 | 0.000 | 0.000 | 0.000 | 0.000 | 0.000 | 0.000 | 0.000 | 0.000 | 0.000 | 0.000 | 0.000 | 0.000 | 0.000 | 0.000 | 0.000 | 0.000 | 0.000 | 2.363 | 0.000 | 0.000 | 0.000 | 0.000 | 0.000 | 0.098 |
| 肉类 Meats | 0.000 | 2.183 | 0.000 | 0.919 | 0.000 | 0.000 | 0.000 | 0.000 | 0.000 | 0.000 | 0.000 | 0.000 | 1.705 | 0.000 | 0.000 | 2.506 | 1.709 | 0.000 | 0.000 | 0.000 | 0.000 | 0.000 | 0.000 | 0.000 | 0.376 |
| 蛋类 Eggs | 0.000 | 2.026 | 0.000 | 0.000 | 0.000 | 0.000 | 0.000 | 0.000 | 0.000 | 0.000 | 0.000 | 0.000 | 0.186 | 0.971 | 0.000 | 0.000 | 0.000 | 0.000 | 0.000 | 0.000 | 0.000 | 0.347 | 0.000 | 0.000 | 0.147 |
| 水产类 Aquatic foods | 0.000 | 0.339 | 0.000 | 0.341 | 0.000 | 0.000 | 0.000 | 0.602 | 0.000 | 0.000 | 0.000 | 0.226 | 3.474 | 1.141 | 0.000 | 1.734 | 2.204 | 0.000 | 1.764 | 0.000 | 0.000 | 2.245 | 1.829 | 0.000 | 0.653 |
| 乳类 Dairy products | 0.000 | 1.474 | 0.000 | 0.911 | 0.000 | 0.000 | 0.000 | 0.425 | 0.000 | 0.000 | 0.000 | 0.000 | 0.000 | 0.371 | 0.257 | 0.629 | 0.319 | 0.000 | 0.091 | 0.000 | 0.000 | 0.474 | 1.356 | 0.000 | 0.272 |
| 蔬菜类 Vegetables | 0.000 | 0.000 | 0.000 | 10.016 | 0.000 | 0.000 | 0.000 | 0.000 | 0.000 | 0.896 | 0.000 | 0.000 | 0.000 | 0.000 | 0.000 | 0.000 | 0.000 | 0.000 | 0.000 | 0.000 | 0.000 | 9.153 | 7.057 | 0.000 | 1.093 |
| 水果类 Fruits | 0.000 | 0.000 | 0.000 | 0.000 | 0.000 | 0.000 | 0.000 | 0.288 | 0.000 | 0.000 | 0.000 | 0.000 | 0.000 | 0.000 | 0.000 | 0.000 | 0.000 | 0.000 | 0.000 | 0.000 | 0.000 | 0.000 | 0.000 | 0.000 | 0.049 |
| 合计 SUM | 0.000 | 6.021 | 0.000 | 12.188 | 0.000 | 0.000 | 0.000 | 1.315 | 0.000 | 0.896 | 0.000 | 0.226 | 5.364 | 2.483 | 0.257 | 4.868 | 4.232 | 0.000 | 4.218 | 0.000 | 0.000 | 12.219 | 10.242 | 0.000 | 2.689 |

附表 7-23　第六次中国总膳食研究的五氯苯膳食摄入量 [单位: ng/(kg bw·d)]

Annexed Table 7-23　Dietary intakes of pentachlorobenzene from the 6$^{th}$ China TDS [Unit: ng/(kg bw·d)]

| 膳食类别<br>Category | 黑龙江<br>HL | 辽宁<br>LN | 河北<br>HE | 北京<br>BJ | 吉林<br>JL | 山西<br>SX | 陕西<br>SN | 河南<br>HA | 宁夏<br>NX | 内蒙古<br>NM | 青海<br>QH | 甘肃<br>GS | 上海<br>SH | 福建<br>FJ | 江西<br>JX | 江苏<br>JS | 浙江<br>ZJ | 山东<br>SD | 湖北<br>HB | 四川<br>SC | 广西<br>GX | 湖南<br>HN | 广东<br>GD | 贵州<br>GZ | 全国平均<br>AVG |
|---|---|---|---|---|---|---|---|---|---|---|---|---|---|---|---|---|---|---|---|---|---|---|---|---|---|
| 谷类 Cereals | 1.566 | 0.977 | 1.559 | 1.388 | 0.836 | 1.812 | 2.421 | 2.934 | 1.365 | 0.918 | 1.703 | 1.307 | 0.855 | 0.803 | 1.300 | 1.852 | 0.703 | 1.738 | 0.755 | 1.693 | 1.941 | 0.916 | 0.652 | 1.928 | 1.413 |
| 豆类 Legumes | 0.115 | 0.174 | 0.091 | 0.129 | 0.120 | 0.143 | 0.250 | 0.197 | 0.073 | 0.057 | 0.012 | 0.150 | 0.131 | 0.087 | 0.070 | 0.158 | 0.112 | 0.075 | 0.117 | 0.182 | 0.034 | 0.104 | 0.031 | 0.258 | 0.120 |
| 薯类 Potatoes | 0.135 | 0.069 | 0.223 | 0.084 | 0.095 | 0.584 | 0.146 | 0.140 | 0.127 | 0.175 | 0.193 | 0.183 | 0.029 | 0.034 | 0.031 | 0.112 | 0.041 | 0.051 | 0.113 | 0.140 | 0.018 | 0.085 | 0.059 | 0.060 | 0.122 |
| 肉类 Meats | 0.133 | 0.148 | 0.256 | 0.085 | 0.148 | 0.131 | 0.074 | 0.325 | 0.319 | 0.093 | 0.169 | 0.069 | 0.387 | 0.273 | 0.298 | 0.204 | 0.244 | 0.185 | 0.060 | 0.327 | 1.246 | 0.356 | 0.132 | 0.237 | 0.246 |
| 蛋类 Eggs | 0.173 | 0.071 | 0.210 | 0.068 | 0.070 | 0.090 | 0.073 | 0.061 | 0.019 | 0.057 | 0.019 | 0.035 | 0.074 | 0.075 | 0.026 | 0.094 | 0.038 | 0.113 | 0.087 | 0.044 | 0.031 | 0.087 | 0.038 | 0.070 | 0.072 |
| 水产类 Aquatic foods | 0.112 | 0.028 | 0.033 | 0.034 | 0.058 | 0.012 | 0.018 | 0.012 | 0.000 | 0.011 | 0.010 | 0.004 | 0.370 | 0.234 | 0.305 | 0.118 | 0.120 | 0.040 | 0.149 | 0.036 | 0.169 | 1.117 | 0.098 | 0.014 | 0.129 |
| 乳类 Dairy products | 0.026 | 0.035 | 0.027 | 0.000 | 0.031 | 0.046 | 0.021 | 0.025 | 0.017 | 0.033 | 0.059 | 0.027 | 0.068 | 0.034 | 0.028 | 0.035 | 0.043 | 0.040 | 0.005 | 0.038 | 0.038 | 0.017 | 0.046 | 0.054 | 0.032 |
| 蔬菜类 Vegetables | 0.458 | 0.311 | 0.979 | 0.373 | 0.616 | 0.295 | 0.410 | 0.397 | 0.322 | 0.286 | 0.444 | 0.709 | 0.636 | 0.567 | 0.932 | 0.743 | 0.634 | 0.580 | 1.249 | 0.817 | 0.505 | 1.017 | 0.225 | 0.583 | 0.587 |
| 水果类 Fruits | 0.130 | 0.134 | 0.000 | 0.090 | 0.098 | 0.000 | 0.060 | 0.023 | 0.000 | 0.197 | 0.012 | 0.032 | 0.105 | 0.085 | 0.063 | 0.043 | 0.064 | 0.069 | 0.021 | 0.012 | 0.092 | 0.070 | 0.028 | 0.043 | 0.061 |
| 合计 SUM | 2.848 | 1.948 | 3.377 | 2.252 | 2.072 | 3.112 | 3.473 | 4.115 | 2.241 | 1.827 | 2.621 | 2.516 | 2.654 | 2.193 | 3.052 | 3.358 | 1.999 | 2.892 | 2.556 | 3.289 | 4.053 | 3.770 | 1.309 | 3.247 | 2.782 |

附表 7-24 第六次中国总膳食研究的六氯苯膳食摄入量 [单位: ng/(kg bw·d)]
Annexed Table 7-24 Dietary intakes of HCB from the 6th China TDS [Unit: ng/(kg bw·d)]

| 膳食类别 Category | 黑龙江 HL | 辽宁 LN | 河北 HE | 北京 BJ | 吉林 JL | 山西 SX | 陕西 SN | 河南 HA | 宁夏 NX | 内蒙古 NM | 青海 QH | 甘肃 GS | 上海 SH | 福建 FJ | 江西 JX | 江苏 JS | 浙江 ZJ | 山东 SD | 湖北 HB | 四川 SC | 广西 GX | 湖南 HN | 广东 GD | 贵州 GZ | 全国平均 AVG |
|---|---|---|---|---|---|---|---|---|---|---|---|---|---|---|---|---|---|---|---|---|---|---|---|---|---|
| 谷类 Cereals | 0.000 | 0.000 | 0.000 | 0.000 | 0.000 | 0.000 | 0.000 | 1.027 | 0.000 | 0.000 | 0.000 | 0.000 | 0.000 | 0.000 | 0.000 | 0.617 | 0.000 | 0.000 | 0.000 | 0.000 | 0.000 | 0.000 | 0.000 | 0.000 | 0.069 |
| 豆类 Legumes | 0.000 | 0.000 | 0.000 | 0.000 | 0.000 | 0.496 | 0.000 | 0.094 | 0.033 | 0.000 | 0.007 | 0.000 | 0.000 | 0.000 | 0.000 | 0.066 | 0.000 | 0.000 | 0.085 | 0.086 | 0.000 | 0.000 | 0.000 | 0.000 | 0.036 |
| 薯类 Potatoes | 0.111 | 0.000 | 0.000 | 0.000 | 0.000 | 0.000 | 0.000 | 0.000 | 0.000 | 0.097 | 0.000 | 0.000 | 0.000 | 0.000 | 0.000 | 0.053 | 0.000 | 0.000 | 0.098 | 0.110 | 0.014 | 0.000 | 0.000 | 0.000 | 0.020 |
| 肉类 Meats | 0.095 | 0.000 | 0.256 | 0.139 | 0.000 | 0.000 | 0.000 | 0.343 | 0.941 | 0.000 | 0.079 | 0.000 | 0.475 | 0.096 | 0.000 | 0.131 | 0.131 | 0.124 | 0.000 | 0.225 | 0.934 | 0.261 | 0.000 | 0.101 | 0.180 |
| 蛋类 Eggs | 0.090 | 0.000 | 0.195 | 0.000 | 0.045 | 0.090 | 0.031 | 0.000 | 0.000 | 0.028 | 0.000 | 0.000 | 0.093 | 0.054 | 0.000 | 0.085 | 0.038 | 0.063 | 0.167 | 0.033 | 0.016 | 0.054 | 0.019 | 0.015 | 0.047 |
| 水产类 Aquatic foods | 0.073 | 0.000 | 0.027 | 0.016 | 0.000 | 0.000 | 0.010 | 0.005 | 0.007 | 0.000 | 0.007 | 0.004 | 0.250 | 0.194 | 0.430 | 0.062 | 0.080 | 0.000 | 0.129 | 0.015 | 0.092 | 2.930 | 0.073 | 0.017 | 0.184 |
| 乳类 Dairy products | 0.013 | 0.000 | 0.019 | 0.000 | 0.000 | 0.026 | 0.015 | 0.000 | 0.012 | 0.000 | 0.034 | 0.018 | 0.000 | 0.000 | 0.017 | 0.022 | 0.000 | 0.022 | 0.000 | 0.012 | 0.000 | 0.000 | 0.000 | 0.000 | 0.009 |
| 蔬菜类 Vegetables | 0.000 | 0.000 | 0.513 | 0.000 | 0.370 | 0.000 | 0.000 | 0.000 | 0.000 | 0.000 | 0.000 | 0.630 | 0.763 | 0.000 | 0.000 | 0.405 | 0.000 | 0.000 | 0.000 | 0.480 | 0.280 | 0.593 | 0.000 | 0.000 | 0.168 |
| 水果类 Fruits | 0.000 | 0.000 | 0.000 | 0.000 | 0.000 | 0.000 | 0.000 | 0.000 | 0.000 | 0.000 | 0.000 | 0.000 | 0.000 | 0.000 | 0.000 | 0.000 | 0.000 | 0.000 | 0.000 | 0.000 | 0.000 | 0.000 | 0.000 | 0.000 | 0.000 |
| 合计 SUM | 0.382 | 0.000 | 1.010 | 0.155 | 0.414 | 0.612 | 0.057 | 1.469 | 0.994 | 0.125 | 0.127 | 0.652 | 1.581 | 0.343 | 0.447 | 1.441 | 0.249 | 0.209 | 0.479 | 0.960 | 1.337 | 3.839 | 0.092 | 0.134 | 0.713 |

附表 7-25　第六次中国总膳食研究的艾氏剂和狄氏剂膳食摄入量 [单位：ng/(kg bw·d)]

Annexed Table 7-25　Dietary intakes of aldrin and dieldrin from the 6<sup>th</sup> China TDS [Unit: ng/(kg bw·d)]

| 膳食类别<br>Category | 黑龙江<br>HL | 辽宁<br>LN | 河北<br>HE | 北京<br>BJ | 吉林<br>JL | 山西<br>SX | 陕西<br>SN | 河南<br>HA | 宁夏<br>NX | 内蒙古<br>NM | 青海<br>QH | 甘肃<br>GS | 上海<br>SH | 福建<br>FJ | 江西<br>JX | 江苏<br>JS | 浙江<br>ZJ | 山东<br>SD | 湖北<br>HB | 四川<br>SC | 广西<br>GX | 湖南<br>HN | 广东<br>GD | 贵州<br>GZ | 全国平均<br>AVG |
|---|---|---|---|---|---|---|---|---|---|---|---|---|---|---|---|---|---|---|---|---|---|---|---|---|---|
| 谷类 Cereals | 0.000 | 0.000 | 0.000 | 0.000 | 0.000 | 0.000 | 0.000 | 0.000 | 0.000 | 0.000 | 0.000 | 0.000 | 0.000 | 0.000 | 0.000 | 0.000 | 0.000 | 0.000 | 0.000 | 0.000 | 0.000 | 0.000 | 0.000 | 0.000 | 0.000 |
| 豆类 Legumes | 0.000 | 0.000 | 0.000 | 0.000 | 0.000 | 0.000 | 0.000 | 0.000 | 0.000 | 0.000 | 0.000 | 0.000 | 0.000 | 0.000 | 0.000 | 0.000 | 0.000 | 0.000 | 0.000 | 0.000 | 0.000 | 0.000 | 0.000 | 0.000 | 0.000 |
| 薯类 Potatoes | 0.000 | 0.000 | 0.000 | 0.000 | 0.000 | 0.000 | 0.000 | 0.000 | 0.000 | 0.000 | 0.000 | 0.000 | 0.000 | 0.000 | 0.000 | 0.000 | 0.000 | 0.000 | 0.000 | 0.000 | 0.000 | 0.000 | 0.000 | 0.000 | 0.000 |
| 肉类 Meats | 0.000 | 0.000 | 0.000 | 0.000 | 0.000 | 0.000 | 0.000 | 0.000 | 0.000 | 0.000 | 0.000 | 0.000 | 0.000 | 0.232 | 0.000 | 0.102 | 0.150 | 0.000 | 0.000 | 0.000 | 0.000 | 0.000 | 0.149 | 0.000 | 0.026 |
| 蛋类 Eggs | 0.000 | 0.058 | 0.000 | 0.000 | 0.041 | 0.000 | 0.000 | 0.000 | 0.000 | 0.000 | 0.000 | 0.000 | 0.000 | 0.000 | 0.000 | 0.054 | 0.027 | 0.000 | 0.000 | 0.000 | 0.000 | 0.000 | 0.000 | 0.000 | 0.006 |
| 水产类 Aquatic foods | 0.000 | 0.049 | 0.000 | 0.000 | 0.000 | 0.000 | 0.000 | 0.000 | 0.000 | 0.000 | 0.000 | 0.000 | 0.000 | 0.000 | 0.042 | 0.062 | 0.000 | 0.000 | 0.000 | 0.000 | 0.000 | 0.000 | 0.000 | 0.000 | 0.004 |
| 乳类 Dairy products | 0.000 | 0.000 | 0.000 | 0.000 | 0.000 | 0.000 | 0.000 | 0.000 | 0.000 | 0.000 | 0.000 | 0.000 | 0.000 | 0.063 | 0.000 | 0.000 | 0.037 | 0.000 | 0.000 | 0.000 | 0.000 | 0.000 | 0.000 | 0.000 | 0.008 |
| 蔬菜类 Vegetables | 0.000 | 0.000 | 0.000 | 0.000 | 0.000 | 0.000 | 0.000 | 0.000 | 0.000 | 0.000 | 0.000 | 0.000 | 0.000 | 0.000 | 0.000 | 0.000 | 0.000 | 0.000 | 0.000 | 0.000 | 0.000 | 0.000 | 0.000 | 0.000 | 0.000 |
| 水果类 Fruits | 0.000 | 0.000 | 0.000 | 0.000 | 0.000 | 0.000 | 0.000 | 0.000 | 0.000 | 0.000 | 0.000 | 0.000 | 0.000 | 0.000 | 0.000 | 0.000 | 0.000 | 0.000 | 0.000 | 0.000 | 0.000 | 0.000 | 0.000 | 0.000 | 0.000 |
| 合计 SUM | 0.000 | 0.108 | 0.000 | 0.000 | 0.041 | 0.000 | 0.000 | 0.000 | 0.000 | 0.000 | 0.000 | 0.000 | 0.000 | 0.295 | 0.042 | 0.217 | 0.214 | 0.000 | 0.000 | 0.000 | 0.000 | 0.000 | 0.149 | 0.000 | 0.044 |

附表 7-26 第六次中国总膳食研究的氯丹膳食摄入量 [单位：ng/(kg bw·d)]

Annexed Table 7-26 Dietary intakes of CHLs from the 6$^{th}$ China TDS [Unit: ng/(kg bw·d)]

| 膳食类别<br>Category | 黑龙江<br>HL | 辽宁<br>LN | 河北<br>HE | 北京<br>BJ | 吉林<br>JL | 山西<br>SX | 陕西<br>SN | 河南<br>HA | 宁夏<br>NX | 内蒙古<br>NM | 青海<br>QH | 甘肃<br>GS | 上海<br>SH | 福建<br>FJ | 江西<br>JX | 江苏<br>JS | 浙江<br>ZJ | 山东<br>SD | 湖北<br>HB | 四川<br>SC | 广西<br>GX | 湖南<br>HN | 广东<br>GD | 贵州<br>GZ | 全国平均<br>AVG |
|---|---|---|---|---|---|---|---|---|---|---|---|---|---|---|---|---|---|---|---|---|---|---|---|---|---|
| 谷类 Cereals | 0.000 | 0.000 | 0.000 | 0.000 | 0.000 | 0.000 | 0.000 | 0.000 | 0.000 | 0.000 | 0.000 | 0.000 | 0.000 | 0.000 | 0.000 | 0.000 | 0.000 | 0.000 | 0.000 | 0.000 | 0.000 | 0.000 | 0.000 | 0.000 | 0.000 |
| 豆类 Legumes | 0.000 | 0.000 | 0.000 | 0.000 | 0.000 | 0.000 | 0.000 | 0.000 | 0.000 | 0.000 | 0.000 | 0.000 | 0.000 | 0.000 | 0.000 | 0.000 | 0.000 | 0.000 | 0.000 | 0.000 | 0.000 | 0.000 | 0.000 | 0.000 | 0.000 |
| 薯类 Potatoes | 0.000 | 0.000 | 0.000 | 0.000 | 0.000 | 0.000 | 0.000 | 0.000 | 0.000 | 0.000 | 0.000 | 0.000 | 0.000 | 0.000 | 0.000 | 0.000 | 0.000 | 0.000 | 0.000 | 0.000 | 0.000 | 0.000 | 0.000 | 0.000 | 0.000 |
| 肉类 Meats | 0.000 | 0.000 | 0.000 | 0.000 | 0.000 | 0.000 | 0.000 | 0.000 | 0.000 | 0.000 | 0.000 | 0.000 | 0.035 | 0.000 | 0.000 | 0.000 | 0.000 | 0.000 | 0.000 | 0.000 | 0.000 | 0.000 | 0.000 | 0.000 | 0.001 |
| 蛋类 Eggs | 0.000 | 0.019 | 0.000 | 0.000 | 0.000 | 0.000 | 0.000 | 0.000 | 0.000 | 0.000 | 0.000 | 0.014 | 0.000 | 0.000 | 0.000 | 0.000 | 0.000 | 0.000 | 0.000 | 0.000 | 0.000 | 0.000 | 0.000 | 0.000 | 0.001 |
| 水产类 Aquatic foods | 0.000 | 0.000 | 0.000 | 0.000 | 0.007 | 0.000 | 0.000 | 0.000 | 0.000 | 0.000 | 0.000 | 0.000 | 0.087 | 0.000 | 0.000 | 0.000 | 0.000 | 0.000 | 0.000 | 0.000 | 0.000 | 0.000 | 0.000 | 0.000 | 0.004 |
| 乳类 Dairy products | 0.000 | 0.000 | 0.000 | 0.000 | 0.005 | 0.000 | 0.000 | 0.000 | 0.000 | 0.000 | 0.000 | 0.000 | 0.034 | 0.000 | 0.000 | 0.000 | 0.016 | 0.000 | 0.000 | 0.000 | 0.000 | 0.000 | 0.000 | 0.000 | 0.002 |
| 蔬菜类 Vegetables | 0.000 | 0.000 | 0.000 | 0.000 | 0.000 | 0.000 | 0.000 | 0.000 | 0.000 | 0.000 | 0.000 | 0.000 | 0.000 | 0.000 | 0.000 | 0.000 | 0.000 | 0.000 | 0.000 | 0.000 | 0.000 | 0.000 | 0.000 | 0.000 | 0.000 |
| 水果类 Fruits | 0.000 | 0.000 | 0.000 | 0.000 | 0.000 | 0.000 | 0.000 | 0.000 | 0.000 | 0.000 | 0.000 | 0.000 | 0.000 | 0.000 | 0.000 | 0.000 | 0.000 | 0.000 | 0.000 | 0.000 | 0.000 | 0.000 | 0.000 | 0.000 | 0.000 |
| 合计 SUM | 0.000 | 0.019 | 0.000 | 0.000 | 0.012 | 0.000 | 0.000 | 0.000 | 0.000 | 0.000 | 0.000 | 0.014 | 0.156 | 0.000 | 0.000 | 0.000 | 0.016 | 0.000 | 0.000 | 0.000 | 0.000 | 0.000 | 0.000 | 0.000 | 0.009 |

附表 7-27 第六次中国总膳食研究的七氯膳食摄入量 [单位: ng/(kg bw・d)]
Annexed Table 7-27 Dietary intakes of heptachlor from the 6th China TDS [Unit: ng/(kg bw・d)]

| 膳食类别 Category | 黑龙江 HL | 辽宁 LN | 河北 HE | 北京 BJ | 吉林 JL | 山西 SX | 陕西 SN | 河南 HA | 宁夏 NX | 内蒙古 NM | 青海 QH | 甘肃 GS | 上海 SH | 福建 FJ | 江西 JX | 江苏 JS | 浙江 ZJ | 山东 SD | 湖北 HB | 四川 SC | 广西 GX | 湖南 HN | 广东 GD | 贵州 GZ | 全国平均 AVG |
|---|---|---|---|---|---|---|---|---|---|---|---|---|---|---|---|---|---|---|---|---|---|---|---|---|---|
| 谷类 Cereals | 0.000 | 0.000 | 0.000 | 0.000 | 0.000 | 0.000 | 0.000 | 0.000 | 0.000 | 0.000 | 0.000 | 0.000 | 0.000 | 0.000 | 0.000 | 0.000 | 0.000 | 0.000 | 0.000 | 0.000 | 0.000 | 0.000 | 0.000 | 0.000 | 0.000 |
| 豆类 Legumes | 0.000 | 0.000 | 0.000 | 0.000 | 0.000 | 0.000 | 0.000 | 0.000 | 0.000 | 0.000 | 0.000 | 0.000 | 0.000 | 0.000 | 0.000 | 0.000 | 0.000 | 0.000 | 0.000 | 0.000 | 0.000 | 0.000 | 0.000 | 0.000 | 0.000 |
| 薯类 Potatoes | 0.000 | 0.000 | 0.000 | 0.000 | 0.000 | 0.132 | 0.000 | 0.000 | 0.000 | 0.000 | 0.000 | 0.000 | 0.000 | 0.040 | 0.000 | 0.000 | 0.000 | 0.000 | 0.000 | 0.000 | 0.000 | 0.000 | 0.000 | 0.000 | 0.007 |
| 肉类 Meats | 0.000 | 0.000 | 0.000 | 0.000 | 0.000 | 0.000 | 0.000 | 0.000 | 0.000 | 0.000 | 0.000 | 0.000 | 0.000 | 0.109 | 0.000 | 0.000 | 0.000 | 0.000 | 0.000 | 0.000 | 0.000 | 0.000 | 0.000 | 0.000 | 0.005 |
| 蛋类 Eggs | 0.000 | 0.000 | 0.000 | 0.037 | 0.000 | 0.000 | 0.000 | 0.000 | 0.000 | 0.000 | 0.000 | 0.000 | 0.000 | 0.027 | 0.000 | 0.000 | 0.000 | 0.000 | 0.000 | 0.000 | 0.000 | 0.000 | 0.000 | 0.000 | 0.003 |
| 水产类 Aquatic foods | 0.000 | 0.000 | 0.000 | 0.000 | 0.000 | 0.000 | 0.000 | 0.000 | 0.000 | 0.000 | 0.000 | 0.000 | 0.000 | 0.061 | 0.000 | 0.000 | 0.000 | 0.000 | 0.000 | 0.000 | 0.000 | 0.000 | 0.000 | 0.000 | 0.003 |
| 乳类 Dairy products | 0.000 | 0.000 | 0.000 | 0.000 | 0.000 | 0.000 | 0.000 | 0.000 | 0.000 | 0.000 | 0.000 | 0.000 | 0.000 | 0.000 | 0.000 | 0.000 | 0.000 | 0.000 | 0.000 | 0.000 | 0.000 | 0.000 | 0.000 | 0.000 | 0.000 |
| 蔬菜类 Vegetables | 0.000 | 0.000 | 0.000 | 0.000 | 0.000 | 0.000 | 0.000 | 0.000 | 0.000 | 0.000 | 0.000 | 0.000 | 0.000 | 0.000 | 0.000 | 0.000 | 0.000 | 0.000 | 0.000 | 0.000 | 0.000 | 0.000 | 0.000 | 0.000 | 0.000 |
| 水果类 Fruits | 0.000 | 0.000 | 0.000 | 0.000 | 0.000 | 0.000 | 0.000 | 0.000 | 0.000 | 0.000 | 0.000 | 0.000 | 0.000 | 0.000 | 0.000 | 0.000 | 0.000 | 0.000 | 0.000 | 0.000 | 0.000 | 0.000 | 0.000 | 0.000 | 0.000 |
| 合计 SUM | 0.000 | 0.000 | 0.000 | 0.037 | 0.000 | 0.132 | 0.000 | 0.000 | 0.000 | 0.000 | 0.000 | 0.000 | 0.000 | 0.238 | 0.000 | 0.000 | 0.000 | 0.000 | 0.000 | 0.000 | 0.000 | 0.000 | 0.000 | 0.000 | 0.017 |

附表 7-28　第六次中国总膳食研究滴滴涕的膳食来源（单位：%）

Annexed Table 7-28　Dietary sources of DDTs from the 6$^{th}$ China TDS (Unit: %)

| 膳食类别<br>Category | 黑龙江<br>HL | 辽宁<br>LN | 河北<br>HE | 北京<br>BJ | 吉林<br>JL | 山西<br>SX | 陕西<br>SN | 河南<br>HA | 宁夏<br>NX | 内蒙古<br>NM | 青海<br>QH | 甘肃<br>GS | 上海<br>SH | 福建<br>FJ | 江西<br>JX | 江苏<br>JS | 浙江<br>ZJ | 山东<br>SD | 湖北<br>HB | 四川<br>SC | 广西<br>GX | 湖南<br>HN | 广东<br>GD | 贵州<br>GZ | 全国平均<br>AVG |
|---|---|---|---|---|---|---|---|---|---|---|---|---|---|---|---|---|---|---|---|---|---|---|---|---|---|
| 谷类 Cereals | 0.0 | 0.0 | 0.0 | 10.1 | 0.0 | 0.0 | 30.2 | 25.8 | 84.1 | 0.0 | 0.0 | 0.0 | 0.0 | 0.0 | 0.0 | 16.7 | 0.0 | 0.0 | 7.1 | 0.0 | 0.0 | 0.0 | 0.0 | 0.0 | 3.4 |
| 豆类 Legumes | 19.3 | 0.0 | 0.0 | 0.0 | 0.0 | 0.0 | 0.0 | 3.5 | 0.0 | 0.0 | 0.0 | 15.1 | 0.6 | 0.0 | 0.0 | 3.6 | 0.0 | 0.0 | 1.3 | 0.0 | 0.0 | 0.0 | 0.0 | 0.0 | 0.9 |
| 薯类 Potatoes | 0.0 | 0.0 | 0.0 | 0.0 | 0.0 | 7.9 | 0.0 | 0.0 | 0.0 | 0.0 | 0.0 | 35.6 | 0.0 | 0.0 | 0.0 | 0.0 | 0.0 | 0.0 | 0.0 | 0.0 | 0.0 | 0.0 | 0.0 | 0.0 | 0.8 |
| 肉类 Meats | 19.8 | 51.2 | 14.4 | 43.5 | 33.1 | 54.8 | 4.3 | 47.9 | 14.2 | 8.6 | 79.7 | 30.0 | 10.2 | 35.9 | 35.3 | 9.8 | 46.1 | 0.0 | 9.1 | 48.7 | 15.8 | 45.5 | 5.8 | 69.9 | 27.6 |
| 蛋类 Eggs | 13.4 | 8.6 | 44.5 | 11.1 | 17.6 | 0.0 | 1.7 | 1.1 | 0.7 | 41.8 | 0.7 | 6.7 | 6.4 | 11.4 | 8.1 | 3.6 | 8.2 | 7.5 | 11.7 | 0.0 | 8.4 | 0.0 | 1.2 | 2.0 | 8.2 |
| 水产类 Aquatic foods | 43.7 | 13.5 | 3.5 | 10.4 | 42.8 | 23.5 | 19.5 | 17.5 | 1.0 | 41.6 | 6.0 | 3.6 | 79.6 | 31.1 | 51.2 | 63.9 | 44.3 | 84.0 | 49.7 | 50.2 | 69.9 | 54.2 | 87.3 | 10.3 | 49.2 |
| 乳类 Dairy products | 3.8 | 17.8 | 2.7 | 18.2 | 6.4 | 13.8 | 44.3 | 4.2 | 0.0 | 8.0 | 13.6 | 9.0 | 1.4 | 12.4 | 5.4 | 2.4 | 1.5 | 8.5 | 1.5 | 1.2 | 5.9 | 0.3 | 5.6 | 17.8 | 5.4 |
| 蔬菜类 Vegetables | 0.0 | 8.9 | 34.9 | 6.7 | 0.0 | 0.0 | 0.0 | 0.0 | 0.0 | 0.0 | 0.0 | 0.0 | 1.9 | 9.2 | 0.0 | 0.0 | 0.0 | 0.0 | 19.5 | 0.0 | 0.0 | 0.0 | 0.0 | 0.0 | 4.7 |
| 水果类 Fruits | 0.0 | 0.0 | 0.0 | 0.0 | 0.0 | 0.0 | 0.0 | 0.0 | 0.0 | 0.0 | 0.0 | 0.0 | 0.0 | 0.0 | 0.0 | 0.0 | 0.0 | 0.0 | 0.0 | 0.0 | 0.0 | 0.0 | 0.0 | 0.0 | 0.0 |
| 糖类 Sugar | 0.0 | 0.0 | 0.0 | 0.0 | 0.0 | 0.0 | 0.0 | 0.0 | 0.0 | 0.0 | 0.0 | 0.0 | 0.0 | 0.0 | 0.0 | 0.0 | 0.0 | 0.0 | 0.0 | 0.0 | 0.0 | 0.0 | 0.0 | 0.0 | 0.0 |
| 水及饮料类 Water and beverages | 0.0 | 0.0 | 0.0 | 0.0 | 0.0 | 0.0 | 0.0 | 0.0 | 0.0 | 0.0 | 0.0 | 0.0 | 0.0 | 0.0 | 0.0 | 0.0 | 0.0 | 0.0 | 0.0 | 0.0 | 0.0 | 0.0 | 0.0 | 0.0 | 0.0 |
| 酒类 Alcohol beverages | 0.0 | 0.0 | 0.0 | 0.0 | 0.0 | 0.0 | 0.0 | 0.0 | 0.0 | 0.0 | 0.0 | 0.0 | 0.0 | 0.0 | 0.0 | 0.0 | 0.0 | 0.0 | 0.0 | 0.0 | 0.0 | 0.0 | 0.0 | 0.0 | 0.0 |

附表 7-29  第六次中国总膳食研究六六六的膳食来源（单位：%）

Annexed Table 7-29  Dietary sources of HCHs from the 6th China TDS (Unit: %)

| 膳食类别 Category | 黑龙江 HL | 辽宁 LN | 河北 HE | 北京 BJ | 吉林 JL | 山西 SX | 陕西 SN | 河南 HA | 宁夏 NX | 内蒙古 NM | 青海 QH | 甘肃 GS | 上海 SH | 福建 FJ | 江西 JX | 江苏 JS | 浙江 ZJ | 山东 SD | 湖北 HB | 四川 SC | 广西 GX | 湖南 HN | 广东 GD | 贵州 GZ | 全国平均 AVG |
|---|---|---|---|---|---|---|---|---|---|---|---|---|---|---|---|---|---|---|---|---|---|---|---|---|---|
| 谷类 Cereals | 0.0 | 0.0 | 59.6 | 0.0 | 0.0 | 0.0 | 0.0 | 0.0 | 0.0 | 0.0 | 0.0 | 0.0 | 0.0 | 0.0 | 0.0 | 0.0 | 0.0 | 0.0 | 0.0 | 0.0 | 0.0 | 0.0 | 0.0 | 0.0 | 9.7 |
| 豆类 Legumes | 2.5 | 27.4 | 3.5 | 0.0 | 31.5 | 0.0 | 0.0 | 0.0 | 3.4 | 0.0 | 0.0 | 3.9 | 0.0 | 0.0 | 0.0 | 0.0 | 0.0 | 0.0 | 0.0 | 0.0 | 0.0 | 0.0 | 7.4 | 0.0 | 4.1 |
| 薯类 Potatoes | 0.0 | 0.0 | 2.8 | 5.0 | 0.0 | 0.0 | 0.0 | 0.0 | 8.7 | 19.6 | 0.0 | 63.0 | 0.0 | 0.0 | 0.0 | 0.0 | 0.0 | 5.5 | 0.0 | 0.0 | 0.0 | 0.0 | 0.0 | 0.0 | 5.3 |
| 肉类 Meats | 11.0 | 30.1 | 5.9 | 19.8 | 11.9 | 76.5 | 7.8 | 51.8 | 85.4 | 5.3 | 37.2 | 25.9 | 9.7 | 35.1 | 0.0 | 38.5 | 17.4 | 11.7 | 4.4 | 68.3 | 56.4 | 23.4 | 0.0 | 25.0 | 24.6 |
| 蛋类 Eggs | 3.3 | 0.0 | 4.2 | 11.4 | 4.8 | 10.6 | 1.6 | 14.7 | 0.3 | 16.2 | 4.4 | 1.5 | 2.8 | 5.2 | 19.0 | 5.6 | 0.0 | 5.3 | 10.8 | 5.4 | 2.2 | 4.5 | 7.9 | 1.4 | 5.1 |
| 水产类 Aquatic foods | 82.4 | 3.4 | 2.7 | 11.9 | 47.3 | 4.7 | 3.2 | 18.4 | 0.5 | 1.5 | 7.5 | 1.0 | 79.1 | 54.9 | 63.0 | 49.1 | 76.8 | 8.4 | 31.2 | 26.3 | 39.9 | 19.1 | 67.8 | 2.2 | 25.9 |
| 乳类 Dairy products | 0.7 | 6.0 | 1.0 | 13.6 | 4.5 | 8.2 | 4.2 | 15.1 | 1.6 | 1.7 | 50.9 | 4.6 | 8.3 | 4.9 | 18.0 | 6.8 | 5.9 | 2.9 | 0.6 | 0.0 | 1.4 | 4.2 | 16.9 | 1.8 | 4.2 |
| 蔬菜类 Vegetables | 0.0 | 33.1 | 20.5 | 38.4 | 0.0 | 0.0 | 83.2 | 0.0 | 0.0 | 55.7 | 0.0 | 1.0 | 0.0 | 0.0 | 0.0 | 0.0 | 0.0 | 66.1 | 53.0 | 0.0 | 0.0 | 48.8 | 0.0 | 69.7 | 21.0 |
| 水果类 Fruits | 0.0 | 0.0 | 0.0 | 0.0 | 0.0 | 0.0 | 0.0 | 0.0 | 0.0 | 0.0 | 0.0 | 0.0 | 0.0 | 0.0 | 0.0 | 0.0 | 0.0 | 0.0 | 0.0 | 0.0 | 0.0 | 0.0 | 0.0 | 0.0 | 0.0 |
| 糖类 Sugar | 0.0 | 0.0 | 0.0 | 0.0 | 0.0 | 0.0 | 0.0 | 0.0 | 0.0 | 0.0 | 0.0 | 0.0 | 0.0 | 0.0 | 0.0 | 0.0 | 0.0 | 0.0 | 0.0 | 0.0 | 0.0 | 0.0 | 0.0 | 0.0 | 0.0 |
| 水及饮料类 Water and beverages | 0.0 | 0.0 | 0.0 | 0.0 | 0.0 | 0.0 | 0.0 | 0.0 | 0.0 | 0.0 | 0.0 | 0.0 | 0.0 | 0.0 | 0.0 | 0.0 | 0.0 | 0.0 | 0.0 | 0.0 | 0.0 | 0.0 | 0.0 | 0.0 | 0.0 |
| 酒类 Alcohol beverages | 0.0 | 0.0 | 0.0 | 0.0 | 0.0 | 0.0 | 0.0 | 0.0 | 0.0 | 0.0 | 0.0 | 0.0 | 0.0 | 0.0 | 0.0 | 0.0 | 0.0 | 0.0 | 0.0 | 0.0 | 0.0 | 0.0 | 0.0 | 0.0 | 0.0 |

附表 7-30　第六次中国总膳食研究混合膳食样品中 PFOA 的含量（单位：μg/kg）

Annexed Table 7-30　Levels of PFOA in food samples from the 6th China TDS (Unit: μg/kg)

| 膳食类别 Category | 黑龙江 HL | 辽宁 LN | 河北 HE | 北京 BJ | 吉林 JL | 山西 SX | 陕西 SN | 河南 HA | 宁夏 NX | 内蒙古 NM | 青海 QH | 甘肃 GS | 上海 SH | 福建 FJ | 江西 JX | 江苏 JS | 浙江 ZJ | 山东 SD | 湖北 HB | 四川 SC | 广西 GX | 湖南 HN | 广东 GD | 贵州 GZ | 全国平均 AVG |
|---|---|---|---|---|---|---|---|---|---|---|---|---|---|---|---|---|---|---|---|---|---|---|---|---|---|
| 谷类 Cereals | ND | ND | ND | ND | ND | ND | 0.09 | ND | 0.03 | ND | ND | ND | ND | ND | 0.02 | ND | ND | ND | ND | ND | ND | ND | ND | ND | 0.01 |
| 豆类 Legumes | ND | ND | ND | ND | ND | ND | ND | ND | ND | ND | ND | ND | 0.02 | ND | 0.06 | 0.02 | ND | ND | ND | ND | ND | ND | ND | ND | 0.01 |
| 薯类 Potatoes | 0.01 | ND | ND | ND | ND | 0.01 | 0.05 | ND | ND | ND | ND | ND | ND | ND | ND | 0.01 | ND | ND | ND | ND | ND | ND | ND | ND | 0.00 |
| 肉类 Meats | 0.04 | 0.03 | 0.07 | ND | 0.05 | ND | 0.02 | ND | ND | 0.05 | 0.02 | 0.03 | 0.04 | 0.07 | 0.03 | 0.07 | 0.12 | 0.15 | 0.05 | 0.02 | ND | ND | ND | 0.02 | 0.04 |
| 蛋类 Eggs | 0.04 | 0.02 | 0.02 | 2.97 | 0.02 | 0.02 | 0.04 | 0.01 | ND | 0.09 | ND | 0.14 | 0.09 | 0.19 | 0.01 | 0.04 | 0.04 | 0.57 | 0.02 | 0.02 | 0.01 | 0.01 | ND | ND | 0.18 |
| 水产类 Aquatic foods | 0.03 | 0.09 | ND | 0.26 | 0.03 | 0.01 | ND | 0.04 | ND | ND | 0.02 | 0.02 | 0.09 | 0.09 | 0.02 | 0.07 | 0.05 | 0.26 | 0.02 | 0.09 | ND | ND | ND | ND | 0.05 |
| 乳类 Dairy products | ND | ND | ND | ND | ND | ND | ND | ND | ND | ND | ND | ND | ND | ND | ND | ND | ND | ND | ND | ND | ND | ND | ND | ND | 0.01 |
| 蔬菜类 Vegetables | ND | ND | ND | ND | ND | 0.01 | ND | ND | ND | ND | ND | ND | 0.04 | ND | 0.01 | 0.01 | 0.03 | ND | ND | ND | ND | ND | ND | ND | 0.01 |
| 水果类 Fruits | ND | ND | ND | ND | ND | ND | ND | ND | ND | ND | ND | ND | ND | ND | ND | ND | ND | ND | ND | ND | ND | ND | ND | ND | 0.00 |

注：未检出（ND）按 1/2 检出限（LOD）计

Note: values not detected (ND) were treated as being equal to half of the detection of limit (LOD)

附表 7-31 第六次中国总膳食研究混合膳食样品中 PFOS 的含量（单位：μg/kg）

Annexed Table 7-31 Levels of PFOS food samples from the 6th China TDS (Unit: μg/kg)

| 膳食类别 Category | 黑龙江 HL | 辽宁 LN | 河北 HE | 北京 BJ | 吉林 JL | 山西 SX | 陕西 SN | 河南 HA | 宁夏 NX | 内蒙古 NM | 青海 QH | 甘肃 GS | 上海 SH | 福建 FJ | 江西 JX | 江苏 JS | 浙江 ZJ | 山东 SD | 湖北 HB | 四川 SC | 广西 GX | 湖南 HN | 广东 GD | 贵州 GZ | 全国平均 AVG |
|---|---|---|---|---|---|---|---|---|---|---|---|---|---|---|---|---|---|---|---|---|---|---|---|---|---|
| 谷类 Cereals | ND | ND | ND | ND | ND | ND | ND | ND | ND | ND | ND | ND | ND | ND | 0.01 | ND | ND | ND | ND | ND | ND | ND | ND | ND | 0.00 |
| 豆类 Legumes | ND | ND | ND | ND | ND | ND | ND | ND | ND | ND | ND | ND | ND | ND | 0.08 | ND | ND | ND | ND | ND | ND | ND | ND | ND | 0.01 |
| 薯类 Potatoes | ND | ND | ND | ND | ND | ND | ND | ND | ND | ND | ND | ND | ND | ND | ND | ND | ND | ND | ND | ND | ND | ND | ND | ND | 0.00 |
| 肉类 Meats | 0.02 | 0.10 | 0.01 | 0.03 | 0.09 | 0.05 | 0.04 | 0.02 | 0.01 | 0.02 | ND | 0.02 | 0.02 | ND | 0.03 | ND | 0.53 | ND | 0.09 | 0.05 | 0.01 | 0.19 | ND | 0.01 | 0.06 |
| 蛋类 Eggs | 0.19 | 0.03 | 0.09 | 0.03 | 0.10 | 0.12 | 0.14 | 0.02 | 0.08 | 0.06 | ND | 0.08 | 0.03 | 0.05 | 0.01 | 0.02 | 0.08 | 0.06 | 0.12 | 0.13 | 0.02 | 0.04 | 0.04 | 0.02 | 0.07 |
| 水产类 Aquatic foods | 4.30 | 0.14 | 0.27 | 0.47 | 0.31 | 0.34 | 0.12 | 0.56 | 0.28 | 0.35 | 0.22 | 0.10 | 0.59 | 0.25 | 0.41 | 0.50 | 0.18 | 0.70 | 0.27 | 0.49 | 0.06 | 0.23 | 0.44 | 0.10 | 0.48 |
| 乳类 Dairy products | ND | ND | ND | ND | ND | ND | ND | ND | ND | ND | ND | ND | ND | ND | ND | ND | ND | ND | ND | ND | ND | ND | ND | ND | 0.00 |
| 蔬菜类 Vegetables | ND | ND | ND | ND | ND | ND | ND | ND | ND | ND | ND | ND | ND | ND | ND | ND | ND | ND | ND | ND | ND | ND | ND | ND | 0.01 |
| 水果类 Fruits | ND | ND | ND | ND | ND | ND | ND | ND | ND | ND | ND | ND | ND | ND | ND | ND | ND | ND | ND | ND | ND | ND | ND | ND | 0.00 |

注：未检出（ND）按 1/2 检出限（LOD）计

Note: values not detected (ND) were treated as being equal to half of the detection of limit (LOD)

附表 7-32　第六次中国总膳食研究 PFOA 的膳食摄入量 [单位: ng/(kg bw·周)]

Annexed Table 7-32　Dietary intakes of PFOA from the 6th China TDS [Unit: ng/(kg bw·week)]

| 膳食类别<br>Category | 黑龙江<br>HL | 辽宁<br>LN | 河北<br>HE | 北京<br>BJ | 吉林<br>JL | 山西<br>SX | 陕西<br>SN | 河南<br>HA | 宁夏<br>NX | 内蒙古<br>NM | 青海<br>QH | 甘肃<br>GS | 上海<br>SH | 福建<br>FJ | 江西<br>JX | 江苏<br>JS | 浙江<br>ZJ | 山东<br>SD | 湖北<br>HB | 四川<br>SC | 广西<br>GX | 湖南<br>HN | 广东<br>GD | 贵州<br>GZ | 全国平均<br>AVG |
|---|---|---|---|---|---|---|---|---|---|---|---|---|---|---|---|---|---|---|---|---|---|---|---|---|---|
| 谷类 Cereals | 0.03 | 0.03 | 0.04 | 0.04 | 0.03 | 0.06 | 7.57 | 0.05 | 2.51 | 0.04 | 0.04 | 0.04 | 0.02 | 0.04 | 1.14 | 0.04 | 0.04 | 0.06 | 0.03 | 0.05 | 0.05 | 0.03 | 0.03 | 0.04 | 0.50 |
| 豆类 Legumes | 0.01 | 0.03 | 0.02 | 0.03 | 0.02 | 0.02 | 0.02 | 0.01 | 0.01 | 0.01 | 0.00 | 0.01 | 0.27 | 0.02 | 0.49 | 0.22 | 0.04 | 0.01 | 0.02 | 0.02 | 0.01 | 0.02 | 0.01 | 0.03 | 0.06 |
| 薯类 Potatoes | 0.07 | 0.00 | 0.00 | 0.00 | 0.01 | 0.19 | 0.66 | 0.00 | 0.01 | 0.01 | 0.01 | 0.01 | 0.00 | 0.00 | 0.00 | 0.04 | 0.00 | 0.00 | 0.00 | 0.00 | 0.00 | 0.00 | 0.00 | 0.00 | 0.04 |
| 肉类 Meats | 0.30 | 0.21 | 0.37 | 0.18 | 0.37 | 0.05 | 0.08 | 0.02 | 0.02 | 0.39 | 0.12 | 0.12 | 0.47 | 0.64 | 0.31 | 0.69 | 1.60 | 1.60 | 0.29 | 0.26 | 0.05 | 0.05 | 0.04 | 0.20 | 0.35 |
| 蛋类 Eggs | 0.16 | 0.09 | 0.07 | 12.80 | 0.07 | 0.05 | 0.10 | 0.05 | 0.00 | 0.31 | 0.00 | 0.33 | 0.41 | 0.40 | 0.03 | 0.12 | 0.11 | 2.84 | 0.05 | 0.04 | 0.01 | 0.02 | 0.00 | 0.00 | 0.75 |
| 水产类 Aquatic foods | 0.08 | 0.16 | 0.00 | 0.47 | 0.03 | 0.01 | 0.00 | 0.02 | 0.00 | 0.00 | 0.01 | 0.00 | 0.66 | 0.63 | 0.10 | 0.30 | 0.28 | 0.65 | 0.09 | 0.09 | 0.01 | 0.01 | 0.01 | 0.00 | 0.15 |
| 乳类 Dairy products | 0.01 | 0.03 | 0.02 | 0.06 | 0.02 | 0.03 | 0.01 | 0.01 | 0.01 | 0.02 | 0.04 | 0.01 | 0.05 | 0.02 | 0.01 | 0.02 | 0.02 | 0.02 | 0.00 | 0.01 | 0.01 | 0.01 | 0.02 | 0.02 | 0.02 |
| 蔬菜类 Vegetables | 0.11 | 0.11 | 0.10 | 0.13 | 0.13 | 0.30 | 0.10 | 0.09 | 0.05 | 0.09 | 0.10 | 0.08 | 1.64 | 0.13 | 0.65 | 0.64 | 1.65 | 0.14 | 0.14 | 0.10 | 0.12 | 0.18 | 0.08 | 0.14 | 0.29 |
| 水果类 Fruits | 0.01 | 0.01 | 0.00 | 0.01 | 0.01 | 0.00 | 0.00 | 0.00 | 0.01 | 0.01 | 0.00 | 0.00 | 0.01 | 0.01 | 0.01 | 0.00 | 0.01 | 0.01 | 0.00 | 0.00 | 0.01 | 0.01 | 0.00 | 0.00 | 0.01 |
| 合计 SUM | 0.77 | 0.67 | 0.61 | 13.73 | 0.70 | 0.70 | 8.54 | 0.27 | 2.61 | 0.89 | 0.32 | 0.61 | 3.52 | 1.90 | 2.73 | 2.07 | 3.74 | 5.32 | 0.63 | 0.58 | 0.28 | 0.33 | 0.18 | 0.42 | 2.17 |

附表 7-33 第六次中国总膳食研究 PFOS 的膳食摄入量 [单位：ng/(kg bw·周)]

Annexed Table 7-33  Dietary intakes of PFOS from the 6th China TDS [Unit: ng/(kg bw·week)]

| 膳食类别 Category | 黑龙江 HL | 辽宁 LN | 河北 HE | 北京 BJ | 吉林 JL | 山西 SX | 陕西 SN | 河南 HA | 宁夏 NX | 内蒙古 NM | 青海 QH | 甘肃 GS | 上海 SH | 福建 FJ | 江西 JX | 江苏 JS | 浙江 ZJ | 山东 SD | 湖北 HB | 四川 SC | 广西 GX | 湖南 HN | 广东 GD | 贵州 GZ | 全国平均 AVG |
|---|---|---|---|---|---|---|---|---|---|---|---|---|---|---|---|---|---|---|---|---|---|---|---|---|---|
| 谷类 Cereals | 0.03 | 0.03 | 0.04 | 0.04 | 0.03 | 0.06 | 0.04 | 0.05 | 0.04 | 0.04 | 0.04 | 0.04 | 0.02 | 0.04 | 0.76 | 0.04 | 0.04 | 0.06 | 0.03 | 0.05 | 0.05 | 0.03 | 0.03 | 0.04 | 0.07 |
| 豆类 Legumes | 0.01 | 0.03 | 0.02 | 0.03 | 0.02 | 0.02 | 0.02 | 0.01 | 0.01 | 0.01 | 0.00 | 0.01 | 0.03 | 0.02 | 0.67 | 0.02 | 0.04 | 0.01 | 0.02 | 0.02 | 0.01 | 0.02 | 0.01 | 0.03 | 0.05 |
| 薯类 Potatoes | 0.01 | 0.01 | 0.01 | 0.01 | 0.01 | 0.01 | 0.01 | 0.01 | 0.01 | 0.01 | 0.01 | 0.02 | 0.00 | 0.00 | 0.00 | 0.00 | 0.00 | 0.01 | 0.01 | 0.01 | 0.00 | 0.01 | 0.00 | 0.00 | 0.01 |
| 肉类 Meats | 0.15 | 0.73 | 0.04 | 0.20 | 0.67 | 0.77 | 0.16 | 0.12 | 0.05 | 0.16 | 0.02 | 0.09 | 0.22 | 0.02 | 0.32 | 0.02 | 7.00 | 0.02 | 0.51 | 0.65 | 0.15 | 3.12 | 0.02 | 0.09 | 0.64 |
| 蛋类 Eggs | 0.85 | 0.13 | 0.33 | 0.14 | 0.45 | 0.27 | 0.35 | 0.05 | 0.12 | 0.20 | 0.00 | 0.19 | 0.14 | 0.11 | 0.03 | 0.07 | 0.20 | 0.32 | 0.34 | 0.21 | 0.04 | 0.10 | 0.11 | 0.04 | 0.20 |
| 水产类 Aquatic foods | 12.98 | 0.25 | 0.29 | 0.85 | 0.38 | 0.24 | 0.05 | 0.29 | 0.08 | 0.40 | 0.09 | 0.03 | 4.48 | 1.81 | 2.01 | 2.15 | 1.03 | 1.57 | 1.19 | 0.45 | 0.64 | 1.67 | 2.48 | 0.04 | 1.48 |
| 乳类 Dairy products | 0.00 | 0.00 | 0.00 | 0.01 | 0.00 | 0.00 | 0.00 | 0.00 | 0.00 | 0.00 | 0.00 | 0.00 | 0.01 | 0.00 | 0.00 | 0.00 | 0.00 | 0.00 | 0.00 | 0.00 | 0.00 | 0.00 | 0.00 | 0.00 | 0.00 |
| 蔬菜类 Vegetables | 0.25 | 0.25 | 0.23 | 0.30 | 0.30 | 0.24 | 0.22 | 0.22 | 0.12 | 0.20 | 0.24 | 0.19 | 0.31 | 0.31 | 0.35 | 0.33 | 0.35 | 0.32 | 0.32 | 0.24 | 0.27 | 0.42 | 0.18 | 0.32 | 0.27 |
| 水果类 Fruits | 0.01 | 0.01 | 0.00 | 0.01 | 0.01 | 0.00 | 0.00 | 0.00 | 0.01 | 0.01 | 0.00 | 0.00 | 0.01 | 0.01 | 0.01 | 0.00 | 0.01 | 0.01 | 0.00 | 0.00 | 0.01 | 0.01 | 0.00 | 0.00 | 0.01 |
| 合计 SUM | 14.28 | 1.46 | 0.96 | 1.59 | 1.88 | 1.62 | 0.88 | 0.76 | 0.43 | 1.04 | 0.41 | 0.57 | 5.23 | 2.32 | 4.15 | 2.65 | 8.67 | 2.31 | 2.43 | 1.63 | 1.17 | 5.37 | 2.84 | 0.55 | 2.72 |

注：摄入量合计时，摄入量 <0.001 的结果按 0 计

Note: values <0.001 were treated as 0

附表 7-34　第六次中国总膳食研究 PFOA 的膳食来源（单位：%）

Annexed Table 7-34　Dietary sources of PFOA from the 6th China TDS (Unit: %)

| 膳食类别 Category | 黑龙江 HL | 辽宁 LN | 河北 HE | 北京 BJ | 吉林 JL | 山西 SX | 陕西 SN | 河南 HA | 宁夏 NX | 内蒙古 NM | 青海 QH | 甘肃 GS | 上海 SH | 福建 FJ | 江西 JX | 江苏 JS | 浙江 ZJ | 山东 SD | 湖北 HB | 四川 SC | 广西 GX | 湖南 HN | 广东 GD | 贵州 GZ | 全国平均 AVG |
|---|---|---|---|---|---|---|---|---|---|---|---|---|---|---|---|---|---|---|---|---|---|---|---|---|---|
| 谷类 Cereals | 3.9 | 5.1 | 6.8 | 0.3 | 4.7 | 8.3 | 88.6 | 19.0 | 96.0 | 4.5 | 13.3 | 6.3 | 0.7 | 1.8 | 41.6 | 2.1 | 0.9 | 1.0 | 4.7 | 9.4 | 19.0 | 9.7 | 13.9 | 8.8 | 23.1 |
| 豆类 Legumes | 1.6 | 5.0 | 2.6 | 0.2 | 3.0 | 2.8 | 0.3 | 5.5 | 0.4 | 1.3 | 0.6 | 1.9 | 7.6 | 1.1 | 17.9 | 10.4 | 1.0 | 0.3 | 2.9 | 3.3 | 4.3 | 6.1 | 4.2 | 6.6 | 2.6 |
| 薯类 Potatoes | 8.5 | 0.6 | 0.6 | 0.0 | 1.0 | 26.8 | 7.7 | 1.7 | 0.2 | 0.8 | 1.8 | 1.3 | 0.1 | 0.1 | 0.1 | 2.0 | 0.1 | 0.0 | 0.8 | 0.6 | 0.3 | 0.9 | 0.8 | 0.4 | 2.0 |
| 肉类 Meats | 38.4 | 30.9 | 59.6 | 1.3 | 53.1 | 6.8 | 1.0 | 7.1 | 0.6 | 44.3 | 37.7 | 19.0 | 13.3 | 33.9 | 11.5 | 33.3 | 42.7 | 30.1 | 46.6 | 45.9 | 18.9 | 15.6 | 19.6 | 47.0 | 16.2 |
| 蛋类 Eggs | 21.1 | 13.4 | 11.0 | 93.2 | 10.6 | 6.6 | 1.2 | 18.3 | 0.0 | 35.3 | 0.1 | 54.9 | 11.5 | 21.2 | 0.9 | 5.6 | 2.9 | 53.3 | 7.2 | 6.3 | 4.0 | 6.0 | 0.2 | 0.1 | 34.6 |
| 水产类 Aquatic foods | 10.5 | 23.3 | 0.2 | 3.4 | 4.7 | 1.4 | 0.0 | 8.3 | 0.0 | 0.1 | 2.7 | 0.8 | 18.6 | 33.3 | 3.5 | 14.7 | 7.6 | 12.3 | 14.8 | 15.3 | 3.9 | 2.2 | 3.1 | 0.1 | 7.0 |
| 乳类 Dairy products | 1.2 | 4.4 | 2.6 | 0.4 | 3.1 | 4.0 | 0.2 | 4.8 | 0.4 | 2.6 | 11.1 | 1.6 | 1.4 | 1.3 | 0.5 | 0.9 | 0.6 | 0.3 | 0.7 | 1.5 | 4.4 | 3.6 | 13.3 | 4.4 | 0.9 |
| 蔬菜类 Vegetables | 13.8 | 16.2 | 15.9 | 1.0 | 18.5 | 42.8 | 1.1 | 34.3 | 2.0 | 9.7 | 32.3 | 13.6 | 46.6 | 7.0 | 23.7 | 30.9 | 44.1 | 2.5 | 21.9 | 17.5 | 42.8 | 53.8 | 43.1 | 32.0 | 13.4 |
| 水果类 Fruits | 0.9 | 1.3 | 0.7 | 0.1 | 1.4 | 0.6 | 0.0 | 1.0 | 0.4 | 1.4 | 0.5 | 0.6 | 0.2 | 0.3 | 0.2 | 0.1 | 0.2 | 0.1 | 0.3 | 0.3 | 2.6 | 2.1 | 1.8 | 0.5 | 0.3 |

附表 7-35　第六次中国总膳食研究 PFOS 的膳食来源（单位：%）

Annexed Table 7-35　Dietary sources of PFOS from the 6th China TDS (Unit: %)

| 膳食类别 Category | 黑龙江 HL | 辽宁 LN | 河北 HE | 北京 BJ | 吉林 JL | 山西 SX | 陕西 SN | 河南 HA | 宁夏 NX | 内蒙古 NM | 青海 QH | 甘肃 GS | 上海 SH | 福建 FJ | 江西 JX | 江苏 JS | 浙江 ZJ | 山东 SD | 湖北 HB | 四川 SC | 广西 GX | 湖南 HN | 广东 GD | 贵州 GZ | 全国平均 AVG |
|---|---|---|---|---|---|---|---|---|---|---|---|---|---|---|---|---|---|---|---|---|---|---|---|---|---|
| 谷类 Cereals | 0.2 | 2.3 | 4.4 | 2.8 | 1.7 | 3.5 | 4.8 | 6.8 | 8.5 | 3.9 | 10.5 | 6.7 | 0.5 | 1.5 | 18.4 | 1.6 | 0.4 | 2.4 | 1.2 | 3.3 | 4.5 | 0.6 | 0.9 | 6.8 | 2.6 |
| 豆类 Legumes | 0.1 | 2.3 | 1.7 | 1.8 | 1.1 | 1.2 | 2.6 | 2.0 | 2.3 | 1.1 | 0.4 | 2.0 | 0.6 | 0.9 | 16.1 | 0.9 | 0.5 | 0.6 | 0.8 | 1.2 | 1.0 | 0.4 | 0.3 | 5.1 | 1.7 |
| 薯类 Potatoes | 0.1 | 0.5 | 0.7 | 0.4 | 0.7 | 0.8 | 1.5 | 1.2 | 2.6 | 1.3 | 2.8 | 2.8 | 0.1 | 0.2 | 0.1 | 0.1 | 0.0 | 0.2 | 0.4 | 0.4 | 0.1 | 0.1 | 0.1 | 0.7 | 0.3 |
| 肉类 Meats | 1.0 | 50.3 | 4.5 | 12.4 | 35.6 | 47.7 | 18.7 | 15.8 | 12.0 | 15.5 | 4.2 | 15.0 | 4.3 | 0.9 | 7.7 | 0.8 | 80.7 | 1.0 | 21.1 | 40.0 | 12.6 | 58.0 | 0.9 | 15.7 | 23.5 |
| 蛋类 Eggs | 5.9 | 9.1 | 34.1 | 8.7 | 23.9 | 16.7 | 40.3 | 7.0 | 26.7 | 19.2 | 0.3 | 33.7 | 2.7 | 4.7 | 0.6 | 2.7 | 2.4 | 13.9 | 14.1 | 12.8 | 3.2 | 1.9 | 3.8 | 6.7 | 7.3 |
| 水产类 Aquatic foods | 90.9 | 17.1 | 30.0 | 53.5 | 20.2 | 14.7 | 6.0 | 38.1 | 17.4 | 38.4 | 21.0 | 5.4 | 85.7 | 78.1 | 48.4 | 81.2 | 11.9 | 67.8 | 49.1 | 27.8 | 54.4 | 31.1 | 87.3 | 6.9 | 54.4 |
| 乳类 Dairy products | 0.0 | 0.3 | 0.2 | 0.4 | 0.1 | 0.2 | 0.2 | 0.2 | 0.3 | 0.3 | 1.1 | 0.2 | 0.1 | 0.1 | 0.0 | 0.1 | 0.0 | 0.1 | 0.0 | 0.1 | 0.1 | 0.0 | 0.1 | 0.4 | 0.1 |
| 蔬菜类 Vegetables | 1.7 | 17.4 | 23.9 | 19.2 | 16.1 | 14.8 | 25.5 | 28.6 | 28.1 | 19.2 | 59.4 | 33.7 | 6.0 | 13.3 | 8.5 | 12.5 | 4.0 | 13.7 | 13.2 | 14.4 | 23.5 | 7.7 | 6.5 | 57.3 | 10.0 |
| 水果类 Fruits | 0.0 | 0.6 | 0.4 | 0.8 | 0.5 | 0.2 | 0.5 | 0.4 | 2.2 | 1.2 | 0.4 | 0.6 | 0.2 | 0.3 | 0.2 | 0.1 | 0.1 | 0.3 | 0.1 | 0.1 | 0.6 | 0.1 | 0.1 | 0.4 | 0.2 |

附表 7-36　第六次中国总膳食研究膳食样品中短链氯化石蜡的含量（单位：ng/g）

Annexed Table 7-36　Levels of SCCPs in food samples from the 6th China TDS (Unit: ng/g)

| 膳食类别 Category | 黑龙江 HL | 辽宁 LN | 河北 HE | 北京 BJ | 吉林 JL | 山西 SX | 陕西 SN | 河南 HA | 宁夏 NX | 内蒙古 NM | 青海 QH | 甘肃 GS | 上海 SH | 福建 FJ | 江西 JX | 江苏 JS | 浙江 ZJ | 山东 SD | 湖北 HB | 四川 SC | 广西 GX | 湖南 HN | 广东 GD | 贵州 GZ | 全国平均 AVG |
|---|---|---|---|---|---|---|---|---|---|---|---|---|---|---|---|---|---|---|---|---|---|---|---|---|---|
| 谷类 Cereals | 265 | 71 | 39 | 29 | 22 | 122 | 36 | 162 | 30 | 43 | 38 | 24 | 21 | 26 | 5 | 9 | 23 | 63 | 11 | 47 | 9 | 38 | 41 | 13 | 49 |
| 豆类 Legumes | 44 | 52 | 162 | 50 | 50 | 19 | 28 | 86 | 89 | 51 | 35 | 43 | 16 | 75 | 12 | 44 | 76 | 18 | 83 | 51 | 69 | 12 | 79 | 93 | 56 |
| 薯类 Potatoes | 12 | 44 | 15 | 30 | 36 | 25 | 14 | 31 | 28 | 28 | 40 | 40 | 17 | 35 | 14 | 17 | 27 | 36 | 17 | 40 | 19 | 23 | 38 | 28 | 27 |
| 肉类 Meats | 31 | 81 | 39 | 25 | 84 | 98 | 58 | 48 | 35 | 49 | 78 | 27 | 39 | 81 | 32 | 116 | 98 | 71 | 80 | 89 | 45 | 80 | 78 | 50 | 63 |
| 蛋类 Eggs | 22 | 11 | 36 | 28 | 53 | 69 | 101 | 14 | 55 | 54 | 73 | 81 | 28 | 69 | 53 | 65 | 70 | 27 | 61 | 102 | 74 | 81 | 27 | 80 | 56 |
| 水产类 Aquatic foods | 44 | 12 | 55 | 22 | 86 | 34 | 62 | 26 | 23 | 77 | 72 | 34 | 40 | 75 | 42 | 56 | 71 | 142 | 87 | 12 | 47 | 36 | 60 | 45 | 53 |
| 乳类 Dairy products | 28 | 50 | 83 | 35 | 18 | 89 | 82 | 69 | 85 | 14 | 71 | 9 | 13 | 34 | 46 | 22 | 43 | 72 | 64 | 53 | 30 | 39 | 117 | 47 | 51 |
| 蔬菜类 Vegetables | 50 | 46 | 73 | 18 | 27 | 43 | 18 | 64 | 70 | 20 | 69 | 66 | 13 | 21 | 12 | 113 | 55 | 40 | 42 | 20 | 24 | 19 | 32 | 34 | 41 |

附表 7-37 第六次中国总膳食研究膳食样品中中链氯化石蜡的含量（单位：ng/g）

Annexed Table 7-37　Levels of MCCPs in food samples from the 6th China TDS (Unit: ng/g)

| 膳食类别 Category | 黑龙江 HL | 辽宁 LN | 河北 HE | 北京 BJ | 吉林 JL | 山西 SX | 陕西 SN | 河南 HA | 宁夏 NX | 内蒙古 NM | 青海 QH | 甘肃 GS | 上海 SH | 福建 FJ | 江西 JX | 江苏 JS | 浙江 ZJ | 山东 SD | 湖北 HB | 四川 SC | 广西 GX | 湖南 HN | 广东 GD | 贵州 GZ | 全国平均 AVG |
|---|---|---|---|---|---|---|---|---|---|---|---|---|---|---|---|---|---|---|---|---|---|---|---|---|---|
| 谷类 Cereals | 306 | 72 | 31 | 23 | 11 | 66 | 29 | 141 | 28 | 38 | 39 | 25 | 6 | 20 | 12 | 21 | 13 | 99 | 10 | 47 | 11 | 21 | 40 | 13 | 47 |
| 豆类 Legumes | 32 | 38 | 202 | 40 | 44 | 14 | 53 | 110 | 104 | 58 | 28 | 46 | 5 | 33 | 12 | 12 | 16 | 16 | 36 | 78 | 34 | 12 | 111 | 35 | 49 |
| 薯类 Potatoes | 12 | 42 | 8 | 12 | 70 | 14 | 7 | 24 | 22 | 17 | 40 | 23 | 10 | 6 | 4 | 11 | 8 | 31 | 10 | 20 | 6 | 6 | 15 | 8 | 18 |
| 肉类 Meats | 35 | 97 | 51 | 30 | 108 | 147 | 114 | 58 | 48 | 62 | 100 | 32 | 13 | 53 | 37 | 103 | 57 | 74 | 95 | 76 | 71 | 67 | 81 | 71 | 70 |
| 蛋类 Eggs | 36 | 29 | 40 | 29 | 65 | 51 | 79 | 97 | 59 | 84 | 177 | 92 | 23 | 48 | 53 | 87 | 23 | 34 | 51 | 47 | 40 | 30 | 31 | 62 | 57 |
| 水产类 Aquatic foods | 46 | 17 | 72 | 33 | 71 | 40 | 61 | 16 | 37 | 86 | 58 | 33 | 12 | 47 | 36 | 17 | 30 | 161 | 72 | 12 | 31 | 26 | 82 | 53 | 48 |
| 乳类 Dairy products | 19 | 71 | 114 | 42 | 33 | 70 | 86 | 111 | 209 | 19 | 54 | 15 | 5 | 13 | 15 | 6 | 17 | 43 | 23 | 39 | 7 | 13 | 104 | 11 | 47 |
| 蔬菜类 Vegetables | 29 | 27 | 70 | 15 | 18 | 30 | 14 | 69 | 72 | 13 | 70 | 80 | 12 | 18 | 10 | 66 | 16 | 25 | 27 | 18 | 19 | 20 | 21 | 20 | 32 |

附表 7-38　第六次中国总膳食研究的短链氯化石蜡膳食摄入量 [单位: ng/(kg bw · d)]
Annexed Table 7-38　Dietary intakes of SCCPs from the 6th China TDS [Unit: ng/(kg bw · d)]

| 膳食类别 Category | 黑龙江 HL | 辽宁 LN | 河北 HE | 北京 BJ | 吉林 JL | 山西 SX | 陕西 SN | 河南 HA | 宁夏 NX | 内蒙古 NM | 青海 QH | 甘肃 GS | 上海 SH | 福建 FJ | 江西 JX | 江苏 JS | 浙江 ZJ | 山东 SD | 湖北 HB | 四川 SC | 广西 GX | 湖南 HN | 广东 GD | 贵州 GZ | 全国平均 AVG |
|---|---|---|---|---|---|---|---|---|---|---|---|---|---|---|---|---|---|---|---|---|---|---|---|---|---|
| 谷类 Cereals | 2305 | 694 | 468 | 366 | 204 | 2009 | 436 | 2377 | 315 | 493 | 462 | 261 | 150 | 261 | 52 | 115 | 231 | 633 | 92 | 724 | 136 | 348 | 297 | 139 | 565 |
| 豆类 Legumes | 32 | 101 | 147 | 81 | 60 | 21 | 37 | 74 | 50 | 32 | 4 | 28 | 30 | 94 | 14 | 58 | 170 | 40 | 88 | 55 | 46 | 14 | 35 | 151 | 61 |
| 薯类 Potatoes | 15 | 50 | 15 | 28 | 69 | 47 | 25 | 40 | 44 | 54 | 64 | 91 | 10 | 23 | 7 | 9 | 16 | 21 | 24 | 40 | 4 | 20 | 15 | 15 | 31 |
| 肉类 Meats | 29 | 86 | 29 | 27 | 89 | 213 | 33 | 42 | 26 | 57 | 88 | 13 | 69 | 111 | 48 | 169 | 184 | 133 | 69 | 182 | 108 | 190 | 129 | 84 | 92 |
| 蛋类 Eggs | 14 | 7 | 18 | 17 | 34 | 23 | 35 | 7 | 11 | 25 | 15 | 29 | 17 | 21 | 18 | 29 | 27 | 10 | 24 | 24 | 16 | 30 | 10 | 20 | 20 |
| 水产类 Aquatic foods | 19 | 3 | 8 | 6 | 15 | 3 | 4 | 2 | 1 | 13 | 4 | 2 | 44 | 76 | 29 | 35 | 56 | 113 | 57 | 2 | 72 | 38 | 49 | 3 | 27 |
| 乳类 Dairy products | 6 | 35 | 32 | 48 | 9 | 59 | 25 | 21 | 21 | 8 | 60 | 2 | 15 | 19 | 16 | 10 | 23 | 38 | 7 | 11 | 9 | 11 | 68 | 21 | 24 |
| 蔬菜类 Vegetables | 254 | 238 | 340 | 112 | 166 | 211 | 82 | 282 | 174 | 82 | 340 | 260 | 83 | 132 | 86 | 762 | 388 | 282 | 276 | 96 | 134 | 161 | 120 | 220 | 220 |
| 合计 SUM | 2675 | 1215 | 1057 | 684 | 646 | 2587 | 678 | 2844 | 642 | 765 | 1038 | 686 | 417 | 738 | 270 | 1187 | 1094 | 1271 | 637 | 1132 | 526 | 812 | 723 | 653 | 1041 |

附表 7-39 第六次中国总膳食研究的中链氯化石蜡膳食摄入量 [单位: ng/(kg bw·d)]

Annexed Table 7-39  Dietary intakes of MCCPs from the 6th China TDS [Unit: ng/(kg bw·d)]

| 膳食类别 Category | 黑龙江 HL | 辽宁 LN | 河北 HE | 北京 BJ | 吉林 JL | 山西 SX | 陕西 SN | 河南 HA | 宁夏 NX | 内蒙古 NM | 青海 QH | 甘肃 GS | 上海 SH | 福建 FJ | 江西 JX | 江苏 JS | 浙江 ZJ | 山东 SD | 湖北 HB | 四川 SC | 广西 GX | 湖南 HN | 广东 GD | 贵州 GZ | 全国平均 AVG |
|---|---|---|---|---|---|---|---|---|---|---|---|---|---|---|---|---|---|---|---|---|---|---|---|---|---|
| 谷类 Cereals | 2662 | 703 | 372 | 290 | 102 | 1087 | 351 | 2068 | 294 | 436 | 474 | 272 | 45 | 201 | 120 | 259 | 131 | 994 | 84 | 724 | 164 | 192 | 290 | 139 | 519 |
| 豆类 Legumes | 23 | 74 | 183 | 65 | 53 | 15 | 70 | 94 | 58 | 37 | 3 | 30 | 9 | 41 | 14 | 16 | 36 | 36 | 38 | 84 | 23 | 14 | 49 | 57 | 47 |
| 薯类 Potatoes | 15 | 48 | 8 | 11 | 133 | 26 | 13 | 31 | 35 | 33 | 64 | 53 | 6 | 4 | 2 | 6 | 4 | 18 | 14 | 20 | 1 | 5 | 6 | 4 | 23 |
| 肉类 Meats | 33 | 103 | 38 | 32 | 114 | 320 | 65 | 51 | 36 | 72 | 113 | 16 | 23 | 72 | 55 | 150 | 107 | 139 | 81 | 155 | 170 | 160 | 134 | 119 | 98 |
| 蛋类 Eggs | 23 | 19 | 20 | 18 | 41 | 17 | 28 | 46 | 12 | 40 | 37 | 32 | 14 | 14 | 18 | 39 | 9 | 13 | 20 | 11 | 9 | 11 | 12 | 16 | 22 |
| 水产类 Aquatic foods | 20 | 4 | 11 | 9 | 13 | 4 | 4 | 1 | 1 | 14 | 3 | 1 | 13 | 48 | 25 | 11 | 24 | 129 | 47 | 2 | 48 | 27 | 67 | 3 | 22 |
| 乳类 Dairy products | 4 | 50 | 44 | 57 | 17 | 46 | 26 | 35 | 51 | 10 | 46 | 3 | 6 | 7 | 5 | 2 | 9 | 23 | 2 | 8 | 2 | 4 | 60 | 5 | 22 |
| 蔬菜类 Vegetables | 148 | 140 | 326 | 93 | 111 | 147 | 64 | 304 | 179 | 53 | 345 | 315 | 76 | 113 | 72 | 445 | 113 | 176 | 177 | 86 | 106 | 170 | 79 | 130 | 165 |
| 合计 SUM | 2927 | 1141 | 1002 | 575 | 584 | 1663 | 620 | 2630 | 666 | 695 | 1085 | 723 | 192 | 502 | 311 | 928 | 432 | 1527 | 465 | 1089 | 524 | 583 | 696 | 473 | 918 |

附表 7-40 第六次中国总膳食研究短链氯化石蜡的膳食来源（单位：%）

Annexed Table 7-40 Dietary sources of SCCPs from the 6$^{th}$ China TDS (Unit: %)

| 膳食类别 Category | 黑龙江 HL | 辽宁 LN | 河北 HE | 北京 BJ | 吉林 JL | 山西 SX | 陕西 SN | 河南 HA | 宁夏 NX | 内蒙古 NM | 青海 QH | 甘肃 GS | 上海 SH | 福建 FJ | 江西 JX | 江苏 JS | 浙江 ZJ | 山东 SD | 湖北 HB | 四川 SC | 广西 GX | 湖南 HN | 广东 GD | 贵州 GZ | 全国平均 AVG |
|---|---|---|---|---|---|---|---|---|---|---|---|---|---|---|---|---|---|---|---|---|---|---|---|---|---|
| 谷类 Cereals | 86.2 | 57.1 | 44.3 | 53.5 | 31.6 | 77.7 | 64.3 | 83.6 | 49.1 | 64.4 | 44.5 | 38.0 | 36.0 | 35.4 | 19.3 | 9.7 | 21.1 | 49.8 | 14.4 | 64.0 | 25.9 | 42.9 | 41.1 | 21.3 | 44.8 |
| 豆类 Legumes | 1.2 | 8.3 | 13.9 | 11.8 | 9.3 | 0.8 | 5.5 | 2.6 | 7.8 | 4.2 | 0.4 | 4.1 | 7.2 | 12.7 | 5.2 | 4.9 | 15.5 | 3.1 | 13.8 | 4.9 | 8.7 | 1.7 | 4.8 | 23.1 | 7.3 |
| 薯类 Potatoes | 0.6 | 4.1 | 1.4 | 4.1 | 10.7 | 1.8 | 3.7 | 1.4 | 6.9 | 7.1 | 6.2 | 13.3 | 2.4 | 3.1 | 2.6 | 0.8 | 1.5 | 1.7 | 3.8 | 3.5 | 0.8 | 2.5 | 2.1 | 2.3 | 3.7 |
| 肉类 Meats | 1.1 | 7.1 | 2.7 | 3.9 | 13.8 | 8.2 | 4.9 | 1.5 | 4.0 | 7.5 | 8.5 | 1.9 | 16.5 | 15.0 | 17.8 | 14.2 | 16.8 | 10.5 | 10.8 | 16.1 | 20.5 | 23.4 | 17.8 | 12.9 | 10.7 |
| 蛋类 Eggs | 0.5 | 0.6 | 1.7 | 2.5 | 5.3 | 0.9 | 5.2 | 0.2 | 1.7 | 3.3 | 1.4 | 4.2 | 4.1 | 2.8 | 6.7 | 2.4 | 2.5 | 0.8 | 3.8 | 2.1 | 3.0 | 3.7 | 1.4 | 3.1 | 2.7 |
| 水产类 Aquatic foods | 0.7 | 0.2 | 0.8 | 0.9 | 2.3 | 0.1 | 0.6 | 0.1 | 0.2 | 1.7 | 0.4 | 0.3 | 10.6 | 10.3 | 10.7 | 2.9 | 5.1 | 8.9 | 8.9 | 0.2 | 13.7 | 4.7 | 6.8 | 0.5 | 3.8 |
| 乳类 Dairy products | 0.2 | 2.9 | 3.0 | 7.0 | 1.4 | 2.3 | 3.7 | 0.7 | 3.3 | 1.0 | 5.8 | 0.3 | 3.6 | 2.6 | 5.9 | 0.8 | 2.1 | 3.0 | 1.1 | 1.0 | 1.7 | 1.4 | 9.4 | 3.2 | 2.8 |
| 蔬菜类 Vegetables | 9.5 | 19.6 | 32.2 | 16.4 | 25.7 | 8.2 | 12.1 | 9.9 | 27.1 | 10.7 | 32.8 | 37.9 | 19.9 | 17.9 | 31.9 | 64.2 | 35.5 | 22.2 | 43.3 | 8.5 | 25.5 | 19.8 | 16.6 | 33.7 | 24.2 |

附表 7-41 第六次中国总膳食研究中链氯化石蜡的膳食来源（单位：%）

Annexed Table 7-41 Dietary sources of MCCPs from the 6th China TDS (Unit: %)

| 膳食类别 Category | 黑龙江 HL | 辽宁 LN | 河北 HE | 北京 BJ | 吉林 JL | 山西 SX | 陕西 SN | 河南 HA | 宁夏 NX | 内蒙古 NM | 青海 QH | 甘肃 GS | 上海 SH | 福建 FJ | 江西 JX | 江苏 JS | 浙江 ZJ | 山东 SD | 湖北 HB | 四川 SC | 广西 GX | 湖南 HN | 广东 GD | 贵州 GZ | 全国平均 AVG |
|---|---|---|---|---|---|---|---|---|---|---|---|---|---|---|---|---|---|---|---|---|---|---|---|---|---|
| 谷类 Cereals | 90.9 | 61.6 | 37.1 | 50.4 | 17.5 | 65.4 | 56.6 | 78.6 | 44.1 | 62.7 | 43.7 | 37.6 | 23.4 | 40.0 | 38.6 | 27.9 | 30.3 | 65.1 | 18.1 | 66.5 | 31.3 | 32.9 | 41.7 | 29.4 | 45.5 |
| 豆类 Legumes | 0.8 | 6.5 | 18.3 | 11.3 | 9.1 | 0.9 | 11.3 | 3.6 | 8.7 | 5.3 | 0.3 | 4.1 | 4.7 | 8.2 | 4.5 | 1.7 | 8.3 | 2.4 | 8.2 | 7.7 | 4.4 | 2.4 | 7.0 | 12.1 | 6.3 |
| 薯类 Potatoes | 0.5 | 4.2 | 0.8 | 1.9 | 22.8 | 1.6 | 2.1 | 1.2 | 5.3 | 4.7 | 5.9 | 7.3 | 3.1 | 0.8 | 0.6 | 0.6 | 0.9 | 1.2 | 3.0 | 1.8 | 0.2 | 0.9 | 0.9 | 0.8 | 3.0 |
| 肉类 Meats | 1.1 | 9.0 | 3.8 | 5.6 | 19.5 | 19.2 | 10.5 | 1.9 | 5.4 | 10.4 | 10.4 | 2.2 | 12.0 | 14.3 | 17.7 | 16.2 | 24.8 | 9.1 | 17.4 | 14.2 | 32.4 | 27.4 | 19.3 | 25.2 | 13.7 |
| 蛋类 Eggs | 0.8 | 1.7 | 2.0 | 3.1 | 7.0 | 1.0 | 4.5 | 1.7 | 1.8 | 5.8 | 3.4 | 4.4 | 7.3 | 2.8 | 5.8 | 4.2 | 2.1 | 0.9 | 4.3 | 1.0 | 1.7 | 1.9 | 1.7 | 3.4 | 3.1 |
| 水产类 Aquatic foods | 0.7 | 0.4 | 1.1 | 1.6 | 2.2 | 0.2 | 0.6 | 0.0 | 0.2 | 2.0 | 0.3 | 0.1 | 6.8 | 9.6 | 8.0 | 1.2 | 5.6 | 8.4 | 10.1 | 0.2 | 9.2 | 4.6 | 9.6 | 0.6 | 3.5 |
| 乳类 Dairy products | 0.1 | 4.4 | 4.4 | 9.9 | 2.9 | 2.8 | 4.2 | 1.3 | 7.7 | 1.4 | 4.2 | 0.4 | 3.1 | 1.4 | 1.6 | 0.2 | 2.1 | 1.5 | 0.4 | 0.7 | 0.4 | 0.7 | 8.6 | 1.1 | 2.7 |
| 蔬菜类 Vegetables | 5.1 | 12.3 | 32.5 | 16.2 | 19.0 | 8.8 | 10.3 | 11.6 | 26.9 | 7.6 | 31.8 | 43.6 | 39.6 | 22.5 | 23.2 | 48.0 | 26.2 | 11.5 | 38.1 | 7.9 | 20.2 | 29.2 | 11.4 | 27.5 | 22.1 |

# 第八章 附 表
# Annexed Tables of Chapter 8

附表 8-1 第六次中国总膳食研究膳食样品中黄曲霉毒素 B1 的含量（单位：μg/kg）

Annexed Table 8-1 Levels of aflatoxin B1 in food samples from the 6th China TDS (Unit: μg/kg)

| 膳食类别<br>Category | 黑龙江<br>HL | 辽宁<br>LN | 河北<br>HE | 北京<br>BJ | 吉林<br>JL | 山西<br>SX | 陕西<br>SN | 河南<br>HA | 宁夏<br>NX | 内蒙古<br>NM | 青海<br>QH | 甘肃<br>GS | 上海<br>SH | 福建<br>FJ | 江西<br>JX | 江苏<br>JS | 浙江<br>ZJ | 山东<br>SD | 湖北<br>HB | 四川<br>SC | 广西<br>GX | 湖南<br>HN | 广东<br>GD | 贵州<br>GZ | 全国平均<br>AVG |
|---|---|---|---|---|---|---|---|---|---|---|---|---|---|---|---|---|---|---|---|---|---|---|---|---|---|
| 谷类 Cereals | ND | ND | ND | 0.051 | ND | 0.034 | ND | 0.070 | ND | ND | 0.029 | ND | ND | ND | ND | 0.265 | 0.065 | 0.017 | 0.089 | 0.029 | 0.394 | 0.131 | 0.023 | ND | 0.051 |
| 豆类 Legumes | ND | 0.220 | 0.126 | ND | ND | 0.270 | ND | 2.681 | ND | ND | 0.019 | ND | ND | ND | 1.005 | 1.261 | ND | 4.804 | 0.206 | 0.155 | 1.473 | 0.503 | 1.566 | ND | 0.596 |
| 薯类 Potatoes | ND | ND | 0.041 | ND | ND | 0.035 | ND | ND | ND | ND | ND | ND | ND | ND | ND | ND | ND | 0.038 | ND | 0.018 | 1.965 | 2.033 | ND | ND | 0.173 |
| 肉类 Meats | ND | ND | 0.046 | 0.029 | ND | 0.047 | ND | ND | ND | ND | ND | ND | ND | ND | ND | ND | ND | 0.043 | ND | 0.013 | 1.666 | 0.012 | 0.067 | ND | 0.081 |
| 蛋类 Eggs | ND | ND | 0.061 | ND | ND | 0.059 | ND | ND | ND | ND | ND | ND | ND | ND | ND | ND | ND | 0.044 | ND | 0.001 | 3.032 | 0.011 | ND | ND | 0.135 |
| 水产类 Aquatic foods | ND | ND | 0.018 | 0.030 | ND | 0.025 | ND | ND | ND | ND | ND | ND | ND | ND | ND | ND | ND | 0.022 | ND | ND | 1.270 | ND | 0.080 | ND | 0.061 |
| 乳类 Dairy products | ND | ND | ND | ND | ND | ND | ND | ND | ND | ND | ND | ND | ND | ND | ND | ND | ND | ND | ND | ND | ND | ND | ND | ND | 0.001 |
| 蔬菜类 Vegetables | ND | ND | 0.041 | ND | ND | 0.041 | ND | ND | ND | ND | ND | ND | ND | ND | ND | ND | ND | 0.035 | ND | ND | 1.728 | ND | 0.071 | ND | 0.081 |
| 水果类 Fruits | ND | ND | ND | ND | ND | ND | ND | ND | ND | ND | ND | ND | ND | ND | ND | ND | ND | ND | ND | ND | ND | ND | ND | ND | 0.001 |

续表

| 膳食类别 Category | 黑龙江 HL | 辽宁 LN | 河北 HE | 北京 BJ | 吉林 JL | 山西 SX | 陕西 SN | 河南 HA | 宁夏 NX | 内蒙古 NM | 青海 QH | 甘肃 GS | 上海 SH | 福建 FJ | 江西 JX | 江苏 JS | 浙江 ZJ | 山东 SD | 湖北 HB | 四川 SC | 广西 GX | 湖南 HN | 广东 GD | 贵州 GZ | 全国平均 AVG |
|---|---|---|---|---|---|---|---|---|---|---|---|---|---|---|---|---|---|---|---|---|---|---|---|---|---|
| 糖类 Sugar | ND | ND | ND | ND | ND | ND | ND | ND | ND | ND | ND | ND | 0.034 | ND | ND | ND | ND | ND | ND | ND | ND | ND | ND | ND | 0.002 |
| 水及饮料类 Water and beverages | ND | ND | ND | ND | ND | ND | ND | ND | ND | ND | ND | ND | ND | ND | ND | ND | ND | ND | ND | ND | ND | ND | ND | ND | 0.001 |
| 酒类 Alcohol beverages | ND | ND | ND | ND | ND | ND | ND | ND | ND | ND | ND | ND | ND | ND | ND | ND | ND | ND | ND | 0.051 | ND | ND | ND | ND | 0.003 |

注：未检出（ND）按 1/2 检出限（LOD）计
Note: values not detected (ND) were treated as being equal to half of the detection of limit (LOD)

附表 8-2　第六次中国总膳食研究膳食样品中黄曲霉毒素 B2 的含量（单位：μg/kg）
Annexed Table 8-2　Levels of aflatoxin B2 in food samples from the 6$^{th}$ China TDS (Unit: μg/kg)

| 膳食类别 Category | 黑龙江 HL | 辽宁 LN | 河北 HE | 北京 BJ | 吉林 JL | 山西 SX | 陕西 SN | 河南 HA | 宁夏 NX | 内蒙古 NM | 青海 QH | 甘肃 GS | 上海 SH | 福建 FJ | 江西 JX | 江苏 JS | 浙江 ZJ | 山东 SD | 湖北 HB | 四川 SC | 广西 GX | 湖南 HN | 广东 GD | 贵州 GZ | 全国平均 AVG |
|---|---|---|---|---|---|---|---|---|---|---|---|---|---|---|---|---|---|---|---|---|---|---|---|---|---|
| 谷类 Cereals | ND | ND | ND | ND | ND | ND | ND | ND | ND | ND | ND | ND | ND | ND | ND | 0.022 | ND | ND | ND | ND | 0.031 | ND | ND | ND | 0.004 |
| 豆类 Legumes | ND | 0.042 | ND | ND | ND | 0.035 | ND | 0.696 | ND | ND | ND | ND | ND | ND | 0.162 | 0.401 | ND | 0.579 | 0.033 | ND | 0.207 | 0.045 | 0.233 | ND | 0.102 |
| 薯类 Potatoes | ND | ND | ND | ND | ND | ND | ND | ND | ND | ND | ND | ND | ND | ND | ND | ND | ND | ND | ND | ND | 0.315 | 0.183 | ND | ND | 0.022 |
| 肉类 Meats | ND | ND | ND | ND | ND | ND | ND | ND | ND | ND | ND | ND | ND | ND | ND | ND | ND | ND | ND | ND | 0.255 | ND | ND | ND | 0.012 |
| 蛋类 Eggs | ND | ND | ND | ND | ND | ND | ND | ND | ND | ND | ND | ND | ND | ND | ND | ND | ND | ND | ND | ND | 0.467 | ND | ND | ND | 0.021 |

续表

| 膳食类别 Category | 黑龙江 HL | 辽宁 LN | 河北 HE | 北京 BJ | 吉林 JL | 山西 SX | 陕西 SN | 河南 HA | 宁夏 NX | 内蒙古 NM | 青海 QH | 甘肃 GS | 上海 SH | 福建 FJ | 江西 JX | 江苏 JS | 浙江 ZJ | 山东 SD | 湖北 HB | 四川 SC | 广西 GX | 湖南 HN | 广东 GD | 贵州 GZ | 全国平均 AVG |
|---|---|---|---|---|---|---|---|---|---|---|---|---|---|---|---|---|---|---|---|---|---|---|---|---|---|
| 水产类 Aquatic foods | ND | ND | ND | ND | ND | ND | ND | ND | ND | ND | ND | ND | ND | ND | ND | ND | ND | ND | ND | ND | 0.182 | ND | ND | ND | 0.009 |
| 乳类 Dairy products | ND | ND | ND | ND | ND | ND | ND | ND | ND | ND | ND | ND | ND | ND | ND | ND | ND | ND | ND | ND | ND | ND | ND | ND | 0.001 |
| 蔬菜类 Vegetables | ND | ND | ND | ND | ND | ND | ND | ND | ND | ND | ND | ND | ND | ND | ND | ND | ND | ND | ND | ND | 0.276 | ND | ND | ND | 0.013 |
| 水果类 Fruits | ND | ND | ND | ND | ND | ND | ND | ND | ND | ND | ND | ND | ND | ND | ND | ND | ND | ND | ND | ND | ND | ND | ND | ND | 0.001 |
| 糖类 Sugar | ND | ND | ND | ND | ND | ND | ND | ND | ND | ND | ND | ND | ND | ND | ND | ND | ND | ND | ND | ND | ND | ND | ND | ND | 0.001 |
| 水及饮料类 Water and beverages | ND | ND | ND | ND | ND | ND | ND | ND | ND | ND | ND | ND | ND | ND | ND | ND | ND | ND | ND | ND | ND | ND | ND | ND | 0.001 |
| 酒类 Alcohol beverages | ND | ND | ND | ND | ND | ND | ND | ND | ND | ND | ND | ND | ND | ND | ND | ND | ND | ND | ND | ND | ND | ND | ND | ND | 0.001 |

注：未检出（ND）按 1/2 检出限（LOD）计

Note: values not detected (ND) were treated as being equal to half of the detection of limit (LOD)

附表 8-3 第六次中国总膳食研究膳食样品中黄曲霉毒素 G1 的含量（单位：μg/kg）

Annexed Table 8-3　Levels of aflatoxin G1 in food samples from the 6<sup>th</sup> China TDS (Unit: μg/kg)

| 膳食类别 Category | 黑龙江 HL | 辽宁 LN | 河北 HE | 北京 BJ | 吉林 JL | 山西 SX | 陕西 SN | 河南 HA | 宁夏 NX | 内蒙古 NM | 青海 QH | 甘肃 GS | 上海 SH | 福建 FJ | 江西 JX | 江苏 JS | 浙江 ZJ | 山东 SD | 湖北 HB | 四川 SC | 广西 GX | 湖南 HN | 广东 GD | 贵州 GZ | 全国平均 AVG |
|---|---|---|---|---|---|---|---|---|---|---|---|---|---|---|---|---|---|---|---|---|---|---|---|---|---|
| 谷类 Cereals | ND | ND | ND | ND | ND | ND | ND | ND | ND | ND | ND | ND | ND | ND | ND | ND | 0.055 | ND | ND | ND | ND | ND | ND | ND | 0.005 |

续表

| 膳食类别<br>Category | 黑龙江<br>HL | 辽宁<br>LN | 河北<br>HE | 北京<br>BJ | 吉林<br>JL | 山西<br>SX | 陕西<br>SN | 河南<br>HA | 宁夏<br>NX | 内蒙古<br>NM | 青海<br>QH | 甘肃<br>GS | 上海<br>SH | 福建<br>FJ | 江西<br>JX | 江苏<br>JS | 浙江<br>ZJ | 山东<br>SD | 湖北<br>HB | 四川<br>SC | 广西<br>GX | 湖南<br>HN | 广东<br>GD | 贵州<br>GZ | 全国平均<br>AVG |
|---|---|---|---|---|---|---|---|---|---|---|---|---|---|---|---|---|---|---|---|---|---|---|---|---|---|
| 豆类 Legumes | ND | ND | ND | ND | ND | ND | ND | ND | ND | ND | ND | ND | ND | ND | ND | ND | ND | ND | ND | ND | ND | ND | ND | ND | 0.002 |
| 薯类 Potatoes | ND | ND | ND | ND | ND | ND | ND | ND | ND | ND | ND | ND | ND | ND | ND | ND | ND | ND | ND | ND | ND | ND | ND | ND | 0.002 |
| 肉类 Meats | ND | ND | ND | ND | ND | ND | ND | ND | ND | ND | ND | ND | ND | ND | ND | ND | ND | ND | ND | ND | ND | ND | ND | ND | 0.002 |
| 蛋类 Eggs | ND | ND | ND | ND | ND | ND | ND | ND | ND | ND | ND | ND | ND | ND | ND | ND | ND | ND | ND | ND | ND | ND | ND | ND | 0.002 |
| 水产类 Aquatic foods | ND | ND | ND | ND | ND | ND | ND | ND | ND | ND | ND | ND | ND | ND | ND | ND | ND | ND | ND | ND | ND | ND | ND | ND | 0.002 |
| 乳类 Dairy products | ND | ND | ND | ND | ND | ND | ND | ND | ND | ND | ND | ND | ND | ND | ND | ND | ND | ND | ND | ND | ND | ND | ND | 0.022 | 0.003 |
| 蔬菜类 Vegetables | ND | 0.112 | ND | ND | ND | ND | ND | ND | ND | ND | ND | ND | ND | ND | ND | ND | 0.022 | ND | ND | ND | ND | ND | ND | 0.022 | 0.009 |
| 水果类 Fruits | ND | ND | ND | ND | ND | ND | ND | ND | ND | ND | ND | ND | ND | ND | ND | ND | ND | ND | ND | ND | ND | ND | ND | ND | 0.002 |
| 糖类 Sugar | ND | ND | ND | ND | ND | ND | ND | ND | ND | ND | ND | ND | ND | ND | ND | ND | ND | ND | ND | ND | ND | ND | ND | ND | 0.002 |
| 水及饮料类 Water and beverages | ND | ND | ND | ND | ND | ND | ND | ND | ND | ND | ND | ND | ND | ND | ND | ND | ND | ND | ND | ND | ND | ND | ND | ND | 0.002 |
| 酒类 Alcohol beverages | ND | ND | ND | ND | ND | ND | ND | ND | ND | ND | ND | ND | ND | ND | ND | ND | ND | ND | ND | ND | ND | ND | ND | 0.022 | 0.003 |

注：未检出（ND）按 1/2 检出限（LOD）计

Note: values not detected (ND) were treated as being equal to half of the detection of limit (LOD)

附表 8-4 第六次中国总膳食研究膳食样品中黄曲霉毒素 M1 的含量（单位：μg/kg）

Annexed Table 8-4　Levels of aflatoxin M1 in food samples from the 6th China TDS (Unit: μg/kg)

| 膳食类别 Category | 黑龙江 HL | 辽宁 LN | 河北 HE | 北京 BJ | 吉林 JL | 山西 SX | 陕西 SN | 河南 HA | 宁夏 NX | 内蒙古 NM | 青海 QH | 甘肃 GS | 上海 SH | 福建 FJ | 江西 JX | 江苏 JS | 浙江 ZJ | 山东 SD | 湖北 HB | 四川 SC | 广西 GX | 湖南 HN | 广东 GD | 贵州 GZ | 全国平均 AVG |
|---|---|---|---|---|---|---|---|---|---|---|---|---|---|---|---|---|---|---|---|---|---|---|---|---|---|
| 谷类 Cereals | ND | ND | ND | ND | ND | ND | ND | ND | ND | ND | 0.005 | ND | ND | ND | ND | ND | ND | ND | ND | ND | ND | ND | ND | ND | 0.003 |
| 豆类 Legumes | ND | ND | ND | 0.024 | ND | ND | ND | ND | ND | ND | ND | ND | ND | ND | ND | 0.026 | ND | 0.087 | ND | ND | ND | 0.055 | 0.038 | ND | 0.011 |
| 薯类 Potatoes | ND | ND | ND | ND | ND | ND | ND | ND | ND | ND | ND | ND | ND | ND | ND | ND | ND | ND | ND | ND | ND | ND | ND | ND | 0.002 |
| 肉类 Meats | ND | ND | ND | ND | ND | ND | ND | ND | ND | ND | ND | ND | ND | ND | ND | ND | ND | ND | ND | ND | ND | ND | ND | ND | 0.002 |
| 蛋类 Eggs | ND | ND | ND | ND | ND | ND | ND | ND | ND | ND | ND | ND | ND | ND | ND | ND | ND | ND | ND | ND | ND | ND | ND | ND | 0.002 |
| 水产类 Aquatic foods | ND | ND | ND | ND | ND | ND | ND | ND | ND | ND | ND | ND | ND | ND | ND | ND | ND | ND | ND | ND | ND | ND | ND | ND | 0.002 |
| 乳类 Dairy products | ND | ND | ND | ND | ND | ND | ND | ND | ND | ND | ND | ND | ND | ND | ND | 0.020 | ND | 0.135 | ND | ND | ND | ND | ND | ND | 0.008 |
| 蔬菜类 Vegetables | ND | ND | ND | 0.023 | ND | ND | ND | ND | ND | ND | ND | ND | ND | ND | ND | ND | ND | ND | ND | ND | ND | ND | ND | ND | 0.003 |
| 水果类 Fruits | ND | ND | ND | ND | ND | ND | ND | ND | ND | ND | ND | ND | ND | ND | ND | ND | ND | ND | ND | ND | ND | ND | ND | ND | 0.002 |
| 糖类 Sugar | ND | ND | ND | ND | ND | ND | ND | ND | ND | ND | ND | ND | ND | ND | ND | ND | ND | ND | ND | ND | ND | ND | ND | ND | 0.002 |
| 水及饮料类 Water and beverages | ND | ND | ND | ND | ND | ND | ND | ND | ND | ND | ND | ND | ND | ND | ND | ND | ND | ND | ND | ND | ND | ND | ND | ND | 0.002 |

续表

| 膳食类别 Category | 黑龙江 HL | 辽宁 LN | 河北 HE | 北京 BJ | 吉林 JL | 山西 SX | 陕西 SN | 河南 HA | 宁夏 NX | 内蒙古 NM | 青海 QH | 甘肃 GS | 上海 SH | 福建 FJ | 江西 JX | 江苏 JS | 浙江 ZJ | 山东 SD | 湖北 HB | 四川 SC | 广西 GX | 湖南 HN | 广东 GD | 贵州 GZ | 全国平均 AVG |
|---|---|---|---|---|---|---|---|---|---|---|---|---|---|---|---|---|---|---|---|---|---|---|---|---|---|
| 酒类 Alcohol beverages | ND | 0.680 | ND | ND | ND | ND | ND | ND | ND | ND | ND | ND | ND | ND | ND | 0.548 | 0.833 | ND | ND | ND | ND | ND | ND | ND | 0.088 |

注：未检出（ND）按1/2检出限（LOD）计

Note: values not detected (ND) were treated as being equal to half of the detection of limit (LOD)

附表 8-5 第六次中国总膳食研究膳食样品中黄曲霉毒素 BG 的含量（单位：µg/kg）

Annexed Table 8-5 Levels of aflatoxin BG in food samples from the 6th China TDS (Unit: µg/kg)

| 膳食类别 Category | 黑龙江 HL | 辽宁 LN | 河北 HE | 北京 BJ | 吉林 JL | 山西 SX | 陕西 SN | 河南 HA | 宁夏 NX | 内蒙古 NM | 青海 QH | 甘肃 GS | 上海 SH | 福建 FJ | 江西 JX | 江苏 JS | 浙江 ZJ | 山东 SD | 湖北 HB | 四川 SC | 广西 GX | 湖南 HN | 广东 GD | 贵州 GZ | 全国平均 AVG |
|---|---|---|---|---|---|---|---|---|---|---|---|---|---|---|---|---|---|---|---|---|---|---|---|---|---|
| 谷类 Cereals | ND | ND | ND | 0.058 | ND | 0.042 | ND | 0.078 | ND | ND | 0.040 | ND | ND | ND | ND | 0.292 | 0.124 | 0.023 | 0.096 | 0.037 | 0.431 | 0.138 | 0.029 | ND | 0.063 |
| 豆类 Legumes | ND | 0.268 | 0.132 | ND | ND | 0.309 | ND | 3.383 | ND | ND | 0.025 | ND | ND | ND | 1.172 | 1.667 | ND | 5.387 | 0.243 | 0.160 | 1.685 | 0.553 | 1.803 | ND | 0.703 |
| 薯类 Potatoes | ND | ND | 0.047 | ND | ND | 0.041 | ND | ND | ND | ND | ND | ND | ND | ND | ND | ND | ND | 0.043 | ND | 0.024 | 2.285 | 2.221 | ND | ND | 0.199 |
| 肉类 Meats | ND | ND | 0.051 | 0.035 | ND | 0.052 | ND | ND | ND | ND | ND | ND | ND | ND | ND | ND | ND | 0.048 | ND | 0.019 | 1.925 | 0.017 | 0.073 | ND | 0.097 |
| 蛋类 Eggs | ND | ND | 0.067 | ND | ND | 0.065 | ND | ND | ND | ND | ND | ND | ND | ND | ND | ND | ND | 0.050 | ND | ND | 3.504 | 0.017 | ND | ND | 0.160 |
| 水产类 Aquatic foods | ND | ND | 0.023 | 0.036 | ND | 0.031 | ND | ND | ND | ND | ND | ND | ND | ND | ND | ND | ND | 0.028 | ND | ND | 1.457 | ND | 0.085 | ND | 0.074 |
| 乳类 Dairy products | ND | ND | ND | ND | ND | ND | ND | ND | ND | ND | ND | ND | ND | ND | ND | ND | ND | ND | ND | ND | ND | ND | ND | 0.026 | 0.007 |

续表

| 膳食类别<br>Category | 黑龙江<br>HL | 辽宁<br>LN | 河北<br>HE | 北京<br>BJ | 吉林<br>JL | 山西<br>SX | 陕西<br>SN | 河南<br>HA | 宁夏<br>NX | 内蒙古<br>NM | 青海<br>QH | 甘肃<br>GS | 上海<br>SH | 福建<br>FJ | 江西<br>JX | 江苏<br>JS | 浙江<br>ZJ | 山东<br>SD | 湖北<br>HB | 四川<br>SC | 广西<br>GX | 湖南<br>HN | 广东<br>GD | 贵州<br>GZ | 全国平均<br>AVG |
|---|---|---|---|---|---|---|---|---|---|---|---|---|---|---|---|---|---|---|---|---|---|---|---|---|---|
| 蔬菜类<br>Vegetables | ND | 0.117 | 0.046 | ND | ND | 0.046 | ND | ND | ND | ND | ND | ND | ND | ND | ND | ND | 0.032 | 0.041 | ND | ND | 2.008 | ND | 0.076 | 0.027 | 0.104 |
| 水果类<br>Fruits | ND | ND | ND | ND | ND | ND | ND | ND | ND | ND | ND | ND | ND | ND | ND | ND | ND | ND | ND | ND | ND | ND | ND | ND | 0.006 |
| 糖类<br>Sugar | ND | ND | ND | ND | ND | ND | ND | ND | ND | ND | ND | ND | 0.039 | ND | ND | ND | ND | ND | ND | ND | ND | ND | ND | ND | 0.007 |
| 水及饮料类<br>Water and beverages | ND | ND | ND | ND | ND | ND | ND | ND | ND | ND | ND | ND | ND | ND | ND | ND | ND | ND | ND | ND | ND | ND | ND | ND | 0.006 |
| 酒类<br>Alcohol beverages | ND | ND | ND | ND | ND | ND | ND | ND | ND | ND | ND | ND | ND | ND | ND | ND | ND | ND | ND | 0.056 | ND | ND | ND | 0.026 | 0.009 |

注：未检出（ND）按 1/2 检出限（LOD）计

Note: values not detected (ND) were treated as being equal to half of the detection of limit (LOD)

附表 Table 8-6 第六次中国总膳食研究的黄曲霉毒 BG 膳食摄入量 [ 单位：ng/(kg bw·d)]

Annexed Table 8-6 Dietary intakes of aflatoxin BG from the 6$^{th}$ China TDS [Unit: ng/(kg bw·d)]

| 膳食类别<br>Category | 黑龙江<br>HL | 辽宁<br>LN | 河北<br>HE | 北京<br>BJ | 吉林<br>JL | 山西<br>SX | 陕西<br>SN | 河南<br>HA | 宁夏<br>NX | 内蒙古<br>NM | 青海<br>QH | 甘肃<br>GS | 上海<br>SH | 福建<br>FJ | 江西<br>JX | 江苏<br>JS | 浙江<br>ZJ | 山东<br>SD | 湖北<br>HB | 四川<br>SC | 广西<br>GX | 湖南<br>HN | 广东<br>GD | 贵州<br>GZ | 全国平均<br>AVG |
|---|---|---|---|---|---|---|---|---|---|---|---|---|---|---|---|---|---|---|---|---|---|---|---|---|---|
| 谷类<br>Cereals | 0.101 | 0.093 | 0.119 | 0.729 | 0.073 | 0.692 | 0.141 | 1.143 | 0.112 | 0.101 | 0.489 | 0.111 | 0.056 | 0.089 | 0.082 | 3.606 | 1.249 | 0.367 | 0.808 | 0.567 | 6.429 | 1.265 | 0.213 | 0.104 | 0.781 |
| 豆类<br>Legumes | 0.006 | 0.519 | 0.120 | 0.011 | 0.010 | 0.340 | 0.009 | 2.898 | 0.004 | 0.004 | 0.003 | 0.004 | 0.013 | 0.008 | 1.371 | 2.195 | 0.014 | 4.488 | 0.258 | 0.172 | 1.133 | 0.638 | 0.799 | 0.012 | 0.626 |
| 薯类<br>Potatoes | 0.009 | 0.009 | 0.045 | 0.006 | 0.011 | 0.078 | 0.014 | 0.008 | 0.011 | 0.012 | 0.010 | 0.014 | 0.003 | 0.004 | 0.003 | 0.004 | 0.004 | 0.032 | 0.009 | 0.024 | 0.466 | 1.890 | 0.002 | 0.004 | 0.111 |

续表

| 膳食类别 Category | 黑龙江 HL | 辽宁 LN | 河北 HE | 北京 BJ | 吉林 JL | 山西 SX | 陕西 SN | 河南 HA | 宁夏 NX | 内蒙古 NM | 青海 QH | 甘肃 GS | 上海 SH | 福建 FJ | 江西 JX | 江苏 JS | 浙江 ZJ | 山东 SD | 湖北 HB | 四川 SC | 广西 GX | 湖南 HN | 广东 GD | 贵州 GZ | 全国平均 AVG |
|---|---|---|---|---|---|---|---|---|---|---|---|---|---|---|---|---|---|---|---|---|---|---|---|---|---|
| 肉类 Meats | 0.007 | 0.008 | 0.039 | 0.038 | 0.006 | 0.114 | 0.004 | 0.005 | 0.005 | 0.007 | 0.007 | 0.003 | 0.011 | 0.008 | 0.009 | 0.009 | 0.012 | 0.074 | 0.005 | 0.038 | 4.611 | 0.039 | 0.121 | 0.010 | 0.216 |
| 蛋类 Eggs | 0.004 | 0.005 | 0.034 | 0.004 | 0.004 | 0.022 | 0.002 | 0.003 | 0.002 | 0.004 | 0.002 | 0.002 | 0.004 | 0.002 | 0.002 | 0.003 | 0.003 | 0.035 | 0.003 | 0.002 | 0.779 | 0.006 | 0.002 | 0.002 | 0.039 |
| 水产类 Aquatic foods | 0.003 | 0.002 | 0.004 | 0.009 | 0.001 | 0.003 | 0.001 | 0.001 | 0.001 | 0.001 | 0.001 | 0.001 | 0.007 | 0.006 | 0.004 | 0.004 | 0.005 | 0.010 | 0.004 | 0.001 | 2.235 | 0.006 | 0.069 | 0.001 | 0.099 |
| 乳类 Dairy products | 0.001 | 0.004 | 0.002 | 0.008 | 0.003 | 0.004 | 0.002 | 0.002 | 0.001 | 0.003 | 0.005 | 0.001 | 0.007 | 0.003 | 0.002 | 0.003 | 0.003 | 0.002 | 0.001 | 0.001 | 0.002 | 0.002 | 0.003 | 0.012 | 0.003 |
| 蔬菜类 Vegetables | 0.038 | 0.605 | 0.216 | 0.038 | 0.037 | 0.227 | 0.028 | 0.027 | 0.015 | 0.025 | 0.030 | 0.024 | 0.038 | 0.038 | 0.043 | 0.042 | 0.226 | 0.264 | 0.039 | 0.029 | 11.264 | 0.052 | 0.287 | 0.175 | 0.575 |
| 水果类 Fruits | 0.006 | 0.008 | 0.004 | 0.012 | 0.008 | 0.003 | 0.004 | 0.002 | 0.009 | 0.011 | 0.002 | 0.003 | 0.007 | 0.006 | 0.005 | 0.003 | 0.006 | 0.005 | 0.002 | 0.002 | 0.006 | 0.006 | 0.003 | 0.002 | 0.005 |
| 糖类 Sugar | 0.001 | 0.001 | 0.001 | 0.001 | 0.001 | 0.001 | 0.004 | 0.001 | 0.001 | 0.001 | 0.001 | 0.001 | 0.005 | 0.001 | 0.001 | 0.001 | 0.001 | 0.001 | 0.001 | 0.001 | 0.001 | 0.001 | 0.001 | 0.001 | 0.001 |
| 水及饮料类 Water and beverages | 0.116 | 0.047 | 0.074 | 0.105 | 0.124 | 0.071 | 0.033 | 0.114 | 0.049 | 0.245 | 0.059 | 0.112 | 0.067 | 0.082 | 0.113 | 0.096 | 0.075 | 0.171 | 0.027 | 0.030 | 0.124 | 0.101 | 0.114 | 0.119 | 0.095 |
| 酒类 Alcohol beverages | 0.002 | 0.003 | 0.001 | 0.003 | 0.001 | 0.001 | 0.001 | 0.001 | 0.001 | 0.002 | 0.001 | 0.001 | 0.002 | 0.001 | 0.002 | 0.004 | 0.006 | 0.011 | 0.001 | 0.005 | 0.003 | 0.002 | 0.001 | 0.001 | 0.002 |
| 合计 SUM | 0.293 | 1.303 | 0.658 | 0.963 | 0.280 | 1.553 | 0.241 | 4.204 | 0.209 | 0.416 | 0.606 | 0.276 | 0.219 | 0.249 | 1.637 | 5.968 | 1.603 | 5.460 | 1.157 | 0.869 | 27.052 | 4.007 | 1.613 | 0.441 | 2.553 |

附表 8-7　第六次中国总膳食研究膳食样品中 T-2、HT-2 总量的含量（单位：μg/kg）

Annexed Table 8-7　Levels of T-2, HT-2 in food samples from the 6$^{th}$ China TDS (Unit: μg/kg)

| 膳食类别 Category | 黑龙江 HL | 辽宁 LN | 河北 HE | 北京 BJ | 吉林 JL | 山西 SX | 陕西 SN | 河南 HA | 宁夏 NX | 内蒙古 NM | 青海 QH | 甘肃 GS | 上海 SH | 福建 FJ | 江西 JX | 江苏 JS | 浙江 ZJ | 山东 SD | 湖北 HB | 四川 SC | 广西 GX | 湖南 HN | 广东 GD | 贵州 GZ | 全国平均 AVG |
|---|---|---|---|---|---|---|---|---|---|---|---|---|---|---|---|---|---|---|---|---|---|---|---|---|---|
| 谷类 Cereals | ND | ND | ND | ND | ND | ND | ND | ND | ND | 0.85 | ND | ND | ND | ND | ND | ND | ND | ND | ND | ND | ND | ND | ND | ND | 0.12 |
| 豆类 Legumes | ND | ND | ND | ND | ND | ND | ND | ND | ND | ND | ND | ND | ND | ND | ND | ND | ND | ND | ND | ND | ND | ND | ND | ND | 0.07 |
| 薯类 Potatoes | ND | ND | ND | ND | ND | ND | ND | ND | ND | ND | ND | ND | ND | ND | ND | ND | ND | ND | ND | ND | ND | ND | ND | ND | 0.07 |
| 肉类 Meats | ND | ND | ND | ND | ND | ND | ND | ND | ND | ND | ND | ND | ND | ND | ND | ND | ND | ND | ND | ND | ND | ND | ND | ND | 0.06 |
| 蛋类 Eggs | ND | ND | ND | ND | ND | ND | ND | ND | ND | ND | ND | ND | ND | ND | ND | ND | ND | ND | ND | ND | ND | ND | ND | ND | 0.07 |
| 水产类 Aquatic foods | ND | ND | ND | ND | ND | ND | ND | ND | ND | ND | ND | ND | ND | ND | ND | ND | ND | ND | ND | ND | ND | ND | ND | ND | 0.06 |
| 乳类 Dairy products | ND | ND | ND | ND | ND | ND | ND | ND | ND | ND | ND | ND | ND | ND | ND | ND | ND | ND | ND | ND | ND | ND | ND | ND | 0.06 |
| 蔬菜类 Vegetables | ND | ND | ND | ND | ND | ND | ND | ND | ND | ND | ND | ND | ND | ND | ND | ND | ND | ND | ND | ND | ND | ND | ND | ND | 0.06 |
| 水果类 Fruits | ND | ND | ND | ND | ND | ND | ND | ND | ND | ND | ND | ND | ND | ND | ND | ND | ND | ND | ND | ND | ND | ND | ND | ND | 0.06 |
| 糖类 Sugar | ND | ND | ND | ND | ND | ND | ND | ND | ND | ND | ND | ND | ND | ND | ND | ND | ND | ND | ND | ND | ND | ND | ND | ND | 0.06 |
| 水及饮料类 Water and beverages | ND | ND | ND | ND | ND | ND | ND | ND | ND | ND | ND | ND | ND | ND | ND | ND | ND | ND | ND | ND | ND | ND | ND | ND | 0.06 |

续表

| 膳食类别<br>Category | 黑龙江<br>HL | 辽宁<br>LN | 河北<br>HE | 北京<br>BJ | 吉林<br>JL | 山西<br>SX | 陕西<br>SN | 河南<br>HA | 宁夏<br>NX | 内蒙古<br>NM | 青海<br>QH | 甘肃<br>GS | 上海<br>SH | 福建<br>FJ | 江西<br>JX | 江苏<br>JS | 浙江<br>ZJ | 山东<br>SD | 湖北<br>HB | 四川<br>SC | 广西<br>GX | 湖南<br>HN | 广东<br>GD | 贵州<br>GZ | 全国平均<br>AVG |
|---|---|---|---|---|---|---|---|---|---|---|---|---|---|---|---|---|---|---|---|---|---|---|---|---|---|
| 酒类<br>Alcohol beverages | ND | ND | ND | ND | ND | ND | ND | ND | ND | ND | ND | ND | ND | ND | ND | ND | 0.16 | ND | ND | ND | ND | ND | ND | ND | 0.06 |

注：未检出（ND）按 1/2 检出限（LOD）计

Note: values not detected (ND) were treated as being equal to half of the detection of limit (LOD)

附表 8-8　第六次中国总膳食研究的 T-2、HT-2 总量膳食摄入量 [ 单位：ng/(kg bw·d)]

Annexed Table 8-8　Dietary intakes of T-2, HT-2 from the 6$^{th}$ China TDS [Unit: ng/(kg bw·d)]

| 膳食类别<br>Category | 黑龙江<br>HL | 辽宁<br>LN | 河北<br>HE | 北京<br>BJ | 吉林<br>JL | 山西<br>SX | 陕西<br>SN | 河南<br>HA | 宁夏<br>NX | 内蒙古<br>NM | 青海<br>QH | 甘肃<br>GS | 上海<br>SH | 福建<br>FJ | 江西<br>JX | 江苏<br>JS | 浙江<br>ZJ | 山东<br>SD | 湖北<br>HB | 四川<br>SC | 广西<br>GX | 湖南<br>HN | 广东<br>GD | 贵州<br>GZ | 全国平均<br>AVG |
|---|---|---|---|---|---|---|---|---|---|---|---|---|---|---|---|---|---|---|---|---|---|---|---|---|---|
| 谷类<br>Cereals | 1.010 | 0.931 | 1.192 | 1.067 | 0.734 | 1.594 | 1.415 | 1.375 | 1.123 | 9.728 | 1.658 | 1.108 | 0.555 | 0.886 | 0.822 | 0.926 | 0.803 | 1.264 | 0.689 | 1.461 | 1.317 | 0.809 | 0.588 | 1.037 | 1.420 |
| 豆类<br>Legumes | 0.063 | 0.159 | 0.065 | 0.105 | 0.097 | 0.073 | 0.089 | 0.073 | 0.039 | 0.041 | 0.007 | 0.040 | 0.129 | 0.076 | 0.080 | 0.092 | 0.143 | 0.053 | 0.071 | 0.074 | 0.041 | 0.090 | 0.030 | 0.115 | 0.077 |
| 薯类<br>Potatoes | 0.088 | 0.089 | 0.068 | 0.065 | 0.114 | 0.141 | 0.135 | 0.083 | 0.109 | 0.119 | 0.101 | 0.141 | 0.034 | 0.044 | 0.031 | 0.038 | 0.036 | 0.046 | 0.085 | 0.062 | 0.016 | 0.069 | 0.025 | 0.040 | 0.074 |
| 肉类<br>Meats | 0.067 | 0.079 | 0.049 | 0.080 | 0.064 | 0.138 | 0.037 | 0.055 | 0.046 | 0.071 | 0.068 | 0.033 | 0.105 | 0.084 | 0.090 | 0.088 | 0.121 | 0.100 | 0.054 | 0.124 | 0.144 | 0.144 | 0.125 | 0.105 | 0.086 |
| 蛋类<br>Eggs | 0.039 | 0.051 | 0.038 | 0.044 | 0.044 | 0.027 | 0.024 | 0.028 | 0.018 | 0.037 | 0.017 | 0.025 | 0.040 | 0.024 | 0.023 | 0.029 | 0.028 | 0.052 | 0.028 | 0.016 | 0.015 | 0.022 | 0.023 | 0.015 | 0.030 |
| 水产类<br>Aquatic foods | 0.026 | 0.022 | 0.010 | 0.017 | 0.011 | 0.007 | 0.004 | 0.005 | 0.002 | 0.010 | 0.004 | 0.003 | 0.065 | 0.064 | 0.042 | 0.038 | 0.050 | 0.023 | 0.039 | 0.008 | 0.093 | 0.064 | 0.051 | 0.004 | 0.027 |
| 乳类<br>Dairy products | 0.013 | 0.042 | 0.023 | 0.082 | 0.031 | 0.040 | 0.018 | 0.019 | 0.015 | 0.033 | 0.051 | 0.013 | 0.068 | 0.034 | 0.021 | 0.026 | 0.032 | 0.022 | 0.006 | 0.012 | 0.017 | 0.017 | 0.035 | 0.027 | 0.029 |

续表

| 膳食类别<br>Category | 黑龙江<br>HL | 辽宁<br>LN | 河北<br>HE | 北京<br>BJ | 吉林<br>JL | 山西<br>SX | 陕西<br>SN | 河南<br>HA | 宁夏<br>NX | 内蒙古<br>NM | 青海<br>QH | 甘肃<br>GS | 上海<br>SH | 福建<br>FJ | 江西<br>JX | 江苏<br>JS | 浙江<br>ZJ | 山东<br>SD | 湖北<br>HB | 四川<br>SC | 广西<br>GX | 湖南<br>HN | 广东<br>GD | 贵州<br>GZ | 全国平均<br>AVG |
|---|---|---|---|---|---|---|---|---|---|---|---|---|---|---|---|---|---|---|---|---|---|---|---|---|---|
| 蔬菜类 Vegetables | 0.376 | 0.334 | 0.282 | 0.377 | 0.373 | 0.300 | 0.282 | 0.267 | 0.149 | 0.252 | 0.296 | 0.236 | 0.382 | 0.382 | 0.430 | 0.422 | 0.516 | 0.472 | 0.394 | 0.290 | 0.343 | 0.524 | 0.232 | 0.401 | 0.346 |
| 水果类 Fruits | 0.060 | 0.080 | 0.036 | 0.115 | 0.084 | 0.033 | 0.038 | 0.023 | 0.093 | 0.109 | 0.015 | 0.032 | 0.070 | 0.059 | 0.054 | 0.026 | 0.064 | 0.052 | 0.018 | 0.016 | 0.061 | 0.060 | 0.028 | 0.023 | 0.052 |
| 糖类 Sugar | 0.002 | 0.001 | 0.001 | 0.002 | 0.001 | 0.001 | 0.036 | 0.001 | 0.001 | 0.001 | 0.001 | 0.001 | 0.007 | 0.001 | 0.001 | 0.001 | 0.001 | 0.001 | 0.001 | 0.001 | 0.001 | 0.001 | 0.001 | 0.001 | 0.002 |
| 水及饮料类 Water and beverages | 1.164 | 0.470 | 0.738 | 1.055 | 1.240 | 0.710 | 0.329 | 1.136 | 0.492 | 2.452 | 0.589 | 1.125 | 0.669 | 0.824 | 1.125 | 0.961 | 0.749 | 1.715 | 0.271 | 0.299 | 1.240 | 1.011 | 1.136 | 1.193 | 0.946 |
| 酒类 Alcohol beverages | 0.021 | 0.032 | 0.010 | 0.026 | 0.009 | 0.001 | 0.002 | 0.003 | 0.001 | 0.020 | 0.004 | 0.003 | 0.021 | 0.014 | 0.021 | 0.036 | 0.156 | 0.108 | 0.014 | 0.005 | 0.030 | 0.016 | 0.001 | 0.002 | 0.023 |
| 合计 SUM | 2.929 | 2.290 | 2.512 | 3.034 | 2.801 | 3.065 | 2.409 | 3.068 | 2.088 | 12.873 | 2.811 | 2.759 | 2.147 | 2.491 | 2.739 | 2.682 | 2.700 | 3.907 | 1.670 | 2.366 | 3.320 | 2.827 | 2.274 | 2.961 | 3.120 |

附表 8-9　第六次中国总膳食研究膳食样品中 DON、3-Ac-DON、15-Ac-DON 总量的含量（单位：μg/kg）
Annexed Table 8-9　The levels of DON, 3-Ac-DON, 15-Ac-DON in food samples from the 6th China TDS (Unit: μg/kg)

| 膳食类别<br>Category | 黑龙江<br>HL | 辽宁<br>LN | 河北<br>HE | 北京<br>BJ | 吉林<br>JL | 山西<br>SX | 陕西<br>SN | 河南<br>HA | 宁夏<br>NX | 内蒙古<br>NM | 青海<br>QH | 甘肃<br>GS | 上海<br>SH | 福建<br>FJ | 江西<br>JX | 江苏<br>JS | 浙江<br>ZJ | 山东<br>SD | 湖北<br>HB | 四川<br>SC | 广西<br>GX | 湖南<br>HN | 广东<br>GD | 贵州<br>GZ | 全国平均<br>AVG |
|---|---|---|---|---|---|---|---|---|---|---|---|---|---|---|---|---|---|---|---|---|---|---|---|---|---|
| 谷类 Cereals | 114.50 | 36.89 | 72.23 | 89.41 | 34.34 | 67.38 | 76.43 | 51.25 | 55.32 | 20.09 | 117.20 | 44.33 | 71.95 | 74.24 | 29.93 | 16.33 | 85.17 | 69.26 | 103.70 | 127.50 | 5.14 | 5.06 | 26.72 | 7.05 | 58.39 |
| 豆类 Legumes | ND | 2.26 | ND | ND | 6.49 | ND | ND | ND | 11.02 | 3.43 | ND | ND | ND | ND | ND | 10.48 | 2.05 | ND | ND | 2.10 | 2.89 | 3.78 | 2.59 | ND | 2.13 |
| 薯类 Potatoes | ND | 6.40 | 3.23 | 26.36 | 1.82 | 5.85 | ND | ND | 6.95 | ND | ND | ND | ND | ND | ND | ND | 2.26 | ND | ND | ND | ND | ND | ND | ND | 2.40 |

续表

| 膳食类别 Category | 黑龙江 HL | 辽宁 LN | 河北 HE | 北京 BJ | 吉林 JL | 山西 SX | 陕西 SN | 河南 HA | 宁夏 NX | 内蒙古 NM | 青海 QH | 甘肃 GS | 上海 SH | 福建 FJ | 江西 JX | 江苏 JS | 浙江 ZJ | 山东 SD | 湖北 HB | 四川 SC | 广西 GX | 湖南 HN | 广东 GD | 贵州 GZ | 全国平均 AVG |
|---|---|---|---|---|---|---|---|---|---|---|---|---|---|---|---|---|---|---|---|---|---|---|---|---|---|
| 肉类 Meats | ND | ND | ND | ND | 2.68 | 8.10 | ND | ND | 7.22 | ND | ND | ND | ND | ND | ND | 6.61 | 2.54 | ND | ND | ND | ND | ND | 2.28 | ND | 1.43 |
| 蛋类 Eggs | ND | ND | ND | ND | ND | ND | ND | ND | ND | ND | ND | ND | ND | ND | ND | ND | ND | ND | ND | ND | 1.74 | ND | ND | ND | 0.36 |
| 水产类 Aquatic foods | ND | ND | ND | 2.12 | ND | 2.31 | ND | 6.63 | ND | ND | 4.32 | ND | 5.52 | ND | 6.41 | 3.10 | 4.18 | ND | ND | ND | 1.81 | 1.48 | 1.14 | ND | 1.77 |
| 乳类 Dairy products | ND | ND | ND | ND | ND | ND | ND | ND | ND | ND | ND | ND | ND | ND | ND | ND | ND | ND | ND | ND | ND | ND | ND | ND | 0.25 |
| 蔬菜类 Vegetables | ND | 2.66 | ND | 2.92 | ND | ND | ND | ND | ND | ND | ND | ND | ND | 1.37 | ND | 4.21 | 2.20 | ND | ND | ND | ND | ND | ND | 0.89 | 0.79 |
| 水果类 Fruits | ND | ND | ND | ND | ND | ND | ND | ND | ND | ND | ND | ND | ND | ND | ND | ND | ND | ND | ND | ND | ND | ND | ND | ND | 0.26 |
| 糖类 Sugar | ND | ND | ND | ND | ND | ND | ND | ND | ND | ND | ND | ND | 9.77 | ND | ND | ND | ND | ND | ND | ND | ND | ND | ND | ND | 0.65 |
| 水及饮料类 Water and beverages | ND | ND | ND | ND | ND | ND | ND | ND | ND | ND | ND | ND | ND | ND | ND | ND | ND | ND | ND | ND | ND | ND | ND | ND | 0.25 |
| 酒类 Alcohol beverages | 2.19 | 13.67 | 0.88 | ND | 2.93 | ND | ND | ND | ND | 3.23 | 1.27 | 2.18 | 6.06 | 3.99 | 1.72 | 17.27 | 15.09 | 1.27 | ND | 2.82 | ND | 1.19 | 2.39 | 11.94 | 3.83 |

注：未检出（ND）按 1/2 检出限（LOD）计

Note: values not detected (ND) were treated as being equal to half of the detection of limit (LOD)

附表 8-10　第六次中国总膳食研究膳食样品中 DON 的含量（单位：μg/kg）

Annexed Table 8-10　Levels of DON in food samples from the 6$^{th}$ China TDS (Unit: μg/kg)

| 膳食类别 Category | 黑龙江 HL | 辽宁 LN | 河北 HE | 北京 BJ | 吉林 JL | 山西 SX | 陕西 SN | 河南 HA | 宁夏 NX | 内蒙古 NM | 青海 QH | 甘肃 GS | 上海 SH | 福建 FJ | 江西 JX | 江苏 JS | 浙江 ZJ | 山东 SD | 湖北 HB | 四川 SC | 广西 GX | 湖南 HN | 广东 GD | 贵州 GZ | 全国平均 AVG |
|---|---|---|---|---|---|---|---|---|---|---|---|---|---|---|---|---|---|---|---|---|---|---|---|---|---|
| 谷类 Cereals | 114.30 | 36.65 | 71.99 | 89.20 | 34.14 | 67.13 | 76.14 | 51.01 | 55.05 | 19.86 | 116.90 | 44.07 | 71.76 | 74.02 | 29.72 | 15.89 | 84.97 | 69.06 | 103.50 | 127.20 | 4.92 | 4.84 | 26.51 | 6.81 | 58.15 |
| 豆类 Legumes | ND | ND | ND | ND | 6.29 | ND | ND | ND | 10.85 | 3.27 | ND | ND | ND | ND | ND | 3.06 | 1.89 | ND | ND | 1.93 | 2.74 | 3.59 | 2.42 | ND | 1.57 |
| 薯类 Potatoes | ND | 6.21 | 3.05 | 26.19 | 1.67 | 5.66 | ND | ND | 6.78 | ND | ND | ND | ND | ND | ND | ND | 2.10 | ND | ND | ND | ND | ND | ND | ND | 2.23 |
| 肉类 Meats | ND | ND | ND | ND | 2.53 | 7.95 | ND | ND | 7.06 | ND | ND | ND | ND | ND | ND | 6.46 | 2.38 | ND | ND | ND | ND | ND | ND | ND | 1.18 |
| 蛋类 Eggs | ND | ND | ND | ND | ND | ND | ND | ND | ND | ND | ND | ND | ND | ND | ND | ND | ND | ND | ND | ND | 1.57 | ND | ND | ND | 0.18 |
| 水产类 Aquatic foods | ND | ND | ND | 1.96 | ND | 2.13 | ND | 6.48 | ND | ND | 4.15 | ND | 5.37 | ND | 6.26 | 2.94 | 4.03 | ND | ND | ND | 1.66 | 1.33 | 0.98 | ND | 1.61 |
| 乳类 Dairy products | ND | ND | ND | ND | ND | ND | ND | ND | ND | ND | ND | ND | ND | ND | ND | ND | ND | ND | ND | ND | ND | ND | ND | ND | 0.10 |
| 蔬菜类 Vegetables | ND | 2.16 | ND | ND | ND | ND | ND | ND | ND | ND | ND | ND | ND | 1.22 | ND | 4.06 | 2.02 | ND | ND | ND | ND | ND | ND | 0.73 | 0.51 |
| 水果类 Fruits | ND | ND | ND | ND | ND | ND | ND | ND | ND | ND | ND | ND | 9.62 | ND | ND | ND | ND | ND | ND | ND | ND | ND | ND | ND | 0.10 |
| 糖类 Sugar | ND | ND | ND | ND | ND | ND | ND | ND | ND | ND | ND | ND | ND | ND | ND | ND | ND | ND | ND | ND | ND | ND | ND | ND | 0.50 |
| 水及饮料类 Water and beverages | ND | ND | ND | ND | ND | ND | ND | ND | ND | ND | ND | ND | ND | ND | ND | ND | ND | ND | ND | ND | ND | ND | ND | ND | 0.10 |

续表

| 膳食类别 Category | 黑龙江 HL | 辽宁 LN | 河北 HE | 北京 BJ | 吉林 JL | 山西 SX | 陕西 SN | 河南 HA | 宁夏 NX | 内蒙古 NM | 青海 QH | 甘肃 GS | 上海 SH | 福建 FJ | 江西 JX | 江苏 JS | 浙江 ZJ | 山东 SD | 湖北 HB | 四川 SC | 广西 GX | 湖南 HN | 广东 GD | 贵州 GZ | 全国平均 AVG |
|---|---|---|---|---|---|---|---|---|---|---|---|---|---|---|---|---|---|---|---|---|---|---|---|---|---|
| 酒类 Alcohol beverages | 2.04 | 11.70 | 0.73 | ND | 2.78 | ND | ND | ND | ND | 3.08 | 1.12 | 2.03 | 5.91 | 2.37 | ND | 17.12 | 13.85 | 1.12 | ND | 2.67 | ND | 1.04 | 2.24 | 11.79 | 3.43 |

注：未检出（ND）按1/2检出限（LOD）计

Note: values not detected (ND) were treated as being equal to half of the detection of limit (LOD)

附表 8-11 第六次中国总膳食研究膳食样品中 3-Ac-DON 的含量（单位：μg/kg）

Annexed Table 8-11 Levels of 3-Ac-DON in food samples from the 6<sup>th</sup> China TDS (Unit: μg/kg)

| 膳食类别 Category | 黑龙江 HL | 辽宁 LN | 河北 HE | 北京 BJ | 吉林 JL | 山西 SX | 陕西 SN | 河南 HA | 宁夏 NX | 内蒙古 NM | 青海 QH | 甘肃 GS | 上海 SH | 福建 FJ | 江西 JX | 江苏 JS | 浙江 ZJ | 山东 SD | 湖北 HB | 四川 SC | 广西 GX | 湖南 HN | 广东 GD | 贵州 GZ | 全国平均 AVG |
|---|---|---|---|---|---|---|---|---|---|---|---|---|---|---|---|---|---|---|---|---|---|---|---|---|---|
| 谷类 Cereals | ND | ND | ND | ND | ND | ND | ND | ND | ND | ND | ND | ND | ND | ND | ND | ND | ND | ND | ND | ND | ND | ND | ND | ND | 0.15 |
| 豆类 Legumes | ND | ND | ND | ND | ND | ND | ND | ND | ND | ND | ND | ND | ND | ND | ND | ND | ND | ND | ND | ND | ND | ND | ND | ND | 0.12 |
| 薯类 Potatoes | ND | ND | ND | ND | ND | ND | ND | ND | ND | ND | ND | ND | ND | ND | ND | ND | ND | ND | ND | ND | ND | ND | ND | ND | 0.11 |
| 肉类 Meats | ND | ND | ND | ND | ND | ND | ND | ND | ND | ND | ND | ND | ND | ND | ND | ND | ND | ND | ND | ND | ND | ND | 2.09 | ND | 0.19 |
| 蛋类 Eggs | ND | ND | ND | ND | ND | ND | ND | ND | ND | ND | ND | ND | ND | ND | ND | ND | ND | ND | ND | ND | ND | ND | ND | ND | 0.12 |
| 水产类 Aquatic foods | ND | ND | ND | ND | ND | ND | ND | ND | ND | ND | ND | ND | ND | ND | ND | ND | ND | ND | ND | ND | ND | ND | ND | ND | 0.11 |
| 乳类 Dairy products | ND | ND | ND | ND | ND | ND | ND | ND | ND | ND | ND | ND | ND | ND | ND | ND | ND | ND | ND | ND | ND | ND | ND | ND | 0.10 |

附录 831

续表

| 膳食类别<br>Category | 黑龙江<br>HL | 辽宁<br>LN | 河北<br>HE | 北京<br>BJ | 吉林<br>JL | 山西<br>SX | 陕西<br>SN | 河南<br>HA | 宁夏<br>NX | 内蒙古<br>NM | 青海<br>QH | 甘肃<br>GS | 上海<br>SH | 福建<br>FJ | 江西<br>JX | 江苏<br>JS | 浙江<br>ZJ | 山东<br>SD | 湖北<br>HB | 四川<br>SC | 广西<br>GX | 湖南<br>HN | 广东<br>GD | 贵州<br>GZ | 全国平均<br>AVG |
|---|---|---|---|---|---|---|---|---|---|---|---|---|---|---|---|---|---|---|---|---|---|---|---|---|---|
| 蔬菜类 Vegetables | ND | ND | ND | 2.77 | ND | ND | ND | ND | ND | ND | ND | ND | ND | ND | ND | ND | ND | ND | ND | ND | ND | ND | ND | ND | 0.22 |
| 水果类 Fruits | ND | ND | ND | ND | ND | ND | ND | ND | ND | ND | ND | ND | ND | ND | ND | ND | ND | ND | ND | ND | ND | ND | ND | ND | 0.10 |
| 糖类 Sugar | ND | ND | ND | ND | ND | ND | ND | ND | ND | ND | ND | ND | ND | ND | ND | ND | ND | ND | ND | ND | ND | ND | ND | ND | 0.10 |
| 水及饮料类 Water and beverages | ND | ND | ND | ND | ND | ND | ND | ND |  | ND | ND | ND | ND | ND | ND | ND | ND | ND | ND | ND | ND | ND | ND | ND | 0.10 |
| 酒类 Alcohol beverages | ND | 1.32 | ND | ND | ND | ND | ND | ND | ND | ND | ND | ND | ND | 1.57 | 1.57 | ND | 1.19 | ND | ND | ND | ND | ND | ND | ND | 0.32 |

注：未检出（ND）按 1/2 检出限（LOD）计

Note: values not detected (ND) were treated as being equal to half of the detection of limit (LOD)

附表 8-12　第六次中国总膳食研究膳食样品中 15-Ac-DON 的含量（单位：μg/kg）

Annexed Table 8-12　Levels of 15-Ac-DON in food samples from the 6$^{th}$ China TDS (Unit: μg/kg)

| 膳食类别<br>Category | 黑龙江<br>HL | 辽宁<br>LN | 河北<br>HE | 北京<br>BJ | 吉林<br>JL | 山西<br>SX | 陕西<br>SN | 河南<br>HA | 宁夏<br>NX | 内蒙古<br>NM | 青海<br>QH | 甘肃<br>GS | 上海<br>SH | 福建<br>FJ | 江西<br>JX | 江苏<br>JS | 浙江<br>ZJ | 山东<br>SD | 湖北<br>HB | 四川<br>SC | 广西<br>GX | 湖南<br>HN | 广东<br>GD | 贵州<br>GZ | 全国平均<br>AVG |
|---|---|---|---|---|---|---|---|---|---|---|---|---|---|---|---|---|---|---|---|---|---|---|---|---|---|
| 谷类 Cereals | ND | ND | ND | ND | ND | ND | ND | ND | ND | ND | ND | ND | ND | ND | ND | 0.313 | ND | ND | ND | ND | ND | ND | ND | ND | 0.088 |
| 豆类 Legumes | ND | 1.986 | ND | ND | ND | ND | ND | ND | ND | ND | ND | ND | ND | ND | ND | 7.304 | ND | ND | ND | ND | ND | ND | ND | ND | 0.440 |
| 薯类 Potatoes | ND | ND | ND | ND | ND | ND | ND | ND | ND | ND | ND | ND | ND | ND | ND | ND | ND | ND | ND | ND | ND | ND | ND | ND | 0.056 |

续表

| 膳食类别 Category | 黑龙江 HL | 辽宁 LN | 河北 HE | 北京 BJ | 吉林 JL | 山西 SX | 陕西 SN | 河南 HA | 宁夏 NX | 内蒙古 NM | 青海 QH | 甘肃 GS | 上海 SH | 福建 FJ | 江西 JX | 江苏 JS | 浙江 ZJ | 山东 SD | 湖北 HB | 四川 SC | 广西 GX | 湖南 HN | 广东 GD | 贵州 GZ | 全国平均 AVG |
|---|---|---|---|---|---|---|---|---|---|---|---|---|---|---|---|---|---|---|---|---|---|---|---|---|---|
| 肉类 Meats | ND | ND | ND | ND | ND | ND | ND | ND | ND | ND | ND | ND | ND | ND | ND | ND | ND | ND | ND | ND | ND | ND | ND | ND | 0.054 |
| 蛋类 Eggs | ND | ND | ND | ND | ND | ND | ND | ND | ND | ND | ND | ND | ND | ND | ND | ND | ND | ND | ND | ND | ND | ND | ND | ND | 0.059 |
| 水产类 Aquatic foods | ND | ND | ND | ND | ND | ND | ND | ND | ND | ND | ND | ND | ND | ND | ND | ND | ND | ND | ND | ND | ND | ND | ND | ND | 0.053 |
| 乳类 Dairy products | ND | ND | ND | ND | ND | ND | ND | ND | ND | ND | ND | ND | ND | ND | ND | ND | ND | ND | ND | ND | ND | ND | ND | ND | 0.050 |
| 蔬菜类 Vegetables | ND | 0.389 | ND | ND | ND | ND | ND | ND | ND | ND | ND | ND | ND | ND | ND | ND | ND | ND | ND | ND | ND | ND | ND | ND | 0.066 |
| 水果类 Fruits | ND | ND | ND | ND | ND | ND | ND | ND | ND | ND | ND | ND | ND | ND | ND | ND | ND | ND | ND | ND | ND | ND | ND | ND | 0.051 |
| 糖类 Sugar | ND | ND | ND | ND | ND | ND | ND | ND | ND | ND | ND | ND | ND | ND | ND | ND | ND | ND | ND | ND | ND | ND | ND | ND | 0.050 |
| 水及饮料类 Water and beverages | ND | ND | ND | ND | ND | ND | ND | ND | ND | ND | ND | ND | ND | ND | ND | ND | ND | ND | ND | ND | ND | ND | ND | ND | 0.050 |
| 酒类 Alcohol beverages | ND | 0.655 | ND | ND | ND | ND | ND | ND | ND | ND | ND | ND | ND | ND | ND | ND | ND | ND | ND | ND | ND | ND | ND | ND | 0.075 |

注：未检出（ND）按 1/2 检出限（LOD）计

Note: values not detected (ND) were treated as being equal to half of the detection of limit (LOD)

附表 8-13 第六次中国总膳食研究膳食样品中 3-Glu-DON 的含量（单位：μg/kg）

Annexed Table 8-13　Levels of 3-Glu-DON in food samples from the 6$^{th}$ China TDS (Unit: μg/kg)

| 膳食类别 Category | 黑龙江 HL | 辽宁 LN | 河北 HE | 北京 BJ | 吉林 JL | 山西 SX | 陕西 SN | 河南 HA | 宁夏 NX | 内蒙古 NM | 青海 QH | 甘肃 GS | 上海 SH | 福建 FJ | 江西 JX | 江苏 JS | 浙江 ZJ | 山东 SD | 湖北 HB | 四川 SC | 广西 GX | 湖南 HN | 广东 GD | 贵州 GZ | 全国平均 AVG |
|---|---|---|---|---|---|---|---|---|---|---|---|---|---|---|---|---|---|---|---|---|---|---|---|---|---|
| 谷类 Cereals | ND | ND | ND | 7.10 | ND | ND | ND | ND | ND | ND | 5.30 | ND | ND | ND | ND | ND | 1.23 | ND | 17.05 | 12.05 | ND | ND | ND | ND | 1.84 |
| 豆类 Legumes | ND | 0.98 | ND | ND | ND | ND | ND | ND | ND | ND | ND | ND | ND | ND | ND | ND | ND | ND | ND | ND | ND | ND | ND | ND | 0.10 |
| 薯类 Potatoes | ND | ND | ND | ND | ND | ND | ND | ND | ND | ND | ND | ND | ND | ND | ND | ND | 0.58 | ND | ND | ND | ND | ND | ND | ND | 0.08 |
| 肉类 Meats | ND | ND | ND | 0.57 | ND | ND | ND | ND | ND | ND | ND | ND | ND | ND | ND | ND | 1.88 | ND | ND | ND | ND | ND | ND | ND | 0.15 |
| 蛋类 Eggs | ND | ND | ND | ND | ND | ND | ND | ND | ND | ND | ND | ND | ND | ND | ND | 1.50 | ND | ND | ND | ND | ND | ND | ND | ND | 0.12 |
| 水产类 Aquatic foods | ND | ND | ND | ND | ND | ND | ND | ND | ND | ND | ND | ND | ND | ND | ND | 0.69 | 5.78 | ND | ND | ND | ND | ND | ND | ND | 0.32 |
| 乳类 Dairy products | ND | 8.03 | ND | ND | ND | ND | ND | ND | ND | ND | ND | ND | ND | ND | ND | ND | ND | ND | ND | ND | ND | ND | ND | ND | 0.38 |
| 蔬菜类 Vegetables | ND | ND | ND | ND | ND | ND | ND | ND | ND | ND | ND | ND | ND | ND | ND | 1.88 | 4.44 | ND | ND | ND | ND | ND | ND | ND | 0.31 |
| 水果类 Fruits | ND | ND | ND | ND | ND | ND | ND | ND | ND | ND | ND | ND | ND | ND | ND | ND | ND | ND | ND | ND | ND | ND | ND | ND | 0.05 |
| 糖类 Sugar | ND | ND | ND | ND | ND | ND | ND | ND | ND | ND | ND | ND | ND | ND | ND | ND | ND | ND | ND | ND | ND | ND | ND | ND | 0.05 |
| 水及饮料类 Water and beverages | ND | ND | ND | ND | ND | ND | ND | ND | ND | ND | ND | ND | ND | ND | ND | ND | ND | ND | ND | ND | ND | ND | ND | ND | 0.05 |

续表

| 膳食类别 Category | 黑龙江 HL | 辽宁 LN | 河北 HE | 北京 BJ | 吉林 JL | 山西 SX | 陕西 SN | 河南 HA | 宁夏 NX | 内蒙古 NM | 青海 QH | 甘肃 GS | 上海 SH | 福建 FJ | 江西 JX | 江苏 JS | 浙江 ZJ | 山东 SD | 湖北 HB | 四川 SC | 广西 GX | 湖南 HN | 广东 GD | 贵州 GZ | 全国平均 AVG |
|---|---|---|---|---|---|---|---|---|---|---|---|---|---|---|---|---|---|---|---|---|---|---|---|---|---|
| 酒类 Alcohol beverages | ND | ND | ND | ND | 3.33 | ND | ND | ND | ND | 2.60 | ND | ND | ND | ND | ND | 1.08 | 0.41 | ND | | | | ND | ND | ND | 0.35 |

注：未检出（ND）按 1/2 检出限（LOD）计
Note: values not detected (ND) were treated as being equal to half of the detection of limit (LOD)

附表 8-14 第六次中国总膳食研究膳食样品中 deepoxy-DON 的含量（单位：μg/kg）
Annexed Table 8-14　Levels of deepoxy-DON in food samples from the 6$^{th}$ China TDS (Unit: μg/kg)

| 膳食类别 Category | 黑龙江 HL | 辽宁 LN | 河北 HE | 北京 BJ | 吉林 JL | 山西 SX | 陕西 SN | 河南 HA | 宁夏 NX | 内蒙古 NM | 青海 QH | 甘肃 GS | 上海 SH | 福建 FJ | 江西 JX | 江苏 JS | 浙江 ZJ | 山东 SD | 湖北 HB | 四川 SC | 广西 GX | 湖南 HN | 广东 GD | 贵州 GZ | 全国平均 AVG |
|---|---|---|---|---|---|---|---|---|---|---|---|---|---|---|---|---|---|---|---|---|---|---|---|---|---|
| 谷类 Cereals | ND | ND | ND | ND | ND | ND | ND | ND | ND | ND | ND | ND | ND | ND | ND | ND | ND | ND | ND | ND | ND | ND | ND | ND | 0.15 |
| 豆类 Legumes | ND | ND | ND | ND | ND | ND | ND | ND | ND | ND | ND | ND | ND | ND | ND | 3.40 | ND | ND | ND | ND | ND | ND | ND | ND | 0.25 |
| 薯类 Potatoes | ND | ND | ND | ND | ND | ND | ND | ND | ND | ND | ND | ND | ND | ND | ND | ND | ND | ND | ND | ND | ND | ND | ND | ND | 0.11 |
| 肉类 Meats | ND | ND | ND | ND | ND | ND | ND | ND | ND | ND | ND | ND | ND | ND | ND | ND | ND | ND | ND | ND | ND | ND | ND | ND | 0.11 |
| 蛋类 Eggs | ND | ND | ND | ND | ND | ND | ND | ND | ND | ND | ND | ND | ND | ND | ND | ND | ND | ND | ND | ND | ND | ND | ND | ND | 0.12 |
| 水产类 Aquatic foods | ND | ND | ND | ND | ND | ND | ND | ND | ND | ND | ND | ND | ND | ND | ND | ND | ND | ND | ND | ND | ND | ND | ND | ND | 0.11 |
| 乳类 Dairy products | ND | ND | ND | ND | ND | ND | ND | ND | ND | ND | ND | ND | ND | ND | ND | ND | ND | ND | ND | ND | ND | ND | ND | ND | 0.10 |

续表

| 膳食类别 Category | 黑龙江 HL | 辽宁 LN | 河北 HE | 北京 BJ | 吉林 JL | 山西 SX | 陕西 SN | 河南 HA | 宁夏 NX | 内蒙古 NM | 青海 QH | 甘肃 GS | 上海 SH | 福建 FJ | 江西 JX | 江苏 JS | 浙江 ZJ | 山东 SD | 湖北 HB | 四川 SC | 广西 GX | 湖南 HN | 广东 GD | 贵州 GZ | 全国平均 AVG |
|---|---|---|---|---|---|---|---|---|---|---|---|---|---|---|---|---|---|---|---|---|---|---|---|---|---|
| 蔬菜类 Vegetables | ND | 1.35 | ND | ND | ND | ND | ND | ND | ND | ND | ND | ND | ND | ND | ND | ND | ND | ND | ND | ND | ND | ND | ND | ND | 0.16 |
| 水果类 Fruits | ND | ND | ND | ND | ND | ND | ND | ND | ND | ND | 2.18 | ND | ND | ND | ND | ND | ND | ND | ND | ND | ND | 0.94 | ND | ND | 0.22 |
| 糖类 Sugar | ND | ND | ND | ND | ND | ND | ND | ND | ND | ND | ND | ND | ND | ND | ND | ND | ND | ND | ND | ND | ND | ND | ND | ND | 0.10 |
| 水及饮料类 Water and beverages | ND | ND | ND | ND | ND | ND | ND | ND | ND | ND | ND | ND | ND | ND | ND | ND | ND | ND | ND | ND | ND | ND | ND | ND | 0.10 |
| 酒类 Alcohol beverages | ND | ND | ND | ND | ND | ND | ND | ND | ND | ND | ND | ND | ND | ND | ND | ND | ND | ND | ND | ND | ND | ND | ND | ND | 0.10 |

注: 未检出 (ND) 按 1/2 检出限 (LOD) 计
Note: values not detected (ND) were treated as being equal to half of the detection of limit (LOD)

附表 8-15　第六次中国总膳食研究的 DON、3-Ac-DON、15-Ac-DON 总量膳食摄入量 [单位: ng/(kg bw · d)]
Annexed Table 8-15　Dietary intakes of DON, 3-Ac-DON, 15-Ac-DON from the 6$^{th}$ China TDS [Unit: ng/(kg bw · d)]

| 膳食类别 Category | 黑龙江 HL | 辽宁 LN | 河北 HE | 北京 BJ | 吉林 JL | 山西 SX | 陕西 SN | 河南 HA | 宁夏 NX | 内蒙古 NM | 青海 QH | 甘肃 GS | 上海 SH | 福建 FJ | 江西 JX | 江苏 JS | 浙江 ZJ | 山东 SD | 湖北 HB | 四川 SC | 广西 GX | 湖南 HN | 广东 GD | 贵州 GZ | 全国平均 AVG |
|---|---|---|---|---|---|---|---|---|---|---|---|---|---|---|---|---|---|---|---|---|---|---|---|---|---|
| 谷类 Cereals | 996.2 | 360.4 | 866.0 | 1128.0 | 319.1 | 1110.0 | 925.2 | 751.7 | 580.8 | 230.5 | 1425.0 | 482.8 | 512.9 | 745.2 | 299.2 | 201.6 | 855.3 | 1095.0 | 869.7 | 1962.0 | 76.8 | 46.4 | 193.6 | 75.5 | 671.2 |
| 豆类 Legumes | 0.261 | 4.375 | 0.270 | 0.439 | 7.768 | 0.306 | 0.370 | 0.306 | 6.154 | 2.171 | 0.030 | 0.169 | 0.536 | 0.318 | 0.332 | 13.799 | 4.582 | 0.222 | 0.295 | 2.252 | 1.945 | 4.360 | 1.148 | 0.480 | 2.204 |
| 薯类 Potatoes | 0.365 | 7.325 | 3.123 | 24.460 | 3.463 | 11.010 | 0.563 | 0.346 | 11.026 | 0.495 | 0.419 | 0.589 | 0.143 | 0.184 | 0.128 | 0.160 | 1.313 | 0.191 | 0.355 | 0.258 | 0.067 | 0.287 | 0.102 | 0.166 | 2.772 |

续表

| 膳食类别<br>Category | 黑龙江<br>HL | 辽宁<br>LN | 河北<br>HE | 北京<br>BJ | 吉林<br>JL | 山西<br>SX | 陕西<br>SN | 河南<br>HA | 宁夏<br>NX | 内蒙古<br>NM | 青海<br>QH | 甘肃<br>GS | 上海<br>SH | 福建<br>FJ | 江西<br>JX | 江苏<br>JS | 浙江<br>ZJ | 山东<br>SD | 湖北<br>HB | 四川<br>SC | 广西<br>GX | 湖南<br>HN | 广东<br>GD | 贵州<br>GZ | 全国平均<br>AVG |
|---|---|---|---|---|---|---|---|---|---|---|---|---|---|---|---|---|---|---|---|---|---|---|---|---|---|
| 肉类 Meats | 0.281 | 0.327 | 0.204 | 0.334 | 2.833 | 17.651 | 0.153 | 0.229 | 5.347 | 0.298 | 0.285 | 0.138 | 0.439 | 0.352 | 0.376 | 9.630 | 4.772 | 0.415 | 0.224 | 0.516 | 0.599 | 0.599 | 3.762 | 0.436 | 2.092 |
| 蛋类 Eggs | 0.163 | 0.214 | 0.160 | 0.181 | 0.183 | 0.114 | 0.102 | 0.118 | 0.076 | 0.155 | 0.072 | 0.102 | 0.168 | 0.098 | 0.096 | 0.119 | 0.117 | 0.218 | 0.117 | 0.066 | 0.386 | 0.092 | 0.096 | 0.065 | 0.137 |
| 水产类 Aquatic foods | 0.108 | 0.094 | 0.042 | 0.553 | 0.044 | 0.234 | 0.016 | 0.488 | 0.010 | 0.041 | 0.244 | 0.011 | 6.006 | 0.265 | 4.444 | 1.917 | 3.341 | 0.094 | 0.162 | 0.033 | 2.780 | 1.563 | 0.925 | 0.017 | 0.976 |
| 乳类 Dairy products | 0.053 | 0.176 | 0.096 | 0.340 | 0.128 | 0.165 | 0.077 | 0.078 | 0.061 | 0.136 | 0.212 | 0.056 | 0.283 | 0.143 | 0.087 | 0.109 | 0.133 | 0.091 | 0.027 | 0.050 | 0.072 | 0.071 | 0.145 | 0.112 | 0.121 |
| 蔬菜类 Vegetables | 1.568 | 13.790 | 1.176 | 18.160 | 1.555 | 1.251 | 1.176 | 1.114 | 0.620 | 1.052 | 1.232 | 0.984 | 1.590 | 8.655 | 1.792 | 28.44 | 15.51 | 1.966 | 1.643 | 1.210 | 1.431 | 2.184 | 0.968 | 5.741 | 4.784 |
| 水果类 Fruits | 0.249 | 0.332 | 0.149 | 0.480 | 0.349 | 0.139 | 0.158 | 0.096 | 0.389 | 0.453 | 0.064 | 0.132 | 0.291 | 0.245 | 0.225 | 0.108 | 0.267 | 0.216 | 0.076 | 0.065 | 0.256 | 0.252 | 0.116 | 0.094 | 0.217 |
| 糖类 Sugar | 0.009 | 0.003 | 0.002 | 0.008 | 0.004 | 0.004 | 0.151 | 0.002 | 0.003 | 0.004 | 0.002 | 0.002 | 1.177 | 0.001 | 0.004 | 0.001 | 0.004 | 0.002 | 0.001 | 0.002 | 0.002 | 0.002 | 0.001 | 0.001 | 0.058 |
| 水及饮料类 Water and beverages | 4.851 | 1.958 | 3.077 | 4.396 | 5.165 | 2.958 | 1.371 | 4.732 | 2.052 | 10.218 | 2.454 | 4.686 | 2.788 | 3.434 | 4.689 | 4.004 | 3.120 | 7.145 | 1.131 | 1.246 | 5.167 | 4.214 | 4.733 | 4.970 | 3.940 |
| 酒类 Alcohol beverages | 0.767 | 7.310 | 0.150 | 0.109 | 0.444 | 0.001 | 0.007 | 0.013 | 0.002 | 1.065 | 0.094 | 0.114 | 2.166 | 0.904 | 0.589 | 10.277 | 15.031 | 2.285 | 0.057 | 0.231 | 0.127 | 0.317 | 0.049 | 0.413 | 1.772 |
| 合计 SUM | 1004.8 | 396.3 | 874.5 | 1177.8 | 341.0 | 1143.5 | 929.4 | 759.2 | 606.6 | 246.6 | 1430.3 | 489.8 | 528.5 | 759.8 | 312.0 | 270.2 | 903.5 | 1107.5 | 873.7 | 1967.8 | 89.6 | 60.3 | 205.7 | 88.0 | 690.3 |

附表 8-16 第六次中国总膳食研究的 DON、3-Ac-DON、15-Ac-DON、3-Glu-DON 总量膳食摄入量 [单位：ng/(kg bw·d)]
Annexed Table 8-16　Dietary intakes of DON, 3-Ac-DON, 15-Ac-DON, 3-Glu-DON from the 6th China TDS [Unit: ng/(kg bw·d)]

| 膳食类别 Category | 黑龙江 HL | 辽宁 LN | 河北 HE | 北京 BJ | 吉林 JL | 山西 SX | 陕西 SN | 河南 HA | 宁夏 NX | 内蒙古 NM | 青海 QH | 甘肃 GS | 上海 SH | 福建 FJ | 江西 JX | 江苏 JS | 浙江 ZJ | 山东 SD | 湖北 HB | 四川 SC | 广西 GX | 湖南 HN | 广东 GD | 贵州 GZ | 全国平均 AVG |
|---|---|---|---|---|---|---|---|---|---|---|---|---|---|---|---|---|---|---|---|---|---|---|---|---|---|
| 谷类 Cereals | 997.0 | 361.3 | 867.0 | 1218.0 | 319.7 | 1111.0 | 926.4 | 752.9 | 581.8 | 231.4 | 1490.0 | 483.8 | 513.3 | 745.9 | 299.9 | 199.3 | 867.6 | 1096.0 | 1013.0 | 2147.0 | 77.9 | 47.1 | 194.1 | 76.4 | 692.408 |
| 豆类 Legumes | 0.313 | 6.285 | 0.324 | 0.527 | 7.849 | 0.367 | 0.444 | 0.367 | 6.186 | 2.205 | 0.035 | 0.202 | 0.644 | 0.382 | 0.399 | 13.880 | 4.701 | 0.266 | 0.353 | 2.314 | 1.979 | 4.435 | 1.173 | 0.576 | 2.342 |
| 薯类 Potatoes | 0.438 | 7.399 | 3.179 | 24.515 | 3.558 | 11.130 | 0.676 | 0.416 | 11.117 | 0.594 | 0.503 | 0.706 | 0.171 | 0.221 | 0.153 | 0.192 | 1.646 | 0.229 | 0.426 | 0.310 | 0.081 | 0.345 | 0.123 | 0.199 | 2.847 |
| 肉类 Meats | 0.337 | 0.393 | 0.245 | 0.935 | 2.886 | 17.770 | 0.184 | 0.275 | 5.385 | 0.357 | 0.342 | 0.166 | 0.527 | 0.422 | 0.452 | 9.704 | 8.285 | 0.498 | 0.269 | 0.619 | 0.719 | 0.719 | 3.866 | 0.523 | 2.328 |
| 蛋类 Eggs | 0.195 | 0.256 | 0.192 | 0.218 | 0.220 | 0.137 | 0.122 | 0.142 | 0.091 | 0.186 | 0.087 | 0.123 | 0.202 | 0.118 | 0.115 | 0.789 | 0.141 | 0.261 | 0.140 | 0.079 | 0.398 | 0.111 | 0.115 | 0.077 | 0.188 |
| 水产类 Aquatic foods | 0.129 | 0.112 | 0.050 | 0.567 | 0.053 | 0.240 | 0.020 | 0.491 | 0.012 | 0.049 | 0.247 | 0.013 | 6.061 | 0.318 | 4.479 | 2.344 | 7.959 | 0.113 | 0.194 | 0.040 | 2.858 | 1.616 | 0.968 | 0.020 | 1.206 |
| 乳类 Dairy products | 0.064 | 5.838 | 0.115 | 0.408 | 0.154 | 0.198 | 0.092 | 0.093 | 0.073 | 0.164 | 0.255 | 0.067 | 0.340 | 0.171 | 0.104 | 0.131 | 0.160 | 0.109 | 0.032 | 0.060 | 0.086 | 0.086 | 0.174 | 0.134 | 0.379 |
| 蔬菜类 Vegetables | 1.881 | 14.070 | 1.411 | 18.480 | 1.866 | 1.502 | 1.411 | 1.337 | 0.744 | 1.262 | 1.479 | 1.181 | 1.908 | 8.973 | 2.150 | 41.100 | 46.800 | 2.360 | 1.972 | 1.452 | 1.717 | 2.621 | 1.161 | 6.075 | 6.871 |
| 水果类 Fruits | 0.299 | 0.398 | 0.179 | 0.576 | 0.418 | 0.166 | 0.190 | 0.115 | 0.467 | 0.543 | 0.077 | 0.158 | 0.350 | 0.294 | 0.270 | 0.130 | 0.321 | 0.259 | 0.091 | 0.078 | 0.307 | 0.302 | 0.140 | 0.113 | 0.260 |
| 糖类 Sugar | 0.011 | 0.004 | 0.002 | 0.009 | 0.005 | 0.005 | 0.181 | 0.002 | 0.004 | 0.005 | 0.002 | 0.002 | 1.183 | 0.001 | 0.005 | 0.001 | 0.005 | 0.002 | 0.001 | 0.002 | 0.002 | 0.002 | 0.001 | 0.001 | 0.060 |
| 水及饮料类 Water and beverages | 5.821 | 2.350 | 3.692 | 5.275 | 6.198 | 3.550 | 1.645 | 5.678 | 2.462 | 12.260 | 2.944 | 5.624 | 3.346 | 4.121 | 5.626 | 4.805 | 3.744 | 8.574 | 1.357 | 1.495 | 6.201 | 5.057 | 5.679 | 5.964 | 4.728 |

续表

| 膳食类别 Category | 黑龙江 HL | 辽宁 LN | 河北 HE | 北京 BJ | 吉林 JL | 山西 SX | 陕西 SN | 河南 HA | 宁夏 NX | 内蒙古 NM | 青海 QH | 甘肃 GS | 上海 SH | 福建 FJ | 江西 JX | 江苏 JS | 浙江 ZJ | 山东 SD | 湖北 HB | 四川 SC | 广西 GX | 湖南 HN | 广东 GD | 贵州 GZ | 全国平均 AVG |
|---|---|---|---|---|---|---|---|---|---|---|---|---|---|---|---|---|---|---|---|---|---|---|---|---|---|
| 酒类 Alcohol beverages | 0.785 | 7.013 | 0.158 | 0.131 | 0.948 | 0.001 | 0.008 | 0.015 | 0.002 | 1.921 | 0.098 | 0.117 | 2.184 | 0.915 | 0.606 | 10.920 | 15.440 | 2.375 | 0.068 | 0.235 | 0.152 | 0.330 | 0.050 | 0.415 | 1.870 |
| 合计 SUM | 1007.3 | 405.3 | 876.6 | 1269.6 | 343.9 | 1146.1 | 931.4 | 761.8 | 608.3 | 250.9 | 1495.7 | 492.1 | 530.3 | 761.8 | 314.2 | 283.3 | 956.8 | 1110.8 | 1017.6 | 2154.1 | 92.4 | 62.7 | 207.6 | 90.5 | 715.4 |

附表 8-17 第六次中国总膳食研究膳食样品中 NIV 的含量（单位：μg/kg）
Annexed Table 8-17 Levels of NIV in food samples from the 6th China TDS (Unit: μg/kg)

| 膳食类别 Category | 黑龙江 HL | 辽宁 LN | 河北 HE | 北京 BJ | 吉林 JL | 山西 SX | 陕西 SN | 河南 HA | 宁夏 NX | 内蒙古 NM | 青海 QH | 甘肃 GS | 上海 SH | 福建 FJ | 江西 JX | 江苏 JS | 浙江 ZJ | 山东 SD | 湖北 HB | 四川 SC | 广西 GX | 湖南 HN | 广东 GD | 贵州 GZ | 全国平均 AVG |
|---|---|---|---|---|---|---|---|---|---|---|---|---|---|---|---|---|---|---|---|---|---|---|---|---|---|
| 谷类 Cereals | ND | ND | ND | ND | ND | ND | ND | ND | ND | ND | ND | ND | ND | ND | ND | 2.03 | 6.58 | ND | 6.63 | ND | ND | ND | ND | ND | 0.704 |
| 豆类 Legumes | ND | ND | ND | ND | ND | ND | ND | ND | ND | ND | ND | ND | ND | ND | ND | 1.15 | ND | ND | ND | ND | ND | ND | ND | ND | 0.104 |
| 薯类 Potatoes | ND | 0.82 | ND | ND | ND | ND | ND | ND | ND | ND | ND | ND | ND | ND | ND | ND | 0.47 | ND | ND | ND | ND | ND | ND | ND | 0.105 |
| 肉类 Meats | ND | ND | ND | ND | ND | ND | ND | ND | ND | ND | ND | ND | ND | ND | ND | ND | 0.69 | ND | ND | ND | ND | ND | ND | ND | 0.080 |
| 蛋类 Eggs | ND | ND | ND | ND | ND | ND | ND | ND | ND | ND | ND | ND | ND | ND | ND | ND | ND | ND | ND | ND | ND | ND | ND | ND | 0.059 |
| 水产类 Aquatic foods | ND | ND | ND | 0.59 | ND | ND | ND | ND | ND | ND | ND | ND | ND | ND | ND | ND | 0.66 | ND | ND | ND | ND | ND | ND | ND | 0.101 |

续表

| 膳食类别 Category | 黑龙江 HL | 辽宁 LN | 河北 HE | 北京 BJ | 吉林 JL | 山西 SX | 陕西 SN | 河南 HA | 宁夏 NX | 内蒙古 NM | 青海 QH | 甘肃 GS | 上海 SH | 福建 FJ | 江西 JX | 江苏 JS | 浙江 ZJ | 山东 SD | 湖北 HB | 四川 SC | 广西 GX | 湖南 HN | 广东 GD | 贵州 GZ | 全国平均 AVG |
|---|---|---|---|---|---|---|---|---|---|---|---|---|---|---|---|---|---|---|---|---|---|---|---|---|---|
| 乳类 Dairy products | ND | ND | ND | ND | ND | ND | ND | ND | ND | ND | ND | ND | ND | ND | ND | ND | ND | ND | ND | ND | ND | ND | ND | ND | 0.050 |
| 蔬菜类 Vegetables | ND | 0.71 | ND | ND | ND | ND | ND | ND | ND | ND | ND | ND | ND | ND | ND | 0.85 | 0.50 | ND | ND | ND | ND | ND | ND | ND | 0.131 |
| 水果类 Fruits | ND | ND | ND | ND | ND | ND | ND | ND | ND | ND | ND | ND | ND | ND | ND | ND | ND | ND | ND | ND | ND | ND | ND | ND | 0.051 |
| 糖类 Sugar | ND | ND | ND | ND | ND | ND | ND | ND | ND | ND | ND | ND | ND | ND | ND | ND | ND | ND | ND | ND | ND | ND | ND | ND | 0.050 |
| 水及饮料类 Water and beverages | ND | ND | ND | ND | ND | ND | ND | ND | ND | ND | ND | ND | ND | ND | ND | ND | ND | ND | ND | ND | ND | ND | ND | ND | 0.050 |
| 酒类 Alcohol beverages | ND | 0.74 | ND | ND | ND | ND | ND | ND | ND | ND | ND | ND | ND | ND | ND | 3.05 | 2.09 | ND | ND | ND | ND | ND | ND | ND | 0.289 |

注：未检出（ND）按 1/2 检出限（LOD）计

Note: values not detected (ND) were treated as being equal to half of the detection of limit (LOD)

附表 8-18 第六次中国总膳食研究的 NIV 膳食摄入量 [单位：ng/(kg bw·d)]

Annexed Table 8-18 Dietary intakes of NIV from the 6th China TDS [Unit: ng/(kg bw·d)]

| 膳食类别 Category | 黑龙江 HL | 辽宁 LN | 河北 HE | 北京 BJ | 吉林 JL | 山西 SX | 陕西 SN | 河南 HA | 宁夏 NX | 内蒙古 NM | 青海 QH | 甘肃 GS | 上海 SH | 福建 FJ | 江西 JX | 江苏 JS | 浙江 ZJ | 山东 SD | 湖北 HB | 四川 SC | 广西 GX | 湖南 HN | 广东 GD | 贵州 GZ | 全国平均 AVG |
|---|---|---|---|---|---|---|---|---|---|---|---|---|---|---|---|---|---|---|---|---|---|---|---|---|---|
| 谷类 Cereals | 0.842 | 0.775 | 0.993 | 0.889 | 0.611 | 1.328 | 1.179 | 1.146 | 0.936 | 0.844 | 1.382 | 0.923 | 0.463 | 0.738 | 0.685 | 25.010 | 66.110 | 1.054 | 55.610 | 1.217 | 1.098 | 0.674 | 0.490 | 0.864 | 6.911 |
| 豆类 Legumes | 0.052 | 0.133 | 0.054 | 0.088 | 0.081 | 0.061 | 0.074 | 0.061 | 0.033 | 0.034 | 0.006 | 0.034 | 0.107 | 0.064 | 0.066 | 1.516 | 0.119 | 0.044 | 0.059 | 0.062 | 0.034 | 0.075 | 0.025 | 0.096 | 0.124 |

续表

| 膳食类别 Category | 黑龙江 HL | 辽宁 LN | 河北 HE | 北京 BJ | 吉林 JL | 山西 SX | 陕西 SN | 河南 HA | 宁夏 NX | 内蒙古 NM | 青海 QH | 甘肃 GS | 上海 SH | 福建 FJ | 江西 JX | 江苏 JS | 浙江 ZJ | 山东 SD | 湖北 HB | 四川 SC | 广西 GX | 湖南 HN | 广东 GD | 贵州 GZ | 全国平均 AVG |
|---|---|---|---|---|---|---|---|---|---|---|---|---|---|---|---|---|---|---|---|---|---|---|---|---|---|
| 薯类 Potatoes | 0.073 | 0.935 | 0.056 | 0.054 | 0.095 | 0.118 | 0.113 | 0.069 | 0.091 | 0.099 | 0.084 | 0.118 | 0.029 | 0.037 | 0.026 | 0.033 | 0.275 | 0.038 | 0.071 | 0.052 | 0.013 | 0.057 | 0.020 | 0.033 | 0.108 |
| 肉类 Meats | 0.056 | 0.065 | 0.041 | 0.067 | 0.053 | 0.115 | 0.031 | 0.046 | 0.039 | 0.060 | 0.057 | 0.028 | 0.088 | 0.070 | 0.075 | 0.076 | 1.301 | 0.083 | 0.045 | 0.103 | 0.120 | 0.120 | 0.105 | 0.087 | 0.122 |
| 蛋类 Eggs | 0.033 | 0.043 | 0.032 | 0.036 | 0.037 | 0.023 | 0.020 | 0.024 | 0.015 | 0.031 | 0.014 | 0.020 | 0.034 | 0.020 | 0.019 | 0.024 | 0.023 | 0.044 | 0.023 | 0.013 | 0.012 | 0.018 | 0.019 | 0.013 | 0.025 |
| 水产类 Aquatic foods | 0.022 | 0.019 | 0.008 | 0.154 | 0.009 | 0.006 | 0.003 | 0.004 | 0.002 | 0.008 | 0.003 | 0.002 | 0.054 | 0.053 | 0.035 | 0.032 | 0.525 | 0.019 | 0.032 | 0.007 | 0.077 | 0.053 | 0.042 | 0.003 | 0.049 |
| 乳类 Dairy products | 0.011 | 0.035 | 0.019 | 0.068 | 0.026 | 0.033 | 0.015 | 0.016 | 0.012 | 0.027 | 0.042 | 0.011 | 0.057 | 0.029 | 0.017 | 0.022 | 0.027 | 0.018 | 0.005 | 0.010 | 0.014 | 0.014 | 0.029 | 0.022 | 0.024 |
| 蔬菜类 Vegetables | 0.314 | 3.690 | 0.235 | 0.314 | 0.311 | 0.250 | 0.235 | 0.223 | 0.124 | 0.210 | 0.246 | 0.197 | 0.318 | 0.318 | 0.358 | 5.720 | 3.539 | 0.393 | 0.329 | 0.242 | 0.286 | 0.437 | 0.194 | 0.334 | 0.784 |
| 水果类 Fruits | 0.050 | 0.066 | 0.030 | 0.096 | 0.070 | 0.028 | 0.032 | 0.019 | 0.078 | 0.091 | 0.013 | 0.026 | 0.058 | 0.049 | 0.045 | 0.022 | 0.053 | 0.043 | 0.015 | 0.013 | 0.051 | 0.050 | 0.023 | 0.019 | 0.043 |
| 糖类 Sugar | 0.002 | 0.001 | 0.001 | 0.002 | 0.001 | 0.001 | 0.030 | 0.001 | 0.001 | 0.001 | 0.001 | 0.001 | 0.006 | 0.001 | 0.001 | 0.001 | 0.001 | 0.001 | 0.001 | 0.001 | 0.001 | 0.001 | 0.001 | 0.001 | 0.002 |
| 水及饮料类 Water and beverages | 0.970 | 0.392 | 0.615 | 0.879 | 1.033 | 0.592 | 0.274 | 0.946 | 0.410 | 2.044 | 0.491 | 0.937 | 0.558 | 0.687 | 0.938 | 0.801 | 0.624 | 1.429 | 0.226 | 0.249 | 1.033 | 0.843 | 0.947 | 0.994 | 0.788 |
| 酒类 Alcohol beverages | 0.017 | 0.396 | 0.008 | 0.022 | 0.008 | 0.001 | 0.001 | 0.003 | 0.000 | 0.016 | 0.004 | 0.003 | 0.018 | 0.011 | 0.017 | 1.814 | 2.079 | 0.090 | 0.011 | 0.004 | 0.025 | 0.013 | 0.001 | 0.002 | 0.190 |
| 合计 SUM | 2.441 | 6.551 | 2.093 | 2.668 | 2.334 | 2.554 | 2.008 | 2.556 | 1.740 | 3.465 | 2.343 | 2.300 | 1.789 | 2.076 | 2.282 | 35.065 | 74.676 | 3.256 | 56.430 | 1.972 | 2.766 | 2.356 | 1.895 | 2.467 | 9.170 |

附录 841

附表 8-19　第六次中国总膳食研究膳食样品中 OTA 的含量（单位：μg/kg）

Annexed Table 8-19　Levels of OTA in food samples from the 6th China TDS (Unit: μg/kg)

| 膳食类别 Category | 黑龙江 HL | 辽宁 LN | 河北 HE | 北京 BJ | 吉林 JL | 山西 SX | 陕西 SN | 河南 HA | 宁夏 NX | 内蒙古 NM | 青海 QH | 甘肃 GS | 上海 SH | 福建 FJ | 江西 JX | 江苏 JS | 浙江 ZJ | 山东 SD | 湖北 HB | 四川 SC | 广西 GX | 湖南 HN | 广东 GD | 贵州 GZ | 全国平均 AVG |
|---|---|---|---|---|---|---|---|---|---|---|---|---|---|---|---|---|---|---|---|---|---|---|---|---|---|
| 谷类 Cereals | ND | ND | ND | ND | ND | ND | ND | ND | 0.038 | 1.262 | ND | ND | ND | ND | ND | 0.132 | ND | ND | ND | ND | ND | ND | ND | ND | 0.062 |
| 豆类 Legumes | ND | ND | ND | ND | ND | 2.173 | ND | ND | ND | ND | ND | ND | ND | ND | ND | ND | ND | ND | ND | ND | ND | ND | ND | ND | 0.093 |
| 薯类 Potatoes | ND | ND | ND | ND | ND | ND | ND | ND | ND | ND | ND | ND | ND | ND | ND | ND | ND | ND | ND | ND | ND | ND | ND | ND | 0.002 |
| 肉类 Meats | ND | ND | ND | ND | ND | ND | ND | ND | ND | ND | ND | ND | ND | ND | ND | ND | ND | ND | ND | ND | ND | ND | ND | ND | 0.002 |
| 蛋类 Eggs | ND | ND | ND | ND | ND | ND | ND | ND | ND | ND | ND | ND | ND | ND | ND | ND | ND | ND | ND | ND | ND | ND | ND | ND | 0.002 |
| 水产类 Aquatic foods | ND | ND | ND | ND | ND | ND | ND | ND | ND | ND | ND | ND | ND | ND | ND | ND | ND | ND | ND | ND | ND | ND | ND | ND | 0.002 |
| 乳类 Dairy products | ND | ND | ND | ND | ND | ND | ND | ND | ND | ND | ND | ND | ND | ND | ND | ND | ND | ND | ND | ND | ND | ND | ND | ND | 0.002 |
| 蔬菜类 Vegetables | ND | ND | ND | ND | ND | ND | ND | ND | ND | ND | ND | ND | ND | ND | ND | ND | ND | ND | ND | ND | ND | ND | ND | ND | 0.002 |
| 水果类 Fruits | ND | ND | ND | ND | ND | ND | ND | ND | ND | ND | ND | ND | ND | ND | ND | ND | ND | ND | ND | ND | ND | ND | ND | ND | 0.002 |
| 糖类 Sugar | ND | ND | ND | ND | ND | ND | ND | ND | ND | ND | ND | ND | ND | ND | ND | ND | ND | ND | ND | ND | ND | ND | ND | ND | 0.002 |
| 水及饮料类 Water and beverages | ND | ND | ND | ND | ND | ND | ND | ND | ND | ND | ND | ND | ND | ND | ND | ND | ND | ND | ND | ND | ND | ND | ND | ND | 0.002 |

续表

| 膳食类别 Category | 黑龙江 HL | 辽宁 LN | 河北 HE | 北京 BJ | 吉林 JL | 山西 SX | 陕西 SN | 河南 HA | 宁夏 NX | 内蒙古 NM | 青海 QH | 甘肃 GS | 上海 SH | 福建 FJ | 江西 JX | 江苏 JS | 浙江 ZJ | 山东 SD | 湖北 HB | 四川 SC | 广西 GX | 湖南 HN | 广东 GD | 贵州 GZ | 全国平均 AVG |
|---|---|---|---|---|---|---|---|---|---|---|---|---|---|---|---|---|---|---|---|---|---|---|---|---|---|
| 酒类 Alcohol beverages | ND | ND | ND | ND | ND | ND | ND | ND | ND | ND | ND | ND | ND | ND | ND | ND | ND | ND | ND | ND | ND | ND | ND | ND | 0.002 |

注：平均值计算中，ND 以 1/2 检出限（LOD）计

Note: in calculation of averages (AVG), values not detected (ND) were treated as being equal to half of the detection of limit (LOD)

附表 8-20 第六次中国总膳食研究膳食样品中 OTB 的含量（单位：μg/kg）

Annexed Table 8-20 Levels of OTB in food samples from the 6th China TDS (Unit: μg/kg)

| 膳食类别 Category | 黑龙江 HL | 辽宁 LN | 河北 HE | 北京 BJ | 吉林 JL | 山西 SX | 陕西 SN | 河南 HA | 宁夏 NX | 内蒙古 NM | 青海 QH | 甘肃 GS | 上海 SH | 福建 FJ | 江西 JX | 江苏 JS | 浙江 ZJ | 山东 SD | 湖北 HB | 四川 SC | 广西 GX | 湖南 HN | 广东 GD | 贵州 GZ | 全国平均 AVG |
|---|---|---|---|---|---|---|---|---|---|---|---|---|---|---|---|---|---|---|---|---|---|---|---|---|---|
| 谷类 Cereals | ND | ND | ND | ND | ND | ND | ND | ND | ND | ND | ND | ND | ND | ND | ND | ND | ND | ND | ND | ND | ND | ND | ND | ND | 0.003 |
| 豆类 Legumes | ND | ND | ND | ND | ND | ND | ND | ND | 0.133 | ND | 4.186 | ND | ND | ND | 6.955 | ND | ND | ND | 0.136 | ND | ND | ND | ND | 0.060 | 0.480 |
| 薯类 Potatoes | ND | ND | ND | ND | ND | ND | ND | ND | ND | ND | ND | ND | ND | ND | ND | ND | ND | ND | ND | ND | ND | ND | ND | ND | 0.002 |
| 肉类 Meats | ND | ND | ND | ND | ND | ND | ND | 4.349 | ND | ND | ND | ND | ND | ND | ND | ND | ND | ND | ND | ND | ND | ND | ND | ND | 0.183 |
| 蛋类 Eggs | ND | ND | ND | ND | ND | ND | ND | ND | ND | ND | ND | ND | ND | ND | ND | ND | ND | ND | ND | ND | ND | ND | ND | ND | 0.002 |
| 水产类 Aquatic foods | ND | ND | ND | ND | ND | ND | ND | ND | 0.016 | ND | ND | ND | ND | ND | ND | ND | ND | 5.185 | ND | ND | ND | ND | ND | ND | 0.219 |
| 乳类 Dairy products | ND | ND | ND | ND | ND | ND | ND | ND | ND | ND | ND | ND | ND | ND | ND | ND | ND | ND | ND | ND | ND | ND | ND | ND | 0.002 |

续表

| 膳食类别<br>Category | 黑龙江<br>HL | 辽宁<br>LN | 河北<br>HE | 北京<br>BJ | 吉林<br>JL | 山西<br>SX | 陕西<br>SN | 河南<br>HA | 宁夏<br>NX | 内蒙古<br>NM | 青海<br>QH | 甘肃<br>GS | 上海<br>SH | 福建<br>FJ | 江西<br>JX | 江苏<br>JS | 浙江<br>ZJ | 山东<br>SD | 湖北<br>HB | 四川<br>SC | 广西<br>GX | 湖南<br>HN | 广东<br>GD | 贵州<br>GZ | 全国平均<br>AVG |
|---|---|---|---|---|---|---|---|---|---|---|---|---|---|---|---|---|---|---|---|---|---|---|---|---|---|
| 蔬菜类<br>Vegetables | ND | ND | ND | ND | ND | ND | ND | ND | ND | ND | ND | ND | ND | ND | ND | ND | ND | ND | ND | ND | ND | ND | ND | 0.097 | 0.006 |
| 水果类<br>Fruits | ND | ND | ND | ND | ND | ND | ND | ND | ND | ND | ND | ND | ND | ND | ND | ND | ND | ND | ND | ND | ND | ND | ND | 0.281 | 0.014 |
| 糖类<br>Sugar | ND | ND | ND | ND | ND | ND | ND | ND | ND | ND | ND | ND | ND | ND | ND | ND | ND | ND | ND | ND | ND | ND | ND | ND | 0.002 |
| 水及饮料类<br>Water and beverages | ND | ND | ND | ND | ND | ND | ND | ND | ND | ND | ND | ND | ND | ND | ND | ND | ND | ND | ND | ND | ND | ND | ND | ND | 0.002 |
| 酒类<br>Alcohol beverages | ND | ND | ND | ND | ND | ND | ND | ND | ND | ND | ND | ND | ND | ND | ND | ND | ND | ND | ND | ND | ND | ND | ND | ND | 0.002 |

注：平均值计算中，ND 以 1/2 检出限（LOD）计

Note: in calculation of averages (AVG), values not detected (ND) were treated as being equal to half of the detection of limit (LOD)

附表 8-21　第六次中国总膳食研究的 OTA 膳食摄入量［单位：ng/(kg bw·d)］

Annexed Table 8-21　Dietary intakes of OTA from the 6$^{th}$ China TDS [Unit: ng/(kg bw·d)]

| 膳食类别<br>Category | 黑龙江<br>HL | 辽宁<br>LN | 河北<br>HE | 北京<br>BJ | 吉林<br>JL | 山西<br>SX | 陕西<br>SN | 河南<br>HA | 宁夏<br>NX | 内蒙古<br>NM | 青海<br>QH | 甘肃<br>GS | 上海<br>SH | 福建<br>FJ | 江西<br>JX | 江苏<br>JS | 浙江<br>ZJ | 山东<br>SD | 湖北<br>HB | 四川<br>SC | 广西<br>GX | 湖南<br>HN | 广东<br>GD | 贵州<br>GZ | 全国平均<br>AVG |
|---|---|---|---|---|---|---|---|---|---|---|---|---|---|---|---|---|---|---|---|---|---|---|---|---|---|
| 谷类<br>Cereals | 0.034 | 0.031 | 0.040 | 0.036 | 0.024 | 0.053 | 0.047 | 0.046 | 0.402 | 14.490 | 0.055 | 0.037 | 0.019 | 0.030 | 0.027 | 1.636 | 0.027 | 0.042 | 0.023 | 0.049 | 0.044 | 0.027 | 0.020 | 0.035 | 0.720 |
| 豆类<br>Legumes | 0.002 | 0.005 | 0.002 | 0.004 | 0.003 | 2.394 | 0.003 | 0.002 | 0.001 | 0.001 | <0.001 | 0.001 | 0.004 | 0.003 | 0.003 | 0.003 | 0.005 | 0.002 | 0.002 | 0.002 | 0.001 | 0.003 | 0.001 | 0.004 | 0.102 |
| 薯类<br>Potatoes | 0.003 | 0.003 | 0.002 | 0.002 | 0.004 | 0.005 | 0.005 | 0.003 | 0.004 | 0.004 | 0.003 | 0.005 | 0.001 | 0.001 | 0.001 | 0.001 | 0.001 | 0.002 | 0.003 | 0.002 | 0.001 | 0.002 | 0.001 | 0.001 | 0.002 |

续表

| 膳食类别<br>Category | 黑龙江<br>HL | 辽宁<br>LN | 河北<br>HE | 北京<br>BJ | 吉林<br>JL | 山西<br>SX | 陕西<br>SN | 河南<br>HA | 宁夏<br>NX | 内蒙古<br>NM | 青海<br>QH | 甘肃<br>GS | 上海<br>SH | 福建<br>FJ | 江西<br>JX | 江苏<br>JS | 浙江<br>ZJ | 山东<br>SD | 湖北<br>HB | 四川<br>SC | 广西<br>GX | 湖南<br>HN | 广东<br>GD | 贵州<br>GZ | 全国平均<br>AVG |
|---|---|---|---|---|---|---|---|---|---|---|---|---|---|---|---|---|---|---|---|---|---|---|---|---|---|
| 肉类 Meats | 0.002 | 0.003 | 0.002 | 0.003 | 0.002 | 0.005 | 0.001 | 0.002 | 0.002 | 0.002 | 0.002 | 0.001 | 0.004 | 0.003 | 0.003 | 0.003 | 0.004 | 0.003 | 0.002 | 0.004 | 0.005 | 0.005 | 0.004 | 0.003 | 0.003 |
| 蛋类 Eggs | 0.001 | 0.002 | 0.001 | 0.001 | 0.001 | 0.001 | 0.001 | 0.001 | 0.001 | 0.001 | 0.001 | 0.001 | 0.001 | 0.001 | 0.001 | 0.001 | 0.001 | 0.002 | 0.001 | 0.001 | <0.001 | 0.001 | 0.001 | 0.001 | 0.001 |
| 水产类 Aquatic foods | 0.001 | 0.001 | <0.001 | <0.001 | <0.001 | <0.001 | <0.001 | <0.001 | <0.001 | <0.001 | <0.001 | <0.001 | 0.002 | 0.002 | 0.001 | 0.001 | 0.002 | 0.001 | 0.001 | <0.001 | 0.003 | 0.002 | 0.002 | <0.001 | 0.001 |
| 乳类 Dairy products | <0.001 | 0.001 | 0.001 | 0.003 | 0.001 | 0.001 | 0.001 | 0.001 | <0.001 | 0.001 | 0.002 | <0.001 | 0.002 | 0.001 | 0.001 | 0.001 | 0.001 | 0.001 | 0.001 | <0.001 | 0.001 | 0.001 | 0.001 | 0.001 | 0.001 |
| 蔬菜类 Vegetables | 0.013 | 0.011 | 0.009 | 0.013 | 0.012 | 0.010 | 0.009 | 0.009 | 0.005 | 0.008 | 0.010 | 0.008 | 0.013 | 0.013 | 0.014 | 0.014 | 0.017 | 0.016 | 0.013 | 0.010 | 0.011 | 0.017 | 0.008 | 0.013 | 0.012 |
| 水果类 Fruits | 0.002 | 0.003 | 0.001 | 0.004 | 0.003 | 0.001 | 0.001 | 0.001 | 0.003 | 0.004 | 0.001 | 0.001 | 0.002 | 0.002 | 0.002 | 0.001 | 0.002 | 0.002 | 0.001 | 0.001 | 0.002 | 0.002 | 0.001 | 0.001 | 0.002 |
| 糖类 Sugar | <0.001 | <0.001 | <0.001 | <0.001 | <0.001 | <0.001 | <0.001 | <0.001 | <0.001 | <0.001 | <0.001 | <0.001 | <0.001 | <0.001 | <0.001 | <0.001 | <0.001 | <0.001 | <0.001 | <0.001 | <0.001 | <0.001 | <0.001 | <0.001 | 0.000 |
| 水及饮料类 Water and beverages | 0.039 | 0.016 | 0.025 | 0.035 | 0.041 | 0.024 | 0.011 | 0.038 | 0.016 | 0.082 | 0.020 | 0.037 | 0.022 | 0.027 | 0.038 | 0.032 | 0.025 | 0.057 | 0.009 | 0.010 | 0.041 | 0.034 | 0.038 | 0.040 | 0.032 |
| 酒类 Alcohol beverages | 0.001 | 0.001 | <0.001 | 0.001 | <0.001 | <0.001 | <0.001 | <0.001 | <0.001 | 0.001 | <0.001 | <0.001 | 0.001 | <0.001 | 0.001 | 0.001 | 0.002 | 0.004 | <0.001 | <0.001 | 0.001 | 0.001 | <0.001 | <0.001 | 0.001 |
| 合计 SUM | 0.098 | 0.076 | 0.084 | 0.101 | 0.093 | 2.493 | 0.080 | 0.102 | 0.434 | 14.593 | 0.094 | 0.092 | 0.072 | 0.083 | 0.091 | 1.695 | 0.087 | 0.130 | 0.056 | 0.079 | 0.111 | 0.094 | 0.076 | 0.099 | 0.876 |

附表 8-22 第六次中国总膳食研究的 OTB 膳食摄入量 [单位: ng/(kg bw·d)]
Annexed Table 8-22 Dietary intakes of OTB from the 6th China TDS [Unit: ng/(kg bw·d)]

| 膳食类别 Category | 黑龙江 HL | 辽宁 LN | 河北 HE | 北京 BJ | 吉林 JL | 山西 SX | 陕西 SN | 河南 HA | 宁夏 NX | 内蒙古 NM | 青海 QH | 甘肃 GS | 上海 SH | 福建 FJ | 江西 JX | 江苏 JS | 浙江 ZJ | 山东 SD | 湖北 HB | 四川 SC | 广西 GX | 湖南 HN | 广东 GD | 贵州 GZ | 全国平均 AVG |
|---|---|---|---|---|---|---|---|---|---|---|---|---|---|---|---|---|---|---|---|---|---|---|---|---|---|
| 谷类 Cereals | 0.034 | 0.031 | 0.040 | 0.036 | 0.024 | 0.053 | 0.047 | 0.046 | 0.037 | 0.034 | 0.055 | 0.037 | 0.019 | 0.030 | 0.027 | 0.031 | 0.027 | 0.042 | 0.023 | 0.049 | 0.044 | 0.027 | 0.020 | 0.035 | 0.035 |
| 豆类 Legumes | 0.002 | 0.005 | 0.002 | 0.004 | 0.003 | 0.002 | 0.003 | 0.002 | 0.074 | 0.001 | 0.431 | 0.001 | 0.004 | 0.003 | 8.138 | 0.003 | 0.005 | 0.002 | 0.144 | 0.002 | 0.001 | 0.003 | 0.001 | 0.097 | 0.372 |
| 薯类 Potatoes | 0.003 | 0.003 | 0.002 | 0.002 | 0.004 | 0.005 | 0.005 | 0.003 | 0.004 | 0.004 | 0.003 | 0.005 | 0.001 | 0.001 | 0.001 | 0.001 | 0.001 | 0.002 | 0.003 | 0.002 | 0.001 | 0.002 | 0.001 | 0.001 | 0.002 |
| 肉类 Meats | 0.002 | 0.003 | 0.002 | 0.003 | 0.002 | 0.005 | 0.001 | 3.821 | 0.002 | 0.002 | 0.002 | 0.001 | 0.004 | 0.003 | 0.003 | 0.003 | 0.004 | 0.003 | 0.002 | 0.004 | 0.005 | 0.005 | 0.004 | 0.003 | 0.162 |
| 蛋类 Eggs | 0.001 | 0.002 | 0.001 | 0.001 | 0.001 | 0.001 | 0.001 | 0.001 | 0.001 | 0.001 | 0.001 | 0.001 | 0.001 | 0.001 | 0.001 | 0.001 | 0.001 | 0.002 | 0.001 | 0.001 | <0.001 | 0.001 | 0.001 | 0.001 | 0.001 |
| 水产类 Aquatic foods | 0.001 | 0.001 | <0.001 | 0.001 | <0.001 | <0.001 | <0.001 | <0.001 | 0.001 | <0.001 | 0.002 | <0.001 | 0.002 | 0.002 | 0.001 | 0.001 | 0.002 | 1.875 | 0.001 | <0.001 | 0.003 | 0.002 | 0.002 | <0.001 | 0.079 |
| 乳类 Dairy products | <0.001 | 0.001 | 0.001 | 0.001 | 0.001 | 0.001 | 0.001 | 0.001 | <0.001 | 0.001 | <0.001 | <0.001 | 0.002 | 0.001 | 0.001 | 0.001 | 0.001 | 0.001 | <0.001 | <0.001 | 0.001 | 0.001 | 0.001 | 0.001 | 0.001 |
| 蔬菜类 Vegetables | 0.013 | 0.011 | 0.009 | 0.013 | 0.012 | 0.010 | 0.009 | 0.009 | 0.005 | 0.008 | 0.010 | 0.008 | 0.013 | 0.013 | 0.014 | 0.014 | 0.017 | 0.016 | 0.013 | 0.010 | 0.011 | 0.017 | 0.008 | 0.626 | 0.037 |
| 水果类 Fruits | 0.002 | 0.003 | 0.001 | 0.004 | 0.003 | 0.001 | 0.001 | 0.001 | 0.003 | 0.004 | 0.001 | 0.001 | 0.002 | 0.002 | 0.002 | 0.001 | 0.002 | 0.002 | 0.001 | 0.001 | 0.002 | 0.002 | 0.001 | 0.093 | 0.006 |
| 糖类 Sugar | <0.001 | <0.001 | <0.001 | <0.001 | <0.001 | <0.001 | <0.001 | <0.001 | <0.001 | <0.001 | <0.001 | <0.001 | <0.001 | <0.001 | <0.001 | <0.001 | <0.001 | <0.001 | <0.001 | <0.001 | <0.001 | <0.001 | <0.001 | <0.001 | 0.000 |
| 水及饮料类 Water and beverages | 0.039 | 0.016 | 0.025 | 0.035 | 0.041 | 0.024 | 0.011 | 0.038 | 0.016 | 0.082 | 0.020 | 0.037 | 0.022 | 0.027 | 0.038 | 0.032 | 0.025 | 0.057 | 0.009 | 0.010 | 0.041 | 0.034 | 0.038 | 0.040 | 0.032 |

续表

| 膳食类别<br>Category | 黑龙江<br>HL | 辽宁<br>LN | 河北<br>HE | 北京<br>BJ | 吉林<br>JL | 山西<br>SX | 陕西<br>SN | 河南<br>HA | 宁夏<br>NX | 内蒙古<br>NM | 青海<br>QH | 甘肃<br>GS | 上海<br>SH | 福建<br>FJ | 江西<br>JX | 江苏<br>JS | 浙江<br>ZJ | 山东<br>SD | 湖北<br>HB | 四川<br>SC | 广西<br>GX | 湖南<br>HN | 广东<br>GD | 贵州<br>GZ | 全国平均<br>AVG |
|---|---|---|---|---|---|---|---|---|---|---|---|---|---|---|---|---|---|---|---|---|---|---|---|---|---|
| 酒类<br>Alcohol beverages | 0.001 | 0.001 | <0.001 | 0.001 | <0.001 | <0.001 | <0.001 | <0.001 | <0.001 | 0.001 | <0.001 | <0.001 | 0.001 | <0.001 | 0.001 | 0.001 | 0.002 | 0.004 | <0.001 | <0.001 | 0.001 | 0.001 | <0.001 | <0.001 | 0.001 |
| 合计<br>SUM | 0.098 | 0.076 | 0.084 | 0.101 | 0.093 | 0.102 | 0.080 | 3.921 | 0.143 | 0.139 | 0.524 | 0.092 | 0.072 | 0.083 | 8.226 | 0.089 | 0.087 | 2.004 | 0.198 | 0.079 | 0.111 | 0.094 | 0.076 | 0.897 | 0.728 |

附表 8-23　第六次中国总膳食研究膳食样品中 ZEN 的含量（单位：μg/kg）

Annexed Table 8-23　Levels of ZEN in food samples from the 6$^{th}$ China TDS (Unit: μg/kg)

| 膳食类别<br>Category | 黑龙江<br>HL | 辽宁<br>LN | 河北<br>HE | 北京<br>BJ | 吉林<br>JL | 山西<br>SX | 陕西<br>SN | 河南<br>HA | 宁夏<br>NX | 内蒙古<br>NM | 青海<br>QH | 甘肃<br>GS | 上海<br>SH | 福建<br>FJ | 江西<br>JX | 江苏<br>JS | 浙江<br>ZJ | 山东<br>SD | 湖北<br>HB | 四川<br>SC | 广西<br>GX | 湖南<br>HN | 广东<br>GD | 贵州<br>GZ | 全国平均<br>AVG |
|---|---|---|---|---|---|---|---|---|---|---|---|---|---|---|---|---|---|---|---|---|---|---|---|---|---|
| 谷类<br>Cereals | 1.01 | 0.21 | 1.38 | 0.52 | 0.48 | 0.31 | 0.22 | 0.76 | 0.21 | 0.35 | 0.59 | 0.24 | 0.59 | 0.28 | 0.30 | 0.22 | 0.99 | 0.21 | 0.55 | 0.19 | 0.25 | ND | 0.36 | 0.02 | 0.43 |
| 豆类<br>Legumes | ND | 2.06 | 0.65 | 0.52 | 0.89 | 0.40 | 0.82 | 0.73 | 0.17 | 0.23 | 0.23 | 0.92 | ND | 0.10 | 0.28 | 0.76 | 0.23 | ND | 1.68 | 3.47 | 0.23 | 0.80 | 0.57 | 0.19 | 0.67 |
| 薯类<br>Potatoes | 0.12 | 0.16 | 0.24 | 0.41 | 1.02 | 0.18 | 0.23 | 0.17 | 0.15 | 0.38 | ND | 0.10 | 1.45 | 0.61 | ND | 0.15 | 2.05 | 0.21 | 0.16 | 0.32 | 0.30 | ND | 0.51 | 0.45 | 0.39 |
| 肉类<br>Meats | 0.13 | 0.16 | 0.32 | 0.14 | 1.24 | 0.20 | 0.15 | 0.43 | 0.21 | 0.35 | ND | 0.13 | ND | ND | 0.20 | ND | 0.52 | 0.11 | 0.47 | ND | 0.12 | ND | 0.27 | ND | 0.22 |
| 蛋类<br>Eggs | 0.11 | 0.18 | 0.23 | ND | 0.96 | 0.25 | 0.19 | 0.34 | 0.18 | 0.84 | ND | ND | 1.28 | 0.12 | 0.25 | ND | 0.14 | 0.20 | 0.44 | ND | 0.15 | ND | ND | ND | 0.25 |
| 水产类<br>Aquatic foods | ND | ND | ND | 0.11 | 1.99 | ND | 0.11 | 0.22 | ND | 0.39 | ND | ND | 1.14 | 0.15 | 0.23 | ND | 0.24 | ND | 0.29 | ND | 0.11 | ND | 0.37 | ND | 0.23 |

续表

| 膳食类别<br>Category | 黑龙江<br>HL | 辽宁<br>LN | 河北<br>HE | 北京<br>BJ | 吉林<br>JL | 山西<br>SX | 陕西<br>SN | 河南<br>HA | 宁夏<br>NX | 内蒙古<br>NM | 青海<br>QH | 甘肃<br>GS | 上海<br>SH | 福建<br>FJ | 江西<br>JX | 江苏<br>JS | 浙江<br>ZJ | 山东<br>SD | 湖北<br>HB | 四川<br>SC | 广西<br>GX | 湖南<br>HN | 广东<br>GD | 贵州<br>GZ | 全国平均<br>AVG |
|---|---|---|---|---|---|---|---|---|---|---|---|---|---|---|---|---|---|---|---|---|---|---|---|---|---|
| 乳类 Dairy products | ND | ND | ND | ND | ND | ND | ND | ND | ND | ND | ND | ND | ND | ND | ND | ND | ND | ND | ND | ND | ND | ND | ND | ND | 0.01 |
| 蔬菜类 Vegetables | ND | 0.18 | 0.23 | ND | 1.00 | 0.10 | ND | 0.25 | ND | 0.28 | ND | 0.23 | 1.29 | ND | 0.17 | ND | 0.24 | 0.12 | 0.27 | ND | 0.11 | ND | 0.43 | ND | 0.21 |
| 水果类 Fruits | ND | ND | ND | ND | ND | ND | 0.13 | ND | 0.17 | ND | ND | ND | ND | 0.10 | ND | ND | ND | ND | ND | ND | ND | ND | ND | ND | 0.03 |
| 糖类 Sugar | ND | ND | ND | ND | ND | ND | ND | ND | ND | ND | ND | ND | 4.99 | ND | ND | ND | ND | ND | ND | ND | ND | ND | ND | ND | 0.22 |
| 水及饮料类 Water and beverages | ND | ND | ND | ND | ND | ND | ND | ND | ND | ND | ND | ND | ND | ND | ND | ND | ND | ND | ND | ND | ND | ND | ND | ND | 0.01 |
| 酒类 Alcohol beverages | ND | ND | ND | ND | ND | ND | ND | ND | ND | ND | ND | 0.12 | 0.12 | ND | ND | ND | ND | ND | ND | ND | ND | ND | ND | ND | 0.02 |

注：平均值计算中，ND 以 1/2 检出限（LOD）计

Note: in calculation of averages (AVG), values not detected (ND) were treated as being equal to half of the detection of limit (LOD)

附表 8-24　第六次中国总膳食研究膳食样品中 ZAN 的含量（单位：μg/kg）

Annexed Table 8-24　Levels of ZAN in food samples from the 6$^{th}$ China TDS (Unit: μg/kg)

| 膳食类别<br>Category | 黑龙江<br>HL | 辽宁<br>LN | 河北<br>HE | 北京<br>BJ | 吉林<br>JL | 山西<br>SX | 陕西<br>SN | 河南<br>HA | 宁夏<br>NX | 内蒙古<br>NM | 青海<br>QH | 甘肃<br>GS | 上海<br>SH | 福建<br>FJ | 江西<br>JX | 江苏<br>JS | 浙江<br>ZJ | 山东<br>SD | 湖北<br>HB | 四川<br>SC | 广西<br>GX | 湖南<br>HN | 广东<br>GD | 贵州<br>GZ | 全国平均<br>AVG |
|---|---|---|---|---|---|---|---|---|---|---|---|---|---|---|---|---|---|---|---|---|---|---|---|---|---|
| 谷类 Cereals | ND | ND | ND | ND | ND | ND | ND | ND | ND | ND | ND | ND | ND | ND | ND | ND | ND | ND | ND | ND | ND | ND | ND | ND | 0.02 |
| 豆类 Legumes | ND | ND | ND | ND | ND | ND | ND | ND | ND | ND | ND | ND | ND | ND | ND | ND | ND | ND | ND | ND | ND | ND | ND | ND | 0.01 |

续表

| 膳食类别<br>Category | 黑龙江<br>HL | 辽宁<br>LN | 河北<br>HE | 北京<br>BJ | 吉林<br>JL | 山西<br>SX | 陕西<br>SN | 河南<br>HA | 宁夏<br>NX | 内蒙古<br>NM | 青海<br>QH | 甘肃<br>GS | 上海<br>SH | 福建<br>FJ | 江西<br>JX | 江苏<br>JS | 浙江<br>ZJ | 山东<br>SD | 湖北<br>HB | 四川<br>SC | 广西<br>GX | 湖南<br>HN | 广东<br>GD | 贵州<br>GZ | 全国平均<br>AVG |
|---|---|---|---|---|---|---|---|---|---|---|---|---|---|---|---|---|---|---|---|---|---|---|---|---|---|
| 薯类 Potatoes | ND | ND | ND | ND | ND | ND | ND | ND | ND | ND | ND | ND | ND | ND | ND | ND | ND | ND | ND | ND | ND | ND | ND | ND | 0.01 |
| 肉类 Meats | ND | ND | ND | ND | ND | ND | ND | ND | ND | ND | ND | ND | ND | ND | ND | ND | ND | ND | ND | ND | ND | ND | ND | ND | 0.01 |
| 蛋类 Eggs | ND | ND | ND | ND | ND | ND | ND | ND | ND | ND | ND | ND | ND | ND | ND | ND | ND | ND | ND | ND | ND | ND | ND | ND | 0.01 |
| 水产类 Aquatic foods | ND | ND | ND | ND | ND | ND | ND | ND | ND | ND | ND | ND | ND | ND | ND | ND | ND | ND | ND | ND | ND | ND | ND | ND | 0.01 |
| 乳类 Dairy products | ND | ND | ND | ND | ND | ND | ND | ND | ND | ND | ND | ND | ND | ND | ND | ND | ND | ND | ND | ND | ND | ND | ND | ND | 0.01 |
| 蔬菜类 Vegetables | ND | ND | ND | ND | ND | ND | ND | ND | ND | ND | ND | ND | ND | ND | ND | ND | ND | ND | ND | ND | ND | ND | ND | ND | 0.01 |
| 水果类 Fruits | ND | ND | ND | ND | ND | ND | ND | ND | ND | ND | ND | ND | ND | ND | ND | ND | ND | ND | ND | ND | ND | ND | ND | ND | 0.01 |
| 糖类 Sugar | ND | ND | ND | ND | ND | ND | ND | ND | ND | ND | ND | ND | 0.15 | ND | ND | ND | ND | ND | ND | ND | ND | ND | ND | ND | 0.02 |
| 水及饮料类 Water and beverages | ND | ND | ND | ND | ND | ND | ND | ND | ND | ND | ND | ND | ND | ND | ND | ND | ND | ND | ND | ND | ND | ND | ND | ND | 0.01 |
| 酒类 Alcohol beverages | ND | ND | ND | ND | ND | ND | ND | ND | ND | ND | ND | ND | ND | ND | ND | ND | ND | ND | ND | ND | ND | ND | ND | ND | 0.01 |

注: 平均值计算中, ND 以 1/2 检出限 (LOD) 计
Note: in calculation of averages (AVG), values not detected (ND) were treated as being equal to half of the detection of limit (LOD)

附表 8-25　第六次中国总膳食研究膳食样品中 α-ZEL 的含量（单位：μg/kg）

Annexed Table 8-25　Levels of α-ZEL in food samples from the 6$^{th}$ China TDS (Unit: μg/kg)

| 膳食类别<br>Category | 黑龙江<br>HL | 辽宁<br>LN | 河北<br>HE | 北京<br>BJ | 吉林<br>JL | 山西<br>SX | 陕西<br>SN | 河南<br>HA | 宁夏<br>NX | 内蒙古<br>NM | 青海<br>QH | 甘肃<br>GS | 上海<br>SH | 福建<br>FJ | 江西<br>JX | 江苏<br>JS | 浙江<br>ZJ | 山东<br>SD | 湖北<br>HB | 四川<br>SC | 广西<br>GX | 湖南<br>HN | 广东<br>GD | 贵州<br>GZ | 全国平均<br>AVG |
|---|---|---|---|---|---|---|---|---|---|---|---|---|---|---|---|---|---|---|---|---|---|---|---|---|---|
| 谷类 Cereals | ND | ND | ND | ND | ND | ND | ND | ND | ND | ND | ND | ND | ND | ND | ND | 0.053 | 0.091 | ND | 0.089 | ND | ND | ND | ND | ND | 0.02 |
| 豆类 Legumes | ND | 0.094 | ND | ND | ND | ND | 4.241 | ND | 3.273 | ND | ND | ND | ND | ND | ND | 0.063 | ND | ND | ND | ND | ND | ND | ND | ND | 0.32 |
| 薯类 Potatoes | ND | ND | ND | ND | ND | ND | ND | ND | ND | ND | ND | ND | ND | ND | ND | ND | 0.054 | ND | ND | ND | ND | ND | ND | ND | 0.01 |
| 肉类 Meats | ND | ND | ND | 0.071 | ND | ND | ND | ND | ND | ND | ND | ND | ND | ND | ND | ND | 0.076 | ND | ND | ND | ND | ND | ND | ND | 0.01 |
| 蛋类 Eggs | ND | 0.058 | ND | ND | ND | ND | ND | ND | ND | ND | ND | ND | ND | ND | ND | 0.056 | 0.084 | ND | ND | ND | ND | ND | ND | ND | 0.01 |
| 水产类 Aquatic foods | ND | ND | ND | ND | ND | ND | ND | ND | ND | ND | ND | ND | ND | ND | ND | ND | 0.057 | ND | ND | ND | ND | ND | ND | ND | 0.01 |
| 乳类 Dairy products | ND | ND | ND | ND | ND | ND | ND | ND | ND | ND | ND | ND | ND | ND | ND | 0.043 | 0.045 | ND | ND | ND | ND | ND | ND | ND | 0.01 |
| 蔬菜类 Vegetables | ND | 0.588 | ND | ND | ND | ND | ND | ND | ND | ND | ND | ND | ND | ND | ND | ND | ND | ND | 1.621 | ND | ND | ND | ND | ND | 0.10 |
| 水果类 Fruits | ND | ND | ND | 0.245 | ND | ND | ND | ND | ND | ND | ND | ND | ND | ND | ND | ND | ND | ND | ND | ND | ND | ND | ND | ND | 0.02 |
| 糖类 Sugar | ND | ND | ND | ND | ND | ND | ND | ND | ND | ND | ND | ND | ND | ND | ND | 0.080 | 0.097 | ND | ND | ND | ND | ND | ND | ND | 0.01 |
| 水及饮料类 Water and beverages | ND | ND | ND | ND | ND | ND | ND | ND | ND | ND | ND | ND | ND | ND | ND | ND | ND | ND | ND | ND | ND | ND | ND | ND | 0.01 |

续表

| 膳食类别 Category | 黑龙江 HL | 辽宁 LN | 河北 HE | 北京 BJ | 吉林 JL | 山西 SX | 陕西 SN | 河南 HA | 宁夏 NX | 内蒙古 NM | 青海 QH | 甘肃 GS | 上海 SH | 福建 FJ | 江西 JX | 江苏 JS | 浙江 ZJ | 山东 SD | 湖北 HB | 四川 SC | 广西 GX | 湖南 HN | 广东 GD | 贵州 GZ | 全国平均 AVG |
|---|---|---|---|---|---|---|---|---|---|---|---|---|---|---|---|---|---|---|---|---|---|---|---|---|---|
| 酒类 Alcohol beverages | ND | ND | ND | ND | ND | ND | ND | ND | ND | ND | ND | ND | ND | ND | ND | ND | ND | ND | ND | ND | ND | ND | ND | ND | 0.01 |

注：平均值计算中，ND 以 1/2 检出限（LOD）计
Note: in calculation of averages (AVG), values not detected (ND) were treated as being equal to half of the detection of limit (LOD)

附表 8-26　第六次中国总膳食研究膳食样品中 β-ZEL 的含量（单位：μg/kg）
Annexed Table 8-26　Levels of β-ZEL in food samples from the 6$^{th}$ China TDS (Unit: μg/kg)

| 膳食类别 Category | 黑龙江 HL | 辽宁 LN | 河北 HE | 北京 BJ | 吉林 JL | 山西 SX | 陕西 SN | 河南 HA | 宁夏 NX | 内蒙古 NM | 青海 QH | 甘肃 GS | 上海 SH | 福建 FJ | 江西 JX | 江苏 JS | 浙江 ZJ | 山东 SD | 湖北 HB | 四川 SC | 广西 GX | 湖南 HN | 广东 GD | 贵州 GZ | 全国平均 AVG |
|---|---|---|---|---|---|---|---|---|---|---|---|---|---|---|---|---|---|---|---|---|---|---|---|---|---|
| 谷类 Cereals | ND | ND | ND | ND | ND | ND | ND | ND | ND | ND | ND | ND | ND | ND | ND | ND | ND | ND | ND | ND | ND | ND | ND | ND | 0.03 |
| 豆类 Legumes | ND | 0.23 | ND | ND | ND | ND | ND | ND | ND | ND | ND | ND | ND | ND | ND | 0.18 | 0.11 | ND | 0.19 | ND | ND | ND | ND | ND | 0.05 |
| 薯类 Potatoes | ND | ND | ND | ND | ND | ND | ND | ND | ND | ND | ND | ND | ND | ND | ND | ND | ND | ND | ND | ND | ND | ND | ND | ND | 0.02 |
| 肉类 Meats | ND | ND | ND | 1.15 | 0.93 | ND | ND | ND | ND | ND | ND | ND | ND | ND | ND | ND | 0.78 | ND | ND | ND | ND | ND | ND | ND | 0.14 |
| 蛋类 Eggs | ND | ND | ND | ND | ND | ND | ND | ND | ND | ND | ND | ND | ND | ND | ND | ND | ND | ND | ND | ND | ND | ND | ND | ND | 0.02 |
| 水产类 Aquatic foods | ND | ND | ND | 0.99 | ND | ND | ND | ND | ND | ND | ND | ND | ND | ND | ND | ND | 0.50 | ND | ND | ND | ND | ND | ND | ND | 0.08 |
| 乳类 Dairy products | ND | ND | ND | ND | ND | ND | ND | ND | ND | ND | ND | ND | ND | ND | ND | ND | ND | ND | ND | ND | ND | ND | ND | ND | 0.02 |

续表

| 膳食类别<br>Category | 黑龙江<br>HL | 辽宁<br>LN | 河北<br>HE | 北京<br>BJ | 吉林<br>JL | 山西<br>SX | 陕西<br>SN | 河南<br>HA | 宁夏<br>NX | 内蒙古<br>NM | 青海<br>QH | 甘肃<br>GS | 上海<br>SH | 福建<br>FJ | 江西<br>JX | 江苏<br>JS | 浙江<br>ZJ | 山东<br>SD | 湖北<br>HB | 四川<br>SC | 广西<br>GX | 湖南<br>HN | 广东<br>GD | 贵州<br>GZ | 全国平均<br>AVG |
|---|---|---|---|---|---|---|---|---|---|---|---|---|---|---|---|---|---|---|---|---|---|---|---|---|---|
| 蔬菜类 Vegetables | ND | 0.23 | ND | ND | ND | ND | ND | ND | ND | ND | ND | ND | ND | ND | ND | ND | ND | ND | ND | ND | ND | ND | ND | ND | 0.03 |
| 水果类 Fruits | ND | ND | ND | ND | ND | ND | ND | ND | ND | ND | ND | ND | ND | ND | ND | ND | ND | ND | ND | 2.46 | ND | ND | ND | ND | 0.12 |
| 糖类 Sugar | ND | ND | ND | ND | ND | ND | ND | ND | ND | ND | ND | ND | ND | ND | ND | ND | ND | ND | ND | ND | ND | ND | ND | ND | 0.02 |
| 水及饮料类 Water and beverages | ND | ND | ND | ND | ND | ND | ND | ND | ND | ND | ND | ND | ND | ND | ND | ND | ND | ND | ND | ND | ND | ND | ND | ND | 0.02 |
| 酒类 Alcohol beverages | ND | 0.20 | ND | 0.28 | ND | ND | ND | ND | ND | ND | ND | ND | ND | ND | ND | ND | ND | ND | ND | ND | ND | ND | ND | ND | 0.04 |

注：平均值计算中，ND 以 1/2 检出限（LOD）计

Note: in calculation of averages (AVG), values not detected (ND) were treated as being equal to half of the detection of limit (LOD)

附表 8-27　第六次中国总膳食研究膳食样品中 α-ZAL 的含量（单位：μg/kg）

Annexed Table 8-27　Levels of α-ZAL in food samples from the 6$^{th}$ China TDS (Unit: μg/kg)

| 膳食类别<br>Category | 黑龙江<br>HL | 辽宁<br>LN | 河北<br>HE | 北京<br>BJ | 吉林<br>JL | 山西<br>SX | 陕西<br>SN | 河南<br>HA | 宁夏<br>NX | 内蒙古<br>NM | 青海<br>QH | 甘肃<br>GS | 上海<br>SH | 福建<br>FJ | 江西<br>JX | 江苏<br>JS | 浙江<br>ZJ | 山东<br>SD | 湖北<br>HB | 四川<br>SC | 广西<br>GX | 湖南<br>HN | 广东<br>GD | 贵州<br>GZ | 全国平均<br>AVG |
|---|---|---|---|---|---|---|---|---|---|---|---|---|---|---|---|---|---|---|---|---|---|---|---|---|---|
| 谷类 Cereals | ND | ND | ND | ND | ND | ND | ND | ND | ND | ND | ND | ND | ND | ND | ND | ND | ND | ND | ND | ND | ND | ND | ND | ND | 0.02 |
| 豆类 Legumes | ND | ND | ND | ND | ND | ND | 0.20 | ND | ND | ND | ND | ND | ND | ND | ND | 0.14 | ND | ND | ND | ND | ND | ND | ND | ND | 0.02 |
| 薯类 Potatoes | ND | ND | ND | ND | ND | ND | ND | ND | ND | ND | ND | ND | ND | ND | ND | ND | ND | ND | ND | ND | ND | ND | ND | ND | 0.01 |

续表

| 膳食类别<br>Category | 黑龙江<br>HL | 辽宁<br>LN | 河北<br>HE | 北京<br>BJ | 吉林<br>JL | 山西<br>SX | 陕西<br>SN | 河南<br>HA | 宁夏<br>NX | 内蒙古<br>NM | 青海<br>QH | 甘肃<br>GS | 上海<br>SH | 福建<br>FJ | 江西<br>JX | 江苏<br>JS | 浙江<br>ZJ | 山东<br>SD | 湖北<br>HB | 四川<br>SC | 广西<br>GX | 湖南<br>HN | 广东<br>GD | 贵州<br>GZ | 全国平均<br>AVG |
|---|---|---|---|---|---|---|---|---|---|---|---|---|---|---|---|---|---|---|---|---|---|---|---|---|---|
| 肉类 Meats | ND | ND | ND | ND | ND | ND | ND | ND | ND | ND | ND | ND | ND | ND | ND | ND | ND | ND | ND | ND | ND | ND | ND | ND | 0.01 |
| 蛋类 Eggs | ND | ND | ND | ND | ND | ND | ND | ND | ND | ND | ND | ND | ND | ND | ND | ND | ND | ND | ND | ND | ND | ND | ND | ND | 0.01 |
| 水产类 Aquatic foods | ND | ND | ND | ND | ND | ND | ND | ND | ND | ND | ND | ND | ND | ND | ND | ND | ND | ND | ND | ND | ND | ND | ND | ND | 0.01 |
| 乳类 Dairy products | ND | ND | ND | ND | ND | ND | ND | ND | ND | ND | ND | ND | ND | ND | ND | ND | ND | ND | ND | ND | ND | ND | ND | ND | 0.01 |
| 蔬菜类 Vegetables | ND | 0.38 | ND | ND | ND | ND | ND | ND | ND | ND | ND | ND | ND | ND | ND | ND | ND | ND | ND | ND | ND | ND | ND | ND | 0.03 |
| 水果类 Fruits | ND | ND | ND | ND | ND | ND | ND | ND | ND | ND | ND | ND | ND | ND | ND | ND | ND | ND | ND | ND | ND | ND | ND | ND | 0.01 |
| 糖类 Sugar | ND | ND | ND | ND | ND | ND | ND | ND | ND | ND | ND | ND | 0.26 | ND | ND | ND | ND | ND | ND | ND | ND | ND | ND | ND | 0.02 |
| 水及饮料类 Water and beverages | ND | ND | ND | ND | ND | ND | ND | ND | ND | ND | ND | ND | ND | ND | ND | ND | ND | ND | ND | ND | ND | ND | ND | ND | 0.01 |
| 酒类 Alcohol beverages | ND | ND | ND | ND | ND | ND | ND | ND | ND | ND | ND | ND | ND | ND | ND | ND | ND | ND | ND | ND | ND | ND | ND | ND | 0.01 |

注：平均值计算中，ND 以 1/2 检出限（LOD）计
Note: in calculation of averages (AVG), values not detected (ND) were treated as being equal to half of the detection of limit (LOD)

附表 8-28 第六次中国总膳食研究膳食样品中 β-ZAL 的含量（单位：μg/kg）

Annexed Table 8-28 Levels of β-ZAL in food samples from the 6$^{th}$ China TDS (Unit: μg/kg)

| 膳食类别<br>Category | 黑龙江<br>HL | 辽宁<br>LN | 河北<br>HE | 北京<br>BJ | 吉林<br>JL | 山西<br>SX | 陕西<br>SN | 河南<br>HA | 宁夏<br>NX | 内蒙古<br>NM | 青海<br>QH | 甘肃<br>GS | 上海<br>SH | 福建<br>FJ | 江西<br>JX | 江苏<br>JS | 浙江<br>ZJ | 山东<br>SD | 湖北<br>HB | 四川<br>SC | 广西<br>GX | 湖南<br>HN | 广东<br>GD | 贵州<br>GZ | 全国平均<br>AVG |
|---|---|---|---|---|---|---|---|---|---|---|---|---|---|---|---|---|---|---|---|---|---|---|---|---|---|
| 谷类 Cereals | ND | ND | ND | ND | ND | ND | ND | ND | ND | ND | ND | ND | ND | ND | ND | ND | ND | ND | ND | ND | ND | ND | ND | ND | 0.008 |
| 豆类 Legumes | ND | ND | ND | ND | ND | ND | ND | ND | ND | ND | ND | ND | ND | ND | ND | ND | ND | ND | ND | ND | ND | ND | ND | ND | 0.006 |
| 薯类 Potatoes | ND | ND | ND | ND | ND | ND | ND | ND | ND | ND | 0.049 | ND | ND | ND | ND | ND | ND | ND | ND | ND | ND | ND | ND | ND | 0.007 |
| 肉类 Meats | ND | ND | ND | ND | ND | ND | ND | ND | 0.258 | ND | 0.078 | 0.129 | ND | ND | ND | ND | ND | ND | ND | ND | ND | ND | ND | ND | 0.024 |
| 蛋类 Eggs | ND | ND | ND | ND | ND | ND | ND | ND | ND | ND | ND | ND | ND | ND | ND | ND | ND | ND | ND | ND | ND | ND | ND | ND | 0.006 |
| 水产类 Aquatic foods | ND | ND | ND | ND | ND | ND | ND | ND | ND | ND | ND | ND | ND | ND | ND | ND | ND | ND | ND | ND | ND | ND | ND | ND | 0.005 |
| 乳类 Dairy products | ND | ND | ND | ND | ND | ND | ND | ND | ND | ND | ND | ND | ND | ND | ND | ND | ND | ND | ND | ND | ND | ND | ND | ND | 0.005 |
| 蔬菜类 Vegetables | ND | 0.068 | ND | ND | ND | ND | ND | ND | 0.074 | ND | ND | ND | ND | ND | ND | ND | ND | ND | ND | ND | ND | ND | ND | ND | 0.011 |
| 水果类 Fruits | ND | ND | 0.090 | ND | 0.140 | ND | 0.397 | ND | 0.329 | ND | ND | ND | 0.117 | 0.229 | 0.683 | ND | ND | 0.261 | 0.405 | 0.647 | ND | 0.303 | ND | 1.188 | 0.202 |
| 糖类 Sugar | ND | ND | ND | ND | ND | ND | ND | ND | ND | ND | ND | ND | 0.122 | ND | ND | ND | ND | ND | ND | ND | ND | ND | ND | ND | 0.010 |
| 水及饮料类 Water and beverages | ND | ND | ND | ND | ND | ND | ND | ND | ND | ND | ND | ND | ND | ND | ND | ND | ND | ND | ND | ND | ND | ND | ND | ND | 0.005 |

续表

| 膳食类别<br>Category | 黑龙江<br>HL | 辽宁<br>LN | 河北<br>HE | 北京<br>BJ | 吉林<br>JL | 山西<br>SX | 陕西<br>SN | 河南<br>HA | 宁夏<br>NX | 内蒙古<br>NM | 青海<br>QH | 甘肃<br>GS | 上海<br>SH | 福建<br>FJ | 江西<br>JX | 江苏<br>JS | 浙江<br>ZJ | 山东<br>SD | 湖北<br>HB | 四川<br>SC | 广西<br>GX | 湖南<br>HN | 广东<br>GD | 贵州<br>GZ | 全国平均<br>AVG |
|---|---|---|---|---|---|---|---|---|---|---|---|---|---|---|---|---|---|---|---|---|---|---|---|---|---|
| 酒类<br>Alcohol beverages | ND | ND | ND | ND | ND | ND | ND | ND | ND | ND | ND | ND | ND | ND | ND | ND | ND | ND | ND | ND | ND | ND | ND | ND | 0.005 |

注：平均值计算中，ND 以 1/2 检出限（LOD）计

Note: in calculation of averages (AVG), values not detected (ND) were treated as being equal to half of the detection of limit (LOD)

附表 8-29 第六次中国总膳食研究的 ZEN 膳食摄入量 [单位：ng/(kg bw·d)]

Annexed Table 8-29 Dietary intakes of ZEN from the 6$^{th}$ China TDS [Unit: ng/(kg bw·d)]

| 膳食类别<br>Category | 黑龙江<br>HL | 辽宁<br>LN | 河北<br>HE | 北京<br>BJ | 吉林<br>JL | 山西<br>SX | 陕西<br>SN | 河南<br>HA | 宁夏<br>NX | 内蒙古<br>NM | 青海<br>QH | 甘肃<br>GS | 上海<br>SH | 福建<br>FJ | 江西<br>JX | 江苏<br>JS | 浙江<br>ZJ | 山东<br>SD | 湖北<br>HB | 四川<br>SC | 广西<br>GX | 湖南<br>HN | 广东<br>GD | 贵州<br>GZ | 全国平均<br>AVG |
|---|---|---|---|---|---|---|---|---|---|---|---|---|---|---|---|---|---|---|---|---|---|---|---|---|---|
| 谷类<br>Cereals | 8.780 | 2.016 | 16.530 | 6.577 | 4.421 | 5.171 | 2.665 | 11.100 | 2.251 | 4.060 | 7.134 | 2.629 | 4.216 | 2.844 | 3.026 | 2.705 | 9.909 | 3.267 | 4.623 | 2.921 | 3.664 | 4.135 | 2.635 | 0.173 | 4.727 |
| 豆类<br>Legumes | 0.010 | 3.994 | 0.585 | 0.842 | 1.060 | 0.441 | 1.076 | 0.625 | 0.094 | 0.148 | 0.024 | 0.603 | 0.021 | 0.127 | 0.327 | 1.006 | 0.525 | 0.009 | 1.779 | 3.718 | 0.155 | 0.917 | 0.251 | 0.307 | 0.777 |
| 薯类<br>Potatoes | 0.149 | 0.183 | 0.232 | 0.378 | 1.941 | 0.343 | 0.427 | 0.218 | 0.244 | 0.742 | 0.017 | 0.229 | 0.829 | 0.411 | 0.005 | 0.081 | 1.194 | 0.154 | 0.227 | 0.320 | 0.061 | 0.011 | 0.200 | 0.244 | 0.368 |
| 肉类<br>Meats | 0.119 | 0.170 | 0.243 | 0.154 | 1.311 | 0.444 | 0.086 | 0.377 | 0.158 | 0.411 | 0.011 | 0.063 | 0.018 | 0.014 | 0.294 | 0.015 | 0.984 | 0.176 | 0.404 | 0.021 | 0.292 | 0.024 | 0.454 | 0.017 | 0.261 |
| 蛋类<br>Eggs | 0.072 | 0.118 | 0.115 | 0.007 | 0.611 | 0.084 | 0.066 | 0.163 | 0.037 | 0.395 | 0.003 | 0.004 | 0.794 | 0.037 | 0.081 | 0.005 | 0.053 | 0.140 | 0.173 | 0.003 | 0.033 | 0.004 | 0.004 | 0.003 | 0.125 |
| 水产类<br>Aquatic foods | 0.004 | 0.004 | 0.002 | 0.029 | 0.351 | 0.001 | 0.007 | 0.016 | <0.001 | 0.064 | 0.001 | <0.001 | 1.246 | 0.158 | 0.160 | 0.006 | 0.189 | 0.004 | 0.187 | 0.001 | 0.166 | 0.011 | 0.299 | 0.001 | 0.121 |
| 乳类<br>Dairy products | 0.002 | 0.007 | 0.004 | 0.014 | 0.005 | 0.007 | 0.003 | 0.003 | 0.002 | 0.005 | 0.008 | 0.002 | 0.011 | 0.006 | 0.003 | 0.004 | 0.005 | 0.004 | 0.001 | 0.002 | 0.003 | 0.003 | 0.006 | 0.004 | 0.005 |

续表

| 膳食类别<br>Category | 黑龙江<br>HL | 辽宁<br>LN | 河北<br>HE | 北京<br>BJ | 吉林<br>JL | 山西<br>SX | 陕西<br>SN | 河南<br>HA | 宁夏<br>NX | 内蒙古<br>NM | 青海<br>QH | 甘肃<br>GS | 上海<br>SH | 福建<br>FJ | 江西<br>JX | 江苏<br>JS | 浙江<br>ZJ | 山东<br>SD | 湖北<br>HB | 四川<br>SC | 广西<br>GX | 湖南<br>HN | 广东<br>GD | 贵州<br>GZ | 全国平均<br>AVG |
|---|---|---|---|---|---|---|---|---|---|---|---|---|---|---|---|---|---|---|---|---|---|---|---|---|---|
| 蔬菜类<br>Vegetables | 0.063 | 0.928 | 1.087 | 0.063 | 6.178 | 0.486 | 0.047 | 1.120 | 0.025 | 1.143 | 0.049 | 0.908 | 8.180 | 0.064 | 1.248 | 0.070 | 1.673 | 0.759 | 1.775 | 0.048 | 0.628 | 0.087 | 1.615 | 0.067 | 1.180 |
| 水果类<br>Fruits | 0.010 | 0.013 | 0.006 | 0.019 | 0.014 | 0.006 | 0.077 | 0.004 | 0.222 | 0.018 | 0.003 | 0.005 | 0.012 | 0.098 | 0.009 | 0.004 | 0.011 | 0.009 | 0.003 | 0.003 | 0.010 | 0.010 | 0.005 | 0.004 | 0.024 |
| 糖类<br>Sugar | <0.001 | <0.001 | <0.001 | <0.001 | <0.001 | <0.001 | 0.006 | <0.001 | <0.001 | <0.001 | <0.001 | <0.001 | 0.601 | <0.001 | <0.001 | <0.001 | <0.001 | <0.001 | <0.001 | <0.001 | <0.001 | <0.001 | <0.001 | <0.001 | 0.025 |
| 水及饮料类<br>Water and beverages | 0.139 | 0.056 | 0.088 | 0.176 | 0.207 | 0.118 | 0.055 | 0.189 | 0.082 | 0.409 | 0.098 | 0.187 | 0.112 | 0.137 | 0.188 | 0.160 | 0.125 | 0.286 | 0.045 | 0.050 | 0.207 | 0.169 | 0.189 | 0.199 | 0.153 |
| 酒类<br>Alcohol beverages | 0.003 | 0.005 | 0.002 | 0.004 | 0.002 | <0.001 | <0.001 | 0.001 | <0.001 | 0.003 | 0.001 | 0.006 | 0.043 | 0.002 | 0.003 | 0.006 | 0.010 | 0.018 | 0.002 | 0.001 | 0.005 | 0.003 | <0.001 | <0.001 | 0.005 |
| 合计<br>SUM | 9.354 | 7.495 | 18.890 | 8.264 | 16.083 | 7.101 | 4.514 | 13.814 | 3.117 | 7.399 | 7.349 | 4.637 | 16.083 | 3.899 | 5.345 | 4.064 | 14.678 | 4.824 | 9.220 | 7.095 | 5.225 | 1.373 | 5.658 | 1.019 | 7.772 |

附表 8-30 第六次中国总膳食研究膳食样品中 FB（FB1+FB2+FB3）的含量（单位：μg/kg）

Annexed Table 8-30　Levels of FBs (FB1+FB2+FB3) in food samples from the 6$^{th}$ China TDS (Unit: μg/kg)

| 膳食类别<br>Category | 黑龙江<br>HL | 辽宁<br>LN | 河北<br>HE | 北京<br>BJ | 吉林<br>JL | 山西<br>SX | 陕西<br>SN | 河南<br>HA | 宁夏<br>NX | 内蒙古<br>NM | 青海<br>QH | 甘肃<br>GS | 上海<br>SH | 福建<br>FJ | 江西<br>JX | 江苏<br>JS | 浙江<br>ZJ | 山东<br>SD | 湖北<br>HB | 四川<br>SC | 广西<br>GX | 湖南<br>HN | 广东<br>GD | 贵州<br>GZ | 全国平均<br>AVG |
|---|---|---|---|---|---|---|---|---|---|---|---|---|---|---|---|---|---|---|---|---|---|---|---|---|---|
| 谷类<br>Cereals | 3.976 | 0.128 | 35.070 | 1.269 | 2.666 | 8.950 | 0.325 | 2.528 | 0.284 | 13.880 | 6.118 | 11.550 | 0.545 | 0.136 | 3.593 | 32.600 | 0.130 | 38.010 | 6.550 | 10.731 | 2.811 | 0.143 | ND | 0.132 | 7.590 |
| 豆类<br>Legumes | ND | 0.278 | 2.079 | 0.330 | ND | 5.846 | 0.621 | ND | 0.177 | ND | 2.138 | ND | ND | ND | ND | 0.646 | 0.180 | ND | 0.549 | 5.373 | 2.336 | 0.297 | ND | 0.370 | 0.896 |

续表

| 膳食类别<br>Category | 黑龙江<br>HL | 辽宁<br>LN | 河北<br>HE | 北京<br>BJ | 吉林<br>JL | 山西<br>SX | 陕西<br>SN | 河南<br>HA | 宁夏<br>NX | 内蒙古<br>NM | 青海<br>QH | 甘肃<br>GS | 上海<br>SH | 福建<br>FJ | 江西<br>JX | 江苏<br>JS | 浙江<br>ZJ | 山东<br>SD | 湖北<br>HB | 四川<br>SC | 广西<br>GX | 湖南<br>HN | 广东<br>GD | 贵州<br>GZ | 全国平均<br>AVG |
|---|---|---|---|---|---|---|---|---|---|---|---|---|---|---|---|---|---|---|---|---|---|---|---|---|---|
| 薯类 Potatoes | ND | 0.347 | 0.701 | 0.158 | ND | 5.255 | 0.121 | 1.059 | 0.029 | ND | 1.016 | 1.353 | ND | 0.853 | ND | 0.114 | 0.081 | 3.283 | 0.091 | 1.332 | ND | 0.286 | ND | 0.938 | 0.717 |
| 肉类 Meats | 2.232 | 0.345 | 2.279 | ND | ND | 10.300 | 0.278 | 2.773 | 0.329 | ND | 3.045 | 1.910 | ND | 0.223 | ND | 0.873 | 0.260 | ND | 0.949 | 0.945 | ND | ND | ND | 0.153 | 1.131 |
| 蛋类 Eggs | ND | ND | ND | ND | ND | ND | ND | ND | ND | ND | ND | ND | ND | ND | ND | 0.096 | ND | ND | 0.083 | ND | ND | 1.105 | ND | 0.200 | 0.087 |
| 水产类 Aquatic foods | 0.606 | ND | ND | ND | ND | 0.571 | ND | ND | 3.808 | ND | ND | ND | 12.110 | ND | ND | ND | ND | ND | 0.922 | ND | ND | ND | ND | 0.387 | 0.787 |
| 乳类 Dairy products | ND | ND | ND | ND | ND | ND | 0.397 | ND | ND | ND | ND | ND | ND | ND | ND | ND | ND | ND | ND | ND | ND | ND | ND | ND | 0.040 |
| 蔬菜类 Vegetables | ND | ND | ND | ND | ND | 1.682 | 0.173 | ND | 0.253 | ND | ND | 1.934 | ND | ND | ND | ND | ND | ND | ND | ND | ND | 0.124 | ND | ND | 0.194 |
| 水果类 Fruits | ND | ND | ND | ND | ND | ND | ND | ND | ND | ND | ND | ND | ND | ND | ND | ND | ND | ND | ND | ND | ND | ND | ND | ND | 0.026 |
| 糖类 Sugar | ND | ND | ND | ND | ND | ND | ND | ND | 0.127 | ND | ND | ND | ND | ND | ND | ND | ND | ND | ND | ND | ND | ND | ND | ND | 0.025 |
| 水及饮料类 Water and beverages | ND | ND | ND | ND | ND | ND | ND | ND | ND | ND | ND | ND | ND | ND | ND | ND | ND | ND | ND | ND | ND | ND | ND | ND | 0.029 |
| 酒类 Alcohol beverages | 3.212 | ND | 0.360 | 0.239 | 2.175 | ND | ND | ND | ND | ND | ND | 1.358 | ND | ND | ND | ND | ND | ND | ND | 16.550 | 2.219 | 1.619 | ND | ND | 1.172 |

注：平均值计算中，ND 以 1/2 检出限（LOD）计

Note: in calculation of averages (AVG), values not detected (ND) were treated as being equal to half of the detection of limit (LOD)

附表 8-31 第六次中国总膳食研究膳食样品中 FB1 的含量（单位：μg/kg）

Annexed Table 8-31 Levels of FB1 in food samples from the 6$^{th}$ China TDS (Unit: μg/kg)

| 膳食类别 Category | 黑龙江 HL | 辽宁 LN | 河北 HE | 北京 BJ | 吉林 JL | 山西 SX | 陕西 SN | 河南 HA | 宁夏 NX | 内蒙古 NM | 青海 QH | 甘肃 GS | 上海 SH | 福建 FJ | 江西 JX | 江苏 JS | 浙江 ZJ | 山东 SD | 湖北 HB | 四川 SC | 广西 GX | 湖南 HN | 广东 GD | 贵州 GZ | 全国平均 AVG |
|---|---|---|---|---|---|---|---|---|---|---|---|---|---|---|---|---|---|---|---|---|---|---|---|---|---|
| 谷类 Cereals | 3.937 | 0.096 | 12.490 | 1.241 | 2.640 | 8.918 | 0.287 | 2.497 | 0.248 | 12.260 | 6.072 | 11.520 | 0.519 | 0.107 | 3.566 | 20.320 | 0.103 | 32.570 | 4.155 | 1.469 | 2.782 | 0.113 | ND | 0.100 | 5.334 |
| 豆类 Legumes | ND | 0.250 | 2.055 | 0.308 | ND | 5.824 | 0.598 | ND | 0.154 | ND | 2.115 | ND | ND | ND | ND | 0.623 | 0.159 | ND | 0.378 | 3.510 | 2.316 | 0.271 | ND | 0.153 | 0.782 |
| 薯类 Potatoes | ND | 0.321 | 0.678 | 0.135 | ND | 5.230 | 0.096 | 1.038 | ND | ND | 0.995 | 1.333 | ND | 0.164 | ND | 0.090 | 0.060 | 1.733 | 0.071 | 1.311 | ND | ND | ND | 0.386 | 0.571 |
| 肉类 Meats | 2.208 | 0.320 | 2.258 | ND | ND | 10.28 | 0.257 | 2.752 | 0.308 | ND | 3.024 | 1.888 | ND | 0.202 | ND | 0.852 | 0.238 | ND | 0.329 | 0.925 | ND | ND | ND | 0.132 | 1.084 |
| 蛋类 Eggs | ND | ND | ND | ND | ND | ND | ND | ND | ND | ND | ND | ND | ND | ND | ND | 0.074 | ND | ND | 0.059 | ND | ND | 0.078 | ND | 0.085 | 0.017 |
| 水产类 Aquatic foods | ND | ND | ND | ND | ND | ND | 0.377 | ND | ND | ND | ND | ND | ND | ND | ND | ND | ND | ND | 0.113 | ND | ND | ND | ND | 0.363 | 0.025 |
| 乳类 Dairy products | ND | ND | ND | ND | ND | ND | 0.152 | ND | ND | ND | ND | ND | ND | ND | ND | ND | ND | ND | ND | ND | ND | ND | ND | ND | 0.020 |
| 蔬菜类 Vegetables | ND | ND | ND | ND | ND | 1.661 | ND | ND | 0.233 | ND | ND | 1.914 | ND | ND | ND | ND | ND | ND | ND | ND | ND | 0.103 | ND | ND | 0.173 |
| 水果类 Fruits | ND | ND | ND | ND | ND | ND | ND | ND | ND | ND | ND | ND | ND | ND | ND | ND | ND | ND | ND | ND | ND | ND | ND | ND | 0.005 |
| 糖类 Sugar | ND | ND | ND | ND | ND | ND | ND | ND | ND | ND | ND | ND | ND | ND | ND | ND | ND | ND | ND | ND | ND | ND | ND | ND | 0.005 |
| 水及饮料类 Water and beverages | ND | ND | ND | ND | ND | ND | ND | ND | ND | ND | ND | ND | ND | ND | ND | ND | ND | ND | ND | ND | ND | ND | ND | ND | 0.005 |

续表

| 膳食类别 Category | 黑龙江 HL | 辽宁 LN | 河北 HE | 北京 BJ | 吉林 JL | 山西 SX | 陕西 SN | 河南 HA | 宁夏 NX | 内蒙古 NM | 青海 QH | 甘肃 GS | 上海 SH | 福建 FJ | 江西 JX | 江苏 JS | 浙江 ZJ | 山东 SD | 湖北 HB | 四川 SC | 广西 GX | 湖南 HN | 广东 GD | 贵州 GZ | 全国平均 AVG |
|---|---|---|---|---|---|---|---|---|---|---|---|---|---|---|---|---|---|---|---|---|---|---|---|---|---|
| 酒类 Alcohol beverages | 3.192 | ND | 0.340 | 0.219 | 2.155 | ND | ND | ND | ND | ND | ND | 1.338 | ND | ND | ND | ND | ND | ND | ND | 1.288 | 2.199 | 1.599 | ND | ND | 0.517 |

注：平均值计算中，ND 以 1/2 检出限（LOD）计

Note: in calculation of averages (AVG), values not detected (ND) were treated as being equal to half of the detection of limit (LOD)

附表 8-32　第六次中国总膳食研究膳食样品中 FB2 的含量（单位：μg/kg）

Annexed Table 8-32　Levels of FB2 in food samples from the 6$^{th}$ China TDS (Unit: μg/kg)

| 膳食类别 Category | 黑龙江 HL | 辽宁 LN | 河北 HE | 北京 BJ | 吉林 JL | 山西 SX | 陕西 SN | 河南 HA | 宁夏 NX | 内蒙古 NM | 青海 QH | 甘肃 GS | 上海 SH | 福建 FJ | 江西 JX | 江苏 JS | 浙江 ZJ | 山东 SD | 湖北 HB | 四川 SC | 广西 GX | 湖南 HN | 广东 GD | 贵州 GZ | 全国平均 AVG |
|---|---|---|---|---|---|---|---|---|---|---|---|---|---|---|---|---|---|---|---|---|---|---|---|---|---|
| 谷类 Cereals | ND | ND | 7.27 | ND | ND | ND | ND | ND | ND | 1.61 | ND | ND | ND | ND | ND | 2.37 | ND | 0.89 | 1.23 | 0.28 | ND | ND | ND | ND | 0.58 |
| 豆类 Legumes | ND | ND | ND | ND | ND | ND | ND | ND | ND | ND | ND | ND | ND | ND | ND | ND | ND | ND | ND | ND | ND | ND | ND | ND | 0.01 |
| 薯类 Potatoes | ND | ND | ND | ND | ND | ND | ND | ND | ND | ND | ND | ND | ND | ND | ND | ND | ND | ND | ND | ND | ND | ND | ND | 0.27 | 0.02 |
| 肉类 Meats | ND | ND | ND | ND | ND | ND | ND | ND | ND | ND | ND | ND | ND | ND | ND | ND | ND | ND | 0.15 | ND | ND | 1.02 | ND | ND | 0.02 |
| 蛋类 Eggs | ND | ND | ND | ND | ND | ND | ND | ND | ND | ND | ND | ND | ND | ND | ND | ND | ND | ND | ND | ND | ND | ND | ND | 0.10 | 0.06 |
| 水产类 Aquatic foods | 0.59 | ND | ND | ND | ND | 0.55 | ND | ND | 3.79 | ND | ND | ND | 12.10 | ND | ND | ND | ND | ND | 0.80 | ND | ND | ND | ND | ND | 0.75 |
| 乳类 Dairy products | ND | ND | ND | ND | ND | ND | ND | ND | ND | ND | ND | ND | ND | ND | ND | ND | ND | ND | ND | ND | ND | ND | ND | ND | 0.01 |

续表

| 膳食类别<br>Category | 黑龙江<br>HL | 辽宁<br>LN | 河北<br>HE | 北京<br>BJ | 吉林<br>JL | 山西<br>SX | 陕西<br>SN | 河南<br>HA | 宁夏<br>NX | 内蒙古<br>NM | 青海<br>QH | 甘肃<br>GS | 上海<br>SH | 福建<br>FJ | 江西<br>JX | 江苏<br>JS | 浙江<br>ZJ | 山东<br>SD | 湖北<br>HB | 四川<br>SC | 广西<br>GX | 湖南<br>HN | 广东<br>GD | 贵州<br>GZ | 全国平均<br>AVG |
|---|---|---|---|---|---|---|---|---|---|---|---|---|---|---|---|---|---|---|---|---|---|---|---|---|---|
| 蔬菜类 Vegetables | ND | ND | ND | ND | ND | ND | ND | ND | ND | ND | ND | ND | ND | ND | ND | ND | ND | ND | ND | ND | ND | ND | ND | ND | 0.01 |
| 水果类 Fruits | ND | ND | ND | ND | ND | ND | ND | ND | ND | ND | ND | ND | ND | ND | ND | ND | ND | ND | ND | ND | ND | ND | ND | ND | 0.01 |
| 糖类 Sugar | ND | ND | ND | ND | ND | ND | ND | ND | ND | ND | ND | ND | ND | ND | ND | ND | ND | ND | ND | ND | ND | ND | ND | ND | 0.01 |
| 水及饮料类 Water and beverages | ND | ND | ND | ND | ND | ND | ND | ND | 0.11 | ND | ND | ND | ND | ND | ND | ND | ND | ND | ND | ND | ND | ND | ND | ND | 0.01 |
| 酒类 Alcohol beverages | ND | ND | ND | ND | ND | ND | ND | ND | ND | ND | ND | ND | ND | ND | ND | ND | ND | ND | ND | 3.50 | ND | ND | ND | ND | 0.16 |

注：平均值计算中，ND 以 1/2 检出限（LOD）计

Note: in calculation of averages (AVG), values not detected (ND) were treated as being equal to half of the detection of limit (LOD)

附表 8-33  第六次中国总膳食研究膳食样品中 FB3 的含量（单位：μg/kg）

Annexed Table 8-33  Levels of FB3 in food samples from the 6$^{th}$ China TDS (Unit: μg/kg)

| 膳食类别<br>Category | 黑龙江<br>HL | 辽宁<br>LN | 河北<br>HE | 北京<br>BJ | 吉林<br>JL | 山西<br>SX | 陕西<br>SN | 河南<br>HA | 宁夏<br>NX | 内蒙古<br>NM | 青海<br>QH | 甘肃<br>GS | 上海<br>SH | 福建<br>FJ | 江西<br>JX | 江苏<br>JS | 浙江<br>ZJ | 山东<br>SD | 湖北<br>HB | 四川<br>SC | 广西<br>GX | 湖南<br>HN | 广东<br>GD | 贵州<br>GZ | 全国平均<br>AVG |
|---|---|---|---|---|---|---|---|---|---|---|---|---|---|---|---|---|---|---|---|---|---|---|---|---|---|
| 谷类 Cereals | ND | ND | 15.30 | ND | ND | ND | ND | ND | ND | ND | ND | ND | ND | ND | ND | 9.92 | ND | 4.55 | 1.17 | 8.98 | ND | ND | ND | ND | 1.68 |
| 豆类 Legumes | ND | ND | ND | ND | ND | ND | ND | ND | ND | ND | ND | ND | ND | 0.68 | ND | ND | ND | ND | 0.16 | 1.85 | ND | ND | ND | 0.21 | 0.10 |
| 薯类 Potatoes | ND | ND | ND | ND | ND | ND | ND | ND | ND | ND | ND | ND | ND | ND | ND | ND | ND | 1.54 | ND | ND | ND | 0.27 | ND | 0.29 | 0.12 |

续表

| 膳食类别 Category | 黑龙江 HL | 辽宁 LN | 河北 HE | 北京 BJ | 吉林 JL | 山西 SX | 陕西 SN | 河南 HA | 宁夏 NX | 内蒙古 NM | 青海 QH | 甘肃 GS | 上海 SH | 福建 FJ | 江西 JX | 江苏 JS | 浙江 ZJ | 山东 SD | 湖北 HB | 四川 SC | 广西 GX | 湖南 HN | 广东 GD | 贵州 GZ | 全国平均 AVG |
|---|---|---|---|---|---|---|---|---|---|---|---|---|---|---|---|---|---|---|---|---|---|---|---|---|---|
| 肉类 Meats | ND | ND | ND | ND | ND | ND | ND | ND | ND | ND | ND | ND | ND | ND | ND | ND | ND | ND | 0.47 | ND | ND | ND | ND | ND | 0.03 |
| 蛋类 Eggs | ND | ND | ND | ND | ND | ND | ND | ND | ND | ND | ND | ND | ND | ND | ND | ND | ND | ND | ND | ND | ND | ND | ND | ND | 0.01 |
| 水产类 Aquatic foods | ND | ND | ND | ND | ND | ND | ND | ND | ND | ND | ND | ND | ND | ND | ND | ND | ND | ND | ND | ND | ND | ND | ND | ND | 0.01 |
| 乳类 Dairy products | ND | ND | ND | ND | ND | ND | ND | ND | ND | ND | ND | ND | ND | ND | ND | ND | ND | ND | ND | ND | ND | ND | ND | ND | 0.01 |
| 蔬菜类 Vegetables | ND | ND | ND | ND | ND | ND | ND | ND | ND | ND | ND | ND | ND | ND | ND | ND | ND | ND | ND | ND | ND | ND | ND | ND | 0.01 |
| 水果类 Fruits | ND | ND | ND | ND | ND | ND | ND | ND | ND | ND | ND | ND | ND | ND | ND | ND | ND | ND | ND | ND | ND | ND | ND | ND | 0.01 |
| 糖类 Sugar | ND | ND | ND | ND | ND | ND | ND | ND | ND | ND | ND | ND | ND | ND | ND | ND | ND | ND | ND | ND | ND | ND | ND | ND | 0.01 |
| 水及饮料类 Water and beverages | ND | ND | ND | ND | ND | ND | ND | ND | ND | ND | ND | ND | ND | ND | ND | ND | ND | ND | ND | ND | ND | ND | ND | ND | 0.01 |
| 酒类 Alcohol beverages | ND | ND | ND | ND | ND | ND | ND | ND | ND | ND | ND | ND | ND | ND | ND | ND | ND | ND | ND | 11.76 | ND | ND | ND | ND | 0.50 |

注：平均值计算中，ND 以 1/2 检出限 (LOD) 计

Note: in calculation of averages (AVG), values not detected (ND) were treated as being equal to half of the detection of limit (LOD)

附表 8-34　第六次中国总膳食研究的 FB（FB1+FB2+FB3）膳食摄入量 [单位：ng/(kg bw·d)]
Annexed Table 8-34　Dietary intakes of FBs (FB1+FB2+FB3) from the 6th China TDS [Unit: ng/(kg bw·d)]

| 膳食类别 Category | 黑龙江 HL | 辽宁 LN | 河北 HE | 北京 BJ | 吉林 JL | 山西 SX | 陕西 SN | 河南 HA | 宁夏 NX | 内蒙古 NM | 青海 QH | 甘肃 GS | 上海 SH | 福建 FJ | 江西 JX | 江苏 JS | 浙江 ZJ | 山东 SD | 湖北 HB | 四川 SC | 广西 GX | 湖南 HN | 广东 GD | 贵州 GZ | 全国平均 AVG |
|---|---|---|---|---|---|---|---|---|---|---|---|---|---|---|---|---|---|---|---|---|---|---|---|---|---|
| 谷类 Cereals | 34.590 | 1.250 | 420.400 | 16.020 | 24.780 | 147.500 | 3.940 | 37.090 | 2.982 | 159.300 | 74.400 | 125.800 | 3.887 | 1.365 | 35.920 | 402.600 | 1.307 | 600.700 | 54.930 | 165.200 | 41.980 | 1.308 | 0.245 | 1.416 | 98.280 |
| 豆类 Legumes | 0.026 | 0.537 | 1.882 | 0.532 | 0.040 | 6.439 | 0.816 | 0.031 | 0.099 | 0.017 | 0.220 | 0.017 | 0.054 | 0.032 | 0.033 | 0.851 | 0.403 | 0.022 | 0.583 | 5.765 | 1.571 | 0.342 | 0.013 | 0.597 | 0.872 |
| 薯类 Potatoes | 0.037 | 0.397 | 0.679 | 0.147 | 0.048 | 9.894 | 0.220 | 1.350 | 0.045 | 0.050 | 1.636 | 3.091 | 0.014 | 0.573 | 0.013 | 0.061 | 0.047 | 2.409 | 0.129 | 1.330 | 0.007 | 0.243 | 0.010 | 0.510 | 0.956 |
| 肉类 Meats | 2.121 | 0.365 | 1.714 | 0.033 | 0.027 | 22.430 | 0.159 | 2.436 | 0.244 | 0.030 | 3.431 | 0.940 | 0.044 | 0.304 | 0.038 | 1.271 | 0.488 | 0.042 | 0.818 | 1.934 | 0.060 | 0.060 | 0.052 | 0.258 | 1.638 |
| 蛋类 Eggs | 0.016 | 0.021 | 0.016 | 0.018 | 0.018 | 0.011 | 0.010 | 0.012 | 0.008 | 0.016 | 0.007 | 0.010 | 0.017 | 0.010 | 0.010 | 0.043 | 0.012 | 0.022 | 0.033 | 0.007 | 0.006 | 0.400 | 0.010 | 0.052 | 0.034 |
| 水产类 Aquatic foods | 0.261 | 0.009 | 0.004 | 0.007 | 0.004 | 0.058 | 0.002 | 0.002 | 0.147 | 0.004 | 0.002 | 0.001 | 13.190 | 0.027 | 0.017 | 0.016 | 0.021 | 0.009 | 0.596 | 0.003 | 0.039 | 0.027 | 0.021 | 0.021 | 0.604 |
| 乳类 Dairy products | 0.005 | 0.018 | 0.010 | 0.034 | 0.013 | 0.016 | 0.122 | 0.008 | 0.006 | 0.014 | 0.021 | 0.006 | 0.028 | 0.014 | 0.009 | 0.011 | 0.013 | 0.009 | 0.003 | 0.005 | 0.007 | 0.007 | 0.014 | 0.011 | 0.017 |
| 蔬菜类 Vegetables | 0.157 | 0.139 | 0.118 | 0.157 | 0.156 | 8.261 | 0.788 | 0.111 | 0.626 | 0.105 | 0.123 | 7.615 | 0.159 | 0.159 | 0.179 | 0.176 | 0.215 | 0.197 | 0.164 | 0.121 | 0.143 | 1.051 | 0.097 | 0.167 | 0.883 |
| 水果类 Fruits | 0.025 | 0.033 | 0.015 | 0.048 | 0.035 | 0.014 | 0.016 | 0.010 | 0.039 | 0.045 | 0.006 | 0.013 | 0.029 | 0.024 | 0.022 | 0.011 | 0.027 | 0.022 | 0.008 | 0.006 | 0.026 | 0.025 | 0.012 | 0.009 | 0.022 |
| 糖类 Sugar | 0.001 | <0.001 | <0.001 | 0.001 | <0.001 | <0.001 | <0.001 | <0.001 | <0.001 | <0.001 | <0.001 | <0.001 | 0.003 | <0.001 | <0.001 | <0.001 | <0.001 | <0.001 | <0.001 | <0.001 | <0.001 | <0.001 | <0.001 | <0.001 | 0.001 |
| 水及饮料类 Water and beverages | 0.485 | 0.196 | 0.308 | 0.440 | 0.516 | 0.296 | 0.137 | 0.473 | 1.043 | 1.022 | 0.245 | 0.469 | 0.279 | 0.343 | 0.469 | 0.400 | 0.312 | 0.715 | 0.113 | 0.125 | 0.517 | 0.421 | 0.473 | 0.497 | 0.429 |

续表

| 膳食类别 Category | 黑龙江 HL | 辽宁 LN | 河北 HE | 北京 BJ | 吉林 JL | 山西 SX | 陕西 SN | 河南 HA | 宁夏 NX | 内蒙古 NM | 青海 QH | 甘肃 GS | 上海 SH | 福建 FJ | 江西 JX | 江苏 JS | 浙江 ZJ | 山东 SD | 湖北 HB | 四川 SC | 广西 GX | 湖南 HN | 广东 GD | 贵州 GZ | 全国平均 AVG |
|---|---|---|---|---|---|---|---|---|---|---|---|---|---|---|---|---|---|---|---|---|---|---|---|---|---|
| 酒类 Alcohol beverages | 1.123 | 0.013 | 0.061 | 0.104 | 0.330 | <0.001 | 0.001 | 0.001 | <0.001 | 0.008 | 0.002 | 0.071 | 0.009 | 0.006 | 0.009 | 0.015 | 0.025 | 0.045 | 0.006 | 1.353 | 1.128 | 0.429 | 0.001 | 0.001 | 0.197 |
| 合计 SUM | 38.84 | 2.98 | 425.23 | 17.54 | 25.96 | 194.83 | 6.23 | 41.52 | 5.24 | 160.65 | 80.09 | 138.03 | 17.71 | 2.86 | 36.72 | 405.43 | 2.87 | 604.18 | 57.38 | 175.85 | 45.48 | 4.31 | 0.95 | 3.54 | 103.94 |

附表 8-35 第六次中国总膳食研究膳食样品中 TeA 的含量（单位：μg/kg）
Annexed Table 8-35　Levels of TeA in food samples from the 6$^{th}$ China TDS (Unit: μg/kg)

| 膳食类别 Category | 黑龙江 HL | 辽宁 LN | 河北 HE | 北京 BJ | 吉林 JL | 山西 SX | 陕西 SN | 河南 HA | 宁夏 NX | 内蒙古 NM | 青海 QH | 甘肃 GS | 上海 SH | 福建 FJ | 江西 JX | 江苏 JS | 浙江 ZJ | 山东 SD | 湖北 HB | 四川 SC | 广西 GX | 湖南 HN | 广东 GD | 贵州 GZ | 全国平均 AVG |
|---|---|---|---|---|---|---|---|---|---|---|---|---|---|---|---|---|---|---|---|---|---|---|---|---|---|
| 谷类 Cereals | 9.27 | 13.23 | 14.87 | 21.37 | 8.50 | 5.03 | 17.22 | 20.44 | 9.84 | 19.63 | 19.28 | 21.53 | 10.20 | 6.44 | 11.03 | 3.25 | 9.03 | 8.33 | 9.36 | 6.83 | 1.79 | 3.21 | 5.42 | 3.49 | 10.77 |
| 豆类 Legumes | ND | 2.39 | 1.03 | ND | ND | 2.33 | 7.63 | 1.14 | 3.42 | 0.67 | 3.59 | 19.58 | 1.38 | ND | 1.49 | 3.24 | ND | ND | ND | 12.01 | 1.96 | 1.22 | ND | ND | 2.67 |
| 薯类 Potatoes | ND | ND | ND | ND | ND | ND | ND | ND | 5.46 | 0.87 | 5.08 | 1.62 | ND | ND | ND | ND | ND | ND | ND | 8.80 | ND | ND | ND | ND | 1.00 |
| 肉类 Meats | 1.63 | ND | ND | ND | 1.30 | ND | ND | 0.71 | ND | 2.43 | 7.96 | 7.29 | 0.96 | ND | 3.15 | ND | ND | ND | ND | 13.87 | ND | 0.90 | ND | ND | 1.74 |
| 蛋类 Eggs | 1.27 | 36.49 | ND | 16.92 | ND | ND | ND | ND | 5.38 | ND | ND | 0.79 | ND | ND | ND | 1.10 | ND | ND | ND | ND | ND | 0.95 | ND | ND | 2.70 |
| 水产类 Aquatic foods | 1.38 | ND | ND | 0.72 | 1.57 | ND | ND | ND | 1.42 | 1.64 | 7.18 | 1.02 | ND | ND | 2.89 | ND | ND | ND | ND | 11.97 | 1.08 | 0.84 | ND | ND | 1.38 |

续表

| 膳食类别 Category | 黑龙江 HL | 辽宁 LN | 河北 HE | 北京 BJ | 吉林 JL | 山西 SX | 陕西 SN | 河南 HA | 宁夏 NX | 内蒙古 NM | 青海 QH | 甘肃 GS | 上海 SH | 福建 FJ | 江西 JX | 江苏 JS | 浙江 ZJ | 山东 SD | 湖北 HB | 四川 SC | 广西 GX | 湖南 HN | 广东 GD | 贵州 GZ | 全国平均 AVG |
|---|---|---|---|---|---|---|---|---|---|---|---|---|---|---|---|---|---|---|---|---|---|---|---|---|---|
| 乳类 Dairy products | 1.11 | ND | ND | 2.06 | 1.54 | 1.09 | 1.92 | 2.60 | 1.37 | 2.03 | ND | 1.99 | 0.75 | 1.64 | 1.24 | 1.93 | 3.00 | ND | ND | 3.30 | ND | 1.25 | ND | ND | 1.23 |
| 蔬菜类 Vegetables | ND | 0.68 | ND | ND | 1.16 | ND | ND | ND | ND | 0.82 | 0.82 | 0.67 | ND | ND | 4.46 | 0.74 | ND | ND | ND | 8.04 | ND | ND | ND | ND | 0.79 |
| 水果类 Fruits | ND | ND | ND | ND | ND | ND | 4.98 | ND | 7.42 | ND | ND | ND | ND | 2.49 | ND | ND | 6.62 | 0.95 | ND | ND | ND | ND | ND | ND | 1.02 |
| 糖类 Sugar | ND | ND | ND | ND | ND | ND | ND | ND | ND | ND | ND | ND | 2.00 | ND | 1.25 | ND | ND | ND | ND | ND | ND | ND | ND | ND | 0.23 |
| 水及饮料类 Water and beverages | ND | ND | ND | ND | ND | ND | ND | ND | ND | ND | ND | ND | ND | ND | ND | ND | ND | ND | ND | ND | ND | ND | ND | ND | 0.10 |
| 酒类 Alcohol beverages | 3.18 | 8.55 | 2.62 | 17.62 | 11.04 | ND | 4.74 | 3.18 | 11.37 | 11.37 | 7.98 | 6.07 | 5.49 | 20.78 | 0.76 | 2.26 | 10.91 | ND | ND | 5.09 | 3.79 | 2.04 | 2.45 | ND | 5.90 |

注：平均值计算中，ND 以 1/2 检出限（LOD）计

Note: in calculation of averages (AVG), values not detected (ND) were treated as being equal to half of the detection of limit (LOD)

附表 Table 8-36　Levels of TEN in food samples from the 6th China TDS (Unit: μg/kg)

| 膳食类别 Category | 黑龙江 HL | 辽宁 LN | 河北 HE | 北京 BJ | 吉林 JL | 山西 SX | 陕西 SN | 河南 HA | 宁夏 NX | 内蒙古 NM | 青海 QH | 甘肃 GS | 上海 SH | 福建 FJ | 江西 JX | 江苏 JS | 浙江 ZJ | 山东 SD | 湖北 HB | 四川 SC | 广西 GX | 湖南 HN | 广东 GD | 贵州 GZ | 全国平均 AVG |
|---|---|---|---|---|---|---|---|---|---|---|---|---|---|---|---|---|---|---|---|---|---|---|---|---|---|
| 谷类 Cereals | 0.973 | 3.615 | 12.750 | ND | 8.263 | 9.544 | 36.860 | 32.610 | 35.810 | 47.110 | 14.620 | 30.290 | 5.085 | 0.948 | 1.716 | 0.272 | 0.159 | 12.690 | 0.993 | 12.350 | 0.413 | 0.573 | 4.659 | ND | 11.35 |
| 豆类 Legumes | ND | 0.270 | ND | ND | 0.580 | 0.604 | 1.249 | 0.524 | 1.560 | 0.471 | 0.249 | 1.014 | 0.598 | ND | 0.382 | 0.326 | ND | 0.264 | ND | 1.997 | 0.622 | 0.270 | 0.322 | ND | 0.479 |

续表

| 膳食类别 Category | 黑龙江 HL | 辽宁 LN | 河北 HE | 北京 BJ | 吉林 JL | 山西 SX | 陕西 SN | 河南 HA | 宁夏 NX | 内蒙古 NM | 青海 QH | 甘肃 GS | 上海 SH | 福建 FJ | 江西 JX | 江苏 JS | 浙江 ZJ | 山东 SD | 湖北 HB | 四川 SC | 广西 GX | 湖南 HN | 广东 GD | 贵州 GZ | 全国平均 AVG |
|---|---|---|---|---|---|---|---|---|---|---|---|---|---|---|---|---|---|---|---|---|---|---|---|---|---|
| 薯类 Potatoes | ND | 1.241 | 0.405 | ND | 0.145 | 0.341 | ND | 0.184 | 3.200 | 0.592 | 0.399 | 1.034 | 0.187 | ND | ND | ND | ND | 0.133 | ND | 0.228 | ND | ND | ND | ND | 0.351 |
| 肉类 Meats | ND | ND | ND | ND | 0.328 | 0.407 | ND | 0.337 | 2.343 | 1.914 | 0.552 | 1.572 | 0.918 | ND | ND | ND | ND | ND | ND | 1.398 | 0.202 | 2.845 | ND | ND | 0.549 |
| 蛋类 Eggs | ND | 36.230 | ND | ND | 0.171 | ND | ND | ND | 2.358 | 0.190 | 0.163 | 0.343 | ND | ND | ND | 0.117 | ND | ND | 0.300 | ND | 0.353 | 0.161 | ND | ND | 1.699 |
| 水产类 Aquatic foods | ND | ND | ND | 0.720 | 0.660 | 0.341 | ND | 1.037 | 1.157 | 3.876 | 1.453 | 0.619 | 0.482 | ND | 0.250 | ND | ND | 0.125 | ND | 1.222 | ND | 0.373 | ND | ND | 0.526 |
| 乳类 Dairy products | ND | ND | ND | ND | ND | ND | ND | ND | ND | ND | ND | ND | ND | ND | ND | ND | ND | ND | ND | ND | 0.258 | ND | ND | ND | 0.035 |
| 蔬菜类 Vegetables | ND | 0.274 | ND | 0.838 | 0.211 | 0.161 | ND | ND | ND | 1.193 | 0.484 | 1.752 | 0.207 | ND | 0.369 | 0.219 | ND | 0.140 | ND | 0.487 | ND | 0.761 | 0.183 | ND | 0.314 |
| 水果类 Fruits | ND | ND | ND | ND | 0.163 | ND | 2.491 | ND | 1.880 | ND | ND | ND | 17.43 | ND | ND | ND | ND | ND | ND | ND | 2.685 | ND | ND | ND | 1.047 |
| 糖类 Sugar | ND | ND | ND | ND | ND | ND | ND | ND | ND | ND | ND | ND | 0.270 | ND | ND | ND | ND | ND | ND | ND | ND | ND | ND | ND | 0.035 |
| 水及饮料类 Water and beverages | ND | ND | ND | ND | ND | ND | ND | ND | ND | ND | ND | ND | ND | ND | ND | ND | ND | ND | ND | ND | ND | ND | ND | ND | 0.025 |
| 酒类 Alcohol beverages | ND | 0.164 | ND | ND | 0.414 | ND | ND | ND | ND | 0.256 | ND | 0.195 | 1.517 | ND | ND | 0.143 | ND | ND | 0.162 | ND | 1.597 | ND | 1.178 | ND | 0.250 |

注：平均值计算中，ND 以 1/2 检出限（LOD）计
Note: in calculation of averages (AVG), values not detected (ND) were treated as being equal to half of the detection of limit (LOD)

附表 8-37　第六次中国总膳食研究膳食样品中 AME 的含量（单位：μg/kg）

Annexed Table 8-37　Levels of AME in food samples from the 6$^{th}$ China TDS (Unit: μg/kg)

| 膳食类别<br>Category | 黑龙江<br>HL | 辽宁<br>LN | 河北<br>HE | 北京<br>BJ | 吉林<br>JL | 山西<br>SX | 陕西<br>SN | 河南<br>HA | 宁夏<br>NX | 内蒙古<br>NM | 青海<br>QH | 甘肃<br>GS | 上海<br>SH | 福建<br>FJ | 江西<br>JX | 江苏<br>JS | 浙江<br>ZJ | 山东<br>SD | 湖北<br>HB | 四川<br>SC | 广西<br>GX | 湖南<br>HN | 广东<br>GD | 贵州<br>GZ | 全国平均<br>AVG |
|---|---|---|---|---|---|---|---|---|---|---|---|---|---|---|---|---|---|---|---|---|---|---|---|---|---|
| 谷类 Cereals | ND | 7.74 | 2.65 | 14.83 | 0.86 | 0.37 | 1.35 | 3.16 | 8.61 | 4.35 | 2.84 | 2.73 | 0.47 | 0.52 | 0.25 | ND | 0.29 | 0.43 | 0.19 | 8.95 | ND | ND | 1.85 | 1.19 | 2.65 |
| 豆类 Legumes | ND | ND | ND | 1.93 | ND | ND | 0.28 | ND | ND | ND | ND | 0.18 | ND | ND | ND | ND | ND | ND | ND | 0.13 | ND | ND | ND | 0.28 | 0.13 |
| 薯类 Potatoes | ND | 0.19 | ND | 2.80 | ND | ND | ND | ND | 1.18 | 0.13 | ND | 0.77 | ND | ND | ND | ND | 0.14 | 0.26 | 0.58 | 0.16 | ND | ND | ND | 0.10 | 0.27 |
| 肉类 Meats | ND | ND | ND | ND | ND | ND | ND | ND | 2.25 | 0.31 | ND | 0.80 | ND | ND | ND | ND | ND | ND | ND | 0.57 | ND | ND | ND | ND | 0.17 |
| 蛋类 Eggs | ND | 1.72 | ND | ND | ND | 0.20 | ND | ND | 1.09 | 1.51 | ND | ND | ND | ND | ND | ND | ND | ND | 0.85 | ND | ND | ND | ND | ND | 0.23 |
| 水产类 Aquatic foods | ND | ND | ND | ND | ND | ND | ND | ND | 0.69 | 0.22 | ND | 0.20 | ND | ND | 0.10 | ND | ND | ND | 0.38 | ND | ND | ND | ND | 0.21 | 0.08 |
| 乳类 Dairy products | ND | ND | ND | ND | ND | ND | ND | ND | ND | ND | ND | ND | ND | ND | ND | ND | ND | ND | ND | ND | ND | ND | ND | ND | 0.01 |
| 蔬菜类 Vegetables | ND | ND | ND | 1.01 | ND | ND | ND | ND | 0.95 | 0.30 | ND | 0.11 | ND | ND | ND | ND | ND | ND | 1.10 | ND | ND | ND | ND | ND | 0.11 |
| 水果类 Fruits | ND | 0.22 | ND | ND | ND | ND | ND | ND | ND | ND | ND | ND | ND | ND | ND | ND | ND | ND | ND | ND | 0.41 | ND | ND | ND | 0.07 |
| 糖类 Sugar | ND | ND | ND | ND | ND | ND | ND | ND | ND | ND | ND | ND | ND | ND | 0.53 | ND | ND | ND | 0.12 | ND | 0.28 | ND | ND | ND | 0.05 |
| 水及饮料类 Water and beverages | ND | ND | ND | 0.16 | ND | ND | ND | ND | ND | ND | ND | ND | ND | ND | 0.21 | ND | ND | ND | ND | ND | ND | ND | ND | ND | 0.02 |

续表

| 膳食类别<br>Category | 黑龙江<br>HL | 辽宁<br>LN | 河北<br>HE | 北京<br>BJ | 吉林<br>JL | 山西<br>SX | 陕西<br>SN | 河南<br>HA | 宁夏<br>NX | 内蒙古<br>NM | 青海<br>QH | 甘肃<br>GS | 上海<br>SH | 福建<br>FJ | 江西<br>JX | 江苏<br>JS | 浙江<br>ZJ | 山东<br>SD | 湖北<br>HB | 四川<br>SC | 广西<br>GX | 湖南<br>HN | 广东<br>GD | 贵州<br>GZ | 全国平均<br>AVG |
|---|---|---|---|---|---|---|---|---|---|---|---|---|---|---|---|---|---|---|---|---|---|---|---|---|---|
| 酒类<br>Alcohol beverages | ND | ND | ND | 1.00 | ND | ND | ND | ND | ND | ND | ND | ND | ND | ND | ND | ND | ND | ND | 0.27 | ND | 0.11 | ND | ND | ND | 0.07 |

注：平均值计算中，ND 以 1/2 检出限（LOD）计
Note: in calculation of averages (AVG), values not detected (ND) were treated as being equal to half of the detection of limit (LOD)

附表 8-38　第六次中国总膳食研究膳食样品中 ALT 的含量（单位：μg/kg）

Annexed Table 8-38　Levels of ALT in food samples from the 6$^{th}$ China TDS (Unit: μg/kg)

| 膳食类别<br>Category | 黑龙江<br>HL | 辽宁<br>LN | 河北<br>HE | 北京<br>BJ | 吉林<br>JL | 山西<br>SX | 陕西<br>SN | 河南<br>HA | 宁夏<br>NX | 内蒙古<br>NM | 青海<br>QH | 甘肃<br>GS | 上海<br>SH | 福建<br>FJ | 江西<br>JX | 江苏<br>JS | 浙江<br>ZJ | 山东<br>SD | 湖北<br>HB | 四川<br>SC | 广西<br>GX | 湖南<br>HN | 广东<br>GD | 贵州<br>GZ | 全国平均<br>AVG |
|---|---|---|---|---|---|---|---|---|---|---|---|---|---|---|---|---|---|---|---|---|---|---|---|---|---|
| 谷类<br>Cereals | ND | ND | ND | ND | ND | ND | ND | ND | ND | ND | ND | ND | ND | ND | ND | ND | ND | ND | ND | ND | ND | ND | ND | 12.74 | 0.68 |
| 豆类<br>Legumes | ND | ND | ND | ND | ND | ND | ND | ND | ND | ND | ND | ND | ND | ND | ND | ND | ND | ND | ND | ND | ND | ND | ND | ND | 0.12 |
| 薯类<br>Potatoes | ND | 2.23 | ND | ND | ND | 0.98 | ND | ND | ND | ND | ND | ND | ND | ND | ND | ND | 1.13 | ND | ND | ND | ND | ND | ND | ND | 0.28 |
| 肉类<br>Meats | ND | ND | ND | ND | ND | 0.53 | ND | ND | ND | ND | 1.12 | 1.24 | ND | ND | ND | ND | ND | ND | ND | ND | ND | ND | ND | ND | 0.21 |
| 蛋类<br>Eggs | ND | ND | ND | ND | ND | ND | ND | ND | 13.10 | ND | ND | ND | ND | ND | ND | ND | ND | ND | ND | ND | ND | ND | ND | ND | 0.66 |
| 水产类<br>Aquatic foods | ND | 12.90 | ND | ND | ND | ND | ND | ND | ND | ND | ND | ND | ND | ND | ND | ND | ND | ND | ND | ND | ND | ND | ND | ND | 0.64 |
| 乳类<br>Dairy products | ND | ND | ND | ND | ND | ND | ND | ND | ND | ND | ND | ND | ND | ND | ND | ND | ND | ND | ND | ND | ND | ND | ND | ND | 0.10 |

续表

| 膳食类别 Category | 黑龙江 HL | 辽宁 LN | 河北 HE | 北京 BJ | 吉林 JL | 山西 SX | 陕西 SN | 河南 HA | 宁夏 NX | 内蒙古 NM | 青海 QH | 甘肃 GS | 上海 SH | 福建 FJ | 江西 JX | 江苏 JS | 浙江 ZJ | 山东 SD | 湖北 HB | 四川 SC | 广西 GX | 湖南 HN | 广东 GD | 贵州 GZ | 全国平均 AVG |
|---|---|---|---|---|---|---|---|---|---|---|---|---|---|---|---|---|---|---|---|---|---|---|---|---|---|
| 蔬菜类 Vegetables | ND | ND | ND | ND | 8.85 | ND | ND | ND | ND | ND | ND | 1.01 | 0.64 | 10.46 | ND | 1.27 | ND | ND | ND | ND | ND | ND | ND | ND | 1.01 |
| 水果类 Fruits | ND | ND | ND | ND | 1.71 | 4.18 | ND | ND | ND | 0.68 | 1.14 | ND | 2.65 | ND | 0.69 | ND | ND | ND | ND | ND | ND | ND | ND | ND | 0.54 |
| 糖类 Sugar | ND | ND | ND | ND | ND | ND | ND | ND | ND | ND | ND | ND | ND | ND | ND | ND | ND | ND | ND | ND | ND | ND | ND | ND | 0.10 |
| 水及饮料类 Water and beverages | ND | ND | ND | ND | ND | ND | ND | ND | ND | ND | ND | ND | ND | ND | ND | ND | ND | ND | ND | ND | ND | ND | ND | ND | 0.10 |
| 酒类 Alcohol beverages | ND | ND | ND | ND | ND | ND | ND | ND | ND | ND | ND | ND | ND | ND | ND | ND | ND | ND | ND | ND | ND | ND | ND | ND | 0.10 |

注：平均值计算中，ND 以 1/2 检出限（LOD）计

Note: in calculation of averages (AVG), values not detected (ND) were treated as being equal to half of the detection of limit (LOD)

附表 8-39 第六次中国总膳食研究的 TeA 膳食摄入量 [单位：ng/(kg bw·d)]

Annexed Table 8-39 Dietary intakes of TeA from the 6th China TDS [Unit: ng/(kg bw·d)]

| 膳食类别 Category | 黑龙江 HL | 辽宁 LN | 河北 HE | 北京 BJ | 吉林 JL | 山西 SX | 陕西 SN | 河南 HA | 宁夏 NX | 内蒙古 NM | 青海 QH | 甘肃 GS | 上海 SH | 福建 FJ | 江西 JX | 江苏 JS | 浙江 ZJ | 山东 SD | 湖北 HB | 四川 SC | 广西 GX | 湖南 HN | 广东 GD | 贵州 GZ | 全国平均 AVG |
|---|---|---|---|---|---|---|---|---|---|---|---|---|---|---|---|---|---|---|---|---|---|---|---|---|---|
| 谷类 Cereals | 80.65 | 129.20 | 178.20 | 269.70 | 79.00 | 82.82 | 208.50 | 299.90 | 103.40 | 225.30 | 234.40 | 234.50 | 72.71 | 64.60 | 110.30 | 40.19 | 90.67 | 131.70 | 78.51 | 105.20 | 26.76 | 29.39 | 39.26 | 37.43 | 123.0 |
| 豆类 Legumes | 0.104 | 4.630 | 0.930 | 0.176 | 0.162 | 2.566 | 10.026 | 0.976 | 1.908 | 0.425 | 0.369 | 12.807 | 2.575 | 0.127 | 1.739 | 4.271 | 0.238 | 0.089 | 0.118 | 12.890 | 1.321 | 1.407 | 0.050 | 0.192 | 2.504 |
| 薯类 Potatoes | 0.146 | 0.149 | 0.113 | 0.108 | 0.190 | 0.235 | 0.225 | 0.139 | 8.656 | 1.687 | 8.177 | 3.703 | 0.057 | 0.074 | 0.051 | 0.064 | 0.061 | 0.076 | 0.142 | 8.787 | 0.027 | 0.115 | 0.041 | 0.066 | 1.379 |

续表

| 膳食类别 Category | 黑龙江 HL | 辽宁 LN | 河北 HE | 北京 BJ | 吉林 JL | 山西 SX | 陕西 SN | 河南 HA | 宁夏 NX | 内蒙古 NM | 青海 QH | 甘肃 GS | 上海 SH | 福建 FJ | 江西 JX | 江苏 JS | 浙江 ZJ | 山东 SD | 湖北 HB | 四川 SC | 广西 GX | 湖南 HN | 广东 GD | 贵州 GZ | 全国平均 AVG |
|---|---|---|---|---|---|---|---|---|---|---|---|---|---|---|---|---|---|---|---|---|---|---|---|---|---|
| 肉类 Meats | 1.554 | 0.131 | 0.082 | 0.134 | 1.375 | 0.229 | 0.061 | 0.628 | 0.077 | 2.830 | 8.971 | 3.587 | 1.682 | 0.141 | 4.688 | 0.147 | 0.202 | 0.166 | 0.090 | 28.374 | 0.240 | 2.124 | 0.209 | 0.174 | 2.412 |
| 蛋类 Eggs | 0.813 | 23.690 | 0.064 | 10.43 | 0.073 | 0.046 | 0.041 | 0.047 | 1.112 | 0.062 | 0.029 | 0.278 | 0.067 | 0.039 | 0.038 | 0.492 | 0.047 | 0.087 | 0.047 | 0.026 | 0.025 | 0.344 | 0.038 | 0.026 | 1.582 |
| 水产类 Aquatic foods | 0.597 | 0.037 | 0.017 | 0.188 | 0.278 | 0.012 | 0.007 | 0.008 | 0.055 | 0.269 | 0.406 | 0.046 | 0.109 | 0.106 | 2.004 | 0.063 | 0.083 | 0.038 | 0.065 | 1.591 | 1.661 | 0.885 | 0.085 | 0.007 | 0.359 |
| 乳类 Dairy products | 0.235 | 0.071 | 0.038 | 2.805 | 0.793 | 0.721 | 0.589 | 0.805 | 0.332 | 1.107 | 0.085 | 0.447 | 0.852 | 0.938 | 0.430 | 0.843 | 1.597 | 0.036 | 0.011 | 0.657 | 0.029 | 0.357 | 0.058 | 0.045 | 0.578 |
| 蔬菜类 Vegetables | 0.627 | 3.523 | 0.470 | 0.628 | 7.123 | 0.501 | 0.470 | 0.446 | 0.248 | 3.334 | 4.035 | 2.630 | 0.636 | 0.636 | 31.977 | 4.983 | 0.860 | 0.787 | 0.657 | 38.606 | 0.573 | 0.874 | 0.387 | 0.668 | 4.403 |
| 水果类 Fruits | 0.100 | 0.133 | 0.060 | 0.192 | 0.139 | 0.055 | 2.998 | 0.038 | 9.969 | 0.181 | 0.026 | 0.053 | 0.117 | 2.361 | 0.090 | 0.043 | 7.071 | 0.818 | 0.030 | 0.026 | 0.102 | 0.101 | 0.047 | 0.038 | 1.033 |
| 糖类 Sugar | 0.004 | 0.001 | 0.001 | 0.003 | 0.002 | 0.002 | 0.001 | 0.001 | 0.001 | 0.002 | 0.001 | 0.001 | 0.241 | <0.001 | 0.019 | <0.001 | 0.002 | 0.001 | <0.001 | 0.001 | 0.001 | 0.001 | <0.001 | <0.001 | 0.012 |
| 水及饮料类 Water and beverages | 1.940 | 0.783 | 1.231 | 1.758 | 2.066 | 1.183 | 0.548 | 1.893 | 0.821 | 4.087 | 0.981 | 1.875 | 1.115 | 1.374 | 1.875 | 1.602 | 1.248 | 2.858 | 0.452 | 0.498 | 2.067 | 1.686 | 1.893 | 1.988 | 1.576 |
| 酒类 Alcohol beverages | 1.111 | 4.573 | 0.444 | 7.664 | 1.674 | <0.001 | 0.125 | 0.160 | 0.082 | 3.748 | 0.592 | 0.318 | 1.963 | 4.702 | 0.260 | 1.347 | 10.866 | 0.180 | 0.023 | 0.416 | 1.927 | 0.541 | 0.051 | 0.004 | 1.782 |
| 合计 SUM | 87.9 | 166.9 | 181.7 | 293.7 | 92.9 | 88.4 | 223.6 | 305.0 | 126.6 | 243.1 | 258.2 | 260.2 | 82.1 | 75.1 | 153.5 | 54.0 | 112.9 | 136.8 | 80.1 | 197.1 | 34.7 | 37.8 | 42.1 | 40.6 | 140.6 |

附表 8-40　第六次中国总膳食研究的 TEN 膳食摄入量 [单位：ng/(kg bw・d)]
Annexed Table 8-40　Dietary intakes of TEN from the 6th China TDS [Unit: ng/(kg bw・d)]

| 膳食类别 Category | 黑龙江 HL | 辽宁 LN | 河北 HE | 北京 BJ | 吉林 JL | 山西 SX | 陕西 SN | 河南 HA | 宁夏 NX | 内蒙古 NM | 青海 QH | 甘肃 GS | 上海 SH | 福建 FJ | 江西 JX | 江苏 JS | 浙江 ZJ | 山东 SD | 湖北 HB | 四川 SC | 广西 GX | 湖南 HN | 广东 GD | 贵州 GZ | 全国平均 AVG |
|---|---|---|---|---|---|---|---|---|---|---|---|---|---|---|---|---|---|---|---|---|---|---|---|---|---|
| 谷类 Cereals | 8.46 | 35.32 | 152.90 | 0.44 | 76.79 | 157.20 | 446.20 | 478.40 | 376.00 | 540.10 | 177.80 | 329.90 | 36.25 | 9.51 | 17.16 | 3.36 | 1.60 | 200.50 | 8.33 | 190.10 | 6.17 | 5.25 | 33.77 | 0.43 | 137.20 |
| 豆类 Legumes | 0.026 | 0.523 | 0.027 | 0.044 | 0.694 | 0.665 | 1.641 | 0.449 | 0.871 | 0.298 | 0.026 | 0.663 | 1.116 | 0.032 | 0.447 | 0.430 | 0.059 | 0.220 | 0.029 | 2.143 | 0.419 | 0.311 | 0.143 | 0.048 | 0.472 |
| 薯类 Potatoes | 0.037 | 1.419 | 0.392 | 0.027 | 0.277 | 0.641 | 0.056 | 0.235 | 5.074 | 1.150 | 0.642 | 2.361 | 0.107 | 0.018 | 0.013 | 0.016 | 0.015 | 0.097 | 0.036 | 0.228 | 0.007 | 0.029 | 0.010 | 0.017 | 0.538 |
| 肉类 Meats | 0.028 | 0.033 | 0.020 | 0.033 | 0.346 | 0.885 | 0.015 | 0.296 | 1.735 | 2.233 | 0.622 | 0.774 | 1.613 | 0.035 | 0.038 | 0.037 | 0.050 | 0.042 | 0.022 | 2.859 | 0.484 | 6.750 | 0.052 | 0.044 | 0.794 |
| 蛋类 Eggs | 0.016 | 23.520 | 0.016 | 0.018 | 0.109 | 0.011 | 0.010 | 0.012 | 0.487 | 0.090 | 0.034 | 0.121 | 0.017 | 0.010 | 0.010 | 0.052 | 0.012 | 0.022 | 0.119 | 0.007 | 0.078 | 0.058 | 0.010 | 0.006 | 1.035 |
| 水产类 Aquatic foods | 0.011 | 0.009 | 0.004 | 0.188 | 0.117 | 0.035 | 0.002 | 0.076 | 0.045 | 0.636 | 0.082 | 0.028 | 0.524 | 0.027 | 0.173 | 0.016 | 0.021 | 0.045 | 0.016 | 0.162 | 0.039 | 0.393 | 0.021 | 0.002 | 0.111 |
| 乳类 Dairy products | 0.005 | 0.018 | 0.010 | 0.034 | 0.013 | 0.016 | 0.008 | 0.008 | 0.006 | 0.014 | 0.021 | 0.006 | 0.028 | 0.014 | 0.009 | 0.011 | 0.013 | 0.009 | 0.003 | 0.005 | 0.074 | 0.007 | 0.014 | 0.011 | 0.015 |
| 蔬菜类 Vegetables | 0.157 | 1.421 | 0.118 | 5.216 | 1.301 | 0.791 | 0.118 | 0.111 | 0.062 | 4.869 | 2.385 | 6.898 | 1.314 | 0.159 | 2.642 | 1.477 | 0.215 | 0.906 | 0.164 | 2.340 | 0.143 | 6.453 | 0.688 | 0.167 | 1.671 |
| 水果类 Fruits | 0.025 | 0.033 | 0.015 | 0.048 | 0.227 | 0.014 | 1.500 | 0.010 | 2.524 | 0.045 | 0.006 | 0.013 | 20.310 | 0.024 | 0.022 | 0.011 | 0.027 | 0.022 | 0.008 | 0.006 | 2.744 | 0.025 | 0.012 | 0.009 | 1.153 |
| 糖类 Sugar | 0.001 | <0.001 | <0.001 | 0.001 | <0.001 | <0.001 | <0.001 | <0.001 | <0.001 | <0.001 | <0.001 | <0.001 | 0.033 | <0.001 | <0.001 | <0.001 | <0.001 | <0.001 | <0.001 | <0.001 | <0.001 | <0.001 | <0.001 | <0.001 | 0.002 |
| 水及饮料类 Water and beverages | 0.485 | 0.196 | 0.308 | 0.440 | 0.516 | 0.296 | 0.137 | 0.473 | 0.205 | 1.022 | 0.245 | 0.469 | 0.279 | 0.343 | 0.469 | 0.400 | 0.312 | 0.715 | 0.113 | 0.125 | 0.517 | 0.421 | 0.473 | 0.497 | 0.394 |

续表

| 膳食类别 Category | 黑龙江 HL | 辽宁 LN | 河北 HE | 北京 BJ | 吉林 JL | 山西 SX | 陕西 SN | 河南 HA | 宁夏 NX | 内蒙古 NM | 青海 QH | 甘肃 GS | 上海 SH | 福建 FJ | 江西 JX | 江苏 JS | 浙江 ZJ | 山东 SD | 湖北 HB | 四川 SC | 广西 GX | 湖南 HN | 广东 GD | 贵州 GZ | 全国平均 AVG |
|---|---|---|---|---|---|---|---|---|---|---|---|---|---|---|---|---|---|---|---|---|---|---|---|---|---|
| 酒类 Alcohol beverages | 0.009 | 0.088 | 0.004 | 0.011 | 0.063 | <0.001 | 0.001 | 0.001 | <0.001 | 0.084 | 0.002 | 0.010 | 0.543 | 0.006 | 0.009 | 0.085 | 0.025 | 0.045 | 0.037 | 0.002 | 0.812 | 0.007 | 0.024 | 0.001 | 0.078 |
| 合计 SUM | 9.3 | 62.6 | 153.8 | 6.5 | 80.4 | 160.5 | 449.6 | 480.1 | 387.0 | 551.1 | 181.9 | 341.2 | 62.1 | 10.2 | 21.0 | 5.9 | 2.4 | 202.6 | 8.9 | 198.0 | 11.5 | 19.7 | 35.2 | 1.2 | 143.4 |

附表 8-41 第六次中国总膳食研究的 AME 膳食摄入量 [单位: ng/(kg bw·d)]
Annexed Table 8-41 Dietary intakes of AME from the 6$^{th}$ China TDS [Unit: ng/(kg bw·d)]

| 膳食类别 Category | 黑龙江 HL | 辽宁 LN | 河北 HE | 北京 BJ | 吉林 JL | 山西 SX | 陕西 SN | 河南 HA | 宁夏 NX | 内蒙古 NM | 青海 QH | 甘肃 GS | 上海 SH | 福建 FJ | 江西 JX | 江苏 JS | 浙江 ZJ | 山东 SD | 湖北 HB | 四川 SC | 广西 GX | 湖南 HN | 广东 GD | 贵州 GZ | 全国平均 AVG |
|---|---|---|---|---|---|---|---|---|---|---|---|---|---|---|---|---|---|---|---|---|---|---|---|---|---|
| 谷类 Cereals | 0.168 | 75.67 | 31.77 | 187.2 | 8.014 | 6.075 | 16.32 | 46.39 | 90.43 | 49.90 | 34.55 | 29.69 | 3.374 | 5.189 | 2.511 | 0.154 | 2.895 | 6.861 | 1.554 | 137.7 | 0.220 | 0.135 | 13.39 | 12.738 | 31.79 |
| 豆类 Legumes | 0.010 | 0.027 | 0.011 | 3.114 | 0.016 | 0.012 | 0.371 | 0.012 | 0.007 | 0.007 | 0.001 | 0.115 | 0.021 | 0.013 | 0.013 | 0.015 | 0.024 | 0.009 | 0.012 | 0.138 | 0.007 | 0.015 | 0.005 | 0.446 | 0.184 |
| 薯类 Potatoes | 0.015 | 0.216 | 0.011 | 2.601 | 0.019 | 0.024 | 0.023 | 0.014 | 1.872 | 0.253 | 0.017 | 1.765 | 0.006 | 0.007 | 0.005 | 0.006 | 0.080 | 0.190 | 0.820 | 0.160 | 0.003 | 0.011 | 0.004 | 0.055 | 0.341 |
| 肉类 Meats | 0.011 | 0.013 | 0.008 | 0.013 | 0.011 | 0.023 | 0.006 | 0.009 | 1.665 | 0.365 | 0.011 | 0.393 | 0.018 | 0.014 | 0.015 | 0.015 | 0.020 | 0.017 | 0.009 | 1.166 | 0.024 | 0.024 | 0.021 | 0.017 | 0.162 |
| 蛋类 Eggs | 0.007 | 1.119 | 0.006 | 0.007 | 0.007 | 0.066 | 0.004 | 0.005 | 0.224 | 0.714 | 0.003 | 0.004 | 0.007 | 0.004 | 0.004 | 0.005 | 0.005 | 0.009 | 0.338 | 0.003 | 0.002 | 0.004 | 0.004 | 0.003 | 0.106 |
| 水产类 Aquatic foods | 0.004 | 0.004 | 0.002 | 0.003 | 0.002 | 0.001 | 0.001 | 0.001 | 0.027 | 0.036 | 0.001 | 0.009 | 0.011 | 0.011 | 0.069 | 0.006 | 0.008 | 0.004 | 0.245 | 0.001 | 0.015 | 0.011 | 0.008 | 0.011 | 0.020 |

续表

| 膳食类别 Category | 黑龙江 HL | 辽宁 LN | 河北 HE | 北京 BJ | 吉林 JL | 山西 SX | 陕西 SN | 河南 HA | 宁夏 NX | 内蒙古 NM | 青海 QH | 甘肃 GS | 上海 SH | 福建 FJ | 江西 JX | 江苏 JS | 浙江 ZJ | 山东 SD | 湖北 HB | 四川 SC | 广西 GX | 湖南 HN | 广东 GD | 贵州 GZ | 全国平均 AVG |
|---|---|---|---|---|---|---|---|---|---|---|---|---|---|---|---|---|---|---|---|---|---|---|---|---|---|
| 乳类 Dairy products | 0.002 | 0.007 | 0.004 | 0.014 | 0.005 | 0.007 | 0.003 | 0.003 | 0.002 | 0.005 | 0.008 | 0.002 | 0.011 | 0.006 | 0.003 | 0.004 | 0.005 | 0.004 | 0.001 | 0.002 | 0.003 | 0.003 | 0.006 | 0.004 | 0.005 |
| 蔬菜类 Vegetables | 0.063 | 0.056 | 0.047 | 6.284 | 0.062 | 0.050 | 0.047 | 0.045 | 0.025 | 1.215 | 0.049 | 0.440 | 0.064 | 0.064 | 0.072 | 0.070 | 0.086 | 0.079 | 7.214 | 0.048 | 0.057 | 0.087 | 0.039 | 0.067 | 0.680 |
| 水果类 Fruits | 0.010 | 0.267 | 0.006 | 0.019 | 0.014 | 0.006 | 0.006 | 0.004 | 1.276 | 0.018 | 0.003 | 0.005 | 0.012 | 0.010 | 0.009 | 0.004 | 0.011 | 0.009 | 0.003 | 0.003 | 0.420 | 0.010 | 0.005 | 0.004 | 0.089 |
| 糖类 Sugar | <0.001 | <0.001 | <0.001 | <0.001 | <0.001 | <0.001 | <0.001 | <0.001 | <0.001 | <0.001 | <0.001 | <0.001 | <0.001 | <0.001 | 0.008 | <0.001 | <0.001 | <0.001 | <0.001 | <0.001 | 0.002 | <0.001 | <0.001 | <0.001 | 0.001 |
| 水及饮料类 Water and beverages | 0.194 | 0.078 | 0.123 | 2.788 | 0.207 | 0.118 | 0.055 | 0.189 | 0.082 | 0.409 | 0.098 | 0.187 | 0.112 | 0.137 | 3.863 | 0.160 | 0.125 | 0.286 | 0.045 | 0.050 | 0.207 | 0.169 | 0.189 | 0.199 | 0.420 |
| 酒类 Alcohol beverages | 0.003 | 0.005 | 0.002 | 0.436 | 0.002 | <0.001 | <0.001 | 0.001 | <0.001 | 0.003 | <0.001 | <0.001 | 0.004 | 0.002 | 0.003 | 0.006 | 0.010 | 0.018 | 0.062 | 0.001 | 0.055 | 0.003 | <0.001 | <0.001 | 0.026 |
| 合计 SUM | 0.49 | 77.46 | 31.99 | 202.45 | 8.36 | 6.38 | 16.84 | 46.68 | 95.61 | 52.93 | 34.74 | 32.61 | 3.64 | 5.46 | 6.58 | 0.45 | 3.27 | 7.48 | 10.30 | 139.31 | 1.02 | 0.47 | 13.67 | 13.54 | 33.82 |

附表 8-42 第六次中国总膳食研究的 ALT 膳食摄入量 [单位：ng/(kg bw·d)]
Annexed Table 8-42 Dietary intakes of ALT from the 6th China TDS [Unit: ng/(kg bw·d)]

| 膳食类别 Category | 黑龙江 HL | 辽宁 LN | 河北 HE | 北京 BJ | 吉林 JL | 山西 SX | 陕西 SN | 河南 HA | 宁夏 NX | 内蒙古 NM | 青海 QH | 甘肃 GS | 上海 SH | 福建 FJ | 江西 JX | 江苏 JS | 浙江 ZJ | 山东 SD | 湖北 HB | 四川 SC | 广西 GX | 湖南 HN | 广东 GD | 贵州 GZ | 全国平均 AVG |
|---|---|---|---|---|---|---|---|---|---|---|---|---|---|---|---|---|---|---|---|---|---|---|---|---|---|
| 谷类 Cereals | 1.684 | 1.551 | 1.986 | 1.778 | 1.223 | 2.656 | 2.358 | 2.292 | 1.871 | 1.688 | 2.764 | 1.846 | 0.926 | 1.476 | 1.370 | 1.544 | 1.339 | 2.107 | 1.149 | 2.434 | 2.196 | 1.348 | 0.979 | 136.500 | 7.378 |

续表

| 膳食类别 Category | 黑龙江 HL | 辽宁 LN | 河北 HE | 北京 BJ | 吉林 JL | 山西 SX | 陕西 SN | 河南 HA | 宁夏 NX | 内蒙古 NM | 青海 QH | 甘肃 GS | 上海 SH | 福建 FJ | 江西 JX | 江苏 JS | 浙江 ZJ | 山东 SD | 湖北 HB | 四川 SC | 广西 GX | 湖南 HN | 广东 GD | 贵州 GZ | 全国平均 AVG |
|---|---|---|---|---|---|---|---|---|---|---|---|---|---|---|---|---|---|---|---|---|---|---|---|---|---|
| 豆类 Legumes | 0.104 | 0.265 | 0.108 | 0.176 | 0.162 | 0.122 | 0.148 | 0.122 | 0.066 | 0.068 | 0.012 | 0.067 | 0.215 | 0.127 | 0.133 | 0.153 | 0.238 | 0.089 | 0.118 | 0.123 | 0.069 | 0.150 | 0.050 | 0.192 | 0.128 |
| 薯类 Potatoes | 0.146 | 2.555 | 0.113 | 0.108 | 0.190 | 1.852 | 0.225 | 0.139 | 0.181 | 0.198 | 0.168 | 0.235 | 0.057 | 0.074 | 0.051 | 0.064 | 0.656 | 0.076 | 0.142 | 0.103 | 0.027 | 0.115 | 0.041 | 0.066 | 0.316 |
| 肉类 Meats | 0.112 | 0.131 | 0.082 | 0.134 | 0.107 | 1.164 | 0.061 | 0.092 | 0.077 | 0.119 | 1.260 | 0.612 | 0.176 | 0.141 | 0.151 | 0.147 | 0.202 | 0.166 | 0.090 | 0.206 | 0.240 | 0.240 | 0.209 | 0.174 | 0.254 |
| 蛋类 Eggs | 0.065 | 0.085 | 0.064 | 0.073 | 0.073 | 0.046 | 0.041 | 0.047 | 2.707 | 0.062 | 0.029 | 0.041 | 0.067 | 0.039 | 0.038 | 0.048 | 0.047 | 0.087 | 0.047 | 0.026 | 0.025 | 0.037 | 0.038 | 0.026 | 0.161 |
| 水产类 Aquatic foods | 0.043 | 3.288 | 0.017 | 0.028 | 0.018 | 0.012 | 0.007 | 0.008 | 0.004 | 0.016 | 0.006 | 0.004 | 0.109 | 0.106 | 0.069 | 0.063 | 0.083 | 0.038 | 0.065 | 0.013 | 0.155 | 0.106 | 0.085 | 0.007 | 0.181 |
| 乳类 Dairy products | 0.021 | 0.071 | 0.038 | 0.136 | 0.051 | 0.066 | 0.031 | 0.031 | 0.024 | 0.055 | 0.085 | 0.022 | 0.113 | 0.057 | 0.035 | 0.044 | 0.053 | 0.036 | 0.011 | 0.020 | 0.029 | 0.029 | 0.058 | 0.045 | 0.048 |
| 蔬菜类 Vegetables | 0.627 | 0.557 | 0.470 | 0.628 | 54.505 | 0.501 | 0.470 | 0.446 | 0.248 | 0.421 | 0.493 | 3.978 | 4.057 | 65.896 | 0.717 | 8.597 | 0.860 | 0.787 | 0.657 | 0.484 | 0.572 | 0.874 | 0.387 | 0.668 | 6.162 |
| 水果类 Fruits | 0.100 | 0.133 | 0.060 | 0.192 | 2.391 | 2.318 | 0.063 | 0.038 | 0.156 | 1.214 | 0.283 | 0.053 | 3.087 | 0.098 | 0.621 | 0.043 | 0.107 | 0.086 | 0.030 | 0.026 | 0.102 | 0.101 | 0.047 | 0.038 | 0.474 |
| 糖类 Sugar | 0.004 | 0.001 | 0.001 | 0.003 | 0.002 | 0.002 | 0.001 | 0.001 | 0.001 | 0.002 | 0.001 | 0.001 | 0.012 | <0.001 | 0.002 | <0.001 | 0.002 | 0.001 | <0.001 | 0.001 | 0.001 | 0.001 | <0.001 | <0.001 | 0.004 |
| 水及饮料类 Water and beverages | 1.940 | 0.783 | 1.231 | 1.758 | 2.066 | 1.183 | 0.548 | 1.893 | 0.821 | 4.087 | 0.981 | 1.875 | 1.115 | 1.374 | 1.875 | 1.602 | 1.248 | 2.858 | 0.452 | 0.498 | 2.067 | 1.686 | 1.893 | 1.988 | 1.576 |
| 酒类 Alcohol beverages | 0.035 | 0.053 | 0.017 | 0.044 | 0.015 | <0.001 | 0.003 | 0.005 | 0.001 | 0.033 | 0.007 | 0.005 | 0.036 | 0.023 | 0.034 | 0.060 | 0.100 | 0.180 | 0.023 | 0.008 | 0.051 | 0.027 | 0.002 | 0.003 | 0.032 |
| 合计 SUM | 4.882 | 9.474 | 4.186 | 5.056 | 60.802 | 9.922 | 3.956 | 5.113 | 6.158 | 7.963 | 6.089 | 8.740 | 9.970 | 69.411 | 5.096 | 12.364 | 4.934 | 6.512 | 2.783 | 3.944 | 5.533 | 4.711 | 3.790 | 139.722 | 16.713 |

附录 873

附表 8-43　第六次中国总膳食研究膳食样品中 BEA 的含量（单位：μg/kg）
Annexed Table 8-43　Levels of BEA in food samples from the 6th China TDS (Unit: μg/kg)

| 膳食类别<br>Category | 黑龙江<br>HL | 辽宁<br>LN | 河北<br>HE | 北京<br>BJ | 吉林<br>JL | 山西<br>SX | 陕西<br>SN | 河南<br>HA | 宁夏<br>NX | 内蒙古<br>NM | 青海<br>QH | 甘肃<br>GS | 上海<br>SH | 福建<br>FJ | 江西<br>JX | 江苏<br>JS | 浙江<br>ZJ | 山东<br>SD | 湖北<br>HB | 四川<br>SC | 广西<br>GX | 湖南<br>HN | 广东<br>GD | 贵州<br>GZ | 全国平均<br>AVG |
|---|---|---|---|---|---|---|---|---|---|---|---|---|---|---|---|---|---|---|---|---|---|---|---|---|---|
| 谷类 Cereals | ND | 1.24 | 0.50 | 2.49 | ND | ND | 1.46 | 0.35 | 10.17 | 0.51 | 0.23 | ND | ND | 0.60 | ND | 2.43 | ND | ND | 0.75 | ND | ND | ND | 0.30 | ND | 0.88 |
| 豆类 Legumes | ND | 0.70 | 0.21 | 5.93 | ND | ND | 0.30 | ND | 0.19 | ND | 0.12 | ND | 0.76 | 0.19 | 0.13 | 0.54 | ND | ND | 3.34 | ND | ND | ND | 1.13 | 3.66 | 0.72 |
| 薯类 Potatoes | ND | ND | 0.29 | 2.59 | 0.19 | ND | 0.37 | ND | ND | ND | ND | ND | ND | 0.55 | ND | ND | ND | ND | 2.60 | ND | ND | ND | 0.42 | 1.64 | 0.37 |
| 肉类 Meats | ND | ND | 0.19 | ND | 0.16 | ND | 0.55 | ND | 0.79 | ND | ND | ND | ND | 1.35 | ND | ND | ND | ND | ND | ND | 0.14 | ND | ND | 1.10 | 0.19 |
| 蛋类 Eggs | ND | 5.05 | 0.34 | 1.50 | ND | ND | 0.66 | ND | 1.32 | ND | 0.15 | ND | ND | 2.73 | ND | 6.89 | ND | ND | 7.88 | 0.16 | ND | ND | ND | 2.45 | 1.22 |
| 水产类 Aquatic foods | ND | ND | ND | 0.34 | 0.33 | ND | 0.17 | ND | 0.31 | ND | ND | ND | ND | 0.52 | 0.10 | ND | ND | ND | 1.02 | 0.27 | ND | ND | ND | 0.59 | 0.16 |
| 乳类 Dairy products | ND | ND | ND | 0.16 | ND | ND | 0.41 | ND | 0.66 | ND | ND | ND | ND | 0.69 | ND | ND | ND | ND | ND | ND | ND | ND | 0.58 | 6.31 | 0.37 |
| 蔬菜类 Vegetables | ND | ND | ND | 1.95 | ND | 0.11 | ND | ND | ND | ND | ND | ND | ND | ND | ND | ND | ND | ND | 1.85 | ND | ND | ND | ND | ND | 0.17 |
| 水果类 Fruits | ND | ND | ND | ND | ND | ND | 0.19 | ND | 0.25 | ND | ND | ND | ND | 0.99 | ND | ND | ND | ND | 0.21 | ND | ND | ND | ND | ND | 0.08 |
| 糖类 Sugar | ND | ND | ND | ND | ND | ND | ND | ND | 0.08 | ND | ND | | 0.82 | ND | ND | ND | ND | ND | ND | ND | ND | ND | ND | ND | 0.05 |
| 水及饮料类 Water and beverages | ND | ND | ND | ND | ND | ND | ND | ND | ND | ND | ND | | ND | ND | ND | ND | ND | ND | ND | ND | ND | ND | ND | ND | 0.01 |

续表

| 膳食类别<br>Category | 黑龙江<br>HL | 辽宁<br>LN | 河北<br>HE | 北京<br>BJ | 吉林<br>JL | 山西<br>SX | 陕西<br>SN | 河南<br>HA | 宁夏<br>NX | 内蒙古<br>NM | 青海<br>QH | 甘肃<br>GS | 上海<br>SH | 福建<br>FJ | 江西<br>JX | 江苏<br>JS | 浙江<br>ZJ | 山东<br>SD | 湖北<br>HB | 四川<br>SC | 广西<br>GX | 湖南<br>HN | 广东<br>GD | 贵州<br>GZ | 全国平均<br>AVG |
|---|---|---|---|---|---|---|---|---|---|---|---|---|---|---|---|---|---|---|---|---|---|---|---|---|---|
| 酒类<br>Alcohol beverages | ND | 0.12 | ND | ND | ND | ND | ND | ND | ND | ND | ND | ND | ND | ND | ND | ND | ND | ND | ND | ND | ND | ND | ND | 4.38 | 0.20 |

注：平均值计算中，ND 以 1/2 检出限（LOD）计

Note: in calculation of averages (AVG), values not detected (ND) were treated as being equal to half of the detection of limit (LOD)

附表 8-44 第六次中国总膳食研究膳食样品中 ENNA 的含量（单位：μg/kg）

Annexed Table 8-44 Levels of ENNA in food samples from the 6th China TDS (Unit: μg/kg)

| 膳食类别<br>Category | 黑龙江<br>HL | 辽宁<br>LN | 河北<br>HE | 北京<br>BJ | 吉林<br>JL | 山西<br>SX | 陕西<br>SN | 河南<br>HA | 宁夏<br>NX | 内蒙古<br>NM | 青海<br>QH | 甘肃<br>GS | 上海<br>SH | 福建<br>FJ | 江西<br>JX | 江苏<br>JS | 浙江<br>ZJ | 山东<br>SD | 湖北<br>HB | 四川<br>SC | 广西<br>GX | 湖南<br>HN | 广东<br>GD | 贵州<br>GZ | 全国平均<br>AVG |
|---|---|---|---|---|---|---|---|---|---|---|---|---|---|---|---|---|---|---|---|---|---|---|---|---|---|
| 谷类<br>Cereals | ND | 1.32 | ND | ND | ND | ND | 1.92 | 0.15 | 5.72 | 0.27 | ND | ND | ND | 0.43 | ND | ND | ND | ND | 0.16 | ND | ND | ND | 0.21 | ND | 0.43 |
| 豆类<br>Legumes | ND | ND | ND | 1.37 | ND | ND | ND | ND | ND | ND | ND | ND | ND | ND | ND | ND | ND | ND | 1.14 | ND | ND | ND | ND | 0.31 | 0.13 |
| 薯类<br>Potatoes | ND | 0.24 | ND | 1.32 | ND | ND | ND | ND | 0.55 | ND | ND | 0.20 | ND | ND | ND | 0.25 | 0.18 | ND | 1.02 | ND | ND | ND | ND | 0.21 | 0.17 |
| 肉类<br>Meats | ND | ND | ND | ND | ND | ND | 0.34 | ND | 1.34 | ND | ND | 0.28 | ND | 0.29 | ND | ND | ND | ND | ND | ND | ND | ND | ND | 0.25 | 0.11 |
| 蛋类<br>Eggs | ND | ND | ND | 1.82 | ND | ND | ND | ND | 0.72 | ND | ND | ND | ND | 0.39 | ND | ND | 0.24 | ND | 1.52 | ND | ND | ND | ND | 0.38 | 0.22 |
| 水产类<br>Aquatic foods | ND | ND | ND | ND | 0.19 | ND | ND | ND | 0.42 | ND | ND | 0.12 | ND | ND | ND | ND | ND | ND | ND | ND | ND | ND | ND | 0.36 | 0.05 |
| 乳类<br>Dairy products | ND | ND | ND | ND | ND | ND | ND | ND | ND | ND | ND | ND | ND | ND | ND | ND | ND | ND | ND | ND | ND | ND | 0.15 | 1.38 | 0.07 |

续表

| 膳食类别<br>Category | 黑龙江<br>HL | 辽宁<br>LN | 河北<br>HE | 北京<br>BJ | 吉林<br>JL | 山西<br>SX | 陕西<br>SN | 河南<br>HA | 宁夏<br>NX | 内蒙古<br>NM | 青海<br>QH | 甘肃<br>GS | 上海<br>SH | 福建<br>FJ | 江西<br>JX | 江苏<br>JS | 浙江<br>ZJ | 山东<br>SD | 湖北<br>HB | 四川<br>SC | 广西<br>GX | 湖南<br>HN | 广东<br>GD | 贵州<br>GZ | 全国平均<br>AVG |
|---|---|---|---|---|---|---|---|---|---|---|---|---|---|---|---|---|---|---|---|---|---|---|---|---|---|
| 蔬菜类 Vegetables | ND | ND | ND | ND | ND | ND | ND | ND | ND | ND | ND | ND | ND | ND | ND | ND | ND | ND | ND | ND | ND | ND | ND | ND | 0.01 |
| 水果类 Fruits | ND | ND | ND | ND | ND | ND | ND | ND | 0.51 | ND | ND | ND | ND | 0.38 | ND | ND | ND | ND | ND | ND | ND | ND | ND | ND | 0.05 |
| 糖类 Sugar | ND | ND | ND | ND | ND | ND | ND | ND | ND | ND | ND | ND | ND | ND | ND | ND | ND | ND | ND | ND | ND | ND | ND | ND | 0.01 |
| 水及饮料类 Water and beverages | ND | ND | ND | ND | ND | ND | ND | ND | ND | ND | ND | ND | ND | ND | ND | ND | ND | ND | ND | ND | ND | ND | ND | ND | 0.01 |
| 酒类 Alcohol beverages | ND | ND | ND | ND | ND | ND | ND | ND | ND | ND | ND | ND | ND | ND | ND | ND | ND | ND | ND | ND | ND | ND | ND | 0.16 | 0.02 |

注：平均值计算中，ND 以 1/2 检出限（LOD）计

Note: in calculation of averages (AVG), values not detected (ND) were treated as being equal to half of the detection of limit (LOD)

附表 8-45　第六次中国总膳食研究膳食样品中 ENNA1 的含量（单位：µg/kg）

**Annexed Table 8-45　Levels of ENNA1 in food samples from the 6$^{th}$ China TDS** (Unit: µg/kg)

| 膳食类别<br>Category | 黑龙江<br>HL | 辽宁<br>LN | 河北<br>HE | 北京<br>BJ | 吉林<br>JL | 山西<br>SX | 陕西<br>SN | 河南<br>HA | 宁夏<br>NX | 内蒙古<br>NM | 青海<br>QH | 甘肃<br>GS | 上海<br>SH | 福建<br>FJ | 江西<br>JX | 江苏<br>JS | 浙江<br>ZJ | 山东<br>SD | 湖北<br>HB | 四川<br>SC | 广西<br>GX | 湖南<br>HN | 广东<br>GD | 贵州<br>GZ | 全国平均<br>AVG |
|---|---|---|---|---|---|---|---|---|---|---|---|---|---|---|---|---|---|---|---|---|---|---|---|---|---|
| 谷类 Cereals | ND | 0.16 | 0.17 | ND | ND | 0.51 | 1.50 | 0.42 | 6.33 | ND | 0.35 | 0.24 | ND | 0.18 | ND | ND | 0.18 | 0.15 | 0.30 | 0.50 | ND | ND | ND | ND | 0.46 |
| 豆类 Legumes | ND | ND | ND | 0.32 | ND | 0.14 | ND | ND | ND | ND | ND | 0.27 | ND | ND | ND | ND | ND | ND | 0.24 | 0.08 | ND | ND | ND | 0.35 | 0.07 |
| 薯类 Potatoes | ND | ND | ND | ND | ND | ND | ND | ND | ND | ND | ND | 0.12 | ND | ND | ND | ND | ND | ND | 0.15 | 0.07 | ND | ND | ND | 0.22 | 0.03 |

续表

| 膳食类别 Category | 黑龙江 HL | 辽宁 LN | 河北 HE | 北京 BJ | 吉林 JL | 山西 SX | 陕西 SN | 河南 HA | 宁夏 NX | 内蒙古 NM | 青海 QH | 甘肃 GS | 上海 SH | 福建 FJ | 江西 JX | 江苏 JS | 浙江 ZJ | 山东 SD | 湖北 HB | 四川 SC | 广西 GX | 湖南 HN | 广东 GD | 贵州 GZ | 全国平均 AVG |
|---|---|---|---|---|---|---|---|---|---|---|---|---|---|---|---|---|---|---|---|---|---|---|---|---|---|
| 肉类 Meats | ND | ND | ND | ND | ND | ND | ND | ND | 0.47 | ND | ND | 0.21 | ND | ND | ND | ND | ND | ND | ND | ND | ND | ND | ND | 0.23 | 0.05 |
| 蛋类 Eggs | ND | ND | ND | 0.61 | ND | ND | ND | ND | ND | ND | ND | ND | ND | ND | ND | ND | ND | ND | 0.36 | ND | ND | ND | ND | 0.24 | 0.06 |
| 水产类 Aquatic foods | ND | ND | ND | ND | 0.18 | ND | ND | ND | ND | ND | ND | ND | ND | ND | ND | ND | ND | ND | ND | ND | ND | ND | ND | 0.25 | 0.03 |
| 乳类 Dairy products | ND | ND | ND | ND | ND | ND | ND | ND | ND | ND | ND | ND | ND | ND | ND | ND | ND | ND | ND | ND | ND | ND | ND | 0.25 | 0.02 |
| 蔬菜类 Vegetables | ND | ND | ND | ND | ND | ND | ND | ND | ND | ND | ND | ND | ND | ND | ND | ND | ND | ND | ND | ND | ND | ND | ND | ND | 0.01 |
| 水果类 Fruits | ND | ND | ND | ND | ND | ND | ND | ND | ND | ND | ND | ND | ND | ND | ND | ND | ND | ND | ND | ND | ND | ND | ND | ND | 0.01 |
| 糖类 Sugar | ND | ND | ND | ND | ND | ND | ND | ND | ND | ND | ND | ND | ND | ND | ND | ND | ND | ND | ND | ND | ND | ND | ND | ND | 0.01 |
| 水及饮料类 Water and beverages | ND | ND | ND | ND | ND | ND | ND | ND | ND | ND | ND | ND | ND | ND | ND | ND | ND | ND | ND | ND | ND | ND | ND | ND | 0.01 |
| 酒类 Alcohol beverages | ND | ND | ND | ND | ND | ND | ND | ND | ND | ND | ND | ND | ND | ND | ND | ND | ND | ND | ND | ND | ND | ND | ND | ND | 0.01 |

注：平均值计算中，ND 以 1/2 检出限（LOD）计

Note: in calculation of averages (AVG), values not detected (ND) were treated as being equal to half of the detection of limit (LOD)

附表 8-46 第六次中国总膳食研究膳食样品中 ENNB 的含量（单位：μg/kg）

Annexed Table 8-46 Levels of ENNB in food samples from the 6$^{th}$ China TDS (Unit: μg/kg)

| 膳食类别 Category | 黑龙江 HL | 辽宁 LN | 河北 HE | 北京 BJ | 吉林 JL | 山西 SX | 陕西 SN | 河南 HA | 宁夏 NX | 内蒙古 NM | 青海 QH | 甘肃 GS | 上海 SH | 福建 FJ | 江西 JX | 江苏 JS | 浙江 ZJ | 山东 SD | 湖北 HB | 四川 SC | 广西 GX | 湖南 HN | 广东 GD | 贵州 GZ | 全国平均 AVG |
|---|---|---|---|---|---|---|---|---|---|---|---|---|---|---|---|---|---|---|---|---|---|---|---|---|---|
| 谷类 Cereals | ND | 1.673 | 1.131 | 0.300 | 0.459 | 17.850 | 9.534 | 2.688 | 42.440 | 7.537 | 1.769 | 1.832 | 1.843 | 1.860 | 0.030 | 0.501 | 0.489 | 1.297 | 0.774 | 1.514 | 0.035 | 0.048 | 0.526 | ND | 4.006 |
| 豆类 Legumes | ND | 0.221 | 0.159 | 0.372 | 0.974 | 1.105 | 0.136 | 0.062 | 0.633 | 0.154 | 0.137 | 1.391 | 0.174 | 0.089 | ND | 0.416 | ND | 0.020 | 0.415 | 0.187 | 0.106 | 0.123 | 0.052 | 2.504 | 0.393 |
| 薯类 Potatoes | ND | 0.464 | 0.334 | 0.511 | 0.306 | 0.051 | 0.164 | 0.038 | 1.036 | ND | 0.534 | 0.458 | 0.052 | ND | ND | 1.045 | ND | 0.033 | 0.213 | 0.096 | 0.045 | 0.040 | ND | 2.900 | 0.347 |
| 肉类 Meats | ND | 0.156 | 0.267 | ND | 0.286 | 0.067 | 0.301 | 0.145 | 3.508 | 0.185 | 0.709 | 0.714 | 0.024 | ND | 0.013 | ND | ND | 0.055 | 0.248 | 0.080 | 0.127 | 0.245 | 0.069 | 3.560 | 0.449 |
| 蛋类 Eggs | ND | ND | 0.260 | 0.543 | 0.079 | 0.067 | 0.081 | 0.079 | 1.161 | 0.024 | 1.135 | 0.095 | ND | ND | ND | 0.162 | 0.748 | 0.054 | 0.355 | ND | 0.077 | 0.327 | ND | 3.745 | 0.375 |
| 水产类 Aquatic foods | ND | ND | 0.080 | 0.325 | 1.329 | 0.018 | 0.146 | 0.225 | 0.901 | 0.135 | 0.612 | 0.208 | 0.029 | ND | 0.067 | 0.668 | ND | 0.045 | 0.286 | 0.023 | 0.090 | 0.301 | 0.108 | 5.881 | 0.479 |
| 乳类 Dairy products | ND | 0.259 | 0.024 | ND | ND | ND | 0.411 | ND | 0.323 | 0.062 | 0.022 | 0.070 | 0.023 | 0.313 | 0.170 | ND | ND | 0.020 | ND | 0.696 | 0.629 | 0.045 | 0.043 | 0.086 | 0.134 |
| 蔬菜类 Vegetables | ND | ND | 0.173 | 0.175 | 0.276 | 0.096 | ND | ND | ND | 0.077 | 0.434 | 0.370 | 0.039 | ND | 0.067 | 0.490 | ND | 0.072 | 0.287 | 0.103 | 0.045 | 0.277 | 0.109 | ND | 0.130 |
| 水果类 Fruits | ND | ND | ND | ND | ND | ND | 0.281 | ND | 1.203 | ND | ND | ND | ND | 0.112 | ND | ND | ND | ND | ND | ND | ND | ND | 0.049 | 0.947 | 0.110 |
| 糖类 Sugar | ND | ND | ND | ND | ND | ND | ND | ND | ND | ND | ND | ND | 0.079 | ND | ND | ND | ND | ND | ND | ND | ND | ND | ND | ND | 0.005 |
| 水及饮料类 Water and beverages | ND | ND | ND | ND | ND | ND | ND | ND | ND | ND | ND | ND | ND | ND | ND | ND | ND | ND | ND | ND | ND | ND | ND | ND | 0.002 |

续表

| 膳食类别 Category | 黑龙江 HL | 辽宁 LN | 河北 HE | 北京 BJ | 吉林 JL | 山西 SX | 陕西 SN | 河南 HA | 宁夏 NX | 内蒙古 NM | 青海 QH | 甘肃 GS | 上海 SH | 福建 FJ | 江西 JX | 江苏 JS | 浙江 ZJ | 山东 SD | 湖北 HB | 四川 SC | 广西 GX | 湖南 HN | 广东 GD | 贵州 GZ | 全国平均 AVG |
|---|---|---|---|---|---|---|---|---|---|---|---|---|---|---|---|---|---|---|---|---|---|---|---|---|---|
| 酒类 Alcohol beverages | ND | ND | ND | ND | 0.132 | ND | ND | ND | ND | 0.007 | ND | ND | 0.024 | 0.025 | ND | ND | ND | ND | ND | ND | ND | ND | ND | ND | 0.009 |

注：平均值计算中，ND 以 1/2 检出限（LOD）计

Note: in calculation of averages (AVG), values not detected (ND) were treated as being equal to half of the detection of limit (LOD)

附表 8-47 第六次中国总膳食研究膳食样品中 ENNB1 的含量（单位：μg/kg）

Annexed Table 8-47 Levels of ENNB1 in food samples from the 6$^{th}$ China TDS (Unit: μg/kg)

| 膳食类别 Category | 黑龙江 HL | 辽宁 LN | 河北 HE | 北京 BJ | 吉林 JL | 山西 SX | 陕西 SN | 河南 HA | 宁夏 NX | 内蒙古 NM | 青海 QH | 甘肃 GS | 上海 SH | 福建 FJ | 江西 JX | 江苏 JS | 浙江 ZJ | 山东 SD | 湖北 HB | 四川 SC | 广西 GX | 湖南 HN | 广东 GD | 贵州 GZ | 全国平均 AVG |
|---|---|---|---|---|---|---|---|---|---|---|---|---|---|---|---|---|---|---|---|---|---|---|---|---|---|
| 谷类 Cereals | ND | 0.53 | 0.35 | ND | ND | 2.95 | 4.08 | 1.17 | 13.71 | 2.93 | 0.70 | 0.69 | 0.37 | 0.30 | ND | 0.13 | 0.28 | 0.44 | 0.48 | 0.81 | ND | ND | 0.13 | 0.16 | 1.26 |
| 豆类 Legumes | ND | ND | ND | 0.39 | 0.19 | 0.42 | ND | ND | 0.95 | ND | ND | 0.74 | ND | ND | ND | ND | ND | ND | 0.40 | ND | ND | ND | ND | 0.87 | 0.17 |
| 薯类 Potatoes | ND | 0.15 | 0.14 | 0.39 | 0.13 | ND | ND | ND | 0.36 | ND | ND | 0.11 | ND | ND | ND | 0.23 | ND | ND | 0.21 | ND | ND | ND | ND | 0.65 | 0.11 |
| 肉类 Meats | ND | ND | 0.12 | ND | ND | ND | ND | ND | 1.06 | ND | 0.13 | 0.20 | ND | ND | ND | ND | ND | ND | ND | ND | ND | ND | ND | 0.67 | 0.10 |
| 蛋类 Eggs | ND | ND | 0.12 | 0.59 | ND | ND | ND | ND | 0.36 | ND | 0.21 | ND | ND | ND | ND | 0.19 | 0.28 | ND | 0.28 | ND | ND | ND | ND | 0.87 | 0.13 |
| 水产类 Aquatic foods | ND | ND | ND | ND | 0.35 | ND | ND | ND | 0.22 | ND | ND | ND | ND | ND | ND | ND | ND | ND | 0.22 | ND | ND | ND | ND | 1.08 | 0.09 |
| 乳类 Dairy products | ND | ND | ND | ND | ND | ND | ND | ND | ND | ND | ND | ND | ND | ND | ND | ND | ND | ND | ND | ND | ND | ND | ND | 0.87 | 0.05 |

续表

| 膳食类别 Category | 黑龙江 HL | 辽宁 LN | 河北 HE | 北京 BJ | 吉林 JL | 山西 SX | 陕西 SN | 河南 HA | 宁夏 NX | 内蒙古 NM | 青海 QH | 甘肃 GS | 上海 SH | 福建 FJ | 江西 JX | 江苏 JS | 浙江 ZJ | 山东 SD | 湖北 HB | 四川 SC | 广西 GX | 湖南 HN | 广东 GD | 贵州 GZ | 全国平均 AVG |
|---|---|---|---|---|---|---|---|---|---|---|---|---|---|---|---|---|---|---|---|---|---|---|---|---|---|
| 蔬菜类 Vegetables | ND | ND | ND | 0.15 | ND | ND | ND | ND | ND | ND | ND | ND | ND | ND | ND | ND | ND | ND | 0.26 | ND | ND | ND | ND | ND | 0.03 |
| 水果类 Fruits | ND | ND | ND | ND | ND | ND | ND | ND | 0.23 | ND | ND | ND | ND | ND | ND | ND | ND | ND | ND | ND | ND | ND | ND | ND | 0.02 |
| 糖类 Sugar | ND | ND | ND | ND | ND | ND | ND | ND | ND | ND | ND | ND | ND | ND | ND | ND | ND | ND | ND | ND | ND | ND | ND | ND | 0.01 |
| 水及饮料类 Water and beverages | ND | ND | ND | ND | ND | ND | ND | ND | ND | ND | ND | ND | ND | ND | ND | ND | ND | ND | ND | ND | ND | ND | ND | ND | 0.01 |
| 酒类 Alcohol beverages | ND | ND | ND | ND | ND | ND | ND | ND | ND | ND | ND | ND | ND | ND | ND | ND | ND | ND | ND | ND | ND | ND | ND | ND | 0.01 |

注: 平均值计算中, ND 以 1/2 检出限 (LOD) 计
Note: in calculation of averages (AVG), values not detected (ND) were treated as being equal to half of the detection of limit (LOD)

附表 8-48  第六次中国总膳食研究的 BEA 膳食摄入量 [单位: ng/(kg bw · d)]
Annexed Table 8-48  Dietary intakes of BEA from the 6$^{th}$ China TDS [Unit: ng/(kg bw · d)]

| 膳食类别 Category | 黑龙江 HL | 辽宁 LN | 河北 HE | 北京 BJ | 吉林 JL | 山西 SX | 陕西 SN | 河南 HA | 宁夏 NX | 内蒙古 NM | 青海 QH | 甘肃 GS | 上海 SH | 福建 FJ | 江西 JX | 江苏 JS | 浙江 ZJ | 山东 SD | 湖北 HB | 四川 SC | 广西 GX | 湖南 HN | 广东 GD | 贵州 GZ | 全国平均 AVG |
|---|---|---|---|---|---|---|---|---|---|---|---|---|---|---|---|---|---|---|---|---|---|---|---|---|---|
| 谷类 Cereals | 0.168 | 12.070 | 5.990 | 31.460 | 0.122 | 0.266 | 17.71 | 5.171 | 106.800 | 5.860 | 2.828 | 0.185 | 0.093 | 6.062 | 0.137 | 30.060 | 0.134 | 0.211 | 6.263 | 0.243 | 0.220 | 0.135 | 2.195 | 0.173 | 9.774 |
| 豆类 Legumes | 0.010 | 1.347 | 0.188 | 9.577 | 0.016 | 0.012 | 0.394 | 0.012 | 0.106 | 0.007 | 0.012 | 0.007 | 1.416 | 0.239 | 0.147 | 0.713 | 0.024 | 0.009 | 3.540 | 0.012 | 0.007 | 0.015 | 0.500 | 5.899 | 1.009 |
| 薯类 Potatoes | 0.015 | 0.015 | 0.281 | 2.405 | 0.363 | 0.024 | 0.682 | 0.014 | 0.018 | 0.020 | 0.017 | 0.024 | 0.006 | 0.369 | 0.005 | 0.006 | 0.006 | 0.008 | 3.658 | 0.010 | 0.003 | 0.011 | 0.163 | 0.890 | 0.376 |

续表

| 膳食类别 Category | 黑龙江 HL | 辽宁 LN | 河北 HE | 北京 BJ | 吉林 JL | 山西 SX | 陕西 SN | 河南 HA | 宁夏 NX | 内蒙古 NM | 青海 QH | 甘肃 GS | 上海 SH | 福建 FJ | 江西 JX | 江苏 JS | 浙江 ZJ | 山东 SD | 湖北 HB | 四川 SC | 广西 GX | 湖南 HN | 广东 GD | 贵州 GZ | 全国平均 AVG |
|---|---|---|---|---|---|---|---|---|---|---|---|---|---|---|---|---|---|---|---|---|---|---|---|---|---|
| 肉类 Meats | 0.011 | 0.013 | 0.139 | 0.013 | 0.169 | 0.023 | 0.313 | 0.009 | 0.584 | 0.012 | 0.011 | 0.006 | 0.018 | 1.843 | 0.015 | 0.015 | 0.020 | 0.017 | 0.009 | 0.021 | 0.347 | 0.024 | 0.021 | 1.864 | 0.230 |
| 蛋类 Eggs | 0.007 | 3.276 | 0.171 | 0.928 | 0.007 | 0.005 | 0.231 | 0.005 | 0.273 | 0.006 | 0.032 | 0.004 | 0.007 | 0.823 | 0.004 | 3.080 | 0.005 | 0.009 | 3.128 | 0.038 | 0.002 | 0.004 | 0.004 | 0.632 | 0.528 |
| 水产类 Aquatic foods | 0.004 | 0.004 | 0.002 | 0.088 | 0.058 | 0.001 | 0.011 | 0.001 | 0.012 | 0.002 | 0.001 | <0.001 | 0.011 | 0.532 | 0.069 | 0.006 | 0.008 | 0.004 | 0.662 | 0.035 | 0.015 | 0.011 | 0.008 | 0.032 | 0.066 |
| 乳类 Dairy products | 0.002 | 0.007 | 0.004 | 0.220 | 0.005 | 0.007 | 0.126 | 0.003 | 0.160 | 0.005 | 0.008 | 0.002 | 0.011 | 0.396 | 0.003 | 0.004 | 0.005 | 0.004 | 0.001 | 0.002 | 0.003 | 0.003 | 0.336 | 2.822 | 0.173 |
| 蔬菜类 Vegetables | 0.063 | 0.056 | 0.047 | 12.130 | 0.062 | 0.557 | 0.047 | 0.045 | 0.025 | 0.042 | 0.049 | 0.039 | 0.064 | 0.064 | 0.072 | 0.070 | 0.086 | 0.079 | 12.140 | 0.048 | 0.057 | 0.087 | 0.039 | 0.067 | 1.085 |
| 水果类 Fruits | 0.010 | 0.013 | 0.006 | 0.019 | 0.014 | 0.006 | 0.116 | 0.004 | 0.331 | 0.018 | 0.003 | 0.005 | 0.012 | 0.943 | 0.009 | 0.004 | 0.011 | 0.009 | 0.065 | 0.003 | 0.010 | 0.010 | 0.005 | 0.004 | 0.068 |
| 糖类 Sugar | <0.001 | <0.001 | <0.001 | <0.001 | <0.001 | <0.001 | <0.001 | <0.001 | 0.001 | <0.001 | <0.001 | <0.001 | 0.099 | <0.001 | <0.001 | <0.001 | <0.001 | <0.001 | <0.001 | <0.001 | <0.001 | <0.001 | <0.001 | <0.001 | 0.004 |
| 水及饮料类 Water and beverages | 0.194 | 0.078 | 0.123 | 0.176 | 0.207 | 0.118 | 0.055 | 0.189 | 0.082 | 0.409 | 0.098 | 0.187 | 0.112 | 0.137 | 0.188 | 0.160 | 0.125 | 0.286 | 0.045 | 0.050 | 0.207 | 0.169 | 0.189 | 0.199 | 0.158 |
| 酒类 Alcohol beverages | 0.003 | 0.065 | 0.002 | 0.004 | 0.002 | <0.001 | <0.001 | <0.001 | <0.001 | 0.003 | 0.001 | 0.001 | 0.004 | 0.002 | 0.003 | 0.006 | 0.010 | 0.018 | 0.002 | 0.001 | 0.005 | 0.003 | <0.001 | 0.151 | 0.012 |
| 合计 SUM | 0.488 | 16.944 | 6.952 | 57.021 | 1.026 | 1.018 | 19.688 | 5.453 | 108.407 | 6.384 | 3.061 | 0.460 | 1.850 | 11.410 | 0.652 | 34.129 | 0.434 | 0.651 | 29.515 | 0.464 | 0.876 | 0.471 | 3.461 | 12.733 | 13.481 |

附表 8-49 第六次中国总膳食研究的 ENNA 膳食摄入量 [单位：ng/(kg bw·d)]

Annexed Table 8-49 Dietary intakes of ENNA from the 6th China TDS [Unit: ng/(kg bw·d)]

| 膳食类别<br>Category | 黑龙江<br>HL | 辽宁<br>LN | 河北<br>HE | 北京<br>BJ | 吉林<br>JL | 山西<br>SX | 陕西<br>SN | 河南<br>HA | 宁夏<br>NX | 内蒙古<br>NM | 青海<br>QH | 甘肃<br>GS | 上海<br>SH | 福建<br>FJ | 江西<br>JX | 江苏<br>JS | 浙江<br>ZJ | 山东<br>SD | 湖北<br>HB | 四川<br>SC | 广西<br>GX | 湖南<br>HN | 广东<br>GD | 贵州<br>GZ | 全国平均<br>AVG |
|---|---|---|---|---|---|---|---|---|---|---|---|---|---|---|---|---|---|---|---|---|---|---|---|---|---|
| 谷类 Cereals | 0.168 | 12.850 | 0.199 | 0.178 | 0.122 | 0.266 | 23.254 | 2.260 | 60.040 | 3.089 | 0.276 | 0.185 | 0.093 | 4.339 | 0.137 | 0.154 | 0.134 | 0.211 | 1.339 | 0.243 | 0.220 | 0.135 | 1.558 | 0.173 | 4.651 |
| 豆类 Legumes | 0.010 | 0.027 | 0.011 | 2.215 | 0.016 | 0.012 | 0.015 | 0.012 | 0.007 | 0.007 | 0.001 | 0.007 | 0.021 | 0.013 | 0.013 | 0.015 | 0.024 | 0.009 | 1.208 | 0.012 | 0.007 | 0.015 | 0.005 | 0.506 | 0.175 |
| 薯类 Potatoes | 0.015 | 0.277 | 0.011 | 1.224 | 0.019 | 0.024 | 0.023 | 0.014 | 0.875 | 0.020 | 0.017 | 0.460 | 0.006 | 0.007 | 0.005 | 0.133 | 0.107 | 0.008 | 1.429 | 0.010 | 0.003 | 0.011 | 0.004 | 0.114 | 0.201 |
| 肉类 Meats | 0.011 | 0.013 | 0.008 | 0.013 | 0.011 | 0.023 | 0.197 | 0.009 | 0.995 | 0.012 | 0.011 | 0.140 | 0.018 | 0.392 | 0.015 | 0.015 | 0.020 | 0.017 | 0.009 | 0.021 | 0.024 | 0.024 | 0.021 | 0.424 | 0.102 |
| 蛋类 Eggs | 0.007 | 0.009 | 0.006 | 1.124 | 0.007 | 0.005 | 0.004 | 0.005 | 0.149 | 0.006 | 0.003 | 0.004 | 0.007 | 0.117 | 0.004 | 0.005 | 0.092 | 0.009 | 0.603 | 0.003 | 0.002 | 0.004 | 0.004 | 0.099 | 0.095 |
| 水产类 Aquatic foods | 0.004 | 0.004 | 0.002 | 0.003 | 0.033 | 0.001 | 0.001 | 0.001 | 0.016 | 0.002 | 0.001 | 0.005 | 0.011 | 0.011 | 0.007 | 0.006 | 0.008 | 0.004 | 0.006 | 0.001 | 0.015 | 0.011 | 0.008 | 0.020 | 0.008 |
| 乳类 Dairy products | 0.002 | 0.007 | 0.004 | 0.014 | 0.005 | 0.007 | 0.003 | 0.003 | 0.002 | 0.005 | 0.008 | 0.002 | 0.011 | 0.006 | 0.003 | 0.004 | 0.005 | 0.004 | 0.001 | 0.002 | 0.003 | 0.003 | 0.089 | 0.617 | 0.034 |
| 蔬菜类 Vegetables | 0.063 | 0.056 | 0.047 | 0.063 | 0.062 | 0.050 | 0.047 | 0.045 | 0.025 | 0.042 | 0.049 | 0.039 | 0.064 | 0.064 | 0.072 | 0.070 | 0.086 | 0.079 | 0.066 | 0.048 | 0.057 | 0.087 | 0.039 | 0.067 | 0.058 |
| 水果类 Fruits | 0.010 | 0.013 | 0.006 | 0.019 | 0.014 | 0.006 | 0.006 | 0.004 | 0.686 | 0.018 | 0.003 | 0.005 | 0.012 | 0.359 | 0.009 | 0.004 | 0.011 | 0.009 | 0.003 | 0.003 | 0.010 | 0.010 | 0.005 | 0.004 | 0.051 |
| 糖类 Sugar | <0.001 | <0.001 | <0.001 | <0.001 | <0.001 | <0.001 | <0.001 | <0.001 | <0.001 | <0.001 | <0.001 | <0.001 | 0.001 | <0.001 | <0.001 | <0.001 | <0.001 | <0.001 | <0.001 | <0.001 | <0.001 | <0.001 | <0.001 | <0.001 | <0.001 |
| 水及饮料类 Water and beverages | 0.194 | 0.078 | 0.123 | 0.176 | 0.207 | 0.118 | 0.055 | 0.189 | 0.082 | 0.409 | 0.098 | 0.187 | 0.112 | 0.137 | 0.188 | 0.160 | 0.125 | 0.286 | 0.045 | 0.050 | 0.207 | 0.169 | 0.189 | 0.199 | 0.158 |

续表

| 膳食类别 Category | 黑龙江 HL | 辽宁 LN | 河北 HE | 北京 BJ | 吉林 JL | 山西 SX | 陕西 SN | 河南 HA | 宁夏 NX | 内蒙古 NM | 青海 QH | 甘肃 GS | 上海 SH | 福建 FJ | 江西 JX | 江苏 JS | 浙江 ZJ | 山东 SD | 湖北 HB | 四川 SC | 广西 GX | 湖南 HN | 广东 GD | 贵州 GZ | 全国平均 AVG |
|---|---|---|---|---|---|---|---|---|---|---|---|---|---|---|---|---|---|---|---|---|---|---|---|---|---|
| 酒类 Alcohol beverages | 0.003 | 0.005 | 0.002 | 0.004 | 0.002 | <0.001 | <0.001 | 0.001 | <0.001 | 0.003 | 0.001 | 0.001 | 0.004 | 0.002 | 0.003 | 0.006 | 0.010 | 0.018 | 0.002 | 0.001 | 0.005 | 0.003 | <0.001 | 0.006 | 0.003 |
| 合计 SUM | 0.488 | 13.341 | 0.419 | 5.033 | 0.498 | 0.511 | 23.61 | 2.542 | 62.876 | 3.613 | 0.469 | 1.036 | 0.358 | 5.448 | 0.456 | 0.574 | 0.622 | 0.651 | 4.713 | 0.394 | 0.553 | 0.471 | 1.922 | 2.228 | 5.534 |

附表 8-50 第六次中国总膳食研究的 ENNA1 膳食摄入量 [单位: ng/(kg bw·d)]

Annexed Table 8-50 Dietary intakes of ENNA1 from the 6th China TDS [Unit: ng/(kg bw·d)]

| 膳食类别 Category | 黑龙江 HL | 辽宁 LN | 河北 HE | 北京 BJ | 吉林 JL | 山西 SX | 陕西 SN | 河南 HA | 宁夏 NX | 内蒙古 NM | 青海 QH | 甘肃 GS | 上海 SH | 福建 FJ | 江西 JX | 江苏 JS | 浙江 ZJ | 山东 SD | 湖北 HB | 四川 SC | 广西 GX | 湖南 HN | 广东 GD | 贵州 GZ | 全国平均 AVG |
|---|---|---|---|---|---|---|---|---|---|---|---|---|---|---|---|---|---|---|---|---|---|---|---|---|---|
| 谷类 Cereals | 0.168 | 1.606 | 2.047 | 0.178 | 0.122 | 8.317 | 18.160 | 6.092 | 66.440 | 0.169 | 4.224 | 2.645 | 0.093 | 1.771 | 0.137 | 0.154 | 1.786 | 2.382 | 2.500 | 7.627 | 0.220 | 0.135 | 0.098 | 0.173 | 5.301 |
| 豆类 Legumes | 0.010 | 0.027 | 0.011 | 0.515 | 0.016 | 0.151 | 0.015 | 0.012 | 0.007 | 0.007 | 0.001 | 0.176 | 0.021 | 0.013 | 0.013 | 0.015 | 0.024 | 0.009 | 0.253 | 0.084 | 0.007 | 0.015 | 0.005 | 0.562 | 0.082 |
| 薯类 Potatoes | 0.015 | 0.015 | 0.011 | 0.011 | 0.019 | 0.024 | 0.023 | 0.014 | 0.018 | 0.020 | 0.017 | 0.273 | 0.006 | 0.007 | 0.005 | 0.006 | 0.006 | 0.008 | 0.216 | 0.069 | 0.003 | 0.011 | 0.004 | 0.119 | 0.038 |
| 肉类 Meats | 0.011 | 0.013 | 0.008 | 0.013 | 0.011 | 0.023 | 0.006 | 0.009 | 0.348 | 0.012 | 0.011 | 0.103 | 0.018 | 0.014 | 0.015 | 0.015 | 0.020 | 0.017 | 0.009 | 0.021 | 0.024 | 0.024 | 0.021 | 0.393 | 0.048 |
| 蛋类 Eggs | 0.007 | 0.009 | 0.006 | 0.373 | 0.007 | 0.005 | 0.004 | 0.005 | 0.003 | 0.006 | 0.003 | 0.004 | 0.007 | 0.004 | 0.004 | 0.005 | 0.005 | 0.009 | 0.141 | 0.003 | 0.002 | 0.004 | 0.004 | 0.062 | 0.028 |
| 水产类 Aquatic foods | 0.004 | 0.004 | 0.002 | 0.003 | 0.031 | 0.001 | 0.001 | 0.001 | <0.001 | 0.002 | 0.001 | <0.001 | 0.011 | 0.011 | 0.007 | 0.006 | 0.008 | 0.004 | 0.006 | 0.001 | 0.015 | 0.011 | 0.008 | 0.014 | 0.006 |

续表

| 膳食类别<br>Category | 黑龙江<br>HL | 辽宁<br>LN | 河北<br>HE | 北京<br>BJ | 吉林<br>JL | 山西<br>SX | 陕西<br>SN | 河南<br>HA | 宁夏<br>NX | 内蒙古<br>NM | 青海<br>QH | 甘肃<br>GS | 上海<br>SH | 福建<br>FJ | 江西<br>JX | 江苏<br>JS | 浙江<br>ZJ | 山东<br>SD | 湖北<br>HB | 四川<br>SC | 广西<br>GX | 湖南<br>HN | 广东<br>GD | 贵州<br>GZ | 全国平均<br>AVG |
|---|---|---|---|---|---|---|---|---|---|---|---|---|---|---|---|---|---|---|---|---|---|---|---|---|---|
| 乳类<br>Dairy products | 0.002 | 0.007 | 0.004 | 0.014 | 0.005 | 0.007 | 0.003 | 0.003 | 0.002 | 0.005 | 0.008 | 0.002 | 0.011 | 0.006 | 0.003 | 0.004 | 0.005 | 0.004 | 0.001 | 0.002 | 0.003 | 0.003 | 0.006 | 0.112 | 0.009 |
| 蔬菜类<br>Vegetables | 0.063 | 0.056 | 0.047 | 0.063 | 0.062 | 0.050 | 0.047 | 0.045 | 0.025 | 0.042 | 0.049 | 0.039 | 0.064 | 0.064 | 0.072 | 0.070 | 0.086 | 0.079 | 0.066 | 0.048 | 0.057 | 0.087 | 0.039 | 0.067 | 0.058 |
| 水果类<br>Fruits | 0.010 | 0.013 | 0.006 | 0.019 | 0.014 | 0.006 | 0.006 | 0.004 | 0.016 | 0.018 | 0.003 | 0.005 | 0.012 | 0.010 | 0.009 | 0.004 | 0.011 | 0.009 | 0.003 | 0.003 | 0.010 | 0.010 | 0.005 | 0.004 | 0.009 |
| 糖类<br>Sugar | <0.001 | <0.001 | <0.001 | <0.001 | <0.001 | <0.001 | <0.001 | <0.001 | <0.001 | <0.001 | <0.001 | <0.001 | <0.001 | <0.001 | <0.001 | <0.001 | <0.001 | <0.001 | <0.001 | <0.001 | <0.001 | <0.001 | <0.001 | <0.001 | 0.000 |
| 水及饮料类<br>Water and beverages | 0.194 | 0.078 | 0.123 | 0.176 | 0.207 | 0.118 | 0.055 | 0.189 | 0.082 | 0.409 | 0.098 | 0.187 | 0.112 | 0.137 | 0.188 | 0.160 | 0.125 | 0.286 | 0.045 | 0.050 | 0.207 | 0.169 | 0.189 | 0.199 | 0.158 |
| 酒类<br>Alcohol beverages | 0.003 | 0.005 | 0.002 | 0.004 | 0.002 | <0.001 | <0.001 | <0.001 | <0.001 | 0.003 | 0.001 | 0.001 | 0.004 | 0.002 | 0.003 | 0.006 | 0.010 | 0.018 | 0.002 | 0.001 | 0.005 | 0.003 | <0.001 | <0.001 | 0.003 |
| 合计<br>SUM | 0.488 | 1.833 | 2.267 | 1.369 | 0.496 | 8.701 | 18.320 | 6.374 | 66.936 | 0.693 | 4.416 | 3.437 | 0.358 | 2.043 | 0.456 | 0.447 | 2.086 | 2.822 | 3.243 | 7.908 | 0.553 | 0.471 | 0.379 | 1.705 | 5.741 |

附表 8-51 第六次中国总膳食研究的 ENNB 膳食摄入量 [ 单位：ng/(kg bw・d)]
Annexed Table 8-51 Dietary intakes of ENNB from the 6th China TDS [Unit: ng/(kg bw・d)]

| 膳食类别<br>Category | 黑龙江<br>HL | 辽宁<br>LN | 河北<br>HE | 北京<br>BJ | 吉林<br>JL | 山西<br>SX | 陕西<br>SN | 河南<br>HA | 宁夏<br>NX | 内蒙古<br>NM | 青海<br>QH | 甘肃<br>GS | 上海<br>SH | 福建<br>FJ | 江西<br>JX | 江苏<br>JS | 浙江<br>ZJ | 山东<br>SD | 湖北<br>HB | 四川<br>SC | 广西<br>GX | 湖南<br>HN | 广东<br>GD | 贵州<br>GZ | 全国平均<br>AVG |
|---|---|---|---|---|---|---|---|---|---|---|---|---|---|---|---|---|---|---|---|---|---|---|---|---|---|
| 谷类<br>Cereals | 0.034 | 16.35 | 13.56 | 3.786 | 4.264 | 294.1 | 115.4 | 39.44 | 445.7 | 86.49 | 21.51 | 19.96 | 13.14 | 18.67 | 0.299 | 6.188 | 4.914 | 20.50 | 6.494 | 23.31 | 0.521 | 0.443 | 3.815 | 0.035 | 48.28 |

续表

| 膳食类别 Category | 黑龙江 HL | 辽宁 LN | 河北 HE | 北京 BJ | 吉林 JL | 山西 SX | 陕西 SN | 河南 HA | 宁夏 NX | 内蒙古 NM | 青海 QH | 甘肃 GS | 上海 SH | 福建 FJ | 江西 JX | 江苏 JS | 浙江 ZJ | 山东 SD | 湖北 HB | 四川 SC | 广西 GX | 湖南 HN | 广东 GD | 贵州 GZ | 全国平均 AVG |
|---|---|---|---|---|---|---|---|---|---|---|---|---|---|---|---|---|---|---|---|---|---|---|---|---|---|
| 豆类 Legumes | 0.002 | 0.428 | 0.144 | 0.600 | 1.166 | 1.217 | 0.178 | 0.053 | 0.353 | 0.097 | 0.014 | 0.910 | 0.324 | 0.111 | 0.003 | 0.548 | 0.005 | 0.017 | 0.440 | 0.201 | 0.071 | 0.142 | 0.023 | 4.041 | 0.462 |
| 薯类 Potatoes | 0.003 | 0.531 | 0.323 | 0.475 | 0.584 | 0.097 | 0.298 | 0.048 | 1.642 | 0.004 | 0.859 | 1.045 | 0.030 | 0.001 | 0.001 | 0.555 | 0.001 | 0.024 | 0.299 | 0.096 | 0.009 | 0.034 | 0.001 | 1.578 | 0.356 |
| 肉类 Meats | 0.002 | 0.165 | 0.201 | 0.003 | 0.302 | 0.147 | 0.172 | 0.128 | 2.599 | 0.216 | 0.799 | 0.351 | 0.043 | 0.003 | 0.019 | 0.003 | 0.004 | 0.085 | 0.214 | 0.163 | 0.304 | 0.581 | 0.113 | 6.016 | 0.526 |
| 蛋类 Eggs | 0.001 | 0.002 | 0.130 | 0.335 | 0.051 | 0.022 | 0.028 | 0.037 | 0.240 | 0.011 | 0.237 | 0.034 | 0.001 | 0.001 | 0.001 | 0.072 | 0.284 | 0.038 | 0.141 | 0.001 | 0.017 | 0.118 | 0.001 | 0.966 | 0.115 |
| 水产类 Aquatic foods | 0.001 | 0.001 | 0.012 | 0.085 | 0.235 | 0.002 | 0.009 | 0.017 | 0.035 | 0.022 | 0.035 | 0.009 | 0.032 | 0.002 | 0.046 | 0.414 | 0.002 | 0.016 | 0.185 | 0.003 | 0.138 | 0.317 | 0.088 | 0.325 | 0.085 |
| 乳类 Dairy products | <0.001 | 0.183 | 0.009 | 0.003 | 0.001 | 0.001 | 0.126 | 0.001 | 0.078 | 0.034 | 0.018 | 0.016 | 0.026 | 0.179 | 0.059 | 0.001 | 0.001 | 0.007 | <0.001 | 0.139 | 0.181 | 0.013 | 0.025 | 0.038 | 0.047 |
| 蔬菜类 Vegetables | 0.013 | 0.011 | 0.806 | 1.087 | 1.699 | 0.473 | 0.009 | 0.009 | 0.005 | 0.316 | 2.139 | 1.458 | 0.249 | 0.013 | 0.482 | 3.311 | 0.017 | 0.466 | 1.886 | 0.494 | 0.255 | 2.345 | 0.410 | 0.013 | 0.749 |
| 水果类 Fruits | 0.002 | 0.003 | 0.001 | 0.004 | 0.003 | 0.001 | 0.169 | 0.001 | 1.616 | 0.004 | 0.001 | 0.001 | 0.002 | 0.107 | 0.002 | 0.001 | 0.002 | 0.002 | 0.001 | 0.001 | 0.002 | 0.002 | 0.023 | 0.315 | 0.094 |
| 糖类 Sugar | <0.001 | <0.001 | <0.001 | <0.001 | <0.001 | <0.001 | <0.001 | <0.001 | <0.001 | <0.001 | <0.001 | <0.001 | 0.010 | <0.001 | <0.001 | <0.001 | <0.001 | <0.001 | <0.001 | <0.001 | <0.001 | <0.001 | <0.001 | <0.001 | <0.001 |
| 水及饮料类 Water and beverages | 0.039 | 0.016 | 0.025 | 0.035 | 0.041 | 0.024 | 0.011 | 0.038 | 0.016 | 0.082 | 0.020 | 0.037 | 0.022 | 0.027 | 0.038 | 0.032 | 0.025 | 0.057 | 0.009 | 0.010 | 0.041 | 0.034 | 0.038 | 0.040 | 0.032 |
| 酒类 Alcohol beverages | 0.001 | 0.001 | <0.001 | <0.001 | 0.020 | <0.001 | <0.001 | <0.001 | <0.001 | 0.002 | <0.001 | <0.001 | 0.008 | 0.006 | 0.001 | 0.001 | 0.002 | 0.004 | <0.001 | <0.001 | <0.001 | 0.001 | <0.001 | <0.001 | 0.002 |
| 合计 SUM | 0.10 | 17.69 | 15.21 | 6.41 | 8.37 | 296.04 | 116.42 | 39.77 | 452.25 | 87.28 | 25.63 | 23.82 | 13.88 | 19.12 | 0.95 | 11.13 | 5.26 | 21.21 | 9.67 | 24.42 | 1.54 | 4.03 | 4.54 | 13.37 | 50.75 |

附表 Table 8-52 第六次中国总膳食研究的 ENNB1 膳食摄入量 [单位: ng/(kg bw·d)]
Annexed Table 8-52　Dietary intakes of ENNB1 from the 6th China TDS [Unit: ng/(kg bw·d)]

| 膳食类别<br>Category | 黑龙江<br>HL | 辽宁<br>LN | 河北<br>HE | 北京<br>BJ | 吉林<br>JL | 山西<br>SX | 陕西<br>SN | 河南<br>HA | 宁夏<br>NX | 内蒙古<br>NM | 青海<br>QH | 甘肃<br>GS | 上海<br>SH | 福建<br>FJ | 江西<br>JX | 江苏<br>JS | 浙江<br>ZJ | 山东<br>SD | 湖北<br>HB | 四川<br>SC | 广西<br>GX | 湖南<br>HN | 广东<br>GD | 贵州<br>GZ | 全国平均<br>AVG |
|---|---|---|---|---|---|---|---|---|---|---|---|---|---|---|---|---|---|---|---|---|---|---|---|---|---|
| 谷类 Cereals | 0.168 | 5.193 | 4.149 | 0.178 | 0.122 | 48.590 | 49.420 | 17.090 | 143.900 | 33.660 | 8.485 | 7.483 | 2.624 | 3.041 | 0.137 | 1.594 | 2.815 | 6.942 | 4.022 | 12.480 | 0.220 | 0.135 | 0.978 | 1.750 | 14.800 |
| 豆类 Legumes | 0.010 | 0.027 | 0.011 | 0.623 | 0.224 | 0.466 | 0.015 | 0.012 | 0.529 | 0.007 | 0.001 | 0.487 | 0.021 | 0.013 | 0.013 | 0.015 | 0.024 | 0.009 | 0.428 | 0.012 | 0.007 | 0.015 | 0.005 | 1.400 | 0.182 |
| 薯类 Potatoes | 0.015 | 0.169 | 0.137 | 0.362 | 0.239 | 0.024 | 0.023 | 0.014 | 0.571 | 0.020 | 0.017 | 0.261 | 0.006 | 0.007 | 0.005 | 0.121 | 0.006 | 0.008 | 0.302 | 0.010 | 0.003 | 0.011 | 0.004 | 0.353 | 0.112 |
| 肉类 Meats | 0.011 | 0.013 | 0.092 | 0.013 | 0.011 | 0.023 | 0.006 | 0.009 | 0.785 | 0.012 | 0.144 | 0.097 | 0.018 | 0.014 | 0.015 | 0.015 | 0.020 | 0.017 | 0.009 | 0.021 | 0.024 | 0.024 | 0.021 | 1.131 | 0.106 |
| 蛋类 Eggs | 0.007 | 0.009 | 0.058 | 0.362 | 0.007 | 0.005 | 0.004 | 0.005 | 0.075 | 0.006 | 0.045 | 0.004 | 0.007 | 0.004 | 0.004 | 0.086 | 0.105 | 0.009 | 0.110 | 0.003 | 0.002 | 0.004 | 0.004 | 0.226 | 0.048 |
| 水产类 Aquatic foods | 0.004 | 0.004 | 0.002 | 0.003 | 0.061 | 0.001 | 0.001 | 0.001 | 0.009 | 0.002 | 0.001 | <0.001 | 0.011 | 0.011 | 0.007 | 0.006 | 0.008 | 0.004 | 0.144 | 0.001 | 0.015 | 0.011 | 0.008 | 0.059 | 0.016 |
| 乳类 Dairy products | 0.002 | 0.007 | 0.004 | 0.014 | 0.005 | 0.007 | 0.003 | 0.003 | 0.002 | 0.005 | 0.008 | 0.002 | 0.011 | 0.006 | 0.003 | 0.004 | 0.005 | 0.004 | 0.001 | 0.002 | 0.003 | 0.003 | 0.006 | 0.389 | 0.021 |
| 蔬菜类 Vegetables | 0.063 | 0.056 | 0.047 | 0.943 | 0.062 | 0.050 | 0.047 | 0.045 | 0.025 | 0.042 | 0.049 | 0.039 | 0.064 | 0.064 | 0.072 | 0.070 | 0.086 | 0.079 | 1.701 | 0.048 | 0.057 | 0.087 | 0.039 | 0.067 | 0.163 |
| 水果类 Fruits | 0.010 | 0.013 | 0.006 | 0.019 | 0.014 | 0.006 | 0.006 | 0.004 | 0.313 | 0.018 | 0.003 | 0.005 | 0.012 | 0.010 | 0.009 | 0.004 | 0.011 | 0.009 | 0.003 | 0.003 | 0.010 | 0.010 | 0.005 | 0.004 | 0.021 |
| 糖类 Sugar | <0.001 | <0.001 | <0.001 | <0.001 | <0.001 | <0.001 | <0.001 | <0.001 | <0.001 | <0.001 | <0.001 | <0.001 | 0.001 | 0.001 | <0.001 | <0.001 | <0.001 | <0.001 | <0.001 | <0.001 | <0.001 | <0.001 | <0.001 | <0.001 | <0.001 |
| 水及饮料类 Water and beverages | 0.194 | 0.078 | 0.123 | 0.176 | 0.207 | 0.118 | 0.055 | 0.189 | 0.082 | 0.409 | 0.098 | 0.187 | 0.112 | 0.137 | 0.188 | 0.160 | 0.125 | 0.286 | 0.045 | 0.050 | 0.207 | 0.169 | 0.189 | 0.199 | 0.158 |

续表

| 膳食类别<br>Category | 黑龙江<br>HL | 辽宁<br>LN | 河北<br>HE | 北京<br>BJ | 吉林<br>JL | 山西<br>SX | 陕西<br>SN | 河南<br>HA | 宁夏<br>NX | 内蒙古<br>NM | 青海<br>QH | 甘肃<br>GS | 上海<br>SH | 福建<br>FJ | 江西<br>JX | 江苏<br>JS | 浙江<br>ZJ | 山东<br>SD | 湖北<br>HB | 四川<br>SC | 广西<br>GX | 湖南<br>HN | 广东<br>GD | 贵州<br>GZ | 全国平均<br>AVG |
|---|---|---|---|---|---|---|---|---|---|---|---|---|---|---|---|---|---|---|---|---|---|---|---|---|---|
| 酒类<br>Alcohol beverages | 0.003 | 0.005 | 0.002 | 0.004 | 0.002 | <0.001 | <0.001 | 0.001 | <0.001 | 0.003 | 0.001 | 0.001 | 0.004 | 0.002 | 0.003 | 0.006 | 0.010 | 0.018 | 0.002 | 0.001 | 0.005 | 0.003 | <0.001 | <0.001 | 0.003 |
| 合计<br>SUM | 0.488 | 5.574 | 4.631 | 2.697 | 0.954 | 49.286 | 49.577 | 17.376 | 146.295 | 34.187 | 8.852 | 8.567 | 2.889 | 3.309 | 0.456 | 2.082 | 3.215 | 7.382 | 6.769 | 12.627 | 0.553 | 0.471 | 1.259 | 5.579 | 15.628 |

附表 8-53 第六次中国总膳食研究膳食样品中 SMC 的含量（单位：μg/kg）
Annexed Table 8-53　Levels of SMC in food samples from the 6<sup>th</sup> China TDS (Unit: μg/kg)

| 膳食类别<br>Category | 黑龙江<br>HL | 辽宁<br>LN | 河北<br>HE | 北京<br>BJ | 吉林<br>JL | 山西<br>SX | 陕西<br>SN | 河南<br>HA | 宁夏<br>NX | 内蒙古<br>NM | 青海<br>QH | 甘肃<br>GS | 上海<br>SH | 福建<br>FJ | 江西<br>JX | 江苏<br>JS | 浙江<br>ZJ | 山东<br>SD | 湖北<br>HB | 四川<br>SC | 广西<br>GX | 湖南<br>HN | 广东<br>GD | 贵州<br>GZ | 全国平均<br>AVG |
|---|---|---|---|---|---|---|---|---|---|---|---|---|---|---|---|---|---|---|---|---|---|---|---|---|---|
| 谷类<br>Cereals | 0.121 | ND | 0.028 | 0.048 | ND | 0.034 | ND | 0.080 | ND | 0.054 | ND | ND | ND | ND | ND | 0.021 | 0.159 | 0.026 | 0.051 | 0.030 | 0.027 | 0.030 | 0.028 | 0.039 | 0.033 |
| 豆类<br>Legumes | ND | 2.183 | ND | 0.370 | ND | ND | ND | ND | ND | ND | ND | ND | ND | 0.067 | ND | 0.111 | 0.039 | 0.162 | 2.072 | ND | 0.087 | 0.065 | 0.059 | ND | 0.218 |
| 薯类<br>Potatoes | ND | 0.033 | 0.120 | 0.140 | ND | 0.071 | ND | ND | ND | 0.054 | 0.034 | ND | ND | 0.104 | ND | ND | ND | 0.061 | 0.128 | 0.011 | 0.150 | 0.072 | ND | 0.131 | 0.047 |
| 肉类<br>Meats | ND | 0.152 | 0.094 | 0.055 | ND | 0.071 | ND | ND | ND | 0.074 | ND | ND | ND | 0.259 | ND | 0.048 | ND | 0.087 | ND | ND | 0.120 | 0.044 | 0.036 | ND | 0.044 |
| 蛋类<br>Eggs | 0.023 | 0.270 | 0.094 | ND | ND | 0.106 | ND | ND | ND | ND | 0.040 | ND | ND | 0.190 | ND | 0.038 | ND | 0.129 | ND | ND | 0.253 | 0.056 | ND | ND | 0.051 |
| 水产类<br>Aquatic foods | 0.012 | ND | ND | 0.047 | ND | 0.067 | ND | ND | ND | 0.056 | ND | ND | ND | 0.120 | ND | ND | ND | ND | ND | ND | 0.108 | 0.204 | ND | ND | 0.026 |

续表

| 膳食类别 Category | 黑龙江 HL | 辽宁 LN | 河北 HE | 北京 BJ | 吉林 JL | 山西 SX | 陕西 SN | 河南 HA | 宁夏 NX | 内蒙古 NM | 青海 QH | 甘肃 GS | 上海 SH | 福建 FJ | 江西 JX | 江苏 JS | 浙江 ZJ | 山东 SD | 湖北 HB | 四川 SC | 广西 GX | 湖南 HN | 广东 GD | 贵州 GZ | 全国平均 AVG |
|---|---|---|---|---|---|---|---|---|---|---|---|---|---|---|---|---|---|---|---|---|---|---|---|---|---|
| 乳类 Dairy products | ND | ND | ND | ND | ND | ND | ND | ND | ND | ND | ND | ND | ND | ND | ND | ND | ND | ND | ND | ND | ND | ND | ND | ND | 0.001 |
| 蔬菜类 Vegetables | ND | 0.087 | 0.098 | 0.091 | ND | 0.064 | ND | ND | ND | ND | ND | 0.116 | ND | ND | ND | 0.085 | ND | 0.102 | 0.171 | ND | 0.155 | 0.056 | 0.089 | ND | 0.047 |
| 水果类 Fruits | ND | ND | ND | ND | ND | ND | ND | ND | ND | ND | ND | ND | ND | ND | ND | ND | ND | ND | ND | ND | ND | ND | ND | ND | 0.001 |
| 糖类 Sugar | ND | ND | ND | ND | ND | ND | ND | ND | ND | ND | ND | ND | 0.052 | ND | ND | ND | ND | ND | ND | ND | ND | ND | ND | ND | 0.003 |
| 水及饮料类 Water and beverages | ND | ND | ND | ND | ND | ND | ND | ND | ND | ND | ND | ND | ND | ND | ND | ND | ND | ND | ND | ND | ND | ND | ND | ND | 0.001 |
| 酒类 Alcohol beverages | ND | ND | ND | ND | ND | ND | ND | ND | ND | ND | ND | ND | ND | ND | ND | ND | ND | ND | ND | ND | ND | ND | ND | ND | 0.001 |

注：平均值计算中，ND 以 1/2 检出限（LOD）计

Note: in calculation of averages (AVG), values not detected (ND) were treated as being equal to half of the detection of limit (LOD)

附表 8-54 第六次中国总膳食研究的 SMC 膳食摄入量 [单位：ng/(kg bw · d)]

Annexed Table 8-54 Dietary intakes of SMC from the 6th China TDS [Unit: ng/(kg bw · d)]

| 膳食类别 Category | 黑龙江 HL | 辽宁 LN | 河北 HE | 北京 BJ | 吉林 JL | 山西 SX | 陕西 SN | 河南 HA | 宁夏 NX | 内蒙古 NM | 青海 QH | 甘肃 GS | 上海 SH | 福建 FJ | 江西 JX | 江苏 JS | 浙江 ZJ | 山东 SD | 湖北 HB | 四川 SC | 广西 GX | 湖南 HN | 广东 GD | 贵州 GZ | 全国平均 AVG |
|---|---|---|---|---|---|---|---|---|---|---|---|---|---|---|---|---|---|---|---|---|---|---|---|---|---|
| 谷类 Cereals | 1.049 | 0.016 | 0.335 | 0.604 | 0.012 | 0.563 | 0.024 | 1.173 | 0.019 | 0.621 | 0.028 | 0.018 | 0.009 | 0.015 | 0.014 | 0.255 | 1.600 | 0.404 | 0.429 | 0.462 | 0.403 | 0.274 | 0.200 | 0.416 | 0.373 |
| 豆类 Legumes | 0.001 | 4.227 | 0.001 | 0.597 | 0.002 | 0.001 | 0.001 | 0.001 | 0.001 | 0.001 | <0.001 | 0.001 | 0.002 | 0.083 | 0.001 | 0.146 | 0.087 | 0.135 | 2.197 | 0.001 | 0.059 | 0.075 | 0.026 | 0.002 | 0.319 |

续表

| 膳食类别 Category | 黑龙江 HL | 辽宁 LN | 河北 HE | 北京 BJ | 吉林 JL | 山西 SX | 陕西 SN | 河南 HA | 宁夏 NX | 内蒙古 NM | 青海 QH | 甘肃 GS | 上海 SH | 福建 FJ | 江西 JX | 江苏 JS | 浙江 ZJ | 山东 SD | 湖北 HB | 四川 SC | 广西 GX | 湖南 HN | 广东 GD | 贵州 GZ | 全国平均 AVG |
|---|---|---|---|---|---|---|---|---|---|---|---|---|---|---|---|---|---|---|---|---|---|---|---|---|---|
| 薯类 Potatoes | 0.001 | 0.038 | 0.116 | 0.129 | 0.002 | 0.134 | 0.002 | 0.001 | 0.002 | 0.105 | 0.054 | 0.002 | 0.001 | 0.070 | 0.001 | 0.001 | 0.001 | 0.045 | 0.180 | 0.011 | 0.031 | 0.061 | <0.001 | 0.071 | 0.044 |
| 肉类 Meats | 0.001 | 0.161 | 0.071 | 0.059 | 0.001 | 0.154 | 0.001 | 0.001 | 0.001 | 0.087 | 0.001 | 0.001 | 0.002 | 0.353 | 0.002 | 0.071 | 0.002 | 0.134 | 0.001 | 0.002 | 0.287 | 0.104 | 0.060 | 0.002 | 0.065 |
| 蛋类 Eggs | 0.015 | 0.175 | 0.047 | 0.001 | 0.001 | 0.035 | <0.001 | <0.001 | <0.001 | 0.001 | 0.008 | <0.001 | 0.001 | 0.057 | <0.001 | 0.017 | <0.001 | 0.091 | <0.001 | <0.001 | 0.056 | 0.020 | <0.001 | <0.001 | 0.022 |
| 水产类 Aquatic foods | 0.005 | <0.001 | <0.001 | 0.012 | <0.001 | 0.007 | <0.001 | <0.001 | <0.001 | 0.009 | <0.001 | <0.001 | 0.001 | 0.122 | 0.001 | 0.001 | 0.001 | <0.001 | 0.001 | <0.001 | 0.166 | 0.215 | 0.001 | <0.001 | 0.023 |
| 乳类 Dairy products | <0.001 | 0.001 | <0.001 | 0.001 | 0.001 | 0.001 | <0.001 | <0.001 | <0.001 | 0.001 | 0.001 | <0.001 | 0.001 | 0.001 | <0.001 | <0.001 | <0.001 | <0.001 | <0.001 | <0.001 | <0.001 | <0.001 | <0.001 | <0.001 | <0.001 |
| 蔬菜类 Vegetables | 0.006 | 0.452 | 0.457 | 0.566 | 0.006 | 0.313 | 0.005 | 0.004 | 0.002 | 0.004 | 0.005 | 0.457 | 0.006 | 0.006 | 0.007 | 0.571 | 0.009 | 0.658 | 1.126 | 0.005 | 0.868 | 0.471 | 0.333 | 0.007 | 0.264 |
| 水果类 Fruits | 0.001 | 0.001 | 0.001 | 0.002 | 0.001 | 0.001 | 0.001 | <0.001 | 0.002 | 0.002 | <0.001 | 0.001 | 0.001 | <0.001 | 0.001 | <0.001 | 0.001 | 0.001 | <0.001 | <0.001 | 0.001 | 0.001 | <0.001 | <0.001 | 0.001 |
| 糖类 Sugar | <0.001 | <0.001 | <0.001 | <0.001 | <0.001 | <0.001 | <0.001 | <0.001 | <0.001 | <0.001 | <0.001 | <0.001 | 0.006 | <0.001 | <0.001 | <0.001 | <0.001 | 0.002 | <0.001 | <0.001 | <0.001 | <0.001 | <0.001 | <0.001 | <0.001 |
| 水及饮料类 Water and beverages | 0.019 | 0.008 | 0.012 | 0.018 | 0.021 | 0.012 | 0.005 | 0.019 | 0.008 | 0.041 | 0.010 | 0.019 | 0.011 | 0.014 | 0.019 | 0.016 | 0.012 | 0.029 | 0.005 | 0.005 | 0.021 | 0.017 | 0.019 | 0.020 | 0.016 |
| 酒类 Alcohol beverages | <0.001 | 0.001 | <0.001 | <0.001 | <0.001 | <0.001 | <0.001 | <0.001 | <0.001 | <0.001 | <0.001 | <0.001 | <0.001 | <0.001 | <0.001 | <0.001 | 0.001 | 0.002 | <0.001 | <0.001 | <0.001 | <0.001 | <0.001 | <0.001 | <0.001 |
| 合计 SUM | 1.100 | 5.079 | 1.041 | 1.989 | 0.047 | 1.221 | 0.040 | 1.202 | 0.035 | 0.871 | 0.107 | 0.499 | 0.042 | 0.722 | 0.046 | 1.079 | 1.715 | 1.499 | 3.940 | 0.487 | 1.891 | 1.239 | 0.641 | 0.518 | 1.127 |

# 第九章 附 表
# Annexed Tables of Chapter 9

附表 9-1 第六次中国总膳食研究膳食样品中高氯酸盐的含量（单位：μg/kg）

Annexed Table 9-1 Levels of perchlorate in food samples from the 6$^{th}$ China TDS (Unit: μg/kg)

| 膳食类别 Category | 黑龙江 HL | 辽宁 LN | 河北 HE | 北京 BJ | 吉林 JL | 山西 SX | 陕西 SN | 河南 HA | 宁夏 NX | 内蒙古 NM | 青海 QH | 甘肃 GS | 上海 SH | 福建 FJ | 江西 JX | 江苏 JS | 浙江 ZJ | 山东 SD | 湖北 HB | 四川 SC | 广西 GX | 湖南 HN | 广东 GD | 贵州 GZ | 全国平均 AVG |
|---|---|---|---|---|---|---|---|---|---|---|---|---|---|---|---|---|---|---|---|---|---|---|---|---|---|
| 谷类 Cereals | 5.47 | 0.74 | 11.55 | ND | 41.19 | 2.14 | 7.01 | 14.69 | 3.09 | 9.80 | 6.44 | 7.30 | 4.19 | 2.86 | 21.61 | 7.01 | 1.25 | 7.02 | 10.09 | 7.13 | ND | 2.08 | 4.09 | 5.31 | 7.60 |
| 豆类 Legumes | 1.08 | 3.33 | 10.91 | 4.83 | 37.60 | 5.51 | 11.82 | 5.49 | 2.47 | ND | 0.29 | 6.06 | 7.17 | 2.63 | 23.26 | 3.20 | 4.87 | 2.80 | 8.50 | 20.85 | 8.22 | 9.10 | 5.25 | 9.98 | 8.14 |
| 薯类 Potatoes | 1.36 | 9.70 | 26.68 | 10.55 | 28.18 | 9.12 | 7.99 | 6.87 | 8.50 | 28.30 | 1.72 | 3.74 | 7.89 | 4.25 | 16.50 | 5.75 | 3.79 | 11.35 | 10.27 | 3.74 | 7.82 | 7.07 | 3.77 | 6.60 | 9.65 |
| 肉类 Meats | 1.37 | ND | 22.63 | 0.66 | 24.71 | 6.32 | 8.41 | 5.23 | 4.08 | 2.87 | 4.23 | 6.60 | 3.23 | 1.30 | 15.84 | 8.72 | 2.55 | 3.10 | 1.88 | 6.16 | 5.34 | 2.71 | 2.78 | 2.59 | 5.98 |
| 蛋类 Eggs | 5.95 | 12.53 | 20.86 | 17.64 | 23.84 | 16.98 | 29.22 | 15.67 | 8.30 | 20.58 | 9.42 | 8.84 | 14.97 | 10.75 | 7.75 | 12.95 | 19.37 | 11.62 | 14.17 | 12.01 | 11.19 | 9.45 | 9.42 | 14.65 | 14.09 |
| 水产类 Aquatic foods | 0.60 | 0.87 | 8.35 | 7.67 | 28.51 | 3.86 | 4.96 | 5.26 | 0.69 | 7.72 | 4.09 | 6.98 | 4.18 | 0.92 | 11.79 | 5.28 | 1.90 | 3.66 | 3.99 | 8.06 | 4.96 | 7.22 | 1.32 | 3.15 | 5.66 |
| 乳类 Dairy products | 6.50 | 8.90 | 12.80 | 5.17 | 11.15 | 5.82 | 6.88 | 5.36 | 6.51 | 9.49 | 4.24 | 7.70 | 4.61 | 8.96 | 7.98 | 2.41 | 9.77 | 7.21 | 11.72 | 6.95 | 9.62 | 7.64 | 8.71 | 5.63 | 7.57 |
| 蔬菜类 Vegetables | 31.66 | 26.54 | 83.79 | 13.89 | 30.69 | 17.55 | 40.56 | 23.74 | 9.50 | 42.17 | 8.94 | 8.09 | 14.45 | 14.55 | 43.39 | 36.80 | 24.15 | 26.83 | 92.87 | 8.90 | 40.28 | 56.81 | 13.06 | 128.88 | 34.92 |

续表

| 膳食类别<br>Category | 黑龙江<br>HL | 辽宁<br>LN | 河北<br>HE | 北京<br>BJ | 吉林<br>JL | 山西<br>SX | 陕西<br>SN | 河南<br>HA | 宁夏<br>NX | 内蒙古<br>NM | 青海<br>QH | 甘肃<br>GS | 上海<br>SH | 福建<br>FJ | 江西<br>JX | 江苏<br>JS | 浙江<br>ZJ | 山东<br>SD | 湖北<br>HB | 四川<br>SC | 广西<br>GX | 湖南<br>HN | 广东<br>GD | 贵州<br>GZ | 全国平均<br>AVG |
|---|---|---|---|---|---|---|---|---|---|---|---|---|---|---|---|---|---|---|---|---|---|---|---|---|---|
| 水果类 Fruits | 4.13 | 1.65 | 2.50 | 2.41 | 3.46 | 6.07 | 0.80 | 1.66 | 1.07 | ND | 2.14 | 1.12 | 1.52 | 6.28 | 1.94 | 7.68 | 2.35 | 1.33 | 6.30 | 7.25 | 15.58 | 1.11 | 1.85 | 2.95 | 3.47 |
| 糖类 Sugar | 0.51 | 2.27 | ND | 0.22 | 0.58 | 0.61 | ND | 0.22 | ND | 0.24 | ND | 14.76 | 14.62 | 0.34 | ND | 1.35 | 0.39 | ND | ND | ND | 1.15 | ND | 1.42 | 0.60 | 1.67 |
| 水及饮料类 Water and beverages | 0.24 | 0.65 | 2.36 | 5.49 | 34.93 | 1.71 | 1.64 | 3.41 | 0.45 | 3.31 | 26.34 | 6.81 | 9.80 | 2.68 | 13.59 | 6.69 | 7.79 | 2.74 | 5.78 | 4.36 | 2.14 | 19.34 | 2.70 | 7.03 | 7.17 |
| 酒类 Alcohol beverages | 0.40 | 0.93 | 0.64 | 1.72 | 1.60 | 0.87 | 0.52 | 3.41 | ND | 0.70 | 0.88 | 2.68 | 3.01 | 4.02 | 2.49 | 2.63 | 3.41 | 2.18 | 4.79 | 1.42 | 5.75 | 6.47 | 4.06 | 0.90 | 2.32 |

注：平均值计算中，ND 以 1/2 检出限（LOD）计

Note: in calculation of averages (AVG), values not detected (ND) were treated as being equal to half of the detection of limit (LOD)

附表 9-2 第六次中国总膳食研究的高氯酸盐膳食摄入量 [单位：μg/(kg bw·d)]

Annexed Table 9-2 Dietary intakes of perchlorate from the 6th China TDS [Unit: μg/(kg bw·d)]

| 膳食类别<br>Category | 黑龙江<br>HL | 辽宁<br>LN | 河北<br>HE | 北京<br>BJ | 吉林<br>JL | 山西<br>SX | 陕西<br>SN | 河南<br>HA | 宁夏<br>NX | 内蒙古<br>NM | 青海<br>QH | 甘肃<br>GS | 上海<br>SH | 福建<br>FJ | 江西<br>JX | 江苏<br>JS | 浙江<br>ZJ | 山东<br>SD | 湖北<br>HB | 四川<br>SC | 广西<br>GX | 湖南<br>HN | 广东<br>GD | 贵州<br>GZ | 全国平均<br>AVG |
|---|---|---|---|---|---|---|---|---|---|---|---|---|---|---|---|---|---|---|---|---|---|---|---|---|---|
| 谷类 Cereals | 0.048 | 0.007 | 0.138 | 0.002 | 0.383 | 0.035 | 0.085 | 0.215 | 0.032 | 0.113 | 0.078 | 0.080 | 0.030 | 0.029 | 0.216 | 0.087 | 0.013 | 0.111 | 0.085 | 0.110 | 0.002 | 0.019 | 0.030 | 0.057 | 0.083 |
| 豆类 Legumes | 0.001 | 0.006 | 0.010 | 0.008 | 0.045 | 0.006 | 0.016 | 0.005 | 0.001 | 0.000 | 0.000 | 0.004 | 0.013 | 0.003 | 0.027 | 0.004 | 0.011 | 0.002 | 0.009 | 0.022 | 0.006 | 0.010 | 0.002 | 0.016 | 0.010 |
| 薯类 Potatoes | 0.002 | 0.011 | 0.026 | 0.010 | 0.054 | 0.017 | 0.015 | 0.009 | 0.013 | 0.055 | 0.003 | 0.009 | 0.004 | 0.003 | 0.008 | 0.003 | 0.002 | 0.008 | 0.014 | 0.004 | 0.002 | 0.006 | 0.001 | 0.004 | 0.012 |

续表

| 膳食类别<br>Category | 黑龙江<br>HL | 辽宁<br>LN | 河北<br>HE | 北京<br>BJ | 吉林<br>JL | 山西<br>SX | 陕西<br>SN | 河南<br>HA | 宁夏<br>NX | 内蒙古<br>NM | 青海<br>QH | 甘肃<br>GS | 上海<br>SH | 福建<br>FJ | 江西<br>JX | 江苏<br>JS | 浙江<br>ZJ | 山东<br>SD | 湖北<br>HB | 四川<br>SC | 广西<br>GX | 湖南<br>HN | 广东<br>GD | 贵州<br>GZ | 全国平均<br>AVG |
|---|---|---|---|---|---|---|---|---|---|---|---|---|---|---|---|---|---|---|---|---|---|---|---|---|---|
| 肉类 Meats | 0.001 | 0.000 | 0.017 | 0.001 | 0.026 | 0.014 | 0.005 | 0.005 | 0.003 | 0.003 | 0.005 | 0.003 | 0.006 | 0.002 | 0.024 | 0.013 | 0.005 | 0.005 | 0.002 | 0.013 | 0.013 | 0.006 | 0.005 | 0.004 | 0.007 |
| 蛋类 Eggs | 0.004 | 0.008 | 0.010 | 0.011 | 0.015 | 0.006 | 0.010 | 0.007 | 0.002 | 0.010 | 0.002 | 0.003 | 0.009 | 0.003 | 0.003 | 0.006 | 0.007 | 0.008 | 0.006 | 0.003 | 0.002 | 0.003 | 0.004 | 0.004 | 0.006 |
| 水产类 Aquatic foods | 0.000 | 0.000 | 0.001 | 0.002 | 0.005 | 0.000 | 0.000 | 0.000 | 0.000 | 0.001 | 0.000 | 0.000 | 0.005 | 0.001 | 0.008 | 0.003 | 0.002 | 0.001 | 0.003 | 0.001 | 0.008 | 0.008 | 0.001 | 0.000 | 0.002 |
| 乳类 Dairy products | 0.001 | 0.006 | 0.005 | 0.007 | 0.006 | 0.004 | 0.002 | 0.002 | 0.002 | 0.005 | 0.004 | 0.002 | 0.005 | 0.005 | 0.003 | 0.001 | 0.005 | 0.003 | 0.001 | 0.001 | 0.003 | 0.002 | 0.005 | 0.003 | 0.003 |
| 蔬菜类 Vegetables | 0.161 | 0.138 | 0.390 | 0.086 | 0.189 | 0.086 | 0.185 | 0.105 | 0.024 | 0.172 | 0.044 | 0.032 | 0.092 | 0.092 | 0.311 | 0.248 | 0.170 | 0.173 | 0.610 | 0.043 | 0.226 | 0.481 | 0.049 | 0.834 | 0.206 |
| 水果类 Fruits | 0.004 | 0.002 | 0.001 | 0.004 | 0.005 | 0.003 | 0.000 | 0.001 | 0.001 | 0.000 | 0.001 | 0.001 | 0.002 | 0.006 | 0.002 | 0.003 | 0.003 | 0.001 | 0.002 | 0.002 | 0.016 | 0.001 | 0.001 | 0.001 | 0.003 |
| 糖类 Sugar | 0.000 | 0.000 | 0.000 | 0.000 | 0.000 | 0.000 | 0.000 | 0.000 | 0.000 | 0.000 | 0.000 | 0.000 | 0.002 | 0.000 | 0.000 | 0.000 | 0.000 | 0.000 | 0.000 | 0.000 | 0.000 | 0.000 | 0.000 | 0.000 | 0.000 |
| 水及饮料类 Water and beverages | 0.005 | 0.005 | 0.029 | 0.097 | 0.722 | 0.020 | 0.009 | 0.064 | 0.004 | 0.135 | 0.259 | 0.128 | 0.109 | 0.037 | 0.255 | 0.107 | 0.097 | 0.078 | 0.026 | 0.022 | 0.044 | 0.326 | 0.051 | 0.140 | 0.115 |
| 酒类 Alcohol beverages | 0.000 | 0.000 | 0.000 | 0.000 | 0.000 | 0.000 | 0.000 | 0.000 | 0.000 | 0.000 | 0.000 | 0.000 | 0.001 | 0.001 | 0.001 | 0.002 | 0.003 | 0.004 | 0.001 | 0.000 | 0.003 | 0.002 | 0.000 | 0.000 | 0.001 |
| 合计 SUM | 0.227 | 0.185 | 0.629 | 0.228 | 1.449 | 0.192 | 0.327 | 0.413 | 0.082 | 0.495 | 0.395 | 0.261 | 0.278 | 0.181 | 0.857 | 0.477 | 0.318 | 0.395 | 0.759 | 0.220 | 0.324 | 0.865 | 0.149 | 1.063 | 0.449 |

附表 9-3 第六次中国总膳食研究高氯酸盐的膳食来源（单位：%）

Annexed Table 9-3 Dietary sources of perchlorate from the 6$^{th}$ China TDS (Unit: %)

| 膳食类别<br>Category | 黑龙江<br>HL | 辽宁<br>LN | 河北<br>HE | 北京<br>BJ | 吉林<br>JL | 山西<br>SX | 陕西<br>SN | 河南<br>HA | 宁夏<br>NX | 内蒙古<br>NM | 青海<br>QH | 甘肃<br>GS | 上海<br>SH | 福建<br>FJ | 江西<br>JX | 江苏<br>JS | 浙江<br>ZJ | 山东<br>SD | 湖北<br>HB | 四川<br>SC | 广西<br>GX | 湖南<br>HN | 广东<br>GD | 贵州<br>GZ | 全国平均<br>AVG |
|---|---|---|---|---|---|---|---|---|---|---|---|---|---|---|---|---|---|---|---|---|---|---|---|---|---|
| 谷类 Cereals | 21.0 | 3.9 | 22.0 | 0.8 | 26.4 | 18.4 | 26.0 | 52.2 | 39.4 | 22.7 | 19.8 | 30.5 | 10.7 | 15.8 | 25.2 | 18.1 | 4.0 | 28.1 | 11.2 | 49.9 | 0.7 | 2.2 | 19.9 | 5.3 | 18.6 |
| 豆类 Legumes | 0.3 | 3.5 | 1.6 | 3.4 | 3.1 | 3.2 | 4.8 | 1.1 | 1.7 | 0.0 | 0.0 | 1.5 | 4.8 | 1.8 | 3.2 | 0.9 | 3.4 | 0.6 | 1.2 | 10.2 | 1.7 | 1.2 | 1.6 | 1.5 | 2.1 |
| 薯类 Potatoes | 0.7 | 6.0 | 4.1 | 4.3 | 3.7 | 8.9 | 4.4 | 2.1 | 16.4 | 11.1 | 0.7 | 3.3 | 1.6 | 1.6 | 1.0 | 0.6 | 0.7 | 2.1 | 1.9 | 1.7 | 0.5 | 0.7 | 1.0 | 0.3 | 2.6 |
| 肉类 Meats | 0.6 | 0.1 | 2.7 | 0.3 | 1.8 | 7.2 | 1.5 | 1.1 | 3.7 | 0.7 | 1.2 | 1.2 | 2.0 | 1.0 | 2.8 | 2.7 | 1.5 | 1.2 | 0.2 | 5.7 | 3.9 | 0.7 | 3.1 | 0.4 | 1.7 |
| 蛋类 Eggs | 1.7 | 4.4 | 1.7 | 4.8 | 1.0 | 2.9 | 3.1 | 1.8 | 2.1 | 2.0 | 0.5 | 1.2 | 3.3 | 1.8 | 0.3 | 1.2 | 2.3 | 2.1 | 0.7 | 1.3 | 0.8 | 0.4 | 2.4 | 0.4 | 1.4 |
| 水产类 Aquatic foods | 0.1 | 0.1 | 0.2 | 0.9 | 0.3 | 0.2 | 0.1 | 0.1 | 0.0 | 0.3 | 0.1 | 0.7 | 1.6 | 0.5 | 1.0 | 0.7 | 0.5 | 0.3 | 0.3 | 0.5 | 2.3 | 0.9 | 0.7 | 0.0 | 0.5 |
| 乳类 Dairy products | 0.6 | 3.4 | 0.8 | 3.1 | 0.4 | 2.0 | 0.6 | 0.4 | 1.9 | 1.0 | 0.9 | 0.7 | 1.9 | 2.8 | 0.3 | 0.2 | 1.6 | 0.7 | 0.2 | 0.6 | 0.9 | 0.3 | 3.4 | 0.2 | 0.8 |
| 蔬菜类 Vegetables | 71.0 | 74.5 | 62.1 | 37.9 | 13.0 | 44.9 | 56.6 | 25.4 | 28.6 | 34.8 | 11.2 | 12.2 | 33.0 | 50.6 | 36.3 | 52.1 | 53.5 | 43.8 | 80.5 | 19.4 | 69.7 | 55.6 | 32.9 | 78.5 | 45.9 |
| 水果类 Fruits | 1.8 | 1.1 | 0.2 | 1.9 | 0.3 | 1.8 | 0.1 | 0.2 | 1.7 | 0.0 | 0.1 | 0.2 | 0.6 | 3.3 | 0.2 | 0.7 | 0.8 | 0.3 | 0.3 | 0.8 | 4.9 | 0.1 | 0.6 | 0.1 | 0.6 |
| 糖类 Sugar | 0.0 | 0.0 | 0.0 | 0.0 | 0.0 | 0.0 | 0.0 | 0.0 | 0.0 | 0.0 | 0.0 | 0.0 | 0.6 | 0.0 | 0.0 | 0.0 | 0.0 | 0.0 | 0.0 | 0.0 | 0.0 | 0.0 | 0.0 | 0.0 | 0.0 |
| 水及饮料类 Water and beverages | 2.0 | 2.8 | 4.6 | 42.3 | 49.8 | 10.6 | 2.7 | 15.6 | 4.4 | 27.4 | 65.5 | 49.0 | 39.3 | 20.3 | 29.7 | 22.5 | 30.6 | 19.8 | 3.4 | 9.9 | 13.7 | 37.7 | 34.4 | 13.1 | 25.7 |
| 酒类 Alcohol beverages | 0.1 | 0.3 | 0.0 | 0.3 | 0.0 | 0.0 | 0.0 | 0.0 | 0.0 | 0.0 | 0.0 | 0.1 | 0.4 | 0.5 | 0.1 | 0.3 | 1.1 | 1.0 | 0.1 | 0.1 | 0.9 | 0.2 | 0.1 | 0.0 | 0.2 |

附表 9-4 第六次中国总膳食研究膳食样品中硝酸盐的含量（单位：mg/kg）

Annexed Table 9-4 Levels of nitrate in food samples from the 6th China TDS (Unit: mg/kg)

| 膳食类别 Category | 黑龙江 HL | 辽宁 LN | 河北 HE | 北京 BJ | 吉林 JL | 山西 SX | 陕西 SN | 河南 HA | 宁夏 NX | 内蒙古 NM | 青海 QH | 甘肃 GS | 上海 SH | 福建 FJ | 江西 JX | 江苏 JS | 浙江 ZJ | 山东 SD | 湖北 HB | 四川 SC | 广西 GX | 湖南 HN | 广东 GD | 贵州 GZ | 全国平均 AVG |
|---|---|---|---|---|---|---|---|---|---|---|---|---|---|---|---|---|---|---|---|---|---|---|---|---|---|
| 谷类 Cereals | 8.9 | 3.1 | 7.4 | 2.2 | 10 | 6.1 | 1 | 11 | 0.4 | 8.1 | 0.68 | 0.026 | 2.6 | 18.2 | 14 | 0.02 | 2.4 | 27 | 1.5 | 7.3 | 0.022 | 0.022 | 7.2 | 0.6 | 5.8 |
| 豆类 Legumes | 13 | 25 | 9.1 | 24 | 35 | 0.017 | 8.7 | 11 | 14 | 4.3 | 0.64 | 12 | 6.9 | 16 | 18 | 6.8 | 13 | 0.021 | 4.1 | 5.2 | 1.5 | 7 | 17 | 9 | 11 |
| 薯类 Potatoes | 4.5 | 127 | 100 | 51 | 60 | 61 | 27 | 74 | 57 | 117 | 11 | 26 | 70 | 25 | 178 | 121 | 61 | 162 | 38 | 60 | 33 | 18 | 66 | 199 | 73 |
| 肉类 Meats | 4.6 | 1.2 | 3.6 | 1 | 5 | 12 | 7.2 | 0.029 | 1.6 | 12 | 0.015 | 12 | 2.2 | 3 | 12 | 0.015 | 9.1 | 0.23 | 7.3 | 1.6 | 0.015 | 0.015 | 0.019 | 3.7 | 4.1 |
| 蛋类 Eggs | 1.2 | 4.7 | 1.7 | 0.018 | 0.017 | 0.021 | 1.4 | 0.015 | 0.67 | 6.9 | 24 | 0.018 | 0.016 | 11 | 0.49 | 0.016 | 0.02 | 3.9 | 0.55 | 0.017 | 0.73 | 0.015 | 3.7 | 3.2 | 2.7 |
| 水产类 Aquatic foods | 4.3 | 5.2 | 3.8 | 4 | 20 | 4.4 | 10 | 2.0 | 5.2 | 14 | 3.3 | 7.5 | 5 | 34 | 11 | 0.86 | 3.1 | 2.3 | 2.7 | 5 | 2.6 | 0.79 | 3.2 | 4.3 | 6.6 |
| 乳类 Dairy products | 68 | 56 | 68 | 43 | 1.8 | 1.9 | 24 | 38 | 18 | 77 | 56 | 73 | 56 | 111 | 69 | 10 | 66 | 72 | 108 | 75 | 9.4 | 58 | 50 | 40 | 52 |
| 蔬菜类 Vegetables | 460 | 327 | 817 | 539 | 584 | 447 | 780 | 569 | 659 | 528 | 1092 | 574 | 833 | 575 | 1308 | 1951 | 889 | 931 | 1842 | 1117 | 1788 | 932 | 1642 | 2622 | 992 |
| 水果类 Fruits | 14 | 0.016 | 27 | 33 | 32 | 20 | 19 | 16 | 19 | 12 | 31 | 22 | 23 | 32 | 0.015 | 20 | 23 | 13 | 18 | 20 | 31 | 29 | 36 | 9.6 | 21 |
| 糖类 Sugar | 14 | 11 | 10 | 24 | 9.9 | 6 | 15 | 33 | 14 | 12 | 2.4 | 6.9 | 92 | 7.5 | 14 | 8.9 | 12 | 0.97 | 20 | 17 | 14 | 5.9 | 22 | 34 | 17 |
| 水及饮料类 Water and beverages | 6.9 | 5 | 6 | 24 | 6.8 | 8 | 5.1 | 3.2 | 13 | 12 | 8 | 5 | 0.88 | 6.5 | 17 | 7.4 | 6.8 | 32 | 4.5 | 12 | 4.9 | 6.1 | 7.7 | 12 | 9.2 |

续表

| 膳食类别 Category | 黑龙江 HL | 辽宁 LN | 河北 HE | 北京 BJ | 吉林 JL | 山西 SX | 陕西 SN | 河南 HA | 宁夏 NX | 内蒙古 NM | 青海 QH | 甘肃 GS | 上海 SH | 福建 FJ | 江西 JX | 江苏 JS | 浙江 ZJ | 山东 SD | 湖北 HB | 四川 SC | 广西 GX | 湖南 HN | 广东 GD | 贵州 GZ | 全国平均 AVG |
|---|---|---|---|---|---|---|---|---|---|---|---|---|---|---|---|---|---|---|---|---|---|---|---|---|---|
| 酒类 Alcohol beverages | 9.4 | 3.1 | 2.5 | 1.7 | 2.2 | 1.5 | 7.4 | 4.3 | ND | 2.9 | 1.6 | 24 | 0.061 | 4.6 | 8.8 | 3.3 | 5.3 | 7.5 | 2.1 | 2.7 | 15 | 3.2 | 2.4 | 1 | 4.9 |

注：平均值计算中，ND 以 1/2 检出限（LOD）计

Note: in calculation of averages (AVG), values not detected (ND) were treated as being equal to half of the detection of limit (LOD)

附表 9-5 第六次中国总膳食研究膳食样品中亚硝酸盐的含量（单位：mg/kg）

Annexed Table 9-5　Levels of nitrite in food samples from the 6$^{th}$ China TDS (Unit: mg/kg)

| 膳食类别 Category | 黑龙江 HL | 辽宁 LN | 河北 HE | 北京 BJ | 吉林 JL | 山西 SX | 陕西 SN | 河南 HA | 宁夏 NX | 内蒙古 NM | 青海 QH | 甘肃 GS | 上海 SH | 福建 FJ | 江西 JX | 江苏 JS | 浙江 ZJ | 山东 SD | 湖北 HB | 四川 SC | 广西 GX | 湖南 HN | 广东 GD | 贵州 GZ | 全国平均 AVG |
|---|---|---|---|---|---|---|---|---|---|---|---|---|---|---|---|---|---|---|---|---|---|---|---|---|---|
| 谷类 Cereals | 0.0097 | 0.0079 | 0.0083 | 0.0070 | 0.031 | 0.0081 | 0.0097 | 0.0078 | 0.0089 | 0.0074 | 0.011 | 0.0085 | 0.0065 | 0.0074 | 0.0068 | 0.0063 | 0.024 | 0.0079 | 0.0068 | 0.0079 | 0.0074 | 0.0074 | 0.0068 | 0.0081 | 0.0095 |
| 豆类 Legumes | 0.0072 | 0.0068 | 0.0060 | 0.0054 | 0.0068 | 0.45 | 0.0056 | 0.0071 | 0.0059 | 0.0054 | 0.0057 | 0.0052 | 0.0057 | 0.0051 | 0.0051 | 0.0058 | 0.0053 | 0.0062 | 0.0056 | 0.0057 | 0.0051 | 0.0065 | 0.0057 | 0.0060 | 0.025 |
| 薯类 Potatoes | 0.0060 | 0.0065 | 0.0058 | 0.0058 | 0.0050 | 0.0063 | 0.0062 | 0.0054 | 0.0057 | 0.0051 | 0.0052 | 0.0052 | 0.0050 | 0.0055 | 0.0050 | 0.0060 | 0.0058 | 0.0053 | 0.0051 | 0.0052 | 0.0066 | 0.0068 | 0.0052 | 0.0061 | 0.0056 |
| 肉类 Meats | 0.0059 | 0.0062 | 0.36 | 0.0063 | 0.0051 | 0.20 | 0.0054 | 0.0052 | 0.0052 | 0.0051 | 0.0051 | 0.0056 | 0.0050 | 0.0052 | 0.0050 | 0.0051 | 0.24 | 0.0054 | 0.0052 | 0.0050 | 0.0050 | 0.0051 | 0.0063 | 0.0052 | 0.038 |
| 蛋类 Eggs | 0.0051 | 0.0066 | 1.7 | 0.0059 | 0.0057 | 0.0068 | 0.0058 | 0.0050 | 0.0073 | 0.85 | 0.0069 | 0.0058 | 0.0054 | 0.0065 | 0.0059 | 0.0053 | 0.0062 | 0.0062 | 0.0059 | 0.0057 | 0.0056 | 0.0051 | 0.0051 | 0.0050 | 0.11 |
| 水产类 Aquatic foods | 0.0050 | 2.8 | 0.0055 | 0.0053 | 0.0050 | 0.0059 | 0.0050 | 0.0052 | 0.0050 | 0.0050 | 0.0056 | 0.49 | 0.0050 | 0.0052 | 0.0050 | 0.0051 | 0.0052 | 0.0059 | 0.0050 | 0.0050 | 0.48 | 0.0051 | 0.0052 | 0.0060 | 0.16 |
| 乳类 Dairy products | 0.005 | 0.005 | 0.005 | 0.005 | 0.005 | 0.005 | 0.005 | 0.005 | 0.005 | 0.005 | 0.005 | 0.005 | 0.005 | 0.005 | 0.46 | 0.005 | 0.005 | 0.005 | 0.005 | 0.005 | 0.59 | 0.005 | 0.005 | 0.005 | 0.048 |

续表

| 膳食类别<br>Category | 黑龙江<br>HL | 辽宁<br>LN | 河北<br>HE | 北京<br>BJ | 吉林<br>JL | 山西<br>SX | 陕西<br>SN | 河南<br>HA | 宁夏<br>NX | 内蒙古<br>NM | 青海<br>QH | 甘肃<br>GS | 上海<br>SH | 福建<br>FJ | 江西<br>JX | 江苏<br>JS | 浙江<br>ZJ | 山东<br>SD | 湖北<br>HB | 四川<br>SC | 广西<br>GX | 湖南<br>HN | 广东<br>GD | 贵州<br>GZ | 全国平均<br>AVG |
|---|---|---|---|---|---|---|---|---|---|---|---|---|---|---|---|---|---|---|---|---|---|---|---|---|---|
| 蔬菜类 Vegetables | 0.0062 | 0.0054 | 0.0050 | 0.0051 | 0.0051 | 0.0051 | 0.0052 | 0.0051 | 0.0050 | 0.0052 | 0.0050 | 0.0050 | 0.0050 | 0.0051 | 0.0050 | 0.0052 | 0.0061 | 0.0051 | 0.0050 | 0.0050 | 0.0051 | 0.0052 | 0.0052 | 0.0052 | 0.0052 |
| 水果类 Fruits | 3.1 | 0.0054 | 0.0050 | 0.0053 | 0.0050 | 0.0050 | 0.0053 | 0.0050 | 0.0058 | 0.0051 | 0.48 | 0.19 | 0.0050 | 0.0052 | 0.0050 | 0.0052 | 0.0050 | 0.0050 | 0.0050 | 0.0055 | 0.0050 | 0.0050 | 0.0050 | 0.0057 | 0.16 |
| 糖类 Sugar | 1.9 | 0.005 | 0.005 | 0.55 | 1.6 | 2.2 | 3.6 | 3.9 | 0.49 | 1.1 | 0.81 | 0.005 | 0.005 | 0.005 | 0.005 | 2.8 | 0.005 | 1.0 | 2.6 | 2.0 | 0.005 | 0.005 | 3.1 | 0.005 | 1.1 |
| 水及饮料类 Water and beverages | 0.0005 | 0.0005 | 0.11 | 0.0005 | 0.0013 | 0.0005 | 0.0005 | 0.0005 | 0.0005 | 0.0005 | 0.0005 | 0.0005 | 0.0005 | 0.0005 | 0.0005 | 0.0005 | 0.0005 | 0.0005 | 0.012 | 0.0005 | 0.18 | 0.0005 | 0.013 | 0.0005 | 0.014 |
| 酒类 Alcohol beverages | 0.0005 | 0.0005 | 0.0005 | 0.0005 | 0.0005 | 0.0005 | 0.0005 | 0.0005 | 0.0005 | 0.0005 | 0.0005 | 0.0005 | 0.0005 | 0.0005 | 0.0005 | 0.0005 | 0.0005 | 0.0005 | 0.0005 | 0.0005 | 0.0005 | 0.0005 | 0.0005 | 0.0005 | 0.0005 |

注：低于检出限的数据以 1/2 检出限计

Note: values below the detection limit (LOD) are expressed as half the LOD

附表 9-6　第六次中国总膳食研究的硝酸盐膳食摄入量 [单位：μg/(kg bw·d)]

Annexed Table 9-6　Dietary intakes of nitrate from the 6$^{th}$ China TDS [Unit: μg/(kg bw·d)]

| 膳食类别<br>Category | 黑龙江<br>HL | 辽宁<br>LN | 河北<br>HE | 北京<br>BJ | 吉林<br>JL | 山西<br>SX | 陕西<br>SN | 河南<br>HA | 宁夏<br>NX | 内蒙古<br>NM | 青海<br>QH | 甘肃<br>GS | 上海<br>SH | 福建<br>FJ | 江西<br>JX | 江苏<br>JS | 浙江<br>ZJ | 山东<br>SD | 湖北<br>HB | 四川<br>SC | 广西<br>GX | 湖南<br>HN | 广东<br>GD | 贵州<br>GZ | 全国平均<br>AVG |
|---|---|---|---|---|---|---|---|---|---|---|---|---|---|---|---|---|---|---|---|---|---|---|---|---|---|
| 谷类 Cereals | 78 | 30 | 89 | 27 | 94 | 101 | 12 | 166 | 4.2 | 93 | 8.3 | 0.28 | 18 | 183 | 136 | 0.24 | 24 | 429 | 12 | 113 | 0.33 | 0.20 | 52 | 6.6 | 70 |
| 豆类 Legumes | 9.0 | 48 | 8.2 | 39 | 41 | 0.018 | 11 | 9.1 | 7.7 | 2.7 | 0.066 | 8.1 | 13 | 20 | 21 | 8.9 | 29 | 0.018 | 4.3 | 5.6 | 1.0 | 8.1 | 7.4 | 15 | 13 |
| 薯类 Potatoes | 5.5 | 145 | 97 | 47 | 114 | 116 | 49 | 95 | 91 | 227 | 18 | 58 | 40 | 17 | 91 | 64 | 36 | 119 | 53 | 60 | 6.8 | 15 | 26 | 108 | 71 |

续表

| 膳食类别<br>Category | 黑龙江<br>HL | 辽宁<br>LN | 河北<br>HE | 北京<br>BJ | 吉林<br>JL | 山西<br>SX | 陕西<br>SN | 河南<br>HA | 宁夏<br>NX | 内蒙古<br>NM | 青海<br>QH | 甘肃<br>GS | 上海<br>SH | 福建<br>FJ | 江西<br>JX | 江苏<br>JS | 浙江<br>ZJ | 山东<br>SD | 湖北<br>HB | 四川<br>SC | 广西<br>GX | 湖南<br>HN | 广东<br>GD | 贵州<br>GZ | 全国平均<br>AVG |
|---|---|---|---|---|---|---|---|---|---|---|---|---|---|---|---|---|---|---|---|---|---|---|---|---|---|
| 肉类 Meats | 4.4 | 1.2 | 2.7 | 1.1 | 5.3 | 25 | 4.1 | 0.025 | 1.2 | 13 | 0.017 | 6.1 | 3.8 | 4.1 | 17 | 0.022 | 17 | 0.36 | 6.3 | 3.3 | 0.036 | 0.036 | 0.031 | 6.2 | 5.2 |
| 蛋类 Eggs | 0.75 | 3.1 | 0.83 | 0.011 | 0.011 | 0.0068 | 0.49 | 0.0071 | 0.14 | 3.2 | 5.1 | 0.0064 | 0.010 | 3.4 | 0.16 | 0.0074 | 0.0074 | 2.8 | 0.22 | 0.004 | 0.16 | 0.0055 | 1.4 | 0.83 | 0.94 |
| 水产类 Aquatic foods | 1.8 | 1.3 | 0.58 | 1.1 | 3.5 | 0.44 | 0.68 | 0.15 | 0.20 | 2.2 | 0.19 | 0.34 | 5.4 | 34 | 7.7 | 0.53 | 2.4 | 0.82 | 1.7 | 0.66 | 4.0 | 0.83 | 2.6 | 0.24 | 3.1 |
| 乳类 Dairy products | 14 | 39 | 26 | 58 | 0.93 | 1.3 | 7.3 | 12 | 4.5 | 42 | 47 | 16 | 63 | 63 | 24 | 4.4 | 35 | 26 | 11 | 15 | 2.7 | 17 | 29 | 18 | 24 |
| 蔬菜类 Vegetables | 2 340 | 1 694 | 3 809 | 3 351 | 3 594 | 2 195 | 3 557 | 2 513 | 1 635 | 2 154 | 5 382 | 2 259 | 5 295 | 3 619 | 9 374 | 13 175 | 6 268 | 6 006 | 12 110 | 5 369 | 10 029 | 7 897 | 6 163 | 16 978 | 5 699 |
| 水果类 Fruits | 14 | 0.020 | 16 | 60 | 45 | 11 | 12 | 6.2 | 25 | 21 | 7.7 | 11 | 27 | 30 | 0.013 | 8.8 | 25 | 11 | 5.5 | 4.7 | 32 | 29 | 17 | 3.2 | 18 |
| 糖类 Sugar | 0.49 | 0.13 | 0.079 | 0.76 | 0.15 | 0.10 | 0.19 | 0.20 | 0.18 | 0.21 | 0.018 | 0.044 | 11 | 0.034 | 0.22 | 0.037 | 0.19 | 0.0076 | 0.056 | 0.11 | 0.10 | 0.047 | 0.08 | 0.15 | 0.61 |
| 水及饮料类 Water and beverages | 134 | 39 | 73 | 420 | 141 | 94 | 28 | 60 | 109 | 492 | 79 | 93 | 9.9 | 90 | 319 | 119 | 85 | 910 | 20 | 57 | 101 | 103 | 147 | 235 | 165 |
| 酒类 Alcohol beverages | 3.3 | 1.7 | 0.42 | 0.76 | 0.33 | 0.0072 | 0.2 | 0.22 | 0.000011 | 0.94 | 0.12 | 1.3 | 0.022 | 1.0 | 3.0 | 2.0 | 5.3 | 14 | 0.47 | 0.22 | 7.6 | 0.86 | 0.05 | 0.036 | 1.8 |
| 合计 SUM | 2 606 | 2 004 | 4 123 | 4 006 | 4 039 | 2 543 | 3 682 | 2 861 | 1 878 | 3 052 | 5 548 | 2 454 | 5 487 | 4 065 | 9 993 | 13 383 | 6 526 | 7 519 | 12 226 | 5 629 | 10 184 | 8 070 | 6 445 | 17 371 | 6 071 |

附表 9-7 第六次中国总膳食研究的亚硝酸盐膳食摄入量 [单位: μg/(kg bw·d)]

Annexed Table 9-7 Dietary intakes of nitrite from the 6th China TDS [Unit: μg/(kg bw·d)]

| 膳食类别 Category | 黑龙江 HL | 辽宁 LN | 河北 HE | 北京 BJ | 吉林 JL | 山西 SX | 陕西 SN | 河南 HA | 宁夏 NX | 内蒙古 NM | 青海 QH | 甘肃 GS | 上海 SH | 福建 FJ | 江西 JX | 江苏 JS | 浙江 ZJ | 山东 SD | 湖北 HB | 四川 SC | 广西 GX | 湖南 HN | 广东 GD | 贵州 GZ | 全国平均 AVG |
|---|---|---|---|---|---|---|---|---|---|---|---|---|---|---|---|---|---|---|---|---|---|---|---|---|---|
| 谷类 Cereals | 0.084 | 0.078 | 0.099 | 0.089 | 0.29 | 0.13 | 0.12 | 0.11 | 0.094 | 0.084 | 0.14 | 0.092 | 0.046 | 0.074 | 0.068 | 0.077 | 0.24 | 0.13 | 0.057 | 0.12 | 0.11 | 0.067 | 0.049 | 0.086 | 0.11 |
| 豆类 Legumes | 0.005 2 | 0.013 | 0.005 4 | 0.008 8 | 0.008 1 | 0.50 | 0.007 4 | 0.006 1 | 0.003 3 | 0.003 4 | 0.000 59 | 0.003 4 | 0.011 | 0.006 4 | 0.006 6 | 0.007 7 | 0.012 | 0.005 1 | 0.005 9 | 0.006 2 | 0.003 4 | 0.007 5 | 0.002 5 | 0.009 6 | 0.027 |
| 薯类 Potatoes | 0.007 3 | 0.007 4 | 0.005 6 | 0.005 4 | 0.009 5 | 0.012 | 0.011 | 0.006 9 | 0.009 1 | 0.009 9 | 0.008 4 | 0.012 | 0.002 9 | 0.003 7 | 0.002 6 | 0.003 2 | 0.003 0 | 0.003 9 | 0.007 1 | 0.005 2 | 0.001 3 | 0.005 7 | 0.002 0 | 0.003 3 | 0.006 2 |
| 肉类 Meats | 0.005 6 | 0.006 5 | 0.27 | 0.006 7 | 0.005 3 | 0.44 | 0.003 1 | 0.004 6 | 0.003 9 | 0.006 0 | 0.005 7 | 0.002 8 | 0.008 8 | 0.007 0 | 0.007 5 | 0.007 4 | 0.44 | 0.008 3 | 0.004 5 | 0.010 | 0.012 | 0.012 | 0.010 | 0.008 7 | 0.054 |
| 蛋类 Eggs | 0.003 3 | 0.004 3 | 0.83 | 0.003 6 | 0.003 7 | 0.002 3 | 0.002 0 | 0.002 4 | 0.001 5 | 0.40 | 0.001 4 | 0.002 0 | 0.003 4 | 0.002 0 | 0.001 9 | 0.002 4 | 0.002 3 | 0.004 4 | 0.002 3 | 0.001 3 | 0.001 2 | 0.001 8 | 0.001 9 | 0.001 3 | 0.053 |
| 水产类 Aquatic foods | 0.002 2 | 0.70 | 0.000 83 | 0.001 4 | 0.000 88 | 0.000 60 | 0.000 33 | 0.000 38 | 0.000 19 | 0.000 82 | 0.000 32 | 0.022 | 0.005 4 | 0.005 3 | 0.003 5 | 0.003 2 | 0.004 2 | 0.002 1 | 0.003 2 | 0.000 66 | 0.73 | 0.005 3 | 0.004 2 | 0.000 33 | 0.063 |
| 乳类 Dairy products | 0.001 1 | 0.003 5 | 0.001 9 | 0.006 8 | 0.002 6 | 0.003 3 | 0.001 5 | 0.001 6 | 0.001 2 | 0.000 27 | 0.004 2 | 0.001 1 | 0.000 57 | 0.002 9 | 0.16 | 0.003 2 | 0.002 7 | 0.001 8 | 0.000 53 | 0.001 0 | 0.17 | 0.001 4 | 0.002 9 | 0.002 2 | 0.016 |
| 蔬菜类 Vegetables | 0.031 | 0.028 | 0.024 | 0.031 | 0.031 | 0.025 | 0.024 | 0.022 | 0.012 | 0.021 | 0.025 | 0.020 | 0.032 | 0.032 | 0.036 | 0.035 | 0.043 | 0.033 | 0.033 | 0.024 | 0.029 | 0.044 | 0.019 | 0.033 | 0.029 |
| 水果类 Fruits | 3.1 | 0.006 6 | 0.003 0 | 0.009 6 | 0.007 0 | 0.002 8 | 0.003 2 | 0.001 9 | 0.007 8 | 0.009 1 | 0.12 | 0.098 | 0.005 8 | 0.004 9 | 0.004 5 | 0.002 2 | 0.005 3 | 0.004 3 | 0.001 5 | 0.001 3 | 0.005 1 | 0.005 0 | 0.002 3 | 0.001 9 | 0.14 |
| 糖类 Sugar | 0.066 | 0.000 059 | 0.000 039 | 0.017 | 0.025 | 0.038 | 0.046 | 0.024 | 0.006 3 | 0.018 | 0.006 1 | 0.000 032 | 0.000 60 | 0.000 023 | 0.000 076 | 0.012 | 0.000 084 | 0.007 8 | 0.007 3 | 0.013 | 0.000 037 | 0.000 040 | 0.011 | 0.000 023 | 0.012 |
| 水及饮料类 Water and beverages | 0.009 7 | 0.003 9 | 1.3 | 0.008 8 | 0.027 | 0.005 9 | 0.002 7 | 0.009 5 | 0.004 1 | 0.020 | 0.004 9 | 0.009 4 | 0.005 6 | 0.006 9 | 0.009 4 | 0.008 0 | 0.006 2 | 0.014 | 0.056 | 0.002 5 | 3.8 | 0.008 4 | 0.24 | 0.009 9 | 0.24 |

续表

| 膳食类别<br>Category | 黑龙江<br>HL | 辽宁<br>LN | 河北<br>HE | 北京<br>BJ | 吉林<br>JL | 山西<br>SX | 陕西<br>SN | 河南<br>HA | 宁夏<br>NX | 内蒙古<br>NM | 青海<br>QH | 甘肃<br>GS | 上海<br>SH | 福建<br>FJ | 江西<br>JX | 江苏<br>JS | 浙江<br>ZJ | 山东<br>SD | 湖北<br>HB | 四川<br>SC | 广西<br>GX | 湖南<br>HN | 广东<br>GD | 贵州<br>GZ | 全国平均<br>AVG |
|---|---|---|---|---|---|---|---|---|---|---|---|---|---|---|---|---|---|---|---|---|---|---|---|---|---|
| 酒类<br>Alcohol beverages | 0.000 17 | 0.000 27 | 0.000 085 | 0.000 22 | 0.000 076 | 0.000 024 | 0.000 013 | 0.000 025 | 0.000 006 | 0.000 16 | 0.000 037 | 0.000 026 | 0.000 18 | 0.000 11 | 0.000 17 | 0.000 3 | 0.000 5 | 0.000 9 | 0.000 11 | 0.000 041 | 0.000 25 | 0.000 13 | 0.000 010 | 0.000 017 | 0.000 16 |
| 合计<br>SUM | 3.3 | 0.85 | 2.6 | 0.19 | 0.41 | 1.2 | 0.22 | 0.19 | 0.14 | 0.58 | 0.31 | 0.26 | 0.13 | 0.14 | 0.30 | 0.16 | 0.76 | 0.21 | 0.18 | 0.19 | 4.9 | 0.16 | 0.35 | 0.16 | 0.74 |

附表 9-8　第六次中国总膳食研究硝酸盐的膳食来源（单位：%）

Annexed Table 9-8　Dietary sources of nitrate from the 6th China TDS (Unit: %)

| 膳食类别<br>Category | 黑龙江<br>HL | 辽宁<br>LN | 河北<br>HE | 北京<br>BJ | 吉林<br>JL | 山西<br>SX | 陕西<br>SN | 河南<br>HA | 宁夏<br>NX | 内蒙古<br>NM | 青海<br>QH | 甘肃<br>GS | 上海<br>SH | 福建<br>FJ | 江西<br>JX | 江苏<br>JS | 浙江<br>ZJ | 山东<br>SD | 湖北<br>HB | 四川<br>SC | 广西<br>GX | 湖南<br>HN | 广东<br>GD | 贵州<br>GZ | 全国平均<br>AVG |
|---|---|---|---|---|---|---|---|---|---|---|---|---|---|---|---|---|---|---|---|---|---|---|---|---|---|
| 谷类<br>Cereals | 3.0 | 1.5 | 2.2 | 0.68 | 2.3 | 4.0 | 0.33 | 5.8 | 0.22 | 3.0 | 0.15 | 0.012 | 0.34 | 4.5 | 1.4 | 0.001 8 | 0.37 | 5.7 | 0.10 | 2.0 | 0.003 2 | 0.002 5 | 0.81 | 0.038 | 1.2 |
| 豆类<br>Legumes | 0.35 | 2.4 | 0.20 | 0.98 | 1.0 | 0.000 72 | 0.31 | 0.32 | 0.41 | 0.089 | 0.001 2 | 0.33 | 0.24 | 0.49 | 0.21 | 0.067 | 0.44 | 0.000 24 | 0.036 | 0.10 | 0.009 9 | 0.10 | 0.11 | 0.084 | 0.22 |
| 薯类<br>Potatoes | 0.21 | 7.2 | 2.4 | 1.2 | 2.8 | 4.5 | 1.3 | 3.3 | 4.8 | 7.5 | 0.33 | 2.4 | 0.72 | 0.42 | 0.91 | 0.48 | 0.55 | 1.6 | 0.44 | 1.1 | 0.067 | 0.19 | 0.40 | 0.62 | 1.2 |
| 肉类<br>Meats | 0.17 | 0.061 | 0.066 | 0.027 | 0.13 | 1.0 | 0.11 | 0.000 88 | 0.065 | 0.44 | 0.000 31 | 0.25 | 0.069 | 0.10 | 0.18 | 0.000 16 | 0.26 | 0.004 8 | 0.051 | 0.059 | 0.000 35 | 0.000 45 | 0.000 49 | 0.036 | 0.085 |
| 蛋类<br>Eggs | 0.029 | 0.15 | 0.020 | 0.000 27 | 0.000 27 | 0.000 27 | 0.013 | 0.000 25 | 0.007 4 | 0.11 | 0.091 | 0.000 26 | 0.000 18 | 0.084 | 0.001 6 | 0.000 053 | 0.000 11 | 0.037 | 0.001 8 | 0.000 070 | 0.001 6 | 0.000 069 | 0.022 | 0.004 8 | 0.016 |
| 水产类<br>Aquatic foods | 0.070 | 0.066 | 0.014 | 0.026 | 0.086 | 0.017 | 0.018 | 0.005 3 | 0.011 | 0.073 | 0.003 4 | 0.014 | 0.099 | 0.84 | 0.077 | 0.004 0 | 0.037 | 0.011 | 0.014 | 0.012 | 0.040 | 0.010 | 0.041 | 0.001 4 | 0.051 |
| 乳类<br>Dairy products | 0.55 | 2.0 | 0.63 | 1.4 | 0.023 | 0.050 | 0.20 | 0.42 | 0.24 | 1.4 | 0.85 | 0.67 | 1.2 | 1.6 | 0.24 | 0.033 | 0.54 | 0.35 | 0.094 | 0.26 | 0.026 | 0.21 | 0.45 | 0.10 | 0.40 |

续表

| 膳食类别 Category | 黑龙江 HL | 辽宁 LN | 河北 HE | 北京 BJ | 吉林 JL | 山西 SX | 陕西 SN | 河南 HA | 宁夏 NX | 内蒙古 NM | 青海 QH | 甘肃 GS | 上海 SH | 福建 FJ | 江西 JX | 江苏 JS | 浙江 ZJ | 山东 SD | 湖北 HB | 四川 SC | 广西 GX | 湖南 HN | 广东 GD | 贵州 GZ | 全国平均 AVG |
|---|---|---|---|---|---|---|---|---|---|---|---|---|---|---|---|---|---|---|---|---|---|---|---|---|---|
| 蔬菜类 Vegetables | 90 | 85 | 92 | 84 | 89 | 86 | 97 | 88 | 87 | 71 | 97 | 92 | 97 | 89 | 94 | 98 | 96 | 80 | 99 | 95 | 98 | 98 | 96 | 98 | 94 |
| 水果类 Fruits | 0.55 | 0.000 99 | 0.39 | 1.5 | 1.1 | 0.43 | 0.31 | 0.22 | 1.3 | 0.68 | 0.14 | 0.47 | 0.50 | 0.75 | 0.000 14 | 0.066 | 0.38 | 0.15 | 0.045 | 0.084 | 0.31 | 0.36 | 0.26 | 0.018 | 0.29 |
| 糖类 Sugar | 0.019 | 0.006 3 | 0.001 9 | 0.019 | 0.003 7 | 0.004 1 | 0.005 1 | 0.007 1 | 0.009 6 | 0.000 67 | 0.000 32 | 0.001 8 | 0.20 | 0.000 85 | 0.002 2 | 0.000 27 | 0.003 0 | 0.000 10 | 0.000 46 | 0.002 0 | 0.001 0 | 0.000 58 | 0.001 2 | 0.000 89 | 0.01 |
| 水及饮料类 Water and beverages | 5.2 | 1.9 | 1.8 | 10 | 3.5 | 3.7 | 0.77 | 2.1 | 5.8 | 16 | 1.4 | 3.8 | 0.18 | 2.2 | 3.2 | 0.89 | 1.3 | 12 | 0.17 | 1.0 | 0.99 | 1.3 | 2.3 | 1.4 | 2.7 |
| 酒类 Alcohol beverages | 0.13 | 0.083 | 0.010 | 0.019 | 0.008 2 | 0.000 28 | 0.005 3 | 0.007 5 | 0.000 058 | 0.031 | 0.002 1 | 0.052 | 0.000 40 | 0.026 | 0.030 | 0.015 | 0.081 | 0.18 | 0.003 8 | 0.003 9 | 0.075 | 0.011 | 0.000 78 | 0.000 21 | 0.030 |

附表 9-9 第六次中国总膳食研究亚硝酸盐的膳食来源 (单位: %)

Annexed Table 9-9 Dietary sources of nitrite from the 6th China TDS (Unit: %)

| 膳食类别 Category | 黑龙江 HL | 辽宁 LN | 河北 HE | 北京 BJ | 吉林 JL | 山西 SX | 陕西 SN | 河南 HA | 宁夏 NX | 内蒙古 NM | 青海 QH | 甘肃 GS | 上海 SH | 福建 FJ | 江西 JX | 江苏 JS | 浙江 ZJ | 山东 SD | 湖北 HB | 四川 SC | 广西 GX | 湖南 HN | 广东 GD | 贵州 GZ | 全国平均 AVG |
|---|---|---|---|---|---|---|---|---|---|---|---|---|---|---|---|---|---|---|---|---|---|---|---|---|---|
| 谷类 Cereals | 2.5 | 9.1 | 3.8 | 47 | 71 | 11 | 54 | 59 | 65 | 15 | 44 | 35 | 36 | 51 | 23 | 48 | 31 | 59 | 32 | 65 | 2.2 | 43 | 14 | 55 | 14 |
| 豆类 Legumes | 0.16 | 1.6 | 0.21 | 4.7 | 2.0 | 43 | 3.4 | 3.2 | 2.3 | 0.59 | 0.19 | 1.3 | 8.4 | 4.4 | 2.2 | 4.8 | 1.6 | 2.4 | 3.3 | 3.3 | 0.070 | 4.7 | 0.72 | 6.1 | 3.6 |
| 薯类 Potatoes | 0.22 | 0.87 | 0.22 | 2.9 | 2.3 | 1.0 | 5.1 | 3.6 | 6.3 | 1.7 | 2.7 | 4.5 | 2.2 | 2.5 | 0.85 | 2.0 | 0.40 | 1.9 | 4.0 | 2.8 | 0.027 | 3.6 | 0.59 | 2.1 | 0.83 |
| 肉类 Meats | 0.17 | 0.77 | 11 | 3.5 | 1.3 | 38 | 1.4 | 2.4 | 2.7 | 1.0 | 1.8 | 1.1 | 6.9 | 4.9 | 2.5 | 4.6 | 58 | 3.9 | 2.5 | 5.5 | 0.25 | 7.6 | 3.0 | 5.5 | 7.3 |

续表

| 膳食类别<br>Category | 黑龙江<br>HL | 辽宁<br>LN | 河北<br>HE | 北京<br>BJ | 吉林<br>JL | 山西<br>SX | 陕西<br>SN | 河南<br>HA | 宁夏<br>NX | 内蒙古<br>NM | 青海<br>QH | 甘肃<br>GS | 上海<br>SH | 福建<br>FJ | 江西<br>JX | 江苏<br>JS | 浙江<br>ZJ | 山东<br>SD | 湖北<br>HB | 四川<br>SC | 广西<br>GX | 湖南<br>HN | 广东<br>GD | 贵州<br>GZ | 全国平均<br>AVG |
|---|---|---|---|---|---|---|---|---|---|---|---|---|---|---|---|---|---|---|---|---|---|---|---|---|---|
| 蛋类 Eggs | 0.098 | 0.50 | 32 | 1.9 | 0.90 | 0.20 | 0.93 | 1.2 | 1.1 | 69 | 0.46 | 0.78 | 2.6 | 1.4 | 0.64 | 1.5 | 0.31 | 2.1 | 1.3 | 0.70 | 0.026 | 1.2 | 0.55 | 0.82 | 7.2 |
| 水产类 Aquatic foods | 0.065 | 82 | 0.032 | 0.73 | 0.22 | 0.051 | 0.15 | 0.20 | 0.13 | 0.14 | 0.10 | 8.4 | 4.3 | 3.7 | 1.2 | 2.0 | 0.55 | 1.0 | 1.8 | 0.35 | 15 | 3.4 | 1.2 | 0.21 | 8.4 |
| 乳类 Dairy products | 0.032 | 0.41 | 0.074 | 3.6 | 0.63 | 0.28 | 0.70 | 0.80 | 0.84 | 0.47 | 1.4 | 0.43 | 4.5 | 2.0 | 53 | 1.4 | 0.35 | 0.86 | 0.30 | 0.53 | 3.5 | 0.90 | 0.83 | 1.4 | 2.1 |
| 蔬菜类 Vegetables | 0.95 | 3.3 | 0.91 | 17 | 7.6 | 2.1 | 11 | 11 | 8.7 | 3.6 | 7.9 | 7.5 | 25 | 22 | 12 | 22 | 5.6 | 15 | 18 | 13 | 0.59 | 28 | 5.6 | 21 | 3.8 |
| 水果类 Fruits | 93 | 0.78 | 0.12 | 5.1 | 1.7 | 0.24 | 1.4 | 0.99 | 5.4 | 1.6 | 38 | 37 | 4.6 | 3.4 | 1.5 | 1.3 | 0.70 | 2.0 | 0.85 | 0.69 | 0.10 | 3.2 | 0.67 | 1.2 | 19 |
| 糖类 Sugar | 2.0 | 0.0069 | 0.0015 | 9.1 | 6.1 | 3.2 | 21 | 12 | 4.4 | 3.1 | 2.0 | 0.012 | 0.47 | 0.016 | 0.025 | 7.2 | 0.011 | 3.7 | 4.1 | 7.0 | 0.00076 | 0.025 | 3.2 | 0.015 | 1.7 |
| 水及饮料类 Water and beverages | 0.29 | 0.46 | 52 | 4.7 | 6.6 | 0.51 | 1.3 | 4.9 | 2.9 | 3.5 | 1.6 | 3.6 | 4.4 | 4.7 | 3.1 | 5.0 | 0.82 | 6.8 | 31 | 1.3 | 78 | 5.3 | 70 | 6.3 | 32 |
| 酒类 Alcohol beverages | 0.0053 | 0.031 | 0.0033 | 0.12 | 0.019 | 0.00020 | 0.0060 | 0.013 | 0.0025 | 0.029 | 0.012 | 0.010 | 0.14 | 0.078 | 0.057 | 0.19 | 0.065 | 0.43 | 0.063 | 0.022 | 0.0052 | 0.084 | 0.0030 | 0.011 | 0.021 |

附表 9-10 第六次中国总膳食研究膳食样品中双酚 A 的含量（单位：μg/kg）
Annexed Table 9-10　Levels of BPA in food samples from the 6$^{th}$ China TDS (Unit: μg/kg)

| 膳食类别<br>Category | 黑龙江<br>HL | 辽宁<br>LN | 河北<br>HE | 北京<br>BJ | 吉林<br>JL | 山西<br>SX | 陕西<br>SN | 河南<br>HA | 宁夏<br>NX | 内蒙古<br>NM | 青海<br>QH | 甘肃<br>GS | 上海<br>SH | 福建<br>FJ | 江西<br>JX | 江苏<br>JS | 浙江<br>ZJ | 山东<br>SD | 湖北<br>HB | 四川<br>SC | 广西<br>GX | 湖南<br>HN | 广东<br>GD | 贵州<br>GZ | 全国平均<br>AVG |
|---|---|---|---|---|---|---|---|---|---|---|---|---|---|---|---|---|---|---|---|---|---|---|---|---|---|
| 谷类 Cereals | 0.26 | 1.45 | 0.16 | 1.34 | ND | 0.20 | 0.87 | 0.98 | 0.30 | 0.30 | 0.36 | 0.17 | 0.27 | 0.24 | 0.17 | 0.27 | 0.16 | 0.18 | 0.18 | ND | 0.26 | 1.45 | 0.16 | 1.34 | 0.47 |

附录　901

续表

| 膳食类别 Category | 黑龙江 HL | 辽宁 LN | 河北 HE | 北京 BJ | 吉林 JL | 山西 SX | 陕西 SN | 河南 HA | 宁夏 NX | 内蒙古 NM | 青海 QH | 甘肃 GS | 上海 SH | 福建 FJ | 江西 JX | 江苏 JS | 浙江 ZJ | 山东 SD | 湖北 HB | 四川 SC | 广西 GX | 湖南 HN | 广东 GD | 贵州 GZ | 全国平均 AVG |
|---|---|---|---|---|---|---|---|---|---|---|---|---|---|---|---|---|---|---|---|---|---|---|---|---|---|
| 豆类 Legumes | ND | 0.20 | 0.87 | 0.98 | 0.30 | 0.30 | 0.36 | 0.17 | 0.27 | 0.24 | 0.17 | 0.27 | 0.16 | 0.18 | 0.18 | ND | 0.21 | ND | 3.39 | 0.51 | 1.17 | 0.56 | 0.19 | 0.72 | 0.48 |
| 薯类 Potatoes | 0.29 | 0.40 | ND | 0.22 | 0.70 | 0.24 | 0.19 | 0.64 | 0.21 | 0.19 | 1.35 | 0.27 | 0.27 | 0.27 | 0.28 | 0.22 | 0.21 | 0.23 | 0.29 | 0.29 | 0.25 | 0.47 | 0.22 | 0.39 | 0.34 |
| 肉类 Meats | 0.21 | 5.82 | 0.38 | 0.36 | 0.45 | 1.10 | 0.18 | 1.74 | 0.23 | 0.78 | 3.63 | 1.67 | 0.93 | 0.25 | ND | 0.90 | 1.03 | 0.18 | 0.26 | 0.47 | 0.85 | 0.48 | 0.39 | 2.21 | 1.02 |
| 蛋类 Eggs | 0.21 | 0.54 | 0.45 | ND | ND | ND | 0.31 | ND | ND | ND | ND | 0.25 | 0.29 | ND | 0.21 | 0.18 | ND | ND | 0.25 | 0.18 | ND | 0.25 | 0.16 | 0.22 | 0.18 |
| 水产类 Aquatic foods | 0.20 | 3.31 | 0.77 | 0.63 | 0.27 | 2.41 | 0.20 | 1.30 | 0.28 | 0.94 | 2.49 | 0.33 | 0.62 | 0.69 | 0.72 | 0.65 | 1.22 | 1.34 | 0.49 | 0.30 | 0.84 | 0.64 | 0.69 | 0.93 | 0.93 |
| 乳类 Dairy products | 0.18 | 0.24 | 0.20 | ND | 0.03 | ND | ND | ND | ND | ND | ND | ND | 0.15 | ND | ND | ND | ND | ND | ND | 0.17 | 0.39 | 0.22 | 0.24 | 0.25 | 0.13 |
| 蔬菜类 Vegetables | 0.15 | 0.20 | 0.17 | 0.45 | ND | 0.28 | 1.09 | 0.35 | 0.19 | 0.48 | 0.23 | 0.24 | 0.19 | 0.30 | 0.29 | 0.30 | 0.58 | 0.29 | 0.19 | 0.33 | 0.31 | 0.34 | 0.39 | 0.94 | 0.35 |
| 水果类 Fruits | 0.43 | 0.25 | 0.61 | 0.47 | 0.26 | 1.50 | 0.22 | 1.06 | 2.60 | 0.38 | ND | 1.43 | 0.41 | 0.26 | 0.18 | 20.00 | 0.15 | 0.55 | 0.48 | 0.25 | 7.93 | 0.18 | 0.54 | ND | 1.68 |
| 糖类 Sugar | 1.65 | 0.65 | 2.03 | 0.52 | 0.78 | 0.53 | ND | 0.78 | 0.20 | 3.26 | 1.07 | 1.52 | 0.25 | 0.54 | 0.39 | ND | 0.67 | 1.51 | 0.34 | 2.70 | 0.85 | 0.55 | 0.36 | 0.54 | 0.91 |
| 水及饮料类 Water and beverages | ND | 0.17 | ND | ND | ND | ND | ND | 1.57 | 1.53 | ND | ND | ND | ND | ND | ND | ND | ND | 0.16 | ND | ND | ND | ND | 0.76 | ND | 0.23 |
| 酒类 Alcohol beverages | 0.21 | 0.19 | ND | ND | 0.17 | ND | ND | 0.40 | 0.36 | 0.61 | ND | ND | ND | ND | ND | 0.48 | ND | ND | 0.16 | ND | ND | ND | ND | 0.17 | 0.16 |

注：平均值计算中，ND 以 1/2 检出限（LOD）计

Note: in calculation of averages (AVG), values not detected (ND) were treated as being equal to half of the detection of limit (LOD)

附表 9-11 第六次中国总膳食研究膳食样品中双酚 S 的含量（单位：μg/kg）

Annexed Table 9-11　Levels of BPS in food samples from the 6th China TDS (Unit: μg/kg)

| 膳食类别 Category | 黑龙江 HL | 辽宁 LN | 河北 HE | 北京 BJ | 吉林 JL | 山西 SX | 陕西 SN | 河南 HA | 宁夏 NX | 内蒙古 NM | 青海 QH | 甘肃 GS | 上海 SH | 福建 FJ | 江西 JX | 江苏 JS | 浙江 ZJ | 山东 SD | 湖北 HB | 四川 SC | 广西 GX | 湖南 HN | 广东 GD | 贵州 GZ | 全国平均 AVG |
|---|---|---|---|---|---|---|---|---|---|---|---|---|---|---|---|---|---|---|---|---|---|---|---|---|---|
| 谷类 Cereals | 0.13 | 0.32 | 1.98 | 0.07 | ND | 0.68 | 0.03 | 0.39 | 0.17 | 1.27 | 0.13 | 0.15 | 0.06 | 0.50 | 0.02 | 6.40 | 0.40 | 0.24 | 0.06 | ND | ND | 0.03 | ND | 0.02 | 0.54 |
| 豆类 Legumes | 1.21 | 1.41 | 1.05 | 0.03 | 0.03 | 0.07 | 1.17 | 0.16 | 2.54 | 1.64 | 0.02 | 0.47 | 0.30 | 3.15 | ND | 0.95 | 0.16 | 1.07 | 1.82 | 4.23 | 0.14 | ND | 1.91 | 0.08 | 0.98 |
| 薯类 Potatoes | 0.11 | 0.24 | 0.16 | 0.03 | ND | 0.15 | 0.16 | 0.47 | 0.04 | 0.65 | 0.02 | 0.18 | 0.06 | 0.12 | 0.14 | 0.27 | 0.26 | 0.12 | 0.15 | 0.03 | ND | 0.20 | 0.15 | 0.21 | 0.16 |
| 肉类 Meats | 0.20 | 8.64 | 6.67 | ND | ND | 2.18 | 4.77 | 16.59 | 0.38 | 2.04 | 0.12 | 0.10 | 11.22 | 67.09 | 0.04 | 6.29 | 3.65 | 2.48 | 4.07 | 0.23 | 0.10 | 0.85 | 0.14 | 1.98 | 5.83 |
| 蛋类 Eggs | 0.07 | 0.04 | 0.62 | 0.31 | 0.03 | 0.03 | ND | 0.04 | 0.21 | 0.02 | 0.04 | 0.07 | 0.64 | 0.22 | 0.23 | 0.11 | 0.02 | 0.15 | 0.02 | ND | ND | 0.07 | 0.03 | 0.02 | 0.13 |
| 水产类 Aquatic foods | 2.16 | 0.60 | 6.34 | 0.74 | 0.09 | 1.92 | 1.50 | 2.62 | 0.03 | 0.76 | 1.51 | 0.13 | 4.59 | 3.13 | 0.02 | 0.51 | 0.09 | 0.64 | 1.62 | 0.37 | 0.03 | 0.43 | ND | 0.16 | 1.25 |
| 乳类 Dairy products | 0.15 | ND | ND | ND | ND | ND | 0.05 | ND | 0.03 | 0.04 | 0.06 | 0.04 | ND | ND | ND | ND | ND | ND | ND | ND | ND | 0.03 | ND | ND | 0.02 |
| 蔬菜类 Vegetables | 0.07 | 0.97 | 0.17 | 0.06 | 0.02 | 0.22 | 0.48 | 0.20 | 0.79 | 1.81 | 0.03 | 0.04 | 0.09 | 0.61 | 0.02 | 1.16 | 0.87 | 0.11 | 0.15 | 0.13 | 0.02 | 0.03 | 0.07 | 0.12 | 0.34 |
| 水果类 Fruits | 0.07 | 1.60 | 0.53 | 0.05 | 0.05 | 0.12 | 0.47 | 0.52 | 0.10 | 1.71 | 0.03 | 0.17 | 0.17 | 0.33 | 0.10 | 0.35 | 0.06 | 0.26 | 0.62 | 0.03 | 0.10 | 0.04 | 0.03 | 0.05 | 0.31 |
| 糖类 Sugar | 0.11 | 0.03 | 0.07 | 0.02 | 0.02 | 0.02 | 0.02 | 0.02 | 0.02 | 0.10 | 0.02 | ND | ND | ND | ND | ND | 0.03 | 0.06 | 0.02 | 0.06 | 0.11 | ND | ND | 0.04 | 0.03 |
| 水及饮料类 Water and beverages | ND | 0.61 | 0.08 | 0.05 | ND | ND | 0.03 | ND | ND | 0.03 | 0.06 | 0.02 | 0.27 | 0.02 | 0.02 | 0.10 | ND | ND | ND | ND | 0.03 | ND | ND | ND | 0.06 |

续表

| 膳食类别<br>Category | 黑龙江<br>HL | 辽宁<br>LN | 河北<br>HE | 北京<br>BJ | 吉林<br>JL | 山西<br>SX | 陕西<br>SN | 河南<br>HA | 宁夏<br>NX | 内蒙古<br>NM | 青海<br>QH | 甘肃<br>GS | 上海<br>SH | 福建<br>FJ | 江西<br>JX | 江苏<br>JS | 浙江<br>ZJ | 山东<br>SD | 湖北<br>HB | 四川<br>SC | 广西<br>GX | 湖南<br>HN | 广东<br>GD | 贵州<br>GZ | 全国平均<br>AVG |
|---|---|---|---|---|---|---|---|---|---|---|---|---|---|---|---|---|---|---|---|---|---|---|---|---|---|
| 酒类<br>Alcohol beverages | 0.02 | 0.03 | 0.02 | 0.02 | ND | ND | 0.02 | 0.02 | 0.08 | ND | ND | 1.54 | ND | ND | ND | ND | ND | 0.02 | 0.03 | ND | 0.02 | ND | 0.03 | ND | 0.08 |

注：平均值计算中，ND 以 1/2 检出限（LOD）计

Note: in calculation of averages (AVG), values not detected (ND) were treated as being equal to half of the detection of limit (LOD)

附表 9-12　第六次中国总膳食研究膳食样品中双酚 F 的含量（单位：μg/kg）

Annexed Table 9-12　Levels of BPF in food samples from the 6th China TDS (Unit: μg/kg)

| 膳食类别<br>Category | 黑龙江<br>HL | 辽宁<br>LN | 河北<br>HE | 北京<br>BJ | 吉林<br>JL | 山西<br>SX | 陕西<br>SN | 河南<br>HA | 宁夏<br>NX | 内蒙古<br>NM | 青海<br>QH | 甘肃<br>GS | 上海<br>SH | 福建<br>FJ | 江西<br>JX | 江苏<br>JS | 浙江<br>ZJ | 山东<br>SD | 湖北<br>HB | 四川<br>SC | 广西<br>GX | 湖南<br>HN | 广东<br>GD | 贵州<br>GZ | 全国平均<br>AVG |
|---|---|---|---|---|---|---|---|---|---|---|---|---|---|---|---|---|---|---|---|---|---|---|---|---|---|
| 谷类 Cereals | ND | ND | ND | ND | ND | ND | ND | ND | ND | ND | ND | ND | ND | ND | ND | ND | ND | ND | ND | ND | ND | ND | ND | 0.17 | 0.01 |
| 豆类 Legumes | ND | 0.18 | ND | 0.16 | ND | 0.44 | 0.38 | ND | ND | ND | ND | 0.62 | ND | ND | ND | 0.29 | ND | 0.16 | ND | 0.19 | 1.06 | ND | ND | ND | 0.15 |
| 薯类 Potatoes | ND | ND | ND | ND | ND | ND | ND | 0.19 | ND | ND | ND | ND | ND | ND | ND | ND | ND | ND | ND | ND | ND | ND | ND | ND | 0.01 |
| 肉类 Meats | ND | ND | ND | 0.26 | ND | ND | ND | ND | 0.21 | 0.28 | ND | ND | ND | ND | ND | ND | ND | ND | ND | ND | 0.17 | 0.21 | ND | ND | 0.05 |
| 蛋类 Eggs | ND | ND | ND | ND | ND | ND | ND | ND | ND | ND | ND | ND | ND | ND | ND | ND | ND | ND | ND | ND | ND | ND | ND | ND | 0.00 |
| 水产类 Aquatic foods | 0.17 | ND | ND | ND | ND | ND | ND | ND | ND | ND | ND | ND | ND | 0.16 | ND | ND | ND | ND | ND | ND | ND | ND | 0.19 | ND | 0.02 |
| 乳类 Dairy products | ND | ND | ND | ND | ND | ND | ND | ND | ND | ND | ND | ND | ND | ND | ND | ND | ND | ND | ND | ND | ND | ND | ND | ND | 0.00 |
| 蔬菜类 Vegetables | ND | ND | ND | ND | ND | ND | ND | ND | ND | ND | ND | ND | ND | ND | ND | ND | ND | ND | ND | ND | 0.19 | ND | ND | ND | 0.01 |

续表

| 膳食类别<br>Category | 黑龙江<br>HL | 辽宁<br>LN | 河北<br>HE | 北京<br>BJ | 吉林<br>JL | 山西<br>SX | 陕西<br>SN | 河南<br>HA | 宁夏<br>NX | 内蒙古<br>NM | 青海<br>QH | 甘肃<br>GS | 上海<br>SH | 福建<br>FJ | 江西<br>JX | 江苏<br>JS | 浙江<br>ZJ | 山东<br>SD | 湖北<br>HB | 四川<br>SC | 广西<br>GX | 湖南<br>HN | 广东<br>GD | 贵州<br>GZ | 全国平均<br>AVG |
|---|---|---|---|---|---|---|---|---|---|---|---|---|---|---|---|---|---|---|---|---|---|---|---|---|---|
| 水果类 Fruits | 0.17 | ND | 0.16 | ND | ND | ND | ND | ND | ND | ND | ND | 0.45 | ND | ND | ND | ND | ND | ND | ND | ND | ND | ND | ND | ND | 0.03 |
| 糖类 Sugar | 0.26 | ND | ND | ND | ND | ND | ND | ND | ND | ND | ND | ND | ND | ND | ND | ND | ND | ND | ND | ND | ND | ND | ND | ND | 0.01 |
| 水及饮料类 Water and beverages | ND | ND | ND | ND | ND | ND | ND | ND | ND | ND | ND | ND | ND | ND | ND | ND | ND | ND | ND | ND | ND | ND | ND | ND | 0.00 |
| 酒类 Alcohol beverages | ND | ND | ND | ND | ND | ND | ND | ND | ND | ND | ND | ND | ND | ND | ND | ND | ND | ND | ND | ND | ND | ND | ND | ND | 0.00 |

注：平均值计算中，ND 以 1/2 检出限（LOD）计

Note: in calculation of averages (AVG), values not detected (ND) were treated as being equal to half of the detection of limit (LOD)

附表 Table 9-13　第六次中国总膳食研究膳食样品中双酚 AF 的含量（单位：μg/kg）

Annexed Table 9-13　Levels of BPAF in food samples from the 6th China TDS (Unit: μg/kg)

| 膳食类别<br>Category | 黑龙江<br>HL | 辽宁<br>LN | 河北<br>HE | 北京<br>BJ | 吉林<br>JL | 山西<br>SX | 陕西<br>SN | 河南<br>HA | 宁夏<br>NX | 内蒙古<br>NM | 青海<br>QH | 甘肃<br>GS | 上海<br>SH | 福建<br>FJ | 江西<br>JX | 江苏<br>JS | 浙江<br>ZJ | 山东<br>SD | 湖北<br>HB | 四川<br>SC | 广西<br>GX | 湖南<br>HN | 广东<br>GD | 贵州<br>GZ | 全国平均<br>AVG |
|---|---|---|---|---|---|---|---|---|---|---|---|---|---|---|---|---|---|---|---|---|---|---|---|---|---|
| 谷类 Cereals | ND | ND | ND | 0.03 | ND | ND | ND | 0.02 | ND | ND | ND | ND | 0.13 | 0.04 | ND | ND | ND | ND | 0.02 | 0.02 | ND | ND | 0.05 | ND | 0.01 |
| 豆类 Legumes | ND | 0.02 | 0.03 | ND | ND | ND | ND | ND | ND | ND | ND | ND | ND | ND | ND | ND | ND | ND | ND | ND | ND | ND | ND | ND | 0.00 |
| 薯类 Potatoes | ND | 0.53 | ND | ND | ND | ND | ND | ND | ND | ND | ND | ND | ND | 0.02 | 0.02 | 0.02 | 0.02 | ND | ND | ND | ND | ND | 0.02 | ND | 0.01 |
| 肉类 Meats | ND | ND | 0.02 | 0.02 | 0.02 | ND | ND | ND | ND | ND | 0.02 | 0.02 | ND | 0.02 | ND | ND | 0.02 | ND | ND | ND | ND | ND | ND | ND | 0.03 |
| 蛋类 Eggs | ND | ND | 0.03 | 0.04 | 0.02 | ND | ND | ND | ND | ND | ND | 0.03 | 0.02 | 0.02 | 0.02 | ND | ND | 0.02 | 0.20 | ND | ND | 0.03 | 0.06 | 0.02 | 0.02 |

附录　905

续表

| 膳食类别 Category | 黑龙江 HL | 辽宁 LN | 河北 HE | 北京 BJ | 吉林 JL | 山西 SX | 陕西 SN | 河南 HA | 宁夏 NX | 内蒙古 NM | 青海 QH | 甘肃 GS | 上海 SH | 福建 FJ | 江西 JX | 江苏 JS | 浙江 ZJ | 山东 SD | 湖北 HB | 四川 SC | 广西 GX | 湖南 HN | 广东 GD | 贵州 GZ | 全国平均 AVG |
|---|---|---|---|---|---|---|---|---|---|---|---|---|---|---|---|---|---|---|---|---|---|---|---|---|---|
| 水产类 Aquatic foods | ND | 0.03 | 0.02 | 0.03 | ND | 0.02 | 0.02 | ND | ND | 0.02 | 0.02 | 0.03 | 0.05 | 0.02 | 0.03 | ND | 0.03 | 0.04 | 0.80 | 0.03 | 0.03 | 1.75 | 0.02 | 0.03 | 0.12 |
| 乳类 Dairy products | ND | ND | 0.02 | ND | ND | ND | 0.03 | ND | ND | ND | 0.02 | ND | ND | ND | ND | ND | ND | ND | ND | ND | ND | ND | ND | ND | 0.00 |
| 蔬菜类 Vegetables | 0.04 | 0.04 | ND | 0.02 | 0.02 | 0.02 | ND | ND | ND | ND | ND | ND | ND | ND | ND | ND | 0.02 | 0.03 | ND | 0.03 | ND | ND | ND | ND | 0.01 |
| 水果类 Fruits | 0.02 | ND | ND | 0.02 | ND | 0.02 | ND | 0.02 | ND | ND | 0.02 | 0.09 | ND | ND | ND | ND | 0.03 | 0.05 | 0.18 | 0.11 | ND | ND | 0.02 | ND | 0.02 |
| 糖类 Sugar | 0.04 | ND | 0.02 | ND | ND | ND | ND | ND | ND | 0.04 | ND | ND | ND | ND | ND | ND | ND | 0.02 | ND | 0.02 | ND | ND | ND | ND | 0.01 |
| 水及饮料类 Water and beverages | ND | ND | ND | ND | ND | ND | ND | ND | ND | ND | ND | ND | ND | ND | ND | ND | ND | ND | ND | ND | ND | ND | ND | ND | 0.00 |
| 酒类 Alcohol beverages | ND | ND | ND | ND | ND | ND | ND | ND | ND | ND | ND | ND | ND | ND | ND | ND | ND | ND | ND | ND | ND | ND | ND | ND | 0.00 |

注：平均值计算中，ND 以 1/2 检出限（LOD）计

Note: in calculation of averages (AVG), values not detected (ND) were treated as being equal to half of the detection of limit (LOD)

附表 9-14 第六次中国总膳食研究的双酚 A 膳食摄入量 [单位：ng/(kg bw·d)]

Annexed Table 9-14 Dietary intakes of BPA from the 6th China TDS [Unit: ng/(kg bw·d)]

| 膳食类别 Category | 黑龙江 HL | 辽宁 LN | 河北 HE | 北京 BJ | 吉林 JL | 山西 SX | 陕西 SN | 河南 HA | 宁夏 NX | 内蒙古 NM | 青海 QH | 甘肃 GS | 上海 SH | 福建 FJ | 江西 JX | 江苏 JS | 浙江 ZJ | 山东 SD | 湖北 HB | 四川 SC | 广西 GX | 湖南 HN | 广东 GD | 贵州 GZ | 全国平均 AVG |
|---|---|---|---|---|---|---|---|---|---|---|---|---|---|---|---|---|---|---|---|---|---|---|---|---|---|
| 谷类 Cereals | 4.31 | 22.41 | 3.10 | 23.83 | 0.92 | 5.39 | 20.60 | 22.35 | 5.52 | 5.01 | 10.00 | 3.12 | 2.54 | 3.48 | 2.29 | 4.22 | 2.17 | 4.62 | 2.04 | 1.83 | 5.62 | 19.47 | 1.53 | 23.16 | 8.31 |

续表

| 膳食类别 Category | 黑龙江 HL | 辽宁 LN | 河北 HE | 北京 BJ | 吉林 JL | 山西 SX | 陕西 SN | 河南 HA | 宁夏 NX | 内蒙古 NM | 青海 QH | 甘肃 GS | 上海 SH | 福建 FJ | 江西 JX | 江苏 JS | 浙江 ZJ | 山东 SD | 湖北 HB | 四川 SC | 广西 GX | 湖南 HN | 广东 GD | 贵州 GZ | 全国平均 AVG |
|---|---|---|---|---|---|---|---|---|---|---|---|---|---|---|---|---|---|---|---|---|---|---|---|---|---|
| 豆类 Legumes | 0.08 | 0.54 | 0.94 | 1.71 | 0.48 | 0.36 | 0.54 | 0.21 | 0.18 | 0.16 | 0.02 | 0.18 | 0.35 | 0.23 | 0.24 | 0.11 | 0.49 | 0.08 | 3.99 | 0.63 | 0.80 | 0.84 | 0.09 | 1.39 | 0.61 |
| 薯类 Potatoes | 0.43 | 0.60 | 0.08 | 0.24 | 1.33 | 0.56 | 0.42 | 0.88 | 0.38 | 0.37 | 2.27 | 0.64 | 0.15 | 0.20 | 0.14 | 0.14 | 0.12 | 0.18 | 0.41 | 0.30 | 0.07 | 0.55 | 0.09 | 0.26 | 0.45 |
| 肉类 Meats | 0.24 | 7.61 | 0.31 | 0.48 | 0.48 | 2.53 | 0.11 | 1.59 | 0.18 | 0.93 | 4.13 | 0.92 | 1.63 | 0.35 | 0.11 | 1.33 | 2.08 | 0.31 | 0.24 | 0.98 | 2.03 | 1.15 | 0.81 | 3.85 | 1.43 |
| 蛋类 Eggs | 0.13 | 0.46 | 0.29 | 0.05 | 0.05 | 0.03 | 0.13 | 0.04 | 0.02 | 0.05 | 0.02 | 0.10 | 0.19 | 0.03 | 0.08 | 0.08 | 0.04 | 0.07 | 0.12 | 0.05 | 0.02 | 0.09 | 0.06 | 0.06 | 0.09 |
| 水产类 Aquatic foods | 0.09 | 1.24 | 0.13 | 0.17 | 0.05 | 0.29 | 0.01 | 0.10 | 0.01 | 0.15 | 0.16 | 0.01 | 0.68 | 0.73 | 0.50 | 0.41 | 1.02 | 0.57 | 0.31 | 0.04 | 1.31 | 0.68 | 0.58 | 0.06 | 0.39 |
| 乳类 Dairy products | 0.04 | 0.17 | 0.08 | 0.10 | 0.05 | 0.05 | 0.02 | 0.02 | 0.02 | 0.04 | 0.06 | 0.02 | 0.17 | 0.04 | 0.03 | 0.03 | 0.04 | 0.03 | 0.01 | 0.03 | 0.11 | 0.06 | 0.14 | 0.11 | 0.06 |
| 蔬菜类 Vegetables | 0.96 | 1.12 | 0.79 | 2.85 | 0.47 | 1.42 | 5.12 | 1.55 | 0.47 | 2.01 | 1.14 | 0.96 | 1.21 | 1.88 | 2.04 | 2.13 | 4.94 | 1.90 | 1.27 | 1.58 | 1.78 | 2.93 | 1.50 | 6.25 | 2.01 |
| 水果类 Fruits | 0.43 | 0.33 | 0.36 | 0.90 | 0.36 | 0.83 | 0.14 | 0.41 | 4.05 | 0.69 | 0.02 | 0.75 | 0.47 | 0.25 | 0.16 | 8.64 | 0.16 | 0.47 | 0.15 | 0.06 | 8.11 | 0.18 | 0.25 | 0.03 | 1.18 |
| 糖类 Sugar | 0.06 | 0.01 | 0.02 | 0.02 | 0.01 | 0.01 | 0.00 | 0.00 | 0.00 | 0.05 | 0.01 | 0.01 | 0.03 | 0.00 | 0.01 | 0.00 | 0.01 | 0.01 | 0.00 | 0.02 | 0.01 | 0.00 | 0.00 | 0.00 | 0.01 |
| 水及饮料类 Water and beverages | 1.46 | 1.32 | 0.92 | 1.32 | 1.55 | 0.89 | 0.41 | 29.70 | 12.59 | 3.07 | 0.74 | 1.41 | 0.84 | 1.03 | 1.41 | 1.20 | 0.94 | 4.60 | 0.34 | 0.37 | 1.55 | 1.26 | 14.44 | 1.49 | 3.53 |
| 酒类 Alcohol beverages | 0.07 | 0.10 | 0.01 | 0.03 | 0.03 | 0.00 | 0.00 | 0.02 | 0.00 | 0.20 | 0.01 | 0.00 | 0.03 | 0.02 | 0.03 | 0.28 | 0.07 | 0.14 | 0.04 | 0.01 | 0.04 | 0.02 | 0.00 | 0.01 | 0.05 |
| 合计 SUM | 8.29 | 35.90 | 7.03 | 31.70 | 5.74 | 12.37 | 27.50 | 56.86 | 23.43 | 12.74 | 18.57 | 8.12 | 8.29 | 8.26 | 7.03 | 18.59 | 12.08 | 12.96 | 8.92 | 5.89 | 21.44 | 27.25 | 19.48 | 36.67 | 18.13 |

附表 9-15 第六次中国总膳食研究的双酚 S 膳食摄入量 [单位：ng/(kg bw·d)]
Annexed Table 9-15 Dietary intakes of BPS from the 6$^{th}$ China TDS [Unit: ng/(kg bw·d)]

| 膳食类别 Category | 黑龙江 HL | 辽宁 LN | 河北 HE | 北京 BJ | 吉林 JL | 山西 SX | 陕西 SN | 河南 HA | 宁夏 NX | 内蒙古 NM | 青海 QH | 甘肃 GS | 上海 SH | 福建 FJ | 江西 JX | 江苏 JS | 浙江 ZJ | 山东 SD | 湖北 HB | 四川 SC | 广西 GX | 湖南 HN | 广东 GD | 贵州 GZ | 全国平均 AVG |
|---|---|---|---|---|---|---|---|---|---|---|---|---|---|---|---|---|---|---|---|---|---|---|---|---|---|
| 谷类 Cereals | 2.17 | 4.89 | 39.38 | 1.21 | 0.10 | 17.93 | 0.77 | 8.88 | 3.16 | 21.42 | 3.52 | 2.80 | 0.56 | 7.31 | 0.27 | 98.83 | 5.36 | 6.05 | 0.68 | 0.19 | 0.18 | 0.43 | 0.08 | 0.36 | 9.44 |
| 豆类 Legumes | 1.27 | 3.73 | 1.13 | 0.05 | 0.04 | 0.09 | 1.73 | 0.20 | 1.67 | 1.12 | 0.00 | 0.31 | 0.65 | 4.00 | 0.01 | 1.45 | 0.38 | 1.10 | 2.14 | 5.21 | 0.10 | 0.01 | 0.96 | 0.15 | 1.15 |
| 薯类 Potatoes | 0.15 | 0.36 | 0.18 | 0.03 | 0.02 | 0.34 | 0.35 | 0.64 | 0.07 | 1.28 | 0.04 | 0.43 | 0.03 | 0.09 | 0.07 | 0.17 | 0.16 | 0.09 | 0.21 | 0.03 | 0.00 | 0.23 | 0.06 | 0.14 | 0.22 |
| 肉类 Meats | 0.23 | 11.30 | 5.45 | 0.01 | 0.01 | 5.00 | 2.93 | 15.18 | 0.29 | 2.43 | 0.14 | 0.06 | 19.71 | 94.42 | 0.06 | 9.26 | 7.37 | 4.12 | 3.66 | 0.47 | 0.25 | 2.03 | 0.29 | 3.44 | 7.84 |
| 蛋类 Eggs | 0.05 | 0.04 | 0.40 | 0.23 | 0.02 | 0.01 | 0.00 | 0.02 | 0.06 | 0.01 | 0.01 | 0.03 | 0.43 | 0.09 | 0.09 | 0.05 | 0.01 | 0.13 | 0.01 | 0.00 | 0.05 | 0.03 | 0.01 | 0.01 | 0.07 |
| 水产类 Aquatic foods | 0.93 | 0.22 | 1.05 | 0.21 | 0.02 | 0.23 | 0.10 | 0.20 | 0.00 | 0.12 | 0.10 | 0.01 | 4.99 | 3.32 | 0.02 | 0.32 | 0.07 | 0.27 | 1.05 | 0.05 | 0.00 | 0.45 | 0.01 | 0.01 | 0.58 |
| 乳类 Dairy products | 0.03 | 0.01 | 0.00 | 0.01 | 0.00 | 0.01 | 0.02 | 0.00 | 0.01 | 0.02 | 0.05 | 0.01 | 0.01 | 0.00 | 0.00 | 0.00 | 0.00 | 0.00 | 0.00 | 0.00 | 0.00 | 0.01 | 0.00 | 0.00 | 0.01 |
| 蔬菜类 Vegetables | 0.45 | 5.39 | 0.81 | 0.35 | 0.12 | 1.11 | 2.27 | 0.89 | 1.97 | 7.60 | 0.16 | 0.14 | 0.59 | 3.87 | 0.16 | 8.13 | 7.47 | 0.69 | 0.97 | 0.63 | 0.11 | 0.26 | 0.28 | 0.83 | 1.89 |
| 水果类 Fruits | 0.07 | 2.12 | 0.32 | 0.10 | 0.07 | 0.07 | 0.29 | 0.20 | 0.16 | 3.10 | 0.01 | 0.09 | 0.20 | 0.32 | 0.09 | 0.15 | 0.06 | 0.22 | 0.19 | 0.01 | 0.10 | 0.04 | 0.01 | 0.02 | 0.33 |
| 糖类 Sugar | 0.00 | 0.00 | 0.00 | 0.00 | 0.00 | 0.00 | 0.00 | 0.00 | 0.00 | 0.00 | 0.00 | 0.00 | 0.00 | 0.00 | 0.00 | 0.00 | 0.00 | 0.00 | 0.00 | 0.00 | 0.00 | 0.00 | 0.00 | 0.00 | 0.00 |
| 水及饮料类 Water and beverages | 0.16 | 4.79 | 0.92 | 0.96 | 0.17 | 0.09 | 0.15 | 0.15 | 0.07 | 1.07 | 0.58 | 0.36 | 2.99 | 0.25 | 0.38 | 1.59 | 0.10 | 0.23 | 0.04 | 0.04 | 0.58 | 0.13 | 0.15 | 0.16 | 0.67 |

续表

| 膳食类别<br>Category | 黑龙江<br>HL | 辽宁<br>LN | 河北<br>HE | 北京<br>BJ | 吉林<br>JL | 山西<br>SX | 陕西<br>SN | 河南<br>HA | 宁夏<br>NX | 内蒙古<br>NM | 青海<br>QH | 甘肃<br>GS | 上海<br>SH | 福建<br>FJ | 江西<br>JX | 江苏<br>JS | 浙江<br>ZJ | 山东<br>SD | 湖北<br>HB | 四川<br>SC | 广西<br>GX | 湖南<br>HN | 广东<br>GD | 贵州<br>GZ | 全国平均<br>AVG |
|---|---|---|---|---|---|---|---|---|---|---|---|---|---|---|---|---|---|---|---|---|---|---|---|---|---|
| 酒类<br>Alcohol beverages | 0.01 | 0.02 | 0.00 | 0.01 | 0.00 | 0.00 | 0.00 | 0.00 | 0.00 | 0.00 | 0.00 | 0.08 | 0.00 | 0.00 | 0.00 | 0.00 | 0.01 | 0.03 | 0.01 | 0.00 | 0.01 | 0.00 | 0.00 | 0.00 | 0.01 |
| 合计<br>SUM | 5.52 | 32.88 | 49.66 | 3.17 | 0.56 | 24.89 | 8.61 | 26.37 | 7.45 | 38.20 | 4.60 | 4.31 | 30.17 | 113.67 | 1.14 | 119.96 | 20.99 | 12.94 | 8.96 | 6.63 | 1.39 | 3.63 | 1.86 | 5.12 | 22.19 |

附表 9-16 第六次中国总膳食研究的双酚 F 膳食摄入量 [单位: ng/(kg bw·d)]

Annexed Table 9-16 Dietary intakes of BPF from the 6th China TDS [Unit: ng/(kg bw·d)]

| 膳食类别<br>Category | 黑龙江<br>HL | 辽宁<br>LN | 河北<br>HE | 北京<br>BJ | 吉林<br>JL | 山西<br>SX | 陕西<br>SN | 河南<br>HA | 宁夏<br>NX | 内蒙古<br>NM | 青海<br>QH | 甘肃<br>GS | 上海<br>SH | 福建<br>FJ | 江西<br>JX | 江苏<br>JS | 浙江<br>ZJ | 山东<br>SD | 湖北<br>HB | 四川<br>SC | 广西<br>GX | 湖南<br>HN | 广东<br>GD | 贵州<br>GZ | 全国平均<br>AVG |
|---|---|---|---|---|---|---|---|---|---|---|---|---|---|---|---|---|---|---|---|---|---|---|---|---|---|
| 谷类<br>Cereals | 0.00 | 0.00 | 0.00 | 0.00 | 0.00 | 0.00 | 0.00 | 0.00 | 0.00 | 0.00 | 0.00 | 0.00 | 0.00 | 0.00 | 0.00 | 0.00 | 0.00 | 0.00 | 0.00 | 0.00 | 0.00 | 0.00 | 0.00 | 2.92 | 0.12 |
| 豆类<br>Legumes | 0.00 | 0.49 | 0.00 | 0.29 | 0.00 | 0.54 | 0.57 | 0.00 | 0.00 | 0.00 | 0.00 | 0.42 | 0.00 | 0.00 | 0.00 | 0.44 | 0.00 | 0.17 | 0.00 | 0.24 | 0.73 | 0.00 | 0.00 | 0.00 | 0.16 |
| 薯类<br>Potatoes | 0.00 | 0.00 | 0.00 | 0.00 | 0.00 | 0.00 | 0.00 | 0.00 | 0.16 | 0.00 | 0.00 | 0.00 | 0.00 | 0.00 | 0.00 | 0.00 | 0.00 | 0.00 | 0.00 | 0.00 | 0.00 | 0.00 | 0.00 | 0.00 | 0.01 |
| 肉类<br>Meats | 0.00 | 0.00 | 0.00 | 0.35 | 0.00 | 0.00 | 0.00 | 0.26 | 0.00 | 0.33 | 0.00 | 0.00 | 0.00 | 0.00 | 0.00 | 0.00 | 0.00 | 0.00 | 0.00 | 0.00 | 0.40 | 0.50 | 0.00 | 0.00 | 0.07 |
| 蛋类<br>Eggs | 0.00 | 0.00 | 0.00 | 0.00 | 0.00 | 0.00 | 0.00 | 0.00 | 0.00 | 0.00 | 0.00 | 0.00 | 0.00 | 0.00 | 0.00 | 0.00 | 0.00 | 0.00 | 0.00 | 0.00 | 0.00 | 0.00 | 0.00 | 0.00 | 0.00 |
| 水产类<br>Aquatic foods | 0.07 | 0.00 | 0.00 | 0.00 | 0.00 | 0.00 | 0.00 | 0.00 | 0.00 | 0.00 | 0.00 | 0.00 | 0.00 | 0.00 | 0.00 | 0.00 | 0.00 | 0.00 | 0.00 | 0.00 | 0.00 | 0.00 | 0.16 | 0.00 | 0.01 |

续表

| 膳食类别<br>Category | 黑龙江<br>HL | 辽宁<br>LN | 河北<br>HE | 北京<br>BJ | 吉林<br>JL | 山西<br>SX | 陕西<br>SN | 河南<br>HA | 宁夏<br>NX | 内蒙古<br>NM | 青海<br>QH | 甘肃<br>GS | 上海<br>SH | 福建<br>FJ | 江西<br>JX | 江苏<br>JS | 浙江<br>ZJ | 山东<br>SD | 湖北<br>HB | 四川<br>SC | 广西<br>GX | 湖南<br>HN | 广东<br>GD | 贵州<br>GZ | 全国平均<br>AVG |
|---|---|---|---|---|---|---|---|---|---|---|---|---|---|---|---|---|---|---|---|---|---|---|---|---|---|
| 乳类<br>Dairy products | 0.00 | 0.00 | 0.00 | 0.00 | 0.00 | 0.00 | 0.00 | 0.00 | 0.00 | 0.00 | 0.00 | 0.00 | 0.00 | 0.00 | 0.00 | 0.00 | 0.00 | 0.00 | 0.00 | 0.00 | 0.00 | 0.00 | 0.00 | 0.00 | 0.00 |
| 蔬菜类<br>Vegetables | 0.00 | 0.00 | 0.00 | 0.00 | 0.00 | 0.00 | 0.00 | 0.00 | 0.00 | 0.00 | 0.00 | 0.00 | 0.00 | 1.02 | 0.00 | 0.00 | 0.00 | 0.00 | 0.00 | 0.00 | 1.09 | 0.00 | 0.00 | 0.00 | 0.09 |
| 水果类<br>Fruits | 0.17 | 0.00 | 0.09 | 0.00 | 0.00 | 0.00 | 0.00 | 0.00 | 0.00 | 0.00 | 0.00 | 0.24 | 0.00 | 0.00 | 0.00 | 0.00 | 0.00 | 0.00 | 0.00 | 0.00 | 0.00 | 0.00 | 0.00 | 0.00 | 0.02 |
| 糖类<br>Sugar | 0.01 | 0.00 | 0.00 | 0.00 | 0.00 | 0.00 | 0.00 | 0.00 | 0.00 | 0.00 | 0.00 | 0.00 | 0.00 | 0.00 | 0.00 | 0.00 | 0.00 | 0.00 | 0.00 | 0.00 | 0.00 | 0.00 | 0.00 | 0.00 | 0.00 |
| 水及饮料类<br>Water and beverages | 0.00 | 0.00 | 0.00 | 0.00 | 0.00 | 0.00 | 0.00 | 0.00 | 0.00 | 0.00 | 0.00 | 0.00 | 0.00 | 0.00 | 0.00 | 0.00 | 0.00 | 0.00 | 0.00 | 0.00 | 0.00 | 0.00 | 0.00 | 0.00 | 0.00 |
| 酒类<br>Alcohol beverages | 0.00 | 0.00 | 0.00 | 0.00 | 0.00 | 0.00 | 0.00 | 0.00 | 0.00 | 0.00 | 0.00 | 0.00 | 0.00 | 0.00 | 0.00 | 0.00 | 0.00 | 0.00 | 0.00 | 0.00 | 0.00 | 0.00 | 0.00 | 0.00 | 0.00 |
| 合计<br>SUM | 0.25 | 0.49 | 0.09 | 0.63 | 0.00 | 0.54 | 0.57 | 0.26 | 0.16 | 0.33 | 0.00 | 0.66 | 0.00 | 1.02 | 0.00 | 0.44 | 0.00 | 0.17 | 0.00 | 0.24 | 2.22 | 0.50 | 0.16 | 2.92 | 0.49 |

附表 Table 9-17 第六次中国总膳食研究的双酚 AF 膳食摄入量 [单位：ng/(kg bw·d)]
Annexed Table 9-17 Dietary intakes of BPAF from the 6<sup>th</sup> China TDS [Unit: ng/(kg bw·d)]

| 膳食类别<br>Category | 黑龙江<br>HL | 辽宁<br>LN | 河北<br>HE | 北京<br>BJ | 吉林<br>JL | 山西<br>SX | 陕西<br>SN | 河南<br>HA | 宁夏<br>NX | 内蒙古<br>NM | 青海<br>QH | 甘肃<br>GS | 上海<br>SH | 福建<br>FJ | 江西<br>JX | 江苏<br>JS | 浙江<br>ZJ | 山东<br>SD | 湖北<br>HB | 四川<br>SC | 广西<br>GX | 湖南<br>HN | 广东<br>GD | 贵州<br>GZ | 全国平均<br>AVG |
|---|---|---|---|---|---|---|---|---|---|---|---|---|---|---|---|---|---|---|---|---|---|---|---|---|---|
| 谷类<br>Cereals | 0.00 | 0.00 | 0.00 | 0.46 | 0.00 | 0.00 | 0.00 | 0.34 | 0.00 | 0.00 | 0.00 | 0.00 | 1.20 | 0.59 | 0.00 | 0.00 | 0.00 | 0.00 | 0.23 | 0.37 | 0.00 | 0.00 | 0.50 | 0.00 | 0.15 |

续表

| 膳食类别<br>Category | 黑龙江<br>HL | 辽宁<br>LN | 河北<br>HE | 北京<br>BJ | 吉林<br>JL | 山西<br>SX | 陕西<br>SN | 河南<br>HA | 宁夏<br>NX | 内蒙古<br>NM | 青海<br>QH | 甘肃<br>GS | 上海<br>SH | 福建<br>FJ | 江西<br>JX | 江苏<br>JS | 浙江<br>ZJ | 山东<br>SD | 湖北<br>HB | 四川<br>SC | 广西<br>GX | 湖南<br>HN | 广东<br>GD | 贵州<br>GZ | 全国平均<br>AVG |
|---|---|---|---|---|---|---|---|---|---|---|---|---|---|---|---|---|---|---|---|---|---|---|---|---|---|
| 豆类 Legumes | 0.00 | 0.00 | 0.00 | 0.00 | 0.00 | 0.00 | 0.00 | 0.00 | 0.00 | 0.00 | 0.00 | 0.00 | 0.00 | 0.00 | 0.00 | 0.00 | 0.00 | 0.00 | 0.00 | 0.00 | 0.00 | 0.00 | 0.00 | 0.00 | 0.00 |
| 薯类 Potatoes | 0.00 | 0.04 | 0.03 | 0.00 | 0.00 | 0.00 | 0.00 | 0.00 | 0.00 | 0.00 | 0.00 | 0.00 | 0.00 | 0.01 | 0.01 | 0.01 | 0.01 | 0.00 | 0.00 | 0.00 | 0.00 | 0.00 | 0.01 | 0.00 | 0.01 |
| 肉类 Meats | 0.00 | 0.69 | 0.00 | 0.03 | 0.00 | 0.00 | 0.00 | 0.00 | 0.00 | 0.00 | 0.03 | 0.01 | 0.00 | 0.02 | 0.00 | 0.00 | 0.04 | 0.00 | 0.00 | 0.00 | 0.00 | 0.00 | 0.00 | 0.00 | 0.03 |
| 蛋类 Eggs | 0.00 | 0.00 | 0.02 | 0.03 | 0.01 | 0.00 | 0.00 | 0.00 | 0.00 | 0.00 | 0.00 | 0.01 | 0.01 | 0.01 | 0.01 | 0.00 | 0.00 | 0.01 | 0.09 | 0.00 | 0.00 | 0.01 | 0.02 | 0.01 | 0.01 |
| 水产类 Aquatic foods | 0.00 | 0.01 | 0.00 | 0.01 | 0.00 | 0.00 | 0.01 | 0.00 | 0.00 | 0.00 | 0.00 | 0.00 | 0.06 | 0.02 | 0.02 | 0.00 | 0.02 | 0.02 | 0.51 | 0.00 | 0.04 | 1.86 | 0.02 | 0.00 | 0.11 |
| 乳类 Dairy products | 0.00 | 0.00 | 0.01 | 0.00 | 0.00 | 0.00 | 0.00 | 0.00 | 0.00 | 0.00 | 0.01 | 0.00 | 0.00 | 0.00 | 0.00 | 0.00 | 0.00 | 0.00 | 0.00 | 0.00 | 0.00 | 0.00 | 0.00 | 0.00 | 0.00 |
| 蔬菜类 Vegetables | 0.26 | 0.20 | 0.00 | 0.15 | 0.14 | 0.09 | 0.00 | 0.00 | 0.00 | 0.00 | 0.00 | 0.00 | 0.00 | 0.00 | 0.00 | 0.00 | 0.17 | 0.17 | 0.00 | 0.14 | 0.00 | 0.00 | 0.09 | 0.00 | 0.06 |
| 水果类 Fruits | 0.02 | 0.00 | 0.00 | 0.04 | 0.00 | 0.01 | 0.00 | 0.01 | 0.00 | 0.00 | 0.00 | 0.05 | 0.00 | 0.00 | 0.00 | 0.00 | 0.03 | 0.04 | 0.05 | 0.03 | 0.00 | 0.00 | 0.00 | 0.00 | 0.01 |
| 糖类 Sugar | 0.00 | 0.00 | 0.00 | 0.00 | 0.00 | 0.00 | 0.00 | 0.00 | 0.00 | 0.00 | 0.00 | 0.00 | 0.00 | 0.00 | 0.00 | 0.00 | 0.00 | 0.00 | 0.00 | 0.00 | 0.00 | 0.00 | 0.00 | 0.00 | 0.00 |
| 水及饮料类 Water and beverages | 0.00 | 0.00 | 0.00 | 0.00 | 0.00 | 0.00 | 0.00 | 0.00 | 0.00 | 0.00 | 0.00 | 0.00 | 1.27 | 0.00 | 0.00 | 0.00 | 0.00 | 0.00 | 0.00 | 0.00 | 0.00 | 0.00 | 0.00 | 0.00 | 0.00 |
| 酒类 Alcohol beverages | 0.00 | 0.00 | 0.00 | 0.00 | 0.00 | 0.00 | 0.00 | 0.00 | 0.00 | 0.00 | 0.00 | 0.00 | 0.00 | 0.00 | 0.00 | 0.00 | 0.00 | 0.00 | 0.00 | 0.00 | 0.00 | 0.00 | 0.00 | 0.00 | 0.00 |
| 合计 SUM | 0.28 | 0.94 | 0.06 | 0.71 | 0.16 | 0.10 | 0.01 | 0.35 | 0.00 | 0.00 | 0.05 | 0.07 | 1.27 | 0.65 | 0.04 | 0.02 | 0.27 | 0.25 | 0.89 | 0.54 | 0.04 | 1.87 | 0.63 | 0.01 | 0.38 |

附表 9-18 第六次中国总膳食研究双酚 A 的膳食来源（单位：%）
Annexed Table 9-18　Dietary sources of BPA from the 6th China TDS (Unit: %)

| 膳食类别<br>Category | 黑龙江<br>HL | 辽宁<br>LN | 河北<br>HE | 北京<br>BJ | 吉林<br>JL | 山西<br>SX | 陕西<br>SN | 河南<br>HA | 宁夏<br>NX | 内蒙古<br>NM | 青海<br>QH | 甘肃<br>GS | 上海<br>SH | 福建<br>FJ | 江西<br>JX | 江苏<br>JS | 浙江<br>ZJ | 山东<br>SD | 湖北<br>HB | 四川<br>SC | 广西<br>GX | 湖南<br>HN | 广东<br>GD | 贵州<br>GZ | 全国平均<br>AVG |
|---|---|---|---|---|---|---|---|---|---|---|---|---|---|---|---|---|---|---|---|---|---|---|---|---|---|
| 谷类 Cereals | 52.0 | 62.4 | 44.1 | 75.2 | 16.0 | 43.6 | 74.8 | 39.3 | 23.6 | 39.3 | 53.9 | 38.4 | 30.6 | 42.2 | 32.6 | 22.7 | 17.9 | 35.6 | 22.9 | 31.0 | 26.2 | 71.5 | 7.8 | 63.2 | 40.3 |
| 豆类 Legumes | 0.9 | 1.5 | 13.4 | 5.4 | 8.3 | 2.9 | 1.9 | 0.4 | 0.8 | 1.3 | 0.1 | 2.3 | 4.2 | 2.8 | 3.4 | 0.6 | 4.1 | 0.6 | 44.8 | 10.6 | 3.7 | 3.1 | 0.5 | 3.8 | 5.1 |
| 薯类 Potatoes | 5.2 | 1.7 | 1.2 | 0.7 | 23.1 | 4.5 | 1.5 | 1.6 | 1.6 | 2.9 | 12.2 | 7.8 | 1.9 | 2.4 | 2.0 | 0.8 | 1.0 | 1.4 | 4.6 | 5.2 | 0.3 | 2.0 | 0.5 | 0.7 | 3.6 |
| 肉类 Meats | 2.9 | 21.2 | 4.4 | 1.5 | 8.4 | 20.5 | 0.4 | 2.8 | 0.8 | 7.3 | 22.2 | 11.3 | 19.6 | 4.2 | 1.6 | 7.2 | 17.2 | 2.4 | 2.6 | 16.6 | 9.5 | 4.2 | 4.1 | 10.5 | 8.5 |
| 蛋类 Eggs | 1.6 | 1.3 | 4.1 | 0.2 | 1.0 | 0.3 | 0.5 | 0.1 | 0.1 | 0.4 | 0.1 | 1.2 | 2.3 | 0.4 | 1.1 | 0.5 | 0.3 | 0.5 | 1.3 | 0.8 | 0.1 | 0.3 | 0.3 | 0.2 | 0.8 |
| 水产类 Aquatic foods | 1.0 | 3.5 | 1.8 | 0.5 | 0.8 | 2.3 | 0.0 | 0.2 | 0.0 | 1.2 | 0.9 | 0.2 | 8.2 | 8.9 | 7.2 | 2.2 | 8.4 | 4.4 | 3.5 | 0.7 | 6.1 | 2.5 | 3.0 | 0.2 | 2.8 |
| 乳类 Dairy products | 0.5 | 0.5 | 1.1 | 0.3 | 0.2 | 0.4 | 0.1 | 0.0 | 0.1 | 0.3 | 0.3 | 0.2 | 2.1 | 0.5 | 0.4 | 0.2 | 0.3 | 0.2 | 0.1 | 0.6 | 0.5 | 0.2 | 0.7 | 0.3 | 0.4 |
| 蔬菜类 Vegetables | 11.6 | 3.1 | 11.2 | 9.0 | 8.1 | 11.5 | 18.6 | 2.7 | 2.0 | 15.8 | 6.1 | 11.8 | 14.6 | 22.8 | 29.1 | 11.4 | 40.9 | 14.6 | 14.2 | 26.8 | 8.3 | 10.8 | 7.7 | 17.0 | 13.7 |
| 水果类 Fruits | 5.2 | 0.9 | 5.2 | 2.8 | 6.3 | 6.7 | 0.5 | 0.7 | 17.3 | 5.4 | 0.1 | 9.2 | 5.7 | 3.1 | 2.3 | 46.5 | 1.4 | 3.6 | 1.6 | 1.1 | 37.8 | 0.7 | 1.3 | 0.1 | 6.9 |
| 糖类 Sugar | 0.7 | 0.0 | 0.2 | 0.1 | 0.2 | 0.1 | 0.0 | 0.0 | 0.0 | 0.4 | 0.0 | 0.1 | 0.4 | 0.0 | 0.1 | 0.0 | 0.1 | 0.2 | 0.0 | 0.3 | 0.0 | 0.0 | 0.0 | 0.0 | 0.1 |
| 水及饮料类 Water and beverages | 17.6 | 3.7 | 13.1 | 4.2 | 27.0 | 7.2 | 1.5 | 52.2 | 53.7 | 24.1 | 4.0 | 17.3 | 10.1 | 12.5 | 20.0 | 6.5 | 7.7 | 35.5 | 3.8 | 6.3 | 7.2 | 4.6 | 74.1 | 4.1 | 17.4 |

续表

| 膳食类别<br>Category | 黑龙江<br>HL | 辽宁<br>LN | 河北<br>HE | 北京<br>BJ | 吉林<br>JL | 山西<br>SX | 陕西<br>SN | 河南<br>HA | 宁夏<br>NX | 内蒙古<br>NM | 青海<br>QH | 甘肃<br>GS | 上海<br>SH | 福建<br>FJ | 江西<br>JX | 江苏<br>JS | 浙江<br>ZJ | 山东<br>SD | 湖北<br>HB | 四川<br>SC | 广西<br>GX | 湖南<br>HN | 广东<br>GD | 贵州<br>GZ | 全国平均<br>AVG |
|---|---|---|---|---|---|---|---|---|---|---|---|---|---|---|---|---|---|---|---|---|---|---|---|---|---|
| 酒类<br>Alcohol beverages | 0.9 | 0.3 | 0.2 | 0.1 | 0.5 | 0.0 | 0.0 | 0.0 | 0.0 | 1.6 | 0.0 | 0.0 | 0.3 | 0.2 | 0.4 | 1.5 | 0.6 | 1.0 | 0.4 | 0.1 | 0.2 | 0.1 | 0.0 | 0.0 | 0.4 |

附表 9-19 第六次中国总膳食研究双酚 S 的膳食来源（单位：%）

Annexed Table 9-19 Dietary sources of BPS from the 6$^{th}$ China TDS (Unit: %)

| 膳食类别<br>Category | 黑龙江<br>HL | 辽宁<br>LN | 河北<br>HE | 北京<br>BJ | 吉林<br>JL | 山西<br>SX | 陕西<br>SN | 河南<br>HA | 宁夏<br>NX | 内蒙古<br>NM | 青海<br>QH | 甘肃<br>GS | 上海<br>SH | 福建<br>FJ | 江西<br>JX | 江苏<br>JS | 浙江<br>ZJ | 山东<br>SD | 湖北<br>HB | 四川<br>SC | 广西<br>GX | 湖南<br>HN | 广东<br>GD | 贵州<br>GZ | 全国平均<br>AVG |
|---|---|---|---|---|---|---|---|---|---|---|---|---|---|---|---|---|---|---|---|---|---|---|---|---|---|
| 谷类<br>Cereals | 39.3 | 14.9 | 79.3 | 38.2 | 17.5 | 72.0 | 8.9 | 33.7 | 42.4 | 56.1 | 76.6 | 65.0 | 1.8 | 6.4 | 23.9 | 82.4 | 25.6 | 46.8 | 7.6 | 2.9 | 12.6 | 11.8 | 4.2 | 7.1 | 32.4 |
| 豆类<br>Legumes | 23.0 | 11.4 | 2.3 | 1.7 | 7.2 | 0.4 | 20.1 | 0.7 | 22.4 | 2.9 | 0.1 | 7.3 | 2.2 | 3.5 | 0.9 | 1.2 | 1.8 | 8.5 | 23.9 | 78.5 | 7.0 | 0.3 | 51.6 | 2.8 | 11.7 |
| 薯类<br>Potatoes | 2.8 | 1.1 | 0.4 | 1.0 | 2.7 | 1.4 | 4.1 | 2.4 | 0.9 | 3.4 | 0.9 | 10.0 | 0.1 | 0.1 | 6.1 | 0.1 | 0.7 | 0.7 | 2.3 | 0.4 | 0.2 | 6.4 | 3.4 | 2.7 | 2.3 |
| 肉类<br>Meats | 4.1 | 34.4 | 11.0 | 0.3 | 1.5 | 20.1 | 33.9 | 57.6 | 3.9 | 6.4 | 3.0 | 1.3 | 65.3 | 83.1 | 5.1 | 7.7 | 35.1 | 31.8 | 40.8 | 7.1 | 18.0 | 56.0 | 15.8 | 67.3 | 25.4 |
| 蛋类<br>Eggs | 0.9 | 0.1 | 0.8 | 7.2 | 3.3 | 0.1 | 0.0 | 0.1 | 0.9 | 0.0 | 0.3 | 0.6 | 1.4 | 0.1 | 7.7 | 0.0 | 0.0 | 1.0 | 0.1 | 0.0 | 0.1 | 0.8 | 0.6 | 0.1 | 1.1 |
| 水产类<br>Aquatic foods | 16.9 | 0.7 | 2.1 | 6.5 | 2.9 | 0.9 | 1.1 | 0.8 | 0.0 | 0.3 | 2.1 | 0.1 | 16.6 | 2.9 | 1.4 | 0.3 | 0.3 | 2.1 | 11.7 | 0.7 | 3.8 | 12.5 | 0.4 | 0.2 | 3.6 |
| 乳类<br>Dairy products | 0.6 | 0.0 | 0.0 | 0.3 | 0.7 | 0.0 | 0.2 | 0.0 | 0.1 | 0.1 | 1.0 | 0.2 | 0.0 | 0.0 | 0.2 | 0.0 | 0.0 | 0.0 | 0.0 | 0.0 | 0.2 | 0.3 | 0.2 | 0.1 | 0.2 |
| 蔬菜类<br>Vegetables | 8.2 | 16.4 | 1.6 | 11.1 | 22.3 | 4.5 | 26.4 | 3.4 | 26.4 | 19.9 | 3.5 | 3.3 | 2.0 | 3.4 | 13.8 | 6.8 | 35.6 | 5.3 | 10.9 | 9.4 | 8.2 | 7.1 | 15.0 | 16.2 | 11.7 |

续表

| 膳食类别<br>Category | 黑龙江<br>HL | 辽宁<br>LN | 河北<br>HE | 北京<br>BJ | 吉林<br>JL | 山西<br>SX | 陕西<br>SN | 河南<br>HA | 宁夏<br>NX | 内蒙古<br>NM | 青海<br>QH | 甘肃<br>GS | 上海<br>SH | 福建<br>FJ | 江西<br>JX | 江苏<br>JS | 浙江<br>ZJ | 山东<br>SD | 湖北<br>HB | 四川<br>SC | 广西<br>GX | 湖南<br>HN | 广东<br>GD | 贵州<br>GZ | 全国平均<br>AVG |
|---|---|---|---|---|---|---|---|---|---|---|---|---|---|---|---|---|---|---|---|---|---|---|---|---|---|
| 水果类<br>Fruits | 1.3 | 6.4 | 0.6 | 3.2 | 12.0 | 0.3 | 3.4 | 0.8 | 2.1 | 8.1 | 0.2 | 2.1 | 0.7 | 0.3 | 7.8 | 0.1 | 0.3 | 1.7 | 2.1 | 0.1 | 7.3 | 1.1 | 0.7 | 0.4 | 2.6 |
| 糖类<br>Sugar | 0.1 | 0.0 | 0.0 | 0.0 | 0.1 | 0.0 | 0.0 | 0.0 | 0.0 | 0.0 | 0.0 | 0.0 | 0.0 | 0.0 | 0.0 | 0.0 | 0.0 | 0.0 | 0.0 | 0.0 | 0.1 | 0.0 | 0.0 | 0.0 | 0.0 |
| 水及饮料类<br>Water and beverages | 2.8 | 14.6 | 1.9 | 30.1 | 29.6 | 0.4 | 1.7 | 0.6 | 0.9 | 2.8 | 12.5 | 8.3 | 9.9 | 0.2 | 32.8 | 1.3 | 0.5 | 1.8 | 0.4 | 0.6 | 41.6 | 3.7 | 8.1 | 3.1 | 8.8 |
| 酒类<br>Alcohol beverages | 0.1 | 0.0 | 0.0 | 0.3 | 0.2 | 0.0 | 0.0 | 0.0 | 0.0 | 0.0 | 0.0 | 1.9 | 0.0 | 0.0 | 0.2 | 0.0 | 0.0 | 0.3 | 0.1 | 0.0 | 0.9 | 0.1 | 0.0 | 0.0 | 0.2 |

附表 9-20　第六次中国总膳食研究双酚 F 的膳食来源（单位：%）

Annexed Table 9-20　Dietary sources of BPF from the 6$^{th}$ China TDS (Unit: %)

| 膳食类别<br>Category | 黑龙江<br>HL | 辽宁<br>LN | 河北<br>HE | 北京<br>BJ | 山西<br>SX | 陕西<br>SN | 河南<br>HA | 宁夏<br>NX | 内蒙古<br>NM | 甘肃<br>GS | 福建<br>FJ | 江苏<br>JS | 山东<br>SD | 四川<br>SC | 广西<br>GX | 湖南<br>HN | 广东<br>GD | 贵州<br>GZ | 全国平均<br>AVG |
|---|---|---|---|---|---|---|---|---|---|---|---|---|---|---|---|---|---|---|---|
| 谷类<br>Cereals | 0.0 | 0.0 | 0.0 | 0.0 | 0.0 | 0.0 | 0.0 | 0.0 | 0.0 | 0.0 | 0.0 | 0.0 | 0.0 | 0.0 | 0.0 | 0.0 | 0.0 | 100.0 | 5.6 |
| 豆类<br>Legumes | 0.0 | 100 | 0.0 | 45.1 | 100 | 100 | 0.0 | 0.0 | 0.0 | 64.0 | 0.0 | 100 | 100 | 100 | 32.9 | 0.0 | 0.0 | 0.0 | 41.2 |
| 薯类<br>Potatoes | 0.0 | 0.0 | 0.0 | 0.0 | 0.0 | 0.0 | 0.0 | 0.0 | 0.0 | 0.0 | 0.0 | 0.0 | 0.0 | 0.0 | 0.0 | 0.0 | 0.0 | 0.0 | 5.6 |
| 肉类<br>Meats | 0.0 | 0.0 | 0.0 | 54.9 | 0.0 | 0.0 | 0.0 | 100 | 100 | 0.0 | 0.0 | 0.0 | 0.0 | 0.0 | 18.1 | 100 | 0.0 | 0.0 | 20.7 |
| 蛋类<br>Eggs | 0.0 | 0.0 | 0.0 | 0.0 | 0.0 | 0.0 | 100.0 | 0.0 | 0.0 | 0.0 | 0.0 | 0.0 | 0.0 | 0.0 | 0.0 | 0.0 | 100 | 0.0 | 0.0 |
| 水产类<br>Aquatic foods | 29.1 | 0.0 | 0.0 | 0.0 | 0.0 | 0.0 | 0.0 | 0.0 | 0.0 | 0.0 | 0.0 | 0.0 | 0.0 | 0.0 | 0.0 | 0.0 | 0.0 | 0.0 | 7.2 |

续表

| 膳食类别<br>Category | 黑龙江<br>HL | 辽宁<br>LN | 河北<br>HE | 北京<br>BJ | 山西<br>SX | 陕西<br>SN | 河南<br>HA | 宁夏<br>NX | 内蒙古<br>NM | 甘肃<br>GS | 福建<br>FJ | 江苏<br>JS | 山东<br>SD | 四川<br>SC | 广西<br>GX | 湖南<br>HN | 广东<br>GD | 贵州<br>GZ | 全国平均<br>AVG |
|---|---|---|---|---|---|---|---|---|---|---|---|---|---|---|---|---|---|---|---|
| 乳类<br>Dairy products | 0.0 | 0.0 | 0.0 | 0.0 | 0.0 | 0.0 | 0.0 | 0.0 | 0.0 | 0.0 | 0.0 | 0.0 | 0.0 | 0.0 | 0.0 | 0.0 | 0.0 | 0.0 | 0.0 |
| 蔬菜类<br>Vegetables | 0.0 | 0.0 | 0.0 | 0.0 | 0.0 | 0.0 | 0.0 | 0.0 | 0.0 | 8.3 | 100 | 0.0 | 0.0 | 0.0 | 49.0 | 0.0 | 0.0 | 0.0 | 8.3 |
| 水果类<br>Fruits | 67.2 | 0.0 | 100 | 0.0 | 0.0 | 0.0 | 0.0 | 0.0 | 0.0 | 36.0 | 0.0 | 0.0 | 0.0 | 0.0 | 0.0 | 0.0 | 0.0 | 0.0 | 11.3 |
| 糖类<br>Sugar | 3.6 | 0.0 | 0.0 | 0.0 | 0.0 | 0.0 | 0.0 | 0.0 | 0.0 | 0.0 | 0.0 | 0.0 | 0.0 | 0.0 | 0.0 | 0.0 | 0.0 | 0.0 | 0.2 |
| 水及饮料类<br>Water and beverages | 0.0 | 0.0 | 0.0 | 0.0 | 0.0 | 0.0 | 0.0 | 0.0 | 0.0 | 0.0 | 0.0 | 0.0 | 0.0 | 0.0 | 0.0 | 0.0 | 0.0 | 0.0 | 0.0 |
| 酒类<br>Alcohol beverages | 0.0 | 0.0 | 0.0 | 0.0 | 0.0 | 0.0 | 0.0 | 0.0 | 0.0 | 0.0 | 0.0 | 0.0 | 0.0 | 0.0 | 0.0 | 0.0 | 0.0 | 0.0 | 0.0 |

附表 9-21 第六次中国总膳食研究双酚 AF 的膳食来源（单位：%）

Annexed Table 9-21 Dietary sources of BPAF from the 6$^{th}$ China TDS (Unit: %)

| 膳食类别<br>Category | 黑龙江<br>HL | 辽宁<br>LN | 河北<br>HE | 北京<br>BJ | 吉林<br>JL | 山西<br>SX | 陕西<br>SN | 河南<br>HA | 内蒙古<br>NM | 青海<br>QH | 甘肃<br>GS | 上海<br>SH | 福建<br>FJ | 江西<br>JX | 江苏<br>JS | 浙江<br>ZJ | 山东<br>SD | 湖北<br>HB | 四川<br>SC | 广西<br>GX | 湖南<br>HN | 广东<br>GD | 贵州<br>GZ | 全国平均<br>AVG |
|---|---|---|---|---|---|---|---|---|---|---|---|---|---|---|---|---|---|---|---|---|---|---|---|---|
| 谷类<br>Cereals | 0.0 | 0.0 | 0.0 | 64.8 | 0.0 | 0.0 | 0.0 | 98.4 | 0.0 | 0.0 | 0.0 | 94.4 | 90.9 | 0.0 | 0.0 | 0.0 | 0.0 | 25.8 | 67.7 | 0.0 | 0.0 | 78.2 | 0.0 | 22.6 |
| 豆类<br>Legumes | 0.0 | 0.0 | 0.0 | 0.0 | 0.0 | 0.0 | 0.0 | 0.0 | 0.0 | 0.0 | 0.0 | 0.0 | 0.0 | 0.0 | 0.0 | 4.0 | 0.0 | 0.0 | 0.0 | 0.0 | 0.0 | 0.0 | 0.0 | 0.0 |
| 薯类<br>Potatoes | 0.0 | 3.8 | 53.8 | 0.0 | 0.0 | 0.0 | 0.0 | 0.0 | 0.0 | 58.5 | 14.3 | 0.0 | 1.8 | 27.7 | 100.0 | 15.5 | 0.0 | 0.0 | 0.0 | 0.0 | 0.0 | 1.2 | 0.0 | 8.4 |
| 肉类<br>Meats | 0.0 | 73.7 | 0.0 | 3.6 | 0.0 | 0.0 | 0.0 | 0.0 | 0.0 | 0.0 | 0.0 | 0.0 | 3.3 | 0.0 | 0.0 | 0.0 | 0.0 | 0.0 | 0.0 | 0.0 | 0.0 | 0.0 | 0.0 | 7.3 |

续表

| 膳食类别 Category | 黑龙江 HL | 辽宁 LN | 河北 HE | 北京 BJ | 吉林 JL | 山西 SX | 陕西 SN | 河南 HA | 内蒙古 NM | 青海 QH | 甘肃 GS | 上海 SH | 福建 FJ | 江西 JX | 江苏 JS | 浙江 ZJ | 山东 SD | 湖北 HB | 四川 SC | 广西 GX | 湖南 HN | 广东 GD | 贵州 GZ | 全国平均 AVG |
|---|---|---|---|---|---|---|---|---|---|---|---|---|---|---|---|---|---|---|---|---|---|---|---|---|
| 蛋类 Eggs | 0.0 | 0.0 | 31.1 | 3.9 | 8.0 | 0.0 | 0.0 | 0.0 | 0.0 | 0.0 | 14.7 | 1.1 | 1.2 | 20.8 | 0.0 | 0.0 | 6.0 | 10.5 | 0.0 | 0.0 | 0.6 | 3.7 | 75.6 | 7.7 |
| 水产类 Aquatic foods | 0.0 | 1.0 | 5.4 | 1.0 | 0.0 | 1.8 | 12.2 | 0.0 | 78.9 | 2.6 | 1.6 | 4.5 | 2.8 | 51.5 | 0.0 | 7.9 | 7.5 | 57.7 | 0.7 | 100 | 99.4 | 2.9 | 24.4 | 20.2 |
| 乳类 Dairy products | 0.0 | 0.0 | 9.4 | 0.0 | 0.0 | 0.0 | 87.8 | 0.0 | 0.0 | 29.1 | 0.0 | 0.0 | 0.0 | 0.0 | 0.0 | 0.0 | 0.0 | 0.0 | 0.0 | 0.0 | 0.0 | 0.0 | 0.0 | 5.5 |
| 蔬菜类 Vegetables | 92.1 | 21.5 | 0.0 | 21.1 | 92.0 | 88.4 | 0.0 | 0.0 | 0.0 | 0.0 | 0.0 | 0.0 | 0.0 | 0.0 | 0.0 | 62.8 | 68.4 | 0.0 | 26.4 | 0.0 | 0.0 | 14.0 | 0.0 | 21.2 |
| 水果类 Fruits | 7.5 | 0.0 | 0.0 | 5.6 | 0.0 | 9.8 | 0.0 | 1.6 | 0.0 | 9.9 | 69.4 | 0.0 | | | 0.0 | 9.8 | 18.1 | 6.0 | 5.2 | 0.0 | 0.0 | 0.0 | 0.0 | 6.2 |
| 糖类 Sugar | 0.5 | 0.0 | 0.3 | 0.0 | 0.0 | 0.0 | 0.0 | 0.0 | 21.1 | 0.0 | 0.0 | 0.0 | | | 0.0 | 0.0 | 0.1 | 0.0 | 0.0 | 0.0 | 0.0 | 0.0 | 0.0 | 1.0 |
| 水及饮料类 Water and beverages | 0.0 | 0.0 | 0.0 | 0.0 | 0.0 | 0.0 | 0.0 | 0.0 | 0.0 | 0.0 | 0.0 | 0.0 | | | 0.0 | 0.0 | 0.0 | 0.0 | 0.0 | 0.0 | 0.0 | 0.0 | 0.0 | 0.0 |
| 酒类 Alcohol beverages | 0.0 | 0.0 | 0.0 | 0.0 | 0.0 | 0.0 | 0.0 | 0.0 | 0.0 | 0.0 | 0.0 | 0.0 | | | 0.0 | 0.0 | 0.0 | 0.0 | 0.0 | 0.0 | 0.0 | 0.0 | 0.0 | 0.0 |

附表 9-22 第六次中国总膳食研究膳食样品中 TCIPP 的含量（单位：ng/g）

Annexed Table 9-22 Levels of TCIPP in food samples from the 6$^{th}$ China TDS (Unit: ng/g)

| 膳食类别 Category | 黑龙江 HL | 辽宁 LN | 河北 HE | 北京 BJ | 吉林 JL | 山西 SX | 陕西 SN | 河南 HA | 宁夏 NX | 内蒙古 NM | 青海 QH | 甘肃 GS | 上海 SH | 福建 FJ | 江西 JX | 江苏 JS | 浙江 ZJ | 山东 SD | 湖北 HB | 四川 SC | 广西 GX | 湖南 HN | 广东 GD | 贵州 GZ | 全国平均 AVG |
|---|---|---|---|---|---|---|---|---|---|---|---|---|---|---|---|---|---|---|---|---|---|---|---|---|---|
| 肉类 Meats | 0.07 | 1.52 | 2.33 | 1.72 | 1.99 | 1.78 | 1.13 | 0.94 | 1.93 | 0.72 | 1.71 | 1.97 | 2.28 | 1.68 | 2.80 | 2.32 | 3.06 | 0.71 | 2.86 | 4.84 | 0.96 | 1.45 | 0.20 | 6.15 | 1.96 |

续表

| 膳食类别<br>Category | 黑龙江<br>HL | 辽宁<br>LN | 河北<br>HE | 北京<br>BJ | 吉林<br>JL | 山西<br>SX | 陕西<br>SN | 河南<br>HA | 宁夏<br>NX | 内蒙古<br>NM | 青海<br>QH | 甘肃<br>GS | 上海<br>SH | 福建<br>FJ | 江西<br>JX | 江苏<br>JS | 浙江<br>ZJ | 山东<br>SD | 湖北<br>HB | 四川<br>SC | 广西<br>GX | 湖南<br>HN | 广东<br>GD | 贵州<br>GZ | 全国平均<br>AVG |
|---|---|---|---|---|---|---|---|---|---|---|---|---|---|---|---|---|---|---|---|---|---|---|---|---|---|
| 蛋类 Eggs | 1.02 | 0.56 | 0.76 | 0.55 | 0.29 | 1.67 | 2.49 | 0.89 | 0.11 | 3.49 | 1.06 | 3.85 | 0.74 | 1.36 | 6.94 | 2.27 | 1.47 | 5.20 | 1.56 | 2.23 | 1.19 | 1.64 | 0.35 | 0.96 | 1.78 |
| 水产类 Aquatic foods | 0.95 | 1.00 | 1.14 | 1.31 | 0.99 | 0.23 | 1.29 | 0.59 | 2.00 | 0.56 | 0.46 | 2.29 | 0.73 | 0.98 | 25.51 | 0.30 | 1.14 | 1.24 | 1.51 | 0.94 | 0.43 | 0.67 | ND | 1.59 | 1.99 |
| 乳类 Dairy products | 0.93 | 0.98 | 0.69 | 0.64 | 0.50 | 0.91 | 0.84 | 0.57 | 0.78 | 0.45 | 0.12 | 0.63 | 0.98 | 0.90 | 0.82 | 0.35 | 0.78 | 0.63 | 1.84 | 1.08 | 0.19 | 0.42 | 0.57 | 0.52 | 0.71 |

注：平均值计算中，ND 以 1/2 检出限（LOD）计

Note: in calculation of averages (AVG), values not detected (ND) were treated as being equal to half of the detection of limit (LOD)

附表 Table 9-23　第六次中国总膳食研究膳食样品中 TCEP 的含量（单位：ng/g）

Annexed Table 9-23　Levels of TCEP in food samples from the 6$^{th}$ China TDS (Unit: ng/g)

| 膳食类别<br>Category | 黑龙江<br>HL | 辽宁<br>LN | 河北<br>HE | 北京<br>BJ | 吉林<br>JL | 山西<br>SX | 陕西<br>SN | 河南<br>HA | 宁夏<br>NX | 内蒙古<br>NM | 青海<br>QH | 甘肃<br>GS | 上海<br>SH | 福建<br>FJ | 江西<br>JX | 江苏<br>JS | 浙江<br>ZJ | 山东<br>SD | 湖北<br>HB | 四川<br>SC | 广西<br>GX | 湖南<br>HN | 广东<br>GD | 贵州<br>GZ | 全国平均<br>AVG |
|---|---|---|---|---|---|---|---|---|---|---|---|---|---|---|---|---|---|---|---|---|---|---|---|---|---|
| 肉类 Meats | 2.04 | 1.26 | 1.38 | 1.61 | 3.00 | 0.52 | 0.51 | 0.51 | 1.19 | 0.86 | 1.00 | 0.39 | 1.64 | 1.85 | 0.37 | 0.94 | 1.23 | 1.13 | 0.90 | 0.86 | 1.12 | 0.51 | 0.97 | 0.87 | 1.11 |
| 蛋类 Eggs | 3.03 | 0.30 | 2.23 | 2.45 | 4.13 | 1.52 | 0.69 | 0.83 | 1.08 | 0.82 | 1.32 | 0.84 | 0.43 | 3.55 | 0.63 | 1.02 | 0.43 | 2.79 | 1.29 | 0.86 | 1.34 | 0.87 | 0.22 | 1.26 | 1.41 |
| 水产类 Aquatic foods | 1.14 | 0.53 | 0.63 | 1.63 | 3.08 | 0.50 | 0.62 | 0.82 | 0.79 | 0.80 | 0.45 | 0.57 | 0.65 | 1.46 | 0.72 | 0.44 | 1.05 | 0.79 | 0.85 | 0.83 | 0.99 | 0.58 | 0.93 | 0.89 | 0.91 |
| 乳类 Dairy products | 0.91 | 0.28 | 0.23 | 0.20 | 0.24 | 0.42 | 0.26 | 0.11 | 0.12 | 0.14 | 0.25 | 0.29 | 0.61 | 0.57 | 0.19 | 0.28 | 0.22 | 0.23 | 0.23 | 0.28 | 0.15 | 0.19 | 0.26 | 0.12 | 0.28 |

附表 9-24 第六次中国总膳食研究膳食样品中 TnBP 的含量（单位：ng/g）
Annexed Table 9-24 Levels of TnBP in food samples from the 6<sup>th</sup> China TDS (Unit: ng/g)

| 膳食类别<br>Category | 黑龙江<br>HL | 辽宁<br>LN | 河北<br>HE | 北京<br>BJ | 吉林<br>JL | 山西<br>SX | 陕西<br>SN | 河南<br>HA | 宁夏<br>NX | 内蒙古<br>NM | 青海<br>QH | 甘肃<br>GS | 上海<br>SH | 福建<br>FJ | 江西<br>JX | 江苏<br>JS | 浙江<br>ZJ | 山东<br>SD | 湖北<br>HB | 四川<br>SC | 广西<br>GX | 湖南<br>HN | 广东<br>GD | 贵州<br>GZ | 全国平均<br>AVG |
|---|---|---|---|---|---|---|---|---|---|---|---|---|---|---|---|---|---|---|---|---|---|---|---|---|---|
| 肉类 Meats | 0.17 | 0.08 | 0.13 | 0.12 | 0.25 | 0.19 | 0.05 | 0.26 | 0.51 | ND | 0.14 | 0.23 | 0.33 | 0.26 | 0.07 | 0.31 | 0.09 | 0.09 | 0.05 | ND | 0.04 | 0.39 | 0.48 | 0.16 | 0.18 |
| 蛋类 Eggs | 0.25 | 0.05 | ND | ND | 0.05 | 0.15 | ND | 0.14 | 0.08 | 0.28 | 0.07 | 0.13 | 0.01 | 0.02 | 0.09 | 0.04 | ND | 0.55 | 0.22 | ND | ND | 0.10 | 0.01 | ND | 0.09 |
| 水产类 Aquatic foods | 0.11 | 0.06 | 0.24 | 0.05 | 0.13 | 0.10 | 0.06 | 0.19 | 0.15 | 0.03 | 0.16 | 0.19 | 0.13 | 0.15 | 0.21 | 0.07 | 0.14 | 0.14 | 0.14 | 0.06 | 0.34 | 0.08 | 0.14 | 0.10 | 0.13 |
| 乳类 Dairy products | 0.09 | 0.21 | 0.13 | 0.02 | 0.06 | 0.04 | 0.16 | 0.54 | 0.32 | 0.07 | 0.04 | 0.18 | 0.07 | 0.04 | 0.12 | 0.09 | 0.03 | 0.11 | 0.17 | 0.04 | 0.01 | 0.12 | 0.07 | 0.36 | 0.13 |

注：平均值计算中，ND 以 1/2 检出限（LOD）计
Note: in calculation of averages (AVG), values not detected (ND) were treated as being equal to half of the detection of limit (LOD)

附表 9-25 第六次中国总膳食研究膳食样品中 TEHP 的含量（单位：ng/g）
Annexed Table 9-25 Levels of TEHP in food samples from the 6<sup>th</sup> China TDS (Unit: ng/g)

| 膳食类别<br>Category | 黑龙江<br>HL | 辽宁<br>LN | 河北<br>HE | 北京<br>BJ | 吉林<br>JL | 山西<br>SX | 陕西<br>SN | 河南<br>HA | 宁夏<br>NX | 内蒙古<br>NM | 青海<br>QH | 甘肃<br>GS | 上海<br>SH | 福建<br>FJ | 江西<br>JX | 江苏<br>JS | 浙江<br>ZJ | 山东<br>SD | 湖北<br>HB | 四川<br>SC | 广西<br>GX | 湖南<br>HN | 广东<br>GD | 贵州<br>GZ | 全国平均<br>AVG |
|---|---|---|---|---|---|---|---|---|---|---|---|---|---|---|---|---|---|---|---|---|---|---|---|---|---|
| 肉类 Meats | 0.63 | 0.02 | 0.20 | 0.63 | 1.33 | 0.03 | 0.03 | 1.38 | 2.06 | 0.55 | 0.16 | 0.14 | 0.07 | ND | 3.23 | 0.81 | 0.04 | 0.09 | 5.56 | 0.15 | 0.05 | 0.26 | 0.08 | 1.69 | 0.80 |
| 蛋类 Eggs | 0.07 | 0.01 | 0.06 | 0.01 | 0.04 | 0.15 | 0.41 | 0.09 | 0.05 | 0.01 | 2.62 | 0.22 | 0.10 | 0.02 | 0.12 | 0.58 | 0.02 | 5.77 | 2.15 | 0.07 | 0.29 | 0.05 | ND | 0.07 | 0.54 |
| 水产类 Aquatic foods | 0.33 | 0.01 | 0.10 | 0.06 | 18.48 | 0.21 | 0.21 | 0.25 | 2.62 | 0.05 | 1.24 | 0.25 | 2.11 | 0.01 | 0.14 | 0.01 | 0.03 | 1.73 | 0.64 | 0.17 | 0.12 | 0.19 | 0.03 | 0.08 | 1.21 |
| 乳类 Dairy products | 0.09 | 0.03 | 0.80 | 0.01 | 2.69 | 0.16 | 0.43 | 4.45 | 0.22 | 0.04 | 0.99 | 0.02 | ND | ND | 0.02 | 3.51 | 0.02 | 1.28 | 0.65 | 0.10 | 1.10 | 3.01 | 0.01 | 0.02 | 0.82 |

附表 9-26 第六次中国总膳食研究膳食样品中 EHDPP 的含量（单位：ng/g）

Annexed Table 9-26 Levels of EHDPP in food samples from the 6th China TDS (Unit: ng/g)

| 膳食类别 Category | 黑龙江 HL | 辽宁 LN | 河北 HE | 北京 BJ | 吉林 JL | 山西 SX | 陕西 SN | 河南 HA | 宁夏 NX | 内蒙古 NM | 青海 QH | 甘肃 GS | 上海 SH | 福建 FJ | 江西 JX | 江苏 JS | 浙江 ZJ | 山东 SD | 湖北 HB | 四川 SC | 广西 GX | 湖南 HN | 广东 GD | 贵州 GZ | 全国平均 AVG |
|---|---|---|---|---|---|---|---|---|---|---|---|---|---|---|---|---|---|---|---|---|---|---|---|---|---|
| 肉类 Meats | 0.04 | 34.28 | 0.09 | 15.84 | 0.13 | 0.23 | 0.00 | 6.69 | 0.09 | 4.89 | 27.31 | 10.99 | 15.68 | 3.48 | 0.54 | 4.17 | 4.26 | 0.61 | 35.50 | 4.32 | 8.37 | 8.61 | 14.48 | 6.22 | 8.62 |
| 蛋类 Eggs | 3.00 | 8.46 | 12.85 | 4.71 | 0.87 | 0.16 | 0.01 | 1.60 | 0.05 | 0.02 | 26.21 | 14.92 | 5.62 | 1.01 | 7.71 | 3.76 | 3.34 | 1.46 | 0.59 | 4.13 | 7.37 | 0.20 | 1.10 | 0.17 | 4.56 |
| 水产类 Aquatic foods | 0.01 | 18.90 | 4.79 | 0.42 | 4.45 | 0.27 | 0.01 | 0.29 | 8.95 | 0.14 | 0.03 | 8.05 | 6.98 | 7.35 | 1.64 | 1.73 | 8.35 | 10.19 | 0.05 | 10.36 | 9.98 | 5.72 | 18.38 | 0.66 | 5.32 |
| 乳类 Dairy products | 1.63 | 1.20 | 1.53 | 0.81 | 3.48 | 0.04 | 1.51 | 0.02 | 16.63 | 0.39 | 1.99 | 0.39 | 0.84 | ND | ND | 0.84 | 8.75 | ND | 4.57 | 0.82 | 0.82 | 0.88 | 1.53 | 0.03 | 2.03 |

注：平均值计算中，ND 以 1/2 检出限（LOD）计

Note: in calculation of averages (AVG), values not detected (ND) were treated as being equal to half of the detection of limit (LOD)

附表 9-27 第六次中国总膳食研究的 TCIPP 膳食摄入量 [单位：ng/(kg bw·d)]

Annexed Table 9-27 Dietary intakes of TCIPP from the 6th China TDS [Unit: ng/(kg bw·d)]

| 膳食类别 Category | 黑龙江 HL | 辽宁 LN | 河北 HE | 北京 BJ | 吉林 JL | 山西 SX | 陕西 SN | 河南 HA | 宁夏 NX | 内蒙古 NM | 青海 QH | 甘肃 GS | 上海 SH | 福建 FJ | 江西 JX | 江苏 JS | 浙江 ZJ | 山东 SD | 湖北 HB | 四川 SC | 广西 GX | 湖南 HN | 广东 GD | 贵州 GZ | 全国平均 AVG |
|---|---|---|---|---|---|---|---|---|---|---|---|---|---|---|---|---|---|---|---|---|---|---|---|---|---|
| 肉类 Meats | 0.07 | 1.99 | 1.91 | 2.29 | 2.12 | 4.07 | 0.69 | 0.86 | 1.50 | 0.86 | 1.95 | 1.09 | 4.01 | 2.36 | 4.21 | 3.41 | 6.18 | 1.18 | 2.56 | 9.98 | 2.30 | 3.48 | 0.43 | 10.72 | 2.93 |
| 蛋类 Eggs | 0.66 | 0.48 | 0.49 | 0.40 | 0.21 | 0.76 | 1.02 | 0.42 | 0.03 | 2.16 | 0.31 | 1.58 | 0.50 | 0.53 | 2.66 | 1.08 | 0.69 | 4.52 | 0.73 | 0.59 | 0.30 | 0.60 | 0.13 | 0.25 | 0.88 |
| 水产类 Aquatic foods | 0.41 | 0.37 | 0.19 | 0.36 | 0.18 | 0.03 | 0.08 | 0.05 | 0.08 | 0.09 | 0.03 | 0.10 | 0.79 | 1.04 | 17.69 | 0.19 | 0.95 | 0.47 | 0.98 | 0.13 | 0.67 | 0.72 | 0.00 | 0.11 | 1.07 |

续表

| 膳食类别 Category | 黑龙江 HL | 辽宁 LN | 河北 HE | 北京 BJ | 吉林 JL | 山西 SX | 陕西 SN | 河南 HA | 宁夏 NX | 内蒙古 NM | 青海 QH | 甘肃 GS | 上海 SH | 福建 FJ | 江西 JX | 江苏 JS | 浙江 ZJ | 山东 SD | 湖北 HB | 四川 SC | 广西 GX | 湖南 HN | 广东 GD | 贵州 GZ | 全国平均 AVG |
|---|---|---|---|---|---|---|---|---|---|---|---|---|---|---|---|---|---|---|---|---|---|---|---|---|---|
| 乳类 Dairy products | 0.20 | 0.69 | 0.26 | 0.87 | 0.26 | 0.60 | 0.26 | 0.18 | 0.19 | 0.25 | 0.10 | 0.14 | 1.11 | 0.51 | 0.29 | 0.15 | 0.42 | 0.23 | 0.20 | 0.22 | 0.06 | 0.12 | 0.33 | 0.23 | 0.33 |
| 合计 SUM | 1.34 | 3.53 | 2.85 | 3.92 | 2.77 | 5.46 | 2.05 | 1.51 | 1.8 | 3.36 | 2.39 | 2.91 | 6.41 | 4.44 | 24.85 | 4.83 | 8.24 | 6.4 | 4.47 | 10.92 | 3.33 | 4.92 | 0.89 | 11.31 | 5.21 |

附表 9-28　第六次中国总膳食研究的 TCEP 膳食摄入量 [ 单位：ng/(kg bw・d)]
Annexed Table 9-28　Dietary intakes of TCEP from the 6$^{th}$ China TDS [Unit: ng/(kg bw・d)]

| 膳食类别 Category | 黑龙江 HL | 辽宁 LN | 河北 HE | 北京 BJ | 吉林 JL | 山西 SX | 陕西 SN | 河南 HA | 宁夏 NX | 内蒙古 NM | 青海 QH | 甘肃 GS | 上海 SH | 福建 FJ | 江西 JX | 江苏 JS | 浙江 ZJ | 山东 SD | 湖北 HB | 四川 SC | 广西 GX | 湖南 HN | 广东 GD | 贵州 GZ | 全国平均 AVG |
|---|---|---|---|---|---|---|---|---|---|---|---|---|---|---|---|---|---|---|---|---|---|---|---|---|---|
| 肉类 Meats | 2.29 | 1.65 | 1.13 | 2.15 | 3.20 | 1.19 | 0.31 | 0.47 | 0.92 | 1.03 | 1.14 | 0.21 | 2.88 | 2.60 | 0.55 | 1.38 | 2.48 | 1.88 | 0.81 | 1.79 | 2.69 | 1.22 | 2.02 | 1.51 | 1.56 |
| 蛋类 Eggs | 1.97 | 0.26 | 1.42 | 1.78 | 3.03 | 0.70 | 0.28 | 0.39 | 0.33 | 0.51 | 0.38 | 0.35 | 0.29 | 1.39 | 0.24 | 0.48 | 0.20 | 2.42 | 0.60 | 0.23 | 0.33 | 0.32 | 0.08 | 0.33 | 0.76 |
| 水产类 Aquatic foods | 0.49 | 0.20 | 0.10 | 0.45 | 0.55 | 0.06 | 0.04 | 0.06 | 0.03 | 0.13 | 0.03 | 0.03 | 0.71 | 1.55 | 0.50 | 0.28 | 0.87 | 0.30 | 0.55 | 0.11 | 1.53 | 0.62 | 0.78 | 0.06 | 0.42 |
| 乳类 Dairy products | 0.19 | 0.20 | 0.09 | 0.28 | 0.12 | 0.28 | 0.08 | 0.03 | 0.03 | 0.08 | 0.22 | 0.07 | 0.69 | 0.33 | 0.07 | 0.12 | 0.12 | 0.08 | 0.02 | 0.06 | 0.04 | 0.06 | 0.15 | 0.06 | 0.14 |
| 合计 SUM | 4.94 | 2.31 | 2.74 | 4.66 | 6.9 | 2.23 | 0.71 | 0.95 | 1.31 | 1.75 | 1.77 | 0.66 | 4.57 | 5.87 | 1.36 | 2.26 | 3.67 | 4.68 | 1.98 | 2.19 | 4.59 | 2.22 | 3.03 | 1.96 | 2.88 |

附表 9-29　第六次中国总膳食研究的 TnBP 膳食摄入量 [单位：ng/(kg bw·d)]
Annexed Table 9-29　Dietary intakes of TnBP from the 6th China TDS [Unit: ng/(kg bw·d)]

| 膳食类别<br>Category | 黑龙江<br>HL | 辽宁<br>LN | 河北<br>HE | 北京<br>BJ | 吉林<br>JL | 山西<br>SX | 陕西<br>SN | 河南<br>HA | 宁夏<br>NX | 内蒙古<br>NM | 青海<br>QH | 甘肃<br>GS | 上海<br>SH | 福建<br>FJ | 江西<br>JX | 江苏<br>JS | 浙江<br>ZJ | 山东<br>SD | 湖北<br>HB | 四川<br>SC | 广西<br>GX | 湖南<br>HN | 广东<br>GD | 贵州<br>GZ | 全国平均<br>AVG |
|---|---|---|---|---|---|---|---|---|---|---|---|---|---|---|---|---|---|---|---|---|---|---|---|---|---|
| 肉类 Meats | 0.19 | 0.11 | 0.11 | 0.16 | 0.27 | 0.44 | 0.03 | 0.24 | 0.40 | 0.00 | 0.15 | 0.13 | 0.58 | 0.37 | 0.10 | 0.45 | 0.19 | 0.15 | 0.04 | 0.00 | 0.09 | 0.95 | 1.00 | 0.28 | 0.27 |
| 蛋类 Eggs | 0.16 | 0.04 | 0.00 | 0.00 | 0.04 | 0.07 | 0.00 | 0.07 | 0.02 | 0.17 | 0.02 | 0.05 | 0.01 | 0.01 | 0.04 | 0.02 | 0.00 | 0.48 | 0.10 | 0.00 | 0.00 | 0.04 | 0.01 | 0.00 | 0.06 |
| 水产类 Aquatic foods | 0.05 | 0.02 | 0.04 | 0.01 | 0.02 | 0.01 | 0.00 | 0.01 | 0.01 | 0.00 | 0.01 | 0.01 | 0.14 | 0.16 | 0.14 | 0.04 | 0.11 | 0.05 | 0.09 | 0.01 | 0.53 | 0.08 | 0.12 | 0.01 | 0.07 |
| 乳类 Dairy products | 0.02 | 0.15 | 0.05 | 0.03 | 0.03 | 0.03 | 0.05 | 0.17 | 0.08 | 0.04 | 0.04 | 0.04 | 0.08 | 0.02 | 0.04 | 0.04 | 0.02 | 0.04 | 0.02 | 0.01 | 0.00 | 0.03 | 0.04 | 0.16 | 0.05 |
| 合计 SUM | 0.42 | 0.32 | 0.2 | 0.2 | 0.36 | 0.55 | 0.08 | 0.49 | 0.51 | 0.21 | 0.22 | 0.23 | 0.81 | 0.56 | 0.32 | 0.55 | 0.32 | 0.72 | 0.25 | 0.02 | 0.62 | 1.1 | 1.17 | 0.45 | 0.45 |

附表 9-30　第六次中国总膳食研究的 TEHP 膳食摄入量 [单位：ng/(kg bw·d)]
Annexed Table 9-30　Dietary intakes of TEHP from the 6th China TDS [Unit: ng/(kg bw·d)]

| 膳食类别<br>Category | 黑龙江<br>HL | 辽宁<br>LN | 河北<br>HE | 北京<br>BJ | 吉林<br>JL | 山西<br>SX | 陕西<br>SN | 河南<br>HA | 宁夏<br>NX | 内蒙古<br>NM | 青海<br>QH | 甘肃<br>GS | 上海<br>SH | 福建<br>FJ | 江西<br>JX | 江苏<br>JS | 浙江<br>ZJ | 山东<br>SD | 湖北<br>HB | 四川<br>SC | 广西<br>GX | 湖南<br>HN | 广东<br>GD | 贵州<br>GZ | 全国平均<br>AVG |
|---|---|---|---|---|---|---|---|---|---|---|---|---|---|---|---|---|---|---|---|---|---|---|---|---|---|
| 肉类 Meats | 0.71 | 0.03 | 0.16 | 0.84 | 1.42 | 0.07 | 0.02 | 1.27 | 1.59 | 0.65 | 0.18 | 0.08 | 0.13 | 0.00 | 4.87 | 1.20 | 0.08 | 0.15 | 4.99 | 0.30 | 0.11 | 0.61 | 0.18 | 2.94 | 0.94 |
| 蛋类 Eggs | 0.05 | 0.01 | 0.04 | 0.01 | 0.03 | 0.07 | 0.17 | 0.04 | 0.01 | 0.01 | 0.76 | 0.09 | 0.06 | 0.01 | 0.05 | 0.28 | 0.01 | 5.02 | 1.00 | 0.02 | 0.07 | 0.02 | 0.00 | 0.02 | 0.33 |
| 水产类 Aquatic foods | 0.14 | 0.00 | 0.02 | 0.02 | 3.27 | 0.03 | 0.01 | 0.02 | 0.10 | 0.01 | 0.08 | 0.01 | 2.29 | 0.01 | 0.10 | 0.01 | 0.02 | 0.65 | 0.42 | 0.02 | 0.18 | 0.21 | 0.03 | 0.01 | 0.32 |

续表

| 膳食类别<br>Category | 黑龙江<br>HL | 辽宁<br>LN | 河北<br>HE | 北京<br>BJ | 吉林<br>JL | 山西<br>SX | 陕西<br>SN | 河南<br>HA | 宁夏<br>NX | 内蒙古<br>NM | 青海<br>QH | 甘肃<br>GS | 上海<br>SH | 福建<br>FJ | 江西<br>JX | 江苏<br>JS | 浙江<br>ZJ | 山东<br>SD | 湖北<br>HB | 四川<br>SC | 广西<br>GX | 湖南<br>HN | 广东<br>GD | 贵州<br>GZ | 全国平均<br>AVG |
|---|---|---|---|---|---|---|---|---|---|---|---|---|---|---|---|---|---|---|---|---|---|---|---|---|---|
| 乳类 Dairy products | 0.02 | 0.02 | 0.31 | 0.01 | 1.38 | 0.10 | 0.13 | 1.38 | 0.05 | 0.02 | 0.84 | 0.00 | 0.01 | 0.00 | 0.01 | 1.53 | 0.01 | 0.47 | 0.07 | 0.02 | 0.32 | 0.86 | 0.01 | 0.01 | 0.32 |
| 合计 SUM | 0.92 | 0.06 | 0.53 | 0.88 | 6.1 | 0.27 | 0.33 | 2.71 | 1.75 | 0.69 | 1.86 | 0.18 | 2.49 | 0.02 | 5.03 | 3.02 | 0.12 | 6.29 | 6.48 | 0.36 | 0.68 | 1.7 | 0.22 | 2.98 | 1.91 |

附表 9-31 第六次中国总膳食研究的 EHDPP 膳食摄入量 [单位：ng/(kg bw·d)]
Annexed Table 9-31 Dietary intakes of EHDPP from the 6th China TDS [Unit: ng/(kg bw·d)]

| 膳食类别<br>Category | 黑龙江<br>HL | 辽宁<br>LN | 河北<br>HE | 北京<br>BJ | 吉林<br>JL | 山西<br>SX | 陕西<br>SN | 河南<br>HA | 宁夏<br>NX | 内蒙古<br>NM | 青海<br>QH | 甘肃<br>GS | 上海<br>SH | 福建<br>FJ | 江西<br>JX | 江苏<br>JS | 浙江<br>ZJ | 山东<br>SD | 湖北<br>HB | 四川<br>SC | 广西<br>GX | 湖南<br>HN | 广东<br>GD | 贵州<br>GZ | 全国平均<br>AVG |
|---|---|---|---|---|---|---|---|---|---|---|---|---|---|---|---|---|---|---|---|---|---|---|---|---|---|
| 肉类 Meats | 0.05 | 44.85 | 0.07 | 21.15 | 0.14 | 0.52 | 0.00 | 6.12 | 0.07 | 5.82 | 31.09 | 6.08 | 27.56 | 4.90 | 0.81 | 6.13 | 8.59 | 1.01 | 31.87 | 8.93 | 20.05 | 20.63 | 30.29 | 10.84 | 11.98 |
| 蛋类 Eggs | 1.95 | 7.23 | 8.22 | 3.42 | 0.64 | 0.07 | 0.01 | 0.76 | 0.02 | 0.01 | 7.59 | 6.12 | 3.78 | 0.40 | 2.95 | 1.79 | 1.57 | 1.27 | 0.28 | 1.09 | 1.84 | 0.07 | 0.42 | 0.04 | 2.15 |
| 水产类 Aquatic foods | 0.00 | 7.08 | 0.80 | 0.12 | 0.79 | 0.03 | 0.00 | 0.02 | 0.35 | 0.02 | 0.00 | 0.36 | 7.60 | 7.80 | 1.14 | 1.09 | 6.95 | 3.84 | 0.03 | 1.38 | 15.46 | 6.09 | 15.56 | 0.04 | 3.19 |
| 乳类 Dairy products | 0.35 | 0.85 | 0.59 | 1.10 | 1.79 | 0.03 | 0.47 | 0.01 | 4.03 | 0.21 | 1.69 | 0.09 | 0.95 | 0.00 | 0.00 | 0.37 | 4.66 | 0.00 | 0.49 | 0.16 | 0.24 | 0.25 | 0.89 | 0.02 | 0.80 |
| 合计 SUM | 2.35 | 60.01 | 9.68 | 25.79 | 3.36 | 0.65 | 0.48 | 6.91 | 4.47 | 6.06 | 40.37 | 12.65 | 39.89 | 13.1 | 4.9 | 9.38 | 21.77 | 6.12 | 32.67 | 11.56 | 37.59 | 27.04 | 47.16 | 10.94 | 18.12 |

附表 9-32 第六次中国总膳食研究 TCIPP 的膳食来源（单位：%）
Annexed Table 9-32  Dietary sources of TCIPP from the 6<sup>th</sup> China TDS (Unit: %)

| 膳食类别 Category | 黑龙江 HL | 辽宁 LN | 河北 HE | 北京 BJ | 吉林 JL | 山西 SX | 陕西 SN | 河南 HA | 宁夏 NX | 内蒙古 NM | 青海 QH | 甘肃 GS | 上海 SH | 福建 FJ | 江西 JX | 江苏 JS | 浙江 ZJ | 山东 SD | 湖北 HB | 四川 SC | 广西 GX | 湖南 HN | 广东 GD | 贵州 GZ | 全国平均 AVG |
|---|---|---|---|---|---|---|---|---|---|---|---|---|---|---|---|---|---|---|---|---|---|---|---|---|---|
| 肉类 Meats | 5.2 | 56.4 | 67.0 | 58.4 | 76.5 | 74.5 | 33.7 | 57.0 | 83.3 | 25.6 | 81.6 | 37.5 | 62.6 | 53.2 | 16.9 | 70.6 | 75.0 | 18.4 | 57.3 | 91.4 | 69.1 | 70.7 | 48.3 | 94.8 | 56.2 |
| 蛋类 Eggs | 49.3 | 13.6 | 17.2 | 10.2 | 7.6 | 13.9 | 49.8 | 27.8 | 1.7 | 64.3 | 13.0 | 54.3 | 7.8 | 11.9 | 10.7 | 22.4 | 8.4 | 70.6 | 16.3 | 5.4 | 9.0 | 12.2 | 14.6 | 2.2 | 16.9 |
| 水产类 Aquatic foods | 30.6 | 10.5 | 6.7 | 9.2 | 6.5 | 0.5 | 3.9 | 3.3 | 4.4 | 2.7 | 1.3 | 3.4 | 12.3 | 23.4 | 71.2 | 3.9 | 11.5 | 7.3 | 21.9 | 1.2 | 20.1 | 14.6 | 0.0 | 1.0 | 20.5 |
| 乳类 Dairy products | 14.9 | 19.5 | 9.1 | 22.2 | 9.4 | 11.0 | 12.7 | 11.9 | 10.6 | 7.4 | 4.2 | 4.8 | 17.3 | 11.5 | 1.2 | 3.1 | 5.1 | 3.6 | 4.5 | 2.0 | 1.8 | 2.4 | 37.1 | 2.0 | 6.3 |

附表 9-33 第六次中国总膳食研究 TCEP 的膳食来源（单位：%）
Annexed Table 9-33  Dietary sources of TCEP from the 6<sup>th</sup> China TDS (Unit: %)

| 膳食类别 Category | 黑龙江 HL | 辽宁 LN | 河北 HE | 北京 BJ | 吉林 JL | 山西 SX | 陕西 SN | 河南 HA | 宁夏 NX | 内蒙古 NM | 青海 QH | 甘肃 GS | 上海 SH | 福建 FJ | 江西 JX | 江苏 JS | 浙江 ZJ | 山东 SD | 湖北 HB | 四川 SC | 广西 GX | 湖南 HN | 广东 GD | 贵州 GZ | 全国平均 AVG |
|---|---|---|---|---|---|---|---|---|---|---|---|---|---|---|---|---|---|---|---|---|---|---|---|---|---|
| 肉类 Meats | 46.4 | 71.4 | 41.2 | 46.1 | 46.4 | 53.4 | 43.7 | 49.5 | 70.2 | 58.9 | 64.4 | 31.8 | 63.0 | 44.3 | 40.4 | 61.1 | 67.6 | 40.2 | 40.9 | 81.7 | 58.6 | 55.0 | 66.7 | 77.0 | 54.2 |
| 蛋类 Eggs | 39.9 | 11.3 | 51.8 | 38.2 | 43.9 | 31.4 | 39.4 | 41.1 | 25.2 | 29.1 | 21.5 | 53.0 | 6.3 | 23.7 | 17.6 | 21.2 | 5.4 | 51.7 | 30.3 | 10.5 | 7.2 | 14.4 | 2.6 | 16.8 | 26.4 |
| 水产类 Aquatic foods | 9.9 | 8.7 | 3.6 | 9.7 | 8.0 | 2.7 | 5.6 | 6.3 | 2.3 | 7.4 | 1.7 | 4.5 | 15.5 | 26.4 | 36.8 | 12.4 | 23.7 | 6.4 | 27.8 | 5.0 | 33.3 | 27.9 | 25.7 | 3.1 | 14.6 |
| 乳类 Dairy products | 3.8 | 8.7 | 3.3 | 6.0 | 1.7 | 12.6 | 11.3 | 3.2 | 2.3 | 4.6 | 12.4 | 10.6 | 15.1 | 5.6 | 5.1 | 5.3 | 3.3 | 1.7 | 1.0 | 2.7 | 0.9 | 2.7 | 5.0 | 3.1 | 4.9 |

附表 9-34 第六次中国总膳食研究 TnBP 的膳食来源（单位：%）
Annexed Table 9-34  Dietary sources of TnBP from the 6th China TDS (Unit: %)

| 膳食类别<br>Category | 黑龙江<br>HL | 辽宁<br>LN | 河北<br>HE | 北京<br>BJ | 吉林<br>JL | 山西<br>SX | 陕西<br>SN | 河南<br>HA | 宁夏<br>NX | 内蒙古<br>NM | 青海<br>QH | 甘肃<br>GS | 上海<br>SH | 福建<br>FJ | 江西<br>JX | 江苏<br>JS | 浙江<br>ZJ | 山东<br>SD | 湖北<br>HB | 四川<br>SC | 广西<br>GX | 湖南<br>HN | 广东<br>GD | 贵州<br>GZ | 全国平均<br>AVG |
|---|---|---|---|---|---|---|---|---|---|---|---|---|---|---|---|---|---|---|---|---|---|---|---|---|---|
| 肉类 Meats | 45.2 | 34.4 | 55.0 | 80.0 | 75.0 | 80.0 | 37.5 | 49.0 | 78.4 | 0.0 | 68.2 | 56.5 | 71.6 | 66.1 | 31.3 | 81.8 | 59.4 | 20.8 | 16.0 | 0.0 | 14.5 | 86.4 | 85.5 | 62.2 | 60.0 |
| 蛋类 Eggs | 38.1 | 12.5 | 0.0 | 0.0 | 11.1 | 12.7 | 0.0 | 14.3 | 3.9 | 81.0 | 9.1 | 21.7 | 1.2 | 1.8 | 12.5 | 3.6 | 0.0 | 66.7 | 40.0 | 0.0 | 0.0 | 3.6 | 0.9 | 0.0 | 13.3 |
| 水产类 Aquatic foods | 11.9 | 6.3 | 20.0 | 5.0 | 5.6 | 1.8 | 0.0 | 2.0 | 2.0 | 0.0 | 4.5 | 4.3 | 17.3 | 28.6 | 43.8 | 7.3 | 34.4 | 6.9 | 36.0 | 50.0 | 85.5 | 7.3 | 10.3 | 2.2 | 15.6 |
| 乳类 Dairy products | 4.8 | 46.9 | 25.0 | 15.0 | 8.3 | 5.5 | 62.5 | 34.7 | 15.7 | 19.0 | 18.2 | 17.4 | 9.9 | 3.6 | 12.5 | 7.3 | 6.3 | 5.6 | 8.0 | 50.0 | 0.0 | 2.7 | 3.4 | 35.6 | 11.1 |

附表 9-35 第六次中国总膳食研究 TEHP 的膳食来源（单位：%）
Annexed Table 9-35  Dietary sources of TEHP from the 6th China TDS (Unit: %)

| 膳食类别<br>Category | 黑龙江<br>HL | 辽宁<br>LN | 河北<br>HE | 北京<br>BJ | 吉林<br>JL | 山西<br>SX | 陕西<br>SN | 河南<br>HA | 宁夏<br>NX | 内蒙古<br>NM | 青海<br>QH | 甘肃<br>GS | 上海<br>SH | 福建<br>FJ | 江西<br>JX | 江苏<br>JS | 浙江<br>ZJ | 山东<br>SD | 湖北<br>HB | 四川<br>SC | 广西<br>GX | 湖南<br>HN | 广东<br>GD | 贵州<br>GZ | 全国平均<br>AVG |
|---|---|---|---|---|---|---|---|---|---|---|---|---|---|---|---|---|---|---|---|---|---|---|---|---|---|
| 肉类 Meats | 77.2 | 50.0 | 30.2 | 95.5 | 23.3 | 25.9 | 6.1 | 46.9 | 90.9 | 94.2 | 9.7 | 44.4 | 5.2 | 0.0 | 96.8 | 39.7 | 66.7 | 2.4 | 77.0 | 83.3 | 16.2 | 35.9 | 81.8 | 98.7 | 49.2 |
| 蛋类 Eggs | 5.4 | 16.7 | 7.5 | 1.1 | 0.5 | 25.9 | 51.5 | 1.5 | 0.6 | 1.4 | 40.9 | 50.0 | 2.4 | 50.0 | 1.0 | 9.3 | 8.3 | 79.8 | 15.4 | 5.6 | 10.3 | 1.2 | 0.0 | 0.7 | 17.3 |
| 水产类 Aquatic foods | 15.2 | 0.0 | 3.8 | 2.3 | 53.6 | 11.1 | 3.0 | 0.7 | 5.7 | 1.4 | 4.3 | 5.6 | 92.0 | 50.0 | 2.0 | 0.3 | 16.7 | 10.3 | 6.5 | 5.6 | 26.5 | 12.4 | 13.6 | 0.3 | 16.8 |
| 乳类 Dairy products | 2.2 | 33.3 | 58.5 | 1.1 | 22.6 | 37.0 | 39.4 | 50.9 | 2.9 | 2.9 | 45.2 | 0.0 | 0.4 | 0.0 | 0.2 | 50.7 | 8.3 | 7.5 | 1.1 | 5.6 | 47.1 | 50.6 | 4.5 | 0.3 | 16.8 |

附表 9-36 第六次中国总膳食研究 EHDPP 的膳食来源（单位：%）
Annexed Table 9-36  Dietary sources of EHDPP from the 6th China TDS (Unit: %)

| 膳食类别 Category | 黑龙江 HL | 辽宁 LN | 河北 HE | 北京 BJ | 吉林 JL | 山西 SX | 陕西 SN | 河南 HA | 宁夏 NX | 内蒙古 NM | 青海 QH | 甘肃 GS | 上海 SH | 福建 FJ | 江西 JX | 江苏 JS | 浙江 ZJ | 山东 SD | 湖北 HB | 四川 SC | 广西 GX | 湖南 HN | 广东 GD | 贵州 GZ | 全国平均 AVG |
|---|---|---|---|---|---|---|---|---|---|---|---|---|---|---|---|---|---|---|---|---|---|---|---|---|---|
| 肉类 Meats | 2.1 | 74.7 | 0.7 | 82.0 | 4.2 | 80.0 | 0.0 | 88.6 | 1.6 | 96.0 | 77.0 | 48.1 | 69.1 | 37.4 | 16.5 | 65.4 | 39.5 | 16.5 | 97.6 | 77.2 | 53.3 | 76.3 | 64.2 | 99.1 | 66.1 |
| 蛋类 Eggs | 83.0 | 12.0 | 84.9 | 13.3 | 19.0 | 10.8 | 2.1 | 11.0 | 0.4 | 0.2 | 18.8 | 48.4 | 9.5 | 3.1 | 60.2 | 19.1 | 7.2 | 20.8 | 0.9 | 9.4 | 4.9 | 0.3 | 0.9 | 0.4 | 11.9 |
| 水产类 Aquatic foods | 0.0 | 11.8 | 8.3 | 0.5 | 23.5 | 4.6 | 0.0 | 0.3 | 7.8 | 0.3 | 0.0 | 2.8 | 19.1 | 59.5 | 23.3 | 11.6 | 31.9 | 62.7 | 0.1 | 11.9 | 41.1 | 22.5 | 33.0 | 0.4 | 17.6 |
| 乳类 Dairy products | 14.9 | 1.4 | 6.1 | 4.3 | 53.3 | 4.6 | 97.9 | 0.1 | 90.2 | 3.5 | 4.2 | 0.7 | 2.4 | 0.0 | 0.0 | 3.9 | 21.4 | 0.0 | 1.5 | 1.4 | 0.6 | 0.9 | 1.9 | 0.2 | 4.4 |

附表 9-37 第六次中国总膳食研究膳食样品中谷氨酸盐的含量（单位：g/kg）
Annexed Table 9-37  Levels of glutamate acid salt in food samples from the 6th China TDS (Unit: g/kg)

| 膳食类别 Category | 黑龙江 HL | 辽宁 LN | 河北 HE | 北京 BJ | 吉林 JL | 山西 SX | 陕西 SN | 河南 HA | 宁夏 NX | 内蒙古 NM | 青海 QH | 甘肃 GS | 上海 SH | 福建 FJ | 江西 JX | 江苏 JS | 浙江 ZJ | 山东 SD | 湖北 HB | 四川 SC | 广西 GX | 湖南 HN | 广东 GD | 贵州 GZ | 全国平均 AVG |
|---|---|---|---|---|---|---|---|---|---|---|---|---|---|---|---|---|---|---|---|---|---|---|---|---|---|
| 谷类 Cereals | 0.74 | 0.75 | 0.85 | 0.26 | 0.14 | 0.16 | 0.20 | 0.22 | 0.77 | 0.02 | 0.45 | 0.05 | 0.71 | 0.41 | 0.13 | 0.03 | 0.03 | 0.15 | 0.36 | 0.26 | 0.28 | 0.78 | 0.15 | 0.41 | 0.34 |
| 豆类 Legumes | 0.21 | 2.55 | 0.45 | 3.31 | 0.25 | 0.02 | 3.06 | 0.05 | 2.25 | 5.15 | 0.63 | 1.72 | 2.11 | 2.30 | 0.13 | 1.18 | 2.61 | 0.11 | 0.22 | 1.07 | 0.69 | 1.71 | 1.21 | 0.08 | 1.38 |
| 薯类 Potatoes | 0.01 | 1.92 | 0.62 | 0.31 | 2.23 | 0.06 | 0.41 | 1.99 | 0.22 | 0.69 | 0.06 | 2.64 | 1.79 | 0.01 | 1.67 | 0.33 | 0.33 | 0.57 | 0.30 | 0.41 | 0.71 | 0.52 | 0.31 | 0.33 | 0.77 |
| 肉类 Meats | 2.48 | 0.22 | 0.75 | 0.34 | 2.53 | 1.78 | 0.34 | 0.13 | 4.80 | 2.48 | 1.10 | 0.01 | 3.23 | 4.90 | 0.54 | 0.23 | 5.77 | 0.66 | 1.24 | 0.02 | 1.31 | 2.21 | 1.34 | 2.68 | 1.71 |
| 蛋类 Eggs | 0.01 | 0.05 | 0.01 | 0.06 | 0.02 | 0.01 | 0.01 | 0.01 | 0.02 | 0.09 | 0.44 | 0.01 | 0.01 | 1.97 | 0.02 | 0.21 | 0.01 | 0.08 | 0.16 | 0.01 | 2.00 | 0.02 | 0.01 | 0.07 | 0.22 |

续表

| 膳食类别<br>Category | 黑龙江<br>HL | 辽宁<br>LN | 河北<br>HE | 北京<br>BJ | 吉林<br>JL | 山西<br>SX | 陕西<br>SN | 河南<br>HA | 宁夏<br>NX | 内蒙古<br>NM | 青海<br>QH | 甘肃<br>GS | 上海<br>SH | 福建<br>FJ | 江西<br>JX | 江苏<br>JS | 浙江<br>ZJ | 山东<br>SD | 湖北<br>HB | 四川<br>SC | 广西<br>GX | 湖南<br>HN | 广东<br>GD | 贵州<br>GZ | 全国平均<br>AVG |
|---|---|---|---|---|---|---|---|---|---|---|---|---|---|---|---|---|---|---|---|---|---|---|---|---|---|
| 水产类<br>Aquatic foods | 1.52 | 8.63 | 2.87 | 4.99 | 1.05 | 0.25 | 1.45 | 0.20 | 6.33 | 1.49 | 0.51 | 0.22 | 0.02 | 5.59 | 1.75 | 1.41 | 6.94 | 0.44 | 0.38 | 3.20 | 0.66 | 1.25 | 3.48 | 0.08 | 2.28 |
| 蔬菜类<br>Vegetables | 3.57 | 1.05 | 1.43 | 0.67 | 1.82 | 0.01 | 0.89 | 4.25 | 0.28 | 2.51 | 0.76 | 1.56 | 2.61 | 0.03 | 2.14 | 1.45 | 0.02 | 0.02 | 1.07 | 0.89 | 2.26 | 1.34 | 1.13 | 2.28 | 1.41 |

注：低于检出限的数据以 1/2 检出限计

Note: values below the detection limit (LOD) are expressed as half the LOD

附表 9-38 第六次中国总膳食研究的谷氨酸盐膳食摄入量 [ 单位：mg/(kg bw · d)]

Annexed Table 9-38 Dietary intakes of glutamate acid salt from the 6th China TDS [Unit: mg/(kg bw · d)]

| 膳食类别<br>Category | 黑龙江<br>HL | 辽宁<br>LN | 河北<br>HE | 北京<br>BJ | 吉林<br>JL | 山西<br>SX | 陕西<br>SN | 河南<br>HA | 宁夏<br>NX | 内蒙古<br>NM | 青海<br>QH | 甘肃<br>GS | 上海<br>SH | 福建<br>FJ | 江西<br>JX | 江苏<br>JS | 浙江<br>ZJ | 山东<br>SD | 湖北<br>HB | 四川<br>SC | 广西<br>GX | 湖南<br>HN | 广东<br>GD | 贵州<br>GZ | 全国平均<br>AVG |
|---|---|---|---|---|---|---|---|---|---|---|---|---|---|---|---|---|---|---|---|---|---|---|---|---|---|
| 谷类<br>Cereals | 6.43 | 7.34 | 10.22 | 3.31 | 1.26 | 2.66 | 2.39 | 3.26 | 8.03 | 0.24 | 5.51 | 0.54 | 5.09 | 4.15 | 1.21 | 0.43 | 0.34 | 2.40 | 3.02 | 4.00 | 4.20 | 7.14 | 1.10 | 4.41 | 3.70 |
| 豆类<br>Legumes | 0.15 | 4.95 | 0.41 | 5.34 | 0.30 | 0.03 | 4.02 | 0.03 | 1.26 | 3.26 | 0.06 | 1.13 | 3.97 | 2.87 | 0.15 | 1.56 | 5.85 | 0.09 | 0.24 | 1.15 | 0.46 | 1.98 | 0.54 | 0.13 | 1.66 |
| 薯类<br>Potatoes | 0.01 | 2.20 | 0.60 | 0.28 | 4.24 | 0.10 | 0.76 | 2.54 | 0.34 | 1.33 | 0.09 | 6.05 | 1.02 | 0.01 | 0.85 | 0.18 | 0.20 | 0.43 | 0.43 | 0.41 | 0.15 | 0.44 | 0.11 | 0.18 | 0.97 |
| 肉类<br>Meats | 2.36 | 0.23 | 0.56 | 0.37 | 2.67 | 3.87 | 0.20 | 0.11 | 3.56 | 2.89 | 1.25 | 0.00 | 5.67 | 6.68 | 0.80 | 0.34 | 10.83 | 1.01 | 1.07 | 0.03 | 3.13 | 5.24 | 2.23 | 4.53 | 2.49 |
| 蛋类<br>Eggs | 0.00 | 0.03 | 0.01 | 0.03 | 0.01 | 0.00 | 0.00 | 0.00 | 0.00 | 0.03 | 0.09 | 0.00 | 0.01 | 0.59 | 0.01 | 0.09 | 0.01 | 0.06 | 0.06 | 0.00 | 0.44 | 0.01 | 0.00 | 0.02 | 0.06 |
| 水产类<br>Aquatic foods | 0.66 | 2.20 | 0.43 | 1.30 | 0.20 | 0.03 | 0.09 | 0.01 | 0.24 | 0.25 | 0.03 | 0.01 | 0.02 | 5.69 | 1.21 | 0.89 | 5.55 | 0.16 | 0.25 | 0.43 | 1.00 | 1.32 | 2.83 | 0.00 | 1.03 |

续表

| 膳食类别 Category | 黑龙江 HL | 辽宁 LN | 河北 HE | 北京 BJ | 吉林 JL | 山西 SX | 陕西 SN | 河南 HA | 宁夏 NX | 内蒙古 NM | 青海 QH | 甘肃 GS | 上海 SH | 福建 FJ | 江西 JX | 江苏 JS | 浙江 ZJ | 山东 SD | 湖北 HB | 四川 SC | 广西 GX | 湖南 HN | 广东 GD | 贵州 GZ | 全国平均 AVG |
|---|---|---|---|---|---|---|---|---|---|---|---|---|---|---|---|---|---|---|---|---|---|---|---|---|---|
| 蔬菜类 Vegetables | 18.17 | 5.43 | 6.66 | 4.13 | 11.18 | 0.03 | 4.03 | 18.76 | 0.69 | 10.23 | 3.71 | 6.14 | 16.57 | 0.20 | 15.34 | 9.78 | 0.16 | 0.13 | 6.99 | 4.26 | 12.69 | 11.44 | 4.25 | 14.74 | 7.74 |
| 合计 SUM | 27.78 | 22.37 | 18.89 | 14.78 | 19.85 | 6.74 | 11.49 | 24.74 | 14.13 | 18.23 | 10.75 | 13.87 | 32.34 | 20.20 | 19.57 | 13.25 | 22.94 | 4.26 | 12.06 | 10.29 | 22.07 | 27.56 | 11.07 | 24.00 | 17.63 |

附表 9-39 第六次中国总膳食研究谷氨酸盐的膳食来源（单位：%）

Annexed Table 9-39 Dietary sources of glutamate acid salt from the 6th China TDS (Unit: %)

| 膳食类别 Category | 黑龙江 HL | 辽宁 LN | 河北 HE | 北京 BJ | 吉林 JL | 山西 SX | 陕西 SN | 河南 HA | 宁夏 NX | 内蒙古 NM | 青海 QH | 甘肃 GS | 上海 SH | 福建 FJ | 江西 JX | 江苏 JS | 浙江 ZJ | 山东 SD | 湖北 HB | 四川 SC | 广西 GX | 湖南 HN | 广东 GD | 贵州 GZ | 全国平均 AVG |
|---|---|---|---|---|---|---|---|---|---|---|---|---|---|---|---|---|---|---|---|---|---|---|---|---|---|
| 谷类 Cereals | 23.16 | 32.86 | 54.10 | 22.38 | 6.38 | 39.50 | 20.82 | 13.20 | 56.83 | 1.30 | 51.30 | 3.86 | 15.73 | 20.54 | 6.19 | 3.20 | 1.55 | 56.11 | 25.05 | 38.91 | 19.01 | 25.89 | 9.95 | 18.39 | 20.96 |
| 豆类 Legumes | 0.55 | 22.12 | 2.16 | 36.18 | 1.51 | 0.43 | 35.01 | 0.17 | 8.91 | 17.86 | 0.60 | 8.13 | 12.23 | 14.24 | 0.77 | 11.81 | 25.48 | 2.16 | 1.96 | 11.18 | 2.10 | 7.17 | 4.85 | 0.56 | 9.44 |
| 薯类 Potatoes | 0.04 | 9.80 | 3.15 | 1.92 | 21.34 | 1.45 | 6.57 | 10.26 | 2.43 | 7.31 | 0.83 | 43.64 | 3.15 | 0.05 | 4.33 | 1.34 | 0.86 | 9.88 | 3.53 | 3.98 | 0.66 | 1.59 | 1.11 | 0.75 | 5.42 |
| 肉类 Meats | 8.49 | 1.04 | 2.97 | 2.49 | 13.46 | 57.59 | 1.69 | 0.47 | 25.22 | 15.86 | 11.59 | 0.02 | 17.54 | 33.08 | 4.11 | 2.55 | 47.20 | 23.74 | 8.90 | 0.37 | 14.18 | 19.01 | 20.15 | 18.86 | 14.09 |
| 蛋类 Eggs | 0.02 | 0.14 | 0.03 | 0.25 | 0.06 | 0.06 | 0.02 | 0.02 | 0.03 | 0.24 | 0.86 | 0.01 | 0.02 | 2.94 | 0.03 | 0.71 | 0.03 | 1.40 | 0.51 | 0.01 | 2.02 | 0.03 | 0.02 | 0.07 | 0.37 |
| 水产类 Aquatic foods | 2.36 | 9.83 | 2.30 | 8.80 | 0.94 | 0.38 | 0.82 | 0.06 | 1.73 | 1.35 | 0.26 | 0.07 | 0.07 | 28.18 | 6.20 | 6.63 | 24.18 | 3.73 | 2.04 | 4.13 | 4.53 | 4.80 | 25.57 | 0.02 | 5.85 |
| 蔬菜类 Vegetables | 65.39 | 24.21 | 35.28 | 27.99 | 56.32 | 0.60 | 35.07 | 75.83 | 4.86 | 56.08 | 34.55 | 44.27 | 51.26 | 0.96 | 78.37 | 73.76 | 0.69 | 2.98 | 58.00 | 41.42 | 57.51 | 41.51 | 38.36 | 61.36 | 43.88 |